Text
Disc

Books are to be returned on or before
the last date below.

2 3 JAN 2004

2 3 JAN 2004

8 April.

2 0 MAY 2005

LIBREX —

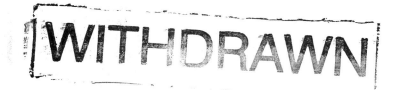

Textbook of Drug Design and Discovery

Third edition

Povl Krogsgaard-Larsen,
Tommy Liljefors and
Ulf Madsen

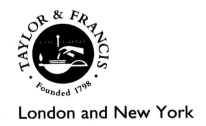
TAYLOR & FRANCIS
Founded 1798

London and New York

First published 2002
by Taylor & Francis
11 New Fetter Lane, London EC4P 4EE

Simultaneously published in the USA and Canada
by Taylor & Francis Inc,
29 West 35th Street, New York, NY 10001

Taylor & Francis is an imprint of the Taylor & Francis Group

© 2002 Povl Krogsgaard-Larsen

Typeset in Baskerville by
Integra Software Services Pvt. Ltd, Pondicherry, India
Printed and bound in Malta by
Gutenberg Press Ltd.

British Library Cataloguing in Publication Data
A catalogue record for this book is available from the British Library

Library of Congress Cataloging in Publication Data
A catalog record for this book has been requested

ISBN 0–415–28287–X HB
ISBN 0–415–28288–8 PB

Contents

6   Receptors: structure, function and pharmacology   156
HANS BRÄUNER-OSBORNE

7   Ion channels: structure, function and pharmacology   173
DAVID J. TRIGGLE

Contributors

Anderson, Paul S.
Chemical and Physical
  Sciences R&D
Bristol-Myers Squibb Company
P.O. Box 80500
Wilmington
DE 19880-0500
USA

Andrews, Peter
Centre for Drug Design and
  Development
The University of Queensland
Brisbane
Queensland 4072
Australia

Bang-Andersen, Benny
H. Lundbeck A/S,
Department of Medicinal
  Chemistry
9, Ottiliavej
DK-2500 Valby
Denmark

Bräuner-Osborne, Hans
Royal Danish School of Pharmacy,
Department of Medicinal
  Chemistry
2, Universitetsparken,
DK-2100 Copenhagen Ø
Denmark

Bøgesø, Klaus P.
H. Lundbeck A/S
9, Ottiliavej
DK-2500 Valby
Denmark

Copeland, Robert A.
Chemical Enzymology
Bristol-Myers Squibb Company
P.O. Box 80400
Wilmington
DE 19880-0400, USA

De Clercq, Erik
Rega Institute
Katholieke Universiteit Leuven
10, Minderbroedersstraat
B-3000 Leuven, Belgium

Dooley, Michael
Centre for Drug Design
  and Development
The University of Queensland
Brisbane
Queensland 4072
Australia

Farver, Ole
Royal Danish School of Pharmacy
Department of Analytical and
  Pharmaceutical Chemistry
2, Universitetsparken
DK-2100 Copenhagen Ø
Denmark

Frydenvang, Karla
Royal Danish School of Pharmacy
Department of Medicinal Chemistry
2, Universitetsparken
DK-2100 Copenhagen Ø
Denmark

Frølund, Bente
Royal Danish School of Pharmacy
Department of Medicinal Chemistry
2, Universitetsparken
DK-2100 Copenhagen Ø
Denmark

Hacksell, Uli
Acadia Pharmaceuticals Inc.
3911 Sorrento Valley Blvd.
San Diego
CA 92121-1402
USA

Halldin, Christer
Department of Clinical NeuroScience
Psychiatry Section
Karolinska Hospital
S-17176 Stockholm
Sweden

Herdewijn, Piet
Rega Institute
Katholieke Universiteit Leuven
10, Minderbroedersstraat
B-3000 Leuven
Belgium

Högberg, Thomas
7TM Pharma A/S
2, Rønnegade
DK-2100 Copenhagen
Denmark

Jane, David E.
Department of Pharmacology
School of Medical Sciences
University of Bristol
University Walk
Bristol BS8 1TD
UK

Kastrup, Jette Sandholm
Royal Danish School of Pharmacy
Department of Medicinal Chemistry
2, Universitetsparken
DK-2100 Copenhagen Ø
Denmark

Kennedy, Ian J.
Department of Pharmacology
School of Medical Sciences
University of Bristol
University Walk
Bristol BS8 1TD
UK

Krogsgaard-Larsen, Povl
Royal Danish School of Pharmacy
Department of Medicinal Chemistry
2, Universitetsparken
DK-2100 Copenhagen Ø
Denmark

Larsen, Claus S.
Royal Danish School of Pharmacy
Department of Analytical and
  Pharmaceutical Chemistry
2, Universitetsparken
DK-2100 Copenhagen Ø
Denmark

Larsen, Ingrid Kjøller
Royal Danish School of Pharmacy
Department of Medicinal Chemistry
2, Universitetsparken
DK-2100 Copenhagen Ø
Denmark

Liljefors, Tommy
Royal Danish School of Pharmacy
Department of Medicinal Chemistry
2, Universitetsparken
DK-2100 Copenhagen Ø
Denmark

Luthman, Kristina
Göteborg University
Department of Chemistry
Medicinal Chemistry
S-412 96 Göteborg
Sweden

Madsen, Ulf
Royal Danish School of Pharmacy
Department of Medicinal Chemistry
2, Universitetsparken
DK-2100 Copenhagen Ø
Denmark

Mitscher, Lester A.
University of Kansas
School of Pharmacy
Department of Medicinal Chemistry
Lawrence, Kansas 66047-2101
USA

Norinder, Ulf
AstraZeneca R&D
Discovery
Medicinal Chemistry
S-15185 Södertälje
Sweden

Pettersson, Ingrid
Novo Nordisk A/S
Novo Nordisk Park G8
DK-2760 Måløv
Denmark

Triggle, David J.
University at Buffalo
State University of New York
415 Capen Hall
Buffalo
NY 14260-1608
USA

Østergaard, Jesper
Royal Danish School of Pharmacy
Department of Analytical and
  Pharmaceutical Chemistry
2, Universitetsparken
DK-2100 Copenhagen Ø
Denmark

Preface

The field of medicinal chemistry and drug design is in a state of swift development and is at present undergoing major restructuring. The molecular biological revolution and the progressing mapping of the human genome have created a new biochemical and biostructural 'world order'. These developments have provided new challenges and opportunities for drug research in general and for drug design in particular. The major objectives of the medicinal chemists are transformation of pathobiochemical and – physiological data into a 'chemical language' with the aim of designing molecules interacting specifically with the derailed or degenerating processes in the diseased organism.

Potential therapeutic targets are being disclosed with increasing frequency, and this exponential growth will continue during the next decades. In this situation, there is a need for rapid and effective target validation and for accelerated lead discovery procedures. Consequently, most industrial medicinal chemistry laboratories have built up new technologies in order to meet these demands. Key words in this regard are construction of compound libraries, high or ultrahigh throughput screening, accelerated ADME and toxicity tests, and automatized cellular assay systems.

In parallel with this development, biostructure-based drug design and intelligent molecular mimicry or bioisosterism are areas of growing importance in the medicinal chemistry 'playing field'. Structural biology is becoming an increasingly important part of molecular biology and biochemistry, and, furthermore, organic chemists are increasingly directing their attention towards synthetic aspects of biomolecules and biologically active compounds biosynthesized by plants and animals. Thus the borderland between biology, biochemistry, and chemistry is rapidly broadening and is becoming the most fruitful working field for innovative and intuitive drug design scientists.

Where are the academic medicinal chemistry and drug design departments in this area of drug research, which is moving towards an increasing degree of integration of scientific disciplines? Furthermore, how should medicinal chemistry teaching programmes be organized and taught in this highly dynamic research area? These burning questions need to be effectively addressed. In order to attract the attention of intelligent students, the creative and fascinating nature of drug design must be the underlying theme of basic and advanced student courses in medicinal chemistry. In relation to industrial screening programmes and 'hit-finding' procedures, students should be taught that the conversions of 'hits' into lead structures and further into drug candidates require advanced synthetic chemistry supported by computational chemistry. Furthermore, these medicinal chemistry approaches should be integrated with molecular pharmacology studies using cloned target receptors, ion channels, or enzymes, expressed in appropriate model systems.

It is beyond doubt that a steadily increasing number of biomolecules will be subjected to X-ray crystallographic structural analysis. The number of enzymes with established three-dimensional structure is now increasing exponentially, and this growth will continue during the next decades. Even oligomeric membrane-bound receptors can now be crystallized and subjected to X-ray crystallographic analysis, but such analyses of mono- or oligomeric receptors are still hampered by major experimental difficulties. In recent years, however, biostructural scientists have succeeded in crystallizing recombinant versions of the binding domains of a G protein-coupled receptor as well as a ligand-gated ion channel. Structural analyses of these binding domains co-crystallized with agonist and antagonist ligands have already provided insight into the structural basis of receptor–ligand interactions and of receptor activation and blockade.

These breakthroughs in biostructural chemistry have opened up new avenues in drug design. Structural information derived from X-ray analyses of enzyme-inhibitor conglomerates has been and continues to be very valuable for the design of new types of inhibitors. Similar pieces of information derived from studies of receptor binding domains co-crystallized with different types of competitive or noncompetitive ligands undoubtedly will be of key importance in receptor ligand design projects. These approaches which are in the nature of drug design on a rational basis will become important parts of student teaching programmes in medicinal chemistry.

In academic research and teaching, biologically active natural products probably will play a progressively important role as lead structures. Not only do such compounds often possess novel structural characteristics, but they also frequently exhibit unique biological mechanisms of action, although naturally occurring 'toxins' typically show nonselective pharmacological effects. By systematic structural modification, including molecular mimicry approaches, it has been possible to 'tame' such 'toxins' and convert them into leads with specific actions on biofunctions of key importance in diseases. Biologically active natural products undoubtedly will continue to be important starting points for academic drug design projects, and such approaches will continue to be exciting case stories in student medicinal chemistry courses.

In this third edition of the textbook, all of these aspects of academic and industrial medicinal chemistry and drug design are dealt with in an educational context.

Povl Krogsgaard-Larsen
Tommy Liljefors
Ulf Madsen

Chapter 1

Drug design and discovery: an overview

Lester A. Mitscher

1.1 INTRODUCTION

Drugs are chemicals that prevent disease or assist in restoring health to diseased individuals. As such they play an indispensable role in modern medicine.

Medicinal chemistry is that branch of science that provides these drugs either through discovery or through design. The classical drugs of antiquity were primarily discovered by empirical observation using substances occurring naturally in the environment. In the last two centuries, drugs increasingly were also prepared by chemical alteration of natural substances. In the century just past many novel drugs were discovered entirely by chemical synthesis. An ever increasing understanding of the nature of disease, how cells work, and how drugs influence these processes has in the last two decades led increasingly to the deliberate design, synthesis and evaluation of candidate drug molecules. In the third millennium, all of these techniques are in use still and the student of drug design and development must appreciate their relative value. Added to this picture are novel opportunities made possible by deeper understanding of cell biology and genetics.

Contemporary medicinal chemistry draws upon many disciplines so that its students and practitioners must have a broad working knowledge above all of organic chemistry but in addition, the student must be comfortable with significant elements of biochemistry, molecular biology, pharmacology, neurobiology, toxicology, genetics, cell biology, biophysics, quantum mechanics, anatomy, physiology, pathology, clinical medicine, computer technology, and the like. This is a tall but manageable order.

The central objective of each branch of chemistry is to possess such an understanding of the relationship between chemical structure and molecular properties that given a set of desired characteristics, a molecule can be proposed and prepared that should come close to possessing them. Next should follow, without undue experimentation, a testing and molecular refining cycle until a satisfactory molecular solution to the problem is at hand. A mature chemical science is efficient in achieving these characteristics. The reader will readily appreciate the complexity of the task in the case of medicinal chemistry and that the subject is still adolescent. A daunting feature is the number of properties that a candidate substance must possess in order to function therapeutically in the human body and so to become a drug. We also have much to learn about pathophysiology. Despite all this, a remarkable range of pharmaceuticals has been developed successfully and the pace of new entity introduction is gratifyingly rapid.

This textbook describes the manner in which medicinal chemists utilize the various fields upon which they draw and the specific stratagems that they employ to advance promising molecules into clinical use for the alleviation of disease and the betterment of mankind. This chapter is intended to introduce briefly some important topics not covered significantly elsewhere in this book and to provide a contextual framework especially for those comparatively new to the study of drug seeking.

1.2   HISTORICAL PERSPECTIVE

From prehistoric times until well into the twentieth century the vast majority of organic drugs originated from natural materials, often in crude mixtures. In early times, there was no possibility of understanding the nature of disease. Rather discoveries were made and preserved based upon observations of natural phenomena and the consequences of consumption of materials that alleviated distress. Of necessity, progress was disjointed and empirical. The use of opium, licorice, ephedra, marijuana, camellia, alcohol, digitalis, coca, quinine and a host of others still in use long predates the rise of modern medicine. It is interesting to note that the uses of these materials often are for diseases that are chronic and prevalent and are based upon responses that are observable in healthy individuals. These natural products are surely not elaborated by plants for our therapeutic convenience. We believe that they have survival value for the plants in dealing with their own ecological challenges and that only a small subset are found to have activity that can be co-opted for human or animal chemotherapy.

About 100 years ago, the mystery of why only certain molecules produced a specific therapeutic response was satisfactorily rationalized by the idea of Langley and Ehrlich that only certain cells contained receptor molecules that served as hosts for the drugs. The resulting combination created a new super molecule that had characteristically new properties producing a response of therapeutic value. One extension of this view was that the drug was a key that fit the target specifically and productively like a corresponding lock. When the fit was appropriate, a positive (agonist) pharmacological action followed analogous to opening a door. In other cases, a different kind of fit blocked the key so that the naturally intended key could not be inserted and antagonist action resulted so that the figurative door could not be opened. Thus, if one had found adventitiously a ligand for a receptor, one could refine its fit by opportunistic and systematic modification of the drug's chemical structure until it functioned very well. This productive idea hardly changed for the next half century and assisted in the preparation of many useful drugs. A less fortunate corollary of this useful picture is that it led to some restriction of imagination in drug design. The drug and its receptor (whose molecular nature was unknown when the theory was promulgated) were each believed to be rigid molecules precrafted to fit one another precisely. Most commonly, receptors are transmembranal glycoproteins accessible from the cell surface whose drug compatible region contains certain specific amino acids arranged in 3D-space.

Since the receptor surface is chiral, it is not surprising that chirality in the drug structure often plays an important role in cellular responses. This important topic is the subject of Chapter 3. Predicting an optimal ligand fit from structure–activity data through mathematical analytical methods is the subject of Chapter 5. These receptor surfaces are often present in molecular clefts such that they create a special local environment that is somewhat protected from the bulk solvent but accessible to substances present in it. The intricacies of interactions in this special environment is treated in Chapter 2. The active site is assembled from non-adjacent amino acid residues as a consequence of the 3D folding of the protein. Non-covalent bonds are formed with the appropriate ligand that indeed produce a temporary new macromolecule that usually signals other macromolecules deeper in the cell that satisfactory occupancy has taken place and the cell responds to this signal by taking the appropriate action.

Further complexities are uncovered continually. For example, a number of receptors are now known that consist of clusters of proteins either preassembled or assembled as a consequence of ligand binding. The component macromolecules can either be homo- or heterocomplexes. The complexity of finding specific ligands for systems of this complexity readily can be imagined (Milligan and Rees 2000).

The main modern difference from the classical picture, other than identifying specifically the chemical nature of the receptor and how it interacts with its ligand, is the realization that neither drug nor receptor need to be rigid. The opposite extreme to lock and key is the zipper model. In this view, a docking interaction takes place (much as the end of a zipper joins the talon piece) and, if satisfactory complementarity is present, the two molecules progressively wrap around each other and accommodate to each others steric needs. The reader will appreciate that all possible intermediate cases (rigid drug/flexible receptor; flexible drug/rigid receptor, etc.) are now known. A consequence of this mutual accommodation is that knowledge of the ground state of a receptor may not be particularly helpful when it adjusts its conformation to ligand binding. Thus, in many cases one now tries to determine the 3D aspects of the receptor–ligand complex. In those cases where X-ray analysis remains elusive, modeling the interactions involved is appropriate. This is the subject of Chapter 4. Further details of this marvelously complex system are presented in Chapter 6.

Earlier it was also noted that enzymes could be modulated for pharmacological benefit. Enzymes share many characteristics with glycoprotein receptors except that they assist in the performance of chemical reactions on their substrates so that the interaction is intrinsically more information rich than is the receptor–ligand interaction (which leaves the ligand unchanged). Until very recently, it was usually only possible to inhibit enzyme action rather than to promote it. Disease frequently results from excessive enzymatic action so selective inhibition of these enzymes is therapeutically useful. These interactions are covered in Chapter 12.

Much later it was discovered that other classes of receptors existed. For example, the highly lipophilic steroid hormones are able to cross the cell membrane and find their receptors in the cytoplasm. Receptor occupation is followed by migration of the new complex into the nucleus followed by selective gene activation. A third class of receptors consists of clusters of proteins assembled such as to create a specific transmembranal central pore. This channel permits the selective directional passage of specific ions in or out of the cell. These ion channels can be ion ligated or current sensitive. The ion flux creates a current that signals for the performance of specific work by the cell. New information involving this complex communication system appears almost daily. Chapter 7 discusses this field.

Over time, it became apparent that DNA and RNA also can be receptors and that the technology needed in order to design ligands for these macromolecules differs in detail from that needed to design ligands for receptors. The earliest applications of DNA liganding lie in inhibiting its formation and function so that cell death was the expected result. Since rapid uncontrolled cell growth is characteristic of cancer, this sort of methodology, starting in about 1940, led to the first successful chemical treatments of this dreaded disease. Revolutionary treatments for cancer are within our grasp based upon novel discoveries in cell biology and genomics. This will be presented in detail in Chapter 17.

Much greater therapeutic safety attends inhibition of the enzymes that are involved in DNA synthesis and its processing. This has led to recent remarkable advances in the chemotherapy of viral diseases. Until quite recent times, viral diseases were extremely difficult to treat but this picture has now changed remarkably as will be described in Chapter 16.

RNA is responsible for the biosynthesis of proteins and use of species specific inhibitory ligands for it results in cell death or stasis. This phenomenon is responsible for the therapeutically useful selective toxicity of many antibiotics.

Interestingly, until the mid 1970s known drug targets were primarily neurotransmitter receptors on cell surfaces. Since that time, a wealth of information has been uncovered and many other choices are now available. In this context, it is interesting therefore to consider the molecular targets for which drugs are contemporarily crafted even though this is shifting rapidly (Drews 2000):

1	Cellular receptors	45%
2	Enzymes	28%
3	Hormones and factors	11%
4	Ion channels	5%
5	DNA	2%
6	Nuclear receptors	2%
7	Unknown	7%

Clearly, cellular receptors and enzymes make up the bulk of the targets favored at this time.

That it took so long to work out the details that we presently understand about drug action is not surprising. When the receptor theory was first advanced, no protein structure would be known for at least 50 years on. Furthermore, in contrast to enzymes, the receptor binds the ligand with temporary non-covalent bonds and does not process its ligand. Thus, one could only infer what intermolecular forces were operating and what could be the molecular and biological consequences of the interaction. Striking advances in molecular spectroscopy have led to the identification of the 3D-structure of many enzymes and their substrates and inhibitors and, indeed, for a few receptors and their ligands. Increasingly nuclear magnetic resonance methods are also producing detailed structural information. The use of computer graphic techniques allows for virtual screening of candidates for synthesis. By this, a given ligand can be subtracted from a 3D-picture of a drug ligand interaction and a new ligand can be fitted in instead. If suggestive, the new ligand can be synthesized and tested. It is also possible to screen actually or virtually through a collection of available molecules to find substances that will fit into the active site in place of a known ligand and then to test it for efficacy. The methodology is still empirical but the time investment is machine time rather than synthesis time so, aside from the cost of the machinery and the development of the sophisticated software, time is saved.

Even this complex picture is greatly simplified. It is now well recognized that most receptors exist as families of subreceptors and that further specificity of action results from ligands that occupy only a specific one of the subreceptors and not the others. Doing this effectively became widely practiced from about 1965. A well-known example of this that illustrates the concept is that norepinephrine exerts a variety of effects in the body by virtue of its occupying all three of the families of adrenergic sub receptors (Figure 1.1). Further complexities arise from there being many subclasses of receptors within each family. Each of these has its own

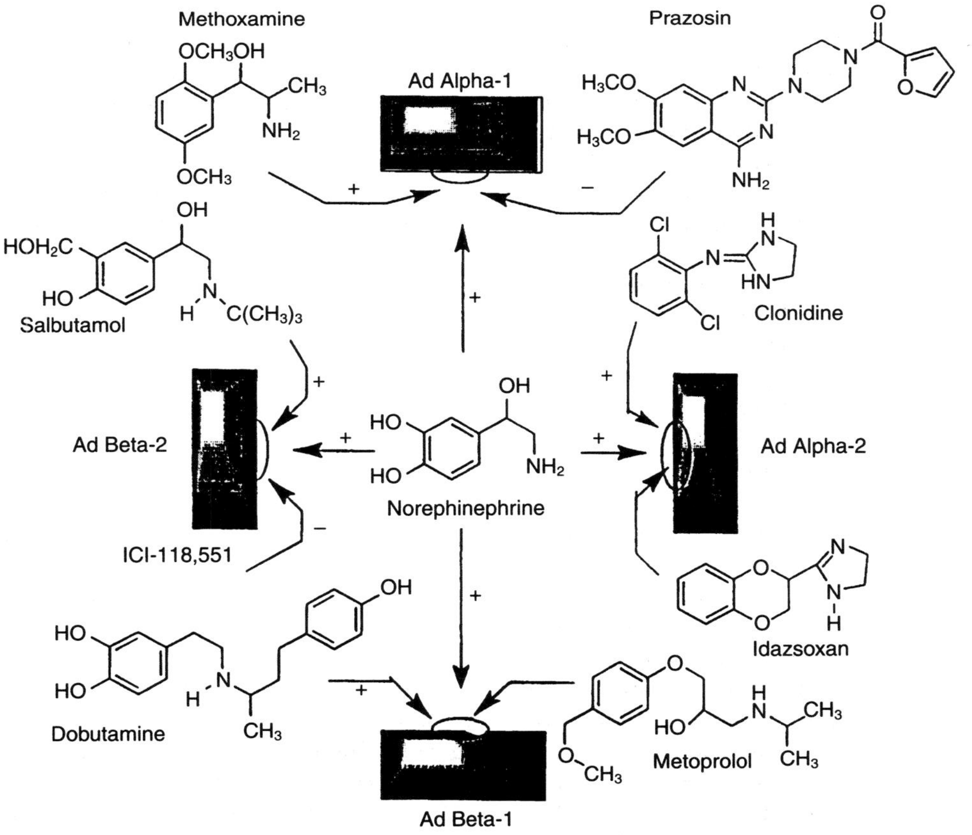

Figure 1.1 Agonists and antagonists for adrenergic receptors.

structural requirements. The body deals with this problem by secreting this neurotransmitter near a specific type of receptor so as to get a specifically desired response and then either destroying the transmitter promptly or reabsorbing it and putting it back into storage for future use once the stimulus that led to neurotransmitter release is over. An added virtue of this means of action is that the action of the drug is temporary so that it has a start point and a stop point of satisfactory length and that it does not migrate far away to occupy unintended receptors and so produce side actions. Through molecular manipulation, specific agonists and antagonists have been prepared for all of these adrenergic subreceptors (Figure 1.1). Thus, through creative analoging fine control of the specific pharmacological response can be obtained.

The devilish complexity of the process of drug design and development will be readily appreciated by considering also that the processes just described deal only with potency and selectivity. Suitable toxicological, pharmacokinetic, pharmacodynamic, pharmaceutical and commercial factors must also be built into the substance before marketing can take place.

Even with the advantage of all this accumulated knowledge it is certain that a great many molecules must be investigated before a marketable version can be found. It is estimated that in 1997 about US$6 billion were spent worldwide on screening technologies and about 100 000 compounds are screened per day. The numbers are truly daunting. Several million compounds must be screened in order to find a thousand or so that have approximately correct characteristics and only a few of these successfully advance through analoging and biotesting to produce a dozen agents suitable for clinical study. Only six of these on average progress into clinical trials and just one reaches the market. Those new to the field may be surprised to learn that terms implying deliberately rational drug design came into general acceptance only in the last 20 years! In this context, the view advanced at that time that X-ray and computer techniques would allow one to prepare only a few dozen substances before finding a marketable substance now appear incredibly naive. It is clear in retrospect that the barriers represented by pharmacokinetic problems had been very significantly underestimated. The appeal of rational drug design is obvious in that it promises to reduce the empiricism of drug seeking enhancing the satisfaction of the practitioners and promising rapid economic returns to their sponsors. Fortunately, the field moves ever closer to the realization of this dream.

The pace of screening has accelerated dramatically in recent years. The application of high throughput screening methods has required rapid synthesis of large arrays of compounds suitable for screening. This in turn has led to the introduction and wide spread acceptance of combinatorial chemical methods.

The remainder of this chapter and, indeed, the book will assume that the reader is familiar with modern synthesis and will therefore address the questions of design and optimization. What molecules should be made, how should they be evaluated, and how should they be advanced to clinical use is our topic. It is important at this stage also to emphasize that priority of discovery is essential not only for very valid commercial reasons but also because drugs relieve suffering and delay is undesirable for humanitarian reasons. Thus, we rarely are able to pursue perfection. We only find it in the dictionary anyhow. The medicinal chemists motto is, instead, 'good enough – soon enough'.

1.3 WHAT KINDS OF COMPOUNDS BECOME DRUGS?

In order to be successful, one should know what gold looks like before panning. Drug seeking is analogous – it is essential to have a good idea of what kind of molecules are likely to become successful drugs before beginning. The normally preferred means of administration of medicaments is oral. Whereas there are no guarantees and many exceptions, the majority of effective oral drugs obey the Lipinski rule of fives. The data upon which this rule rests is drawn from 2500 entries extracted from the US Adopted Names, the World Drug lists, and the internal Pfizer compound collections. There are four criteria:

1   The substance should have a molecular weight of 500 or less.
2   It should have fewer than five hydrogen-bond donating functions.
3   It should have fewer than ten hydrogen-bond accepting functions.
4   The substance should have a calculated $\log P$ ($c \log P$) between approximately −1 to +5.

In short, the compound should have a comparatively low molecular weight, be relatively non-polar and partition between an aqueous and a particular lipid phase in favor of the lipid phase but, at the same time, possess perceptible water solubility. There are many biologically active compounds that satisfy these criteria that fail to become drugs but there are comparatively few successful orally active drugs that fail to fit (Lipinski *et al.* 2001). Thus, this is a helpful guide but not a law of nature.

These criteria put in semi-quantitative terms a great deal of accumulated observations and rationalizations. For absorption and tissue distribution, a drug must be absorbed through a succession of lipid bilayers before reaching its target. Drugs must be able to pass through these barriers rapidly enough to allow therapeutic concentrations to build up. As diffusion is a logarithmic function of size and shape, comparatively compact molecules of modest molecular weight are most suitable. There must, in addition, be sufficient water solubility for dissolution and transport to take place. This correlates reasonably well with the capacity to donate and to accept a moderate number of hydrogen bonds. There must also be sufficient lipid solubility to allow the drug to enter and pass out of a lipid environment. The semi-quantitative aspects of the Lipinski rules address the question of how much is enough. In this sense, the rules embody useful aspects of the Hansch quantitative structure–activity equations that will be covered extensively in Chapter 5. It is also apparent that the pK_a of the molecule in question is also critical because it reflects the polarity of a substance as a function of the pH of its environment. Acids, bases and amphoteric molecules have strong polarities, hence partitioning behavior, that are strongly influenced by this. The more salt-like they become the poorer is their ability to be absorbed through lipid bilayers. Likewise, if they are too non-polar they will dissolve in the lipid bilayers and remain there.

Some of these considerations can be made clearer by the use of a simple cartoon (Figure 1.2). (1) Some small and rather water soluble substances pass in and out of cells through water lined transmembrane pores. Many salts fit into this category. (2) Other agents that are significantly polar are conducted into

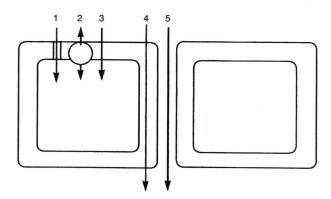

Figure 1.2 Means of cellular uptake and passage by drugs: (1) Passage through porins; (2) active uptake/ejection; (3) passive diffusion into cytoplasm; (4) passive diffusion through the cell; and (5) pericellular passage.

or out of cells by membrane associated and energy consuming proteins. Polar nutrients that the cell requires, such as glucose and many amino acids fit into this category. More recently drug resistance by cells has been shown to be mediated in many cases by analogous protein importers and exporters. (3) Those molecules that are partially water soluble and partially lipid soluble can pass through cell membranes by passive diffusion and are driven in the direction of the lowest concentration. (4) In cells lining the intestinal tract, it is possible for such molecules to pass into the body through the cell membrane alone. (5) Finally, it is also possible for molecules with suitable water solubility, small size and compact shape to pass into the body between cells. This last route is generally not available for passage into the central nervous system (CNS) because the cells are pressed closely together closing off these junctions. This tight capillary junction in aggregate is known as the blood–brain barrier. (6) If all else fails, hypodermic injection is the answer.

For drugs to become successful parenteral agents administered by hypodermic needle, satisfactory water solubility is an overridingly important criterion and a low to moderate molecular weight is much less important. Insulin and some glycopeptide antibiotics such as vancomycin exemplify these substances.

Other routes of administration (transdermal, sublingual, pulmonary, vaginal, rectal, e.g.) are much less frequently used. Each has special features requiring adjustment of molecular properties for optimization. Unfortunately, this fascinating topic would require too much space to explore here.

1.4 PREPARATION AND ORGANIZATION FOR DRUG SEEKING

Flowchart 1.1 synopsizes the stages through which the work passes from inception to marketing and beyond in drug seeking. From this the complexity of the task of finding new medications is readily apparent.

COMMON STAGES IN THE DRUG SEEKING CAMPAIGN

Year 0–1	Identify a suitable disease; Assemble a multi-disciplinary team; Select a promising approach; Obtain a satisfactory budget
	Start the chemistry (collect natural product sources; synthesize or purchase chemicals)
	Start the pharmacology (devise and perfect a suitable screen; select 'hits')
Year 1–2	Confirm potential utility of 'hits' in animals (potency; selectivity; acceptable toxicity)
Year 3–5	Analog around the most promising 'hits'; Ascertain freedom to operate (examine patents/literature); Detailed pharmacology (potency; mode of action; acute and chronic toxicity; reproductive toxicity; genotoxicity); Adjust absorption, distribution, metabolism and excretion characteristics; Devise large scale synthesis; Formulation studies; Stability studies; Apply for patent protection
Year 4–9	Phase I clinical studies (Safety; Dosage; Blood Levels)
	Phase II clinical studies (Effectiveness; Side Effects)
	Phase III clinical studies (Range of effectiveness; Long-term and rare side effects)
Year 8–11	Regulatory review
Year 10–15	Marketing and Phase IV clinical studies (Monitor safety; Very large scale chemistry; Distribution; Advertising; Education)
Year 17–20	Patent protection expires; Generic competition

Flowchart 1.1 The time course and the various stages through which a drug seeking campaign usually passes.

Once organizational and fiscal considerations have been accomplished the project can begin. These decisions are non-trivial and are usually made by committee. They require a great deal of judgement because there are rarely enough resources and talent to do all of the things one would like to do. Whereas the rewards for success are great, the consequences of failure are often devastating. This is a heavy responsibility.

Contemporarily important disease targets are typically CNS derangements, cancer, infectious diseases, degenerative diseases and cardiovascular problems. The pharmaceutical industry is still in the process of centripetal separation into fewer but much larger firms on the one hand and a number of much smaller specialized firms on the other. The large firms carry on drug discovery and development the whole way from inception to marketing. They become increasingly risk averse as a consequence and only drugs promising to earn major sales can be justified to the share holders. One consequence is that the category of orphan diseases, that is diseases with too fewer affluent sufferers to warrant attention, is expanding rapidly and increasingly includes diseases present in the developed countries where big pharma lies. The smaller firms lack the resources to accomplish this by themselves so specialize in serving the process through specialization in a narrower range of higher risk research. Development of novel screens, production of compound collections for screening, exploration of unusual means of administration, and the like, characterize their activity. They must of necessity pursue niche markets unattractive to big pharma, identify partners with deeper pockets, or be absorbed by them in order to survive.

The project team must examine the theories of disease causation and pick a likely approach that has not been thoroughly examined already, for which suitable therapy is not already available, and which one believes one has the resources to address. As an increasingly common alternative, a novel gene or gene product is selected that appears to be involved in the pathology of a disease. Successful knock-out mouse studies often enhance confidence that a novel cause-and-effect relationship exists involving the selected target and that the patient could tolerate the treatment.

With this in hand, it is possible to assemble a team of scientists with all of the necessary skills needed to address the problem. The team will then select an interesting molecule from which to proceed or will devise a suitable high through-put molecular screen to detect molecules with the needed characteristics and collect molecules to screen from which these can reasonably be expected to emerge. From the compounds found to be active in the screen, suitable molecules will be selected to advance. These 'hits' may be substances that are in the literature, a collection of compounds in one's retained sample collection, a collection of molecules available for purchase (often a diverse combinatorial library), a collection of extracts of natural origin, or a series of molecules speculatively synthesized on the belief that one or more might be active, and the like. This selection is often a very challenging part of the whole process.

Proof of concept is obtained from animal studies when the hit substance is shown to be active in whole cell or organ systems in model diseases. Next the initial lead molecules are modified synthetically to identify the pharmacophore and to enhance potency and selectivity. Then, other imperfections in the lead are solved by synthetic modification to elevate the lead into candidate drug status. The many problems beyond potency, selectivity and safety that must be overcome are listed in Section 1.6 of this chapter. Next, detailed pharmacological study in more than one species identify the likely utility and safety of the candidate drug in model diseases. Suitable back-up substances are prepared and brought forward as insurance against unexpected failure of the candidate to survive the development sequence. This happens all too often and then an alternative candidate must be brought forward. It is prudent to have more than one such back-up substance available and it is wise if their chemical structures differ significantly from the structure of the primary candidate. Suitable formulations and an economically attractive chemical synthesis is developed. Finally, clinical trials are undertaken.

This listing implies that these stages are completed in sequence. Unfortunately, however, it is often the case that difficulties in a later stage require the group to retreat to an earlier stage and bring alternative molecules forward again. As much of the early work as possible is carried out in parallel. This back and forth work is frustrating and consumes considerable time. Overall completion of the process normally consumes 8–12 years and costs between 0.3–0.5 billion dollars. At an estimated average profit return, firms often expect approximately 5 years of sales before the first profit is returned. With this extraordinary level of investment and commitment it is not surprising that drug houses merge with regularity and that they are intensely interested in methods promising to reduce the risks involved and in shortening the time between conception and marketing. Commercial viability contemporarily requires the introduction of 1–3 such substances each year and stock valuation is significantly affected by guesstimates of the quality and quantity of a firm's pipeline of promising molecules.

1.5 SOURCES OF HITS, LEADS AND CANDIDATE DRUGS

Once suitable biological screens have been set up, collections of promising molecules are passed through them. The initial screens often have high throughput but limited information content. Molecules which attach themselves significantly to selected enzymes or receptor preparations are called 'hits'. A necessary gating level of affinity is usually settled upon. This is often 50 micromolar or stronger. From the list of hits, drug-like molecules are selected that appear free from potentially toxic moieties, untoward reactivity or other undesirable features. The survivors of this screen are then tested in ever more elaborate biological assays, usually involving whole cell systems, to verify that affinity reflects potentially useful activity. Those surviving molecules that warrant the time, costs and effort of analog preparation to further enhance their desirable properties are called 'leads'. One generally tries to reach single digit micromolar potency or stronger with such compounds. When the leads have been refined further so that satisfactory potency, selectivity, freedom from toxicity, chemical novelty, suitable pharmacokinetic and pharmacodynamic properties, etc. are present in animal models of disease, the survivors are elevated to the status of 'candidate drugs' suitable for extensive biological evaluation up to and including clinical trials in humans. Single digit nanomolar potency is usually sought for these compounds. It will be seen that the biological tests become ever more content rich, challenging, and time consuming. The costs escalate dramatically as the experimentation proceeds. It is also clear that the number of substances that satisfy these ever more stringent requirements falls off dramatically with time. It is often estimated that for each 7000 substances that start, only one comes through to the end and that up to a dozen years often elapses from start to finish. The statistics are even more discouraging in the age of combinatorial chemistry where the numbers of compounds screened for each success is even larger.

Knowing what kinds of molecules make useful drugs, one needs to know where to find them. The possibilities are in theory infinite. In practice, however, suitable sources are well recognized.

1.5.1 Natural products

1.5.1.1 Higher plant and animal products

As described in Section 1.2, prehistoric drug discovery started with higher plant and animal substances and this continues to this day to be a fruitful source of biologically active molecules belonging to unanticipated structural types. Adding to the long list of classical plant products that have survived into modern medicine, one can list many substances of more recent origin including the antibiotics (penicillins, cephalosporins, tetracyclines, aminoglycosides, glycopeptides, etc.), anticancer agents (taxol, camptothecin, vinca alkaloids, doxorubicin, bleomycin, etc.), the immunosuppressant drugs cyclosporin and tacrolimus, and a variety of other pharmacological agents such as compactin, asperlicin, etc. In addition, natural products have provided the structural pattern that has led to the synthesis of valuable medications (snake venom peptides that led to orally active angiotensin converting enzyme inhibitors, cocaine which led to local anesthetics, willow bark glycosides led to aspirin and then to the COX-II inhibitors, and so on). The continuing encroachment of human habitation raises legitimate fears of extinction of important potential sources of drugs that are yet to be discovered in tropical regions. In many cases, as in traditional Chinese medicine and Ayurveda, a great deal of ethnobotanical medicine also exists to be mined. There is reason for haste in bioprospecting. These materials have the potential advantage of having had informal clinical trials before analoging begins. This lessens the chance that a nasty toxicological surprise awaits, as too often it does, at the end of long and expensive evaluation of a synthetic substance. The current commerce in herbal medicines in Europe and the United States of America is very substantial. Some of these herbals will in time be the source of new medications, some will remain in use in their present form and some will fade away as a consequence of scientific scrutiny. It is most likely that the successful materials will be suitable for chronic or preventative medicine rather than for rapid cure of florid conditions.

Animal products have also led to important medications. Porcine insulin, for example, is only one of a variety of hormones used in replacement therapy or, in modified form, for other therapeutic purposes. Genetic engineering techniques have had a significant impact here. Human insulin is now readily available from fermentation sources following transfection of the genes needed for its production and development of techniques for expression, excretion and isolation. Likewise available is human growth hormone. This list will expand dramatically in the years just ahead. A somewhat analogous promising developing technology is the production of genetically modified crops as a source of pharmaceuticals. This promises to be an economic resource at least partially divorced from national boundaries (Gruber and Theisen 2000).

One can also cite the anti-inflammatory uses of analogs of cortical hormones when given in suprahormonal doses made possible as a consequence of partial synthesis. The antifertility and anticancer properties of sex hormone analogs, and the like, have also benefitted from this work.

One of the primary values of natural products in drug seeking is the impressive molecular complexity and novelty that they possess. Very few chemists are imaginative enough to compete successfully with the structural diversity found in nature. Indeed, few synthesis chemists would be bold enough to make them if nature had not provided the pattern first. This process of drug discovery is useful but slow. It can, however, stimulate an enormous additional effort when a useful new structural type is identified. Large scale directed industrial screening of natural products from fermentations and the deliberate search for anticancer chemotherapy under the sponsorship of federal agencies represent modern variants of this ancient process.

A promising future avenue for drug discovery using natural products lies in the new field of combinatorial biosynthesis. Here manipulation of the genes involved in biosynthetic pathways are assembled in novel combinations leading to forced evolution and the artificial generation of novel structures that have yet to be found in nature.

Whereas the use of animal products in medicine is easy to rationalize, the reader may wonder how it is that higher plant products have useful pharmacological properties. In those comparatively few cases where we have convincing evidence, it appears that plant products occasionally have sufficient topographic similarity to indigenous mammalian chemicals that they can substitute topologically for them at their receptors. One cites ephedrine and epinephrine, morphine and enkephalins, and tetrahydrocannabinol and anandamide as pairs that illustrate this point. Thus, we believe that plants make these compounds for their own purposes but their biological activity is sufficiently broad that they can be co-opted for human medicinal chemical purposes also. As far as is known, the human receptors have no obvious counterpart in plants so the mutual fit is fortuitous.

1.5.1.2 Arthropod and insect products

Arthropod and insect products have yet to produce many significant medicinal agents but they show significant promise. The alkaloids in the skin of certain colorful tropical tree frogs show profound biological activity (rationalizing their ethnic use as arrow and dart poisons) and batracotoxin, for example, is under serious study for its cardiovascular properties. Intensive study has shown that these compounds are not produced directly by the frogs but rather are accumulated from digestion of arthropods that make up much of their diet. The florid appearance of the frogs seems to be an advertisement. Rather than seeking concealment they are clearly visible so that potential predators are warned not to eat them by mistake.

1.5.1.3 Fermentation products

Soil micro-organisms produce a wide variety of compounds when grown on complex media. This takes advantage of their versatile natural role in converting dead plants and animals into compost and their ability to exist on soil detritus as a consequence of their amazing intrinsic biosynthetic versatility. The first medicinal products from soil streptomycetes, bacteria and fungi, aside from alcohol, were powerful antibiotics that provided them with safety in their natural habitat but could also be used to combat human infections. Some of the more cytotoxic agents found are used in treatment of tumors. More recently, they have proven a valuable source of a wide variety of structures with general physiological activity that does not depend upon killing cells for their action. The use of fermentation products related to mevalonin and compactin, for example, to inhibit 3-hydroxy-3-methyl-glutaryl coenzyme A reductase and so reduce plasma cholesterol levels is a striking example. These and related agents have generated billions of dollars in revenue to their discoverer's firms.

1.5.1.4   Marine products

The Seven Seas were among the last regions of the earth to see extensive natural product exploration and have proven to be a rich source of unusual chemical structures. Most have proven to be too toxic or too narrow in spectrum to find use in human medicine but some, such as briostatin and dolestatin, have astonishing potency as cytotoxic agents and are under intensive clinical examination as potential antitumor agents. More recent compounds of this type showing anticancer promise include eleutherobin (a microtubule stabilizing compound from a soft coral), discodermolide and the sponge product mycalamide B. Marine gorgonians have proven to be comparatively rich sources of prostaglandins although other sources have proven to be more convenient in practice. The search goes on and practical results seem probable.

1.5.1.5   Pre-existing substances

Hundreds of thousands of organic chemicals have been synthesized for non-drug purposes. A number of these, when examined in appropriate test systems turn out to have useful pharmacological properties. For example, p-aminobenzenesulfonamide, found to be an antimicrobial agent of sufficient value to earn a Nobel prize in the 1930s had actually been synthesized in 1908 by Gelmo in Vienna but was not known at the time to be a biologically active substance. It is probably not useful to speculate about the toxicity and morbidity that could have been avoided during the First World War years if only it had been suitably tested in a timely manner! A more recent example involves the non-neutrative sweetner aspartame. The great economic utility of this compound as a sucrose substitute was discovered serendipitously when it was found to be exceptionally sweet tasting in the course of being weighed as a chemical intermediate in a synthetic project having a very different objective.

1.5.1.6   Compounds prepared by speculative syntheses

Once a popular avenue towards drug discovery, many compounds of unusual but suggestive structure have been synthesized so that they could be evaluated as potential drugs. Historically these were provided to pharmacologists in the hope that a useful biological property would be found during the course of general biological evaluation. The benzodiazepines were made in this mode and were found to be of outstanding medicinal value in the treatment of psychoses. This was not suspected in advance of their preparation and evaluation. An instructive and entertaining account of the work that led to this wonderful discovery is available (Sternbach 1979). This mode of drug discovery fell very much out of favor during the computer assisted drug design decades but is making a strong come back in the days of combinatorial chemistry.

1.5.1.7   Compound collections

Most firms archive samples of unsuccessful substances prepared in various drug-seeking campaigns. These are then subjected to each new screen that is developed and it is remarkable how often this turns up unsuspected activities that ultimately lead to useful new agents following further structural manipulation.

1.5.1.8 Combinatorial libraries

Because this methodology has become so prominent in such a short time, it deserves more extensive treatment than the other topics in this section can receive. Classically, chemists have prepared substances one at a time and took pride in using novel reactions and reactants to obtain the highest possible yield in the greatest possible purity. No matter how satisfying this is to its practitioners it is time consuming and expensive. As long as the rate of construction of new substances was faster than the time required for biological evaluation, there was no motivation for change. The development of many new tests and of high throughput screening methods in the 1980s, however, created a demand for more compounds to test. Chemists responded to this need by developing methods for multiple parallel synthesis and combinatorial chemistry. Now it is possible in favorable cases to prepare hundreds to thousands of compounds in very short time and synthesis and testing are back in phase with each other.

Combinatorial chemistry has consequently become a method of choice for the rapid construction of large arrays of drug-like molecules. It had its beginnings with the Merrifeld resin-based peptide syntheses which were so useful that they were rewarded with a Nobel prize. The iterative nature of protein synthesis and the ready availability of the component parts made this methodology particularly apt and the explosion of information in cell biology made it particularly timely. Given that there are approximately the same number of amino acids commonly found in proteins as there are letters in the Latin alphabet and how many languages have been constructed from this alphabet, one readily appreciates the astronomical numbers of peptides that could in principle be prepared in a combinatorial mode by assembling all conceivable combinations of amino acids into peptides. To be sensible, smaller combinatorial arrays are made. By single compound synthesis, just making all of the possible tripeptides alone would be a life-time labor. Use of combinatorial methodology to be explicated below makes this a reasonably trivial undertaking.

Biochemists rapidly embraced this resin-based chemistry as did firms developing bioassays that did not have chemical libraries on hand or synthetic chemists to prepare them. Peptides are the normal means with which cells conduct their inter- and intracellular business. They are often biosynthesized near the site of their action so specificity of action is managable. The situation is different when they must be administered to patients for they must survive digestive processes and have a long way to travel and many cell membranes to cross before they reach their site of action. They often make satisfactory drugs if one is prepared to inject, but their polarity and digestibility make them poor drugs for oral therapeutic purposes. An enormous effort has been expended to overcome these natural drawbacks but the results have not yet been impressive. Still, they make convenient hits and methods for converting peptides into more drug-like molecules (peptidomimetics) are gradually being developed. This topic is treated extensively in Chapter 15.

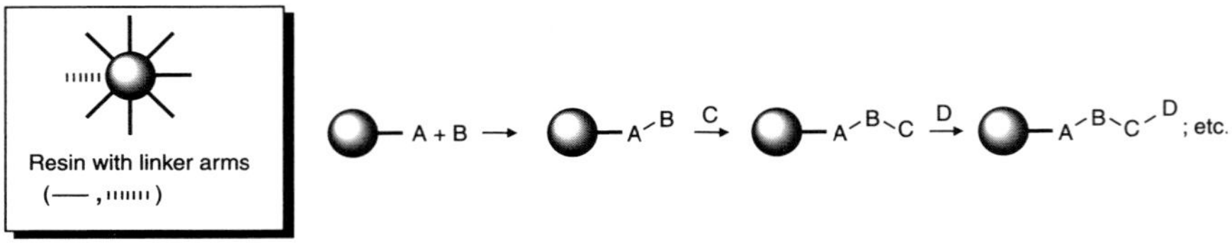

Figure 1.3 Single resin/single peptide (Merrifeld style) methodology.

Generally speaking only microgram to milligram quantities of peptides are prepared for biological evaluation using resin methods because of the limited loading capacity of the resins. These are often tested in mixtures that must be deconvoluted later to identify the active components. Many ingenious methods have been developed to tag these resin bound peptides so that their chemical history (and putative structures) can be determined without needing to separate them from the resin and determine their chemical structure by laborious micro methods.

Some of the methodologies used for the construction of very large arrays (libraries) of compounds preparable by iterative chemistry can be illustrated by the following examples.

1.5.1.8.1   Single resin/single peptide (Merrifeld style)

In this case (Figure 1.3), an insoluble resin (r) contains a number of linker arms (—), functionalized at the end so that an amino acid, represented by a capital letter (A, B, C, etc.) can be attached to each one and then reacted sequentially with additional amino acids to form peptide bonds. A different linker arm (----) can be present to which a signal sequence can be attached. The chemical nature of the two different types of linker arms differs so that they can be individually reacted and their contents detached independently from each other. At the end of the reaction sequence, the linker arm in most cases is selectively severed to release the peptide for analysis and testing and the resin and its arm can be recycled.

1.5.1.8.2   Combinatorial mode: mix and split style

In this case (Figure 1.4), an amino acid is linked to arms on a reaction inert resin and then split into two equal portions. One of these is reacted with amino acid A and the other with B to produce resins with two different dipeptides attached.

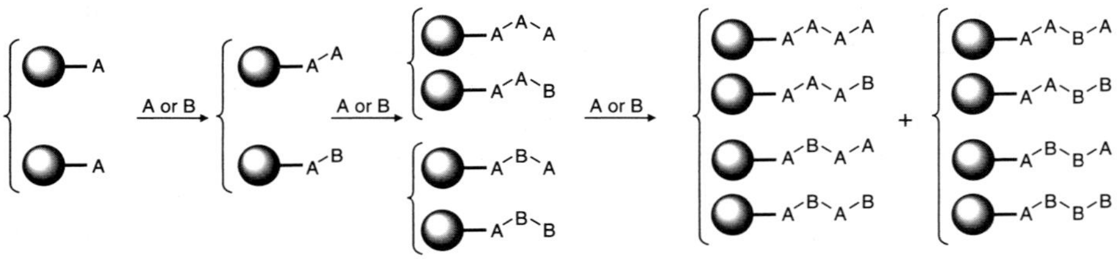

Figure 1.4 Combinatorial synthesis. Mix and split style.

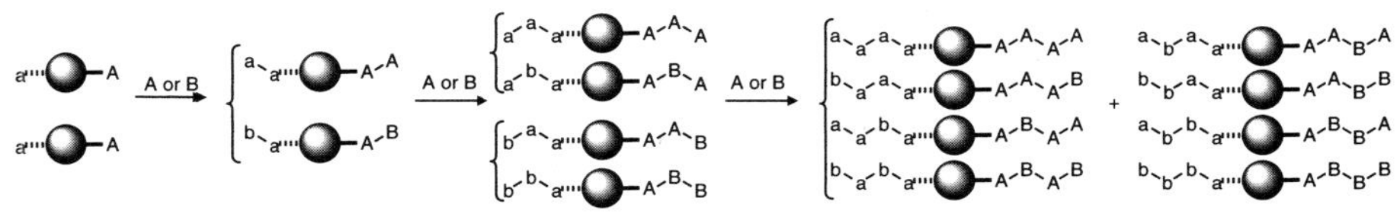

Figure 1.5 Combinatorial synthesis. Label, mix, and split style.

These are mixed and split again into two equal piles. Amino acid A is added to the first pile and B to the second. This produces two mixtures each containing two different tripeptides. Repetition produces two different resin mixtures each containing four different tetrapeptides. This process can be repeated indefinitely.

1.5.1.8.3   Combinatorial mode: label, mix and split style

In this example (Figure 1.5), the capital letters stand for one of two different amino acids while the small letters stand for one of two different but corresponding nucleotide or some other type of monomer. Each time amino acid A is added, code nucleotide a is also added. Likewise with B and b. The two kinds of linker arms are chemically distinct so that the code sequence and the peptide sequence can be removed independently for analysis. In this way, the history of the bead can be ascertained. Knowing this one knows what peptide should be on the bead.

1.5.1.8.4   Radiofrequency detection

It is possible to place a tunable radio signal-generator in the resin. In this way, the active compound on a resin can be determined by identifying the signal that it generates.

1.5.1.8.5   Deconvolution

The chemical labor of adding a signal sequence, detaching it and analyzing it can be avoided by use of biological deconvolution methods.

1.5.1.8.6   Iterative deconvolution

In this process, one does not mix the resins after the last reaction but keeps the resins terminating in A separate from those terminating in B and then mixes these into groups (Figure 1.6a). Each of these is tested separately and let us say that the mixture of tetrapeptides terminating in A is active (boxed in the figure). Next one synthesizes two mixed resins in which the penultimate amino acid is A in one and B in the other (Figure 1.6b). These are tested separately and, say, the group with amino acid B in the third position is active (boxed in the figure). Another iteration in which **r**-A-A-B-A and **r**-A-B-B-A are individually prepared and tested reveals that the active component responsible for activity in this whole series was **r**-A-B-B-A. This process is dependent on biological rather than chemical analysis for success. The more complex the library of compounds is, the more useful this process is.

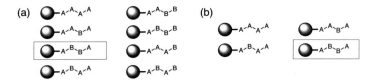

Figure 1.6 Iterative convolution: first (a) and second phase (b).

1.5.1.8.7   Positional deconvolution

In this process (Figure 1.7a), a series of sublibraries are prepared whose composition is systematically varied. In this manner, all C-terminal amino acids are the same whereas the remaining positions can have any of the possible compositions. If tripeptides consisting of all possible combinations of three amino acids are involved, 27 different peptides will be produced. In the example given (Figure 1.7a), the first amino acid is A, B, or C. One presumes that activity is found for this library. In this case, a second library (Figure 1.7b) is produced which contains A, B, or C as the first amino acid but always contains A as the last amino acid. Next (Figure 1.7c), a third library is produced which contains only A as the second amino acid. The fourth library (Figure 1.7d) has all the cases in which only A is the first amino acid. The fifth library (Figure 1.7e) has all the cases in which the third amino acid is B. The sixth library (Figure 1.7f) has all the cases in which the second amino acid is B. The seventh library (Figure 1.7g) has all the cases in which the first amino acid is B. The eighth library (Figure 1.7h) has all the cases in which the third amino acid is C. The ninth library (Figure 1.7i) has all the cases in which the second amino acid is C. The tenth and last library (Figure 1.7j) has all the cases in which the first amino acid is C.

Each of these libraries is tested. In this example libraries one, three, seven and eight are active. The only way in which this result could be obtained is if the sequence of the one active constituent is B-A-C. This example looks more laborious than it actually is although complex libraries with many components require the preparation and testing of a large number of sublibraries.

1.5.1.8.8   Omission and tester libraries

Another deconvolution method is to make a set of sublibraries where no component contains amino acid A, another without B and another without C. These omission libraries are tested. A tester library contains all of the peptides missing from the tester libraries. One of these has A peptides added, another B added and a third has C added. Testing of these libraries reveals the active sequence.

1.5.1.8.9   The Pasteur-like method

In a limited number of cases where the peptide still bound to the resin is biologically active in this form and the result of the activity is generation of a color or a zone of inhibition, it is possible to distribute the individual resin particles on a seeded solid surface such as an agar plate. After the test is complete the active

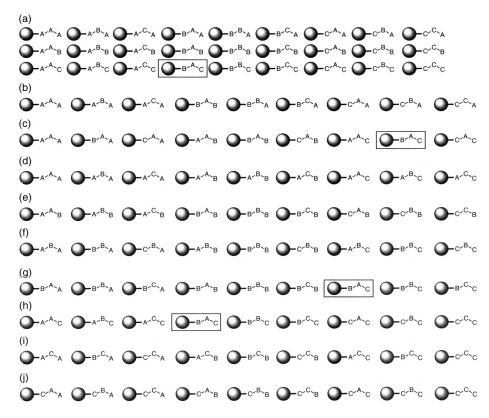

Figure 1.7 (a) Positional deconvolution; (b) Sequences ending with A; (c) Sequences with A in the middle; (d) Sequences starting with A; (e) Sequences ending with B; (f) Sequences with B in the middle; (g) Sequences starting with B; (h) Sequences ending with C; (i) Sequences with C in the middle; and (j) Sequences beginning with C.

resins are visible on inspection of the plate and can be picked off of the agar surface using tweezers and analyzed. Alternatively, the active beads may become colored in solution as a consequence of their activity and can be picked out on this basis. Another method involves the presence of a code residue that is colored. When tested in collections of beads in wells, the ones that are active are associated with a particular color. The components of that well can be tested individually in a separate series and the one that produces that color is the active one. This provides a confirmatory test and reveals the identity of the active product.

1.5.1.8.10 *Spatially addressed libraries*

PHOTOLITHOGRAPHIC METHOD

In this method (Figure 1.8), the resin is affixed to a solid support so as to form a coated layer, analogous to the surface of a credit card or a thin layer plate. The amino

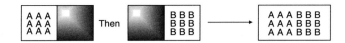

Figure 1.8 Photolithographic synthesis of peptide arrays. In this illustration, one field is covered while the other is reacted with A. Next, the mask is shifted and the uncovered field is reacted with B. Many different patterns can be used so that at the end of an iterative process each location has a different peptide. Thousands of different peptides can be generated in an amazingly small area.

acids to be affixed are derivatized with a photolabile protecting group. The surface of the resin bed is partially protected by a series of opaque filters. Irradiation with light deprotects the amino acid in question which is then bound to the surface of the resin bed. A second amino acid can be bound to a different region by use of another opaque filter protecting another region. A second amino acid can be joined to each of these first amino acids to form a group of dipeptides and this process can be repeated many times. The nature of the peptides found depends upon the number and the pattern of the successive filters. The result is that each address on the resin bed surface can be occupied by a different peptide whose identity is revealed by its *X/Y* co-ordinates. Testing consists of washing the surface with the test solution and observing a visible response.

PIN METHOD

In this experiment, a different peptide is generated on the end of each of a rank of pins affixed to a block. The peptide-containing pins can then be inserted in a 96 well plate (or larger) such that a single or a collection of different peptides is present in each well. Testing ensues and the identity of the actives comes from the identity of the peptide generated on the tip of the corresponding pin.

TEA BAG METHOD

In this method, a collection of resins is placed in each of a collection of porous plastic bags whose holes are sufficiently small to retain the resins but large enough to allow access to solutions into which the bags can be dipped. In this way, each bag can be made to contain an individual peptide or a collection of peptides whose identity is ascertained from the label on the bag.

The previous examples are but a selection of the many ingenious methods that have been developed for solid phase organic synthesis (SPOS) in a combinatorial or multiple parallel synthesis mode. For simplicity, the reactions have been illustrated using amino acid conversions to peptides. Oligonucleotides, oligosaccharides and many other kinds of organic molecules can be made in a similar manner. The power of the methodology is clear.

The reactions are generally driven to completion by use of excess reagents and long reaction times so that deletion errors are minimized. The excess reactants are removed by filtration and washing away the unwanted materials. Several components can be attached to each resin so as to saturate all of the available attachment

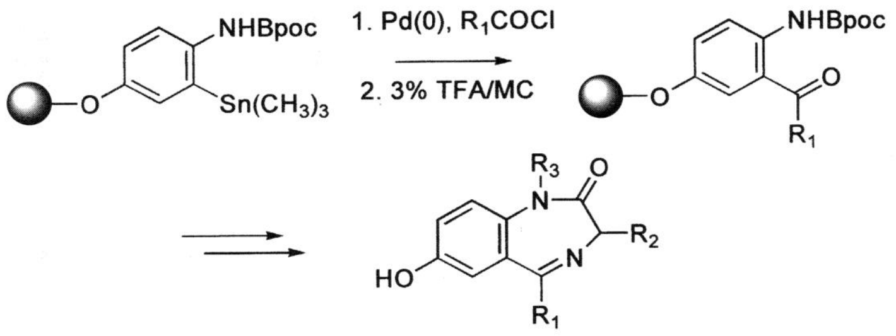

Figure 1.9 Combinatorial mode synthesis of hydroxylated benzodiazepines.

arms. This loading, however, is limited by the need to avoid interference with the chemistry by adjacent molecules. In principle, porous beads can be more heavily loaded than solid beads. In some instances, the compounds can be evaluated while still attached to the beads but in many cases, the compounds must be detached for analysis/identification and for pharmacological testing. For this to work, obviously the chemistry involved in linking the first component to the resin must differ from that involved in linking subsequent molecules to the first component. This kind of chemistry is termed 'orthogonal'.

Before long combinatorial libraries of DNA and RNA molecules were also prepared by iterative methods. Carbohydrate libraries have been the slowest of the informational macromolecules to be synthesized successfully by combinatorial methods. A principal barrier to be solved here is the necessity of controlling the stereochemistry of the anomeric center and its comparative chemical fragility.

The first drug-like heterocycles to be made in a combinatorial resin-based mode were the benzodiazepines (Figure 1.9). In this work, three different small organic molecules were combined using resin technology to produce a modest library of benzodiazepines which were screened for biological activity. The initial benzodiazepine libraries suffered from the defect that the attachment point to the resin arm required that the final products have a polar phenolic hydroxyl group following removal from the resin. The polarity of this functional group would inhibit penetration into the CNS (Bunin and Ellman 1992). Subsequent modifications led to the development of traceless linkers wherein the attachment point to the resin was lost upon cleavage from the resin without leaving behind a function in the products (Figure 1.10). The final benzodiazepines were therefore identical with those prepared previously one at a time in solution. Indeed, this chemistry could have been performed in solution if preferred. Gratifyingly, biotesting revealed that classic medicinal chemistry had identified the most active compounds already, albeit more slowly. This and related works opened a flood gate and within 5 years examples of most common drug-like molecules were synthesized and the methodology became increasingly divorced from resin methods and solution based methods, often termed multiple parallel synthesis (MPS), became increasingly popular. It was somewhat slow to take hold in drug preparation because the chemistry involved in the construction of small non-peptides is often much more idiosyncratic than peptide chemistry. By the year 2001, an average of three papers a day devoted to combinatorial and multiple parallel synthesis methods appeared in the chemical

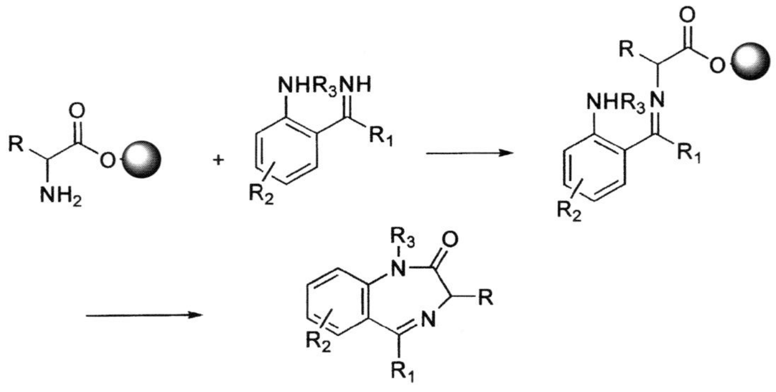

Figure 1.10 Combinatorial mode of traceless linker synthesis of benzodiazepines.

literature (not all of it devoted to drug seeking) and hundreds of different chemical libraries have been reported (Bunin, Dener and Livingston, 1999).

The combinatorial nature of this chemistry can be seen in that four variable positions are involved. Considering that the position of aromatic substitution involving R_2 is also variable, the reader can appreciate that thousands of analogs can be prepared quickly by simple variants of this process. Additional features of interest highlight the particular aptness of this example and illustrate important considerations in doing analogous work. The basic nucleus/core/centroid, where $R=R_1=R_2=R_3=H$, has a molecular weight of 160. This leaves 340 a.m.u. (500 − 160) to distribute amongst the four variable parts or an average of 85 a.m.u. that can be attached to each without getting the molecular weight too high. This would allow six methylenes or a benzene ring, etc. at each place. The projections from the centroids cover roughly the four cardinal points of the compass allowing significant exploration of space. The functional groups to which the R groups are attached are rather different from one another allowing flexibility and orthogonality in construction chemistry. The final products can readily be prepared so that they satisfy all of the Lipinski-rule characteristics and they are accordingly drug-like. The centroid has an amide and an imine function that can contribute to pharmacokinetic properties and even contribute to receptor binding so the centroid does not represent dead weight.

The speed with which a great number of analogs can be constructed can be illustrated by considering the result of starting with just 10 different variations of the R_2 in the aromatic ring. Ten different acyl side chains raises the number of analogs to 100 (10×10) and ten different groups attached to the anilino nitrogen leads to 1000 ($10 \times 10 \times 10$) variants. Use of 10 different amino acids in the condensation step produces 10 000 members in this small library alone. If each analog is chosen with some care using medicinal chemical logic, an enormous amount of useful knowledge emerges from testing such a library. Of course, if one does dumb things, then a large number of useless molecules emerge! Doing the work in successive pulses – that is, making smaller probing libraries, testing and using the results to define what should be in the next small library – is safer and more efficient than making all the possible analogs at once. Many hundreds of additional examples could be presented, including many in which the chemistry is performed in solution in individual reactors but there is not space enough for this.

The term combinatorial implies all conceivable arrangements of the available units. Since this would be very inefficient, but take nothing for granted, it is the antithesis of structure-based drug design where one presumes to understand the task sufficiently that only one or at most a few analogs need to be made in order to be successful. Neither extreme turns out to be realistic at this time. In fact, current trends show that the partisans for these extremes are coming ever closer in their views. Focused libraries, that is, smaller collections of promising molecules are now increasingly the objective of work in this field and it is becoming ever more intellectually satisfying to pursue.

In terms of speed, one can ask what one is talking about. The traditional mode of drug preparation is one at a time (usual speed analoging = usa) and the compound is not tested until available in significant quantity and demonstrable purity. A skilled medicinal chemist in a forgiving series can generally prepare between 50 and 100 compounds yearly. When drug evaluation was comparatively slow, this was sufficient to keep one's pharmacological colleagues quite busy. In the days of high throughput screening, this disincentive to preparing more compounds in unit time has been swept away. A combinatorial or multiple parallel synthesis chemist can now prepare this many analogs in a matter of a few days. Having made this analysis, however, one must point out that this is true but somewhat misleading. What is not stated is the time required to develop and rehearse the chemistry to be employed. This can take a matter of a few days to a year or more depending upon the state of the literature and the complexity of the targets. Nonetheless, the point is clear. Employment of combinatorial chemistry is essential for success in a competitive world.

Another factor which is not much discussed in the literature is the comparative costs of making combinatorial libraries. The purchase or synthesis of the component parts is often rather steep if very large libraries consisting of palpable quantities of each product are required. In industry, this is often less than the labor costs so may actually not be a major factor. The cost of automated equipment and the housing of complex synthesizers with large 'footprints' is itself not trivial. In talking with various firms, the number of about US$20 per analog seems not unreasonable. Thus making quite large libraries is expensive. The effective cost is reduced somewhat by archiving the materials and testing them in subsequent drug seeking campaigns when novel tests become available. The relative price of time and the value of the products appears to be the key consideration in judging the comparative value of this methodology.

Another important question is the level of purity one should aim for. In earlier times, this factor was all too often neglected and many examples have been discussed informally where worthless biological results were obtained from grossly impure products. Sometimes, in fact, the activity came from the impurity, or even that the substance in the vial was not the one on the label. Much greater care is now expended on quality assurance and commonly one expects at least 80–90% purity for each library component.

The question often arises as to how many compounds should be in a drug-seeking library. The ideal answer would be one. This is almost always impossible to realize. On the other hand, a skillful medicinal chemist who must make a hundred thousand compounds in order to get a candidate drug should be shot for incompetence. The usual answer is that somewhere between a hundred and a thousand substances will generally suffice. This is particularly true when uses the technique of pulsed libraries. Here one makes a limited number of structurally diverse molecules whose properties give them a chance of having useful pharmacokinetic and pharmacodynamic properties. The testing results suggest the next group to be prepared and evaluated. Each pulse then leads to a progressively more suitable collection of molecules from which the winners emerge expeditiously.

The question of whether to perform combinatorial or MPS chemistry on resins or in solution is partly a question of taste. Resin chemistry is not as familiar to the average chemist and requires attachment–detachment sequences analogous to protection–deprotection sequences resulting in unavoidable lengthening of the construction chemistry. The chemistry of the various attachments also must be compatable with the various linkers and the detachments must take place in the appropriate sequence. The resins must also be stable to the reagents and the reaction conditions and should not leave traces in the final products. Precedent chemistry is usually optimized in solution and so the reactions have to be adapted to the solid phase environment's needs. These disadvantages are balanced in part by the ease of purification of the products. Resin methodology is particularly useful for long sequences (more than five steps) and for very large libraries of comparatively small quantities (mgs at most) prepared by iterative processes. Solution methods are less limited in quantities to be prepared and conditions to be employed. They are also more familiar to the average chemist and many choices of reaction chambers are now available from which to choose.

Special applications of resins in solution phase organic synthesis (SnPOS) have also proven popular. For example, reagents can be present on resins. Following reaction, the excess or exhausted reagents can be removed by filtration and washing thereby simplifying workup. The synthesis of the adrenergic β-blocker propranolol serves as an example (Figure 1.11). Here, a six-step sequence was employed in which three of the steps utilized resin supported reagents. To start an amberlyst supported carbonate ion and iodine reacted with isopropylvinylamine salt and the resulting halide was transformed to the corresponding acetate ester with amberlyst supported acetate salt resin. Hydrolysis with potassium carbonate and ether formation with mesyl chloride was followed by a nucleophilic displacement with amberlyst-1-naphthoate resin and the carbonate protecting group was removed by KOH hydrolysis to produce propranolol. Obvious variants could be used to produce a library of analogs. Many other reactions have been performed with solid supported reagents (SSR) and this area has been nicely reviewed.

Resins can also be used to capture reaction by-products (e.g. basic resins to absorb acidic products) which can be separated by simple filtrations. These reactions can be worked up and the product isolated in pure form often by simple filtration and evaporation of solvents. Because the isolation of a large number of products resulting from combinatorial chemistry or multiple parallel synthesis can be exceedingly laborious and time consuming if performed in the traditional way, the convenience and time saving by using resin capture technology can be very

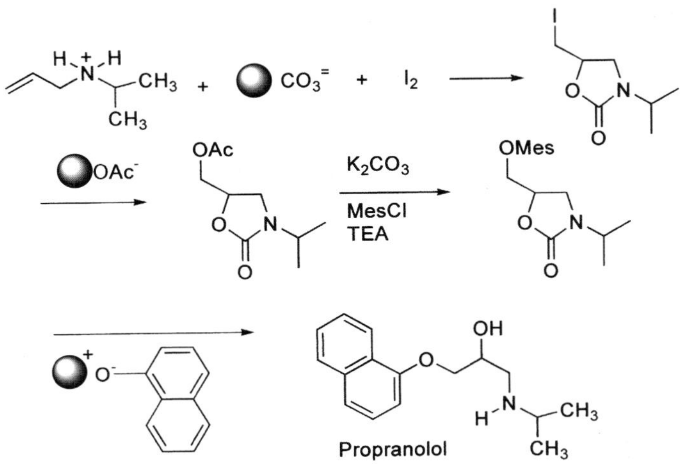

Figure 1.11 Solid phase organic synthesis of propranolol.

impressive. One certainly does not want to give back the time saved in construction by employing tedious separation operations! As an example of the utility of resin capture, a large collection of ureas was made by reacting an amine in solution with an excess of a substituted isocyanate to force the reaction to completion (Figure 1.12). The excess of isocyanate was captured by addition of a resin-immobilized amine to form an insoluble urea. The insoluble urea was removed by filtration and the desired urea in solution was obtained in pure form in high yield by filtration and washing.

In order for the combinatorial methods on resins to be useful, it is essential that suitable assays be developed and appropriate data handling methods be applied. In some cases, affinity chromatography using immobilized receptors/enzymes serves to separate beads containing active ligands. In others, soluble receptor/ enzyme preparations bind to the tethered ligands on beads. Finally, one uses traditional solution methods in which soluble compounds are assayed alone or in

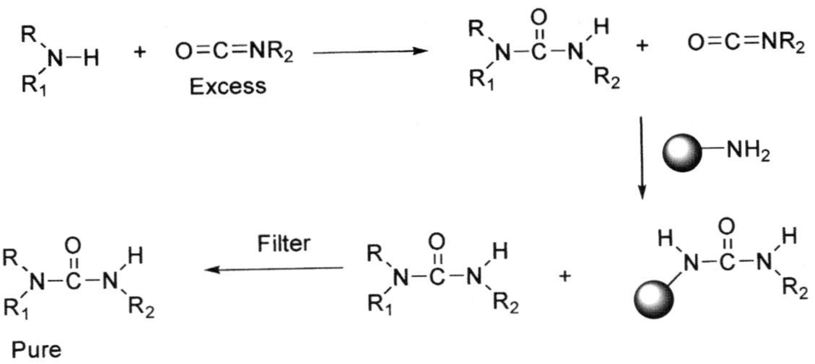

Figure 1.12 Resin capture methodology in the combinatorial synthesis of urea arrays.

combination with established ligands. Each of these devices possesses different requirements for success and must discriminate between specific and non-specific binding. Following up combinatorial hits in this way and progressing to candidate drugs is a form of chemical evolution and requires a combination of opportunism and the skillful application of drug design elements!

1.6   LEAD OPTIMIZATION

If potency, efficacy and selectivity were the only needed characteristics of a drug, the work of the medicinal chemist would be dramatically simplified. However, these characteristics are just the opening chapters in a long and complex saga. Many other factors must be built in before the job is done. The most important of these are summarized in the useful acronym ADME-To (absorption, distribution, metabolism and excretion as well as toxicity). Clearly, the drug must reach the site of action in a timely manner and in sufficient concentration to produce the desired effect.

The most common means of administration is oral and in this drug taking mimics eating. A degree of water solubility is required as only dissolved drug has a chance of being absorbed. Only highly lipophilic substances such as nitroglycerine and cocaine are significantly absorbed during the comparatively short time that substances are present in the mouth. The drug must next survive the acidic environment of the stomach and pass into the small intestine where the bulk of absorption takes place. Here the pH is neutral to slightly acidic. Although the upper part of the small intestine is fairly short, it is highly convoluted and highly vascularized. These factors promote absorption. Metabolism can take place here as a consequence of digestive enzymes (which create a particular problem for polypeptides) and because the gut wall is fairly rich in oxidative enzymes. As time for absorption is fairly short as the gut contents pass downstream, lipophilic small molecules are better absorbed than large molecules reflecting their comparative ease of diffusion. The pH of the small intestine is nearly neutral and the cells lining it are surrounded by the lipid bilayer of the cell surface. Thus, unless the drug benefits from active energy-requiring uptake mechanisms that primarily facilitate uptake of amino acids and glucose, the drug must be significantly unionized to penetrate into the body. Neutral substances and tertiary amines benefit from this. The Lipinski rule of fives puts this requirement into semi-quantitative terms.

Following absorption, the blood rapidly presents the drug to the liver. The liver is like a grease trap in the sense that it retards passage of lipophilic molecules and is rich in metabolizing enzymes that enhance the polarity of many foreign bodies. This causes their release as metabolically transformed molecules into the general circulation and facilitates their subsequent excretion in the urine. Oxidation, hydrolysis, reduction, etc. are Class I metabolic transformations introducing polar functions into many lipid molecules. When this is still insufficiently polarizing, Phase II metabolic transformations take place in which glucuronidation, sulfation and the like take place rendering the molecule still more polar. In some cases, the drug or its metabolite(s) are excreted in the bile back into the small intestine.

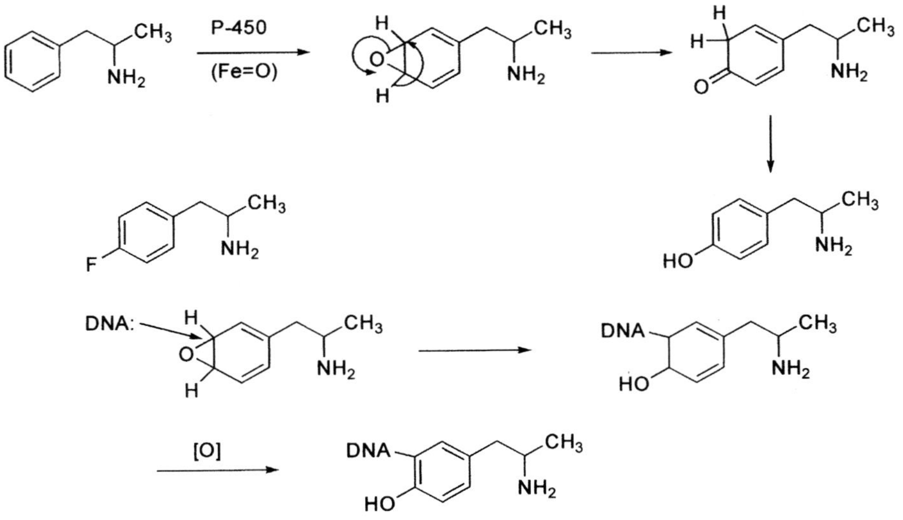

Figure 1.13 Oxidative metabolism of tyrosine.

In many cases, the drug then is excreted in the feces. In some cases, however, it undergoes further intestinal metabolism or in its own right is reabsorbed and presented again to the liver. This process is not common but is known as entero-hepatic cycling. An illustrative example of the process of polarizing metabolism is provided by amphetamine (Figure 1.13). This substance is hydroxylated to a more polar phenol by action of a heme containing P-450 enzyme. The intermediate is an arene oxide which undergoes rearrangement to the isolated product. This process can be blocked by installation of a p-fluoro substituent that deadens the aromatic ring to electrophilic substitution.

Occasionally, this well meant physiological process results in toxicity instead. Arene oxides are reactive species that can if long-lived, alkylate DNA, for example. If such adducts are not repaired in a timely manner, mutations can occur. Reactions of this type rationalize how apparently inert molecules such as certain polycyclic aromatic hydrocarbons (Figure 1.14) present in incompletely combusted materials present in chimney condensates, tobacco smoke, automobile exhausts, etc. can be carcinogenic. Epoxide hydrolase is but one of the mechanisms cells employ to intercept and detoxify such reactive molecules. Glutathione is yet another.

After release from the liver into the general circulation, the drug may or may not be bound to serum proteins. Molecules that undergo this binding are often acidic and lipophilic and in this are similar in properties to fatty acids. This is a normal means of transporting fatty acids without their salts (soaps) causing hemolysis of the fragile red-blood corpuscles. Drugs bound to serum proteins are often inhibited thereby from reaching their receptors in a timely manner although they are in equilibrium with them. They also remain longer in the body than otherwise as the

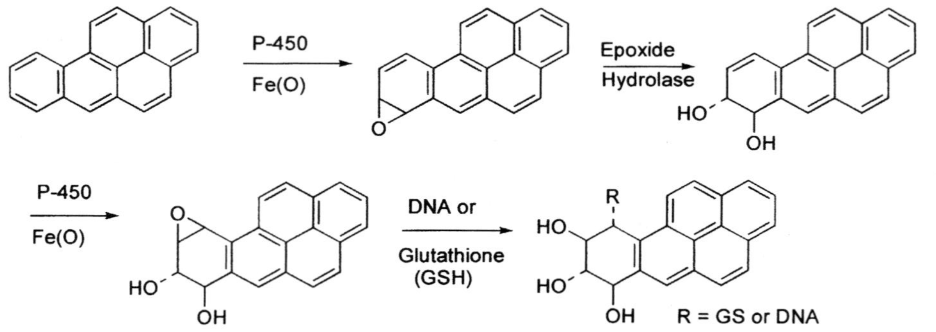

Figure 1.14 Oxidative metabolism of a polycyclic aromatic hydrocarbon (PAH).

urine is a protein-free filtrate. Most drugs, however, are not seriously protein bound so readily reach their receptors and interact with them. Organs are not uniformly supplied with blood but all organs and tissues are accessible, so most drugs can reach the site of action. The brain is unusual in that whereas it is richly supplied with blood, it is protected from the general circulation by the blood–brain barrier. In contrast to other organs where cells do not press closely together and therefore some passage of drugs can take place between cells, the cells lining the capillaries of the brain are tightly pressed together. The practical consequence of this is that drugs targeted to the brain are generally required to be more lipophilic than drugs targeted to other organs.

The kidneys serve to filter the blood and to retain essential molecules (certain salts and especially water) and to excrete waste materials. Thus, it is a selective clearing organ. This is the principal route of excretion of drugs and their metabolites. The product of the rate of absorption of drugs, their degree of metabolic transformation, their distribution in the body, and their rate of excretion is called pharmacokinetics. This is in effect the influence of the body on a drug as a function of time. The interaction of the drug with its receptors and the consequences of this as a function of time are pharmacodynamics. Both of these characteristics are strongly influenced by chemical structure and the skillful medicinal chemist must be able to optimize them through analoging. It is important to note in this respect that in doing this the parts of the drug molecule that are in direct contact with the receptor/enzyme may not be altered covalently without dramatically altering the potency of the molecule. This part of the molecule is defined as the pharmacophore. The rest of the molecule is molecular scaffolding and its structure is much less specifically demanding. It is in this part of the molecule that adjustments in ADME-To properties are more likely to be successful.

In favorable cases, it is possible to adjust molecular properties in a temporary manner by covering a misbehaving functional group by a moiety that is removed enzymically in the body once the problem area is bypassed. For example, a polar carboxylic acid moiety can be converted to an ester so that the resulting product undergoes enzymic hydrolysis in the liver or blood following efficient absorption. The product is the active drug which then proceeds to the receptor or target enzyme and functions as intended. This methodology is known as prodruging and is the topic of Chapter 14.

The medicinal chemist is expected to remedy any shortcomings by molecular manipulation. Bitter experience has shown that it is often easier to achieve potency, efficacy and selectivity in a molecule than it is to satisfy the ADME-To characteristics. Thus, it is usual to start with molecules that appear to be drug-like at the outset rather than to make a hit drug-like later. In addition to ADME-To, a number of other characteristics must also be satisfactory. These are listed below:

- Freedom from mutagenicity (in most cases mutagenicity is a show stopper if it is series general rather than molecule specific)
- Freedom from teratogenicity
- Chemical stability
- Synthetic or biological accessibility
- Acceptable cost
- Ability to patent
- Clinical efficacy
- Solubility
- Satisfactory taste
- Ability to formulate satisfactorily for administration
- Freedom from an idiosyncratic problem.

Toxicity is often difficult to control other than by the avoidance of the presence of functional groups that are known to be bad actors. Thioureas, aromatic nitro groups, furan rings, and electrophilic functions are well known to be problematic. This is not to say that there are no successful drugs with these functions present, but they always raise a red flag and require close examination in the testing phases because there are many precedent cases that engender concern. Functional groups that alter DNA are special problems. Flat three-ring containing aromatic molecules intercalate into DNA and are troublesome as they often cause frame shift mutations that, if not repaired, are self perpetuating when the DNA molecules are replicated. The resulting cells are transformed and will usually function poorly if not die or be cancerous.

Since the thalidomide disaster, drugs are closely monitored for safety in pregnant animals. This is particularly important for drugs that are likely to be administered chronically.

Failure to pass any of these challenges can be a show stopper. Getting a drug through to the market is equivalent to winning a lottery. All of the numbers must be correct and in the right sequence or one comes away only with a piece of non-negotiable paper.

Some insight into the popularity of particular drug design methods can be gained by considering just what chemists do when faced with the need to solve these problems. The following table results from an analysis of the frequency of particular drug design methods importantly utilized in the articles published in *The Journal of Medicinal Chemistry* during 1999 (Volume 21).

Technique	Number of articles wherein used
Bioisosteres	56
Natural product leads	49
Structure-based drug design	41
Prodrugs	32
Metabolism	31
Molecular rigidification	31
Peptidomimetics	27
Absolute configuration	26
Screening	21
Combinatorial libraries	19
DNA as a target	18
COMFA	15
Computer assisted drug design	12
Conformation	12

Some of these methods are under represented because of the existence of specialized journals dealing with particular methodologies (for example, several journals deal with combinatorial methods alone although these do not always focus specifically on drug discovery). The members of the list and the rank ordering varies from year to year but the practicing medicinal chemist must know when these methods are appropriate and when they are not and how to employ and to evaluate them.

Interestingly, the classical method of bioisosterism (or molecular mimicry) has led the list for nearly two decades so is worth singling out briefly. Bioisosteric atoms and groupings are those that have approximately the same size or molecular volumes so their interchange results in similarity in chemical, physical and notably biological properties of the resulting analogs. Classical isosteres include interchange of atoms in the same row of the periodic chart such as $-CH_2-, -NH-, -O-$ and $-F$. Note that hydrogen atoms are added to compensate for valence differences. This is known as the Grimm hydride displacement rule. Over time the definition of isosterism has broadened to include some isoelectronic interchanges as well. Examples of this phenomenon include $-S-$ and $-O-$ as well as $-F, -Cl$ and $-Br$. Bioisosteres include the classical isosteres, but bioisosteric atoms or groups of atoms do not nescessarily overlap. However, bioisosteres show sufficient steric, electronic or other properties to ensure biological activity similar to the parent. This widely employed drug design technique is covered in extenso in Chapters 9 and 10 to which the interested reader is directed.

Important additional insight can be gained from compilations of the reasons drugs fail in the clinic. Although there has not been a recent survey, experience indicates that the information that is available is not very different today. The data described in the following table comes from England and covers the years 1964–1985 (Prentis *et al.* 1988).

Problem	Instance	Percentage
Pharmacokinetic problems	78	39
Efficacy not proven	58	29
Toxicity	22	11
Adverse effects	20	10
Limited commercial interest	10	5
Replaced by improved candidate	4	2
Budget exhausted	2	1
Chemical problem	1	0.5
Unknown reason	3	1.5
Sum	198	100

Prudence requires that due attention be paid prospectively to avoiding structures likely to fall into one of these categories. One notes in particular the primacy of pharmacokinetic and toxicity problems.

1.7   CELL BIOLOGY AND GENOMICS AS A SOURCE OF DRUG TARGETS

The classical means of drug discovery involved finding a chemical that had a favorable influence on disease and, using this as a tool, eventually sorting out what its cellular target was and then figuring out how this could produce the observed effect. This has the character of a very involved detective story associated with few useful clues. Gradually this changed, as the result of increasing knowledge of cellular physiology, to understanding how a cell or organ system actually functioned and then finding a defective bit of cellular physiology associated with the cause of disease and then to searching for molecules that might rectify the situation. Clearly, this was a more gratifying and focused intellectual exercise but was by no means much simpler. In more recent years, increasing knowledge of cell biology converted an alphabet soup of vaguely characterized cellular factors into palpable molecules identified with particular signaling pathways involved in cellular responses to various external or internal stimuli. This led to the crafting of agents that could increase or decrease these signals in a therapeutically useful way.

New possibilities of increasing complexity continually open up as our knowledge of cell function and pathology becomes ever sophisticated. At the moment of this writing, the complete genome of *Homo sapiens* has just been published in two versions (The human genome, *Science* (2001) **291**; *Nature* (2001) **409**). We now know the 30 000 or so genes that lead to all of the proteins of which we are composed. Even with the added complication of post-translation modifications this is an unexpectedly finite number of informational macro-molecules with which to deal. Hurtful to our pride is the knowledge that genetically we are not much more complicated than a nematode! Many of the gene products made using these genes are receptors and enzymes of whose function we are presently unaware. This powerful new knowledge promises to define many new molecular targets for chemotherapy and gives us powerful tools for advancements in medicine undreamed of until very recent times. Indeed, this reverses the classical mode of drug seeking. Instead of proceeding from agent to target to knowledge of cellular physiology at the molecular level, we now are prepared to begin with knowledge of cellular factors, to trace their function, to determine what role, if any, they play in particular disease states, to devise molecular cures and then to search for molecules that will have these properties.

The days when a medicinal chemist need only have a knowledge of synthesis are rapidly passing away and contemporary drug seeking requires a knowledge of at least the application of high level chemistry to very sophisticated biological phenomena. The future involves mastery of important aspects of very new sciences.

Genomics is the comprehensive study of the interrelationships among families of genes. We already have at our disposal gene chips containing the mRNA produced by very large numbers of different DNA molecules in response to various cellular treatments. When quantitated as a function of time, this gives us powerful insights into how cells respond to particular stimuli and how they differ from diseased cells. Tracing back to the DNA involved and forward to the gene products increases our repertoire of targets for chemotherapy.

Functional genomics is the study of genomes to determine the biological function of all the genes and their products.

Proteomics is the study of the full set of proteins encoded by a genome.

Informatics is the study of the information storage and retrieval of information gathered from genomic and proteomic studies.

1.8   FUTURE DEVELOPMENTS

It is always perilous to predict the future in turbulent times. The unprecedented capabilities made possible by decoding of the genome not only for humans but for other life forms as well will surely transform the face of modern biology. Whereas for the majority of the century just past by and large chemistry put the ball in play in drug seeking, clearly the current century will be dominated as far as can be seen at this moment by biology. Medicinal chemistry lies at the interface between these two and cannot fail to be transformed as well. The art and science of medicine in the last century has been strongly influenced by the properties of small molecules. The years ahead will see a strong overlay associated with large molecules. In order to be functional, chemical education for those to practice medicinal chemistry must retain its traditional ability to predict the properties of molecules and to construct them efficiently but be expanded at the same time to include much more serious treatment of biological topics as well. The strain on the traditional curriculum will be substantial. Medicinal chemistry departments have made a strong start in this direction. Chemistry departments will need to join.

During the last century, every advance in organic chemistry has rapidly been incorporated into medicinal chemistry. One can cite advances in the understanding of reaction mechanisms, conformational analysis, host–guest interactions, quantum mechanics, spectroscopy, and so on. This is unlikely to change.

It is safe to predict that a more profound understanding of the factors involved in ADME-To lies just ahead. Understanding more perfectly the relationship between chemical structure and these factors will greatly facilitate drug design and discovery. Increasing use of structure-based drug design techniques will doubtless also take place enhancing our ability to craft more potent and more specific agents. These prospects are exhilarating.

The unraveling of the genome leads us to the identification of targets for chemotherapy not previously suspected and even allows us to dream of the possibility of correcting genetic defects, enhancing our prospects for a longer and more healthy life, and for devising drugs for specific individuals! Explanations for the perplexing phenomena of significantly varying responses of different individuals to the same treatment are likely to come from a better understanding of differing gene patterns in patients. Presuming that individual variations in response may often have a genetic basis, dividing populations into subgroups with similar genetic characteristics could allow us to prescribe drugs and even dosages within these groups so that a larger percentage would respond favorably. This form of individual gene typing is possible even now but would be very expensive. The costs could become manageable with time and effort. It is doubtful, however, if this could in the foreseeable future be brought within the reach of the very poor. The moral implications of this must be anticipated and settled. It is also likely that perplexing species differences in response to chemotherapy that complicate drug development may also be understood when the genomes of more species become available. Means of dealing with multidrug resistance will also depend upon this knowledge. Determination of the genome of pathogens, such as *Mycobacterium tuberculosis*, leads to the identification of novel targets for chemotherapy with the possibility of reducing resistance development and also to gene products that are associated with infection and pathogenicity.

The new biological capabilities raise many new prospects and problems for society. These not only open great scientific possibilities but also raise perplexing moral issues for which we are not yet prepared. Scientific knowledge by itself is morally neutral. What is done with it is not. It is imperative that we chose wisely and are reasonably tolerant when we occasionally put our feet wrong.

It is probably true that the majority of medicinal chemists who have ever lived are active when these lines are being written and it is certainly true that there has never been a more exciting time to take up the study of medicinal chemistry. In 1900, even far seeing geniuses such as Ehrlich could hardly imagine a small percentage of the wonders that are common place in 2000. It is very likely that wonders unimaginable today will be recounted in 2100. The techniques recounted in the remainder of this book represent the cutting edge of modern technology and represent the launching pad from which the wonders that lie ahead will be reached.

FURTHER READING

Annual Reports in Medicinal Chemistry. A yearly compilation of reviews on medicinal chemical topics organized by the Medicinal Division and published by The American Chemical Society. The current volume is no. 35.

Baichwal, V.R. and Baeuerle, P.A. (1998) Kinases in pro-inflammatory signal transduction pathways: new opportunities for drug discovery. *Annu. Repts. Med. Chem.*, **33**, 233.

Bailey, D.S. (1999) Pharmacogenomics and its impact on drug design and optimization. *Annu. Repts. Med. Chem.*, **34**, 339.

Black, J.W. (1989) Drugs from emasculated hormones: the principle of syntopic antagonism. *Science*, **245**, 486.

Brown, F.K. (1998) Chemoinformatics: what is it and how does it impact drug discovery. *Annu. Repts. Med. Chem.*, **33**, 375.

Flam, F. (1994) Chemical prospectors scour the seas for promising drugs. *Science*, **266**, 1324.

Gallop, M. *et al.* (1994) Applications of combinatorial technologies. I. Background and peptide combinatorial libraries. *J. Med. Chem.*, **37**, 1233.

Gordon, E. *et al.* (1994) Applications of combinatorial technologies. II. Combinatorial organic synthesis, library screening strategies and future directions. *J. Med. Chem.*, **37**, 1385.

Greer, J. *et al.* (1994) Application of the three-dimensional structures of protein target molecules in structure-based drug design. *J. Med. Chem.*, **37**, 1035.

Lau, K.F. and Sakul, H. (2000) Pharmacogenomics. *Annu. Repts. Med. Chem.*, **35**, 261.

Murcko, M.A., Caron, P.R.l. and Charifson, P.S. (1999) Structure-based drug design. *Annu. Repts. Med. Chem.*, **34**, 297.

Oldenberg, K.R. (1998) Current and future trends in high throuput screening for drug discovery. *Annu. Repts. Med. Chem.*, **33**, 301.

Stewart, B.H., Wang, Y. and Surendran, N. (2000) *Ex vivo* approaches to predicting oral pharmacokinetics in humans. *Annu. Repts. Med. Chem.*, **35**, 299.

Sweetnam, P.M. *et al.* (1993) The role of receptor binding in drug discovery. *J. Natural Products*, **56**, 441.

Trainor, G.L. (2000) Privileged structures – an update. *Annu. Repts. Med. Chem.*, **35**, 289.

Trivedi, B.K., Low, J.E., Carson, K. and LaRosa, G.J. (2000) Chemokines: targets for novel therapeutics. *Annu. Repts. Med. Chem.*, **35**, 191.

Weisbach, J. and Moos, W.H. (1995) Diagnosing the decline in major pharmaceutical research laboratories: a prescription for drug companies. *Drug Dev. Research*, **34**, 243.

REFERENCES

Bunin, B.A. and Ellman, J.A. (1992) A general and expedient method for the solid-phase synthesis of 1,4-benzodiazepine derivatives. *J. Am. Chem. Soc.*, **114**, 10997.

Drews, J. (2000) *Science*, **287**, 1962.

Gelmo, P. (1908) Über Sulfonamide der p-Amidobenzolsulfonsäure. *J. Pr. Chem.*, **N.S. 77**, 369–382.

Gruber, V. and Theisen, M. (2000) Genetically modified crops as a source for pharmaceuticals. *Annu. Repts. Med. Chem.*, **35**, 357.

Lipinski, C.A., Lombardo, F., Dominy, B.W. and Feeney, P.J. (2001) Experimental and computational approaches to estimate solubility and permeability in drug discovery and development settings. *Adv. Drug Deliv. Rev.*, **46**, 3.

Milligan, G. and Rees, S. (2000) Oligomerisation of G protein coupled receptors. *Annu. Repts. Med. Chem.*, **35**, 271.

Prentis, R.A., Lis, Y. and Walker, S.R. (1988) Pharmaceutical innovation by the seven UK-owned pharmaceutical companies. *British J. Clin. Pharmacol.*, **25**, 387.

Sternbach, L. (1979) The benzodiazepine story. *J. Med. Chem.*, **22**, 1.

Chapter 2

Role of molecular recognition in drug design

Peter Andrews and Michael Dooley

2.1 INTRODUCTION

Molecular recognition underpins every aspect of life, from the replication of the genome through genetic transcription and protein translation to the assembly and integrity of complex multicellular organisms such as humans. Drugs, which may modify any of these processes, also derive their actions by the absolute control of molecular recognition. Understanding the underlying physical basis for an association between drugs and their receptors is paramount to the ultimate task of drug design, that of *predicting* affinities of new drugs. This is a formidable challenge requiring a detailed knowledge of the physical forces that comprise drug–receptor interactions, and an understanding of the thermodynamic backdrop of the association, to ultimately determine the strength of drug–receptor interactions.

This chapter gives a basic understanding of the various types of non-bonded drug–receptor interactions and associated entropy terms, including a discussion of the various levels of approximation commonly used to calculate the overall strengths of the resulting intermolecular interactions from these components. It details some of the successes and pitfalls that go along with the use of various approximations in the prediction of drug affinity. It should leave the reader with no doubt that while the principles of molecular recognition are reasonably well understood, the business of predicting binding affinities between drugs and receptors is still far from an exact science.

2.2 THERMODYNAMIC CONSIDERATIONS OF DRUG BINDING

The interaction of a drug with its receptor may be written in the form of equation (2.1)

$$L{:}S_l + R{:}S_r + S_{bulk} \rightleftharpoons L^*{:}R^*{:}S_{lr} + S^*_{bulk} \tag{2.1}$$

where $L{:}S_l$ is the free ligand in solution surrounded by a perturbed solvation shell, $R{:}S_r$ is the free receptor together with a perturbed solvation shell and S_{bulk} is the bulk solvent. On the right hand side of the equilibrium, $L^*{:}R^*{:}S_{lr}$ represents the complex of ligand and receptor and a perturbed solvation shell and S^*_{bulk}

represents the bulk solvent. The ligand and receptor states and the solvation structure are all modified therefore nothing on the left hand and right hand sides can be considered equivalent (designated by *). The position of the equilibrium and therefore the affinity of the ligand are determined by the free energy difference (ΔG) between the two sides and this can be formally expressed in terms of equation (2.2). Here R is the gas constant, T is the temperature in Kelvin and K_d is the dissociation constant for the ligand. Optimally, in the context of drug design, there is a large negative free energy change in the right-hand direction of equation (2.1).

$$\Delta G = RT \ln K_d \tag{2.2}$$

The great challenge for drug design is to determine the free energy change by computational means and therefore *predict* the binding affinity of a new drug. Calculation of the free energy change resulting from a ligand–receptor interaction can be used to predict the K_d of the ligand by equation (2.2). However, there is a very narrow margin for error since small variations in ΔG lead to large errors in K_d. Therefore, accurate predictions of affinity will require very accurate calculation of ΔG.

Free energy perturbation techniques are used to determine relative binding energies of ligands, however this method suffers from computational expense and the limitation that only very closely related ligands can be studied. Since the free energy change can also be related to the enthalpy (ΔH) and entropy changes (ΔS) for the equilibrium by equation (2.3), methods which approximate the free energy change by summing the component parts of molecular interactions have become popular.

$$\Delta G = \Delta H - T\Delta S \tag{2.3}$$

The components of molecular interactions have typically been divided into entropic and enthalpic terms. The entropic contributions include the cost of reducing the rotational and translational entropy of the ligand, restricting rotation of internal rotors of the ligand and the receptor and the entropic cost or benefit of solvent reorganization. The enthalpic terms include the contributions of favorable and unfavorable non-bonded interactions and penalties for binding high-energy conformers. Several studies have used equations of a form similar to equation (2.4) to estimate ΔG

$$\Delta G = \Delta G_{t+r} + \Delta G_r + \Delta G_x + \Delta G_{conf} \tag{2.4}$$

where ΔG_{t+r} is the cost of binding the ligand into the receptor, ΔG_r is the cost of restricting internal rotations, ΔG_x is the sum of the contributions of individual functional groups X, including weak intermolecular bonds such as hydrogen bonds and the free energy change associated with solvent reorganization (the hydrophobic effect), and ΔG_{conf} is the energy penalty for binding a high energy conformer.

2.3 THE PHYSICAL BASIS OF INTERMOLECULAR INTERACTIONS

2.3.1 Enthalpic contributions

2.3.1.1 *Electrostatic interactions*

Electrostatic interactions are the net result of the attractive forces between the positively charged nuclei and the negatively charged electrons of the two molecules. The attractive force between these opposite charges leads to three main bond types: charge–charge, charge–dipole and dipole–dipole interactions. The reader is directed to useful reviews on this topic by Bongrand (1999) and Glusker (1998).

2.3.1.1.1 *Ionic bonds*

The strength of any electrostatic (coulombic) interaction can be calculated from equation (2.5), where q_i and q_j are two charges separated by a distance r_{ij} in a medium of dielectric constant ε. This equation applies equally to ionic interactions, where the charges q_i and q_j are integer values, or to polar interactions, in which the total energy is summed over the contributions calculated from the partial charges on all the individual atoms.

$$E = \frac{q_i q_j}{\varepsilon r_{ij}} \tag{2.5}$$

It follows from equation (2.5) that the strength of an ionic interaction is inversely proportional to the distance separating the two charges and to the dielectric constant ε of the surrounding medium. The strength of an ionic interaction is thus dependent on its environment. In hydrophobic environments, like the interior of a protein molecule, the dielectric constant may be as low as 4, whereas in bulk phase water the corresponding value is 80. In other environments, intermediate values are appropriate e.g. for interactions occurring near the surface of a protein, an ε value of 28 is commonly used. Since the strength of coulombic interactions decays proportionally to the distance between the charges whereas other electrostatic interactions are even more sensitive to distance (decaying with the square, cube or sixth power of distance), they frequently dominate the initial long-range interactions between ligands and receptors. However, association does not require the ligand and receptor to have opposite net charges. For example, dihydrofolate reductase from *Escherichia coli* and superoxide dismutase from various species and their respective ligands each carry net negative charges.

2.3.1.1.2 *Charge–dipole and dipole–dipole interactions*

Although charge–dipole and dipole–dipole interactions are weaker than ionic bonds, they are nevertheless key contributors to the overall strengths of ligand–receptor interactions, since they occur in any molecule in which electronegativity differences between atoms result in significant bond, group or molecular dipole moments.

The key differences between ionic and dipolar interactions relate to their dependence on distance and orientation. For charge–dipole interactions, the strength of the interaction depends inversely on the square of the distance, while for dipole–dipole interactions, it reduces with the cube of the distance separating the dipoles. These interactions are also inversely proportional to the dielectric constant ε and they are therefore environmentally dependent.

Dipolar interactions may be either attractive or repulsive, depending on the relative orientation of the dipole moments. That is, there is a geometric dependence to the interaction.

2.3.1.1.3   Higher order multipole interactions

Ion–quadrupole and dipole–quadrupole interactions are known to be quite strong in the gas-phase and ion–quadrupole interactions in solution can be as strong as ion–dipole interactions (Dougherty 1996). As an example, interactions between aromatic rings and amine groups are observed in several crystal structures from the protein databank e.g. a thrombin complex (1uma), Lao-binding protein complexed with ornithine (1lah) and oligopeptide binding protein (2olb). Favorable interactions also arise from quadrupole–quadrupole interactions between aromatic rings. It has been shown that there is a statistical preference for particular contact geometries between aromatic rings that maximize this interaction (Hunter 1994).

2.3.1.1.4   Inductive interactions

The formation of a ligand–receptor complex is often accompanied by intramolecular and/or intermolecular redistributions of charge. In the intramolecular case, this redistribution is referred to as an induced polarization, whereas a redistribution of charge between two molecules is described as a charge transfer interaction. In either case, the resulting interactions are always attractive and strongly dependent on the distance separating the two molecules.

2.3.1.1.5   Dispersion forces

Dispersion or London forces are the universal forces responsible for attractive interactions between non-polar molecules. Their occurrence is due to the fact that any atom will, at any given instant, be likely to possess a finite dipole moment as a result of the movement of electrons around the nuclei. Such fluctuating dipoles tend to induce opposite dipoles in adjacent molecules, thus resulting in a net attractive force. Although the individual interactions between pairs of atoms is relatively weak and is inversely proportional to the sixth power of the distance between the atoms, the total contribution to binding from dispersion forces can be very significant if there is a close fit between ligand and receptor. The quality of the steric match is thus the dominant factor in nonpolar interactions.

2.3.1.1.6   Hydrogen bonds

Hydrogen bonds are a complicated mix of electrostatic (coulombic) character, which makes them important in long range interactions, and dipolar character, which play an important role in aligning molecular components of biological systems. They are responsible for maintaining the tertiary structure of proteins and nucleic acids, as well as the binding of many ligands. The strongest hydrogen bonds are formed between groups with the greatest electrostatic character. Thus carboxylates are better acceptors than amides, ketones or unionized carboxyls, whilst substituted ammonium ions are better donors than unsubstituted ammonium ions or trigonal donors.

There is considerable evidence that burying unsatisfied hydrogen bond partners can be unfavorable. For example, McDonald and Thornton (1994) have performed a statistical analysis of high-resolution protein structures, which indicates that only 1.3% of amide NH groups and 1.8% of amide carbonyl groups are buried without forming hydrogen bonds. In the context of ligand–receptor interactions, Fersht *et al.* (1985) have shown that burying an unsatisfied donor or acceptor results in a $16\,\mathrm{kJ\,mol^{-1}}$ destabilization of the complex for a charged group and $4\,\mathrm{kJ\,mol^{-1}}$ for a neutral group.

N-methylacetamide has been used for some time as a prototypic model of protein backbone for the calorimetric and theoretical study of hydrogen bond formation during protein folding. The results of these studies may also be applicable where hydrogen bonds are formed between protein and ligand. Theoretical and experimental (Ben-Tal *et al.* 1997) studies both indicate that hydrogen bond formation between peptide bonds where the partners move from a solvated environment to a desolvated environment (either the interior of a protein or the interface between a ligand and the active-site) is energetically *unfavorable* (ΔG_8, Figure 2.1). The energetics of the system are best viewed as a thermodynamic cycle, as illustrated in Figure 2.1. A hydrogen bond is marginally stable in an aqueous environment (ΔG_4), but considerably more stable in a non-polar environment (ΔG_7). The result is that whilst burying a hydrogen bond might be energetically unfavorable, the burial of an unpaired hydrogen bond partner is around $5.7\,\mathrm{kJ\,mol^{-1}}$ *more unfavorable* ($\Delta G_5{}^*, \Delta G_7{}^*, \Delta G_8{}^*$) than burying the hydrogen bond. If these results are generally applicable to various types of neutral hydrogen bond partners, then the implications for drug design are that while desolvating and burying a neutral hydrogen bond may be energetically *unfavorable*, failure to pair a hydrogen bond partner on the protein with one on the ligand, i.e. burying an unpaired hydrogen bond partner, may be even more energetically unfavorable. This is clearly an issue of ongoing debate in the field.

2.3.1.2   Steric interactions

2.3.1.2.1   Short-range repulsive forces

The short-range repulsive forces resulting from the overlap of the electron clouds of any two molecules increase exponentially with decreasing internuclear

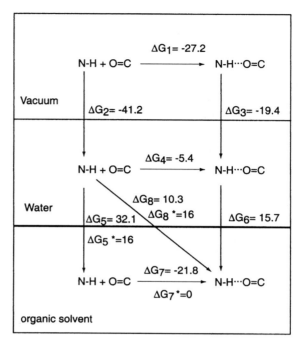

Figure 2.1 Thermodynamic cycle of hydrogen bond formation between N–H and C=O groups in different phases.

separation. The balance between these repulsive interactions and the dispersion forces thus determines both the minimum and the most favorable non-bonded separation between any pair of atoms. The equilibrium distance can be determined from crystal data, and is equivalent to the sum of the van der Waals radii of the two interacting atoms.

For non-polar molecules this balance between the attractive dispersion forces and the short range repulsive forces is generally defined in terms of the Buckingham (6-exp) potential given in equation (2.6) or the alternative Lennard-Jones 6–12 potential, given in equation (2.7). The extreme repulsive forces that develop as atoms approach closer than the sum of their van der Waals radii are perhaps the single most decisive influence on whether a molecule will bind to a receptor since very small steric clashes between molecules will abolish affinity.

$$E = \frac{Ae^{-Br}}{r^d} - \frac{C}{r^6} \tag{2.6}$$

$$E = \frac{A}{r^{12}} - \frac{C}{r^6} \tag{2.7}$$

2.3.2   Entropic contributions

2.3.2.1   *Translational and rotational entropy*

The formation of any ligand–receptor complex is accompanied by the replacement of the three rotational and three translational degrees of freedom of the ligand by six vibrational degrees of freedom in the complex ('residual motion'). The extent of this change is primarily dependent on the relative 'tightness' of the resulting complex. For a typical ligand–protein complex, the estimated change in free energy resulting from the loss of entropy on binding (at 310 K) ranges from 9 kJ mol^{-1} for a loose interaction to 45 kJ mol^{-1} for a tightly bound complex (Searle and Williams 1992).

In addition to this loss of rotational and translational freedom, there is a further entropy loss due to the conformational restriction that accompanies binding of flexible ligands. Based on the observed entropy changes accompanying cyclization reactions, the extent of this entropy loss is estimated at 5–6 kJ mol^{-1} per internal rotation, although the actual figure again depends on how tight a complex is formed between the ligand and the receptor. For bimolecular interactions that do not involve covalent bonds, a range of 1.6–3.4 kJ mol^{-1} per internal rotor has been proposed (Searle and Williams 1992). In the case of rigid analogs, for which there is no loss of conformational entropy on binding, this factor provides a free energy advantage relative to more flexible ligands and this is the basis of one of the central tenets of medicinal chemistry, that of conformational restriction.

In some cases, the bound conformation of a flexible molecule may also be its lowest energy conformation, in which the penalty for the resulting conformational constraint will be restricted to the loss of internal rotational entropy described above. In other cases, however, the optimal interaction between ligand and receptor will require a higher energy conformation, and this energy penalty will further reduce the net binding energy observed (for further discussions of conformational energy penalties see Chapter 4).

2.3.2.2   *Hydrophobic effect*

When a non-polar molecule is placed in water, stronger water–water interactions are formed around the solute molecule to compensate for the weaker interactions between solute and water. This results in an increasingly ordered arrangement of water molecules around the solute and thus a negative entropy of dissolution. The decrease in entropy is roughly proportional to the non-polar surface area of the molecule. The association of two such non-polar molecules in water reduces the total non-polar surface area exposed to the solvent, thus reducing the amount of structured water, and therefore providing a favorable entropy of association.

Although it can be determined theoretically from statistical mechanics calculations or free energy simulations, the hydrophobic effect is commonly estimated empirically. One of the methods used is measurement of the solubility of simple hydrocarbons in water (solvent transfer method). Estimates of the free energy required to transfer hydrocarbons from water into a hydrophobic environment range from 0.1 to 0.14 kJ mol^{-1} for every square angstrom of solvent-accessible hydrocarbon surface removed from exposure to water by the binding process (Williams and Bardsley 1999).

2.3.2.3 Solvent reorganization

In principle, the entropic component of the hydrophobic effect described in the previous section might be applied to a broad range of hydropathic types, not just non-polar molecules and surfaces. Thus, Klotz (1997) has made a theoretical derivation that electrostatic interactions (not only ionic) in water would have a large favorable entropic component. Intuitively this may be rationalized as similar to the entropic component of the hydrophobic effect. The solvation shell of the polar groups would be more ordered than the bulk solvent, and an interaction between two such polar groups would eliminate some of that water back to the bulk solvent with a favorable entropy gain. Klotz used the dissociation of acetic acid in water (ΔG 6.5 kcal mol^{-1} at 300 K, $\Delta H \sim 0$, $\Delta S - 22$ cal mol^{-1} K^{-1}) as an example. Negative entropies of transfer of ions and molecules from the gas phase to water also support this.

2.4   THE TOTAL ENERGY OF INTERMOLECULAR INTERACTION

2.4.1   Free energy perturbation

Free energy perturbation techniques are used to determine the difference in the free energy of binding between two ligands and a common receptor, or between the same ligands and solvent, by utilizing the concept of a thermodynamic cycle. This method has proved astoundingly accurate in predicting relative binding energies of ligand series, but still suffers from problems of computational expense. Its use is also limited to narrow structural changes between the two ligands. It does not require any partitioning of individual energetic components of the free energy change (Kollman 1993; Pang and Kollman 1995).

2.4.2   Partitioning methods

As noted earlier, the total free energy change ΔG resulting from a ligand–receptor interaction is the sum of the free energy changes associated with all of the electrostatic, inductive, non-polar and hydrophobic interactions listed in the previous sections, less any conformational energy and rotational, translational or conformational entropy costs associated with the interaction. Some of these terms can be calculated relatively simply using the equations given in the preceding pages. Others, such as the entropy terms, are much more complex, and are frequently handled empirically. It is important to avoid double counting these terms. The total free energy change can be calculated in a variety of ways, and the reader is directed to the review by Ajay and Murcko (1995), which gives a detailed account of the various methods.

Ultimately, a complete theoretical description of all of the energy contributions described above would require quantum mechanical treatment of the entire system, including solving the time-dependent Schrödinger equation for ligand, receptor, surrounding solvent and any other relevant solutes. The resulting free energy of interaction would be directly comparable, and hopefully in close agreement, with the observed dissociation constant for the ligand–receptor interaction. It is doubtful, however, if there is real benefit for the 3D QSAR or drug design practitioner in pursuing the calculation of intermolecular interactions to this level of complexity. The real question for us is not 'What is the total electrostatic or van der Waals, enthalpic or entropic, H-bond or hydrophobic, contribution to the intermolecular interaction?'. Rather, we want to know the answers to questions like 'What increase in binding could I expect if I add this functional group to my ligand?'.

2.5 ESTIMATING INDIVIDUAL GROUP COMPONENTS IN LIGAND–RECEPTOR INTERACTIONS AND CO-OPERATIVITY

The total free energy of interaction between a ligand and its receptor provides a measure of the strength of the association between the two molecules, but tells us little or nothing about the overall quality of their match. Does the observed binding reflect a composite of interactions between every part of the ligand and its recep-tor, or is it a case of one or two strong interactions contributing sufficient energy to disguise an otherwise mediocre fit? Is the observed increase in interaction energy resulting from the addition of a new functional group consistent with what might have been anticipated? To answer these questions we need some means of estimat-ing the intrinsic binding strengths of individual functional groups, i.e. the free energy changes resulting (after allowance for any loss in translational or rotational entropy) when the specified functional groups are aligned optimally and without strain with corresponding functional groups in the receptor (Jencks 1981).

2.5.1 Intrinsic binding energies

Recall that the free energy of binding, ΔG, can be defined in terms of the binding energies for the individual functional groups which make up the ligand according to equation (2.4). The fourth term in equation (2.4) is the sum of the binding energies ΔG_x associated with each functional group X. In the ideal case, when the specified functional group is aligned optimally and without strain with the corres-ponding functional group in the receptor, ΔG_x is referred to as the intrinsic binding energy (Jencks 1981). In other cases, the term apparent binding energy is used. Page (1977) referred to this as the 'anchor principle', on the premise that the difference in binding of a ligand with or without the particular functional group incorporates only the factors associated with that group, i.e. the intrinsic binding energy ΔG_x of that group.

It should be noted that each binding energy ΔG_x incorporates a number of terms in addition to the obvious enthalpy of interaction between the functional group and its corresponding binding site on the receptor. These include the enthalpy changes associated with the removal of water of hydration from the functional group and its target site and the subsequent formation of bonds between the displaced water molecules, and the corresponding entropy terms associated with the displacement and subsequent bonding of water molecules.

The anchor principle assumes that intrinsic binding energies are properties of the functional group and are independent of the groups to which the particular functional group is attached. Such intrinsic binding potentials might thus reasonably be used in an additive manner to provide an overall estimate of the ligand–receptor interaction. The original application of the anchor principle described by Page (1977) related to data on the selectivity of amino acid-tRNA synthetases, from which he estimated intrinsic binding energies for the methylene group in the range 12–$14\,kJ\,mol^{-1}$, and for carboxyl and amino groups of 18 and $>28\,kJ\,mol^{-1}$ respectively.

Intrinsic binding energies are not rigorously accurate, they are only useful approximations. If a molecule containing a particular functional group binds with a higher affinity than the corresponding molecule lacking that functional group, by definition there is a higher entropy cost to be paid by the higher affinity molecule. This is paid off against the intrinsic binding energy of the functional group resulting in an underestimation of the intrinsic binding. Conversely, the additional binding energy of the functional group may increase the enthalpy of neighboring interactions. This is paid into the intrinsic binding energy, leading to an overestimation. Other factors such as solvent effects and the conformational effect (Wiley and Rich 1993; Epps *et al.* 1990) of the functional group on the ligand are also buried in the intrinsic binding energy value and may not be easily predicted. Thus Williams and Bardsley (1999) showed that the enthalpy of interaction of a functional group is strengthened by an adjacent functional group in a manner that is separate from the well known entropically driven chelate effect. They suggest that this precludes the derivation of free energies of binding characteristic of common functional groups since these values must always be context dependent i.e. dependent on the molecular architecture of the ligand and probably the receptor.

The Williams and Bardsley (1999) study involved a series of ligands for the vancomycin antibiotics, which differ only by the presence or absence of a methyl group. The binding of *N*-acetyl-D-ala-D-ala, (**2.1**) (the truncated natural ligand for the vancomycin antibiotics from bacterial cell walls) was compared with ligands lacking methyl groups, i.e. glycine–alanine replacements of either or both positions (**2.2**, **2.3** and **2.4**). To a first approximation, the differences in binding affinities were attributed to the difference in hydrophobic surface area between the ligands: other factors such as conformational states were considered to be equivalent. The contribution of the hydrophobic effect was calculated to be 0.18–$0.24\,kJ\,mol^{-1}\,\text{Å}^{-2}$, which is larger than the values determined by solvent transfer. This inconsistency was traced to enthalpy–entropy compensation, which can negate prediction of binding affinities using partitioning of enthalpic and entropic components of the free energy change. At the molecular level, the motional restriction imposed by the favorable burial of the hydrophobic methyl group was transferred to a neighboring carboxylate, which strengthened the hydrogen bond this group made to the antibiotic. For systems that are networks of weak co-operative interactions (like ligand–protein interactions), any strengthening of one interaction necessarily strengthens linked interactions and essentially renders meaningless attempts to rigorously partition free energy. The same effect was noted for another series of vancomycin ligands (**2.5**, **2.6**, **2.1**) where the strength of the hydrogen bond

(2.1)   (2.2)

(2.3)   (2.4)

(2.5)   (2.6)

between the carboxylate of the ligand and vancomycin was found to increase through the series as adjacent co-operative networks of interactions increased.

Solvent effects may complicate derivation of intrinsic binding energies using the anchor principle. This is best illustrated by example. Morgan *et al.* (1991) has reported a series of thermolysin inhibitors in which a substrate peptide linkage is replaced by a phosphinate linkage $(-PO_2-CH_2-)$ and phosphonamide (PO_2-NH-) linkages. The crystal structures of the complexes between thermolysin and these two inhibitors show that they are essentially identical except for the presence of a single hydrogen bond from the phosphonamidate NH to the carbonyl oxygen of Ala 113. The methylene group of the phosphinate is unable to make this hydrogen bond. Surprisingly, the binding affinity of these two series is identical, resulting in a calculated intrinsic binding energy of $0\,kJ\,mol^{-1}$ for a neutral hydrogen bonding pair. In this case, it appears that any beneficial enthalpic component of the hydrogen bond is completely offset by other costs. It is likely that a major cost is desolvation energy that the phosphonamide must pay, but that the phosphinate does not (see Chapter 4). Recall from the discussion on hydrogen bond contributions above, that the phosphinate should be more unstable than the phosphonate since it buries the unpaired carbonyl oxygen of Ala 113. This example clearly illustrates that even if you can 'see' at atomic level the interface between ligand and receptor, indeed between a ligand series and a receptor, it is still very difficult to infer the important contributions to the ligand's affinity or predict the consequences of structural change on binding affinity.

Notwithstanding the above evidence that the anchor principle gives functional group contributions that are a complicated mix of enthalpic and entropic contributions that are context dependent, they are still useful in drug design. For example, the limiting contribution for a methyl group in many different systems appears to be a maximum of around $12–14\,kJ\,mol^{-1}$ which can be used to assess the effectiveness of the introduction of a methyl group into a drug.

2.5.2   Active site mutagenesis

Another measure of intrinsic binding energy based on the anchor principle is the impact of a single amino acid substitution in the active site of an enzyme on transition state stabilization, as determined by the change in either catalytic efficiency or inhibitor binding. As before, comparison of reaction rates or inhibitor dissociation constants with and without a single functional group in the active site will tend to overestimate the intrinsic binding energy (defined as including desolvation energies of the functional group and its partner in the transition state or an analogous inhibitor), but may nevertheless provide a useful measure of the increase in binding that might be targeted by the drug designer.

2.5.3   'Average' functional group contributions

An alternative to the anchor principle approach was developed by Andrews *et al.* (1984), who sought to average the contributions of individual functional groups to the observed binding energies of 200 ligand–protein interactions in aqueous solution. In effect, this approach combined the ideas of Page and Jencks (1971) with those of Beddell *et al.* (1979), who had earlier used a simple regression analysis to estimate the strengths of covalent (Schiff base) and ionic interactions between hemoglobin effector molecules and a variety of hemoglobin mutants lacking the corresponding binding groups.

Although the fit obtained by Beddell *et al.* (1979) was remarkably good, the calculated energies were much lower than those estimated using the anchor principle, primarily because no account was taken of the entropic costs of the interaction. In the subsequent work by Andrews *et al.*, this factor was taken into account, with the average loss of overall rotational and translational entropy accompanying ligand–receptor binding, ΔG_{t+r}, being estimated at $58.5\,kJ\,mol^{-1}$ ($14\,kcal\,mol^{-1}$) at $310\,K$. Regression analysis led to the 'average' values of the binding energies associated with each functional group in the 200 ligands, as follows: C(sp^2 or sp^3), $3\,kJ\,mol^{-1}$; O, S, N, or halogen, $5\,kJ\,mol^{-1}$; OH and C=O, 10 and $14\,kJ\,mol^{-1}$, respectively; and CO_2^-, OPO_3^{2-}, and N^+, 34, 42 and $48\,kJ\,mol^{-1}$, respectively.

It should be stressed that these values are not intrinsic binding energies in the sense defined above: this would be the case only if each functional group in each ligand in the series was optimally aligned with a corresponding functional group in the receptor. In fact, since every functional group of every ligand was included in the analysis, the calculated values are averages of apparent binding energies, including those for some groups which may not interact with the receptor. This may apply particularly to the sp^2 or sp^3 carbons, many of which provide the structural framework for the ligands but are shielded from interaction with receptor groups by intervening functional groups of the ligand. The calculated averages might thus be expected to be smaller than the corresponding intrinsic binding energies, although the assumption of a constant rotational and translational entropy loss appropriate to a tightly bound complex will tend to operate in the other direction. In general, the magnitudes of the values for particular functional groups are in accord with the ranges derived from application of the anchor principle for different bond types (see below).

A further outcome of the preceding analysis was the finding of a negative coefficient for n_r, the number of degrees of internal rotational freedom. The loss of each internal rotation on receptor binding results in an entropy loss that reduces the free energy of binding by an average of 3 kJ mol^{-1}, which may be compared to the estimated value for the total loss of conformational freedom around a single bond of $5–6 \text{ kJ mol}^{-1}$ (Page and Jencks 1971). The smaller number obtained empirically implies that conformational freedom is not fully lost for all the bonds in an average ligand–receptor interaction, and is consistent with experimental estimates of $1.6–3.6 \text{ kJ mol}^{-1}$ for the entropic cost of restricting rotations in hydrocarbon chains (Searle and Williams 1992).

These values have been used by Andrews (1986) and others to determine the quality of fit of a ligand to its receptor. This is done by comparing the observed binding constant to the average binding energy calculated from equation (2.4) by summing the binding energies of the component groups and then subtracting the two entropy related terms. Ligands that match their receptors exceptionally well have a measured binding energy that substantially exceeds this calculated average value. Conversely, if the observed binding energy is very much less than the calculated average value, then the ligand either matches its receptor less well than average, or binds to the receptor in a comparatively high energy conformation.

Although clearly useful guides, the application of these numbers in drug design is restricted by the fact that they are averages of apparent binding energies, rather than true measures of intrinsic binding activity. There are also concerns as to the statistical validity of the use of multiple regression to extract average values from the raw data, particularly with respect to the inclusion of the constant rotational and translational entropy term rather than an adjustable parameter.

In view of these problems, it would obviously be more useful if the true intrinsic binding energies of specified binding groups could be calculated directly from observations on well-defined interactions, including proper allowance for the rotational, translational and other entropy losses associated with the interaction.

2.5.4   The role of ΔG_{t+r}

The theoretical limit for the complete loss of rotational and translational entropy on the formation of a bimolecular complex in solution at a standard state of 1 mol^{-1} and 298 K has been calculated by several authors (Page 1977; Finkelstein and Janin 1989; Williams *et al.* 1991). For a ligand of average molecular weight (say 200 dalton) this figure is approximately 60 kJ mol^{-1}. The question is, how much of this rotational and translational entropy is really lost on binding?

Calculations and experimental data cited by Page (1977) suggest that the net loss of rotational and translational entropy on formation of a 'tight' bimolecular complex, including allowance for residual motion, would be on the order of

45 kJ mol^{-1} at 310 K, compared to 12 kJ mol^{-1} for a very 'loose' complex. It follows that the net loss of rotational and translational entropy (including residual motion) on bimolecular complex formation cannot be regarded as a constant for any but the tightest ligand–receptor interactions, and even then the actual entropy loss is significantly less than the corresponding entropy of the free ligand. Much of the rotational and translational entopy is converted to vibrational entropy in the bound ligand. Based on the data of Williams and others, a reasonable estimate of ΔG_{t+r} for 'tight' complexes would appear to be about 75% of the entropy of the unbound ligand, in agreement with the original figure proposed by Page (1977) of 45 kJ mol^{-1} for an average-sized ligand. Williams argues that the overall loss of entropy of a bimolecular interaction is related to the enthalpy of interaction by a curve of the general form of Figure 2.2. Whatever the exact form of this curve, it clearly shows that ΔG_{t+r} should be a variable value that increases up to a limiting value of 45–50 kJ/mol at 298 K as the enthalpy of interaction increases. A sliding value for ΔG_{t+r} rather than the fixed value used in most approximation methods may be more useful and strictly more accurate.

The use of a constant figure of 58.5 kJ mol^{-1} (14 kcal mol^{-1}) rather than 45 kJ mol^{-1} for the average functional group binding energies calculated by Andrews *et al.* means these values are likely to be overestimated. Furthermore, the use of a constant rotational and translational entropy term to calculate average molecular binding energies from equation (2.4) will lead to a systematic error that underestimates weak interactions (for which a smaller value of ΔG_{t+r} should be used) and may overestimate stronger ones (for which a larger ΔG_{t+r} value may

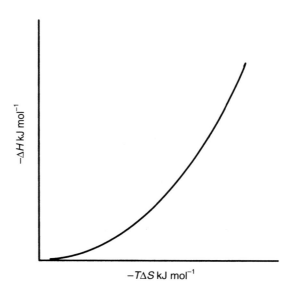

Figure 2.2 The general form of the relationship between enthalpy of association and the entropic cost of the interaction at room temperature. There is a limiting entropic cost that may be approached even when intermolecular associations are mediated by non-bonded interactions (Williams and Westwell 1998). The curve suggests that a sliding scale for ΔG_{t+r} (−TS) would be more appropriate than a constant value.

Table 2.1 Functional group contributions to ligand–receptor interactions (kJ mol^{-1})

Group type	Technique employed to determine contribution			
	Anchor principle	Site-directed mutagenesis	Average energy	Partition energy
Nonpolar (per CH$_2$)	12–14	1–3	3–6	
H-bond (uncharged)	16	2–6	5–14	1–12
H-bond (charge assisted)	20–42	15–19		
Ionic bond	18–28+	12–25	34–48	
ΔG_{t+r} (translation/rotation)	12–45		58.5*	
ΔG_r (internal rotation)	5–6		3	2–4

Note
* Assumed value.

be appropriate). Nevertheless, the numbers do provide the basis for some simple 'rules-of-thumb' that may be used by drug designers to answer practical design questions.

2.6   SOME RULES OF THUMB

The apparent contributions of different functional groups and/or bond types to overall binding energies derived from the various studies reviewed above are summarized in Table 2.1. Also included are corresponding values used or suggested for the overall loss of rotational and translational entropy, ΔG_{t+r}, and the loss of conformational entropy resulting from restriction of free rotation, ΔG_t.

Which of these numbers can most appropriately be used to explain the observed affinities of known ligands, or to *predict* the affinities of new ligands? The answer really depends on the question being asked.

2.6.1   What should this functional group do for my ligand?

If we wish to know what incremental binding contribution we might expect upon the addition of a functional group which is optimally aligned with a corresponding group in the receptor, then the numbers based on the anchor principle are probably the best bet, though co-operativity has to be born in mind. In particular, Wolfenden and Kati's (1991) observations in adenosine deaminase inhibitors of incremental binding energies of up to 42 kJ mol^{-1} (7 orders of magnitude increase in binding affinity) must be near the limit for charge-assisted hydrogen bonding by a hydroxyl group. As noted above, this and most other figures based on the anchor principle are not true intrinsic binding energies but a complicated mix of additional enthalpic and entropic terms. This is observed in the case of the adenosine deaminase study, where the hydroxyl not only forms a charge assisted hydrogen bond to a carboxylate, but also forms an additional charge interaction with a zinc atom and displaces a tightly bound water molecule already engaged in similar interactions with the enzyme. As an indication of potential incremental binding, however, these apparent binding energies are entirely appropriate, since they are then being applied in precisely the same way that they were derived. This was born out by the more recent example of cytidine deaminase ligands, where introduction of a particular hydroxyl also resulted in a seven orders of magnitude improvement in affinity. Observation of the crystal structure of the cytidine deaminase–ligand complex shows that there is a very similar network of interactions between the hydroxyl and both adenosine deaminase and cytidine deaminase. A more conservative estimate of the value of a charge-assisted hydrogen bond would be in the range of 16–$20\,\mathrm{kJ\,mol^{-1}}$, based on the work of Fersht *et al.* (1985). Page's estimate of 12–$14\,\mathrm{kJ\,mol^{-1}}$ per CH_2 group, having been derived from observations on highly selective t-RNA synthetases, is probably also approaching the limit for an attractive interaction between non-polar groups.

The corresponding figures for charged groups, 18–$28\,\mathrm{kJ\,mol^{-1}}$, are not based on examples where they are the primary determinants of specificity, and may be underestimates. An indication of this likelihood may be obtained using simple observations on the interactions of individual charged groups with appropriate enzymes. The phosphate ion, for example, binds alkaline phosphatase with a dissociation constant of $2.3 \times 10^{-6}\,\mathrm{M}$, equivalent to a ΔG value of approximately $33\,\mathrm{kJ\,mol^{-1}}$. Taking the most conservative estimate for the loss of rotational and translational entropy associated with this interaction, $12\,\mathrm{kJ\,mol^{-1}}$ for a loosely bound complex, equation (2.4) then gives a lower estimate for binding of the phosphate ion of $45\,\mathrm{kJ\,mol^{-1}}$. If the same value of ΔG_{t+r} is applied to the binding of oxalate ion to transcarboxylase, for which the dissociation constant is $1.8 \times 10^{-6}\,\mathrm{M}$ (Northrop and Wood 1969) ($33\,\mathrm{kJ\,mol^{-1}}$), equation (2.4) gives an apparent binding energy of $24\,\mathrm{kJ\,mol^{-1}}$ per carboxylate group after allowance for a minimal conformational entropy loss of $3\,\mathrm{kJ\,mol^{-1}}$.

2.6.2 How well does my ligand fit the receptor?

Summation of the average contributions of individual binding groups, including allowance for conformational, rotational and translational entropy terms as shown in equation (2.4), provides a simple back-of-the-envelope calculation of the strength of binding which might be expected for a ligand forming a typical interaction with a receptor. This figure, when compared to the observed affinity of the ligand for the target receptor, gives a direct indication of the relevance of the structure in 3D QSAR. If the observed binding is stronger than anticipated, it is reasonable to expect that the structure offers a reasonable fit to the receptor in a reasonably low energy conformation. If, on the other hand, the observed binding is significantly weaker than anticipated then it is likely that the ligand either matches its receptor less well than average, or binds to the receptor in a comparatively high energy conformation.

For this purpose, the optimal binding contributions determined from highly specific applications of the anchor principle are not appropriate, since the absence of detailed structural data means that the summation in equation (2.4) is necessarily done over all the functional groups in the ligand, regardless of whether or not they are directly involved in binding to the receptor. For those groups which make up the molecular framework, including most notably the sp^2 or sp^3 carbons, the average contribution should thus be much less than that derived from the anchor principle, while the contribution of substituents positioned to interact with corresponding receptor groups may be of similar magnitude.

Comparison with the other data in Table 2.1 suggests that the average values derived previously by Andrews *et al.* (1984) are a reasonable starting point for goodness of fit calculations. Clearly, they could be improved by adjusting the entropy terms to account for the extent to which rotational, translational and conformational entropy are lost in individual complexes, or even by employing a smaller entropy cost rather than 58.5 kJ mol^{-1} for ΔG_{t+r}. Either of these modifications would lead to a reduction in the size of the average functional group contributions, and this would be most significant for charged substituents.

Meanwhile, the two most extreme cases from the original set of 200 ligand–protein interactions studied by Andrews *et al.* (1984) offer simple examples of the application of the original 'average' numbers.

Substitution of these numbers into equation (2.4) for biotin suggested that it bound to the protein avidin almost 70 kJ mol^{-1} more tightly than anticipated on the basis of its constituent functional groups, implying an exceptional match to the structure of the protein. It has since been established that this is indeed the case, with polarization of the biotin molecule by the protein actually leading to an ionic interaction where a neutral hydrogen bonding interaction had been assumed.

At the opposite extreme is the case of methotrexate, for which equation (2.4) shows that the molecule binds to dihydrofolate reductase some 74 kJ mol^{-1} less tightly than anticipated, suggesting that despite its exceptional affinity for the enzyme the ligand does not offer a good overall fit to the active site of the enzyme. Again, the direct evidence of the crystal structure verifies this suggestion, with substantial parts of the structure, including one of the carboxylic acid groups, being exposed to solvent rather than utilized in binding to the enzyme.

2.6.3 Conclusion

It will be evident from the preceding discussion that the magnitudes of the intrinsic binding energies associated with different functional groups, or even types of interactions, are far from being precisely defined. The uncertainty in the numbers arises for two reasons.

First, the experimental data rarely provide any real degree of confidence that the observed change in binding energy actually reflects a single interaction between the target functional group and its binding partner in the receptor. Even in cases where there are structural data to show the binding interface with and without the additional functional group, as in the case of the phosphinate/phosphonamide inhibitor pairs described in Section 2.5.1, it is very difficult to predict the consequences of structural change on binding affinity. Binding affinity is a property of the state changes from the left-hand side to the right-hand side of equation (2.1), it is not attributable to the nature of the binding interface alone. It has become quite apparent that the task of predicting the state changes involved in ligand–receptor interactions is daunting. The medicinal chemist's traditional rigid receptor hypothesis is long since dead. Receptors have been shown to be capable of unpredictable conformational changes in response to different ligands, which may bring different ensembles of functional group interactions into play at the interface, further complicating the extraction of meaningful contributions (Davis and Teague 1999).

Second, the interpretation of the observed numbers invariably involves juggling differences between rather large entropy and enthalpy contributions in order to finally deduce the relatively small contribution due to the target binding group. The problem is akin to the legendary technique for weighing the ship's captain by weighing the ship before and after he comes aboard – except that in this case there is the additional complication of an unknown and variable number of stowaways!

The eventual solution to these uncertainties will require much more detailed analyses of structurally well-defined interactions, preferably including estimates of the extent to which each individual functional group is actually participating in the overall interaction (lengths and orientations of bonds, tightness of match between surfaces, states of ionization of binding groups, etc.) and the extent to which rotational, translational and conformational entropy have been lost in the process. With the increase in high-resolution structural details of intermolecular complexes and the rise of accurate calorimetric techniques (to independently calculate equilibrium constants, ΔH and ΔS) (Ladbury and Chowdhry 1996) improving our underlying knowledge, the goal of accurately predicting affinities may yet be achievable.

REFERENCES AND FURTHER READING

Ajay and Murcko, M.A. (1995) Computational methods to predict binding free energy in ligand–receptor complexes. *J. Med. Chem.*, **38**, 4953–4967.

Andrews, P.R., Craik, D.J. and Martin, J.L. (1984) Functional group contributions to drug–receptor interactions. *J. Med. Chem.*, **2**, 1648–1656.

Andrews, P. (1986) Functional groups, drug–receptor interactions and drug design. *Trends Pharmacol. Sci.*, **7**, 148–151.

Beddell, C.R., Goodford, P.J., Stammers, D.K. and Wootton, R. (1979) Species differences in the binding of compounds designed to fit a site of known structure in adult haemoglobin. *Br. J. Pharmacol.*, **65**, 535–543.

Ben-Tal, N., Sitkoff, D., Topol, I.A., Yang, A.-S., Burt, S.K. and Honig, B. (1997) Free energy of amide hydrogen bond formation in vacuum, in water, and in liquid alkane solution. *J. Phys. Chem. B.*, **101**, 450–457.

Bongrand, P. (1999) Ligand–receptor interactions. *Rep. Prog. Phs.*, **62**, 921–968.

Davis, A.M. and Teague, S.J. (1999) Hydrogen bonding, hydrophobic interactions, and the failure of the rigid receptor hypothesis. *Angew. Chem. Int. Ed.*, **38**, 736–749.

Dougherty, D.A. (1996) Cation-π-interactions in chemistry and biology: a new view of benzene, Phe, Tyr and Trp. *Science*, **271**, 163–168.

Epps, D.E., Cheney, J., Schostarez, H., Sawyer, T.K., Prairie, M., Krueger, W.C. and Mandel, F. (1990) Thermodynamics of the interaction of inhibitors with the binding site of recombinant human renin *J. Med. Chem.*, **33**, 2080–2086.

Fersht, A.R., Shi, J.-P., Knill-Jones, J., Lowe, D.M., Wilkinson, A.J., Blow, D.M. *et al.* (1985) Hydrogen bonding and biological specificity analysed by protein engineering. *Nature*, **314**, 235–238.

Finkelstein, A.V. and Janin, J. (1989) The price of lost freedom: entropy of bimolecular complex formation. *Protein Eng.*, **3**, 1–3.

Glusker, J.P. (1998) Directional aspects of intermolecular interactions. In *Design of Organic Solids*, edited by E. Weber, pp. 3–53. Berlin: Springer-Verlag.

Hunter, C.A. (1994) Meldola Lecture – the role of aromatic interactions in molecular recognition. *Chem. Soc. Rev.*, **23**, 101–109.

Jencks, W.P. (1981) On the attribution and additivity of binding energies. *Proc. Natl. Acad. Sci. USA*, **78**, 4046–4050.

Klotz, I.M. (1997) *Ligand–receptor energetics: a guide for the perplexed*, pp. 95–96. New York: John Wiley & Sons, Inc.

Kollman, P. (1993) Free energy calculations – applications to chemical and biochemical phenomena. *Chem. Rev.*, **93**, 2395–2417.

Ladbury, J.E. and Chowdhry, B.Z. (1996) Sensing the Heat: the application of isothermal titration calorimetry to thermodynamic studies of biomolecular interactions. *Chemistry & Biology*, **3**, 791–801.

McDonald, I.K. and Thornton, J.M. (1994) Satisfying hydrogen bonding potentials in proteins. *J. Mol. Biol.*, **238**, 777–793.

Morgan, B.P., Scholtz, J.M., Ballinger, M.D., Zipkin, I.D. and Bartlett, P.A. (1991) Differential binding-energy – a detailed evaluation of the influence of hydrogen-bonding and hydrophobic groups on the inhibition of thermolysin by phosphorus-containing inhibitors. *J. Am. Chem. Soc.*, **113**, 297–307.

Northrop, D.B. and Wood, H.G. (1969) Transcarboxylase VII. Exchange reactions and kinetics of oxalate inhibition. *J. Biol. Chem.*, **244**, 5820–5827.

Page, M.I. and Jencks, W.P. (1971) Entropic contributions to rate accelerations in enzymic and intramolecular reaction and the chelate effect. *Proc. Natl. Acad. Sci. USA*, **68**, 1678–1683.

Page, M.I. (1977) Entropy, binding energy and enzyme catalysis. *Angew. Chem. Int. Ed. Engl.*, **16**, 449–459.

Pang, Y.P. and Kollman, P.A. (1995) Applications of free energy derivatives to analog design. *Perspectives in Drug Discovery*, **3**, 106–122.

Searle, M.S. and Williams, D.H. (1992) The cost of conformational order: entropy changes in molecular associations. *J. Am. Chem. Soc.*, **114**, 10690–10697.

Wiley, R.A. and Rich, D.H. (1993) Peptidomimetics derived from natural-products. *Med. Res. Rev.*, **13**, 327–384.

Williams, D.H. and Bardsley, B. (1999) Estimating binding constants – the hydrophobic effect and cooperativity. *Perspectives in Drug Discovery and Design*, **17**, 43–59.

Williams, D.H., Cox, J.P.L., Doig, A.J., Gardner, M., Gerhard, U., Kaye, P.T., Lal, A.R., Nicholls, I.A., Salter, C.J. and Mitchell, R.C. (1991) Towards the semiquantitative estimation of binding constants. Guides for peptide–peptide binding in aqueous solution. *J. Am. Chem. Soc.*, **113**, 7020–7030.

Williams, D.H. and Westwell, M.S. (1998) Aspects of weak interactions. *Chem. Soc. Rev.*, **27**, 57–63.

Wolfenden, R. and Kati, W.M. (1991) Testing the limits of protein–legand binding discrimination with transition-state analog inhibitors. *Acc. Chem. Res.*, **24**, 209–215.

Chapter 3

Stereochemistry in drug design

Ian J. Kennedy and David E. Jane

3.1 INTRODUCTION

In the year 2000, the sales of chiral drugs reached $120 billion representing almost one-third of all drug sales world-wide (Figure 3.1), a fact which reinforces the importance of the link between chirality and drug design. In turn, this stems from the often overlooked reality that the biological targets for which these drugs are designed to interact with are themselves chiral. Therefore, dramatic differences are often witnessed in the action of one enantiomer over another in biological systems, ultimately in humans.

This raises the questions of why these drugs need to be chiral and how can such compounds be synthesized? In this chapter, we attempt to answer these questions by providing an overview of the rationale behind synthesizing asymmetric biologically active compounds and the methods that can be employed to obtain them. However, this is merely an introduction to this vast subject, individual points of

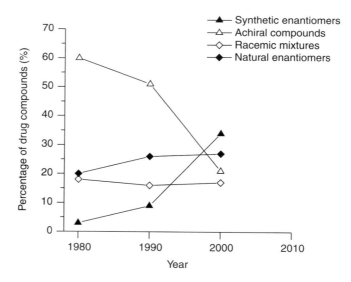

Figure 3.1 The sales of synthetic drugs as single enantiomers at the expense of achiral compounds.

which are described in more detail in the references listed at the end of the chapter.

In summary, the first section gives an overview of the fundamental principles behind stereochemistry, merely intended as a brief review. Should it be required, further information can be found in standard textbooks (Robinson 2000). Following on from this a rationale is presented as to why chiral drugs are needed from a molecular recognition perspective and how they may be obtained. Included within this are several examples of how these methodologies have been adopted in the synthesis of known drugs. The final section outlines analytical methods for the assessment of the purity of chiral drugs.

3.2 WHAT ARE STEREOISOMERS?

There are a number of different types of isomerism that can be divided as shown in Figure 3.2. Although both geometric and conformational isomers are by definition classed as stereoisomers, optical isomers are probably the most significant in terms of drug design and it is this type of isomerism that is discussed in this chapter.

Such molecules that can possess optical activity are said to be chiral. Chirality is simply a symmetry property of an object that describes its inability to be superimposed upon its mirror image i.e. it lacks reflectional symmetry. This generally arises because of substitution around a tetrahedral carbon atom (the stereogenic center) of four different groups, although other atoms such as nitrogen or phosphorous may also behave as stereogenic centers. The important point is that such substitutions lead to the loss of symmetry and this is the prerequisite for a compound to be chiral. Such compounds can exist as two different stereoisomers, or enantiomers, which are related as object to image through a reflectional plane. For example, Figure 3.3 shows one of the simplest chiral molecules, lactic acid, produced by the body as a result of anaerobic respiration. It has a central stereogenic center and no internal symmetry plane and thus can exist in one of two chiral enantiomeric forms. However, propanoic acid possesses a symmetry plane down the center of the molecule and so is achiral.

An important point concerning the enantiomers of a chiral molecule is that they are identical except for two properties. First, they are chemically different only in

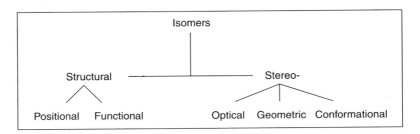

Figure 3.2 The different classes of isomerism. Stereoisomers are isomers that have the same constitution but differ only in their 3D arrangement.

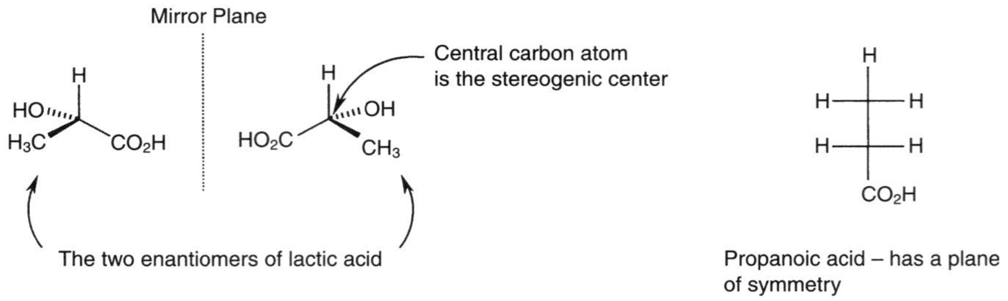

Figure 3.3 The two enantiomers of lactic acid are mirror images of each other. However, propanoic acid is achiral as it has a plane of symmetry through the center of the molecule.

the way that they react with other chiral molecules. This is a key attribute – the importance of which is discussed in more detail in the following sections. Second, their physical properties differ solely in the way in which they interact with plane polarized light, hence the term optical activity. All other properties such as melting point, solubility and spectroscopic data are identical.

The aforementioned differences in optical activity of chiral molecules can be simply explained by their lack of internal symmetry. When ordinary light is passed through a polarizer, the resultant light beam possesses electromagnetic waves that oscillate only in a single plane that is perpendicular to the direction of travel. If this light were to then pass through a solution containing a symmetrical molecule, collisions with the molecule in a particular orientation are canceled out by encounters with the mirror image molecular orientation. However, if this were to be repeated with a sample containing unequal amounts of enantiomers of a chiral compound then the plane of polarization will be altered. This is because there will be no 'canceling effect' and the net amount of rotation can then be measured. If a 50:50 (racemic) mixture of two enantiomers were to be examined, again there would be a net overall effect of zero rotation as each enantiomer would cancel out the rotation caused by the other.

The degree of rotation caused by a chiral molecule is easily measured using a polarimeter. If a molecule is seen to rotate the light anticlockwise it is labeled as *laevorotatory*, or if it is clockwise it is called *dextrorotatory*. The abbreviated labels (−) or L for laevo- and (+) or D for dextrorotatory are also used. Since this net rotation, termed $[\alpha]_D$ (or specific rotation), is an intrinsic property of an optically active molecule it can be used to quantify the amount or purity of a chiral molecule. This value is dependent on the wavelength of light used, the length of the sample tube through which the light is passed, temperature, solvent and sample concentration. The light source most often used for such determinations is that emitted by a sodium lamp at 589 nm (the so-called sodium D line).

The specific rotation at 20 °C can therefore be expressed as:

$$[\alpha]_D^{20} = \frac{\text{observed rotation (degrees)}}{\text{length of sample tube (dm)} \times \text{concentration (g/ml)}}$$

Optical purity can be defined as the ratio of the specific optical rotation of the enantiomeric mixture and the specific optical rotation of the pure enantiomer and is usually expressed as a percentage.

The observed optical rotation (D or L) was the earliest method of distinguishing between enantiomers, but this method gives no indication as to the actual spatial geometry of a molecule i.e. the configuration about the stereogenic centre. This was rectified by the introduction of the Fischer convention which labelled such centres as having either D or L configuration based on an arbitrary standard, (+)-glyceraldehyde. However, this system has now been superseded by the Cahn–Ingold–Prelog (or 'sequence rule') system which can be used to unambiguously assign any stereogenic center as possessing either (R) or (S) stereochemistry. This is deduced using a set of rules that assign priorities to the substituents attached to the stereogenic centre, the details of which are outside the scope of this review. A detailed discussion of these rules is available in any general organic chemistry textbook (e.g. Robinson 2000). Once the priorities of the substituents have been assigned, enantiomers are readily classified as being the (R) or (S) isomers. This is done by first viewing the molecule from the opposite group of lowest priority. If the remaining groups are seen to go from lowest to highest priority in a clockwise direction then the center is labeled as (R), and vice versa for (S). Lactic acid is again used as an example to demonstrate this (Figure 3.4).

Molecules such as lactic acid are relatively simple in that they only have one stereogenic center, but what are the implications if multiple stereogenic centers are present? As an example, the drug ephedrine has two stereogenic centers and thus there are four possible isomers (Figure 3.5). Since there can only be two possible enantiomers of a chiral compound then the relationship between these two pairs must be a

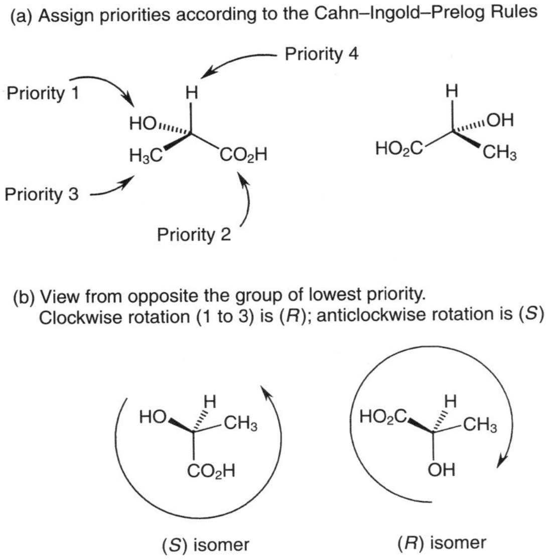

Figure 3.4 Procedure for assigning stereogenic centers as possessing either (R) or (S) configuration.

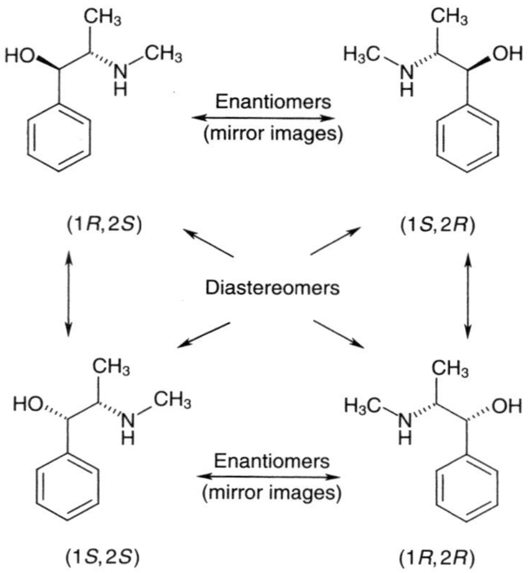

Figure 3.5 The relationship between enantiomers and diastereomers. The biologically active forms of ephedrine are those with the (1R, 2S) and (1S, 2S) configurations, which are diastereomers of each other.

non-mirror image one. Such stereoisomers that are non-superimposable, non-mirror images of each other are known as diastereomers.

Therefore, although enantiomers must have an opposite configuration at all stereogenic centers, diastereomers must be opposite at only some, but may be the same at the others. As previously described, two enantiomers of a racemate have identical chemical properties in an achiral environment. However, an extremely important property of diastereomers is that unlike enantiomers, they will (unless by coincidence) have non-identical physical and chemical properties such as boiling point, solubility and spectral properties. The potential applications of this are discussed in Sections 3.5.1 and 3.5.2.

As a general rule, the total number of isomers of any given molecule is also given by the rule:

Number of isomers $= 2^n$

where n is the total number of stereogenic centers.

So, as in ephedrine, a compound with two centers will have four isomers, three centers leads to eight isomers and so on. However, there are examples where this rule does not hold true because some isomers may be *meso* compounds. These can be described as isomers that contain stereogenic centers but are achiral due to the presence of a symmetry plane. This generally arises when the three groups attached to one stereogenic center are the same as those attached to another. All of this implies that a *meso* compound will be superimposable on its mirror image hence will be optically inactive. These principles are demonstrated well using

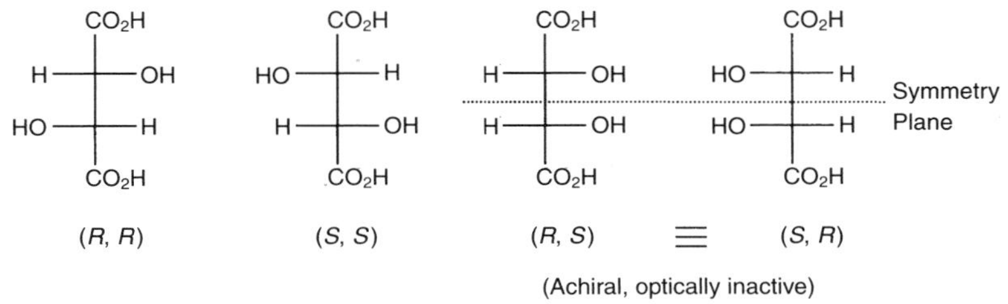

Figure 3.6 Tartaric acid has two stereogenic centers but only three stereoisomers.

tartaric acid. This compound has two stereogenic centers and so should have four isomers – two pairs of enantiomers. However, the (R, S) and (S, R) configurations are superimposable since they have a plane of symmetry. Therefore, tartaric acid has three isomers – a pair of enantiomers and a *meso* isomer (Figure 3.6).

The definition of optical purity discussed above has been largely superseded by two related terms enantiomeric excess (ee) and diastereomeric excess (de). Enantiomeric excess can be defined as the proportion of the major enantiomer less that of the minor enantiomer whereas de is defined as the proportion of the major diastereomer less that of the minor one. Both ee and de are usually expressed as percentages.

Should the only difference between enantiomers be their interaction with plane polarized light then their existence would be little more than academic. However, as described above stereochemistry has important implications in terms of biological activity. The origin and nature of these phenomena are described in the following section.

3.3   THE ORIGIN OF STEREOSPECIFICITY IN MOLECULAR RECOGNITION

In 1896, Emil Fischer proposed that the substrates of an enzyme must have a complementary shape to the active site, this theory being known as the lock and key hypothesis (Figure 3.7). This was the first attempt to explain the specificity of enzyme action. However, this theory was erroneous as it suggested that enzymes only have one optimal substrate and all others fit less well and therefore the catalyzed reaction is less efficient. This is not the case as some enzymes can catalyze reactions on a range of different substrates. In order to take this observation into account, Koshland later proposed that the enzyme is forced to change shape to some extent in order to take up the optimal shape to accommodate the binding of substrates to the active site. This induced fit model (Figure 3.8) explains why enzymes can accommodate a range of substrates. However, it is now thought that not only the enzyme can change shape, the substrate can also alter its shape to fix it in the optimal conformation for the reaction catalyzed by the enzyme.

Although the induced fit model was proposed for enzymes, it has also been proposed that it may also explain drug–receptor interactions. Receptors are made

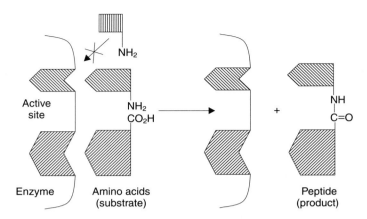

Figure 3.7 The lock and key hypothesis – the enzyme and substrate must have a complementary shape.

up of chiral building blocks and are themselves chiral and would therefore be expected to be enantioselective in their interactions with chiral drugs. In order to explain the stereoselective action of drugs on receptors, the three-point receptor theory was proposed (Figure 3.9). In this theory, only one enantiomer has the optimal spatial disposition of the three groups A, B and C to interact with the complementary sites on the receptor. The less active enantiomer binds less effectively with the receptor, as the groups on the ligand cannot align favorably with the corresponding sites on the receptor. This theory is successful in explaining stereoselectivity of drug action although it must be born in mind that there may be more than three interactions of a drug with a receptor. In addition, these interactions are not necessarily all ionic or hydrogen bonds; hydrophobic or steric interactions may also suffice.

The three-point receptor theory has been useful in understanding the mechanism of enzyme action and also in the rational design of inhibitors. An example of an

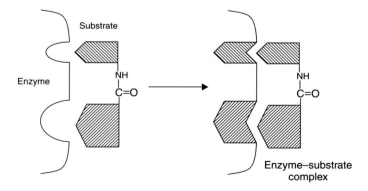

Figure 3.8 The induced fit model – the enzyme is forced to change shape to interact optimally with the substrate.

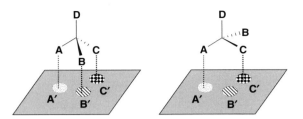

Figure 3.9 The three-point receptor theory.

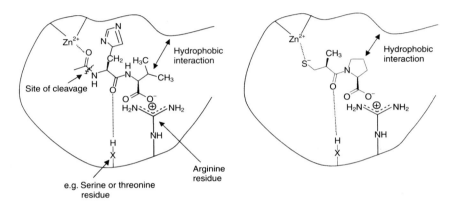

Figure 3.10 Left panel: Interaction of the terminal dipeptide sequence of angiotensin I with ACE showing site of peptide cleavage. Right panel: Note Captopril interacts with ACE in a similar fashion to angiotensin I.

inhibitor designed by such rational drug design is the angiotensin converting enzyme (ACE) inhibitor captopril, which is marketed as an antihypertensive drug. Captopril was developed by taking into account a model of the mechanism by which ACE converts angiotensin I into angiotensin II (Figure 3.10). It is worth noting that captopril has two stereogenic centers and despite this was developed and marketed as a single enantiomer. Only one of the four possible isomers of captopril can bind optimally with the active site (Figure 3.10) illustrating the usefulness of the three-point receptor theory (note, however, that captopril has four areas of contact with the active site).

The three-point receptor theory has also been used for understanding chromatographic resolution of mixtures of enantiomers on chiral stationary phases, which can be thought of as artificial receptors (see Section 3.5.2).

3.4 WHY IS STEREOCHEMISTRY IMPORTANT IN DRUG DESIGN?

The sale of single enantiomer drugs shot past the $120 billion mark in the year 2000 and is projected to increase further over the next few years. Thus, chiral drugs whether sold as racemates or as the active enantiomer are likely to dominate drug markets in the near future. There are a number of reasons for the growth of chiral drug sales. Pharmaceutical companies see it as a way of prolonging the patent life of their existing racemic drugs by patenting and then marketing the active enantiomer, thereby undercutting competition from generic drug sales (Agranat and Caner 1999). In addition, some companies see this switching from racemate to single active enantiomer as a way into the drug market. One such company, Sepracor synthesizes the individual enantiomers of racemic drugs that are already on the market. If the activity resides in a single enantiomer then Sepracor patents the drug and will then either licence the drug back to the original company or market the drug itself. There are problems associated with this approach, Sepracor obtained a patent claiming the use of (S)-fluoxetine (Prozac) and (R)-fluoxetine (Figure 3.11) for the treatment of migraine and depression, respectively. Eli Lilly, the company responsible for the initial discovery of Prozac had already determined that the individual enantiomers of fluoxetine had almost equal activity as serotonin reuptake inhibitors and did not patent the individual enantiomers. Eli Lilly therefore took out a licence on the Sepracor patent allowing them sole rights to market (R)-fluoxetine as an antidepressant. This was seen as a strategy for extending the fluoxetine program until 2015. However, Lilly have terminated the agreement with Sepracor as clinical data showed a statistically significant negative cardiac side effect of the (R)-enantiomer at the highest dose tested. The underlying reason for this is likey to involve the differences in rates of metabolism of the two enantiomers, which means that only 25% of the fluoxetine in the plasma is the (R)-enantiomer. Thus, higher doses of the (R)-enantiomer were needed in clinical trials to give an equivalent therapeutic effect. Another strategic reason may also have played a part in the decision as fluoxetine would be competing with a new generation of antidepressants with multiple modes of action rather than relying on only serotonin reuptake (Thayer 2000).

The Food and Drug Administration (FDA) strongly urges companies to evaluate both the racemates and the corresponding individual enantiomers as new drugs. Thus, even if a drug is to be sold as a racemate the individual enantiomers need to be evaluated which increases the cost and timescale of drug development. Increasingly, drug companies are developing single enantiomer drugs to avoid these unnecessary costs. This strategy has been aided by the considerable increase in the methodology available for the synthesis and the assessment of purity of chiral drugs.

However, these are not the only reasons for testing individual enantiomers of chiral drugs, lessons learned from mistakes made by marketing racemic drugs also

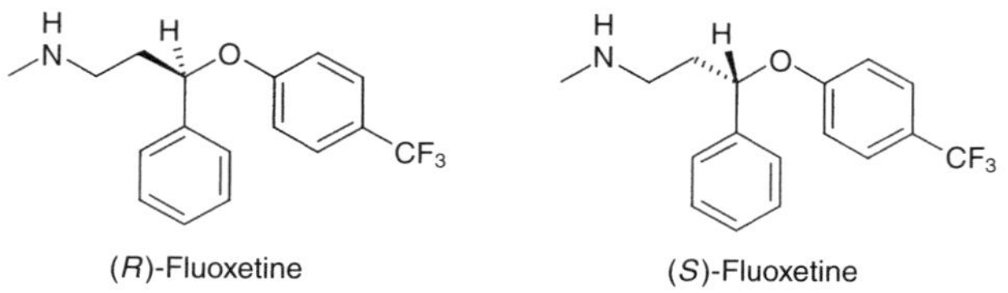

(R)-Fluoxetine   (S)-Fluoxetine

Figure 3.11 The structure of the serotonin reuptake inhibitor fluoxetine.

play a part such as in the tragic case of thalidomide (Figure 3.14). Racemic thalidomide was developed in the 1950s and was used as a sleeping pill and to treat morning sickness, but only outside the USA as FDA approval was not given. Unfortunately, the drug had serious side effects as it was found to be teratogenic causing foetal abnormalities. It was later discovered in tests with mice that the (S)-enantiomer possessed the teratogenic activity whilst the (R)-enantiomer possessed the sedative activity. However, subsequent studies using rabbits revealed that the enantiomers racemise under physiological conditions. Recently, thalidomide has hit the headlines again as the use of the racemate for treatment of leprosy has been approved by the FDA but only under the strictest of guidelines. It appears that thalidomide may also have therapeutic utility in the treatment of AIDS related disorders and tuberculosis.

The origin of the rising number of chiral drugs lies in the rational drug design process as medicinal chemists are now targeting receptors and enzymes, which are thought to be involved in the disease process. As these targets are themselves chiral, it is not surprising that the individual enantiomers of a drug may have differential activity. Indeed, Pfeiffer's rule states that 'the lower the effective dose of a drug the greater the difference in the pharmacological effect of the optical isomers'. This is simply stating that for drugs which potently interact with a receptor, it is unlikely that the individual enantiomers would both fit into the binding site. It should be noted that not only the pharmacodynamic aspects are important in the discussion of the activity of chiral drugs. Pharmacokinetics are also affected as the absorption and clearance of drugs involves interaction with enzymes and transport proteins. Thus, the individual enantiomers of a chiral drug may be metabolized by enzymes at different rates and may be transformed into different chemical entities. As a result of these considerations, it is very important that individual enantiomers of chiral drugs are tested in the clinic.

Ariëns (1986), a pioneer in the field of enantioselective drug actions, has proposed that the active enantiomer of a chiral drug be termed the eutomer whilst the less active enantiomer should be termed the distomer. The eudismic ratio (ER) is defined as the ratio of the activity of the eutomer to that of the distomer. The presence of the distomer in the racemic drug can have a number of consequences on the biological activity.

3.4.1 The distomer is inactive (high eudismic ratio)

In this case, the distomer is either inactive or displays no undesirable side effects. In the case of the antihypertensive agent (β-blocker) propranolol (Figure 3.12), the (S)-enantiomer is 130-fold more potent than the (R)-enantiomer as a β-adrenoceptor antagonist (i.e. ER = 130). A number of other β-blockers based on this structure show high eudismic ratios. These drugs are therefore marketed as racemates as the distomer displays no side effects. Despite this, there would have been advantages in marketing the (S)-enantiomer if only to extend patent life. Some drugs show even greater enantioselectivity, dexetimide has 10 000-fold greater affinity for the muscarinic acetylcholine receptor than levetimide (Figure 3.12). The distomer in these cases has been termed isomeric ballast by Ariëns (1986) as at the very least marketing racemic drugs is wasteful of resources.

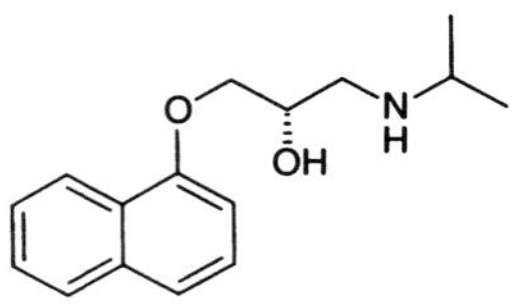

(S)-Propranolol (Eutomer, ER = 130) 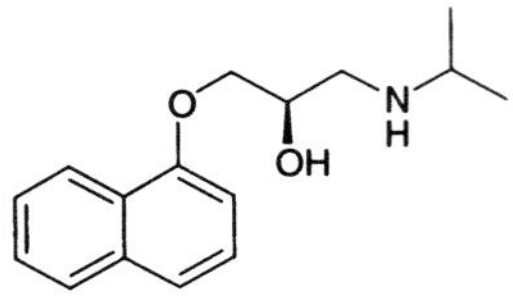   (R)-Propranolol (Distomer)

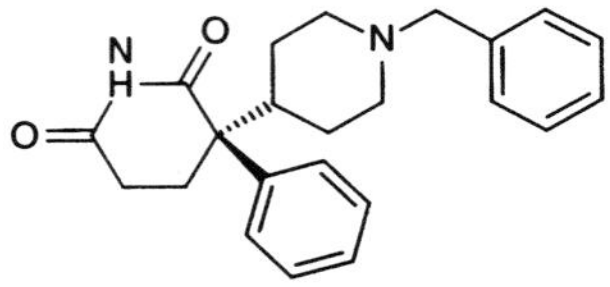

(S)-(+)-Dexetimide (Eutomer, ER = 10 000) 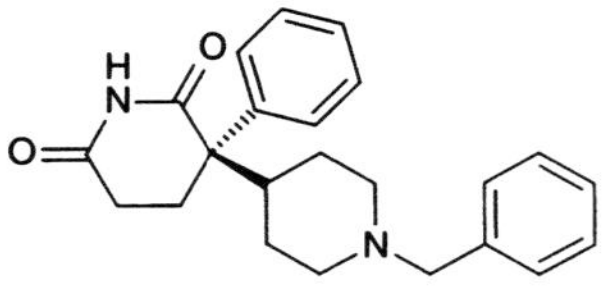   (R)-(–)-Levetimide (Distomer)

Figure 3.12 Examples of drugs where the distomer is weak/inactive.

3.4.2 Both enantiomers have independent therapeutic benefits

In some instances, both enantiomers of a drug may have different therapeutic value. The classical example of this behavior is quinine and quinidine (Figure 3.13). Quinine, which was originally obtained from the bark of cinchona trees was for centuries the only treatment for malaria. The first stereoselective synthesis of quinine has recently been published by Stork and co-workers (2001). Quinidine,

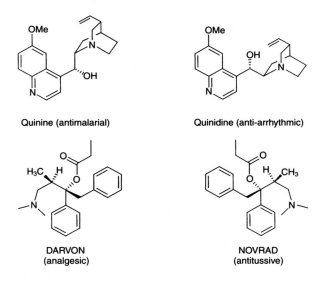

Quinine (antimalarial)   Quinidine (anti-arrhythmic)

DARVON
(analgesic)

NOVRAD
(antitussive)

Figure 3.13 Examples of drugs where both enantiomers possess therapeutic benefits.

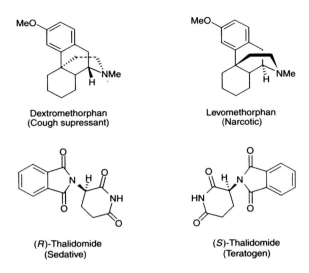

Dextromethorphan
(Cough supressant)

Levomethorphan
(Narcotic)

(*R*)-Thalidomide
(Sedative)

(*S*)-Thalidomide
(Teratogen)

Figure 3.14 Examples of drugs where the distomer possesses harmful effects.

on the other hand, is used as a Class 1A anti-arrhythmic agent and acts by increasing action potential duration.

The drug dextropropoxyphene marketed by Eli Lilly has trade names reflecting the different activities of the enantiomers. Thus the (2*R*, 3*S*)-enantiomer, DARVON has analgesic properties whilst the (2*S*, 3*R*)-enantiomer NOVRAD (Figure 3.13) is an antitussive (prevents or relieves coughing).

3.4.3   Distomer possesses harmful effects

In some cases, it is known that the distomer produces harmful or undesirable side effects. Thus, dextromethorphan is used as a cough suppressant, whereas levomethorphan has antitussive properties it is also an opioid narcotic (Figure 3.14). The harmful teratogenic side effects of the (*S*)-enantiomer of thalidomide have already been discussed (Section 3.4).

3.4.4   The eutomer and the distomer have the opposite biological activity

It is sometimes observed that the enantiomers of a chiral drug may have opposite biological activity. One example of this is (−)-dobutamine, which is an agonist at α-adrenoceptors whereas (+)-dobutamine is an antagonist (Figure 3.15). However, (+)-dobutamine is ten-fold more potent than the (−)-isomer as a β_1-adrenoceptor agonist and is used to treat cardiogenic shock.

The individual enantiomers of the 1,4-dihydropyridine analog BayK8644 (Figure 3.15) have opposing effects on L-type calcium channels with the (*S*)-enantiomer being an activator and the (*R*)-enantiomer being an antagonist (see also Section 7.4.3).

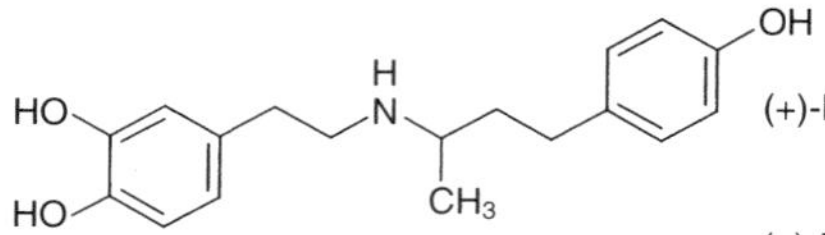

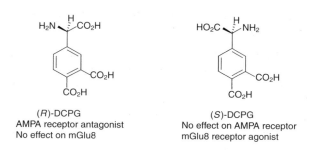

(+)-Dobutamine – β-adrenoceptor agonist
α-adrenoceptor antagonist

(–)-Dobutamine – β-adrenoceptor agonist
α-adrenoceptor agonist

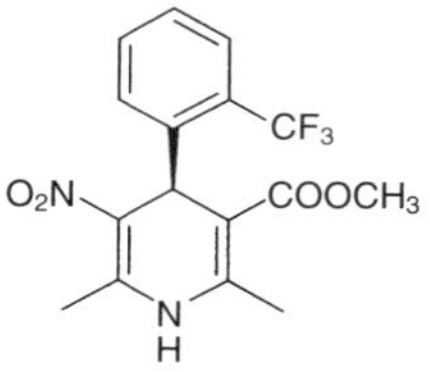

(S)-BayK8644
(activator of L-type Ca^{2+} channel)

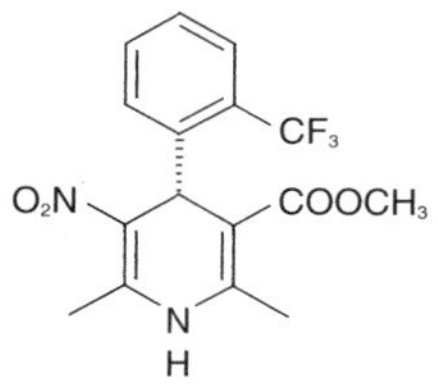

(R)-BayK8644
(antagonist of L-type Ca^{2+} channel)

Figure 3.15 Examples of drugs where the eutomer and the distomer have the opposite biological activity.

3.4.5   The racemate has a therapeutic advantage over the individual enantiomers

Both enantiomers may contribute to the therapeutic effect though examples of chiral drugs exhibiting this phenomenon are quite rare. We have recently reported that racemic 3,4-dicarboxyphenylglycine (DCPG, Figure 3.16) displays a greater potency in preventing sound-induced seizures in an experimental model of generalized epilepsy seizures than either enantiomer alone (Moldrich *et al.* 2001). The (R)-enantiomer of DCPG has antagonist activity at the AMPA receptor subtype of ionotropic glutamate receptors whereas the (S)-enantiomer has agonist activity at the mGlu8 receptor subtype of metabotropic glutamate receptors (Thomas *et al.* 2001) (glutamate receptors; see also Section 9.3). Thus, combining an AMPA receptor antagonist with a mGlu8 receptor agonist leads to a potentiation of anti-epileptic activity. Interestingly, the racemate exhibited lower potency in the

(R)-DCPG
AMPA receptor antagonist
No effect on mGlu8

(S)-DCPG
No effect on AMPA receptor
mGlu8 receptor agonist

Figure 3.16 Both (R)- and (S)-3,4-DCPG have potential therapeutic value, the racemate, however, is more potent as an anti-epileptic agent.

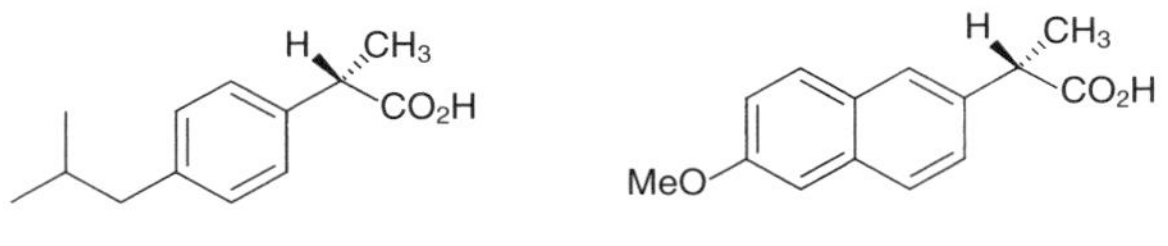

(S)-Ibuprofen (eutomer)   (S)-Naproxen (eutomer)

Figure 3.17 Examples of drugs where one enantiomer is converted into the other in the body.

rotarod test than the individual enantiomers suggesting that it did not impair motor performance beyond that experienced with either of the isomers alone.

3.4.6   One enantiomer converted into the other in the body

The inter-conversion of the enantiomers of thalidomide under physiological conditions has already been discussed. Another group of drugs which are known to exhibit this phenomenon are the α-arylpropionic acids, which are non-steroidal anti-inflammatory drugs (NSAIDs). These drugs are used to treat rheumatoid arthritis and as analgesics. It is known in the case of naproxen and ibuprofen (Figure 3.17) that the desired activity resides in the (S)-enantiomer while the (R)-enantiomer undergoes metabolic inversion to the (S)-enantiomer. Ostensibly, these drugs are safe to give in the racemic form as the distomer is converted to the eutomer in the body, however, it is known that in the course of the metabolism of the (R)-enantiomer, ibuprofen accumulates in fatty tissue in the body. The (S)-enantiomer is not metabolized in the same fashion and therefore marketing the biologically active (S)-enantiomer is advantageous.

Hopefully, these examples have persuaded the reader of the necessity of careful pharmacological testing of the individual enantiomers as well as the racemic mixture before marketing a chiral drug.

3.5   METHODS OF OBTAINING PURE STEREOISOMERS

Unfortunately, the preparation of pure stereoisomers is not trivial, arising from the fact that a reaction between two achiral starting materials, in an achiral environment, cannot generate a chiral product. This is essentially a description of the paradigm that chirality cannot just be created from nowhere. For example, the reaction between but-1-ene and hydrogen bromide (Figure 3.18) produces a compound containing a stereogenic center, so is it possible to generate a single enantiomer? The answer to this is no as the intermediate secondary carbocation contains a sp^2 hybridized carbon. It is therefore planar, has a plane of symmetry and is achiral.

As a result, subsequent attack by bromide ion can occur equally well from either the top or the bottom face. So, although the final product contains a stereogenic center, equal amounts of each isomer are produced leading to an achiral racemic mixture. So, how are pure chiral compounds obtained? Essentially, the answer to this is that there are three main methods: (1) resolution of racemates; (2) use

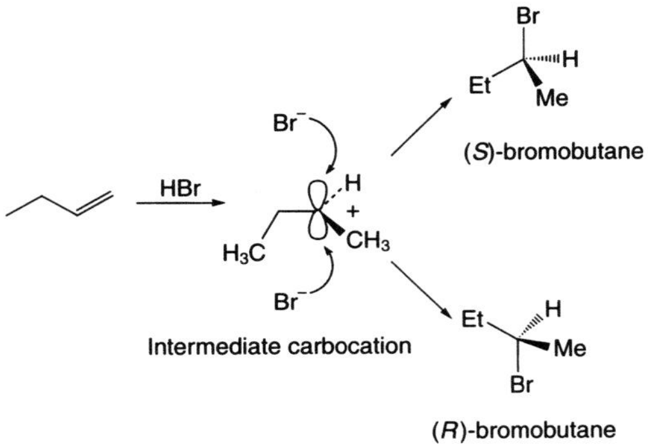

Figure 3.18 The reaction of achiral reagents in an achiral environment cannot produce an optically active product.

of naturally available chiral compounds (the chiral pool); or (3) stereoselective synthesis. These are described in more detail below, each of these methodologies being illustrated by examples taken from commercially available therapeutic agents.

3.5.1 Resolution of racemates by crystallization of diastereomers

Resolution is perhaps the oldest and most often used method of obtaining separation of a pair of enantiomers, and it is still widely used in the pharmaceutical industry for preparing optically active drugs. Although direct crystallizations of racemic mixtures can sometimes be performed in a chiral medium, the most common procedure utilizes the previously described principle that two diastereomers of a compound possess different chemical and physical properties. Of these, solubility disparities are widely used in order to produce differential crystallizations. The most common method of achieving this is to react a free carboxylic acid group of the racemate with a chiral base such as brucine, strychnine or basic amino acids such as lysine or arginine to produce diastereomeric salts (Figure 3.19). Other functional groups on the molecule such as bases, alcohols or aldehydes can also be used equally well. The resolving agents used have traditionally been derived from natural sources such as the alkaloid bases, but more recently advances have been made in the use of synthetic 'designer resolving agents'.

If the racemic mixture were reacted in this way with a pure optically active reagent then only two diastereomers are produced. These can then be crystallized and the initial precipitate should contain a higher proportion of one diastereomer (due to solubility differences), but usually this crystallization procedure needs to be repeated several times as the difference in solubility of the two isomers is rarely that pronounced. As the theoretical yield of this procedure is only 50% the racemization and recycling of the unwanted isomer is often performed in order to increase the economic viability of the procedure. This is

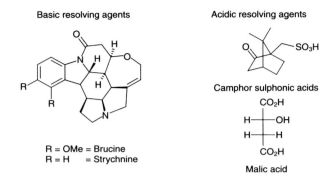

Basic resolving agents

Acidic resolving agents

Camphor sulphonic acids

R = OMe = Brucine
R = H   = Strychnine

Malic acid

Figure 3.19 Some commonly used resolving agents.

obviously of particular importance if this methodology is being used in large scale pharmaceutical production. Once the desired purity of the diastereomer has been achieved, the chiral auxiliary can then be removed to furnish the enantiomerically pure compound (Figure 3.20).

Although the predictability of success of such classical resolutions is not easy, a number of criteria for the choice of resolving agent have been proposed:

1 The asymmetric center should be in close proximity to the group used for salt formation.
2 The resultant salt should have a rigid structure.
3 Stronger acids and bases are preferential to weaker.
4 The resolving agent must be stable under the reaction conditions but be easily recovered after crystallization.

Despite this, the choice of which resolving agent to use often comes from trial and error experience. Overall, the disadvantages of this procedure are that it can be laborious and without recycling, it often results in a poor overall yield of the required diastereomer. There is also the requirement that the product needs to be

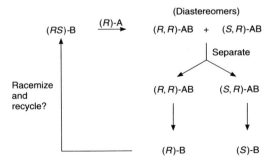

Figure 3.20 Schematic procedure for resolution of a racemate by crystallization of its diastereomeric salt.

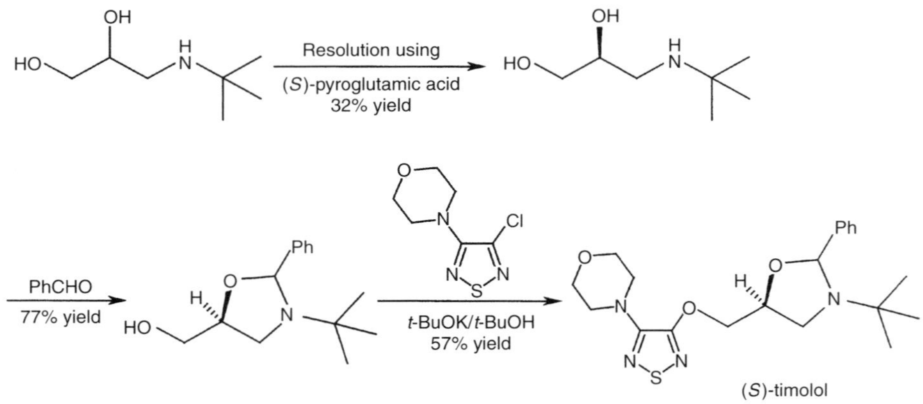

Figure 3.21 Synthesis of (S)-timolol using classical resolution.

a solid in order to be recrystallized! However, it is an inexpensive, well-established procedure, applicable to a variety of compounds on a large scale and requires no or little technical expertise or special equipment. There is also good availability and choice of chiral reactants from which to form the diastereomer. An example of the use of this technique can be found in the synthesis of (S)-timolol, a β-blocker antihypertensive drug (Figure 3.21).

3.5.2 Enantioselective chromatography

The preparative separation of the enantiomers of chiral drugs using chromatography is now an established procedure both in the pharmaceutical industry and in academic medicinal chemistry laboratories. Indeed, in some cases HPLC separation technology has been applied instead of synthesis or resolution to separate the individual enantiomers of chiral drugs, particularly at the development stage of drug discovery. New technology such as simulated moving bed (SMB) chromatography allows in some instances the resolution of chiral drugs up to 0.5–1.5 kg of racemate per kilogram of chiral stationary phase (CSP) per day. Separation of chiral drugs by chromatography relies on the formation of diastereomeric complexes. There are two main methods of accomplishing this either by precolumn derivatization using a chiral derivatizing agent followed by separation using conventional reversed-phase chromatography or separation using a column containing an immobilized CSP or via inclusion of a chiral mobile phase additive. There are a number of problems associated with precolumn derivatization, notwithstanding the inconvenience of having to perform a reaction before analysis. It is necessary to establish that the chiral derivatizing agent is enantiomerically pure and that racemization of either of the stereogenic centers of the diastereoisomer does not occur during the derivatization process. In addition, differential reaction rates of the sample with the derivatizing agent may lead to enantiomeric enrichment and racemization or enrichment may occur during the isolation and purification of the derivative. Addition of a chiral mobile phase additive (such as a cyclodextrin, or a (S)-proline copper complex) has met with success and has some advantages over CSPs such as the ability to use less expensive non-chiral columns. However, the direct separation of enantiomers using columns containing immobilized CSPs is usually the method of choice. Methodology for the resolution of chiral drugs on CSPs is now well developed and a number of different columns are commercially available. A brief overview of this methodology will be discussed. For a more detailed review see Francotte (2001).

3.5.2.1 Ligand-exchange

Chiral ligand-exchange chromatography relies on the covalent binding of an optically active ligand to the solid support. This type of separation is mainly used for the separation of amino acids using a CSP consisting of (S)-proline bound to the silica gel solid support. In order to separate racemic amino acids, copper (II) ions are first passed through the column to form a complex with the (S)-proline. The racemic mixture is then passed down the column and the (R)- and (S)-isomers displace one of the (S)-proline ligands from the copper complex resulting in the formation of transient diastereomeric complexes. These complexes formed with the two enantiomers of the amino acid of interest and immobilized (S)-proline have different stabilities resulting in one isomer of the amino acid being retained on the column for longer than the other.

3.5.2.2 Crown ethers

Chiral crown ethers have been immobilized on solid supports in order to affect the separation of both underivatized amino acids containing a primary amino group and chiral primary amines. The commercially available Crownpak column consists of a single enantiomer of a chiral dinaphthyl crown ether (Figure 3.23) immobilized on a stationary phase. Chiral separation using crown ether CSPs relies on the formation of a diastereomeric inclusion complex formed between the ammonium ion of the primary amino group and the oxygen atoms of the crown ether. In order to ensure protonation of the primary amino group separations are usually carried out in dilute acid solution such as aqueous perchloric acid. A preparative separation of the enantiomers of (RS)-3,4-DCPG (mentioned in Section 3.4.5) was obtained using the CR(+) column (see Figure 3.22 and Thomas et al. 2001).

For natural amino acids resolved on the Crownpak CR(+) column the D (or in most cases R) enantiomer is eluted before the L enantiomer. It has been claimed that the absolute configuration of an amino acid can be inferred from the elution order of the isomers from the CR(+) column. A CR(−) column which has the reverse enantioselectivity to the CR(+) column is also commercially available. One disadvantage of using this column is that mobile phases containing more than 15% methanol results in leaching of the chiral crown ether from the column and deterioration of CSP performance. Recently, a CSP bearing structural similarity to the crown ether found in the Crownpak column has been developed that has additional functionality allowing covalent immobilization on silica gel (Hyun et al. 2001).

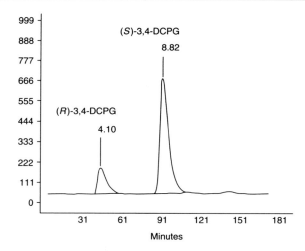

Figure 3.22 A mixture of (R)- and (S)-3,4-DCPG resolved on a Crownpak CR(+) column. Chromatography conditions: aqueous perchloric acid, pH 2, 20 °C, flow rate 0.4 ml/min. Detected at 230 nM.

3.5.2.3   Pirkle columns

These columns were mainly the result of the work of Pirkle and co-workers. There are two main types: (1) a π acceptor phase based mainly on N-(3,5-dinitrobenzoyl)-phenylglycine bonded via a linker to the silica (Figure 3.23); and (2) a π donor phase typically based on naphthylamino acid derivatives bonded to silica. The separation is achieved by the formation of a strong three-point interaction with only one enantiomer of a chiral drug. These interactions include the formation charge–transfer complexes, π–π bonding and steric effects. These types of column are commercially available and can be used for preparative separations. The main disadvantage of these columns is that they only separate aromatic compounds and therefore precolumn derivatization of the drug of interest may be necessary. Recently modified versions of these columns

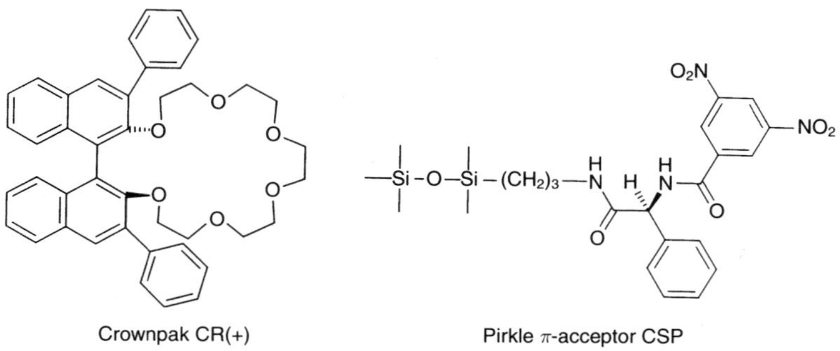

Crownpak CR(+)   Pirkle π-acceptor CSP

Figure 3.23 Examples of crown ether and Pirkle chiral stationary phases.

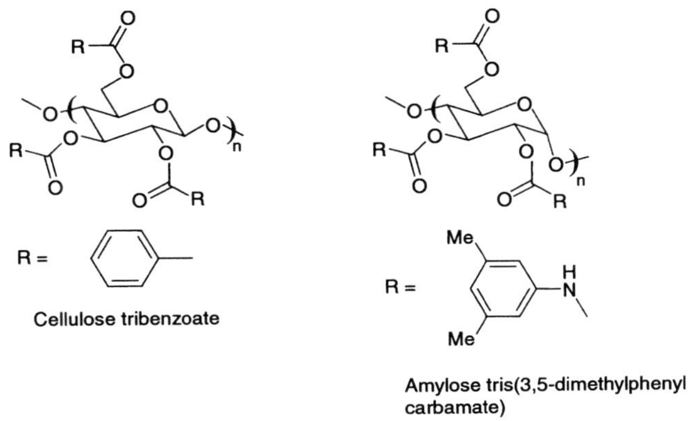

Figure 3.24 Examples of cellulose and amylose chiral stationary phases.

such as Whelk-O1 and α-Burke 1 have been used to separate β-blockers and NSAIDs.

3.5.2.4 Cellulose and amylose phases

A number of cellulose derivatives have been used as chiral stationary phases (e.g. cellulose tribenzoate marketed as Chiralcel OB). The amylose bonded phases are exemplified by amylose *tris*-(3,5-dimethylphenylcarbamate) marketed as Chiralpak AD (Figure 3.24). Both these types of column have been used to effect both analytical and preparative resolutions of a wide variety of chiral drugs. The current trend is to prepare immobilized polysaccharide-based stationary phases as these columns can be used with a wider variety of organic solvents in the mobile phase due to their low solubility in such solvents. This improves the resolution and also allows the use of more polar mobile phases thus increasing the solubility of the racemic drug (Francotte 2001).

3.5.2.5 Miscellaneous phases

Cyclodextrin based CSPs have also been used for both analytical and preparative separations. Cyclodextrins are cyclic oligosaccharides consisting of interlinked α-D-glucose units. The most commonly used cyclodextrins are comprised of 6, 7 or 8 glucose units, α-, β- and γ-cyclodextrin, respectively, arranged in a doughnut-shaped structure and differ in the size of the hydrophobic cavity and thus, the types of molecules that can be separated. Compounds can form inclusion complexes by binding inside the cavity and this forms the basis of the enantioselectivity.

Macrocyclic antibiotics such as vancomycin and teicoplanin have been incorporated into stationary phases. However, these phases are mostly used in analytical rather than preparative separations though separations of a few milligrams of material have been demonstrated. These phases have shown greatest applicability to the resolution of racemic amino acids.

3.5.2.6   *Simulated moving bed chromatography*

Large-scale separation of chiral drugs is now possible using CSPs and this methodology is now seen as a viable alternative to more established procedures for preparation of single enantiomers of chiral drugs. Two main procedures in use are (1) batch chromatography; and (2) simulated moving bed chromatography (SMBC). Batch chromatography consists of applying the sample (up to 100 g) to the top of the column (with a diameter of 5–30 cm for larger separations) and eluting with an appropriate mobile phase. The alternative method SMBC is finding increasing favor in the pharmaceutical industry. In SMBC 6–12 columns containing a CSP are joined in a ring and fluid is circulated using 4–5 pumps. As the racemate travels through the columns, a zone of one enantiomer leads the rest of the injected sample while a zone of the opposite enantiomer lags behind. Using a computer controlled system, some of the leading enantiomer and independently some of the trailing enantiomer is withdrawn at intervals. There are a number of reasons for the success of SMBC such as the fact that the separation is run in overload conditions. In addition, as the process is continuous solvent consumption is considerably reduced. The SMBC has an additional advantage over batch chromatography in that the whole stationary phase is used in the separation process rather than a small section, as is the case for the batch process. As polysaccharide-based columns have a high loading capacity they have been widely used for chiral SMBC separations of up to 1.5 kg of racemate per kilogram of CSP per day. The SMBC has been applied to the separation of a number of chiral drugs and intermediates such as propranolol, the analgesic tramadol, the anti-asthmatic agent formoterol and of the antitussive agent guaifenesine (Francotte 2001).

3.5.3   Asymmetric synthesis

Whilst a conventional synthetic sequence followed by isolation of the required enantiomers is usually successful for compounds containing single stereogenic centers, multiple centers in a target molecule often make this process difficult. It would be more beneficial and less wasteful if a synthesis could be achieved in which all centers were produced in only their correct geometry. Asymmetric synthesis to obtain chiral molecules has been one of the most widely investigated and rapidly growing areas of organic chemistry in the last 30 years. It can be defined as:

> A synthesis in which an achiral unit of a substrate molecule is converted to a chiral unit such that the possible stereoisomers are formed in unequal amounts.
> (Aitken and Kilenyi 1994)

In essence, this statement describes the previously discussed rule that optically active materials cannot be created from inactive starting materials or conditions, but in the presence of anything asymmetric the products need not be formed in equal amounts. The predominant ways in which this can be achieved are described in the following sections.

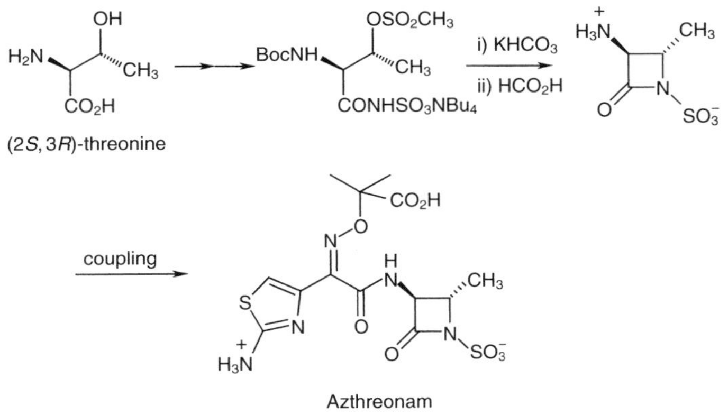

Figure 3.25 Synthesis of Azthreonam using (2S, 3R)-threonine as the chiral template.

3.5.3.1 The chiral pool

This is often referred to as 'first generation' methodology as it is perhaps the most obvious, involving the use of a chiral starting material obtained from the vast diversity of nature itself. The particular unit is usually chosen as it closely resembles and has the required stereochemistry as a fragment of the desired product. Therefore, the chosen molecule is providing a 'chiral template' from which the target compound can be assembled. The chiral unit itself may also be capable of exerting a degree of inductive stereocontrol in subsequent steps of the synthesis (see below). In order to be of use, these natural products must be readily available and moderately inexpensive. There are numerous examples of the usage of a wide variety of compounds including alkaloids, terpenes and carbohydrates, but the most commonly utilized group are the naturally occurring amino acids. These are widely used as they have a relatively simple structure containing only one or two stereogenic centers, are relatively amenable to chemical transformation and are readily available at low cost. Their particular utility is demonstrated in the example below in which (2S, 3R)-threonine is used as the chiral template in the synthesis of the antibiotic Azthreonam (Figure 3.25).

3.5.3.2 Stereoselective synthesis

Methodologies of asymmetric synthesis have evolved rapidly but essentially involve forming new stereogenic centers in the substrate via the presence of another asymmetric group (ultimately derived from the chiral pool). This is now a huge subject area, but can essentially be divided into a number of broad areas, which are briefly described in the following sections. Additional information can be found in the reviews in the further reading section.

3.5.3.2.1 The use of a chiral auxiliary

This second generation methodology is similar to using a chiral pool reagent to achieve the desired configuration. However, instead of selecting a chiral starting material that resembles the skeleton of the target, the 'chiral group' is purposefully attached to the achiral substrate solely for the purpose of controlling the stereo-chemical outcome of subsequent reactions. The unit chosen is not an integral part of the target compound, but instead is removed once it has performed its function. Therefore, the three steps can be depicted as:

1   Appendage of the enantiomerically pure chiral auxiliary to the substrate;
2   Reaction with the achiral reagent producing two diastereomers with induction hopefully providing these in greatly unequal amounts; and
3   Removal of the auxiliary, avoiding conditions that may cause racemization.

The advantage of this methodology is that reaction of the chiral substrate (i.e. with auxiliary attached) produces a diastereomer. Therefore, even if a high level of induction in subsequent reactions is not produced the products can potentially still be separated to isolate the required material in good enantiomeric purity. But what is it that causes this induction to provide unequal amounts of diastereomers?

Virtually all reactions of this type can be explained in terms of kinetics. If the rate constant leading to the (R) product is different to that leading to the (S) product then these two isomers will be formed in different amounts and the enantiomeric ratio of products formed will reflect this. This rate constant is directly linked to the activation energy of the reaction by the Arrhenius equation so the greater the difference in activation energy to form the two isomers then the greater the selectivity. Conversely, if the two activation energies are the same then no selectivity is observed. This difference in activation energy can be explained by the fact that the transition states leading to the product are in themselves diastereo-meric and thus not equivalent and have different energies. As an example, the reaction between 4-methylhex-1-ene and hydrogen bromide, produces a chiral molecule containing a new stereogenic centre (Figure 3.26). This is because the carbocation intermediate has no symmetry plane and so attack by bromide ion from either the top or bottom faces is not equally favorable.

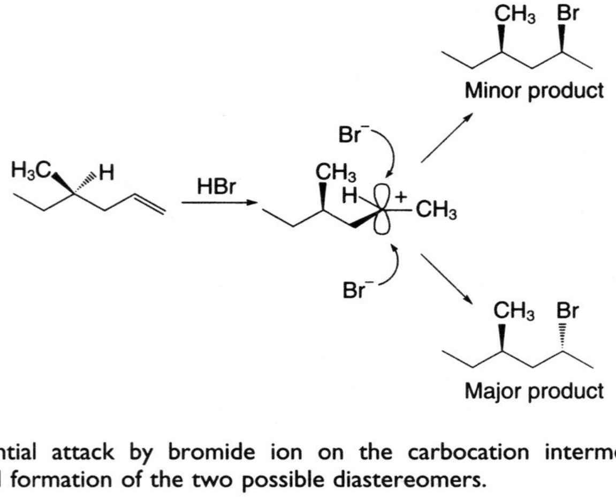

Figure 3.26 Preferential attack by bromide ion on the carbocation intermediate leads to dif-ferential formation of the two possible diastereomers.

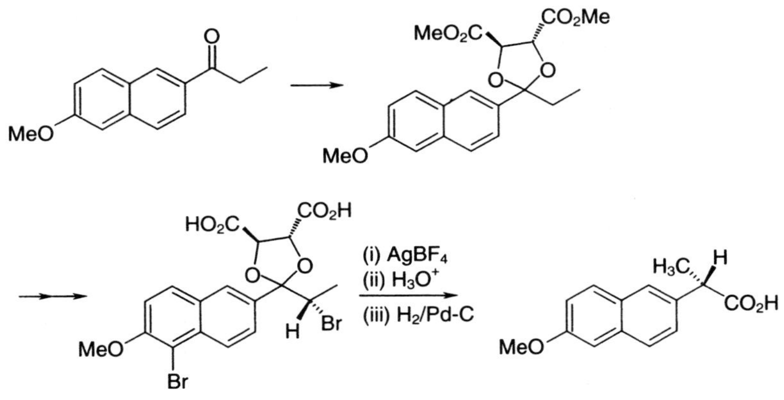

Figure 3.27 Synthesis of (S)-Naproxen using tartaric acid as a chiral auxiliary.

In this case, the non-equivalence is the result of steric interference, and this is generally the basis for first and second-generation asymmetric methods, although other factors such as chelation, hydrogen bonding and electrostatic interactions may also be important. A good example of this is the synthesis of the anti-inflammatory agent (S)-Naproxen. In this route, (2R, 3R)-tartaric acid is used as the chiral auxiliary which can be recovered in the penultimate step (Figure 3.27).

3.5.3.2.2 *The use of chiral reagents and catalysts (third and fourth generation methodology)*

The main disadvantage of using a chiral auxiliary is that additional steps are required in the synthesis for appendage and removal of the chiral group. However, if the chiral product is formed directly from an achiral starting material using a chiral reagent then this is avoided. An added advantage to this methodology over first and second generation methods is that the choice of starting material is now far wider as it now no longer needs to be derived from the chiral pool. However, although the number of chiral reagents is increasing, there are no comprehensive literature reviews covering the availability of chiral reagents for particular synthetic transformations. In order to overcome the additional problem of also requiring a stoichiometric amount of reagent, chiral catalysts have been developed. This is the most recent and perhaps pivotal area of asymmetric synthesis and essentially involves using a chiral catalyst to promote the reaction of an achiral starting material into a chiral product. By definition, the advantage is that only a small molar ratio of catalyst is required (often less than 0.05 equivalents being used), which can be recovered and reused.

One of the most widely exploited areas of catalytic asymmetric synthesis is hydrogenation using a chiral transition metal complex. Two important ligands in this area are (1) BINAP; and (2) DIPAMP, (Figure 3.28) which are often

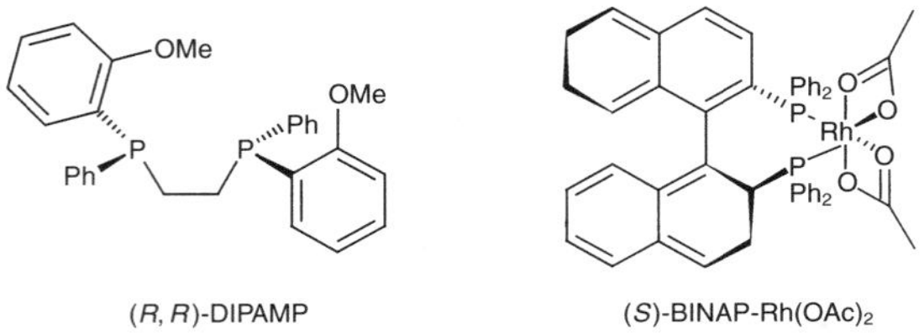

(R, R)-DIPAMP   (S)-BINAP-Rh(OAc)₂

Figure 3.28 Two commonly utilized chiral catalysts for performing asymmetric hydrogenations. BINAP (right) is shown as its octahedral rhodium acetate complex.

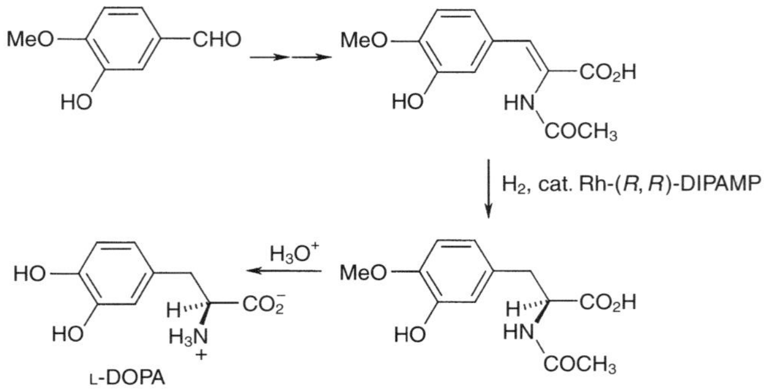

Figure 3.29 Synthesis of L-DOPA using asymmetric hydrogenation.

complexed to rhodium (II) or ruthenium (II) acetate. These are particularly effective because of the rigid structure of the complex, which is octahedral and can exist in two enantiomeric forms.

The DIPAMP is used in the industrial synthesis of (S)-3,4-dihydroxyphenylalanine (L-DOPA), an anti-Parkinson's agent (Figure 3.29). This compound is of particular interest as the actual active drug, dopamine, is the decarboxylated product of L-DOPA, but this cannot cross the blood–brain barrier to reach the target site. However, the prodrug DOPA can do this and after reaching the site of action it is only the L-isomer, which is stereoselectively decarboxylated by the enzyme DOPA decarboxylase. Therefore, it is essential to administer the prodrug in only the L-configuration in order to avoid a potentially dangerous build up of the D-isomer.

3.5.3.2.3   Use of enzymes and whole organisms

Enzymes are nature's chiral catalysts which are extremely versatile catalyzing almost every known chemical reaction. Common misconceptions about enzyme specificity following on from the Lock and Key hypothesis have hampered the development of the use of enzymes in enantioselective synthesis. This has been exacerbated due to the wrongly held view that aqueous conditions were needed for enzyme function and that only one enantiomer could be produced due to the stereospecificity of enzyme action. However, it is now generally agreed that enzymes can accommodate a variety of structurally diverse substrates and in some cases can be used under a wide variety of temperature, pressure and pH conditions. This being particularly applicable to the so-called extremophile class of enzyme isolated from microbes capable of surviving in extreme environments. Most enzymes can also carry out their function in organic solvents as long as they are not totally anhydrous.

Enzymes catalyzing a wide variety of chemical reactions are available for enantioselective synthesis and thanks to the advent of molecular biological techniques, the choice of enzyme is not restricted to those found in nature. It is now a relatively straightforward process to manipulate enzyme structure using mutagenesis and recombinant technology allowing the stability, activity and substrate specificity of enzymes to be controlled. High throughput screening methods used in the discovery phase of drug development can be used to discover an appropriate enzyme for a particular chemical synthesis and also to adapt the enzyme to the reaction conditions.

One of the first decisions to make when considering an enantioselective synthesis using an enzyme is whether to use whole cells or a cell-free enzyme preparation. Cell-free enzyme preparations offer advantages in simplicity of use, as well as tolerance to harsh conditions such as the use of organic solvents but suffer from the disadvantage of being expensive and may also need additional co-factors to function correctly. On the other hand, whole cells are relatively cheap and all necessary co-factors are present but product isolation can be complex and side reactions may also occur due to the presence of other enzymes in the cells.

A comprehensive review of the use of enzymes in drug synthesis is beyond the scope of this chapter and therefore only selected examples are given. Readers are referred to more detailed reviews given in the reading list for further information (see Sheldon 1993; Roberts 1999; Schulze and Wubbolts 1999; McCoy 2001). Enzymes from all six major classes (see Table 3.1) have been used either in the production of chiral drugs or intermediates used in their synthesis.

The cardiovascular drug diltiazem (see Sections 7.3.3 and 7.5.3) is manufactured on a multihundred tonne scale from a chiral phenylglycidyl ester which is in turn produced via a lipase catalyzed resolution (Figure 3.30). Only the $(2S, 3R)$-isomer

Table 3.1 The classification of enzymes

Enzyme class	Examples of enzymes	Reactions catalyzed
Oxidoreductase	Dehydrogenases, oxidases, peroxidases	Oxidation/reduction reactions
Transferase	Aminotransferases	Group transfer reactions (e.g. methyl, acyl, phosphate)
Hydrolase	Lipases/esterases, proteases, amidopeptidases, acylases, hydantoinases	Hydrolysis (e.g. esters, amides, hydantoins)
Lyase	Decarboxylases, dehydratases, aldolases, oxynitrilases	Additions to, or formation of, C=C, C=O or C=N bonds
Isomerase	Racemases, epimerases	Structural and geometric rearrangements
Ligase	DNA ligase	Formation of C—C, C—N, C—O or C—S bonds

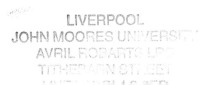

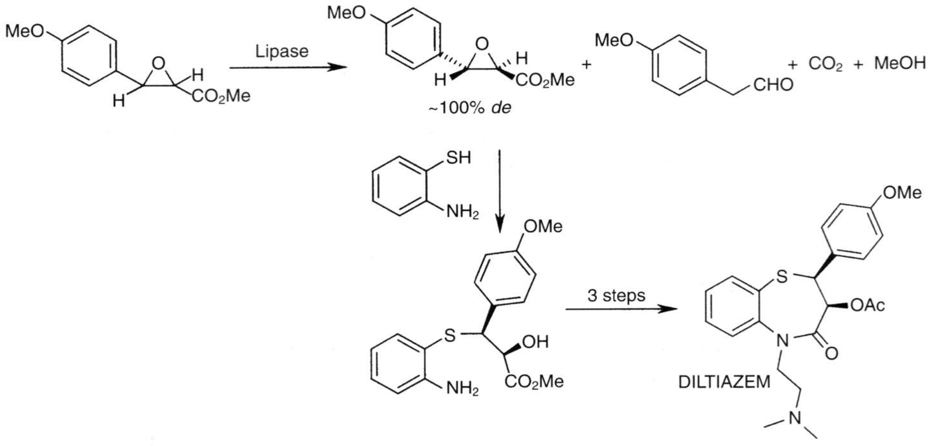

Figure 3.30 Route to diltiazem involving a lipase catalyzed resolution.

of the phenylglycidyl ester is hydrolyzed to the corresponding carboxylic acid which is unstable and decomposes to the corresponding phenylacetaldehyde.

Several antibiotics based on the penicillin or cephalosporin structure contain (R)-4-p-hydroxyphenylglycine as the acyl side-chain. This amino acid is produced on a multithousand tonne scale by dynamic kinetic resolution of the corresponding hydantoin (Figure 3.31). In resolutions of racemates using hydrolases, the maximum theoretical yield is 50% (one enantiomer is unaffected by the hydrolase). However, by allowing racemization to occur simultaneously the theoretical yield can be increased to 100%, this process being known as dynamic kinetic resolution. In the aforementioned hydantoin hydrolysis, racemization of the unchanged (S)-hydantoin is achieved either by carrying out the process at alkaline pH or by the inclusion of a hydantoin racemase.

Fermentation has also been used for the bulk preparation of a number of pharmaceutical and related compounds (for more details see Sheldon 1993). Fermentation is distinct from enzymatic transformations using whole cells as the

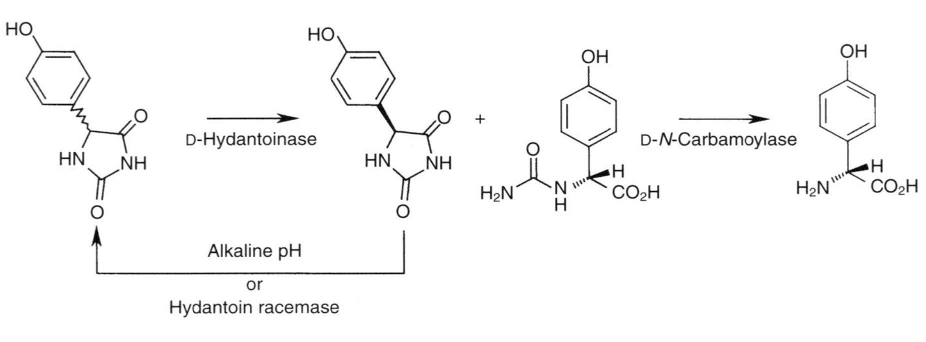

Figure 3.31 Industrial process for the production of (R)-p-hydroxyphenylglycine.

former involves the use of growing cells. In relation to pharmaceutical products, fermentation has been mainly used in the production of β-lactam antibiotics (cephalosporins and penicillins), steroid drugs (market value >$1 billion), ephidrene, pseudoephidrine, and intermediates for the manufacture of β-blockers. Fermentation is the most cost-effective or in some cases the only way to produce complex chiral molecules such as cyclosporin (immunosuppressant agent), avermectins (anthelmintic agents) and vitamin B_{12}.

3.6 ANALYTICAL METHODS OF DETERMINING PURITY OF STEREOISOMERS

A number of methodologies are now available for the accurate assessment of enantiomeric purity, which are critical for all phases of the drug discovery process. In the drug development phase, it is vital to know the purity of individual enantiomers to understand the structure–activity relationships of drug candidates while in the pharmacokinetic phase, it is necessary to determine the levels of drug enantiomers in biological fluids. It should be a standard practice to use more than one analytical method to determine enantiomeric purity. Fortunately, a wide variety of analytical methods have been developed. One of the main methods of determining the purity of the individual enantiomers of chiral drugs concerns the use of HPLC using chiral stationary phases as discussed in Section 3.5.2. In this Section, some of the main alternative methods available for determining enantiomeric purity will be discussed.

3.6.1 Optical rotation

One of the oldest and most commonly used methods available for the assessment of enantiomeric purity involves measuring optical rotation using a polarimeter (for details of how this is measured see Section 3.2). The main advantage of this method is that it is quick and can be performed without the need for costly apparatus. However, there are problems associated with this method of purity assessment; care must be taken to remove chiral impurities from the sample and to ensure that it was isolated without accidental enantiomeric enrichment. This is particularly a problem with crystallization as enantiomers crystallize at different rates in a chiral medium (see Section 3.5.1). In the case of novel compounds, the maximum optical rotation of the pure enantiomer will not be known and in these cases pure samples of each enantiomer will be needed before using this form of purity assessment. When comparing optical rotations, it is essential to compare samples of the same concentration in the same solvent and to carry out the reading at the same temperature as used from the standard as all these factors can affect the sign and magnitude of the rotation. For water soluble compounds such as amino acids, optical rotation also depends on pH.

Empirical rules have been devised which allow the correlation of the sense of optical rotation with absolute configuration. However, these should be used with caution as closely related compounds with the same absolute configuration can rotate plane-polarized light in different directions. Thus, it is unlikely that such correlations will replace X-ray crystallography as the method of choice for determining absolute configuration.

3.6.2   NMR spectroscopy

Nuclear magnetic resonance (NMR) spectroscopy has been widely used to determine enantiomeric purity. Enantiomers cannot be distinguished by NMR spectroscopy and so this method relies on the formation of diastereoisomers by the addition of a chiral agent to the mixture of enantiomers. There are three main methods of forming diastereomeric mixtures, via a chiral derivatizing agent (CDA), a chiral lanthanide shift reagent or the use of a chiral solvent.

The formation of diastereomeric mixtures using a chiral derivatizing reagent suffers from the same disadvantages as highlighted in Section 3.5.2 covering precolumn derivatization of samples for HPLC analysis. Despite these limitations CDAs are still widely used. One CDA, α-methoxy-α-trifluoromethylphenylacetic acid (MTPA, Figure 3.32) developed by Mosher has been used to analyze enantiomeric purity of amino acids and α-hydroxy acids. Using ^{1}H NMR spectroscopy, the purity of the original enantiomer can be estimated by taking the ratio of the integral of the peaks due to the methoxy groups of the diastereoisomers formed via MTPA derivatization. The MTPA has the advantage over previously reported reagents such as O-methylmandelic acid (Figure 3.32) of being stable to racemization as it lacks an α-hydrogen atom. In addition, as MTPA contains a trifluoromethyl group, ^{19}F NMR spectroscopy can be used thus considerably simplifying the NMR spectrum.

A non-derivatizing method involves using a chiral lanthanide shift reagent which when complexed with the sample of interest shifts some of the signals in the NMR spectrum. As the lanthanide shift reagent is chiral, diastereomeric complexes are formed with the mixture of enantiomers in the analytical sample and these exhibit different shifts in the NMR spectrum. The europium shift reagents illustrated in Figure 3.32 have been used to analyze the purity of chiral compounds containing a wide range of functional groups such as alcohols, esters, ketones and sulphonamides.

Chiral solvating agents (CSAs) have been used to analyze the enantiomeric purity of a range of chiral compounds. This is illustrated by the use of 1-(9-anthryl)-2,2,2-trifluoroethanol to analyze chiral amines, alcohols, α-amino acid esters and lactones. This methodology involves the addition of 1–10 mol equivalents of the CSA to the bulk NMR solvent and relies on the formation of diastereomeric solvation complexes with the chiral analytical sample. The major drawback of this method is that there is

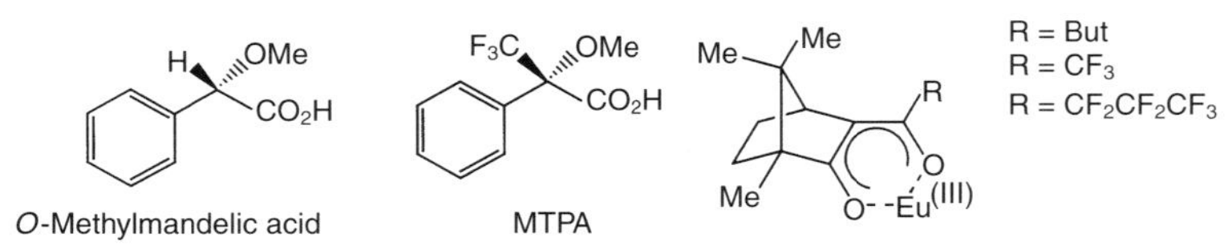

Figure 3.32 Examples of chiral reagents used for the determination of enantiomeric purity by NMR spectroscopy.

not one resolving agent that is applicable to all chiral compounds. The use of NMR for the analysis of the purity of chiral drugs is limited by the fact that non-polar solvents usually give optimal peak separations and this excludes the use of polar solvents such as DMSO, which are required to dissolve a number of polar pharmacologically active compounds. Analytical methods based on HPLC, GC and capillary electrophoresis are now used more often than those relying on NMR spectroscopy for determining enantiomeric purity of chiral drugs.

3.6.3 Gas chromatography

Chiral gas chromatography (GC) has emerged as an extremely efficient and sensitive method for the determination of the enantiomeric purity of chiral drugs (for a comprehensive review see Schurig 2001). In addition, it is now possible to effect preparative separations of volatile racemic compounds. The main limitation of this technique is that the sample needs to be readily vaporized without decomposition. However, there are a number of advantages to the use of chiral GC such as the ability to analyze multicomponent mixtures of enantiomers and to separate the enantiomers away from trace contaminants. It is possible to extend the detection of enantiomeric impurities down to the picogram level enabling the reliable determination of enantiomeric excess to levels >99.9%.

Chiral GC relies on the use of a CSP of high enantiomeric purity to effect resolution of mixtures of enantiomers. There are three main types of CSPs available for GC analysis:

1   Those using chiral amino acid derivatives, which resolve mixtures of enantiomers via the formation of diastereomeric complexes involving hydrogen bond interactions.
2   Phases including chiral metal complexes, which separate mixtures of enantiomers via the formation of diastereomeric metal complexes.
3   Phases including cyclodextrin derivatives, which separate mixtures of enantiomers via formation of inclusion complexes.

These phases are usually linked to polysiloxanes, which produces columns with enhanced thermal stability and separation efficiency.

In the case of the chiral inhalation anaesthetics enflurane (CHF_2OCF_2CHFCl), isoflurane and desflurane efficient separation on chiral GC, CSPs has allowed preparative scale resolution of the enantiomers which have been subsequently tested in biomedical trials. Using analogous methodology to that used in simulated moving bed (SMB) HPLC, the enantiomers of enflurane have been separated by enantioselective GC SMB on a large scale.

3.6.4 Capillary electrophoresis (CE)

A relatively new method of enantioseparation involves the use of capillary electromigration techniques, which have been developed over the past 15 years (for a review see Chankvetadze and Blaschke 2001). In common with chiral GC and HPLC, the origin of the enantioseparation lies in the non-covalent intermolecular interactions between the analyte and the chiral selector and is not based on electrophoretic mobility, as enantiomers possess the same charge densities. In HPLC, the CSP is usually chemically bonded to the silica gel, however, CE is usually carried out with bare silica capillaries. For this reason, the chiral selector is added to the electrolyte in order to form diastereomeric complexes with the analyte thereby effecting chiral discrimination.

In common with HPLC, a number of chiral selectors have been used to effect enantioseparation such as cyclodextrins, polysaccharides, macrocyclic antibiotics and proteins. In an elegant study, it has been shown that the enantiomers of N-derivatized amino acids such as (RS)-3,5-dinitrobenzoylleucine can be resolved in non-aqueous CE using t-butylcarbamoylquinine as a chiral selector. Conversely, t-butylcarbamoylquinine and t-butylcarbamoylquinidine can be separated using (R)- or (S)-3,5-dinitrobenzoylleucine as a chiral selector.

3.6.5   Mass spectrometry

A newly emerging technology for the rapid analysis of chiral drugs involves the use of mass spectroscopy (Tao *et al.* 2001; Jacoby 2001). Four main methods are available for mass spectrometry-based analysis of mixtures of enantiomers:

1   Generation of diastereomeric adducts using chiral reference compounds and chemical ionization, fast atom bombardment, or electrospray mass spectrometry. In this method, one enantiomer of the analyte is isotopically labeled so that the corresponding diastereomeric mixture can be mass resolved.
2   Using exchange reactions. A diastereomeric adduct typically generated from the chiral ligand and a chiral host such as a β-cyclodextrin is mass selected and allowed to exchange the chiral ligand with a neutral gas. Resolution is achieved as exchange rates vary with the chirality of the analyte incorporated into the adduct ion.
3   Collision-induced dissociation of diastereomeric adducts formed from the analyte and a chiral reference substance in a tandem mass spectrometry experiment.
4   Kinetic method using tandem mass spectrometry.

A recent report illustrating the application of the kinetic method describes the use of diastereomeric copper (II) complexes with a drug and a chiral reference compound (in this case (S)-amino acids) to analyze the enantiomeric purity of a range of chiral drugs (propranolol, DOPA, norepinephrine, ephedrine, isoproterenol and atenolol). Using electrospray mass spectroscopy these trimeric complex ions (three ligands – one of the analyte and two of the reference (S)-amino acid) are collisionally activated leading to loss of either a neutral reference or a neutral drug molecule. The ratio of these two competitive dissociation rates is then related via the kinetic method to the enantiomeric composition of the analyte. The advantage of this method over other previously described methods is that isotopic labeling is avoided and commercially available instruments can be used. In addition, the method is sensitive enough to allow analysis of mixtures with a few percent enantiomeric contamination (2–4% ee). Another advantage of using mass spectroscopy for analysis is that it can be coupled to other separation methods such as HPLC and GC.

FURTHER READING

Agranat, I. and Caner, H. (1999) Intellectual property and chirality of drugs. *Drug Discovery Today*, **4**, 313–321.

Aitken, R.A. and Kilenyi, S.N. (1994) *Asymmetric synthesis*, 1st edition. London: Chapman and Hall.

Ariëns, E.J. (1986) Chirality in bioactive agents and its pitfalls. *Trends Pharmacol. Sci.*, **7**, 200–205.

Chankvetadze, B. and Blaschke, G. (2001) Enantioseparations in capillary electromigration techniques: recent developments and future trends. *J. Chromatography A*, **906**, 309–363.

Francotte, E.R. (2001) Enantioselective chromatography as a powerful alternative for the preparation of drug enantiomers. *J. Chromatography A*, **906**, 379–397.

Hyun, H.H., Han, S.C., Lipshutz, B.H., Shin, Y.-J. and Welch, C.J. (2001) New chiral crown ether stationary phase for the liquid chromatographic resolution of α-amino acid enantiomers. *J. Chromatography A*, **910**, 359–365.

Jacoby, M. (2001) Fast separations for drugs. *Chemical & Engineering News*, **79** (21), 68–69.

McCoy, M. (2001) Making drugs with little bugs. *Chemical & Engineering News*, **79** (21), 37–43.

Moldrich, R.X., Beart, P.M., Jane, D.E., Chapman, A.G. and Meldrum, B.S. (2001) Anticonvulsant activity of 3,4-dicarboxyphenylglycines in DBA/2 mice. *Neuropharmacology*, **40**, 696–699.

Roberts, S.M. (1999) Preparative biotransformations. *J. Chem. Soc., Perkin Trans. 1*, 1–21.

Robinson, M.J.T. (2000) *Organic stereochemistry*. New York: Oxford University Press.

Schulte, M. and Strube, J. (2001) Preparative enantioseparation by simulated moving bed chromatography. *J. Chromatography A*, **906**, 399–416.

Schulze, B. and Wubbolts, M.G. (1999) Biocatalysts for industrial production of fine chemicals. *Current Opinion in Biotechnology*, **10**, 609–615.

Schurig, V. (2001) Separation of enantiomers by gas chromatography. *J. Chromatography A*, **906**, 275–299.

Sheldon, R.A. (1993) *Chirotechnology, industrial synthesis of optically active compounds*. New York: Marcel Decker.

Stork, G., Niu, D., Fujimoto, A., Koft, E.R., Balkovec, J.M., Tata, J.R. and Dake G.R. (2001) The first stereoselective total synthesis of quinine. *J. Am. Chem. Soc.*, **123**, 3239–3242.

Tao, W.A., Gozzo, F.C. and Cooks, R.G. (2001) Mass spectrometric quantitation of chiral drugs by the kinetic method. *Anal. Chem.*, **73**, 1692–1698.

Thayer, A. (2000) Eli Lilly pulls the plug on Prozac isomer drug. *Chemical & Engineering News*, **78** (40), 8.

Thomas, N.K., Wright, R.A., Howson, P.A., Kingston, A.E., Schoepp, D.D. and Jane, D.E. (2001) (S)-3,4-DCPG a potent and selective mGlu8a receptor agonist activates metabotropic glutamate receptors on primary afferent terminals in the neonatal rat spinal cord. *Neuropharmacology*, **40**, 311–318.

Triggle, D.J. (1997) Stereoselectivity of drug action. *Drug Discovery Today*, **2**, 138–147.

Chapter 4

Computer-aided development and use of three-dimensional pharmacophore models

Tommy Liljefors and Ingrid Pettersson

4.1 STRUCTURE- AND PHARMACOPHORE-BASED LIGAND DESIGN

The explosive development of computer technology and methodologies to calculate molecular properties have increasingly made it possible to use computer techniques to aid the drug discovery process. The use of computer techniques in this context is often called *computer-aided drug design (CADD)*, but since the development of a drug involves a large number of steps in addition to the development of a high-affinity ligand (bioavailability, toxicity and metabolism must also be taken into account as discussed in Chapter 1), a more appropriate name is *computer-aided ligand design (CALD)*.

If the 3D-structure of the target enzyme or receptor is available from X-ray crystallography, preferentially with a co-crystallized ligand so that the binding site and binding mode of the ligand is known, it is feasible to study the biomacromolecule–ligand complex in a direct way by interactive computer graphics techniques and computational chemistry. In this way, a detailed knowledge of the interactions between the ligand and the enzyme/receptor may be obtained. New candidate ligands may be 'docked' into the binding site in order to study if the new structure can interact with the receptor in an optimal way. This procedure is known as *structure-based ligand design*. An example of the use of this type of ligand design in the development of new high-affinity ligands for dihydrofolate reductase (DHFR) is discussed in Chapter 17.

It may seem straightforward to develop new ligands for known enzyme or receptor structures, but there are many difficult problems involved. For instance, conformational changes of the ligand and/or the biomacromolecule may be necessary for an optimal binding. In addition, conformational energies, multiple binding modes and differential solvation effects must be taken into account. However, much progress in this field have been made in recent years and several successful examples of the use of structure-based ligand design in a drug development process have been reported.

Many target receptors of high interest in connection with drug development, e.g. seven trans-membrane (7-TM) neurotransmitter receptors (see Chapter 6), are membrane-bound and all attempts to crystallize and determine the structure of these receptors by X-ray crystallography have so far been unsuccessful. In the absence of an experimentally determined 3D-structure for the receptor, ligand design may be performed by the use of a *pharmacophore model* based on the analysis and comparison of molecular properties and receptor binding data for known receptor ligands. In the present chapter, the development and use of 3D-pharmacophore models will be discussed.

In 3D-pharmacophore studies, the concept of *pharmacophore* is employed in an attempt to deduce the spatial relationships between those parts of the ligand which are essential for its binding to the receptor – the *3D-pharmacophore*. On the basis of this, a comparison of the molecular volumes of active and inactive compounds may additionally give information about the dimensions of the binding cavity. High-affinity ligands are characterized by being capable of assuming a conformation which positions those parts of the ligand which are crucial for the affinity in such a way that they are complementary to the 3D-arrangement of their binding partners (e.g. amino acid residues) in the binding cavity. An additional requirement for high affinity is that the ligand in this bioactive conformation does not display steric repulsions with the receptor.

A well-developed 3D-pharmacophore model, preferentially including information about the dimensions of the receptor binding cavity, may be employed to design new ligands which fit the model and/or to search databases for new compounds which are compatible with the model. It should be noted that a 3D-pharmacophore model in general does not yield quantitative predictions of receptor affinities. The main use of such models is restricted to the prediction of candidate ligands as active or inactive (high or low affinity). Such a classification may be fruitfully used in the selection of new molecules to be synthesized in a drug discovery project. However, 3D-pharmacophore models are starting points for the 3D-QSAR methodology (see Chapter 5) by which quantitative predictions may be made.

The development of a 3D-pharmacophore model and its use for ligand design is necessarily an iterative and multidisciplinary process. The initial model, based on known ligands, is used to design new compounds to test the model and the outcome of receptor binding studies of the new compounds is used to validate, refine (or discard) the model.

4.2   THE PHARMACOPHORE CONCEPT

Nineteenth century organic chemists developing organic dyes introduced the concept of *chromophore* for those parts of a molecule which are responsible for its color. In analogy, Paul Ehrlich in the early 1900s, introduced the term *pharmacophore* to describe those parts of a molecule which are responsible for its biological activity. Pharmacophore and pharmacophore elements are central concepts in medicinal chemistry. The idea behind these concepts comes from the common observation that variations of some parts of the molecular structure of a compound drastically influence the activity at a target receptor, whereas variations of other parts only cause minor activity changes. (In the following, the term receptor is used in a general sense for the biomacromolecular target and no distinction between enzymes and receptors is made).

A *pharmacophore element* is traditionally defined as an atom or a group of atoms (a functional group) common for active compounds with respect to a receptor and essential for the activity of the compounds. However, the concept of pharmacophore element may fruitfully be extended to include representations of interactions of functional groups with receptor sites as discussed in Section 4.4. The pharmacophore is a collection of pharmacophore elements and the concept of *3D-pharmacophore* may be used when the relative spatial positions of the pharmacophore elements are included in the analysis. Thus, a 3D-pharmacophore consists of a specific 3D-arrangement of pharmacophore elements. The pharmacophore concept has been used for a long time in medicinal chemistry in a topological sense (2D), however, the use of computer techniques has enormously facilitated the topographical (3D) use of the concept.

4.3   BASIC PRINCIPLES AND A STEP-BY-STEP PROCEDURE

The basic principles of the development of a 3D-pharmacophore model are illustrated in Figure 4.1. On the basis of conformational analysis of a set of active molecules with pharmacophore elements A, B and C, a conformation of each molecule is selected for which the pharmacophore elements of the molecules overlap in space as shown in the figure. The selected conformations are the putative bioactive conformations of the molecules and the overlapping pharmacophore elements and their spatial positions make up the 3D-pharmacophore. It is useful for the following discussion to separate the 3D-pharmacophore identification process into a number of discrete steps.

Step 1. A set of high-affinity ligands for the target receptor is collected and pharmacophore elements are selected. The molecules in the set should have as diverse structural frameworks as possible. Pharmacophore elements and their representations are discussed in Sections 4.4. In order to facilitate the next step in the process, the conformational analysis, the selected compounds should have as few torsional degrees of freedom as possible. The receptor binding data for the

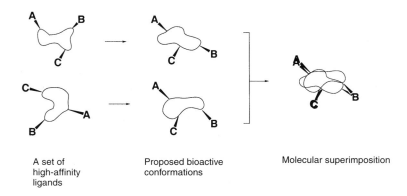

A set of
high-affinity
ligands

Proposed bioactive
conformations

Molecular superimposition

Figure 4.1 The basic principles of 3D-pharmacophore identification.

selected compounds, preferentially obtained by a radioligand binding assay, should be of high quality and preferably from the same laboratory.

Step 2.   An exhaustive conformational analysis is performed for each compound in the set in order to identify low-energy conformations for each active molecule. Conformational properties and conformational analysis are discussed in Section 4.5.

Step 3.   Molecular superimposition techniques are used to identify low-energy conformations of each molecule in the set, conformations for which the selected pharmacophore elements superimpose (see Section 4.6). The aim of this step is to identify the bioactive conformation of each molecule and a common 3D-pharmacophore for all high-affinity compounds.

Step 4.   When a common 3D-pharmacophore for all high-affinity compounds have been identified, inactive or low-affinity compounds which fit the 3D-pharmacophore in a low-energy conformation may be used to explore the dimensions of the receptor cavity and to identify receptor-excluded and receptor-essential volumes. This is discussed in Section 4.7.

In addition, it may be necessary to take differential solvent properties into account in the interpretation of the affinity data and in the design of new compounds. This is discussed in Section 4.8.

4.4   PHARMACOPHORE ELEMENTS AND THEIR REPRESENTATIONS

The selection of pharmacophore elements is generally based on experimental observations about parts (atoms, functional groups) of a set of active molecules which are common for these molecules and essential for the activity. Pharmacophore elements used in the development of 3D-pharmacophore models are most often atoms or functional groups (or derived from atoms or functional groups) which may interact with receptor binding sites via hydrogen bonds, electrostatic forces or van der Waals forces (for a discussion of such interactions see Chapter 2). Thus, heteroatoms such as oxygens and nitrogens and polar functional groups such as carboxylic acids, amides and hydroxy groups are commonly found to be pharmacophore elements. Drug molecules frequently include aromatic ring systems. Since such ring systems may strongly interact with, for instance, aromatic side-chains of the receptor or hydrophobic receptor regions they are very often essential for the activity and therefore selected as pharmacophore elements.

Many potent dopamine D_2 receptor agonists are derived from the structure of dopamine itself (**4.1**). Thus, their structures often include an *ortho*-dihydroxy phenyl (catechol) moiety and a nitrogen atom as exemplified by (**4.2**). However, only the *meta*-hydroxy group is necessary for activity as shown by the active compound (**4.3**). Furthermore, it has been demonstrated that the catechol/phenol moiety may be bioisosterically replaced by, for instance, an indole ring (**4.4**) or a pyrazole ring (**4.5**). Considering these experimental observations, suitable pharmacophore elements for dopamine D_2 receptor agonists may include the

(4.1)   (4.2)   (4.3)

(4.4)   (4.5)

nitrogen atom corresponding to the one in (**4.1**), the aromatic ring and the *meta*-hydroxy group or its bioisosteric equivalent. A closer analysis of the structures suggests that it may be desirable to include the hydrogen bond donating and/or accepting properties of the hydroxy group in the pharmacophore. Similarly, explicit inclusion of the direction of the nitrogen atom-lone pair, or in the protonated case the N–H bond vectors, may extend the usefulness of the pharmacophore. Although, the pharmacophore concept originally was formulated in terms of atoms and functional groups it is often, as will be discussed in the next section, a great advantage to represent the functional group in terms of its possible interactions with the receptor.

4.4.1 Representation of pharmacophore elements as ligand points and site points

If we consider a hydroxy group as a pharmacophore element, the important properties of this functional group in connection with its binding to the receptor are its hydrogen bond donating and accepting properties. The hydroxy group pharmacophore element may be represented in various ways as shown in Figure 4.2.

The representation in Figure 4.2a does not specify any particular properties of the hydroxy group and a pharmacophore built on the selection of such a

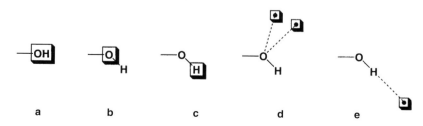

Figure 4.2 Various representations of a hydroxy group as a pharmacophore element.

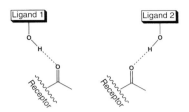

Figure 4.3 A hydroxy group may interact equally well with a carbonyl group in a ligand–receptor interaction without the requirement that the atoms of the hydroxy group in different ligands superimpose.

pharmacophore element merely requires that a hydroxy group is present at a particular location in 3D-space in all active compounds.

In Figures 4.2b,c, the hydrogen bond accepting and donating properties, respectively, are indirectly specified. The use of the oxygen or the hydrogen atom as a pharmacophore element (a *ligand point*) implies that the corresponding atoms should superimpose in space in all active compounds. However, this does not take into account that a hydroxy group of a set of ligands may bind equally well to the receptor, even if the atoms of the functional group in different ligands have different locations in space. For instance, as illustrated in Figure 4.3, the hydroxy group may bond hydrogen equally well to a carbonyl group of a receptor binding site without requiring that the hydroxy hydrogen atom or oxygen atom in all active compounds are located in the same positions in space.

The extension of the pharmacophore concept to include *site points* as shown in Figure 4.2d,e is a great advance in 3D-pharmacophore development. The dashed line between the site point and the ligand functional group represents a hydrogen bond interaction with a receptor site and the site point itself represents the interacting part of the receptor (e.g. an atom in an amino acid residue, see Section 4.4.2). Suitable site-points for some nitrogen and oxygen containing functional groups are shown in Figure 4.4. The site points for amines, ammonium groups and the imidazole group simulate possible hydrogen bonding interactions with

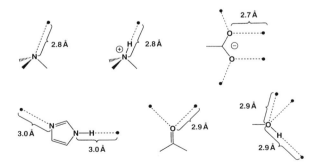

Figure 4.4 Site points for some oxygen and nitrogen containing functional groups.

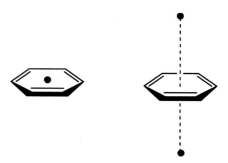

Figure 4.5 Ligand point and site points commonly used to represent a phenyl ring or other aromatic systems.

a receptor site. The site points are placed in the direction of the N–lone pair or N–H bond at typical hydrogen-bonding distances.

Depending on the structures and the structural diversity of the set of molecules to be analyzed, various combinations of site points and ligand points may be used. The use of the site point *and* the nitrogen atom as pharmacophore elements implies that not only the amino group as such is important, but that a specific direction of the interaction between the amine and the receptor is crucial for the activity. If *only* the site point is used and not the nitrogen atom, the implication is that the interaction with the receptor site represented by the site point may take place from different directions with different positions of the nitrogen atom.

An aromatic system such as a phenyl group is often represented by a ligand point positioned at the center of the aromatic ring (Figure 4.5). Specification of all carbon atoms in the ring will give such a ring an unrealistically large weight in a subsequent molecular least-squares superimposition (see Section 4.6). In some applications, it is useful to employ site points for an aromatic system located on the normal passing through the centroid of the aromatic system, above and below the ring plane (Figure 4.5). Such points may represent electrostatic and van der Waals interactions between the aromatic group and amino acid residues in the receptor binding site. They may also be used to enforce co-planarity of aromatic ring systems.

4.4.2   Comparison of site-points with experimentally observed ligand–protein interactions

Figure 4.6a shows the amino acid arginine including site points constructed according to the principles in Figure 4.4. These site points describe possible (optimal) hydrogen bond interactions between arginine and a receptor. The experimental structure of the complex between arginine and the amino acid transport protein LAO (lysine, arginine, ornithine-binding protein) is displayed in Figure 4.6b. On comparing the positions of the site-points in Figure 4.6a with the receptor atoms (including an oxygen of a water molecule) to which arginine is hydrogen bonded in the experimental structure (Figure 4.6b), it is clear that the site-points closely correspond to these hydrogen bonded receptor atoms. Only one out of the

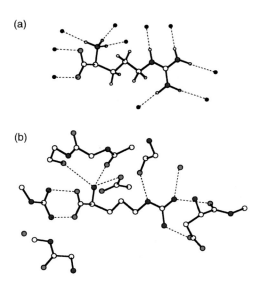

Figure 4.6 (a) The amino acid arginine with site points describing possible optimal hydrogen bonding interactions; and (b) arginine bound to the LAO transport protein.

ten site-points in Figure 4.6a does not correspond to a receptor atom in the experimental structure. (It may, however, correspond to a crystallographically unresolved water oxygen.) Other molecules may now be designed whose site points are able to overlap those of arginine. If this can be accomplished by a low-energy conformation of the designed molecule (see Section 4.5 for a discussion on conformational energies), it is predicted that the new molecule may bind to the protein in the same way as arginine.

4.4.3   Representation of pharmacophore elements by explicit molecular properties

As an alternative to (and extension of) the representations of pharmacophores elements by ligand points or site points, as described above, molecules may be analyzed in terms of ensembles of explicit molecular properties as hydrogen bond donors and acceptors, hydrophobic areas, charged groups etc. A computer-program which analyzes molecules in this way is CATALYST. Predefined properties are hydrogen-bond acceptor, hydrogen-bond donor, hydrophobic (aliphatic or aromatic), negative or positive charge, negatively or positively ionizable, and ring aromatic. In order to allow for variations in the geometry of the interaction between a molecule and its receptor, distance variation as well as angle variation is taken into account in this approach. For instance, a hydrogen bond acceptor is defined by a distance from the atom which accepts a hydrogen bond to the site which donates the hydrogen bond with an allowed variation at both ends. These

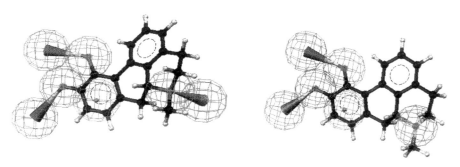

Figure 4.7 Two alternative pharmacophore models generated manually by using the program CATALYST.

allowed variations are defined by spheres and the optimal interaction is defined by the midpoint of the spheres.

CATALYST may be employed to generate a pharmacophore in a manual or in an automatic mode. Examples of *manually* generated pharmacophore models are shown in Figure 4.7. In the manual mode, a compound with a high biological activity in a proposed bioactive conformation is used and the user manually assign properties (pharmacophore elements) to the molecule. In this example, different properties proposed to be important for the dopaminergic activity of apomorphine have been assigned to the functional groups. As apomorphine is a very rigid molecule, the global energy minimum conformation is proposed to be the biological active one. In both alternatives in Figure 4.7, the hydroxyl groups are proposed to be hydrogen-bond donors (magenta colored spheres). In the Figure, it can be seen that there is a tolerance both at the start and end of the hydrogen bond. One of the aromatic rings has been assigned to be an essential hydrophobic group (blue sphere). Two different ways to treat the basic nitrogen are shown. To the left, the nitrogen is shown as a hydrogen bond acceptor (green spheres). To the right, the nitrogen atom is considered to be positively ionizable (red sphere). In order to add further constraints to the pharmacophore model, spheres representing volumes of steric repulsive interactions with the receptor (receptor essential volumes, see Section 4.7) may be added.

In order to generate a pharmacophore model by using CATALYST in an *automatic* mode (for an example, see Section 4.9.4), a set of compounds with measured biological activities is required. In the order of 20 compounds with activities covering 4–6 orders of magnitude is recommended for this approach. For each molecule, a set of conformations representing the available conformational space of the molecule is generated by the software. During the subsequent generation of the pharmacophore model, all conformations and relevant properties of the functional groups are being considered. The automatic procedure includes a QSAR calculation (for a discussion on QSAR, see Chapter 5). The software returns the ten best models in terms of fit of the compounds to the model and the ability of the model to account for the biological activities of the compounds.

Pharmacophore models generated by CATALYST either automatically or manually may be used in searching of large databases for new compounds which fit the model and which may be developed into new drugs (for an example, see Section 4.9.4). It should be noted, that in the databases used for such searching each compound is represented by a number of different conformations. This is necessary as it cannot be known in advance which (if any) conformation of a compound fits the pharmacophore model.

4.5   THE RECEPTOR-BOUND OR 'ACTIVE' CONFORMATION

4.5.1   Thermodynamic considerations

The great majority of drug molecules are flexible, which means that they through rotations about bonds and/or inversions about atomic centers may adopt a large number of conformations, giving the molecule a correspondingly large number of different 3D-shapes. In the context of the pharmacophore concept, this means that a ligand in general may exhibit a large number of possible spatial relationships between its pharmacophore elements. The pharmacophore hypothesis implies that for an active molecule, one of these conformations is optimally complementary to the receptor binding site and that the ligand, when bound to the receptor is characterized by a specific molecular conformation.

The single most important (and certainly most difficult) problem in 3D-pharmacophore identification is the identification of the *receptor-bound (bioactive) conformation*. If this can be accomplished, the spatial relationships of the pharmacophore elements in this conformation defines the 3D-pharmacophore (see Figure 4.1) and new candidate ligands may be tested to investigate if they fit this 3D-pharmacophore. Inactive molecules which fit the 3D-pharmacophore are of special interest since they may contain extra molecular volume which can be used for mapping of the dimensions of the receptor cavity (see Section 4.7).

The ligand–receptor interaction is characterized by the equilibrium (4.1), as illustrated in Figure 4.8.

$$\text{ligand} + \text{receptor} \overset{K}{\rightleftharpoons} \text{ligand–receptor complex} \tag{4.1}$$

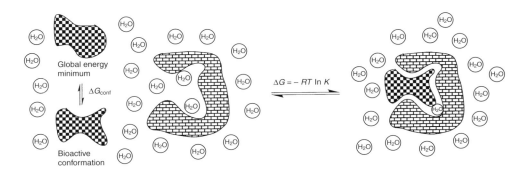

Figure 4.8 The equilibrium characterizing the ligand–receptor interaction.

The free energy difference ΔG is given by equation (4.2) where K is the equilibrium constant, R the gas constant $(8.314\,J\,K^{-1}mol^{-1})$, T the absolute temperature in Kelvin (K_d is the dissociation constant).

$$\Delta G = -RT \ln K, \quad K_d = \frac{1}{K} \tag{4.2}$$

Neglecting for the moment conformational changes of the protein and the difference in solvation energy of the ligand–protein complex and the uncomplexed protein, the overall free energy of binding may be separated into three components as shown in equation (4.3).

$$\Delta G = \Delta G_{inter} + \Delta G_{conf} - \Delta G_{solv} \tag{4.3}$$

ΔG_{conf} is the free energy required for the ligand to adopt the bioactive conformation (the conformational energy penalty), ΔG_{inter} corresponds to the intermolecular interaction of this conformation with the receptor and ΔG_{solv} is the solvation free energy of the unbound ligand (these solvation effects are discussed in Section 4.8). In terms of the pharmacophore concept, ΔG_{inter} is due to binding interactions between the pharmacophore elements and the complementary binding sites of the receptor (e.g. amino acid residues and backbone atoms).

When ΔG_{conf} increases, equation (4.3) shows that ΔG becomes more positive and consequently, the equilibrium in equation (4.1) is shifted to the left, i.e. the affinity of the ligand decreases.

The factor of decrease in affinity (K_{conf}) corresponding to a conformational energy penalty (ΔG_{conf}) for the bioactive conformation may be calculated from equation (4.4) ($T = 310\,K$).

$$\Delta G_{conf} = RT \ln K_{conf} = 5.9 \log K_{conf} \tag{4.4}$$

Thus, if the active conformation has a conformational energy penalty of $5.9\,kJ\,mol^{-1}$ the decrease in the affinity is a factor of 10 due to this 'conformational effect'. For each additional $5.9\,kJ\,mol^{-1}$ of conformational free energy, the affinity decreases by a further factor of 10.

An example of the relationship between conformational energy of the bioactive conformation and the affinity is shown in Figure 4.9. Compound (**4.6**) is a potent dopamine D_2 receptor agonist. The receptor-bound conformations of the related compounds (**4.6**)–(**4.9**) have been deduced by using (**4.9**) as a template and the conformational energies of the bioactive conformations have been calculated by molecular mechanics (see Section 4.5.3.1). These conformations are labeled

(4.6)   (4.7)   (4.8)   (4.9)

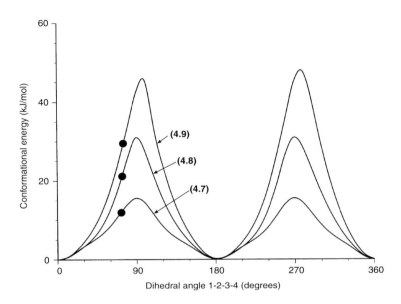

Figure 4.9 Calculated potential energy curves for rotation about the central bond in (**4.7**)–(**4.9**). The bullets denote the deduced bioactive conformations of the compounds.

by bullets in Figure 4.9. The affinities as well as the agonist activities of (**4.7**)–(**4.9**) are significantly lower than that of (**4.6**). Furthermore, the affinities and the agonist activities of (**4.7**)–(**4.9**) are in order (**4.7**)>(**4.8**)>(**4.9**). These data are nicely accounted for by the calculated conformational energies of the bioactive confor- mations of (**4.7**)–(**4.9**) as shown in Figure 4.9. A higher conformational energy corresponds to a lower activity. Note that the deduced bioactive conformations of (**4.7**)–(**4.9**) are not energy minimum conformations.

4.5.2 The conformational energy of the bioactive conformation

As shown above by equations (4.3) and (4.4), the affinity of a ligand decreases when the conformational energy required to adopt the bioactive conformation (the conformational energy penalty) increases. Thus, a question of great practical importance in the development of 3D-pharmacophore models is how much above the global energy minimum we must go to be sure to include the bioactive conformation of a high-affinity ligand. In other words, which energy cut-off should we use in the conformational search for possible candidates for the bioactive conformation of a ligand? The conformational energies reguired for ligands to adopt their bioactive conformations have been calculated for a large number of experimentally determined ligand–protein complexes (Boström *et al.* 1998). It was found that for the great majority of ligand–protein complexes studied, the conformational energies for the bioactive conformations were calculated to be less

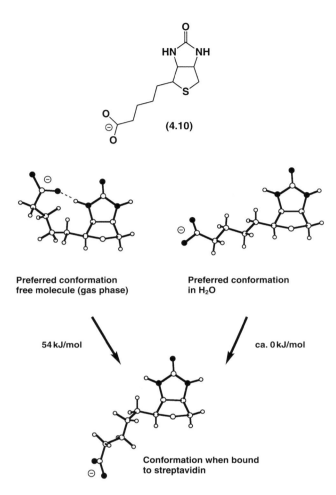

Figure 4.10 Calculated preferred conformations of biotin (**4.10**) in the gas phase and in aqueous solution and the bioactive conformation of (**4.10**) when it binds to streptavidin.

than $13 \, \text{kJ mol}^{-1}$. Thus, the bioactive conformation of a high-affinity ligand most probably has a low conformational energy penalty ($\leq 13 \, \text{kJ mol}^{-1}$). It is important to note, that the conformational energy for the bioactive conformation must be calculated with reference to the internal energy of the ligand in *aqueous solution* (i.e. the energy of the ligand in aqueous solution excluding the solvation energy) (Boström *et al.* 1998). A conformational search performed for the 'free' ligand *in vacuo* may result in an unrealistically high calculated conformational energy for the bioactive conformation. An example of this is illustrated in Figure 4.10. Biotin (**4.10**) binds with very high affinity to the enzyme streptavidin. The experimentally observed bioactive conformation is shown in the figure. A conformational search *in vacuo* results in a preferred conformation with a strong hydrogen bond between the carboxylate group and the NH of the ureido group. The energy difference between the bioactive conformation and this global energy minimum conformation of the 'free' ligand is calculated to be very high, $54 \, \text{kJ} \, \text{mol}^{-1}$. Considering equation (4.4), such a high conformational energy penalty is clearly not compatible with the high affinity of (**4.10**). However, the global energy minimum conformation of (**4.10**) in aqueous solution (Figure 4.10) is similar to the observed bioactive conformation. In particular, the strong hydrogen bond displayed by the preferred conformation in gas phase is not present in the preferred conformation in aqueous phase. The internal energy difference between the bioactive conformation and the preferred conformation in aqueous solution is calculated to be essentially zero as expected from the high affinity of (**4.10**).

4.5.3 Conformational analysis

The bioactive conformation is not necessarily the lowest energy conformation of the molecule in solution, in the crystal or in the gas phase. (It may not even correspond to an energy minimum structure in any of these phases as shown by the example in the Section 4.5.2). Thus, experimental data on structures and conformational equilibria alone are of limited use in attempts to identify the bioactive conformation. A computational approach is required and the entire conformational space must be investigated.

There are two groups of methods which may be used for the calculation of conformational properties of molecules: (i) quantum chemical methods; and (ii) molecular mechanics or force field methods. In the quantum chemical methods (an approximation of) the Schrödinger equation is solved, treating the molecule as a collection of positively charged nuclei and negatively charged electrons moving under the influence of Coulombic potentials.

A hierarchy of quantum chemical methods at different levels of approximation are being used in computational chemistry. In the *ab initio* methods, all electrons are included in the calculations, whereas in the *semi-empirical methods* only the outer (valence) electrons are explicitly included in the calculations and many terms are not calculated but fitted to experimental data. Although several of these methods are being increasingly used in connection with problems in medicinal chemistry, the levels of theory necessary to yield reliable results are at the present time in general much too time-consuming to be of practical use for the extensive search of conformational space which is needed in connection with 3D-pharmacophore identification. These methods will thus not be considered here.

The other group of computational methods, molecular mechanics or force field methods, are well suited for extensive calculations on conformational properties of molecules of interest in medicinal chemistry and may also be used for calculations on biomacromolecules.

4.5.3.1 Molecular mechanics (force field) calculations

Molecular mechanics is a method for the calculation of molecular structures, conformational energies and other molecular properties using concepts from classical mechanics. A molecule is considered as a collection of atoms held together by classical forces. These forces are described by potential energy functions of structural features like bond lengths, bond angles, torsional (dihedral) angles, etc.

The energy (E) of the molecule is calculated as a sum of terms as in equation (4.5).

$$E = E_{\text{stretching}} + E_{\text{bending}} + E_{\text{torsion}} + E_{\text{van der Waals}} + E_{\text{electrostatic}}$$
$$+ E_{\text{hydrogen bond}} + \text{cross terms} \qquad (4.5)$$

The first four terms in the sum are the energies due to deviations of bond lengths, bond angles, torsional angles and non-bonded distances, respectively, from their reference or 'ideal' values. $E_{\text{electrostatic}}$ gives the electrostatic attraction or repulsion between bond dipoles or partial atomic charges. Although a large part of the hydrogen bonding is included in the electrostatic energy component, many molecular mechanics methods include an additional hydrogen bonding term ($E_{\text{hydrogen bond}}$) to fine-tune the energies and geometries of a hydrogen bond interaction. More advanced force fields include cross terms such as stretch–bend, bend–bend, torsion–stretch etc. These terms are of importance for the accurate calculation of geometric properties of small rings (stretch–bend term) or for the calculation of vibrational frequencies (bend–bend term).

The energies are calculated using analytical potential energy functions similar to those used in classical mechanics. For a more comprehensive discussion on molecular mechanics see Burkert and Allinger (1982) in Further reading.

The molecular mechanics method calculates the energy as a function of the nuclear co-ordinates and energy minimization is an integral part of the method. A trial molecular geometry is constructed, most often by using computer graphics techniques, and the atoms are iteratively moved (without breaking bonds) using an energy minimization technique until the net forces on all atoms vanish and the total energy of the molecule reaches a minimum. The 3D-structure of the molecule corresponding to this energy minimum is one of the stable conformations of the molecule but *not necessarily* the most stable one (Figure 4.11). Since the energy minimization methods cannot move the molecule across energy barriers, the minimization of a trial molecule continues until the first *local energy minimum* is

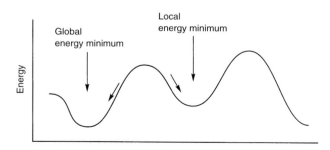

Figure 4.11 Energy minimization proceeds downhill to the nearest energy minimum.

found. Other local energy minima including the lowest energy one (the *global energy minimum*) may be found by repeating the calculation with another start geometry or more efficiently by the use of a conformational search method (see Section 4.5.3.2).

In general, the calculated results from a molecular mechanics calculation refer to the isolated molecule (*in vacuo*). However, the importance of including solvation in the conformational analysis was stressed in Section 4.5.2. Several methods are currently available by which solvent effects may be included in the calculation. In the present context, the most useful of these methods are the dielectric continuum methods (Cramer and Truhlar 1999).

4.5.3.2 *Conformational search methods*

As described in Section 4.5.3.1, the energy minimization procedure moves the molecule from the initial (trial) geometry to the *closest* local energy minimum. Many methods for conformational search have been devised but only the major ones, systematic search in torsional space and the random search methods, are described here. If well implemented, both methods are of similar efficiency and may be feasible for up to 10–15 rotatable bonds with current computer resources.

The systematic conformational search methodology is in principle simple and straightforward. New structures are generated using all combinations of torsional angle values at a preset resolution (angle increment) which gives a uniform grid search in torsional space. In the one-dimensional (one rotatable bond) or 2D (two rotatable bonds) cases, so-called *torsional driving* is feasible. Each torsional angle is incremented by a user defined value and the dihedral value is then kept fixed while the molecule is energy-minimized with respect to all other degrees of freedom. The result of a calculation using torsional driving is a potential energy curve or a potential energy (conformational) map which displays not only energy minima but also energy barriers and pathways for conformational interconversions. This type of calculations is very time consuming and is therefore seldom used for problems involving more than two rotatable bonds. Examples of potential energy curves calculated by the torsional driving method are shown in Figure 4.9 and in Section 4.9.2.

For three and more rotatable bonds, conformational search methods in general focus on finding energy minima. In random conformational search methods, random numbers are used to determine how many and which torsional angles to be incremented and by how much. A trial conformation generated in this way by the computer program is then energy minimized and the resulting conformation is compared with those already stored. If it is a new conformation, it is added to the storage. The procedure is repeated a large number of times and the completeness of the search may be estimated by how many times each stored conformation have been found. An advantage of this methodology is that it can be halted at any time and restarted and the results from repeated runs may be combined. For a thorough discussion on conformational search methods see Further reading (Leach 1991).

4.6   MOLECULAR SUPERIMPOSITION

4.6.1   Least-squares superimposition, flexible fitting and template forcing

A 3D-pharmacophore model is characterized by a particular 3D-arrangement of pharmacophore elements. Active (high affinity) ligands are able to assume a low-energy conformation in which the pharmacophore elements are positioned at closely similar relative positions in space as those of the 3D-pharmacophore model. During the development of a pharmacophore model, molecular super-imposition techniques are used to investigate similarities and differences between the accessible conformations of different molecules with respect to the spatial positions of their pharmacophore elements. When a 3D-pharmacophore model has been developed, molecular superimpositions are used to investigate if new molecules fit the model.

The most commonly used molecular superimposition method is the rigid-body *least-squares superimposition* of pharmacophore elements represented as ligand points or site points. The root mean square deviation (rms) between selected points in the test molecule and the corresponding points in the reference molecule is minimized by displacing and rotating the test molecule as a rigid body. The rms value of the resulting least-squares fit is given by equation (4.6).

$$\text{rms} = \sqrt{\left(\frac{\sum_{i=1}^{N} R_i^2}{N}\right)} \tag{4.6}$$

R_i in equation (4.6) is the distance between the ith pair of ligand or site points and N is the number of such pairs. The rms value is zero (Å) for a perfect fit and increases as the fit is decreased. For examples of superimpositions see Section 4.9.2.

It may not always be possible to obtain an optimal fit between two molecules in local energy conformations. Deviations of torsional angles from the values for a stable conformation of the molecule may be necessary for a good fit. Molecular superimposition algorithms often include possibilities to perform *flexible fitting* by automatic variations of the torsional angles of user defined rotatable bonds until an optimal fit between fitting points (pharmacophore elements) are found.

An alternative to the least-squares superimposition method is to connect the fitting points to be superimposed by an isotropic spring, which by the use of an energy minimization procedure forces the test molecule to be fitted to the reference molecule ('template forcing').

Molecular superimposition techniques have been developed in which molecular properties and fields are being fitted instead of ligand points and site points. The most interesting of these methods are based on the fact that in addition to shape complementarity, electronic complementarity is important for molecular recognition. That is, positively and negatively charged parts of the molecular surface should interact with oppositely charged parts in the receptor binding cavity. Thus, methods have been devised to identify a common charge pattern or even better a common pattern of electrostatic potentials on or just outside the molecular surface of low-energy conformations of a set of high-affinity ligands. (The electrostatic potential is the potential energy between a unitary positive charge placed at a position in space and the molecular charge distribution.)

4.6.2 The use of molecular superimposition techniques

The ultimate use of a 3D-pharmacophore model is for the design of new ligands. Molecular superimposition techniques are then indispensable tools for testing if newly designed ligands fit the model in low-energy conformations. Molecular superimpositions and their use are exemplified in Section 4.9.2. However, an equally important use of molecular superimposition techniques is to investigate if inactive (low affinity) compounds fit the model. If such a compound does not fit the model in any conformation, the obvious rationalization of its low affinity is its inability to present the pharmacophore elements in a correct way (see Section 4.3). If the compound fits the model but in a high-energy conformation, the equally straightforward rationalization of its lack of affinity is that the energy penalty for binding to the receptor is too high (see Section 4.5). However, if the inactive compound fits the model in a low-energy conformation, there are three possibilities to rationalize its inactivity: (i) the compound is too voluminous in some direction(s) causing steric repulsive interactions with the receptor (see Section 4.7); (ii) the compound has a very unfavorable free energy of solvation (see Section 4.8); or (iii) the electronic properties of the ligand are not complementary to the receptor binding site (see Section 4.6.1). If none of the cases is probable, the 3D-pharmacophore model is seriously in doubt and should be reconsidered. Thus, molecular superimposition studies may corroborate or discard a 3D-pharmacophore model. Testing of the 3D-pharmacophore model with all available high- and low-affinity ligands should be done before design of new molecules based on the model is attempted.

4.7 RECEPTOR-EXCLUDED AND RECEPTOR-ESSENTIAL VOLUMES

The volume of a molecule may be computed and graphically displayed in terms of the sum of atomic van der Waals radii. For a superimposed set of high-affinity ligands for the target receptor, the *combined volume* may be calculated as the union of the volumes for all the molecules in the set (Figure 4.12). This volume should be readily accomodated by the receptor and the combined volume gives an estimate of the lower bound of the receptor volume available for binding of ligands (the *receptor-excluded volume*). The volume occupied by the receptor is called the *receptor-essential volume* and is not available for ligand binding (Figure 4.12). The analysis of molecular volumes on the basis of a 3D-pharmacophore model may give valuable information about the dimensions of the receptor cavity. An inactive or low-affinity compound which fits the 3D-pharmacophore model in a low-energy conformation may have a van der Waals volume larger than the combined volume of

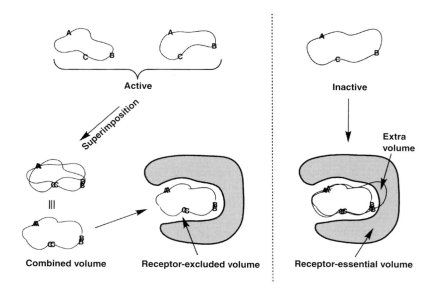

Figure 4.12 The *combined volume* gives an estimate of the lower-bound of receptor volume available for ligand binding (*receptor-excluded volume*). Inactive compounds may have an *extra volume* which overlaps the *receptor-essential volume* and thus causes steric repulsive interactions between the ligand and the receptor.

the high-affinity set of molecules (*extra volume*). For a valid 3D-pharmacophore model, the extra volume of the inactive compound indicates positions in space, where the ligand volume is in conflict with the receptor-essential volume (Figure 4.12). This information is extremely valuable in connection with design of new ligands based on a 3D-pharmacophore model as it provides knowledge about volumes in space where ligand fragments should not be present.

The potent GABA$_A$ receptor agonist muscimol ((**4.11**), Figure 4.13) displays an affinity for the GABA$_A$ receptor of 6 nM (IC$_{50}$, ^{3}H[GABA]). The affinity of the 4-methyl analog (**4.12**) is drastically lower, 26 000 nM. An analysis of the molecular properties of (**4.11**) and (**4.12**) strongly indicates that the large decrease in the affinity of (**4.12**) compared to (**4.11**) is solely due to steric repulsive interactions between the methyl group in (**4.12**) and the receptor. In the superimposition of (**4.11**) and (**4.12**) in their deduced bioactive conformations shown in Figure 4.13, the 'extra volume' of the methyl group is displayed. Thus, in the design of new ligands for the GABA$_A$ receptor, care should be taken so that no parts of the ligands occupy this 'disallowed' volume in space.

4.8 SOLVATION EFFECTS

In Section 4.5.2, it was demonstrated that the conformational properties of a molecule may be strongly influenced by the solvent and that it is important to take

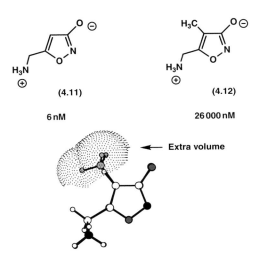

Figure 4.13 A superimposition of muscimol (**4.11**) and 4-methyl muscimol (**4.12**) illustrating the extra volume due to the 4-methyl group in (**4.12**).

solvation effects into account in the calculation of the conformational energy penalty of a bioactive conformation. In addition to its influence on the conformational properties, the aqueous environment in terms of the free energies of solvation (hydration) of the molecular species involved in the equilibrium in equation (4.1) and Figure 4.8 must also be taken into account. A larger stabilization of the ligand by the aqueous environment (i.e. a more negative free energy of hydration), shifts the equilibrium in Figure 4.8 to the left and the affinity for the receptor becomes lower.

As an example of this effect of the solvent, compound (**4.13**) binds to the enzyme thermolysin with a K_i-value of 9.1 nM. X-ray crystallography of the ligand–enzyme complex shows that the NH group indicated by an arrow interacts with a carbonyl oxygen of the enzyme binding site via a hydrogen bond. However, compound (**4.14**) binds equally well to the enzyme ($K_i = 10.6$ nM) in spite of the fact that the CH_2 group in (**4.14**), replacing the NH group in (**4.13**), cannot form a hydrogen bond to the enzyme. Computer simulations of the ligand–protein equilibrium show that (**4.14**) interacts less well with the enzyme than (**4.13**) by 10 kJ mol^{-1} ($\Delta\Delta G_{inter}$ in equation 4.3, Section 4.5.1). However, (**4.14**) is less well stabilized by the solvent than (**4.13**) by $11\,kJ\,mol^{-1}$ ($\Delta\Delta G_{solv}$). The net effect is that $\Delta\Delta G$ is close to zero and that (**4.13**) and (**4.14**) have essentially the same affinities for the enzyme (Merz Jr. and Kollman 1989).

In the development of 3D-pharmacophore models and in the design of new ligands based on such models, the free energies of hydration of the ligand must be taken into account. This may be done by only including compounds with similar free energies of solvation in the set on which the model is built. Otherwise such effects must be qualitatively estimated or explicitly calculated.

4.9   EXAMPLES OF 3D-PHARMACOPHORE MODELS AND THEIR USE

In this section, examples of development of 3D-pharmacophore models and their use are discussed. In addition to these examples, it should be noted that Chapter 11 includes a discussion on a pharmacophore model for the serotonin transporter.

4.9.1   Apomorphine congeners: conformational energies vs. agonist activities

An often used strategy in the structural elaboration of a lead compound is a simplification of the lead structure by ring-cleavage and/or deletion of rings. Compounds (**4.16**)–(**4.25**) are examples of such compounds, derived from the structure of the potent dopamine D_2 receptor agonist apomorphine (**4.15**).

Figure 4.14 displays a simple 3D-pharmacophore model for dopamine D_2 receptor agonists of the catechol type, based on three ligand points and a site point. Topologically (2D), compounds (**4.16**)–(**4.25**) all may display the same relative positions of the pharmacophore elements as (**4.15**). However, when

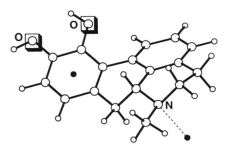

Figure 4.14 A 3D-pharmacophore model for dopamine D_2 agonists of the catechol type. The oxygen atoms, the center of the catechol ring and a site point 2.8 Å from the nitrogen atom in the direction of the nitrogen lone electron pair are selected as pharmacophore elements.

(**4.16**)–(**4.25**) are subjected to conformational analysis by molecular mechanics, it is found that most of the compounds require high conformational energies to fit the 3D-pharmacophore defined in Figure 4.14 (Pettersson and Liljefors 1987). Figure 4.15 displays the relationship between calculated conformational energies for the bioactive conformations of (**4.16**)–(**4.25**) and their obeserved agonist activities. The highly active compounds (**4.18**) and (**4.24**) have conformational energies of less

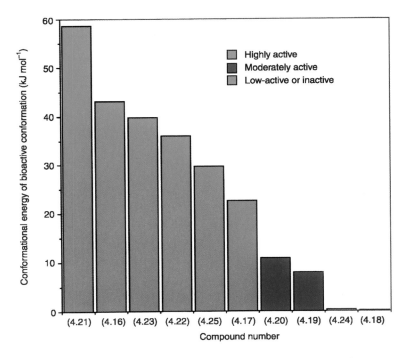

Figure 4.15 Calculated conformational energies of the deduced active conformations of compounds (**4.16**)–(**4.25**) vs. their dopamine receptor agonist activities.

than $2\,kJ\,mol^{-1}$, whereas the moderately active compounds (**4.20**) and (**4.19**) display conformational energies of 8 and $11\,kJ\,mol^{-1}$ respectively. All low active or inactive compounds have conformational energies in excess of $20\,kJ\,mol^{-1}$. This clearly demonstrates that conformational energies must be taken into account in the design of new ligands from a template structure.

4.9.2   A 3D-pharmacophore model for dopamine D_2 receptor antagonists

$(1R, 3S)$-Tefludazine (**4.26**) and (S)-octoclothepin (S)-(**4.27**) are high-affinity dopamine D_2 receptor antagonists (Figure 4.16). On the basis of these compounds, a 3D-pharmacophore for D_2 receptor antagonists has been developed (Liljefors and Bøgesø 1988). The pharmacophore elements chosen are the centers of the aromatic rings, the nitrogen atoms encircled in Figure 4.16, and a site point in each molecule, $2.8\,\text{Å}$ from the nitrogen atom in the direction of the nitrogen lone pair (Figure 4.16).

Based on exhaustive conformational analysis of the two compounds by molecular mechanics and molecular least-squares superimposition studies, the superimposition shown in Figure 4.17 was obtained (rms $= 0.23\,\text{Å}$). A closer inspection of this superimposition reveals that a simultaneous rotation in (**4.26**) and (S)-(**4.27**) about the C–N bond connecting the piperazine ring to the tricyclic ringsystem, preserves the excellent superimposition of the pharmacophore elements. However, such a simultaneous rotation generates an infinite number of possible 3D-pharmacophore candidates. It will be demonstrated below that calculated conformational energies may be used to select among these candidates.

Figure 4.18 displays calculated potential energy curves for different orientations of the piperazine rings in (**4.26**) and (S)-(**4.27**). The two curves are slightly displaced so that the pair of dihedral angles giving an optimal fit of the pharmacophore elements are placed directly above each other. The superimposition shown in Figure 4.17 corresponds to dihedral angles of $290°$ for (S)-(**4.27**) and $300°$ for (**4.26**).

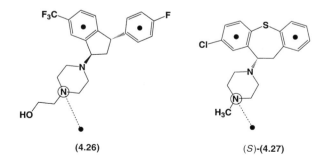

(4.26)   (S)-(4.27)

Figure 4.16 Pharmacophore elements used in the development of a 3D-pharmacophore model for dopamine D_2 receptor antagonists.

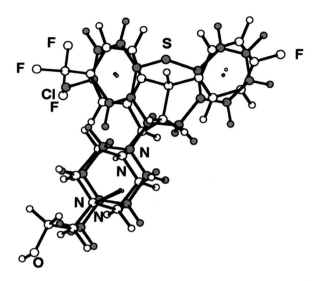

Figure 4.17 A least-squares molecular superimposition of compounds (**4.26**) (unfilled atoms) and (*S*)-(**4.27**) (green atoms). Note that the trifluoromethly group in (**4.26**) and the chloro substituent in (*S*)-(**4.27**) (the 'neuroleptic substituents') are very similarily positioned in space.

The potential energy curve for (**4.26**) displays several low-energy regions corresponding to possible receptor-bound conformations. However, the potential energy curve for (*S*)-(**4.27**) displays only a few such regions – only a small region with dihedral angles in the range of 260–315°, lies below $13\,\mathrm{kJ\,mol}^{-1}$ (see Section 4.5.2). Since the corresponding region in the potential energy curve of (**4.26**) (270–325°) has conformational energies well below $10\,\mathrm{kJ\,mol}^{-1}$, the receptor-bound conformations for (**4.26**) and (*S*)-(**4.27**) are most probably to be found for dihedral angles in these regions. The conformations for (**4.26**) and (*S*)-(**4.27**) displayed in the superimposition in Figure 4.17 correspond to the lowest-energy conformations in these regions.

The enantiomers of (**4.27**) may be used to test the proposed receptor-bound conformation for (*S*)-(**4.27**) (Bøgesø *et al.* 1991). The conformational properties of (*S*)- and (*R*)-(**4.27**) are such that it is possible to find a conformation for (*R*)-(**4.27**) for which the pharmacophore elements superimpose extremely well with those of the proposed receptor-bound conformation of (*S*)-(**4.27**). This superimposition is shown in Figure 4.19. Note that in the superimposition, the two enantiomers have different conformations of their tricyclic ring systems.

The very high degree of similarity displayed by the two enantiomers in their proposed bioactive conformations (Figure 4.19) implies that energy contributions due to intermolecular interactions with receptor sites should be essentially the same for the enantiomers. $\Delta\Delta G$ should consequently be determined by the difference in conformational energies of the conformations shown in Figure 4.19, as discussed in Section 4.5.1. Experimentally, (*S*)-(**4.27**) binds stronger to the receptor than

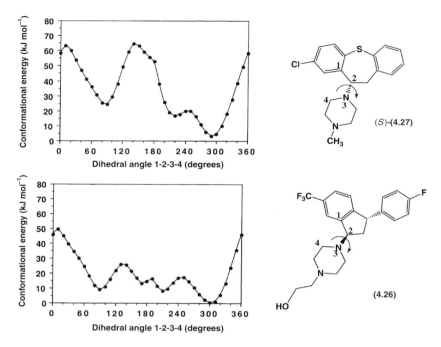

Figure 4.18 Potential energy curves calculated using molecular mechanics for the rotation about the C2–N3 bond in (**4.26**) and (*S*)-(**4.27**). Note that the global energy conformation for (*S*)-(**4.27**), (corresponding to a conformational energy of 0.0 kJ mol^{-1}) is not included in the potential energy curve. The global energy conformation has another conformation of the tricyclic ring system.

(*R*)-(**4.27**) by 4.2 kJ mol^{-1}. The conformational energy difference calculated by molecular mechanics is 5.8 kJ mol^{-1} in favor of (*S*)-(**4.27**). Since energy contributions due to desolvation, hydrophobicity, loss of entropy etc. are identical for enantiomers, the calculated energy may be directly compared with the experimental one. The very good agreement between calculated and experimental results strongly supports the proposed receptor-bound conformation for (*S*)-(**4.27**) (and thus for (**4.26**)). This analysis demonstrates that enantiomers having such conformational properties that pharmacophore elements are able to superimpose may be valuable tools in 3D-pharmacophore identification and validation.

A representation of the 3D-pharmacophore in terms of disconnected fragments derived from the superimposition in Figure 4.17 is shown in Figure 4.20.

4.9.3 3D-pharmacophore models for the design of selective 5-HT$_{2A}$ vs. D$_2$ receptor antagonists

On the basis of analyses of a large number of dopamine D$_2$ receptor antagonists and their receptor affinities, the basic pharmacophore model displayed in Figure 4.20 was extended to include further pharmacophore elements and, most importantly, receptor essential volumes (sterically disallowed regions). The final

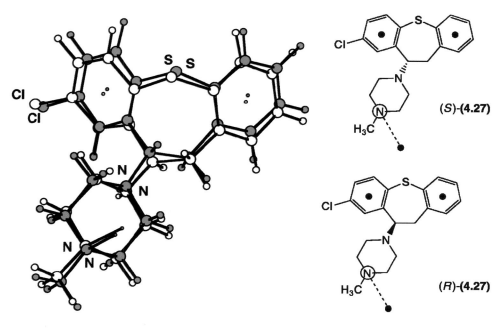

Figure 4.19 A molecular least-squares superimposition (rms = 0.28 Å) of (*S*)-(**4.27**) (green atoms) and (*R*)-(**4.27**) (unfilled atoms). The pharmacophore elements used in the superimposition are included in the structural formulas.

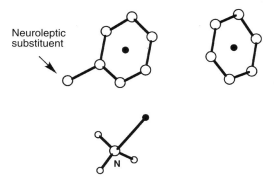

Figure 4.20 A representation of the basic 3D-pharmacophore model for dopamine D_2 receptor antagonists. The position of the 'neuroleptic substituent' which generally increases the affinity of the molecule for the dopamine D_2 receptor is included in the model.

model is displayed in Figure 4.21 (upper left part). The receptor essential volumes were identified by analyses of compounds with low affinity for the D_2 receptor as described in Section 4.7 and are represented by tetrahedrons in Figure 4.21. In order to study if differences in pharmacophoric features may be employed for the design of compounds selective for the serotonin 5-HT$_{2A}$ receptor with respect to

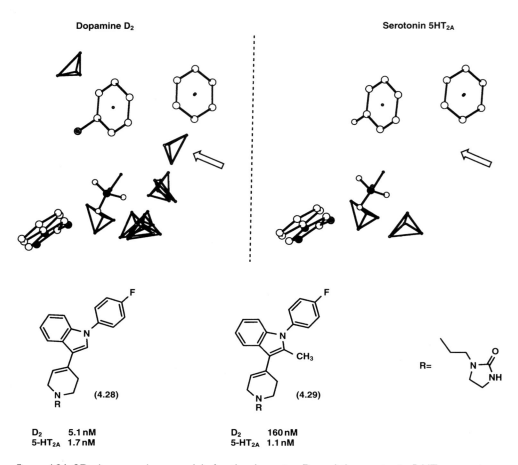

Figure 4.21 3D-pharmacophore models for the dopamine D_2 and the serotonin 5-HT$_{2A}$ receptors. The tetrahedrons represent receptor essential volumes. The arrow points at one of the differences between the pharmacophore models. The effect of the indicated pharmacophore difference is illustrated for compounds (**4.28**) and (**4.29**). The D_2 and 5-HT$_{2A}$ affinity data are IC$_{50}$-values obtained by using [^{3}H]-spiroperidol and [^{3}H]-ketanserin, respectively, as radioligands.

the D_2 receptor, a 3D-pharmacophore model for 5-HT$_{2A}$ receptor antagonists was developed using the same methodology as described in Section 4.9.2 for D_2 receptor antagonists (Andersen *et al.* 1994). The final 3D-pharmacophore model for 5-HT$_{2A}$ antagonists is displayed in Figure 4.21 (upper right part). The two models are in many respects very similar. However, on comparing the receptor essential volumes in the two models, it is clear that the D_2 receptor causes steric repulsions between ligands and the receptor in a significantly larger number of volumes in space than the 5-HT$_{2A}$ receptor. One important difference is indicated by an arrow in Figure 4.21.

Compound (**4.28**) is a high affinity but essentially non-selective D_2 and 5-HT_{2A} receptor antagonist (Figure 4.21). This compound fits very well to both pharmacophore models in a low-energy conformation and there are no conflicts between (**4.28**) and the receptor essential volumes in either of the models. These findings are compatible with the high afffinity and non-selectivity of (**4.28**) .

Compound (**4.29**) can also be fitted to the two pharmacophore models in a low-energy conformation. However, the methyl group in (**4.29**) is in strong conflict with the sterically disallowed region indicated by an arrow in the D_2 pharmacophore model. This is reflected by its decreased affinity for the D_2 receptor (Figure 4.21). In contrast, the methyl group in (**4.29**) as may be predicted from the pharmacophore model does not have any effect on the affinity for the 5-HT_{2A} receptor. As a result, compound (**4.29**) displays selectivity for the 5-HT_{2A} receptor with respect to the D_2 receptor (by a factor of 145).

This example illustrates the importance of receptor essential volumes in the context of 3D-pharmacophore models and their usefulness for the design of new ligands. For further discussions on dopamine and serotonin receptor ligands, see Chapter 11.

4.9.4 A pharmacophore based database searching for new antimalarial drugs

Artemisinin (**4.30**), a naturally occurring compound isolated from the chinese plant *Artemisia annua* displays potent antimalarial activity. Since (**4.30**) is a quite complex molecule, structurally simpler 1,2,4-trioxanes have been synthesized and tested for antimalarial activity. Five structural classes of such analogs (**4.31**)–(**4.35**) have been used to develop a pharmacophore model for antimalarial activity with the aim of using the pharmacophore model for database searching for leads which may be developed into new antimalarial drugs (Grigorov *et al.* 1997).

On the basis of 23 compounds from the five structural classes of 1,2,4-trioxanes, pharmacophore models were developed by using the automatic pharmacophore generation capabilities of the CATALYST software (see Section 4.4.3). By using *in vitro* as well as *in vivo* data, two pharmacophore models corresponding to the

(4.30) (4.31) (4.32)

(4.33) (4.34) (4.35)

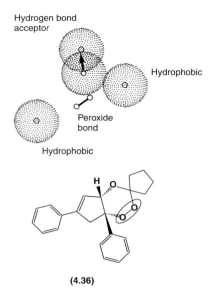

(4.36)

Figure 4.22 A schematic illustration of a CATALYST pharmacophore model used as a query for database searching.

(4.37)   **(4.38)   R=H**
                    (4.39)   R=OOH

two series of biological data were developed. The two models turned out to be very similar. A schematic illustration of the resulting *in vivo* pharmacophore model is shown in Figure 4.22. The model is made up by two hydrophobic pharmacophore elements corresponding to one of the phenyl groups and the cyclopentane ring system in (**4.36**), a representative of the compounds in the structural class (**4.34**). In addition, a hydrogen bond acceptor is included corresponding to the hydrogen accepting properties of the ether oxygen in (**4.36**). Finally, a peroxide moiety in an appropriate position was added to the pharmacophore model as this moiety is crucial for the antimalarial activity.

The pharmacophore was then used for searching the NCI (National Cancer Institute) database transferred by the CATALYST software into a multiconformational database (version 4.6 of the NCI database contains 98868 compounds). The database search resulted in four hits. Artemisinin (**4.30**) was one of the hits, the other three were (**4.37**)–(**4.39**). By using the QSAR capabilites of the

CATALYST software to estimate the activities of these compounds, compounds (**4.38**) and (**4.39**) were both predicted to be less active than artemisinin (**4.30**) by a factor of more than one hundred. However, compound (**4.37**) was predicted to have an antimalarial activity only ca. ten times lower than that of artemisinin which makes it an interesting lead for the development of new antimalarial drugs.

REFERENCES

Andersen, K., Liljefors, T., Gundertofte, K., Perregaard, J. and Bøgesø, K.P. (1994) Development of a receptor-interaction model for serotonin 5-HT$_2$ receptor antagonists. Prediction of selectivity with respect to dopamine D$_2$ receptors. *J. Med. Chem.*, **37**, 950–962.

Bøgesø, K.P., Liljefors, T., Arnt, J., Hyttel, J. and Pedersen, H. (1991) Octoclothepin Enantiomers. A reinvestigation of their biochemical and pharmacological activity in relation to a new model for dopamine D-2 receptor antagonists. *J. Med. Chem.*, **34**, 2023.

Grigorov, M., Weber, J., Tronchet, J.M.J., Jefford, C.W., Milhous, W.K. and Maric, D. (1997) A QSAR study of the antimalarial activity of some synthetic 1,2,4-trioxanes. *J. Chem. Inf. Comput. Sci.*, **37**, 124–130.

Liljefors, T. and Bøgesø, K.P. (1988) Conformational analysis and structural comparisons of 1R,3S-(+)-, 1S,3R-(−)-tefludazine, S-(+)-octoclothepin and (+)-dexclamol in relation to dopamine receptor antagonism and amine-uptake inhibition. *J. Med. Chem.*, **31**, 306–312.

Pettersson, I. and Liljefors, T. (1987) Structure–activity relationships for apomorphine congeners. Conformational energies vs. biological activities. *J. Computer-Aided Mol. Design*, **1**, 143–152.

FURTHER READING

Boström, J., Norrby, P.-O. and Liljefors, T. (1998) Conformational energy penalties of protein-bound ligands. *J. Computer-Aided Mol. Design*, **12**, 383–396.

Burkert, U. and Allinger, N. L. (1982) *Molecular Mechanics, ACS Monograph 177*. Washington D.C.: American Chemical Society.

Cramer, C.J. and Truhlar, D.G. (1995) Continuum solvation models: classical and quantum mechanics implementations. In *Reviews in Computational Chemistry*, Vol. 6, edited by K.B. Lipkowitz and D.B. Boyd, pp. 1–72. New York: VCH Publishers.

Cramer, C.J. and Truhlar, D.G. (1999) Implicit solvation models: equilibria, structure, spectra and dynamics. *Chem. Rev.*, **99**, 2161–2200.

Golender, V.E. and Vorpagel, E.R. (1993) Computer-assisted pharmacophore identification. In *3D QSAR in Drug Design. Theory Methods and Applications*, edited by H. Kubinyi, pp. 137–149. Leiden: Escom Science Publishers.

Güner, O.F. (ed.) (2000) *Pharmacophore Perception, Development, and Use in Drug Design*. La Jolla: International University Line.

Leach, A.R. (1991) A survey of methods for searching the conformational space of small and medium-sized molecules. In *Reviews in Computational Chemistry*, Vol. 2, edited by K.B. Lipkowitz and D.B. Boyd, pp. 1–55. New York: VCH Publishers.

Marshall, G.R. (1993) Binding site modeling of unknown receptors. In *3D QSAR in Drug Design. Theory, Methods and Applications*, edited by H. Kubinyi, pp. 80–116. Leiden: Escom Science Publishers.

Merz Jr., K.M. and Kollman, P.A. (1989) Free energy perturbation simulations of the inhibition of thermolysin. Prediction of the Free Energy of Binding of a New Inhibitor. *J. Med. Chem.*, **111**, 5649–5658.

Ripka, W.C. and Blaney J.M. (1991) Computer graphics and molecular modeling in the analysis of synthetic targets. In *Topics in Stereochemistry*, Vol. 20, edited by E.L. Eliel and S.H. Wilen, pp. 1–85. New York: J. Wiley & Sons.

Siebel, G.L. and Kollman, P.A. (1990) Molecular mechanics and the modeling of drug structures. In *Comprehensive Medicinal Chemistry*, Vol. 4, edited by C. Hansch, P.G. Sammes, J.B. Taylor and C.A. Ramsden, pp. 125–138. Oxford: Pergamon Press.

Sprague, P.W. and Hoffmann, R. (1997) CATALYST pharmacophore models and their utility as queries for searching 3D databases. In *Computer-Assisted Lead Finding and Optimization. Current Tools for Medicinal Chemistry*, edited by H. van der Waterbeemd, B. Testa and G. Folkers, pp. 225–240. Basel: Verlag Helvetica Chimica Acta.

Still, W.C., Tempczyk, A., Hawley, R.C. and Hendrickson, T. (1990) Semianalytical treatment of solvation for molecular mechanics and dynamics. *J. Amer. Chem. Soc.*, **112**, 6127–6129.

Wermuth, C.-G. and Langer, T. (1993) Pharmacophore identification. In *3D QSAR in Drug Design. Theory Methods and Applications*, edited by H. Kubinyi, pp. 117–136. Leiden: Escom Science Publishers.

Chapter 5

Quantitative structure–activity relationships and experimental design

Ulf Norinder and Thomas Högberg

5.1 INTRODUCTION

Pharmacophoric mapping is of great value in generating new chemical lead structures, especially when a limited number of compounds are available or when different chemical classes are used (see Chapter 4). A structural fit, reflected by the 3-D geometry of a structure in its active conformation is a necessary but not sufficient cause of activity, since electronic and hydrophobic forces between ligand and receptor are required for the response. An inherent limitation with pharmacophoric modeling techniques like the active analog approach is their inability to quantitatively describe the biological effect, i.e. one can usually only distinguish active from inactive compounds. In the process of optimizing a lead structure, it is necessary to utilize the information from quantitative activity data and from other structural properties in a more efficient way in order to predict more active congeners. Furthermore, quantitative structure–activity relationships (QSAR) can provide a great deal of information regarding the nature of ligand–target protein interactions. In series of homologous derivatives, various quantitative structure–activity analyses utilizing linear free energy relationships, multiple linear regression, and pattern recognition techniques have been applied. Furthermore, recent progress has been made in combining molecular modeling and statistical models, which allows for handling of non-congeneric series.

5.2 HANSCH ANALYSIS

5.2.1 Hydrophobic correlations

The biological activity can be regarded as a function of the physico-chemical and structural properties of the ligand. Already at the turn of the century, Meyer and Overton observed independently of each other that the anesthetic potency of simple organic molecules increases linearly with their oil/water partition coefficients (P). Four decades later Ferguson connected the narcotic activity and partition coefficients with thermodynamic principles. He stated that under equilibrium conditions, narcotic activity was correlated to the relative saturation of membranes by the gaseous narcotic substance. However, Hansch reasoned that too lipophilic molecules will partition into the first line of lipid membranes and be retained there.

Likewise, too hydrophilic molecules will not readily partition from the first aqueous compartment into the lipid of a membrane. Accordingly, Hansch and co-workers observed in the 1960s that the biological activity for several sets of congeners conformed with a parabolic dependence on lipophilicity ($\log P$) according to equation (5.1). Thus, an optimal $\log P$ value would correspond to the maximum probability of a compound to reach a receptor protein on a random walk between various lipophilic and hydrophilic compartments. The optimal lipophilic value, $\log P_o = a/2b$, is obtained from the derivative $d(\log 1/C)/d \log P$ being equal to zero. The biological activity is usually expressed as the logarithm of the inverse concentration or dose [$\log (1/C)$ or pC] which produces some standard response, e.g. $\log (1/\text{IC}_{50})$ or $\log (1/\text{ED}_{50})$.

$$\text{biological activity} \left(\log \frac{1}{C} \right) = a \log P - b(\log P)^2 + c \tag{5.1}$$

Phenomena involved in the transport of the ligand to its site of action and the hydrophobic interactions with the receptor are mainly determined by equation (5.1). For several classes of CNS active substances it has been found that the activity and thus the penetration over the blood–brain barrier (BBB) is optimal for $\log P_o$ (octanol) values in the range of 1.5–2.7, with a mean value of 2.1 (see also Section 5.4.5 for a more recent view). A linear dependence on $\log P$ might be expected up to a point where the hydrophobic region of the receptor is filled out and thereafter the activity decreases due to steric hindrance during the interaction of ligand and receptor. In several cases, the whole lipophilicity range may not have been investigated and, thus, only a linear dependence is revealed.

5.2.2   Multifactorial correlations

In order to take other types of molecular interactions into account, Hansch and Fujita included descriptors for steric, electronic and hydrophobic (= lipophilic) properties in the QSAR equation (5.2), which is based on the fact that the variables can be related to free energies in a linear free energy relationship (LFER). In the literature you will find the expressions parameter, descriptor or variable used with the same meaning.

$$\log \left(\frac{1}{C} \right) = a(\text{parameter}) + b(\text{electronic parameter})$$
$$+ c(\text{steric parameter}) + d(\text{other descriptor}) + e \tag{5.2}$$

where a, b, c, d and e are the regression coefficients determined by a least squares regression analysis (multiple linear regression, MLR), often referred to as a Hansch analysis. Different physico-chemical parameters have been used to describe the global properties of the molecule or the contribution from individual substituents. The most commonly used substituent parameters are shown in Table 5.1. These independent variables (parameters and descriptors) can be collinear, i.e. the same information is carried by the parameters, which will lead to false correlations. By including indicator variables, one can for example describe the presence or

Table 5.1 Physico-chemical parameters used in QSAR

Parameter	Symbol
Hydrophobic parameters	
Partition coefficient	$\log P$, CLOGP, Prolog P
Substituent constant	π
Hydrophobic fragmental constant	f, f'
Distribution coefficient	$\log D$
Apparent partition coefficient (fixed pH)	$\log P'$, $\log P_{app}$
Capacity factor in HPLC	$\log k$, $\log k_w$
Solubility parameter	δ
Electronic descriptors	
Hammett constants	σ, σ^-, σ^+
Taft's inductive (polar) constants	σ^*, σ_I
Swain and Lupton field parameter	$\mathfrak{I}$
Swain and Lupton resonance parameter	$\mathfrak{R}$
Ionization constant	pK_a, ΔpK_a
Chemical shifts (^{13}C and ^{1}H)	δ
Theoretical parameters	
Atomic net charge	q^σ, q^π
Superdelocalizability	S^N, S^E, S^R
Energy of highest occupied molecular orbital	E_{HOMO}
Energy of lowest unoccupied molecular orbital	E_{LUMO}
Electrostatic potentials	$V(r)$
Steric descriptors	
Taft's steric parameter	E_S, E^c
Molar volume	MV
Molecular weight	MW
Van der Waals radius	r
Van der Waals volume	V_W
Molar refractivity	MR
Parachor	P_r
STERIMOL parameters	L, B_1, B_5 (B_2, B_3, B_4)

absence of a certain substituent or other structural characteristics. In the ideal case, the biological data and physico-chemical parameters should be spread evenly and over a large range as will be discussed in the following Section 5.7 on experimental design.

The number of compounds (n) in the correlation must be considerably larger than the number of parameters used, i.e. four to six compounds (data points) per variable for medium-sized data sets in order to avoid chance correlations. In the PLS method described in Section 5.5, this is not a limitation even if redundant variables should be avoided. The correlation coefficient r, the relative measure of the quality of fit, should be around 0.9 for *in vitro* data, i.e. the explained variance r^2 should be over 80%, for acceptable regression equations. The standard deviation s, the absolute measure of the quality of fit, should not exceed the standard deviation in the biological data set too much. The regression coefficients (a, b, c, d etc.) should make sense from a physico-chemical standpoint (cf. ρ-values in physical organic chemistry) and be justified by confidence intervals at the 95% level (not shown in the following equations).

Importantly, the physico-chemical descriptors contain information that will give direct insight about properties essential for the transport to the site of action and for the interaction with the target protein required for the biological activity. Thus, one should select and statistically justify independent (low intercorrelation coefficients) variables, which describe different structural properties. In the analysis, one should aim for the simplest model to describe the data (principle of parsimony).

5.3   PHYSICO-CHEMICAL PROPERTIES

5.3.1   Electronic descriptors

The first and still most widely used electronic substituent parameter σ was developed by Hammett 1935 on the basis of ionization constants for benzoic acid derivatives. The Hammett equation (5.3) is expressed as

$$\rho\sigma = \log K_X - \log K_H \tag{5.3}$$

where K_H and K_X are the ionization constants for benzoic acid and a *para* or *meta* substituted derivative, respectively, and $\rho = 1$ for measurements in water at 25 °C. Positive σ values represent electron withdrawing properties ($X = CN, NO_2, CF_3$) and negative σ values electron donating properties ($X = NH_2, CH_3$).

A number of related Hammett parameters applicable for special circumstances, e.g. σ_p^-, σ_p^+, σ_m and σ_p, can provide mechanistic insight on the nature of the interaction if a considerably better correlation is obtained with a particular constant (cf. equation (5.18) below).

The inductive field (polar) component of the electronic substituent effect could be separated from the resonance part. Swain and Lupton described the Hammett σ constant as a linear combination of a resonance effect $\mathfrak{R}$ and a field effect $\mathfrak{F}$. These parameters are not position-dependent, which makes them useful and easy to handle in QSAR (cf. equation (5.20)). The Hammett constant σ is related to the $\mathfrak{F}$ and $\mathfrak{R}$ values as expressed in equation (5.4)

$$\sigma = f\mathfrak{F} + r\mathfrak{R} \tag{5.4}$$

where f and r are weighting factors.

5.3.2   Hydrophobic parameters

Analogous to the derivation of the Hammett constant, the substituent constant π for hydrophobic effect can be described by equation (5.5),

$$\pi = \log P_X - \log P_H \tag{5.5}$$

where P_X is the partition coefficient of a substituted derivative and P_H that of the parent compound. The distribution is measured between an organic solvent and water and the partition coefficient P is the ratio of the same solute in the two immiscible solvents. Octanol is the accepted standard system used and it has been justified as a suitable model for lipid constituents in biomembranes by the slightly amphiphilic nature introduced by the hydroxyl group in the long alkyl chain. The hydrogen bond donating and accepting properties facilitate the interaction with several types of solutes and octanol also dissolves an appreciable amount of water during equilibrium conditions. The partitioning to other solvent systems can be calculated by the Collander equation (5.6). This linear relationship between $\log P$ obtained in different systems makes it reasonable to apply one arbitrary standard system (octanol) even if limitations have been pointed out.

$$\log P_1 = a \log P_2 + c \tag{5.6}$$

A positive π corresponds to a lipophilic character and negative π to a hydrophilic character relative to hydrogen. In the case of ionizable solutes, $\log P$ for the non-ionized species can be determined from the distribution coefficient D, which is dependent on pH, by inclusion of the ionization constant(s) in the calculation (e.g. equations (5.7) and (5.8)). Partition through membranes is usually regarded to be associated with the non-ionized molecules.

$$\log D_{acid} = \log P - \log[1 + 10^{(pH - pK_a)}] \tag{5.7}$$

$$\log D_{base} = \log P - \log[1 + 10^{(pK_a - pH)}] \tag{5.8}$$

However, the determination of partition coefficients by the classical shake flask technique is connected with several practical problems, e.g. disturbances from minor impurities, effects of ions in aqueous buffers, difficulties to analyze solutes in both phases especially for compounds with extreme $\log P$ values, necessity to work with very low concentrations of solute to diminish aggregation, and establishment of equilibrium conditions. These problems to determine $\log P$ values can largely be overcome by use of HPLC-derived hydrophobicity data. The HPLC methodology can also be applied to small and impure amounts of material and gives accurate data by frequent use of calibration standards. Furthermore, no quantitative methods for the determination of the solutes are required. The chromatographically derived values are not unique, but they can be converted into the familiar octanol/water partition coefficients. This makes HPLC the method of choice for experimental determination of $\log P$ values.

The slope a in equation (5.1) has been found to have values in the range from about 0.2 to 1.4. It has been argued that a-values of about unity implies complete desolvation and binding deep into a lipophilic pocket (cf. equations (5.13), (5.14), (5.17) and (5.25)), whereas a-values of about 0.5 reflects only partial desolvation and binding along the surface of a protein (cf. equations (5.12) and (5.15)). However, this view is under debate, since binding to a highly structured membrane reduces the freedom of an alkyl chain, which will diminish the slope a and the π values.

The additive properties of the π values make it possible to estimate $\log P$ of a new compound, either completely from tables or by combination of experimental values and tabulated data. For example, the $\log P$ value for xylene can be estimated with a high degree of accuracy from the $\log P$ values of benzene and toluene by the following simple calculation.

$$\pi_{Me} = \log P_{Ph-Me} - \log P_{Ph-H} = 2.69 - 2.13 = 0.56$$

$$\log P_{xylene} = \log P_{Ph-Me} + \pi_{Me} = 2.69 + 0.56 = 3.25 \text{ (Experimental 3.20)}$$

However, in several cases, especially for aliphatic compounds, large differences between observed $\log P$ values and partition coefficients calculated from π values are found. To overcome these limitations, Rekker introduced the concept of fragmental constants f, which are related to the π values according to equation (5.9). The fragmental constants, which were statistically derived from over thousand $\log P$ determinations, measure the absolute lipophilicity contribution of a given structural fragment i, which occurs a_i number of times in a structure. Interaction factors F were also introduced in order to correct for intramolecular electronic, steric or hydrogen bond interactions between fragments according to equation (5.10).

$$f_X = f_H + \pi_X \tag{5.9}$$
$$\log P = \Sigma a_i f_X + \Sigma F_i \tag{5.10}$$

The fragmental constant system has been modified by Leo and Hansch based on a small number of accurately determined $\log P$ values instead of the statistical approach used by Rekker. Based on this concept a computer program CLOGP was developed, which allows for more facile calculations of $\log P$ values.

5.3.3   Steric descriptors

The description of steric bulk of a substituent is difficult to assess, since the conformation may vary among the ligands in the test series as well as for the target protein. However, several parameters have been successfully applied. The steric effect has been described by Taft's steric parameter E_S, derived from acidic hydrolysis of esters (X-CH$_2$COOR). E_S is more negative for larger groups [t-Bu, CCl$_3$] and more positive for smaller groups (H, F, OH).

In order to better account for the shape of the substituents, Verloop has developed a set of parameters using the STERIMOL program based on CPK-models. The length parameter L and the four width parameters B_1, B_2, B_3, and B_4 which describe the dimensions of the group along fixed axes, were originally used. However, different possibilities may result for the B_2–B_4 parameters depending on the selection of B_1, which is not a very satisfactory situation. Because of this and also because of reported statistical chance correlations in the literature using the original STERIMOL parameters a new set of descriptors was developed by Verloop. These second generation parameters retained the STERIMOL length parameter L and the minimum width parameter B_1 but introduced a new width parameter B_5, which represents the largest width orthogonal to L but is independent of any angle between B_1 and B_5 (cf. equation (5.14)).

1 To determine the STERIMOL parameters one proceeds in the following manner: Determine the bond between the parent skeleton and the substituent and place that bond in the plane of the paper (or screen). Project the vdW surface of the substituent onto the same plane. Measure the length from the point of attachment (P) to the projected vdW surface along the bond of attachment. This value constitutes the STERIMOL parameter L.

2 Rotate the structure 90° to see the structure along the bond between the parent skeleton and the substituent. Project the vdW surface of the substituent onto the plane of the paper (or screen). Measure the shortest length as well as the longest length from the point of attachment (P) to the projected vdW surface. These two values constitute the STERIMOL parameters B_1 and B_5, respectively.

The definitions of the second generation STERIMOL parameters of L, B_1 and B_5 are shown in Figure 5.1. The parameters B_1 and B_5 are orthogonal to L as a consequence of the procedure described above. By using ratios of L/B_1 and B_5/B_1 one might get information on any directionality of importance for the receptor interaction.

Alternatively, the van der Waals radii and the molar volume $MV = MW/d$ have been used. The molar refractivity (MR) is related to the molar volume by the Lorentz–Lorenz equation (5.11).

$$MR = \left[\frac{(n^2 - 1)}{(n^2 + 2)}\right]\left(\frac{MW}{d}\right) \tag{5.11}$$

where n is the refraction index, d is the density and MW is the molecular weight. Fragment values have been calculated since MR is an additive property of the molecule. A larger MR value for a substituent corresponds to a larger steric

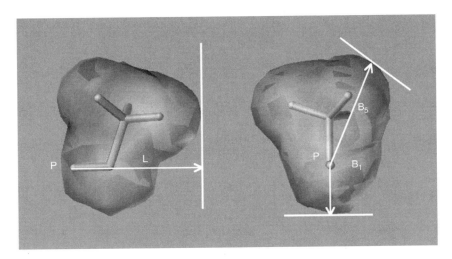

Figure 5.1 Definition of the second generation STERIMOL parameters used in QSAR work exemplified by a methoxy group substituent.

Table 5.2 Commonly used aromatic substituent parameters and principal properties (PP) calculated from the complete set of parameters by principal component analysis (Section 5.5)

Subst.	σ_m	σ_p	$\mathfrak{I}$	$\mathfrak{R}$	π	MR	L	B_1	B_5	PP_1	PP_2	PP_3
H	0.00	0.00	0.00	0.00	0.00	1.03	2.06	1.00	1.00	1.35	−3.00	−0.39
F	0.34	0.06	0.43	−0.34	0.14	0.92	2.65	1.35	1.35	2.38	−1.95	0.45
Cl	0.37	0.23	0.41	−0.15	0.71	6.03	3.52	1.80	1.80	2.22	−0.15	−0.57
Br	0.39	0.23	0.44	−0.17	0.86	8.88	3.82	1.95	1.95	2.08	0.38	−0.74
I	0.35	0.18	0.40	−0.19	1.12	13.94	4.23	2.15	2.15	1.49	1.00	−1.21
NO₂	0.71	0.78	0.67	0.16	−0.28	7.36	3.44	1.70	2.44	4.12	1.12	0.87
CH₃	−0.07	−0.17	−0.04	−0.13	0.56	5.65	2.87	1.52	2.04	0.25	−1.84	−1.36
CCH	0.21	0.23	0.19	0.05	0.40	9.55	4.66	1.60	1.60	1.30	−0.01	−0.60
CHCH₂	0.05	−0.02	0.07	−0.08	0.82	10.99	4.29	1.60	3.09	−0.09	−0.18	−0.65
C₂H₅	−0.07	−0.15	−0.05	−0.10	1.02	10.30	4.11	1.52	3.17	−0.71	−0.65	−0.90
C₃H₅	−0.07	−0.21	−0.03	−0.19	1.14	13.53	4.14	1.55	3.24	−1.02	−0.56	−0.83
C₃H₇	−0.07	−0.13	−0.06	−0.08	1.55	14.96	4.92	1.52	3.49	−1.35	0.15	−0.78
CH(CH₃)₂	−0.07	−0.15	−0.05	−0.10	1.53	14.98	4.11	1.90	3.17	−0.87	0.16	−1.89
C₄H₉	−0.08	−0.16	−0.06	−0.11	2.13	19.59	6.17	1.52	4.54	−2.43	1.22	−0.32
CH₂CH(CH₃)₂	−0.10	−0.20	−0.07	−0.13	1.98	19.62	4.92	1.52	4.45	−2.16	0.61	−0.55
C(CH₃)₃	−0.10	−0.20	−0.07	−0.13	1.98	19.62	4.11	2.60	3.17	−1.03	1.20	−3.70
C₅H₁₁	−0.08	−0.15	−0.06	−0.09	2.67	24.25	7.17	1.52	5.23	−3.22	2.21	−0.03
C₆H₅	0.06	−0.01	0.08	−0.08	1.96	25.36	6.28	1.71	3.11	−1.51	1.73	−0.64
C₆H₁₁	−0.15	−0.22	−0.13	−0.10	2.51	26.69	6.17	1.91	3.49	−2.68	1.67	−1.83
CF₃	0.43	0.54	0.38	0.19	0.88	5.02	3.30	1.99	2.61	2.83	1.00	−1.10
CN	0.56	0.66	0.51	0.19	−0.57	6.33	4.23	1.60	1.60	3.59	0.57	0.52
CHO	0.35	0.42	0.31	0.13	−0.65	6.88	3.53	1.60	2.36	2.51	−0.13	0.05
CH₂OH	0.00	0.00	0.00	0.00	−1.03	7.19	3.97	1.52	2.70	0.62	−1.22	−0.44
COCH₃	0.38	0.50	0.32	0.20	−0.55	11.18	4.06	1.60	3.13	2.13	0.73	0.42
COC₆H₅	0.34	0.43	0.30	0.16	1.05	30.33	5.81	1.60	5.98	−0.71	3.40	1.37
CONH₂	0.28	0.36	0.24	0.14	−1.49	9.81	4.06	1.50	3.07	1.90	−0.12	0.63
COOH	0.37	0.45	0.33	0.15	−0.32	6.93	3.91	1.60	2.66	2.36	0.28	0.17
COOCH₃	0.37	0.45	0.33	0.15	−0.01	12.87	4.73	1.64	3.36	1.60	1.21	0.42
COOC₂H₅	0.37	0.45	0.33	0.15	0.51	17.47	5.95	1.64	4.41	0.62	2.33	0.88
NH₂	−0.16	−0.66	0.02	−0.68	−1.23	5.42	2.78	1.35	1.97	−0.36	−3.85	−0.12
NCH₃	−0.30	−0.84	−0.11	−0.74	−0.47	10.33	3.53	1.35	3.08	−2.03	−3.29	−0.18
N(CH₃)₂	−0.15	−0.83	0.10	−0.92	0.18	15.55	3.53	1.35	3.08	−1.97	−2.76	0.46
NHC₄H₉	−0.34	−0.51	−0.28	−0.25	1.45	24.26	6.88	1.35	4.87	−4.18	0.46	−0.11
N(C₂H₅)₂	−0.23	−0.90	0.01	−0.91	1.18	24.85	4.83	1.35	4.39	−3.76	−1.37	0.66
NHC₆H₅	−0.12	−0.40	−0.02	−0.38	1.37	30.04	4.53	1.35	5.95	−3.30	0.53	0.82
NHCOCH₃	0.21	0.00	0.28	−0.26	−0.97	14.93	5.09	1.35	3.61	0.23	−0.27	1.54
NHCONH₂	−0.03	−0.24	0.04	−0.28	−1.30	13.72	5.06	1.35	3.61	−0.74	−1.11	0.84
OH	0.12	−0.37	0.29	−0.64	−0.67	2.85	2.74	1.35	1.93	0.96	−3.02	0.54
OCF₃	0.38	0.35	0.38	0.00	1.04	7.86	4.57	1.35	3.61	1.25	0.71	1.04
OCH₃	0.12	−0.27	0.26	−0.51	−0.02	7.87	3.98	1.35	3.07	0.06	−1.57	0.85
OC₂H₅	0.10	−0.24	0.22	−0.44	0.38	12.47	4.80	1.35	3.36	−0.57	−0.78	0.88
OCH(CH₃)₂	0.10	−0.25	0.22	−0.45	1.05	17.06	6.05	1.35	4.42	−1.62	0.37	1.31
OC₄H₉	0.10	−0.32	0.25	−0.55	1.55	21.66	6.86	1.35	4.79	−2.40	0.97	1.62
OCH(CH₃)₂	0.10	−0.45	0.30	−0.72	0.36	17.06	4.80	1.35	4.10	−1.33	−0.85	1.53
OC₆H₅	0.25	−0.03	0.34	−0.35	2.08	27.68	4.51	1.35	5.89	−1.64	1.63	1.74
SH	0.25	0.15	0.28	−0.11	0.39	9.22	3.47	1.70	2.33	1.47	−0.31	−0.48
SCF₃	0.40	0.50	0.35	0.18	1.44	13.81	4.89	1.70	3.94	1.16	2.11	0.17
SCH₃	0.15	0.00	0.20	−0.18	0.61	13.82	4.30	1.70	3.26	0.17	0.15	−0.28
SO₂NH₂	0.46	0.57	0.41	0.19	−1.82	12.28	4.02	2.04	3.05	3.04	1.08	−0.04

bulk and a greater tendency to interact via dispersion forces. A compilation of commonly used parameters for aromatic substituents is shown in Table 5.2.

5.3.4   Biological relevance

Recently, the relevance of several statistical correlations on enzyme inhibitors have been supported by computer modeling in cases where the solid-state structure of the enzymes have been determined (cf. equation (5.25)). For example, binding with substituents in certain positions correlated with hydrophobicity (π) whereas in other positions with molar refractivity (*MR*). The significance of the π terms in the correlation equations could be rationalized by van der Waals contacts with hydrophobic regions, where desolvation is the major driving force. On the other hand, correlations of substituents with *MR* appeared in polar regions of the protein where binding mainly involves dispersion forces. This means that it is possible not only to retrospectively correlate the data and predict more active congeners but also to gain mechanistic information on the nature of the interactions between the ligand/substrate and the receptor/enzyme.

5.4   APPLICATIONS OF HANSCH EQUATIONS

5.4.1   Hydrophobic and steric factors

A wide range of biological activities has been correlated with linear free energy-related parameters and a selection of examples will be given to show some of the information that can be obtained. For simple *in vitro* systems, e.g. enzyme inhibition data, simpler and more accurate relationships may be derived than for more complex biological systems, which involve a combination of transport, distribution and receptor-interaction phenomena.

Protein binding is a non-specific interaction to hydrophobic areas of serum proteins and linear relationships between $\log K$ (binding constant) and $\log P$ has indeed been found. Equation (5.12) shows the relationship for binding of sulfony-lurea derivatives to bovine serum albumin (BSA) and the small (0.33) regression coefficient indicates binding of an only partly desolvated compound.

$$\log K = 0.33 \log P + 0.24 \, pK_a + 1.48$$
$$n = 15, \quad r^2 = 0.90, \quad s = 0.090 \tag{5.12}$$

In concordance with the Meyer-Overton findings, the narcotic effect on tadpoles of a set of structurally diverse compounds was simply explained by the lipophilicity according to equation (5.13), which supports a non-specific interaction. In this case, the regression coefficient is close to unity, which is in line with a complete accumulation of the molecules in a lipophilic bioenvironment similar to that in octanol.

$$\log\left(\frac{1}{C}\right) = 0.94 \log P + 0.87$$
$$n = 51, \quad r^2 = 0.94 \tag{5.13}$$

(5.1)   (5.2)

The muscarinic effect of a series of *meta*-substituted benzyltrimethylammonium derivatives (**5.1**) investigated on isolated rat jejunum could be modeled by equation (5.14), which indicates binding of the *meta*-substituent X into a lipophilic pocket (large regression coefficient for the hydrophobic parameter π) of limited size (negative coefficient for the STERIMOL parameter B_5).

$$\log\left(\frac{1}{ED}\right) = 1.30\pi - 0.41\,B_5 + 5.68$$

$$n = 10, \quad r^2 = 0.90, \quad s = 0.186$$

(5.14)

The displacement of the benzodiazepine [^{3}H]flunitrazepam from bovine brain membranes of a series of quinolinones (**5.2**) was significantly correlated to steric and hydrophobic parameters, however for different positions, according to equation (5.15). The positive coefficient of Taft's steric constant for the *ortho*-positions ($E_S(2,6)$) might indicate a required co-planar arrangement of the phenyl ring during the receptor binding, which is abolished by too much bulk in these positions. However, lipophilic (and large) groups are favorable in other positions and the intermediate size of the π coefficient reflects a partial desolvation during the hydrophobic interaction of the *meta*-substituents ($\pi(3,5)$).

$$\log\left(\frac{1}{IC_{50}}\right) = 0.481\,E_S(2,6) + 0.606\pi(3,5) + 4.81$$

$$n = 20, \quad r^2 = 0.76, \quad s = 0.278$$

(5.15)

5.4.2 Influence of electronic and other factors

The *in vivo* activity of a series of 17 tricyclic antipsychotics (**5.3**) related to octoclothepin (X = Cl) have been correlated with the electronic and steric parameters of the X substituent according to equation (5.16).

$$\log\left(\frac{1}{ED_{50}}\right) = 0.698\,\sigma_p + 0.347\,E_S + 0.0458\,MV - 0.00059\,MV^2 + 0.297$$

$$n = 17, \quad r^2 = 0.93, \quad s = 0.128$$

(5.16)

An electron-withdrawing X group will enhance the activity as shown by the positive value of the coefficient for σ_p. The parabolic dependence on MV indicate that a too large X group could be detrimental for the activity by steric interference

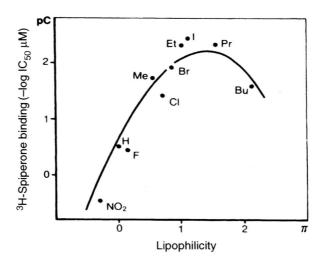

(5.3)   **(5.4)**

but smaller substituents interact favorably with the dopamine receptor, which is believed to mediate the antipsychotic activity. The latter aspect is also supported by the positive coefficient of E_S. In this case, the lipophilic parameters π and π^2 were not significantly involved.

The influence of the aromatic substituent X in a series of 12-mono-substituted potential antipsychotic salicylamides (**5.4**) on their ability to displace [³H]spiperone from the dopamine D_2 receptors *in vitro* has been investigated (Figure 5.2). The parabolic dependence on lipophilicity is clear from equation (5.17), which indicates that a limited size of the substituent X can be tolerated by the dopamine D_2 receptor since transportation effects should be negligible in this type of assay.

$$\log\left(\frac{1}{IC_{50}}\right) = 1.28\pi - 0.518\pi^2 - 0.692\sigma_m + 1.495$$

$$n = 12, \quad r^2 = 0.94, \quad s = 0.399$$

(5.17)

The fungicidal activity against *Cladosporium cucumerinum* of a series of arylethyn-sulfones (**5.5**) could be explained by electronic, lipophilic and steric descriptors in

Figure 5.2 Relationship between the inhibition of [³H]spiperone binding and lipophilicity (π) of the 3-substituent (X) of 6-methoxysalicylamides (**5.4**). Reproduced with permission of the American Chemical Society.

equation (5.18). A favorable correlation was obtained with σ^-, which is based on ionization of substituted phenols in water and used for correlation of reactions having an electron-rich reaction center in conjugation with electron with drawing substituents. The correlation with this electronic substituent with a positive coefficient (ρ value) argues for a nucleophilic attack on the triple bond to be of importance for the biological action.

$$pC = 1.10\sigma^- + 0.84\pi - 0.07\pi^2 + 2.10\,E_S + 4.17$$
$$n = 25, \quad r^2 = 0.89, \quad s = 0.248 \tag{5.18}$$

5.4.3   Ionization constants

The acidity of the phenolic group in the antipsychotic 6-methoxysalicylamides (**5.6**) has been considered to be of importance for the biological activity. To better understand, the effects of the substituents on the acidity a number of models with steric and electronic descriptors were investigated. The most significant regression equation (5.19) was obtained with a σ parameter for the *ortho*-substituent X and the modified Taft parameter E^c for the *para*-substituent Y. The regression coefficient of σ_0 is in accordance with the well-known stabilization of anionic forms by electron withdrawing *ortho*-substituents. The steric effect induced by the *para*-substituent can be rationalized by the influence on the conformation of the methoxy substituent. A more perpendicular orientation of the methoxy group inflicted by a more bulky Y substituent could lead to a weakening of the $OH-O=C$ hydrogen bond, an effect which increases the acidity of the phenol.

$$pK_{a1} = -1.66\sigma_0 - 1.36\,E_p^c + 7.98$$
$$n = 9, \quad r^2 = 0.92, \quad s = 0.37 \tag{5.19}$$

5.4.4   Predictions from equations

A series of substituted benzamides (**5.7**) of the clebopride ($4 = NH_2, 5 = Cl, 6 = H$) type containing both phenols ($n = 12$) and non-phenols ($n = 10$) with substituents in the 3-, 4-, and 5-positions were treated in a Hansch analysis. The indicator variable I_{OH} is set to unity for phenols and zero for non-phenols (cf. example on PLS analysis of benzamides with pyrrolidine side chains in Section 5.5). The affinity for the [³H]spiperone binding site could be modeled by a small number of substituents describing electronic properties, e.g. Swain and Lupton resonance parameters for the substituent in the 4-position ($\Re_4$) and the sum for the 3- and 5-substituents ($\Re_{(3+5)}$) as shown in equation (5.20).

(5.5)   (5.6)

$$\log\left(\frac{1}{IC_{50}}\right) = -1.75\,\mathfrak{R}_4 - 3.69\,\mathfrak{R}_{(3+5)} + 0.80\,I_{OH} + 0.04 \tag{5.20}$$

$$n = 22, \quad r^2 = 0.82, \quad s = 0.321, \quad F = 27.1$$

The equation (5.20) could be used to predict that compound (**5.8**) should have an IC_{50} value of 0.45 nM, i.e. ten-fold more active than the previous most potent member of the series. Synthesis and testing of this compound showed that the activity ($IC_{50} = 0.36$ nM) conformed with the predicted value to a degree we had not dare to expect. Figure 5.3 shows the new potent benzamide (**5.8**) included in the regression equation (5.21). Notably, the regression coefficients are virtually unchanged compared to equation (5.20), which is in accordance with the good prediction.

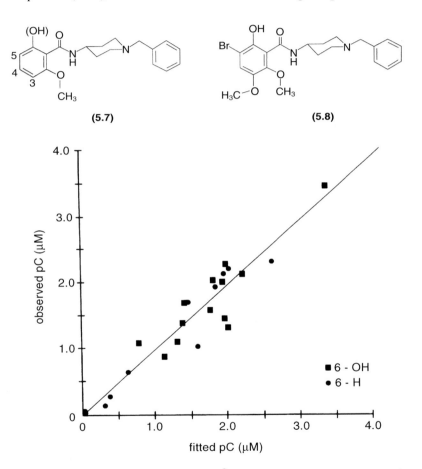

Figure 5.3 Found pC ($\log 1/IC_{50}$; μM) values for [^{3}H]spiperone binding shown as a function of data calculated according to the equation (5.21):

$$\log\left(\frac{1}{IC_{50}}\right) = -1.76\,\mathfrak{R}_4 - 3.75\,\mathfrak{R}_{(3+5)} + 0.81\,I_{OH} + 0.02 \tag{5.21}$$

$$n = 23, \quad r^2 = 0.87, \quad s = 0.313, \quad F = 41.8$$

It should be emphasized, however, that extrapolation outside the data set most often leads to large differences between predicted and found values, since the original model does not necessarily take the descriptors properly into account. In this case, we had included all the substituents used in the original test set, but the combinations of substituents were different in the predicted compound.

5.4.5   Blood–brain barrier penetration

As mentioned in Section 5.2.1, the optimal $\log P$ for penetration of the BBB is around 2.1 for a wide range of compounds. In a study aiming for centrally acting histamine H_2 antagonists, the physico-chemical properties of importance for the brain penetration was investigated in detail by Young and co-workers. A good correlation was found between the logarithms of the equilibrium brain/blood concentration ratios in the rat and the partition parameter $\Delta \log P$ (equation (5.22)) but not for $\log P$ in octanol (equation (5.23)).

$$\log\left(\frac{C_{\text{brain}}}{C_{\text{blood}}}\right) = -0.604\, \Delta \log P + 1.23$$
$$n = 6, \quad r^2 = 0.96, \quad s = 0.249$$
(5.22)

$$\log\left(\frac{C_{\text{brain}}}{C_{\text{blood}}}\right) = 0.150 \log P_{\text{oct}} - 0.96$$
$$n = 6, \quad r^2 = 0.026, \quad s = 1.241$$
(5.23)

Seiler introduced the $\Delta \log P$ parameter, as the difference between the octanol/water and cyclohexane/water $\log P$ values, which is related to the overall hydrogen-bonding capacity of a compound by equation (5.24).

$$\Delta \log P = \log P_{\text{oct}} - \log P_{\text{cyh}} = \Sigma I_{\text{H}} - 0.16$$
$$n = 195, \quad r^2 = 0.94, \quad s = 0.333$$
(5.24)

where I_{H} is the hydrogen-bonding ability for a given substituent. The larger the I_{H} value the more prone a substituent is to donate or accept a hydrogen bond, e.g. 2.60 for Ar–OH, 1.18 for Ar–NH$_2$, 0.45 for –NO$_2$, 0.31 for C=O, and 0.11 for ether –O–. Thus, the BBB penetration can be increased by lowering the overall hydrogen-bonding ability of a compound by, for example, encouraging intramolecular hydrogen bonding, shielding with non-polar groups and by making less polar prodrugs. The principles could be utilized in the design of potent histamine H_2 antagonists, which readily cross the BBB, such as zolantidine (**5.9**) with a $\Delta \log P$ of 1.69 and a $\log P_{\text{oct}}$ of 5.41.

5.4.6   Relations to molecular modeling

In a classical paper from the Hansch and Langridge groups (1982), the QSAR models for papain hydrolysis of phenyl hippurates (**5.10**) were compared with X-ray crystallography-based molecular modeling. Papain is a cystein protease

(5.9)   **(5.10)**

which hydrolyzes a number of esters, amides and peptides. A QSAR with the equation (5.25) was derived for a set of substituted phenyl hippurates.

$$\log \frac{1}{K_{\mathrm{m}}} = 0.57\sigma + 1.03\pi'_3 + 0.61\ MR_4 + 3.80$$

$$n = 25, \quad r^2 = 0.82, \quad s = 0.208$$

(5.25)

where σ refers to substituents in any positions, MR_4 (scaled with 0.1 to be comparable with the other parameters) for the *para*-substituents and π'_3 indicates that only π for the most hydrophobic group in the *meta*-position is considered significant. The latter parameter makes mechanistic sense, since substituents that are hydrophobic ($\pi > 0$) partition into the enzyme, whereas those with negative values cause a rotation around the phenyl ring to place the less hydrophilic hydrogen onto the enzyme while the X-substituent is oriented into the aqueous phase. The term MR_4 cannot be replaced with π, which indicates that the *para*-substituent does not contact a lipophilic surface. On the other hand, the most lipophilic *meta*-substituent is making a hydrophobic interaction with complete desolvation as indicated by the correlation coefficient (1.03).

The solid-state structure has been determined for an enzyme–inhibitor complex between (benzyloxycarbonyl->L-phenylalanyl->L-alanylmethylene-papain, ZPA-papain), which allows for a proper orientation of the phenyl hippurates in the active site. The derived model was used to validate the QSAR equation (5.25) and indeed all terms could be shown to accommodate the modeling data. Thus, the 4-substituents collide with a highly polar amide moiety in Gln-142 and remain exposed to solvent. The hydrophobic *meta*-substituent is completely buried (desolvated) within a shallow hydrophobic pocket, whereas the other *meta*-position is oriented into the solvent as shown in Figure 5.4.

5.5   PATTERN RECOGNITION

5.5.1   PCR and PLS methods

In some cases where a structure–activity model is to be derived there are more variables, i.e. characteristics of the structures under investigation, than there are compounds. In such instances, traditional methods such as MLR (see previous Section 5.2) cannot be used since there are more unknown variables than available equations (one equation for each compound in the test set). This situation is especially true for the 3D-QSAR models (see Section 5.6) where the number of variables typically exceeds the number of compounds by a factor of a 100. Pattern

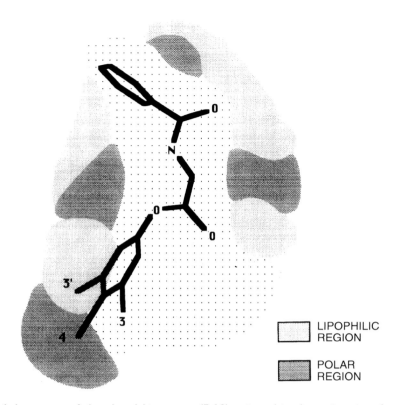

LIPOPHILIC
REGION

POLAR
REGION

Figure 5.4 A cartoon of the phenyl hippurates (**5.10**) oriented in the active site of papain. The different shadings indicating hydrophobic and polar regions have been adopted by Magnus Jendbro according to the original modeling work by Hansch, Langridge and co-workers.

recognition methods, such as PLS (Partial least squares projections to latent structures), PCR (Principal component regression) and PCA (Principal component analysis), can be used to analyze these kinds of problems. All three methods contract (reduce) the original description of each molecule into a few descriptive dimensions, so-called principal components (PCs). Thus, these methods re-express the original matrix of data (X) for the compounds under investigation as a mean vector (X_m) plus the product of a score matrix T and a loading matrix P' (Figure 5.5). The scores, where each investigated compound has a computed set of score values, give the best summary of X and can be seen as the underlying factors of the studied system. Furthermore, the scores are, using the method described above, linear combinations of the original variables (equation (5.26)).

$$t_1 = C_1 V_1 + C_2 V_2 + C_3 V_3 + \ldots + C_n V_n \tag{5.26}$$

where C_n are the weighting constants (loadings), V_n the original variables and t_1 is the first score value for a molecule (see Figure 5.5).

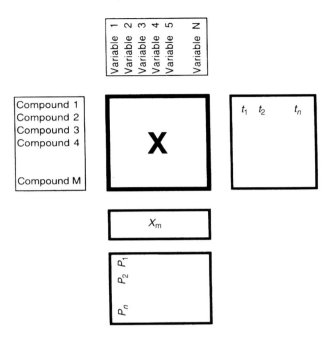

Figure 5.5 Schematic representation of the deconvolution of the structural descriptor matrix X into a score vector T ($t_1, t_2, \ldots, t_n$) and a loading vector P' ($P_1, P_2, \ldots, P_n$).

How are the principal components then calculated? Starting from the description of the investigated compounds (the mean centered data matrix X; see below for further explanation) the first PC is computed with the objective to explain as much information as possible in matrix X. This gives rise to the first score vector t_1 and the first row vector P'_1. The information contained in the first PC is then subtracted from the matrix X by subtracting the $t_1 P'_1$ matrix from X. A second PC with the same objective as that of the first PC, i.e. to explain as much information as possible in the new, updated matrix X is then calculated and so on for additional PCs. A mathematical consequence of the way the PCs are computed makes each PC orthogonal (independent) to all other PCs and that the first PC (PC1) contains the largest part of explained variance (information content) in the data. Subsequent PCs contain decreasingly smaller amounts of explained variance. It is desirable to first center the data matrix by subtracting the mean value of each column from the respective column (mean centering of the data matrix). Otherwise, the first PC will contain no interesting structural information but will instead represent a vector from origo to the point represented by the mean values.

How many components should then be calculated (extracted), i.e. used to describe the properties of the investigated compounds? Certainly one should only extract relevant information and stop when the amount of noise becomes too large in a calculated component. The term 'extracted' is mostly used in the literature instead of 'calculated', when dealing with PCs. A cross-validation (CV) procedure described by Wold (1979) is used to determine the stoppage point.

In CV, a portion of the data is left out, a PC is extracted and a model is created with the remaining data. The left out data are then predicted by the model. As long as the prediction of the left out data becomes better, the extracted component is judged to be significant and is kept in the model. When the prediction of the left out data does not improve any more, the extraction of components is stopped and the resulting model is based on the previously extracted significant components.

There is a fundamental difference between PLS and PCR in deriving the PCs. The PCR is composed of two steps. In the first step, a PCA is applied to the description of the structures (the X matrix; see Figure 5.5) and a relevant number of PCs are extracted. These PCs are then, in a second step, correlated against the biological activity using MLR. In PLS, a correlation between the chemical descriptors (variables) and biological activity (or other properties) is obtained where PLS uses the available biological information (biological activity) during the extraction of PCs. Thus, PLS tries to derive PCs that explain as much as possible of the biological information while PCR in the first step, the PCA, tries to explain as much as possible of the structural description of the molecules and then, in the second step, uses the derived PCs to derive a good model with respect to the measured activities. This means that the PCs from PLS and PCR differ from each other. Since PLS is targeted at explaining the activities this also means that PLS usually produces somewhat better QSARs compared with PCR. Some of the advantages of using PLS/PCR compared with multiple regression techniques are the following:

1   The number of compounds in the analysis can be significantly smaller than the number of variables used.
2   There are no collinearities between final variables since PLS/PCR is PC based, which means that addition of relevant variables will improve the relationship.
3   The original data set of chemical descriptor may contain 'missing data', i.e. a number of variables have not been assigned a value for some reason and are missing. The PLS/PCR tolerates a certain number of such data depending on the distribution in the data matrix X.

All evidence suggest that PLS gives at least as good relationships (predictions) as other linear regression techniques and sometimes much better.

5.5.2 Application of PLS

Partial least squares has been used by Norinder and Högberg to study the QSAR between the *in vitro* affinity to [³H]spiperone binding sites of mono- and disubstituted benzamides (**5.11**) with a large number of physico-chemical descrip-

(5.11)

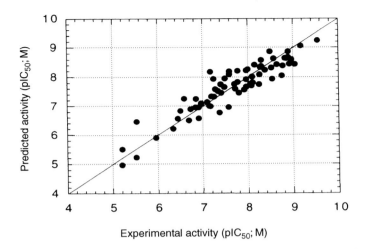

Figure 5.6 Plot of predicted vs. experimental [^{3}H]spiperone displacing activity (pIC$_{50}$; M) of substituted salicylamides (**5.11**). The QSAR was made with the PLS method as described in Section 5.5.

tors for size, lipophilicity and electronic characteristics. Each of the 3- and 5-substituents were described by the original physico-chemical parameters ($\sigma_m, \sigma_p, \mathfrak{J}, \mathfrak{R}, \pi, MR, L, B_1$ and B_5 in Table 5.1) and the corresponding squared values. Since only two choices exist for position 2($R_2 = H, OH$) a so-called indicator variable (I_2) was used. This variable can assume two values; $I_2 = 0$ for $R_2 = H$ and $I_2 = 1$ for $R_2 = OH$. A similar indicator variable (I_S) was also used to represent the stereochemistry of the side chain (I_S; $R = -1$, $S = 1$, racemate $= 0$). In total, 38 variables were used to describe each compound.

The PLS analysis resulted in 4 PCs which explained 86% of the variance (information) in binding affinity (see Figure 5.6). The analysis pointed out the major importance of size, lipophilicity and electronic properties of the 3-substituent as well as a (S)-configuration of the side chain.

5.6   3D-QSAR METHODOLOGIES

5.6.1   Methods and strategy

Structure–activity relationships of traditional type, e.g. Hansch analysis or pattern recognition methods as discussed above, usually do not take the 3D structures of the investigated compounds into account in an explicit manner. Instead, they use substituent parameters and indicator variables to describe the structural variations.

Today it is well recognized that, at the molecular level, the interactions that produce an observed biological effect are usually non-covalent and that such steric and electrostatic interactions can account for many of the observed molecular properties. Extensions to the traditional QSAR approaches have been developed which explicitly uses the 3D geometry of the structures during the development of a QSAR model. These new technologies, commonly referred to as 3D-QSAR methodologies, include approaches such as the HASL method (Doweyko 1988), REMOTEDISC (Ghose *et al.* 1989) and GRID/GOLPE (Cruciani and Watson 1994). The presently most used technique, CoMFA (Comparative Molecular Field Analysis), was developed by Cramer and co-workers (Cramer *et al.* 1988).

The following steps have to be considered when trying to develop a 3D-QSAR model:

1   Identification of active conformation(s)
2   Alignment rule
3   3D-grid construction
4   Calculation of field values
5   Selection of training set compounds
6   PLS analysis
7   Interpretation of results (contour maps)
8   Predictions of new compounds.

One of the most fundamental problems when trying to develop a good and predictive 3D-QSAR model is the identification of the bioactive conformation(s) (cf. the detailed discussion in Chapter 4) of the investigated compounds and how to align them (steps 1 and 2). This becomes especially critical when one is dealing with a set of structurally diverse compounds. Considerable effort has been devoted to investigate and develop better protocols for alignment of compounds (see Norinder 1998 for a recent review). There are several available methods, such as SEAL, Catalyst and DISCO, by which atoms or molecular properties are super-imposed onto a reference compound or a set of reference compounds (Section 5.6.2). Fitting the interaction fields of the investigated compounds onto the corresponding fields of a reference compound (field fitting, see Section 5.6.3) as well as experimental geometries from X-ray crystallography (see Section 5.6.4) can also be used for alignment purposes. However, for flexible molecules there is usually not one unique 'best' way of identifying bioactive conformations and super-imposing the geometries. Attempts have been made to device iterative schemes where a number of conformations and alignments are investigated in order to find a self-consistent 3D-QSAR model. Examples of such programs are COMPASS (Jain *et al.* 1994) and TDQ (Norinder 1996). However, in the end the researcher must in most cases decide which superimpositioning scheme to use for the 3D-QSAR model. If a predictive model can be successfully be developed, then this may serve as an indication that the choice of alignment scheme was a reasonable one.

Once the choice of molecular alignments and conformations is made, then a 3D-grid box is spanned around the molecules under investigation. The box is filled with grid points (see Figure 5.7) with an internal distance of usually between 1 and 3 Å (step 3).

A probe atom with, in the cases used here as examples (see below), the van der Waals properties of a sp^3 carbon and a charge of $+1$ is placed at each grid point and two forces (interactions) related to steric and charge interactions are calculated for each molecule (step 4). Thus, all the computed values become a 'fingerprint' for each molecule. All values are stored in a large data matrix (see Figure 5.5) where each

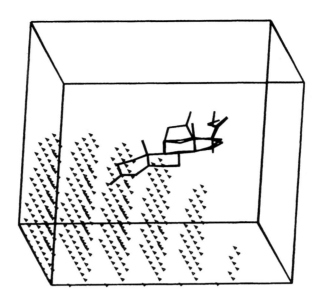

Figure 5.7 The 3D box, with partially depicted grid points, used in the 3D-QSAR example in Section 5.6. Steroids I and II are shown with hydrogens omitted for clarity.

row is related to a compound. Each of the two sets of calculated forces (steric and electrostatic, respectively) are usually referred to as a field. Thus, in this example we have a steric field and an electrostatic field. To delineate the relationship between biological activity and structural description, where the number of variables greatly exceeds the number of compounds, the method of PLS is used (step 6). Again, CV is used to judge the predictivity and statistical quality of the derived 3D-QSAR model by leaving a portion of the compounds out from the data set and building a model with the remaining compounds (see Section 5.5 for more details on CV). The results of a 3D-QSAR model are usually depicted as 3D contour maps. Each grid point in the box spanned around the molecules is associated with, in this case, two coefficients from the PLS analysis. One coefficient is related to the steric field and the other coefficient is related to the electrostatic field. Each of the two sets of coefficients are displayed as iso-contour maps (step 7). In most cases, it is not a trivial task to choose the appropriate iso-contour level in order to create a meaningful picture. The interpretation of contour maps are discussed in the following examples.

5.6.2   Application to steroids

Here the 3D-QSAR methodology will be exemplified by a data set of 30 steroids with affinities for human corticosteroid-binding globulins (CBG) where $\log(K)$ have been used as dependent variable which means that higher values indicate higher affinity for the receptor:

$$\log(K) = c_i E_{\text{steric}}(i) + c_j E_{\text{elec}}(j)$$

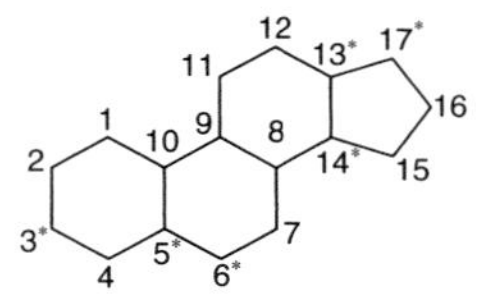

Figure 5.8 Steroid skeleton with atomic numbering system. Atoms indicated with an asterisk were used to superimpose steroids 2–30 in Figure 5.9 onto steroid 1.

where c_i and c_j are coefficients for grid points i and j, respectively, and E_{steric} and E_{elec} are the corresponding steric and electrostatic interaction energies.

This example is often used as a benchmark in 3D-QSAR investigations. Since all the compounds possess a common substructure, the steroid skeleton, the numbered atoms containing an asterisk in Figure 5.8 were used to superimpose compounds 2–30 onto compound 1 (see Figure 5.9).

Compounds 1–21 were used as training set (step 5) and the remaining steroids (22–30) were used as test set for which the affinities should be predicted by the derived 3D-QSAR model (step 8). A 3D-grid with an internal separation of $2.0\,\text{Å}$ between grid points was constructed based on the training set. Two fields (steric and electrostatic) were computed. Each steroid was defined by 1600 variables. A so-called leave-one-out CV scheme was used to determine the number of relevant PLS components. In a leave-one-out procedure one compound is held out and the remaining compounds are used to develop a model. The activity of the held-out compound is then predicted by the model. Then, all but the second molecule are used to generate a model that predicts the activity of the second molecule and so on. This procedure resulted in two significant PLS components. The Q^2 value was 0.791 for the training set and Q^2 is defined in equation (5.27).

$$Q^2 = 1.0 - \left\{ \frac{\Sigma(\text{Pred}_i - \text{Exp}_i)^2}{\Sigma(\text{Exp}_i - \text{Exp}_m)^2} \right\} \tag{5.27}$$

where Pred_i and Exp_i are the predicted and experimental activity for the held-out compound i, respectively. Exp_m is the mean value of the experimental activities of all compounds and the summation in equation (5.27) runs over all compounds.

The R^2 value, where R^2 is defined analogous to Q^2, for the training set compounds was 0.901, and RMSE (root mean squared error) = 0.361. For the test set compounds 22–30, the RMSE was 0.471, which is a value indicating that the model has fair predictivity. The contours for the electrostatic interactions are here displayed as an iso-contour map depicting the 25% most influential areas (Figure 5.10).

How can these iso-contour maps (Figure 5.10) be interpreted and used for the development of new compounds? Let us examine the resulting negative electrostatic contour map (colored red) from the 3D-QSAR model based on steroids 1–21. The red region is mainly concentrated around (outside) the three position of the steroids. This location coincides very well with the keto moiety present in a large number of the steroids in the training set. Thus changing the electrostatic nature of this oxygen atom into something less negative or, to some extent, the direction of the oxygen atom, as in steroids 2, 3, 5, 9, 16, 17 and 18, will result in compounds with lower affinity. The steric iso-contour maps can be interpreted in a similar manner. Thus areas of positive steric regions (green), mainly centered around position 21 (the position at the end of the substituent on position 17) indicate that

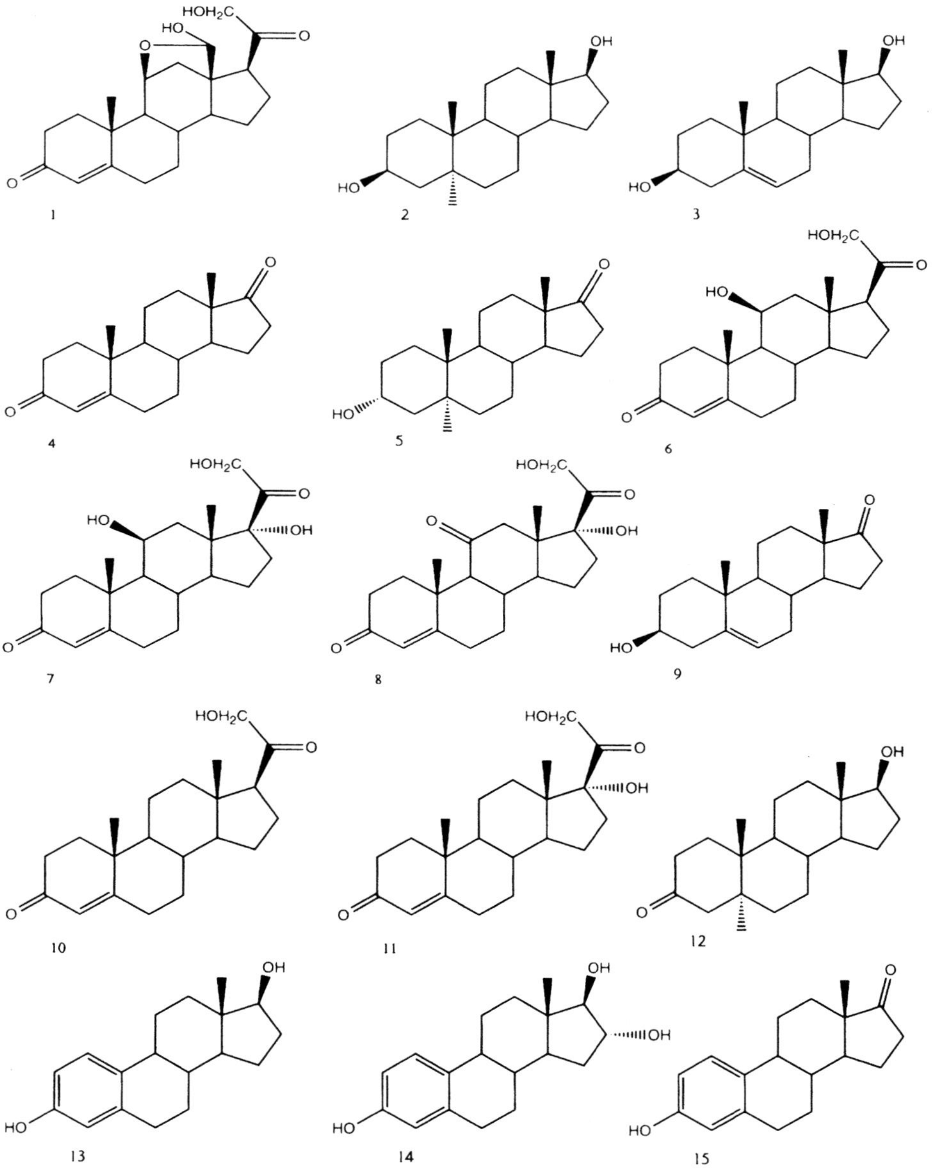

Figure 5.9 (Continued)

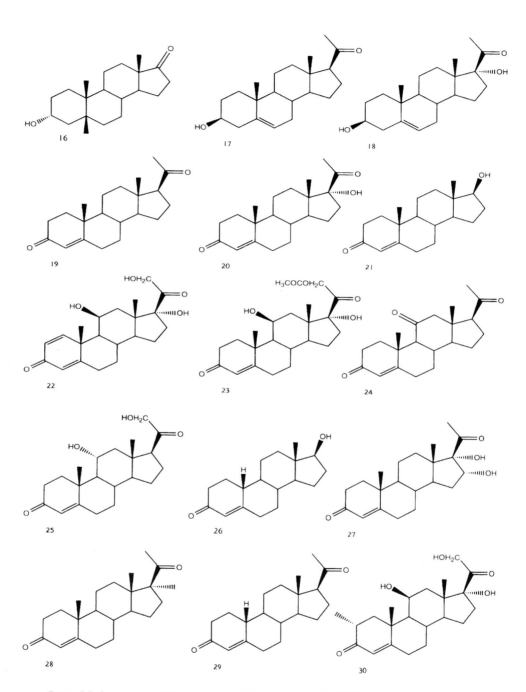

Figure 5.9 Structures of the steroids 1–30 used in the 3D-QSAR analysis in Section 5.6.

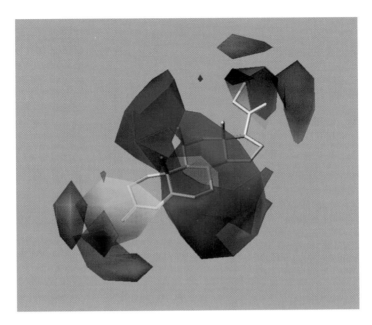

Figure 5.10 Contour map resulting from the 3D-QSAR analysis of steroids 1–21. The contours depict the 25% most influential areas (red and blue colors correspond to negative and positive electrostatic areas, respectively, while the yellow and green colors correspond to negative and positive steric areas). Steroids 1 and 11 are shown with hydrogens omitted for clarity.

it is favorable to have a substituent or substructure present close to these regions, e.g. steroids 6–8, 10–11 and 17–20.

5.6.3 Application to dopamine D_1 agonists

In the previous section, all compounds possessed a common substructure and the alignment procedure was not a problem. In this section, the investigated compounds are much more diverse (Figure 5.11) although they all contain two common elements that are of crucial importance for dopamine D_1 activity, namely an non-aromatic nitrogen atom and its electron lone-pair and an aromatic centre (Wilcox *et al.* 1998). With this knowledge at hand one may align the compounds in reasonable manner for a 3D-QSAR analysis. However, since we do not know the exact positions of the compounds, a field-fit method will be used here to construct the final alignments for the compounds in relation to a reference compound. The most potent compound is selected (in this case compound 6-Br-APB) as reference. The field-fit method operates in the following way. For each compound A:

1   The sum of the squared differences between the calculated interactions energies (steric and electrostatic) at each grid point for the investigated

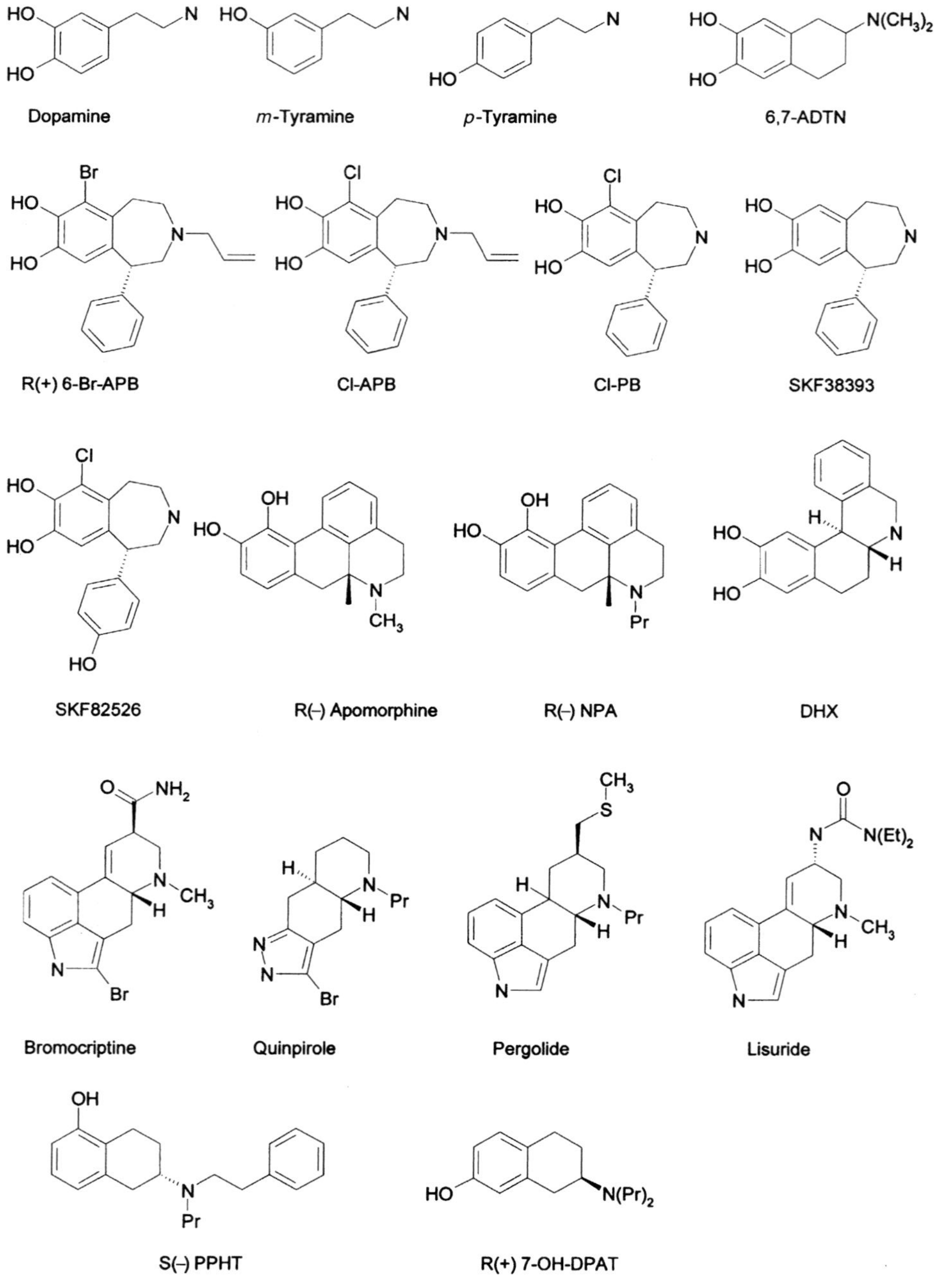

Figure 5.11 Structures of dopamine D$_1$ agonists.

compound and the corresponding values of the reference compound (in this case 6-Br-APB) are computed:

$$\text{Error(A)} = \sum_i (E_{\text{steric}}(i, \text{compound A}) - E_{\text{steric}}(i, \text{ref. compound}))^2$$
$$+ \sum_j (E_{\text{elec}}(j, \text{compound A}) - E_{\text{elec}}(j, \text{ref. compound}))^2$$

2   Compound A is then translated in the x, y and z directions of the co-ordinate system as well as rotated around the x-, y- and z-axis so that the computed error (Error(A)) is minimized.
3   The orientation of compound A corresponding to the smallest error is then used for the subsequent development of a 3D-QSAR model.

The training set of 12 compounds was selected using a field-based dissimilarity method. Thus, after the field-based alignment of the compounds, a PCA was performed on the two fields (steric and electrostatic) and 5 PCs were calculated. The 5-score values from the PCs of each compound were then used to select 12 compounds that were the farthest apart and, consequently, covered the field properties of the investigated data set most uniformly. The remaining 6-test set compounds were predicted with a RMSE value of 0.547, which implies that the derived model can predict new compounds with reasonable accuracy. The final 3D-QSAR model (4 PLS components) based on all 18 compounds had a good correlation ($Q^2 = 0.803, R^2 = 0.990, \text{RMSE} = 0.141$). In this example, the logarithm of the affinity to the D_1 receptor was used, i e. $-\log(K_i)$, which means that higher values indicate higher affinity to the receptor:

$$-\log(K_i) = c_i E_{\text{steric}}(i) + c_j E_{\text{elec}}(j)$$

Figure 5.12 shows the contour map of the model and indicates some interesting areas of importance. Negative electrostatic charge (colored red) in the region around the hydroxy groups, which can be attributed most certainly to hydrogen-bonding, favors high affinity. With respect to steric interactions, the area around the phenyl substituent of the 7-membered ring (colored green) is favorable with respect to steric bulk while the region around the non-aromatic nitrogen atom is not suited for placement of large substituents (yellow area).

5.6.4   Application to human rhinovirus

Sometimes uncertainties with respect to alignments of the ligands under investigation may be eliminated, or at least greatly reduced, with the existence of ligand/protein complexes. In this example of some antiviral compounds of human rhinovirus 14, there are complexes available from X-ray crystallography. Originally, Klebe and Abraham (1993) investigated this set of eight compounds using CoMFA.

The X-ray geometries of the ligands show that the four compounds (top set) with an 8 atom side-chain connecting the oxazole ring with the phenyl ring have opposite orientations compared with the four compounds (bottom set) with

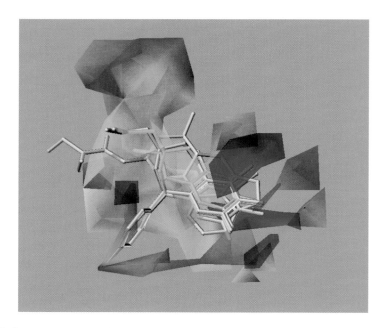

Figure 5.12 Contour map resulting from the 3D-QSAR analysis of the dopamine D_1 agonists. The contours depict the most influential areas (red and blue colors correspond to negative and positive electrostatic areas, respectively, while the yellow and green colors correspond to negative and positive steric areas). Compounds 6,7-ADTN, Cl-APB, Cl-PB, 6-Br-APB (bold structure), LISURIDE and SKF82526 are depicted.

a 6 atom side-chain connecting the corresponding rings (Figure 5.13). Without knowledge of the X-ray geometries of these compounds it is rather unlikely that the researcher would have suggested the X-ray orientation mode (Figure 5.14). Rather, the investigator would probably have tried to superimpose some 'obvious' pharmacophoric groups, such as the three rings present in all eight structures, or some maximum common substructure, such as the moiety consisting of the oxazoline ring and the pentyl phenyl ether group (Figure 5.15). In this example, we shall examine both choices of alignment and try to derive models for both orientations in order to see the consequences of our choices of alignment.

It is possible to derive a CoMFA model for the eight compounds based on the X-ray orientation mode (Figure 5.14) that have a $Q^2 = 0.515$ (leave-one-out validation, 3 PLS components) and an appreciable $R^2 = 0.997$. However, on the other hand, it is also possible to derive a corresponding model based on the maximum common substructure mode (Figure 5.15) of orientation: $Q^2 = 0.514$ (leave-one-out validation, 2 PLS components) and $R^2 = 0.976$. Furthermore, dividing the compounds into a training set and a test set each consisting of four compounds one can develop 2 CoMFA models that have quite reasonable predictive ability considering the very small training and test sets that we have available. The RMSE values for the test set are 1.260 and 1.280 for the X-ray and maximum common substructure orientation-mode, respectively. So, from this perspective, it

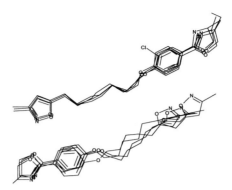

Figure 5.13 Structures of the human rhinovirus 14 antiviral compounds.

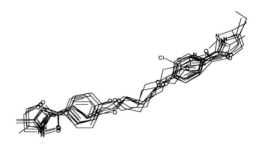

Figure 5.14 Superimpositioning of the human rhinovirus 14 antiviral compounds according to X-ray crystallography.

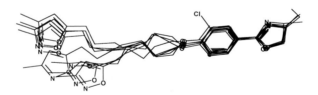

Figure 5.15 Superimpositioning of the human rhinovirus 14 antiviral compounds using atomistic substructure fitting.

would not have been possible either to distinguish between the two alternatives. Only further predictions of new compounds with failures and successes would, in the absence of the X-ray structure information, possibly give the researcher enough insight into the orientation problem to understand that the two series of compounds orient in opposite manners.

This example highlights that models can be developed with good statistical quality and predictive ability, but predict 'correct' observations from an 'incorrect' basis or understanding of the problem. Thus, it is important also to design experiments that challenges the models rather than confirms them.

5.6.5   Pros and cons

One advantage with 3D-QSAR studies is that the same protocol, i.e. steps 1–8 mentioned in Section 5.6.1, can be used for every new problem of interest. Also, the method can handle data sets to be investigated that contain structurally different compounds and predict new compounds of potential interest containing slightly different scaffolds than originally present among the training set compounds.

A limitation of the technique is that the models are only predictive in 3D space, which have been covered by substructures of sufficient variation. Thus, if in a certain position only a methyl-, ethyl-, and a propyl group have been present in the investigated structures, the 3D-QSAR model cannot make a reasonable prediction for the longer alkyl side chains such as butyl, pentyl and so on. A QSAR model based on some physico-chemical description, such as the 3D-dimensions of the side chain, can at least make a prediction for the latter group of substituents even though it represents an extrapolation. One interesting aspect of the contour maps of the derived 3D-QSAR models is their relationship to important drug–receptor interactions. Let us consider a case where the 3D-structure of the active site in a receptor is known. The compounds investigated in the study have been aligned by docking them into the active site. Each drug–receptor complex has then been brought into a common reference system by superimposing the receptor protein in each case onto each other. The compounds in their aligned orientations have then been taken out from the complex and used to derive a 3D-QSAR model. When the contour maps, which have the investigated compounds as reference, are overlaid on the drug–receptor complexes the spacial positioning of the most important parts of the contour maps may, in favorable cases, be located onto certain amino acid residues of the receptor protein. Then, this provides a description of the importance of various drug–receptor interactions. Thus, protein chemistry and biology, biotechnology, molecular modeling, conformational analysis, computational chemistry (to derive charges and other descriptors) and QSAR form a closely interlinked interdisciplinary entity in drug development.

5.7   EXPERIMENTAL DESIGN

5.7.1   Factorial design and principal properties

In order to be able to create a useful QSAR with good predictability, one wants the compounds included in the model (usually called the training set) to cover a large number of substituents and/or structural variation. However, at the same time it is desirable to keep the number of compounds to be synthesized and tested at a minimum. To obtain as much information as possible with a minimum of observations, one needs a protocol (experimental or statistical design) where the structures are varied in a carefully selected manner. Such protocols are found in the field of experimental design. There are several different types of protocols available but most often are factorial design schemes used due, in part, to the ease of evaluating these set-ups.

In a factorial design, each variable is assigned to a certain number of levels. A two level factorial design, which is most frequently used in chemistry, with four variables (a, b, c, d) involves 16 experiments (2^4). Each variable is designated a high level $(+)$ and a low level $(-)$ and the protocol is given in Table 5.3. The outcome of the 16 experiments may then be evaluated by some least squares method (like PLS).

Chemical substituents, however, are characterized by a large number of physico-chemical properties. To perform a complete two-level factorial or fractional factorial (reduced scheme) design using the original variables would involve too many compounds and be practically impossible. One method to circumvent this problem involves utilization of so called 'principal properties' (PPs), which are principal component derived variables (scores) from the original physico-chemical parameters. However, since the PPs are not continuous due to a limited number of substituents, it is not possible to construct a factorial design with exactly defined high and low levels. Instead, the substituents are classified according to the size and sign of their PPs. Table 5.2 shows the three first PPs of a number of aromatic substituents.

Practically, however, PPs are usually derived separately for each study since the objective is to span the chemical property space of the available substituents for the investigated compounds as effectively as possible. This will then, in turn, help to select compounds having a large variation in the mentioned physico-chemical property space. However, since different sets of substituents are used for different investigations and the purpose of each PCA is to explain as much information as possible with each PC the numerical values of the PPs may differ considerably between different PCAs (see Tables 5.2 and 5.4). Again, one must look upon these values (PPs) as guidance when selecting substituents having a large difference and variation in physico-chemical properties and pay less attention to the exact numerical values. The QSAR equations that are subsequently

Table 5.3 Experimental design protocol for a two level factorial design

#	a	b	c	d
1	+	+	+	+
2	−	+	+	+
3	+	−	+	+
4	−	−	+	+
5	+	+	−	+
6	−	+	−	+
7	+	−	−	+
8	−	−	−	+
9	+	+	+	−
10	−	+	+	−
11	+	−	+	−
12	−	−	+	−
13	+	+	−	−
14	−	+	−	−
15	+	−	−	−
16	−	−	−	−

derived from the selected compounds, the training set, are based on the original physico-chemical variables. However, an alternative approach is to use the PPs directly as variables in the QSAR model. In this case, all substituents must have the same framework. Thus, one must include all the substituents to be used both for the training set compounds as well as for those compounds that are to be predicted from the derived QSAR model in the PCA when one calculates the PPs, since the exact numerical values will be used in this case to derive the QSAR equation.

5.7.2   Applications of factorial design

An example of using PPs as design variables for some substituted benzamides (**5.11**) (the same compounds as used in Section 5.5) is given below. The number of different available 3- and 5-substituents were few (F, CN, NO_2, Cl, H, OH, NH_2, Me, OMe, I, Br, Et, n-Pr, n-Bu) in this retrospective study and the PPs derived for this subset are shown in Table 5.4.

The fractional factorial design protocol and the choice of substituents are listed in Table 5.5. The 16 selected compounds were then used to construct a model by which the activities of the remaining 54 benzamides were predicted using PLS.

Three significant components were extracted. They explained 89% of the variance in binding affinity. The model explained 61% of the variance of the biological data for the test set of 54 benzamides (**5.11**). Figure 5.16 shows a plot a calculated vs. experimental activities. The substituents R_3 and R_5 were described by a total of 38 variables, i.e. the parameters σ_m, σ_p, $\mathfrak{I}$, $\mathfrak{R}$, π, MR, L, B_1 and B_5 (cf. Table 5.1), the corresponding squared values and indicator values for R_2 and stereochemistry (*), in the same way as in the PLS analysis in Section 5.5. As can be seen in Figure 5.16, the small training set predicts the activity quite well and covers a large activity

Table 5.4 Design levels for the R_3- and R_5-substituents used in retrospective study of some benzamides (**5.11**)

Substituent	PP_1	PP_2	FDL^a
F	2.17	0.16	++
CN	0.79	2.51	
NO_2	0.56	2.94	
Cl	0.35	1.34	
H	2.46	−0.65	+−
OH	2.11	−1.46	
NH_2	1.92	−2.56	
Me	0.52	−0.62	
OMe	0.09	−1.29	
I	−1.34	1.65	−+
Br	−0.28	1.57	
Et	−1.30	−0.72	−−
n-Pr	−2.56	−0.69	
n-Bu	−4.38	−0.93	

Note
a   FDL = factorial design levels.

Table 5.5 Experimental design protocol and selected substituents for the benzamides (**5.11**)[a]

#	R_3		R_5		R_2	R_3	R_5	R_2
	a	b	c	d	abcd			
1	+	+	+	+	+	Cl	Cl	OH
2	−	+	+	+	−	Br	OH	H
3	+	−	+	+	(−)	OMe	Cl	OH
4	−	−	+	+	+	Pr	Cl	OH
5	+	+	−	+	(−)	NO_2	Br	OH
6	−	+	−	+	(+)	Br	Br	H
7	+	−	−	+	+	Me	Br	OH
8	−	−	−	+	−	Et	Br	H
9	+	+	+	−	−	Br	OMe	H
10	−	+	+	−	(+)	I	OMe	H
11	+	−	+	−	(+)	Me	OMe	H
12	−	−	+	−	(−)	Pr	Me	OH
13	+	+	−	−	+	Cl	Pr	OH
14	−	+	−	−	(−)	Br	Et	OH
15	+	−	−	−	(−)	H	Et	OH
16	−	−	−	−	+	Et	Et	OH

Note
a   Parenthesis indicate a deviation from the protocol in selecting the substituent.

span which is quite frequently the consequence of the experimental design procedure. The model also predicts the remaining 54 benzamides in the test set reasonably well.

The second example is related to a set of β-adrenergic blockers analyzed by Norinder. The 101 compounds available are of the phenoxypropanolamine type (**5.12**) with a reasonable structural variation. Again a two-level PP fractional factorial design was applied and eight compounds were selected according to the design protocol (Table 5.8). Substituents R_1 and X were treated with indicator variables since only two choices existed in each case $\{R_1 = t\text{-Bu}(+1), i\text{-Pr}(-1);$ X $=$ direct attached $(-1), NH (+1)\}$. Substituents R and R_2 were characterized by the following physico-chemical variables: R $= MR, L, B_1, B_5$; $R_2 = \mathfrak{F}, \mathfrak{R}, \pi, MR, L, B_1, B_5$. See Tables 5.6 and 5.7 for the calculated PPs of R- and R_2-substituents, respectively, using PCA on the original physico-chemical parameters.

The PLS analysis resulted in three significant components which explained 92% of the variance of the biological data in the training set (the eight compounds in Table 5.9). The model explained 67% of the variance of the biological data of the remaining 93 compounds. The model predicts compounds A–D (Table 5.9) to be interesting new structures with high activity.

If one uses all of the 101 available compounds to derive a model the same four compounds (A–D) are predicted by this model to possess high activity. Thus, not very much new information was added to the model by incorporating an additional 93 compounds, which is also indicated by the fact that the PLS regression coefficients were virtually the same for both models. This further proves the power of using experimental design to cover the available structural variation by a small number of compounds in a good manner.

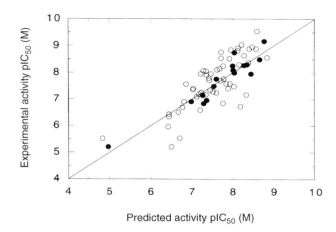

Figure 5.16 Plot of predicted vs. experimental [³H]spiperone displacing activity (pIC₅₀; M) of substituted salicylamides (**5.11**). The QSAR was made with the PLS method as described in Section 5.5. Solid and open circles represent the training set and test set compounds, respectively.

Table 5.6 Calculated score vectors for R-substituents in phenoxypropanolamine derivatives (**5.12**)

Substituent	PC_1	PC_2	FDL^a
H	−4.06	−1.00	−−
$(CH_2)_2OCH_3$	−0.42	−0.73	
CH_2CHCH_2	−0.33	−0.36	
$(CH_2)_2CH_3$	−0.30	−0.23	
CH_3	−2.60	0.18	−+
CH_2CH_3	−1.24	−0.13	
$CH(CH_2)_2$	−0.95	−0.04	
$CH(CH_3)_2$	−0.52	0.98	
$(CH_2)_3CH_3$	1.02	−0.53	+−
$CH_2C_6H_5$	1.83	−0.46	
$(CH_2)_4CH_3$	2.15	−0.72	
$(CH_2)_5CH_3$	3.31	−0.93	
$CH_2CH(CH_3)_2$	0.45	2.99	++
C_6H_5	0.80	0.18	
$CH(CH_2)_4$	0.86	0.81	

Note
a   Designated factorial design levels.

Thus, using the predictive power of these models one can design compounds with the desired potency in a very efficient way, which is advantageous in the drug development phase. This also shows the usefulness of statistical design whereby structural variation is performed in an organized manner. These methods provide a broad basis for constructing a QSAR with good predictability, which makes it possible to keep the number of compounds to be synthesized and tested at a minimum.

Table 5.7 Calculated score vectors for R_2-substituents in phenoxypropanolamine derivatives (**5.12**)

Substituent	PC_1	PC_2	FDL^a
CH_2CHCH_2	−3.10	−0.92	− −
$(CH_2)_2CH_3$	−3.04	−0.76	
CH_2CH_3	−1.62	−1.09	
OCH_2CH_3	−1.20	−0.52	
SCH_3	−1.43	0.44	− +
I	−0.92	2.21	
$COCH_3$	0.00	1.28	
OCH_3	0.19	−0.79	+ −
CH_3	0.42	−1.52	
OH	2.46	−1.28	
H	2.58	−2.48	
Br	0.27	1.75	+ +
Cl	0.91	1.20	
NO_2	1.65	2.75	

Note
a Designated factorial design levels.

Table 5.8 Fractional factorial design protocol and choice of training set compounds of phenoxypropanolamine derivatives (**5.12**)

#	R		R_1^a	R_2		X^b	R	R_2
	a	b	c	abc	ab	bc		
1	+	+	+	+	+	(+)	$CH(CH_2)_4$	Cl
2	−	+	+	−	−	+	CH_2CH_3	CH_2CHCH_2
3	+	−	+	−	−	−	$(CH_2)_5CH_3$	CH_2CHCH_2
4	−	−	+	+	(+)	(−)	H	H
5	+	+	−	(−)	+	−	C_6H_5	Cl
6	−	+	−	+	−	−	$(CH_2)_2CH_3$	OCH_3
7	+	−	−	+	−	+	$(CH_2)_3CH_3$	CH_3
8	−	−	−	(−)	(+)	+	CH_2CHCH_2	CH_3

Parenthesis indicate a choice for the training set of a substituent which deviates from the protocol.
Notes
a R_1 has only two choices: (+) = $C(CH_3)_3$, (−) = $CH(CH_3)_2$.
b X has only two choices: (+) = −NH−, (−) = (da).

Table 5.9 Predicted activities for compounds A–D of phenoxypropanolamine derivatives (**5.12**)

Compound	R	R_1	R_2	X	Pred. Act.
A	$(CH_2)_3CH_3$	$C(CH_3)_3$	I	NH	7.54
B	$(CH_2)_3CH_3$	$C(CH_3)_3$	Br	NH	7.42
C	$(CH_2)_3CH_3$	$C(CH_3)_3$	$(CH_2)_2CH_3$	NH	7.43
D	$(CH_2)_3CH_3$	$C(CH_3)_3$	Cl	NH	7.34

(5.12)

5.7.3   Combinatorial chemistry and experimental design

Nature manages to make large numbers of diverse compounds, e.g. proteins, from a limited number of building blocks. Combinatorial chemistry, mimicking this process, has evolved from producing large libraries of complex mixtures of oligomers to producing single drug-like molecules by parallel synthesis. Thus, it might be argued that combinatorial chemistry nowadays can eliminate synthetic capacity as a limitation in the lead finding and optimization once synthesis, isolation, analysis and data handling has effectively been automated. The number of possible endproducts increases rapidly with the number of building blocks and the number of positions varied which, in turn, effects resources like available physical space, time and money that all put limits to the size of a combinatorial library in practice (Figure 5.17).

A number of objectives may be envisaged for a combinatorial library:

1   Create a focused library of limited size with pure compounds for lead optimization.
2   Create a diverse library complementing already existing libraries in sparsely populated chemical space ('hole-filling').
3   Create a highly diverse general library, possibly as mixtures, for lead identification.

Experimental design can reinforce the utility and effectiveness of combinatorial chemistry to make it more than a 'numbers game'. The products obtained should have the properties needed for efficacy as well as for acceptable bioavailability and low toxicity. The reagents (building blocks) used should be available at reasonable costs and have the required reactivity for the specific chemistries. The following question comes to mind: Should one make the diversity selection in reagent chemical space or in the final product space (cf. Figure 5.17)? There are distinct advantages in diversity selection using the former set, namely, that, in most cases, the reagents are smaller compounds, both with respect to size and molecular weight, which permits easier, faster and more extensive characterization using quantum chemical calculations, should this be necessary. Besides, optimized diverse sets of reagents of different classes (Y_n, Z_m, etc.) can be utilized in reactions with several scaffolds (X) to produce many libraries, which makes the effectiveness even larger. Also, the combinatorial explosion is kept under control, i.e. there is no need for an explicit enumeration (creation) of all the compounds of the library, which simplifies the diversity analysis. Investigations have been performed that suggest that indeed it is possible to work in reagent (building block) chemical space without loosing diversity in product space.

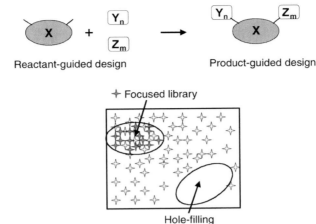

Reactant-guided design   Product-guided design

Figure 5.17 Combinatorial synthesis by reaction of scaffold X with reagents Y_n and Z_m to produce a library of n·m products by n + m reactions. Below is shown the product space with examples of a focused library and the need for hole-filling of the library.

Think of creating a library consisting of three building blocks A, B and C. Let us assume that we, at our disposal, have 50 different A:s, 100 different B:s and 75 different C:s. Evaluation in reagent space is rather trivial, but diversity selection in product space would involve calculating descriptors for $50 \times 100 \times 75 = 375\,000$ compounds. In many cases, the size of such a library would not permit us to perform adequate analysis using available software and techniques.

Thus, experimental design is as important as before considering the magnitude of compounds that potentially can be synthesized and tested by current high throughput techniques.

FURTHER READING

Box, G.E.P., Hunter, W.G. and Hunter, J.S. (1978) *Statistics for Experimenters*. New York: Wiley.

Cramer, R.D., Patterson, D.E. and Bunce, J.D. (1988) Comparative molecular field analysis (CoMFA). I. Effect of shape on binding of steroids to carrier proteins. *J. Am. Chem. Soc.*, **110**, 5959–5967.

Cruciani, G. and Watson, K.A. (1994) Comparative molecular field analysis using GRID force-field and GOLPE variable selection methods in a study of inhibitors of glycogen phosphorylase b. *J. Med. Chem.*, **37**, 2589–2601.

de Paulis, T., Hall, H., Kumar, Y., Rämsby, S., Ögren, S.O. and Högberg, T. (1990) Potential antipsychotic agents. 6. Synthesis and antidopaminergic properties of substituted N-(1-benzyl-4-piperidinyl)salicylamides and related compounds. QSAR based design of more active members. *Eur. J. Med. Chem.*, **25**, 507–517.

Dean, P.M. (1987) *Molecular foundations of drug–receptor interaction*. Cambridge: Cambridge University Press.

Doweyko, A.M. (1988) The hypothetical active site lattice. An approach to modelling sites from data on inhibitor molecules. *J. Med. Chem.*, **31**, 1396–1406.

Fauchére, J.L. (ed.) (1989) *QSAR: Quantitative Structure–Activity Relationships in Drug Design.* New York: Alan R. Liss.

Ghose, A., Crippen, G., Revankar, G., McKernan, P., Smee, D. and Robbins, R. (1989) Analysis of the in vitro activity of certain ribonucleosides against parainfluenza virus using a novel computer-aided molecular modeling procedure. *J. Med. Chem.*, **32**, 746–756.

Gupta, S.P. (1989) QSAR studies on drugs acting at the central nervous system. *Chem. Rev.*, **89**, 1765–1800.

Hansch, C. and Leo, A.J. (1979) *Substituent Constants for Correlation Analysis in Chemistry and Biology.* New York: Wiley.

Jain, A.N., Koile, K. and Chapman, D. (1994) Compass: Predicting biological activities from molecular surface properties. Performance comparisons on a steroid benchmark. *J. Med. Chem.*, **37**, 2315–2327.

Klebe, G. and Abraham, U. (1993) On the prediction of binding properties of drug molecules by comparative molecular field analysis. *J. Med. Chem.*, **36**, 70–80.

Kubinyi, H. (1993) QSAR: Hansch analysis and related approaches. In *Methods and Principles in Medicinal Chemistry*, edited by R. Mannhold., P. Krogsgaard-Larsen and H. Timmermann. Weinheim: VCH. This book provides an excellent overview of the different techniques in the field.

Kubinyi, H. (ed.) (1993) *3D QSAR in Drug Design. Theory, Methods and Applications.* Leiden: ESCOM Science Publishers.

Kubinyi, H. (ed.) (1998) *3D QSAR in Drug Design. Volume 2 Ligand–Protein Interactions and Molecular Similarity.* Dordrecht: Kluwer Academic Publishers.

Kubinyi, H. (ed.) (1998) *3D QSAR in Drug Design. Volume 3 Recent Advances.* Dordrecht: Kluwer Academic Publishers.

Linusson, A., Gottfries, J., Lindgren, F. and Wold, S. (2000) Statistical molecular design of building blocks for combinatorial chemistry. *J. Med. Chem.*, **43**, 1320–1328.

Nelson Smith, R., Hansch, C., Kim, K.H., Omiya, B., Fukumura, G., Dias Selassie, C., Jow, P.Y.C., Blaney, J.M. and Langridge, R. (1982) The use of crystallography, graphics, and quantitative structure–activity relationships in the analysis of the papain hydrolysis of X-phenyl hippurates. *Arch. Biochem. Biophys.*, **215**, 319–328.

Norinder, U. (1991) An experimental design based quantitative structure–activity relationship study on β-adrenergic blocking agents using PLS. *Drug. Des. Discov.*, **8**, 127–136.

Norinder, U. and Högberg, T. (1991) QSAR on substituted salicylamides using PLS with implementation of 3D-MEP descriptors. *Quant. Struct.-Act. Relat.*, **10**, 1–5.

Norinder, U. and Högberg, T. (1992) A quantitative structure–activity relationship for some dopamine D_2 antagonists of benzamide type. *Acta Pharm. Nord.*, **4**, 73–78.

Norinder, U. (1996) 3D-QSAR investigation of the tripos benchmark steroids and some protein-tyrosine kinase inhibitors of styrene type using the TDQ approach. *J. Chemometrics*, **10**, 533–545.

Norinder, U. (1998) Recent progress in CoMFA methodology and related techniques. *Perspec. Drug. Des. Dis.*, **12/14**, 25–39.

Perun, T.J. and Propst, C.L. (1989) *Computer-Aided Drug Design. Methods and Applications.* New York: Marcel Dekker.

Pliska, V., Testa, B. and van de Waterbeemd, H. (1996) Lipophilicity in drug action and toxicology. In *Methods and Principles in Medicinal Chemistry*, edited by R. Mannhold and H. Kubinyi. Weinheim: VCH.

Ramsden, C.A. (ed.) (1990) Quantitative drug design. In *Comprehensive Medicinal Chemistry*, Vol. 3, edited by C. Hansch, P. G. Sammes and J. B. Taylor. Oxford: Pergamon

Press. This book provides a full and critical account of all aspects of QSAR by experts in the field.

Tsai, R.-S., Carrupt, P.-A., Testa, B., Gaillard, P., El Tayar, N. and Högberg, T. (1993) Effects of solvation on the ionization and conformation of raclopride and other antidopaminergic 6-Methoxysalicylamides: insight into the pharmacophore. *J. Med. Chem.*, **36**, 196–204.

Wermuth, C.G. (ed.) (1993) *Trends in QSAR and Molecular Modeling 92*. Leiden: ESCOM Science Publishers.

Wilcox, R.E., Tseng, T., Brusniak, M.-Y. K., Ginsburg, B., Pearlman, R.S., Teeter, M., DuRand, Starr, C.S. and Neve, K.A. (1998) CoMFA-based prediction of agonist affinities at recombinant D1 vs. D2 dopamine receptors. *J. Med. Chem.*, **41**, 4385–4399.

Wold, S. (1979) Cross-validatory estimation of the number of components in factor and principal components models. *Technometrics*, **20**, 379–405.

Wold, S. and Dunn III, W.J. (1983) Multivariate quantitative structure–activity relationships (QSAR). Conditions for their applicability. *J. Chem. Inf. Comp. Sci.*, **23**, 6–13.

Young, R.C., Mitchell, R.C., Brown, T.H., Ganellin, C.R., Griffiths, R., Jones, M., Rana, K.K., Saunders, D., Smith, I.R., Sore, N.E. and Wilks, T.J. (1988) Development of a new physicochemical model for brain penetration and its application to the design of centrally acting H_2 receptor histamines antagonists. *J. Med. Chem.*, **31**, 656–671.

Chapter 6

Receptors: structure, function and pharmacology

Hans Bräuner-Osborne

6.1 INTRODUCTION

Communication between cells are mediated by compounds such as neurotransmitters and hormones which upon release will activate a receptor in the target cells. This communication is of pivotal importance for many physiological functions and dysfunction in cell communication pathways often have severe consequences. Many diseases are thus caused by dysfunction in the pathways and in these cases, drugs designed to act at the receptors have beneficial effects. Receptors are thus very important drug targets.

The definition of receptors is constantly debated, in particular as a consequence of the ever increasing knowledge of the many varying ways cells communicate. However, in general it is agreed that a receptor consist of one or more macromolecule(s) which upon binding of a signaling molecule will cause a cellular response. As will be exemplified in Chapters 9–11, the structural requirements for the signaling molecules are very specific. The receptor–ligand interaction has often been described by the 'lock and key' model. Likewise, the cellular responses mediated by the receptors are also very specific. Accordingly, receptors are classified by the signaling molecule, e.g. 'glutamate receptor', and by the signaling pathway. The latter is divided into four major superfamilies: (1) G-protein coupled receptors; (2) ligand-gated ion channels; (3) tyrosine kinase receptors; and (4) nuclear receptors. The structure and function of these families will be discussed in detail in this chapter.

The first receptors were cloned in the mid-eighties and since then hundreds of receptor genes have been identified. Based on the sequence of the human genome it is currently estimated that more than one thousand human receptors exist. Almost all receptors are heterogeneous, meaning that several receptor subtypes are activated by the same signaling molecule. One such example is the excitatory neurotransmitter glutamate for which 23 receptors have been cloned. As shown in Figure 6.1, the amino acid sequence of these receptors vary and the receptors form subgroups which, as will be discussed in Chapter 9, share pharmacology.

As can also be seen in Figure 6.1, the same signaling molecule can act on both G-protein coupled receptors and ligand-gated ion channels. One of the reasons for the heterogeneity is that it allows cells to be regulated in subtle ways. For example, whereas the fast synaptic action potential is initiated by glutamate receptors of the ligand-gated ion channel family, these receptors are by themselves regulated

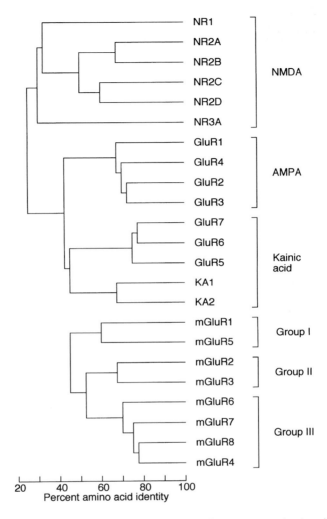

Figure 6.1 Phylogenetic tree showing the amino acid sequence identity between cloned mammalian glutamate receptors. The subgroups according to receptor pharmacology has been noted. The NMDA, AMPA, and kainic acid receptors belong to the superfamily of ligand-gated ion channels whereas the metabotropic glutamate receptors (mGluR1-8) belong to the superfamily of G-protein coupled receptors (Adapted from Bräuner-Osborne *et al.*, *J. Med. Chem.*, **43**, 2000, 2621).

by the slower and longer acting glutamate receptors from the G-protein coupled receptor family. The action on these two receptor families is actually shared by a number of other neurotransmitters such as GABA (Chapter 9), acetylcholine (Chapter 10) and serotonin (Chapter 11).

The receptor is activated upon release of the signaling molecule and it is evidently equally important to stop the signaling again. This is often achieved by transporters situated in the vicinity of the receptor which will remove the signaling molecule from the extracellular to the intracellular space, where it is either stored or degraded. Blockade of a transporter will cause an elevation of the extracellular concentration of the signaling molecule and thus lead to increased receptor activation, and transporters can thus be viewed as indirect receptor targets. However, in the strict sense, transporters are not receptors, but medicinal chemistry related to the two targets are very similar (Chapter 11). As a matter of fact, molecules acting on receptors, such as serotonin receptors, often also act on the transporters, such as serotonin transporters, which in some cases is desirable and in other cases not.

6.1.1   Synaptic processes and mechanisms

As exemplified above, receptors are located in a complex, integrated and highly interactive environment which can be further illustrated by the processes and mechanisms of synapses (Figure 6.2). The synapses are key elements in the interneuronal communication in the peripheral and the CNS. In the CNS, each neuron has been estimated to have synaptic contact with several thousand other neurones, making the structure and function of the CNS extremely complex.

Each neurotransmitter system operates through a characteristic set of synaptic processes and mechanisms (Figure 6.2), which are highly regulated and with distinct requirements for activation. In principle, each of these steps in the neurotransmission process is susceptible to specific pharmacological intervention. Synaptic functions may be facilitated by stimulation of the neurotransmitter biosynthesis, for example by administration of a biochemical precursor, or by inhibition of the metabolism/degradation pathway(s). There are several examples of therapeutically successful inhibitors of enzymes catalyzing intra- or extracellular metabolic processes. Similarly, it has been

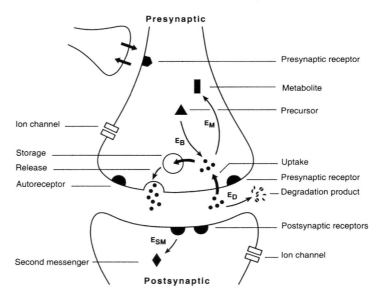

Figure 6.2 Generalized schematic illustration of processes and mechanisms associated with an axosomatic synapse in the CNS. E, enzymes; metabolic (E_M), biosynthetic (E_B), degradation (E_D), second messenger (E_{SM}); •, neurotransmitter.

shown in a number of cases that neurotransmitter function can be stimulated in a therapeutically beneficial manner via stimulation of neurotransmitter release or via inhibition of neuronal transport systems. It is possible that transport mechanisms in synaptic storage vesicles (Figure 6.2) also are potential sites for effective pharmacological intervention. Autoreceptors normally play a key role as a negative feedback mechanism regulating the release of certain neurotransmitters, making this class of presynaptic receptors therapeutically interesting.

Pharmacological stimulation or inhibition of the above mentioned synaptic mechanisms are, however, likely to affect the function of the entire neurotransmitter system. Activation of neurotransmitter receptors may, in principle, represent the most direct and selective approach to stimulation of a particular neurotransmitter system. Furthermore, activation of distinct subtypes of receptors operated by the neurotransmitter concerned may open up the prospect of highly selective pharmacological intervention. This principle may apply to pre- as well as post-synaptic receptors and also to ion channels associated with or independent of receptors (Figure 6.2) (see also Chapter 7).

Direct activation of receptors by full agonists may result in rapid receptor desensitization (insensitive to activation). Partial agonists are much less liable to induce receptor desensitization and may therefore be particularly interesting for neurotransmitter replacement therapies. Whereas desensitization may be a more or less pronounced problem associated with pharmacological or therapeutic use of receptor agonists, receptor antagonists, which in many cases have proved useful therapeutic agents, may inherently cause receptor supersensitivity. The presence of allosteric binding sites at certain receptor complexes, which may function as physiological modulatory mechanisms, offer unique prospects of selective and flexible pharmacological manipulation of the receptor complex concerned. Whilst some receptors are associated with ion channels, others are coupled to second messenger systems. Key steps in such enzyme-regulated multistep intracellular systems (Figure 6.2), which also include regulation of gene transcription by second messengers, represent targets for therapeutic interventions.

There is an urgent need for novel psycho-active drugs with specific actions. This demand is particularly pronounced in the field of neurologic disorders, where effective drugs in many cases are not yet available, even for symptomatic treatments. In terms of receptors, the heterogeneity offers opportunities to develop new ligands with increased receptor subtype selectivity and corresponding decrease of side effects. On the other hand, it simultaneously becomes a challenge to generate ligands with selectivity for one of many closely related targets.

6.2 RECEPTOR STRUCTURE AND FUNCTION

As mentioned in the previous section, receptors have been divided into four major superfamilies: (1) G-protein coupled receptors; (2) ligand-gated ion channels; (3) tyrosine kinase receptors; and (4) nuclear receptors. The three first receptor superfamilies are located in the cell membrane and the latter family is located intracellularly.

Our understanding of ligand–receptor interactions and receptor structure has increased dramatically during the last couple of years, not least due to the rapidly growing number of 3D-crystallographic structures that have been determined of either full receptors or isolated ligand binding domains. Thus today, structures of partial or full receptors of all four receptor superfamilies have been determined. Clearly, the information obtained from 3D-structures of ligand binding domains in the presence of ligands is very valuable for rational drug design. Likewise, knowledge of how the receptor functions can be used to e.g. design antagonists targeted to block mechanisms by which the receptor is activated (such as a conformational change).

6.2.1   G-protein coupled receptors

The G-protein coupled receptors (GPCRs) is the largest of the four superfamilies with some estimated 600 human receptor genes. A large fraction of these are taste and odor sensing receptors which are not of immediate interest for the pharmaceutical industry but are of interest, for e.g. fragrance manufactures. Nevertheless, it is estimated that 50% of all currently marketed drugs act on GPCRs and the superfamily thus remains a very important target for drug research. It is fascinating to note the very broad variety of signaling molecules which are able to act via this receptor superfamily, which, as already noted, include tastes and odors and for example light (photons), ions, monoamines, nucleotides, amino acids, peptides, proteins and pheromones.

The receptors are also referred to as 7TM receptors due to the seven α-helical transmembrane segments found in all GPCRs (Figure 6.3). The GPCRs have been further subdivided into family A, B and C based on their amino-acid sequence homology. Thus receptors within family A are closer related to each other than to receptors in family B and C etc. This grouping also coincides with the way ligands binds to the receptors. Thus, as illustrated in Figure 6.3, the endogenous signaling molecules bind to the transmembrane region of family A receptors (e.g. acetylcholine, histamine, dopamine and serotonin GPCRs, Chapters 10–11), to both the extracellular loops and amino-terminal domain of family B receptors (e.g. glucagon

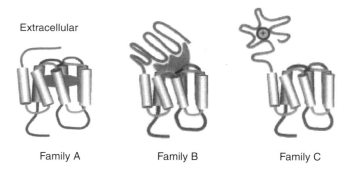

Family A   Family B   Family C

Figure 6.3 The three families of G-protein coupled receptors. All G-protein coupled receptors contain seven α-helical transmembrane segments and are thus also called 7TM receptors. Note the difference in agonist binding in the three families; family A receptors bind the agonist in the 7TM region, family B receptors bind the agonist in both the 7TM region and the extracellular amino-terminal domain, and family C receptors bind the agonist exclusively in the extracellular amino-terminal domain. (Adapted from Ji *et al.*, *J. Biol. Chem.*, **273**, 1998, 17299).

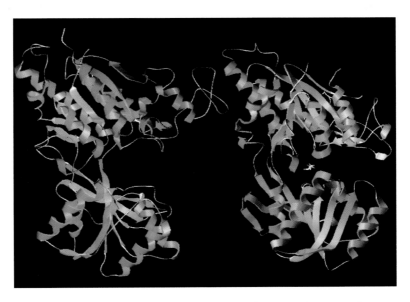

Figure 6.4 The structure of the amino-terminal domain of the metabotropic glutamate receptor
subtype mGluR1 in the open inactive form (left) and the closed active form with
glutamate bound in the cleft (right). The structures were generated using the program
'Swiss PDB viewer 3.5' with co-ordinates from Brookhaven Protein Data Base.

and secretin GPCRs) and exclusively to the extracellular amino-terminal domain of
family C receptors (e.g. glutamate and GABA GPCRs, Chapter 9).

It is known that agonist binding to family A and presumably family B receptors
cause a conformational change in the 7TM domain which is then relayed to the
intracellular loops causing G-protein activation. It has yet to be fully elucidated
how agonist binding to the amino-terminal domain of family C receptors is
brought through the 7TM domains. The structure of the isolated amino-terminal
domain of the glutamate GPCR subtype mGluR1 has recently been determined
in the absence and presence of glutamate. As shown in Figure 6.4, the domain
consist of two globular lobes forming an agonist-binding cleft which close upon
agonist binding. The initial event in family C receptor activation is thus closure
of the cleft which then induces a conformational change in the 7TM domain
probably by direct interaction of the closed amino-terminal domain and the extracellular loops as illustrated in Figure 6.13.

As already eluted to above, the intracellular loops of GPCRs interact with
G-proteins. The G-proteins are trimeric and consist of G_{α}, G_{β} and G_{γ} subunits
(Figure 6.5). Receptor activation will cause an interaction of the receptor with the
trimeric $G_{\alpha\beta\gamma}$-protein, catalyzing an exchange of GDP for GTP in the G_{α} subunit
whereupon the G-protein disassociate into activated G_{α} and $G_{\beta}\gamma$ subunits. Both
of these will then activate effector molecules such as adenylate cyclase and potassium
channels (Figure 6.5). 27 G_{α}, 5 G_{β} and 13 G_{γ} subunits have been identified in humans
and like the receptors they form groups based on the amino acid homology and the

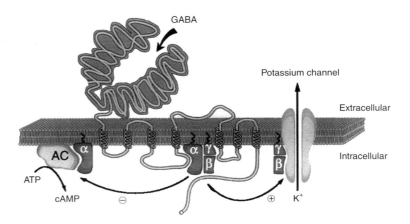

Figure 6.5 Cartoon of the family C receptor subtype GABA$_B$R1 interacting with an intracellular trimeric G-protein consisting of α-, β- and γ-subunits. Receptor activation will catalyze an exchange of GDP for GTP in the α-subunit which leads to activation and separation of the α- and $\beta\gamma$-subunits. Both of these will modulate downstream effectors such as inhibition of adenylate cyclase (AC) by the α-subunit and activation of potassium channels. (Adapted from Bettler *et al.*, *Curr. Opin. Neurobiol.*, **8**, 1998, 345).

effectors they interact with. For example, the G$_\alpha$ proteins have been divided into the G$_{\alpha i}$ class (inhibits adenylate cyclase), the G$_{\alpha s}$ class (stimulates adenylate cyclase), the G$_{\alpha q}$ class (stimulates phospholipase C) and the G$_{\alpha 12}$ class (function not fully eluci-dated). The GPCRs are classified as to which class of G$_\alpha$ proteins they mainly interact with. Thus, the GABA$_B$ receptor shown in Figure 6.5 would be termed a G$_{\alpha i}$ coupled receptor. Given that receptors prefer a given subset of G-proteins which again preferentiall interact with a given subset of effector proteins, each of which are differentially expressed in cell types, it is clear that the response of the same receptor might not be exactly the same in all cells. For example, the GABA$_B$ receptor shown in Figure 6.5 will inhibit adenylate cyclase and potassium channels in some cells but only inhibit adenylate cyclase in others where the potassium channel is not expressed. This will of course lead to different cellular effects in the two cell types which exemplifies the dynamic complexity of GPCR function and pharmacology.

6.2.2   Ligand-gated ion channel receptors

Ligand-gated ion channels can both be excitatory (e.g. ionotropic glutamate receptors and nicotinic acetylcholine receptors) or inhibitory (e.g. glycine and GABA$_A$ receptors) by conduction of Na$^+$/Ca^{2+} or Cl$^-$ ions which will hypo- or hyperpolarize the cell, respectively (see Chapter 7 for further details). The nicotinic acetylcholine receptor, at the nerve-muscle synapse, is the best understood ligand-gated ion channel which upon acetylcholine binding allow as many as 10 000 potas-sium and sodium ions per millisecond to pass through the channel. As shown in Figure 6.6, the receptor consist of two acetylcholine binding α_1 subunits and three other subunits (β_1, γ and δ) which form a pentameric pore in the cell membrane.

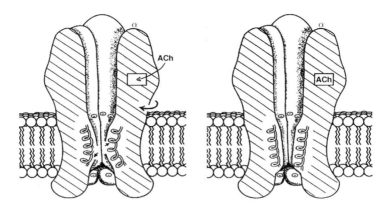

Figure 6.6 Cartoon based on the actual 3D-structure of the neuromuscular nicotinic acetyl-choline receptor which belong to the superfamily of ligand gated ion channels. The receptor consists of five subunits (two α-, one β-, one γ- and one δ-subunit). The receptor is shown in the inactive form where the ion channel pore is closed by five α-helices with kinks pointed toward the channel pore (left). Agonist binding to the α-subunits cause a conformational change relayed to the pore lining α-helices which rotate and thereby open the channel (right). (Adapted from Unwin, *J. Struc. Biol.*, **121**, 1998, 181).

A low-resolution 3D-structure of the nicotinic acetylcholine receptor has been determined in the absence and presence of acetylcholine (Figure 6.6). The pore itself is lined with five α-helices, one from each of the five receptor subunits, which have a kink in the middle of the membrane spanning part. This bend is the gate of the receptor, which in the closed state points toward the channel. Agonist binding to the extracellular part of the α-subunits induces local conformational changes which are then relayed to the three additional subunits and ultimately leads to rotation of the pore-lining α-helices whereby the channels opens.

Nicotinic acetylcholine receptors are also present in the central nervous system. In humans, these receptors consist of at least one of five different acetylcholine binding α-subunits (α_2–α_6) and at least one of three different β-subunits (β_2–β_4). The number of subunit combinations forming functional receptors is thus staggering high, but in reality only certain combinations are present. Furthermore, even fewer combinations such as the $\alpha_4\beta_2$ receptor, has therapeutic interest. Finally, a homopentameric α_7-subunit receptor has been identified in humans which has also been of significant therapeutic interest. Other ligand-gated ion channels also consist of four or five homo- or heteromeric subunits.

High-resolution 3D structures of the isolated ligand binding domain of the ionotropic glutamate receptor subunit GluR2 (Figure 6.1) has been determined. As shown in Figure 6.7, the overall structure and function of this domain show a striking resemblance with the domain from the mGluR1 receptor (Figure 6.4). Thus, the agonist binding cleft of both GluR2 and mGluR1 close around the agonist upon binding, which in the case of GluR2 is relayed to the membrane spanning part of the receptor causing an opening of the channel pore (Figure 6.7).

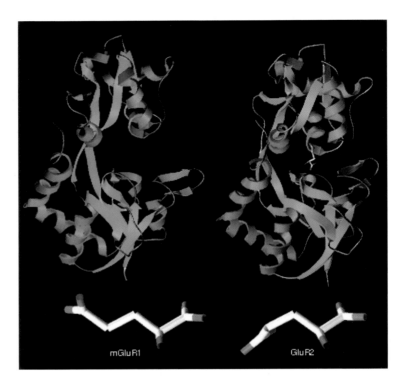

Figure 6.7 Structure of the agonist binding domain of the ionotropic glutamate receptor subtype GluR2 which belong to the superfamily of ligand gated ion channels. The domain is shown in the open inactive form (upper left) and the closed active form with glutamate bound in the cleft (upper right). Note the similarity in the overall structure of the agonist binding domain of GluR2 and mGluR1 (compare with Figure 6.4). The difference in conformation of glutamate bound to mGluR1 and GluR2 are also shown. The structures were generated using the program 'Swiss PDB viewer 3.5' with co-ordinates from Brookhaven Protein Data Base.

The conformation of glutamate bound to GluR2 and mGluR1 is quite different as illustrated in Figure 6.7. Such information is very valuable in the design of glutamate receptor subtype selective compounds which is discussed in further detail in Chapter 9.

6.2.3   Tyrosine kinase receptors

The tyrosine kinase receptors (TKR) have a large extracellular agonist binding domain, one transmembrane segment and an intracellular domain. The receptors can be divided into two groups: (1) those that contain the tyrosine kinase as an integral part of the intracellular domain; and (2) those that are associated with a Janus kinase (JAK). Examples of the former group are the insulin receptor family, the fibroblast growth factor (FGF) receptor family and examples of the latter are the cytokine receptor family such as the erythropoietin (EPO) receptor and the thrombopoietin (TPO) receptor. However, both groups share the same mechanism of activation: Upon agonist binding two intracellular kinases are brought together which will initiate autophosphorylation of tyrosine residues of the intracellular tyrosine kinase domain (Figure 6.8). This will attract other proteins (e.g. Shc/Grb2/Sos and STAT for the two receptor groups, respectively) which are also phosphorylated and this will initiate protein cascades which will ultimately lead to regulation of transcriptional factors (e.g. Elk-1, Figure 6.8) and thus regulation of genes involved in e.g. cell proliferation and differentiation. As described for the G-protein coupled receptors, all the proteins in the intracellular activation cascades are heterogeneous leading to individual responses (i.e. regulation of different subset of genes) in individual cell types.

Some of the receptors exist as monomers in the absence of agonist whereas other exist as covalently linked dimers (the insulin receptor family) or non-covalently linked dimers. In case of the monomers, the agonist will bring the two receptor subunits together by binding to both subunits simultaneously and thereby initiate

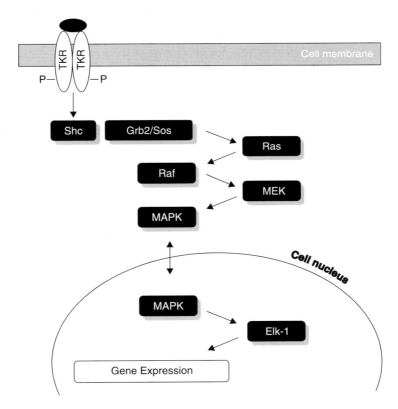

Figure 6.8 Cartoon of a protein cascade initiated by agonist binding to two tyrosine kinase receptors (TKR) causing autophosphorylation of the dimerized intracellular receptor domains. This cause activation of a cascade of intracellular proteins (abbreviated Shc, Grb2/Sos, Ras, Raf, MEK and MAPK), which ultimately leads to activation of transcription factors (e.g. Elk-1) and thus regulation of gene expression. (Adapted from Campbell *et al.*, *Oncogene*, **17**, 1998, 1395).

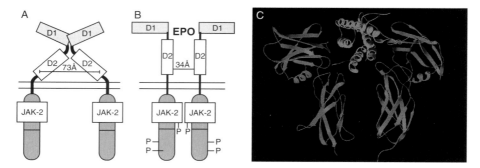

Figure 6.9 Cartoon of the activation mechanism of the EPO receptor which belong to the JAK/STAT receptor class of the superfamily of TKR: (A) The receptor is dimerized in the inactive conformation by interaction of amino acids which are similar to those involved in binding of EPO and the intracellular JAK kinases are kept too far apart to initiate autophosphorylation; (B) binding of EPO to the dimer interface tilts the structure and brings the JAK kinases in close proximity which initiates the autophosphorylation; and (C) the actual structure of EPO (in cyan) bound to the extracellular receptor domains of the EPO receptor (in green). (Adapted from Wilson *et al.*, *Curr. Opin. Struc. Biol.*, **9**, 1998, 696. The structure was generated using the program 'Swiss PDB viewer 3.5' with co-ordinates from Brookhaven Protein Data Base).

the autophosphorylation. In case of the preformed inactive dimers, agonist binding will cause a conformational change in the receptor, which brings the two intracellular kinases together and thus initiate the autophosphorylation. The best understood example in this regard is the EPO receptor of which the 3D-structure of the extracellular agonist binding domain has been determined in the absence and presence of EPO (Figure 6.9). In the absence of EPO, the domain is a dimer in which the ends are too far apart for the JAK's to reach each other. The EPO binds to the same amino acids on the receptor that forms the dimer interface and thereby tilts the two receptor subunits. This brings the JAK's close together and initiate the autophosphorylation (Figure 6.9).

6.2.4   Nuclear receptors

Nuclear receptors are cellular proteins and are thus not embedded in the membrane like the previously described receptors. In contrast to the membrane bound receptors, they bind small lipophilic hormones and function as ligand modulated transcription factors. The nuclear receptors have been classified according to the type of hormone they bind. Thereby, receptors have been divided into those which bind steroids (glucocorticoids, progestestins, mineralocorticoid androgens and estrogens) and steroid derivatives (vitamin D_3), non-steroids (thyroid hormone, retinoids, prostaglandins), and orphan receptors for which the physiological agonist has yet to be discovered. The receptor family is relatively small (~ 70 subtypes) of which the majority actually still belongs to the group of orphan receptors.

The nuclear receptors consist of a ligand binding domain and a DNA binding domain. Upon activation, the two receptors dimerize, as homo- or heterodimers, and bind to specific recognition sites on the DNA. Co-activators will then associate with the dimeric receptor and initiate transcription of the target gene(s). Each receptor recognize specific DNA sequences, also known as the hormone response elements, which are located upstream of the genes that are regulated.

A 3D high-resolution structures of both ligand and DNA binding domains have been determined. In drug research the main focus has been on the structures of the ligand binding domains which for several receptors have been determined in absence and presence of ligands. One such example is shown in Figure 6.10 which illustrate the mechanism of agonism and antagonism of the superfamily of nuclear receptors. The ligand binding site is a hydrophobic pocket in the center of the protein which in the absence of ligand is partially filled with hydrophobic residues from α-helix H11. Upon agonist binding, H11 is displaced by the agonist and α-helix H12 folds back over the binding pocket. The co-activators binds to and recognize residues in α-helices H3, H4 and H12, and agonist binding thus reposition H12 such that the co-activator binding motif is generated. This also explains how some antagonists work at the molecular level. The antagonist BMS614 is larger than the physiological hormone and thus pushes H12 away from the ligand binding pocket. In this way, H12 now occupies the space between H3 and H4 and thus prevent the co-activator from binding (Figure 6.10).

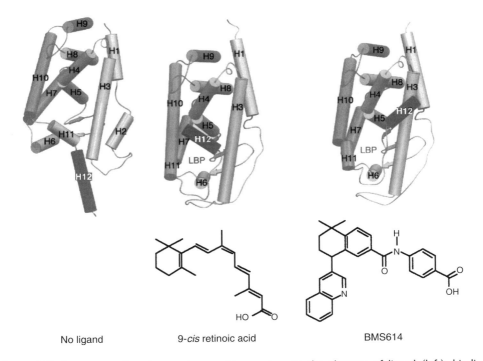

No ligand   9-*cis* retinoic acid   BMS614

Figure 6.10 Structures of nuclear retinoic acid receptors in the absence of ligand (left), binding the agonist 9-*cis* retinoic acid (middle) or the antagonist BMS614 (right) in the ligand binding pocket (LBP). Note the difference in location of α-helix H12 which is the key player in the activation mechanism (see text for further details). (From Bourguet *et al.*, *Trends Pharmacol. Sci.*, **21**, 2000, 381).

6.3   RECEPTOR PHARMACOLOGY

6.3.1   Recombinant vs. *in situ* assays

The last decade has had a profound impact on how receptor pharmacology is performed. As mentioned in the introduction, receptor cloning was initiated in the mid-eighties and today the majority of receptors have been cloned. Thus, it is now possible to determine the effect of ligands on individual receptor subtypes expressed in recombinant systems rather than a mixture of receptors in e.g. an organ. This is very useful given that receptor selectivity is a major goal in terms of decreasing side effects of drugs and development of useful pharmacological tools which can be used to elucidate the physiological function of individual receptor subtypes. Furthermore, recombinant assay systems allow one to assay cloned human receptors which is otherwise often not possible to obtain. Although most receptors are more than 95% identical between humans and rodents, there have been cases of drugs developed for rats rather than for humans due to the fact that the compounds were active on the rat receptor but not on the human receptor due to the small differences in primary amino acid sequence.

It should be noted that the use of organ and whole animal pharmacology is still required. As previously noted, the cellular effects of receptor activation depends on the intracellular contents of the proteins involved in e.g. the signaling cascades. These effects can only be determined when the receptor is situated in its natural environment rather than in a recombinant system. In most situations, both recombinant and *in situ* assays are thus used to fully evaluate the pharmacological profile of new ligands. Furthermore, once a compound with the desired selectivity profile has been identified in the recombinant assays, it is important to confirm that this compound has the predicted physiological effects in e.g. primary non-recombinant cell lines which express the receptor, in organs and/or in whole animals.

6.3.2   Binding vs. functional assays

Binding assays used to be the preferred choice of method for pharmacological evaluation which was mainly due to the ease of these assays compared to functional assays which generally required more steps than binding assays. However, several factors have changed this perception: (1) biotechnological functional assays have evolved profoundly and have decreased the number of assay steps and increased the throughput; (2) functional assay equipment has been automated; (3) ligand binding requires a high-affinity ligand which for many targets identified in genome projects simply does not exist; (4) binding assays are unable to discriminate between agonists and antagonists; and (5) binding assays will only identify compounds binding to the same site as the radioactively labeled tracer.

The Fluorometric Imaging Plate Reader (FLIPR^{TM}) illustrates this development towards functional assays. Cells transfected with a receptor coupled to increase in intracellular calcium levels (e.g. a $G_{\alpha q}$ coupled GPCR or a Ca^{2+} permeable ligand-gated ion channel) are loaded with the dye Fluo-3 which in itself is not fluorescent. However, as shown in Figure 6.11, the dye becomes fluorescent when exposed to Ca^{2+} in the cell in a concentration dependent manner. In this manner, ligand

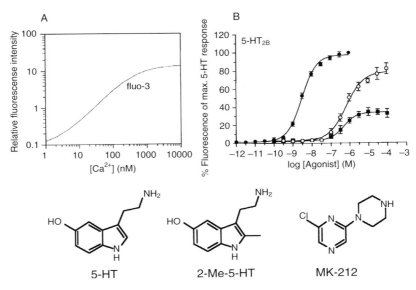

Figure 6.11 (A) Relation between Ca^{2+} concentration and relative fluorescence intensity of the fluorescent probe fluo-3. (B) The $5\text{-}HT_{2B}$ receptor subtype belong to the superfamily of G-protein coupled receptors and are coupled to increase in inositol phosphates and intracellular Ca^{2+}. Cells expressing $5\text{-}HT_{2B}$ receptors were loaded with fluo-3 and the fluorescence was determined upon exposure to the endogenous agonist 5-HT and the partial agonists 2-Me-5-HT and MK-212 on a FLIPR™. (Adapted from Jerman *et al.*, *Eur. J. Pharmacol.*, **414**, 2001, 23).

concentration–response curves can be generated on the FLIPR™ very fast as it reads all wells of a 384-well tissue culture plate simultaneously. Many other functional assays along these lines have been developed in recent years.

6.3.3 Partial and full agonists

Agonists are characterized by two pharmacological parameters, potency and maximal response. The most common way of describing the potency is by measurement of the agonist concentration which elicit 50% of the compounds own maximal response (the EC_{50} value). The maximal response is commonly described as per cent of the maximal response of the endogenous agonist. The maximal response is also often described as efficacy or intrinsic activity which were defined by Stephenson and Ariëns, respectively. Compounds, such as 2-Me-5-HT and MK-212 in Figure 6.11, which show a lower maximal response than the endogenous agonist 5-HT are termed partial agonists. The parameters potency and maximal response are independent of each other and on the same receptor it is thus possible to have e.g. a highly potent partial agonist and a low potent full agonist. Both parameters are important for drug research, and it is thus desirable to have a pharmacological assay system which is able to determine both the potency and maximal response of the tested ligands.

6.3.4 Antagonists

Antagonists do not activate the receptors but block the activity elicited by agonists and accordingly they are only characterized by the parameter affinity. The most common way of characterization of antagonists is by competition with an agonist (functional assay) or a radioactively labeled ligand (binding assay). In both cases, the antagonist concentration is increased and the agonist or radioligand, which are being displaced, are held at a constant concentration. It is then possible to determine the concentration of antagonist which inhibits the response/binding to 50% (the IC_{50} value). The IC_{50} value can then be transformed to affinity (K) by the Cheng–Prusoff equation.

Functional assay:

$$K = \frac{IC_{50}}{\left(1 + \dfrac{[\text{Agonist}]}{EC_{50}}\right)} \tag{6.1}$$

where [Agonist] is the agonist concentration and EC_{50} is for the agonist in the particular assay.

Binding assay:

$$K = \frac{IC_{50}}{\left(1 + \dfrac{[\text{Radioligand}]}{K_D}\right)} \tag{6.2}$$

Where [Radioligand] is the radioligand concentration and K_D is the affinity of the radioligand.

It is important to observe that the Cheng–Prusoff equation is only valid for competitive antagonists.

The Schild analysis is often used to determine whether an antagonist is competitive or non-competitive. In the Schild analysis, the antagonist concentration is kept constant while the agonist concentration is varied. For a competitive antagonist, this will cause a rightward parallel shift of the concentration–response curves without a reduction of the maximal response (Figure 6.12A). The degree of rightshifting is determined as the dose ratio (DR), which is the concentration of agonist giving a particular response in the presence of antagonist divided by the concentration of agonist that gives the same response in the absence of antagonist. Typically one will choose the EC_{50} values to calculate the DR. In the Schild analysis, the log $(DR - 1)$ is depicted as a function of the antagonist concentration (Figure 6.12B). When the slope of the curve equals 1 it is a sign of competitive antagonism and the affinity can then be determined by the intercept of the abscissa. When the slope is significantly different from 1 or the curve is not linear it is a sign of non-competitive antagonism which invalidates the Schild analysis.

As shown in the example in Figure 6.12, five concentration–response curves are generated to obtain one antagonist affinity determination and it can thus be seen that the Schild analysis is rather work intensive compared to e.g. the transformation by the Cheng–Prusoff equation where one inhibition curve generates one antagonist affinity determination. However, the latter cannot be used to determine whether an antagonist is competitive or non-competitive which is the advantage of the Schild analysis.

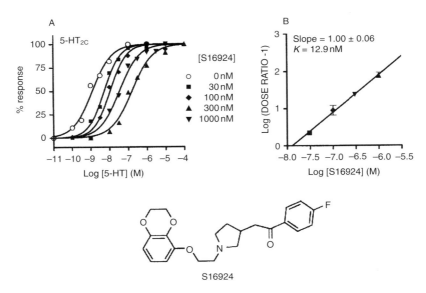

Figure 6.12 Schild analysis of the competitive antagonist S16924 on cells expressing the 5-HT$_{2C}$ receptor. (A) Concentration–response curves of the agonist 5-HT were generated in the presence of varying concentrations of S16924. Note the parallel right shift of the curves and the same level of maximum response; and (B) dose ratios are calculated and plotted as a function of the constant antagonist concentration generating a straight line with a slope of 1.00 ± 0.06. These results and the observations from (A) are in agreement with a competitive interaction and the antagonist affinity can thus be determined by the intercept of the abscissa; $K = 12.9$ nM. (Adapted from Cussac *et al.*, *Naunyn Schiedbergs Arch. Phamacol.*, **361**, 2000, 549).

When testing a series of structurally related antagonists one would thus often determine the nature of antagonism with the Schild analysis for a couple of representative compounds. If these are competitive antagonists, it would then be reasonable to assume that all compounds in the series are competitive and thus determine the affinity by use of the less work intensive Cheng–Prusoff equation.

6.3.5 **Allosteric modulators**

Allosteric modulators can both be stimulative or inhibitory (non-competitive antagonists) and typically these compounds bind outside the endogenous agonist binding site. This class of compounds modulate the effect of agonist and accordingly they show no activity in the absence of agonist. Well-known examples are the benzodiazepines which enhance the effect of GABA on GABA$_A$ receptors and PCP which inhibit the effect of glutamate on NMDA receptors (Chapter 9).

As noted in Section 6.3.4, the Schild analysis is very useful to discriminate between competitive and non-competitive antagonists, and an example of the latter is shown in Figure 6.13. The ligand CPCCOEt is a selective antagonist at the mGluR1 receptor, and the Schild analysis clearly demonstrate that the antagonism is non-competitive due to the depression of the maximal response (compare Figure 6.12A and 6.13).

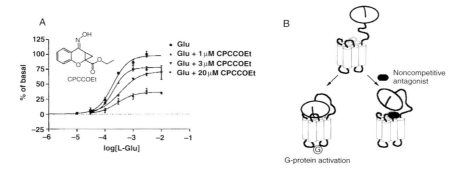

Figure 6.13 Schild analysis of the non-competitive antagonist CPCCOEt on cells expressing the metabotropic glutamate receptor subtype mGluR1: (A) Concentration–response curves of the agonist glutamate (Glu) were generated in the presence of varying concentrations of CPCCOEt. In contrast to the Schild analysis shown in Figure 6.12, a clear depression of the maximal response is seen with increasing antagonist concentrations. This shows that the antagonist is non-competitive; and (B) cartoon showing the interaction between the closed glutamate bound amino terminal domain of mGluR1 and the seven transmembrane domain (lower left). Receptor mutagenesis studies have shown that CPCCOEt binds to the 7TM domain of mGluR1 and thus act by obstructing the intramolecular agonist-induced interaction (lower right). (Adapted from Litschig *et al.*, *Mol. Pharmacol.*, **55**, 1999, 453 and Bräuner-Osborne *et al.*, *J. Med. Chem.*, **43**, 2000, 2621).

As noted previously, glutamate binds to the large extracellular amino-terminal domain whereas CPCCOEt has been shown to bind to the extracellular part of the 7TM domain (Figure 6.13B). CPCCOEt thus blocks the intramolecular communication between the amino-terminal domain and the 7TM domain.

FURTHER READING

Bourguet, W., Germain, P. and Gronemeyer, H. (2000) Nuclear receptor ligand-binding domains: three-dimensional structures, molecular interactions and pharmacological implications. *Trends Pharmacol. Sci.*, **21**, 381–388.

Bräuner-Osborne, H., Egebjerg, J., Nielsen, E.Ø., Madsen, U. and Krogsgaard-Larsen, P. (2000) Ligands for glutamate receptors: design and therapeutic prospects. *J. Med. Chem.*, **43**, 2609–2645.

Egea, P.F., Klaholz, B.P. and Moras, D. (2000) Ligand–protein interactions in nuclear receptors of hormones. *FEBS Lett.*, **476**, 62–67.

Ji, T.H., Grossmann, M. and Ji, I. (1998) G-protein-coupled receptors. I. Diversity of receptor–ligand interactions. *J. Biol. Chem.*, **273**, 17299–17302.

Kenakin, T.P. (1997) *Pharmacologic analysis of drug–receptor interaction*, 3rd edition. London: Lippincott Williams & Wilkins.

Schlessinger, J. (2000) Cell signalling by receptor tyrosine kinases. *Cell*, **103**, 211–225.

Unwin, N. (1998) The nicotinic acetylcholine receptor of the *Torpedo* electric ray. *J. Struct. Biol.*, **121**, 181–190.

Wilson, I.A. and Jolliffe, L.K. (1999) The structure, organization, activation and plasticity of the erythropoietin receptor. *Curr. Opin. Struct. Biol.*, **9**, 696–704.

Chapter 7

Ion channels: structure, function and pharmacology

David J. Triggle

7.1 INTRODUCTION

7.1.1 Ion channels and cellular function

'*The grave's a fine and private place*', wrote the Elizabethan poet Andrew Marvel, but the cell is not. Ions moving through the ion channels of the cell's membranes are both an integral component of the music of life and a constant reminder of the cellular traffic that defines cellular excitability. Ion channels serve as one of the mechanisms through which cells respond to informational inputs. Under physiological conditions ion channels permit the orderly movement of ions across cellular membranes – both plasma membranes and the membranes of cellular organelles. Under pathological conditions ion channels generate disorderly ionic traffic and cellular death.

7.1.2 Ion channels as membrane effectors

Excitable cells respond to a variety of informational inputs, chemical and physical, including neurotransmitters, hormones, pheromones, heat, light and pressure. These informational inputs are coupled to cellular response through transduction systems that include enzyme activation, substrate internalization and ion channel opening and closing (Figure 7.1). Ion channels are one class of biological effectors. They function to permeate ions, including the physiological cations Na^+, K^+, Ca^{2+} and Mg^{2+} and the anion Cl^-, in response to diverse cell stimuli. The resultant ionic current may itself be the end consequence as in the maintenance of membrane potential or the discharge of potential in electric fish. More commonly, the ion current is coupled to other events, including the alteration of cellular sensitivity to other stimuli and the major generic processes of excitation–contraction coupling and stimulus–secretion coupling. In the latter examples, there is a dual function for calcium since it both carries current and serves as a cellular messenger coupling cell excitation to the calcium-dependent events of contraction and secretion.

The cell maintains a highly asymmetric distribution of ions across its membranes. Na^+, Ca^{2+} and Cl^- are maintained at low intracellular levels and K^+ at high intracellular level relative to the extracellular environment. Maintenance of this asymmetric distribution depends upon the selective permeability of cell membranes and the work of ionic pumps including Na^+, K^+-ATPase and Ca^{2+}-ATPase

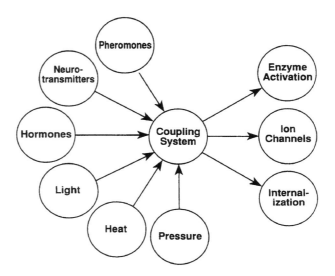

Figure 7.1 Ion channels as one of several mechanisms by which informational inputs are translated through intermediate coupling devices into cellular responses.

that maintain ionic gradients in the face of constant leakage and to restore these gradients subsequent to dissipation by channel activating stimuli.

The lipid bilayer of the cell is essentially impermeable to ions and ion channels (or an equivalent function) are therefore necessary components of cellular membranes and likely arose relatively early during cellular evolution. Uncontrolled movements of ions represent toxic or lethal stimuli and ion channels are, therefore, regulated species. The processes of channel regulation of opening and closing are thus critical to any understanding of the physiologic and pharmacologic control of channel activity.

7.1.3   Ion channels and ion distribution

The relationship between ion concentrations, membrane potential and ion chemical and electrical gradients is depicted in Figure 7.2. At a typical resting cellular potential of 70 mV (by convention negative interior) both electrical and concentration gradients combine to provide a net inward driving force for Na^+ entry of 120 mV. When the membrane potential is maintained at the equilibrium potential for Na^+ (positive interior) the inwardly directed concentration gradient is exactly balanced by the outwardly directed electrical gradient and there is no net movement of Na^+ ions. A representative comparison of the equilibrium potentials for Na^+, K^+, Ca^{2+} and Cl^- is presented in Table 7.1. Quite generally, the opening of Na^+ and Ca^{2+} channels will dissipate membrane potential – depolarize – to mediate cellular excitation. In contrast, opening of K^+ or Cl^- channels will maintain or elevate membrane potential – hyperpolarize – to mediate inhibitory responses. Conversely, the closing of K^+ or Cl^- channels will be disinhibitory in nature leading to cell excitation and the blockade of Na^+ or Ca^{2+} channels will prevent

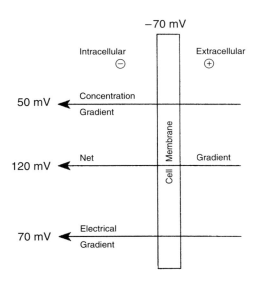

Figure 7.2 Ion movements across a cell membrane are determined by the net product of the concentration gradient and the electrical gradient. In the example where the net membrane potential is $-70\,mV$ both concentration and electrical gradients favor Na^+ entry into the cell. If the membrane potential is set at the equilibrium potential for Na^+, $\sim +50\,mV$, then these gradients will balance and there will be no net movement of Na^+.

Table 7.1 Ionic concentrations and equilibrium potentials in excitable cells

Ion	$[X]_{ext}$ mM	$[X]_{int}$ mM	Equilibrium potential mV (approximate)
Na^+	145	12	$+70$
K^+	4	155	-90
Ca^{2+}	1.5	$<10^{-4}$	$>+120$
Cl^-	123	4	-90

depolarization and thus mediate inhibitory responses. When two or more ion channels open or close together the resultant membrane potential, and response, will represent the sum of these events.

There are very important implications to this elementary analysis of ion movements for the actions of drugs on ion channels. Drugs that open Na^+ or Ca^{2+} channels will tend to depolarize cells and to be excitatory in nature while drugs that open K^+ or Cl^- channels will hyperpolarize cells and be inhibitory in nature. A similar, but opposing relationship, will apply to antagonists at these channels (Figure 7.3). However, the control of ion channels must not be viewed in isolation or as one channel at a time, but rather should be seen as linked events whereby channels are multiply involved in the control of cellular function. Thus, the influx of Ca^{2+} through Ca^{2+} channels – an excitatory event – can lead to the activation of Ca^{2+}-dependent K^+ channels – an inhibitory event. This is depicted in Figure 7.4

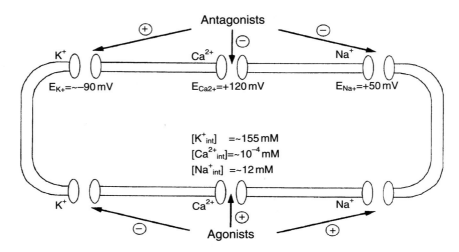

Figure 7.3 The equilibrium potentials for Na^+, K^+ and Ca^{2+} and the effects of drugs that open or close selectively these channels (see text for additional details). $(+)$ indicates excitatory event and $(-)$ indicates an inhibitory event.

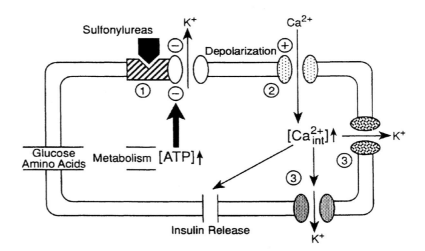

Figure 7.4 Ion channels frequently function in co-operation or sequentially. In this insulin-secreting β-cell of the pancreas ATP derived from metabolic input blocks K_{ATP}^+ channels (1) thus depolarizing the cell. This K^+ channel is the target for the hypoglycemic sulfonylurea antidiabetic drugs that block the channel at a specific receptor site. Depolarization activates Ca^{2+} channels (2) that causes an influx of Ca^{2+} into the cell to stimulate the release of insulin. The elevation of intracellular Ca^{2+} also activates Ca^{2+}-dependent K^+ channels (3) that open to restore membrane potential. Thus, the net balance of electrical activity in the cell will be determined by the combined activities of the three types of ion channels.

where in an insulin-secreting pancreatic β-cell, there exist both ATP-sensitive K^+ channels and voltage-gated Ca^{2+} channels. When the ATP levels are elevated in response to rising glucose or amino acid concentrations post-feeding the K^+ channel closes: the resultant depolarization activates the voltage-gated Ca^{2+} channel and the resultant Ca^{2+} influx promotes insulin release. Subsequently, the activation of Ca^{2+}-sensitive K^+ channels serves to repolarize the cell.

7.1.4   Activation and inactivation of ion channels

The schematized depiction of impulse conduction in a nerve fiber indicates the association between different ionic processes and the different behavior of distinct ion channels (Figure 7.5). The depolarization of a nerve axon by a step depolarization results in the rapid activation of Na^+ channels to permit a fast inward and depolarizing current that is carried virtually exclusively by Na^+ ions and a later outward and repolarizing current carried by K^+ ions. Two important differential properties of ion channels are illustrated in Figure 7.5. Channels may open rapidly or slowly and they may stay open in response to a constant stimulus or they may open and close in a relatively transient manner. Thus, the rates and properties of activation and inactivation are important characteristics of ion channels and these differential properties are increasingly being linked to specific components of channel molecular structure. Figure 7.5 also illustrates the principle of the voltage clamp procedure whereby the application of a specific voltage step or 'clamp' permits the magnitudes, directions and kinetics of ion currents to be measured. This may be achieved at the macroscopic level where large number of channels

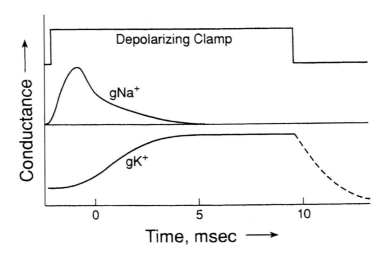

Figure 7.5 Schematic representation of Na^+ and K^+ conductance changes during the period of maintained depolarization ('depolarizing clamp'). The Na^+ conductance (gNa^+) activates and inactivates rapidly and the K^+(gK^+) conductance activates less rapidly and does not inactivate over the period of the clamp depicted.

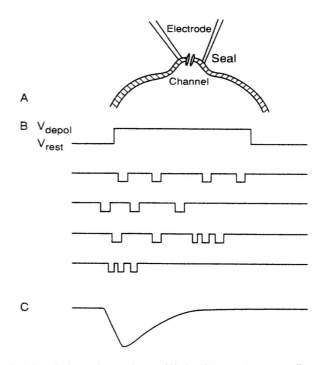

Figure 7.6 The principle of the voltage clamp: (A) In this version a small piece of membrane containing a single ion channel is clamped between two electrodes; (B) The opening and closing of single channels is observed as an all-or-none stochastic event and the sum of these events is depicted under (C).

are studied simultaneously (tissue or whole cell), with a few channels and even with single ion channels in patch-clamp techniques that study small patches of native or reconstituted membranes (Figure 7.6).

7.2   STRUCTURE AND FUNCTION OF ION CHANNELS

7.2.1   Ion channels as efficient and regulated species

Ion channels are discriminating cellular entities. Ion channels translocate ions on the basis of ion type – cations vs. anions – on the basis of ion charge – monovalent vs. divalent – and on the basis of ion size – Na^+ vs. K^+. Channels permeate ions very efficiently at rates $>10^7$ ion/sec, that approach diffusion-controlled limits. Enzymes and carriers operate generally at orders of magnitude lower efficiency. To charge a membrane of capacity $1\,\mu F/cm^2$ by $100\,mV$ requires the transfer of some 6000 ions per square micrometer and with a channel of conductance $20\,pS$ this can be accomplished in $0.5\,sec$. Because of this efficiency ion channels are frequently relatively minor components of excitable cells. Channels

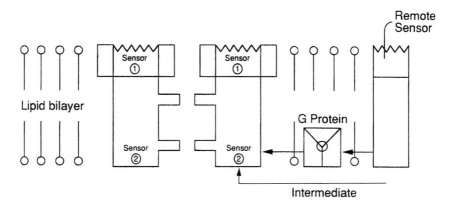

Figure 7.7 The fundamental architecture of ion channels depicting sensors (integral and remote), gates in the channel pore and both G protein and cytoplasmic routes for messenger modulation of the channel.

are also regulated species, regulated most frequently by changes in chemical or electrical potential, and hence must possess a certain minimal organization structure (Figure 7.7). It is helpful to regard ion channels through an analogy to allosteric enzymes, functioning to accelerate ion transit across an essentially impermeable membrane barrier, through changes in chemical or electrical potential recognized at sites distal to the channel pore itself.

7.2.2   The structure of ion channels

The structure of Figure 7.7 includes sensors that function as the regulatory components ('allosteric sites') and that are responsive to chemical or physical stimuli, gates that open and close in response to these stimuli, a pore through which ions pass and a 'selectivity filter' that confers upon the channel its ionic selectivity. In principle, the ionic selectivity of a channel may be mediated through two very different mechanisms. The channel may discriminate on the basis of ionic size through 'molecular sieving' or may discriminate through a process of selective ionic binding with components of the channel pore. There is increasing evidence that the latter is the dominant mechanism and that ions do bind with channel components during transit and, moreover, that ion channels have multiple ion binding sites and that multiple occupancy of these sites facilitates ion transit. The 2D representation of an ion channel depicted in Figure 7.7 was derived from indirect evidence obtained during a century of biophysical, largely electrophysiological, investigations. The essential validity of this model has now been confirmed through a direct structure determination of a K^+ channel (Figure 7.8). Although this is a structure of a bacterial ion channel and one that is gated by changes in pH, rather than voltage or chemical transmitters, there is general agreement that the underlying molecular details are generally applicable to other ion channels.

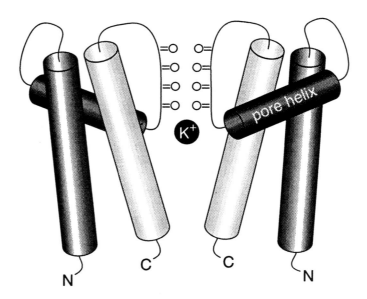

Figure 7.8 Schematic representation of two of the four subunits that make up the functional bacterial K^+ channel. The 'selectivity filter' comprises the aligned carbonyl residues and the pore helices (two are shown) project a dipole field that lowers the energy barrier for K^+ ion entry into the pore of the channel. One K^+ ion is shown in the pore region.

7.2.3   Families of ion channels

Structural studies indicate that there are at least two major families of ion channels. This structural classification into the voltage-gated and ligand-gated families parallels the functional classification established from biophysical and pharmacologic studies. The primary sequences and subunit organization of a large number of channels are now available and with the determination of the 3D-structure of a K^+ channel (Figure 7.8) there is a good foundation upon which to analyze drug–channel interactions.

Each of these major channel families is internally homologous, but both families share fundamental structural and topological similarities. This common structural plan consists of an approximately symmetric disposition of homologous subunits or domains surrounding a central pore. Ligand-gated channels are composed of a set of subunits which, though substantially homologous, bear individually specialized functions including the receptor and regulatory drug binding sites. Thus, the typical ligand-gated ion channel is a heteromeric expression of these subunits – typically a pentameric arrangement as in the nicotinic acetylcholine receptor-channel of skeletal muscle – $\alpha_2\beta\gamma\delta$ – where the α-subunits bear the acetylcholine binding sites. However, homomeric expression does occur as in neuronal nicotinic receptors that can be made up of α- and β-subunits or exclusively of α-subunits. Each of the five homologous subunits of the acetylcholine receptor ion channel has four transmembrane helices and the five subunits are arranged around a central transmembrane pore that is lined with the polar residues of the M2 helices. Concentrations of negative charge are to be found at the top and the bottom of the channel.

Voltage-gated channels for Na^+ and Ca^{2+} are also of subunit organization, but the principal channel functions are associated with a large subunit of approximately 200 kDA and which is made up of four homologous domains – I–IV. This major subunit carries the drug binding sites and makes up the architecture of the channel pore. This subunit is associated with other subunits that can regulate both the expression of the channel and its functional properties (Figure 7.9). Each of the domains of the voltage-gated Na^+ and Ca^{2+} channels is composed of six transmembrane helices and the pore is composed up of residues between S5 and S6. Helix S4 contains a sequence of positively charged residues and these confer voltage-sensing upon the channel. In contrast, the voltage-gated K^+ channel is comprised of a smaller peptide that is homologous to one of the domains of the Na^+ or Ca^{2+} channels: a functional K^+ channel is formed as tetrameric association of these individual subunits. The smaller size of the K^+ channel suggests that it may be ancestral to the Na^+ and Ca^{2+} channels and, consistent with this argument, there are more variations on the structure of the K^+ channel including those with six transmembrane helices – voltage-gated, Ca^{2+}-activated and HERG (human ether-a-go-go related gene) channels, the latter contributing to important human cardiac arrhythmias. K^+ channels with two transmembrane helices include the inwardly rectifying channel family that includes K_{ATP}^+ channels.

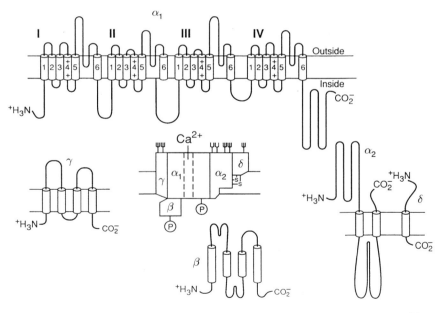

Figure 7.9 Schematic arrangement of the subunits that comprise the voltage-gated Ca^{2+} channel and their organization. The α_1 subunit is the major structural and functional component and bears the permeation machinery and the principal drug binding sites. The cytosolic β-subunit is of particular importance in facilitating the expression of the α_1 subunit and for modifying its gating properties upon activation. Channel diversity arises from the presence of distinct α, β, γ and δ subtypes.

Quite generally, ion channels show remarkable conservation across species – from *Drosophila* to man. This serves as eloquent testimony to the cellular importance of ion channels and to the fitness of design once achieved.

7.2.4   Structure–function correlations

Increasingly, knowledge of the sequences of the channels, their subunit organizations and, most recently, their 3D structures makes it possible to assign specific structural motifs to defined functions, including the sites of drug action and aberrant function as in 'ion channel diseases'. A detailed exposition of these findings lies outside the scope of this chapter, but some illustrative examples may be illustrative of the advances that are being made.

The GABA-gated Cl⁻ channel is a heteromeric organization of homologous subunits. The pentameric association is derived dominantly from the α-, β-and γ-subunits and the opening of this channel by GABA which leads to inhibitory responses is potentiated by benzodiazepines; this action is the basis for their therapeutic effectiveness as sedatives, anxiolytics, muscle relaxants and anti-epileptics (Chapter 9). The benzodiazepines bind to a regulatory site located between the α- and γ-subunits. Depending upon the type of α-subunit, α_1–α_6, the GABA receptor may be sensitive or insensitive to benzodiazepines. Only the α_1, α_2, α_3 and α_5 subunits confer sensitivity to benzodiazepines in the GABA receptor channel. These subunits all contain histidine at position 101 and its replacement by arginine abolishes benzodiazepine sensitivity. Furthermore, selective replacement of histidine by arginine in only the α_1-subunit abolishes the sedating effects of benzodiazepines, but leaves the anxiolytic actions unchanged.

The nicotinic acetylcholine receptor channel is a pentameric association of subunits with the α-subunit bearing the acetylcholine receptor site. The pore of the channel is formed from the lining of the M2 helices and is comprised of polar residues with non-polar leucine side chains intruding into the pore at rest ('closed gate'). During activation by acetylcholine the M2 helices twist, rotating away the leucine residues and replacing them with smaller polar residues, and permit ions to flow through the channel pore (Figure 7.10).

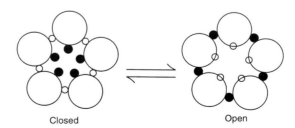

Closed   Open

Figure 7.10 The opening of the nicotinic acetylcholine receptor channel complex subsequent to binding of two molecules of acetylcholine to the α-subunits. Twisting of the M2 helices rotates the non-polar leucine residues (dark circles) away from the pore and replaces them with smaller polar residues (open circles) that permits ion flow through the pore.

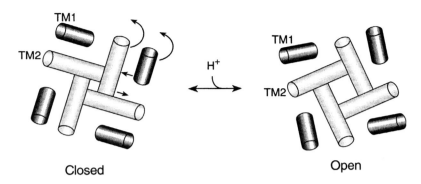

Closed   Open

Figure 7.11 The transition between the closed and open states of the bacterial K^+ channel that is activated by a change in pH. Anticlockwise rotation of the MI and M2 helices opens the channel to K^+ ions.

Voltage-gated ion channels present a similar transmembrane profile, but have six transmembrane helices designated S1 to S6 (Figure 7.9). The S4 helix has a common sequence in all voltage-gated channels being composed of positively charged lysine or arginine residues separated by two non-polar residues. Each helix thus carries five or six positive charges and serves as the voltage sensor for the channel. As the membrane depolarizes, this helix unscrews by breaking and remaking hydrogen bonds to adjacent helices and thus effectively transfers one gating charge. Progressive replacement of these positive charges by neutral residues shifts the voltage-dependence of the channel activation process. Other components of the sequence can be identified with other functions. The intracellular sequence linking domains II and IV of the Na^+ channel is critical to channel inactivation. Although the primary biophysical and pharmacological properties for Na^+ and Ca^{2+} channels are carried within the major α-subunit, other subunits notably the β-subunits play major roles. In the voltage-gated Ca^{2+} channel, the β-subunit interacts specifically with the α-subunit in the cytoplasmic loop between domains I and II.

Finally, the actual direct determination of the structure of a K^+ channel (Figure 7.8) permits explanation of the channel activation mechanisms for voltage-gated ion channels. In the model of Figure 7.11, a counter-clockwise rotation of the two transmembrane domains of each subunit of the tetrameric complex leads to pore opening.

7.3   THE CLASSIFICATION OF ION CHANNELS

7.3.1   Criteria for ion channel classification

Ion channels may be classified according to a variety of criteria. The nature of the permeant ion serves as one scheme to designate Cl^-, Na^+, K^+ and Ca^{2+} channels. Although appropriately descriptive this classification is extremely broad, since it is now clear that multiple classes of channels exist for single ions. Additionally, few channels are totally selective for a single ion and ionic selectivity can be altered, sometimes dramatically so, by differing experimental conditions. Channels may be classified according to the nature of the regulatory signal – as potential-dependent channels, activated by changes in membrane potential or as ligand-gated channels, activated by interaction with specific physiological chemical signals. Most recently, mechanically-dependent channels, activated by changes in cellular pressure or tension, have been described: these are important in hair cells of the ear and in cells, such as cardiac cells, where changes in pressure occur during contraction.

The differentiation of voltage-gated and ligand-gated channels (Table 7.2) has been of particular value and has been confirmed by structural studies (Section 7.2.3). The former class responds primarily to changes in membrane potential over defined ranges of electrical activity, and the latter to changes in chemical potential through drug–receptor interactions. Ligand-gated channels may have the chemical sensor as an integral component of the channel or as a remote component (Figure 7.12). Thus in Figure 7.12a which represents the nicotinic acetylcholine receptor–channel complex (and proteins of the same family) the channel and receptor functions are clearly part of the same heteromeric protein assembly, whereas in Figures 7.12b and c, they are clearly quite separate. An example of the latter process is the activation of voltage-gated cardiac Ca^{2+} channels through interaction of norepinephrine at the β-adrenoceptor. The activating ligand is actually an intermediate soluble second messenger, c-AMP.

The distinction at the molecular level between voltage- and ligand-gated ion channels is, however, less than absolute. All channels exhibit sensitivity to endogenous or exogenous chemical species, both naturally occurring and synthetic, and potential-dependent channels are well recognized to exhibit remarkable chemical sensitivity and ligand-gated channels are not insensitive to changes in membrane potential. The basis for channel activation by a signal lies in an understanding that the ion channel is a stochastic molecular device that opens and closes in a probabilistic manner:

$$I = N_f P_o i$$

where I is the total current through the channel, N_f is the total number of functional ion channels, P_o is the opening probability and i is the unitary current. Changes in chemical or electrical potential can increase or decrease P_o or N_f (or both) and thus change the total current through the channel.

Table 7.2 Summary of channel classes

Voltage-gated	Ligand-gated	Mechano-gated	pH
Na^+	GABA	Various ions	K^+
K^+	Glycine		
Ca^{2+}	n-AchR		
	c-AMP		
	Purines		
	Glutamate		

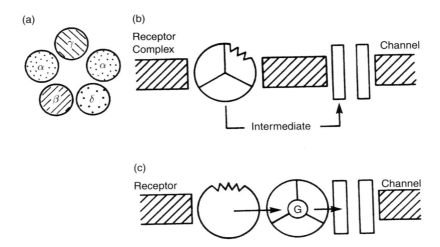

Figure 7.12 Schematic arrangements of ligand-gated ion channels depicting: (a) An oligomeric association of subunits which contain both the channel machinery and the drug receptor; (b) a separate assembly where the drug binding site and the channel machinery are linked through an intermediate (soluble) messenger; and (c) a separate assembly where the drug binding site and the channel machinery are coupled through an intermediate guanine nucleotide (G) binding protein.

7.3.2 Ion channel classification by electrophysiologic criteria

Channels are also classified according to their electrophysiologic characteristics – conductance (current carried) and kinetics and completeness of activation and inactivation. Such distinctions can be seen clearly in the currents of Figure 7.5 where the Na^+ current activates rapidly and inactivates rapidly and the K^+ current activates slowly and does not inactivate during the time course of the trace.

7.3.3 Ion channel classification by drug action

Ion channels may also be classified according to the drugs with which they interact. This classification is obviously in place for ligand-gated channels such as the nicotinic acetylcholine receptor or the GABA and glycine receptors, but it is also applicable to voltage-gated channels that demonstrate a remarkable degree of sensitivity to chemical ligands. Thus, the Na^+ and K^+ currents of Figure 7.5 are sensitive to tetrodotoxin (**7.1**) and tetraethylammonium (**7.2**) that serve as inhibitors of Na^+ and K^+ channels, respectively (Figure 7.13). The actions of tetrodotoxin (**7.1**), a toxin from the puffer fish, underlies its lethal effects and the occasional fatalities from individuals who dine on this delicacy. The 1,4-dihydropyridine nifedipine (**7.3**) (Figure 7.13) blocks voltage-gated Ca^{2+} channels and these actions underlie its clinical cardiovascular uses.

Naturally occurring toxins and synthetic chemicals continue to be of major utility in both the classification of ion channels and in the generation of therapeutic agents.

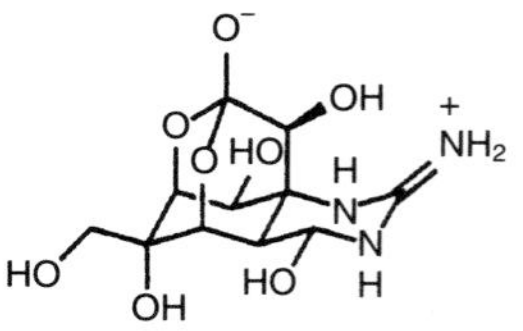

Figure 7.13 Drugs that interact with ion channels: tetrodotoxin (7.1) at Na$^+$ channels and tetraethylammonium (7.2) at K$^+$ channels. Nifedipine (7.3), verapamil (7.4) and diltiazem (7.5) are the first generation Ca^{2+} channel anatagonists. These drugs interact potently and selectively with the L-type voltage-gated Ca^{2+} channel.

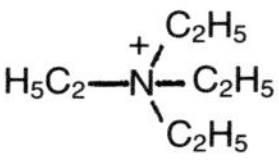

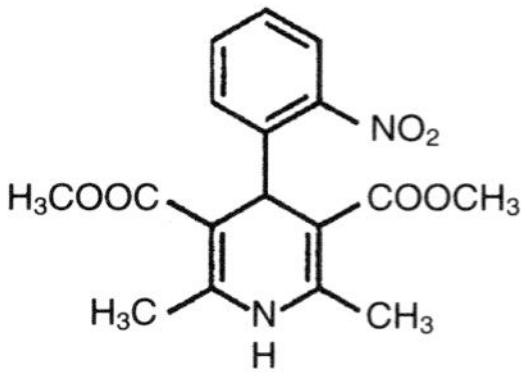

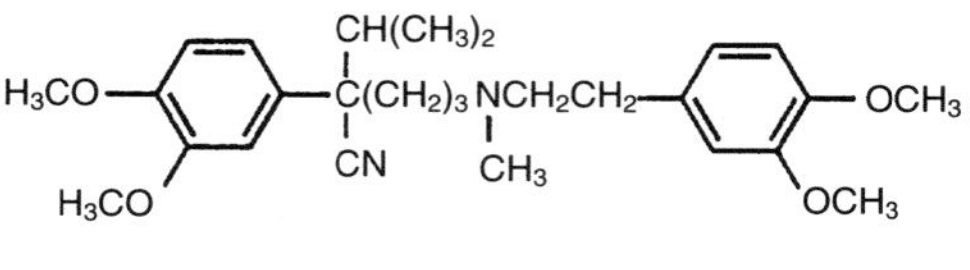

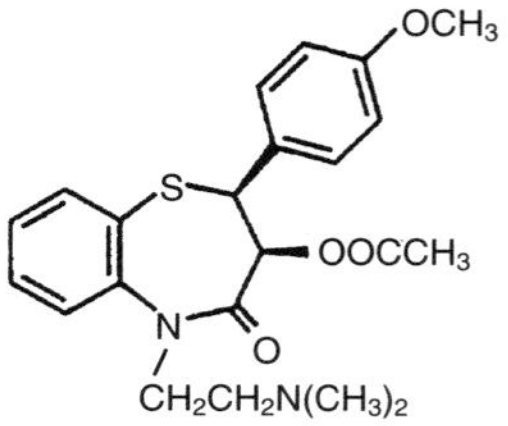

Thus, lidocaine, procaine and related agents owe their local anesthetic and anti-arrhythmic properties to their selective interactions with Na$^+$ channels. Similarly, the heterogeneous group of agents depicted in the lower portion of Figure 7.13, including the 1,4-dihydropyridine nifedipine (7.3), the phenylalkylamine verapamil (7.4) and the benzothiazepinone diltiazem (7.5) are all used as molecular tools with which to classify Ca^{2+} channels and as major cardiovascular drugs (Table 7.3).

In practice, all of these properties of ion channels – ion selectivity, electrophysiological properties, pharmacological sensitivity, and location – are used to classify ion channels. This is illustrated in Table 7.4 for voltage-gated Ca^{2+} channels and in Table 7.5 for K$^+$ channels, a particularly diverse group. The application of molecular biologic techniques has added a particularly fundamental base – classification according to sequence. Collectively, these techniques have

Table 7.3 Therapeutic uses of Ca^{2+} channel antagonists

Uses	Verapamil	Nifedipine	Diltiazem
Angina pectoris	+++	++	+++
PSVT	+++	−	++
Atrial fibrillation and flutter	++	−	++
Hypertension	++	+++	++
Hypertrophic cardiomyopathy	+	−	−
Raynaud's disease	++	++	++

Notes
+ + +, most common use; ++, common use; +, less common use; −, not indicated.

Table 7.4 Classification of voltage-gated Ca^{2+} channels

Nomenclature	Channel class				
	T	L	N	P/Q	R
Sequence, CaV	3.1–3.3	1.1–1.3	2.2	2.1	2.3
Current	I_T	I_L	I_N	$I_{P/Q}$	I_R
Conductance, pS	5–10	25	20	10–20	–
Activation threshold	low	high	high	high	high
Inactivation rate	fast	slow	moderate	rapid	
Permeation	$Ba^{2+} > Ca^{2+}$	$Ba^{2+} > Ca^{2+}$	$Ba^{2+} > Ca^{2+}$	$Ba^{2+} > Ca^{2+}$	$Ba^{2+} = Ca^{2+}$
Function and location	Cardiac SA node, neurons, rep. spiking, spike activity	E-coupling in muscle cells, neurons	------------------neurons only------------------ neurotransmitter release		
Pharmacology blockers	mibefradil flunarizine kurotoxin	nifedipine verapamil diltiazem	ω-CTXGVIA	ω-AGAIVA	–
Agonist		BayK8644			
Subunit composition (α subunits only)	$\alpha_1 G$, $\alpha_1 H$, $\alpha_1 I$	$\alpha_1 S$, $\alpha_1 C$, $\alpha_1 D$, $\alpha_1 F$	$\alpha_1 B$	$\alpha_1 A$	$\alpha_1 E$

Table 7.5 Classification of K^+ channels

Class	Type	Pharmacology	Properties
Voltage-gated			
K_V	delayed rectifier (delayed outward)	TEA, 4-AP PCP, 9-AA	Delayed activation; slow inactivating
K_{VR}	rapid delayed rectifier	dofetilide, sotalol quinidine, tedisamil	rapidly activating component of cardiac current
K_{VS}	slow delayed rectifier		very slow activating component of cardiac current
K_A	transient outward current	4-AP, quinidine PCP, dendrotoxin	activated by hyperpolarization following depolarization
K_{IR}	inward rectifier	TEA, gaboon Viper venom	channel conductance highest when hyperpolarized
Calcium-activated			
BK_{Ca}	high-conductance (maxi-K)	TEA, charybdotoxin noxius toxin, iberatoxin	activated by Ca^{2+}_{int}
IK_{Ca}	intermediate-conductance	TEA, quinine, charybdotoxin	activated by Ca^{2+}_{int}
SK_{Ca}	small conductance	quinine, mepacrine, Apamin, leiurotoxin I	activated by Ca^{2+}_{int}
Receptor-coupled			
K_M	muscarinic-inactivated K^+ channel	W.7	slow to activate at negative potentials, nn-inactivating
Other			
K_{ATP}	ATP-sensitive K^+ channel	glibenclamide, tolbutamide pinacidil, nicorandil	inhibited by $[ATP_{int}]$

revealed that ion channels fall into a limited number of families and that within each family substantial homology exists. Additionally, it is clear that ion channels of apparently fundamentally different characteristics exhibit considerable similarities in their proposed membrane topologies. One of the most important questions now in active resolution is that of relating ion channel structure and function and of generating mechanisms for channel opening and closing processes.

7.4   ION CHANNELS AS PHARMACOLOGICAL RECEPTORS

7.4.1   Receptor properties of ion channels

The pharmacological properties of ion channels indicate that they may be considered as pharmacological receptors with the following overall properties:

1   Channels should exist as homologous protein families.
2   Channels should posses specific drug binding sites which exhibit defined structure–activity relationships, including stereoselectivity, for interacting ligands.
3   Both activator and antagonist drugs should exist.
4   Channels should be regulated by drug and hormone action and by pathological states.
5   Channels should contribute to specific molecular disease states by virtue of aberrant expression or mutated channel structure.

These expectations have been fully realized for many ion channels, including the voltage-gated Ca^{2+} channels where drug interactions have been studied with particular intensity. However, ion channels also exhibit a number of specific and distinctive properties of ligand interaction.

7.4.2   State-dependent interactions of ion channels

Ion channels exist in a number of states or families of states where, quite generally, they are resting and activatable, open and permeant and, in the case of voltage-gate channels, inactivated following the activation process (Figure 7.14). Each of these states represents a different channel conformation and, in principle, a different conformation of, or access pathway to the drug binding site. In the scheme of Figure 7.14, a drug may exhibit higher affinity for the inactivated state of the channel and will thus serve as an antagonist. In contrast, an agent may stabilize the open state of a channel and thus serve as a channel activator or agonist. Alternative pathways of drug access to a binding site may exist. A hydrophilic drug with preferential affinity for the inactivated state may access its binding site through the open state of the channel (pathway A, Figure 7.14), whereas a hydrophobic species that partitions extensively into the membrane may access the site through the lipid bilayer pathway of the membrane (pathway B, Figure 7.14). Similar considerations dictate the pathways through which these drugs leave their binding sites. According to this 'modulated receptor' hypothesis:

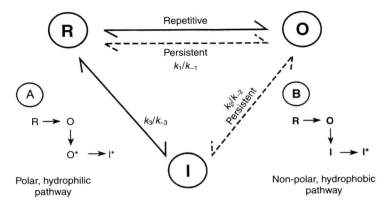

Figure 7.14 The 'modulated receptor' mechanism of drug action at ion channels. Drugs may bind to or access preferentially receptors in the channel in the resting, open or inactivated states of the channel. Each of the states can have a different affinity for a drug. The equilibrium between the channel states will be determined by the physiologic, pathologic or experimental conditions prevailing and hence the apparent drug affinity will vary according to this equilibrium. Repetitive depolarization defines a frequency-dependent process and persistent depolarization defines a voltage-dependent process as in cardiac and vascular smooth muscle, respectively, and thus the action of the Ca^{2+} channel antagonists (see text for further details).

1 Different channel states have different affinities for drugs.
2 Drugs may exhibit quantitatively and qualitatively different structure–activity relationships for different channel states.
3 Drugs stabilize different channel states.
4 Drugs alter the kinetics of channel state inter-conversion.

These considerations apply both to voltage-gated and ligand-gated ion channels and examples of drugs that exhibit such state-dependent interactions are readily available for both channel classes. In a simple two-state model where two states of the channel, A and B, have dissociation constants K_A and K_B for a drug, then K_{app}, the observed dissociation constant, will be given by:

$$K_{app} = \frac{1}{\left[\dfrac{h}{K_A}\right] + \left[1 - \dfrac{h}{K_B}\right]}$$

where h is the fraction of the channel in state A and $1 - h$ is the fraction in state B.

These state-dependent interactions are illustrated in a number of ways. The local anesthetic lidocaine demonstrates enhanced affinity by a factor of several hundred-fold for the depolarized (inactivated) state of the Na^+ channel (Figure 7.15). Access to and from binding sites associated with the ion channel will also control drug–receptor interactions. Interaction of local anesthetics with Na^+ channels reveals a clear dependency of potency upon stimulation frequency. This frequency-dependent property is consistent with a process whereby drug binding requires

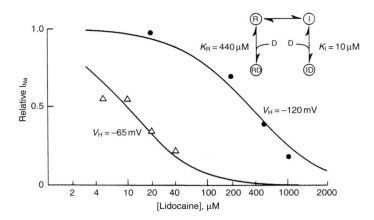

Figure 7.15 The voltage-dependent binding of lidocaine at the Na$^+$ channel. Dose–response curves for lidocaine inhibition of the Na$^+$ current (I_{Na^+}) are measured at holding potentials of -120 mV (when the channels are essentially all in the resting R state) and at -65 mV when the channels are in the inactivated I state. (Reproduced with permission from Bean, Cohen and Tsien, *J. Gen. Physiol.*, **8**, 1983, 613–642).

channel opening, whereas drug dissociation can occur during stimulus-free intervals. Thus, with increasing frequency of stimulation – increased channel opening – drug progressively accumulates at drug binding sites to produce greater block. With a decrease in frequency, channel block decreases correspondingly. Such state-dependent interactions define the anti-arrhythmic actions of a number of drugs.

Quaternary ammonium ions block K$^+$ channels and reveal further complexities in channel–drug interaction schemes (Figure 7.16). Quaternary ammonium ions applied intracellularly to excitable cells will enter and block the channel only

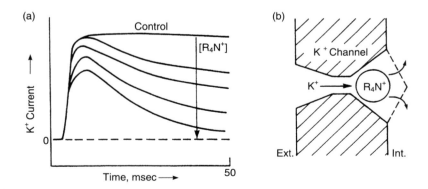

Figure 7.16 (a) Time-dependent blockade of K$^+$ current by quaternary ammonium ion. The extent of block is dependent upon time and progressively increases with increasing duration of channel open time. This indicates that the drug accesses its binding site *only* when the channel is open; (b) schematic representation of a quaternary ammoniumion being trapped in the pore after channel closure. K$^+$ ion movement and channel opening serve to displace the blocker.

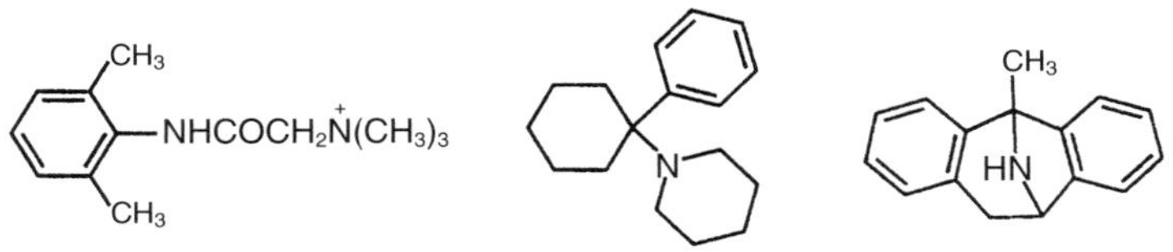

Figure 7.17 Structural formulae of drugs that show selective interaction with the open state of the Na^+ channel [QX-222 (**7.6**)] or the ligand-gated NMDA channel [PCP (**7.7**) and MK-801 (**7.8**)].

during the open state. The channel may close with drug trapped at the binding site from which it cannot escape until the channel is reopened.

Similarly, drugs that function as non-competitive antagonists in ligand-gated channels may interact at sites associated with the channel rather than the receptor component of the receptor-channel complex (Figure 7.17). The quaternary ammonium local anesthetic QX 222 (**7.6**) interacts preferentially with the open state of the channel, and at the N-methyl-D-aspartate class of excitatory amino acid receptors the agents phencyclidine (**7.7**) and MK-801 (**7.8**) also bind with highest affinity to the open channel state (see Chapter 9).

These state-dependent aspects of drug interactions are important from at least three perspectives. They are important in the determination of the selectivity of drug action. The voltage- and frequency-dependent actions of local anesthetics define their utility as Class 1 anti-arrhythmic agents, whereby the very efficacy of the drug is enhanced by the pathological condition and minimized by the physiologic condition. The state-dependent interactions also serve as valuable molecular probes of channel structure and function by revealing subtleties of interactions and access pathways. Finally, these interactions are important to the determination and analysis of structure–activity relationships of drugs active at ion channels.

7.4.3 Structure–activity relationships and state-dependent interactions

The interpretation of structure–activity relations for channel-active drugs is complex since it may depend significantly upon the choice of experimental conditions. These conditions may best be controlled through electrophysiologic studies. These may not generate large data bases, but they can establish the fundamental mode of interaction of lead compounds. Accordingly, comparisons of drug activities obtained under different conditions or in different preparations must be interpreted with caution. Differences in activity may indicate the existence of channel subtypes, but may be equally consistent with the existence of state-dependent interactions. The comparisons of pharmacologic and radioligand binding activities in a series of 1,4-dihydropyridine Ca^{2+} channel antagonists depicted in Figure 7.18 is illustrative of this issue. Clearly, the higher pharmacologic activity of this series in smooth muscle relative to cardiac muscle may be consistent with different channel

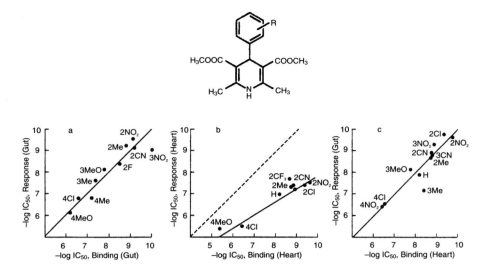

Figure 7.18 Comparison of the binding and pharmacologic affinities of a series of 1,4-dihydropyridines in smooth and cardiac muscle. The 1,4-dihydropyridines are all analogs of nifedipine (**7.3**) with the indicated phenyl ring substituents. Binding and pharmacologic affinities were measured in (a) intestinal smooth muscle, and (b) cardiac muscle. A comparison of the binding affinities in the two preparations is depicted in panel (c). The filled line represents the line of best fit and the dashed line 1:1 equivalence.

subtypes and there is evidence for this (Section 7.5.3). However, the equal binding affinities of the same compounds obtained from depolarized membrane preparations are also consistent with the existence of voltage-dependent binding as defining the different structure–function relationships. Binding affinity increases with increasing and maintained depolarization: this will be the situation with smooth muscle where maintained depolarization is the stimulus mode, rather than the repetitive depolarization observed for cardiac muscle.

A further example from the 1,4-dihydropyridine series, derives from the enantiomeric pair of Figure 7.19. In this series, the *S*- and *R*-enantiomers show activator and antagonist properties respectively. However, if the *S*-enantiomer interacts with the voltage-gated Ca^{2+} channel in the depolarized state it shows

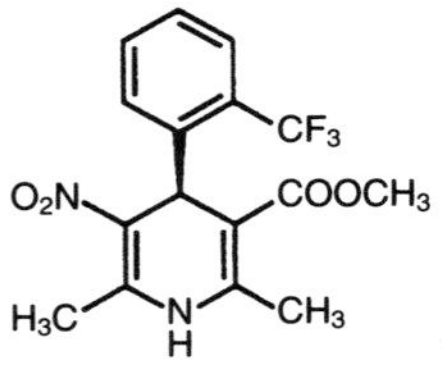

(7.9) 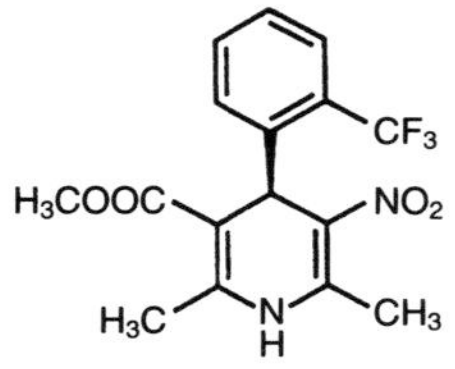   **(7.10)**

Figure 7.19 The enantiomers of a 1,4-dihydropyridine that show activator, (*S*)-BayK8644 (**7.9**), and antagonist, (*R*)-BayK8644 (**7.10**), properties.

antagonist activity. Thus, state–dependent interactions may generate both quantitative and qualitative changes in structure–activity relationships for drugs active at ion channels.

7.5 DRUGS ACTING AT SPECIFIC ION CHANNELS

7.5.1 Multiple sites for drug action

A principal feature of ion channels and drug action is the presence of multiple, discrete sites of action. These sites or receptors are frequently linked one to the other and to the functional machinery of the channel by complex allosteric interactions. Thus, binding of a drug to one channel receptor site may alter not only the ion permeation characteristics but may also simultaneously alter the interactions of drugs at other, but allosterically, linked receptor sites. These interactions render complex the interpretation of the actions of drugs at ion channels. Useful examples of this complexity are provided by drugs that act at voltage-gated Na^+, Ca^{2+} and K^+ channels and at the K_{ATP}^+ and NMDA receptors as examples of ligand-gated ion channels.

7.5.2 Drugs acting at Na^+ channels

At least nine major classes of drugs interact at the Na^+ channel at discrete receptors where they mediate distinct responses (Table 7.6). The guanidinium toxins, tetrodotoxin and saxitoxin, are generally assumed to block the permeation pathway of the channel. However, structure–activity relationships in these molecules are extremely limited, principally because of their complex synthetic chemistry. However, both the guanidinium group and the hydroxyl functions do appear necessary for activity. The other structural classes of Na^+ channel drugs exhibit more complex interactions with their interaction properties being profoundly state-dependent. Veratridine (**7.12**) and the lipid-soluble alkaloid toxins (Figure 7.20)

Table 7.6 Drug interactions at voltage-gated Na^+ channels

Site	Toxin or drug	Activity
1	Tetrodotoxin, saxitoxin	block activation
2	Batrachotoxin, veratridine grayanotoxin	persistent activation
3	α-Scorpion toxins	block activation
	sea anemone II toxin	persistent activation
4	β-Scorpion toxins	shift voltage-dependence
5	Brevetoxins	repetitive firing
6	δ-Conotoxins	block inactivation
7	DDT, pyrethroids	block activation shift voltage-dependence
8	Coral toxin	block activation
9	Local anesthetics anticonvulsants	block activation

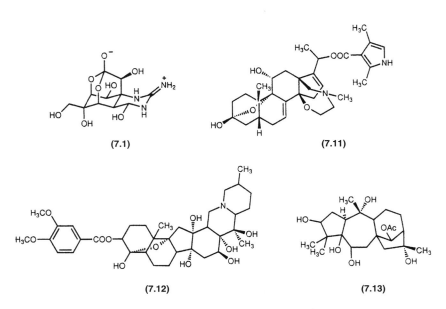

Figure 7.20 Structural formulae of toxins that interact at the Na$^+$ channel. Tetrodotoxin (**7.1**), batrachotoxin (**7.11**), veratridine (**7.12**) and grayanotoxin (**7.13**).

have the common property of activating the Na$^+$ channels and maintaining their open state. Although, consistent with their very different chemical structures, these agents do not interact at identical binding sites, they do share and the net consequence of their interaction to produce a state of persistent activation of the Na$^+$ channel. This activation occurs through an allosteric stabilization of the channel open state. Accordingly, drug-bound channels are activatable at membrane potentials far more negative than unmodified channels: the action of the drug is effectively to shift the voltage-activation curve for the Na$^+$ channel leftward to more negative membrane potentials.

A variety of peptide toxins also interact at Na$^+$ channels and are derived from scorpions, sea anemones and fish hunting cone snails of the *Conus* genus. These polypeptide toxins all contain several disulfide bridges that serve to maintain a relatively rigid structure. The toxins from sea anemones and scorpions are small proteins of 45–50 and 60–70 residues, respectively, while the conotoxins (Figure 7.21) are significantly smaller in size with some 20 residues. Although they are all disulfide-bridged entities they appear to interact in different ways. The conotoxins act in a manner similar to tetrodotoxin (**7.1**) and saxitoxin, whereas the sea anemone and scorpion toxins have more complex modes of interaction that appear to involve shifts of the channel activation curves to more negative membrane potentials in a manner similar to that of veratridine (**7.12**).

Other examples of drugs that interact at Na$^+$ channels include the pyrethroid insecticides, analogs of the pyrethroid neurotoxins isolable from *Chrysanthemums*. These agents (Figure 7.22) also interact allosterically with the channel and bind

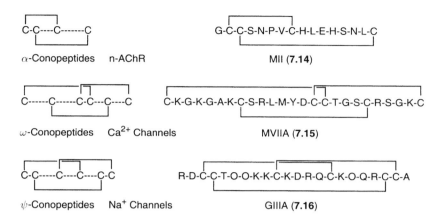

Figure 7.21 Structural formulae of representative examples of the conotoxin (derived from cone snails) series of peptide toxins. The α-, ω- and ψ-conopeptides are illustrated by general formulae with specification of cysteine disulfide bridges and one example from each group (**7.14–7.16**) with the amino acid sequence given by one-letter abbreviations.

preferentially to the open state causing a persistent channel activation: this underlies their neurotoxic properties. Local anesthetics, including lidocaine and procaine, also interact with the Na⁺ channel and this forms the basis for their anesthetic actions and for their anti-arrhythmic properties.

Currently, therapeutic attention at the Na⁺ channel is directed to the search for new anticonvulsants, neuroprotective agents and analgesia. The principal compounds available are the anticonvulsants phenytoin (**7.21**) and carbamazepine (**7.22**), lamotrigine (**7.23**) for neuropathic pain and riluzole (**7.24**) for the neuro-degeneration observed in amyotrophic lateral sclerosis (Figure 7.23).

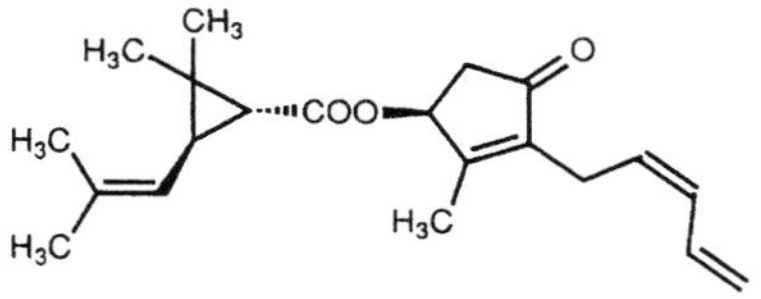

(7.17)

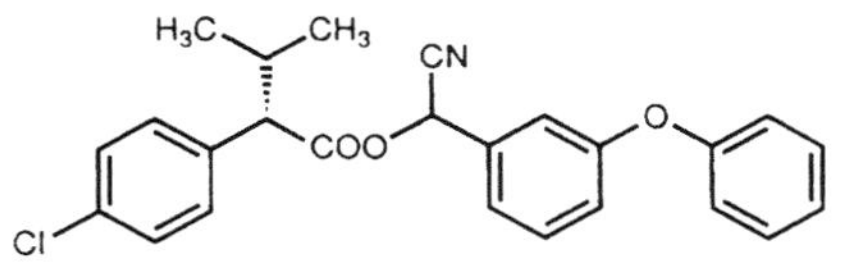

(7.18)

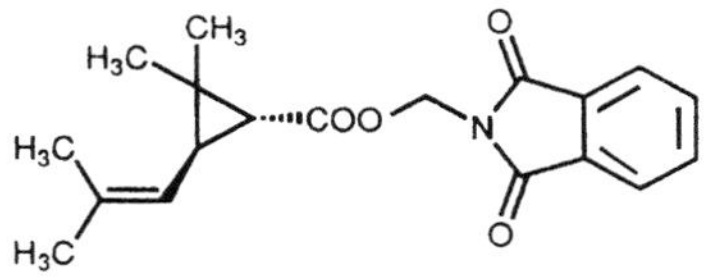

(7.19)

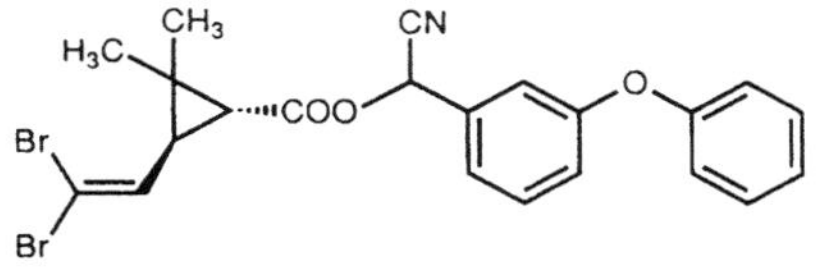

(7.20)

Figure 7.22 Pyrethrins (**7.17–7.20**) active at the Na⁺ channel.

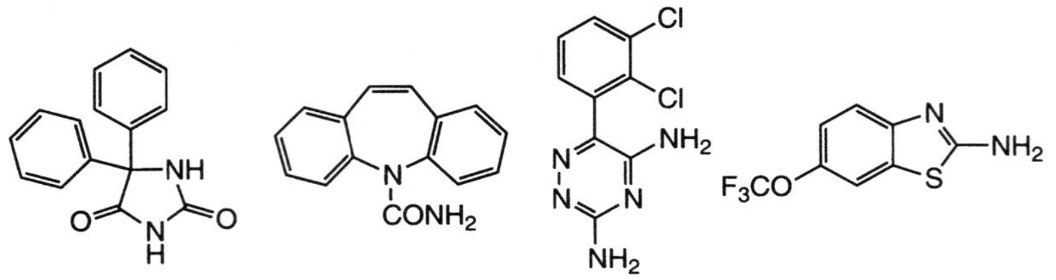

Figure 7.23 Clinically useful Na$^+$ channel antagonists. Phenytoin (**7.21**), carbamazepine (**7.22**), lamotrigine (**7.23**) and riluzole (**7.24**).

7.5.3   Drugs acting at Ca^{2+} channels

In contrast to the situation with K$^+$ channels, the pharmacology of the voltage-gated Ca^{2+} channels has been dominated by synthetic agents of the 1,4-dihydro-pyridine, benzothiazepinone and phenylalkylamine classes (Figure 7.13). These agents have served simultaneously as major therapeutic agents for cardiovascular diseases (Table 7.3) including hypertension and angina, and as molecular tools with which to analyze channel structure and function. The structures depicted in Figure 7.13 are inhibitors of Ca^{2+} influx through one particular class of Ca^{2+} channel – the L-type channel that functionally dominates the cardiovascular system – but there is considerable interest in drugs that may selectively modulate other classes of Ca^{2+} channels (Table 7.4) since such drugs may have prominent effects in neuronal and other disorders. Some drugs that act on these channel types are depicted in Figure 7.24.

The drugs of Figure 7.13 interact at separate and discrete sites on the L-type channel as shown in Figure 7.25 which demonstrates schematically the arrangement of these sites and the allosteric linkages that exist. The drug–receptor interactions depicted all show state-dependent properties with preferential drug interaction at the open and/or the inactivated states of the channel. Thus, depolarizing conditions that favor the formation of these states enhances the activity of these agents. However, verapamil (**7.4**) and diltiazem (**7.5**), are protonated species at physiological pH, exhibit frequency-dependent interactions, whereas the neutral nifedipine (**7.3**) exhibits voltage-dependent interactions. This difference in mechanism may reflect hydrophilic and hydrophobic access pathways for these drugs and may also underlie their different therapeutic applications with verapamil being an effective Class IV anti-arrhythmic agent and nifedipine (and all other 1,4-dihydropyridines) lacking such properties.

Consistent with their different chemical classes and their interaction at discrete receptor sites there is a separate structure–activity relationship that exists for each of the chemical classes. That for the 1,4-dihydropyridines has been particularly well described and is of interest since both activator and antagonist drugs exist. The overall structure–activity relationship is depicted in Figure 7.26. In a QSAR approach the activity of nifedipine analogs bearing substituents in the 4-phenyl ring could be described by:

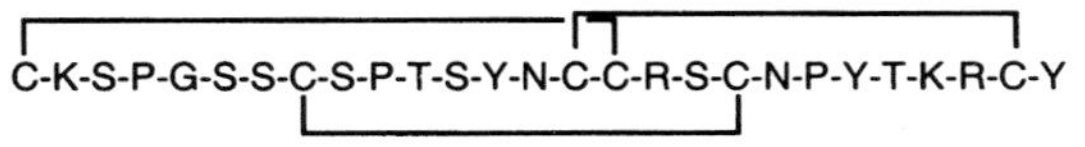
C-K-S-P-G-S-S-C-S-P-T-S-Y-N-C-C-R-S-C-N-P-Y-T-K-R-C-Y

(7.25)

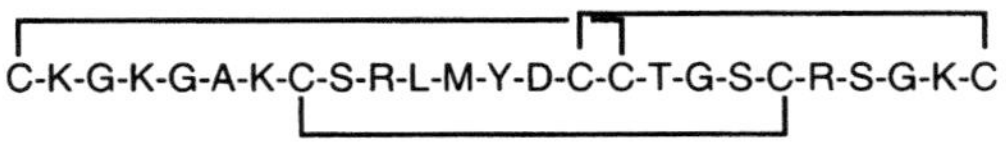
C-K-G-K-G-A-K-C-S-R-L-M-Y-D-C-C-T-G-S-C-R-S-G-K-C

(7.15)

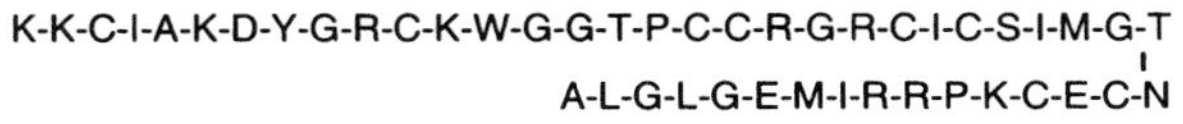
K-K-C-I-A-K-D-Y-G-R-C-K-W-G-G-T-P-C-C-R-G-R-C-I-C-S-I-M-G-T
A-L-G-L-G-E-M-I-R-R-P-K-C-E-C-N

(7.26)

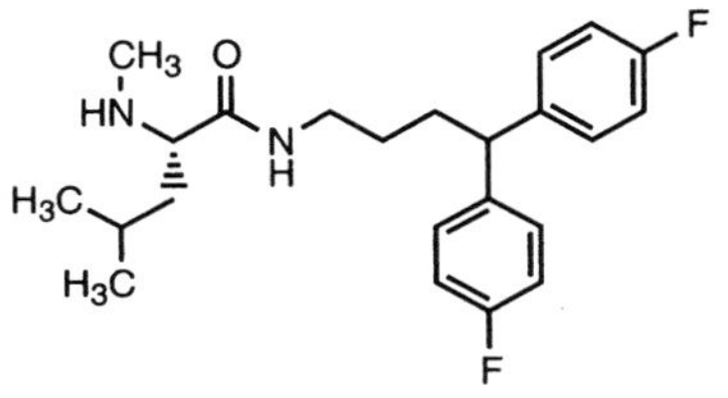
CH3
O
HN
N
H
H3C
H3C
F
F

(7.27)

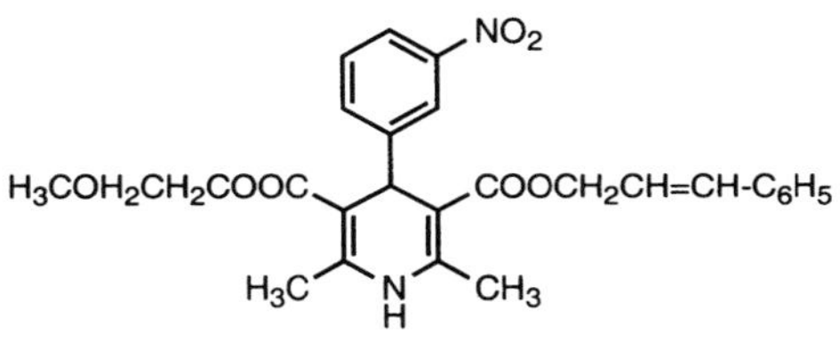
NO2
H3COH2CH2COOC
COOCH2CH=CH-C6H5
H3C
N
H
CH3

(7.28)

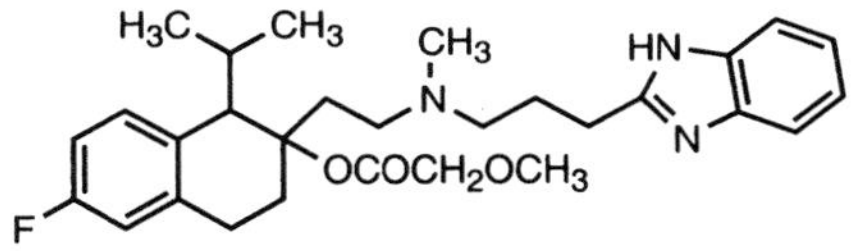
H3C
CH3
CH3
N
HN
N
OCOCH2OCH3
F

(7.29)

Figure 7.24 Drugs that interact with non-L-type voltage-gated Ca^{2+} channels. ω-Conotoxin GVIA (**7.25**, N-type channels); ω-Conotoxin MVIIA (**7.15**, N-type channels); ω-Agatoxin IVA (**7.26**, P-type channels), **7.27** (N-type channels), cilnidipine (**7.28**, N-type channels) and mibefradil (**7.29**, T-type channels).

$$\log 1/\mathrm{IC}_{50} = 0.62\pi + 1.96\delta m - 0.44L_{\mathrm{meta}} - 3.26B_{1\mathrm{para}} - 1.51L_{\mathrm{meta'}} + 14.23$$

$$n = 46, \quad r = 0.90, \quad s = 0.67, \quad F = 33.93$$

where δm is the electronic parameter, π a hydrophobicity index, and L and B_1 are steric parameters. The stereochemical requirements for interaction at the 1,4-dihydropyridine receptor have been examined in considerable detail through the synthesis of rigid analogs, the determination of solid state and solution conformations, and the application of computational techniques. There is general agreement that optimum activity of the 1,4-dihydropyridines requires a flattened boat conformation for the 1,4-dihydropyridine ring and a pseudoaxial phenyl ring oriented orthogonally to the 1,4-dihydropyridine ring with the aryl substituents

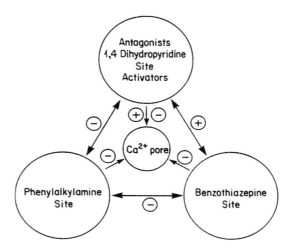

Figure 7.25 Representation of three primary pharmacologic receptors at the voltage-gated Ca^{2+} channel depicting their linkage to the permeation and gating machinery of the L-type channel and the allosteric linkages between these discrete receptors (+, positive allosteric interaction: −, negative allosteric interaction).

oriented away (antiperiplanar) from the 1,4-dihydropyridine ring (Figure 7.26). Additionally, there is an interesting stereochemical discrimination of pharmacological activity where, in appropriately substituted 1,4-dihydropyridines, there is activator activity in the *S*-enantiomer and antagonist activity in the *R*-enantiomer

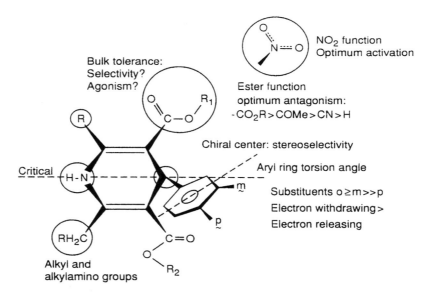

Figure 7.26 The structure–activity relationship for 1,4-dihydropyridine antagonists and activators at the L-type voltage-gated Ca^{2+} channel.

(Figure 7.19). Furthermore, because the interactions of the 1,4-dihydropyridines with their receptor site are voltage-dependent the S-enantiomer can transition from activator to antagonist as the membrane potential becomes progressively less polarized.

The 1,4-dihydropyridines also provide a series of second generation drugs, including nimodipine (**7.30**), nitrendipine (**7.31**), nicardipine (**7.32**), amlodipine (**7.33**), felodipine (**7.34**) and isradipine (**7.35**) (Figure 7.27). These agents have greater vascular selectivity than the parent 1,4-dihydropyridine, and this originates, in part, from their greater degree of voltage-dependence of interaction.

Molecular biology studies have defined both the location of the 1,4-dihydropyridine, benzothiazepinone and phenylalkylamine binding sites in the major $\alpha 1$ subunit of the L-type Ca^{2+} channel and the residues that are involved in binding the drugs. The 1,4-dihydropyridine binding site is located on the IIS5, the IIS6 and the IVS6 domains with critical contributions from tyrosine-1152 (IIIS6), isoleucine-1156 (IIIS6), methionine-1161 (IIS6) and asparagine-1472 (IVS6). A schematic arrangement of the binding sites at the α_1 subunit of the L-type Ca^{2+} channel is sketched in (Figure 7.28).

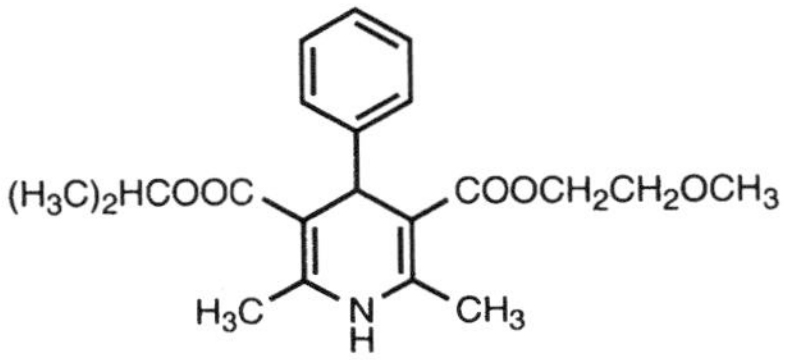

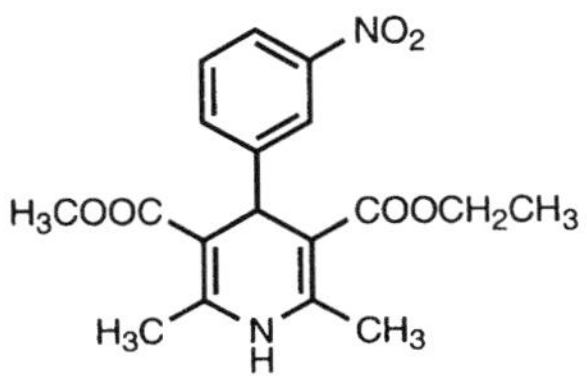

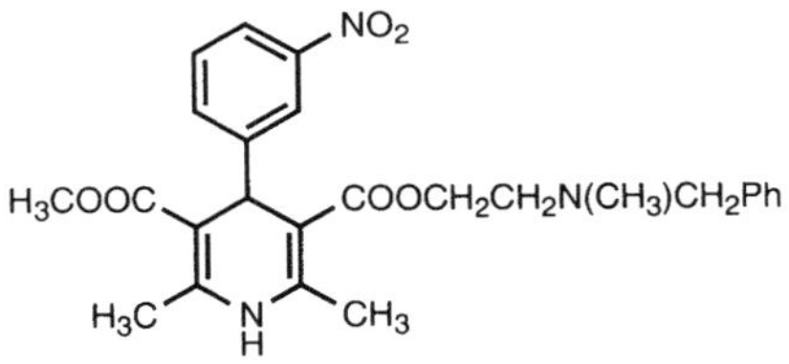

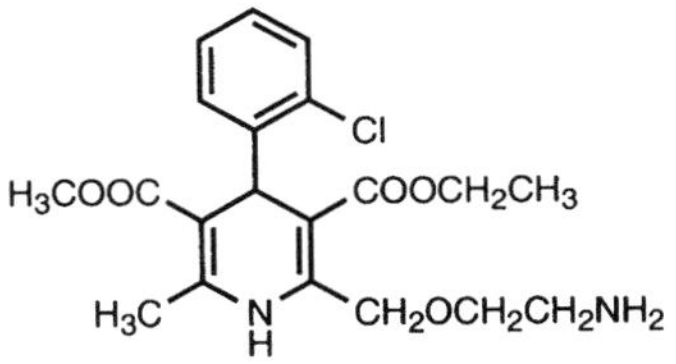

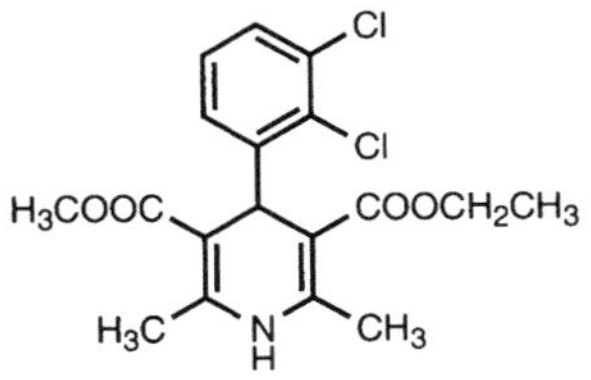

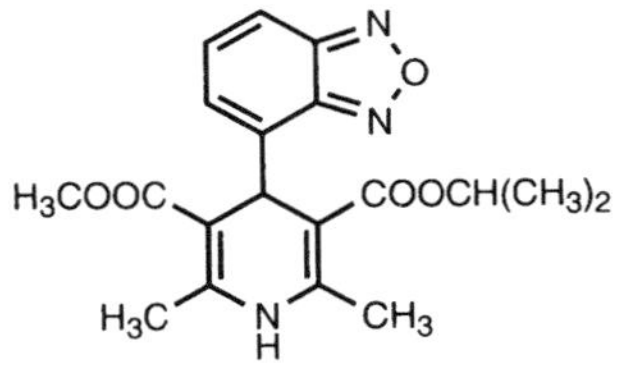

Figure 7.27 Structural formulae of second generation 1,4-dihydropyridines: Nimodipine (**7.30**), Nitrendipine (**7.31**), Nicardipine (**7.32**), Amlodipine (**7.33**), Felodipine (**7.34**) and Isradipine (**7.35**).

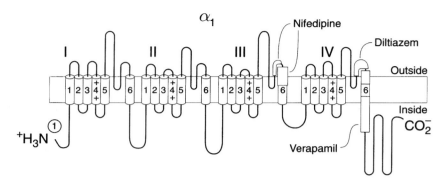

Figure 7.28 The α_1 subunit of the L-type voltage-gated Ca^{2+} channel showing the location of the principal binding sites for the antagonists nifedipine (**7.3**), verapamil (**7.4**) and diltiazem (**7.5**).

7.5.4   Drugs acting at K⁺ channels

K^+ channels constitute a remarkably diverse molecular group of excitable proteins and their pharmacology is correspondingly diverse (Table 7.5). Quaternary ammonium ions, including tetraethylammonium, are channel blockers acting through pore mechanisms but are not very discriminating with respect to channel type. The specific pharmacology of the voltage-gated channels (K_V) is dominated by toxins from scorpions including agitoxin, charybdotoxin and kaliotoxin that block the channel pore as well as by toxins from sea anemone, snails of the *Conus* genus and from spiders including tarantulas. The scorpion toxins are globular miniproteins that share a common scaffold with 29–39 amino acid residues and three or four disulfide bridges with a common motif – G26-K27-C28-M/I29-N/G30-X31-K32-C33-(n)34-C35 where (n) represents a charged residue. The lysine residue at position 27 (K27) appears to be of critical significance and it is suggested that it may 'plug' the pore acting as a surrogate K^+ ion.

From a clinical perspective the ATP-sensitive K^+ channels are of particular importance. These were first recognized in the heart, but are now known to be of widespread distribution and to exist as several major subtypes. They serve to couple the cell metabolic state to membrane potential: with an increase in the cellular ATP levels the channel is blocked and membrane potential decreases. The structure of the channel is a subunit organization consisting of an inward rectifier channel K_{ir} with an sulfonylurea receptor (SUR) subunit that interacts with the synthetic sulfonylurea hypoglycemic agents. The sulfonylurea receptor family are large transmembrane proteins that contain 15 transmembrane sequences and two large cytoplasmic loops (Figure 7.29). The sulfonylurea receptors are members of the ABC transporter superfamily of proteins, which also includes the cystic fibrosis transmembrane regulator gene product. It is the combination of K_{ir} and SUR as an octameric complex that constitutes the active K^+ATP channel: expression of either subunit alone does not generate channel activity. This channel is the location for the hypoglycemic sulfonylureas (Figure 7.30), including the first- and second generation tolbutamide (**7.36**) and glibenclamide (**7.37**) that function

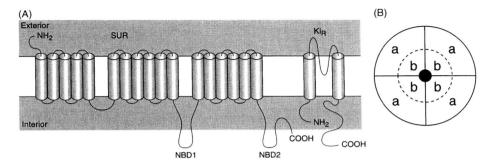

Figure 7.29 (A) The linear sequence of the SUR and its association with the K_{ir} channel subunit; and (B) a functional K^+_{ATP} channel is an octamer consisting of four channel subunits (b) and four SUR subunits (a).

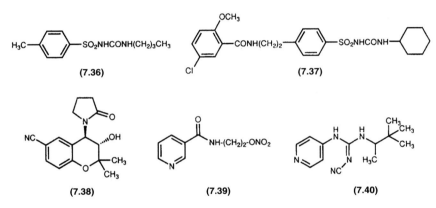

Figure 7.30 Drugs active at the K^+_{ATP} channel (see also Figure 7.4). Antagonists: tolbutamide (**7.36**) and glibenclamide (**7.37**). Activators: cromakalim (**7.38**), nicorandil (**7.39**) and pinacidil (**7.40**).

as antagonists, as well as the K^+ channel activators including cromakalim (**7.38**), nicorandil (**7.39**) and pinacidil (**7.40**). The K^+ channel activators continue to attract attention because of their potential as selective cardiovascular (hypertension, angina), non-cardiovascular (asthma, urinary incontinence) and central nervous system (anticonvulsant, antineurodegenerative) therapeutic roles.

7.6 ION CHANNELS AND DISEASES

As benefits, their status as a class of pharmacological receptors ion channels are associated with defined molecular diseases that arise from specific mutations in channel proteins and that are associated with aberrant function or altered expression. A very partial list of such diseases and mutations is presented in Table 7.7.

Hyperkalemic periodic paralysis is a dominant mutation of the α-subunit of the skeletal muscle voltage-gated Na^+ channel. Mutations in this subunit are associated with a group of diseases referred collectively to 'potassium-aggravated myotonias'. Enhanced serum K^+ brought on by exercise or K^+-rich foods brings about a non-life-threatening muscle paralysis.

Long QT syndrome is a cardiac disease associated with arrhythmias and sudden death. It can arise from mutations in either voltage-gated Na^+ or K^+ channels. A severe form of the disease associated with Na^+ channels arises from a three amino acid deletion in the cytoplasmic loop between domains III and IV of the α-subunit. This produces a non-inactivating current and increases the QT interval of the electrocardiogram. The most common form of the disease is associated with mutations in the K^+ channel. The LQT syndrome has become an area of considerable importance to drug development since drugs that can induce such behavior either directly or by interfering with the P450 drug metabolism system are obviously to be avoided prior to clinical introduction. A number of drugs, including the antihistamines terfenadine and astemizole, the gastric motility agent cisapride and the antihypertensive agent mibefradil, have all been withdrawn from clinical use because of this occurrence.

In persistent hyperinsulinaemia there is an unregulated secretion of insulin with consequent profound hypoglycemia. The disease can arise from mutations in either the SUR or the K_{ir} subunits and activity of the channel is lost leading to a persistent depolarization of the cell and insulin release.

A number of molecular diseases are associated with defects in voltage-gated Ca^{2+} channels. Murine muscular dysgenesis involves a lack of excitation–contraction coupling in skeletal muscle with an absence of functional α_1-subunits: the protein is truncated at the C-terminal and expression of this aberrant protein is reduced. Familial hemiplegic migraine is associated a migraine aura and involves paralysis of one-half of the body during an attack. Several mutations within the α_1-subunit have been associated with this disease.

Cystic fibrosis is the most common molecular disease associated with the Caucasian population and involves defects in the epithelial Cl^- channel with

Table 7.7 Ion channel diseases

Channel	Disease
Voltage-gated Na^+	Hyperkalemic periodic paralysis
	Long QT syndrome
	Generalized epilepsy with fever
Voltage-gated K^+	Episodic ataxia
	Long QT syndrome
Inward rectifier K^+ (K_{ATP}^+)	Familial persistent hyperinsulineamia
	Hypoglycemia of infancy
Voltage-gated Ca^{2+}	Muscular dysgenesis (murine)
	Hypokalemic periodic paralysis
	Familial hemiplegic migraine
Chloride channels, CFTR	Cystic fibrosis

associated defects in the excretion of NaCl (high salt concentration in the sweat), pathological abnormalities in the lung, intestine and male reproductive system. Although some 400 separate mutations have been described in the cystic fibrosis transmembrane regulator, the most common defect arises from a single amino acid deletion, phenylalanine, at position 508.

7.7 ION CHANNELS AS LETHAL SPECIES

The focus on ion channels thus far has been on ion channels as integral and endogenous protein species. However, there are exogenous proteins that when incorporated into the cell membrane form ion channels and these can serve as lethal species by disrupting ion and solute flow. There are some 40 families of pore- and channel-forming proteins and peptides, including a number of bacterial toxins. This toxin family includes diphtheria, botulinum, tetanus, α-hemolysin and insecticidal δ-toxins. Many species produce amphiathic, bioactive and pore-forming peptides. Frogs generate the magainins that serve virucidal, bactericidal and fungicidal actions thus serving to defend frogs against infections. Melittin, a 26 amino acid peptide, is produced by bees and defensins, 35–95 residues, are produced by mammals and have anti-infective functions. Such agents are likely to be of value in the search for new antibiotics.

7.8 FUTURE DEVELOPMENTS

Ion channels continue to represent both a major challenge and a major opportunity to the discipline of medicinal chemistry. They are a major challenge because of the complex kinetic interconversions that are integral to channel function, because of the multiplicity of subtypes and because determination of structure–function relationships of drug action has been more difficult than with other classes of receptors. The opportunities arise because these difficulties are being approached at the very time that molecular biology is making available detailed information about the structure and function of ion channels, including 3D structure. Ion channels, of course, serve as major integrating loci of cells where many different signals are integrated to modulate the health and welfare of the cell. Ion channel drugs are important to human therapy and are likely to become increasingly so in the twenty-first century.

FURTHER READING

Alexander, S.P.H. and Peters, J.A. (eds.) (2000) Receptor and ion channel nomenclature supplement. *Trends Pharmacol. Sci. Suppl.*

Anger, T., Madge, D.J., Mulla, M. and Riddall, D. (2001) Medicinal chemistry of neuronal voltage-gated sodium channel blockers. *J. Med. Chem.*, **44**, 115–137.

Ashcroft, F.M. (2000) *Ion Channels and Disease*. London and San Diego: Academic Press.

Endo, M., Kurachi, Y. and Mishina, M. (eds.) (1999) *Pharmacology of Ionic Channel Function. Activators and Inhibitors*. Berlin and Heidelberg: Springer.

Gura, T. (2001) Innate immunity: ancient system gets new respect. *Science*, **291**: 2068–2071.

Hille, B. (1992) *Ionic Channels in Excitable Membranes*, 2nd edition. Sinauer Associates, Sunderland, MA.

Hofmann, F., Lacinova, L. and Klugbauer, N. (1999) Voltage-dependent calcium channels: from structure to function. *Rev. Biochem. Physiol.*, **139**, 33–88.

Mulvaney, A.W., Spencer, C.I., Culliford, S., Borg, J.J., Davies, S.G. and Kazlowski, R.Z. (2000) Cardiac chloride channels: physiology, pharmacology and aproaches for identifying novel modulators of activity. *Drug Discovery Today*, **5**, 492–505.

Narahashi, T (2000) Neuroreceptors and ion channels as the basis for drug action: past, present and future. *J. Pharmacol. Exp. Therap.*, **294**, 1–26.

Rudy, B. and Seeburg, P. (eds.) (1999) Molecular and functional diversity of ion channels and receptors. *Ann. New York Acad. Sci.*, **868**.

Saier, M.H., Jr. (2000) Families of proteins forming transmembrane channels. *J. Membrane Biol.* **175**, 165–180.

Triggle, D. J. (1990) Drugs acting on ion channels. In *Comprehensive Medicinal Chemistry*, Vol. 3, edited by C. Hansch, J.C. Emmett, P.D. Kennewell, C.A. Ramsden, P.G. Sammes and J.B. Taylor, pp. 647–899. Oxford, UK: Pergamon Press.

Watling, K.J. (ed.) (2001) *The RBI Handbook of Receptor Classification and Signal Transduction*. RBI, Natick, Maine.

Chapter 8

Radiotracers: synthesis and use in imaging

Christer Halldin and Thomas Högberg

8.1 INTRODUCTION

Molecules labeled with radioactive isotopes (radionuclides) have been used extensively to study transformations and distributions of endogenous compounds and pharmaceuticals, since it allows for detection of very low levels of materials. Thus, it is a useful technique to track transformed compounds with a common origin without the need for development of specific analytical methods for each of the constituents. Recently, this field has entered a new area with the development of techniques to measure and display radioactivity in 3D by computerized tomography.

The chapter illustrates the synthesis of radioactive compounds. It is divided in sections depending upon the half-life of the radionuclides used, since this will have a profound influence on the synthetic strategy. It is not a comprehensive treatment, but it will give the reader some insight into this special discipline of organic chemistry. The second part of the chapter illustrates the use of different types of imaging.

Compounds radiolabeled with long-lived radionuclides such as ^{14}C, ^{3}H and ^{125}I are commonly used in *in vitro* imaging autoradiographic studies. Several imaging techniques are available for the *in vivo* visualization of morphology or biochemical processes in the human body, i.e. X-ray CT (Computed Tomography), MRI (Magnetic Resonance Imaging), SPECT (Single Photon Emission Computed Tomography) and PET (Positron Emission Tomography). X-ray CT provides anatomical information based on the differential absorption of X-rays by tissue. The MRI uses magnetic and radiofrequency fields to afford anatomical information based on the proton relaxation properties and proton density of tissue. The SPECT is used to visualize and measure the relative concentration of radioactivity in tissue after injection of compounds labeled with a relatively short-lived single photon emitting radionuclide such as ^{123}I. The PET has been widely used to visualize and quantify different biochemical processes such as metabolic processes and receptor densities. The PET technique utilizes radiotracers labeled with relatively short-lived positron emitting radionuclides such as ^{18}F or ^{76}Br or ultrashort-lived radionuclides such as ^{11}C, ^{13}N and ^{15}O. With this technique, minute amounts of radiotracers can be used due to the very high specific radioactivity obtainable by the short-lived radionuclides.

Biochemical changes can be determined by PET and SPECT in order to monitor pathological conditions in living humans even before any anatomical defects occur.

This has a great diagnostic value and gives new information about disease states and their potential therapeutic treatments. Radiolabeling of endogenous compounds such as glucose, amino acids and acetate have been used in studies on metabolism and synthesis of various human tissues such as tumor, cardiac and brain tissue. Receptor selective radioligands which display a high affinity for the receptor and a minimal metabolic degradation are used to probe receptor status. Imaging of CNS receptors in the human brain is a rapidly expanding area which previously was restricted to postmortem binding studies. While both PET and SPECT can detect radiotracer distribution, the SPECT technique is more readily available than PET. The development of a new generation of SPECT cameras, coincidence positron imaging using a gamma camera should significantly increase PET utilization. The PET requires a cyclotron to generate the radionuclides in close connection to the radiochemistry laboratory and the PET camera. However, the PET technique offers several advantages such as the ability to measure the concentration of the tracer quantitatively, a greater sensitivity, a higher resolution and chemically more diverse radiotracers.

8.2   NUCLEAR CHEMISTRY

An array of precursors and compounds labeled with the long-lived radionuclides ^{14}C, ^{3}H and ^{125}I are commercially available. These radiolabeled compounds have been used for a long time in biochemical and pharmaceutical research, e.g. metabolic, receptor binding and autoradiographic studies. The SPECT uses γ-emitting radionuclides such as ^{123}I, ^{99m}Tc, ^{67}Ga and ^{111}In. The former radionuclide is commercially available and can be produced by the $^{121}Sb(\alpha,2n)^{123}I$ reaction (Table 8.1), i.e. by bombardment of α-particles on a target containing the stable isotope ^{121}Sb to produce the radionuclide ^{123}I and two neutrons. Iodine-123 has a half-life of 13 h and can easily be incorporated with a sufficient level of

Table 8.1 Preparation and some physical properties of commonly used radionuclides

Nuclide	Half-life	Reaction[a]	Mode of decay	Maximum specific radioactivity (Ci/mmol)
^{15}O	2 min	$^{14}N(d,n)^{15}O$	β^+ (100%)	9.1×10^7
^{11}C	20 min	$^{14}N(p,\alpha)^{11}C$	β^+ (100%)	9.2×10^6
^{13}N	10 min	$^{16}O(p,\alpha)^{13}N$	β^+ (100%)	1.9×10^7
^{18}F	110 min	$^{18}O(p,n)^{18}F$	β^+ (97%)	1.7×10^6
^{76}Br	16 h	$^{5}As(d,n)^{76}Br$	β^+ (57%)	1.9×10^5
^{99m}Tc	6 h	$^{99}Mo(generator)^{99m}Tc$	γ (89%)	–
^{123}I	13 h	$^{121}Sb(\alpha,2n)^{123}I$	E.C. (100%)	2.4×10^5
^{125}I	60 days	$^{124}Xe(n,\gamma)^{125}I$	E.C. (100%)	2.2×10^3
^{3}H	12 years	$^{6}Li(n,\alpha)^{3}H$	β^- (100%)	29
^{14}C	5730 years	$^{14}N(n,p)^{14}C$	β^- (100%)	6.2×10^{-2}

Notes

a   The nuclear reactions indicate the target isotope and the bombarding particle, e.g. $^{14}N(d,n)^{15}O$: nitrogen-14 produce, upon bombardment with one deuteron, oxygen-15 and eject a neutron. d = deuteron; n = neutron; p = proton; α = alpha particle.

radioactivity into several types of organic molecules such as receptor radioligands. The transportation of ^{123}I from the cyclotron to the laboratory/hospital should be rapid and the experimental logistics effective. Compounds labeled with the short-lived PET radionuclides ^{18}F and ^{76}Br (half-lives 110 min and 16 h) and the ultrashort-lived ^{11}C, ^{13}N and ^{15}O (half-lives 20, 10 and 2 min) are not commercially available and must be prepared in the vicinity of a cyclotron, even if ^{76}Br potentially should be able to handle in a similar fashion as ^{123}I.

In a PET facility, the cyclotron, the radiochemistry laboratory and the PET camera constitute the three main operative units. Today, most centers employing PET are using low or medium energy sized cyclotrons to produce one or more of the positron-emitting radionuclides: ^{11}C, ^{13}N, ^{15}O and ^{18}F. The ultrashort half-lives of ^{11}C, ^{13}N and ^{15}O, implies that they must be produced immediately prior to use by an adjacent cyclotron. They are formed by means of nuclear reactions that occur on bombardment of target mediums with charged particles (Table 8.1). The production of ^{11}CO$_2$ is demonstrated in Figure 8.1 as an example of this special type of chemistry. The irradiated materials can be either in a solid, liquid or gaseous state. Radiochemical yields are dependent on factors including target shape, design of target foil and efficiency of target cooling. The amount of radioactivity that can be obtained is regulated by the energy of the accelerated particles and the beam current imposed on target.

Labeling of a compound without affecting its biochemical properties is possible by exchange of stable atoms present in the parent molecule. For instance, carbon-12 (^{12}C) or oxygen-16 (^{16}O) is replaced with the corresponding positron emitting radionuclides ^{11}C or ^{15}O. The small kinetic isotope effect that may occur is considered negligible for most applications. The ultrashort half-lives of especially ^{11}C or ^{15}O make them advantageous for sequential investigations with short time intervals in the same individual (animal or human), thereby allowing the subject to be its own control. The use of radionuclides with relatively longer half-lives such as ^{18}F or ^{76}Br provides an opportunity to follow the radioactivity from the radiolabeled compound for a longer period of time, but leads to use of analogs rather than that of natural compounds.

The specific radioactivity is defined as the ratio of radioactivity per mole of the labeled compound with a maximum specific radioactivity inversely related to the physical half-lives of the radionuclide. The maximum theoretically possible specific radioactivity for ^{11}C is 10^7 Ci/mmol (Table 8.1), but due to the difficulties of completely eliminating external sources of ^{12}C this high specific radioactivity is never obtained. A specific radioactivity higher than 1000 Ci/mmol (37 GBq/μmol), is sufficient for most of the radioligands in use in PET investigations of receptors. In addition, when highly potent radioligands are used an even higher specific radioactivity should be used to avoid mass effect on the receptor.

8.3 LONG-LIVED RADIONUCLIDES

Access to ^{14}C-, ^{3}H- or ^{125}I-labeled precursors or common compounds for biological work can in most cases be obtained from commercial sources. This is especially the case for ^{14}C- and ^{3}H-labeled materials with the longest half-life. The simpler the structure

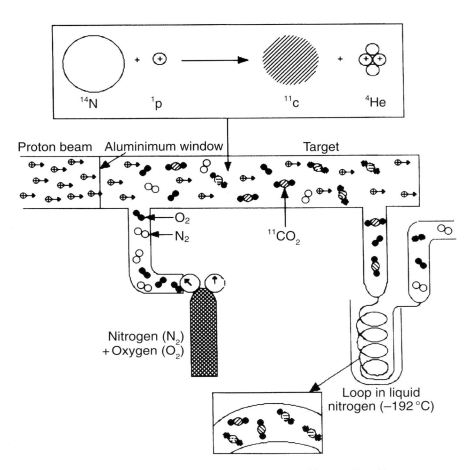

Figure 8.1 The production of ^{11}C via the nuclear reaction $^{14}N(p,\alpha)^{11}C$. ^{11}C is produced by proton bombardment of N_2 which is reacting with trace amounts of O_2 to give $^{11}CO_2$. The prepared $^{11}CO_2$ is trapped in a loop cooled with liquid nitrogen until further use.

the lower the price, i.e. in many situations it is preferable to make the target structure via a lengthy sequence from very simple compounds. For example, $[^{14}C]CH_3I$, $[^{14}C]BaCO_3$, $[^{14}C]KCN$, $[^{3}H]H_2$ and $[^{3}H]CH_3I$ are commonly used sources for the introduction of these long-lived radionuclides. Some representative examples of the synthesis of labeled compounds will be given to show what the effect of considerations such as price, availability and half-life will have on the synthetic strategy.

8.3.1 ^{14}C-labeled compounds

Studies of metabolism and disposition of drugs in animals are preferably made with ^{14}C-labeled derivatives in order to avoid exchange of labile tritium for hydrogens *in vivo* (cf. Section 8.3.2), which is a common problem with tritium-labeling, and to give more easily identified metabolites. However, synthetic limitations or the low obtainable specific radioactivity may necessitate other labeling protocols especially with tritium as discussed in 8.3.2. Depending upon the structure, the radiolabel should be introduced in the part of the structure that will provide most of the expected metabolites in radioactive form. One should for example avoid synthetically attractive choices like methylation of a heteroatom (e.g. N-$^{14}CH_3$), which is likely to be lost via P450 mediated α-oxidation to form radioactive formaldehyde instead of the radioactive desmethyl metabolite needed for the identification work.

NNC 756 (**8.8**) is a potent dopamine D_1 receptor ligand, which was needed in radiolabeled form for studies on the distribution and metabolic fate. The obvious way to label the nitrogen with $^{14}CH_3$ was not used for reasons outlined above. Instead, the label was introduced in the ring via a six step sequence shown in Scheme 8.1. The radioactive precursor (**8.1**) was made with tetrafluoroborate as counteranion and reacted with 7-benzofurancarbaldehyde to produce the epoxide (**8.2**), which was reacted with N-methyl-3-chloro-4-methoxyphenethylamine. Opening of the epoxide produced two compounds (**8.3**) and (**8.4**) in a ratio of 9:1, with the desired isomer (**8.3**) in excess. Separation by reversed-phase chromatography and acid catalyzed ring closure with sulphuric acid in trifluoroacetic acid of (**8.3**) gave (**8.5**), which was resolved as dibenzoyl-D-tartrate (DBDT) salt to yield (**8.6**). Demethylation with boron tribromide gave optically pure (**8.7**). Finally, the hydrogenation over Rh/C gave [^{14}C]NNC 756 ([^{14}C]**8.8**) with a specific radioactivity of 24 mCi/mmol and an enantiomeric purity of >97%.

8.3.2 ^{3}H-labeled compounds

Tritium is the most commonly used radionuclide for radiolabeling in biology and medicine. Often the introduction of tritium is made at a late stage in the sequence via exchange or synthetic techniques, which are associated with certain limitations:

1   Exchange reactions with tritiated water or acetic acid (CH_3COOT) under acid, base or metal-catalyzed conditions often produce compounds with a low-specific radioactivity;

2   hydrogenation reactions are restricted by the availability of multiple C–C bond precursors and the required chemoselectivity in the reactions (e.g. interference from reactions with other multiple bonds and halogens);

3   hydrogenolysis of aryl-halogen derivatives (especially Ar-I and Ar-Br) has similar selectivity problems as hydrogenation;

4   methylation reactions require a desmethyl precursor and an applicable structure; and

5   hydride reductions are limited by the availability and quality of commercial hydride reagents, i.e. [^{3}H]NaBH$_3$ has often a lower specific activity than theoretically possible.

Since the frequent loss of tritium as tritiated water renders the data more difficult to interpret, non-specific equilibration and exchange of labile hydrogens for tritium is less suitable when the tracer will be used for *in vivo* work. Besides, the degree of labeling with tritium in the different positions is usually not known, which can be of importance in studies where metabolic transformations may occur

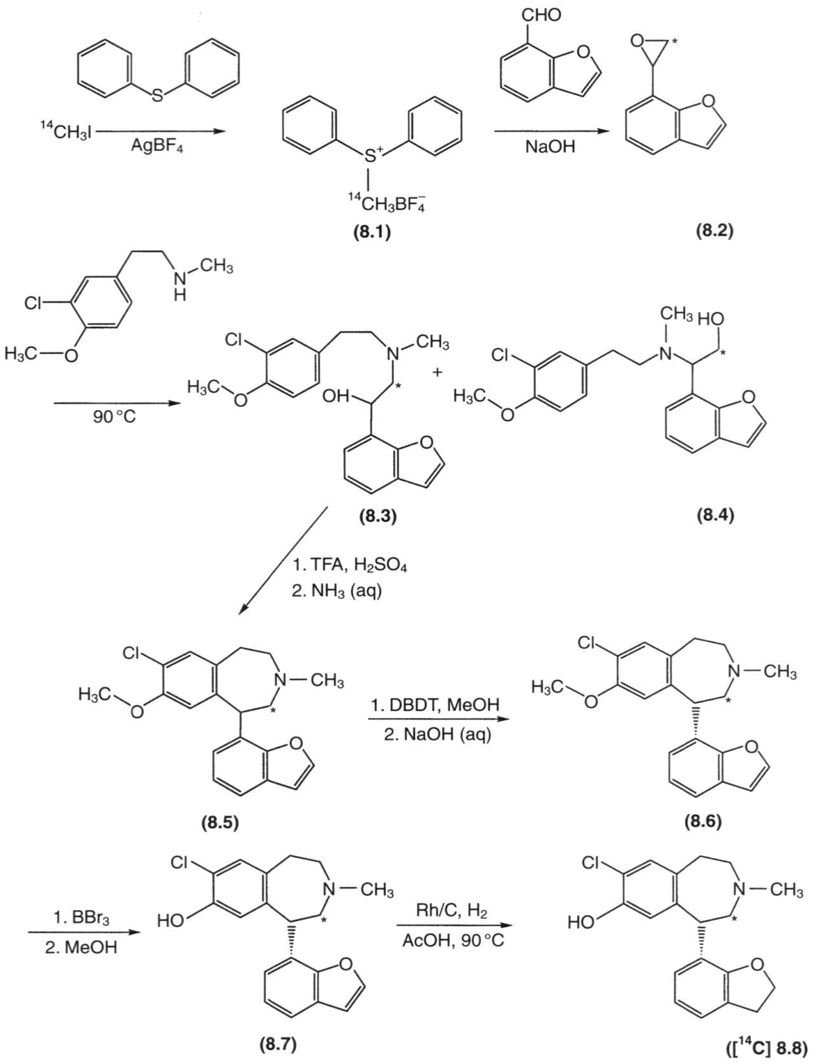

Scheme 8.1

(cf. Section 8.3.1). The development of transition metal catalyzed exchange reactions with tritium gas in which heteroatoms (oxygen and nitrogen) in the target structure can co-ordinate to the metal and promote insertion of tritium in a C–H bond offers a possibility to introduce tritium in positions that are not equally prone to uncatalyzed loss of tritium.

Reduction of olefins will lead to a well-defined regiochemistry even if the stereochemistry could be characterized to a lesser degree. The choice of catalyst will have a large effect on the obtained specific radioactivity, since hydrogen adsorbed on many

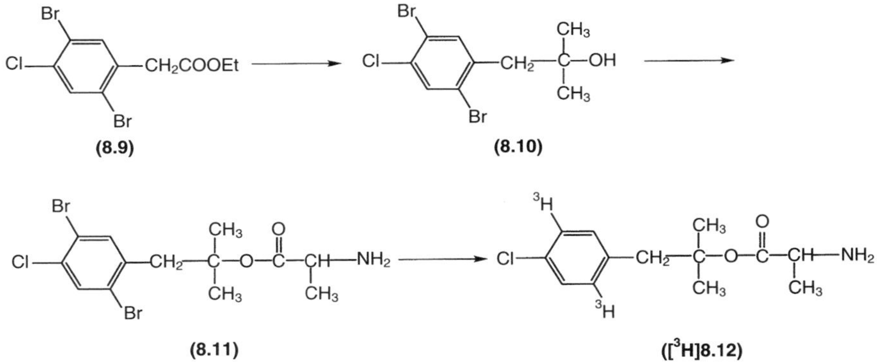

Scheme 8.2

catalysts will equilibrate with tritium if the reaction is too slow. Alternatively, hydrogenolysis of halogen derivatives can be applied to ascertain a well defined labeling. Many studies of receptor binding, especially at low-affinity binding sites, require high degree of specific radioactivity which translates into two tritium atoms per molecule.

Alaproclate (**8.12**) was developed as a selective synaptic serotonin uptake inhibitor. It also possessed affinity for other unknown receptor sites which prompted the preparation of a derivative with two tritium atoms in positions resistant to metabolic attack (Scheme 8.2). The 2,5-dibromo-4-chlorophenylacetate ester (**8.9**), prepared from 4-chlorotoluene, was subjected to a Grignard reaction with methyl magnesium iodide to give (**8.10**). The alanine ester (**8.11**) was obtained by acylation of (**8.10**) with 2-bromopropionyl bromide followed by amination. After optimization of the conditions, the two bromine atoms could selectively be hydrogenolyzed with tritium gas over Pd/C as catalyst in DMF and one equivalent triethylamine. The positions of the tritium atoms in ([^{3}H]**8.12**) can be established by ^{3}H-NMR, which shows *ortho* and *meta* ^{1}H–^{3}H couplings in a fully coupled spectrum and the expected *para* substitution of the tritium atoms as two uncoupled peaks of equal intensity in a proton decoupled spectrum.

The glucocorticosteroid budesonide (**8.13**) is used in the treatment of asthma, rhinitis and inflammatory bowel diseases. It has been made in tritiated form by an efficient reductive and oxidative sequence (Scheme 8.3). Thus, hydrogenation with tritium gas of budesonide gives the corresponding 1,2-ditritio derivative (**8.14**). The following oxidation provides [^{3}H]budesonide containing different levels of tritium in the 1- and 2-positions. In the case of (**8.14**), the hydrogens in the α-position are labile due to the possibility of enolization, which will lead to loss of tritium, in contrast to ([^{3}H]**8.13**) which is not subject to a facile tritium–hydrogen exchange.

8.3.3 ^{125}I-labeled compounds

In order to obtain higher specific radioactivity, than is possible with ^{3}H, the radionuclide ^{125}I can be used in applicable cases, which is especially advantageous for

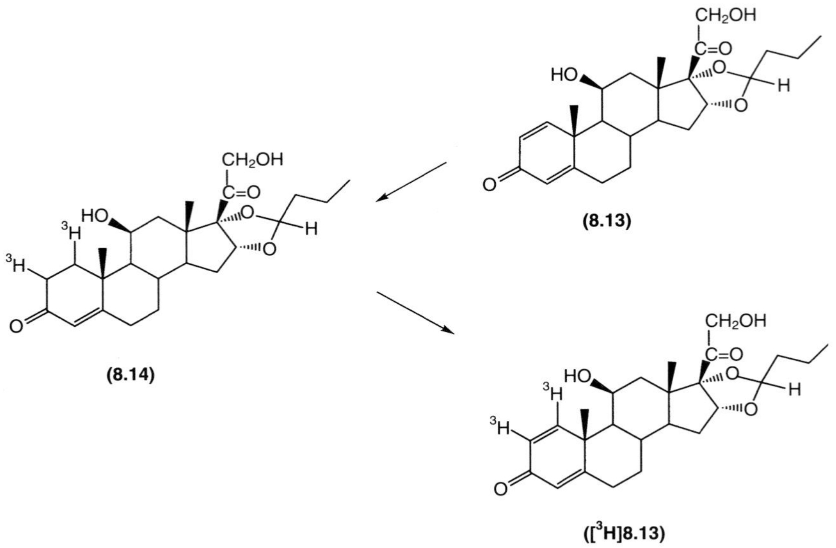

Scheme 8.3

autoradiographic studies. The gamma emitting radionuclide ^{125}I has a half-life of 60 days which enables work during a reasonable time span. Tritium ligands can be made with a specific radioactivity up to 29 Ci/mmol per tritium, compared to 2200 Ci/mmol for ^{125}I-labeled ligands. One reason for the high specific radio-activity of ^{125}I is that the preparation is carrier-free with no dilution of stable iodine. For the development of ^{123}I-labeled radioligands for SPECT (see Sections 8.4.1 and 8.6.2), the use of ^{125}I-labeled radioligands provides essential initial information about the binding properties of the ligand *in vitro* and *in vivo* in animals.

It is common to make non-specific labeling of proteins with this radionuclide. Several types of radioligands for use in receptor binding studies have been designed with ^{125}I substituents. The synthetic work with iodine is, however, more demanding with respect to safety aspects than synthesis with tritium.

NCQ 298 (**8.18**) is a highly selective and potent ligand, developed in our laboratories, for labeling of dopamine D_2 receptors. The regiospecific synthesis of [^{125}I]NCQ 298 ([^{125}I]**8.18**) from the dimethoxy compound (**8.15**) is shown in Scheme 8.4. The desiodo compound (**8.17**) is made by *ortho*-lithiation of the benzamide to produce the doubly chelated intermediate (**8.16**), which is reacted with tributyl borate and oxidized with hydrogen peroxide. Carrier-free ^{125}I was oxidized by chloramine-T in dilute hydrochloric acid and reacted with (**8.17**) to produce the radioligand ([^{125}I]**8.18**) in high radiochemical yield and purity. Notably, the direct halogenation reaction proceeds with full regiocontrol.

On the other hand, if the 2,3-dimethoxybenzamide (**8.15**) is iodinated or brominated (see Section 8.4.2) a mixture of halogenated isomers will be formed. In order to achieve a regioselective introduction, one can for example use the *ipso*-directing effect of silicon or use a halogen-metal exchange reaction by starting

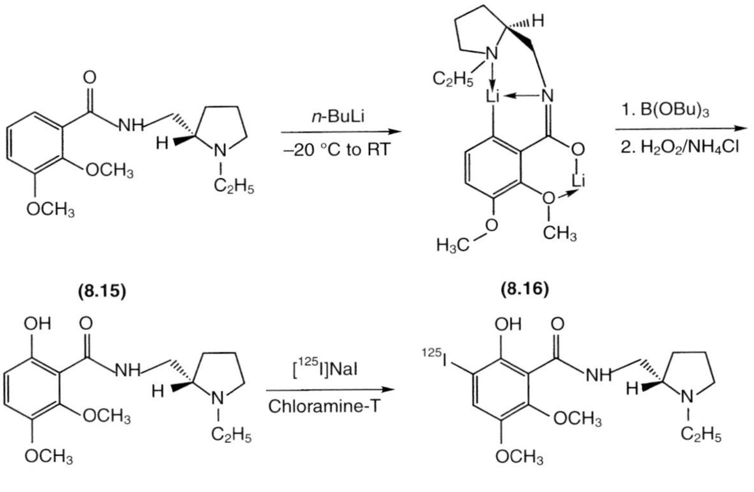

Scheme 8.4

with the corresponding trialkyltin-derivative (**8.22**), as exemplified in Scheme 8.6 in the synthesis of [^{76}Br]FLB 457.

8.4   SHORT-LIVED RADIONUCLIDES

8.4.1 ^{123}I- and ^{99m}Tc-labeled compounds

The most widely used gamma emitting radionuclides in SPECT are ^{99m}Tc and ^{123}I. A number of successful ligands labeled with ^{123}I for SPECT imaging of various receptors have been developed during the past 10 years. Introduction of ^{123}I is usually carried out in a similar way as for ^{125}I, i.e. by electrophilic substitution of an electron-rich aromatic ring by reaction with [^{123}I]NaI in the presence of oxidation agents such as chloramine-T or peracetic acid.

An example of preparation of a ^{123}I SPECT tracer is given by the cocaine analogs [^{123}I]β-CIT ([^{123}I]**8.19**) (Scheme 8.5), which has been used for examination of Parkinson's disease as demonstrated in Section 8.6.2. The introduction of iodine-123 in the phenyl ring, which is not electron-rich enough to permit an efficient direct oxidative iodination analogous to the one used in the synthesis of ([^{125}I]**8.18**), requires a different strategy. Thus, a trimethyltin precursor (**8.20**) was made by a palladium catalyzed reaction using hexamethylditin in the presence of palladium-tetrakis-triphenylphosphine of the parent iodo compound (**8.19**) as shown in Scheme 8.5. This reaction is an efficient chemoselective way (note the ester and tertiary amine functions) to set up the molecule for a mild iodostannyl-ation reaction. The trimethyltin precursor (**8.20**) is treated with no-carrier-added

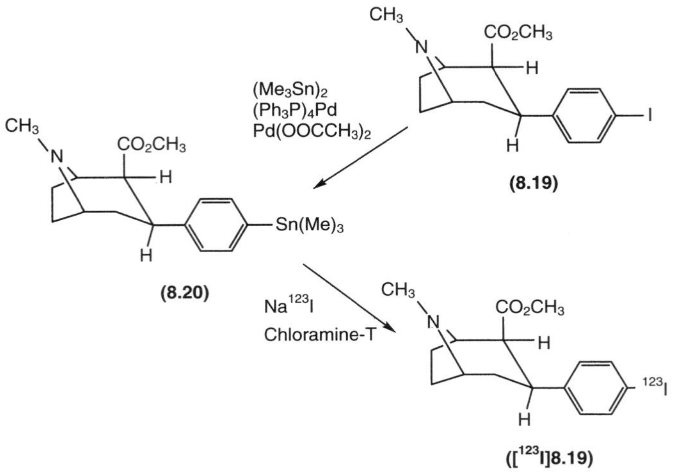

Scheme 8.5

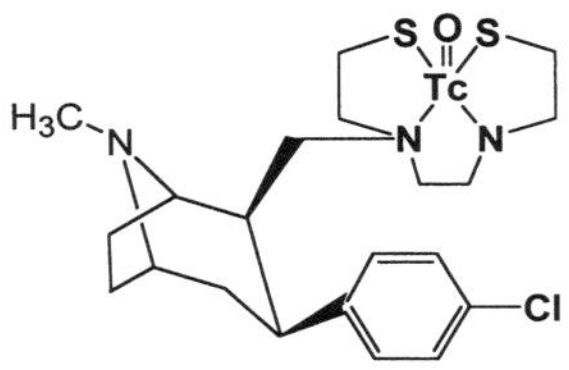

([^{99m}Tc]8.21)

(no dilution with stable iodine) [^{123}I]NaI to form [^{123}I]β-CIT ([^{123}I]**8.19**) with high specific radioactivity (usually >12000 Ci/mmol). When using this labeling method careful purification of the trimethyltin precursor must be performed to ensure a precursor which is free from unlabeled (^{127}I)β-CIT. Presence of carrier β-CIT will reduce the specific radioactivity of the final product and may also result in undesired pharmacological effects for the patient. The advantages of the iodostannylation method are a rapid reaction, high yield, mild radioiodination conditions and a regiospecific incorporation of the iodine. Alternatively, one can use a Cu(I) assisted reaction starting from the corresponding bromo precursor or a method based on direct iodination of the desiodo precursor at oxidative conditions. An advantage with the latter method is facile access to the precursor and elimination of the risk for unlabeled β-CIT in the final solution. Disadvantages are, however, that the direct iodination is not regiospecific, requires heating and results in lower yields. The nuclide ^{99m}Tc is often chelated to the molecule, which can be a suitable tagging technique for studies of e.g. formulations of pharmaceuticals or vascular perfusion (e.g. [^{99m}Tc]hexamethylpropyleneamine oxime) ([^{99m}Tc]

HMPAO). Imaging of dopamine transporters in human with ^{99m}Tc labeled TRODAT–1([^{99m}Tc]**8.21**), a tropane analog, has recently been performed.

8.4.2 ^{76}Br-labeled compounds

The positron emitting radionuclide ^{76}Br has a half-life of 16 h, which makes it possible to follow the radioligand distribution for more than 24 h, if the biological half-life of the compound is long enough. However, the limited access to ^{76}Br and the relatively high doses of radiation to target organs, when ^{76}Br is injected into the body, are disadvantages compared to other PET radionuclides with shorter half-lives. Several substituted benzamides and salicylamides developed at the Astra laboratories have high affinity and selectivity for central dopamine D$_2$ receptors. These properties and a low level of non-specific binding are reasons for their suitability as radioligands for PET.

One recently developed ligand, FLB 457 (**8.23**) has an extremely high affinity for the dopamine D$_2$ receptors, which makes it possible to also study regions containing low densities of receptors outside the striatum. This ligand has also been prepared in carbon-11 labeled form by a reaction analogous to the one described for raclopride ([^{11}C]**8.41**) in Section 8.5.1. Scheme 8.6 shows the preparation of the bromine-76 labeled benzamide FLB 457 ([^{76}Br]**8.23**) as well as the corresponding salicylamide FLB 463 ([^{76}Br]**8.24**). In the former case, a bromostannylation reaction of the tributyltin derivative (**8.22**) is required in order to establish full regiocontrol, whereas the bromination of (**8.17**) provides only one regioisomer (cf. the synthesis of the corresponding iodo derivative ([^{125}I]**8.18**)).

8.4.3 ^{18}F-labeled compounds

Compared to ^{11}C, the half-life of 110 min of ^{18}F allows for a relatively long synthesis and transportation of the radiotracer over moderate distances as well as studies

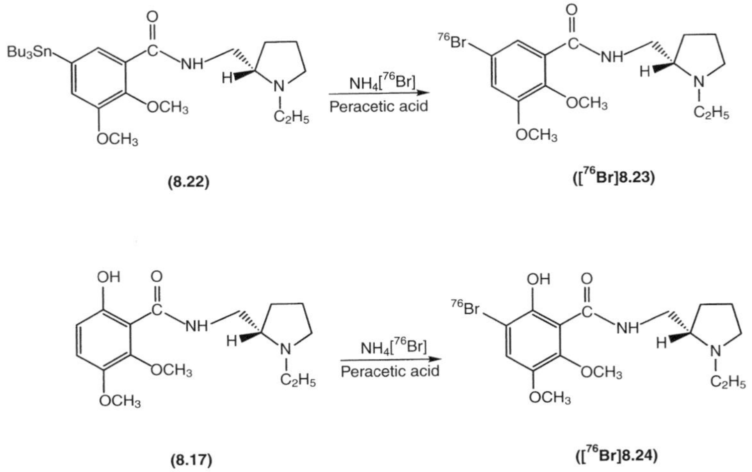

Scheme 8.6

([^{18}F]8.25)

of relatively slow biological processes. The labeling of radiotracers with radioactive halogen nuclides usually implies synthesis of analogs rather than of the natural molecules. However, the small size of fluorine makes it possible to replace a hydrogen in many cases without distorting the properties. Accordingly, ^{18}F is a widely used tag in PET of naturally occurring molecules and therapeutic agents. However, the unique electronic properties of fluorine may lead to compounds with deviating properties, which must be investigated prior to the use. For example, a profound influence on the pK_a of amines substituted with fluorine in α- or β-position has been shown to affect the binding affinities of ligands. There are also possibilities to take advantage of the slightly altered properties inflicted by fluorine incorporation in the design of the tracer, e.g. in the most extensively used tracer 2-[^{18}F]fluoro-2-deoxyglucose ([^{18}F]FDG) ([^{18}F]8.25). [^{18}F]FDG has been widely used in metabolic studies of the brain and the heart. After intravenous administration, [^{18}F]FDG is phosphorylated to FDG-6-phosphate mediated by hexokinase. Because FDG-6-phosphate is not a substrate for glycolysis and does not undergo further metabolism, it remains trapped in the cell over the course of several hours. [^{18}F]FDG is usually prepared from [^{18}F]fluoride which can be produced from ^{18}O(p,n)^{18}F using H_2 ^{18}O as target (Table 8.1). [^{18}F]Fluoride can be separated by an anion-exchange column and allowed to react with 1,3,4,6-tetra-O-acetyl-2-O-trifluoromethanesulphonyl-β-D-mannopyranose in the presence of an aminopolyether such as Kryptofix[2.2.2] to enhance the nucleophilicity of fluoride to yield [^{18}F]FDG in about 50% total yield.

Another example of fluorine labeling is the preparation of [^{18}F]NCQ 115 ([^{18}F]8.30) (Scheme 8.7) which is a selective dopamine D_2 receptor antagonist. Notably, the affinity of this N-benzyl pyrrolidine (8.30) for the receptor resides in the opposite stereoisomer compared to the other mentioned benzamides with N-ethyl pyrrolidine side chains, e.g. (8.18), (8.23) and (8.24). NCQ 115 has a fluorine in a synthetically accessible position in the parent compound and was therefore suggested as a potential ^{18}F-labeled radioligand for PET. [^{18}F]4-Fluorobenzyl iodide (8.28) was prepared in a 3-step synthesis from potassium [^{18}F]fluoride. The first critical step relies upon a nucleophilic displacement of the quaternary anilinium group which proceeds with regiocontrol due to the influence of the electron-withdrawing aldehyde para-substituent. The nucleophilicity of the fluoride ion is enhanced by using the aminopolyether cryptand Kryptofix[2.2.2] to complex the potassium counterion. N-4-Fluorobenzylation of the corresponding secondary

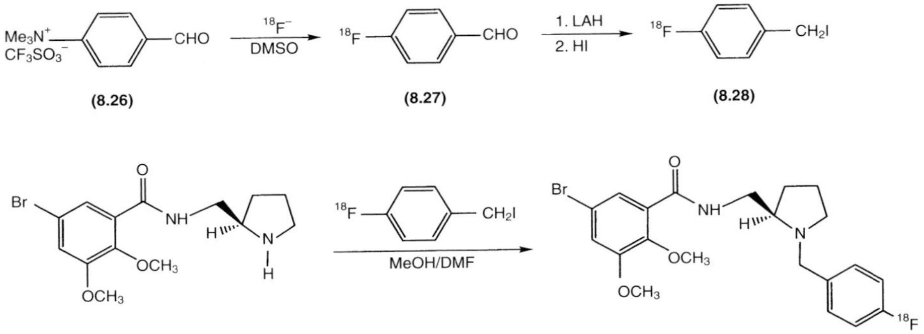

Scheme 8.7

pyrrolidine precursor (**8.29**) was performed giving (\[^{18}F\]**8.30**) with a total synthesis time of 90 min including purification with semi-preparative HPLC (Scheme 8.7).

8.5   ULTRASHORT-LIVED RADIONUCLIDES

In the preparation of compounds labeled with radionuclides such as ^{11}C, ^{13}N or ^{15}O (half-lives 20, 10 and 2 min) a series of requirements related to the ultrashort half-life of the radionuclide must be considered. When optimizing the radio-chemical yield of a reaction, influence of conventional parameters such as sub-strate and reagent concentrations, temperature, pH and solvent compositions are considered. However, the most critical parameter in the synthesis of these ultra-short-lived tracers is time. Even if a reaction is completed within two half-lives of the radionuclide, it may be favorable to stop the reaction earlier since the radioactivity decay has also to be considered (Figure 8.2).

8.5.1 ^{11}C-labeled compounds

The radioactivity must be introduced by readily accessible radiolabeled precursors. Examples of ^{11}C-labeled precursors that can either be produced directly in the target or obtained via rapid on-line reactions starting from ^{11}CO$_2$ are shown in Scheme 8.8. The most widely used labeled ^{11}C-labeled precursor today is \[^{11}C\]methyl iodide. Recently, a more reactive precursor \[^{11}C\]methyl triflate was shown to give higher yields in the synthesis of some commonly used PET radioligands.

The labeling reactions must occur rapidly and in high yields. The complete procedure, from the production of the labeled precursor to the delivery of the purified labeled compound should not exceed more than three half-lives of the radionuclide. A typical total synthesis time for a ^{11}C-labeled radioligand including purification is 30 min. The principal strategy is to introduce the labeled precursor as late as possible, followed by none or just a few additional reactions before the final purification. In addition, handling of high levels of radioactivity on a routine

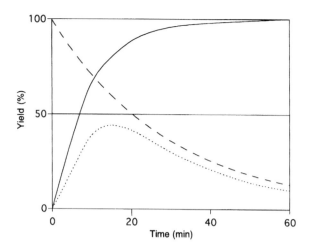

Figure 8.2 The radiochemical yield of a hypothetical ^{11}C-reaction as a function of time (dotted line). Dashed line: the decay curve of the radionuclide. Solid line: the chemical yield of the reaction.

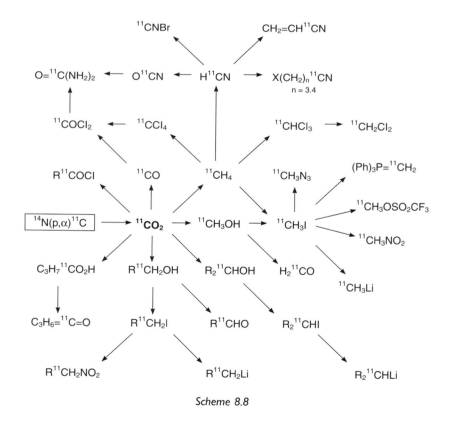

Scheme 8.8

basis requires an automated/remote-controlled experimental set-up installed in a lead-shielded hot-cell to ensure maximal radiation protection. On-line and one-pot reactions shorten the total synthesis time and reduce radioactivity losses.

The stoichiometry of a radiolabeling reaction differs from that of an ordinary chemical synthesis. The amount of the radionuclide produced in the cyclotron is in the nanomolar range. With such small amounts, all other substrates or reactants used are necessarily in large excess. This condition will favor a fast incorporation of the labeled precursor. However, because of the small amounts of the labeled precursor a general problem is that even small amounts of impurities might disturb the reaction. The various steps for the synthesis and PET-application of a radiotracer are presented in Figure 8.3. Efficient PET investigations require an

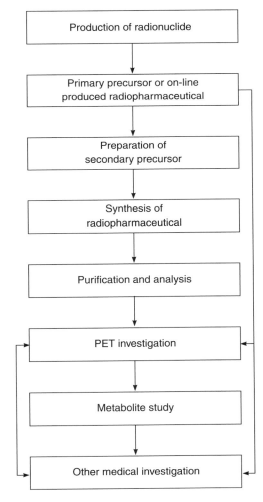

Figure 8.3 Various steps involved before and during medical investigations using positron-emitting radionuclides.

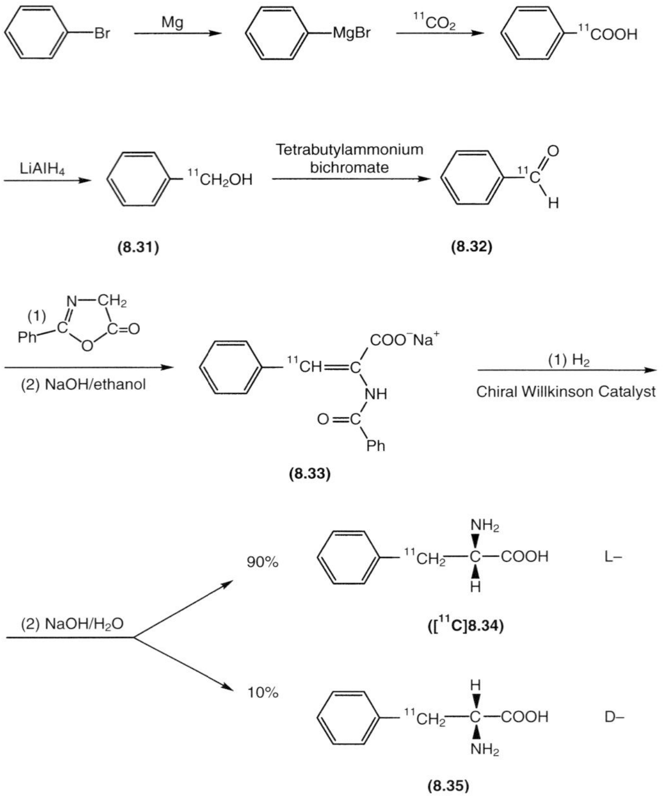

Scheme 8.9

unusually high degree of interdisciplinary collaboration and co-ordination set in a very tight time frame. Thus, PET centers have been established to optimize all steps in this sequence of events and to be cost-effective units. At the end of 1994, the number of PET research centers has reached more than 120 compared to only about 30 centers 10 years ago.

An example of a multi-step synthesis that can be performed with ^{11}C is the seven-step synthesis of optically enriched L-[3-^{11}C]phenylalanine ([^{11}C]8.34) from [^{11}C] carbon dioxide via [^{11}C]benzaldehyde (8.32) (Scheme 8.9). The labeled benzaldehyde was prepared by a selective oxidation of [^{11}C]benzylalcohol (8.31). The three steps from [^{11}C]CO_2 to (8.32) were accomplished within 5 min. [^{11}C]Benzaldehyde was condensed with a 2-phenyl-5-oxazolone to give the [α-^{11}C]-4-benzylidene-2-phenyl-5-oxazolone which was opened by sodium hydroxide in ethanol to give the amide protected α-aminocinnamic acid (8.33). Asymmetric catalytical hydrogenation was performed using a chiral Wilkinson catalyst to obtain the L-form of the amino acid ([^{11}C]8.34) in 80% e.e. The total synthesis time for this seven-step synthesis was 50 min including HPLC purification.

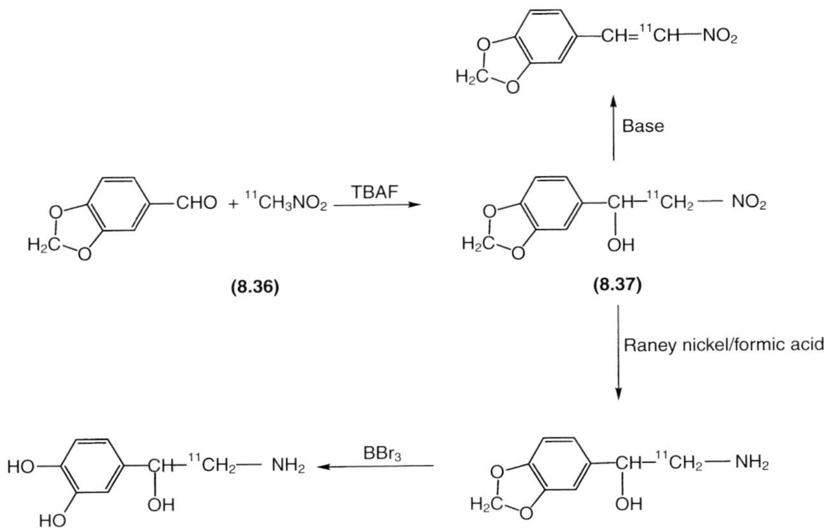

Scheme 8.10

Many analogs of norepinephrine have been radiolabeled for investigation of presynaptic binding sites of the heart. In order to investigate the sympathetic nerve terminal and the noradrenaline metabolism it may be of advantage to use the endogenous transmitter norepinephrine itself and not an analog. A synthetic approach has been developed for the preparation of racemic [^{11}C]norepinephrine ([^{11}C]8.39) starting from [^{11}C]nitromethane (8.36) (Scheme 8.10). In the first step, piperonal is reacted with [^{11}C]nitromethane with the mild base tetrabutylammonium fluoride (TBAF) as catalyst to give 80–90% of the initial condensation product (8.37). Usual bases employed in Knovenagel reactions, such as sodium hydroxide or secondary amines, lead to the nitrostyrene derivative after dehydration of (8.37). Reduction of the nitro group is accomplished with Raney nickel/formic acid to give (8.38), which is deprotected with boron tribromide.

The salicylamide [^{11}C]raclopride ([^{11}C]8.41) is the most extensively used PET radioligand for the quantitative examination of dopamine D$_2$ receptors in striatum by PET. Both enantiomers, [^{11}C]raclopride ([^{11}C]8.41) and the inactive isomer C[^{11}C]8.43), have been labeled with ^{11}C by O-methylation with [^{11}C]methyl iodide from the corresponding desmethyl precursors (Scheme 8.11). Both enantiomerically pure precursors were obtained by resolving 2-aminomethyl-1-ethylpyrrolidine by fractional crystallization of the ditartrates. The enantiomeric excess of both enantiomers was over 99.8% according to gas chromatographic analysis of the diastereomeric O-methylmandelic amides. Coupling of the resolved pyrrolidine amines with 3,5-dichloro-2,6-dimethoxybenzoyl chloride followed by bisdemethylation gave the enantiomerically pure and symmetrical precursors

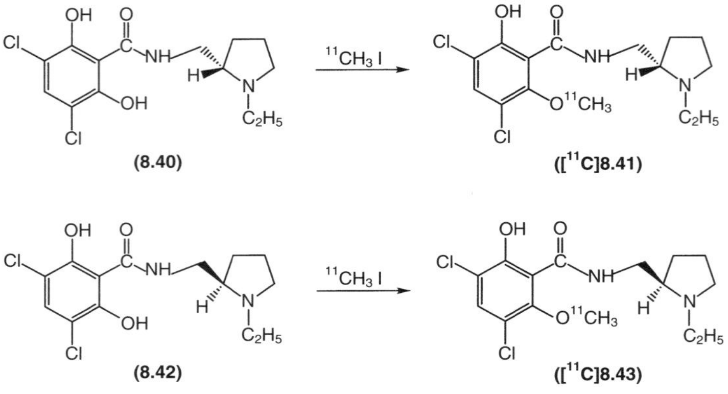

Scheme 8.11

(8.40) and (8.42). The O-methylation with [^{11}C]methyl iodide was performed by use of 5 M NaOH as the base in dimethylsulphoxide (DMSO) (Scheme 8.11).

8.5.2 ^{13}N-labeled compounds

The half-life of 10 min of ^{13}N limits the reaction time available and gives an unusual challenge for the development of synthesis methods and strategy for its incorporation into suitable PET tracers. Both synthetic and enzymatic approaches have been applied to the preparation of ^{13}N labeled radiotracers. Nitrogen-13 can be produced by the ^{16}O(p,α)^{13}N reaction. [^{13}N]NH$_3$ is a blood flow tracer, which can be produced by reduction of [^{13}N]nitrate and nitrite in the presence of a mixture of NaOH and TiCl$_3$, with a radiochemical purity greater than 99%. An alternative method is the deuteron irradiation of methane from which [^{13}N] ammonia is collected in an acidic water solution.

A number of enzymatically synthesized L-[^{13}N]amino acids, such as alanine, leucine, aspartic acid, valine, tyrosine and phenylalanine, have been reported. The general reaction used is glumatic acid dehydrogenase catalyzed formation of L-[^{13}N]amino acids from [^{13}N]NH$_3$ and an α-keto acid. Alternatively, [^{13}N]glutamic acid is synthesized and the ^{13}N amino group is transferred to an α-keto acid in a transaminase reaction catalyzed by glutamate–pyruvate or glutamate–oxaloacetate transferase. A variety of ^{13}N-labeled tracers has thus been synthesized, but the half-life limits the number of tracers used routinely today.

8.5.3 ^{15}O-labeled compounds

Preparation of oxygen-15 tracers for PET provides the ultimate challenge in organic synthesis due to the ultrashort half-life of 2 min. Despite the short half-life of ^{15}O the following tracers are used routinely worldwide today:

1 $[^{15}O]O_2$ is produced by the $^{14}N(d,n)^{15}O$ or $^{15}N(p,n)^{15}O$ reaction. $[^{15}O]O_2$ has been used to determine blood flow, oxygen extraction fraction and oxygen metabolism after administration to patients by inhalation.

2 $[^{15}O]CO_2$ is produced by passing $[^{15}O]O_2$ over activated charcoal heated at $400\,°C$ to $600\,°C$.

3 $[^{15}O]H_2O$ is prepared by bubbling $[^{15}O]CO_2$ into water or by direct action of $[^{15}O]O_2$ with hydrogen. Cerebral blood flow is measured routinely with $[^{15}O]H_2O$.

4 $[^{15}O]$butanol, a new tracer for blood flow, is produced by the reaction between tri-n-butyl borane and $[^{15}O]O_2$. The yield is high, and more than $100\,mCi$ of $[^{15}O]$butanol can be prepared with intervals of $10\,min$.

8.6 IMAGING TECHNIQUES

8.6.1 Autoradiography

The use of radioligands in autoradiographic imaging studies of small animals can give valuable information on distribution, density and kinetics. Slices of the human post-mortem brain can also be incubated with radioligands in order to map the distribution of different receptors. For autoradiography the brain is cryosectioned using a cryomicrotome into $100\,\mu m$ whole hemisphere sections. The tissue sections are transferred to glass plates, put into specially designed incubation chambers and incubated with radiolabeled compounds. The sections are then put into X-ray cassettes together with beta radiation sensitive film for exposure, 4 days for ^{125}I labeled compounds and 4 weeks for ^{3}H-labeled compounds. The films are developed and fixed using conventional techniques. The autoradiograms can be analyzed using computerized densitometry and with a high resolution video camera. Also ^{11}C- and ^{18}F-labeled compounds can be used with exposure times of only 1–4 h. Because of the differences in the range of the radiation, higher resolution is obtained with radioligands labeled with ^{3}H ($0.0072\,mm$ in H_2O) and ^{125}I than with ^{11}C ($4.12\,mm$ in H_2O) or ^{18}F.

An example of an autoradiogram of a whole hemisphere section of a human brain post mortem is given in Figure 8.4. It illustrates the binding of the highly selective and potent serotonin 5-HT$_{1A}$ receptor radioligand $[^{3}H]$WAY-100635. The image of the whole hemisphere demonstrates a high uptake of radioactivity in the hippocampus, raphe nuclei and neocortex regions known to have a high density of serotonin 5-HT$_{1A}$ receptors.

8.6.2 SPECT

The most common SPECT systems consists of a gamma camera with one or three NaI detector heads mounted on a gantry, an on-line computer for acquisition and processing of data, and a display system. The detector head rotates around the axis of the patient at small angle increments ($3°$–$10°$) for $180°$ or $360°$ angular sampling. The data are collected at each angular position and normally stored in the computer for later reconstruction of the images of the planes of interest.

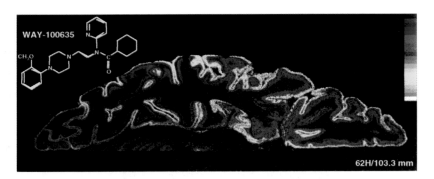

Figure 8.4 [³H]WAY-100635 binding to serotonin 5-HT₁A receptors in a post-mortem human brain using whole hemisphere autoradiography. The figure was kindly provided by Dr Håkan Hall, Karolinska Institutet, Sweden.

Multi-head gamma cameras collect data in several projections simultaneously and reduce the time of imaging. The best SPECT cameras of today have a resolution of 5–6 mm.

The SPECT radiopharmaceuticals are used for detecting radioactivity in the whole body. For brain imaging, there exists a large number of tracers for monitoring blood–brain barrier transport, cerebral perfusion, receptor binding and binding to monoclonal antibodies. A perfusion tracer which is widely used for detection of a number of diseases is [^{99m}Tc]hexamethylpropyleneamine oxime ([^{99m}Tc]HMPAO, [^{99m}Tc]**8.21**).

The SPECT tracer [^{123}I]β-CIT ([^{123}I]**8.19**) is an analog to cocaine with a high affinity for the dopamine transporter ($K_d = 0.11$ nM). This recently developed radioligand has proven to be useful for studies of Parkinson's disease. Figure 8.5 shows a 52-year-old control subject (upper images) and a 55-year-old patient with Parkinson's disease (lower images). The patient had recieved no medication before this study. A reduced uptake of [^{123}I]β-CIT was demonstrated in the Parkinson's patient in a brain region normally having a high density of dopamine transporters (localized by arrows). This finding is of high diagnostic value in the examination of Parkinson's patients.

8.6.3 PET

The influence of the biological system on the radioligand *in vivo* cannot easily be simulated *in vitro*. Several conditions such as protein binding in plasma and the extracellular fluids, radioligand metabolism and ligand transport across the blood–brain barrier cannot be explored *in vitro*. By use of imaging techniques such as PET, *in vivo* visualization of biochemical processes can be performed in the human body.

While SPECT is more readily available than PET, the PET technique offers advantages such as the ability to measure the concentration of the tracer quantiatively, a greater sensitivity, a higher resolution and more diverse types of

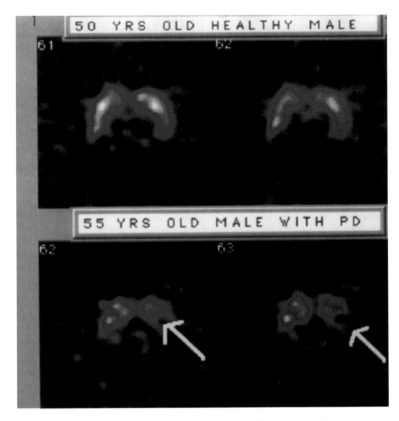

Figure 8.5 SPECT images taken 21 h after injection of $[^{123}I]\beta$-CIT ($[^{123}I]$**8.19**) in a healthy male (top) and a patient with Parkinson's disease (bottom). The images demonstrate highly reduced uptake in the patient with Parkinson's disease (arrow). The figure was kindly provided by Dr Jyrki Kuikka, Kuopio University Hospital, Finland.

radiotracers. The use of short-lived radionuclides and PET gives a low radiation dose to the subject. In addition, repeated investigations can be performed within short-time intervals.

The principles of the PET technique is demonstrated in Figure 8.6. Positron emitting radionuclides disintegrate and emit positrons (positively charged electrons, β^+), that interact with the corresponding antiparticle, an electron (β^-) after traveling in tissue for 1–2 mm. The mass of the two particles is converted to gamma (γ) radiation (annihilation) and two 511 keV photons are emitted simultaneously in opposite directions. The rays emitted are detected externally by a ring of scintillation detectors placed around the subject. The two γ-signals have to be registered by two coincidence coupled detectors within a time window to be counted as originating from the same disintegration. The last generation of PET-systems is used for data acquisition and image reconstruction of 47 slices in the 3D mode with a spatial resolution of 3–4 mm where 2 mm is the maximum theoretical resolution.

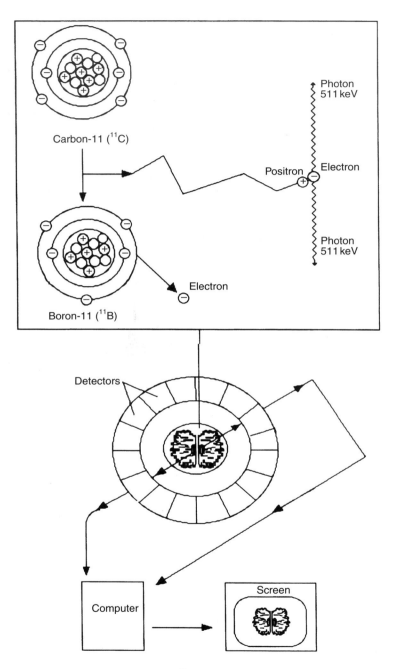

Figure 8.6 The positron-emitting radionuclide ^{11}C decays to form a positron, which annihilates with an electron. The resulting gamma energy, two photons traveling in opposite directions, can be detected externally by a ring of scintillation detectors placed around the subject in the PET camera.

Several PET radiopharmaceuticals are today used as standard tools for investigations of various disease states and control of treatment effects with drugs. The following examples can be mentioned:

1   2-[^{18}F]fluoro-2-deoxyglucose ([^{18}F]FDG, ([^{18}F]**8.25**) is the most frequently used tracer. It measures the glucose metabolism in tumors, heart and especially brain in various disease conditions.

2   [1-^{11}C]acetate, which enters the Krebs tricarboxylic acid cycle at the last possible step by binding to coenzyme-A, can be used as a tracer to reflect the oxygen consumption in the heart. It is prepared from methylmagnesium bromide and [^{11}C]CO$_2$.

3   [^{13}N]ammonia is a precursor that can be incorporated into biomolecules. However, it is a readily diffusible tracer and it enters tissues and metabolic processes, which will reflect the regional blood flow.

4   L-[^{11}C]methionine reflects the amino acid utilization, i.e. transport, protein synthesis, transmethylation and other metabolic processes. It can be easily prepared from the sulfide anion of L-homocysteine and [^{11}C]CH$_3$I.

5   n-[^{15}O]butanol and [^{15}O]H$_2$O are used to study blood flow in the brain and other organs. The partition coefficient of n-[^{15}O]butanol is 1.0, which is an advantage compared to [^{15}O]H$_2$O.

6   [^{11}C]raclopride ([^{11}C]**8.41**) is a selective antagonist for the dopamine D$_2$ receptors that has been used to measure the receptor occupancy in patients treated with different antipsychotics. The preparation is shown in Scheme 8.11.

7   [carbonyl-^{11}C]WAY-100635 is a selective antagonist for the serotonin 5-HT$_{1A}$ receptors which is used to measure receptor density in diseases such as depression, schizophrenia and epilepsy.

Besides [^{11}C]raclopride ([^{11}C]**8.41**) and [carbonyl-^{11}C]WAY-100635, a large number of receptor radioligands have been developed during the past 10 years. Selective radioligands are prepared and widely used in PET for visualization of dopamine, benzodiazepine, muscarinic and serotonin receptors.

Several PET radioligands have been developed for the presynaptic norepinephrine uptake system in the heart. Most of them are, however, analogs labeled with either ^{18}F or ^{76}Br. Recently, the endogenous compound itself, [^{11}C]norepinephrine ([^{11}C]**8.39**), has been synthesized and evaluated in the monkey with PET. Figure 8.7 shows two PET experiments in the monkey heart. The first experiment is a control study (left). In the second pretreatment experiment (right), the selective norepinephrine uptake inhibitor desipramine was given 30 min before injection of [^{11}C]norepinephrine. The results demonstrate that a major part of the radioactivity visualized by PET results from neuronal uptake of racemic ([^{11}C]**8.39**) in the monkey heart.

The preparation and PET examination of radiolabeled stereoisomers are important in radioligand development. Stereospecificity has been demonstrated for drug binding to plasma proteins to a moderate degree. Active transport across membranes is also stereospecific, whereas passive diffusion is primarily related to lipophilicity, which is identical for enantiomers. Stereospecificity is a basic criterion for specific binding to a receptor, an enzyme or a transport mechanism. The active enantiomer (sometimes called eutomer) with specific binding should have a higher

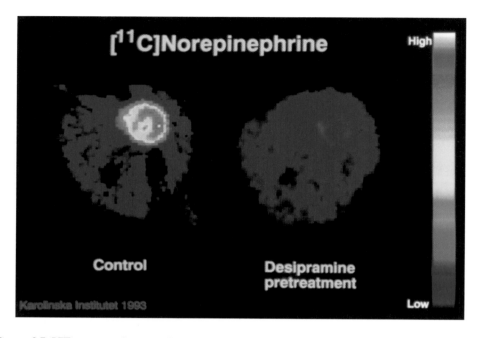

Figure 8.7 PET images showing distribution of radioactivity in the chest of a monkey after injection of [^{11}C]norepinephrine ([^{11}C]**8.39**) in a control experiment (left) and a pretreatment experiment with desipramine (right). The figure was kindly provided by Dr Lars Farde, Karolinska Institutet, Sweden.

accumulation in a target region *in vivo* than the inactive enantiomer (distomer). Comparative PET studies with enantiomers have been suggested as a method to differentiate specific from non-specific binding, which is the key problem in quantitative determination of receptor binding. The usefulness of this method has been demonstrated by PET for several enantiomeric pairs and is exemplified here with the dopamine D_2 receptor antagonist [^{11}C]raclopride ([^{11}C]**8.41**) and its inactive enantiomer ([^{11}C]**8.43**).

Enantiomers have identical physicochemical properties, such as partion coefficient, in a symmetrical environment. In general, if there is no involvement of chiral transport processes across the blood–brain barrier, then the identical partition coefficient of the enantiomers will result in an identical distribution ratio (radioactivity in brain/radioactivity in plasma). Accordingly, it may be possible in PET studies to use the measured brain radioactivity after the injection of an inactive enantiomer as an estimate of the background concentration of radioactivity obtained after the injection of an active enantiomer (Figure 8.8). In radioligand binding experiments *in vitro*, the background level is reduced by simply washing away the free radioligand before the radioactivity is measured. This cannot be accomplished in *in vivo* experiments with PET, because the free radioligand concentration adds to the non-specific binding and increases the background.

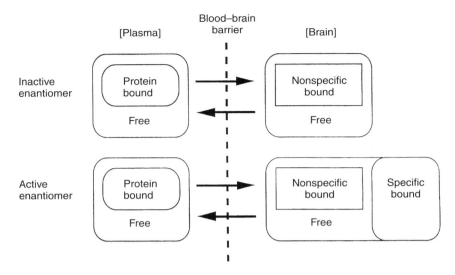

Figure 8.8 Compartments for the distribution of enantiomers.

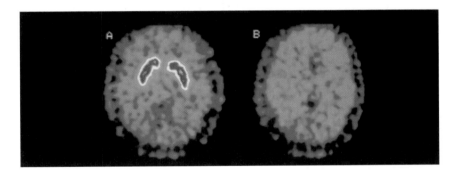

Figure 8.9 PET images showing distribution of radioactivity in the brain after injection of [^{11}C]raclopride ([^{11}C]**8.41**) (A) and the inactive enantiomer ([^{11}C]**8.43**) (B). The figure was kindly provided by Dr Lars Farde, Karolinska Institutet, Sweden.

After the injection of ([^{11}C]**8.41**), there was a high accumulation of radioactivity in the dopamine-rich basal ganglia, whereas the concentration of radioactivity in any other regions could not be differentiated reliably from the background level (Figure 8.9). After the injection of ([^{11}C]**8.43**), there was no such accumulation of radioactivity. Thus, the binding of [^{11}C]**8.41**) is stereoselective.

It is generally assumed that the antipsychotic effect of neuroleptic drugs is mediated by blockade of dopamine receptors. By the use of this *in vivo* technique, it is possible to relate clinical drug effects to receptor binding data obtained in the same living subjects. New information of relevance for the identification of tentative target regions for the antipsychotic drug effect may be found by a regional examination of radioligand binding *in vivo* in the human brain.

FURTHER READING

Aquilonius, S.-M., Eckernäs, S.-Å. and Gillberg, P.-G. (1983) Large section cryomicrotomy in human neuroanatomy and neurochemistry. In *Brain Microdissection Techniques*, edited by A.C. Cuello, pp. 155–170. New York: Wiley.

Bengtsson, S., Gawell, L., Högberg, T. and Sahlberg, C. (1985) Synthesis and ^{3}H NMR of ^{3}H alaproclate of high specific activity. *J. Labelled Compd. Radiopharm.*, **22**, 427–435.

Coenen, H.H. (1986) Radiohalogenation methods: an overview. In *Progress in Radiopharmacy*, edited by P.H. Cox, S.J. Mather, C.B. Sampson and C.R. Lazarus, pp. 196–220. Dordrecht: Kluwer Academic Publishers.

Coenen, H.H., Moerlein, S.M. and Stöcklin, G. (1983) No-carrier-added radiolabelling methods with heavy halogens. *Radiochemica Acta*, **34**, 47–68.

Farde, L., Hall, H., Ehrin, E. and Sedvall, G. (1986) Quantitative analysis of dopamine D_2 receptor binding in the living human brain by positron emission tomography. *Science*, **231**, 258–261.

Farde, L., Halldin, C., Någren, K., Suhara, T., Karlsson, P., Schoeps, K.-O., Swahn, C.-G. and Bone, D. (1994) PET shows high specific [^{11}C]norepinephrine binding in the primate heart. *Eur. J. Nucl. Med.*, **21**, 345–347.

Farde, L., Pauli, S., Hall, H., Eriksson, L., Halldin, C., Högberg, T., Nilsson, L., Sjögren, I. and Stone-Elander, S. (1988) Stereoselective binding of [^{11}C]raclopride in living human brain – a search for extrastriatal central D_2-dopamine receptors by PET. *Psychopharmacology*, **94**, 471–478.

Fleming, J.S., Goatman, K.A., Julyan, P.J., Boivin, C.M., Wilson, M.J., Barber, R.W., Bird, N.J. and Fryer T.D. (2000) A comparison of performance of three gamma camera systems for positron emission tomography. *Nucl. Med. Commun.*, **21**, 1095–1102.

Foged, C., Hansen, L. and Halldin, C. (1993) ^{14}C-Labelling of NNC 756, a new dopamine D_1 antagonist. *J. Labelled Compd. Radiopharm.*, **33**, 747–757.

Fowler, J.S. and Wolf, A. (1986) Positron emitter-labelled compounds: priorities and problems. In *Positron Emission Tomography and Autoradiography: Principles and Applications for the Brain and Heart*, edited by M. Phelps, J. Mazziotta and H. Schelbert, pp. 391–450. New York: Raven Press.

Hall, H., Högberg, T., Halldin, C., Köhler, C., Ström, P., Ross, S.B., Larsson, S.A. and Farde, L. (1991) NCQ 298, A new selective iodinated salicylamide ligand for the labelling of dopamine D_2 receptors. *Psychopharmacology*, **103**, 6–18.

Hall, H., Lundkvist, C., Halldin, C., Farde, L., Pike, V.W., McCarron, J.A., Fletcher, A., Cliffe, I.A., Barf, T. and Sedvall, G. (1997) Autoradiographic localization of 5-HT1A receptors in the post-mortem human brain using [^{3}H]WAY-100635 and [^{11}C]WAY-100635. *Brain Research*, **745**, 96–108.

Hall, H., Sedvall, G., Magnusson, O., Kopp, J., Halldin, C. and Farde, L. (1994) Distribution of D_1- and D_2-dopamine receptors, dopamine and its metabolites in the human brain. *Neuropsychopharmacology*, **11**, 245–256.

Halldin, C. (1991) Radioligands for dopamine receptor PET studies: benzamides and ligands for dopamine D_1-receptors. In *Brain Dopaminergic Systems: Imaging with Positron Tomography*, edited by J.C. Baron, D. Comar, L. Farde, J.L. Martinot and B. Mazoyer, pp. 23–38. Dordrecht: Kluwer Academic Publishers.

Halldin, C. (1995) Dopamine receptor radioligands. *Med. Chem. Res.*, **5**, 127–149.

Halldin, C., Farde, L., Högberg, T., Hall, H., Ström, P., Ohlberger, A. and Solin, O. (1991) A comparative PET-studies of five carbon-11 or fluorine-18 labelled salicylamides. Preparation and *in vitro* dopamine D_2 receptor binding. *Nucl. Med. Biol.*, **18**, 871–881.

Halldin, C., Högberg, T. and Farde, L. (1994) Fluorine-18 labelled NCQ 115, a selective dopamine D_2 receptor ligand. Preparation and positron emission tomography. *Nucl. Med. Biol.*, **21**, 627–631.

Halldin, C. and Långström, B. (1985) Asymmetric synthesis of L-[3-^{11}C]phenylalanine using chiral hydrogenation catalysts. *Int. J. Appl. Radiat. Isot.*, **35**, 945–948.

Halldin, C. and Nilsson, S.-O. (1992) Carbon-11 radiopharmaceuticals – radiopharmacy aspects. In *Progress in Radiopharmacy*, edited by P.A. Schubiger and G. Westera, pp. 115–129. Dordrecht: Kluwer Academic Publishers.

Halldin, C., Suhara, T., Farde, L. and Sedvall, G. (1995) Preparation and examination of labelled stereoisomers *in vivo* by PET. In *Chemist's Views of Imaging Centers*, edited by A.M. Emran, pp. 497–511. New York: Plenum.

Högberg, T. (1993) The development of dopamine D$_2$-receptor selective antagonists. *Drug Design and Discovery*, **9**, 333–357.

Högberg, T., Ström, P., Hall, H., Köhler, C., Halldin, C. and Farde, L. (1990) Synthesis of [^{123}I], [^{125}I]- and unlabelled (S)-3-iodo-5,6-dimethoxy-N-((1-ethyl-2-pyrrolidinyl) methyl) salicylamide (NCQ 298), selective ligands for the study of dopamine D$_2$ receptors. *Acta Pharm. Nord.*, **1**, 53–60.

Kuikka, J., Bergström, K., Vanninen, E., Laulumaa, V., Hartikainen, P. and Länsimies, E. (1993) Initial experience with single-photon emission tomography using iodine-123 labelled 2β-carbomethoxy-3β-(4-iodophenyl)tropane in human brain. *Eur. J. Nucl. Med.*, **20**, 783–786.

Kung, H.F. (1990) Radiopharmaceuticals for CNS receptor imaging with SPECT. *Nucl. Med. Biol.*, **17**, 85–92.

Kung, H.F., Kim, H.-J., Kung, M.-P., Meegalla, S.K., Plössl, K. and Lee, H.-K. (1996) Imaging of dopamine transporters in humans with technetium-99m TRODAT-1. *Eur. J. Nucl. Med.*, **23**, 1527–1530.

Långström, B., Antoni, G., Gullberg, P., Halldin, C., Malmorg, P., Någren, K., Rimland, A. and Svärd, H. (1987) Synthesis of L- and D-[methyl-^{11}C]methionine. *J. Nucl. Med.*, **28**, 1037–1040.

Loch, C., Halldin, C., Bottleander, M., Swahn, C.-G., Moresco, R.-M., Maziere, M., Farde, L. and Maziere, B. (1994) Preparation and evaluation of [^{76}Br]FLB 457, [^{76}Br]FLB 463 and [^{76}Br]NCQ 115, three selective benzamides for mapping dopamine D$_2$ receptors with PET. *J. Labelled Compd. Radiopharm.*, **35**, 437–438.

Maziere, B. and Delforge, J. (1994) Contribution of positron emission tomography to pharmacokinetic studies. In *Pharmacokinetics of Drugs*, edited by P.G. Welling and L.P. Balant, pp. 455–480. New York: Springer-Verlag.

Maziere, B., Coenen, H.H., Halldin, C., Någren, K. and Pike, V.W. (1992) PET radioligands for dopamine receptors and re-uptake sites: chemistry and biochemistry. *Nucl. Med. Biol.*, **19**, 497–512.

Någren, K., Schoeps, K.-O., Halldin, C., Swahn, C.-G. and Farde, L. (1994) Selective synthesis of racemic 1-^{11}C-labelled norepinephrine, octopamine and phenethylamine and *in vivo* study of [1-^{11}C]norepinephrine in the heart with PET. *Appl. Radiat. Isot.*, **45**, 515–521.

Pike, V.W., Halldin, C. and Wikström, H. (2000) Radioligands for the study of brain 5-HT1A receptors *in vivo*. *Progr. Med. Chem.*, **38**, 189–247.

Saha, G.B. (1993) *Physics and Radiobiology of Nuclear Medicine*, 1st edition. New York: Springer-Verlag.

Saha, G.B., MacIntyre, W.J. and Raymundo, T.G. (1994) Radiopharmaceuticals for brain imaging. *Seminars in Nuclear Medicine*, **24**, 324–349.

Stöcklin, G. (1992) Tracers for metabolic imaging of brain and heart. Radiochemistry and radiopharmacology. *Eur. J. Nucl. Med.*, **19**, 527–551.

Stöcklin, G. and Pike, V.W. (eds) (1993) *Radiopharmaceuticals for Positron Emission Tomography. Methodological Aspects*. Dordrecht: Kluwer Academic Publishers.

Chapter 9

Excitatory and inhibitory amino acid receptor ligands

Ulf Madsen and Bente Frølund

9.1 THERAPEUTIC PROSPECTS FOR EXCITATORY AND INHIBITORY AMINO ACIDS

γ-Aminobutyric acid (GABA) and (S)-glutamic acid (Glu) are the major inhibitory and excitatory neurotransmitters, respectively, in the CNS. The balance between the activity of the two are of utmost importance for CNS functions, and dysfunctions of either of the two can be related to various neurologic disorders in the CNS.

9.1.1 Neurodegenerative diseases

In relation to the development of a number of neurodegenerative diseases, hypoactivity of GABA and/or hyperactivity of Glu neuronal functions seem to be involved. Neurodegenerative disorders such as epilepsy, Huntington's chorea, Parkinson's disease, AIDS dementia and amyotrophic lateral sclerosis are examples of progressive diseases, where compounds interacting with the GABAergic and/or glutamatergic receptor systems may be of therapeutic value. Analysis of brain tissue samples from sites near seizure foci in epileptic patients or from animal models of epilepsy have revealed severe impairment of the GABAergic system. Reduction in the level of the GABA-synthesizing enzyme, Glu decarboxylase (GAD) (Figure 9.2) has been reported as well as reduction in the number of and/or efficiency of GABA transporters in models of epilepsy. Pharmacological studies have shown compounds enhancing GABA levels to be anticonvulsive and compounds with the reverse action to be convulsive. Similar studies using Glu receptor active compounds have shown the opposite effects in animal seizure models, convulsive action of agonists and anticonvulsive action of antagonists.

The primary causes of such neurodegenerative diseases are far from being fully elucidated. Several factors may play important roles, including genetic factors, free radicals and autoimmune mechanisms. Studies in recent years have, however, been focused on the role of Glu in the processes causing neurone injury and, ultimately, death. The view that hyperactivity of Glu neurones is an important causative factor in neurodegenerative processes is supported by *in vitro* and *in vivo* studies in a variety of model systems.

Focus has also been put on the function of GABA. The neurodegenerative process probably depends on the balance between excitatory and inhibitory mechanisms. Thus, inhibition of central glutamatergic activity represent one therapeutic strategy, whereas enhancement of central GABAergic activity represents another. Such strategies may, at least, slow down the progress of these very severe chronic disorders, and/or be used as symptomatic treatment, correcting the level of neuronal GABA and/or Glu activity. The question is whether such interventions can be performed without unwanted side effects. A general activation of inhibitory amino acid receptors or a general blockade of excitatory amino acid receptors may cause severe adverse effects due to the many physiological functions of these receptors. Development of selective agents interacting with specific subtypes of receptors involved in the neurodegenerative processes may be a possible therapeutic strategy.

9.1.2   CNS ischemia

Extensive neurodegeneration can also be observed in the brain after ischemic insults such as stroke or cardiac arrest. The neurodegeneration is, at least in part, caused by an excessive efflux of Glu, which is closely related to a compromised energy supply. Similarly, elevated extracellular levels of GABA are observed after ischemic insults. Data from experimental models of stroke shows that stimulation of GABA functions results in neuroprotection and suggests an increase of GABA activity to be a therapeutic approach. Stimulation of GABAergic activity should in any event, decrease glutamatergic activity. An immediate treatment with Glu antagonists may also be of beneficial value, and the concern towards side effects will be less strict for a short-term treatment compared to chronic administration. In numerous animal models of focal and global ischemia, various Glu receptor antagonists have shown promising neuroprotective properties, and several Glu antagonists have been subjected to clinical trials. In spite of effective blockade of Glu neurotoxicity, these compounds have all been withdrawn due to serious unwanted effects. However, different types of Glu antagonists are still being tested, in the search for candidates with fewer or no side effects.

9.1.3   Alzheimer's disease

In Alzheimer's disease an especially complicated neuropathological pattern is observed. Brain tissue from Alzheimer patients is characterized by extensive degeneration of especially cholinergic neurones. The prominent symptoms of Alzheimer patients are cognitive impairment and memory deficits, and a progressive, inevitable fatal, neurodegeneration. Hyperactivity of Glu neurones are believed to be involved in the development of the disease. However, neurodegeneration of Glu neurones are also observed at a certain stage of the disease.

The cause for this degeneration is not known, but the concomitant reduction of Glu neuronal function may be part of the learning and memory deficits observed in Alzheimer patients. The dual role of Glu neurones, involving both hypo- and hyperactivity, is illustrated in Figure 9.1. A Glu antagonist, capable of preventing the neurotoxicity due to Glu hyperactivity (Figure 9.1B), may simultaneously aggravate the hypoactivity observed at other Glu synapses (Figure 9.1C). On the other hand, a Glu agonist, administered in order to restore activity in the latter situation, may enhance the neurotoxicity observed in the hyperactivity situation.

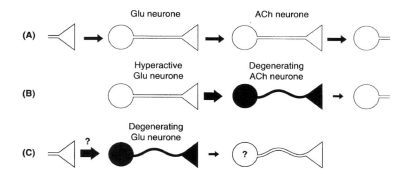

Figure 9.1 Schematic illustration of the interaction between a glutamatergic (Glu) and a cholinergic (ACh) neurone; (A) normal condition; (B) hyperactive; and (C) hypoactive Glu neurones, the two latter representing situations in Alzheimer's disease.

A possible therapeutic solution, at least in theory, may be the use of a partial agonist (see Section 6.3.3). A partial Glu agonist with an appropriately balanced agonist/ antagonist profile may partially block the hyperactivity in certain brain areas, whereas in areas of hypoactivity a certain level of activity may be maintained due to the intrinsic activity, although reduced, of the partial agonist itself. It is not known whether such a strategy can be exploited therapeutically, but it does focus pharmacological attention on partial agonists (see Section 9.3.2.4).

9.1.4 Other neurologic disorders

The GABAergic compounds, notably benzodiazepines (see Section 9.2.5.3) have been successfully used for treatment of anxiety. Recent animal studies have also shown inhibitors of Glu activity to be anxiolytic. However, clinical application of Glu antagonists for this indication will require development of compounds with very limited or no side effects.

Increasing evidence from animal studies support the proposal that GABA as well as Glu receptors are involved in pain transmission and the plasticity which accompanies sensitization to pain. Thus, enhancement of GABA activity or inhibition of Glu activity may be used in the treatment of chronic pain.

Finally, abnormal inhibitory and/or excitatory amino acid neurotransmission seems to play a role in schizophrenia. Apart from the well-established imbalance observed for dopaminergic and cholinergic neurotransmission, there has been some controversy as to whether hypo- or hyperactivity at GABA and Glu receptors are implicated in the neurologic pattern of schizophrenia. Activation of the GABAergic system produce psychotomimetic effects in normal human beings and stimulate the psychotic symptoms in schizophrenic patients, and drug abuse of a Glu antagonist (PCP, see Section 9.3.1.3) has caused schizophrenic symptoms. These observations have been interpreted as indicative of GABA hyper- and Glu hypoactivity, respectively, to be part of schizophrenia. However, recent contradictory results seem to indicate that Glu hyperactivity is involved, and clinical trials are going on with both an antagonist as well as with a positive modulator of AMPA receptors.

9.2 GABA: INHIBITORY NEUROTRANSMITTER

The role of the neutral amino acid GABA (**9.1**) as the major inhibitory neurotransmitter in the CNS is fully established. Furthermore, GABA is involved in the regulation of a variety of physiological mechanisms in the periphery. GABA is present in high concentrations in many brain regions and the majority of central neurones are sensitive to GABA and receive synaptic input from GABAergic neurones. The major role of the GABAergic neurotransmitter system is to balance neuronal excitability. Imbalance due to impaired operation of the GABA-mediated inhibitory synapses may be an important factor in several neurologic disorders as described in Section 9.1. These aspects have focused interest on the various processes and mechanisms associated with GABA-mediated neurotransmission in the CNS as potential targets for clinically useful drugs.

9.2.1 Therapeutic targets

The GABAergic neurotransmitter system involves a number of synaptic processes and mechanisms, which have been studied pharmacologically and constitute potential therapeutic targets. GABA is formed in the presynaptic nerve terminals

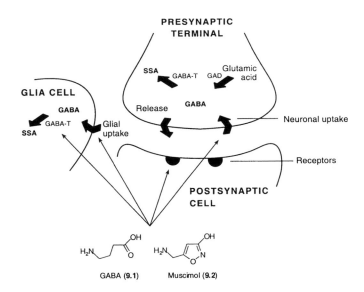

Figure 9.2 Schematic illustration of the biochemical pathways, transport mechanisms, and receptors at a GABA-operated axo-somatic synapse. GAD: (S)-glutamic acid decarboxylase; GABA-T: GABA:2-oxoglutarate aminotransferase; SSA: succinic acid semi-aldehyde. The interactions with various GABA synaptic mechanisms of GABA and the heterocyclic GABA analog muscimol (**9.2**), is indicated.

and released into the synaptic cleft, where it activates the postsynaptic GABA receptors (Figure 9.2). This activation causes an opening of the chloride channels, resulting in hyperpolarization of the nerve membrane potential. GABA is taken up by presynaptic nerve terminals and glial cells, and subsequently, it is enzymatically metabolized to form succinic acid semialdehyde (SSA).

Many drugs with effects in the brain, such as anxiolytics, anticonvulsants, myo-relaxants, sedatives and general anaesthetics have been shown to interact with the GABA neurotransmitter system. Possible targets of action of these drugs include direct GABA receptor agonism/antagonism, allosteric modulation of the GABA receptors or interference with GABA reuptake or metabolism.

9.2.2   The GABA molecule

The structural requirements for activation of the different targets in the GABA neurotransmitter system have been extensively studied using GABA as a lead compound.

The GABA molecule has a very high degree of flexibility and there is strong evidence supporting the view that GABA adopts dissimilar active conformations at different synaptic recognition sites. Thus, pharmacological studies of GABA analogs with restricted conformations may lead to compounds with selective actions. Synthesis and structure–activity studies of GABA analogs, in which the conformational and electronic parameters have been systematically changed, have shed much light on the molecular pharmacology of the GABA synaptic mechanisms.

Muscimol (**9.2**), a constituent of the mushroom *Amanita muscaria*, is a very potent GABA$_A$ (see Section 9.2.5 for receptor classification) agonist but muscimol is also an inhibitor of neuronal and glial GABA uptake and a substrate for the GABA-metabolizing enzyme GABA transaminase (GABA-T) (Figure 9.2). Muscimol has been used as a lead for the design of different classes of GABA analogs, and systematic variation of the molecular structure of muscimol in order to separate the multiple affinities of this compound, has provided a number of specific GABA$_A$ receptor agonists and GABA uptake inhibitors (Figure 9.3). Conversion of muscimol into THIP (**9.3**) and the isomeric compound THPO (**9.4**) effectively separated GABA$_A$ receptor and GABA uptake affinity; THIP proved to be a specific GABA$_A$ agonist, whereas THPO is a GABA uptake inhibitor. Further development led to the monoheterocyclic compounds isonipecotic acid (**9.5**), isoguvacine (**9.6**), nipecotic acid (**9.7**) and guvacine (**9.8**), where **9.5** and **9.6** were shown to be specific GABA$_A$ agonists and **9.7** and **9.8** GABA uptake inhibitors (Figure 9.3).

The degree of stereoselectivity of the GABA transport mechanisms has been compared with that of the GABA$_A$ receptor binding sites using the *S*- and *R*-forms of chiral GABA analogs as test compounds (Figure 9.4). The *S*- and *R*-forms of the flexible GABA analog 4-aminopentanoic acid (**9.9**) are equally effective at GABA$_A$ receptor sites, and both interact with the neuronal as well as the glial GABA uptake systems. Conformational restriction of the C2-C3 bonds of the enantiomers of 4-aminopentanoic acid as in (*S*)- and (*R*)-*trans*-4-amino-2-pentenoic acid (**9.10**) has quite dramatic effects on the pharmacological profiles. Thus, the *S*-form of this

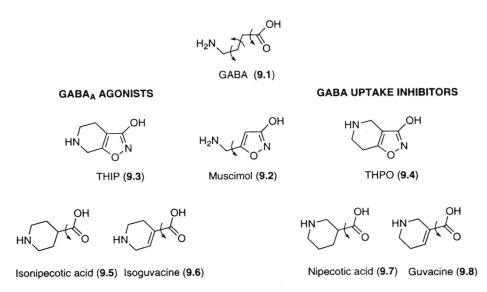

Figure 9.3 Structures of some GABA_A agonists and GABA uptake inhibitors illustrating the structural requirements for activation of GABA_A receptors and for inhibition of GABA uptake.

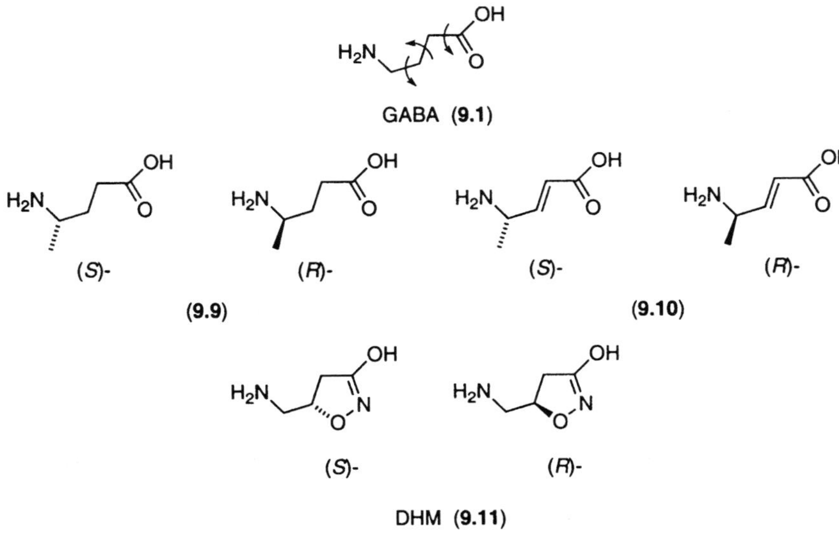

Figure 9.4 Structures of S- and R-forms of GABA analogs.

conformationally restricted GABA analog specifically binds to and activates GABA_A receptors, whereas its R-isomer interacts with neuronal and glial GABA uptake systems without showing detectable affinity for GABA_A receptor sites. These results show that the degree of stereoselectivity of GABA synaptic mechanisms depends on the conformational mobility of the chiral GABA analog tested. Thus, enantiomers of semi-rigid, chiral GABA analogs show markedly different pharmacological profiles.

Studies on chiral analogs of muscimol have supported these structure–activity relationships. Thus, the S-form of dihydromuscimol (DHM, **9.11**) is an extremely potent and highly selective $GABA_A$ agonist and (R)-DHM is a selective inhibitor of GABA uptake.

9.2.3 GABA biosynthesis and metabolism

The biochemical pathways underlying the synthesis and catabolism of GABA, have largely been mapped out and the key enzymes are identified and characterized. The main pathway for GABA synthesis is decarboxylation of Glu catalyzed by GAD which uses pyridoxal-5'-phosphate (PLP) as a cofactor (Figure 9.2). GABA is released via a specific release system into the synaptic cleft by depolarization of the presynaptic neurone. The initial step of the degradation of GABA is transformation into SSA. This transamination step, which is catalyzed by the PLP-dependent GABA-T, takes place within presynaptic GABA terminals as well as in surrounding glia cells (Figure 9.2). Extracellular enzymatic degradation does not seem to play any role in the inactivation of GABA.

The crystal structure of GABA-T has recently been reported, which undoubtedly will assist the development of new inhibitors on a more rational basis. The compounds discussed in the following section have all, however, been developed prior to the determination of the crystal structure of the enzyme.

9.2.3.1 Inhibitors of GABA metabolism

A number of mechanism-based inactivators of GABA-T has been developed and has been shown to work *in vitro* and *in vivo*. These compounds are typically analogs of GABA, containing appropriate functional groups at C4 of the GABA backbone. The functional group are converted by GABA-T into electrophiles, which react with nucleophilic groups at or near the active site of the enzyme and thereby inactivate the enzyme irreversibly. Although GABA-T, like other PLP-dependent enzymes, does not show strict stereospecificity with respect to inactivation by mechanism-based inactivators, such inhibitors do react with the enzyme in a stereoselective manner. Thus, the S-forms of the GABA-T inhibitors 4-amino-5-hexenoic acid (Vigabatrin) (**9.12**), 4-amino-5-hexynoic acid (**9.13**) and the fluoromethyl derivative (**9.14**) are more active as GABA-T inactivators than the respective R-isomers (Figure 9.5). These observations are in good agreement with results obtained from modeling studies of the inhibitors using the reported crystal structure of the enzyme. Selective inactivation of GABA-T using Vigabatrin is successfully applied in treatment of epilepsy. In this regard, it is interesting and fortunate that the active S-isomer of Vigabatrin is actively taken up by the neuronal as well as the glial transport mechanisms, whereas the R-isomer is not transported.

A number of conformationally rigid analogs of Vigabatrin and 4-amino-5-halopentanoic acid has recently been developed. The saturated 5-fluoro analog **9.16** exhibit inactivation of GABA-T similar to, although not as potent

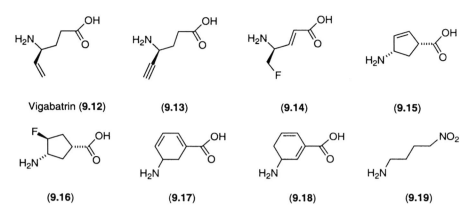

Vigabatrin (9.12)   (9.13)   (9.14)   (9.15)

(9.16)   (9.17)   (9.18)   (9.19)

Figure 9.5 Structures of some GABA-T inhibitors, compound **9.15** being inactive.

as, the corresponding open-chain analogs. This is in contrast to the unsaturated conformationally constrained Vigabatrin analog **9.15**, which does not inactivate GABA-T. Gabaculine (**9.17**), a naturally occurring neurotoxin isolated from *Streptomyces toyacaensis* and isogabaculine (**9.18**) are potent irreversible inactivators of GABA-T. In contrast to Vigabatrin (**9.12**), the cyclic analogs of GABA do not alkylate the enzyme. As a result of enzymatic processing by GABA-T these compounds are converted into aromatic pyridoxamine-5-phosphate adducts, which do not desorb from the active site of the enzyme. 4-Nitro-1-butanamine (**9.19**) is a GABA-T inhibitor, in which the weakly acidic nitromethylene group participates in the inactivation of the enzyme (see Scheme 9.2).

The mechanism for inactivation of GABA-T by Vigabatrin (**9.12**) is outlined in Scheme 9.1. As shown, a Schiff base (**9.20**) is formed between the co-factor PLP and the terminal amino group from a lysine residue. Transamination with **9.12** generates a new iminium ion **9.21**, which undergoes rate-determining enzyme-catalyzed deprotonation to give the iminium ion **9.23** after reprotonation. In analogy with transamination reaction on GABA, **9.23** could be hydrolyzed to give the SSA analog **9.25** and pyridoxamine-5-phosphate **9.24**. However, **9.23** is a Michael acceptor electrophile, which undergoes conjugate addition by an active-site nucleophile X⁻ and the inactivated enzyme **9.26** is produced.

The initial steps in the inactivation of GABA-T by the naturally occurring inhibitor, gabaculin (**9.17**) (Scheme 9.2, upper part), are analogous with those described for Vigabatrin (**9.12**) (Scheme 9.1). Gabaculine (**9.17**) is recognized by GABA-T and is coupled to PLP to give the Schiff base **9.27**. Although **9.28**, formed by deprotonation of **9.27**, contains a dihydrobenzene ring showing some electrophilic character, **9.28** is not sufficiently reactive to alkylate GABA-T. As shown in Scheme 9.2, one of the highly activated protons at C2 in the dihydrobenzene ring of **9.28** is removed. Subsequent reprotonation of the complex by a protonated nucleophile on the enzyme (GABA-T) gives compound **9.29**, which inactivates GABA-T via tight, but non-covalent binding to the active site. A major driving

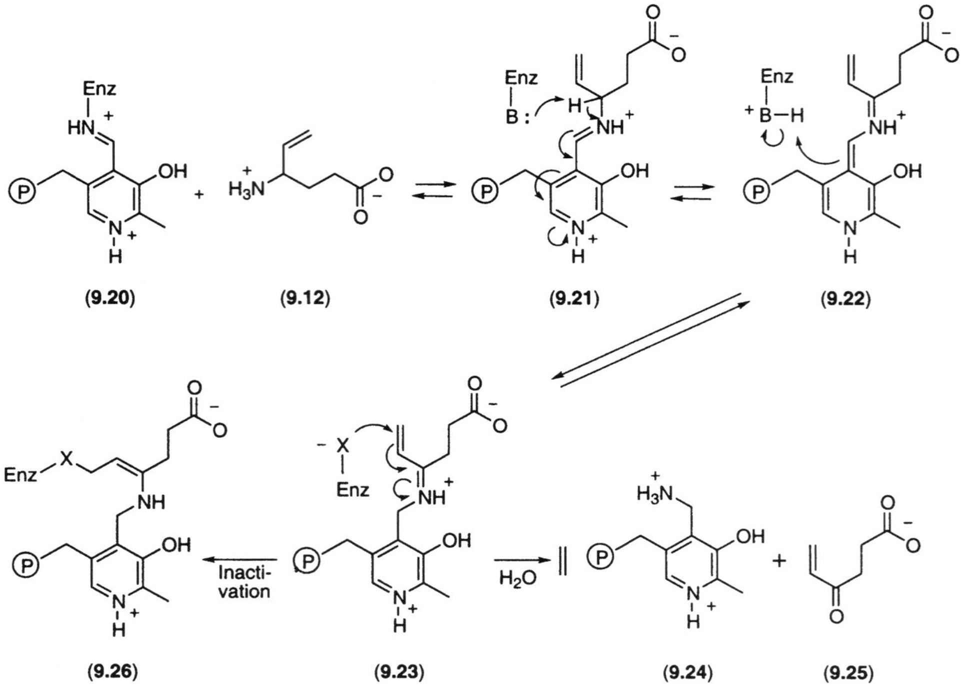

Scheme 9.1 Proposed inactivation mechanism of GABA-T by Vigabatrin (9.12).

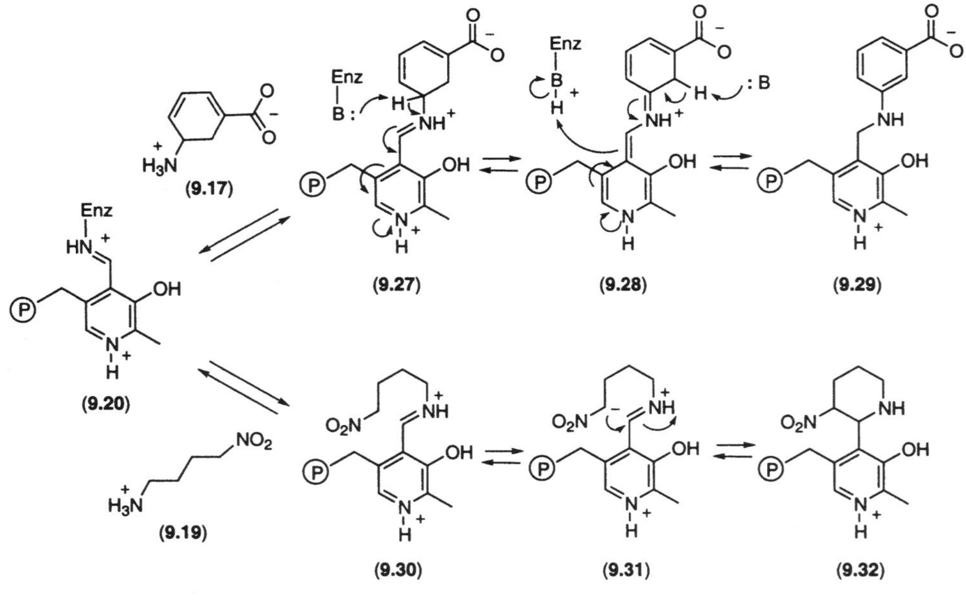

Scheme 9.2 Proposed inactivation mechanism of GABA-T by gabaculine (9.17) (upper part) and by 4-nitro-1-butanamine (9.19) (lower part).

force in the conversion of **9.28** into **9.29** is the aromatization of the dihydrobenzene ring of **9.28**.

The mechanism of action of the GABA-T inhibitor **9.19** is outlined in Scheme 9.2 (lower part). Like gabaculine (**9.17**), **9.19** reacts with PLP. This reaction produces **9.32**, which inhibits the action of GABA-T in a manner analogous with that described for compound **9.29**. The key step in the formation of **9.32** is the intramolecular nucleophilic reaction between the anionic nitromethylene and iminium group of **9.31**.

9.2.4   GABA uptake

The action of GABA at the synapses is terminated by reuptake into both pre-synaptic nerve terminals and surrounding glial cells (Figure 9.2). The GABA taken up into nerve terminals is available for reutilization, whereas GABA taken up in glial cells is metabolized to SSA by GABA-T and cannot be resynthesized to afford GABA again since glial cells lack GAD. The uptake process is catalyzed by sodium-coupled transport systems located in plasma membranes of nerve endings and glial cells and it has been demonstrated that both sodium and chloride ions are cotrans-ported with GABA by the transporter. The GABA uptake data obtained from studies using cultured cells from mammalian CNS are consistent with heterogen-eity of both neuronal and glial transport mechanisms. Molecular cloning studies have also shown that the GABA transporters are heterogenous and four different GABA transporter have, until now, been cloned. The four subtypes, which are homologs for the human and rat transporters, have been termed GAT-1, GAT-2, GAT-3 and BGT-1 (the betaine/GABA transporter). Studies of the neuronal vs. glial localization of GABA transporter mRNA have disclosed that whereas GAT-1, GAT-3 and BGT-1 mRNAs are present in both neurones and glial cells, GAT-2 is the only transporter being selectively expressed in non-neuronal cells.

9.2.4.1   Inhibitors of GABA uptake

A logical approach for increasing GABA neurotransmission would be blockade of the uptake systems in order to enhance the amount of GABA in the synaptic cleft. A selective blockade of glial uptake would be optimal, as this would ensure an elevation of the GABA concentration in the presynaptic nerve terminals. It has been established that neuronal and glial uptake mechanisms have dissimilar substrate specificities. The structural requirements for uptake inhibitors are also different from what is required for interaction with postsynaptic GABA receptors, as described in Section 9.2.2. Thus, selective interaction with the different GABA uptake sites is possible. Nipecotic acid (**9.7**) is an effective inhibitor of neuronal as well as glial GABA uptake, being twice as potent at the latter system. Furthermore, nipecotic acid has been shown to be a substrate for neuronal as well as glial GABA transport carriers making analyses of the pharmacology of this compound difficult. A number of cyclic amino acids structurally related to nipecotic acid, including guvacine (**9.8**) show a profile very similar to that of nipecotic acid. Whereas introduction of small substituents on the amino groups of nipecotic acid (**9.7**) or guvacine (**9.8**) results in compounds with reduced affinity for the GABA transport

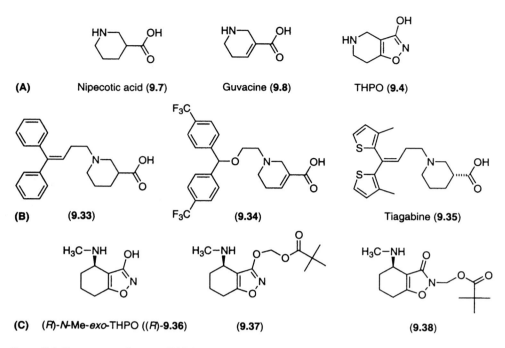

Figure 9.6 Structures of some GABA uptake inhibitors: (A) nipecotic acid, guvacine and THPO; (B) lipophilic analogs, (**9.33–9.35**); and (C) (R)-N-Me-exo-THPO ((R)-**9.36**) and two prodrugs of (R)-**9.36**.

carriers, N-(4,4-diphenyl-3-butenyl)nipecotic acid (**9.33**) and structurally related analogs, such as **9.34** (Figure 9.6B), are much more potent than the parent amino acids. In contrast to **9.7** and **9.8**, these lipophilic compounds are able to cross the blood–brain barrier and are potent anticonvulsants in animal models. Tiagabine (**9.35**) (Figure 9.6B), a structurally related compound, is now marketed as an add-on therapeutic agent for treatment of epilepsy.

The molecular mechanism underlying the interaction of the lipophilic analogs with GABA uptake systems is unknown. In contrast to the N-unsubstituted amino acids, these analogs do not seem to be substrates for the GABA transporters, although the competitive nature of action strongly suggest that they do interact directly with the carrier binding site. Molecular pharmacological studies of nipecotic acid (**9.7**) and guvacine (**9.8**) disclose high affinity for GAT-1 and GAT-2 and rather low affinity for GAT-3, whereas the lipophilic analogs, including tiagabine (**9.35**) interact selectively with GAT-1. A few compounds with moderate potency and selectivity for GAT-3 and BGT-1 have been identified. The GAT subtypes have different distribution in the brain and subtype selective compounds would be useful tools for studies of the physiological and pharmacological importance of the GAT subtypes, and may explain the different anticonvulsant profiles observed for different compounds.

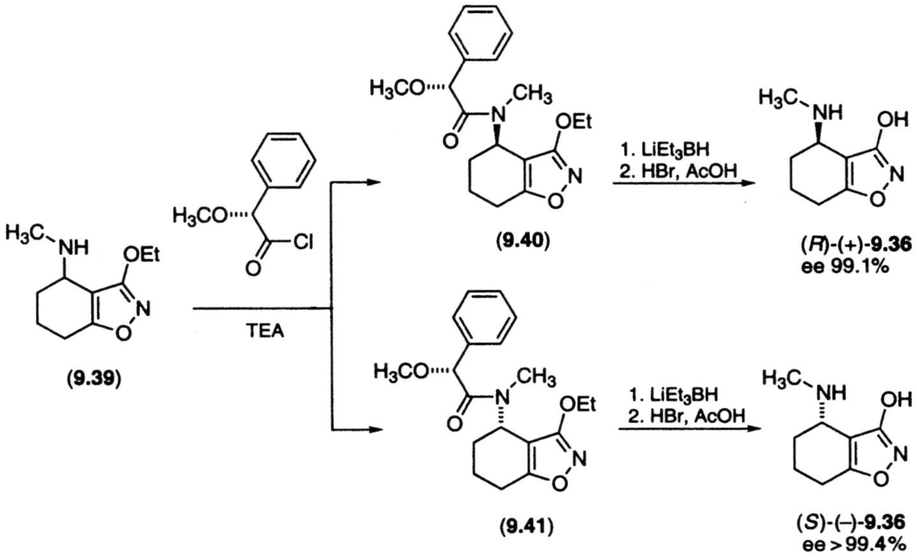

Scheme 9.3 Separation of the two enantiomers of N-Me-exo-THPO (**9.36**).

THPO has been used as a lead in the search for more glia-selective inhibitors. N-Me-*exo*-THPO (**9.36**) (Figure 9.6C) was developed as a GABA uptake inhibitor and the R-enantiomer of **9.36** has shown the highest degree of selectivity for the glial GABA transport system so far observed, with the S-form being inactive. Removal of the methyl group of (R)-N-Me-*exo*-THPO or replacement of this group by larger groups lead to pronounced loss of activity on the GABA transport. Since **9.36** is not active in mice after systemic administration, the prodrug approach was used to study the *in vivo* pharmacology of this compound. The O- and N-pivaloyl-oxymethyl derivatives, **9.37** and **9.38** (Figure 9.6C), respectively, were shown to be bioreversible derivatives of (R)-N-Me-*exo*-THPO ((R)-**9.36**) and showed potent anticonvulsant effect after subcutaneous administration in mice. These results underline the importance of the glial GABA uptake system as a potential therapeutic target in convulsive disorders.

The enantiomers of N-Me-*exo*-THPO (**9.36**) were synthesized, as shown in Scheme 9.3, from **9.39** via the diastereomeric α-methoxyphenylacetamides, **9.40** and **9.41**, which were separated using preparative HPLC. The absolute configuration of the R-enantiomer of **9.36** was established by an X-ray crystallographic analysis (Figure 9.7). In the low-energy conformation, as shown in Figure 9.7, (R)-nipecotic acid ((R)-**9.7**) adopts a chair conformation with the carboxylate group in equatorial orientation. The depicted conformation of THPO (**9.4**) is derived from the X-ray structure of its O-methyl derivative. THPO is much weaker than (R)-nipecotic acid as a GABA uptake inhibitor, but both compounds show a low degree of selectivity for glial vs. neuronal GABA uptake. The similarity of the conformations of THPO and of (R)-nipecotic acid may indicate that the two compounds interact with the GABA transport carriers in conformations similar to

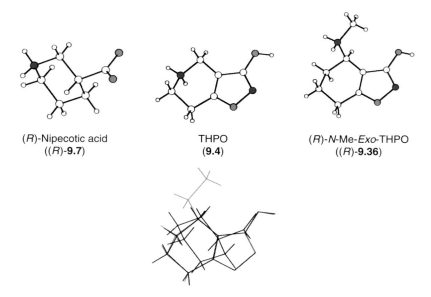

Figure 9.7 Comparison and superimposition of low-energy conformations of the GABA uptake inhibitors (R)-nipecotic acid ((R)-**9.7**) (blue), THPO (**9.4**) (green) and (R)-N-Me-exo-THPO ((R)-**9.36**) (red). The molecular structure of zwitterionic (R)-**9.7** was determined by an X-ray crystallographic analysis. The depicted molecular structure of cationic **9.4** is derived from the structure of O-Me-THPO hydrochloride, determined by an X-ray crystallographic analysis. The illustrated molecular structure of cationic ((R)-**9.36**) is based on an X-ray crystallographic analysis of the hydrobromide salt of ((R)-**9.36**).

those illustrated in Figure 9.7. The low-energy conformation of (R)-N-Me-*exo*-THPO ((R)-**9.36**) obviously is different from those of (R)-nipecotic acid and THPO. Since (R)-N-Me-*exo*-THPO shows a 13-fold higher selectivity as an inhibitor of glial vs. neuronal GABA uptake, this particular conformation of (R)-N-Me-*exo*-THPO may represent an important structural determinant for glia-selective GABA uptake inhibition.

9.2.5   GABA receptors

The GABA receptors have been divided into two main groups: (1) the ionotropic GABA$_A$ and GABA$_C$ receptors, which produce fast synaptic inhibition; and (2) the metabotropic (G-protein coupled) GABA$_B$ receptors, which produce slow and prolonged inhibitory signals. The classification of GABA receptors based on pharmacological characterization using selective ligands is outlined in Figure 9.8. Whereas BMC (**9.42**) and SR 95531 (**9.43**) are the classical antagonists at GABA$_A$ receptors, isoguvacine (**9.6**) and THIP (**9.3**) are specific GABA$_A$ receptor agonists. (R)-baclofen (**9.44**) is the classical GABA$_B$ receptor agonist and the corresponding phosphonic acid analog, (R)-phaclofen (**9.45**), was the first GABA$_B$ antagonist to be characterized. The GABA$_C$ receptors are insensitive to both BMC and baclofen, but

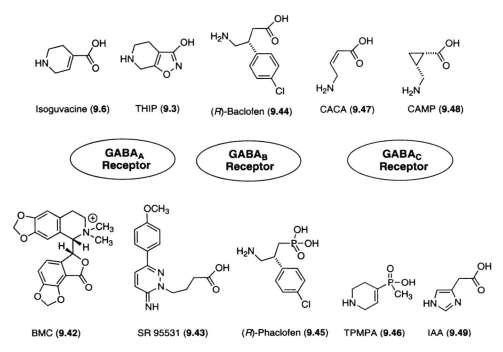

Figure 9.8 Schematic illustration of the different classes of GABA receptors and the structures of standard agonists (upper part) and antagonists (lower part) used for pharmacological characterization of these receptors.

are selectively antagonized by TPMPA (**9.46**), whereas CACA (**9.47**) and CAMP (**9.48**) are GABA$_C$ receptor agonists. Interestingly, the partial GABA$_A$ agonist, IAA (**9.49**) has been shown to be a potent antagonist at GABA$_C$ receptors.

The heterogeneity of GABA$_A$ receptors in the brain is large, because of the large number of different GABA$_A$ receptor subunits. At least 17 different subunits ($\alpha_{1-6}, \beta_{1-4}, \gamma_{1-4}, \delta, \varepsilon,$ and π) have been identified. The GABA$_A$ receptors are formed as a pentameric assembly of different subunits, making the existence of a very large number of such heteromeric GABA$_A$ receptors possible. The assembly, which in most receptors includes two α subunits, two β subunits and one γ or δ subunit, determines the pharmacology of the functional receptor. The GABA$_C$ receptors are the least characterized of the GABA receptors, but the membrane topology is assumed to be very similar to that of GABA$_A$ receptors. However, GABA$_C$ receptors are derived exclusively of ρ subunits (ρ_{1-3}) expressed primarily in the retina. The various isoforms of the ρ subunits can assemble into homomeric chloride channels showing a pharmacology different from the GABA$_A$ receptors.

The metabotropic GABA$_B$ receptors belong to the family of G-protein coupled receptors and more particularly to the subfamily C which comprises the metabotropic Glu receptors (see also Chapter 6). Two isoforms, GBR1 and GBR2, of the receptor protein have been isolated and more recent it has been shown that the two isoforms exist as a heterodimer and form a fully functional GABA$_B$ receptor.

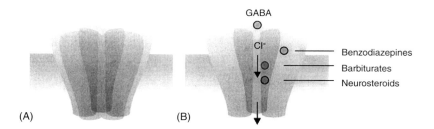

Figure 9.9 (A) Schematic model of the pentameric structure of the GABA$_A$ receptor complex; and (B) a schematic illustration of the GABA$_A$ receptor complex indicating the chloride ion channel and additional binding sites.

9.2.5.1   The GABA$_A$ receptor complex

The postsynaptic GABA$_A$ receptor is a receptor complex containing a number of modulatory binding sites for drugs such as benzodiazepines, barbiturates, and neurosteroids (Figure 9.9). The GABA$_A$ receptor regulates the influx of chloride ions in such a way that receptor activation causes hyperpolarization of the cell membrane and, thus, decreased sensitivity of the neurone to excitatory input. The complexity of the GABA$_A$ receptor function is comparable to that of the NMDA subtype of Glu receptor channels (see Section 9.3.1.3).

Site-directed mutagenesis studies have shown that the binding site for benzodiazepines is located at the interface between the α and γ subunit in the GABA$_A$ receptor complex, whereas the binding site for GABA and GABA$_A$ agonists is located at the interface between the α and β subunit. The potency and maximal response of ligands for the GABA binding site is highly subunit dependent. At some subunit combinations certain compounds may act as agonists and at other subunit combinations as antagonists or low efficacy partial agonists. Despite the fact that the GABA binding site is located at the interface between the α and β subunit, the pharmacological profile of the receptor seems to be determined by the interaction of all subunits present in the receptor. To study this in more detail more GABA$_A$ agonists, partial agonists and antagonists are needed with specific effects at the physiologically relevant GABA$_A$ receptors of different subunit compositions.

9.2.5.2   GABA$_A$ receptor ligands

The conformationally restricted analogs of GABA, muscimol (**9.2**), thiomuscimol (**9.50**) and DHM (**9.11**), are highly potent GABA$_A$ agonists (Figure 9.10). These compounds indicate that the 3-isoxazolol, the 3-isothiazolol and the 2-isoxazoline-3-ol heterocyclic systems are bioisosteres of the carboxyl group of GABA with respect to GABA$_A$ receptors. Whereas muscimol (**9.2**) interacts more effectively than GABA with GABA$_A$ receptors *in vivo* and *in vitro*, it binds less tightly than GABA to GABA$_B$ receptor sites and to GABA transport mechanisms. Thiomuscimol (**9.50**) does not affect GABA uptake *in vitro*, but as muscimol it is metabolized by GABA-T, and this metabolism reduces the value of these potent GABA$_A$ agonists for *in vivo* pharmacological studies.

A number of analogs of the structurally constrained GABA$_A$ agonist THIP (**9.3**) have been synthesized. As for the muscimol series, the 3-isoxazolol ring system has been replaced by other heterocyclic systems (Figure 9.10). With the exception of thio-THIP (**9.51**), which is a very weak GABA$_A$ agonist, none of these THIP analogs show significant GABA$_A$ receptor affinities, emphasizing the strict structural requirement for activation of GABA$_A$ receptors. THIP, which undergoes very limited metabolic decomposition *in vivo*, penetrates the brain–blood barrier. THIP shows non-opioid analgesic and anxiolytic effect and appears to improve the quality of sleep.

In general, the availability of antagonists with specific or highly selective effects on receptors is essential for elucidation of the physiological role of the receptors concerned. The fact that all GABA$_A$ antagonists, so far studied pharmacologically, are convulsants, makes it highly unlikely that such compounds are going to play an important role in future therapy. In certain diseases, where a reduction in the GABA$_A$ function is desired, low-efficacy partial GABA$_A$ agonists may have therapeutic interest (see Section 9.1.4).

4-PIOL (**9.53**) and the isothiazole analog (**9.54**) (Figure 9.11) have been shown to be low-efficacy partial agonists, with dominating antagonist profiles on brain tissue *in vitro*. In contrast to the desensitization observed after direct activation of GABA$_A$ receptors by full agonists, repeated administration of 4-PIOL (**9.53**) to cerebral cortical neurones did not cause significant desensitization of the GABA$_A$ receptors studied.

A number of analogs containing different substituent in the 4-position of the 3-isoxazolol ring of 4-PIOL (**9.53**) (Figure 9.11) has been synthesized in order to investigate the effect on the pharmacological profile. The results from these studies are listed in Figure 9.12 where the receptor pharmacology is represented by the K_i values from [^{3}H]muscimol binding studies and by IC$_{50}$ values from an electrophysiological model. Substituents in the 4-position of 4-PIOL analogs seem to be allowed in contrast to what has been found for the corresponding muscimol analogs. Introduction of a methyl or an ethyl group in the 4-position of muscimol to give **9.55** and **9.56** (Figure 9.11), respectively, leads to virtually inactive compounds. The methyl, ethyl and benzyl analogs of 4-PIOL (**9.57–9.59**)

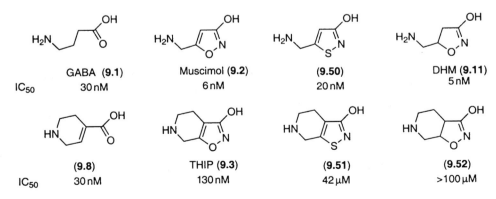

Figure 9.10 Structures of some GABA$_A$ receptor ligands with IC$_{50}$ values from [^{3}H]GABA binding.

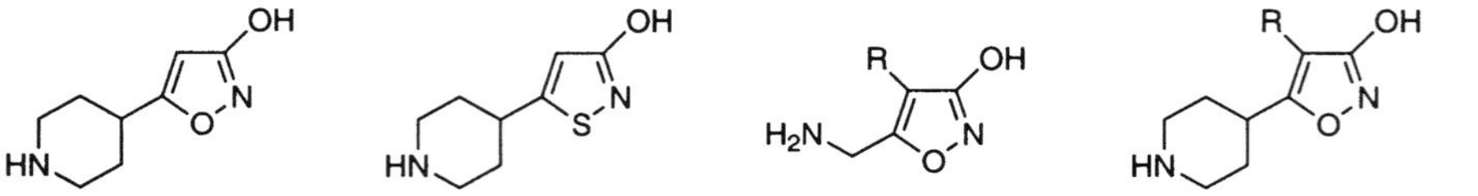

4-PIOL (**9.53**) (**9.54**) (**9.55, 9.56**) R = Me, Et (**9.57–9.61**) R = Me, Et, Bn, 2-naphthylmethyl, 2-(2-naphthyl)ethyl

Figure 9.11 Structures of the partial $GABA_A$ receptor agonists 4-PIOL (**9.53**) and the thia analog (**9.54**), muscimol analogs (**9.55**, **9.56**) and 4-PIOL analogues (**9.57–9.61**).

(Figure 9.12) show that larger substituents in the 4-position of the 3-isoxazolol ring of 4-PIOL affords compounds with higher affinity for the $GABA_A$ receptors. Extension of the aromatic system from a phenyl to a naphthyl group to give **9.60** markedly increases the affinity, with a corresponding increase in potency, whereas extension of the linker joining the 2-naphthyl group and the 3-isoxazolol ring to give compound **9.61** resulted in a 10-fold reduction in affinity relative to **9.60**.

Using whole-cell patch-clamp techniques on cultured cerebral cortical neurones in the electrophysiological testing, the functional properties of the 4-PIOL analogs (**9.57–9.61**) in the absence or in the presence of the specific $GABA_A$ receptor agonist isoguvacine (**9.6**) (Figure 9.8), were studied. The study showed that the structural modifications led to a change in the pharmacological profile of the compounds from low-efficacy partial $GABA_A$ receptor agonist activity to potent and selective antagonist effect. The 2-naphthylmethyl analog **9.60** showed an antagonist potency comparable with that of the standard $GABA_A$ antagonist SR 95531 (**9.43**) (Figure 9.12). These structure–activity studies seem to indicate that the binding modes of 4-PIOL (**9.53**) and muscimol (**9.2**) are different, as illustrated in Figure 9.13A. In this model illustrating the possible $GABA_A$ receptor interactions the 3-isoxazolol rings do not overlap (Figure 9.13B), implying that the 4-position in 4-PIOL does not correspond to the 4-position in muscimol. Thus, a large cavity at the 4-PIOL recognition site of the $GABA_A$ receptor seems to exist.

9.2.5.3 *Benzodiazepines and neurosteroids*

The GABAergic compounds acting at the benzodiazepine site or at the barbiturate site have been used as hypnotics for several decades. Agonists at these binding sites increase the chloride flux by modulation of the receptor response to GABA stimulation. Benzodiazepines increase the frequency of channel opening in response to GABA and barbiturates act by increasing mean channel open time. In the absence of GABA, the modulatory ligands do not produce any effect on the channel opening.

Not only drugs that have a benzodiazepine structure such as diazepam (**9.62**) and **9.63** can interact with the high-affinity benzodiazepine binding sites in the CNS, but also compounds such as β-carboline (**9.64**), imidazopyridine (**9.65**) and triazolopyridazine (**9.66**) as illustrated in Figure 9.14. The pharmacological profile of ligands binding to the benzodiazepine site spans the entire continuum from full and partial agonists, through antagonists, to partial and full inverse agonists.

Compound	R-	[³H]muscimol binding K_i (μM)	Electro-physiology IC_{50} (μM)
9.53	H-	9.1	110
9.57	CH_3-	10	26
9.58	CH_3CH_2-	6.3	10.3
9.59	CH_2- (benzyl)	3.8	4.0
9.60	CH_2- (naphthylmethyl)	0.049	0.37
9.61	$(CH_2)_2$- (naphthylethyl)	0.49	0.89

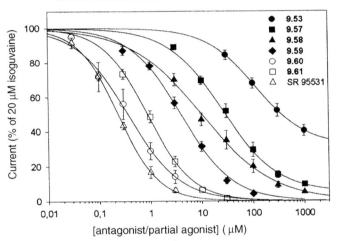

Figure 9.12 (Top) Receptor binding affinity (K_i values from [³H]muscimol binding on rat brain synaptic membranes) and *in vitro* electrophysiological activity (IC_{50} values from whole-cell patch clamp recording from cerebral cortical neurons) for a number of 4-PIOL analogs; (Bottom) effect of the partial agonists or antagonists on the response to 20 μM isoguvacine using whole-cell patch clamp recordings from cultured cerebral cortical neurons. 20 μM isoguvacine and varying concentrations of antagonist/partial agonist were applied simultaneously to the cells. The response to 20 μM isoguvacine alone has been set to 100%, and the other responses are expressed relative to this.

Antagonists do not influence GABA-induced chloride flux, but antagonize the action of benzodiazepine site agonists as well as of inverse agonist. The compounds with different efficacies produce a wide variety of behavioral pharmacological effects. The full benzodiazepine agonists show anxiolytic, anticonvulsant, sedative,

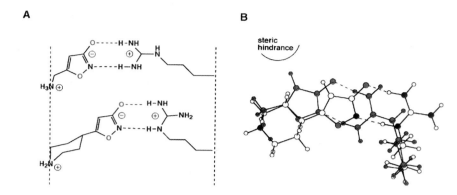

Figure 9.13 (A) Hypothetical model for the binding of muscimol and 4-PIOL to the GABA$_A$ receptor; (B) a superimposition of the proposed bioactive conformations of muscimol (9.2) and 4-PIOL (9.53) binding to two different conformations of an arginine residue at the agonist binding site.

Diazepam (9.62)   Ro15-4513 (9.63)   DMCM (9.64)

Zolpidem (9.65)   CL218872 (9.66)

Figure 9.14 Structures of some ligands for the benzodiazepine site.

and muscle relaxant effects, whereas the inverse agonists produce anxiety and convulsions. Of particular therapeutic interest are the reports of compounds, which are partial agonists at the benzodiazepine site, displaying potent anxiolytic and anticonvulsive effects with markedly less sedation and muscle relaxation compared to conventional benzodiazepines.

The relationship between GABA$_A$ receptor subunit composition and molecular pharmacology of benzodiazepines has been extensively studied and, as for GABA$_A$

ligands, the benzodiazepines show highly subunit dependent pharmacological profiles. From such studies it may be possible to identify and localize distinct subtypes of GABA_A receptors associated with different physiological and patho-physiological functions enabling development of novel compounds with more specific actions.

Neuroactive steroids are a novel class of positive allosteric modulators of the GABA_A receptor that interact with a specific steroid recognition site on the receptor–ion channel complex. Neurosteroids are synthesized in the brain, whereas other neuroactive steroids with pharmacological effects in the CNS are not necessarily synthesized in the CNS tissue. Neurosteroids and neuroactive steroids are important endogenous agents for influencing brain function by modulation of the activation of GABA_A receptors. They include pregnenolone (**9.67**) and reduced metabolites such as (**9.68**) and its 5β epimer (**9.69**) (Figure 9.15A). These steroids are rapidly biotransformed when administered exogenously due to metabolism of the 3-α-OH group at the 3-position. Thus, they exhibit rapid onset and short duration of action. Several synthetic analogs such as alphaxolone (**9.70**), ganaxolone (**9.71**) and **9.72** (Figure 9.15B) have been developed and show promising therapeutic effects. In general neuroactive steroids produce effects in animal models of CNS disorders similar to those of other positive allosteric modulators of the GABA_A receptor without significant side-effects.

9.2.5.4 GABA_B receptor ligands

Of the two GABA receptor classes insensitive to BMC (**9.42**), the GABA_B receptors have been most extensively studied. The GABA_B receptors are coupled to G-proteins, which upon activation cause a decrease in calcium and an increase in potassium membrane conductance. The GABA_B receptors seem to be pre-

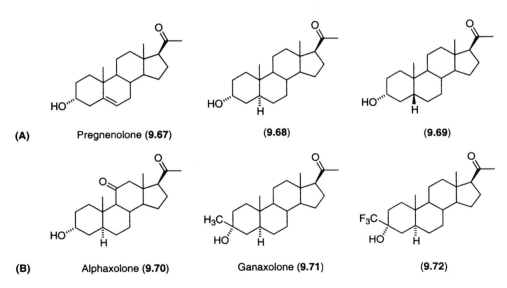

(A) Pregnenolone (**9.67**)   (**9.68**)   (**9.69**)

(B) Alphaxolone (**9.70**)   Ganaxolone (**9.71**)   (**9.72**)

Figure 9.15 Structures of some (A) neurosteroids; and (B) neuroactive steroids.

dominantly located presynaptically and they modulate synaptic transmission by depressing neurotransmitter release, including Glu release. These receptors are activated by GABA and, in contrast to $GABA_A$ receptors, also by the GABA analog (*R*)-baclofen (**9.44**). Baclofen was developed as a lipophilic derivative of GABA, in an attempt to enhance the blood–brain barrier penetrability of the endogenous ligand. (*R*)-Baclofen is effective in certain types of spasticity and has been in clinical use as an antispastic agent before discovery of the $GABA_B$ receptor. The clinical effect is believed to be related to $GABA_B$ receptor mediated inhibition of the release of Glu from hyperactive Glu terminals.

Although, a number of phosphinic acid-based $GABA_B$ receptor agonists have been synthesized, the number of selective and potent agonists for the $GABA_B$ receptor is limited and (*R*)-baclofen remains one of the more potent and selective agonists for the $GABA_B$ receptor. Among the agonists synthesized, the phosphinic acid analog of GABA (**9.73**) and its methyl analog (**9.74**) (Figure 9.16A) are the most active, being 3- and 7-fold more potent than (*R*)-baclofen, respectively.

The phosphonate analog of (*R*)-baclofen, (*R*)-phaclofen (**9.45**) as well as saclofen (**9.75**) and 2-OH-saclofen (**9.76**) (Figure 9.16B) were introduced as the first $GABA_B$ antagonists with peripheral as well as central activity. In attempt to improve the pharmacology of the $GABA_B$ receptor agonist **9.73**, a new series of selective and potent $GABA_B$ antagonists, capable of penetrating the blood–brain

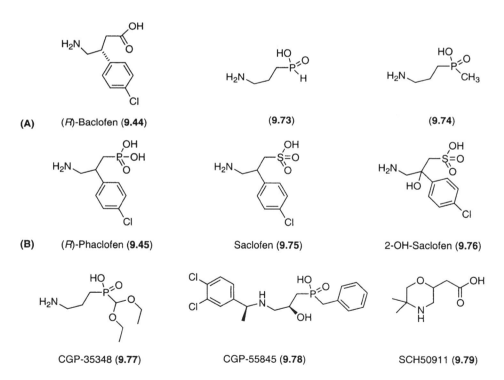

Figure 9.16 Structures of (A) $GABA_B$ receptor agonists and some examples of (B) $GABA_B$ receptor antagonists.

barrier after systemic administration, was discovered. One of the initial compounds in this series CGP-35348 (**9.77**) was succeeded by compound **9.78** (Figure 9.16B), showing very high affinities for the GABA$_B$ receptor. 2,5-Disubstituted-1,4-morpholines, exemplified by compound **9.79**, represent another structural class of GABA$_B$ receptor antagonists, which has been shown to be systemically active.

9.2.5.5 *GABA$_C$ receptor ligands*

The GABA$_C$ receptors do not respond to either BMC (**9.42**) or baclofen (**9.44**) (Figure 9.8). CACA (**9.47**) is a selective agonist for GABA$_C$ receptors but inactive at GABA$_A$ receptors, whereas the *trans*-isomer TACA (**9.80**) (Figure 9.17A) shows no preference. CAMP (**9.48**) is a selective GABA$_C$ agonist being inactive at GABA$_A$ receptors. All other known GABA$_A$ agonists seem to have some agonist/antagonist action at GABA$_C$ receptors, exemplified by THIP (**9.3**) and P4S (**9.81**) (Figure 9.17B), which are partial agonists at GABA$_A$ receptors and competitive antagonists at GABA$_C$ receptors. TPMPA (**9.46**) is a selective antagonist for GABA$_C$ receptors, at least 100 times more potent as an antagonist at GABA$_C$ receptors than at GABA$_A$ receptors. In contrast to the GABA$_A$ receptors the GABA$_C$ receptors are insensitive to barbiturates, benzodiazepines and neurosteroids.

9.3 GLUTAMIC ACID: EXCITATORY NEUROTRANSMITTER AND EXCITOTOXIN

Glu and a number of other endogenous acidic amino acids show excitatory effects when applied on central neurones. These excitatory amino acids also show neurotoxic properties when administered locally either at high concentrations for short periods or at lower concentrations for longer periods of time. This combination of neuroexcitatory activity and neurotoxic properties have been termed 'excitotoxicity' and seems to be a general phenomenon for excitatory amino acids.

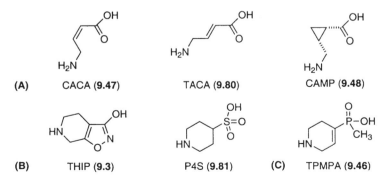

Figure 9.17 Structures of GABA$_C$ receptor (A) agonists; (B) partial agonists; and (C) an antagonist.

Glu is ubiquitously distributed in the CNS in high concentrations, and in addition to being the major excitatory neurotransmitter Glu participates in many metabolic processes and it is a precursor for the inhibitory neurotransmitter GABA. The high concentrations of Glu found in the CNS initially made it difficult to accept a transmitter role of Glu. Specific release and uptake mechanisms have, however, been identified and characterized, and these mechanisms can explain how the concentration-levels of Glu in the synaptic cleft is regulated. These highly efficient systems control the synaptic activity and prevent the above mentioned neurotoxicity of Glu in the normal mature brain. It is still unclear to what extent other acidic amino acids, such as (S)-aspartic acid or (S)-homocysteic acid, serve as endogenous neurotransmitters. Glu receptors are present in high numbers on most neurones in the CNS, reflecting the, atleast indirect, influence of Glu on virtually all physiological functions. Glu receptors play an important role in the synaptic plasticity associated with learning and memory functions, and these aspects open interesting therapeutic possibilities for Glu receptor agonists or other agents enhancing synaptic excitatory activity. Such agents may be used for improving cognition, learning and memory in certain pathological situations.

9.3.1 Classification of and ligands for Glu receptors

9.3.1.1 Receptor multiplicity

The Glu receptors are divided into two main classes (Figure 9.18, see also Figure 6.1) comprising a group of receptor-operated ion channels and a group of G-protein coupled receptors. Three types of ionotropic receptors have been identified, named N-methyl-D-aspartic acid (NMDA), 2-amino-3-(3-hydroxy-5-methyl-4-isoxazolyl)propionic acid (AMPA) and kainic acid (Kain) receptors. The group of metabotropic receptors (G-protein coupled receptors) is a very large and heterogeneous group of receptors subdivided into Group I, II and III. All receptor types are activated by Glu (**9.82**), and the three ionotropic receptors are named after selective agonists, whereas the metabotropic receptors have been classified according to pharmacology of ligands, second messenger coupling and sequence homology.

Figure 9.18 illustrates the number of subunits cloned within each class of receptors. At present, six NMDA receptor subunits (NR1, NR2A-NR2D, and NR3A), four AMPA-preferring subunits (GluR1-4) and five Kain preferring subunits (GluR5-7, KA1 and KA2) have been identified. The stoichiometry of subunits forming the functional ionotropic receptor complexes in vivo is still not clarified, but it is believed to be tetra- or pentameric structures of heteromeric nature. For the metabotropic receptors each circle in Figure 9.18 represents a single receptor protein (mGluR1-8). Each receptor protein is a functional unit, possibly with homo-dimers as the functional assembly in vivo.

In the following sections (9.3.1.2–9.3.1.7), some of the important ligands and characteristics of the individual receptor classes will be briefly covered. Examples covering more detailed medicinal chemistry studies are discussed in Section 9.3.2.

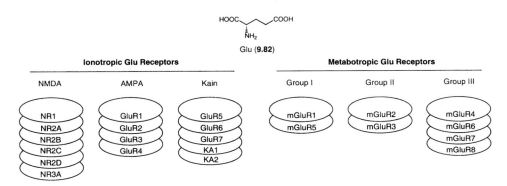

Figure 9.18 Schematic illustration of the multiplicity of excitatory amino acid receptors and the structure of Glu (**9.82**).

9.3.1.2 *Structure of ionotropic Glu receptors*

Cloning of the ionotropic Glu receptor subunits has disclosed the amino acid sequences of the receptor proteins, and the topology of these has been a matter of discussion. Studies defining the extra- and intracellular surfaces have now led to a model of the topology of the ionotropic Glu receptor comprising: a very large extracellular N-terminal domain, three transmembrane domains, one re-entry loop and an intracellular C-terminal (Figure 9.19). This model is based on a structure obtained from an X-ray crystallographic analysis of a soluble GluR2 binding domain consisting of the colored parts in Figure 9.19A (see also Figure 6.6). This soluble protein is formed by expression of a truncated form of the extracellular domain with the transmembrane domains, M1, M3 and the re-entry loop replaced by a hydrophilic linker (not shown). The protein exerts binding characteristics similar to the intact receptor protein. The binding site from this crystal structure is shown in Figure 9.19B, and the amino acid residues in the receptor protein binding to the Kain molecule (Figure 9.19C). The publication of this crystal structure with a ligand included has opened up new possibilities for structure-based design of ligands for these receptors.

In the following sections, important ligands for the different Glu receptors will be described. Most of these ligands have been developed prior to the appearance of the above mentioned crystal structure.

9.3.1.3 *NMDA receptor ligands*

The NMDA receptors have been characterized extensively and have been shown to be a receptor complex comprising a number of different binding sites (Figure 9.20), which can be manipulated pharmacologically. The NMDA receptor ion channel fluxes Na^+, K^+ and Ca^{2+} ions. Ca^{2+} ions have important intracellular functions as a second messenger, and Ca^{2+} also is implicated in the neurotoxicity observed after excessive receptor stimulation. NMDA (**9.83**), (*R*)-2-amino-2-(3-hydroxy-5-methyl-4-isoxazolyl)acetic acid [(*R*)-AMAA, **9.84**], (2*S*, 3*R*, 4*S*)-CCG (**9.85**) and (1*R*, 3*R*)-ACPD (**9.86**) (Figure 9.20A) are potent and selective agonists

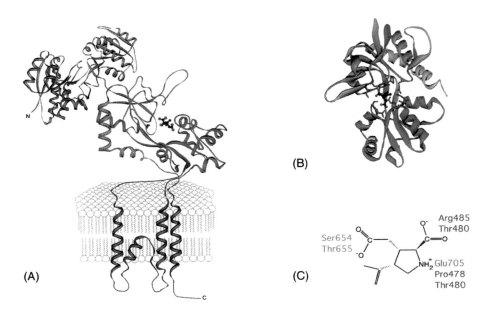

Figure 9.19 (A) Illustration of a single ionotropic Glu receptor subunit with a large extracellular amino-terminal domain, three transmembrane domains, a re-entry loop and an intracellular carboxy-terminal. The colored extracellular segments including Glu in the binding site is based on the crystal structure obtained of the soluble GluR2 binding core (see also Figure 6.6). (B) Model of the Glu binding core based on the crystal structure of the soluble binding core of GluR2 with the residues from the two extracellular segments involved in ligand binding indicated in blue and red. (C) Structure of Kain with numbers on interacting amino acid residues.

at the NMDA receptor. A great number of competitive NMDA receptor antagonists have been developed, most of which are analogs of (*R*)-2-amino-5-phosphono-valeric acid [(*R*)-AP5, **9.87**] or (*R*)-4-(3-phosphonopropyl)-2-piperazinecarboxylic acid [(*R*)-CPP, **9.88**] (Figure 9.20B). Most of these NMDA antagonists are phosphono amino acids, in which the carboxy and phosphono groups are separated by four or six atoms, and for most of the compounds resolved, the activity resides in the *R*-form. (±)-*Cis*-LY233053 (**9.89**) represents an example of an NMDA antagonist with a tetrazole ring functioning as the distal acidic moiety.

Glycine (**9.90**) has been shown to be a co-agonist at the NMDA receptors. Thus, in order to get a response at the NMDA receptors, both the NMDA receptor site and the glycine site have to be activated simultaneously by agonists. Electrophysiological studies seem to indicate that a high extracellular glycine concentration, perhaps a saturating concentration, is normally found in the synapse. Thus, release and uptake of Glu seem to be the determining factor for triggering excitatory responses at NMDA receptors, whereas a more slow change in the glycine concentration may modulate the level of activity at these receptors. (*R*)-HA-966 (**9.91**) is a partial agonist at the glycine site, and the quinoxalinedione ACEA-1021 (**9.92**) represents a large group of competitive glycine site antagonists. It is important to note that this glycine site/receptor (sometimes referred to as the Glycine$_B$ receptor) is excitatory in nature,

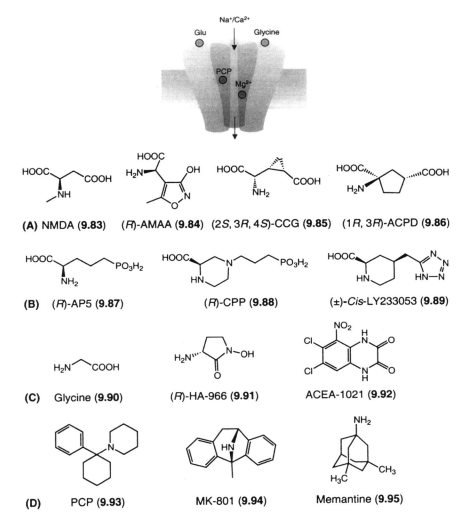

Figure 9.20 Schematic model of the NMDA receptor complex and structures of some selective (A) agonists; (B) competitive antagonists; (C) glycine site ligands; and (D) non-
competitive antagonists.

and not to be mistaken for the inhibitory, strychnine sensitive Glycine$_A$ receptor,
primarily found in the spinal cord.

Apart from a strict requirement for both Glu and glycine to activate the NMDA
receptors, another unusual factor is observed for this ligand gated ion channel. At
normal resting potentials, the NMDA receptors are blocked by Mg^{2+}, probably
binding to a site within the ion channel. When the neurone is partially depolarized,
e.g. by activation of other ionotropic Glu receptors on the same neurone, the Mg^{2+}
blockade is released, and the NMDA receptor ion channel can be activated to give
further depolarization. Thus, in some respects the NMDA receptors seem to function
as an amplification system working only at certain levels of activity of the neurones.

A site for non-competitive NMDA antagonists has been characterized, most often referred to as the phencyclidine (PCP, **9.93**) site. The action of PCP, MK-801 (**9.94**) (Figure 9.20D) and other non-competitive NMDA antagonists are use-dependent, meaning that repeated activation of the NMDA receptors by an agonist is needed to obtain effective antagonist activity of these antagonists. The interpretation of this phenomenon has been that these agents require access to the open ion channel in order to exert their use-dependent antagonism. The mechanism of use-dependency seems very interesting in relation to the treatment of neurodegenerative disorders. In principle, such non-competitive antagonists should elicit therapeutically useful antagonism at synapses with hyperactivity, as observed in neurodegenerative situations (Section 9.1), whereas less efficient antagonism are to be expected at synapses with normal synaptic activity. This would be expected to lead to reduced side effects of non-competitive NMDA antagonists as compared to competitive antagonists. Unfortunately, most non-competitive antagonists studied so far, have shown severe psychotomimetic side effects, which have prevented therapeutic applications. The amantadine analog Memantine (**9.95**), which show a low affinity to the PCP site compared to MK-801, is however very well tolerated in man. Memantine has been used for a number of years in the treatment of Parkinson's disease and is at present in the clinic for other indications, e.g. Alzheimer's disease.

Other binding sites, including at least two different binding sites for polyamines (blockade inside the ion channel and blockade or stimulation outside the ion channel), and a site for Zn^{2+} have also been identified at the NMDA receptor complex, but these sites are not further described here.

9.3.1.4 *AMPA receptor ligands*

Originally, the AMPA receptors were named Quis receptors after the naturally occurring compound quisqualic acid (Quis, **9.96**). Quite early it was however realized, that Quis is a non-selective Glu receptor agonist. Quis receptors were renamed to the AMPA receptors on the basis of the very potent and specific agonist activity of (*S*)-AMPA (**9.97**). Tritiated AMPA is used as the standard ligand for AMPA receptor binding studies. (*S*)-ACPA (**9.98**) is an analog of AMPA with even higher potency than AMPA. (*S*)-ACPA show very limited desensitization of AMPA receptors compared to AMPA itself. Willardiine is like Quis a naturally occurring compound with AMPA agonist activity and (*S*)-F-Willardiine (**9.99**) show potent and selective activity at AMPA receptors (Figure 9.21).

A very large and important group of competitive AMPA receptor antagonists is constituted by analogs of quinoxalinedione, with NBQX (**9.100**) being one of the early examples and still widely used as a pharmacological agent. Two more recent quinoxalinedione AMPA antagonists, Ro 48-8587 (**9.101**) and LY293558 (**9.102**), are systemically active. **9.101** has been radiolabeled as a tool for studies of the antagonist binding site. The isoxazole (*S*)-2-amino-3-[5-*tert*-butyl-3-(phosphono-methoxy)-4-isoxazolyl]propionic acid [(*S*)-ATPO, **9.103**], represents a group of selective AMPA antagonists derived from the structure of AMPA itself. More detailed structure activity studies on AMPA receptor agonists and antagonists are described in Sections 9.3.2.1 and 9.3.2.2, respectively.

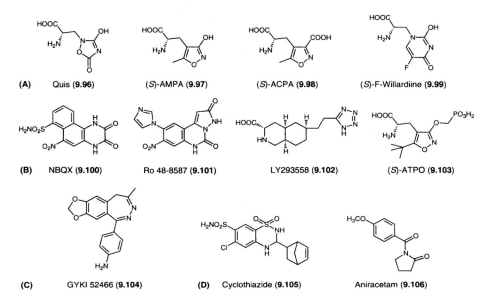

Figure 9.21 Structures of some selective AMPA receptor: (A) agonists; (B) competitive antagonists; (C) non-competitive antagonist; and (D) modulatory agents.

A number of compounds with non-competitive antagonist effects at AMPA receptors have been identified. GYKI 52466 (**9.104**) and other 2,3-benzodiaze-pines show potent and selective antagonist effects at AMPA receptors by interaction with an allosteric site. The rapid desensitization observed after application of agonists at AMPA receptors can be modulated by compounds such as the diuretic cyclothiazide (**9.105**) and the nootropic agent aniracetam (**9.106**). These compounds essentially block desensitization to agonists, thereby enhancing the excitatory activity, in some cases several-fold, depending on the initial level of desensitization observed for the individual agonist.

The AMPA receptors mediate fast excitatory activity, and AMPA antagonists have shown neuroprotective properties in numerous animal models. It is as yet unknown, whether such antagonists can be administered to man without severe side effects. In agreement with the previous discussions, AMPA receptors may have particular therapeutic interest (see also Section 9.3.2.4).

9.3.1.5   Kain receptor ligands

Studies using molecular cloning techniques have shown AMPA and Kain receptors to be closely related at the molecular level. Furthermore, these receptors show similar pharmacology, and only a limited number of selective Kain agonists are known. Kain (**9.107**) has been the standard agonist of choice for many years despite its non-selective action, and [³H]Kain is the ligand generally used for binding studies of Kain receptors (Figure 9.22). Kain also shows relatively potent

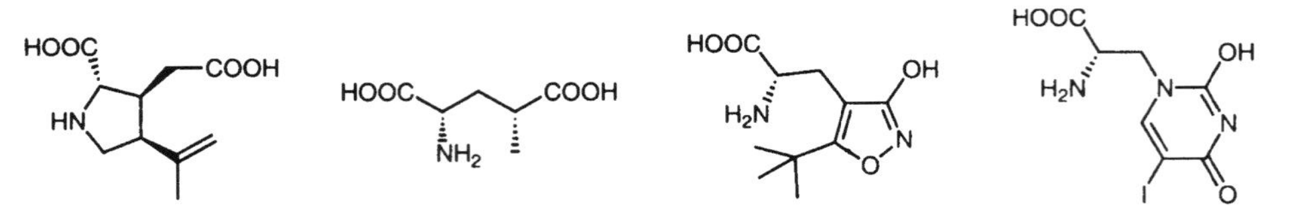

(A) Kain (**9.107**) (2*S*,4*R*)-4-Me-Glu (**9.108**) (*S*)-ATPA (**9.109**) (*S*)-I-Willardiine (**9.110**)

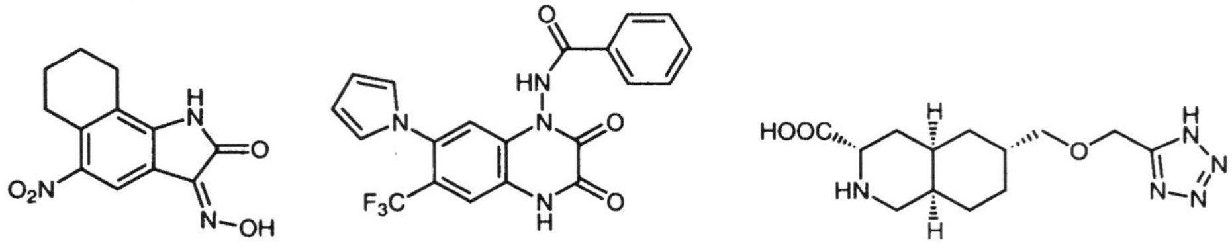

(B) NS-102 (**9.111**) LU97175 (**9.112**) LY294486 (**9.113**)

Figure 9.22 Structures of some Kain receptor (A) agonists and (B) antagonists.

interaction with AMPA receptors as well, and it is frequently used as agonist for studies of AMPA receptors, because Kain, in contrast to AMPA itself, does not desensitize AMPA receptors. (2*S*, 4*R*)-4-Me-Glu (**9.108**) shows selective affinity for the [^{3}H]Kain binding site and potent agonist activity at recombinant GluR5 and GluR6 receptors. More recently the AMPA derivative (*S*)-ATPA (**9.109**) has shown, apart from fairly weak AMPA agonist activity (Section 9.3.2.1), highly potent GluR5 agonist activity. Similarly does (*S*)-I-Willardiine (**9.110**), in contrast to (*S*)-F-Willardiine (**9.99**), show selective activity at GluR5. The agonist pairs AMPA/ATPA and F-/I-Willardiine indicate that in spite of close similarity in the structural requirements for activation of AMPA and Kain receptors, relatively small differences in at least the bulk tolerance can be used for the design of selective compounds.

Only a few antagonists at Kain receptors have been developed. NS-102 (**9.111**) has been reported to have affinity for [^{3}H]Kain binding site and antagonist activity at homomeric GluR6, but solubility problems limits its utility. LU97175 (**9.112**) and LY294486 (**9.113**) represent newer compounds with promising antagonist activities, at GluR5-7 and GluR5, respectively.

9.3.1.6 *Structure of metabotropic Glu receptors*

The metabotropic Glu receptors belong to family C of G-protein coupled receptors. The metabotropic Glu receptors have in analogy to the ionotropic Glu receptors a very large extracellular N-terminal domain, comprising the binding site for Glu and seven transmembrane spanning domains (see Section 6.2.1 and Figures 6.2 and 6.3). The binding of Glu in the extracellular domain lead to a closing of the two binding lopes, a concomitant conformational change of the receptor protein, and, by a yet unknown mechanism, to activation of the G-protein coupled to the receptor protein at the intracellular domains (see also Section 6.2.1 and Figures 6.3 and 6.12). An X-ray crystallographic structure of the extracellular ligand-binding region has been published for one of the subtypes of the metabotropic receptors (mGluR1). In analogy with the ionotropic Glu receptors (Section 9.3.1.2) this has furnished detailed new knowledge about the receptor binding site, which will be of importance for the development of new ligands.

Based on pharmacology, transduction pathways and amino acid sequences the metabotropic receptors has been divided into three groups: Group I consisting of mGluR1,5 stimulating phospholipase C and Group II (mGluR2,3) and Group III (mGluR4,6-8) both inhibiting the formation of cyclic AMP. This means that agonist stimulation of Group I receptors leads to cell excitation, whereas agonist stimulation of Group II and Group III receptors leads to cell inhibition. However, some of the metabotropic receptors are located presynaptically, and may function as autoreceptors. Thus, activation of such receptors inhibit the presynaptic release of Glu. The responses obtained through metabotropic receptors are generally slower than ionotropic receptor responses, and may be regarded as modulation of the fast excitatory tone set by the ionotropic Glu receptors.

9.3.1.7 Metabotropic receptor ligands

Characterization of metabotropic Glu receptors did not really proceed until after the cloning of the different subtypes in the early nineties. Thus, the research within this group of receptors has been going on for much shorter time than for the ionotropic Glu receptors. The focus on metabotropic receptors has however been enormous in recent years, among other things because of the little therapeutic success obtained after many years of research within the ionotropic area. Apart from Glu itself, (1*S*,3*R*)-ACPD (**9.114**), ibotenic acid (**9.115**) and Quis (**9.96**) were among the first potent metabotropic agonists (Figure 9.23A), though they are fairly non-selective.

Synthesis of the homologs of these and other Glu analogs (Figure 9.23B) did however afford compounds with more selective activity at metabotropic Glu receptors. Thus, (*S*)-2-aminoadipic acid [(*S*)-2-AA, **9.116**], was shown to be a

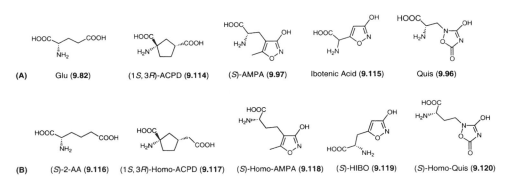

Figure 9.23 Structures of (A) Glu (**9.82**) and some Glu analogs and (B) corresponding homologs compounds showing activity at metabotropic Glu receptors.

mGluR2 and mGluR6 agonist, (1*S*, 3*R*)-Homo-ACPD (**9.117**) a Group I agonist, whereas (*S*)-Homo-AMPA (**9.118**) showed specific activity at mGluR6, and no activity at neither ionotropic Glu receptors or at other metabotropic Glu receptors. A number of homoibotenic acid (HIBO) analogs, including HIBO (**9.119**) itself show Group I antagonist activity and (*S*)-Homo-Quis (**9.120**) is a mixed Group I antagonist/Group II agonist. The activity of these and other Glu homologs indicate that Glu is interacting with the metabotropic receptors in an extended conformation. The effect of backbone extension of different Glu analogs is often unpredictable, but chain length are nevertheless a factor of utmost importance. A more detailed structure–activity study on HIBO analogs as Group I antagonists is described in Section 9.3.2.3.

Conformationally restricted analogs containing a Glu backbone or acidic phenylglycine analogs are two very important groups of compounds, which have afforded many analogs with selective activity at metabotropic receptors, including agonists as well as antagonists (Figure 9.24). The two Group I agonists ABHxD-I (**9.121**) (non-selective) and (*S*)-3,5-DHPG (**9.122**), are representatives of the two groups, and the two Group I antagonists (*S*)-4-CPG (**9.123**) and (*RS*)-AIDA (**9.124**) belong to the latter group.

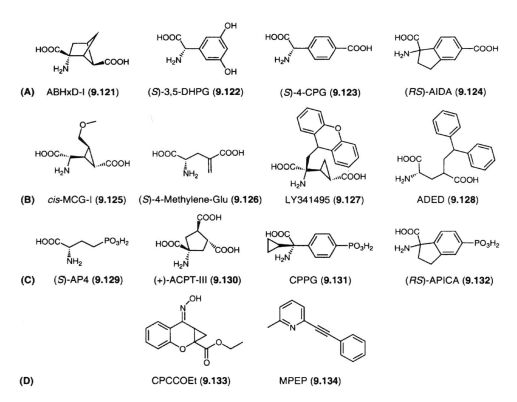

(A)   ABHxD-I (**9.121**)   (*S*)-3,5-DHPG (**9.122**)   (*S*)-4-CPG (**9.123**)   (*RS*)-AIDA (**9.124**)

(B)   *cis*-MCG-I (**9.125**)   (*S*)-4-Methylene-Glu (**9.126**)   LY341495 (**9.127**)   ADED (**9.128**)

(C)   (*S*)-AP4 (**9.129**)   (+)-ACPT-III (**9.130**)   CPPG (**9.131**)   (*RS*)-APICA (**9.132**)

(D)   CPCCOEt (**9.133**)   MPEP (**9.134**)

Figure 9.24 Structures of some metabotropic receptor ligands showing selectivity towards (A) Group I; (B) Group II or (C) Group III; and (D) noncompetitive antagonists.

The two Glu analogs *cis*-MCG-I (**9.125**) and (*S*)-4-Methylene-Glu (**9.126**) have shown fairly selective activity as Group II agonists, whereas the two related Glu analogs containing large lipophilic substituents LY341495 (**9.127**) and ADED (**9.128**) are converted into Group II antagonists.

At Group III metabotropic receptors the phosphonate Glu analog (*S*)-AP4 (**9.129**) and (+)-ACPT-III (**9.130**) are selective agonists, whereas CPPG (**9.131**) and (*RS*)-APICA (**9.132**) are selective antagonists.

The pharmacology of metabotropic ligands has evolved with the availability of the cloned receptors and thus, many subtype selective ligands have been discovered compared to ionotropic ligands. However, many of the above mentioned ligands have not been fully tested on all metabotropic (or ionotropic) subtypes, and the selectivity is therefore not fully investigated yet.

More recently a number of non-competitive antagonists at metabotropic Glu receptors has been discovered by high-throughput screening of compound libraries. These antagonists, represented by CPCCOEt (**9.133**) (see also Section 6.3.3 and Figure 6.12) and MPEP (**9.134**), are selective mGluR1 and mGluR5 antagonists, respectively, and show very high potency compared to the competitive antagonists.

The metabotropic receptors affect the activity of neurones and indirectly affect the activity of ion channels. Studies on animal models have shown both neuroprotective and neurotoxic properties of metabotropic agonists. This is related to the signal transduction mechanisms for the different subtypes, as mentioned in Section 9.3.1.6. Group I receptors being excitatory and Group II and III inhibitory, and also that some metabotropic receptors are presynaptically located, whereas other subtypes are postsynaptic in nature.

9.3.2 Ibotenic acid: a naturally occurring excitotoxin and lead structure

Many naturally occurring acidic amino acids have shown activity at excitatory amino acid receptors and have been used extensively as lead structures in the search for new and better ligands. The *Amanita muscaria* constituent ibotenic acid (**9.115**) shows potent activity at both NMDA receptors and certain metabotropic receptor subtypes, and it is a weak agonist at AMPA/Kain receptors. It is used as a pharmacological and neurotoxic agent, although chemical instability limits the utility in experimental pharmacology.

It is believed that Glu (**9.82**) interacts with the various Glu receptors in different conformations, suggesting that development of Glu analogs with restricted conformations may lead to compounds with selective action. Ibotenic acid is a conformationally restricted analog of Glu in which the 3-hydroxyisoxazole moiety functions as a bioisostere to the distal carboxyl group of Glu. Glu as well as ibotenic acid exist primarily on their fully ionized forms at physiological pH as illustrated in Figure 9.25. The similarity observed for the delocalization of charge on the distal carboxylate group of Glu and of the deprotonated 3-isoxazolol may explain the utility of this bioisosteric replacement.

Ibotenic acid has been used as the lead structure for the design of many compounds of importance in medicinal chemistry studies of different Glu receptors.

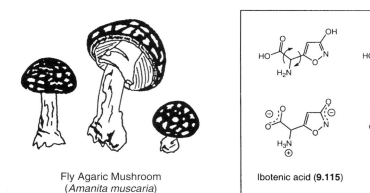

Fly Agaric Mushroom
(*Amanita muscaria*)

Ibotenic acid (**9.115**)   Glu (**9.82**)

Figure 9.25 Illustration of the structural flexibility of ibotenic acid (**9.115**) (isolated from the fly agaric mushroom) and of Glu (**9.82**), and delocalization of the three charges existing at physiological pH (pK_a values: Ibotenic acid, 3.0, 5.0 and 8.2; Glu, 2.2, 4.3 and 10.0).

In the subsequent sections such structure–activity studies are illustrated for AMPA receptor agonists (Section 9.3.2.1), AMPA receptor antagonists (Section 9.3.2.2), Group I metabotropic antagonists (Section 9.3.2.3) and finally the principle of functional partial agonism (Section 9.3.2.4).

9.3.2.1   5-Substituted AMPA analogs

The tolerance for bulk in the 5-position of the isoxazole ring of AMPA analogs has been investigated by synthesis of a number of analogs with different substituents. Two series of compounds with 5-alkyl or 5-aryl substituents, respectively, are listed in Table 9.1. The influence on AMPA receptor pharmacology is represented by the IC_{50} values from [^{3}H]AMPA binding studies and by the EC_{50} values from an *in vitro* electrophysiological model. (*RS*)-AMPA (**9.136**) is obviously a very potent agonist, but the pharmacology of AMPA analogs is very dependent on the substituent in the 5-position of the isoxazole ring.

For the 5-alkyl substituted analogs a fairly simple structure–activity relationship seems to exist. Analogs with an increasing size of the substituent generally seem to lose activity. The compounds with small substituents are fairly potent (**9.136**–**9.138**), the butyl analog (**9.139**) is somewhat weaker, and the loss of activity is more dramatic for the analogs with branched substituents compared to the analogs with unbranched substituents. This is obvious from the isopentyl (**9.142**), neopentyl (**9.144**) and 4-heptyl (**9.145**) analogs, being very weak or inactive as AMPA agonists, indicating that there is a fairly strict limit for the size of the 5-substituent. On the basis of these compounds, the existence of a hydrophobic pocket at the receptor binding site capable of accommodating small substituents has been hypothesized. The demethylated analog (**9.135**) is an exception in terms of activity. It does show fairly high affinity for AMPA receptors, but is unexpectedly weak in the cortical slice preparation. However,

Table 9.1 Receptor affinity (IC_{50} values from [3H]AMPA binding) and *in vitro* electrophysiological activity (EC_{50} values from the rat cortical slice preparation) for 5-alkyl and 5-aryl substituted AMPA analogs

	R	IC_{50} (µM)	EC_{50} (µM)			IC_{50} (µM)	EC_{50} (µM)
(9.135)	—H	0.27	900	(9.146)		35	390
(9.136)	-CH₃	0.04	3.5	(9.147)		0.57	7.4
(9.137)	-CH₂-CH₃	0.03	2.3	(9.148)		>100	>1000
(9.138)	-CH₂-CH₂-CH₃	0.09	5.0	(9.149)		5.5	96
(9.139)	-CH₂-CH₂-CH₂-CH₃	1.0	32	(9.150)		1.2	11
(9.140)	-CH(CH₃)CH₃	0.19	9.0	(9.151)		72	>1000
(9.141)	-CH₂-CH(CH₃)CH₃	0.61	23	(9.152)		54	>1000
(9.142)	-CH₂-CH₂-CH(CH₃)CH₃	>100	>1000	(9.153)		0.03	0.92
(9.143)	-C(CH₃)₃ *(RS)-ATPA*	11	48	(9.154)		0.28	5.8
(9.144)	-CH₂-C(CH₃)₃	55	420	(9.155)		3.5	43
(9.145)	-CH(CH₂-CH₂-CH₃)(CH₂-CH₂-CH₃)	99	>1000	(9.156)		0.09	2.3

electrophysiological experiments performed on dissociated neurones did show potent activity of **9.135**. This indicates that **9.135** may be a substrate for Glu uptake systems, which lead to low activity in intact test systems such as the cortical slice preparation. Glu itself is also found to be a very weak agonist in this electrophysiological model.

The picture concerning the structure–activity relationship is less clear for the 5-aryl substituted AMPA analogs. The 5-phenyl analog (APPA, **9.146**) is a fairly weak agonist, indicating that a phenyl group is too big a substituent in order to have potent AMPA agonist activity. However, APPA is pharmacologically interesting because it functions as a partial agonist, with an intrinsic activity of approximately 60% compared to other agonists. This aspect will be further discussed in Section 9.3.2.4. When the three pyridyl analogs 2-, 3-, and 4-pyridyl-AMPA (**9.147–9.149**) were examined, a very dramatic effect depending on the position of the pyridine nitrogen was observed. The 2-pyridyl analog **9.147** being a very potent agonist, **9.148** inactive and **9.149** fairly weak. The pyrazine analog **9.150** was also fairly potent, whereas the tetrazole analog (**9.151**) was quite weak. The tetrazole is obviously smaller in size, but it is however a quite acidic substituent, which may be unfavorable. The 2-methyl and 3-methyl-tetrazole analogs (**9.152** and **9.153**) were also very different in activity, **9.153** being the most potent AMPA agonist known so far. Also the 2-thienyl (**9.154**) and the 2-thiazole (**9.156**) analogs are very potent AMPA agonists, whereas the 3-thienyl (**9.155**) analog is fairly weak. These structures indicate that a heteroatom in the 2 position of the 5-substituent is of importance for the activity. The mechanism behind this dramatic effect of the heteroatom is not known. The heteroatoms may be involved in intra- and/or intermolecular hydrogen bonding to the receptor protein. These compounds also show that the size of the substituent is by no means the only factor of importance for potent receptor interaction.

9.3.2.2   Isoxazole based AMPA receptor antagonists

The AMPA receptor antagonists have been, and still are, of great interest as pharmacological tools and potential therapeutic agents, especially in relation to neurodegenerative disorders. In the search for compounds with AMPA antagonist activity many derivatives of AMPA itself have been prepared. Among the competitive NMDA receptor antagonists many acidic amino acids with a backbone longer than Glu have successfully been developed (Section 9.3.1.3). In analogy with this strategy the compound AMOA (**9.157**) was synthesized. This AMPA derivative is a selective AMPA receptor antagonist, though of fairly low potency. In order to improve the potency a number of analogs with different substituents and different distal acidic groups was synthesized. The *tert*-butyl analog ATOA (**9.158**) was found to be somewhat more potent than AMOA, and in analogy with the NMDA antagonists, the phosphonate analogs **9.159** and **9.160** proved to be significantly more potent than the carboxylate analogs. ATPO was shown to be the most potent analog, with a significant improvement of potency compared to AMOA and selective activity for AMPA receptors (Figure 9.26).

Due to the improved potency of ATPO, the compound was resolved by chiral HPLC to give the two enantiomers. The absolute configuration of the obtained enantiomers was established by an X-ray crystallographic analysis of the *R*-form (Figure 9.27A). The pharmacology of the two enantiomers was investigated on recombinant AMPA (GluR1, GluR1+2, GluR3 and GluR4) and Kain receptors (GluR5, GluR6 and GluR6+KA2) expressed in *Xenopus* oocytes. All activity was shown to reside in the *S*-form (**9.103**), with the *R*-form (**9.161**) being very weak or inactive on all receptor subtypes (Figure 9.27B–D). (*S*)-ATPO (**9.103**) was a fairly selective agonist at AMPA receptors, being approximately equipotent on GluR1-4, whereas it was somewhat weaker on the Kain preferring subtype GluR5. At GluR6 or GluR6+KA2 no activity was observed. GluR5 has previously shown pharmacology

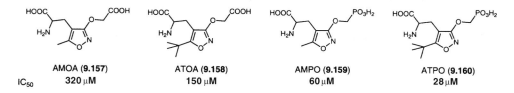

AMOA (**9.157**)	ATOA (**9.158**)	AMPO (**9.159**)	ATPO (**9.160**)
IC_{50} 320 μM	150 μM	60 μM	28 μM

Figure 9.26 Structures of some competitive AMPA receptor antagonists with antagonist potencies from the rat cortical slice preparation (IC_{50} values).

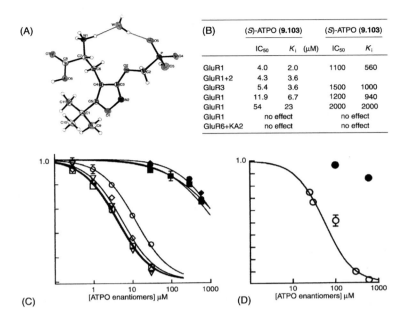

Figure 9.27 (A) Perspective drawing of (R)-ATPO·H$_2$O (**9.161**) obtained from an X-ray crystal-lographic analysis. Hydrogen bonds to the water molecule are indicated by thin lines. (B) Table with antagonist effects determined for the enantiomers of ATPO towards Kain induced activation of homo- and heteromeric Glu receptors expressed in *Xenopus* oocytes. (C) Concentration-dependent inhibition by (S)-ATPO (**9.103**) (open symbols) and (R)-ATPO (**9.161**) (closed symbols) of Kain induced responses in *Xenopus* oocytes expressing GluR1 (□), GluR1 + 2 (▽), GluR3 (◇), GluR4 (○) or (D) GluR5.

related to the AMPA receptor subtypes, in spite of its clear structural relationship to Kain receptor subtypes.

Development of subtype selective compounds is of importance in the under-standing of the physiological and pathological importance of the receptor subtypes and may lead to valuable therapeutic compounds. The number of such com-pounds is still very limited and many of the older compounds have not been investigated on recombinant receptors at all. With the increasing knowledge on the structure of the receptor proteins and the availability of recombinant receptors for pharmacological testing, the issue of subtype pharmacology will be of great importance in the work to come.

9.3.2.3 Homoibotenic acid analogs as metabotropic antagonists

A number of 4-substituted analogs of (S)-HIBO (**9.119**) has been synthesized and was originally found to be selective and fairly potent AMPA receptor agonists. (S)-HIBO itself did, in analogy to the demethylated AMPA analog (**9.135**), show fairly high-affinity for AMPA receptors, but quite low activity in the functional test (Table 9.2). Other analogs with small substituents, (S)-methyl-(**9.162**) and

Table 9.2 Receptor binding affinity (IC_{50} values from [^{3}H]AMPA binding), *in vitro* electrophysiological activity (EC_{50} values from the rat cortical slice preparation) and activity at metabotropic Glu receptors (K_b values at cloned mGluRs expressed in chinese hamster ovary cells) of 4-alkyl-HIBO analogs

		[^{3}H]AMPA	Electrophys.	mGluR1	mGluR5	mGluR2	mGluR4
		IC_{50} (μM)	EC_{50} (μM)	K_b (μM)			
(S)-HIBO	(9.119)	0.80	330	250	490	>1000	>1000
(S)-Methyl-HIBO	(9.162)	0.32	18	190	180	>1000	>1000
(S)-Butyl-HIBO	(9.163)	0.48	17	110	97	>1000	>1000
Octyl-HIBO	(9.164)	>100	>500	>100	nd	>1000	>1000
Pentyl-HIBO	(9.165)	11	630	140	190	>1000	>1000
Hexyl-HIBO	(9.166)	>100	>1000	140	110	>1000	>1000
Heptyl-HIBO	(9.167)	>100	>500	160	990	>1000	>1000

(S)-butyl-HIBO (**9.163**) were fairly potent agonists, whereas the octyl-analog (**9.164**) was inactive (Table 9.2). These findings are in good agreement with the structure–activity relationships described for the 5-substituted AMPA analogs.

Testing on recombinant metabotropic receptors disclosed that these HIBO analogs also had antagonist activity at group I metabotropic receptors. The activity of (S)-Methyl-HIBO and (S)-Butyl-HIBO on mGluR1 and mGluR5 were approximately the same. This was interesting from a pharmacological point of view and also of potential therapeutic interest. The inactivity of Octyl-HIBO at AMPA receptors showed that there certainly is a size-limit for AMPA agonists, however the low solubility of Octyl-HIBO did not allow a full investigation in the metabotropic assays. In the search for compounds with selective activity on metabotropic receptors, Pentyl-, Hexyl- and Heptyl-HIBO (**9.165–9.167**) was synthesized. For Pentyl-HIBO a dramatic loss of activity on AMPA receptors was observed, and for Hexyl- and Heptyl-HIBO no AMPA agonist activity was left at all. However, all three compounds showed antagonist activity at metabotropic receptors, **9.165** and **9.166** with approximately the same activities at mGluR1 and mGluR5. Thus, Hexyl-HIBO can be characterized as a selective Group I receptor antagonist. Interestingly Heptyl-HIBO (**9.167**) show the same potency at mGluR1 as **9.165** and **9.166**, but a significantly lower activity at mGluR5. Thus, **9.167** is an antagonist selective for this mGluR1. *In vivo* studies in mice has shown Hexyl-HIBO to antagonize NMDA-induced convulsions. Unfortunately this antagonism was only observed when Hexyl-HIBO was given i.c.v., whereas peripheral administration (i.v.) did not lead to protection against the NMDA induced convulsions. This indicate that Hexyl-HIBO do not penetrate the blood–brain barrier, or alternative it may be metabolized systemically to an extent preventing blood–brain barrier penetration. The results does however, show that such metabotropic antagonists may have therapeutic potential.

9.3.2.4   Functional partial agonism

The partial agonism observed for racemic APPA (**9.146**) (Section 9.3.2.1) greatly stimulated the interest in this compound and a resolution procedure was developed to furnish the two enantiomers. Resolution was accomplished by diastereomeric salt formation using racemic APPA and (*R*)- or (*S*)-phenylethylamine (PEA). When (*RS*)-APPA was mixed with (*S*)-PEA and recrystallized from ethanol, the diastereomeric salt consisting of (*R*)-APPA and (*S*)-PEA precipitated and could be purified by repeated recrystallization, affording (*R*)-APPA after liberation from the salt. Analogously, (*S*)-APPA was obtained using (*R*)-PEA for the salt formation.

In contrast to the racemate, originally characterized as a partial agonist, (*S*)-APPA proved to be a full agonist at AMPA receptors, slightly more potent than the racemate (Figure 9.28A). (*R*)-APPA had no intrinsic activity at AMPA receptors when applied alone, but when co-applied with AMPA or (*S*)-APPA it antagonized the excitation evoked by these agonists. The dose–response curves of these two AMPA agonists could be shifted to the right in a parallel fashion, indicating that (*R*)-APPA was a competitive AMPA receptor antagonist (Figure 9.28A). These results reveal that the original partial agonism observed for (*RS*)-APPA was due to the interaction of a full agonist [(*S*)-APPA] and a competitive antagonist [(*R*)-APPA].

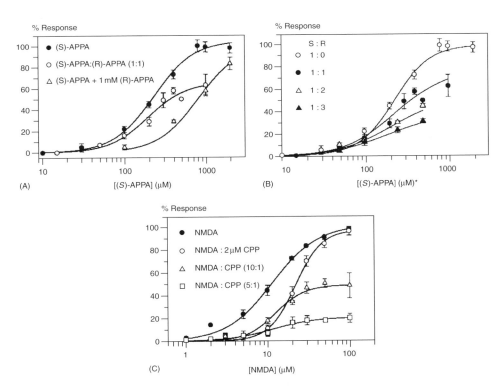

Figure 9.28 Dose–response curves from the rat cortical slice preparation. (A) (*S*)-APPA, (*RS*)-APPA (**9.146**) and parallel shift of the (*S*)-APPA curve with 1 mM (*R*)-APPA. (B) Curves obtained with fixed molar ratios of (*S*)- and (*R*)-APPA; 1:0, 1:1 (racemate), 1:2 and 1:3. *The *X*-axis represents the concentration of (*S*)-APPA, whereas the concentration of (*R*)-APPA is 0, 1, 2 or 3 times the concentration of (*S*)-APPA in the four different experiments. (C) Curves obtained with NMDA (**9.83**), fixed molar ratios of NMDA and CPP (**9.88**) (10:1 and 5:1) and rightward shift of the NMDA curve with 2 μM CPP.

Subsequently, dose–response curves were obtained using different ratios of (*R*)- and (*S*)-APPA. This is shown in Figure 9.28B for (*S*)-APPA alone and for different ratios of (*S*)-APPA/(*R*)-APPA [(1:1) (racemic APPA), (1:2) and (1:3)]. It is seen that with an increasing amount of the antagonist, the maximum response is depressed. The curves have not been extended further due to the rather low potency of the enantiomers. The figure illustrates the principle of functional partial agonism. This principle implicates that, in theory, any desired level of intrinsic activity can be obtained when mixing an agonist and a competitive antagonist in a fixed molar ratio. Functional partial agonism can be achieved using any pair of agonist and competitive antagonist. Furthermore, this principle can be applied not only to AMPA receptor ligands, but also to ligands of other ionotropic Glu receptors or other ionotropic neurotransmitter systems in general. The maximal activity attainable will depend on the relative potency of the two agents. It is important to notice the difference between these experiments using agonists and competitive antagonists, to achieve functional partial agonism, and the conventional pharmacological experiment designed to demonstrate competitive antagonism. In the latter case, a dose response curve for the agonist is determined in the presence of a fixed concentration of a competitive antagonist, which will shift the dose–response curve for the agonist to the right in a parallel fashion. In contrast to this, functional partial agonism is established using fixed molar ratios of the two components, i.e. the curves are obtained using increasing doses, at a fixed ratio, of both agonist and antagonist.

Another example of the principle of functional partial agonism is shown in Figure 9.28C using NMDA (**9.83**) and the competitive NMDA antagonist CPP (**9.88**). The high potency of these two compounds makes it possible to obtain full curves. Again, the figure shows the possibility of reaching any level of activity between 0 and 1, by choosing appropriate ratios of agonist and competitive antagonist.

Partial agonists may be therapeutically valuable in relation to Alzheimer's disease as described in Section 9.1.3 and may also prove to have therapeutic application in other disorders. For *in vivo* studies of functional partial agonism, a number of factors will have to be carefully considered. First of all, the level of efficacy desired for the disease in question is not known, and will have to be determined. If the two compounds, the agonist and the appropriate competitive antagonist, are administered systemically it is important to make sure that both compounds actually reach the site of action in the necessary concentrations. This means that absorption, metabolism, penetration and other factors will have to be taken into consideration for both compounds. At this point, the principle of functional partial agonism has been introduced – the future will show the applicability.

9.4   FUTURE DEVELOPMENTS

The cloning of the many GABA and Glu receptor subtypes and their pharmacological characterization has speeded up the development of selective ligands. More recently crystal structure determinations of binding cores has increased the structural knowledge about the receptor proteins and about the amino acid residues in the binding sites, and this has opened up the possibility of structure-based design. This may lead to a better understanding of the ligand–receptor interactions, receptor mechanisms and to the developments of more selective compounds. Many ligands have been developed as experimental tools and have been important for the understanding of many brain functions and pathophysiological aspects. However, the success as therapeutic agents, especially within the Glu area, is still very limited. The subtypes of receptors involved in the disorders described in Section 9.1 are still largely unknown, and thus, whether subtype-selective agents will be of therapeutic utility is also unknown. Determination of what subunits combinations are present *in vivo* and the physiological significance of these, combined with development of better subtype selective ligands may eventually lead to new therapeutic agents.

FURTHER READING

Armstrong, N. and Gouaux, E. (2000) Mechanisms for activation and antagonism of an AMPA-sensitive glutamate receptor: crystal structures of the GluR2 ligand binding core. *Neuron*, **28**, 165–181.

Bowery, N.G. and Enna, S.J. (2000) γ-Aminobutyric acid$_B$ receptors: first of the functional metabotropic heterodimers. *Perspectives Pharmacol.*, **292**, 2–7.

Bräuner-Osborne, H., Egebjerg, J., Nielsen, E.Ø., Madsen, U. and Krogsgaard-Larsen, P. (2000) Ligands for glutamate receptors: design and therapeutic prospects. *J. Med. Chem.*, **43**, 2609–2645.

Chebib, M., Johnston, G.A.R. (2000) GABA-activated ligand gated ion channels: Medicinal chemistry and molecular biology. *J. Med. Chem.*, **43**, 1427–1447.

Ebert, B., Madsen, U., Lund, T.M., Lenz, S.M. and Krogsgaard-Larsen, P. (1994) Molecular pharmacology of the AMPA agonist, (S)-2-amino-3-(3-hydroxy-5-phenyl-4-isoxazolyl)-propionic acid [(S)-APPA] and the AMPA antagonists, (R)-APPA. *Neurochem. Int.*, **24**, 507–515.

Enna, S.J. and Bowery, N.G. (eds.) (1997) *The GABA Receptors*. New Jersey: Humana Press Inc.

Frølund, B., Tagmose, L., Liljefors, T., Stensbøl, T.B., Engblom, C., Kristiansen, U. and Krogsgaard-Larsen, P. (2000) A novel class of potent 3-isoxazolol GABA$_A$ antagonists: design, synthesis, and pharmacology. *J. Med. Chem.*, **43**, 4930–4933.

Gasior, M., Carter, R.B. and Witkin, J.M. (1999) Neuroactive steroids: potential therapeutic use in neurological and psychiatric disorders. *Trends Pharmacol. Sci.*, **20**, 107–112.

Krogsgaard-Larsen, P., Frølund, B. and Frydenvang, K. (2000) GABA uptake inhibitors. Design, molecular pharmacology and therapeutic aspects. *Curr. Pharm. Design*, **6**, 1193–1209.

Kunishima, N., Shimada, Y., Tsuji, Y., Sato, T., Yamamoto, M., Kumasaka, T., Nakanishi, S., Jingami, H. and Morikawa, K. (2000) Structural basis of glutamate recognition by a dimeric metabotropic glutamate receptor. *Nature*, **407**, 971–977.

Madsen, U., Bräuner-Osborne, H., Frydenvang, K., Hvene, L., Johansen, T.N., Nielsen, B., Sánchez, C., Stensbøl, T.B., Bischoff, F., Krogsgaard-Larsen, P. (2001) New class of selective antagonists at Group I metabotropic glutamic acid receptors. *J. Med.Chem.*, **44**, 1051–1059.

Moroni, F., Nicoletti, F. and Pellegrini-Giampietro, D.E. (eds.) (1998) *Metabotropic glutamate receptors and brain functions*. London: Portland Press.

Nanavati, S.M. and Silverman, R.B. (1989) Design of potential anticonvulsant agents: mechanistic classification of GABA aminotransferase inactivators. *J. Med. Chem.*, **32**, 2413–2421.

Schoepp, D.D., Jane, D.E. and Monn, J.A. (1999) Pharmacological agents acting at subtypes of metabotropic glutamate receptors. *Neuropharmacology*, **38**, 1431–1476.

Zhang, D., Pan, Z.-H., Awobuluyi, M. and Lipton, S.A. (2001) Structure and function of GABA$_C$ receptors: a comparison of native versus recombinant receptors. *Trends Pharmacol. Sci.*, **22**, 121–132.

Chapter 10

Acetylcholine and histamine receptors and receptor ligands: medicinal chemistry and therapeutic aspects

Povl Krogsgaard-Larsen and Karla Frydenvang

10.1 ALZHEIMER'S DISEASE

Alzheimer's disease (AD) is a degenerative disorder of the human CNS that normally manifests in mid to late adult life with progressive cognitive, memory and intellectual impairment. The clinical features of the disease are accompanied by widespread loss of neocortical neurones (causing cerebral atrophy), by the presence of neurofibrillary tangles (composed, among other things, of paired helical filaments) in large pyramidal neurones, and by the presence of amyloid or senile plaques (extracellular fibrous protein deposits composed of a number of proteins including the amyloid β (Aβ) peptide).

The etiology of AD is complex. Epidemiological surveys have shown that genetic factors account for approximately 50% of the population variance for AD. These studies have also indicated that non-genetic factors including possibly head injury, reduced amounts of early childhood education, environmental exposure, etc. may be associated risk factors.

To date, no effective curative or preventive treatment for AD exists. However, since the central cholinergic neurones, which use acetylcholine (ACh) as neurotransmitter, for unknown reasons are particularly vulnerable in AD, and since these neurones play a key role in learning and memory processes in the brain, the synaptic processes associated with these neurones are potential therapeutic targets in AD (see subsequent sections). Partial and temporary symptomatic improvement of the cognitive deficits in AD actually can be achieved by the administration of inhibitors of the ACh-hydrolyzing enzyme acetylcholinesterase (AChE) (see Section 10.2.7).

In parallel with the attempts to develop cholinergic therapies for symptomatic treatment of Alzheimer patients, the biological mechanisms underlying AD are being extensively studied with the object of disclosing alternative targets for curative or preventive therapeutic interventions in the disease.

Recent insights from molecular genetic, molecular biological, and cell biological experiments have suggested that abnormalities in the processing of the membrane-bound β-amyloid precursor protein (β-APP) of unknown physiological function (Figure 10.1) are central to the pathogenesis of AD. This knowledge therefore provides a number of potential therapeutic targets for drug development.

There is a substantial body of evidence that the Aβ peptide formed by abnormal decomposition of β-APP is toxic to nerve cells, although it is an unresolved question,

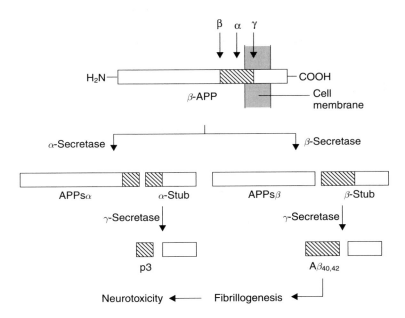

Figure 10.1 An outline of the enzymatic processes involved in the proteolytic cleavage of the membrane-bound β-APP leading to the formation of the toxic Aβ40 and Aβ42 peptides and other peptide fragments.

whether there are specific receptors for the Aβ peptide. It has been shown that exposure to the Aβ peptide activates apoptosis cell death pathways and potentiates the cytotoxic effects of excitatory amino acid neurotransmitters (see Chapter 9). However, one paradox that has not yet been resolved is that the neurotoxic effects of Aβ peptide, when examined *in vitro*, are acute (within hours or days), whereas the progress of AD appears to be very slow, over many years.

In spite of this and a number of other unanswered questions, the enzymes involved in the proteolytic cleavage of β-APP have been, and continue to be, extensively studied as potential therapeutic targets in AD. In one pathway, β-APP is cleaved after amino acid residue 687 by a putative membrane-bound protease termed α-secretase at or near the cell membrane (Figure 10.1). This enzymatic pathway generates a soluble N-terminal fragment (APPsα) that may have a mild neurotrophic activity. The residual membrane-bound C-terminal fragment (α-stub) is then subsequently cleaved by a putative enzyme, γ-secretase, which is not yet fully characterized. This enzymatic cleavage, which takes place in the transmembrane domain of the α-stub, generates the 3-kDa fragment termed p3.

The alternate pathway involves an initial cleavage of β-APP by β-secretase at amino acid residue 671. This hydrolytic reaction generates a 99-amino acid C-terminal fragment (β-stub) and APPsβ, and the former peptide then undergoes a second cleavage in the transmembrane domain by γ-secretase at either residue 711 or 713 to liberate, respectively, Aβ peptide of 40 amino acid residues (Aβ40) or of 42 residues (Aβ42) in length. Both of these peptides show neurotoxic effects.

(10.1)

The protein β-APP and its decomposition products (Figure 10.1) accumulate in pathological structures in the brains of Alzheimer patients. Sequencing of the β-APP gene, which is encoded on chromosome 21, led to the discovery of mutations at codons 670/671, 692, 715, 716, and 717 in families with the very rare early-onset forms of familial AD. All of these mutations alter β-APP processing. Thus, the codons 670/671 mutation increases the production of both $A\beta_{40}$ and $A\beta_{42}$, and similar effects are observed for some of the other mutations indicated. These observations have provided a biological clue by indicating that one way, although rare, to develop AD is to alter β-APP processing and increase the generation of $A\beta$ peptides.

As a result of an intense search for inhibitors of β-secretase and, in particular, γ-secretase (Figure 10.1), compound **10.1** (DAPT; AN-37124; LY-374973) was recently identified as a potent inhibitor of γ-secretase. In animal studies, subcutaneous administration of **10.1** was shown to markedly reduce the level of total $A\beta$ in several brain regions, and this compound is now in development as a potential therapeutic agent in AD.

10.2 CHOLINERGIC SYNAPTIC MECHANISMS AS THERAPEUTIC TARGETS

It was mentioned in the previous section that the most prominent neurochemical observation in the brains of Alzheimer patients is the loss of cholinergic neurones. Thus, biopsy and autopsy brain material from AD patients show loss of the presynaptic marker enzyme, acetyl-CoA:choline-O-acetyltransferase (ChAT), which is catalyzing the synthesis of ACh from choline (Figure 10.2). Furthermore, these neurochemical examinations disclosed reduced levels of the ACh-metabolizing enzyme, acetylcholinesterase (AChE) and of the presynaptic muscarinic autoreceptor sites of the M_2 subtype (see Section 10.2.1), correlating with dementia score of severity of neurohistopathology. Postsynaptic muscarinic receptor sites, which primarily are of the M_1 subtype do, however, to a large extent seem to survive the loss of cholinergic nerve terminals in different brain regions, although the functional state of these postsynaptic receptors, which are loosing their neurotransmitter input, has not been fully elucidated.

These neurochemical observations obviously have focused much pharmacological and therapeutic interest on central cholinergic synapses (Figure 10.2). In AD, there is a need for ACh replacement therapies, and ideally such therapeutic approaches should be selectively targeted at cholinergic synapses in the brain areas containing the degenerating ACh systems.

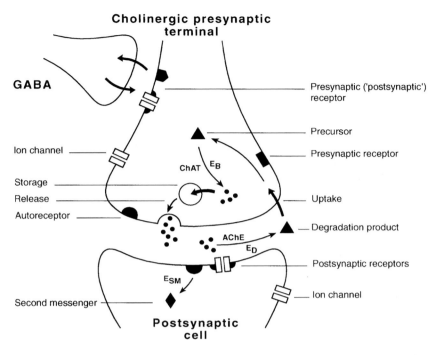

Figure 10.2 A schematic illustration of the receptors, ion channels, transporters and enzymes associated with a cholinergic synapse.

Administration of the ACh precursor choline or the lipidic choline derivative, lecithin, would be expected to stimulate indiscriminately all ACh systems in the brain and, perhaps predominantly, in the periphery with virtually unpredictable pharmacological consequences. These aspects may explain the very limited success, so far, of clinical studies on lecithin in AD.

In contrast to all other neurotransmitter systems using small molecules as signaling substances, the transmission process at cholinergic synapses is not terminated by reuptake of ACh into presynaptic terminals. The ACh is decomposed to choline and acetic acid in the synaptic cleft, a reaction which is catalyzed by AChE. Choline is subsequently taken up by specific transporters in the presynaptic cell membrane and converted intracellularly into transmitter ACh. Thus, in order to enhance cholinergic transmission processes, the enzyme AChE, rather than transporter systems, should be inhibited, and since such inhibitors are expected to stimulate all cholinergic functions in the brain and the periphery, they would seem to have limited therapeutic potential (see Section 10.2.7). The therapeutic prospects of pharmacological manipulation of ACh storage or release mechanisms (Figure 10.2) have not been thoroughly investigated.

As indicated in Figure 10.2, the release of ACh is under inhibitory control by presynaptically located GABA receptors of the $GABA_A$ as well as the $GABA_B$ subtypes (see Chapter 9). Whereas activation of these receptors results in reduced release of ACh, full or partial GABA receptor blockade is expected to stimulate ACh release. In animal experiments, administration of $GABA_A$ receptor agonists or antagonists actually have been shown to impair or facilitate, respectively, learning and memory processes. The clinical implications of these observations are at present under investigation.

So far, the cholinergic synaptic receptors have been most extensively studied as therapeutic targets in AD, and the heterogeneity of muscarinic as well as nicotinic ACh receptors in the CNS may make it possible to identify subtypes of these receptors, which are of particular pharmacological relevance in AD (see subsequent section). On the basis of neurochemical evidence so far available, the post-synaptic M_1 receptors seem to be of primary therapeutic interest (Figure 10.2). Partial agonists at M_1 receptors probably have less predisposition to cause receptor desensitization than full agonists, making the former type of agonists more interesting from a therapeutic point of view. As a result of degeneration of ACh nerve terminals, such agents might be expected to act as agonists at the virtually 'empty' and, thus, presumably supersensitive postsynaptic M_1 receptors. In other brain regions, where the muscarinic synapses are normosensitive, partial M_1 agonists may have weak or, ideally, no effects.

Antagonists at presynaptic M_2 receptors, which function as autoreceptors mediating negative feed-back regulation of ACh release, might be useful drugs at the early stages of AD, and compounds with mixed M_1 agonist/M_2 antagonist profiles may prove to be of particular interest.

The presynaptically located nicotinic ACh receptors (Figure 10.2) are involved in a positive feed-back regulation of ACh release. Thus, activation of these receptors stimulates ACh release, and agonists, or preferentially partial agonists, at these receptors obviously have therapeutic interest in the early stages of AD, where ACh neurones are still functioning, though at reduced levels.

10.2.1　Muscarinic and nicotinic acetylcholine receptors and receptor ligands

As for other neurotransmitters, multiple receptors exist for ACh in the periphery as well as in the CNS (see Chapter 6). The ACh receptors are classified into two main groups: (1) the muscarinic; and (2) the nicotinic receptors (Figure 10.3). Whereas, the muscarinic acetylcholine receptors (mAChRs) belong to the group of G protein-coupled receptors, nicotinic acetylcholine receptors (nAChRs) are ligand-gated ion channels containing five subunits, which may be identical (homomeric receptors) or different (heteromeric receptors).

Muscarine (**10.3**), which like muscimol and ibotenic acid (see Chapter 9) is a constituent of *Amanita muscaria*, to some extent reflects the structure of ACh (**10.2**) (Figure 10.3). The quaternary ammonium group is essential for the interaction of **10.3** with mAChRs, and the ether group appears to be strongly involved in the receptor binding of **10.3**. However, the relative importance of the other structural elements of **10.3** for receptor binding and activation has not yet been fully elucidated. The structure of nicotine (**10.4**), on the other hand, is very different from that of ACh (**10.2**), and the molecular basis of the very tight binding of **10.4** to nAChRs is still under investigation.

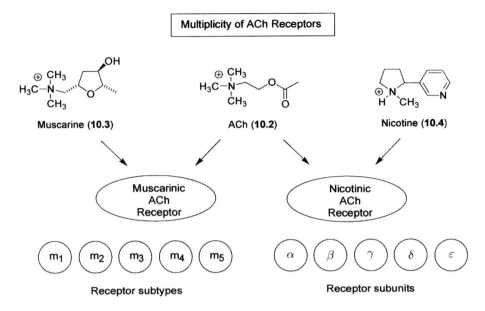

Figure 10.3 Structures of ACh (**10.2**) and the classical muscarinic and nicotinic ACh receptor agonists, muscarine (**10.3**) and nicotine (**10.4**), respectively, and an indication of the heterogeneity of ACh receptors.

Molecular cloning studies have revealed a high degree of heterogeneity of mAChRs (Figure 10.3). Five subtypes of such receptors (m_1-m_5) have been cloned and expressed in different model systems. So far, the correlation between these receptor subtypes, cloned from different tissues, and the mAChRs characterized using classical pharmacological methods (M_1-M_3) is not entirely clear, although m_1-m_3 are generally accepted to have pharmacological characteristics very similar to those of M_1-M_3, respectively (Figure 10.4).

Knockout animals, which typically are mice, are experimental animals, in which one, or perhaps two or three, genes have been deleted. In cases, where the deleted genes are coding for proteins of vital importance, the knockout mice only survive for short periods of time. However, in a number of cases, it has been possible to produce knockout mice lacking certain receptor or ion channel subtypes or enzymes as the results of deletion of the corresponding genes. Studies of the function and behavior of such animal models may provide important information about the physiological role of the particular biomechanisms.

In order to shed light on the functional roles of the mAChRs, knockout mice lacking one of the receptor subtypes m_1-m_5 have been produced. Mice lacking m_1 receptors had lost the ability to develop seizures after administration of muscarinic agonists and showed reduced hippocampal-based memory and learning as the most prominent behavioral alterations, as expected from pharmacological studies. In agreement with important roles of m_2 receptors in heart tissue and as cholinergic autoreceptors in the CNS (Figure 10.2), mice lacking m_2

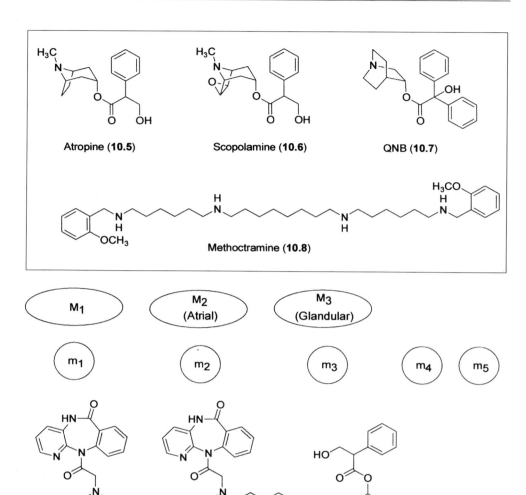

Figure 10.4 Multiplicity of muscarinic ACh receptors and structures of a number of non- or subtype-selective antagonists.

receptors did not show bradycardia or autoreceptor-mediated regulation of ACh release after administration of m_2-selective agonists (see Section 10.2.3). A prominent feature of m_3 receptor knockout mice was decreased mAChR-mediated salivation and smooth muscle contraction *in vitro*. Mice without m_4 receptors showed increased basal locomotor activity and reduced capacity to express mAChR-mediated analgesia, whereas m_5 receptor knockout animals, among other alterations, showed a pronounced decrease in mAChR-mediated dopamine release in the CNS.

These knockout animals are being intensively studied behaviorally and pharmacologically in order to validate these receptor subtypes as potential therapeutic targets.

Advances in molecular biology and selective probe design have resulted in the discovery of nine nAChR subunits expressed in the human CNS, and these receptor subunits are designated $\alpha_2-\alpha_7$ and $\beta_2-\beta_4$. Five additional nAChR subunits, which are expressed in the peripheral nervous system (PNS), are designated α_1, β_1, γ, δ, and ε (Figure 10.3). As mentioned previously, nAChR subunits oligomerize into both homopentameric and heteropentameric receptor subtypes. Each of these pentameric nAChRs possesses distinct ligand selectivity, pharmacological profile, and distribution in the CNS and the PNS. In the CNS and ganglia, α and β subunits assemble to form subtypes with the $(\alpha)_2(\beta)_3$ stoichiometry. Of major interest is the $\alpha_4\beta_2$ subtype, which exhibits very high affinity for the nAChR agonists nicotine (**10.4**), cytisine (**10.36**), and epibatidine (**10.37**) (see Section 10.2.5). Ganglionic nAChRs are known to consist of the following subtypes: $\alpha_3\beta_4$, $\alpha_3\alpha_5\beta_4$, and $\alpha_3\alpha_7\beta_x$. Finally, PNS nAChRs at the neuromuscular junction take the form of $\alpha_1\beta_1\delta\gamma$ or $\alpha_1\beta_1\delta\varepsilon$.

From the point of view of drug design, the region- or tissue-selective localizations of nAChRs are interesting, since nAChRs of different subunit composition will show more or less different affinities for structurally dissimilar nAChR agonists and antagonists, as exemplified for **10.4**, **10.36**, and **10.37**. These observations have greatly stimulated drug design programs in the nAChR field.

10.2.2 Muscarinic antagonists as pharmacological tools and therapeutic agents

The discovery that the alkaloids atropine (**10.5**) and scopolamine (**10.6**) (Figure 10.4) block the actions of ACh at muscarinic receptors and produce a number of therapeutically useful actions, including antispasmodic and antiparkinsonian effects, led to an extensive search for synthetic analogs of these natural products. Among various potent synthetic muscarinic receptor antagonists, quinuclidinyl benzilate (QNB, **10.7**) is used as a radioactive ligand for studies of muscarinic receptor sites. Like **10.5** and **10.6**, compound **10.7** does, however, bind tightly to all subtypes of muscarinic receptors, and this lack of selectivity makes these compounds inapplicable for studies of muscarinic receptor subtypes.

In contrast to these classical muscarinic receptor antagonists, pirenzepine (**10.9**) shows major affinity variations in different tissues. It binds weakly to muscarinic receptors in the heart but interacts strongly with such receptors in the cerebral cortex and sympathetic ganglia, whereas it shows intermediate affinity for receptors in salivary glands and in stomach fundic mucosa. Based on these pharmacological and binding studies, the muscarinic receptors were subdivided into two main classes: (1) M_1 receptors showing high affinity for **10.9**; and (2) a heterogeneous class of receptors (M_2) having much lower affinity for **10.9**.

The antagonist **10.9** did, however, not clearly distinguish between the muscarinic receptors previously classified together as M_2. An analog of **10.9**,

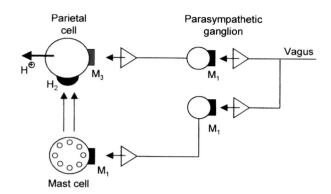

Figure 10.5 A schematic illustration of the muscarinic (M_1 and M_3) and histaminergic (H_2) receptors involved in acid secretion from parietal cells.

(11-[[2-[(diethylamino)methyl]-1-piperidinyl]acetyl]-5,11-dihydro-6*H*-pyrido[2,3-*b*]-benzodiazepin-6-one) (AF-DX 116, **10.10**) has, however, been shown to discriminate between M_2 receptor subtypes in peripheral tissues, showing high affinity for the M_2 receptors in the heart (M_2 atrial) and low affinity for the non-M_1 receptors in endocrine glands (M_3 glandular).

Whereas glandular M_3 receptors display low affinity for **10.9** as well for **10.10**, they are effectively blocked by compound **10.11** and related compounds, which show limited affinity for M_1 and for atrial M_2 receptors. These studies emphasize the different pharmacological characteristics of M_2 and M_3 receptors, and this difference has been supported by the observation that methoctramine (**10.8**) and related polyamines selectively block M_2 receptors (Figure 10.4).

Muscarinic antagonists were once the most widely used drugs for the management of peptic ulcer. Whereas the non-selective muscarinic antagonists atropine (**10.5**) or scopolamine (**10.6**) produce pronounced side effects, notably dry mouth, loss of visual accomodation and difficulty in urination, the M_1-selective antagonist pirenzepine (**10.9**) can be more safely used in the treatment of ulcer. Nevertheless, side effects do occur after administration of **10.9** to patients, and **10.9** has now largely been replaced by histamine H_2 antagonists (see Section 10.3.2) and, in particular, by proton pump inhibitors as antiulcer drugs.

According to our current knowledge, the antiulcer effects of **10.9** are based on different mechanisms of action. The main contribution results from the inhibition of acid secretion (Figure 10.5). Within the parasympathetic pathway, acid secretion is controlled by excitatory M_1 and M_3 receptors. M_1 receptors are located in the parasympathetic ganglion and at the histamine-containing mast cells. M_3 receptors, on the other hand, are located directly on the acid-producing parietal cells. A selective blockade of M_1 receptors therefore induces an inhibition of acid secretion via direct (ACh-mediated) and indirect (histamine-mediated) pathways. Selective M_3 antagonists obviously would be much less effective inhibitors of acid secretion, but compounds showing potent antagonist effects at M_1 as well as M_3 receptors would seem to be interesting as antiulcer agents. Such compounds actually have been developed but apparently have not been sufficiently effective

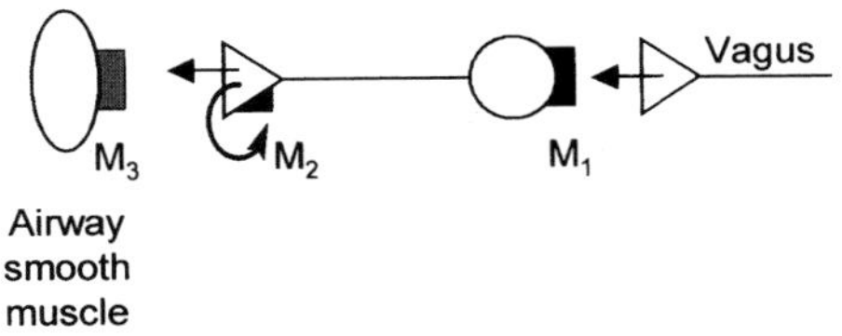

Figure 10.6 A schematic illustration of the muscarinic receptors (M_1, M_2 and M_3) involved in the regulation of the function of airway smooth muscles.

and safe to compete with histamine H_2 antagonists or proton pump inhibitors as drugs for the treatment of peptic ulcer.

There is a growing interest in mAChR antagonists for the treatment of broncho-pulmonary diseases. The airways receive a rich cholinergic innervation, and M_1 receptors are widely distributed in the respiratory tract. The cholinergic innervation of airway smooth muscle tissue contains M_1, M_2 and M_3 receptors (Figure 10.6). M_1 receptors located in the parasympathetic ganglia probably exert a facilitatory effect on neurotransmission, which is primarily under control of nAChRs (not illustrated). The release of ACh during vagal stimulation is controlled by a negative feed-back mechanism utilizing M_2 autoreceptors. Contraction of airway smooth muscle is primarily mediated by M_3 receptors.

Several clinical studies have disclosed that the M_1-selective antagonist pirenzepine (**10.9**) is not sufficiently effective for the treatment of chronic bronchitis or asthma because of its insufficient blockade of M_3 receptors located in the smooth muscle tissue. These aspects prompted the development of compounds showing high affinity for M_1 as well as M_3 receptors, but showing little, or preferentially no, antagonist effect at M_2.

Using pirenzepine (**10.9**) as lead structure, a series of analogs were synthesized and pharmacologically characterized. Within this group of compounds, BIBO 126 (**10.12**) showed the desired, though not the optimal, pharmacological profile being 40-fold more potent at the M_1 than at the M_2 receptor and showing

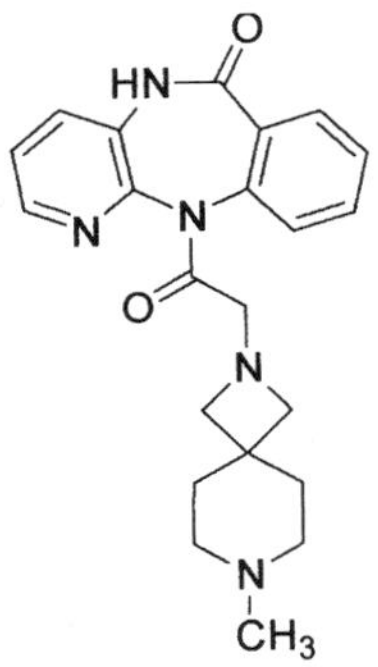

BIBO 126 (**10.12**)

similar affinity for M_1 and M_3 receptors. Compound **10.12** contains a spiro-diamino sidechain with protolytic properties similar to those of **10.9**, which has pK_a 2.1 and 8.2.

Compounds **10.12** and **10.9** have been subjected to comparative pharmacological studies in animals, and although these two compounds show significantly different receptor affinity profiles, their effects in functional assay system were similar. Nevertheless, the search for compounds showing the desired selectivities at M_1, M_2 and M_3 receptors continue in order to develop muscarinic antagonist drugs for the treatment of chronic bronchitis and nocturnal asthma.

10.2.3   Muscarinic agonists and partial agonists: bioisosteric design

The quaternary structure of ACh (Figure 10.7) and the rapid hydrolysis of its ester moiety in biological systems make ACh inapplicable for most types of pharmacological experiments and, of course, for clinical studies. Removal of one or more of the *N*-methyl groups of ACh with the object of obtaining cholinergic compounds capable of penetrating the blood–brain barrier (BBB) results in pronounced loss of activity.

Arecoline (**10.13**) which is a constituent of areca nuts, the seeds of *Areca catechu*, is a cyclic 'reverse ester' bioisostere of ACh, containing a tertiary amino group. In contrast to the findings for ACh, **10.13** is approximately equipotent with its quaternized analog, *N*-methylarecoline, as a muscarinic ACh receptor agonist.

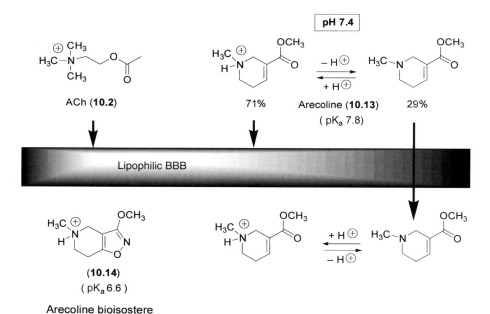

Figure 10.7 Structures of ACh (**10.2**) and the muscarinic agonists arecoline (**10.13**) and the isoxazole arecoline bioisostere **10.14**. The ability of **10.13** to penetrate the BBB is illustrated.

At pH 7.4, **10.13** is partially protonated, and using equation (10.1) the percentage ionization of **10.13** can be calculated to be 71 (Figure 10.7). Whilst **10.13** is assumed to bind to and activate muscarinic ACh receptors in its protonated form, the presence of a fraction of unionized molecules (29%) allows **10.13** to penetrate the BBB.

Analogously, the percentage of unionized acid in aqueous solution can be calculated using this equation. Thus, equation (10.1) can be used to calculate the percentage on acidic form of bases (ionized form) as well as acids (unionized form).

$$\%\mathrm{Ionized} = \frac{100}{[1 + \mathrm{antilog(pH - pK_a)}]} \tag{10.1}$$

Compound **10.13**, which actually is a partial agonist at both M_1 and M_2 receptors, has been shown to improve cognitive functions significantly when infused (i.v.) in Alzheimer patients, and **10.13** facilitates learning in normal young humans. These effects of **10.13** are, however, shortlived reflecting rapid *in vivo* hydrolysis of the ester group of this compound. Furthermore, the pronounced side effects of **10.13** probably reflect the ability of this muscarinic agonist to activate peripheral and central M_2 receptors in addition to the desired partial agonist effect on central M_1 receptors.

Bioisosteric replacements of the carboxyl group of GABA analogs by the 3-isoxazolol group or structurally related heterocyclic units with protolytic properties similar to that of the carboxyl group have led to a number of specific and very potent GABA$_A$ agonists. Similar bioisosteric replacements in the molecule of glutamic acid have led to heterocyclic amino acids with specific actions at subtypes of central glutamic acid receptors (see Chapter 9). These findings prompted the development of the arecoline bioisostere 3-methoxy-5-methyl-4,5,6,7-tetrahydro-isoxazolo[4,5-*c*]pyridine (**10.14**) containing the hydrolysis-resistant ester isostere 3-methoxyisoxazole (Figure 10.7).

Like **10.13**, the isoxazole bioisostere **10.14** interacts potently with central M_1 as well as M_2 receptors, but the latter compound is a more selective ligand for M_1 receptor sites than is **10.13**, and the partial agonist character of **10.14** is more pronounced than that of the lead compound, **10.13**. Compared with **10.13**, the bicyclic bioisostere **10.14** has a lower pK_a value (6.6) and a higher $\log P$ value, and these physico-chemical properties can explain why **10.14** very easily penetrates the BBB.

Compound **10.14** has been used as a 'second lead' for the design and development of a number of effective muscarinic agonists showing different degrees of M_1 selectivity and pharmacological profiles ranging from antagonists through low-efficacy agonists to full agonists. Like **10.14**, 3-methoxy-5,6,7,8-tetrahydro-4*H*-isoxazolo[4,5-*c*]azepine (**10.21**) is a partial muscarinic agonist, **10.21** being markedly more potent than **10.14**. The 'pharmacological importance' of the *O*-alkyl groups of these compounds is reflected by the observation that the *O*-ethyl analog (**10.22**) is a competitive muscarinic antagonist, whereas the *O*-isopropyl analog (**10.23**) shows the characteristics of a non-competitive antagonist.

Oxotremorine (**10.15**) is a very potent partial muscarinic agonist, which shows some selectivity for autoreceptors of the M_2 type. Extensive structural modifications of **10.15** have led to compounds with a broad spectrum of pharmacological

(10.15)   (10.16)   (10.17)   (10.18)

(10.19)   (10.20)   (10.14)   (10.21)

(10.22)   (10.23)   (R)-(10.24)   (S)-(10.24)

(S)-(10.25)   (10.26)

effects ranging from full agonists to antagonists at central and/or peripheral muscarinic receptors.

The potent peripheral actions of **10.15**, including the effects on cardiovascular mechanisms, probably reflect its preferential activation of M_2 receptors. Attempts have been made to design analogs of **10.15** with pharmacological profiles relevant to AD. One of these analogs (BM5, **10.16**) has been characterized as an M_1 agonist/ M_2 antagonist (see Section 10.2). An evaluation of the potential of **10.16** as a therapeutic agent in AD must await further behavioral pharmacological studies.

The naturally occurring heterocyclic cholinergic agonist pilocarpine (**10.17**) is widely used as a topical miotic for the control of elevated intraocular pressure associated with glaucoma. The bioavailability of pilocarpine is, however, low, and based on studies in animal models it has been suggested that this compound does not easily penetrate the BBB. Compound **10.17** is a partial muscarinic agonist showing an *in vitro* pharmacological profile very similar to that of arecoline (**10.13**).

Impairments of position discrimination learning in animals could be overcome by systemically administered **10.13** as well as **10.17** at doses lower than those producing marked autonomic effects. These observations are interesting in relation to AD and have focused behavioral pharmacological interest on prodrugs of **10.17** showing improved bioavailability (see Chapter 14).

The compounds **10.18–10.20** show very high affinity for mAChRs. The 3-amino-1,2,4-oxadiazole **10.18**, which interacts non-selectively with mAChR subtypes, probably is the most potent muscarinic agonist known. The arecoline (**10.13**) bioisosteres, the 2-ethyltetrazole (**10.20**) and the 3-hexyloxy-1,2,5-thiadiazole (**10.19**) analogs have been reported to preferentially activate M_1 receptors vs. M_2 receptors. Compound **10.19** has been evaluated clinically as a potential drug for the treatment of AD.

Compound **10.19** did improve the symptoms of Alzheimer patients but only after administration of doses, which also provoked cholinergic side effects. During the clinical studies of **10.19** it was, quite surprisingly, observed that the compound was capable of reducing the psychotic symptoms of AD patients, which in addition suffered from schizophrenia. These observations disclosed an involvement of the central mAChRs in schizophrenia, possibly reflecting an interaction between cholinergic and dopaminergic neurones.

Thus, whereas treatment of AD patients with muscarinic agonists or partial agonists has been shown not to be straightforward due to apparently unavoidable peripheral cholinergic side effects, such compounds are potential therapeutic agents in schizophrenia.

More recently, the (R)- and (S)-forms of 5,7-dimethyl-3-propargyloxy-4,5,6,7-tetrahydroisothiazolo[4,5-c]pyridine (**10.24**) were synthesized (see Scheme 10.1) and characterized as mAChR ligands *in vitro*. Both of these enantiomers of **10.24** bind tightly to muscarinic receptor sites, and they were both shown to be approximately an order of magnitude more potent at M_1 than at M_2 receptors. (R)-**10.24** typically showed a 3–5 fold higher affinity for muscarinic receptor sites than (S)-**10.24**. This surprisingly low degree of stereoselectivity may reflect that the part of these molecules carrying the chiral center does not bind tightly to the receptor proteins during the interactions with the mAChRs.

Although the propargyloxy side chain present in **10.24** and **10.25** appears to be optimal for binding of this group of compounds to mAChRs, the triple bond can be reduced to a double bond (**10.33** and **10.35** in Scheme 10.1) without significant loss of receptor affinity. Furthermore, compound **10.26**, in which the triple bond of **10.25** has been replaced by a nitrile group, binds tightly to muscarinic receptors, though weaker than **10.25**.

10.2.4 Muscarinic agonists and partial agonists: synthetic and structural aspects

The syntheses of a number of partial muscarinic agonists containing the bicyclic 4,5,6,7-tetrahydroisothiazolo[4,5-c]pyridine heterocyclic system are outlined in Scheme 10.1. The synthetic strategy has been to first build up the six-membered rings containing the nitrogen atoms, which become the basic groups of the target compounds **10.24–10.26**, **10.33**, and **10.35**, and containing functional groups

Scheme 10.1 (i) CH$_2$=CH-CN, C$_2$H$_5$OH; (ii) KOC(CH$_3$)$_3$, toluene, ClCOOC$_2$H$_5$; (iii) H$_2$SO$_4$ (85%), 60–70 °C; (iv) C$_6$H$_5$CH$_2$NH$_2$, xylene, reflux; (v) H$_2$S, DMF, Br$_2$; (vi) CH$_2$=CH-CH$_2$Br, (C$_4$H$_9$)$_4$N·HSO$_4$, K$_2$CO$_3$, KOH/CH$_3$OH; (vii) HCOOH, CH$_2$O, reflux; (viii) HBr/ AcOH (33%); (ix) (Boc)$_2$O, K$_2$CO$_3$; (x) CN-CH$_2$-Cl, (C$_4$H$_9$)$_4$N·HSO$_4$, K$_2$CO$_3$; (xi) HCl, ether, NaOH; (xii) CH≡C-CH$_2$Br, (C$_4$H$_9$)$_4$N·HSO$_4$, K$_2$CO$_3$; (xiii) HCOOH, CH$_2$O, reflux.

suitable for the construction of the 3-isothiazolol unit annulated with the six-membered ring.

Nucleophilic addition of the amino group of the starting material **10.27** to acrylonitrile gives the dinitrile **10.28**. In the presence of the strong base potassium *tert*-butoxide, a carbanion in the α-position of the unsubstituted chain is formed, and this anion attacks the nitrile group of the methylated chain to form a cyclic product containing an imino group. This imino group is hydrolyzed under mild conditions to give the keto group of **10.29**, and partial hydrolysis of the nitrile group of **10.29** under more drastic conditions gives compound **10.30**. Treatment of **10.30** with benzylamine converts the keto group into an enamino group with the double bond conjugated with the amide group, and this intermediate, **10.31**, can now be transformed into the bicyclic compound, **10.32**. Thus, by treatment of **10.31** with hydrogen sulfide, the benzylamino group is replaced by a mercapto group, and this group and the amide group undergo an oxidative cyclization reaction in the presence of bromine to give **10.32**. The hydroxy groups of **10.32** or the corresponding Boc-protected derivative, **10.34**, are alkylated using the appropriate alkylation reagents, and acid hydrolyses of the alkylation products remove the N-protecting groups to give the final compounds **10.24–10.26**, **10.33**, and **10.35**.

(R)-**10.25** and (S)-**10.25** were prepared by optical resolution of **10.25** using (2R, 3R)-O,O'-dibenzoyltartaric acid and (2S, 3S)-O,O'-dibenzoyltartaric acid, respectively, for diastereomeric salt formation. The absolute stereochemistry of

(S)-**10.25** was established by an X-ray crystallographic analysis of its (2S, 3S)-O,O'-dibenzoyltartaric acid salt (Figure 10.8). Since (R)-**10.24** and (S)-**10.24** were synthesized from (R)-**10.25** and (S)-**10.25**, respectively, by N-methylation, these chemical transformations unequivocally established the absolute configuration of the enantiomers of **10.24**. In the crystals of the (2S, 3S)-O,O'-dibenzoyltartaric acid salt of (S)-**10.25**, two conformationally different forms of the cation of (S)-**10.25** were observed (Figure 10.8), probably reflecting a low-energy barrier for rotating the propargyloxy side chain of the molecule.

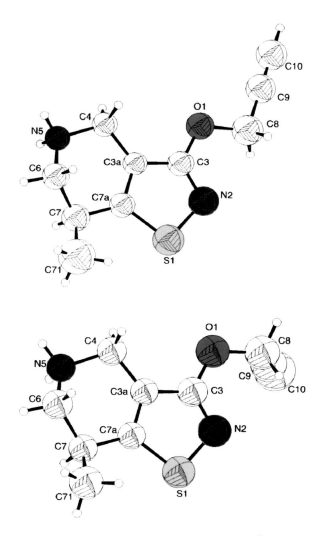

Figure 10.8 Perspective drawings of the two conformationally different cations of compound (S)-**10.25** crystallized as a salt with (2S,3S)-O,O'-dibenzoyltartaric acid. Spheres representing the isotropic or equivalent isotropic displacement parameters of the non-hydrogen atoms are shown at the 50% probability level. Hydrogen atoms in calculated positions are represented by spheres of arbitrary size.

10.2.5   Nicotinic agonists and partial agonists: bioisosteric design

A large number of naturally occurring alkaloids interact potently with nAChRs in the CNS and the PNS, and many of these compounds are generally described as very toxic compounds. The toxicological, or rather pharmacological, effects of these toxins are mediated by nAChRs with different subunit composition (see Section 10.2.1). The classical nAChR agonists, nicotine (**10.4**) and cytisine (**10.36**) show particularly high affinity for the $\alpha_4\beta_2$ subtype of nAChRs, which comprise the majority of nicotinic cholinergic receptors in the brain. Thus radiolabeled **10.4** and **10.36** (^{3}H-nicotine and ^{3}H-cytisine) are useful tools for studies of this class of nAChRs.

Epibatidine (**10.37**) was isolated from the skin of the poisonous frog, *Epipedobates tricolor*, and represents a new class of amphibian alkaloids, which probably serves the role in nature to protect the frog from potential predators. Compound **10.37** is a non-opioid analgesic, which is several hundred times more potent than morphine. **10.37** binds strongly to central nAChRs of the $\alpha_4\beta_2$ subtype, which mediate its analgesic effects, and **10.37** therefore is a very potent inhibitor of the receptor binding of ^{3}H-nicotine and ^{3}H-cytisine. The concentration of **10.37** in the frog skin is low, and less than 0.5 mg of this compound was isolated from the skin of 750 frogs, emphasizing the need for the development of effective methods for the synthesis of this compound (see Section 10.2.6).

Anatoxin-a (**10.38**) was first isolated from the freshwater blue-green algae, *Anabaena flosaquae*. This toxin, which possesses a 9-azabicyclo[4.2.1]nonane skeleton, is a highly potent nAChR agonist and an effective inhibitor of the receptor binding of ^{3}H-nicotine. The high potency of this nAChR ligand and its unique structural characteristics make **10.38** a useful tool for studies of nAChRs.

Bioisosteric replacements of the pyridine ring of nicotine (**10.4**) have been reported, and the 3-methylisoxazole bioisostere ABT-418 (**10.39**) has been shown to be a potent nAChR agonist. This compound has been extensively characterized in different *in vitro* assay systems and animal models, and it shows beneficial effects in

Nicotine
(**10.4**)

Cytisine
(**10.36**)

Epibatidine
(**10.37**)

Anatoxin-a
(**10.38**)

ABT-418
(**10.39**)

Altinicline
(**10.40**)

(**10.41**)

(**10.42**)

Alzheimer patients. Like nicotine (**10.4**), the analog, (*S*)-5-ethynyl-3-(1-methyl-2-pyr-rolidinyl)pyridine (altinicline, **10.40**), is a potent agonist at the $\alpha_4\beta_2$ nAChR subtype, but shows less effects than **10.4** at the peripheral and ganglionic $\alpha_3\beta_4$ nAChR subtype. This subtype-selectivity of **10.40** may explain its limited peripheral side effects, and **10.40** is undergoing clinical trials for the treatment of Parkinson's disease.

A large number of analogs of the naturally occurring potent nAChR ligands have been synthesized and pharmacologically characterized, as exemplified by **10.41** and **10.42**. Compound **10.41**, which is a ring homolog of **10.37** binds effectively to nAChRs, though somewhat weaker than **10.37**. Compound **10.42**, which is a conformationally restrained analog of **10.4** is essentially inactive, indicating that the conformations attainable by the nicotine structural element of **10.42** apparently do not reflect the receptor-active conformation(s) of nicotine (**10.4**). In structure–activity studies along these lines, it must, however, be kept in mind that the additional structure element incorporated into the nicotine analog **10.42** may interfere with its binding to the active site of the receptor.

10.2.6 Nicotinic agonists: synthetic aspects

The pronounced pharmacological interest in epibatidine (**10.37**) has prompted the development of several synthetic methods for the preparation of this unique compound. The synthetic sequence outlined in Scheme 10.2 is an effective route to **10.37**, which has been optimized for the production of the target compound on large scale.

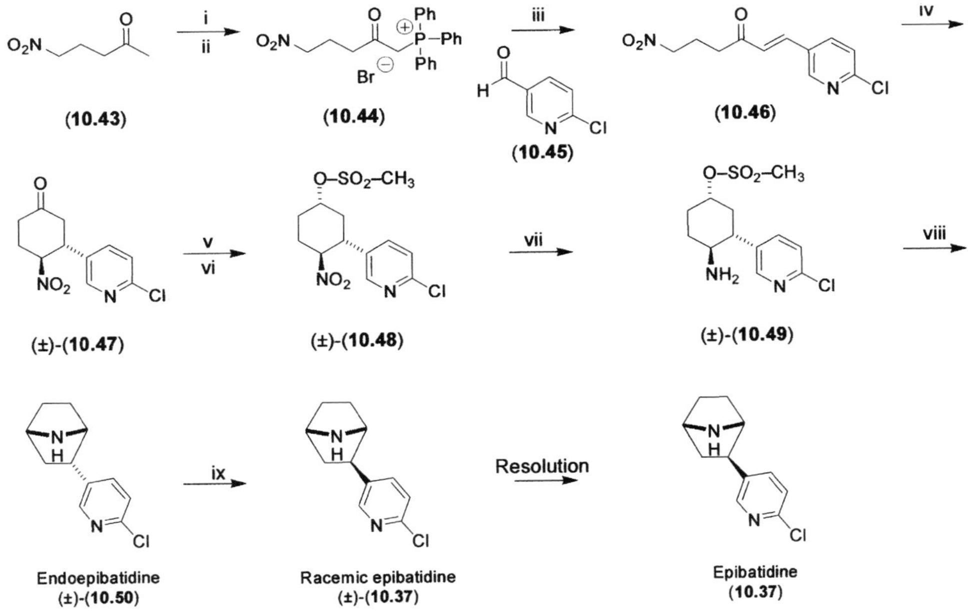

Scheme 10.2 (i) Br$_2$, CH$_3$OH; (ii) (Ph)$_3$P, benzene; (iii) CH$_2$Cl$_2$, NaOH; (iv) KF/Al$_2$O$_3$, THF, 25 °C; (v) NaBH$_4$, C$_2$H$_5$OH; (vi) CH$_3$SO$_2$Cl, CH$_2$Cl$_2$, pyridine; (vii) SnCl$_2$·2H$_2$O, C$_2$H$_5$OH; (viii) toluene; (ix) KOC(CH$_3$)$_3$, HOC(CH$_3$)$_3$.

The methyl group of the starting material **10.43** was selectively brominated, and treatment of the bromomethyl ketone intermediate with triphenylphosphine gave the quaternized salt **10.44**. A Wittig reaction of the phosphorane, generated from **10.44**, with the chloropyridine aldehyde **10.45** provided the α, β-unsaturated ketone **10.46**. Under weakly basic conditions, the anion, formed at the carbon α to the nitro group, underwent a nucleophilic addition to the double bond, producing the cyclized compound **10.47** with the indicated relative stereochemistry. Reduction of the keto group of **10.47** to give a secondary alcohol group proceeded in a stereoselective manner, and after treatment of the alcohol intermediate with methanesulfonyl chloride, compound **10.48** was obtained. Reduction of the nitro group of **10.48** provided amine **10.49**, still as a racemate but with the relative stereochemistry shown. Compound **10.49** easily underwent an intramolecular nucleophilic substitution reaction, with methanesulfonate as the leaving group, to give the *endo* isomer of epibatidine, endoepibatidine (**10.50**). Treatment of **10.50** with strong base induced epimerization to give the corresponding *exo* isomer, which is epibatidine (**10.37**), obtained in the racemic form but with the correct relative stereochemistry. Using different optically active carboxylic acids, racemic **10.37** was resolved to give epibatidine (**10.37**), which was shown to be identical with **10.37** isolated from frog skin (see Section 10.2.5).

10.2.7 Acetylcholinesterase inhibitors

Inhibitors of AChE allow a build up of ACh at the nerve endings resulting in a prolonged activation of cholinergic receptors. Treatment with such inhibitors has been useful in myasthenia gravis, a disease associated with the rapid fatigue of

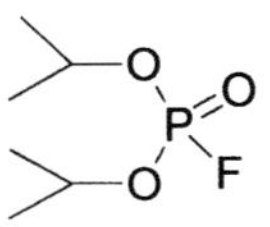

(10.51)

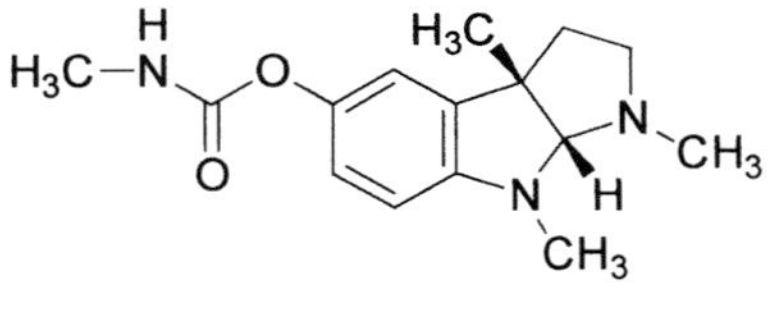

Physostigmine **(10.52)**
(pK_a 1.8; 7.9)

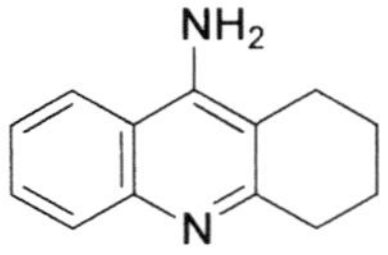

Tacrine **(10.53)**
(pK_a 10.0)

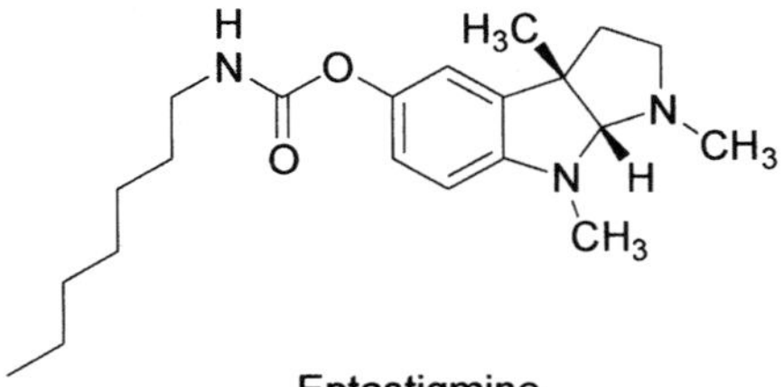

Eptastigmine
(10.54)

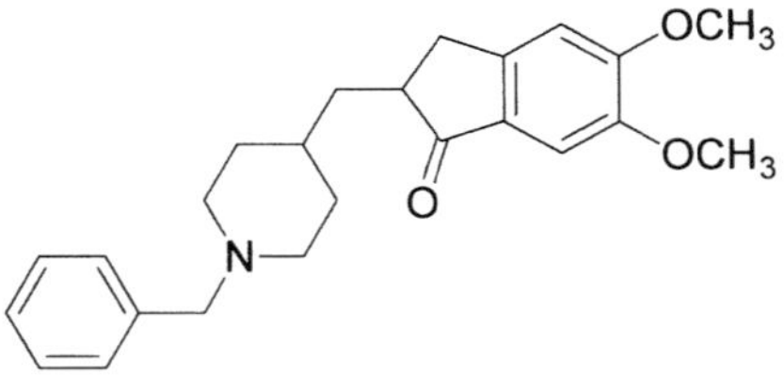

Donepezil
(10.55)

muscles and also in the treatment of glaucoma, where stimulation of the ciliary body improves drainage from the eye and, thus, decreases intraocular pressure.

Two main classes of AChE inhibitors have been developed: (1) irreversible organophosphorus inhibitors, such as dyflos (**10.51**); and (2) carbamoylating, but reversible, inhibitors, such as physostigmine (eserine, **10.52**). The former class of compounds has a long duration of action in the body, and after a single dose of drug the activity of AChE only returns after resynthesis of the enzyme. Due to dangers of overdosage they are only used therapeutically for the treatment of a limited number of glaucoma patients. A variety of volatile organophosphorus AChE inhibitors have been produced on large scales for use as nerve gasses in war, whereas other less volatile compounds of this category have been used as insecticides.

Inhibitors of the latter class including **10.52** are protonated at physiological pH and are bound at the anionic site of AChE. The relative positions of the ammonium and carbamate groups allow a transfer of the carbamoyl group onto the serine hydroxyl group at the esteratic site of the enzyme. The carbamoylated enzyme is hydrolyzed to regenerate the enzyme with a half-life of less than one hour. Kinetic studies originally gave the impression that **10.52** and related carbamates were acting as simple reversible competitive inhibitors of AChE.

Inhibitors of AChE, notably **10.52**, have been studied clinically in AD. Treatment of Alzheimer patients with **10.52** have marginally improved learning and memory, but these positive effects have been accompanied by unacceptable side effects. Although amines like **10.52** are capable of penetrating the BBB (see Figure 10.7), they are likely to enhance the activity at virtually all cholinergic synapses in the periphery and the CNS. Thus, stimulation of all nicotinic and muscarinic ACh receptors may explain the complex therapeutic effect/side effect profiles observed after administration of **10.52** to AD patients.

9-Amino-1,2,3,4-tetrahydroacridine (tacrine, THA, **10.53**) is a non-selective but reversible inhibitor of AChE. In spite of its strongly basic character (pK$_a$ 10.0) and, thus, high degree of protonation at physiological pH, **10.53** is capable of penetrating the BBB to some extent, probably as a result of the lipophilic character of its phenyl and cycloalkyl ring structures.

Clinical studies of **10.53** in Alzheimer patients have shown improvements in learning and memory, at least in certain groups of patients. These promising effects have been proposed to reflect selective effects of **10.53** on brain AChE. Since **10.53** also has pharmacological effects unrelated to the inhibition of AChE, the mechanism(s) underlying its clinical effects in AD are not fully understood.

Eptastigmine (**10.54**) is more lipophilic than **10.52**, and **10.54** actually showed very promising effects in AD patients. However, the development of this derivative of **10.52** as a therapeutic agent was stopped after two patients developed aplastic anemia during the phase III clinical trials. Donepezil (**10.55**) is structurally unrelated to **10.52** and is described as a 'second-generation' AChE inhibitor. In clinical trials, **10.55** has been shown to be devoid of the problems associated with the administration of tacrine (**10.53**) to AD patients, and **10.55** offered modest improvement in cognitive processes for at least a few months in almost 50% of the patients studied. These data illustrate the limited therapeutic effects in AD of AChE inhibitors.

10.3   HISTAMINE RECEPTORS

Histamine (2-(imidazole-4-yl)ethylamine) (**10.64**), which is biosynthesized by decarboxylation of the basic amino acid histidine, is involved as a chemical messenger in a variety of complex biological actions. In mammals, it is mainly stored in an inactive bound form in many body tissues, from which it is released by different stimuli and mechanisms. Histamine exerts its biological functions via activation of specific receptors, and during the past 2–3 decades three pharmacologically distinct histamine receptors designated H_1, H_2 and H_3 have been characterized (Figure 10.9). Like the H_1 and H_2 receptors, the H_3 receptor, and also the very recently cloned H_4 receptor, have been shown to belong to the group of G protein-coupled receptor (see Chapter 6).

Activation of H_1 receptors stimulates the contraction of smooth muscles in many organs such as the gut, the uterus, and the bronchi. Contraction of the bronchi leads to restriction of the passage of air into and out of the lungs as in asthma. Stimulation of H_1 receptors on smooth muscles in for example fine blood vessels does, however, cause muscle relaxation, and the resulting vasodilation may result in severe fall in blood pressure. Furthermore, histamine increases the permeability of the capillary walls so that more of the plasma constituents can escape into the tissue space, leading to the formation of oedema. This series of events is manifest in the well-known redness and wheal associated with histamine release, the so-called 'triple response'. Histamine is also involved in the removal of the products of cell

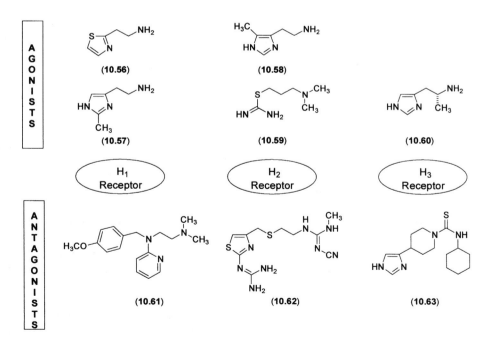

Figure 10.9 A schematic illustration of the multiplicity of histamine receptors and the structures of a number of subtype-selective agonists and antagonists.

damage during inflammation. Under these circumstances, the liberation of histamine is accompanying the production of antibodies and their interaction with foreign proteins. Under extreme circumstances, however, the effects of histamine can become pathological, leading to exaggerated responses with distressing results, as may occur in some allergic conditions.

A number of selective and very potent antagonists at H_1 receptors are now available. Such compounds, including mepyramine (**10.61**), are structurally very different from histamine. These 'antihistamines' are typically developed via lead optimization of accidentally discovered compounds capable of blocking the effects of histamine on the perfused lung or the isolated ileum or trachea from guinea pigs or on human bronchi. A number of these competitive H_1 antagonists are used clinically.

Compounds showing selective agonist activity at subtypes of histamine receptors are essential as tools for pharmacological studies of histamine receptors. In order to develop such agonists, the molecule of histamine has been subjected to extensive structural modifications. Most of these histamine analogs, in which the imidazole ring and/or the 2-aminoethyl side chain have been alkylated or otherwise structurally modified, show very weak histamine agonist activity. These systematic structural variations of histamine have, however, led to receptor subtype-selective agonists. Thus, 2-methylhistamine (**10.57**) and, in particular, 2-(thiazol-2-yl)ethylamine (**10.56**) are selective agonists at H_1 receptors, though weaker than histamine itself. On the other hand, 5-methylhistamine (**10.58**) selectively activates H_2 receptors. Similarly, S-[3-(N,N-dimethylamino)propyl]isothiourea (dimaprit, **10.59**), in which the imidazole ring of histamine has been bioisosterically replaced by an S-alkylisothiourea group showing similar protolytic properties, is a highly selective H_2 receptor agonist. These two H_2 agonists have been useful tools in connection with the elegant design and development of selective H_2 receptor antagonists such as **10.62** (see Section 10.3.2).

Studies in recent years have established that histamine is acting as a neurotransmitter in the CNS. Whilst H_1 and H_2 receptors seem to be predominantly localized on postsynaptic membranes of central neurones, H_3 receptors appear to function predominantly as presynaptic receptors, possibly as histamine autoreceptors. Although H_3 receptors have also been detected in some peripheral organs, this class of histamine receptors exists primarily in the CNS. Very recently, a fourth G protein-coupled histamine receptor, H_4, has been identified and pharmacologically characterized. This H_4 receptor exhibits a very restricted localization and is found primarily in intestinal tissue, spleen and immune active cells, such as T cells, suggesting a therapeutic potential for H_4 receptor ligands in allergic and inflammatory diseases. The H_4 receptor shows signal transduction mechanisms and pharmacological characteristics similar to those of H_3 receptors.

The physiological role of the central histamine neurotransmitter system is far from being elucidated, but it has been suggested that it plays a role in cerebral circulation, energy metabolism, and states of wakefulness. These aspects have focused pharmacological interest on agonists as well as antagonists at H_3 receptors. Interestingly, stereoselectivity of agonists is much more pronounced at H_3 receptors than either H_1 or H_2 receptors, and (R)-α-methylhistamine (**10.60**) has been shown to be a selective and very potent H_3 receptor agonist (Figure 10.9). Whilst a number of H_2 antagonists interact potently with H_3 receptors, highly selective H_3 antagonists, notably thioperamide (**10.63**), have recently been described. The availability of such compounds is likely to stimulate studies of the precise role of histamine in the CNS.

10.3.1　Protolytic properties of histamine and histamine analogs

Studies of the protolytic properties of histamine have played an important part in the design of selective H_2 antagonists (see subsequent section) and in the interpretation of structure–activity relationships for subtype-selective histamine receptor agonists. At physiological pH (7.4) the primary amino group (pK_a 9.8) of histamine is almost fully ionized, whereas the monobasic imidazole ring (pK_a 6.0) is only about 4% protonated (see equation (10.1), Section 10.2.3). Thus, in aqueous solution at physiological pH only ca. 4% of histamine exists as the resonance-stabilized dication **10.65**. The ionized side chain of **10.65** exerts a negative inductive ($-I$) effect on the protonated imidazole ring. This electron-withdrawing effect reduces the electron density at the nearest ring nitrogen atom (N3) and, thus, facilitates the dissociation of a proton from this atom to form the monocation **10.66**, named the N^τ–H tautomer. The methyl group of the H_2 receptor-selective agonist **10.58** exerts a positive inductive ($+I$) effect on the heterocyclic ring. This electron-repelling effect of the methyl group, which increases the electron density at N1, further stabilizes the N1–H bond in **10.67** and, consequently, the N^τ–H tautomer **10.68** after dissociation of a proton from the dication **10.67**.

Based on extensive structure–activity studies of histamine analogs, it is assumed that the monocationic N^τ–H tautomer **10.66** is the active form of histamine at H_1 as well as H_2 receptors. The protonated primary amino group and the lone pair of electrons at N3 in **10.66** are essential for the binding of histamine to H_1 receptors, whereas the protonated primary amino group and the N1–H group are essential molecular components for the binding of **10.66** to H_2 receptors.

10.3.2　H_2 and H_3 receptor antagonists: design and therapeutic aspects

Histamine (**10.64**) has a physiological function in regulating the secretion of acid in the stomach where, acting on the H_2 receptor, it stimulates the parietal cells to

Histamine (**10.64**)　　　(**10.65**)　　　(**10.66**)

(**10.58**)　　　(**10.67**)　　　(**10.68**)

produce hydrochloric acid (see Figure 10.5). This probably is a protective mechanism, since the acid controls the local bacterial population. Under different conditions, the regulation of acid secretion by histamine or other chemical messengers may run out of control, and under such circumstances excessive acid secretion can lead to the formation of gastric and/or duodenal ulcers.

These aspects prompted the design and development of selective antagonists at H_2 receptors, and this field of drug research has been one of the most active and successful areas in medicinal chemistry. Systematic structural modifications of histamine led to the discovery of burimamide (**10.69**) as a selective but relatively weak H_2 receptor antagonist. The low activity of **10.69** was explained in terms of non-optimal protolytic properties of its imidazole ring, which is substantially more basic (pK$_a$ 7.2) than is the ring of histamine. Consequently, the degree of protonation of the imidazole ring of **10.69** is more than an order of magnitude higher than that of histamine at physiological pH. This increased basic character of the ring of **10.69** reflects a $+I$ effect of the alkyl side chain, and, furthermore, this electron-repelling effect favors the dissociation of the proton from N1 in **10.70** by increasing the electron density at N3. Thus, the N^π–H tautomer **10.71** will be the dominating neutral form of burimamide. Since burimamide appears to bind to the H_2 receptor in a neutral form, and since the imidazole ring of burimamide is assumed to bind to the site of the H_2 receptor, which binds the imidazole ring of histamine, the N^π–H tautomer **10.71** of burimamide was considered nonoptimal for effective receptor binding.

This reasoning prompted modifications of the structure of burimamide in order to obtain compounds, which more closely resembled histamine. Introduction of a sulphur atom into the side chain and a methyl group into position 5 of the ring of burimamide gave metiamide (**10.72**), which showed greater potency and selectivity as an H_2 receptor antagonist than did burimamide. Introduction of the sulphur atom converted the $+I$ effect of the side chain of burimamide into a $-I$ effect, whereas the C5 methyl group exerts a $+I$ effect. As a consequence of these structural modifications, the electron densities at C5-N1 and at C4-N3 in metiamide were, respectively, increased and decreased as compared with burimamide. Thus, the facilitated dissociation of the N3-H proton from protonated metiamide (**10.73**) gives the desired N^τ–H tautomer (**10.72** or **10.74**) as the dominating neutral form of metiamide.

(10.69)   (10.70)   (10.71)

(10.72)   (10.73)   (10.74)

Cimetidine (**10.75**)

Ranitidine (**10.76**)

Side effects, such as agranulocytosis, of metiamide (**10.72**) led to the replacement of its thiourea unit by the structurally related cyanoguanidine group to give cimetidine (**10.75**), which is more active than **10.72** as an H_2 antagonist and less toxic. Cimetidine turned out to be a successful drug, and, since its introduction some two decades ago, several million patients suffering from diseases caused by unnaturally high gastric secretion of hydrochloric acid have derived benefit from its therapeutic use. In recent years, a wide variety of other H_2 antagonists, notably ranitidine (**10.76**), have been introduced in the human clinic. The structural basis of the proposed interaction of the 2-guanidinothiazole and the 2-dimethylamino-methylfuran groups of **10.62** and **10.76**, respectively, with the imidazole-binding part of the H_2 receptor is not fully understood.

The cloning of the H_3 receptor, and its proposed involvement in a number of diseases and pathological conditions such as asthma, migraine, hypertension, septic shock, and in learning and memory degenerative disorders like AD have prompted an intense search for H_3 receptor ligands, primarily H_3 antagonists.

Since the discovery of thioperamide (**10.63**) as a potent and selective H_3 antagonist, a number of 4(5)-substituted imidazole derivatives have been designed,

GT-2016 (**10.77**)

GR 175737 (**10.78**)

Verongamine (**10.79**)

(**10.80**)

(**10.81**)

synthesized and pharmacologically evaluated. Some of the more prominent new H$_3$ receptor antagonists are GT-2016 (**10.77**) and GR 175737 (**10.78**) which show receptor affinities in the low nanomolar range.

Verongamine (**10.79**) is, so far, the only natural product that has been reported to possess H$_3$ antagonist effect. **10.79** only binds to H$_3$ receptors with moderately high affinity (IC$_{50}$ = 500 nM), and due to the presence of polar groups in the molecule, **10.79** does not easily penetrate the BBB. Based on molecular modeling studies, the compounds **10.79** and **10.80** were shown to adopt very similar energy-minimized conformations, and based on these studies, a series of lipophilic and highly potent H$_3$ antagonists were designed. Within this group of acetylenic imidazole derivatives, compound **10.81** turned out to be almost three orders of magnitude more potent than the lead compound, **10.79**. These compounds are undergoing further pharmacological evaluation as potential therapeutic agents.

FURTHER READING

Ali, S.M., Tedford, C.E., Gregory, R.,Yates, S.L. and Phillips, J.G. (1998) New acetylene based histamine H$_3$ receptor antagonists derived from the marine natural product verongamine. *Bioorg. Med. Chem. Lett.*, **8**, 1133–1138.

Arneric, S.P. and Brioni, J.D. (1999) *Neuronal Nicotinic Receptors: Pharmacology and Therapeutic Opportunities*. New York: Wiley-Liss.

Birdsall, N.J.M., Nathanson, N.M. and Schwarz, R.D. (2001) Muscarinic receptors: it's a knockout. *Trends Pharmacol. Sci.*, **22**, 215–219.

Brown, J.H. (ed.) (1989) *The Muscarinic Receptors*. Clifton, New Jersey: The Humana Press.

Cooper, D.G., Young, R.C., Durant, G.J. and Ganellin, C.R. (1990) Histamine receptors. In *Comprehensive Medicinal Chemistry*, Vol. 3, edited by C. Hansch, P.G. Sammes, J.B. Taylor and J.C. Emmett, pp. 323–421. Oxford: Pergamon Press.

Eberlein, W.G., Engel, W., Hasselbach, K.M., Mayer, N., Mihm, G., Rudolf, K. and Doods, H. (1992) Tricyclic compounds as selective muscarinic antagonists: structure activity relationships and therapeutic implications. In *Trends in Receptor Research*, edited by P. Angeli, U. Gulini and W. Quaglia, pp. 231–249. Amsterdam: Elsevier.

Fisher, A. (ed.) (1996) *Muscarinic Agonists and the Treatment of Alzheimer's Disease*. Heidelberg: Springer-Verlag.

Kovalainen, J.T., Christiaans, J.A.M., Kotisaari, S., Laitinen, J.T., Männistö, P.T., Tuomisto, L. and Gynther, J. (1999) Synthesis and *in vitro* pharmacology of a series of new chiral histamine H$_3$-receptor ligands: 2-(R and S)-amino-3-(1H-imidazol-4(5)-yl)propyl ether derivatives. *J. Med. Chem.*, **42**, 1193–1202.

Leurs, R., Watanabe, T. and Timmerman, H. (2001) Histamine receptors are finally 'coming out'. *Trends Pharmacol. Sci.*, **22**, 337–339.

Pedersen, H., Bräuner-Osborne, H., Ball, R.G., Frydenvang, K., Meier, E., Bøgesø, K.P. and Krogsgaard-Larsen, P. (1999) Synthesis and muscarinic receptor pharmacology of a series of 4,5,6,7-tetrahydroisothiazolo[4,5-c]pyridine bioisosteres of arecoline. *Bioorg. Med. Chem.*, **7**, 795–809.

Schmitt, J.D. and Bencherif, M. (2000) Targeting nicotinic acetylcholine receptors: advances in molecular design and therapies. *Annu. Rep. Med. Chem.*, **35**, 41–51.

St George-Hyslop, P.H., McLaurin, J. and Fraser, P.E. (2000) Neuropathological, biochemical and genetic alterations in AD. *Drug News Perspect.*, **13**, 281–288.

Szántay, C., Kardos-Balogh, Z., Moldvai, I., Szántay, C. Jr., Temesvári-Major, E. and Blaskó, G. (1996) A practical enantioselective synthesis of epibatidine. *Tetrahedron*, **52**, 11053–11062.

Timmerman, H. (1990) Histamine H_3 ligands: just pharmacological tools or potential therapeutic agents? *J. Med. Chem.*, **33**, 4–11.

Wess, J., Buhl, T., Lambrecht, G. and Mutschler, E. (1990) Cholinergic receptors. In *Comprehensive Medicinal Chemistry*, Vol. 3, edited by C. Hansch, P.G. Sammes, J.B. Taylor and J.C. Emmett, pp. 423–491. Oxford: Pergamon Press.

Chapter 11

Dopamine and serotonin receptor and transporter ligands

Klaus P. Bøgesø and Benny Bang-Andersen

11.1 RECEPTORS AND TRANSPORTERS FOR DOPAMINE AND SEROTONIN

Dopamine (DA) and serotonin (5-hydroxytryptamine, 5-HT) are both important neurotransmitters in the human brain. A schematic drawing of a neurotransmitter synapse representative for both DA and serotonin is shown in Figure 11.1. Neurotransmitters are released from vesicles into the synaptic cleft where they subsequently can activate a number of postsynaptic receptors (PR). The neurotransmitters may also activate a number of autoreceptors (AR) which regulate the synthesis and release of the transmitters, and generally, activation of autoreceptors leads to inhibition of neurotransmitter synthesis and release. The autoreceptors can be localized both presynaptically or somatodendritically (on the cell bodies). The concentration of neurotransmitter in the synapse may also be regulated by active reuptake into the presynaptic terminal by transporters (T).

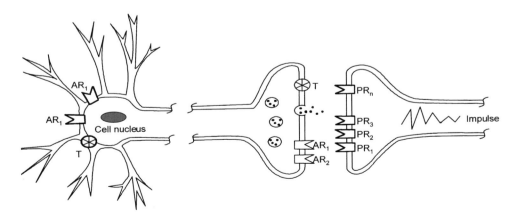

Figure 11.1 Neurotransmitter synapse. PR: Postsynaptic receptor; AR: Autoreceptor; T: Transporter.

11.2   DOPAMINE AND SEROTONIN RECEPTOR LIGANDS

11.2.1   Molecular biology and structure of receptors for dopamine and serotonin

Subtypes of DA receptors were not known until Kebabian and Calne in 1979 suggested that the DA receptor, which stimulated adenylyl cyclase, and the receptor that did not stimulate adenylyl cyclase were distinct categories of receptors and should be designated D-1 and D-2, respectively. The same year, Peroutka and Snyder suggested the existence of two different serotonin receptor subtypes based on differential drug potencies for serotonin receptor sites labeled with [^{3}H]5-HT and [^{3}H]spiroperidol, respectively. In both of these cases, the subtypes were identified by the use of classical pharmacological techniques, but since the late 1980s, the application of molecular biological techniques has had a major impact on the identification of additional subtypes of these receptors.

The DA and serotonin receptor subtypes known today are shown in Figures 11.2 and 11.3, respectively. All of these receptors are putative 7-TM G-protein-coupled receptors (see Chapter 6) except for the 5-HT$_3$ receptor, which is a ligand-gated ion channel regulating the permeability of Na$^+$ and K$^+$ ions. Selective ligands have been developed for the majority of these receptors of which the 7-TM receptors in particular have proven to be drug targets for a number of psychiatric disorders.

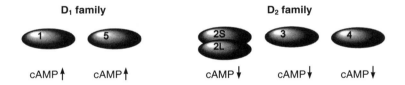

Figure 11.2 Dopamine (DA) receptor classification. cAMP↑: Activation of receptor stimulates adenylyl cyclase which results in an increase in the intracellular concentration of cyclic adenosine monophosphate (cAMP); cAMP↓: Activation of receptor inhibits adenylyl cyclase which results in a decrease in the intracellular concentration of cAMP.

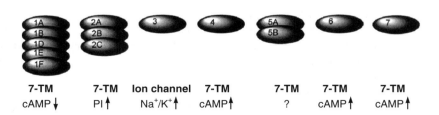

Figure 11.3 Serotonin (5-hydroxytryptamine, 5-HT) receptor classification. 7-TM and ion channel: Classification of receptor type; cAMP↑ and cAMP↓: see legend to Figure 11.2; PI↑: Activation of receptor stimulates phospholipase C which results in an increase in the intracellular turnover of phosphatidylinositol (PI) biphosphate; Na$^+$/K$^+$: Activation of receptor increases the permeability of sodium and potassium ions into the cell.

The 7-TM receptors are 350–550 amino acid peptides that have seven regions consisting of 20–25 hydrophobic amino acids, which form helices through the nerve cell membrane. Between the helices there are loops of varying length (three extracellular and three intracellular). The third intracellular loop is longer and is believed to interact with the G-protein. The N-terminal end is extracellular, while the carboxy terminal end is intracellular (for further discussions on 7-TM receptors, see Chapter 6).

11.2.1.1 Dopamine receptor subtypes

The DA receptor subtypes are divided into two families based on structural and pharmacological similarities (Figure 11.2): The D_1 family (D_1 and D_5 receptors) and the D_2 family (D_2, D_3 and D_4 receptors). Activation of D_1 and D_5 receptors leads generally to stimulation of adenylyl cyclase while inhibition is observed after D_2, D_3 and D_4 receptor activation. In addition, there are two isoforms of the D_2 receptor named D_{2S} (short) or D_{2L} (long).

Dopamine D_1 and D_2 receptors are expressed in regions associated with motor, limbic and neuroendocrine function, and D_2 antagonists and agonists are used in the treatment of schizophrenia and Parkinson's disease, respectively. The more recently identified receptor subtypes D_3, D_4, and D_5 have more restricted distributions. D_3 and D_4 receptors are primarily localized in limbic regions of the brain associated with emotion, whereas little to no expression is seen in striatal regions associated with motor function. The D_5 receptor has very limited distribution in the human brain. The involvement of the different DA receptor subtypes in the treatment of schizophrenia will be discussed in more detail in the following.

11.2.1.2 Serotonin receptor subtypes

A total of 14 serotonin receptor subtypes grouped in seven families are known (Figure 11.3). The receptors of the $5-HT_1$ family are all negatively coupled to adenylyl cyclase, while the $5-HT_4$, $5-HT_6$ and $5-HT_7$ receptors are all positively linked to adenylyl cyclase. All members of the $5-HT_2$ family are linked to phosphatidylinositol (PI) turnover (i.e. stimulation leads to an increased production of inositol phosphates and increased concentration of intracellular Ca^{2+}). Signal transduction pathways for $5-HT_5$ receptors remain to be defined unequivocally.

All of the serotonin receptor subtypes are expressed in the human brain but several of the subtypes are also found in the periphery. The $5-HT_{1A}$ receptor is involved in modulation of emotion and mood, and partial $5-HT_{1A}$ agonists such as buspirone have anxiolytic and antidepressant activity. The $5-HT_{1B}$ and $5-HT_{1D}$ (formerly called $5-HT_{1D\beta}$ and $5-HT_{1D\alpha}$ in humans) receptors are autoreceptors that regulate neurotransmitter release, and they may prove to be interesting targets for antidepressant or anxiolytic drugs. The $5-HT_{2A}$ receptor is found both in the CNS and the periphery. In the periphery, it is widely distributed and mediates contractile responses in bronchial, gastrointestinal, urinary, uterine and vascular smooth muscle. Platelet aggregation and increased capillary permeability are also $5-HT_{2A}$ mediated actions. Therefore, $5-HT_{2A}$ antagonists such as ketanserin have shown potential as antihypertensive and antiplatelet aggregating drugs. In the brain, the 5-HT$_{2A}$ receptor is found in cortical areas, in parts of the limbic system and in the basal ganglia. Therefore, 5-HT$_{2A}$ receptors are important targets for development of antipsychotic drugs. The 5-HT$_{2C}$ (formerly called 5-HT$_{1C}$) receptor is predominantly localized in the brain, and their dysregulation may contribute to particular symptoms of anxiety and depression. In addition, antagonism of 5-HT$_{2C}$ receptors may be important for the effect of antipsychotic drugs and may also be responsible for their potential to increase weight gain. The 5-HT$_3$ receptor is widely distributed in the periphery (cardiovascular and gastrointestinal systems) but it is also found in the brain. The nausea and gastrointestinal discomfort often seen in the first weeks of treatment of depressed patients with Selective Serotonin Reuptake Inhibitors (SSRIs, see also Section 11.3.2.2) is probably caused by activation of 5-HT$_3$ receptors. Along similar lines antagonists for the 5-HT$_3$ receptor are used to control vomiting in e.g. cancer patients. Interestingly, 5-HT$_3$ antagonists are effective in certain animal models of schizophrenia and anxiety. The 5-HT$_6$ and 5-HT$_7$ receptors are mainly expressed in the brain. Several antidepressant and antipsychotic drugs bind with high affinity to these receptors but no clear picture has been found between the affinity of these compounds for these receptors and their clinical profile.

As already mentioned, selective ligands have been described for many of the dopamine and serotonin receptor subtypes but it is not within the scope of this chapter to review all of these ligands. In the following, we have chosen to concentrate on ligands which have shown a potential as antipsychotic or antidepressant drugs or which have been important in the discovery of these drugs.

11.2.2   Antipsychotic drugs

11.2.2.1   Classical antipsychotic drugs

Antipsychotic drugs are primarily used to treat schizophrenia and a number of other psychotic disorders, such as e.g. schizoaffective disorder. These disorders are distinguished from each other on the basis of characteristic clusters of symptoms and, in the case of schizophrenia, the characteristic symptoms can be arranged into two broad categories – positive and negative. The positive symptoms appear to reflect an excess or distortion of normal function (i.e. delusion, hallucinations, disorganized thinking, disorganized behavior and catatonia), whereas the negative symptoms appear to reflect a diminution or loss of normal functions (i.e. affective flattening, poverty of speech and an inability to initiate and persist in goal-directed activities). However, in recent years, more and more interest has been devoted to the importance of cognitive deficits as the core of schizophrenia, and in future the diagnostic schema for schizophrenia may very well also include cognitive symptoms (i.e. impairment of memory, executive function and attention).

Reserpine (**11.1**, Figure 11.4), which is the principal active indole alkaloid of the roots of *Rauwolfia serpentina*, was first described as an antihypotentive and tranquillizing agent, whereas chlorpromazine (**11.2**, Figure 11.5) was described as an antihistaminergic agent. It was subsequently discovered in the 1950s that both reserpine and chlorpromazine were effective in the treatment of mainly the

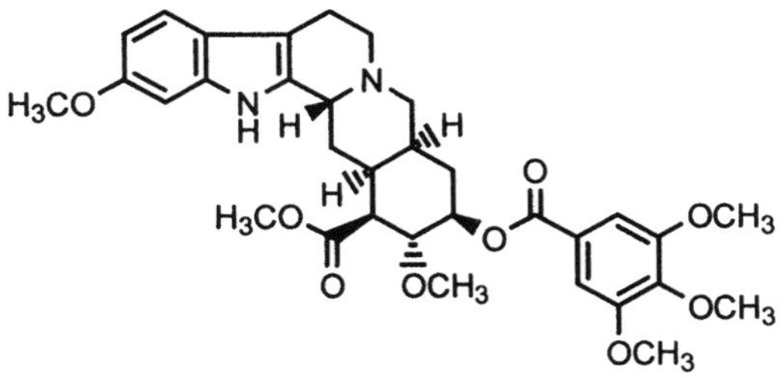

Reserpine (11.1)

Figure 11.4 Reserpine.

positive symptoms of schizophrenia. However, the use of both compounds was associated with severe side effects such as parkinsonian symptoms (i.e. tremor, muscle rigidity and akinesia), dystonia, akathisia and tardive dyskinesia, which subsequently were known as extrapyramidal symptoms (EPS). It was later shown that the two compounds had very different mechanisms of action despite their similar clinical effects. Reserpine blocks unselectively the accumulation of the monoamines norepinephrine (NE), DA and 5-HT by synaptic vesicles (vesicular pool). The monoamines will subsequently leak out of the vesicles and into the presynaptic neurone, where the enzymes monoamine oxidase-A and -B (MAO-A and MAO-B) will deaminate them. As a result, the synaptic cleft will be depleted for any of these monoaminergic neurotransmitters. On the contrary, chlorpromazine is a postsynaptic dopamine receptor antagonist. However, the net effect of both reserpine and chlorpromazine is the same – no or reduced neurotransmission in dopaminergic synapses.

Observations along these lines resulted in the 1960s in the formulation of the 'dopamine hypothesis of schizophrenia', which has provided a theoretical framework for understanding the biological mechanisms underlying this disorder. In its simplest form, the DA hypothesis states that schizophrenia is associated with a hyperdopaminergic state. The hypothesis is still valid today although a number of other hypotheses have been formulated during the years, which focus on other neurotransmitter systems or which in addition to the dopamine system includes other neurotransmitter systems (see Sections 11.2.2.2 and 11.2.2.3). It is believed that reserpine and chlorpromazine exert their effect on positive symptoms by reducing the dopamine hyperactivity in limbic areas of the brain, whereas the EPS results from the reduction of dopaminergic neurotransmission in striatal areas. The striatum is known as the motor system of the brain and is, e.g. closely related to parkinsonism. The neurochemical origin of this disease is also linked to reduced neurotransmission in dopaminergic synapses although due to degeneration of the cells.

Today, the term classical antipsychotic drugs is linked to compounds that show effect in the treatment of the positive symptoms of schizophrenia at similar doses that induce EPS. In addition, the classical antipsychotic drugs are without effect on negative and cognitive symptoms, and today it is generally agreed that these compounds may even worsen these symptoms. It has been argued that the

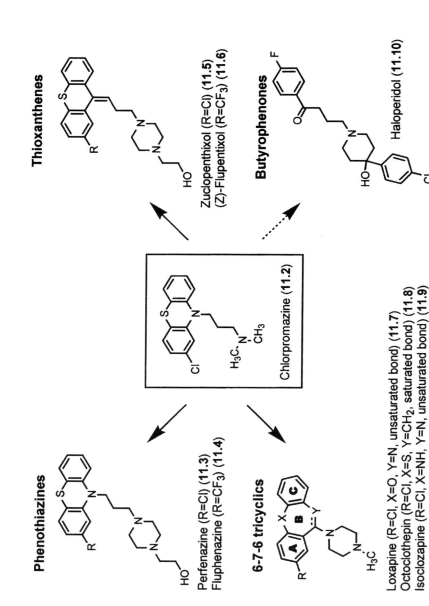

Thioxanthenes

Zuclopenthixol (R=Cl) (11.5)
(Z)-Flupentixol (R=CF₃) (11.6)

Butyrophenones

Haloperidol (11.10)

Chlorpromazine (11.2)

Phenothiazines

Perfenazine (R=Cl) (11.3)
Fluphenazine (R=CF₃) (11.4)

6-7-6 tricyclics

Loxapine (R=Cl, X=O, Y=N, unsaturated bond) (11.7)
Octoclothepin (R=Cl, X=S, Y=CH₂, saturated bond) (11.8)
Isoclozapine (R=Cl, X=NH, Y=N, unsaturated bond) (11.9)

Figure 11.5 Classical antipsychotic drugs.

worsening of negative and cognitive symptoms may be a consequence of EPS, and the separation of the dose–response curves for antipsychotic action and EPS is the foremost important property of the newer antipsychotic drugs (see Section 11.2.2.2).

The use of reserpine as an antipsychotic drug was, in addition to EPS, limited by its hypotensive action. Furthermore, the complicated structure of reserpine made it a rather poor target for structural manipulation in order to make an antipsychotic drug without EPS and hypotensive action, and today, reserpine is mainly used as an experimental tool.

However, the structure of chlorpromazine with its phenothiazine backbone was an excellent lead for medicinal chemists (Figure 11.5). After the discovery of chlorpromazine in the beginning of the 1950s, medicinal chemists modified the structure of chlorpromazine without changing the phenothiazine backbone, and these modifications led to a number of drugs such as perphenazine (**11.3**) and fluphenazine (**11.4**) (Figure 11.5). Medicinal chemists around the world also replaced the phenothiazine backbone with other tricyclic structures, and these modifications led to other classes of classical antipsychotic drugs such as the thioxanthenes and the 6-7-6 tricyclics. The thioxanthene backbone was in particular investigated by H. Lundbeck A/S, and this work has resulted in drugs such as zuclopenthixol (**11.5**) and (Z)-flupentixol (**11.6**) (Figure 11.5). The 6-7-6 tricyclic backbone has also led to a number of classical antipsychotic drugs such as loxapine (**11.7**), octoclothepin (**11.8**) and isoclozapine (**11.9**) (Figure 11.5). The R group, which is found in all of these compounds, is called the 'neuroleptic substituent'. For further discussions on the 'neuroleptic substituent' see Chapter 4, Section 4.9.2.

In the late 1950s, researchers at Janssen discovered an entirely new class of classical antipsychotic drugs without a tricyclic structure, namely the butyrophenones. Haloperidol (**11.10**, Figure 11.5) is the most prominent representative of this class of compounds, and today haloperidol is considered the archetypical classical antipsychotic drug for both preclinical experiments and clinical trials.

The classical antipsychotic drugs were all discovered by the use of *in vivo* (animal) models, because today's knowledge about receptor multiplicity and receptor-binding techniques as screening models were not available at that time. However, many of the *in vivo* models, which were used at that time, would today be considered to be predictive of various side effects. For example, antagonism of methyl phenidate-induced stereotypies was used as a model predictive of antipsychotic action whereas catalepsy, which is the syndrome in rats that corresponds to EPS in humans, was used to predict EPS. However, today it is known that both stereotypies and catalepsy are mediated via antagonism of striatal D_2 receptors, and both models are therefore essentially EPS models. With only these models available at that time, it was difficult to find new antipsychotic drugs without the potential to induce EPS.

Examination of the classical antipsychotic drugs by today's range of receptor-binding techniques and other more advanced biochemical methods has revealed that these drugs are postsynaptic D_2 receptor antagonists, and this accounts for both their antipsychotic action and their potential to induce EPS. However, these drugs also display affinity for a large number of other sites and receptors, which may contribute to their antipsychotic action and to some extent to their adverse effects.

11.2.2.2 Newer antipsychotic drugs

Isoclozapine (**11.9**, Figure 11.5), which has the 'neuroleptic chloro substituent' in benzene ring **A**, is a classical antipsychotic drug. On the contrary, clozapine (**11.11**, Figure 11.6), which has the chloro substituent in benzene ring **C** (Figure 11.5), has revolutionized the pharmacotherapy of schizophrenia. In the middle of the 1960s, it was shown that clozapine was effective in the treatment of the positive symptoms

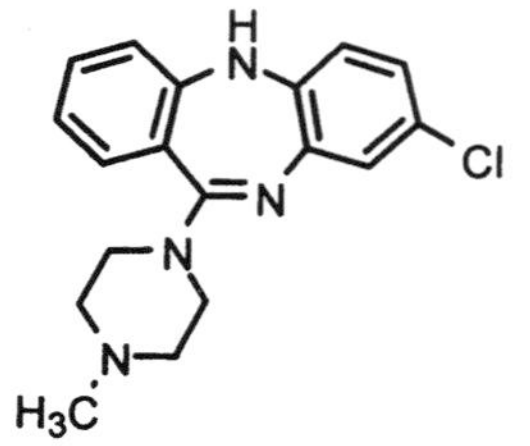

Clozapine (11.11)

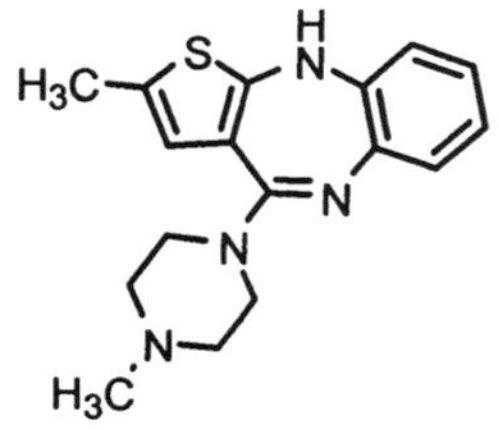

Olanzapine (11.12)

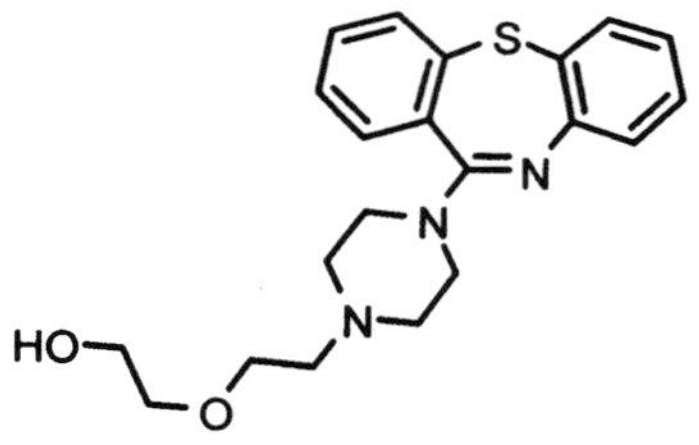

Quetiapine (11.13)

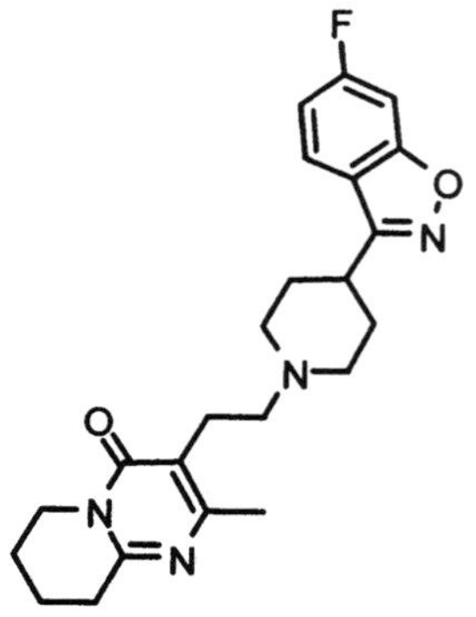

Risperidone (11.14)

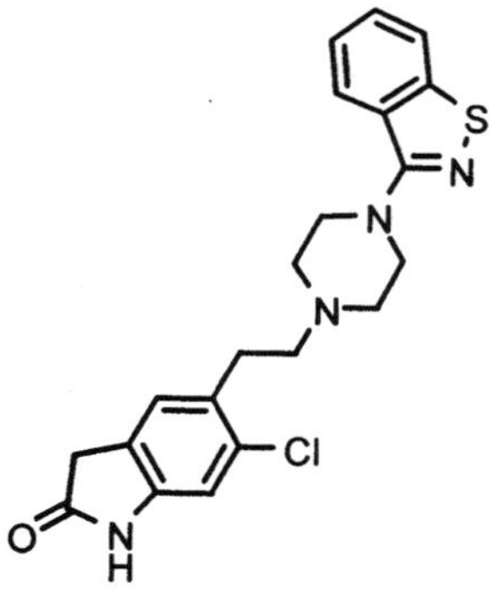

Ziprasidone (11.15)

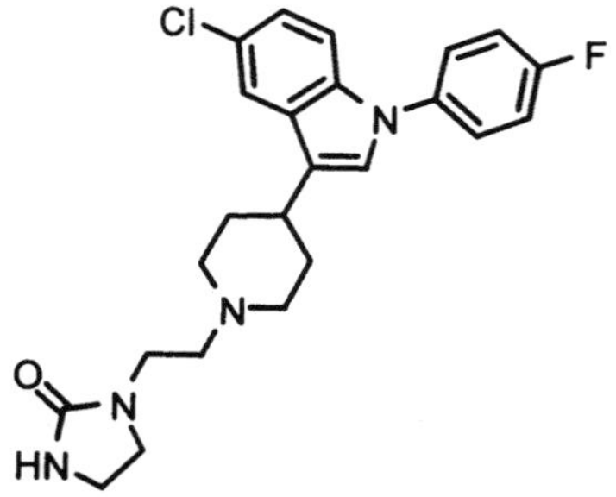

Sertindole (11.16)

Figure 11.6 Newer antipsychotic drugs.

of schizophrenia and free of inducing EPS in humans. However, the judgement at that time among pharmacologists and clinicians was that a compound without EPS could not be an effective antipsychotic drug. It was not until its 'second' discovery in the 1980s by clinicians in the United States of America that clozapine was judged to be the drug of the future, and this view was further substantiated in the years to come. Very importantly, it was shown that clozapine to some extent was effective in the treatment of negative and cognitive symptoms, and also in the treatment of refractory schizophrenia (individuals who do not respond adequately to classical antipsychotic drugs which is estimated to be as high as one-third of the treated). Unfortunately, clozapine can cause potentially fatal agranulocytosis in a small percentage of individuals (1–2%), which necessitates periodic monitoring of the blood picture of individuals undergoing treatment with the drug. Therefore, much effort has been directed toward the identification of new antipsychotic drugs with a clozapine-like clinical profile but without the potential to cause agranulocytosis.

This search has resulted in a number of new antipsychotic drugs such as olanzapine (**11.12**), quetiapine (**11.13**), risperidone (**11.14**), ziprasidone (**11.15**) and sertindole (**11.16**) (Figure 11.6). A closer look at the structure of these compounds reveals that olanzapine and quetiapine were obtained by structural modification of clozapine, whereas risperidone and ziprasidone were obtained from the butyrophenones. However, sertindole is quite different in chemical structure, and the discovery of sertindole are discussed in Section 11.2.2.2.1.

Binding profiles and catalepsy data for the newer antipsychotic drugs as well as for the classical antipsychotic drug haloperidol are shown in Table 11.1. All compounds have 'mixed' receptor profiles except for quetiapine, which in our hands is a relative selective α_1 ligand (others find it to be a more balanced 5-HT$_2$/α_1 ligand). With this exception, the general tendency is that these drugs like all classical antipsychotics display relatively high affinity for D$_2$ receptors (classical and newer antipsychotics are antagonists at D$_2$ receptors). However, when compared to

Table 11.1 Receptor profile and EPS potential of antipsychotic drugs

Compound	Receptor binding K_i(nM)							In vivo ED$_{50}$ (μmol/kg)
	D_1	D_2	D_3	D_4	5-HT$_{2A}$	5-HT$_{2C}$	α_1	Catalepsy max., sc
Classical antipsychotic drug								
Haloperidol (**11.10**)	15	0.82	1.1	2.8	28	1500	7.3	0.37
Newer antipsychotic drugs								
Risperidone (**11.14**)	21	0.44	14	7.1	0.39	6.4	0.69	20
Olanzapine (**11.12**)	10	2.1	71	32	1.9	2.8	7.3	37
Quetiapine (**11.13**)	390	69	1100	2400	82	1500	4.5	>80
Ziprasidone (**11.15**)	9.5	2.8	n.t.	73	0.25	0.55	1.9	>97
Sertindole (**11.16**)	12	0.45	2.0	17	0.20	0.51	1.4	>91
Clozapine (**11.11**)	53	36	310	30	4.0	5.0	3.7	460

Sources: Data from Arnt, J. and Skarsfeldt, T. (1998) Do Novel Antipsychotics Have Similar Pharmacological Characteristics? A Review of the Evidence. *Neuropsychopharmacology*, **18**, 63–101 and Lundbeck Screening Database; n.t. not tested.

haloperidol, these newer antipsychotics display an increased affinity for 5-HT$_2$ (5-HT$_{2A/2C}$) receptors and α_1-adrenoceptors relative to their D$_2$ affinity, and this difference in affinity for D$_2$ and 5-HT$_2$ receptors has been used to rationalize their different propensity to induce EPS at therapeutic doses. Another argument, which has proven to distinguish classical and newer antipsychotic, is that all of these compounds to some extent have a preference for limbic as compared to striatal regions of the brain (see also below). In line with this evidence, the newer antipsychotics are either inactive or much weaker than haloperidol in the catalepsy model, and it has subsequently been shown that this tendency correlate quite well with their different propensity to induce EPS in humans.

Clozapine and the other new antipsychotic drugs are often called 'atypical antipsychotics' but the term 'newer antipsychotics' is preferred, as they cannot be seen as a homogeneous class. Although a number of common limitations have become apparent for these drugs, they have their own advantages and limitations. For example, all the drugs except clozapine display limited effect in the treatment of refractory schizophrenia. Several of the drugs have also a strong tendency to increase weight gain. But whereas clozapine and olanzapine are known to increase weight gain rather dramatically, ziprasidone is more or less without this effect. Some of the drugs but in particular ziprasidone and sertindole exert some prolonging effect on the QT interval in the surface electrocardiogram. A prolonged QT-interval is a reflection of abnormally prolonged repolarization of cardiac tissue and has been associated with a risk for development of ventricular arrhythmias. Thus, there is still room for improved antipsychotic drugs for the treatment of schizophrenia as none of these newer antipsychotics are perfect.

11.2.2.2.1   Sertindole discovery

In the 1970s, H. Lundbeck A/S had successfully marketed a number of what is today known as classical antipsychotic drugs, and the medicinal chemistry program at H. Lundbeck A/S was still aimed at finding new antipsychotic drugs by manipulation of the phenothiazine or thioxanthene structures. However, in 1975 the first compounds were synthesized in a project aimed at finding new NSAIDs (nonsteroidal anti-inflammatory drugs), and fortunately the compounds were also examined in a few *in vivo* models predictive of antipsychotic and antidepressant action. It was found that the two racemic *trans*-1-piperazino-3-phenylindanes **11.17** and **11.18** (Figure 11.7) were relative potent in the methyl phenidate model, which as already mentioned was seen as a model predictive of antipsychotic action but today mostly is seen as a model for EPS and *in vivo* D$_2$ antagonism. However, when at the same time it was found that these compounds were about a factor of ten weaker in the catalepsy model (predictive of EPS), these compounds were seen as prototypes of a new class of antipsychotic drugs with a promising side effect profile, notably with respect to EPS.

In 1980, the *trans*-racemate tefludazine (**11.19**, Figure 11.7) was selected from this series as a development candidate with potential antipsychotic action. Tefludazine displayed a similar ratio as the two lead compounds in the methyl phenidate vs. the catalepsy model but tefludazine was at least a factor of 100 more potent in these *in vivo* models. After the discovery of the multiplicity of dopamine

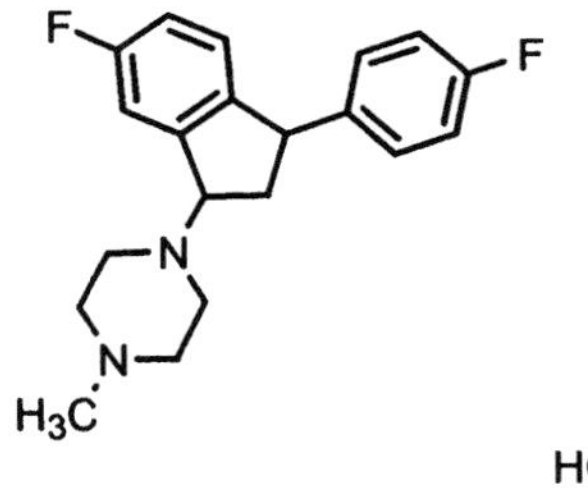

11.17 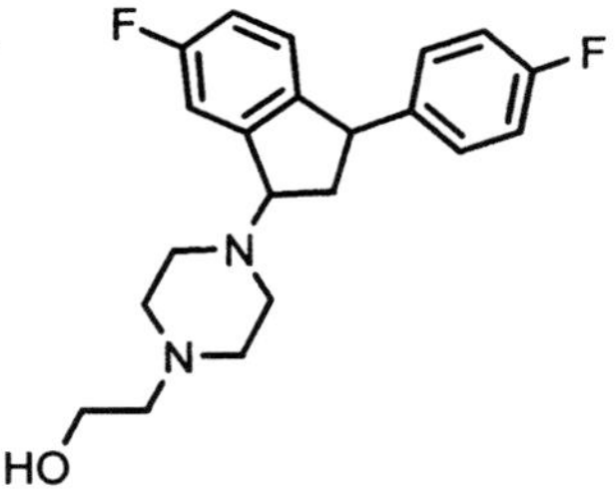   **11.18**

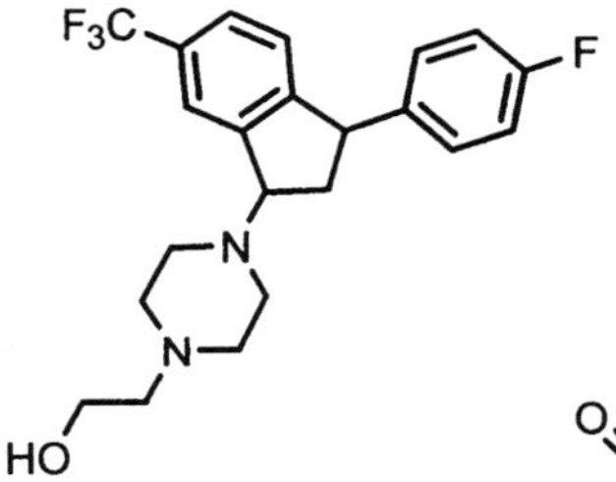

Tefludazine (11.19) 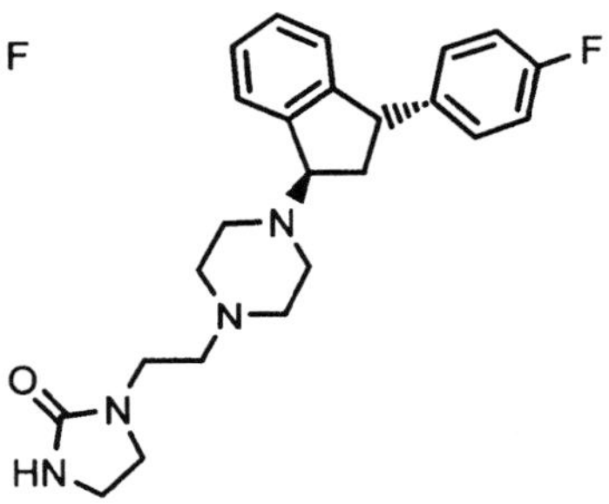   Irindalone (11.20)

Figure 11.7 Selected *trans*-1-piperazino-3-phenylindanes.

and serotonin receptors in 1979, many pharmaceutical companies around the world, including H. Lundbeck A/S, implemented receptor-binding assays for D_1, D_2, 5-HT_1, 5-HT_2 receptors. Thus, it was subsequently shown that the most prominent feature of tefludazine was its high affinity for D_2 and 5-HT_2 receptors. It was also shown that tefludazine was a potent *in vivo* D_2 antagonist (methyl phenidate model) and an extremely potent and long-acting *in vivo* 5-HT_2 antagonist (quipazine model).

During the 1980s, an electrophysiological *in vivo* model for evaluation of limbic vs. striatal selectivity was introduced at H. Lundbeck A/S. This was a chronic model where rats were treated with a drug for three weeks before the number of active dopamine neurones were measured in the ventral tegmental area (VTA) and in substantia nigra pars compacta (SNC) from where neurones project to limbic and striatal areas, respectively. After treatment with classical antipsychotic drugs such as chlorpromazine and haloperidol, neurones in both areas were completely inhibited (by equal doses), whereas clozapine selectively inactivated the dopamine neurones in the VTA. At H. Lundbeck A/S, it was demonstrated that this model had the potential to predict the therapeutic window between antipsychotic action and EPS of putative new antipsychotic drugs. It was subsequently shown that tefludazine displayed some selectivity in this model. The dose–response curves for inhibiting the neurones in the VTA as compared to the SNC were separated by a factor of three, which substantiated the preclinical evidence for tefludazine as a development candidate. Unfortunately, due to toxicological findings in dogs, the development of this compound was discontinued in Phase I.

It was subsequently discovered that removal of the 'neuroleptic substituent' in the indan benzene ring (i.e. the trifluoromethyl group in **11.19**), reduced the D_2 antagonism, whereas the 5-HT$_2$ antagonism was retained. Concurrent replacement of the hydroxyethyl side chain with the more bulky 1-ethyl-2-imidazolidinone side chain, resulted in irindalone (**11.20**, Figure 11.7), which was a very potent and selective 5-HT$_2$ antagonist. Irindalone was developed as a potential antihypertensive drug, but in 1989 the development was discontinued in Phase II for strategic reasons. Irindalone was, in contrast to tefludazine, developed as the pure (1R, 3S)-enantiomer. This configuration of the 1-piperazino-3-phenylindanes is generally associated with receptor antagonistic properties, while other stereoisomers are uptake inhibitors (see Section 11.3.3 and Figure 11.17).

A general disadvantage of the piperazinoindanes is their stereoisomerism, which complicates all stages of drug discovery and development process. Therefore, the corresponding piperazino-, tetrahydropyridino- and piperidino-indoles were designed, but their synthesis was not straightforward. These compounds could eventually be synthesized, and it was discovered that the piperidinoindole moiety bioisosterically substituted for the *trans*-piperazinoindan moiety with respect to D_2 and 5-HT$_2$ antagonism. One of the compounds synthesized in this series was sertindole (**11.16**, Figure 11.6), which incorporates structural elements from both tefludazine (neuroleptic substituent) and irindalone (imidazolidinone side chain). Despite high affinity for both D_2 and 5-HT$_2$ receptors, sertindole displayed the *in vivo* profile of a selective 5-HT$_2$ antagonist. Therefore, it was very surprising that sertindole in the VTA/SNC model displayed very selective inhibition of dopamine neurones in the VTA as compared to the SNC. It was found that the dose–response curves were separated by a factor of 100, and sertindole was subsequently pushed through development and marketed in 1996 for the treatment of schizophrenia. Sertindole was temporarily withdrawn in 1998 because of uncertainties regarding the connection between QT prolongation and the ability to induce potentially fatal cardiac arrhythmias in humans. The suspension was lifted early 2002.

11.2.2.3 Future perspectives

Clozapine (**11.11**) still remains the golden standard of the industry with respect to clinical effect, and much effort has been put into trying to understand the mechanisms behind the superiority of clozapine. It has been shown that clozapine displays affinity for a large number of receptor subtypes in the human brain such as a substantial number of the DA and the serotonin receptor subtypes. Thus, besides the newer antipsychotics already discussed, which are 'mixed' D_2/5-HT$_2$ antagonists displaying affinity for quite a few other receptor subtypes as well, one of the important strategies of the industry has been to develop more selective ligands. One of the goals has been to retain antipsychotic action but diminish adverse effects, and this approach has resulted in a number of development candidates (most prominent representative in parentheses) with the following profiles (Figure 11.8): Selective D_1 antagonists (SCH-23390, **11.21**), D_2/D_3

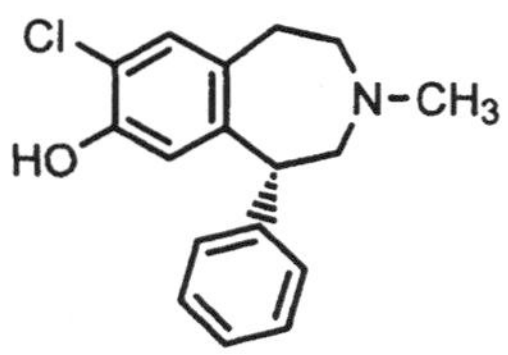

SCH-23390 (**11.21**) 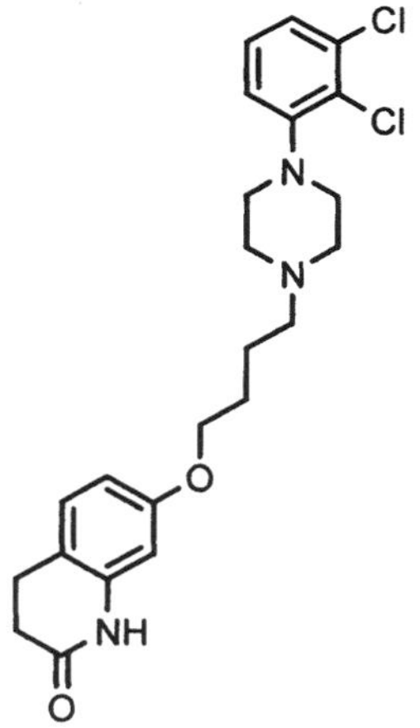   Aripiprazole (**11.22**) 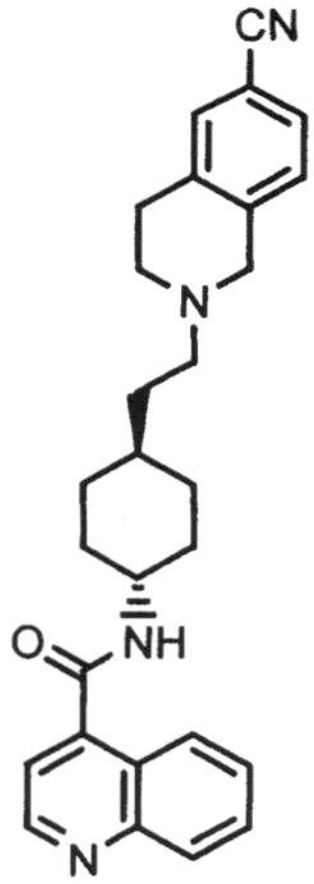   SB-277011-A (**11.23**)

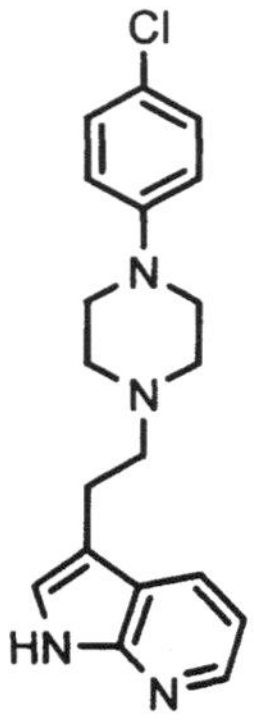

L-745,870 (**11.24**) 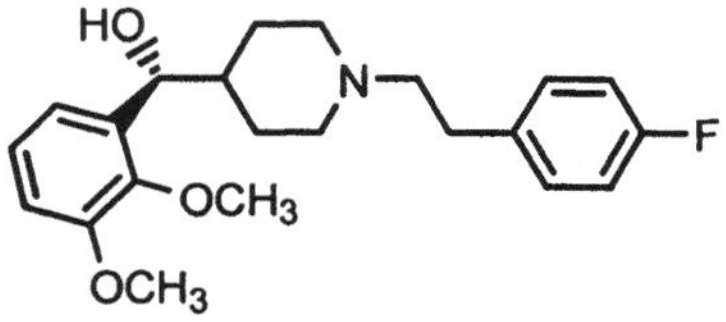   M-100,907 (**11.25**) 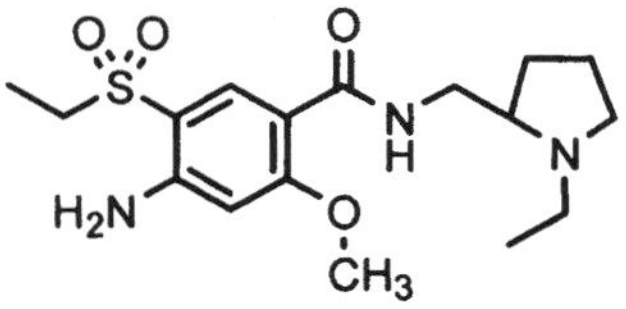   Amisulpride (**11.26**)

Figure 11.8 Selective dopamine and serotonin ligands developed as potential antipsychotics.

(partial) agonists (aripiprazole, **11.22**), selective D_3 antagonists (SB-277011-A, **11.23**), selective D_4 antagonists (L-745,870, **11.24**) and selective 5-HT$_{2A}$ antagonists (M-100,907, **11.25**). Years ago, the industry also aimed at selective D_2 antagonists but today there are no signs of such compounds in the pipeline of pharmaceutical companies. The benzamide class of antipsychotics was developed as selective D_2 antagonists, and today amisulpride (**11.26**) is probably the most interesting compound from this class as it has been shown to be effective against both positive and negative symptoms of schizophrenia. Other compounds from this class include raclopride and remoxipride, of which the latter has been marketed but withdrawn because of fatal aplastic anemia. It has later been shown that the benzamides often have affinity for D_3 and D_4 receptors, too, but that they are rather selective for DA vs. serotonin receptors.

The next generation of marketed antipsychotics may very well be a presynaptic D_2/D_3 (partial) agonist or a subtype selective DA antagonist possibly combined with some 5-HT_{2A} antagonism. Aripiprazole and M-100,907 are currently undergoing Phase III clinical trials for the treatment of schizophrenia, and whereas positive results have been published for aripiprazole, it has recently been shown that M-100,907 was without effect in the treatment of acute schizophrenia, although it may still be effective as an add-on in chronic treatment. Aripiprazole is actually a partial D_2/D_3 agonist, which in functional *in vivo* models manifests itself as presynaptic D_2 agonism and postsynaptic D_2 antagonism but the hypothesis behind this is not discussed here. Furthermore, a number of D_1 antagonists have undergone clinical trials during the years but there are still no drugs on the market from this class of compounds, whereas selective D_3 antagonists still undergo clinical trials, and no results have yet been published. The D_4 antagonists will receive a little more attention, as the D_4 receptor probably has been the most investigated target for schizophrenia during the 1990s.

The 'dopamine D_4 hypothesis of schizophrenia' is based on two principal observations, namely the localization of D_4 receptors in limbic areas of the brain (the site of antipsychotic action) and the 'selective' affinity of clozapine for D_4 receptors over D_2 receptors. In our hands, clozapine is not found to be selective for D_4 receptors (Table 11.1), and also other groups have questioned the selectivity. However, manipulation of D_4 receptors could be beneficial in the treatment of schizophrenia and would not be expected to cause EPS.

It has recently been shown that clozapine is a silent antagonist at D_4 receptors whereas a number of D_4 ligands, which initially were postulated to be selective D_4 antagonists, notably L-745,870 (**11.24**), indeed are partial D_4 agonists in some *in vitro* efficacy assays. Thus, L-745,870 may not have been the most appropriate compound for the clinical evaluation of D_4 antagonism in the treatment of schizophrenia. In the future, more will be learned about the efficacy (intrinsic activity) at DA and serotonin receptors of the different compounds which have undergone clinical trials during the years, and this may foster new medicinal chemistry programs in order to make new and better antipsychotic drugs. Also non-dopaminergic and/or non-serotonergic targets have attracted attention over the years, and certainly the glutamatergic system will be in focus in the future. However, these new targets still have to prove that they may give drugs with antipsychotic action in the clinic.

11.3 DOPAMINE AND SEROTONIN TRANSPORTER LIGANDS

11.3.1 Molecular biology and structure of transporters for biogenic amines

Termination of the neurotransmission in the dopaminergic and serotonergic synapses is effected by the rapid reuptake of the neurotransmitters into the presynaptic terminal (Figure 11.1). The knowledge regarding the structure and function of the transporter molecules has increased dramatically in recent years

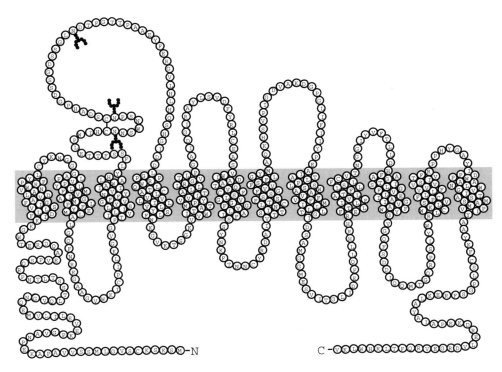

Figure 11.9 Illustration of the human DA transporter showing the amino acid sequence and the putative 12 transmembrane α-helices. N- and C-terminal ends are intracellular. By courtesy of Lene Nørregaard, University of Copenhagen.

following the cloning of the 5-HT and DA transporters (5-HTT and DAT) from several species. These transporters, as well as the norepinephrine transporter (NET), are important drug targets notably for antidepressant drugs. But they are also the target for the psychostimulant drug cocaine, and it is possible that both environmental and endogenous toxins are transported into the neurone by the transporters.

The transporter molecules for the biogenic amines are peptides consisting of 600–700 amino acids. They all contain 12 stretches of 20–24 hydrophobic residues, and it is therefore suggested that they have 12 membrane-spanning helices.

Both the N- and C-terminal ends are believed to be located intracellularly. All the loops are relatively short except the second extracellular loop, which is long. While the secondary structure of these proteins is known, their tertiary structure is still unknown due to lack of X-ray crystallographic data.

The highest homology among the cloned human transporters is found between DAT (Figure 11.9) and NET. This is not surprising considering the close structural resemblance of the transmitters DA and NE, and this has clear implications for the design of selective DA uptake inhibitors (see below).

The localization of the transporters generally parallels the localization of the DA, NE and serotonin neurones, respectively. Subtypes of the three transporters are not known. However, polymorphic variants are known of both the DAT and the 5-HTT genes.

Inhibition of reuptake of the biogenic amines is either studied by measuring the inhibition of the uptake of the tritiated amines in brain slices, in synaptosomes or in suitable cell lines expressing cloned transporters, alternatively, by displacement of tritiated selective inhibitors of the transporters.

11.3.2   Antidepressant drugs

11.3.2.1   First generation drugs

The pharmacotherapy of depression started in the late 1950s with the introduction of the two drugs iproniazid (**11.27**) and imipramine (**11.29**, Figure 11.10). Iproniazid was originally an antituberculosis drug, but it was noticed that the drug had an antidepressant effect. Structural modifications of the tricyclic antipsychotic drugs (with chlorpromazine (**11.2**, Figure 11.5) as a prototype) led to the 6-7-6 tricyclic compound imipramine. It was subsequently discovered that iproniazid was an unselective, irreversible inhibitor of the enzymes MAO-A and MAO-B which

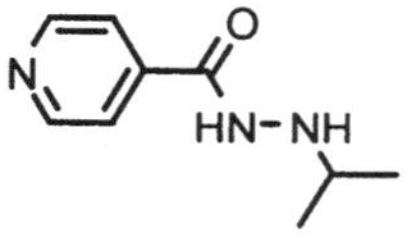

Iproniazid (**11.27**) 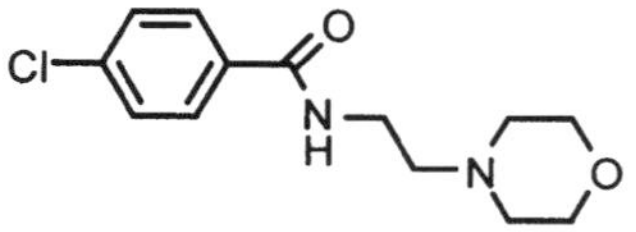   Moclobemide (**11.28**)

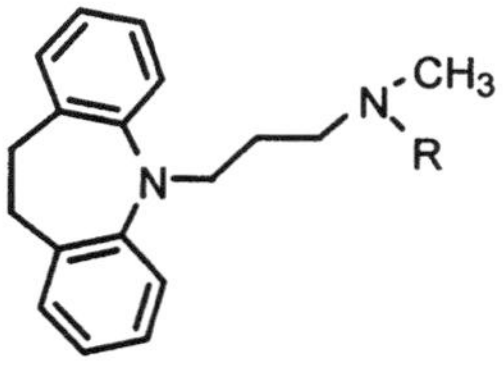

Imipramine (R=CH₃) (**11.29**)   Amitriptyline (R=CH₃) (**11.31**)
Desipramine (R=H) (**11.30**)   Nortriptyline (R=H) (**11.32**)

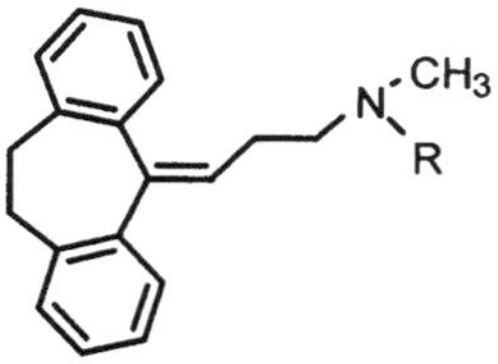

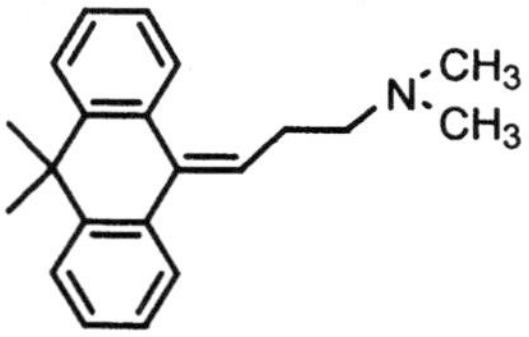

Melitracen (**11.33**)

Figure 11.10 Antidepressant drugs from MAO-inhibitor and tricyclic classes.

deaminate the monoamines NE, DA and 5-HT. Imipramine was found to block the transporters for NE and 5-HT. Both mechanisms led to an increase of the concentrations of NE and 5-HT in the synapse. These observations led to the so-called 'amine hypothesis of depression', saying that, for unknown reasons, there is a decreased availability of these neurotransmitters in depression.

Although the discovery of these two different classes of drugs was of major therapeutic importance, it quickly turned out that both types had serious side effects. Treatment with MAO inhibitors could induce a hypertensive crisis because of a fatal interaction with foodstuffs such as cheese, containing tyramine. It was therefore necessary to introduce dietary restrictions during treatment with MAO inhibitors. Reversible MAO-A (responsible for the breakdown of NE and 5-HT) inhibitors have been developed later (such as moclobemide (**11.28**)), but such drugs are still not totally devoid of the 'cheese-effect' because the tyramine potentiation is inherent to blockade of MAO-A in the periphery. The MAO inhibitors are therefore only used to a small extent in the antidepressant therapy of today.

A major problem with the tricyclic antidepressants such as imipramine (**11.29**), desipramine (**11.30**), amitriptyline (**11.31**), nortriptyline (**11.32**) and melitracen (**11.33**) is that, due to their fundamental tricyclic structures, in addition to their blockade of 5-HTT and/or NET, they also block a number of postsynaptic receptors notably for NE, acetylcholine and histamine (Figure 11.11). Therefore, they may induce a number of anticholinergic and cardiovascular side effects, such as dryness of the mouth, constipation, confusion, dizziness, orthostatic hypotension, tachycardia or arrhytmia, and sedation. Moreover, they are toxic in overdose.

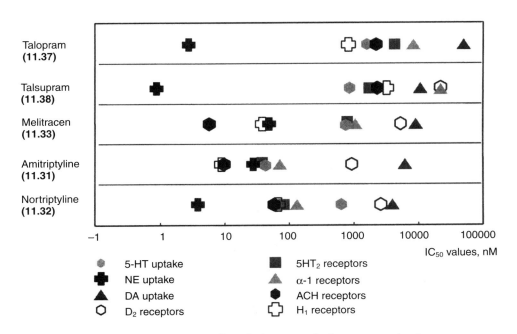

Figure 11.11 Receptor profiles of talopram and talsupram vs. tricyclics.

So, even if these drugs represented a major therapeutic break-through, it quickly became clear that there was a need for better and more safe drugs.

11.3.2.2   The selective serotonin reuptake inhibitors (SSRIs)

As can be seen from Figure 11.11, nortriptyline (**11.32**) is a relative selective NE uptake inhibitor, while the corresponding dimethyl derivative, amitriptyline (**11.31**), is a mixed 5-HT/NE uptake inhibitor with concomitant high affinity for the postsynaptic receptors mentioned above. The same is true for the corresponding pair imipramine/desipramine. Paul Kielholz coupled these observations to the clinical profiles of these drugs, and Arvid Carlsson noticed that the tertiary amine drugs, which were mixed 5-HT and NE uptake inhibitors, were 'mood elevating', while the secondary amines, being primarily NE uptake inhibitors, increased more 'drive' in the depressed patients. Because the foremost quality of an antidepressant drug should be mood elevation (elevation of drive before mood could induce a suicidal event), Carlsson advocated for the development of selective serotonin reuptake inhibitors. Consequently, a number of companies started discovery programmes aimed on designing such drugs in the early 1970s.

11.3.2.2.1   Citalopram discovery

In the middle of the 1960s, chemists at H. Lundbeck A/S were looking for more potent derivatives of the tricyclic compounds amitriptyline, nortriptyline and melitracen which the company had developed and marketed in the years before. The trifluoromethyl group had in other in-house projects proved to increase potency in thioxanthene derivatives with antipsychotic activity (see Figure 11.5), and it was therefore decided to attempt to synthesize the 2-CF$_3$ derivative (**11.35**) of melitracen (Figure 11.12). The precursor molecule **11.34** was readily synthesized, but attempts to ring-close it in a manner corresponding to the existing melitracen method, using concentrated sulfuric acid, failed. However, another product was formed which through meticulous structural elucidation proved to be the bicyclic phthalane (or dihydroisobenzofuran) derivative **11.36**. Fortunately, this compound was examined in test models for antidepressant activity, and was very surprisingly found to be a selective NET inhibitor. Some derivatives were synthesized, among them two compounds that later got the INN (International Nonproprietary Name), names talopram (**11.37**) and talsupram (**11.38**). These compounds are still among the most selective NE uptake inhibitors (SNRIs) ever synthesized (Figure 11.11 and Table 11.3).

Both talopram and talsupram were investigated for antidepressant effect in clinical trials but were stopped in Phase II for various reasons, among which were an activating profile in accordance with their potent NE uptake inhibition and the suggestion from Carlsson of rather looking for selective serotonin uptake inhibitors. A project was therefore started in early 1971 with the aim of developing an SSRI from the talopram structure.

It may look strange to use an SNRI as template structure for an SSRI. However, in the first series synthesized, two compounds (**11.40** and **11.41**, Table 11.2) without dimethylation of the phthalane ring showed a tendency for increased 5-HT uptake, and in accordance with the structure–activity relationships mentioned above

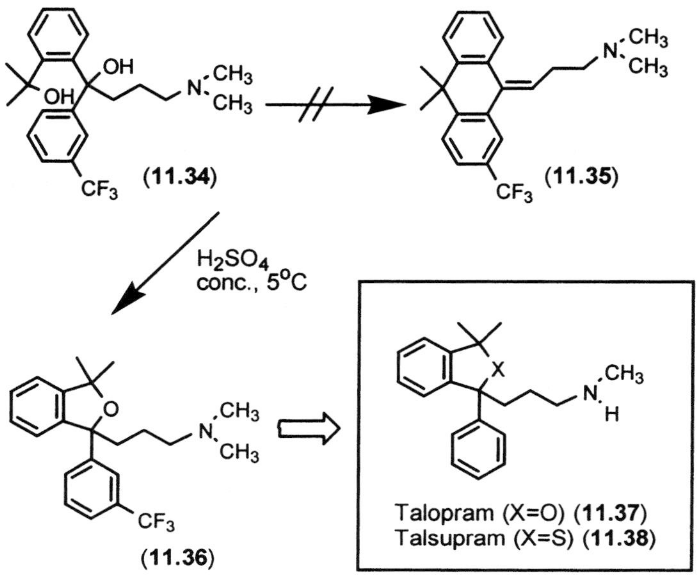

Figure 11.12 Discovery of phenylphthalane antidepressants.

Table 11.2 5-HT and NE uptake inhibition of selected talopram derivatives

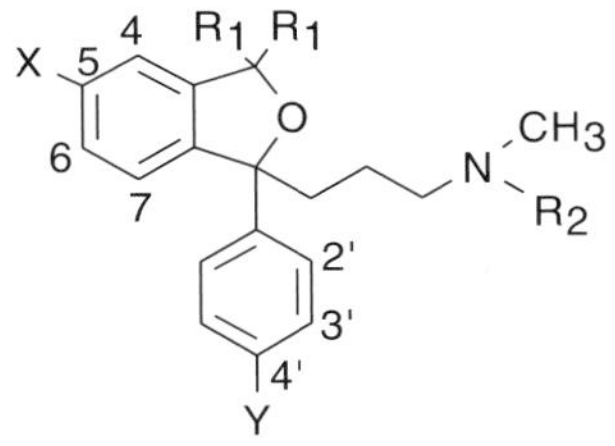

Compound	R_1	R_2	X	Y	5-HT uptake (in vitro) Rabbit blood pl. IC_{50} (nM)	NE uptake (in vivo) Mouse heart ED_{50} (μmol/kg)
Talopram (11.37)	CH_3	H	H	H	3400	2.2
(11.39)	CH_3	CH_3	H	H	53000	5
(11.40)	H	H	H	H	1300	43
(11.41)	H	CH_3	H	H	600	66
(11.42)	H	CH_3	H	Cl	110	170
(11.43)	H	CH_3	Cl	H	220	>200
(11.44)	H	CH_3	Cl	Cl	24	>80
(11.45)	H	CH_3	H	Br	310	NT
(11.46)	H	CH_3	H	CN	54	23
(11.47)	H	CH_3	CN	Cl	10	>80
Citalopram (11.48)	H	CH_3	CN	F	38	>40

Source: Data from Lundbeck Screening Database.

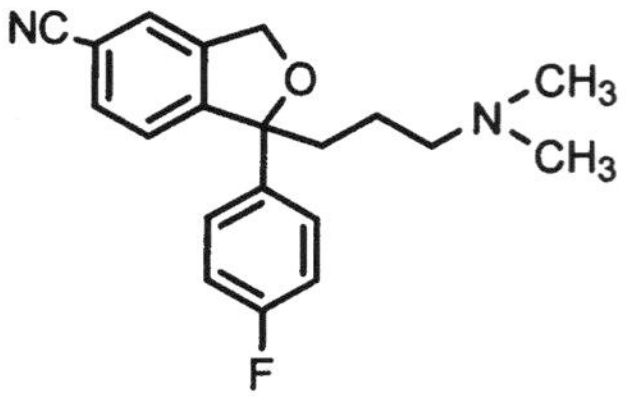

Citalopram (**11.48**)
14.1.1976

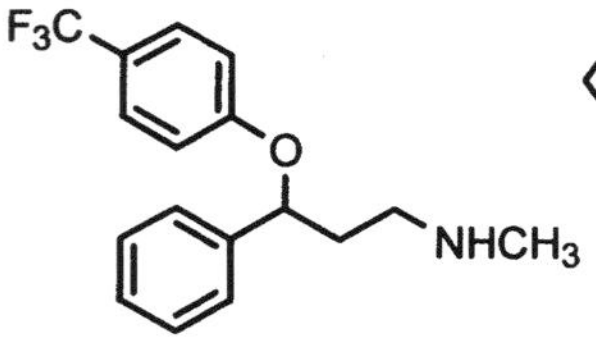

Fluoxetine (**11.49**)
10.1.1974

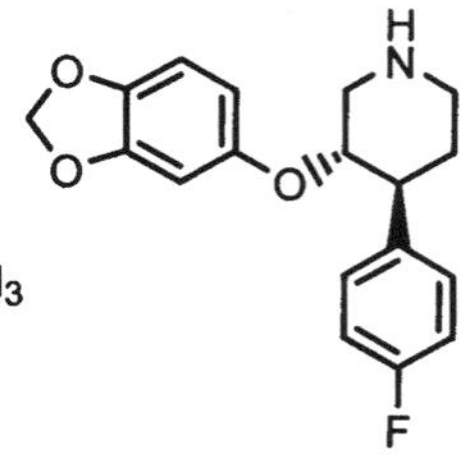

Paroxetine (**11.50**)
30.1.1973

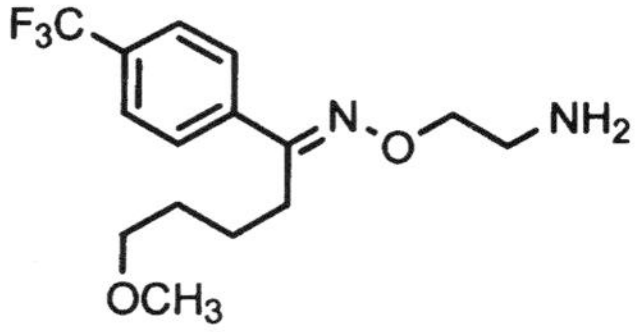

Fluvoxamine (**11.51**)
20.3.1975

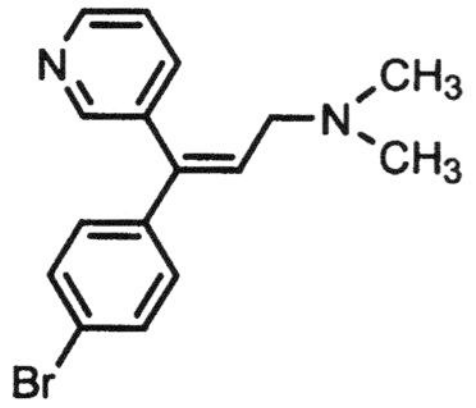

Zimelidine (**11.52**)
28.04.1971

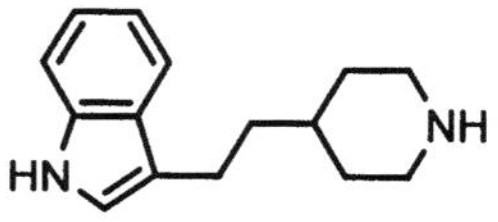

Indalpine (**11.53**)
12.12.1975

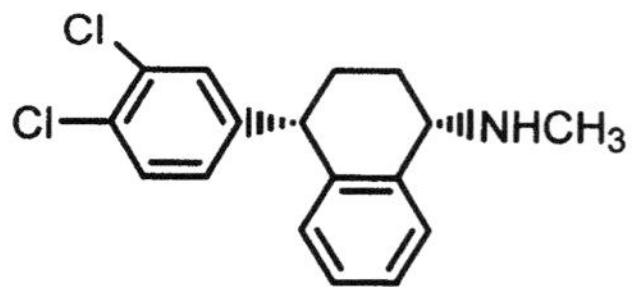

Sertraline (**11.54**)
1.11.1979

Figure 11.13 Selective serotonin reuptake inhibitors (SSRIs).

for tricyclics, the *N,N*-dimethyl derivative **11.41** was the more potent. Therefore, compound **11.41** became a template structure for further structural elucidation.

In this phase of the project, test models for measuring neuronal uptake were not available, so 5-HT uptake inhibition was measured as inhibition of tritiated 5-HT into rabbit blood platelets, while inhibition of NE uptake was measured *ex vivo* as inhibition of tritiated NE into the mouse heart (Table 11.2). Although these models were not directly comparable, they were acceptable as long as the goal was development of selective compounds.

Chlorination of the template structure **11.41**, further increased 5-HT uptake and decreased NE uptake inhibition (**11.42** and **11.43**), again in accordance with observations by Carlsson that halogenation both in zimelidine (**11.52**, Figure 11.13) (see below) derivatives and in the 2-chloro derivative of imipramine (clomipramine) increased 5-HT uptake. And indeed, the dichlorinated **11.44** derivative proved to be a selective 5-HT uptake inhibitor! So the goal of obtaining an

SSRI from an SNRI was actually achieved very fast (in 1971), when less than 50 compounds had been synthesized.

Structure–activity relationships were further explored, and it was established that high activity generally was found in 5, 4'-disubstituted compounds where both substituents were halogen or other electron-withdrawing groups. Cyano-substituted compounds were obtained by reaction of the bromo precursors (e.g. **11.45**) with CuCN. One of the cyano-substituted compounds was (**11.48**), later known as citalopram. The compound was synthesized for the first time in August 1972. It was feared that the cyano group might be metabolically labile, but this was subsequently shown not to be the case neither in animals nor in humans. Citalopram displayed the best overall preclinical profile and was consequently selected for development. The 5-cyano substituent in citalopram also proved to be surprisingly chemically stable, e.g. it was not attacked by Grignard reagents, which led to a new and patentable process for its production.

Citalopram was launched in Denmark in 1989, and it has since been registered in 73 countries worldwide. Citalopram is a racemate, having an asymmetric carbon at the 1-position. When it was synthesized in 1972, classical resolution via diastereomeric salts was the only realistic alternative for separation of the enantiomers. However, it is generally difficult to make salts of citalopram, and the few salts which were successfully prepared from chiral acids showed no resolution after recrystallizations. Finally, an intermediate was resolved in this way, and the resolved intermediate could then be transformed into the pure S- and R-enantiomers. Subsequent testing showed that all the 5-HT uptake inhibition resided in the S-enantiomer. The high stereospecificity was later rationalized in the 5-HTT pharmacophore model discussed in Section 11.3.2.2.3. The pure S-enantiomer has subsequently been developed (INN name escitalopram) and is successfully produced by Simulated Moving Bed (SMB) separation of enantiomers.

11.3.2.2.2 Other SSRIs

In Figure 11.13 are shown the seven SSRIs that have reached the market. The dates are the priority dates of the first patent applications. However, the two first compounds on the market were both withdrawn due to serious, although rare, side effects. Zimelidine (**11.52**) was found to induce an influenza-like symptom in 1–2% of the patients, which in rare cases (1/10 000) resulted in the so-called Guillain-Barré syndrome. The drug was withdrawn in 1983 after $1\frac{1}{2}$ years on the market. Indalpine (**11.53**) induced agranulocytosis in 1/20 000 patients and was withdrawn in 1984.

As it appears from Figure 11.13, all the marketed SSRIs (except sertraline) was discovered in the first half of the 1970s, meaning that the companies had no detailed information regarding the structural classes their competitors were developing. Accordingly, rather diverse (at least at first sight) structures were developed. However, they were all selective serotonin inhibitors (Table 11.3), although their selectivity ratios vary significantly, citalopram/escitalopram being the most selective compounds. The SSRIs generally have low affinity for receptors for DA, NE and 5-HT and other neurotransmitters, although exceptions exist. With regard to interaction with P450 enzymes there are important differences, e.g. paroxetine and fluoxetine having significant affinity for CYP2D6.

Table 11.3 The effect of SSRIs, talopram and talsupram on the inhibition of uptake of 5-HT, NE and DA

Compound	Uptake inhibition IC_{50} (nM)			Ratio	
	5-HT	NE	DA	NE/5-HT	DA/5-HT
Citalopram (**11.48**)	3.9	6100	40000	1560	10300
Escitalopram (S)-(**11.48**)	2.1	2500	65000	1200	31000
R-citalopram (R)-(**11.48**)	275	6900	54000	25	200
Indalpine (**11.53**)	2.1	2100	1200	1000	570
Sertraline (**11.54**)	0.19	160	48	840	250
Paroxetine (**11.50**)	0.29	81	5100	280	17600
Fluvoxamine (**11.51**)	3.8	620	42000	160	11000
Zimeldine (**11.52**)	56	3100	26000	55	460
Fluoxetine (**11.49**)	6.8	370	5000	54	740
Talopram (**11.37**)	1400	2.5	44000	0.0017	0.00006[a]
Talsupram (**11.38**)	770	0.79	9300	0.0010	0.00008[a]

Note

a   NE/DA; Data from Hyttel, J. (1994) Pharmacological Characterization of Selective Serotonin Reuptake Inhibitors (SSRIs). *Int. Clin. Psychopharmacology*, **9** Suppl. 1, 19–26 and Lundbeck Screening Database.

11.3.2.2.3   *The 5-HTT pharmacophore model*

Despite very different molecular structures, the SSRIs all bind to the serotonin transporter. As information about the 3D-structure of the transporter was lacking, development of a pharmacophore model was of major interest. Generally, published pharmacophoric models for 5-HT-uptake inhibitors only include one aromatic moiety and the basic nitrogen atom in the construction of the pharmacophore. The distance between these pharmacophoric elements is comparable to the distance found in serotonin itself. The second phenyl ring found in many 5-HT-uptake inhibitors shows no spatial correlation in these models.

Recently, we have developed a pharmacophore model of the 5-HT uptake site based on extensive conformational studies and superimpositions of SSRIs and other uptake inhibitors (Figure 11.14). In contrast to previous models, this model operates with two aromatic ring binding sites, and a site point 2.8 Å away from the nitrogen atom in the direction of the lone pair as fitting points. This site point mimics a hypothetical hydrogen-binding site on the 5-HT transporter. The basic nitrogen atom of the SSRIs is not always superimposable. However, when the site points are used instead, very good superimpositions are obtained. Many SSRIs have aromatic substituents (cyano, trifluoromethyl, chloro, methylendioxo etc.), and these substituents all occupy the volume marked with yellow on Figure 11.14.

The model has been validated with a number of 5-HT-uptake inhibitors in addition to the compounds in Figure 11.13. However, importantly the model explains the more than 100-fold stereoselectivity of citalopram enantiomers. It is possible to find a conformation of R-citalopram that is superimposable on the active conformation of S-citalopram, however, the energy penalty is 2.8 kcal/mol. This corresponds closely to a 100-fold affinity difference. The enantiomers of fluoxetine show no stereoselectivity and this is explained in a similar way.

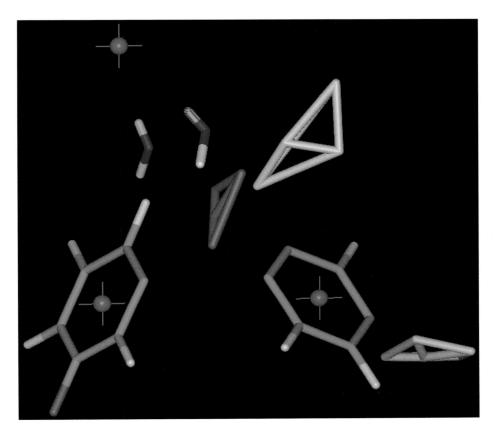

Figure 11.14 Pharmacophore model of the 5-HT uptake site. Green: Phenyl ring binding sites. Blue: Nitrogen atoms. Pink: Transporter interaction site-point. Yellow: Allowed volume for SSRI substituents. White: Forbidden volume at 5-HTT, allowed at NET. Red: Possible hydrogen bond acceptor site. For further discussions on pharmacophore models see Chapter 4.

As mentioned above, the SNRI talopram was transformed into the SSRI, citalopram, by making relatively small changes in the molecule. A similar observation was made by researchers at Eli Lilly in their fluoxetine series, because the SSRI profile of this compound could be changed into an SNRI profile by replacing the *p*-trifluoromethyl group of fluoxetine with an *O*-methyl (tomoxetine) or an *O*-methoxy (nisoxetine (**11.55**)) substituent (Figure 11.15). Later other SNRIs such as reboxetine (**11.56**) and viloxazine (**11.57**) were developed. Talopram, nisoxetine and tomoxetine can be acccomodated without problems in the SSRI model in low-energy conformations, leading to the conclusion that the change in profile must be due to unfavorable steric interactions of the SNRIs substituents at the 5-HTT site. Superimposition studies confirmed that the 3,3-dimethyl substituents of talopram, the methyl and methoxy groups of tomoxetine and nisoxetine, and the ethoxy groups of reboxetine and viloxazine all occupy the same volume (marked as the

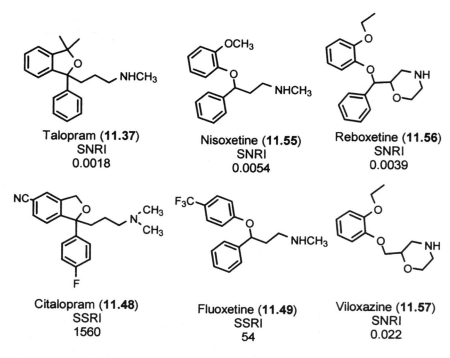

Figure 11.15 Structurally related SNRIs and SSRIs. NET/5-HTT IC_{50} ratio shown.

white pyramidal structure on Figure 11.14) in space. This volume is therefore 'forbidden' at the 5-HTT site.

Certain aspects, such as the original observation of a change from mixed inhibitors in tricyclics with dimethylamino group to NE uptake inhibitors in corresponding monomethyl derivatives still remain to be explained. The amine group in SSRIs varies from primary to secondary and tertiary amines, including heterocyclic amines.

11.3.2.3 Unmet needs and new treatment strategies

Due to their high safety in use, the SSRIs have been extremely successful, and a number of new indications (e.g. panic disorder, obsessive compulsive disorder, social phobia) have been registered for many of the drugs in addition to major depression. However, there are still two major problems in the treatment of depression: Slow onset-of-action (4–6 weeks) in the patients and treatment resistance in up to 30% of the patients.

While the reasons for treatment resistance remain unclear, hypotheses regarding the slow onset of SSRIs have been formulated. The SSRIs exert their antidepressant effect through the stimulation of various postsynaptic receptors by the serotonin that is accumulating as a consequence of the uptake inhibition. However, extracellular 5-HT will not only increase in projection areas but also in the cell body region (the raphé region). The resulting stimulation of somatodendritic 5-HT$_{1A}$ receptors here (see Figure 11.1, T = 5-HTT and AR$_1$ = 5-HT$_{1A}$ receptors) will inhibit synaptic 5-HT release, thereby counteracting the acute effect of SSRIs. These receptors desensitize over a time period congruent with the delay in antidepressant effect of SSRIs. 5-HT uptake inhibition with concomitant 5-HT$_{1A}$ blockade may therefore result in a faster onset of action of SSRIs. Animal experiments with combinations of SSRIs and 5-HT$_{1A}$ antagonists, and preliminary clinical trials with combinations of SSRIs and pindolol (a β-blocker with additional 5-HT$_{1A}$ antagonistic effect) seem to confirm this hypothesis.

11.3.3 Dopamine uptake inhibitors

In relation to drug development, there has been less focus on dopamine uptake inhibitors than on 5-HT and NE uptake inhibitors. This is due to their inherent stimulatory effect that may complicate development and may lead to a risk of drug addiction and abuse. However, compounds with a different pharmacokinetic profile than cocaine (which is a mixed DA, NE and 5-HT uptake inhibitor) may on the other hand be useful for treatment of the same conditions in cocaine abusers. Moreover, in certain conditions (e.g. Parkinson's disease) and as an additional element in antidepressants DA uptake inhibition may be useful. In fact, two antidepressants, nomifensine (**11.58**) and bupropion (**11.65**) (Figure 11.16) has significant DA uptake inhibition, although nomifensine is an even more potent NE uptake inhibitor, and bupropion is a relatively weak DA/NE uptake inhibitor. Nomifensine did have a stimulant antidepressant profile, but was withdrawn in 1986 due to induction of acute haemolytic anemia. Bupropion is both used as antidepressant and for the treatment of smoking cessation. Another mixed uptake inhibitor is mazindol (**11.61**) that is used in the treatment of obesity.

11.3.3.1 *Structural considerations*

Besides nomifensine, bupropion and mazindol, a number of pharmaceutical companies developed mixed inhibitors of DA, NE and 5-HT uptake in the 1980s (Figure 11.16). However, these efforts did not lead to new drugs in any of the cases, probably due to the problems with development of stimulating drugs mentioned above.

All of these compounds are potent inhibitors of DA and NE uptake, and with the exception of nomifensine, bupropion and **11.64** they are also 5-HT-uptake inhibitors. Optimum activity is invariably found in compounds with 3′,4′-dichloro-substitution. Furthermore, it was reported that the 3′,4′-dichlorophenyl ring had a similar spatial orientation in the more potent enantiomer (*S*-configuration in all cases). Based on these facts, we proposed a 'qualitative' pharmacophore model for DA-uptake inhibitors consisting of a phenyl ring (ring A, with an optimal 3′,4′-dichloro-substitution) and a nitrogen atom held by a molecular framework in a position to each other that mimics the fully extended (antiperiplanar) conformation of DA. A further common structural element is the second phenyl ring 'B', held in an optimal position to ring 'A' and the nitrogen atom by the molecular framework.

The 3-phenyl-1-indanamines is a rare example of how a single scaffold by extensive substitution and stereo SAR studies can be used for drug development

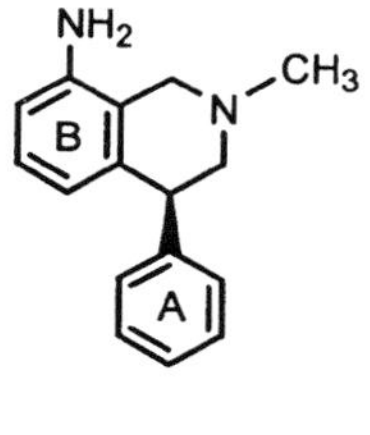

Nomifensine (**11.58**) 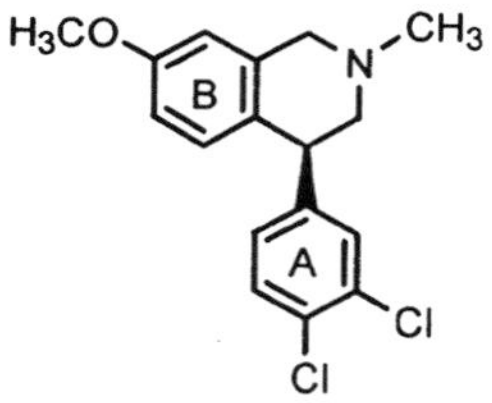   Diclofensine (**11.59**) 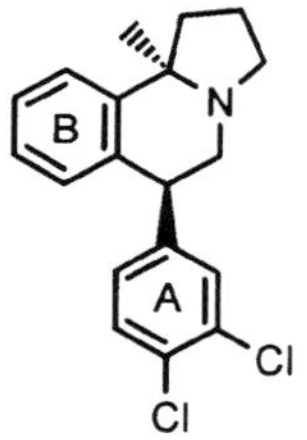   (**11.60**) 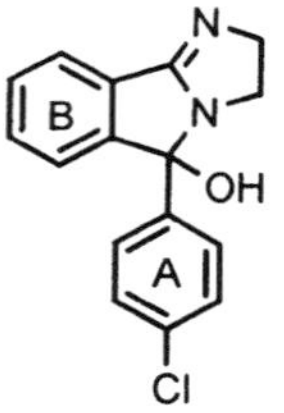   Mazindol (**11.61**)

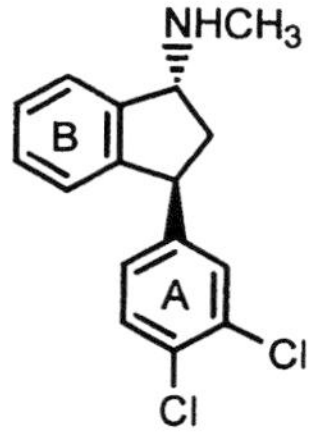

Indatraline (**11.62**)   (**11.63**) 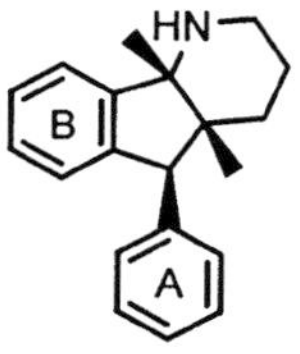   (**11.64**) 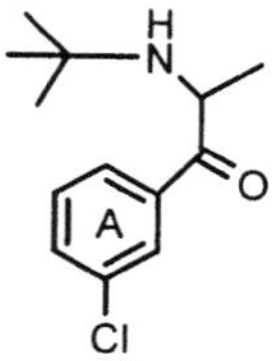   Bupropion (**11.65**)
(1*R*,3*S*)-enantiomer

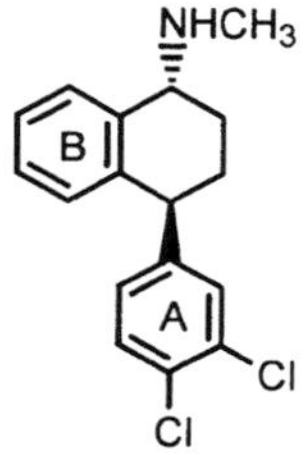

Figure 11.16 Dopamine uptake inhibitors.

on both transporters and receptors for the same neurotransmitters. The 3-D SAR of this class of compounds is shown in Figure 11.17, and has been described in detail elsewhere (Bøgesø, further reading). Briefly, small amine derivatives (notably dimethyl or monomethyl) are inhibitors of 5-HT, NE and DA uptake with *cis*-isomers being predominantly 5-HT (and NE) uptake inhibitors, while *trans*-isomers such as indatraline (**11.62**) are potent inhibitors of all three transporters (note that a corresponding SAR is observed in the tetralines where sertraline is an SSRI, while the *trans*-isomer, **11.63**, Figure 11.16, is a mixed inhibitor of all three transporters). (1*R*, 3*S*)-3-Phenyl-1-piperazinoindans are potent antagonists of DA, 5-HT$_2$ and α_1 receptors with the highest activity confined to 6, 4′-disubstituted compounds (see also Section 11.2.2.2.1 and Chapter 4). The (1*S*, 3*R*)- and (1*R*, 3*R*)-enantiomers are potent DA and NE uptake inhibitors (maximal activity in 3,4-dichloro substituted derivatives), while the (1*S*, 3*S*)-enantiomers are inactive.

As mentioned, cocaine (**11.66**, Figure 11.18) is an equally potent inhibitor of the uptake of DA, NE and 5-HT. Although its euphorigenic effects are mainly believed to be associated with its DA potentiating effects, it is possible that the increased levels of NE and 5-HT also contribute both to the positive (euphoric) and to the negative (anxiogenic effect) of cocaine in humans. Another element, which has been suggested to be important for cocaine euphoria, is the rapid (and short-lasting) rate of DAT occupancy and the resulting DA increase that follows cocaine intake. The DA-uptake inhibitors have, therefore, been in focus in the treatment of cocaine abuse. An ideal drug would bind to the cocaine binding site without affecting the transport of DA itself. A way to search for such a compound could

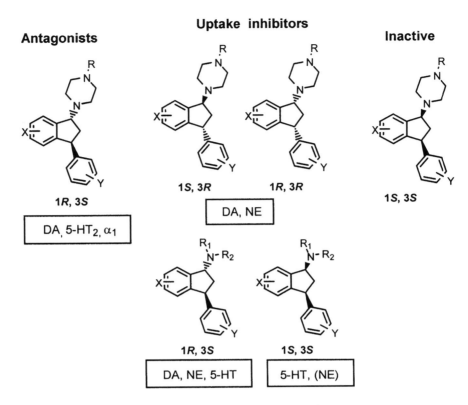

Figure 11.17 Stereo SAR of 3-phenyl-1-indanamines.

be to look for compounds with a high affinity for the binding site of a cocaine ligand and a low potency for inhibiting uptake of tritiated DA.

The cocaine scaffold has therefore, especially in recent years, also been subject to extensive SAR studies, including syntheses of an abundance of derivatives. Many groups have found that the ester bond between the phenyl ring and the tropane amine can be deleted, thus increasing stability and also potency. One of these compounds is WIN 35,428 (**11.67**) which is also used as a binding ligand for DAT in a tritiated form. Further increase in potency and stability is obtained in brasofensine (**11.68**) which has the optimal 3,4-dichloro-substitution and where the methylester is replaced by an methyl oxime ether. This compound is in development for the treatment of Parkinson's disease. Very interesting studies have shown that the basic nitrogen of the tropane ring, which was considered to be an essential pharmacophoric element, can be replaced with both oxygen (O-914, **11.69**) and carbon (O-1414, **11.70**) without consequence for DAT uptake inhibition. Whether a similar replacement is possible in other DAT inhibitors still remains to be shown.

Finally, straight chain analogs of the piperazinoindans are also potent and selective DA uptake inhibitors. One of these compounds (vanoxerine, GBR 12,909, **11.71**) has been investigated in depression, but with negative results, implicating

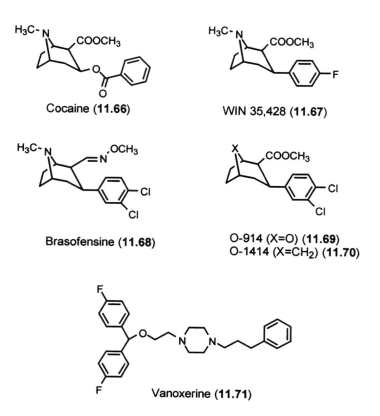

Cocaine (11.66)

WIN 35,428 (11.67)

Brasofensine (11.68)

O-914 (X=O) (11.69)
O-1414 (X=CH$_2$) (11.70)

Vanoxerine (11.71)

Figure 11.18 Dopamine uptake inhibitors derived from cocaine and vanoxerine.

that concomitant 5-HT and/or NE uptake inhibition probably is a prerequisite for antidepressant action.

FURTHER READING

Arnt, J. and Skarsfeldt, T. (1998) Do novel antipsychotics have similar pharmacological characteristics? A review of the evidence. *Neuropsychopharmacology*, **18**, 63–101.

Barnes, N.M. and Sharp, T. (1999) A review of central 5-HT receptors and their function. *Neuropharmacology*, **38**, 1083–1152.

Bøgesø, K.P. (1998) *Drug Hunting: The Medicinal Chemistry of 1-Piperazino-3-Phenylindanes and Related Compounds*. Copenhagen, Denmark. Copy may be obtained from author.

Emilien, G., Maloteaux, J.-M., Geurts, M., Hoogenberg, K. and Cragg, S. (1999) Dopamine receptor-physiological understanding to therapeutic intervention potential. *Pharmacology & Therapeutics*, **84**, 133–156.

Hrib, N.J. (2000) The dopamine D$_4$ receptor: a controversial therapeutic target. *Drug of the Future*, **25**, 587–611.

Kinon, B.J. and Lieberman, J.A. (1996) Mechanisms of action of atypical antipsychotic drugs: a critical analysis. *Psychopharmacology*, **124**, 2–34.

Meador-Woodruff, J.H., Damask, S.P., Wang, J., Haroutunian, V., Davis, K.L. and Watson, S.J. (1996) Dopamine receptor mRNA expression in human striatum and neucortex. *Neuropsychopharmacology*, **15**, 17–29.

Pinder, R.M. and Wieriga, J.H. (1993) Third-generation antidepressants. *Medicinal Research Reviews*, **13**, 259–325.

Rowley, M., Bristow, L.J. and Hutson, P.H. (2001) Current and novel approaches to the drug treatment of schizophrenia. *J. Med. Chem.*, **44**, 477–501.

Snyder, S.H. (1996) *Drugs and the Brain*. New York: Scientific American Library; 18, W.H. Freeman and Company.

Chapter 12

Enzymes and enzyme inhibitors

Robert A. Copeland and Paul S. Anderson

12.1 INTRODUCTION

Every aspect of cell biology, from intermediate metabolism to protein synthesis to catabolism, requires the chemistry of bond forming and bond breaking reactions at various steps. The majority of these common chemical reactions, however, proceed at spontaneous rates that are too slow to support life. Hence, all living organisms rely on the catalytic power of enzymes to accelerate reaction rates, and thus sustain life.

While the importance of enzymatic catalysis in normal physiology cannot be overstated, aberrant catalysis can also play an important role in a variety of human diseases. A significant number of genetic disorders, for example, result in the overexpression or mutation-based gain of function for key enzymes of metabolic pathways. Other diseases, such as cancers and inflammatory diseases, involve aberrant hyperproliferation of specific cell types. The metabolic pathways that fuel cell proliferation all involve enzyme catalysis, making the enzymes of these pathways attractive targets for chemotherapeutic intervention. Enzymatic catalysis is required not only for human life, but also for life in micro-organisms (e.g. viral, bacterial and protozoan life) and larger parasites that infect human beings. Hence, essential enzyme functions within these organisms are also attractive targets for infectious disease therapies.

It is not surprising, then, that the abolition of aberrant enzyme activity, through the administration of small molecule enzyme inhibitors, is a common strategy for pharmaceutical intervention in human diseases. In fact, a recent survey demonstrates that nearly 30% of all drugs in current clinical use elicit their pharmacological effects by inhibition of specific enzyme targets. As new targets are identified through the recent advances in genomic and proteomic sciences, the proportion of drugs that act through enzyme inhibition is likely to increase further. Hence, a significant effort is put forth by the pharmaceutical community to target key enzymes for inhibition by small molecular weight, orally bioavailable drugs. Table 12.1 gives some sense of the breadth of enzyme targets that are currently being pursued for this purpose.

A critical step towards the identification and optimization of small molecule inhibitors of specific enzymes is a thorough understanding of the reaction mechanism of the target enzyme, and of the chemical and structural basis for ligand interactions with the enzyme. In this chapter, we present an introduction to some of the key features of enzymatic catalysis and enzyme–inhibitor interactions that

Table 12.1 Some examples of enzymes that are targets for current drugs and experimental therapeutic agents

Compound	Target enzyme	Clinical use
Acetazolamide	Carbonic anhydrase	Glaucoma
Acyclovir	Viral DNA polymerase	Herpes
AG7088	Rhinovirus 3C protease	Common Colds
Allopurinol	Xanthine oxidase	Gout
Argatroban	Thrombin	Heart disease
Aspirin	Cyclooxygenases	Inflammation
Amoxicillin	Penicillin binding proteins	Bacterial infections
Captopril, Enalapril	Angiotensin converting enzyme	Hypertension
Carbidopa	Dopa decarboxylase	Parkinson's disease
CELEBREX, VIOXX	Cyclooxygenase-2	Inflammation
Clavulinate	β-lactamase	Bacterial resistance
Digoxin	Sodium, potassium ATPase	Heart disease
Efavirenz, Nevirapine	HIV-1 reverse transcriptase	AIDS
Epristeride, Finasteride	Steroid 5α-reductase	Benign prostate hyperplasia, Male pattern baldness
Fluorouracil	Thymidylate synthase	Cancer
Leflunomide	Dihydroorotate dehydrogenase	Inflammation
Lovastatin	HMG-CoA reductase	Cholesterol lowering
Methotrexate	Dihydrofolate reductase	Cancer, Inflammation
Nitecapone	Catechol-O-methyltransferase	Parkinson's disease
Norfloxacin	DNA gyrase	Urinary tract inflections
Omeprazole	H^+, K^+-ATPase	Peptic ulcers
PALA	Aspartate transcarbamoylase	Cancer
Sorbinol	Aldose reductase	Diabetic retinopathy
Trimethoprim	Bacterial Dihydrofolate reductase	Bacterial Infections
VIAGRA	Phosphodiesterase	Erectile Dysfunction

Source: Adapted and expanded from Copeland, R.A. (2000) *Enzymes: A Practicle Introduction to Structure, Mechanism and Data Analysis*, 2nd edition. New York: Wiley-VCH.

form the basis of enzymology-based drug discovery. We shall see that enzymes function to accelerate specific chemical reactions through common thermo-dynamic mechanisms. These mechanisms involve a sequential series of enzyme–ligand binding interactions that facilitate the chemical transformations of the substrate molecule to the reaction product. Small molecules that mimic these specific binding interactions prove to be high-affinity ligands for the enzyme, and thus provide a basis for inhibitor design. We shall see further that to facilitate the chemical transformations of the substrate, enzymes often undergo dynamic structural changes during catalysis. These conformational transitions, within the ligand binding site and elsewhere on the enzyme molecule, create novel structural features that can be targeted by small molecule inhibitors.

12.2 CHEMICAL MECHANISMS OF ENZYME CATALYSIS

Speed and reaction fidelity are two requirements of biochemical reactions for the sustainment of life. Hence, enzymes have evolved to facilitate these reactions by greatly accelerating the reaction rates and by acting on specific reactant molecules (referred to as substrates). In this section, we shall explore the structural and chemical mechanisms by which enzymes achieve reaction rate acceleration and substrate specificity. In all of the discussion that follows, it is important for the reader to recognize that enzymes, like all other catalysts, cannot alter the thermo-dynamics of chemical reactions; rather they can only accelerate the rates at which these reactions occur. Recall that the Gibb's free energy of a reaction is a path-independent function, depending only on the initial and final states of the reaction system. Since the reactants (substrates) and products of the uncatalyzed and enzyme–catalyzed reactions are identical, it must be true that ΔG of both reactions is the same:

$$\Delta G_{\text{uncatalyzed}} = \Delta G_{\text{enzyme-catalyzed}} \tag{12.1}$$

Thus, as stated above, the catalytic power of enzymes results from their ability to recognize specific substrates and to accelerate the rate at which these molecules are converted to reaction products. These common features of enzyme catalysis can be understood in terms of the reaction pathway through which enzyme reactions proceed, and particularly in terms of the attainment of the transition state of the reaction.

12.2.1   Transition-state theory in enzyme catalysis

All chemical reactions proceed through a high energy, short-lived virtual state commonly referred to as the *transition state* of the reaction. This concept is well illustrated by the reaction of an alkyl halide with a hydroxide ion to form an alcohol (Figure 12.1A). As the reaction proceeds the carbon–halide bond is ruptured and a new carbon–oxygen bond is formed. One can imagine that at some moment during the reaction, the reactive carbon exists in a pseudo-pentacoordinate state in which partial bonds exist simultaneously with both the halide and the oxygen atoms; this species is the transition state. Clearly, such a state would be extremely unstable, occurring at a very high free energy and for a very short time (typical transition state half-lives are ca. 10^{-13} s). Nevertheless, the reaction must attain this transition state to proceed to products. As illustrated in the free energy diagram in Figure 12.1B, attainment of the transition state represents the most energetically costly step in the reaction pathway, and thus limits the rate at which the system proceeds from the reactant state to the product state.

   All enzymes accelerate the rates of chemical reactions by a common mechanism: by lowering the energy barrier to attaining the reaction transition state. Let us consider a simple enzymatic reaction in which a single substrate molecule is converted into a single product. The enzyme catalyzed reaction proceeds through a number of intermediate states. First, the free enzyme and substrate molecules must encounter one another,

$$E + S \underset{K_S}{\rightleftharpoons} ES$$

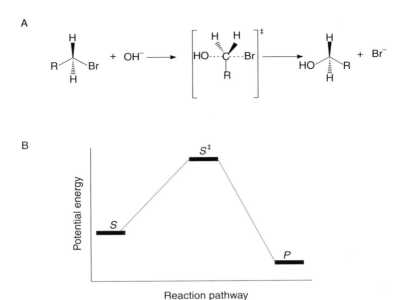

Figure 12.1 (A) Reaction of an alkyl halide with hydroxide ion, illustrating the reaction transition state; and (B) free energy diagram for the reaction profile of a simple chemical reaction.

through diffusion-controlled collision, and bind each other to form an initial encounter complex. This binary complex is referred to as the *ES* or Michaelis complex. Under equilibrium conditions the formation of the *ES* complex is governed by the concentrations of the free enzyme and substrate in solution and by the dissociation constant for the binary complex, K_S.

$$K_S = \frac{[E][S]}{[ES]} \qquad (12.2)$$

Under physiological and most laboratory conditions, the equilibrium favors the *ES* complex, so that there is a net stabilization of the system. This gain in binding energy can in part contribute to the energetic cost of attaining the transition state. After formation of the Michaelis complex, structural rearrangements of the enzyme active site (i.e. the binding pocket where substrate binds) induce changes in the bound substrate, transforming the substrate molecule into its transition state structure. The bound transition state is greatly stabilized within the context of the enzyme bound state, relative to the free form, by a combination of effects to be discussed in Section 12.2.3. The overall effect, however, is to diminish the energy barrier (referred to as the *activation energy*, $\Delta G^{\ddagger}$). From the bound transition state, the system may proceed directly, or through intervening intermediate states, to the bound product state, *EP*, and finally to release of the product molecule and recovery of the free enzyme. Each step subsequent to *ES* formation represents a microequilibrium characterized by a forward and reverse rate constant. These individual steps are often difficult to measure experimentally. Hence, a single forward rate constant, referred to as k_{cat}, is used to collectively represent the rate of forward progress from the ES state to the final free product and free enzyme state. Thus, a minimum reaction scheme for a simple, single substrate enzymatic reaction is as follows:

$$E + S \underset{K_S}{\rightleftharpoons} ES \xrightarrow{k_{cat}} E + P$$

The term K_S represents the dissociation constant for the binary enzyme–substrate complex and can be related to the free energy of binding, ΔG_{ES} as follows:

$$\Delta G_{ES} = -RT \ln\left(\frac{1}{K_S}\right) \tag{12.3}$$

where R is the ideal gas constant and T represents temperature in degrees Kelvin. The term k_{cat} reflects the rate of transition from the bound substrate ground state to the transition state, and can be related to a free energy difference between these two states as:

$$\Delta G_{k_{cat}} = RT\left(\ln\left(\frac{k_B T}{h}\right) - \ln(k_{cat})\right) \tag{12.4}$$

where k_B is the Boltzman constant and h is Planck's constant. The overall activation energy is the energy difference between the free enzyme and substrate state and the transition state, which is given by combining equations (12.3) and (12.4):

$$\Delta G^{\ddagger} = -RT \ln\left(\frac{k_{cat}}{K_S}\right) + RT \ln\left(\frac{k_B T}{h}\right) \tag{12.5}$$

From equation (12.5) we see that the ratio k_{cat}/K_S, which has units of a second order rate constant, is a good measure of the overall rate of the enzyme–catalyzed reaction. The catalytic efficiency of an enzyme is thus measured by the ratio of this second-order rate constant to the second order rate constant for the uncatalyzed reaction ([k_{cat}/K_S]/[$k_{uncatalyzed}$]). By this measure, some enzymes achieve a rate enhancement of some 10^{17} over the uncatalyzed reaction! We also see from equation (12.5) that the binding energy associated with formation of the ES complex is used to offset partially the energetic cost of attainment of the transition state. One strategy that enzymes use to lower the activation barrier of reaction is to partition the energy among several binding complexes, including the ES complex, the EP complex and various intermediate species (Figure 12.2). As we shall see in the next section, however, enzymes also use specific chemical strategies to stabilize the transition state itself. The overall effect, from a combination of factors, is to substantially lower the reaction activation energy, as schematically illustrated in Figure 12.2.

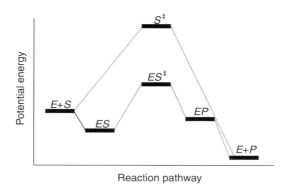

Figure 12.2 Free energy diagram for a simple enzyme–catalyzed reaction, illustrating the reduction in activation energy required to reach the transition state.

In the laboratory, it is most often the case that enzyme reactions are studied under conditions of low concentrations of enzyme and high concentrations of substrate ($[S] \gg [E]$). Under these conditions, product formation is linear with time early in the reaction, until about 10–20% of the substrate has been consumed. During this initial linear phase, the reaction rate or velocity is measured as the slope of the linear product vs. time progress curve. The reaction velocity depends on the concentration of *ES* complex in the system. In the early phase of the reaction, the velocity is constant (i.e. the progress curve is linear) because the system is at a steady state with respect to the concentration of *ES* complex, rather than at equilibrium (i.e. the rate of formation of the *ES* complex is the same as its rate of disappearance so that the concentration remains constant for the duration of the measurement period). Because the system is not in equilibrium under these conditions, the thermodynamic dissociation constant in the above equations must be replaced with a steady-state kinetic term, K_M (also known as the Michaelis constant). If one were to measure the steady-state velocity as a function of substrate concentration for a simple enzyme reaction under these laboratory conditions, the results would appear as illustrated in Figure 12.3A. At low substrate concentrations the velocity increases quasi-linearly with increasing substrate concentration. However, the system saturates at higher substrate concentrations, eventually reaching a maximum velocity, V_{max}, at infinite substrate concentration. This saturable, hyperbolic behavior was first described by Michaelis and Menten and later adapted for a steady-state treatment by Briggs and Haldane. The following equation describes the dependence of steady-state enzyme velocity on substrate concentration, and is known as the Michaelis–Menten equation in honor of the scientists who first defined it.

$$v = \frac{V_{max}[S]}{K_M + [S]} \tag{12.6}$$

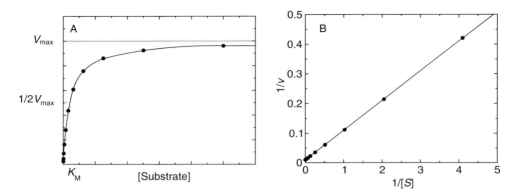

Figure 12.3 (A) Reaction velocity as a function of substrate concentration for a simple enzyme catalyzed reaction; and (B) the same data as in (A) plotted in double reciprocal form.

The term K_M, like K_S, has units of molarity as does the substrate concentration. If we were to fix the substrate concentration at the same numerical value as K_M, and rearrange equation (12.6), we would obtain:

$$v = \frac{V_{max}[S]}{2[S]} = \frac{1}{2}V_{max} \tag{12.7}$$

Equation (12.7) provides a working definition of K_M: K_M is that substrate concentration that yields a velocity equal to half of the maximum velocity under steady-state conditions. Hence, this kinetic term relates to the concentration of substrate required to half saturate the system under steady-state conditions, even though it cannot be equated with a true equilibrium dissociation constant.

The term V_{max} in the above equations can be related to k_{cat} as follows:

$$k_{cat} = \frac{V_{max}}{[E]} \tag{12.8}$$

Thus, enzyme reactions can be quantified in terms of the kinetic parameters k_{cat}, K_M and k_{cat}/K_M. These kinetic constants are obtained by experimentally measuring the reaction velocity as a function of substrate concentration at a fixed, known concentration of enzyme. The resulting data are fit directly to the Michaelis–Menten equation by non-linear regression analysis to obtain estimates of K_M and V_{max}. Alternatively, the data are plotted in double reciprocal form with $1/v$ plotted on the y-axis and $1/[S]$ on the x-axis, producing a linear function. The slope of the linear fit in such plots provides an estimate of the ratio K_M/V_{max} while the y-intercept provides an estimate of $1/V_{max}$ (Figure 12.3B). These double reciprocal plots (also known as Lineweaver–Burk plots) were commonly used in the days prior to the widespread use of personal computers with non-linear curve fitting capacity, and they remain popular today.

As described above, the kinetic constant K_M provides a measure of ground state substrate affinity for the enzyme, while the second order rate constant k_{cat}/K_M provides a measure of the efficiency of transition state lowering by the enzyme, hence a measure of overall catalytic efficiency.

12.2.2   Active site structure stabilizes the transition state

Almost all enzymes in biology are proteins and are thus composed of polypeptide chains of the 20 natural amino acids. The specific details of the 3D-structure into which the polypeptide chain folds defines the tertiary structure of the protein and, in the case of enzymes, also defines the structural details of the binding pocket into which the substrate molecule binds and is chemically transformed into product. This chemically reactive ligand binding pocket is referred to as the enzyme active site. The detailed structure of this active site determines the range of ligand structures that can be bound and the types of chemical transformations that can take place. Generally, the active sites of enzymes are small, mainly hydrophobic pockets that are well shielded from bulk solvent. Initial substrate binding to the active site is generally reversible and is mediated by common reversible chemical interactions with amino acid side chains and main chain atoms within the active site; these interactions include hydrogen bonding, hydrophobic interactions, van der Waals forces, etc. The topology and nature of the amino acid side chains contained within the active site also dictate the chemical reactivity of the enzyme. In many cases, the repertoire of chemical reactivities provided by the natural amino acids is augmented by incorporation of a non-protein co-factor (e.g. hemes, flavins, metal ions, pyridoxal phosphate, etc.) within the enzyme active site. These co-factors provide additional electrophilic, nucleophilic and redox chemistry components for catalysis.

One of the hallmarks of enzymes·is that they catalyze very specific chemical reaction of particular substrate molecules. This high degree of substrate specificity was recognized early in the development of enzymology, and led to the suggestion that there is a complementary structural relationship between the substrate molecule and the enzyme active site. The earliest version of this hypothesis was articulated by Emil Fisher and is referred to as the 'lock and key' model of enzyme catalysis. In this model, the enzyme active site is viewed as a static structure that has evolved to exactly complement the structure of the substrate – in terms of molecular volume, 3D shape and electrostatic distribution – in much the same way that the disposition of tumblers in a lock exactly complement the structure of the correct key. The original version of this model views the enzyme active site as complementary to the ground-state structure of the substrate, as the model was formulated prior to the development of transition state theory. Today, however, it is clear that the active site structure of enzymes, while demonstrating binding affinity for ground-state substrate, have evolved to best complement the structure of the reaction transition state. Indeed, this is well illustrated by studies of substrate specificity for a variety of enzymes. For example, Table 12.2 summarizes the results of steady-state measurements of peptide hydrolysis by the protease pepsin for a series of synthetic peptides of varying amino acid sequence. What is clear from these data is that the K_M varies very little throughout the range of peptide

Table 12.2 Substrate specificity of pepsin for synthetic peptides demonstrating selectivity based on transition state, rather than ground-state structure

Peptide[a]	K_M (mM)	k_{cat} (s^{-1})	k_{cat}/K_M (mM^{-1}s^{-1})
Cbz-G-H-F-F-OEt	0.8	2.4300	3.04000
Cbz-H-F-W-OEt	0.2	0.5100	2.55000
Cbz-H-F-F-OEt	0.2	0.3100	1.55000
Cbz-H-F-Y-OEt	0.2	0.1600	0.80000
Cbz-H-Y-F-OEt	0.7	0.0130	0.01860
Cbz-H-Y-Y-OEt	0.2	0.0094	0.04700
Cbz-H-F-L-OMe	0.6	0.0025	0.00417

Source: Data from Bender M.L., Bergeron, R.J. and Komiyama, M. (1984) *The Bioorganic Chemistry of Enzymatic Catalysis.* New York: Wiley.
Note
a   One letter code for amino acid residues is used here. Cbz is carbobenzyloxy, OEt is an ethyl ester of the carboxyl terminus of the peptide and OMe is a methyl ester of the carboxyl terminus of the peptide.

structures studied; yet there is almost a 1000-fold variation in the efficiency of catalysis among these peptidic substrates. Hence, the enzyme is discriminating among these potential substrates not on the basis of their ground state structures, but rather on the basis of best fit between the enzyme active site and the transition-state structure of the substrate.

Thus, the enzyme active site is structurally adapted to facilitate the bond distortions of the substrate that lead to strong interactions between the enzyme and the reaction transition-state. To achieve this transition-state complementarity, hence transition-state stabilization, enzymes use a number of structural and chemical strategies. A few of the more common of these strategies are described briefly in the following sections.

12.2.3   Strategies for transition-state stabilization

There is a variety of strategies used by enzymes to stabilize the transition state-structure and thus accelerate the reaction rate. Four common strategies that are discussed are approximation, covalent catalysis, acid/base catalysis and conformational distortions.

12.2.3.1   *Approximation*

The term approximation refers to the bringing together of the substrate molecules and reactive groups of the enzyme active site into the required proximity and orientation for facile catalysis. Consider a reaction involving bond formation between two substrate molecules, A and B to form a single product, A-B. For this reaction to occur in solution the two substrate molecules must encounter one another through diffusion-controlled collisions. Not only must the two substrates encounter one another, they must do so in an orientation that allows the appropriate bond distortions to occur so that the reaction transition state can be attained. In solution, both substrate molecules will be solvated, and at least some, energetically costly, desolvation will need to occur before bond formation can ensue.

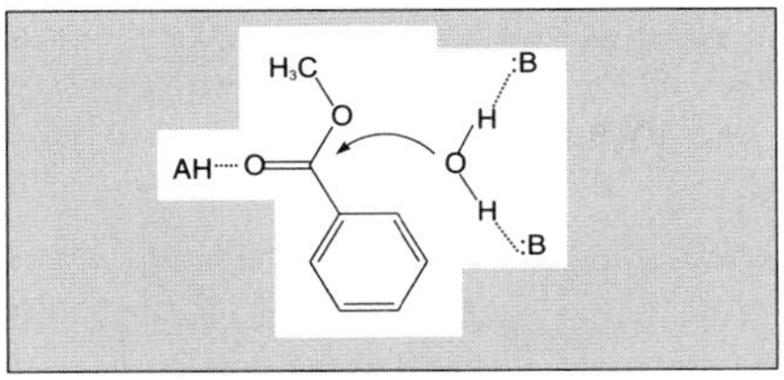

Figure 12.4 Schematic representation of an enzyme active site for a two substrate $(A + B)$ reaction illustrating the orbital alignments that take place within the active site. In this illustration, a water molecule is positioned properly for nucleophilic attack of an ester substrate. Two basic groups (:B) from the enzyme anchor the water molecule in the proper orientation for reaction.

Binding to the enzyme active site ameliorates all of these effects. The mere act of binding brings the two substrate molecules into close proximity with one another within the enzyme active site. The specific set of interactions between the enzyme and substrate molecule that stabilize the *ES* complex also ensure a specific orientation of the bound substrate that best favors the molecular orbital distortions that lead to the transition-state structure. For a bisubstrate reaction as we are considering here, binding of A and B within the enzyme active site not only brings the two molecules into proximity with one another, but also aligns them in a specific orientation to facilitate catalysis (Figure 12.4). The cost of desolvation is offset in the enzyme–catalyzed reaction by the favorable binding energy associated with *ES* complex formation. Thus, a number of energetic advantages are realized by bringing the substrate molecules together within the solvent-shielded environment of the enzyme active site. These advantages are collectively referred to as approximation effects, and provide some means of overcoming the energy barrier to transition-state formation.

12.2.3.2 *Covalent catalysis*

Another mechanism for promoting bond distortions that lead to the transition-state structure is to form a covalent bond between an atom of the substrate and a reactive group within the enzyme active site. The resulting covalent intermediate resembles the transition-state structure of the substrate, thus helping to overcome a significant portion of the activation barrier to catalysis. The covalent species formed during catalytic turnover must be transient, so that both a bond forming and bond breaking step must occur along the reaction pathway. Often one finds that the overall reaction rates of enzymes that utilize covalent catalysis are rate limited by one of these two reaction steps; i.e. either covalent intermediate formation or breakdown is the slowest step in catalysis. Hence, the covalent intermediates formed by these enzymes are relatively long-lived and can often be trapped and studied by crystallographic and other biophysical methods. Covalent catalysis in enzymes is generally mediated by nucleophilic and electrophilic catalysis, and more rarely by redox chemistry.

Nucleophilic catalysis refers to the situation where electrons are donated from an active site nucleophile to a substrate atom, resulting in bond formation. Amino acid side chains that can act as reactive nucleophiles include: serine, cysteine, aspartate, lysine, histidine and tyrosine; examples of enzymes forming covalent intermediates between substrates and each of these active site residues are known. A good example of nucleophilic catalysis comes from the reaction mechanism of the family of hydrolytic enzymes known as the serine proteases. These enzymes hydrolyze amide bonds within peptides and proteins through a mechanism involving acylation and deacylation of the active site serine. Serine is not a particularly good nucleophile by itself, but the serine proteases have evolved a specific mechanism for enhancing the nucleophilicity of this amino acid side chain. Within the active sites of all serine proteases is a triad of amino acids made up of aspartic acid, histidine and serine, as illustrated for α-chymotrypsin in Figure 12.5A. The hydroxyl group of the serine forms a hydrogen bond with one of the ring nitrogens of the histidine residue. The other ring nitrogen of this histidine forms a hydrogen bond with the

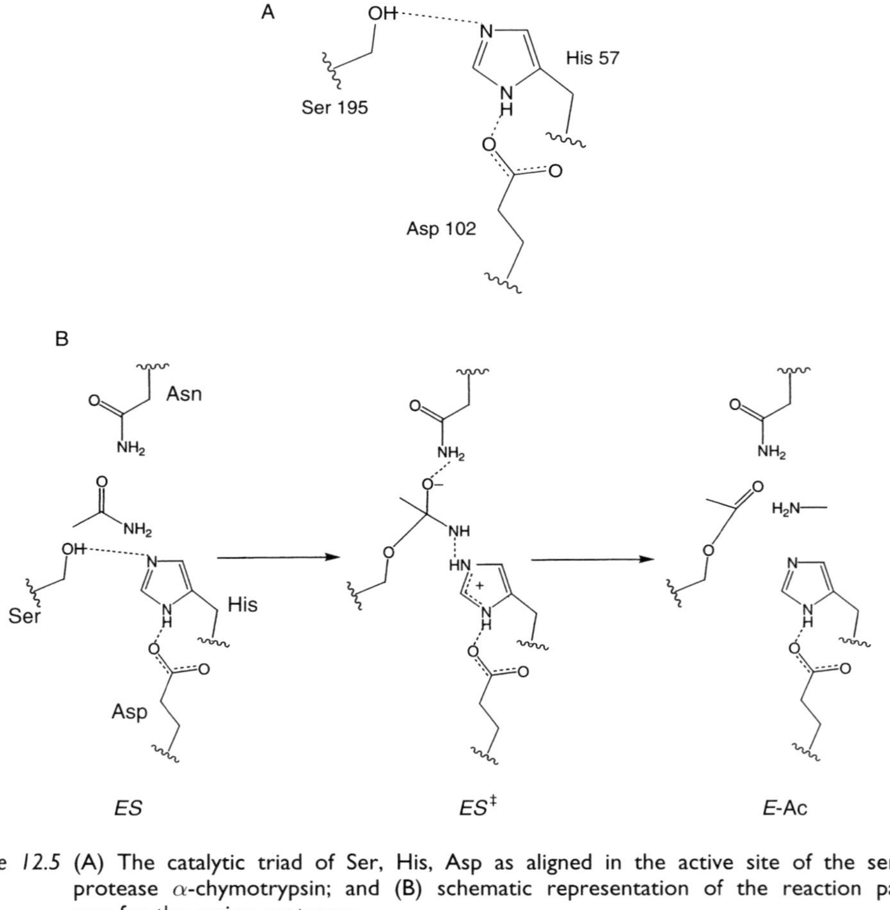

Figure 12.5 (A) The catalytic triad of Ser, His, Asp as aligned in the active site of the serine protease α-chymotrypsin; and (B) schematic representation of the reaction pathway for the serine proteases.

aspartic acid residue. In this way, the side chain oxygen atom of the serine is made much more nucleophilic and is able to attack the amide bond of the substrate peptide. This is a good example of the concept, described above, of active site topography dictating chemical reactivity for enzymes. The mechanism of acyl transfer for the serine proteases is illustrated in Figure 12.5B. The peptide substrate binds within the enzyme active site to form the initial Michaelis complex. This is followed by nucleophilic attack of the scissile peptide bond by the active site serine, resulting in formation of a tetrahedral transition state containing a charged oxygen species (an oxyanion). The oxyanionic nature of the transition state requires specific charge neutralizing interactions with other amino acid residues within the enzyme active site (another example of active site structure designed to stabilize the transition state). The transition state next decays with proton donation from the active site histidine residue to the newly formed amine of the C-terminal peptide fragment of the substrate. This C-terminal product is released from the enzyme, but the N-terminal fragment remains covalently bound to the active site serine. The departure of the C-terminal peptide product creates a cavity through which a water molecule can enter and attack the remaining acyl-serine group within the active site. This leads to deacylation of the enzyme, release of the N-terminal peptide product, and recovery of the free enzyme species.

Electrophilic catalysis involves covalent intermediate formation between cationic electrophiles in the enzyme active site and electron-rich atoms in the substrate or co-factor molecule. None of the natural amino acids are good electrophiles, so enzymatic electrophilic catalysis is generally mediated by enzyme co-factors, especially metal ions. Other co-factors that are common in electrophilic catalysis include pyridoxal phosphate and *in situ* formation of lysine-substrate Schiff bases. As with nucleophilic catalysis, the main advantage to covalent adduct formation is that the resulting intermediate resembles the structure of the reaction transition state, and thus helps to overcome the activation barrier to transition-state formation. In some cases, the enzymatic electrophile does not directly attack the substrate molecule, but rather serves to enhance the nucleophilicity of an attacking co-factor. This is a common strategy for many zinc metalloenzymes where a metal-co-ordinated water molecule serves as the attacking species. In the matrix metalloproteases, for example, the active site zinc ion serves two roles in catalysis of peptide bond hydrolysis. First, it serves to enhance the nucleophilicity of a co-ordinated water molecule that attacks the peptidic substrate. Second, the zinc ion helps to neutralize the oxyanion formed during bond rupture by forming a partial co-ordinate bond, as illustrated in Figure 12.6.

12.2.3.3   Acid/base chemistry

Enzyme reactions generally require some proton transfer step(s) during turnover, and these are facilitated by acidic and basic groups within the enzyme active site. Most often these acid/base functionalities are derived from the amino acid side chains of aspartic acid, glutamic acid, histidine, cysteine, tyrosine and lysine, and from the free amino and carboxyl termini of the protein. Acid/base groups can participate directly in critical proton donation or abstraction from substrate molecules, as we have already seen for the active site histidine of the serine proteases (Figure 12.5B).

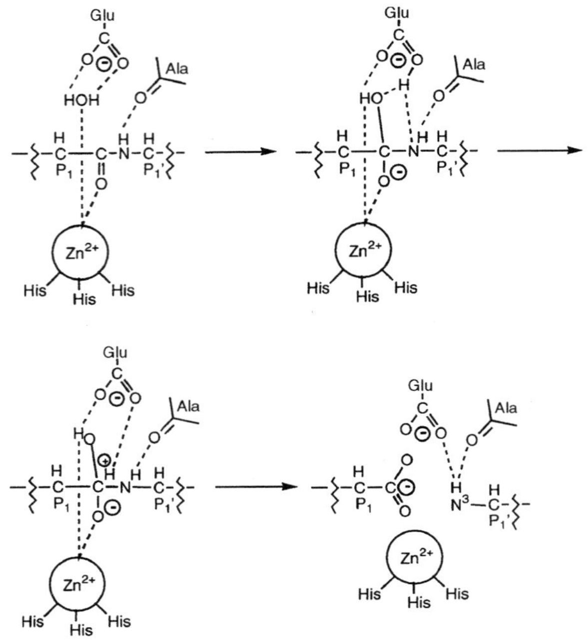

Figure 12.6 Role of the active site zinc in the reaction mechanism of the matrix metalloproteases. Redrawn and modified from Whittaker, M., Floyd, C.D., Brown, P., and Gearing, A.J.H. (1999) *Chem. Rev.*, **99**, 2735–2776. Figure kindly provided by Dr Carl P. Decicco.

These groups can also play more subtle roles in stabilizing transition-state structures by helping to polarize specific chemical bonds, as seen, for example, for the active site glutamic acid of the matrix metalloproteases (Figure 12.6).

12.2.3.4 *Conformational distortions*

As already discussed, the bond distortions required to bring the ground-state substrate molecule to the transition-state structure represent the highest energetic barrier to reaction progress. Once bound in the enzyme active site, the ground-state substrate molecule must be forced to adopt the transition-state structure. One way that enzymes accomplish this is by introducing strain into the system through conformational distortions of the enzyme active site. There is clear experimental evidence for enzyme conformational adjustments subsequent to substrate binding. How can these conformational changes be used to stabilize the bound transition-state? One hypothesis for this is known as the induced strain model. In this model, the most stable form of the enzyme is one in which the active site topography is most complementary to the transition-state structure of the reaction (i.e. in its lowest energy conformation, the active site is preorganized to best complement the reaction transition-state structure). Substrate binds to the enzyme active site in its ground-state configuration. To accommodate this ligand, the enzyme adjusts its conformation to maximize favorable contacts with the bound substrate. However, this altered conformation of the enzyme is thermodynamically unfavorable, occurring at a higher potential energy than the resting state of the enzyme. Hence, the system relaxes back to the lowest energy state of the enzyme and in so doing forces bond distortions of the bound substrate that lead to the transition state. Product formation and release then follow and the enzyme is returned to its un-ligated lowest energy conformation. These concepts are schematically illustrated in Figure 12.7.

The conformational distortions associated with transition-state stabilization typically involve a number of steric and electronic changes in the active site structure. Thus, changes not only in protein packing but also in hydrogen bonding patterns, van der Waals interactions, and charge distribution can participate in the induction of strain to the ground-state substrate and/or in the stabilization of the transition-state structure. The serine proteases again offer a good example of this latter concept. Acylation of the active site serine and formation of the bound transition state produces an oxyanion from an uncharged peptidic substrate. Conformational adjustments of the active sites of serine proteases involve movements of key residues to produce new hydrogen bonding interactions that help to stabilize this developing charge on the oxygen atom. Thus, hydrogen bonding patterns, hydrophobic interactions, charge distribution, etc. within the enzyme active site may appear unfavorable for substrate interactions, but are in fact situated for optimal interactions with the transition state.

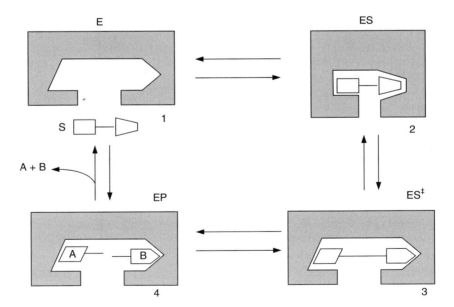

Figure 12.7 Schematic representation of the induced strain model of enzyme catalysis. Figure reprinted from Copeland, R.A. (2000) *Enzymes: A Practical Introduction to Structure, Mechanism and Data Analysis*, 2nd edition. New York: Wiley-VCH. With permission of the publisher.

The strategies discussed here for transition state stabilization are commonly used in concert with one another to optimize enzyme–transition state interactions. As we shall see in the following sections, some of these same strategies can be exploited in ligand design to enhance the binding affinity of small molecule inhibitors.

12.3   REVERSIBLE ENZYME INHIBITORS

The majority of enzyme inhibitors that are used as drugs in human medicine are simple reversible inhibitors of their target enzyme. The term reversible inhibitor implies that there is a reversible equilibrium established between the enzyme and inhibitor that can be characterized by a rate constant for binary enzyme–inhibitor complex formation, a rate constant for binary complex dissociation, and an equilibrium dissociation constant for the enzyme–inhibitor complex. The dissociation constant for an enzyme–inhibitor complex is often represented by the special symbol K_i to indicate that we are dealing with an inhibitory ligand. If we consider a simple, one substrate enzyme reaction we find that there are a number of potential ways that an inhibitor could interact with an enzyme species. The various equilibria associated with these potential interactions are summarized in Figure 12.8.

In Figure 12.8, the free enzyme (E) can combine with substrate to form the ES complex with a corresponding dissociation constant, K_S. The ES complex can then go on to form product through a series of chemical steps collectively described by k_{cat}. Alternatively, the free enzyme can combine with the inhibitor molecule (I) to form the binary EI complex with dissociation constant K_i. The EI complex can potentially bind substrate to form the ternary ESI complex. The dissociation constant for substrate release from the ESI complex is, however, not necessarily the same as for release from the ES complex. Hence, in our illustration the substrate dissociation constant for the ESI complex is modified by the term α. The ESI ternary complex could also be formed by inhibitor binding to the binary ES complex. In this case, the inhibitor dissociation constant would be modified by the same α term as just described. In principle, the ESI complex could go on to form product at a reduced rate relative to the uninhibited enzyme, a situation referred to as partial inhibition. However, most of the enzyme inhibitors that are used as drugs are not of this type, and for the remainder of our discussion we shall assume that saturation of the appropriate enzyme species with inhibitor leads to a complete loss of catalytic activity.

Thus K_i represents the inhibitor dissociation constant for the EI complex while αK_i represents the inhibitor dissociation constant for the ESI complex. The various equilibria illustrated in Figure 12.8 lead to three potential kinetic modes of enzyme inhibition: competitive inhibition; non-competitive inhibition; and uncompetitive inhibition (Figure 12.9). The nature and characteristics of these three inhibitor modalities are discussed next.

12.3.1   Competitive inhibition

An inhibitor that binds exclusively to the free enzyme, displaying no affinity for the binary ES complex, is referred to as a competitive inhibitor. The terminology comes

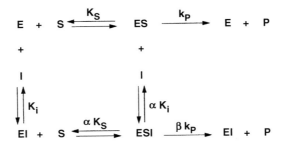

Figure 12.8 Equilibrium scheme for enzyme turnover in the presence and absence of reversible inhibitors. Figure reprinted from Copeland, R.A. (2000) *Enzymes: A Practical Introduction to Structure, Mechanism and Data Analysis*, 2nd edition. New York: Wiley-VCH. With permission of the publisher.

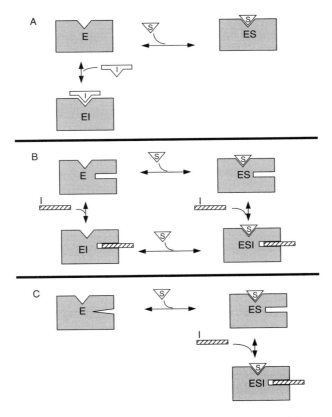

Figure 12.9 Cartoon representations of the three major modes of inhibitor interactions with enzymes: (A) competitive inhibition; (B) non-competitive inhibition; (C) uncompetitive inhibition. Figure reprinted from Copeland, R.A. (2000) *Enzymes: A Practical Introduction to Structure, Mechanism and Data Analysis*, 2nd edition. New York: Wiley-VCH. With permission of the publisher.

from the fact that the free enzyme can combine with either inhibitor or substrate molecules, but not both simultaneously. Hence, the inhibitor and substrate compete for the same form of the enzyme, and bind in a mutually exclusive fashion.

The competitive relationship between inhibitor and substrate binding in this case suggests to many researchers that the two molecules share a common binding site on the enzyme; i.e. that competitive inhibitors bind within the enzyme active site, sterically blocking substrate binding, as illustrated schematically in Figure 12.9A. Structural analysis of enzyme–inhibitor complexes often confirms this inference for competitive inhibitors. However, it is important to realize that it is also possible for a competitive inhibitor to bind to the enzyme in a binding pocket distal to the active site and to affect substrate binding through induction of a conformational change that is propagated to the active site (an allosteric mechanism). Hence, although often the case, kinetic determination of competitive inhibition alone cannot be viewed as *prima facie* evidence for a commonality of binding sites for the inhibitor and substrate molecules.

In the presence of a competitive inhibitor, the velocity equation (i.e. the Michaelis–Menten equation) is modified as follows:

$$v = \frac{V_{max}[S]}{[S] + K_M\left(1 + \frac{[I]}{K_i}\right)} \tag{12.9}$$

We see from equation (12.9) that as the concentration of a competitive inhibitor is increased, the apparent value of K_M is increased by the term $(1 + [I]/K_i)$ with no concomitant effect on V_{max}. Thus, if one were to generate a double reciprocal plot of velocity as a function of substrate concentration at several concentrations of a competitive inhibitor, one would expect that the slopes (K_M/V_{max}) of the lines would be influenced by the presence of inhibitor but not the y-intercepts $(1/V_{max})$. The resulting plot would therefore be characterized by a series of lines that intersect at the y-axis, as illustrated in Figure 12.10A; this is the classical signature of a competitive inhibitor. The value of the dissociation constant K_i is determined by fitting the untransformed velocity data (as in Figure 12.3A) to equation (12.9). Alternatively, K_i can also be determined from the x-intercept obtained by linear fitting of a replot of the apparent K_M value (determined by fitting the velocity data to equation (12.6)) as a function of $[I]$.

A general way to assess the effects of any inhibitor on enzyme activity is to plot the fractional activity (v/v_0) as a function of inhibitor concentration (under conditions of fixed enzyme and substrate concentrations) on a semi–log scale, in what is commonly referred to as a dose-response plot. The diminution of activity with increasing inhibitor concentration can be fit to a Langmuir isotherm as follows:

$$\frac{v}{v_0} = \frac{1}{1 + \frac{[I]}{IC_{50}}} \tag{12.10}$$

where v is the velocity observed at inhibitor concentration $[I]$, v_0 is the velocity observed in the absence of inhibitor, and IC_{50} is the concentration of inhibitor

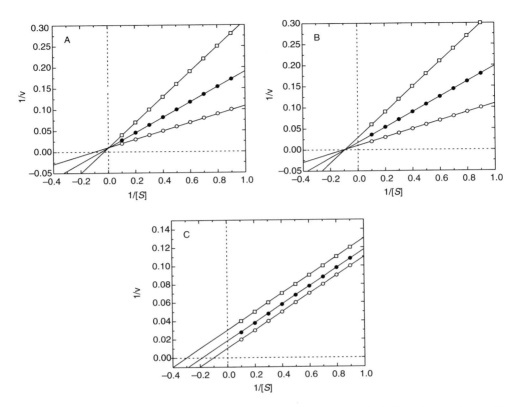

Figure 12.10 Double reciprocal plots for the three major modes of inhibitor interactions with enzymes: (A) competitive inhibition; (B) non-competitive inhibition (with $\alpha = 1$); and (C) uncompetitive inhibition.

required to reduce the observed velocity to half of that seen in the absence of inhibitor (i.e. $0.5v_0$). The IC_{50} value is related to the inhibitor K_i in different ways, depending on the inhibitor modality. For competitive inhibitors the relationship is:

$$IC_{50} = K_i \left(1 + \frac{[S]}{K_M}\right) \tag{12.11}$$

Thus, from equation (12.11) we see that the IC_{50} of a competitive inhibitor increases with increasing concentration of substrate. This is another classic signature of competitive inhibition that can be used to diagnose this form of inhibition. Figure 12.11 illustrates this concept, demonstrating the shift in IC_{50} for a competitive inhibitor studied at substrate concentrations of $0.1\,K_M$ and $10\,K_M$.

Because they bind in the enzyme active site, structural analogs of substrates, products, reaction intermediates and transition-state species generally behave as competitive inhibitors. These molecules provide good starting points for drug design, and numerous examples of active site-directed competitive inhibitors can be found among the drugs in clinical use.

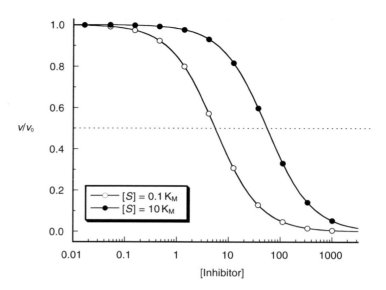

Figure 12.11 Concentration–response plots for competitive inhibition of an enzyme-catalyzed reaction studied at two fixed concentrations of substrate: $[S] = 0.1\,K_M$ (open circles) and $[S] = 10\,K_M$ (closed circles). The dashed line at $v/v_0 = 0.5$ indicates the level at which 50% inhibition of enzymatic activity is achieved.

The antiproliferative drugs methotrexate and trimethoprim are good examples of active-site directed, competitive enzyme inhibitors. Both compounds inhibit the enzyme dihydrofolate reductase (DHFR), which catalyzes a critical step in the biosynthesis of deoxythymidine. Inhibition of DHFR blocks deoxythymidine biosynthesis, which in turn blocks cellular proliferation. Hence, inhibitors of DHFR are useful as inhibitors of cellular proliferation for cancer, inflammatory diseases, and as antibiotics.

The chemical structure of the substrate of DHFR, dihydrofolate, is illustrated in Figure 12.12A. Hoping to engage similar sets of active site interactions, initial attempts to identify inhibitors of this enzyme focused on compounds that were structural analogs of this substrate. From these efforts, the antiproliferative drug methotrexate (Figure 12.12B) was discovered. Kinetic analysis revealed methotrexate to be a competitive inhibitor of DHFR with a K_i of <1 nM ($<1 \times 10^{-9}$ M). Indeed, when the crystal structures of DHFR with dihydrofolate and methotrexate were solved, they revealed a very similar binding mode for the two ligands, with a remarkable number of common interactions within the enzyme active site (Figure 12.13). For example, hydrogen bonds are formed between the side chain carboxylate of Asp 27 and two amine groups of the ligands. A network of hydrogen bonds connects Trp 22 with heteroatom interactions within the ligand through an intervening active site water molecule. Another active site water interacts with a ligand amine and with active site residues Thr 113, Trp 30, and Tyr 111.

The crystal structure of the DHFR-methotrexate complex reveals that the majority of enzyme–inhibitor interactions are localized to the first ring (i.e. the

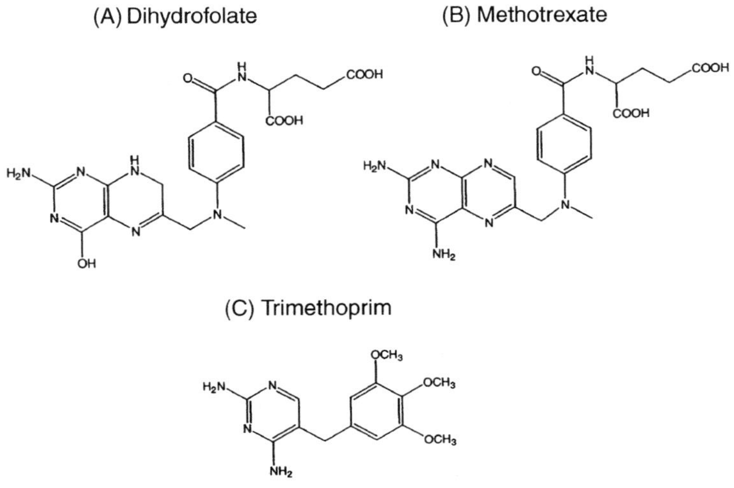

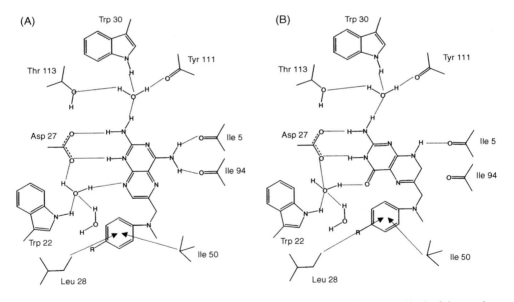

(A) Dihydrofolate

(B) Methotrexate

(C) Trimethoprim

Figure 12.12 Chemical structures of ligands of the enzyme dihydrofolate reductase: (A) the substrate dihydrofolate; (B) the inhibitor methotrexate; and (C) the inhibitor trimethoprim.

Figure 12.13 Schematic representations of the active site interactions between dihydrofolate reductase and the ligands (A) methotrexate; and (B) dihydrofolate. Figure adapted and redrawn from data in Klebe, G. (1994) *J. Mol. Biol.*, **237**, 212–235.

2,4-diaminopyrimidine) of the pteridine ring system. This conclusion was also drawn prior to the crystal structure on the basis of structure–activity relationship (SAR) studies, in which the structure of the lead inhibitor is systematically varied to define the minimum structural unit required for inhibition (this minimal structure is referred to as the *pharmacophore*). Once the 2,4-diaminopyrimidine system was identified as the pharmacophore for DHFR inhibition, systematic substitutions off this ring system were investigated, leading to the discovery of trimethoprim (Figure 12.12C). Trimethoprim is a very potent inhibitor of the DHFR from *E. coli* ($K_i = 1.35$ nM; 1.35×10^{-9} M). Testing of this compound with mammalian forms of DHFR revealed that trimethoprim was a selective inhibitor of the bacterial enzyme (e.g. the K_i for the human enzyme is 170 000 nM). Today both methotrexate and trimethoprim are prescribed as antiproliferative agents. Methotrexate is used in cancer and inflammatory disease therapies, while trimethoprim is used for treatment of infectious diseases.

Another example of a clinically relevant competitive enzyme inhibitor is lovastatin, a drug that is used to control cholesterol levels in the blood. Cholesterol is a major constituent of the atherosclerotic plaques that can build up on the inner walls of arteries, leading to coronary heart disease. Controlling circulating cholesterol levels is a valuable method for preventing plaque buildup. About half of the cholesterol in the body comes from dietary intake, and the other half results from *de novo* biosynthesis in the liver. The biosynthesis of cholesterol, starting from acetyl-coenzyme A, requires 20 enzymatic steps. The rate-limiting step in the overall synthetic pathway is the conversion of 3-hydroxy-3-methylglutaryl coenzyme A (HMG-CoA) to mevalonic acid by the enzyme 3-hydroxy-3-methylglutaryl coenzyme A reductase (HMG-CoA reductase). Inhibition of HMG-CoA reductase blocks *de novo* cholesterol biosynthesis, thus leading to a significant reduction in total body cholesterol.

The reaction mechanism of HMG-CoA reductase is illustrated in Figure 12.14A. The enzyme binds HMG-CoA (**12.1**: $K_M = 10$ µM; 1×10^{-5} M) and reduces the

Figure 12.14 (A) Reaction mechanism of the enzyme HMG-CoA reductase; (B) ring opening reaction of lovastatin leading to the active enzyme inhibitor. Note the structural similarity between the active inhibitor and intermediate **2** of the HMG-CoA reductase mechanism.

thiolester to intermediate **12.2**, using NADPH as a redox co-factor. This is followed by base-catalyzed elimination of the coenzyme A thiol, leaving behind the aldehyde, **12.3**. The aldehyde is then reduced to the alcohol by another equivalent of NADPH, leading to the product, mevalonic acid (**12.4**).

Lovastatin (also known as mevinolin) is a natural product that was isolated from a number of fungi by different laboratories. The Merck group, for example, isolated lovastatin from *Aspergillus terreus* and demonstrated that this molecule was a potent inhibitor of cholesterol biosynthesis *in vitro*. Lovastatin turns out to be a prodrug (i.e. an inactive species that is metabolically converted to an active compound) that undergoes a ring-opening reaction to form the active species illustrated in Figure 12.14B. This active form of lovastatin bears a striking resemblance to the intermediate species **12.2** of the reaction pathway of HMG-CoA reductase (Figure 12.14A). The compound was indeed found to be a very potent competitive inhibitor of HMG-CoA reductase with a K_i value of 0.64 nM (6.4×10^{-10} M).

Structural mimics of reaction pathway intermediates and transition states, such as lovastatin, are generally found to be extremely potent (i.e. tight binding) enzyme inhibitors. This is not surprising since, as discussed above, the enzyme active site is evolved to best compliment the structure of the reaction transition state. A number of enzyme inhibitors have been developed on the basis of this concept. Additional examples of clinically relevant reaction intermediate-based inhibitors are the drugs captopril and enalapril, two inhibitors of angiotensin-converting enzyme (ACE) which are used in the treatment of hypertension.

The octapeptide angiotensin II is a powerful modulator of hypertension, acting to increase blood pressure in two distinct ways: (1) the peptide is itself a vasoconstrictor; and (2) it stimulates the release of the hormone aldosterone which facilitates the excretion of potassium ions and the retention of sodium and water in cells. Both the electrolyte changes and vasoconstriction caused by angiotensin II contribute to raising blood pressure. Angiotensin II is generated *in vivo* by proteolytic cleavage of the C-terminal dipeptide His-Lys from the decapeptide precursor angiotensin I. The conversion of angiotensin I to angiotensin II is catalyzed by the zinc metalloenzyme ACE. The ACE proteolytic activity additionally contributes to hypertension by hydrolyzing, thus inactivating, the vasodilating nonapeptide, bradykinin. Hence, inhibition of ACE would reduce blood pressure by blocking the pressure raising effects of angiotensin II and by sparing the pressure lowering peptide bradykinin from proteolytic inactivation.

Angiotensin-converting enzyme, like other zinc carboxypeptidases, catalyzes peptide bond cleavage by forming a co-ordinate bond between the zinc ion and the oxygen atom of the carbonyl group of the amide bond to be hydrolyzed (an example of electrophilic catalysis). This co-ordination to zinc polarizes the carbonyl bond, making it more susceptible to nucleophilic attack by an active site water molecule, whose nucleophilicity is itself enhanced by a near-by active site base. The zinc co-ordinated intermediate then leads to a transition state in which the carbonyl carbon is tetrahedral, making bonds to both the zinc co-ordinated oxygen and the oxygen of the attacking water molecule (Figure 12.15A). Both captopril and enalapril inhibit ACE by mimicking the zinc-co-ordinated transition-state structure. The sulphydryl group of captopril (Figure 12.15B) co-ordinates to the active site zinc. Additional active site interactions are made with the methyl,

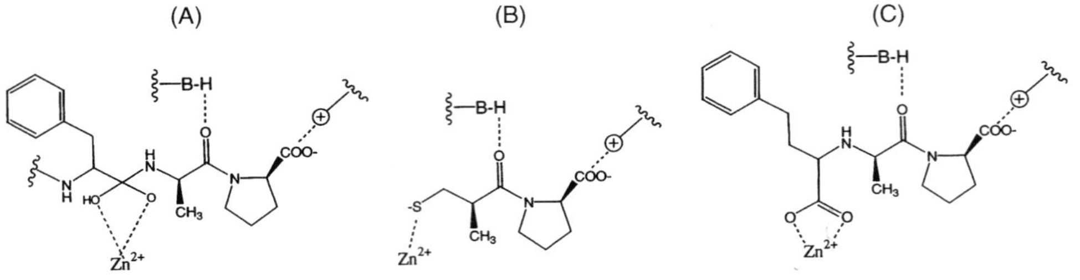

Figure 12.15 Schematic representation of the ACE active site interactions with (A) the substrate tetrahedral intermediate; (B) captopril; and (C) enalaprilate.

carbonyl and carboxylate groups as illustrated in Figure 12.15B. These combined interactions mimic the structure of the reaction intermediate leading to a tight binding enzyme–inhibitor complex with a K_i of 1.7 nM (1.7×10^{-9} M). Captopril was the first selective ACE inhibitor to be used as an antihypertension drug. However, uncomfortable side effects, such as rashes and loss of taste, were found with captopril, owing to the sulphydryl group within this molecule. This sulphydryl group was replaced by a carboxyl group, and other groups were added to make additional interactions with the enzyme active site in the molecule known as enalaprilate (Figure 12.15C). Enalaprilate is a very potent inhibitor of ACE, displaying a K_i of 0.18 nM (1.8×10^{-10} M). The free carboxylate of enalaprilate, however, limits membrane transport of the molecule into cells. To overcome this limitation, the drug is administered as the ethyl ester form, known as enalapril, which is converted to enalaprilate *in vivo* by the enzymatic action of various esterases (this is another example of a prodrug). Today both captopril and enalapril are prescribed for the treatment of hypertension.

12.3.2   Non-competitive inhibition

Non-competitive inhibition refers to the situation where the inhibitory molecule has binding affinity for both the free enzyme and the enzyme–substrate binary complex. Hence, it is possible to form a ternary *ESI* complex with a non-competitive inhibitor. Here the affinity of the inhibitor for the free enzyme is quantified in terms of the dissociation constant K_i and the affinity for the *ES* complex is quantified in terms of αK_i (see Figure 12.8). If the inhibitor has equal affinity for both *E* and *ES*, the value of α is 1. If the inhibitor binds preferentially to *E* or to *ES* then the value of α is greater than or less than 1, respectively (these latter two cases are sometimes referred to as *mixed inhibition* in some of the biochemical literature). The general velocity equation for non-competitive inhibition is given by:

$$v = \frac{V_{\max}[S]}{[S]\left(1 + \dfrac{[I]}{\alpha K_i}\right) + K_M\left(1 + \dfrac{[I]}{K_i}\right)} \tag{12.12}$$

The apparent values of both V_{max} and K_M are affected by the presence of a non-competitive inhibitor. Hence, double reciprocal plots at varying non-competitive inhibitor concentration results in a nest of lines that converge beyond the y-axis above, on, or below the x-axis, depending on whether α is >1, equal to 1, or <1, respectively (Figure 12.10B). Since non-competitive inhibitors can bind to the ES complex, the IC_{50} for these inhibitors is not significantly influenced by substrate concentration. Non-competitive inhibitors that display similar affinity for the free enzyme and ES complex can offer a pharmacological advantage over competitive inhibitors in situations where the cellular concentrations of substrates are high relative to K_M. In such cases, the cellular effect of the inhibitor is not diminished by a need to compete with high concentrations of substrate for the free enzyme. Also, some enzymes bind macromolecular substrates and catalyze multiple turnover events without substrate dissociation (this is referred to as precessive catalysis). An example of a precessive enzyme reaction is the sequential addition of nucleotides to a growing nucleic acid strand by DNA and RNA polymerases. For enzymes like these, the ES complex, rather than the free enzyme, may be the predominant species in cells. Hence, non-competitive inhibitors might show an advantage over competitive inhibitors in these situations.

Examples of clinically useful non-competitive enzyme inhibitors come from the class of AIDS (Acquired Immune Deficiency Syndrome) drugs known as non-nucleoside reverse transcriptase inhibitors (NNRTI's). The HIV virus has been clearly established as the causative agent in AIDS. The HIV belongs to a family of viruses referred to as *Retroviridae*, which contain an RNA-based genetic system. To replicate the virus must reverse-transcribe its RNA into DNA by the action of an enzyme known as reverse transcriptase (RT), and then incorporate this DNA into the genome of the infected host cell. Hence, the viral life cycle is critically dependent on the enzymatic activity of the RT, and inhibition of this enzyme should block replication.

The HIV RT is a member of the DNA polymerase family of enzymes. It consists of a heterodimer of two protein subunits, p51 and p66. Each of these subunits folds into a classic polymerase structure consisting of three subdomains that are arranged in a way that resembles a human hand; the three subdomains are referred to as the fingers, palm and thumb subdomains (Figure 12.16). Under *in vitro* conditions HIV RT utilizes an RNA or DNA template to direct complementary base incorporation into a small DNA primer strand. Deoxynucleotide triphosphates (dNTP; ATP, TTP, GTP, CTP) are utilized as the source of bases for DNA primer extension; which dNTP is used for a particular turnover cycle depends on the next base to be incorporated into the growing DNA strand, dictated by the next base of the complementary template. Thus, the enzyme utilizes two substrates *in vitro*: a template–primer complex (TP) and the four dNTP's. Results of kinetic studies suggest that these substrates bind to the enzyme in a preferred order, leading to the following reaction sequence:

$$E + TP \underset{K_{TP}}{\rightleftharpoons} E{-}TP \underset{K_{dNTP}}{\rightleftharpoons} E{-}TP{-}dNTP \xrightarrow{k_{cat}} E{-}TP_{(n+1)}$$

The enzyme is highly precessive so that $TP_{(n+1)}$ release does not readily occur. Thus, multiple rounds of dNTP incorporation occur on the enzyme-bound primer

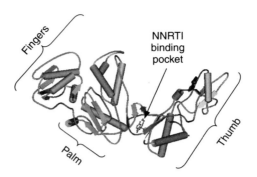

Figure 12.16 Crystal structure of HIV-1 reverse transcriptase with the inhibitor efavirenz bound to the NNRTI binding pocket. The structure of the p66 subunit only is shown. Note the three subdomains referred to as the fingers, palm and thumb subdomains. Structural data from Ren, J. Milton, J., Weaver, K.L., Short, S.A., Stuart, D.I. and Stammers, D.K. (2000) *Structure (London)*, **8**, 1089–1094.

until the full length of the template has been complimented. The rate limitation on k_{cat} can be either the chemistry of phosphodiester bond formation itself, or a rate-limiting conformational change of the enzyme that is required for dNTP incorporation. Competitive inhibitors can block binding of *TP* or of dNTP. Non-competitive inhibitors can act subsequent to substrate binding by: (1) disrupting the chemistry of phosphodiester bond formation; (2) blocking a catalytically required conformational transition of the enzyme; or (3) altering the reaction pathway so as to change the rate-limiting step in catalysis.

Early attempts to inhibit HIV RT relied on competitive inhibitors that were nucleoside analogs. Some of these compounds were clinically useful, but these inhibitors generally lack specificity for the viral polymerase over mammalian nucleoside-utilizing enzymes. Hence, side effects associated with the use of these inhibitors limited their clinical utility. Random screening of compound libraries identified several non-nucleoside-based inhibitors of RT that were non-competitive with respect to both TP and dNTP's; two of these compounds, nevirapine (Viramune) and efavirenz (Sustiva) have been studied in detail and are currently used in the treatment of AIDS patients (see Figure 12.17 for the chemical structures of these molecules).

Nevirapine is a selective inhibitor of HIV RT, showing no ability to inhibit the polymerases from mammalian cells. The K_i for nevirapine inhibition of RT has been reported to range from 19 to 400 nM, depending on assay conditions and *TP* composition. All of the kinetic studies reported in the literature agree, however, that nevirapine is a non-competitive inhibitor of RT, displaying equal affinity for the free enzyme (E), the enzyme–TP binary complex (E–TP) and the E–TP–dNTP ternary complex (E–TP–dNTP). The crystal structure of HIV RT complexed to nevirapine has been solved. The structure reveals that the inhibitor binds in a deep hydrophobic pocket close to, but not overlapping, the active site of polymerization. The binding site contains two tyrosine residues, Tyr 181 and Tyr 188, that make hydrophobic contact with the inhibitor. These hydrophobic interactions contribute

A Nevirapine   B Efavirenz

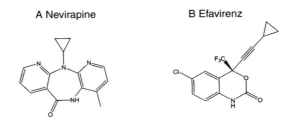

Figure 12.17 Chemical structures of the HIV-1 reverse transcriptase inhibitors (A) nevirapine; and (B) efavirenz.

to the binding energy for the inhibitor; as expected mutation of Tyr 181 to Ile disrupts this hydrophobic interaction resulting in a large reduction in inhibitor affinity. The binding pocket for nevirapine exists on the p66 subunit of the enzyme only. This observation is consistent with equilibrium binding data that suggest a single inhibitor binding site per heterodimer. The binding pocket is situated near the interface between the 'palm' and 'thumb' subdomains of the p66 subunit and may therefore play a role in conformational changes that affect the disposition of these subdomains during catalysis. This observation led to the speculation that the NNRTI's inhibit RT by blocking a catalytically required conformational transition of the enzyme. Subsequent presteady-state kinetic studies suggest that it is more likely that these inhibitors slow down, but do not block entirely the chemical steps in primer extension. The main effect of the NNRTI's may be to alter the nature of the rate-limiting step in catalysis subsequent to substrate binding.

Efavirenz is also an NNRTI that acts as a non-competitive inhibitor of HIV RT. Kinetic and equilibrium binding studies suggest that efavirenz binds to the same pocket on the enzyme as nevirapine. This suggestion has recently been verified by crystallographic determination of the structure of the RT-efavirenz complex. The structure reveals interactions between efavirenz and Tyr 181 and Tyr 188, as with nevirapine. Additional hydrophobic interactions with efavirenz are made with Trp 229, Phe 227, Leu 100 and Val 106. The inhibitor also makes ring-edge contacts with Tyr 318 and Val 179 and hydrogen bonding interactions with the mainchain carbonyl of Lys 101. All of these interactions contribute to the binding energy for this inhibitor. Unlike nevirapine, efavirenz shows a preference for binding to the ternary $E–TP–dNTP$ complex over the free enzyme. The K_d values for efavirenz complexes of the various enzyme forms are as follows: $K_E = 170 \pm 5$ nM; $K_{E–TP} = 30 \pm 2$ nM; $K_{E–TP–dNTP} = 4 \pm 0.5$ nM. Therefore, efavirenz is best described as a mixed-type non-competitive inhibitor.

Today both nevirapine and efavirenz are used in combination with other AIDS drugs to control viral levels in AIDS patients. Both inhibitors are well tolerated by patients and are very effective in blocking viral replication. The rapidity of viral replication and the infidelity of the HIV replication system result in a high rate of mutation in all HIV proteins including the RT. Mutations that confer resistance to inhibition are a significant problem for all AIDS drugs, including the NNRTI's. In this regard efavirenz appears to have some advantage over other NNRTI's. In clinical trials and in patient treatment with NNRTI's the most common mutation found to develop in RT is a change of Lys 103 to Asn. This residue is within the NNRTI binding pocket and makes van der Waals contacts with some inhibitors. The K103N mutation results in a 40-fold reduction in nevirapine affinity for the enzyme. In contrast, the affinity of efavirenz for the K103N mutant enzyme is reduced by only six-fold. The crystal structure of the RT-efavirenz complex may provide a structural rationale for the reduced resistance against this inhibitor. The topography of the inhibitor binding pocket is altered by the mutation. The binding configuration of efavirenz appears to be more adaptable to these structural changes than that of nevirapine and other NNRTI's. Thus tight binding interactions are maintained by efavirenz with this pocket in the mutant form of RT where similar interactions are lost by the other NNRTI's. Nevertheless, continued research will be required to provide additional drugs, hopefully ones that are more refractory to target mutations, for the treatment of this devastating disease.

12.3.3   Uncompetitive inhibition

An uncompetitive inhibitor is one that binds exclusively to the *ES* complex, displaying no affinity for the free enzyme. The inhibitor binding pocket is only revealed in the presence of enzyme-bound substrate. This can occur due to conformational changes in enzyme structure that accompany substrate binding, opening up a previously occluded binding pocket (Figure 12.9C). Alternatively, the inhibitor binding pocket could be composed of structural elements from both the enzyme and the substrate molecules, so that the binding pocket, *per se*, does not exist except in the context of the *ES* complex.

The velocity equation for uncompetitive inhibition is as follows:

$$v = \frac{V_{\max}[S]}{[S]\left(1 + \frac{[I]}{\alpha K_i}\right) + K_M} \tag{12.13}$$

Algebraic rearrangement of equation (12.13) demonstrates that both $V_{\max}$ and K_M are influenced by the same factor $(1 + [I]/\alpha K_i)$. In double reciprocal plots, the y-intercept $(1/V_{\max}(1 + [I]/\alpha K_i))$ varies with uncompetitive inhibitor concentration, but the slope $(K_M(1 + [I]/\alpha K_i)/V_{\max}(1 + [I]/\alpha K_i))$ is unaffected, since the inhibitor concentration term cancels. Thus, the classic signature of an uncompetitive inhibitor is a double reciprocal plot composed of parallel lines (Figure 12.10C).

Because uncompetitive inhibitors bind exclusively to the *ES* complex, the IC_{50} of these inhibitors decreases with increasing substrate concentration as follows:

$$IC_{50} = \alpha K_i\left(1 + \frac{K_M}{[S]}\right) \tag{12.14}$$

Thus, in the exact opposite direction as for competitive inhibitors, the IC_{50} of uncompetitive inhibitors shifts to lower values with increasing substrate concentrations.

As with non-competitive inhibitors, uncompetitive inhibitors can have pharma-cological advantages for target enzymes that catalyzed precessive reactions or for which cellular substrate concentrations are high relative to K_M.

The steroid 5α-reductase inhibitor episteride provides a clinically interesting example of uncompetitive enzyme inhibition. The androgen dihydrotestosterone (DHT) mediates a number of male sexual characteristics. The DHT is produced by the reduction of testosterone by the enzyme steroid 5α-reductase. A genetic deficiency in this enzyme was identified in association with a population of pseudo-hermaphrodites in the Dominican Republic. These individuals do not display normal male genitalia until the onset of puberty; hence they are raised as females until then. Other phenotypical characteristics of these individuals include no male pattern baldness, mild or no acne, and underdeveloped prostates. These observa-tions led to the suggestion that inhibitors of steroid 5α-reductase might be clinically useful in the treatment of benign prostate hyperplasia, a non-cancerous enlargement of the prostate that affects a significant proportion of men over 50 years old.

The reaction mechanism of steroid 5α-reductase is illustrated in Figure 12.18. The enzyme binds the redox co-factor NADPH first and then binds testosterone to form a ternary enzyme-NADPH-testosterone complex. Hydride transfer to the β-carbon of the testosterone double bond then occurs; the enolate intermediate thus formed is stabilized by an acid group within the enzyme active site. The α-carbon of the enolate is then protonated by an active site base, leading to

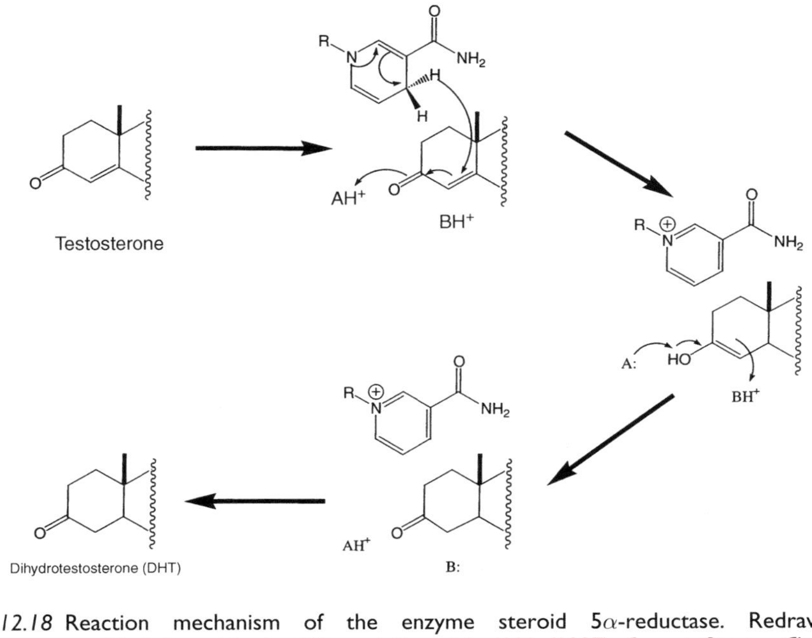

Figure 12.18 Reaction mechanism of the enzyme steroid 5α-reductase. Redrawn and modified from Harris, G.S. and Kozarich, J.W. (1997) Current Opinion Chem. Biol., 1, 254–259.

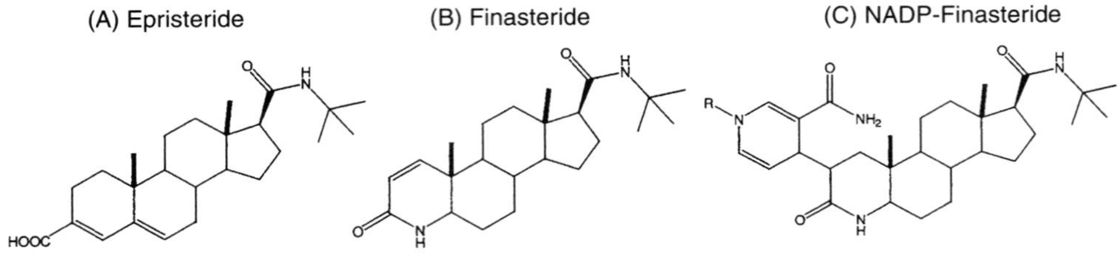

Figure 12.19 Chemical structures of inhibitors of steroid 5α-reductase: (A) epristeride; (B) finasteride; and (C) the covalent NADP-finasteride complex.

the product, DHT. The DHT and then the $NADP^+$ co-factor are released to regenerate the free enzyme.

Epristeride (Figure 12.19A) was designed to mimic the testosterone enolate intermediate of the steroid 5α-reductase reaction pathway. The carboxylate functionality of the inhibitor electronically resembles the enolate. The pK_a of the carboxylate is 4.8, so that it is the anion form that is responsible for inhibition under physiological conditions. Kinetic and equilibrium binding studies demonstrated that epristeride is an uncompetitive inhibitor with respect to the NADPH co-factor, binding to the enzyme only after formation of the NADPH–enzyme binary complex, with a K_d of ca. 25 nM (2.5×10^{-8} M). This is expected from the reaction mechanism if the inhibitor is indeed functioning as a reaction intermediate mimic. Surprisingly, the inhibitor was also found to be uncompetitive with respect to testosterone. The interpretation of this observation is that the inhibitor binds to the enzyme form that results from release of the DHT product, prior to $NADP^+$ release.

Epristeride demonstrated the expected lowering of DHT levels upon oral dosing. In healthy volunteers this compound reduced circulating levels of DHT by 25–54%. The drug was not pursued in further clinical trials, however, most likely because more potent inhibitors of steroid 5α-reductase, such as finasteride (see below), were contemporaneously identified.

12.4   OTHER TYPES OF INHIBITORS

While many drugs behave as simple reversible enzyme inhibitors, compounds that inhibit enzyme by other mechanisms can also demonstrate clinical utility. Space does not permit an exhaustive review of all forms of enzyme inhibition. However, three other inhibitor modes that have led to a number of clinically useful drugs are slow, tight-binding inhibitors, covalent enzyme modifiers, and mechanism-based enzyme inhibitors. Examples of these inhibition modes will be described here.

12.4.1   Slow, tight-binding inhibitors

Simple, reversible inhibitors bind to enzymes rapidly, typically at diffusion-limited rates, and likewise dissociate from the enzyme on a relatively fast time scale. Some inhibitors, however, bind slowly to enzymes either because their rate of binding is limited by a chemical event or because binding is associated with a rate-limiting conformational change of the enzyme. There are a number of examples of inhibitors that bind to the enzyme initially with modest affinity but then induce a conformational change in the enzyme leading to much tighter binding affinity (the inhibitor equivalent of the induced fit model discussed above for substrate interactions). In this case, the onset of inhibition is slow relative to the rate of enzyme turnover so that the product progress curve for the enzyme goes from a linear function in the absence of inhibitor, to a curvilinear form in the presence of the inhibitor. The non-linear character of the progress curve results from an initial rate of turnover characteristic of the weak, initial enzyme interaction with the inhibitor, and a second rate of turnover that results from the final inhibitor binding species (Figure 12.20). Hence, the accumulation of product with time is a function of three parameters: the initial velocity of reaction, the final velocity of reaction, and a rate constant associated with the transition between these enzyme–inhibitor complexes. The true affinity of the inhibitor for the enzyme can thus only be assessed after this final equilibrium has been established.

The selective inhibitors of cyclooxygenase-2 (COX2) are excellent contemporary examples of drugs in clinical use that function by slow, tight-binding enzyme inhibition. The COX2 is one of two isozymes of cyclooxygenase that catalyze the conversion of arachidonic acid to prostaglandin H_2. Prostaglandin H_2 and its metabolites serve a protective function in the GI and kidneys but also stimulate the pain, swelling, and fever associated with inflammation. The activity of the COX1 isozyme is mainly responsible for the protective functions of prostaglandin production while COX2 activity is associated with inflammatory response. Traditional anti-inflammatory drugs, such as aspirin and ibuprofen, inhibit both COX1

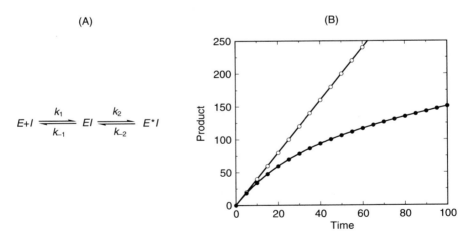

Figure 12.20 (A) A two-step reaction mechanism involving initial inhibitor binding to an enzyme followed by a conformational transition of the enzyme that results in much tighter inhibitor binding. The symbols E and E^* represent the two distinct conformational states of the enzyme. (B) Product appearance time courses for an enzyme in the absence (open circles) and presence (closed circles) of an inhibitor conforming to the mechanism illustrated in (A).

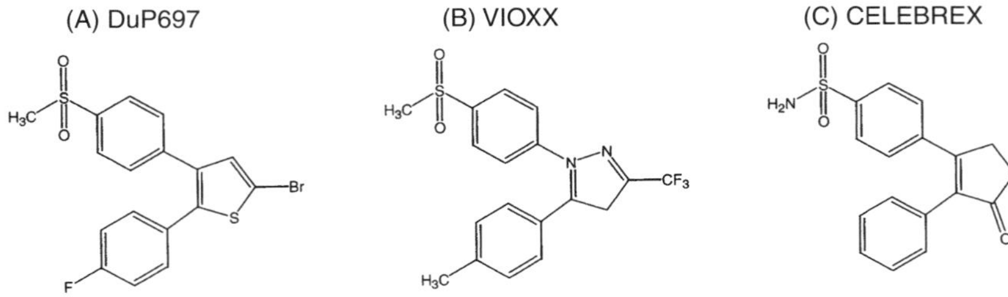

Figure 12.21 Chemical structures of COX-2 selective inhibitors that function by a slow, tight-binding mechanism: (A) DuP697; (B) VIOXX; and (C) CELEBREX.

and COX2. Prolonged use of these drugs is associated with GI and renal ulceration as a result of COX1 inhibition. Hence, selective inhibitors of COX2 provide a clear mechanism for anti-inflammatory therapy without untoward side effects.

The first selective COX2 inhibitor to be described was the experimental compound DuP697 (Figure 12.21A). This compound proved to be an excellent anti-inflammatory agent in animal models without associated ulcerogenicity. Detailed kinetic analysis of DuP697 inhibition of COX1 and COX2 demonstrated an unexpected mechanism for isozyme selectivity. The compound binds to both COX1 and COX2 with equal, modest affinity ($K_i \sim 5\,\mu$M). Inhibitor binding induces a slow conformational change in COX2, but not COX1, that increases inhibitor affinity by >10-fold. Thus, the isozyme-selective induction of a conformational change in the enzyme leads to potent inhibition of COX2 that is not seen for COX1. This observation led several groups to investigate structural analogs of DuP697, resulting in improved potency and selectivity based on this same isozyme-selective conformational transition. Ultimately, two COX2 selective inhibitors, based on this inhibition mechanism, have been brought to the clinic for the treatment of inflammatory diseases: VIOXX and CELEBREX (Figure 12.21B and C). Both compounds are structurally related to DuP697 and both demonstrate the same slow, tight-binding inhibition of COX2 but not COX1. These compounds have quickly become the standard of care for anti-inflammatory therapies and provide a great benefit to patients due to the amelioration of GI and renal side effects with these new medicines.

12.4.2   Covalent enzyme modifiers

Many chemically reactive compounds can interact with specific amino acid side chains within proteins to covalently modify them, in a process referred to as affinity labeling. When the amino acid side chain is critical to the catalytic mechanism of the enzyme, covalent modification leads to irreversible inactivation. Generally, compounds that covalently modify enzymes in this way do so too indiscriminately to be useful as drugs. In some cases, however, covalent modifiers (also referred to as affinity labels) have been discovered that are highly selective for a specific enzyme active site. A classical example of this is the anti-inflammatory drug aspirin.

Aspirin (acetylsalicylic acid) and its analogs have been used, in one form or another, to treat pain, fever and general inflammation since the time of Hippocrates. The anti-inflammatory activity of aspirin results from its ability to block prostaglandin biosynthesis by inhibiting the cyclooxygenase isozymes COX1 and COX2 (see above). Aspirin irreversibly inactivates these enzymes by acetylation of an active site serine residue within the arachidonic acid binding pocket. The additional bulk added to the serine by acetylation sterically blocks arachidonic acid entry into this binding pocket, thus acting as an irreversible competitive inhibitor.

A more recent example of a enzyme-selective covalent modifier is the compound AG7088, an experimental drug that inhibits the 3C protease of human rhinovirus, the causal agents of common colds in humans.

Rhinovirus are members of the *picornavirus* family of RNA viruses that rely on proteolytic processing of a viral polyprotein for replication. One viral protease that is critical for replication is the 3C protease. This enzyme is a cysteine protease, using an active site cysteine as the attacking nucleophile for peptide bond hydrolysis. Inhibition of this enzyme will therefore block viral replication, potentially leading to a rapid resolution of the infection.

The Agouron group solved the crystal structure of the rhinovirus 3C protease and used this structural information for inhibitor design. The first inhibitor to be designed was based on a short peptide representing the canonical substrate sequence on the N-terminal side of the 3C protease cleavage site. The last residue in this peptide (i.e. the group immediately preceding the scissile bond of the substrate) was replaced by an aldehyde group that binds to the active site cysteine to create a tetrahedral carbon structure resembling the transition state of the reaction. This proved to be a potent inhibitor of the enzyme, with a K_i of 6 nM. Reduction of the aldehyde to the corresponding alcohol resulted in a complete loss of binding affinity. This suggested that small molecule, non-covalent inhibitors were unlikely to be effective against this enzyme. Based on these results the Agouron group focused their efforts on finding better, irreversible modifiers of the active site cysteine. Replacement of the aldehyde group with an α,β-unsaturated ethyl ester provided the peptide with a Michael acceptor that could readily undergo nucleophilic attack by the active site cysteine. Optimization of the rest of the peptide led to compound AG7088 (Figure 12.22A). The kinetics of AG7088 inhibition of the protease indicated that the compound first binds reversibly and then more slowly inactivates the enzyme by forming a covalent species. Thus, the compound acts as a slow binding, irreversible inhibitor, conforming to the mechanism:

$$E + I \underset{k_{\text{off}}}{\overset{k_{\text{on}}}{\rightleftharpoons}} EI \xrightarrow{k_{\text{inact.}}} E - I$$

The affinity of such compounds cannot be measured by an equilibrium dissociation constant, as there is no back reaction. Instead, affinity is quantified in terms of the second order rate constant obtained from the ratio $k_{\text{obs}}/[I]$, where k_{obs} is the observed pseudo-first order rate constant for inactivation (measured as described above for slow, tight-binding inhibitors); the second order rate constant for AG7088

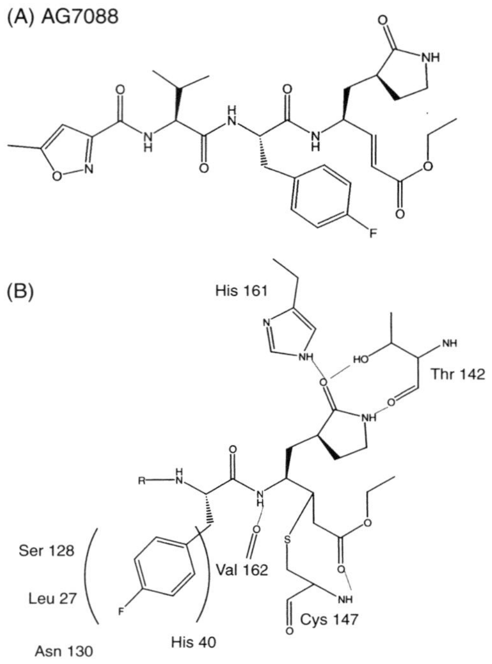

Figure 12.22 (A) Chemical structure of the rhinovirus 3C protease inhibitor AG7088; and (B) schematic representation of the covalent species formed between AG7088 and the active site cysteine of the rhinovirus 3C protease.

inactivation of the 3C protease is $1\,470\,000\,\text{s}^{-1}\,\text{M}^{-1}$. The crystal structure of AG7088 bound to the 3C protease confirmed the expected mechanism of covalent inhibition. The side chain sulfur of the active site cysteine forms a covalent bond to the β-carbon of the formerly unsaturated ethyl ester group (see Figure 12.22). The affinity of the inhibitor is further augmented by hydrophobic interactions with leucine and asparagine residues and by hydrogen bonding interactions with histidine, threonine and serine side chains, as well as with mainchain heteroatoms of a valine and the active site cysteine in the binding pocket. AG7088 not only shows activity as an enzyme inactivator *in vitro*, it also demonstrates good inhibition of viral replication in cellular assays. In HeLa and MRC-5 cells the mean EC_{50} for inhibition of viral replication was 23 nM, while the compound showed no toxicity for these cells at concentrations as high as $100\,\mu\text{M}$. This compound has now entered human clinical trials to determine its safety and effectiveness at treating common colds.

12.4.3   Mechanism-based enzyme inhibitors

Mechanism-based inhibitors are molecules that themselves are inactive as enzyme inhibitors, but resemble the substrate or product of the enzyme reaction enough to be recognized and acted upon by the enzyme. The chemical transformation of the molecule within the enzyme active site results either in covalent modification of the enzyme or of a cofactor, leading to inactivation, or *in situ* formation of an extremely tight-binding non-covalent inhibitor. This form of inhibition is distinct from affinity labeling in that mechanism-based inhibition relies on the normal chemistry of enzymatic catalysis to transform the compound into an active inhibitor. Affinity labels, on the other hand, rely on the inherent chemical reactivity of the labeling molecule itself. Mechanism-based inhibitors, therefore, are usually very specific for a particular target enzyme, making this form of inhibition attractive for drug applications (see Chapter 9).

A recent example of a clinically useful mechanism-based enzyme inhibitor is the drug finasteride, an inhibitor of steroid 5α-reductase. Inhibitors of this enzyme, as described earlier, have potential application in the treatment of benign prostate hyperplasia, male pattern baldness, and severe acne. Finasteride (Figure 12.19B) is a structural analog of testosterone and binds to the enzyme within the testosterone binding pocket. The compound was initially described as a reversible slow, tight-binding inhibitor of steroid 5α-reductase. More detailed kinetic and chemical studies, however, revealed that the molecule actually functions through an unusual form of mechanism-based inhibition. Like testosterone, finasteride binds to the enzyme–NADPH binary complex to form a ternary complex. The NADPH reduction of and hydride transfer to finasteride then occurs within the active site of the enzyme with formation of a lactam enolate of finasteride, analogous to the testosterone enolate reaction intermediate. This species then attacks the electrophilic pyrimidine of the $NADP^+$ cofactor, leading to a covalent NADP-finasteride adduct (Figure 12.19C). This adduct occupies both the NADPH and testosterone binding pockets simultaneously as a bisubstrate inhibitor. The favorable binding interactions with both substrate binding pockets leads to very high affinity inhibition; the estimated K_d for the NADP-finasteride adduct is $0.3\,pM$ ($3 \times 10^{-13}\,M$) with an estimated half-life for dissociation of >30 days! Hence, in practice finasteride acts essentially as an irreversible inactivator of steroid 5 α-reductase.

Finasteride demonstrates good efficacy for the treatment of benign prostate hyperplasia. Patients treated with this drug for 36 months had a median reduction in prostate volume of 27% (relative to pretreatment volume) with correlated improvements in urinary flow rates and other symptoms. The drug is currently prescribed for this indication and is also undergoing clinical trials for the treatment of prostate cancer. Finasteride has also demonstrated clinical efficacy in the treatment of male pattern baldness, promoting hair growth in a significant portion of treated men. The drug is currently prescribed for this indication as well.

12.5 SUMMARY

In this chapter, we have briefly introduced the chemical mechanisms by which enzymes catalyze the critical biochemical reactions of life. Strategies for substrate recognition and transformation to the reaction transition state were discussed in the context of achieving reactant specificity and reaction rate acceleration. Blocking the pathogenic activity of enzymes with small molecular weight inhibitors forms the mechanistic basis for a large proportion of currently prescribed drugs. We saw that the same structural determinants of substrate binding and chemical transformation can be exploited to design potent enzyme inhibitors that compete with the natural substrate for the free enzyme. Other modes of reversible enzyme inhibition were also introduced and clinically relevant examples of each inhibitor modality were discussed. Examples of other types of enzyme inhibitors, such as slow, tight-binding inhibitors, covalent modifiers and mechanism-based inhibitors were also presented. These examples give some sense of the diversity of strategies available for the chemotherapeutic use of enzyme inhibition. As we enter the twenty-first century, new technologies are enhancing our ability to identify pathogenic targets associated with human diseases. A significant portion of these to-be-discovered targets is likely to be enzymes. Hence, continued study of the catalytic mechanisms and methods for inhibition of these proteins will remain a mainstay of pharmaceutical science for the foreseeable future.

FURTHER READING

Chan, C.-C., Boyce, S., Brideau, C., Charleson, S., Cromlish, W., Ethier, D., Evans, J., Ford-Hutchinson, A.W., Forrest, M.J., Gauthier, J.Y., Gordon, R., Gresser, M., Guay, J., Kargman, S., Kennedy, B., Leblanc, Y., Leger, S., Mancini, J., O'Neill, G.P., Ouellet, M., Patrick, D., Percival, M.D., Perrier, H., Prasit, P., Rodger, I., Tagari, P., Therien, M., Vickers, P., Visco, D., Wang, Z., Webb, J., Wong, E., Xu, L.-J., Young, R.N., Zamboni, R. and Riendeau, D. (1999) Rofecoxib [Vioxx, MK-0966; 4-(4'-methylsulfonylphenyl)-3-phenyl-2-(5H)-furanone]: A potent and orally active cyclooxygenase-2 inhibitor. Pharmacological and biochemical profiles. *J. Pharmacol. Exp. Ther.*, **290**, 551–560.

Copeland, R.A. (2000) *Enzymes: A Practical Introduction to Structure, Mechanism and Data Analysis*, 2nd edition. New York: Wiley-VCH.

Copeland, R.A., Williams, J.M., Giannaras, J., Nurnberg, S., Covington, M., Pinto, D., Pick, S. and Trzaskos, J.M. (1994) Mechanism of selective inhibition of the inducible isoform of prostaglandin G/H synthase. *Proc. Natl. Acad. Sci. USA*, **91**, 11202–11206.

Drews, J. (2000) Drug discovery: A historical perspective. *Science*, **287**, 1960–1964.

Fersht, A. (1999) *Structure and Mechanism in Protein Science*. New York: Freeman.

Harris, G.S. and Kozarich, J.W. (1997) Steroid 5α-reductase inhibitors in androgen-dependent disorders. *Current Opinion Chem. Biol.*, **1**, 254–259.

Levy, M.A., Brandt, M., Heys, R., Holt, D.A. and Metcalf, B.W. (1990) Inhibition of rat liver steroid 5α-reductase by 3-androstene-3-carboxylic acids: mechanism of enzyme–inhibitor interactions. *Biochemistry*, **29**, 2815–2824.

Mathews, D.A., Dragovich, P.S., Webber, S.E., Fuhrman, S.A., Patick, A.K., Zalman, L.S., Hendrickson, T.F., Love, R.A., Prins, T.J., Marakovits, J.T., Zhou, R., Tikhe, J., Ford, C.E., Meador, J.W., Ferre, R.A., Brown, E.L., Binford, S.L., Brothers, M.A., DeLisle, D.M. and Worland, S.T. (1999) Structure-assisted design of mechanism-based irreversible inhibitors of human rhinovirus 3C protease with potent antiviral activity against multiple rhinovirus serotypes. *Proc. Natl. Acad. Sci. USA*, **96**, 11000–11007.

Purich, D.L. (ed.) (1996) *Contemporary Enzyme Kinetics and Mechanism*, 2nd edition. San Diego: Academic Press.

Ren, J., Milton, J., Weaver, K.L., Short, S.A., Stuart, D.I. and Stammers, D. K. (2000) Structural basis for the resilience of efavirenz (DMP-266) to drug resistance mutations in HIV-1 reverse transcriptase. *Structure (London)*, **8**, 1089–1094.

Segel, I.H. (1975) *Enzyme Kinetics*, 2nd edition. New York: Wiley.

Silverman, R.B. (1992) *The Organic Chemistry of Drug Design and Drug Action*. San Diego: Academic Press.

Spence, R.A., Kati, W.M., Anderson, K.S. and Johnson, K.A. (1995) Mechanism of inhibition of HIV-1 reverse transcriptase by nonnucleoside inhibitors. *Science*, **267**, 988–993.

Chapter 13

Metals in medicine: inorganic medicinal chemistry

Ole Farver

13.1 INTRODUCTION

Bioinorganic chemistry lies in the interface between inorganic chemistry and biology, and although biology is generally associated with organic chemistry, in fact most of the chemical elements from hydrogen to bismuth bear potential in drug design (Figure 13.1). Thus, inorganic chemistry is beginning to have a larger impact on modern medicine. Given the enormous variety and range in reactivity of inorganic compounds, the application of inorganic chemistry in improving human health opens for a whole new research field. While still in its infancy, bioinorganic chemistry is destined to play an increasingly important role in modern medicinal chemistry since essential as well as non-essential and toxic elements can be utilized in drug design.

Pharmaceuticals may control metabolism of essential elements in two ways:

1   Supply of specific drugs with target properties may enable delivery or removal of elements to/from specific sites.
2   The natural physiological pathways may be blocked by the drug.

A general problem associated with the use of inorganic compounds as pharmaceuticals is the poor characterization of the compounds with respect to toxicity *in vivo*. The issues of understanding the reaction mechanisms and identification

IA	IIA	IIIB	IVB	VB	VIB	VIIB	VIIIB	VIIIB	VIIIB	IB	IIB	IIIA	IVA	VA	VIA	VIIA	VIIIA
H																	He
Li	Be											B	C	N	O	F	Ne
Na	Mg											Al	Si	P	S	Cl	Ar
K	Ca	Sc	Ti	V	Cr	Mn	Fe	Co	Ni	Cu	Zn	Ga	Ge	As	Se	Br	Kr
Rb	Sr	Y	Zr	Nb	Mo	Tc	Ru	Rh	Pd	Ag	Cd	In	Sn	Sb	Te	I	Xe
Cs	Ba	*La*	Hf	Ta	W	Re	Os	Ir	Pt	Au	Hg	Tl	Pb	Bi	Po	At	Rn
Fr	Ra	*Ac*	Th	Pa	U												

Figure 13.1 The periodic table of the elements. Selected elements which are important in bioinorganic chemistry are highlighted: **bulk biological elements**; *essential elements*; **possibly essential trace elements**. Other elements may be used in drugs or as probes.

of target centers are together with the toxicity problem central aspects that have to be addressed before potential new drugs can be applied. This underlines the major point: *Specific biological activity of inorganic compounds can be achieved by proper design.*

Metals are commonly found as natural constituents in proteins where they perform a wide spectrum of specific functions associated with biological processes. Metalloproteins with catalytic properties are called metalloenzymes. They implement chemical transformations of certain molecules called substrates, and it is interesting to note that almost half of all enzymes in the human organism are depending on the presence of one or more metal ions. Obviously, these metal ions are key pharmaceutical targets for drugs. Inorganic chemistry thus has a huge potential in modern pharmacology as it introduces a new realm of compounds. It is noteworthy that metal ions control some of the fundamental biochemical processes such as RNA and DNA replication. From an 'inorganic' point of view co-ordination chemistry in biological systems (metalloproteins and -enzymes) is particularly interesting, and this applies to both the thermodynamic (structure and binding) and the kinetic (reactivity) aspects.

13.1.1 Essential and non-essential elements

Elements are called essential if their absence causes irreversible damage to the organism or if the optimal function of the organism is impaired. Otherwise they are labeled non-essential. The chemistry behind the way the human body utilizes the elements is fascinating, but even the mechanisms of how essential elements are supplied from the diet are poorly understood.

Which elements are essential or beneficial and which are non-essential or even toxic for a certain organism? These questions are continuously being discussed. The elements as such are not good or evil and we recognize a general concentration dependence of the action of all elements. As the diagram in Figure 13.2 indicates, there is a dose/effect response curve different for each element. Many substances may even have an ambivalent effect which illustrates the saying of Paracelsus: *The dose makes the poison.*

Homeostasis which means maintenance of an optimal concentration of beneficial elements, as well as detoxification, i.e. transport of non-beneficial elements out of the system, require a delicate balance between processes of uptake, utilization, and excretion. As far as the essential elements are concerned, too low concentrations will result in deficiency diseases. Excess of an otherwise beneficial element as well as addition of a toxic compound will cause poisoning of the organism (Figure 13.2). This could either be due to unwanted redox reactions where damaging byproducts such as the hydroxyl radical is formed or by non-specific binding to certain centers which may lead to inhibition of the normal physiological processes.

As far as the non-essential (or toxic) elements are concerned, the concentration region in the left-hand side of Figure 13.2 (a) can be applied since these elements show no toxic effect in a certain limited concentration range. This provides us with an opportunity to apply the compounds pharmacologically, e.g. killing certain cell

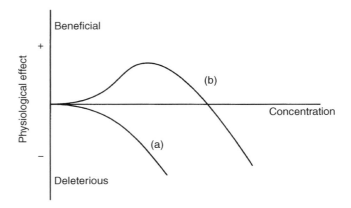

Figure 13.2 Dose/effect diagram. An organism's response to (a) non-essential or toxic and (b) essential elements. Note that at sufficiently small concentrations, toxic compounds are tolerated. Essential elements become toxic at elevated concentrations.

types or micro-organisms that are more sensitive to a particular element. Examples are drugs based on Pt(II) and Au(I) complexes. These metal ions are otherwise highly toxic and should be administered with the utmost care. The toxicity may also depend on a certain oxidation state. Arsenic, for example is generally considered being a highly toxic substance, but As(III) compounds are much more toxic than As(V) compounds.

13.1.2   History

Inorganic compounds have been applied in medicine for thousands of years. The ancient Egyptians and Hebrews are supposed to have utilized copper for sterilization of water (3000 years B.C.E.). About the same time the Chinese used gold for medical purposes – including the noble purpose of obtaining a state of immortality (youth elixir). Calomel (Hg_2Cl_2) has been a well-known diureticum since the renaissance and was used until the 1950s. P. Ehrlich's arsenic compounds were the first successful pharmaceuticals for treating syphilis. Another drug worth mentioning is AuCN which was used as a relatively efficient drug against tuberculosis. Gold therapies are applied even today in treatment of rheumatoid arthritis, both as injections of gold thiolates and orally as aurarofin (Section 13.8.6). It is, however, noteworthy that serendipity has played a major role in the discovery of all these treatments. Introduction of Pt(II) complexes that have revolutionized treatment of several malignant tumor species is an excellent example. Platinum compounds and their mechanism of action (as far as they are known today) will be discussed in Section 13.8.5.

For modern rational drug design and development, it is of utmost importance to understand the reaction mechanism of the inorganic compounds, including identification of the target centers. And indeed, a huge world of inorganic drugs, which have not yet been explored is now slowly opening.

13.2 CLASSIFICATION OF INORGANIC PHARMACEUTICALS

Inorganic drugs may be divided into three different categories (Figure 13.3):

1 *Active complexes*: In this case, it is the entire complex, metal ion and ligands, which determines the action. Many inert positively charged co-ordination compounds act as neurotoxins by blocking acetylcholine receptors. *Cis*-platinum and other uncharged Pt(II) and Ru(II) complexes are active as antitumor drugs (Section 13.8.5). Bi(III) complexes with sulphur containing ligands are used in the treatment of gastrointestinal diseases. These compounds will be dealt with later in more detail (Section 13.8.8). Insoluble salts of certain heavy metals can be applied as X-ray contrast compounds, such as $BaSO_4$. The rare earth gadolinium (Gd) is used in NMR diagnostics. The $[Xe]4f^7$ electron configuration of Gd^{3+} with its 7 unpaired electrons makes the ion highly paramagnetic. However, due to pronounced toxicity gadolinium compounds are administered as chelate compounds protecting the organism, e.g. as the $GdEDTA^-$ complex. Tin co-ordinated to protophorphyrin inhibits heme oxygenase degradation of a certain iron-heme product to bilirubin. The latter compound is the most frequent cause of neonatal jaundice.

Active complexes
- Cr, Co, Rh (neuromuscular blockers)
- Pt, Ru (anticancer drugs)
- Gd (NMR probes)
- Co (vitamin B_{12})
- Al, Zr (antiperspirant)
- Ba (x-ray contrast)
- Sn (jaundice)
- Bi (antiulcer and -bacterial agents)

Active elements
- Li (manic-depressive psychosis)
- F (tooth paste)
- Ag, Hg (antimicrobial compounds)
- ^{99m}Tc, ^{111}In (radiodiagnostica)
- Au (rheumatoid arthritis)

Active ligands
- *Delivered by a metal ion*
  - Ca, Mg, Al (antacid compounds)
  - Fe (antihypertensiva)
  - Ti, Au (anticancer)
- *Delivered to a metal ion*
  - Bleomycin (Fe)
  - Penicillamine (Cu)
  - Desferrioxamine (Fe, Al)
  - Bisphosphonates (Ca)

Figure 13.3 Classification of inorganic drugs. Adapted from P.J. Sadler (1991).

2   *Active elements*: In this case, the metal ion is decisive for the action of the drug while the anion or ligand only serves to keep the metal ion in solution or simply as a counter ion. The effect of lithium in the manic-depressive psychosis is well known even if not fully understood. Interestingly, the lithium ion is counteracting both phases of the cyclic course of this disease (Section 13.8.1). The cariostatic effect of fluoride is well established although the mechanism is still unclear. Formation of a particularly resistant crystalline layer of tooth enamel (fluoroapatite) is one possibility. Inhibition of caries-promoting enzymes by fluoride ions is another widely accepted idea. Silver(I) and mercury(II) are potential antibacterial agents, and silver sulfadiazene is still used clinically (Section 13.8.6). Technetium (the ^{99m}Tc isotope) is applied in radiodiagnostics. The γ-active isotope has a half-life of 6 h. Tc is mainly administered as a $Tc^{VII}(CNR)_6^+$ complex. The significance of gold in treating rheumatoid arthritis is discussed further in Section 13.8.6.

3   *Active ligands*: Many ligands can be delivered to or from a metal ion in the organism. The classic iron(III) co-ordination compound, nitroprusside $[Fe^{III}(CN)_5NO]^{2-}$, with its $[Ar]d^5$ electron configuration, relatively easily releases NO which functions as an hypotensive agent causing smooth muscle relaxation. The half life of the very reactive NO radical is only 6 sec. Some selected chelates are presented in Section 13.6.

13.3   THE HUMAN BODY AND BIOINORGANIC CHEMISTRY

The living organism may be considered being an open system in a steady state where energy input and output maintain a dynamic flow equilibrium (a dissipative system). Besides energy flux, life requires a constant exchange of material, which in principle could comprise all elements of the periodic table (Figure 13.1). The occurrence of a given element in an organism depends on several factors. First of all, how available the element is in nature, i.e. abundance and accessibility. But elements which are rarer or more difficult to obtain may be accumulated actively by the organism, nonetheless. In the latter case, energy consuming processes are required. The composition of elements in the human body is given in Table 13.1.

Table 13.1 requires some comments: The large quantities of hydrogen and oxygen simply reflect the amount of 'inorganic' water. 'Organic' carbon comes in second. Calcium is the first metallic element to be encountered, and its primary function is stabilization of the skeleton. The table also demonstrates rather large quantities of the metals potassium, sodium, and magnesium, and furthermore the non-metallic elements nitrogen, sulfur, phosphorous, and chlorine are abundant.

Now follows iron and zinc as the first representatives of the transition metals, though in much smaller quantities. They constitute together with the non-metallic elements fluorine and silicon, which are important for our bone structure, the transition to the genuine trace elements. Here we set the boundary, quite arbitrarily, to less than 1 g per 70 kg body weight. Many trace elements are essential, which as stated above, means that the organism will be irreversibly damaged by eliminating them from the food. Elements in Table 13.1 which are marked by an asterix, some of

Table 13.1 Constitution of the human organism (adult 70 kg)

Element	Mass (g)	Recommended daily dose (mg)
oxygen	45500	
carbon	12600	
hydrogen	7000	
nitrogen	2100	
calcium	1050	800–1200
phosphorous	700	800–1200
sulfur	175	10
potassium	140	2000–5500
chlorine	105	3200
sodium	105	1100–3300
magnesium	35	300–400
iron	4.2	10–20
zinc	2.3	15
silicon	1.4	
rubidium*	1.1	
fluorine	0.8	1.5–4.0
bromine*	0.2	
strontium*	0.14	
copper	0.11	1.5–3
aluminium*	0.1	
lead*	0.08	
antimony	0.07	
cadmium*	0.03	
tin*	0.03	
iodine	0.03	0.15
manganese	0.03	2–5
vanadium*	0.02	
selenium	0.02	0.05–0.07
barium*	0.02	
arsenic*	0.01	
boron*	0.01	
nickel*	0.01	
chromium	0.005	0.05–0.2
cobalt	0.003	0.2
molybdenum	<0.005	ca. 0.1

Source: Recommended Dietary Allowance, RDA.
Note
* The elements marked by * are either non-essential or their function is unknown.

which occurring in rather large concentrations, probably are not essential like rubidium, strontium, bromium, and aluminium. The reason why these elements occur is their close chemical resemblance with essential ones: $Rb^+ \sim K^+$, $Br^- \sim Cl^-$, $Al^{3+} \sim Fe^{3+}$. Certain elements which are known to be toxic, even in very small quantities, like arsenic, lead, and cadmium require special attention. It has been discussed whether these elements in minimal amounts (Figure 13.2 (a)) could be, if not essential to the organism, then at least beneficial. It is not inconceivable at all that during evolutionary pressure all elements have obtained some physiological function.

It is also noteworthy that elements like silicon and titanium which are found in abundance in many minerals forming the earth's crust play such a marginal role in biological systems. The reason is, of course, that these elements are practically non-available in aqueous solution at pH 7. On the other hand, a rather exotic metal like molybdenum is relatively soluble at neutral pH as $Mo^{VI}O_4^{2-}$, and molybdenum has found an important function as an essential metal in certain enzymes (Section 13.8.3).

Now, which elements are essential, which are beneficial without being indispensable, and which are exclusively toxic? From the previous section this seems to be a difficult question. And it is! Maybe the best answer is given by Paracelsus, referred to above, that it is the amount which determines the effect.

The diagram in Figure 13.2 demonstrates that too low concentration of essential elements will cause deficiency effects. The same element in too large quantity, however, will lead to poisoning whether this is caused by excessive uptake or excretion failure. Toxication of this nature can be treated by 'inorganic' chemistry using e.g. chelate therapy. Synergistic processes where one chelate binds the unwanted element while another transports it out of the organism has proven particularly effective. Menkes' and Wilson's diseases are caused by impaired copper uptake and defect copper excretion, respectively. In both cases, chelate therapy is used in treatment of the patients.

Since the human body functions by uptake, accumulation, transport, and storage of chemical compounds the arbitrary differentiation between 'organic' and 'inorganic' matter is irrelevant and just a historical relic. The double helix structure of DNA, for instance, could not be stabilized without the presence of mono- and divalent cations that compensate for the electrostatic repulsion between the negatively charged phosphate groups. Electric nerve impulses as well as more complex trigger mechanisms are initiated by rapid bursts of ions across membranes. Particularly Na^+, K^+, and Ca^{2+} ions are used to trigger cellular responses. Degradation of organic molecules requires acid and base catalysis which at physiological pH could not take place without the presence of either Lewis acids like the zinc(II) ion or Lewis bases that could be inorganic anions. Electron transfer is essential for all energy conversion processes in organisms, and here redox active transition metals like iron and copper become indispensable. The metal ions may be bound in small proteins and undergo redox transformations without catalyzing chemical changes in substrates. Instead the current carriers pass electrons to or from redox active iron and copper containing enzymes which are involved in specific biological functions. The reduction potentials of the metal ions co-ordinated to biological ligands embedded in a protein will usually differ markedly from potentials of the particular metal ion complexes in aqueous solution.

From the previous, it is evident that all fundamental biological processes proceed in reactions that often involve inorganic substances in central roles. It is thus obvious that inorganic chemistry holds a huge potential for developing new pharmaceuticals which may influence physiological processes. All this requires a detailed knowledge of interactions between metal ions and organic molecules; a field also known as co-ordination chemistry. Stability and kinetics of metal ion complexes will therefore be a central subject in this chapter describing inorganic drugs.

13.4 CO-ORDINATION CHEMISTRY

According to Lewis' definition, all metal ions as such are Lewis acids since they can co-ordinate to free electron pairs (i.e. Lewis bases). The outcome of this reaction is called a co-ordination compound or a complex between the central metal ion (Lewis acid) and the electron donor (Lewis base). A complex is thus composed of ions or molecules which may exist individually in solution, but in combination they produce the co-ordination compound. The ions or molecules co-ordinated to the central metal ion are called ligands and make up the co-ordination sphere. The number of points at which ligands are attached to the metal ion is called the co-ordination number. The different categories of ligands are shown in Table 13.2.

13.4.1 Chelate effect

Ligands (Lewis bases) with several binding sites are called polydentate ligands (chelates) and form particularly stabile complexes: metal-chelates. The most advantageous situation occurs when 5- or 6-membered rings can be formed. One of the important factors controlling the stability of a complex is the chelate effect: The stability of a co-ordination compound increases with the number of binding centers of the ligands. Amino acids, peptides and proteins contain many metal binding groups which make them excellent chelates. Besides peptide NH and C=O groups, many side chains may serve as complexing agents for metal ions. These include thiolate in cysteine, the imidazole ring of histidine, carboxylates of glutamic acid and aspartic acid, and the amino side chain of lysine.

The rationale behind the chelate effect is quite straightforward. As soon as a metal ion co-ordinates to one of the binding centers in a multidentate ligand, the chance for co-ordination of other potential donor groups enhances since these cannot get very far away and only need to swing into position. If two independent molecules having access to much larger volume of the solution should bind, the second ligand must find its way to the metal ion by diffusion in a bimolecular

Table 13.2 Ligand types

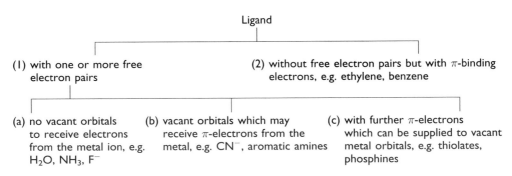

Ligand

(1) with one or more free electron pairs

(2) without free electron pairs but with π-binding electrons, e.g. ethylene, benzene

(a) no vacant orbitals to receive electrons from the metal ion, e.g. H_2O, NH_3, F^-

(b) vacant orbitals which may receive π-electrons from the metal, e.g. CN^-, aromatic amines

(c) with further π-electrons which can be supplied to vacant metal orbitals, e.g. thiolates, phosphines

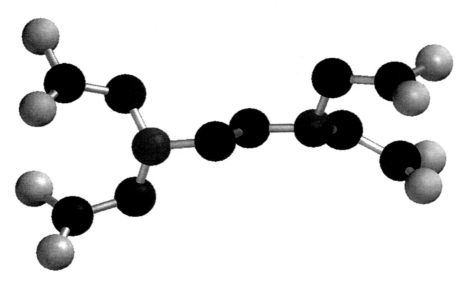

Figure 13.4 Structure of the free EDTA molecule. Carbon atoms are black, oxygen light gray, and nitrogen dark gray. Hydrogen atoms are not shown.

process. The difference in rates between the two processes, uni- vs. bimolecular, would typically be of an order of 10^4. A favorable entropic factor further adds to the stability since chelation is accompanied by release of non-chelating ligands like water from the co-ordination sphere. An example of a good chelate is shown in Figure 13.4, where the six possible donor groups in EDTA are all more or less in the correct position for metal ion co-ordination.

A closely related effect is termed the macrocyclic effect. It simply relates to the notion that a complex with a cyclic polydentate ligand has greater thermodynamic stability when compared with a similar non-cyclic ligand. Important examples are afforded by the porphyrin and corrin rings. As a consequence, macrocyclic complexes provide bioinorganic groups of widespread occurrence and utility in nature, being found in e.g. crown ethers, cryptands (alkali metals), cytochromes (iron), chlorophyll (magnesium), and coenzyme-B_{12} (cobalt).

Based on a large number of experimental data on the stability of divalent metal ion complexes with a given ligand, a certain trend has been demonstrated which is relatively insensitive to the choice of ligands. This variation is also known as the Irving–Williams series:

$$Ca^{2+} < Mg^{2+} < Mn^{2+} < Fe^{2+} < Co^{2+} < Ni^{2+} < Cu^{2+} > Zn^{2+}$$

The order is partly related to the decrease in ionic radii across the series which leads to stronger electrostatic effects and in addition to changes in crystal field stabilization energies. The latter is discussed in Section 13.4.3.

13.4.2 Hard and soft acids and bases (HSAB principle)

Metal ions may be divided into two categories:

1 Those which bind strongly to bases binding strongly to the proton; i.e. bases in the ordinary sense of the word (Class a metals).
2 Those binding preferentially to large polarizable or unsaturated bases that usually show insignificant basicity towards the proton (Class b metals).

This division is obviously not absolute and intermediate examples exist. Nevertheless, the division is reasonably distinct and has proven to be quite useful. We may now divide the bases into two categories: (1) Those which are polarizable or 'soft' bases; and (2) those which are not, the 'hard' bases. There are cases where a base is soft and at the same time binds to the proton with high affinity, e.g. the sulfide ion. However, generally it is true that hardness of a base is correlated with good proton binding. Among the bases with the central atom from main groups V, VI, and VII of the periodic table (which constitute the majority of all bases), those with nitrogen, oxygen, and fluorine are the hardest in their respective groups and at the same time the most basic towards the proton (F^-, OH^-, NH_3).

For Class a metal ions the order of complex stability is the following:

$$F^- > Cl^- > Br^- > I^-$$
$$O \gg S > Se > Te$$
$$N \gg P > As > Sb > Bi$$

while for Class b metal ions the order is virtually the opposite:

$$F^- < Cl^- < Br^- < I^-$$
$$O \ll S \sim Se \sim Te$$
$$N \ll P > As > Sb > Bi$$

It is now obvious that Class a metal ions co-ordinate best to the least polarizable (hardest) atoms of the group while Class b metal ions prefer the more polarizable (softer) atoms within the same family. It is also noteworthy that the softest (most polarizable) atom from a group does not necessarily form the most stable complexes with Class b metal ions. The reason is that many bases in general are poor ligands for all metal ions. Still, complexes between soft bases with Class b metal ions will in all cases be far more stable than their complexes with class a metals.

In Table 13.3, all metal ions which exhibit some importance in the bioinorganic chemistry are classified. The division of these Lewis acids was performed using the above mentioned criterion by comparing the stability of complexes with bases containing nitrogen vs. phosphorus, oxygen vs. sulfur, and fluorine vs. iodine.

It is quite straightforward to catagorize the two types of Lewis acids as in Table 13.3. The general feature of a Class a metal ion is a small ionic radius, high positive charge, and/or valence electrons that cannot be distorted easily. Class b metal ions are in contrast associated with low oxidation state, large ionic radius,

Table 13.3 Classification of Lewis acids

Hard	Soft
H^+, Li^+, Na^+, K^+	$Cu^+, Ag^+, Au^+, Tl^+, Hg_2^{2+}$
$Mg^{2+}, Ca^{2+}, Sr^{2+}, Mn^{2+}$	$Pd^{2+}, Cd^{2+}, Pt^{2+}, Hg^{2+}$
$Al^{3+}, La^{3+}, Gd^{3+}, Cr^{3+}, Co^{3+}, Fe^{3+}, As^{3+}$	Tl^{3+}, Au^{3+}
$Si^{4+}, Ti^{4+}, Os^{4+}$	
Borderline	
$Fe^{2+}, Co^{2+}, Ni^{2+}, Cu^{2+}, Zn^{2+}, Sn^{2+}, Pb^{2+}, Sb^{3+}, Bi^{3+}, Ru^{2+}, Os^{2+}$	

and/or relatively easily distorted outer electrons. Since features of Class a metals thus may be characterized by small polarizability they are called hard (Lewis) acids while Class b type metal ions having higher polarizability are called soft (Lewis) acids. This leads to a useful corollary which is as simple as it is useful:

Hard acids prefer to coordinate to hard bases, while soft acids prefer soft bases

This rule has proven to be extremely useful for estimating the stability of co-ordination compounds including complex formation between metal ions and biomolecules. Obviously other properties like the net charge of the ligand, steric factors, and resonance effects will influence the stability of the complex. Nonetheless, the stability order for soft acid complexes with Lewis bases is as follows:

$$S \sim C > I > Br > Cl > N > O > F$$

For hard acids, the division is even sharper since generally only complexes with oxygen or fluorine donor atoms will exist in aqueous solution. It should also be noted that the order of the above Lewis bases is exactly the same as the one for increasing electronegativity.

In the classification, polarizability was used as the decisive property, but other effects that are correlated with polarizability could well be responsible. For example, high ionization potentials are usually identified with small polarizability while a low ionization potential gives rise to larger polarization, and further the ionization potential is directly related to electronegativity. Also unsaturated bases which may accept π-electrons from the Lewis acid or easily reducible bases which could promote electron transfer to the metal ion are associated with a high degree of polarizability.The Hard and Soft Acid and Base (HSAB) principle will be widely applied in the following.

13.4.3   Kinetics: inert and labile complexes

Any complex formation takes place in a substitution reaction by replacement of one ligand by another. Following the terminology for organic reactions, we use the terms nucleophilic and electrophilic substitution. A nucleophilic reagent is one which donates electrons while an electrophilic reagent receives electrons.

These terms are synonymous with Lewis' base and acid definition, respectively. In a kinetic process, a good nucleophile is one which reacts rapidly with electrophilic reagents like a metal ion, and vice versa. Thus, any substitution reaction is fundamentally an acid–base reaction.

What primarily determines the rate of a substitution reaction, is the ratio between charge and size (charge density) of the metal ion, but when transition metals are involved also the d-electron structure should be taken into account. The term labile will be used for very reactive complexes while less reactive ones are called inert. Obviously, there is no sharp division between inert and labile co-ordination compounds. A useful definition of a labile system is one where the reaction is complete within the time of mixing (i.e. <1 min). The term inert is used for complexes that react sufficiently slow to be monitored by traditional spectroscopic methods, or which react too slowly to be studied at all. Care should be taken not to confuse the term labile (kinetic) with the thermodynamic designation, stable. It is often true that thermodynamically stable compounds react slowly whereas unstable compounds react rapidly. However, this is not an absolute requirement. Hg(II) as well as Fe(II) form very stable complexes with cyanide, $Hg(CN)_4^{2-}$ and $Fe(CN)_6^{4-}$ but the mercury complex exchanges its ligands extremely rapidly and must be categorized as labile. The iron complex, on the other hand, is inert. Other pertinent examples are many cobalt(III) complexes which are rather unstable but will nevertheless persist in solution for weeks and must thus be categorized as inert.

Knowledge of the kinetic properties of complexes will obviously be decisive in the design of drugs. If a pharmaceutical in form of an organic molecule is transferred to a target site by means of a metal ion, it is not advantageous to choose a metal ion that forms highly inert complexes. On the other hand, it is an absolute necessity that a complex formation between Pt(II) and DNA bases must lead to products sufficiently inert in order to have the adequate time to affect the division of tumor cells.

From information about the electronic structure of metal ion complexes, some general rules for the reactivity of these compounds can be stated. What characterizes transition metals is the partial occupancy of the d-orbitals. Following the crystal field theory the five d-orbitals split in the presence of the electrostatic field provided by the ligands (crystal field). Those orbitals lying in the direction of the ligands are raised in energy compared to the orbitals pointing away from the ligands. In an octahedral field the d-orbitals split as follows from Figure 13.5.

The doubly degenerate energy levels are denominated e while the triply degenerate levels are called t_2. The energy difference, Δ_O, is called the ligand field splitting. The two high energy d-orbitals of an octahedral complex are thus type e-orbitals while the three lower lying orbitals are of the t_2 type. The first three d electrons will go into each of the three t_2-orbitals (Hund's rule). The next electrons will enter either into the e-orbitals or pair up with electrons of the t_2-orbitals. The choice depends on the magnitude of the energy separating the two levels, Δ_O, and the energy required for pairing electrons in the same orbital. If the ligand field splitting is small, the electrons will preferentially occupy different orbitals with parallel spin and form a high-spin complex. If the splitting is large, the electrons will enter the t_2-orbitals forming a low-spin complex. For an octahedral iron(II) co-ordination compound, i.e. a d^6 system, there are thus two possibilities: $t_2^4 e^2$ (high spin) and t_2^6 (low spin) depending upon the magnitude of Δ_O. For aqua complexes

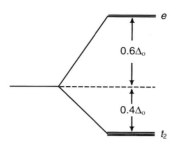

Figure 13.5 Crystal splitting of the *d*-orbitals. The diagram shows the splitting of a set of *d*-orbitals in a metal ion complex having an octahedral symmetry. The energy difference between the *e* and t_2 orbitals is designated Δ_O.

of divalent metal ions from the first transition series, the value of Δ_O is about 100 kJ/mol while the energy difference becomes twice as large for the trivalent aqua ions from the same series. When other ligands replace water, Δ_O changes as well, i.e. Δ_O is also a function of the ligands. The order of increasing splitting is called the spectrochemical series and is empirically found to be:

$$I^- < Br^- < Cl^- < F^- < OH^- < H_2O < NH_3 < NO_2^- < CO < CN^-$$

Those ligands associated with high splitting are called strong-field ligands, and those that give rise to low splitting energies are called weak-field ligands. For octahedral complexes with divalent metal ions of the first transition series the borderline between high-spin and low-spin complexes may be found after ammonia. Weak-field ligands from iodide to ammonia thus give rise to high-spin complexes while the remaining co-ordination compounds will be of the low-spin type. For trivalent metal ions of the same series, the border between strong-field and weak-field ligands lies between water and ammonia. From ammonia to cyanide the octahedral complexes will be of the low-spin type. For the transition metals of the second and third transition series the situation is much simpler. Due to the much larger ligand field splitting no high-spin octahedral complexes have ever been encountered with these elements. Tetrahedral complexes of the first transition series are always of the high spin type, as the result of a much smaller crystal field splitting, $\Delta_T (= 4/9 \times \Delta_O)$.

By preferentially filling up the lower lying t_2-orbitals the *d* electrons will stabilize the system relative to an average arrangement of the electrons among all available orbitals. The gain in binding energy obtained by distributing the charges in a non-symmetrical way is called crystal field stabilization energy (CFSE). The reason becomes quite obvious when looking at Figure 13.5. The *e*-orbitals clearly have higher energy than the t_2-orbitals. Taking an arbitrary zero when each orbital is randomly occupied, i.e. a spherically symmetric distribution, we may assign an energy of $-2/5 \times \Delta_O$ to the three t_2-orbitals and $+3/5 \times \Delta_O$ to the *e*-orbitals. We can now calculate the stabilization energies for complexes with any number of *d* electrons by assigning the appropriate energy to each electron. For example a d^5 high-spin octahedral complex will acquire a CFSE of $(-3 \times 2/5 + 2 \times 3/5) \times \Delta_O$

equal to 0. On the other hand, the corresponding low-spin d^5 complex will be stabilized by $-5 \times 2/5 \times \Delta_O$ or $-2 \times \Delta_O$. Thus, the latter will be considerably less reactive than the former.

The reactivity of octahedral complexes may now be predicted quite simply: The main group metal ions (alkali and alkaline earth metals) with d^0 electron structure together with the d^{10}-systems have no CFSE and in general thus exchange ligands extremely rapidly. Also d^1, d^2 and d^9 complexes having only a slight excess of electrons in the t_2-orbitals are expected to react fast. The same applies to high-spin d^4, d^5, d^6, and d^7 complexes. The d^3 system and low-spin complexes with d^4, d^5, and d^6 configuration are predicted to be substitution inert with d^6 being the least reactive. Finally, the d^8 configuration deserves a special comment since this system leads to very stable and inert square planar compounds. Platinum(II) complexes belong to this group and are discussed in detail in Section 13.4.5.

It was mentioned earlier that the thermodynamically stable $Hg(CN)_4^{2-}$ complex is substitution labile. It follows nicely the above notion, since Hg(II) has d^{10} electron configuration (CFSE = 0). In the corresponding inert $Fe(CN)_6^{4-}$ low-spin complex the Fe(II) iron has d^6 configuration (CFSE = $-12/5 \times \Delta_O$), and the reactivity is once more in accordance with the prediction based on CFSE. Cu(II) (d^9) and Zn(II) (d^{10}) co-ordination compounds are found frequently in enzyme systems where their large reactivity is fully exploited.

13.4.4   Redox reactions

The classical definition of oxidation is a process in which oxygen has been gained, while a reduction reaction is one where oxygen has been lost. This definition has now been replaced with the concepts electron loss (oxidation) and electron uptake (reduction). A reduction–oxidation (redox) reaction is thus a process in which changes in oxidation states or oxidation numbers take place, and the alleged electron transfer is a sort of book-keeping for balancing the equations. Mechanistically, it is often difficult to discern between atom or group transfer and plain electron transfer processes.

Many transition metals exist in several stable oxidation states which render them particularly interesting also in biological redox chemistry. Redox reactions play a central role in biochemistry; pertinent examples are photosynthesis and respiration where cascades of electron transfer reactions are coupled to synthesis of high-energy molecules like adenosine triphosphate (ATP) and similar compounds. The photosynthetic turnover of CO_2 is quite impressive with production of about 200 billion tons of carbohydrate annually. This production of reduced carbon compounds is accompanied by evolution of oxygen (O_2) following oxidation of two water molecules. However, one of the expenses for living under oxygen rich conditions is the danger of unwanted radical formations. Oxygen easily gets reduced to hydrogen peroxide, and in the presence of reducing metal ions like Fe^{2+} or Cu^+ further reactions may take place like the Fenton reaction, generating hydroxyl radicals:

$$Fe^{2+} + HO_2^- \rightarrow FeO^+ + {}^{\cdot}OH$$

In the presence of other reductants, this hydroxyl radical production can even become a catalytic reaction, promoting DNA strand scission through attack on the sugar–phosphate backbone. Free metal ions with redox properties should be avoided, and supplement of e.g. iron(II) as nutritional additive is therefore not unproblematic. Fortunately, the organism possesses numbers of effective chelates, proteins like albumin, transferrin, etc. that to a certain limit will sequester redox-active iron- and copper ions. Other major biochemical targets of oxygen seem to be lipids and proteins. Thus, elevated levels of oxygen are clearly toxic for mammals leading first to coughing and soreness of the throat and eventually to pulmonary edema and irreversible lung and other tissue damage.

13.4.5   The *trans*-effect

As mentioned in Section 13.4.3, Pt(II) (low-spin d^8 electron configuration) preferentially forms square planar complexes which are both stable and inert. Many other low-spin d^8 systems also form square planar complexes, e.g. Ni(II), Pd(II), Au(III), and Ir(I). The kinetics of this type of co-ordination compounds have been investigated thoroughly, and it was shown that all of these complexes generally undergo nucleophilic substitution.

That these four-co-ordinated complexes are square planar rather than tetrahedral, which is otherwise the preferred geometry, was observed early in the twentieth century. The fact that a compound like $Pt(NH_3)_2Cl_2$ could be produced in two forms demonstrated that the geometry could not be tetrahedral. One form was produced by reacting $PtCl_4^{2-}$ with ammonia while the other form could be obtained by heating solid $[Pt(NH_3)_4]Cl_2$. Since the complexes were monomeric, it was concluded that they were *cis/trans* isomers. Further studies demonstrated that the first reaction led to a *cis* configuration and the latter to the *trans* isomer. The rationale behind this behavior which also applies to the function of '*cis*-platinum' as an antitumor agent is called the *trans*-effect, and the concept correlates many of the reactions of square planar Pt(II) complexes.

The utility of this *empirical* rule can be illustrated by the synthesis of *cis*- and *trans*-$Pt(NH_3)_2Cl_2$ which is in keeping with the concept of the *trans*-effect (Figure 13.6). In the upper row, we begin with $PtCl_4^{2-}$; in the second row the starting material is $Pt(NH_3)_4^{2+}$. The negatively charged chloride ion has a greater labilizing effect on a group sitting opposite to it (*trans* position) than on a group in *cis* position. Also, this labilizing effect is usually larger for a negative ligand than it is for a neutral σ-bonding molecule like ammonia. In the upper reaction scheme of Figure 13.6, the second ammonia molecule will enter in a *cis* position since the chloride ion has a larger *trans* directing effect than that of ammonia. In the lower reaction series, the ammonia molecule opposite the chloride ion will be the most labile one and the result will be that Cl^- ion number two enters into the *trans* position. The empirical rule is thus quite useful, and in the section on *cis*-platinum (13.8.5) we shall see why the *trans* form is inactive as a cytostatic drug.

Briefly the *trans*-effect can be outlined as follows: The rate of substitution of a ligand is determined by the nature of the substituent at the opposite end of the diagonal (in *trans* position). Thus, while the chemical bond between the metal ion and any substituent is little affected by the character of neighboring

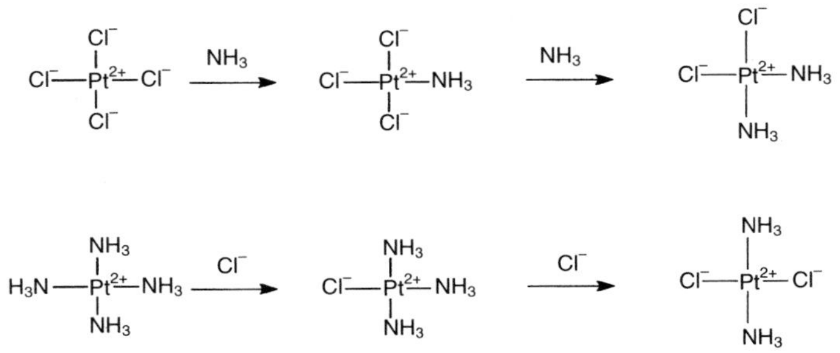

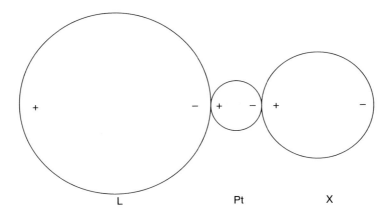

Figure 13.6 Illustration of the *trans*-effect. Synthesis of *cis*- and *trans*-[PtCl$_2$(NH$_3$)$_2$]. In the upper reaction, the second ammonia molecule enters a *cis*-position because the *trans*-directing influence of the chloride ion is larger than that of ammonia. In the lower process, a chloride ion replaces the most labile ammine ligand which is opposite, the chloro group.

molecules (*cis* position), it is greatly influenced by those farther away in the *trans* position. The approximate order of increasing *trans*-effect for typical ligands is

$$H_2O < OH^- < NH_3 < Cl^- < Br^- < I^- < NO_2^- < NO < CO < CN^-$$

It is worth emphasizing that the *trans*-effect is an empirical rule and based on kinetic effects and thus does not reflect the thermodynamic stability of a complex. The effect can nevertheless be dramatic. A complex containing a ligand with a large *trans*-directing effect may undergo substitution at rates a factor of 10^6 or higher compared with a ligand lower in the *trans*-effect series.

The *trans*-effect is relatively easily explained in terms of ligand polarizability (Figure 13.7). It is therefore not surprising that the above series of *trans*-directing

L   Pt   X

Figure 13.7 Trans-effect. Distribution of charge-induced dipoles in L-Pt-X of *trans*-[PtA$_2$LX]. The two A ligands are not depicted.

ligands correlate with the classification of Lewis bases presented in Section 13.4.2. We consider the *trans*-effect of L on the ligand X in *trans*-PtA$_2$LX (the A ligands are not shown). The primary positive charge on the platinum(II) ion induces a dipole in L, which in turn induces a dipole in the metal ion. However, this dipole is oriented in such a way to repel donor electrons on the Lewis base, X. Thus, the Pt-X bond will be weakened (and lengthened). The theory explains immediately the correlation between *trans*-influence of L and its polarizability, e.g. Cl$^-$ < I$^-$ < CN$^-$. Further, it predicts that the effect will be larger if the metal ion is itself polarizable. This agrees with the observation that Pt(II) is stronger influenced than e.g. Ni(II) or Pt(IV).

13.4.6   Plasma mobilization index

It will often be of interest to predict how a given pharmaceutical influences the metal ion balance in an organism. This may, however, be quite complicated as several potential chelates usually are present, as for example amino acids, proteins, and inorganic anions in the blood plasma. In principle, the effect can be calculated by simulation of the multiple equilibria present in the biological fluid from known stability constants for the metal ion with the different ligands together with the ligands' acid–base properties. The useful concept of a plasma mobilization index (PMI) was introduced by May and Williams in 1977, but we shall define the concept in a slightly different manner. The metal ions in a biological system are assumed to be distributed among states involving metal–protein and metal–small molecule complexes, all in equilibrium. We now let [M_{TOT}] indicate the concentration of all forms in which a given metal ion exists in the biological fluid containing some chelating drug, while [M_P] denotes the total concentration of the metal ion in normal fluid. The PMI is now defined as

$$PMI = \frac{[M_{TOT}]}{[M_P]} \tag{13.1}$$

An example, using computer simulation based on known stability constants, is shown in Figure 13.8 where PMI curves are calculated for copper(II) and Zn(II) in plasma in the presence of the strongly chelating agent, *d*-penicillamine (D-PEN (see Section 13.6.2)). Here it is obvious that administrating even very small amounts of D-PEN (concentration ~1 µM) the PMI for copper(II) is increased by a factor of 10 ($\log_{10} PMI = 1$) and there will be a ten-fold increase in mobilizing copper(II) ions with a possibility of either passing it on to some tissue or excreting it. Zinc(II) ions, in contrast, are influenced to a much smaller degree by D-PEN as can be seen from Figure 13.8. More complicated schemes involving several protein and small molecule complexes can of course be calculated in a similar way.

It is, however, often possible to perform a good estimate by the following simple approximate considerations. Let us as an example take Fe(III) in blood plasma (pH 7.4). Here the iron(III) is primarily bound to transferrin (Tr) which is present in a concentration of 10^{-8} M. The stability constant for the Fe(III) transferrin complex is 10^{20} M^{-1}. Suppose now that some iron(III) chelating drug (L) is

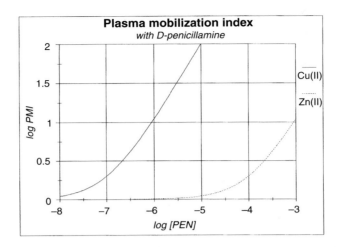

Figure 13.8 Plasma mobilization index curves. Simulated PMI curves calculated for d-penicillamine (D-PEN) using stability constants from the literature. Full line: Cu(II); broken line: Zn(II).

introduced which is essentially fully deprotonated at physiological pH ($pK_a < 6$) with a binding constant, K_L. We now have the following competing processes:

$$Fe(III) + Tr \rightleftarrows Fe(III)Tr \qquad K_{Tr} = 10^{20} \ M^{-1}$$
$$Fe(III) + L \rightleftarrows Fe(III)L \qquad K_L$$

and may calculate the ratio between the concentrations of Fe(III)Tr and Fe(III)L:

$$\frac{[Fe(III)Tr]}{[Fe(III)L]} = \frac{K_{Tr} \cdot [Tr]}{K_L \cdot [L]} \tag{13.2}$$

where [Tr] and [L] are concentrations of free transferrin and drug, respectively. If this is inserted into the expression for PMI we find:

$$PMI = \frac{K_L \cdot [L]}{K_{Tr} \cdot [Tr]} + 1 \tag{13.3}$$

In order for the drug to perturb the metal ion balance, the product $K_L \cdot [L]$ should be larger than $K_{Tr} \cdot [Tr]$. In the present example, the latter product is 10^{12} so if the stability of the drug–metal ion complex for example is $10^{10} \ M^{-1}$ the drug will play no role whatsoever in affecting the Fe(III) ion distribution in the plasma. Realistically, a concentration of a given pharmaceutical cannot exceed 1 mM. Thus, in this simplified example the iron(III) balance will only become perturbed if chelating agents with binding constants above 10^{15} are involved. Such drugs are known and used under certain circumstances (see Section 13.8.4).

For metal ions like calcium(II) which do not bind as strongly to chelates in the plasma (stability constants around $10^6 \, M^{-1}$) the situation can be quite critical. Administrating drugs like tetracycline (Section 13.7.1) may affect the physiological calcium ion balance seriously.

13.5   CHELATE THERAPY

As demonstrated in Figure 13.2, inadequate supply of essential elements will lead to deficiency symptoms. However, the same elements will in excess be directly toxic irrespective of whether the excess is caused by insufficient excretion or extravagant intake. That heavy metals constitute a hazard to the health is well known. Both types of toxication can be treated by using antagonists (chelate therapy) which involves complex binding (sequestration) and transport of acutely poisonous elements by means of polydentate ligands (Table 13.4). When realizing the number of essential elements found in the organism, it is obvious that selectivity plays a vital role and thus constitutes a fundamental challenge in bioinorganic chemistry. Development of chelating pharmaceuticals that selectively sequester the undesired (heavy) metal ions becomes imperative; and here our knowledge of co-ordination chemistry becomes profitable. The most successful ligands demonstrate selectivity by (i) exclusive fitting to ions of definite size and charge; (ii) comprising donor atoms that prefer Lewis acids of certain hardness or softness (Section 13.4.2). Further, the chelates must (iii) form thermodynamically stable and kinetically inert co-ordination compounds (Section 13.4.1–13.4.5); and finally (iv) be able to excrete the undesired metal ion rapidly and effectively.

13.5.1   Synergistic chelate therapy

The purpose of chelate therapy is to couple proper sequestration with effective excretion; thus, combining several ligands is often exploited. In order to transfer a target metal across the membrane and out of the cell, the complex should be lipophilic and neutrally charged. Conversely, in the extracellular environment, it would be advantageous if the metal ion is co-ordinated in an electrically charged complex which is water soluble in order to be excreted through the kidneys. An example of synergistic chelate therapy is treatment of mercury(II) poisoning. Hg(II) ions will chelate strongly to the thiolate groups in BAL (Section 13.6.1) forming an electrically neutral compound. Since the complex is lipophilic, it is soluble in the membrane, and thus can be effectively conducted out of the cell by a

Table 13.4 Chelating ligands towards toxic metal ions

Ligand	Commercial or trivial name	Preferred metal ions
2,3-dimercapto-1-propanol	Dimercaprol (BAL)	$Hg^{2+}, As^{3+}, Sb^{3+}, Ni^{2+}$
D-β, β-dimethylcysteine	D-penicillamine, (D-PEN)	Cu^{2+}, Hg^{2+}
Ethylenediaminetetraacetic acid	EDTA	Ca^{2+}, Pb^{2+}
Desferrioxamine	DFO, desferral	Fe^{3+}, Al^{3+}

passive transport. Outside the cell, EDTA might sequester the Hg(II) ions in a charged Hg(II)EDTA^{2-} complex that may gently be excreted with the urine. Due to the high electrical charge, anionic forms of EDTA as such cannot pass the cell membrane. Another example of synergism is the enhanced elimination of iron when treatment with desferrioxamin is combined with addition of ascorbic acid.

13.6   SELECTED CHELATES

13.6.1   BAL

The first example of chelate therapy was performed during World War II when BAL (2,3-dimercapto-1-propanol; British Anti Lewisite (Figure 13.9)) was applied as antagonist against arsenic containing poison gas. BAL, being a very soft Lewis base, will preferentially co-ordinate to soft heavy metal ions. Thus, aside from As, the chelate will be highly efficient in treatment of mercury toxication. Today, however, BAL is exclusively utilized in connection with acute gold poisoning in patients undergoing treatment with gold containing pharmaceuticals (Section 13.8.6). BAL is a yellowish liquid with only limited solubility in water and with a very unpleasant odor. An advantage of BAL is its lipophilic character which facilitates transport into the cells. However, the drug itself is toxic and must be administered with great care.

A related chelate is unithiol (2,3-dimercaptopropanesulphonic acid) which is a derivative of BAL. This compound is water soluble and so are the stable heavy metal ion complexes. Unithiol may be used extracellularly in the treatment of acute toxication with the soft heavy metals like copper, lead, mercury, and cadmium.

13.6.2   D-penicillamine

The structure of D-penicillamine (D-PEN) is shown in Figure13.9 where the three different donor groups should be noticed: Two hard donor atoms (amine-*N* and carboxylate-*O*) together with the soft thiolate (−SH) group. This makes the chelate a universal drug for both soft and hard Lewis acids but showing limited ion selectivity, however. D-PEN is water soluble and, in contrast to BAL, not inherently toxic. Nevertheless, the L-isomer is a vitamin-B$_6$ antagonist and thus harmful to the organism. D-PEN has found wide application and may in most cases replace BAL. It is often applied simultaneously with EDTA as in the treatment of lead poisoning and is also effective sequestering gold and mercury. Of particular interest is the administration of D-PEN to patients suffering from Wilson's disease (Section 13.8.6).

13.6.3   EDTA

Ethylenediaminetetraacetic acid (EDTA) (Figure 13.4), and its analogs are all excellent chelates sequestering most metal ions, but for this same reason not very

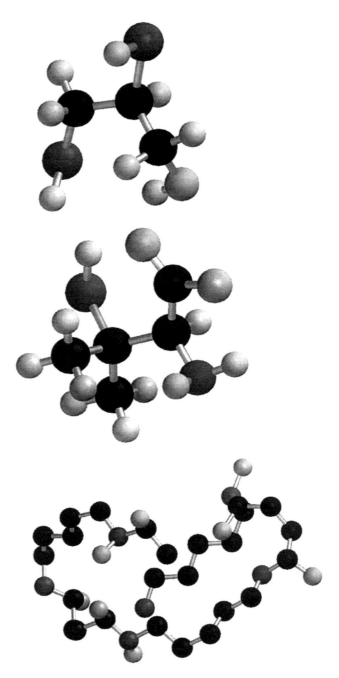

Figure 13.9 Selected ligands from Table 13.4. Structures of BAL (upper), D-PEN (center), and DFO (lower). Carbon atoms are black, oxygen light gray, nitrogen and sulfur dark gray. Hydrogen atoms (light) are only shown in the two former structures. The structure of EDTA is illustrated in Figure 13.4.

selective. EDTA co-ordinates preferentially to hard metal ions (Section 13.4.2) and due to the large chelate effect quite stable complexes are formed. EDTA is only slowly metabolized in the organism with a biological half-life of 1 h. Since EDTA is only inadequately absorbed from the gastrointestinal tract, it is usually administered by intravenous injections. But due to the low degree of selectivity the hazard of eliminating essential metal ions is high. Adding the drug as Na_2H_2EDTA, the serum concentration of calcium ions will be lowered (Section 13.4.6), possibly with severe muscle spasms as a result. Instead, the CaH_2EDTA salt is recommended, and in general the diet should be supplemented with essential metal ions during EDTA treatment.

13.6.4   Desferrioxamine

The siderophores are naturally occurring small molecule chelates secreted by many micro-organisms in order to extract iron from the surroundings. One important example of a siderophore is desferrioxamine (DFO, desferral) (Table 13.4 and Figure 13.9). The molecule is seen to contain a large amount of (hard) oxygen donor atoms which in an octahedral geometry render it highly specific towards iron(III), with a stability constant of not less than $10^{31}\,M^{-1}$ for the chelate. Other siderophores show stability constants for Fe(III) complexation up to $10^{50}\,M^{-1}$. The chelate is used in the treatment of acute iron poisoning and in certain cases of anaemia where iron is accumulated in liver and heart. The binding constants for the corresponding Fe(II) complexes are much smaller due to larger ionic radius and smaller charge of this ion, and release of iron can be induced simply by reduction of the Fe(III) ion. Since the co-ordination chemistry of Al^{3+} is quite similar to that of Fe^{3+}, DFO can also be used in cases of aluminum poisoning (Section 13.8.4). Incidentally, chelate formation also lies behind the body's strategy of producing fever in cases of infections. The higher temperature kills bacteria by reducing their ability to synthesize particular iron chelating ligands.

DFO and other siderophores have also been exploited as potential antimalarial chemotherapeutics. As free ligands they may block the iron metabolism, but the pharmacological prospects are not ideal (see Section 13.8.4).

13.7   DRUG–METAL ION INTERACTION

Many pharmaceuticals are inherently excellent chelates and may as such interact with metal ions, intra- as well as extracellularly. This interaction can be beneficial but also injurious. Favorable effects are seen where complex formation induces better uptake or transport of the drug while detrimental consequences occur if drug uptake is precluded. The effect is determined by a number of factors like charge, structure, and presence of hydrophobic or hydrophilic groups. The HSAB principle (Section 13.4.2) and knowledge of the chemistry of co-ordination compounds (Section 13.4.3) become useful in this context. Some examples are given in the following sections.

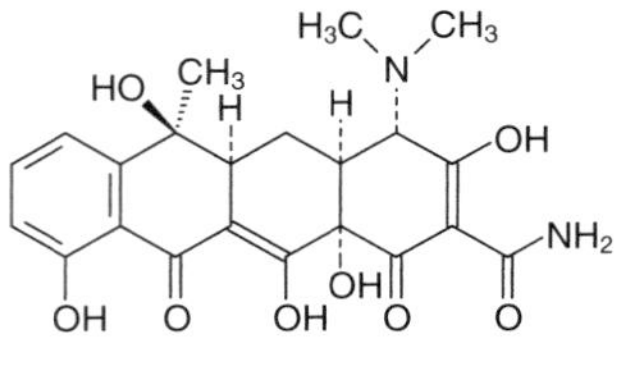

Figure 13.10 Drawing of the tetracycline molecule. Notice the abundance of oxygen atoms (hard bases).

13.7.1 Undesirable interactions

A well-known example of a harmful drug–metal ion interaction is inhibition of tetracycline uptake in the organism by calcium, zinc, and iron ions. The structure of the drug is shown in Figure 13.10, and it is seen that the molecule comprises a large number of (hard) donor atoms, first and foremost oxygen. Thus, it comes as no surprise that many hard metal ions will bind to this drug. Incidentally, the action of tetracycline seems to be related to its chelating ability to Mg^{2+} ions.

13.7.2 Beneficial interactions

Copper complexes with biological macromolecules will be treated in a later Section (13.8.6). But copper also co-ordinates to many pharmaceuticals and the anti-inflammatory effect of salicylic acid derivatives and also of other drugs involved in tissue repair seems to be related to Cu(II) chelation. The copper-containing enzyme lysyl oxidase catalyzes cross lacing of connective tissue, and copper ions are mobilized by co-ordination to smaller organic ligands. The same strategy of copper mobilization occurs with superoxide dismutase (Section 13.8.6), another important copper containing enzyme which catalyzes degradation of the superoxide radical, O_2^-:

$$2O_2^- + 2H^+ \rightarrow O_2 + H_2O_2$$

A Fe(II) chelate isolated from a *Streptomyces* fungus, bleomycin (Chapter 17) is exploited as an antitumour drug due to its ability to cleave DNA molecules (Section 13.8.4). A final important example of beneficial complex formation is related to zinc(II) ions. Zinc is found in the enzyme carbonic anhydrase which catalyzes the hydration of carbon dioxide (Section 13.8.7). Certain anti-epileptica, like acetazole-amide, co-ordinate to the zinc(II) ion directly in the enzyme and thus obstruct the catalytic transformation of carbon dioxide.

13.8 INORGANIC CHEMISTRY AND PHARMACEUTICALS

So far, the pharmaceutical industry has concentrated its effort mainly on developing drugs based upon organic chemistry and on natural products. However, the remaining part of the periodic table is manifesting itself with an ever increasing offering of diagnostics and genuine pharmaceuticals.

Table 13.5 Content of Na^+, K^+, and Cl^- (concentrations in mM)

	Na^+	K^+	Cl^-
Sea water	460	10	550
Red blood cells	11	92	50
Blood plasma	160	10	100

13.8.1 Alkali metals

Sodium and potassium are found in large concentrations both in sea water and in the earth's crust. Thus, it is not surprising that all living organisms exploit these metal ions in relatively high quantities. In Table 13.5, some examples of Na^+, K^+, and Cl^- (counter ion) content are presented.

The most important biological roles of sodium and potassium are (a) to stabilize cell membranes and enzymes by electrostatic effects and osmosis. Many biomolecules will thus denature when subjected to distilled water. Secondly, (b) these ions transmit electrical signals by diffusion through a certain concentration gradient.

Ions can be pumped actively across biological membranes against a concentration gradient, while the diffusion controlled concentration equilibrium proceeds passively through ion channels that are regulated chemically or electrostatically.

The most important difference between the chemistry of the individual alkali metals is due to their ionic radii and consequently the radius/charge ratio. Thus, the metal ions may possess individual functions in conjunction with specific ligands; the larger the radius the higher the co-ordination number becomes.

Lithium, sodium, and potassium exist in aqueous solution as labile hydrates (Section 13.4.3) which exchange water molecules extremely rapidly ($10^9 \, s^{-1}$ or faster). Many chelates form stable complexes with the alkali metals, such as EDTA. Lately, highly effective and specific ligands (ionophores) have been synthesized, like 'crown ethers' and 'cryptands'. Figure 13.11 shows a crown ether with a potassium ion attached.

In these compounds, the metal ions become co-ordinated to strategically positioned heteroatoms (O, N), and the size of the rings can be designed to adjust to certain metal ion radii. The biologically important aspect here is that the ion binds to heteroatoms on the inside of the macromolecule while the surface is more lipophilic. Consequently, such complexes will comfortably be transported across phospholipid double layers (5–6 nm) in biological membranes. Pharmacologically active natural products of this kind will function as antibiotics since they may transfer alkali metals in and out of the cells and thereby perturb the natural metal ion balance. Examples are valinomycin (Figure 13.12) and nonactin. The latter is, due to its size and number of binding centers, optimal for K^+ co-ordination (Table 13.6).

Another efficient method for controlled cation transport through lipid double layers involves incorporation of ionic channels in membranes. The gramicidins are relatively small peptides which have been used as antibiotics for more than 50 years. Dimers of the peptide form a tube that is 3 nm in length and with an inner diameter of about 0.4–0.5 nm. Thus, two dimers are needed to span inner to outer

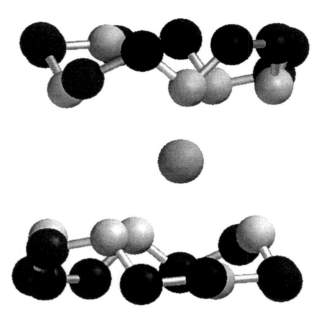

Figure 13.11 Crown ether with potassium. The potassium ion is seen squeezed in between the two ring systems and is co-ordinated to 8 oxygen atoms. Hydrogen atoms are not shown. Co-ordinates are taken from the Cambridge Crystallographic Data Centre.

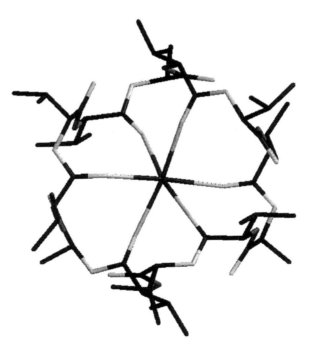

Figure 13.12 Potassium complex with valinomycin. Potassium is co-ordinated to 6 oxygen atoms. Co-ordinates are taken from the Cambridge Crystallographic Data Centre.

Table 13.6 Characteristic properties of alkali and alkaline earth metal ions

	Li^+	Na^+	K^+	Mg^{2+}	Ca^{2+}
Ionic radius (pm)	60	102	138	72	100
Co-ordination number	4	6	6–8	6	7–8
Preferred donor	oxygen	oxygen	oxygen	oxygen nitrogen phosphate	oxygen nitrogen

side of the membrane. The size of the hole restricts passage of ions to those with certain limited radii.

Lithium salts play a particular role in treatment of manic-depressive psychosis, and a large number of people take about 1 g of lithium carbonate each day. The effective plasma concentration is 1 mM while 2 mM exhibits toxic side effects, and already 3 mM is a lethal dose. The Li^+ ion has approximately the same radius as the Mg^{2+} ion, and both metal ions demonstrate high affinity phosphate binding. Lithium ions inhibit the enzymatic function of inositol monophosphatase thereby preventing release of phosphate from the active site. Inositol phosphatases are magnesium-dependent, and structural studies have shown that Li^+ may bind to one of the catalytic Mg(II) sites. Co-ordination of lithium ions to phosphate-containing messenger molecules could further perturb the *trans*-cellular communication which may be another rationale for its antipsychotic effect. Inositol phosphates are responsible for mobilizing calcium ions, and Li^+ will therefore influence the calcium ion level in cells, which makes it imperative to monitor the calcium concentration carefully in the patients during lithium treatment.

13.8.2 Alkaline earth metals

Among the essential metals, the magnesium ion, Mg^{2+}, has the smallest ionic radius which distinguishes it proficiently from Ca^{2+}. The high charge/radius ratio results in the Mg^{2+} ion being a particularly good Lewis acid with a preferred co-ordination number of 6. Binding (stability) constants for some representative complexes are given in Table 13.7.

Magnesium has an important role in stabilizing cell walls since it cross-laces the residing carboxylate and phosphate groups. The free magnesium ion concentration is typically 1 mM inside the cell. Deficiency in magnesium will induce accumulation of calcium ions as charge compensation intracellularly and eventually cause myospasms.

Table 13.7 Stability constants ($\log K$) of some typical Mg^{2+} and Ca^{2+} complexes at 25 °C and I = 0 M

	$\log K$	
	Mg^{2+}	Ca^{2+}
Acetate	1.3	1.1
EDTA	8.7	11
Glycine	3	1.5

Serious Mg^{2+} deficiency will result in mental and physical retardation, since magnesium is involved in the energy production (phosphate transport) and protein synthesis. The role of the magnesium ion seems to be essentially charge compensation for the negative charges of phosphate groups at pH 7. Mg^{2+} constitutes an essential part (prosthetic group) in a series of enzymes and in most cases phosphate seems to be involved. It is interesting to note that in spite of its great importance the concentration level of the magnesium(II) ion in the body is not controlled by some sophisticated physiological mechanism. It seems to be dictated solely by the solubility of the magnesium compounds with the anions present.

The calcium ion is probably the most important and ambidextrous of the essential metal ions in biology. The majority of this metal is found in the skeleton (about 1.0 kg in an adult person) while 10 g is engaged in a series of fundamental physiological processes from cell division and coagulation of blood to immune responses and muscle contraction. Deviations from the normal metabolism of the biominerals may lead to pathological effects, including deposition of calcium salts in blood vessels or in kidney stones. Also undesirable demineralization processes such as dental caries and bone resorption (osteoporosis) are commonly observed.

Contrary to magnesium, the concentration of Ca^{2+} inside the cell is vanishingly small, about 10^{-7} M, while the extracellular concentration is in the mM range. This requires very effective and specific calcium pumps in order to sustain this huge concentration gradient. Calcium is taken up in the small intestine bound to the active form of vitamin-D, in a yield of 50%. Excess of calcium is excreted through the kidneys.

Due to the larger size of the Ca^{2+} ion relative to that of Mg^{2+} (Table 13.6), calcium is often found attached to proteins with a co-ordination number of 7 or 8. Proteins with many acidic groups are particularly effective ligands for calcium ions, and a well-known example is parvalbumin (Figure 13.13) a protein located in smooth muscles. This protein is related to the extended family of the structurally flexible calmodulins which also co-ordinate to certain enzymes thereby activating them. Calmodulins are monomeric proteins consisting of a chain of 148 amino acids which are capable of binding up to four calcium ions. The 3D-structure was first determined for parvalbumin and termed the EF hand, where the letters E and F signify alpha helices. Another conformationally flexible class of calcium binding proteins, annexins, are important in cell regulation and blood coagulation.

Calcium ion release from storage proteins is the basis for the messenger function of Ca^{2+} ions which trigger liberation of a neurotransmitter, leading to opening of potassium ion channels. Calcium ion activation of phosphate transferring kinases should also be mentioned, due to its central role in muscle contraction and other Ca^{2+} controlled processes.

In association with membranes one finds some highly acidic calcium storage proteins called calsequestrines that bind up to 50 Ca^{2+} ions per molecule and release the metal ions through interactions with other macromolecules or by electrical impulses from nerve cells.

Barium sulphate (baryt) is used as X-ray contrasting agent and should as such not be confounded with barium carbonate which is dissolved in the acidic environment of the stomach. Ba^{2+} is highly toxic since it has an ionic radius similar to that of potassium and therefore will affect the cellular potassium transport.

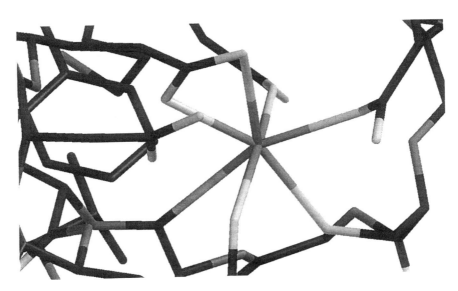

Figure 13.13 Molecular structure of parvalbumin. The metal ion center of parvalbumin. The calcium ion is shown seven-co-ordinated to peptide carbonyl and carboxylate oxygen atoms. A water molecule may further bind to the calcium ion. Co-ordinates are taken from the Protein Data Bank (1A75).

13.8.3 The chromium group

The chromate ion, CrO_4^{2-}, is carcinogenic but precisely why is not known. The ion shows resemblance to sulfate and indeed is carried inside the cell by the sulfate transporting system. In the cytoplasm, the chromate ion will react with sulfur-containing peptides like glutathione whereby Cr(VI) becomes reduced to Cr(V). In this oxidation state chromium reacts with DNA molecules, and oxidation of DNA is probably the reason for the mutagenic action.

Several decades ago, it was observed that vanadium(V) as the vanadate anion, VO_4^{3-}, could stimulate glucose uptake and glycogen synthesis. However, vanadate is too toxic for the human organism to be a useful insulin-mimetic. A new class of vanadium complexes have been synthesized with certain organic ligands and they seem to be less toxic to humans.

Cr(III) is, in contrast to Cr(VI), not carcinogenic. Indeed, it has been proposed that chromium in this oxidation state is of biological importance. It was earlier suggested that the glucose tolerance factor was a chromium(III) complex with nicotinamide and glutathione as ligands. This idea has now been abandoned, however. Still, it has been documented that diabetes mellitus can be affected in a positive manner by addition of Cr(III) compounds. The high level of chromium(III) in the plant, shepherd's bag, has been known and utilized by nature healers, but nowadays a water soluble chromium(III) nicotinamide complex is applied. The intrinsic problem with Cr(III) compounds is, as in the case of Fe(III), the inherently low solubility at pH 7. A tripicolinatochromium(III) complex is now marketed as a

Table 13.8 Distribution of group VIB metals in the earth's crust and in sea water (concentrations in ppm)

	Earth's crust	Sea water
Cr	100	$5 \cdot 10^{-4}$
Mo	1.5	0.01
W	1.5	$1 \cdot 10^{-4}$

nutritional supplement although its long-term biological effects on humans have not been fully characterized. The complex stimulates the activity of membrane spanning protein tyrosine kinases activated by insulin, but the mechanism is not fully understood and requires further examination.

There is no doubt about the importance of molybdenum being an essential trace element, which may derive from its relatively large abundance in sea water (Table 13.8). Mo is a constituent part of a series of enzymes all catalyzing biological oxidation- and reduction processes: N_2 reduction to NH_3 (nitrogen fixation); reduction of NO_3^- to NO_2^-; oxidation of SO_3^{2-} to SO_4^{2-}; oxidation of aldehydes to carboxylic acids; etc. All of these molybdenum-containing enzymes are exceedingly complex and contain other metal ions as well, often iron. The function of molybdenum is connected to its redox chemistry where, besides the stable Mo(VI) state, also complexes in the oxidation state (IV) have been characterized. Since molybdenum is generally found co-ordinated in poly-oxyanions, Mo is capable of mediating oxygen atom transfer as exemplified in some of the above processes. In Figure 13.14 is shown the prosthetic group in a Mo-containing enzyme, xanthine oxidase. Besides co-ordination to the protein by two thiolate side chains, Mo(VI) is also connected to two oxygen ligands.

Tungsten would seem to be precluded as an essential trace element. Nevertheless, some bacteria have been discovered that exploit W in the same manner as other species utilize Mo. It is interesting that both molybdate and tungstate oxyanions also demonstrate insulin-like effects.

13.8.4   Iron and cobalt

When oxygen, O_2, made its first appearance on the earthly scene about 2 billion years ago most of the living organisms probably perished. A few species survived by strictly isolating themselves in oxygen free pockets, becoming what nowadays would be labeled anaerobic organisms. New forms of life evolved, however, that were capable of exploiting the highly oxidizing property of dioxygen (aerobic organisms). Almost 20 times as much energy can be extracted from glucose in the presence of oxygen than in its absence. Thus, the need for oxygen transport as well as for the development of protective measures against undesirable redox processes (antioxidants) emerged.

Iron (together with copper) plays the leading role in all biological processes wherein oxygen turnover takes place. Iron(II) co-ordinates to a certain type of porphyrin and forms a complex labeled heme (Figure 13.15). Vertebrates utilize

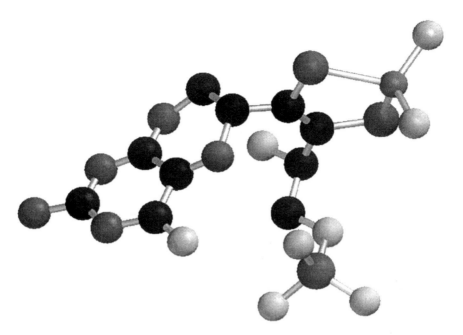

Figure 13.14 The prosthetic group in xanthine oxidase. The molybdenum ion is seen in the upper right corner co-ordinated in a tetrahedral arrangement to two thiolate sulfur atoms (dark gray) and two oxygen atoms (light gray). Co-ordinates are taken from the Protein Data Bank (1FIQ).

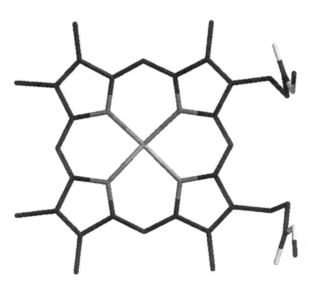

Figure 13.15 Heme. The heme prosthetic group consisting of an iron(II) ion complexed in a square planar geometry to four pyrrole nitrogen atoms of a substituted porphyrin ligand.

two such heme proteins for reversible O_2 transport and storage: Hemoglobin in red blood cells and myoglobin in muscle tissue. Anaemia results from insufficient dioxygen supply usually due to a low hemoglobin blood level. The oxygen molecule is co-ordinated axially to the heme group which contains a high spin (d^6) Fe(II) ion. The resulting oxo compound is, however, a low spin complex which stabilizes the Fe(II) state (Section 13.4.3) and thus prevents oxidation to Fe(III).

Cytochromes are heme proteins but here the shift between Fe(III) and Fe(II) is exploited in order to take up and deliver electrons. The reduction potentials extend over a huge range (+400 to −400 mV vs. the standard hydrogen electrode) which is brought about by exchanging the axial ligands. Anions stabilize Fe(III) and cause lowering of the standard potentials while co-ordination of aromatic and hydrophobic groups will cause an increase in the stability of the Fe(II) state.

Cytochromes are further part of the important respiration enzyme, cytochrome c oxidase which catalyzes the reduction of O_2 to H_2O. The enzyme activates and reduces 95% of the dioxygen we consume and couples exergonic O_2 reduction to endergonic proton pumping to drive ATP (adenosine triphosphate) synthesis. The organism is applying ATP for synthesizing important macromolecules (carbohydrates, proteins, lipids, etc.). There is now a rather good understanding of the reaction cycle of this large protein and the 3D-structure is also known with high precision.

Another significant heme enzyme is cytochrome P-450 which as a dioxygen activating metalloporphyrin catalyzes a series of important biological oxidation processes. Enzymatic monooxygenation reactions, e.g. the conversion of vitamin-D or transformation of drugs like morphine are examples of such processes. Unwanted reactions like epoxidation of benzene to produce carcinogenic derivatives or oxidation of nitrosamines to form reactive radicals are examples of a toxicological function of cytochrome P-450. An iron(V) oxo complex is the favored model for the activation of oxygen during the catalytic turnover.

Peroxidase and catalase are further illustrations of heme containing enzymes (antioxidants) which scavenge undesirable peroxides. There are also examples of other Fe-containing proteins which do not accommodate the heme group but where iron is co-ordinated in a cave-like complex together with sulfur. Some of these proteins possess a catalytic action and constitute part of redox enzymes.

Malaria is a devastating infectious disease killing close to 2 million children annually. The commonly used antimalarial therapy has become increasingly ineffective due to chloroquinone resistance. However, a new series of drugs based on tervalent metal ion co-ordination compounds like the ethylenediamine-*bis* [propylbenzylimino] Fe(III) complex exhibit highly selective activity, ironically particularly against chloroquinone resistant parasites. Heme, released from hemoglobin in the parasite, is very toxic to eukaryotic cells due to lysing of the membranes. In order to prevent this action the parasite polymerizes heme, but the above imino complexes inhibit this protective process thereby destroying the host.

Iron is the most abundant transition metal in biological chemistry, and transport and storage of this metal have been studied assiduously. The big challenge here is that Fe(II) easily becomes oxidized to Fe(III) and that the products formed generally are highly insoluble at pH 7. The solubility product of $Fe(OH)_3$ is thus 10^{-38} M^4 which implies that at neutral pH the concentration of Fe^{3+} is only 10^{-17} M, unless

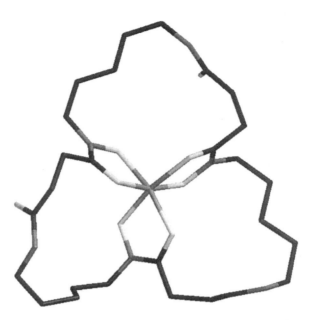

Figure 13.16 Structure of a siderophore. A siderophore iron(III) complex with hydroxamate groups (ferrioxamine). Fe(III) is co-ordinated to six oxygen atoms.

Fe(III) is sequestered to some chelate. Among the naturally occurring chelates we find the siderophores (Section 13.6.4). These compounds are either catecholates or hydroxamates (Figure 13.16) which form exceedingly stable complexes with Fe(III). The salmonella bacteria produce a siderophore which binds iron(III) with a stability constant of not less than $10^{50}\,M^{-1}$. Another siderophore, desferrioxamine (Section 13.6.4) produced by the *Streptomyces* fungus is used in order to prevent iron poisoning in connection with blood transfusion. Pathogenic micro-organisms rely on a constant supply of iron, and therefore the availability of iron to bacteria invading the organism plays an important role in many diseases like cholera and tuberculosis where a decrease in iron content in the blood is invariably observed. The micro-organisms have to mobilize iron, but cannot exploit tightly bound iron in the blood serum. The heme–iron complex is very stable and iron can be liberated only by enzymatic degradation of the ligand. Effective iron scavenging chelates will thus act as potent antibiotics and naturally occurring iron complexing agents are therefore of great interest in medicine both as antibiotics and as drug delivery agents.

Iron as nutrient generally occurs by means of simple Fe(II) compounds although iron uptake is much more advantageous through the heme complex. Higher animals do not apply siderophores in the transport system but another protein called transferrin in which the metal ions are tightly bound to phenolate, carboxylate, and imidazole groups as well as to inorganic carbonate. Secured in this protein, Fe^{3+} is transferred into the cells where a concomitant hydrogen ion release takes place. Under these circumstances, the complex is much less stable and the iron(III) ions are released to the cytoplasm. Iron is immediately stored intracellularly (as FeO(OH) i.e. rust) in other non-heme proteins like ferritin and hemosiderin. The latter storage protein is particularly active during iron overload. When needed, iron ions are mobilized from ferritin by reduction of Fe(III) to Fe(II). Iron compounds are found in many redox processes including less desirable ones like free radical reactions. It is therefore of utmost importance that iron transport is carefully controlled. Chronic iron poisoning (hemochromatosis) usually originates from digestion of excess of the metal supplied from cooking utensils and results in corrosion of the gastrointestinal tract.

Other trivalent metal ions will also co-ordinate to transferrin, like Al(III) for instance. But since Al^{3+} cannot be reduced inside the cells, the process becomes irreversible and this is one rationale for the toxic effect of aluminium. Throughout the last decade it has been discussed whether aluminium is involved in Alzheimer's disease (see Chapter 10) where amyloid protein containing plaques concentrate in certain sections of the brain, e.g. the hippocampus. It has been demonstrated that Al^{3+} can cross link polynucleotides and that Alzheimer patients apparently have reduced transferrin activity. It also appears that exposure to aluminium in drinking water correlate with higher risk of attaining the disease. But this correlation does of course not necessarily mean causality, and a significant role of aluminium in the pathophysiology of Alzheimer's disease is unlikely.

Bleomycin (see Chapter 17) is an antitumor agent which is isolated from the *Streptomyces* fungus. Bleomycin couples to DNA with iron(II) ions co-ordinated to the peptide and, in the presence of dioxygen, a catalytic process is induced in which a phosphorous carbohydrate bond is broken. The mechanism is not fully comprehended but probably a Fe(V)-oxo compound is formed which may scavenge hydrogen atoms from the deoxyribose ring.

'Sodium nitroprusside', $Na_2[Fe(CN)_5NO]$ (Figure 13.17) is an active hypotensive agent used in treatment of heart infarct and in control of blood pressure during

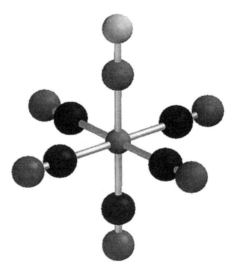

Figure 13.17 Nitroprusside. The 'nitroprusside' anion, $[FeCN_5NO]^{2-}$. The NO group is pointing upwards.

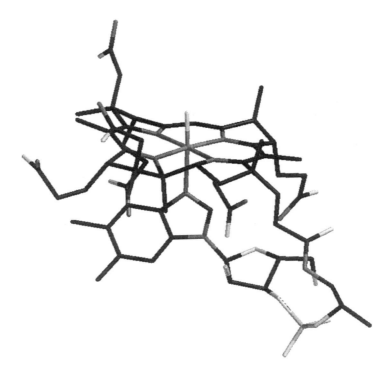

Figure 13.18 Coenzyme B_{12}. The prosthetic group in vitamin B_{12}. Besides co-ordinating to four corrin nitrogen atoms the cobalt(III) ion is also bound to an axial ligand, nitrogen from a benzimidazole group. Notice the vacant sixth position. This is the binding site for substrates. A phosphate group is seen in the lower right corner. Co-ordinates are taken from the Protein Data Bank (1CB7).

heart surgery. Release of NO causes relaxation of the muscles surrounding the blood vessels, probably by co-ordination of nitric oxide to an iron porphyrin receptor within the guanylate cyclase enzyme which converts guanine triphosphate to cyclic guanine monophosphate. NO is also synthesized in the human body in a process where an iron containing (heme) enzyme catalyzes oxidation of the amino acid, arginine, to nitric oxide.

The role of cobalt as essential trace element is confined to one function only, namely as the redox active metal ion in coenzyme-B_{12} which contains a Co–C (adenosyl) bond. As early as in the 1920s, it was well established that pernicious anaemia could be cured with injections of extracts from liver samples, and trace element analysis demonstrated later that these extracts contained cobalt. A derivative of the co-enzyme, vitamin B_{12}, is the only essential cobalt compound known. One could term vitamin B_{12} a natural drug since we cannot produce it ourselves. Co co-ordinates as Co^{3+} (low spin d^6) to a 15-membered corrin ring system reminiscent of the 16-membered porphyrin ring (compare Figure 13.15 with Figure 13.18), except that the ring has been diminished by one bond which coerces the ring system, in contrast to heme, to be non-planar.

The surprising observation upon examining the coenzyme-B$_{12}$ structure is that one of the axial ligands can be an alkyl residue: -C$_n$H$_{2n+1}$. This is the only known example of a naturally occurring metal–carbon (metalloorganic) bond. The trivalent Co^{3+} ion in a low-spin d^6 hexaco-ordinated state becomes stabilized in a square planar geometry upon two electron reduction to Co$^+$ (d^8) (Section 13.4.3). The bond between cobalt and carbon is thus disrupted and the released ligand may be transferred to a substrate linked to the enzyme. With the coenzyme-B$_{12}$ coupled to the right enzyme the rate of alkylation is accelerated up to 10^{10} times.

13.8.5   Platinum and ruthenium

The square planar 'cis-platinum' (cis-diamminedichloroplatinum(II); cisDDP) (Figure 13.19) is one of the most effective antitumor agents known. The detailed mechanism of its function is discussed in Chapter 17.

cisDDP is administered intravenously as an aqueous salt solution. Due to the large chloride ion concentration ($\sim$0.1 M) in the plasma the complex retains its composition and as an uncharged molecule it can diffuse (passively) across the cell membrane and enter the cell. However, here the chloride concentration is considerably smaller ($\sim$3 mM) and the complex is rapidly transformed into the cationic aqua complex, [Pt(NH$_3$)$_2$(H$_2$O)$_2$]$^{2+}$ (a thermodynamic effect). Since water molecules, as discussed in Section 13.4.5, have a lower *trans*-directing effect than ammonia they are easily substituted by other and better co-ordinating groups, e.g. base molecules like guanine from DNA. An equivalent complex can for steric reasons not be formed with the *trans*-isomer. In Figure 13.20, a model complex with two neighboring guanine bases is displayed. The co-ordination of platinum to guanosine in cis[Pt(NH$_3$)$_2${d(pGpG)}] destroys the stacking of the bases and causes a sharp bend in the DNA helix structure (70–90° in contrast to the typical 10° in DNA).

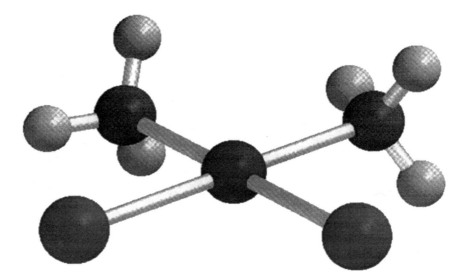

Figure 13.19 cis-Platinum. The square planar cis-diamminedichloroplatinum(II) complex.

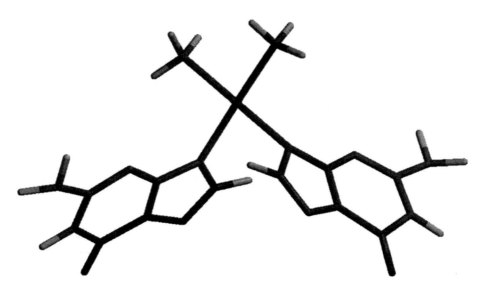

Figure 13.20 Platinum-DNA model complex. Square planar complex of platinum(II) with two ammine and two guanine ligands.

A pertinent question is now why the *cis*DDP drug (to some degree) selectively destroys tumor cells rather than normal healthy cells. Certain proteins have been isolated in human cells, 'high mobility group' proteins (HMG) which function as transcription factors. It has been observed that HMG proteins recognize and bind to the *cis*-platinum-DNA adduct. A consequence of such binding is inhibition of nucleotide excision which means that the adduct may block the *in vivo* repair in these cells. Apparently, the HMG proteins are expressed predominantly in tumor cells. This repair-shielding hypothesis would explain why tumor cells are particularly sensitive to *cis*-platinum. Figure 13.21 shows binding of HMG to DNA containing *cis*[Pt(NH$_3$)$_2${d(pGpG)}].

Tumor cells are known to contain a large concentration of transferrin receptors. This can be utilized in targeting strategies either by blocking iron uptake or for transfer and release of cytotoxic metals complexes inside the cells. Ruthenium(III) shows a very large affinity towards the imidazole side chain of histidine and by co-ordinating to one of the Fe(III) binding sites (His) in transferrin, Ru(III) is taken up by the cells. Ru(III) complexes with heterocyclic ligands like imidazole, indazole and bipyridine all show high activity against tumor metastases. Like for *cis*-platinum, aquation of the complex seems to be an important step. Ru(III) complexes are probably prodrugs which are reduced inside the cell to the more reactive Ru(II) species. The complexes bind to DNA, preferentially to N-7 of guanine bases.

13.8.6   Copper, silver, and gold

Copper and iron constitute the most important redox active transition metals in bioinorganic chemistry, and they seem to complement each other. Both

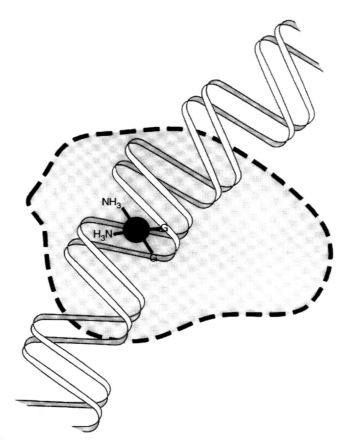

Figure 13.21 Binding of HMG to *cis*[Pt(NH₃)₂{d(pGpG)}]. Schematic drawing of how the high-mobility-group protein may bind to *cis*-platinum modified DNA.

copper- and iron proteins are involved in oxygen transport and charge transfer. But while the iron containing proteins and enzymes are always found intracellularly copper proteins and enzymes operate outside the cells. Molluscs (snails, clams, etc.) and arthropods (arachnids, crustaceans, etc.) utilize an extracellular copper protein, hemocyanin for oxygen transport, i.e. an analog to the intracellular iron containing heme protein, hemoglobin.

In humans, most copper is found in the brain and in heart and liver. The high metabolic rate of these organs requires relative large concentrations of copper containing enzymes, some of which are presented below. Not surprisingly, copper deficiency leads to brain diseases and anaemia.

Copper is also found in many oxygenating enzymes, i.e. proteins which catalyze the incorporation of oxygen into organic substrates. An important example is dopamine-β-hydroxylase which catalyzes an insertion of oxygen into the β-carbon of the side chain of dopamine to produce norepinephrine. This enzyme contains

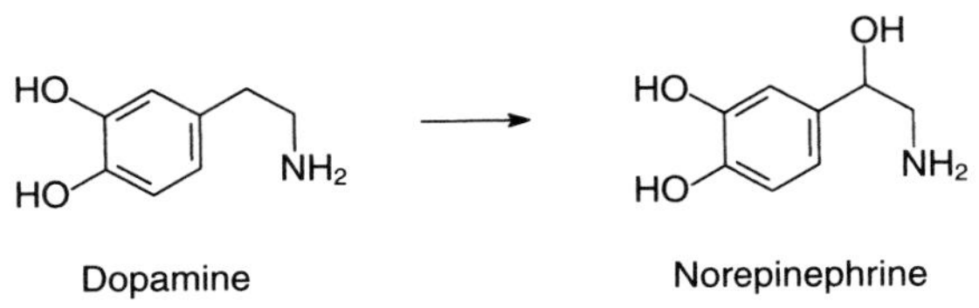

Dopamine   Norepinephrine

Figure 13.22 Dopamine-β-hydroxylase oxygenation of dopamine (left) to norepinephrine (right). The reducing substrate, ascorbate, reduces both Cu(II) ions to Cu(I) in the enzyme, one of which then binds to the oxidizing substrate, O_2.

one pair of Cu(II) ions per active center. Ascorbate reduces the copper(II) ions to Cu^+ which bind O_2 whereupon the hydroxylation takes place (Figure 13.22). The two copper ions in this enzyme are at least 0.4 nm apart and hence catalysis is unlikely to involve a binuclear copper center. Instead a model has been proposed in which the two copper ions perform different functions; one copper is involved in electron transfer from ascorbate while the other binds dioxygen and performs the substrate hydroxylation. Another member of this class of proteins, peptidyl-α-amidase catalyzes the conversion of C-terminal glycine extended peptides to their bioactive amidated forms, and hence is responsible for the biosynthesis of essential neuropeptide hormones like vasopressin and oxytocin.

Copper is also integrated into the so-called oxidases that catalyze the reduction of dioxygen to water. Here we find the very important enzyme, cytochrome c oxidase which besides two Fe-heme groups include three copper ions in two distinct centers. This enzyme has already been discussed in Section 13.8.4. Many other oxidases exclusively contain copper and often in functional groups of 4 metal ions at a time. Ceruloplasmin is a 130 kDa multicopper oxidase which is widely distributed in vertebrates. It occurs in plasma and plays an important role in iron homeostatis. Other functions include its participation in antioxidant defence and in processes related to metabolism of copper, biogenic amines, and nitric oxide. Its main physiological function seems to be the ferroxidase activity, and inherited mutations or targeted disruption of the ceruloplasmin gene leads to impaired iron efflux from cells. Oxidation of Fe(II) released from cells and its subsequent incorporation into apotransferrin is the mechanism wherby ceruloplasmin is involved in mediating iron from cellular stores.

The human variant of the antioxidant enzyme, superoxide dismutase, contains both copper and zinc (13.7.2). The toxic superoxide anion, O_2^-, is sometimes deliberately produced by organisms for particular objectives. Thus, some phagocytes which are part of the immune system in higher organisms produce large quantities of superoxide together with peroxide and hypochlorite by means of oxidases in order to kill invading micro-organisms. In unfortunate cases this protection system may fail giving rise to certain autoimmune diseases like rheumatoid arthritis. Under these circumstances superoxide dismutase is administered as an anti-inflammatory pharmaceutical. The same therapy is consistently applied during open heart surgery in order to protect the tissue against oxidative attack by the superoxide radical. Also the process of aging and neurodegenerative diseases like amylotropic lateral sclerosis have been linked to O_2^- production.

A large group of electron transfer proteins is found in which a single copper ion is co-ordinated per molecule. They partake in e.g. the photosynthesis and in the bacterial respiration system.

Copper is a potent poison for any cell and thus proteins of the metallothionein type (Section 13.8.7) exist which will transport excessive copper ions out of the cells. Due to the delicate balance between plethora and deficiency of copper a tight control of uptake and excretion of this metal is needed. Excess of copper leads to copper accumulation in liver and brain which untreated leads to severe damage of these organs and results in early death (Wilson's disease). Therapy with powerful copper chelates like d-penicillamine (Section 13.6.2) can keep the copper concentration on a suitable level. Deficiency in copper is just as serious since it leads to grave mental and physical illnesses (e.g. Menkes' disease). Like in Wilson's disease it involves a hereditary dysfunction in copper metabolism. The gene is localized on the X chromosome and both the intact and the defect gene have been cloned. The corresponding Cu-containing ATPase has been shown to posses a large content of cysteines which tightly bind the soft Cu(I) ions.

Certain copper complexes also exhibit antitumor activities. The compounds should be uncharged (lipophilic) and co-ordination compounds between Cu(II) and phenanthroline, thiosemicarbazone and salicylic acid derivatives have proven effective in treatment of certain forms of leukemia.

The term 'prions' is used to describe proteins involved in certain neuro-degenerative maladies like the Creutzfeld–Jacob disease. In the primary sequence of a prion protein an octapeptide sequence ProHisGlyGlyGlyTrpGlyGln, repeated up to 10 times in certain pathologies has been identified. These octapeptides are gaining much attention as potential copper co-ordination sites, as this copper binding may induce conformational changes/oligomerization, responsible for the pathological forms of the prions.

Silver is of little interest in a bioinorganic context except that many silver(I) compounds can be used as effective antibacterial drugs, like silver sulfadiazene which is used clinically in ointments as an antimicrobial agent in instances of severe burns. Also silver nitrate has been applied in dilute solutions in cases of eye infections due to its antiseptic property. Small concentrations (<1%) of silver nitrate show low toxicity.

Gold, on the other hand, has been applied in certain contexts during history. Already the ancient Chinese several thousand years ago produced an elixir containing colloidal gold which should ensure eternal life. The benefit of this treatment has never been fully documented, however. Nevertheless, gold(I) compounds are currently the only class of drugs known to halt the progression of rheumatoid arthritis. Initially, gold compounds like gold sulfide and gold thiomalate were painfully administered as intramuscular injections. Later it was discovered that triethylphosphinegold(I) tetra-O-acetylthioglucose (auranofin, Figure 13.23) was equally effective and could be administered orally. As is seen, in this drug gold is co-ordinated as Au(I) to sulfur- and phosphorous containing ligands.

The mode of action of gold(I) compounds is still not explained satisfactorily. As an extremely soft metal ion Au(I) shows a large affinity towards soft bases like sulfur (thiolates) and phosphorous (phosphines) while the affinity towards

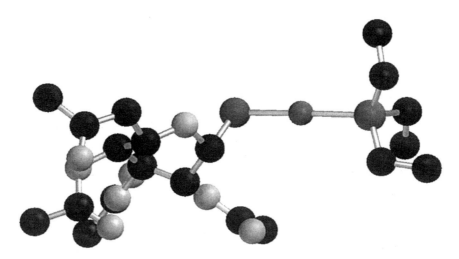

Figure 13.23 Auranofin. Gold(I) is co-ordinated linearly to a phosphine group (right) and a thiolate (left).

oxygen- and nitrogen containing ligands is small. Most Au(I) complexes have a co-ordination number of two and with a linear geometry. The Au(I) co-ordination in auranofin is shown in Figure 13.23. Several explanations have been propounded for the mechanism of gold(I) compounds in treatment of rheumatoid arthritis. In this context, it is interesting to note that the copper level is directly related to the extent of the disease. This has lead to proposals that anti-arthritic drugs like D-PEN and auranofin operate by affecting the center of co-ordination for copper ions, like the one found in human serum albumin. Albumin is the most abundant protein in plasma, with an approximate concentration ~0.6 mM. It consists of a single polypeptide chain including 585 amino acids one of which, in position 34, is a cysteine with a free thiolate side chain. As demonstrated by NMR studies, auranofin co-ordinates to this site and induces a conformational change in the protein. This affects the copper binding center in albumin (imidazole from a histidine group) whereby the copper homeostasis becomes perturbed. It has been suggested that the damage of the joints due to tissue inflammation is the result of lipid oxidation caused by free radicals such as O_2^-. This notion provides a link from gold to copper. Yet, in another hypothesis gold(I) complexes are suggested to inhibit formation of undesired antibodies in the collagen region.

It seems like the soft Lewis base, cyanide, plays a significant role in gold metabolism since patients who are in auranofin treatment excrete $[Au(CN)_2]^-$ in the urine. Cyanide ions are natural metabolites in the human organism and are formed by oxidation of thiocyanate by means of the myeloperoxidase enzyme. The dicyanoaurate(I) complex in itself possesses an anti-arthritic function and might be the proper active component. Thus, the ligand in auranofin (and in analogous gold(I) preparations) might just serve as binding and transport agent. The cyano complex has also been reported to exhibit anticancer and anti-HIV activity.

Gold-based pharmaceuticals unfortunately possess unpleasant side effects which include allergic reactions as well as gastrointestinal and renal problems. These side effects may be linked to the production of gold(III) metabolites which are strongly oxidizing. Patients with gold-related dermatitis exhibit an intense reaction to Au(III) exposure but not to Au(I). Strong oxidants as peroxide and hypochlorite, the latter synthesized *in vivo* from chloride by the myeloperoxidase enzyme in phagocytic cells, oxidize gold(I) to gold(III). Thus, a better understanding of the mechanism of gold preparations is indeed needed in order to produce more effective and less toxic gold-based drugs.

13.8.7   Zinc, cadmium, and mercury

Zinc is involved in a large number of biological processes and today more than 200 proteins containing Zn^{2+} are known. Among these, many essential enzymes are found which catalyze the transformation or degradation of proteins, nucleic acids, lipids, etc. Besides, the zinc ion stabilizes many different proteins like insulin. Thus, it is not very surprising that zinc deficiency will lead to severe pathological effects. The recommended daily intake of zinc is $\sim$15 mg (Table 13.1) only half of which is absorbed. Although food generally contains sufficient zinc to maintain this level, zinc deficiency occurs, producing effects like poor appetite, growth retardation, and skin lesions to mention but a few. The most affected enzymes are alkaline phosphatase and carboxypeptidase.

There is no ligand stabilization energy associated with the d^{10} Zn^{2+} ion which makes the metal ion quite tolerant to severe distortions of the preferred tetrahedral co-ordination. An important reason for cadmium, mercury, and lead poisoning is the ability of these ions to substitute for zinc in vital enzymes. The chemical advantage of zinc is first and foremost the high ionization potential of Zn^{2+} that makes it an excellent Lewis acid under physiological conditions at pH $\sim$7. When a substrate co-ordinates to Zn(II) in an enzyme, it becomes polarized and this includes both water, peptides, esters, and other molecules. The zinc ion thus manifests similar catalytic effect as strong acids, only at neutral pH. The pK_a value of a water molecule bound to zinc in an enzyme is typically less than 7.

Carbonic anhydrase is an enzyme which catalyzes the hydrolysis of CO_2:

$$CO_2 + H_2O \rightleftarrows H^+ + HCO_3^-$$

and is of fundamental significance in respiration. The catalytic process occurs 10^7 times faster in the presence of the zinc enzyme compared with the uncatalyzed reaction. The process is delineated in Figure 13.24. Certain anti-epileptic pharmaceuticals like acetazil amide co-ordinate, as described earlier, directly to the zinc(II)

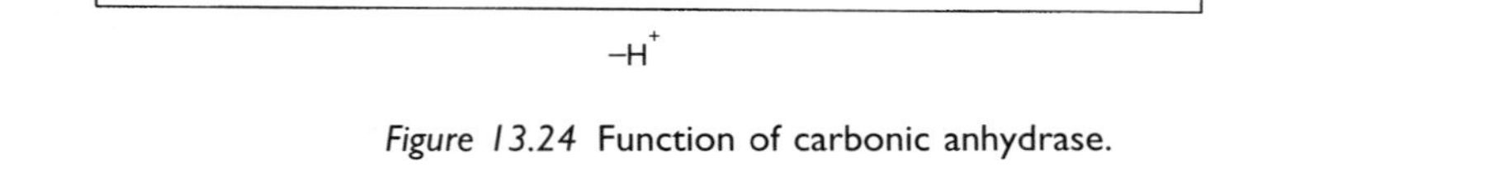

$$\left[E-Zn-OH\right]^+ \xrightarrow{CO_2} \left[E-Zn(OH)CO_2\right]^+ \longrightarrow \left[E-Zn-HCO_3\right]^+ \xrightarrow{H_2O} \left[E-Zn-H_2O\right]^{2+} + HCO_3^-$$

$$-H^+$$

Figure 13.24 Function of carbonic anhydrase.

ion in the active center of the enzyme and thus obstructs the catalytic transformation of carbon dioxide. With accumulation of CO_2 in the blood stream pH drops, and it has been suggested that this perturbs the GABA concentration in brain cells, either by increasing the GABA synthesis or by blocking the process of degradation (see Chapter 9).

In the same manner zinc-containing enzymes do for example catalyze cleaving of peptides (carboxypeptidase) and transformation of alcohols into aldehydes (alcohol dehydrogenase). Primary and secondary alcohols are rapidly and reversibly oxidized to aldehydes and ketones, respectively, by alcohol dehydrogenase, which is therefore responsible for the large concentrations of acetaldehyde accumulating after oxidation of ethanol and leading to effects ranging from the 'hangover' syndrome to liver damages. The process involves NAD^+ dependent oxidation of the alcohol and is thus a redox reaction. The zinc(II) ion being redox inactive serves to bind and activate the substrate.

Collagenases, in which zinc is co-ordinated to three histidine ligands are essential for development of the embryo and for wound healing. Zinc dependent tissue-dissolving enzymes are also involved in degradation of amyloid proteins in AD (see Chapter 10). Another interesting aspect related to zinc containing proteases is snake toxin which contains enzymes that effectively dissolve connective tissue and inhibit blood clotting. These toxins, however, completely loose their effect by sequestration of the metal ion. Neurotoxins produced by the tetanus and botulinum bacteria also contain zinc dependent proteases which specifically destroy synaptic membrane proteins.

Insulin consists of two relatively short peptide chains, and in the pancreas the hormone is stored in different hexamer modifications which besides calcium contain two or four zinc ions. Insulin is mobilized by reversible removal of zinc ions by chelating agents. While Zn^{2+} only plays a structural role here, thiolate co-ordinated Zn(II) is found in the DNA repair protein where it recognizes mutagenic methylated forms of guanine bases and removes the methyl group.

A relatively new field involving zinc bioinorganic chemistry is the so-called zinc fingers, small proteins which recognize DNA base sequences and thereby contribute to regulation of the genetic transcription. The reason for their name, zinc fingers, is obvious as shown in Figure 13.25. Zinc(II) is co-ordinated in a tetrahedral geometry to two thiolates (from cysteine) and two imidazoles (from histidine) in the protein while neighboring amino acid residues (the fingers) protrude into the DNA molecule where they couple specifically to DNA base pairs by wrapping closely around the double stranded DNA, featuring several protein/base pair contacts and thus securing multiple recognition. Zinc co-ordination to thiolate cysteines has also been observed in proteins with repair function as well as in nucleic acid binding proteins of the HIV retrovirus.

Cadmium exhibits many chemical similarities to zinc and therefore binds to the same proteins. Cadmium, however, being a 'softer' Class b metal (Section 13.4.2) co-ordinates with higher affinity to sulfur containing amino acid residues. But since the Cd^{2+} ion is a much poorer Lewis acid than Zn^{2+}, cadmium incorporation into enzymes will impede any catalytic action. Thereby cadmium becomes significantly more poisonous than e.g. lead. Cadmium is absorbed through the food particularly from animal organs and from mushrooms. Certain small cysteine rich proteins,

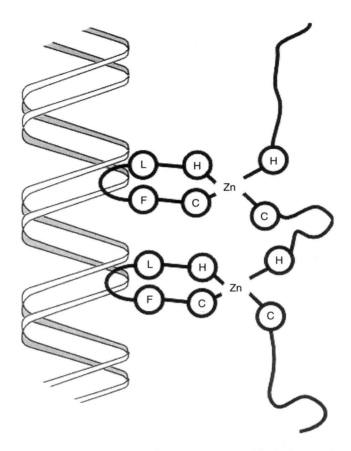

Figure 13.25 Zinc fingers. Zn(II) is co-ordinated to two cysteine (C) thiolates and two histidine (H) imidazoles in a tetrahedral geometry. Neighboring hydrophobic amino acids, leucine (L) and phenylalanine (F) form contact with DNA bases.

called metallothionein (Figure 13.26), are found in liver and kidneys. These proteins bind Cd^{2+}, Hg^{2+}, and Cu^+ (the soft metal ions) with very high affinity and thus serve in detoxication.

Mercury is even more toxic than cadmium due to the high solubility of the Hg^{2+} salts at physiological pH. Besides, metal organic mercury(II) compounds are easily formed (e.g. CH_3Hg^+, methyl mercury) which as chlorides are soluble in biological membranes and comfortably penetrate into the cells. Organic mercury compounds may be produced by bio-alkylation, i.e. the process catalyzed by vitamin B_{12} (Section 13.8.4). Cadmium and mercury compounds should under no circumstances be exposed to the environment, and notwithstanding the possible industrial usefulness, these metal ions should be operated in minimum amount and with great care.

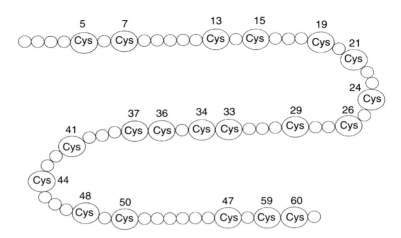

Figure 13.26 Metallothionein. Amino acid sequence of the metallothionein protein. Notice that approximately 1/3 of the amino acids are cysteine residues which will bind avidly to soft heavy metal ions.

13.8.8   Antimony and bismuth

As seen in Figure 13.1, arsenic might be an essential trace element while antimony and bismuth are not. However, the latter two elements have been applied in medicine for centuries. The early arsenic drugs developed by P. Ehrlich have already been mentioned (Section 13.1.2). As with arsenic the lower oxidation state of antimony(III) is the most toxic one, and only Sb(V) is used in pharmaceuticals. Presently, drugs based on antimony(V) complexes with polyhydroxy (carbohydrate) ligands are applied against diseases caused by certain parasites. Although the mechanism of action is not fully understood there are strong indications that Sb(V) is transferred to the particular site of attack where it becomes reduced to the more toxic Sb(III) which then destroys the parasite.

Bismuth compounds have been used extensively in treatment of gastrointestinal diseases. Due to the rather strong oxidizing properties of Bi(V), only drugs based on the 'softer' bismuth(III) ion are used, however. A potent antiulcer pharmaceutical is a colloidal Bi(III) citrate complex. Again, the mechanism of action is poorly understood, but polymers of the compound might be deposited in the ulcer wound forming a protective coating.

Some bismuth(III) complexes with sulfur containing ligands show high activity against the *Heliobacter pylori* bacteria. In this case inhibition of the nickel(II) containing enzyme, urease, that catalyzes the degradation of urea into carbon dioxide and ammonia, seems a plausible rationale for the antibacterial action. The ammonia produced from urea will neutralize the environment of the bacteria and help them to survive under the acidic conditions of the gastric lumen and mucosa (pH $\sim$ 2). The antiulcer effect of the Bi(III) thiolate complexes is higher than for the thiolates alone, indicating that bismuth is more than just delivering the sulfur containing ligand to the target. A noteworthy feature of the complex

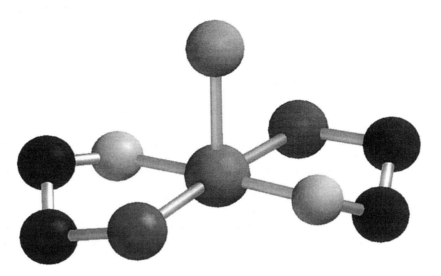

Figure 13.27 Bismuth antiulcer complex. Bismuth(III) complex with two chelating 2-mercapto-ethanol ligands and an axial chloride ion. Sulfur atoms are dark gray, oxygen atoms are light gray and carbon atoms black. Hydrogen atoms are not shown. The sixth position is occupied by an electron lone pair.

(Figure 13.27) is the position of a lone pair on one side of the bismuth co-ordination sphere. This may have an important bearing on the inhibitory function of the compound.

13.9   CONCLUDING REMARKS

As has hopefully come out of this chapter, the inorganic chemistry plays an increasingly important role in modern drug development. There are more than 25 elements with unambiguous importance for biological processes and in future pharmacology research, studies of uptake, metabolism, and excretion of these elements ought to be included. Besides, many compounds with other elements in the periodic table possess potential possibilities in development of biologically active complexes. In many cases, it will be possible to control metabolism of essential metal ions by means of organic pharmaceuticals since an intimate synergism exists between the function of inorganic elements and organic compounds of the body. As is well established, metal ions control some of the fundamental biochemical processes such as DNA and RNA replication, and many enzymes hereby hold a key position as pharmaceutical targets. A large need for development of new methods and strategies exists for testing inorganic compounds, and new techniques are further needed in modern pharmacological experimentation with inorganic molecules all the way from analytical tools to examination of co-ordination compounds in intact biological material. A larger emphasis should be put on kinetics rather than stability of inorganic compounds, since the most interesting biological processes, more often than not, take place rapidly and far from equilibrium. Hereby, a new and exciting field of research with a variety of challenges has opened in bioinorganic chemistry.

FURTHER READING

Cotton, F.A., Wilkinson, G. and Gaus, P.L. (1995) *Basic Inorganic Chemistry*. New York: J. Wiley.

Guo, Z. and Sadler, P.J. (2000) Medicinal inorganic chemistry. *Adv. Inorg. Chem.*, **49**, 183–306.

Kaim, W. and Schwederski, B. (1994) *Bioinorganic Chemistry: Inorganic Elements in the Chemistry of Life*. New York: J. Wiley.

Lippard, S.J. and Berg, J.M. (1994) *Principles of Bioinorganic Chemistry*. Mill Valley, California: University Science Books.

Sadler, P.J. (1991) Inorganic chemistry and drug design. *Adv. Inorg. Chem.*, **36**, 1–48.

Williams, R.J.P. and Frausto da Silva, J.J.R. (1996) *The Natural Selection of the Chemical Elements. The Environment and Life's Chemistry*. Oxford: Clarendon Press.

Chapter 14

Design and application of prodrugs

Claus S. Larsen and Jesper Østergaard

14.1 THE PRODRUG CONCEPT

14.1.1 Definition

As a result of rational drug design or the employment of combinatorial chemistry in combination with high throughput screening, a huge number of novel active molecules emerges. However, many such potential leads exhibiting high affinities towards a variety of molecular targets (i.e. receptors, enzymes, etc.) are, *per se*, prevented from becoming real drug candidates due to their inherent physico-chemical properties. This being based on the fact that only seldomly an active agent with optimal structural configuration for eliciting the desired therapeutic response at the target site possesses the best molecular form and properties for its delivery to the site of ultimate action (see Section 14.1.2).

There are several approaches that potentially can be taken in dealing with poor drug delivery characteristics. It is possible to circumvent some drug delivery problems by dosage form design. A second approach is to make a new drug analog of the original drug. In this approach, entirely new molecules exhibiting the desired physicochemical properties are designed; but changes in the pharmacological profile, as compared to the original drug, may be the outcome resulting in the demand for further expensive and time consuming biological testing. Often poor delivery characteristics of potential drug candidates are efficiently overcome by exploitation of bioreversible chemical derivatization or in other words the prodrug approach.

Prodrug design comprises an area of drug research devoted to optimization of drug delivery where the pharmacologically inactive prodrug requires transformation within the body in order to release the active drug. This approach has many advantages. First, the changes in physicochemical properties and the pharmacological profile of the drug are transient since the well-characterized parent drug molecule is regenerated from the prodrug *in vivo*. Second, introduction of a number of chemical transient changes in the drug molecule is possible allowing prodrug derivatives with a broad spectrum of physicochemical properties to be synthesized. The prodrug approach can be illustrated as shown in Figure 14.1. In this example, a drug molecule exhibits poor membrane permeability due to suboptimal physicochemical properties. By covalent attachment of a pro-moiety (or transport-moiety) to the active compound, a prodrug is formed, which overcomes the barrier for the clinical use of the drug. Once past the barrier, ideally, the

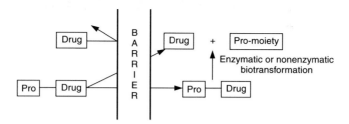

Figure 14.1 Schematic illustration of the prodrug concept.

prodrug undergoes quantitative chemical or enzymatic conversion to the parent compound (and a nontoxic transport-moiety). Prodrug formation can thus be considered as a means to mask temporarily undesirable physicochemical properties of the parent molecule.

14.1.2   Barriers to drug action

Administration of a prodrug is one of the avenues when attempting to control drug delivery and generate predictable drug concentration vs. time profiles at specific drug receptors. The rationale behind the prodrug approach is that the prodrug is capable of overcoming one or more of the barriers to drug delivery more efficiently than the parent drug. Some of the potential barriers related to the pharmaceutical and pharmacokinetic phase, respectively, are depicted in Scheme 14.1. The former phase comprises (i) incorporation of a potential drug entity into a convenient drug delivery system or a dosage form; and (ii) release of the active from the formulation whereas the pharmacokinetic phase embraces the absorption, distribution, metabolism, and excretion of the drug.

Major drug formulation barriers resulting from the physicochemical properties of the drug include

- Poor aqueous solubility
  – preventing the drug from being administered in form of injectables
  – giving rise to dissolution rate-limited (and variable) oral bioavailability
- Low lipophilicity
  – limiting the design of lipid-based formulations
- Chemical instability
  – preventing the drug from being incorporated into adequate dosage forms

In the pharmacokinetic phase, major barriers limiting the therapeutic value of an active agent, are

- Incomplete absorption across biological membranes such as the gastrointestinal mucosa and the blood–brain barrier
- Low and variable bioavailability due to extensive first-pass metabolism

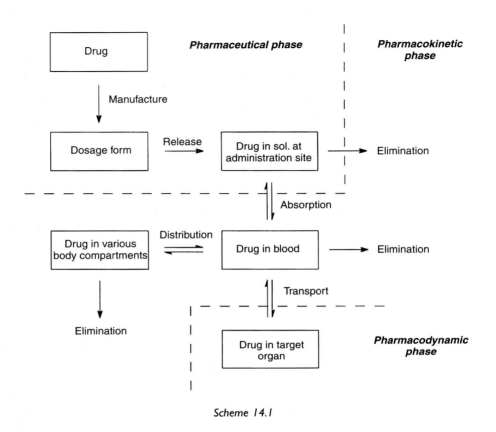

Scheme 14.1

- Too rapid absorption or excretion when a longer duration of action is desired
- Lack of site-specificity

14.1.3 Prodrug design in an industrial setting

An application for marketing authorization of a new chemical entity (NCE) is granted on basis of adequate demonstration of the quality, safety and efficacy of the drug. This comprehensive documentation comprises a compilation of the results obtained from a large number of multifaceted activities many of which are interrelated in such a manner that delay in one area may influence the momentum of other activities significantly. In order to minimize the time to marketed drug, it is therefore important to select the lead candidate early in the development process. A prerequisite for selecting the right candidate is that the appropriate amount of information is available at this decision point. Traditionally, lead selection has been based almost exclusively on target activities with little attention paid to the physicochemical and pharmacokinetic behavior of the potential leads.

In recent years, however, preliminary data related to the latter two areas have been included in the selection criteria.

The regulatory authorities consider a prodrug of a lead as a NCE. Thus, already performed studies (for example toxicity studies) using such a lead have to be repeated in case the prodrug is to be introduced in the development programme. From the above, proper exploitation of the prodrug approach appears most realistic if prodrug design constitutes, at least partly, an integral part of the drug design process. Attempts to identify suitable prodrug derivatives to improving drug therapy are obvious when recognized that the physicochemical characteristics of a highly interesting lead compound constitute an impediment to further development. In addition, utilization of prodrug design should also be considered in relation to (i) development of two or more dosage forms of the drug candidate; (ii) improved competitiveness of the drug in the marketplace accomplished by optimization of parameters like bioavailability or pharmacokinetic profile; and (iii) strategies in the areas of patent life time and product life circle management.

14.2   CHOICE AND FUNCTION OF THE PRO-MOIETY

Drug candidates may possess a variety of functional groups available for bioreversible chemical derivatization (see Section 14.3). Simple prodrug derivatives are obtained by direct attachment of a functional group of the pro-moiety to a functional group of the active agent. The types of sufficiently labile drug pro-moiety linkages formed in this way are limited for each chemical functional group as for example a carboxyl group. On the other hand, within a particular type of prodrug linkage bioreversible derivatives of a drug candidate such as carboxylic acid esters exhibiting significantly different properties might be designed dependently on the transport-moieties chosen (Figure 14.2). Thus, the desired rate and mechanism of cleavage of the prodrug bond might be accomplished by selection of an appropriate transport-moiety. In addition, the chemical nature of the applied pro-moiety influences the physicochemical and pharmacokinetic characteristics of the designed

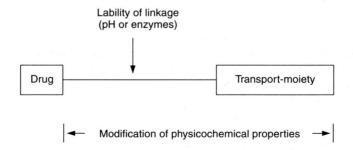

Figure 14.2 Function of transport-moiety to provide control of lability of prodrug bond and to optimize physicochemical properties.

prodrug as outlined below. Rational prodrug design, therefore, consists of three basic steps:

(1) Identification of the drug delivery problem
(2) Identification of the physicochemical properties required for maximum efficacy or delivery
(3) Selection of a transport-moiety providing a prodrug derivative exhibiting the proper physicochemical characteristics and which can be cleaved in the desired biological compartment

14.2.1   Cleavability of the prodrug bond

A basal prerequisite for the prodrug approach to be useful in solving drug delivery problems is the availability of chemical derivative types satisfying the prodrug requirements, the most prominent of these being reconversion of the prodrug to the parent drug *in vivo*. This prodrug–drug conversion process may take place before absorption, after entrance into the systemic circulation or at the specific site of drug action in the body, all dependent upon the specific goal for which the prodrug is designed. Whereas prodrugs designed to overcome solubility problems in formulating intravenous (i.v.) injectables should be converted immediately after i.v. administration, the rate of conversion should be lower in case a prodrug is aimed at providing a sustained drug action through rate-limiting cleavage of the prodrug bond.

Conversion or activation of prodrugs to the parent drug molecules in the body is the result of enzyme-mediated cleavage or pH-dependent hydrolysis of the established prodrug linkage. Within a homologous series of derivatives of the same drug (for example different carboxylic acid esters) the chemical nature of the pro-moiety may give rise to both electronic and steric effects influencing the lability of the prodrug bond. Prediction of chemical reactivity through substituent effects is often possible from empirical linear free energy relationships (LFERs). In the present context simple LFERs considered are linear correlations of the general form

$$\log k_{x} = \log k_{H} + \rho \sigma_{x} \tag{14.1}$$

where k_{H} is the rate constant for hydrolysis of the prodrug derivative possessing a hydrogen atom at the substitution site, and k_{x} refers to the rate constant for the derivative in which the hydrogen atom at the substitution site has been replaced by the substituent X. The substituent constant σ_{x} refers to the electronic (or steric) effect of the substituent. While the substituent constant is a parameter which in essence is dictated by the chemical nature of the substituent, the reaction constant ρ varies with the type of reaction and external conditions such as the solvent. In other words ρ is a quantitative measure of the sensitivity of the given reaction to polar or steric substituent effects. In rational prodrug design facile identification of suitable pro-moieties providing feasible chemical lability of the prodrug linkage is often possible from such linear correlations established by using tabulated values of, for example, Hammett's or Taft's polar substituent constants (reflecting electronic

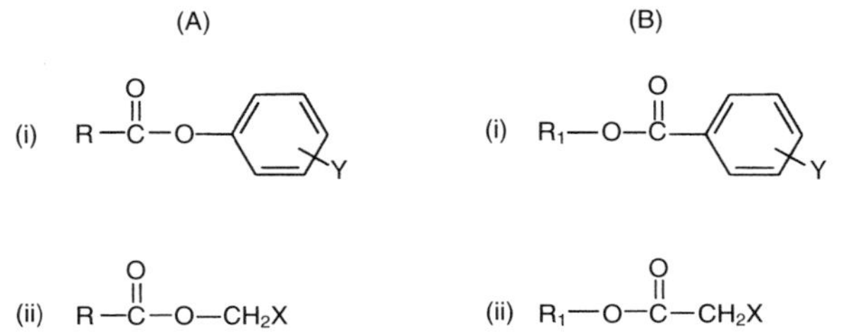

(A)

(i)   R—C(=O)—O—⟨aryl⟩Y

(ii)   R—C(=O)—O—CH₂X

(B)

(i)   R₁—O—C(=O)—⟨aryl⟩Y

(ii)   R₁—O—C(=O)—CH₂X

Figure 14.3 Types of ester derivatives: (A) Drug containing a carboxylic acid group; and (B) Drug containing a hydroxy functional group.

effects resulting from substitution in aromatic and aliphatic structures, respectively) and Charton's steric parameters.

For drug substances containing a carboxyl group, ester derivatives can be obtained from aliphatic alcohols and phenol type compounds (Figure 14.3A). Similarly, if the drug possesses an OH-group, different types of ester derivatives might be synthesized (Figure 14.3B). Neutral or alkaline hydrolysis of ester functions are facilitated by low electron density at the carbonyl carbon atom. Such an electron deficiency at the reaction site is accomplished by introducing an electronegative substituent in (i) the *meta-* or *para-*position of the aromatic ring (substituent Y) or (ii) aliphatic structures (substituent X). The majority of prodrugs to be activated by non-enzymatic processes is characterized by a high chemical instability at physiological pH (7.4) while preferably exhibiting a higher stability at lower pH. As will be discussed below an example of such prodrug types is *N*-Mannich bases (Section 14.3.2.1). A serious drawback of prodrugs requiring chemical (non-enzymatic) release of the active agent is the inherent lability of the compounds, raising some stability issues at least in cases of liquid dosage forms. In particular situations, such formulation problems have been overcome by using a more sophisticated approach involving double prodrugs where use is made of an enzymatic release mechanism prior to the spontaneous reaction (Section 14.3.1).

Prodrugs might be designed to be cleaved by action of enzymes to ensure fast regeneration of the drug once the barrier to efficient drug delivery has been overcome. In addition, site-specific drug delivery through site-specific prodrug activation may be accomplished exploiting that a target tissue contains specific enzymes or high concentrations of particular enzymes relative to non-target tissues (Section 14.4.2.2). Although examples of drug substances regenerated from their prodrugs by biochemical reductive or oxidative processes are available, the most common prodrugs are those requiring a hydrolytic cleavage mediated by hydrolases such as esterases and lipases. Rates of enzyme hydrolysis can to some degree be described as a function of some combination of electronic, steric, and hydrophobic parameters. However, application of LFERs to reactions catalyzed by hydrolytic enzymes appears less straightforward. For example, while the chemical reactivity of ester derivatives is readily predictable on basis of the steric and electronic properties of the substituents in both the acyl and alcohol moieties, this does not apply for enzyme-facilitated hydrolysis. In general, steric effects alter non-enzymatic and enzymatic ester hydrolysis rates in the same direction. For enzymatic ester hydrolysis, the hydrophilic property and charge of the ester may play a major role and consequently non-enzymatic hydrolysis cannot be used as a reliable guide to enzyme-catalyzed reactions. Thus, initial assessment of the susceptibility of prodrug candidates to undergo enzyme-mediated cleavage might be achieved by measurement of the stability of the derivatives after incubation in plasma or a homogenate from liver, intestine, skin or cornea, dependent on the intended route of administration of the prodrug. To this end, it should be emphasized that enzyme capacities might be subject to significant interspecies variation. For example, esters are usually hydrolyzed markedly faster in rat plasma than in human plasma whereas dog plasma often is less efficient than human plasma.

The influence of chemical structure on the chemical and enzymatic lability of a homologous series of potential prodrug candidates can be illustrated by the data obtained (Table 14.1) for various esters of the model drug compound benzoic acid. The rate of hydroxide ion-catalyzed hydrolysis of these esters is primarily determined by the polar (electronic) effects exhibited by the alcohol moieties of the esters since the steric effects in these portions can be considered to be almost constant due to the presence of a methylene group connected to oxygen in all the derivatives. Omitting the rate data for compound 8, where intramolecular catalysis by the carboxylate anion occurs, and compound 11, the hydrolysis rates of these esters are correlated by the following expression

$$\log k_{OH} = 0.54\sigma^* + 0.74 \quad (n = 16; \ r = 0.962) \tag{14.2}$$

Table 14.1 Rate data for the alkaline and enzymatic hydrolysis of various benzoic acid esters at 37 °C

Compound	R	σ^* for R	k_{OH} (M^{-1} min^{-1})	80% Human plasma	
				k(min^{-1})	$t_{1/2}$ (min)
1	H	0.49	13.6	6.4×10^{-3}	108
2	CH$_3$	0.00	6.59	3.3×10^{-3}	210
3	C$_2$H$_5$	−0.10	5.52	1.5×10^{-2}	46
4	C$_3$H$_7$	−0.12	4.50	1.7×10^{-2}	40
5	C$_4$H$_9$	−0.25	5.33	2.9×10^{-2}	24
6	C$_6$H$_5$	0.75	13.0	3.7×10^{-2}	19
7	CH$_2$C$_6$H$_5$	0.27	4.63	4.7×10^{-2}	15
8	(C=O)O$^-$	−1.06	6.28	$<10^{-4}$	>100 h
9	(C=O)OCH$_3$	2.00	70.1	2.0×10^{-1}	3.5
10	(C=O)OC$_2$H$_5$	2.26	60.3	4.4×10^{-2}	16
11	(C=O)CH$_2$C$_6$H$_5$	–	55.7	2.7×10^{-1}	2.6
12	(C=O)NH$_2$	1.68	69.9	1.7×10^{-2}	40
13	(C=O)N(CH$_3$)$_2$	1.94	19.2	>5.0	<8 s
14	SCH$_3$	1.56	24.4	3.1×10^{-2}	22
15	(S=O)CH$_3$	2.88	274	5.9×10^{-1}	1.2
16	(O=S=O)CH$_3$	3.68	592	5.8×10^{-1}	1.2
17	CH$_2$N(CH$_3$)$_2$	0.49	9.83	>8.0	<5 s
18	CH$_2$N(CH$_3$)$_3^+$	1.90	95.1	>8.0	<5 s

where k_{OH} is the 2nd order rate constant for specific base catalysis of hydrolysis ($M^{-1}\,min^{-1}$) and the Taft polar substituent constant σ^* refers to R in RCH_2OH for the alcohols. This LFER may be useful for prediction of the reactivity of a benzoate ester derivative solely on basis of the σ^* value of the appropriate alcohol substituent. A large number of σ^* values are compiled in the literature. The variation of rate of hydrolysis can also be accounted for in terms of the different stabilities of the leaving alcohol groups as expressed by the pK_a values of the alcohols.

In contrast, the plasma-catalyzed hydrolysis (pH 7.4) of the esters cannot be correlated in the same manner. It is apparent that by increasing the chain length in the alkyl esters, the enzymatic reactivity increases except when going from methyl to ethyl. The *N,N*-dimethylglycolamide ester 13 is seen to be cleaved extremely fast in human plasma although being chemically highly stable. The rapid rate of hydrolysis of compound 13 has been attributed to a pseudocholinesterase present in plasma. The protonated esters 17 and 18 are also cleaved very rapidly in plasma in contrast to the benzoylglycolic acid (compound 8). The high resistance of the latter derivative towards enzymatic hydrolysis is most likely caused by its negative charge at physiological pH due to the observation that various other esters with an ionized carboxylate group such as hemisuccinate esters are poor substrates for hydrolytic plasma enzymes.

14.2.2 Modification of physicochemical properties

Prodrug design has been used to improve the performance of drugs by overcoming various barriers to drug delivery (Section 14.1.2). In most cases, this has been accomplished by formation of prodrug derivatives altering the basic physicochemical characteristics of a drug substance which in addition to chemical stability encompasses (i) lipophilicity; and (ii) aqueous solubility. The fraction of a drug which reaches the receptor for therapeutic response is largely governed by dissolution and transport processes. These processes are primarily dependent on the latter two fundamental physicochemical properties. Due to this fact several more or less successful attempts to create tools for estimating aqueous solubility and lipophilicity of prodrugs have been made as outlined in the following sections.

14.2.2.1 Lipophilicity

Probably the most successful application of bioreversible derivatization is in the area of improving the passive drug transport across various biological membranes. In general, the transport rate is usually enhanced by attachment of a hydrophobic group to a drug substance, e.g. by formation of a more lipophilic derivative. Initially, the rate of diffusion across the membrane will increase exponentially with increasing lipophilicity of prodrug derivatives of a given compound. At higher lipophilicities, the transport rate levels off reaching a maximum value. Since an increase in lipophilicity, with a few exceptions, is accompanied by a comparable or greater decrease in aqueous solubility further increment in lipophilicity will ultimately result in a decrease in the flux over the membrane due to poor aqueous solubility. Thus, it is apparent that both solubility and lipophilicity constitute the most important factors in passive drug absorption. Drugs, which are too polar or hydrophilic often exhibit poor transport properties, whereas those that are too non-polar or lipophilic frequently have low bioavailability as a consequence of insufficient aqueous solubility. Although being the subject of some debate as to which *in vitro* partitioning system best mimics biological membranes, lipophilicity most often is expressed by the *n*-octanol-water partition coefficient (P_{oct}) given as the ratio of the activities (or in dilute solution the concentrations) of the solute in the two phases at equilibrium. A $\log P_{oct}$ value of 1 expresses that the solute concentration in the octanol phase, at equilibrium, is ten times higher than in the aqueous phase. However, the equilibrium constant *per se* does not give insight into the absolute magnitude of the concentration of a solute in the two respective phases. Therefore, two compounds having the same P_{oct} value may vary with respect to membrane transport properties since significant difference in size of intermolecular cohesive forces of the two substances (for example hydrogen bonding) will result in different absolute affinities for the two almost immiscible phases. The optimal balance between aqueous solubility and $\log P_{oct}$ to ensure good absorption depends on the nature of the biomembrane and the volume of the aqueous phase adjacent to the membrane. If dissolution phenomena are not rate-limiting, a $\log P_{oct}$ of about 2 appears optimal for gastrointestinal absorption.

In the area of parenteral oil depot formulations the prodrug approach has been extensively exploited to generate prodrug derivatives with feasible lipophilicities (see Section 14.4.3). For this type of formulations the rate of prodrug release from the oil vehicle, and thus the duration of action, is at least partly dictated by the partition coefficient of the entity between the oil and the tissue fluid after intramuscular (i.m.) injection.

Since many drugs are either weak acids or bases or salts hereof, dissociation constitutes a factor in determining absorbability. It is generally accepted that the unionized and thus most lipophilic form of an acidic or basic drug is absorbed far more efficiently than the ionic species. Assuming that partitioning only takes place for unionized species, the partition coefficient of a weak acid at a given pH can be expressed by

$$P_{pH} = P_{HA} f_{HA} \tag{14.3}$$

where P_{HA} is the intrinsic partition coefficient of the weak acid and f_{HA} is the fraction of the undissociated acid at the particular pH value ($f_{HA} = [H^+]/[H^+] + K_a$). Equation 14.3 can also be written in the form

$$\log P_{pH} = \log P_{HA} - \log (1 + 10^{(pH-pK_a)}) \tag{14.4}$$

where K_a is ionization constant of the acid. The analogous expression for a weak base is

$$\log P_{pH} = \log P_B - \log (1 + 10^{(pK_a-pH)}) \tag{14.5}$$

where P_B is the intrinsic partition coefficient of the weak base.

Partition coefficients of chemical entities can be predicted reasonably well by several group contribution approaches. In prodrug design, the lipophilicity (expressed as the *n*-octanol-water partition coefficient) of members of a homologous series of derivatives are generally estimated with acceptable accuracy by using tabulated values of the Hansch substituent constant Π_X defined as

$$\Pi_X = \log P_{RX} - \log P_{RH} \tag{14.6}$$

where P_{RX} is the partition coefficient for the derivative RX which is obtained from the derivative RH by substitution of a hydrogen atom with the group or atom X.

14.2.2.2 Solubility

In spite of the great importance of aqueous solubility in the pharmaceutical and other applied chemical disciplines, it is a very poorly understood phenomenon. There are no generally useful guidelines for estimating the solubility of a drug substance in water based on consideration of its structure and physicochemical properties. One reason for the lack of predictability of the solubility of crystalline compounds is that it is not a simple equilibrium, but it rather consists of a combination of equilibria.

Intermolecular interactions in the crystalline state constitute important factors in determining the aqueous solubility of a drug, due to their influence on the thermodynamic activity of the solid drug. The melting point (*MP*) and the thermodynamic activity of a drug in its solid phase are two distinct parameters, but are related to a certain degree. Both properties have been used as indicators of the strength of interactions in the crystalline phase. Quantitative relationships between molecular structure and melting point are generally not found. Qualitatively, melting points within a series of structurally similar compounds increase with increasing molecular weight (*MW*), compactness, rigidity, and symmetry, and the number of polar, particularly hydrogen bonding, groups in the molecule. Thus, for closely related series of compounds linear correlations in melting points have occasionally been observed although linearity of such correlations cannot be accounted for thermodynamically.

Although based on many assumptions and approximations a rough estimate of the ideal solubility of non-electrolytes at 25 °C from chemical structure and *MP* (in Celcius degrees) is provided by the expression

$$\log X_{id} = -\frac{\Delta S_f}{2.303\, R\, 298.15}(MP - 25) \tag{14.7}$$

where $\log X_{id}$ is the logarithm of the mole fraction solubility, ΔS_f is the entropy of fusion and R refers to the gas constant. Assuming that $\Delta S_f = 13.5\,\text{cal K}^{-1}\,\text{mol}^{-1}$ for rigid molecules equation (14.7) might be written

$$\log X_{id} = -0.0099(MP - 25) \tag{14.8}$$

revealing an apparent linearity between ideal solubility and *MP*. The anti-epileptic agent phenytoin (**14.1**) is a high melting, weakly acidic, and sparingly water-soluble drug. Phenytoin exhibits poor oral bioavailability after administration in various dosage forms. In order to disrupt the major intermolecular interactions in the crystal lattice responsible for the undesired physicochemical properties, a series of 3-acyloxymethyl derivatives of phenytoin (**14.2a–j**) was synthesized. The derivatives

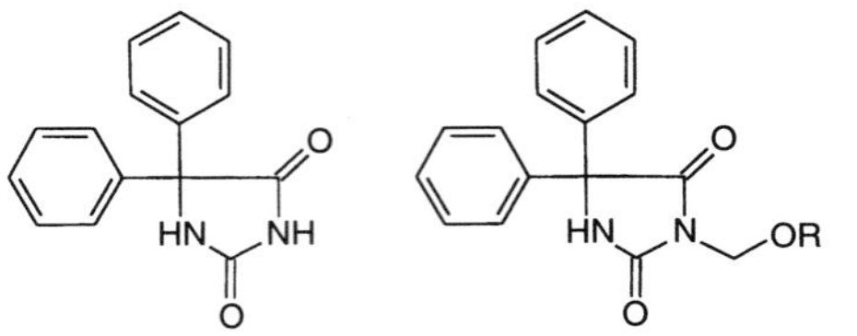

(14.2a)	R= (C=O)CH$_3$
(14.2b)	R= (C=O)C$_2$H$_5$
(14.2c)	R= (C=O)C$_3$H$_7$
(14.2d)	R= (C=O)C$_4$H$_9$
(14.2e)	R= (C=O)C(CH$_3$)$_3$
(14.2f)	R= (C=O)C$_5$H$_{11}$
(14.2g)	R= (C=O)C$_6$H$_{13}$
(14.2h)	R= (C=O)C$_7$H$_{15}$
(14.2i)	R= (C=O)C$_8$H$_{17}$
(14.2j)	R= (C=O)C$_9$H$_{19}$

Scheme 14.2

were reasonable soluble in various metabolizable glycerol esters such as tributyrin and triolein allowing the prodrugs to be incorporated in soft gelatine capsules. The prodrug 3-pentanoyloxymethyl-5,5-diphenylhydantoin (**14.2f**) when administered in tributyrin gave superior oral phenytoin bioavailability in rats when compared to sodium phenytoin administered as an aqueous solution. Some physicochemical data for the derivatives are presented in Table 14.2. As seen from Figure 14.4 a reasonable linearity between the logarithm of molar solubility of the prodrug derivatives in ethyl oleate and their *MPs* was established implying that crystal lattice energy differences, as indicated by *MP* behavior, appear to influence the solubility of the esters in this organic solvent.

The approach represented by equations (14.7) and (14.8) has been extended to provide approximate predictions of aqueous solubility of non-electrolytes. The real solubility of crystalline drugs involves the consideration of the aqueous activity coefficient as well as the ideal solubility. In this case, a relationship between molar aqueous solubility (*S*) (25 °C), and the partition coefficient P_{oct} and the *MP* might be established according to the semi-empirical expression

$$\log S \cong -a \log P_{oct} - b\, MP + c \tag{14.9}$$

Table 14.2 Melting point (*MP*), molecular weight (*MW*), and molar solubility (*S*) at 25 °C of various esters of 3-hydroxymethyl-5,5-diphenylhydantoin in ethyl oleate. **14.2a–j** refer to the chemical structures presented in Scheme 14.2

Compound	MP (°C)	MW	$10^3 \times S$(M)
14.2a	158–159	324.3	4.63
14.2b	172–174	338.4	5.02
14.2c	134–135	352.4	13.1
14.2d	89–92	366.4	111.4
14.2e	134–135	366.4	25.9
14.2f	107–108	380.4	52.3
14.2g	87–88	394.5	74.5
14.2h	67.5–68.0	408.5	257.0
14.2i	78.5–80.0	422.5	129.0
14.2j	56–57	436.5	281.8

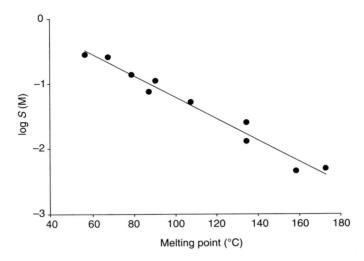

Figure 14.4 Plot of the logarithm of the molar solubility S of various 3-acyloxymethyl-5,5-diphenylhydantoins in ethyl oleate at 25 °C against their melting points.

where a, b and c are constants varying slightly depending on the basic chemical structure of the series of compounds investigated. For rigid and short molecules $\Delta S_f = 13.5\ \mathrm{cal\ K^{-1}\ mol^{-1}}$ and equation (14.9) becomes

$$\log S \cong -1 \log P_{\mathrm{oct}} - 0.01\ MP + 1.05 \tag{14.10}$$

In attempt to improve the therapeutic value of the anticancer agent 5-fluorouracil (5-FU) (**14.3**) several prodrug types have been evaluated. Among these, various N_1- and N_3-monosubstituted bioreversible derivatives of 5-FU have been investigated (Scheme 14.3). The physicochemical characterization of the derivatives included determination of MP, S, and P_{oct} with the latter two parameters determined for the undissociated forms of the derivatives. By multiple-regression analysis of the parameters of this series of 5-FU derivatives, covering a considerable range of MPs, $\log P$, and $\log S$ values, the following relationship between the parameters were found

$$\log S = -0.98\ (\pm 0.13)\ \log P - 0.009\ (\pm 0.002)\ MP + 0.12\ (\pm 0.33)$$
$$(n = 15;\quad r = 0.914) \tag{14.11}$$

which is in surprisingly good agreement with the theoretical correlation given by equation (14.10). Although semi-empirical of nature such relationships may be valuable for the prediction of aqueous solubilities of congeneric series of prodrug derivatives from the knowledge of the MP and P_{oct}, the latter being easily estimated *a priori* by group contribution approaches.

Aqueous solubility limitations are critical for the development of parenteral and oral drug products. For poorly soluble non-electrolytes the prodrug approach

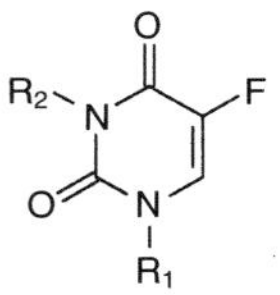

(14.3)

Compound:		
5-Fluorouracil (5-FU) **(14.3)**	$R_1 = H$	$R_2 = H$
1-acyloxymethyl-5-FU	$R_1 = CH_2O-acyl$	$R_2 = H$
3-acyloxymethyl-5-FU	$R_1 = H$	$R_2 = CH_2O-acyl$
3-acyl-5-FU	$R_1 = H$	$R_2 = acyl$
3-alkoxycarbonyl-5-FU	$R_1 = H$	$R_2 = (C=O)O-alkyl$
3-aryloxycarbonyl-5-FU	$R_1 = H$	$R_2 = (C=O)O-aryl$
1-alkylcarbamoyl-5-FU	$R_1 = (C=O)N-alkyl$	$R_2 = H$

Scheme 14.3

has been applied to circumvent solubility problems by using transport-moieties possessing an ionizable functional group, e.g. phosphate esters, amino acid esters and hemiesters of dicarboxylic acids (see Section 14.4.3), allowing various salts of such prodrug derivatives to be formed. In spite of the fact that salt formation is routinely employed, quantitative relationships between chemical structure and physicochemical properties of salts are virtually non-existing. In qualitative terms, however, it is recognized that increased compactness, symmetry, and rigidity of the ions would be expected to decrease escape tendencies of the salts. Likewise, it is generally observed that increasing lipophilicity of the counterion decreases water solubility. In thermodynamic terms the molar free energy change when a salt is dissolved in water, ΔG_{sol} can be expressed as

$$\Delta G_{sol} = \Delta G_+ + \Delta G_- - \Delta G_{lattice} \tag{14.12}$$

where ΔG_+, ΔG_-, and $\Delta G_{lattice}$ are the energies of hydration of the cation, hydration of the anion, and the crystal lattice energy, respectively. Consequently, the solubility will depend on which terms, the hydration energies or the lattice energy, are most sensitive to changes in structure. In optimization of aqueous solubility by prodrug design both of the latter two parameters therefore have to be taken into consideration. Significant increase in aqueous solubility has been achieved via simple bioreversible modifications which result in disruption of the crystal lattice. To this end, the use of the prodrug approach can be illustrated by considering the antiviral agent vidarabine (**14.4**). The poor aqueous solubility of the drug substance (0.0018 M) at 25 °C is most likely caused by strong intermolecular hydrogen bonding in the crystalline state as reflected in its *MP* (260 °C). The significantly enhanced solubility of the 5′-formate ester (**14.5**), corresponding to approximately 0.12 M (25 °C), has been attributed to disruption of the strong intermolecular interactions in the crystal as judged by the decrease in *MP* of the derivative

(14.4) R= H

(14.5) R= $\overset{\overset{\displaystyle O}{\displaystyle \|}}{C}$—H

(175 °C). Thus, a 60-fold increase in solubility is the result of incorporation of the small, polar formyl group in **14.4**. The 5′-formate ester prodrug is rapidly hydrolyzed in human blood with a half-life of 6–8 min, and it appears to be a useful parenteral delivery form of vidarabine, although the solution stability is rather limited.

14.2.3 Macromolecular transport vectors

Most drug candidates have *MWs* of about 200–500 dalton. A bioreversible derivative obtained by covalent attachment of a pro-moiety of similar size to such therapeutic agents can be referred to as a low molecular weight prodrug. In ophthalmic drug delivery, for example, where the active agent only has to pass one biological barrier (cornea) before reaching the target area, it is possible by proper selection of the transport-moiety to synthesize prodrug derivatives endowed with feasible membrane transport properties and *in vivo* labilities. In case the target site only can be reached after transport via the systemic circulation the *in vivo* fate of the drug is affected by drug distribution, protein binding, tissue storage, and excretion, not to mention the enormous range of metabolic reactions that drugs may undergo. The latter processes are also influenced by the physicochemical properties of the drug or prodrug derivative, however in a less preditive manner limiting the use of the low molecular weight prodrug approach to optimize systemic site-specific drug delivery or drug targeting (Section 14.4.2). Drug targeting is especially attractive for highly toxic compounds and for drugs having a narrow therapeutic window. In its simplest sense, targeted drug delivery is achieved by enhancing drug availability at the target or response site while minimizing its availability at other sites, especially those that manifest toxicity.

The chemotherapeutic utility of macromolecular prodrugs, in which a drug is attached to a macromolecule through a bioreversible linkage, to provide drug targeting has been the focus of intense research for decades. Although an account on low molecular weight prodrugs is the subject of the present chapter, a brief description of the potential utility of the macromolecular prodrug approach is given below. The rationale behind this approach is that the transport properties of the macromolecular prodrug should be dictated predominantly by the macromolecular transport vector. In the field of cancer, chemotherapy design

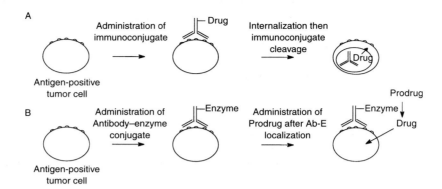

Figure 14.5 (A) Simplified scheme of the site-directed drug delivery to and activation of a monoclonal antibody-drug conjugate in a tumor cell; (B) simplified scheme of the site-specific activation of a prodrug at a tumor cell using the ADEPT concept.

of macromolecular prodrugs has received considerable interest since anticancer agents tend to be highly toxic and their effectiveness limited by a very small therapeutic ratio. Thus, macromolecular conjugates obtained by a bioreversible attachment of anticancer agents to a wide array of macromolecules endowed with intrinsic target receptor affinities such as monoclonal antibodies (mAB) and hormones have been evaluated *in vitro* and *in vivo* (Figure 14.5). Despite the tremendous efforts devoted to the design of parenteral site-specific soluble macromolecular drug carrier systems, the current level of success has been rather disappointing. There are at least three major reasons for this: (i) the multitude of physiological barriers the macromolecular prodrug has to fight against on its way from the administration site to the ultimate target of the drug entity; (ii) the task of accomplishing the correct timing of the events leading to optimal drug action, e.g. selective regeneration and suitable maintenance of the active agent at the target site; and (iii) potential immunogenicity and loss of the intrinsic receptor affinity upon covalent linkage of the cytotoxic agent to the macromolecular transport vector.

An interesting principle bearing some resemblance to antibody-based macromolecular prodrugs is the so-called ADEPT concept (antibody-directed enzyme prodrug therapy) (Figure 14.5). In the ADEPT approach, an enzyme, which catalyzes the conversion of a low molecular weight prodrug to the active cytotoxic drug, is covalently linked to a monoclonal antibody that binds antigen preferentially expressed on the surface of tumor cells, or in tumor interstitium. In the first step, the mAB-enzyme complex is administered and accumulates at the tumor site. Enough time is allowed for clearance of the complex from normal (non-target) tissue before the prodrug of the anticancer agent is administered. This leads to enzyme-catalyzed regeneration of the cytotoxic parent drug specifically at the tumor site. Although drawbacks to the use of the ADEPT approach are similar to those mentioned above for antibody-based macromolecular prodrugs, the concept appears potentially attractive due to the possibility of using enzymes which have catalytic properties different from those of any endogenous enzyme.

Besides drug targeting, other important objectives may be achieved by using soluble macromolecular prodrugs, including:

(1) Stabilization of the therapeutic agent
(2) Enhancement of drug solubility
(3) Improvement of circulation life time
(4) Extended duration of action

The latter objectives may be obtained by employing biodegradable macromolecular pro-moieties without any apparent specificity for discrete cell-surface receptors encompassing proteins, polypeptides, polysaccharides as well as synthetic polymers. The composition of such macromolecular prodrugs can be created in a more or less sophisticated way as evident from the schematic presentation given in Figure 14.6. Prodrug derivatives, in which the drug is linked directly to the macromolecular backbone, may act as a depot releasing the active agent in a predictable manner. In most cases, regeneration rates of the parent drug are exclusively governed by pH-dependent hydrolysis due to the bulky polymer matrix rendering the hydrolytic center inaccessible to enzymatic attack.

Intercalation of a spacer arm between the drug and the carrier may serve three purposes. First, the terminal functional group of the spacer arm can be varied, thus allowing covalent drug fixation to be established through a variety of chemical bonds. Second, steric hindrance of enzyme activation of the liganded drug might be circumvented by augmenting the distance between the drug and the carrier backbone. By proper selection of the spacer arm encompassing both the length and the chemical structure, and the spacer to drug bond, a localized effect may be obtained in case the spacer-drug link is designed to be cleaved selectively by enzymes secreted extracellularly by the target pathological cells. Third, sequentially labile macromolecular prodrugs can be constructed in such a way that the pH-dependent hydrolysis only liberates the spacer-drug derivative, i.e. the corresponding low molecular weight prodrug. After parenteral administration, the macromolecular derivative might

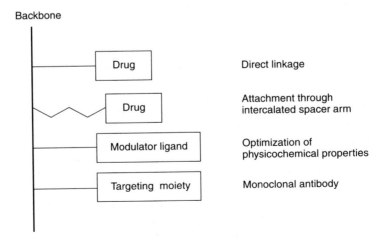

Figure 14.6 Schematic presentation of possible macromolecular prodrug structures.

therefore act as a depot releasing the low molecular weight prodrug, which after extravasation or diffusion from the injection site is activated at the diseased tissue.

The disposition and persistance of the macromolecular conjugate might be altered or improved by employing different types of ligands. Linkage of, *per se*, inactive chemical entities to the polymeric carrier can modify the overall physicochemical characteristics of the derivatives resulting in for example a diminished liver uptake. Of a more speculative utility is the incorporation of a target specific moiety in order to guide the prodrug selectively to the target area.

14.3 BIOREVERSIBLE DERIVATIVES FOR VARIOUS FUNCTIONAL GROUPS

The most common type of prodrugs are esters derived from hydroxy or carboxyl groups present in the parent drug molecules. In a number of cases, however, other strategies are required, since the drug to be modified does not contain such groups readily amenable to esterification. Therefore, bioreversible derivatives of a variety of functional groups have been investigated in the design of potentially useful prodrug types, some of which are presented in Table 14.3. An outline of the more commonly used types of derivatives is given in the following sections.

Table 14.3 Prodrug forms of various functional groups in drug substances

Functional group	Prodrug form	
-COOH	$-\overset{O}{\overset{\|}{C}}-OR$	Esters
	$-\overset{O}{\overset{\|}{C}}-O-\overset{R_1}{\overset{\|}{C}H}-O-\overset{O}{\overset{\|}{C}}-R_2$	α-Acyloxyalkyl esters
	$-\overset{O}{\overset{\|}{C}}-NHR$	Amides
-OH	$-O-\overset{O}{\overset{\|}{C}}-R$	Esters
	$-O-\overset{O}{\overset{\|}{C}}-OR$	Carbonate esters
	$-O-\overset{O}{\overset{\|}{P}}\overset{OH}{\underset{OH}{}}$	Phosphate esters
	$-OR$	Ethers
	$-O-\overset{R_1}{\overset{\|}{C}H}-O-\overset{O}{\overset{\|}{C}}-R_2$	α-Acyloxyalkyl ethers
-SH	$-S-\overset{O}{\overset{\|}{C}}-R$	Thioesters

Functional group	Derivative structure	Name
	$-S-CH(R_1)-O-C(=O)-R_2$	α-Acyloxyalkyl thioethers
	$-S-S-R$	Disulphides
$\mathord{>}C=O$	$-C(OR_1)(OR_2)-$	Ketals
	$\mathord{>}C=N-R$	Imines
	$\mathord{>}C{=}{\cdots}-O-C(=O)-R$	Enol esters
	(ring: C with O and N — oxazolidine)	Oxazolidines
	(ring: C with S and N — thiazolidine)	Thiazolidines
$-NH_2$	$-NH-C(=O)-R$	Amides
	$-NH-C(=O)-O-R$	Carbamates
	$-N=C(R_1)(R_2)$	Imines
	$-NH-C(R)=C(R_1)-R_2$	Enamines
	$-NH-CH_2-N(R_1)-C(=O)-R_2$	N-Mannich bases
	$-NH-C(=O)-O-CH(R_1)-O-C(=O)-R_2$	N-Acyloxyalkoxycarbonyl derivatives
$\mathord{>}N-$	$-\overset{+}{N}(CH(R_1)-O-C(=O)-R_2)$	N-Acyloxyalkyl derivatives
$R_1-C(=O)-OR_2$	$R-SO_2-N=C(R_1)(O-R_2)$	N-Sulphonyl imidates
$-SO_2NH_2$	$-SO_2NH-CH_2O-R$	N-Sulphonyl imidates
NH-Acidic group	$-C(=O)-N(R)-CH_2-N(R_1)(R_2)$	N-Mannich bases
e.g. $-C(=O)-HN$	$-C(=O)-N(R)-CH_2OH$	N-Methyols
or heterocyclic amine	$-C(=O)-N(R)-CH(R_1)-O-C(=O)-R_2$	N-Acyloxyalkyl derivatives

14.3.1   Esters as prodrugs for compounds containing carboxyl or hydroxy groups

The popularity of using esters as a prodrug type for drugs containing carboxyl or hydroxy functions (or thiol groups) stems primarily from the fact that the organism is rich in enzymes capable of hydrolyzing ester bonds. The distribution of esterases is ubiquitous and several types are found in the blood, liver, and other organs or tissues. In addition, by appropriate esterification it is possible to obtain derivatives with almost any desirable aqueous solubility or lipophilicity as well as *in vivo* lability, the latter being dictated by electronic and steric factors (Section 14.2.1). Accordingly, a significant number of carboxylic acid drugs and drugs containing alcohol groups have been modified for a multitude of reasons employing the ester prodrug approach. Examples of applications of the latter prodrug type are found in Section 14.4.

The pH-dependent rate of hydrolysis of simple ester derivatives *in vitro* can often be described by the general rate equation

$$k_{\mathrm{obs}} = k_{\mathrm{H^+}} a_{\mathrm{H^+}} + k_{\mathrm{o}} + k_{\mathrm{OH^-}} a_{\mathrm{OH^-}} \tag{14.13}$$

where k_{obs} is the observed pH-dependent pseudo-1st order rate constant for hydrolytic cleavage of the ester bond, and $k_{\mathrm{H+}}$ and $k_{\mathrm{OH-}}$ represent the 2nd order rate constants for specific acid and base catalysis, respectively. k_{o} is the apparent 1st order rate constant for the spontaneous degradation. $a_{\mathrm{H+}}$ and $a_{\mathrm{OH-}}$ refer to the hydrogen and hydroxide ion activity, respectively. Plots of $\log k_{\mathrm{obs}}$ against pH yield the characteristic U-shaped pH-rate profile or a V-shaped profile in case the contribution of the spontaneous reaction to k_{obs} becomes insignificant. Although differing with respect to stability in aqueous solution the chemical instability of ester derivatives may be high and aqueous dosage forms can therefore be difficult to formulate. In attempt to improve the aqueous solubility of metronidazole (**14.6**), the solubility of which is about 1% w/v, eight amino acid esters of the drug were prepared and evaluated for their feasibility as water-soluble parenteral delivery forms of metronidazole. As seen from Table 14.4 the ester prodrugs exhibit poor stability in aqueous buffer pH 7.4 (37 °C). Even at lower pH the esters are too unstable to be formulated as a ready-to-use injection formulation. Table 14.4 also illustrates that the rate of regeneration of **14.6** from the prodrugs mediated by plasma enzymes depends strongly on the chemical structure of the pro-moiety. For further information about different ester types introduced to improve the aqueous solubility of drugs containing a hydroxy group (Drug-OH) see Section 14.4.3.

Not only steric effects within the alcohol portion have influence on the enzymatic hydrolysis of esters. Enzyme-mediated hydrolysis might also be highly sensitive to steric hindrance caused by the acyl portion. In penicillins, for example, the environment around the carboxyl group is sterically hindered, and simple aliphatic

(14.6)

Table 14.4 Half-lives for the hydrolysis of various amino acid esters of metronidazole (**14.6**) in 80% human plasma (pH 7.4) and 0.05 M phosphate buffer (pH 7.40) at 37 °C

Ester	$t_{1/2}$ in human plasma (min)	$t_{1/2}$ in buffer (min)
N,N-dimethylglycinate	12	250
Glycinate	41	115
N-Propylglycinate	8	90
3-Aminopropionate	207	315
3-Dimethylaminopropionate	46	52
3-Dimethylaminobutyrate	334	580
4-Morpholinoacetate	30	1880
4-Methyl-1-piperazinoacetate	523	1720

or aromatic esters are not sufficiently labile *in vivo* to function as prodrugs. This shortcoming can be overcome by preparing a double ester prodrug type, acyloxyalkyl or alkoxycarbonyloxyalkyl esters, in which the terminal ester group is accessible to enzymatic cleavage. The first step in regeneration of the parent drug from this type of esters is enzyme-catalyzed hydrolysis of the terminal ester bond with the formation of a highly unstable α-hydroxyalkyl ester which rapidly dissociates by a spontaneous reaction to yield the parent acidic drug and an aldehyde (Scheme 14.4). By a similar mechanism, alkoxycarbonyloxyalkyl esters (containing a terminal carbonate ester function) release an alcohol, carbon dioxide and an aldehyde upon hydrolysis. Double prodrugs might be the result of chemical structures different from the above mentioned double esters and refer, in general, to prodrugs where activation of the drug is initiated by enzymatic cleavage of a terminal functional group under formation of an unstable intermediate which undergoes a fast, spontaneous rearrangement to the active agent.

The applicability of α-acyloxyalkyl esters as biologically reversible transport forms has also been extended to include the phosphate group, phosphonic acids and phosphinic acids. An example is compound **14.7**, an angiotensin converting enzyme (ACE) inhibitor, where the phosphinic acid group has been *O*-α-acyloxyalkylated to yield fosenopril (**14.8**) which is better absorbed orally than the parent active compound as a consequence of its greater lipophilicity.

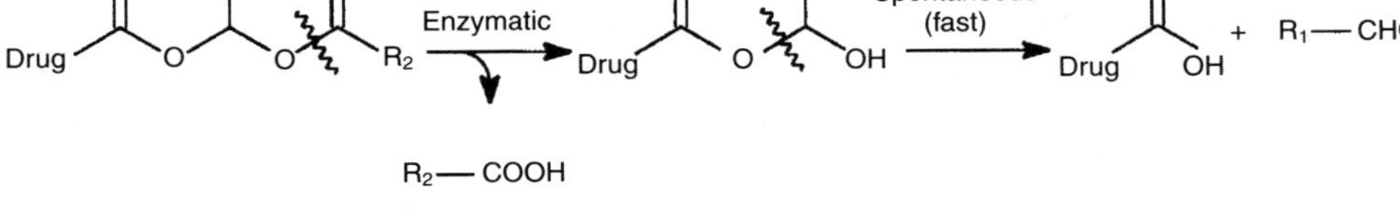

Scheme 14.4

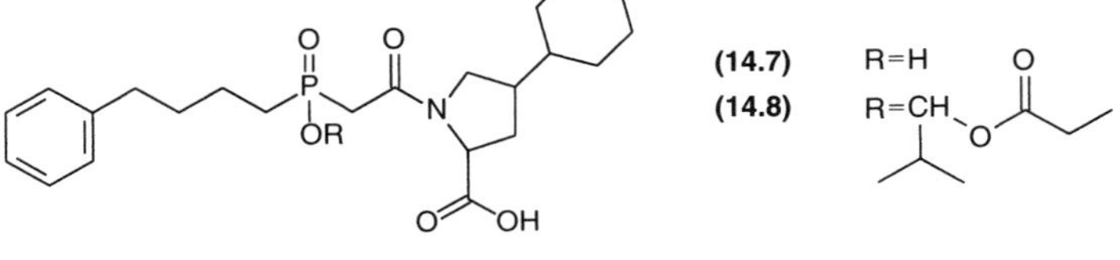

(14.7)   R=H
(14.8)   R=CH

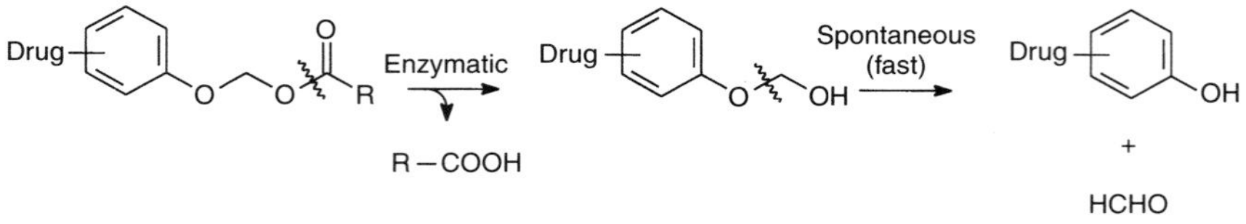

Scheme 14.5

O-α-Acyloxyalkyl ethers may constitute a useful prodrug type for compounds containing a phenol group. Such derivatives are hydrolyzed by a sequential reaction involving formation of an unstable hemiacetal intermediate (Scheme 14.5). Like normal phenol esters, they are susceptible to enzymatic hydrolysis by e.g. human plasma enzymes. This type of ethers are, however, more stable against hydroxide ion-catalyzed hydrolysis than phenolate esters, a feature which makes them potentially more favorable in prodrug design.

14.3.2   Prodrugs for amides, imides and other NH-acidic compounds

14.3.2.1   N-Mannich bases

N-Mannich bases can function as prodrug candidates for NH-acidic compounds like various amides, imides, and hydantoins as well as for aliphatic and aromatic amines (see Section 14.3.3.3). They are generally formed by reacting an NH-acidic compound with formaldehyde, or, in very rare cases, other aldehydes and a primary or secondary aliphatic or aromatic amine (Scheme 14.6).

   N-Mannich bases are readily hydrolyzed in aqueous solution. The rate of hydrolysis usually increases with increasing pH resulting in a sigmoidal (S-shaped) pH-rate profile. The shape of the pH-rate profile can be accounted for by assuming spontaneous decomposition of the free *N*-Mannich base (B) and the protonated form (BH$^+$). The expression of the pH-dependent pseudo-1st order rate constant (k_{obs}) is

$$k_{obs} = k_1 f_B + k_2 f_{BH^+} = k_1 \left(\frac{K_a}{a_{H^+} + K_a} \right) + k_2 \left(\frac{a_{H^+}}{a_{H^+} + K_a} \right) \tag{14.14}$$

where f_B and f_{BH^+} are the fractions of the *N*-Mannich species on basic and acidic form, respectively. K_a is the apparent ionization constant for the protonated *N*-Mannich base, and k_1 and k_2 represent the 1st order rate constants for the spontaneous degradation of B and BH$^+$, respectively.

   The reaction mechanism proposed for the decomposition involves as rate-limiting step an unimolecular N–C bond cleavage with formation of an amide (or imide) anion and an immonium cation. In subsequent fast steps, a solvent molecule

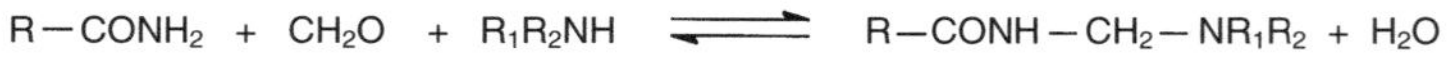

$$R-CONH_2 + CH_2O + R_1R_2NH \rightleftharpoons R-CONH-CH_2-NR_1R_2 + H_2O$$

Scheme 14.6

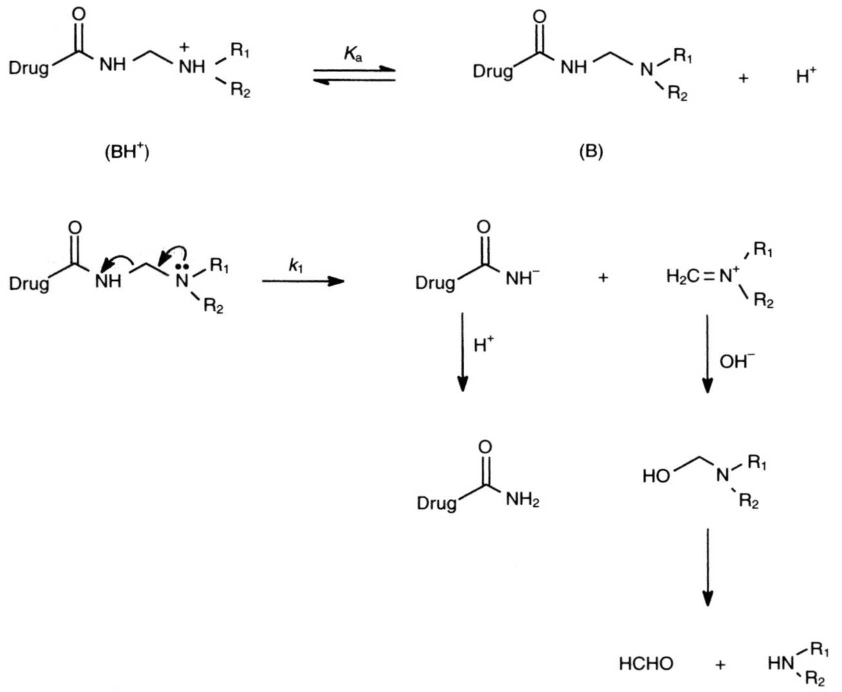

Scheme 14.7

transfers a proton to the anion and a hydroxide ion to the immonium ion, giving methylolamin which rapidly dissociates to formaldehyde and amine (Scheme 14.7). The structural effects on the decomposition rate of N-Mannich bases derived from carboxamides, sulphonamides or imides, and aliphatic or aromatic amines involve (i) steric effects; (ii) basicity of the amine component; and (iii) acidity of the amide component. The effect of these factors are most pronounced with respect to the rate constant k_1 and, accordingly, to the degradation rate in weakly acidic to basic aqueous solution. The rates of hydrolysis of unprotonated N-Mannich bases are accelerated strongly by (i) increasing steric effects within the amine substituent; (ii) increasing basicity of the amine component; and (iii) increasing acidity of the parent amide-type compound. For some N-Mannich bases of benzamide and various amines the rate constant k_1 can be expressed by the following equation

$$\log k_1 = 2.30v - 3.50 \quad (k_1 \text{ in min}^{-1}; \ 37\,^{\circ}\text{C}) \tag{14.15}$$

where v is Charton's steric substituent constant for alkyl amino groups. The marked influence of the steric effect on k_1 is evident from comparison of the k_1 values for benzamide N-Mannich bases of diethylamine (0.52 min^{-1}) and ethylamine (0.0084 min^{-1}).

For amines having the same steric properties but differing in basicity, the rate constants k_1 for degradation of the respective N-Mannich bases increase almost

10-fold with an increase of unity of the pK_a of the amines. Further, the reactivity of this prodrug type increases strongly with increasing acidity of the parent amide-type compound. Thus, for N-Mannich bases derived from morpholine the following relationship has been observed

$$\log k_1 = -1.15\,pK_a + 13.9 \quad (k_1 \text{ in min}^{-1};\ 37\,^\circ\text{C}) \tag{14.16}$$

where pK_a refers to the ionization constant for the parent amide-type compound. For benzamide, for example, pK_a is about 14.5. From the above it appears that by suitable selection of the amine component, it should be possible to obtain prodrugs of a given amide-type drug varying significantly with respect to *in vivo* lability. Furthermore, other physicochemical properties such as aqueous solubility, dissolution rate, and lipophilicity can be modified for the parent drug compound.

Transformation of an amide into an N-Mannich base introduces a readily ionizable amino function which may allow the preparation of derivatives with greatly enhanced water solubility at slightly acidic pH values where, fortunately, the stability often is sufficiently high. The concept of N-Mannich base formation of NH-acidic compounds to yield more soluble prodrugs has been utilized in the case of clinically used rolitetracycline (**14.10**). This water-soluble N-Mannich base of tetracycline and pyrrolidine is decomposed quantitatively to tetracycline (**14.9**) in neutral aqueous solution, the half-life being 40 min at pH 7.4 and 37 °C. Breakdown of this prodrug is not catalyzed by enzymes, a feature generally observed for N-Mannich bases.

Several biologically active peptides have been identified, including small peptides consisting of only two amino acids. The clinical utility of such chemical entities is, however, seriously hampered by substantial delivery problems. Peptides are highly polar compounds and do not easily pass biological membranes by passive diffusion. In addition, they suffer from considerable metabolic lability. An α-aminoamide moiety is found in many peptides, and a potentially useful and broadly applicable prodrug type for this group may be 4-imidazolidinones formed by reacting such peptides with ketones or aldehydes (Scheme 14.8). Such imidazolidinyl peptides, which may be regarded as cyclic N-Mannich bases, undergo a complete hydrolysis in the pH range 1–10 with maximum rates normally occurring at pH > 4.

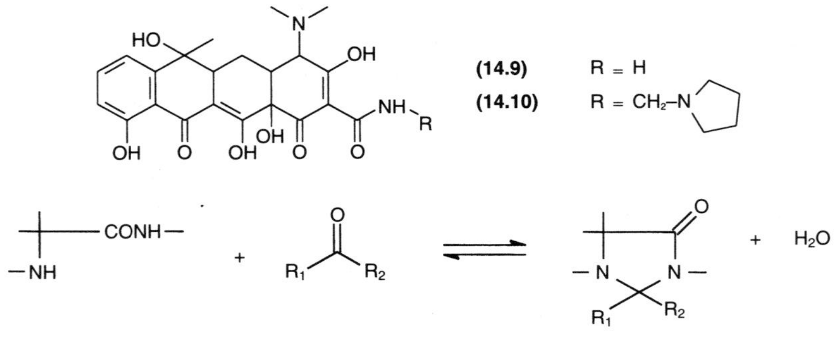

Scheme 14.8

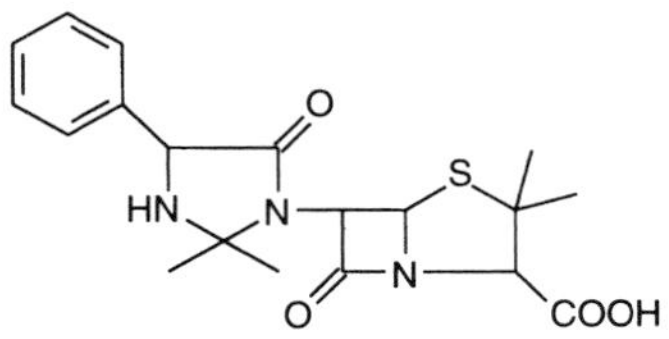

(14.11)

Another example of cyclic *N*-Mannich base-type prodrugs is clinically used hetacillin (**14.11**) which is formed by condensation of ampicillin with acetone. The prodrug is readily hydrolyzed to yield the active ampicillin and acetone, $t_{1/2}$ being 15–20 min at pH 4–8 (35 °C). An advantage of hetacillin is its higher stability in concentrated aqueous solutions compared to ampicillin sodium, which undergoes a facile intermolecular aminolysis by attack of the side-chain amino group in one molecule on the β-lactam moiety of a second molecule.

14.3.2.2   *N*-α-acyloxyalkyl derivatives

N-α-acyloxyalkylation is a commonly used approach to provide prodrugs of various secondary amides, imides, hydantoins, uracils, and tertiary or *N*-heterocyclic amines. By variation of the acyl portion of this type of derivatives it is possible to control the rate of regeneration of the parent drug and to obtain prodrugs with varying physicochemical properties. Whereas, the derivatives which can be referred to as double prodrugs, exhibit reasonable stability in aqueous solution *in vitro* comparable to that of other esters, they are in general rapidly cleaved *in vivo* by virtue of enzyme-mediated hydrolysis. The activation of the parent NH-acidic compound is accomplished by a two-step reaction (Scheme 14.9). The enzymatic cleavage of the ester bond results in the formation of an intermediate *N*-α-hydroxyalkyl derivative which instantaneously decomposes to yield the parent NH-acidic compound and the corresponding aldehyde. Thus, the rate of drug formation is solely dependent on the rate of the initial ester cleavage which as previously mentioned can be controlled by predominantly steric factors.

N-α-acyloxymethylation is most commonly employed, providing derivatives from which formaldehyde is released from the *N*-hydroxymethyl intermediate. In this case, instantaneous decomposition of the formed intermediate requires that the pK_a of the NH-acidic agent is lower than about 10.5 as evident from the established linear relationship between the rate of hydrolysis (expressed in terms

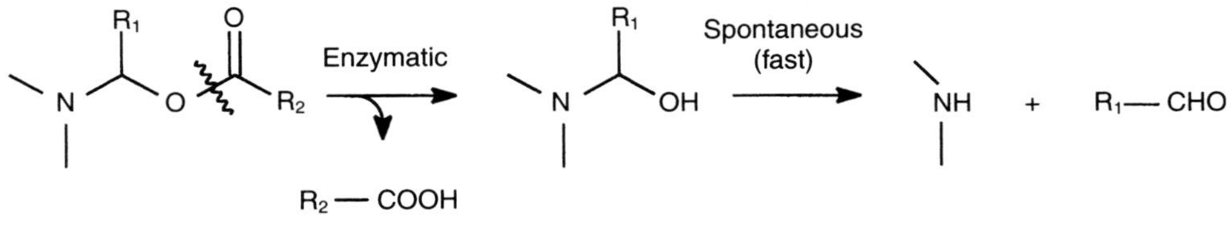

Scheme 14.9

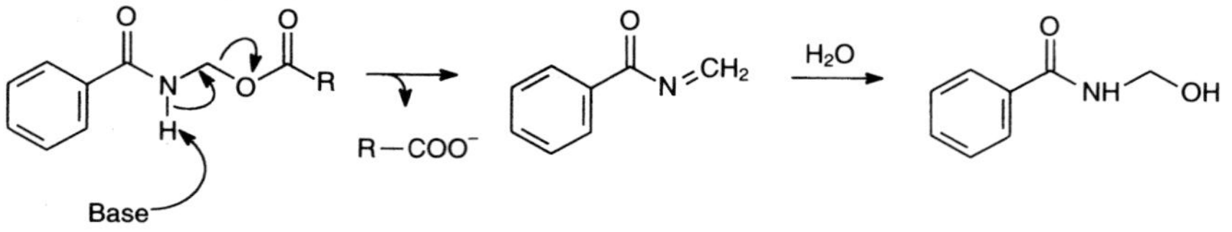

Scheme 14.10

of the half-life) at pH 7.4 of such *N*-hydroxymethyl derivatives and the pK_a of the parent NH-acidic chemical entity

$$\log t_{1/2} = 0.77 pK_a - 8.34 \quad (t_{1/2} \text{ in min; } 37\,°C) \tag{14.17}$$

However, by using other aldehydes than formaldehyde, the *N*-α-alkylol intermediates thus formed would be more unstable than the *N*-methylol analog, hence expanding the applicability of *N*-α-acyloxyalkylation to NH-acidic drugs possessing pK_a values above 11. It should be emphasized that *N*-α-acyloxyalkylation of NH-acidic compounds like primary amides, carbamates, and sulphonamides is not feasible due to the *in vitro* instability of the derivatives. The latter type of derivatives is extremely unstable in aqueous solution decomposing by an elimination–addition mechanism involving a reactive *N*-acylimine intermediate as illustrated in Scheme 14.10 for *N*-α-acyloxymethyl derivatives of benzamide. In similar derivatives derived from secondary amides the nitrogen atom has no hydrogen attached, and the formation of an *N*-acylimine by a base-catalyzed process is thereby not possible.

14.3.2.3   *N*-acyl derivatives

N-acylation of amide- and imide-type compounds may be a useful prodrug approach in some particular cases. In assessing *N*-acylated amides or imides as potential prodrugs it is important to consider the possibility of drug regeneration afforded by enzyme-catalyzed hydrolysis. Thus, N_3-acetyl-5-fluorouracil (**14.12**) and N_1-ethoxycarbonyl-5-fluorouracil (**14.13**) hydrolyze with half-lives of 40 and 550 min, respectively, at pH 7.4 and 37 °C. In 80% human plasma, however, half-lives of about 2–4 min have been observed. As a result of their altered physicochemical properties and easy bioconversion, these prodrug derivatives of 5-FU have shown improved ocular and rectal absorption as compared to the parent drug.

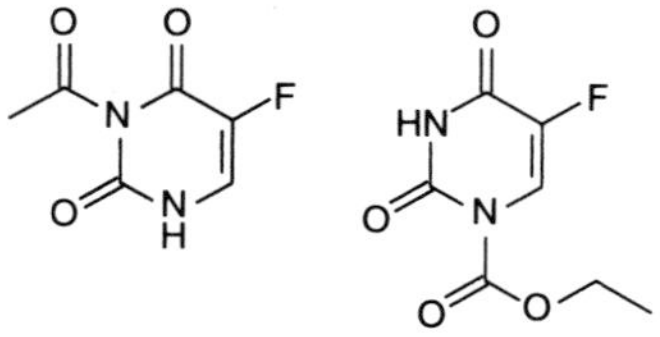

(14.12)   (14.13)

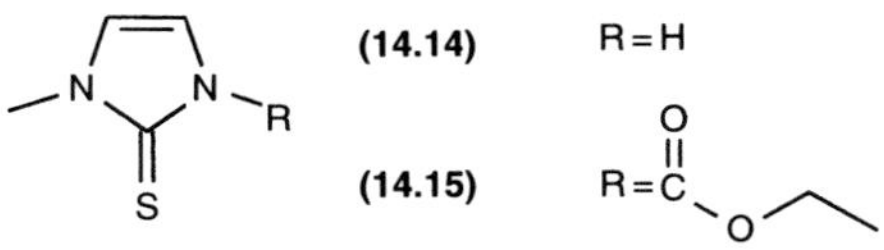

(14.14)   R=H

(14.15)   R=C(=O)O ethyl (ethoxycarbonyl)

Carbimazole (**14.15**) is a widely used prodrug of the antithyroid methimazole (**14.14**). In the presence of serum enzymes, the ethoxycarbonyl group is rapidly cleaved.

14.3.3   Prodrugs for amines

14.3.3.1   Amides

In prodrug design, *N*-acylation of amines to yield amides has been used only to a limited extent due to the relatively high stability of amides *in vivo*. However, certain activated amides are sufficiently chemically labile including the *N*-L-isoleucyl derivative of dopamine and the *N*-glycyl derivative midodrin (**14.17**) which is an orally absorbable prodrug of compound (**14.16**).

14.3.3.2   N-acyloxyalkoxycarbonyl derivatives

The utility of carbamates as prodrug derivatives for amines ($R–NH–(C=O)–OR_1$) is limited due to the general resistance of carbamates to undergo enzymatic cleavage *in vivo*. By introduction of an enzymatically labile ester function in the carbamate structure it is, however, possible to circumvent this problem. Thus, *N*-acyloxyalkoxycarbonyl derivatives of primary and secondary amines may be readily transformed to the parent amine *in vivo*. Enzymatic hydrolysis of the ester moiety in such derivatives leads to an unstable hydroxyalkoxycarbonyl intermediate which spontaneously decomposes into the parent amine via a labile carbamic acid (Scheme 14.11). Such acyloxyalkyl carbamates may be promising biolabile

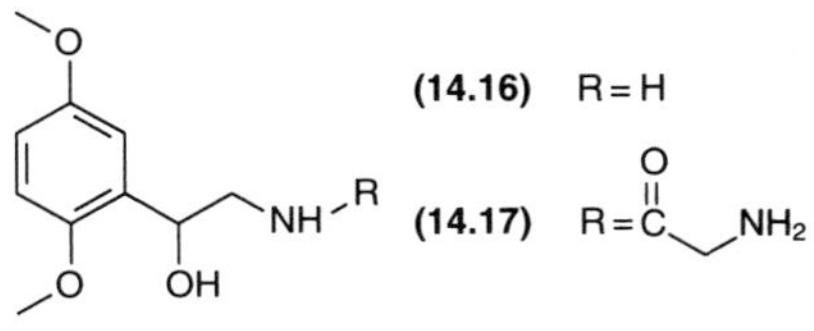

(14.16)   R = H

(14.17) $R = C(=O)NH_2$

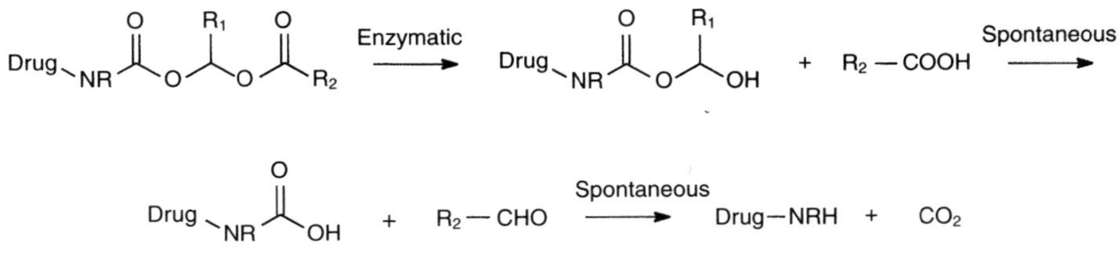

Scheme 14.11

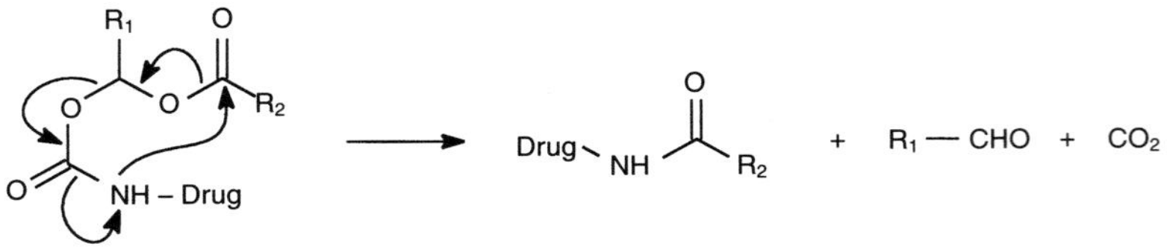

Scheme 14.12

prodrugs for amino functional drugs since they are neutral compounds and combine a high stability in aqueous solution with a high susceptibility to undergo enzymatic reconversion to the active agent initiated by hydrolysis of the terminal ester function. In case of primary amines, it should be noticed that an intramolecular acyl transfer reaction, leading to the formation of a stable N-acylated parent amine (Scheme 14.12), may compete with the reaction sequence presented in Scheme 14.11 at physiological pH and thus diminish the amount of amine regenerated. Such intramolecular N-acylation is structurally impossible in derivatives obtained from secondary amines.

14.3.3.3   N-Mannich bases

Besides being considered as a potential approach of derivatizing amide-type drugs (see Section 14.3.2.1), N-Mannich base formation can also be thought as a means of forming prodrugs of primary and secondary amines in which case the amide-type component constitutes the transport-moiety. By N-Mannich base formation, the pK_a value of the corresponding acid of the amine component is lowered by about 3 units. Thus, compared to the parent amines the derivatives are much less protonated at physiological pH, resulting in enhanced biomembrane-passage ability. This expectation of increased lipophilicity has been confirmed for e.g. the N-Mannich base derived from benzamide and phenylpropanolamine (α-(1-aminoethyl)benzylalcohol). The partition coefficient of the derivative between n-octanol and phosphate buffer pH 7.4 is about 100-times higher than that of the parent amine. By benzamidomethylation, the pK_a of phenylpropanolamine decreases from 9.4 to 6.2 revealing that the derivative is predominantly unprotonated at pH 7.4, a major contributing factor to the enhanced P value of the latter compound.

The availability of biologically acceptable amide-type pro-moieties affording an appropriate cleavage rate of a N-Mannich base of a given amine at pH 7.4 is limited. In search for useful candidates, it has been found that N-Mannich bases of salicylamide (**14.20**) and different aliphatic amines including amino acids show an unexpectedly high cleavage rate at neutral pH, thus indicating the utility of this transport group (Scheme 14.13). Although the salicylamide N-Mannich bases are more stable in weakly acidic solution (pH 2–5) than at pH 7.4, a drawback to the use of this prodrug type still is its limited *in vitro* stability. Improved stability may be achieved by further derivatization of the latter type of N-Mannich bases under formation of double prodrugs. Since the hydroxy group is responsible for the high reactivity of these derivatives, presumably through intramolecular catalysis, protection of this

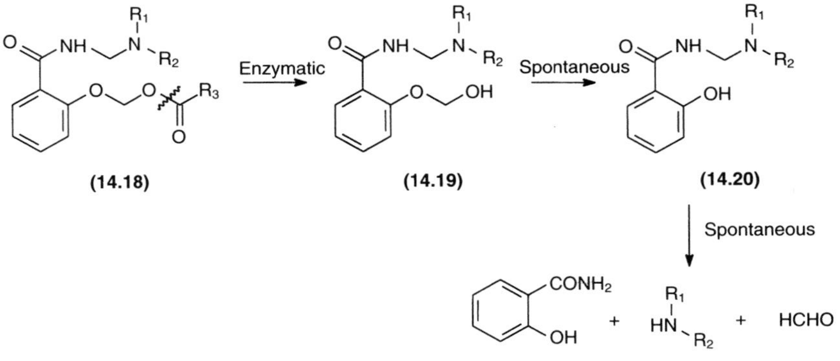

Scheme 14.13

group can afford derivatives exhibiting enhanced *in vitro* stability. This is actually achievable by acyloxymethylation of the phenolic hydroxy group. The *O*-acyloxymethyl derivative (**14.18**) is significantly more stable than (**14.20**) in the pH range 2–8. In the presence of human plasma, the ester group is rapidly hydrolyzed by virtue of enzymatic catalysis yielding (**14.19**) which spontaneously degrades to (**14.20**) (Scheme 14.13). In addition to providing an *in vitro* stabilizing effect, the concept of *O*-acyloxymethylation makes it possible to obtain prodrug derivatives of a given amine possessing varying physicochemical properties of importance for drug delivery, such as water solubility and lipophilicity. This can simply be effected by selection of an appropriate acyloxymethyl group (varying the R_3 group).

14.3.4   Prodrugs for compounds containing carbonyl groups

Despite the existence of a fairly large number of drugs containing a carbonyl group only a few bioreversible derivatives have been explored for molecules containing an aldehydic or ketonic functional group. Potential prodrug types include Schiff bases, oximes and enol esters, however, only oxazolidines and thiazolidines are briefly considered in the following section.

14.3.4.1   Oxazolidines and thiazolidines

In addition to constituting a possible approach of derivatizing β-aminoalcohols (see Section 14.3.6), oxazolidine formation can also be thought as a means of achieving prodrugs of aldehydes and ketones in which case the β-aminoalcohol component acts as the transport-moiety (Scheme 14.14). In considering oxazolidines as prodrug candidates for carbonyl-containing chemical entities, their weakly basic character (pKa 5–7) may be advantageous since such derivatives are protonated at acidic pH and may thus exhibit a desired aqueous solubility at low pH.

Thiazolidines have been applied as prodrug derivatives for various steroids containing a 3-carbonyl group to improve their topical anti-inflammatory activity. Thiazolidines (spirothiazolidines) of hydrocortisone and hydrocortisone 21-acetate

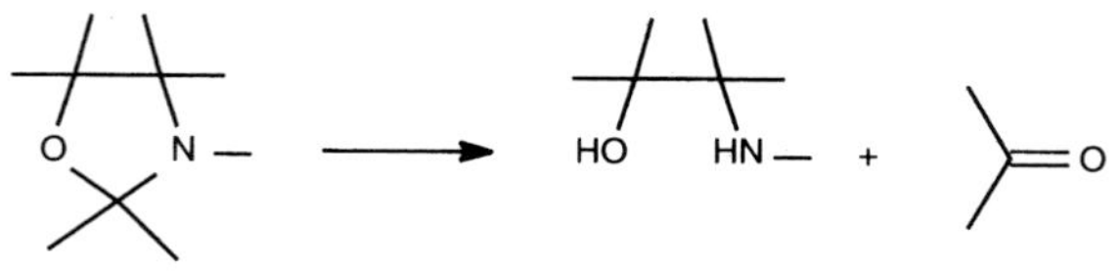

Scheme 14.14

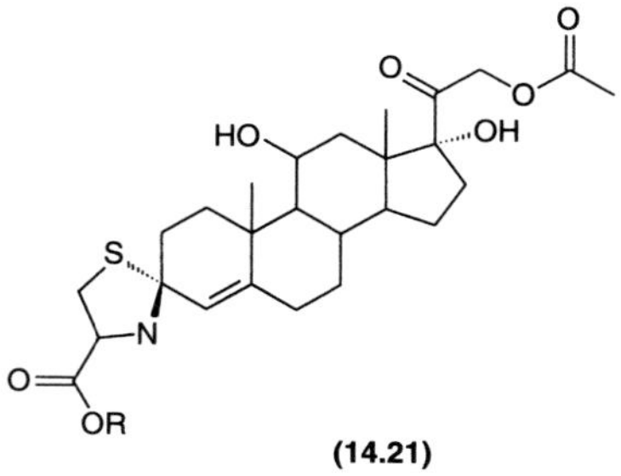

(14.21)

(**14.21**), prepared with cysteine esters or related β-aminothiols, have been shown to be readily converted to the parent corticosteroids at conditions similar to those prevailing in the skin, thus meeting the requirement for a prodrug. Thiazolidine ring opening proceeds by a spontaneous S_N1 cleavage of the carbon–sulphur bond to give a Schiff base intermediate which then is hydrolyzed. In particular, cysteine derivatives may be attractive as pro-moieties due to release of cysteine as a by-product. Also, the carboxyl group of cysteine is easily esterifiable, thus providing a convenient method for changing the lipophilicity/hydrophilicity of the spirothiazolidine prodrugs.

14.3.5 Drug activation from intramolecular cyclization reactions

14.3.5.1 *Ring-opened derivatives as prodrugs for cyclic drugs*

Pilocarpine (**14.22**) is used as a typical miotic agent for controlling the elevated intraocular pressure associated with glaucoma. Its ocular bioavailability is low and the duration of action is short, thereby necessitating frequent dosing corresponding to 3–6 times a day. This leads to transient peaks and valleys in pilocarpine concentration in the eye, which in turn result in dose-related ocular side effects such as myopia and miosis. There is, therefore, a high incidence of patient non-compliance, which has been suspected to be responsible for inadequate pressure control and deterioration of vision. A useful prodrug of pilocarpine should (i) exhibit a higher lipophilicity than pilocarpine in order to enable an efficient corneal membrane transport; (ii) possess adequate solubility and stability for formulation as eyedrops; (iii) be converted to the active within cornea or once the membrane has been passed; and (iv) lead to a controlled release and hence prolonged duration of action of pilocarpine.

Pilocarpic acid esters may be promising prodrug candidates with the above mentioned desired attributes. A series of alkyl and aralkyl esters of pilocarpic acid (**14.23**)

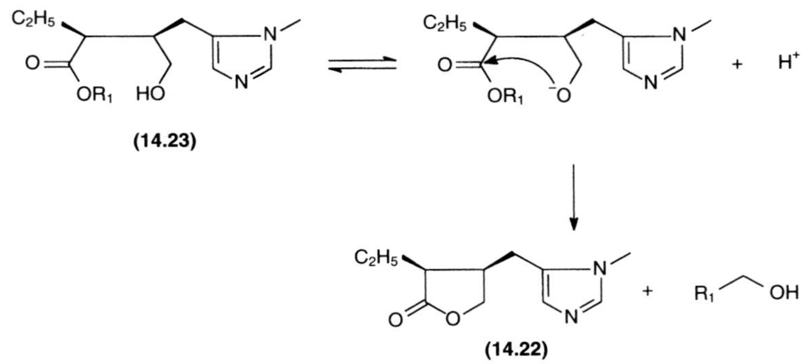

Scheme 14.15

has been shown to function as prodrugs of pilocarpine both *in vitro* and *in vivo*. In aqueous solution, the esters undergo quantitative and apparent specific base-catalyzed lactonization to pilocarpine (Scheme 14.15). As appears from the rate data shown in Table 14.5, the various esters differ greatly in their rates of cyclization, the variation being fully accounted for in terms of polar effects exerted by the alcohol portion of the esters. An LFER was found between the logarithm of half-time of pilocarpine formation (pH 7.4; 37 °C) and the Taft polar substituent constant σ^*, the latter referring to R in RCH_2OH for the alcohols according to the expression

$$\log t_{1/2} = -1.44\sigma^* + 2.73 \ (t_{1/2} \text{ in min}) \ (n = 9; \ r = 0.998) \tag{14.18}$$

It is apparent that by appropriate variation of the alcohol portion of the esters, there are possibilities to vary and predict the rate of ring closure and hence to

Table 14.5 Rate data for the conversion of pilocarpic acid monoesters to pilocarpine in aqueous solution (37 °C), Tafts polar substituent constant σ^* refering to R in the alcohols RCH_2OH, and partition coefficients for the compounds

Compound	R	σ^* for R	$t_{1/2}^a$ (min)	$\log P^b$
Pilocarpine				−0.15
Pilocarpic acid esters:				
Methyl	H	0.49	95	0.07
Ethyl	CH_3	0.00	510	0.58
Butyl	$CH_2CH_2CH_3$	−0.12	820	1.58
Hexyl	$(CH_2)_4CH_3$	−0.23	1105	2.56
Benzyl	C_6H_5	0.75	50	1.82
4-Chlorobenzyl	C_6H_4-4-Cl	0.87	30	2.54
4-Methylbenzyl	C_6H_4-4-CH_3	0.59	77	2.31
4-*tert*-butylbenzyl	C_6H_4-4-$C(CH_3)_3$	0.52	87	3.52
Phenetyl	CH_2-C_6H_5	0.27	227	2.16

Notes
a Half-live of lactonization at pH 7.40.
b Logarithm of the partition coefficients between octanol and 0.05 M phosphate buffer solution at pH 7.40.

control and modify the rate of pilocarpine generation. Likewise, by proper selection of the alcohol moiety it is possible to confer a wide range of lipophilicities on the prodrug derivatives (Table 14.5).

The rate of cyclization of the monoesters to yield pilocarpine increases proportionally with the hydroxide ion concentration in the pH range 3.5–10. The main drawback of these derivatives is their limited solution stability, making it difficult to prepare ready-to-use solutions with a not too low pH and an acceptable shelf-life. This problem can, however, be totally overcome by blocking the free hydroxy group in the monoesters by further esterification. The double esters (**14.24**) or double prodrugs thus obtained are highly stable in aqueous solution even at pH 6–7 (predicted shelf-lives exceeding 5 years at 25 °C). In addition these, double prodrugs are subject to facile enzymatic hydrolysis at the *O*-acyl bond. In human plasma or rabbit eye tissue homogenate, pilocarpine is formed from the double prodrugs in quantitative amounts through a sequential process (Scheme 14.16). Besides solving the stability problem of the monoester derivatives, the pilocarpic acid diesters were found to possess even better ocular delivery characteristics including enhanced absorption and longer lasting pilocarpine activity. Although highly lipophilic at pH 7.4, the basic character of the imidazole moiety in the compounds (pK$_a$ about 7) allows for the preparation of sufficiently water-soluble salts, e.g. nitrates or fumarates.

Similar ring-opened double prodrugs are peptide derivatives of 2-aminobenzophenones (**14.25**) which may be water-soluble prodrugs of diazepam and related slightly soluble 1,4-benzodiazepines, suitable for parenteral administration. The derivatives are stable *in vitro*, but are cleaved *in vivo* by aminopeptidases with formation of a 2-aminoacetamidobenzophenone (**14.26**) which subsequently undergoes a spontaneous cyclization to the corresponding benzodiazepine (**14.27**) (Scheme 14.17).

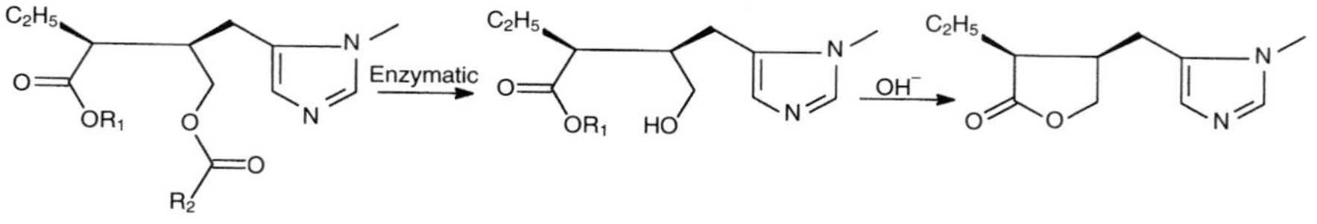

Scheme 14.16

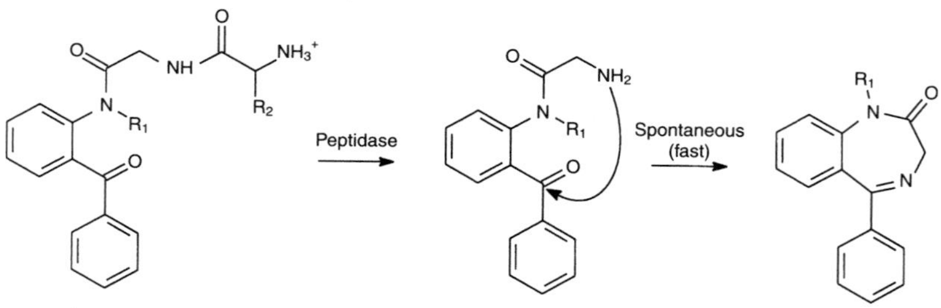

Scheme 14.17

The rate of *in vivo* hydrolysis of the peptide linkage depends markedly upon the L-amino acid attached to the 2-aminoacetamidobenzophenone where peptide derivatives from Phe and Lys are cleaved much faster than those from Gly and Glu. Whereas the benzophenone derived from diazepam cyclizes almost immediately, that of demethyldiazepam shows a half-life of conversion of 15 min at pH 7.4 and 37 °C.

14.3.5.2   Drug release facilitated by intramolecular cyclization reactions

Many bioreversible derivates rely on enzymatic hydrolysis of the prodrug bond for achievement of useful regeneration rates of the active agent. However, these conditions are not always attainable or may be subject to considerable inter- or intra-species variability. A prodrug strategy to overcome this problem takes advantage of facile intramolecular cyclization reactions where a latent nucleophile is unmasked by different biological or chemical triggering mechanisms that in turn initiate the cyclization reaction to release the parent drug (Figure 14.7). Generally, intramolecular nucleophilic catalysis is favored by formation of five- or six-membered cyclic transition states. In addition to the character of the nucleophile and the type of carboxylic acid derivative, the rate of an intramolecular reaction is dependent on the degrees of freedom of the intercalated alkyl chain. Thus, steric factors resulting in less flexible molecules may lead to increased reaction rates.

Alkylaminoethyl carbamate prodrugs (**14.28**) have been developed using a terminal free amino group as a nucleophile to facilitate the release of the melanocytotoxic agent 4-hydroxyanisole (**14.29**) (Scheme 14.18). These prodrugs were developed to release the parent drug in a non-enzymatic fashion and, therefore, to avoid the potential variation in release rates due to variable enzyme activities among individuals. At pH 7.4 (37 °C) the most labile prodrug ($R_1=CH_3$, $R_2=CH_3$) released the drug with a half-life of 36 min. In comparison, the related derivative only differing by an extension of the carbon chain between the two nitrogen atoms to 3 methylenes was much less reactive exhibiting a $t_{1/2}$ of 942 min.

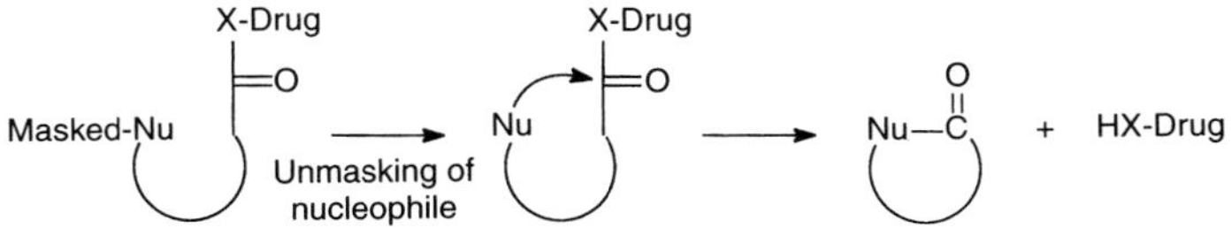

Nu = nucleophile; X = O, NH, S

Figure 14.7 Prodrug strategy that takes advantage of intramolecular cyclization reactions.

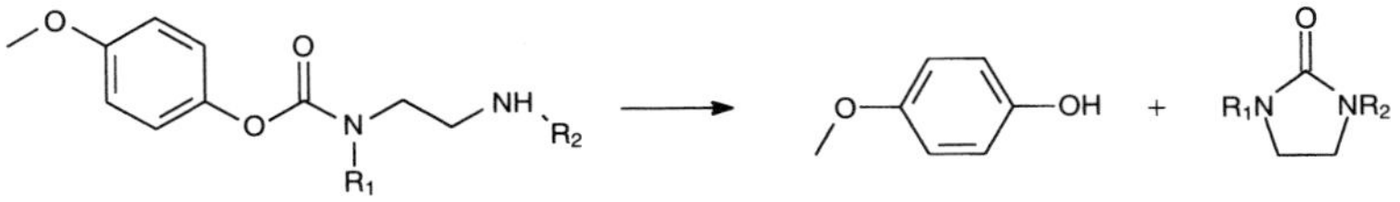

(14.28)   (14.29)

Scheme 14.18

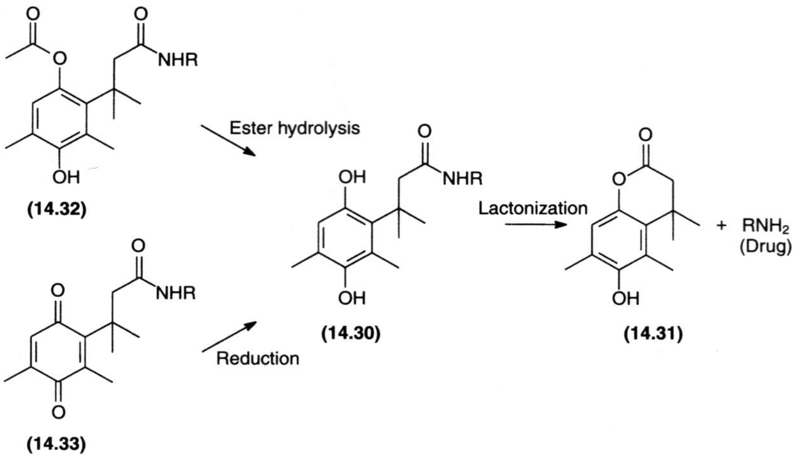

Scheme 14.19

The chemically highly reactive phenolamide derivative **14.30** can function as a prodrug for an amine drug. The intramolecular lactonization reaction, affording the parent amine drug and the lactone (**14.31**), proceeds with a half-life of about 1 min at physiological pH and temperature. The reactivity of this compound is attributed to the presence of the 'trimethyl lock' (methyl groups in positions 3, 3 and 6′). The half-life is, however, too short for practical use. In order to transform (**14.30**) into a chemically more stable and yet enzymatically labile prodrug the double prodrugs (**14.32**) and (**14.33**) have been developed. The parent amine is regenerated via a two-step process. The initial enzymatic step may be catalyzed by esterases or reductive mechanisms, the ester portion in (**14.32**) and the quinone portion in (**14.33**) being transformed to (**14.30**), respectively, followed by the non-enzymatic lactonization (Scheme 14.19).

14.3.6   Cyclic prodrugs involving two functional groups of the drug

Bioreversible cyclization of the peptide backbone may constitute a promising approach in small peptide drug delivery. Backbone cyclization caps the C- and N-terminal functionalities and may result in conformationally restricted cyclic peptides possessing a higher stability toward proteolysis as compared to their corresponding linear peptides. Further advantages of this cyclization strategy can be reduction in charge of the peptide, creation of solution structures that may allow for intramolecular hydrogen bonding and reduction in hydrodynamic volume. The latter characteristics may all add to improved membrane transport properties of such cyclized derivatives. Methodologies reported for linking the N-terminal amino group to the C-terminal carboxyl group include the use of (i) an acyloxyalkoxy pro-moiety (**14.34**); (ii) a 3-(2′-hydroxy-4′,6′-dimethylphenyl)-3,3-dimethylpropionic acid pro-moiety (**14.35**); and (iii) a coumaric acid pro-moiety (**14.36**) (Figure 14.8).

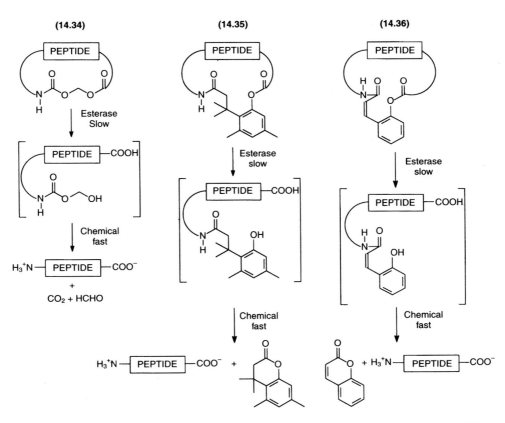

Figure 14.8 Proposed pathway of conversion of acyloxyalkoxy-based cyclic prodrugs (**14.34**), 3-(2′-hydroxy-4′,6′-dimethylphenyl)-3,3-dimethyl-propanoic acid-based cyclic prodrugs (**14.35**), and coumaric acid-based cyclic prodrugs (**14.36**) to the parent peptide in esterase containing media.

Using a model hexapeptide, H-Trp-Ala-Gly-Gly-Asp-Ala-OH, cyclic prodrugs have been obtained by employing the above methodologies (i) and (ii). These derivatives were designed to be susceptible to esterase metabolism (slow step) leading to a series of consecutive chemical reactions by which the linear peptide was regenerated. In aqueous buffer at pH 7.4 (37 °C) both prodrugs degraded quantitatively to the hexapeptide. Hydrolysis of the cyclic derivatives proceeded much faster in human blood than in the buffer solution. *In vitro* transport studies (Caco-2 cells) have revealed that in comparison with the hexapeptide, both cyclic prodrugs showed at least a 70-fold higher capacity of permeating this cell culture model of the intestinal mucosa.

Oxazolidines (see Section 14.3.4.1) can be prodrug candidates for the β-amino-alcohol function which is present in several drugs, e.g. various sympathomimetic amines and β-blockers. By varying the carbonyl moiety, oxazolidines exhibiting different stabilities can be obtained. Thus, the following half-lives of hydrolysis of

(14.37)

various (–)-ephedrine oxazolidines (**14.37**) have been found at pH 7.4 and 37 °C: 5 min (benzaldehyde), 5 sec (salicylaldehyde), 30 min (pivaldehyde), and 6 min (cyclohexanone).

14.4 APPLICATIONS OF THE PRODRUG APPROACH

The prodrug approach has been successfully applied to a wide variety of drugs. Most applications have aimed at (i) enhancing biomembrane transport and bio-availability; (ii) increasing site-specificity; and (iii) improving drug formulation.

14.4.1 Biomembrane passage and bioavailability

Therapeutic agents have to permeate one or more biological membrane(s) in order to reach the target site. Although drugs are administered by a number of quite different routes, this section primarily deals with the use of prodrug design to solve delivery problems related to some of the most widely used routes of administration, e.g. oral, dermal and ocular drug delivery.

14.4.1.1 Oral absorption

For orally administered drugs one major challenge of reaching their sites of action is that they have to cross the intestinal epithelial cells to enter the systemic circulation. Poor transport properties may lead to low bioavailability which may also result from low water solubility, low stability in the gastrointestinal juices or extensive first-pass metabolism.

Well-known examples of transiently increasing the lipophilicity to enhance absorption of polar drugs by prodrug modification include various ampicillin derivatives. Being zwitterionic in the pH range of the gastrointestinal tract, ampicillin (**14.38**) possesses a low lipophilicity and the absorption fraction after oral administration amounts to about 30%. Altering the polarity of the penicillin by esterification of the free carboxyl group to form the prodrugs pivampicillin (**14.39**) and bacampicillin (**14.40**) has proven successful, resulting in essentially complete absorption of (**14.38**). During or after entering into the systemic circulation, these prodrugs are cleaved by enzymes to yield the active antibiotic. A discussion of the mechanism of cleavage of such double ester prodrugs is given in Section 14.3.1. Recently, it has been realized that some orally administered peptidomimetic drugs are absorbed through the intestinal peptide transport systems. One of these transport systems accepts various β-lactam antibiotics, including ampicillin, and acts as

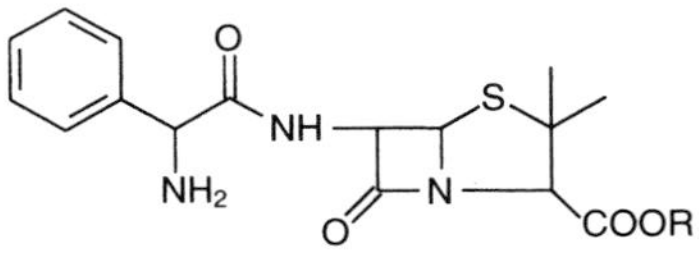

(14.38)   R = H

(14.39) 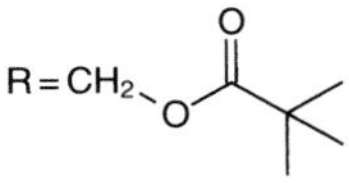   R = CH₂

(14.40)   R = CH

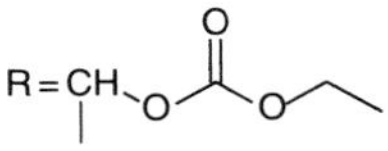

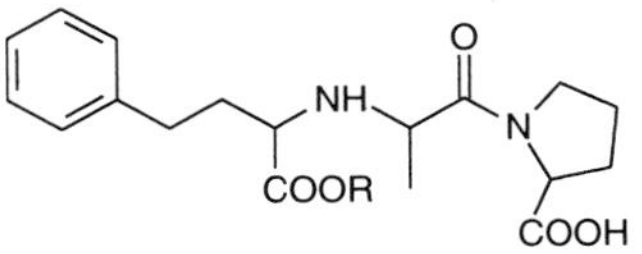

(14.41)   R = H
(14.42)   R = C₂H₅

a carrier for their absorption. The enhanced lipophilicity of the ampicillin pro-drugs favors passive membrane transport but the improved bioavailability could also reflect that the ester derivatives are better substrates for the carrier system than ampicillin. Also various peptidic ACE inhibitors like enalapril (**14.42**) are substrates for peptide transport systems. Enalapril is the ethyl ester of the active acid (**14.41**). Although the ethyl ester is much better absorbed than the active acid, it is rather slowly cleaved in the organism by liver hydrolases.

The intestinal peptide transport systems have been a key target for prodrug approaches. According to this approach, prodrugs appropriately designed in the form of di- or tripeptide analogs (the di- or tripeptide constituting the 'functionally based' pro-moiety) can be absorbed across the intestinal brush border membrane via a peptide transport system. The prodrug may be targeted to the epithelial membrane and hydrolyzed on the apical surface of the epithelium prior to absorption by the transporter or may be absorbed intact and hydrolyzed intracellularly by peptidases or esterases prior to exit from the cell. A dipeptidyl prodrug derivative of L-α-methyldopa, L-α-methyldopa-L-phenylalanine (**14.43**) has been prepared. This prodrug displayed up to 20 times increase in intestinal permeability compared to the parent compound in *in situ* single pass rat intestinal perfusion studies. Experiments have shown the occurrence of hydrolysis of the prodrug in intestinal cell homogenates, suggesting liberation of the parent compound after intestinal uptake.

Several drugs show poor and variable oral absorption characteristics as a result of insufficient water solubility (less than about 0.1% w/v) leading to dissolution rate-limited absorption. An example of a prodrug used to increase the aqueous solubility and to improve dissolution behavior is the water-soluble dipotassium salt of clorazepate (**14.44**) which is marketed as a prodrug of the slightly soluble

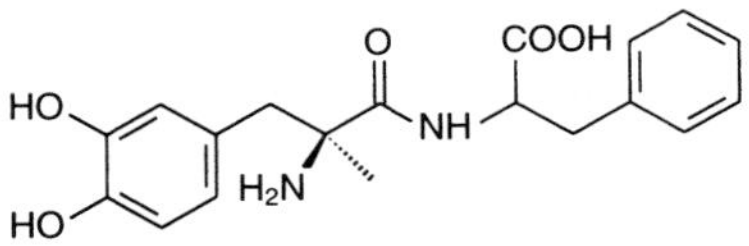

(14.43)

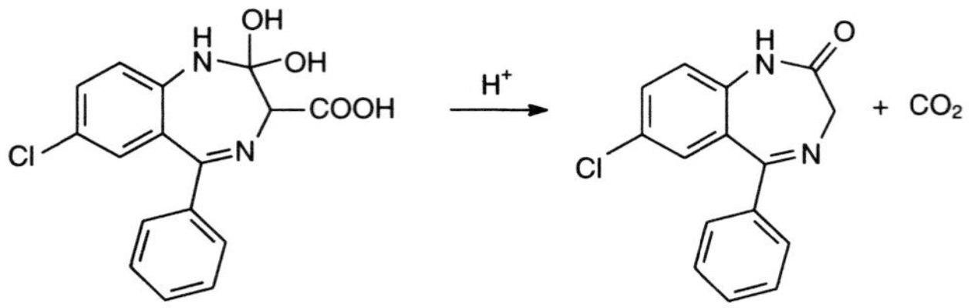

(14.44)   **(14.45)**

Scheme 14.20

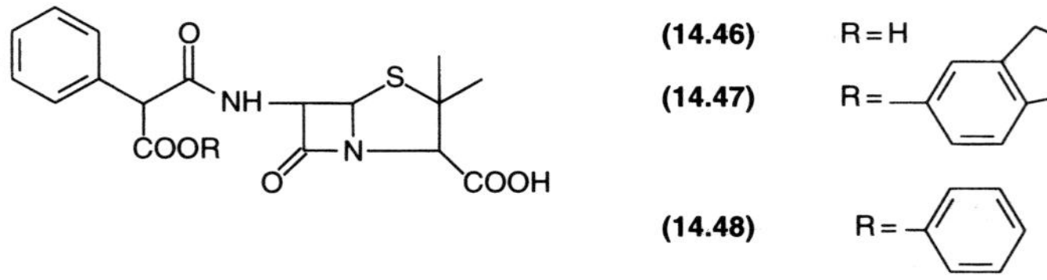

(14.46)	R = H
(14.47)	R = (indane group)
(14.48)	R = (phenyl group)

demethyldiazepam (**14.45**). In acidic solution clorazepate spontaneously decarboxylates to the parent drug constituting the form absorbed (Scheme 14.20). Prodrug strategies to enhance aqueous solubility is further dealt with in Section 14.4.3.

The poor gastrointestinal absorption of carbenicillin (**14.46**) is due to acid-catalyzed degradation of the drug in the stomach as well as to its strongly polar character. By bioreversible esterification of the side-chain carboxyl group, the more acid-stable and lipophilic derivatives carindacillin (**14.47**) and carfecillin (**14.48**) are obtained. Following absorption carbenicillin is released in the blood by enzymatic hydrolysis of these clinically used prodrugs.

14.4.1.2 Dermal absorption

The potential of various prodrug types to enhance the delivery of drugs through the skin (transdermal delivery) and into the skin (dermal delivery) have been investigated. Most drugs diffuse poorly through the skin, in particular through stratum corneum, because of unfavorable physicochemical properties. Several studies have demonstrated biphasic solubility as being an important determinant of the flux across the skin, i.e. in order to diffuse readily through the skin a compound should possess adequate water as well as lipid solubility. This can often be achieved by the prodrug approach and, in fact, the dermal delivery of several drug molecules such as steroids, antiviral, and antipsoriasis agents have been improved by this approach.

Levonorgestrel (**14.49**) is a very potent, lipophilic contraceptive drug which is very poorly soluble in water (1µg/ml at 25°C), and does not permeate through the skin at a sufficient rate. Two carbonate ester prodrugs containing hydroxy functional groups in the alkyl portion of the pro-moiety **14.50** and **14.51** were synthesized. Although the prodrugs were more soluble in aqueous ethanol than the parent steroid, their $\log P_{oct}$ values were close to that of levonorgestrel indicating that the

(14.49)	R = H
(14.50)	R = (C=O)OCH₂CH(OH)CH₂OH
(14.51)	R = (C=O)O(CH₂)₄CH(OH)CH₂OH

$$R = H$$
$$R = (C=O)OCH_2CH(OH)CH_2OH$$
$$R = (C=O)O(CH_2)_4CH(OH)CH_2OH$$

(14.52)	R = H
(14.53)	R = CH₂O(C=O)CH₃
(14.54)	R = CH₂O(C=O)CH(CH₃)₂

$$R = H$$
$$R = CH_2O(C=O)CH_3$$
$$R = CH_2O(C=O)CH(CH_3)_2$$

octanol solubility of the esters also exceeded that of the steroid. Thus, the carbonate ester prodrugs (14.50) and (14.51) exhibit greater biphasic solubility than levonorgestrel and were found to enhance the transdermal delivery of total levonorgestrel 30 and 15 times, respectively.

Nalidixic acid (14.52) is a relatively high melting solid which is poorly soluble in water and isopropyl myristate, but has shown some promise in the topical treatment of psoriasis. By esterifying the carboxyl group by *O*-acyloxymethylation, prodrug derivatives 14.53 and 14.54 being both more lipid- and water-soluble have been obtained. Diffusion studies *in vitro* using human skin have shown that the isobutyryloxymethyl derivative affords a 5–6 fold enhanced delivery of nalidixic acid from both polar and non-polar vehicles relative to application of nalidixic acid itself.

14.4.1.3   Ocular absorption

A major problem in ocular therapeutics is the attainment of an optimal drug concentration at the site of action. The difficulty is largely due to the fact that all of the existing drugs, many of which were originally developed for systemic use, lack the physicochemical properties for overcoming the severe constraints imposed by the eye on drug absorption. These constraints include precorneal factors that rapidly remove the drug from the conjunctival sac where it is applied and a well-designed corneal structure that restricts the passage of drug molecules. The net result is that less than 10%, and often 1% or less, of the instilled dose is ocularly absorbed. Corneal drug penetration is inefficient owing to a mismatch of the physicochemical properties of the drug with those of the cornea. Optimal $\log P_{oct}$ values of 2–3 for transcellular corneal drug permeation have been suggested. This observation has formed the basis for bioreversible modification of hydrophilic ophthalmic drugs, the first of which was epinephrine. Since then, several other ophthalmic drugs have been investigated for prodrug derivatization including timolol, pilocarpine, and terbutaline.

Epinephrine (14.55) has long been used for the treatment of glaucoma although its corneal absorption is poor because of its high polarity and rapid metabolic destruction. Originally, epinephrine solutions were manufactured with a pH of about 3.5 due to the high instability of the ophthalmic agent in aqueous solution.

(14.55)   (14.56)   (14.57)

Optimum stability is observed in the pH range 3–4. In addition to acid-catalyzed racemization, epinephrine is extremely sensitive to oxidation, a reaction which is base-catalyzed. Even at low pH levels, oxidation occurs rapidly and such formulations exhibited short shelf-lives. Later, it was observed that such ophthalmic solutions could be stabilized by incorporation of boric acid which forms a 1:1 complex (14.56) with epinephrine thereby masking the labile *ortho*-diphenol structure. In the presence of the antioxidant sodium bisulfite this complex was much less sensitive to oxidation allowing the preparation of a reasonably stable ophthalmic solution with a pH close to 7.

Thus, two problems – ocular irritation and instability in solution – were solved by this formulation approach. However, bioavailability of (14.55) from the latter formulation type was still very poor. The development of the prodrug, dipivefrin (14.57) has lead to a markedly improved ocular delivery of epinephrine. This dipivalate ester prodrug is much more lipophilic than epinephrine and esterification of the phenolic hydroxy groups gives rise to a derivative exhibiting significantly better chemical and metabolic stability than the parent drug. These properties coupled with a sufficiently high susceptibility to undergo enzymatic hydrolysis in the eye during and after absorption are responsible for the approximately 20 times higher antiglaucoma activity of dipivefrin in comparison with parent epinephrine upon local administration in humans. In addition, undesirable cardiotoxic side effects due to epinephrine absorption from the tear duct overflow are diminished because lower doses of the prodrug can be used.

14.4.1.4   Prevention of first-pass metabolism

Extensive presystemic metabolism may exclude a pharmacologically interesting lead candidate, intended for the oral route, from further development due to formation of unwanted metabolites and variable bioavailability. This metabolic inactivation of chemical entities may take place in the intestinal lumen, at the brush border of the intestinal cells, in the mucosal cells lining the gastrointestinal tract, the liver, or the lung. Although liver first-pass metabolism is avoided by using alternative routes of administration such as the sublingual and transdermal route, oral administration is most convenient and generally preferred for most drug substances.

The prodrug approach may be useful in reducing or circumventing first-pass metabolism where the obvious approach is to transiently mask the metabolic labile

(14.58)   R = H

(14.59)   R = C(=O)— (2-aminophenyl)   H₂N

(14.60)   R = C(=O)— (2-hydroxyphenyl)

(14.61)   R = C(=O)— phenyl

functionalities in the drug molecule. The latter approach, however, requires regeneration of the drug after the prodrug has entered the systemic circulation. Many drugs containing phenolic hydroxy groups undergo extensive first-pass metabolism. Rapid inactivation of such drugs (e.g. morphine, isoprenaline, naltrexone, and various steroids) is the result of sulphate conjugation, glucuronidation or methylation of the phenolic moieties. By masking the metabolizable phenol group of the opioid antagonist naltrexone (**14.58**) in the form of the anthranilate ester (**14.59**) and the salicylate ester (**14.60**), prodrugs with significantly enhanced oral bioavailability have been obtained. Oral administration of (**14.59**) and (**14.60**) to dogs resulted in a bioavailability of the parent drug of 49 and 31%, respectively. In comparison, the bioavailability of naltrexone was about 1% whereas the unsubstituted benzoate ester (**14.61**) did not improve the absorption fraction. Hydrolysis data revealed that the esters (**14.59**) and (**14.60**) are more stable toward enzymatic hydrolysis than the benzoate ester, indicating that these esters survive presystemic hydrolysis to a greater extent.

Orally administered drugs can gain access to the systemic circulation via two separate and functionally distinct absorption pathways – the portal blood and the intestinal lymphatics, with the former representing the major absorption path for the vast majority of orally administered drugs. The intestinal lymphatics are a specialized absorption and transport pathway for lipids and highly lipophilic compounds ($\log P > 5-6$). Drug delivery opportunities associated with intestinal lymphatics include the bypass of hepatic first-pass metabolism after oral dosing. The overall lipophilicity of the drug or prodrug constitutes the major factor governing the extent of lymphatic absorption. Two approaches have been explored for achieving sufficiently lipophilic, bioreversible derivatives encompassing the formation of simple ester derivatives and the design of prodrugs involving 'functionally based' pro-moieties. The latter approach to enhance lymphatic absorption has arisen from an understanding of the processes associated with the absorption and subsequent intracellular processing of absorbed lipid digestion products. Intestinal lymphatic delivery of a variety of glyceride prodrugs have been investigated in which the drug has been conjugated to either mono- or diglycerides.

Testosterone (**14.62**) undergoes almost quantitative first-pass metabolism after oral administration. Various depot injectables consisting of esters of testosterone dissolved in vegetable oils are available for the treatment of androgen deficiency syndromes. In addition, an oral formulation containing testosterone undecanoate (**14.63**) is marketed. It has been shown that the latter highly lipophilic ester is almost exclusively transported via the intestinal lymphatics. Oral bioavailability of testosterone after administration of (**14.62**) and (**14.63**) to humans of 3.6 and 6.8%,

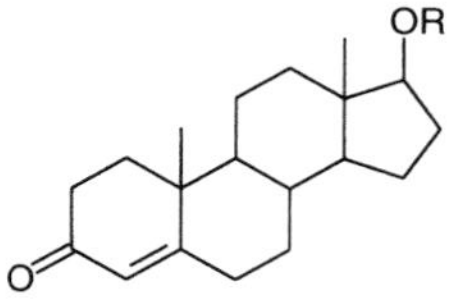

| (14.62) | R = H |
| (14.63) | R = (C=O)C$_{10}$H$_{21}$ |

respectively, have been found in a comparative bioavailability study. The far from quantitative absorption of the ester prodrug might reflect that the ester is partly hydrolyzed in the intestinal lumen or might be due to a limited transport capacity of the gastrointestinal lymphatics.

An alternative way to protect a phenolic moiety against presystemic metabolism is to prepare an ester derivative endowed with a built-in esterase inhibiting function. In this case, the prodrug can diminish its own rate of hydrolysis, and thereby pass intact through the gut wall and liver. This strategy has been employed for the bronchodilator agent terbutaline (**14.67**). *N,N*-disubstituted carbamate esters are generally very stable against both chemical and enzymatic hydrolysis and have, in addition, esterase-inhibiting properties. The prodrug bambuterol (**14.64**) was found to possess these properties, being a potent inhibitor of pseudocholinesterase. Upon oral administration most of the dose given reaches the systemic circulation in intact form. Reconversion to parent terbutaline proceeds through consecutive reactions involving an initial enzyme-mediated oxidation to give *N*-hydroxymethyl carbamates (**14.65**), which subsequently are decomposed spontaneously to formaldehyde and *N*-monomethyl carbamates (**14.66**). The latter derivative is hydrolyzed by virtue of pseudocholinesterase (Scheme 14.21). This enzyme is selectively inhibited by bambuterol. Thus, the prodrug inhibits its own

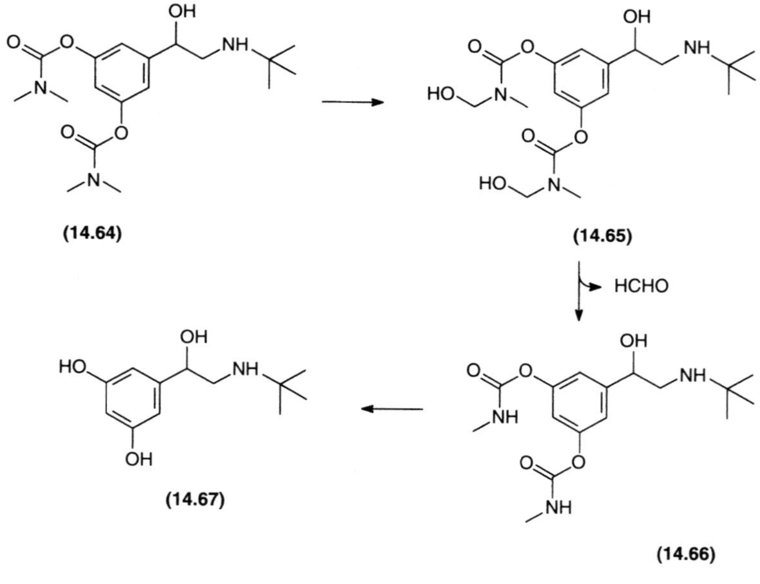

Scheme 14.21

hydrolysis resulting in a slow formation of the active drug. In addition to these desirable gains in bioavailability and duration of action, bambuterol affords enhanced delivery of the parent drug to its site of action, the lungs, with concomitant reduction of side effects due to lower plasma levels of free terbutaline.

14.4.2 Site-specific drug delivery

Although the concept of targeted or site-specific drug delivery has been evolving for quite some time, the routine attainment of targeted delivery is still one of the most elusive pharmaceutical challenges. Site-specific drug delivery might be achieved by site-directed drug delivery or site-specific bioactivation. The former concept relates to design of prodrugs that afford an increased or selective transport of the parent drug to the site of action. Site-directed delivery can further be divided into localized site-directed and systemic site-directed drug delivery. The objective of the second approach is to accomplish bioreversible derivatives that are distributed throughout the organism but undergo bioactivation only in the vicinity of the target area. In the following, examples will be given to illustrate the possible utilization of these principles to achieve drug targeting.

14.4.2.1 Site-directed drug delivery

Up to now, successful site-directed drug delivery has been achieved in the field of localized drug delivery where the prodrug is applied directly to the target organ which is the case in dermal and ocular delivery (see Sections 14.4.1.2 and 14.4.1.3).

Compared to localized drug delivery, systemic site-directed delivery constitutes a much more difficult task (see also Section 14.2.3), since the drug has to be transported via the systemic circulation to the desired organ or tissue, passing various complex and not easily predictable barriers on the way. Besides various attempts to accomplish drug targeting in cancer chemotherapy, an interesting approach to obtain site-directed delivery to the brain has been investigated. The drug (D), which is aimed to be delivered to the brain, is coupled to a quaternary carrier (i.e. N-methylnicotinic acid) $(QC)^+$ to yield $D-QC^+$ which is reduced to the neutral, lipophilic dihydro form (dihydrotrigonelline) (D-DHC) (Scheme 14.22). After administration, this compound is distributed throughout the body including the brain. D-DHC is then enzymatically oxidized back to the original quaternary

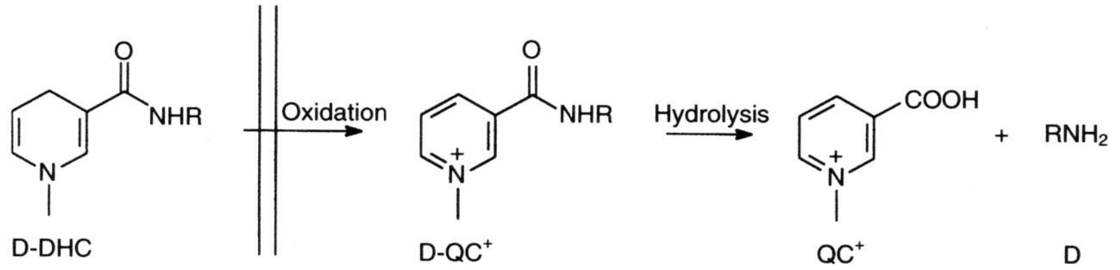

Scheme 14.22

entity (D-QC)$^+$. The latter hydrophilic compound is prevented from passing through the blood–brain barrier. Thus, the ionic form is trapped in the brain and undergoes slow enzymatic cleavage releasing the active agent. Because of the facile elimination of D-QC$^+$ from the circulation only small amounts of the free drug are released in the blood. This concept has been applied to several drugs including dopamine, phenytoin, and penicillins.

14.4.2.2 Site-specific bioactivation

Quantitative or qualitative differences between the target site and non-target sites might be exploited in prodrug design to activate or release the active agent in the vicinity of the target area. Differences in pH or more often in enzyme levels have founded the platform for synthesis of bioreversible derivatives which after the distribution phase are selectively activated in the desired organ within the body.

Site-specific activation can be exemplified by the action of the antiviral agent acyclovir (**14.68**) where the herpesvirus encoded enzyme, pyrimidine deoxy-nucleoside (thymidine) kinase, is responsible for converting acyclovir to its phosphate monoester (Figure 14.9). Subsequently, cellular enzymes catalyze the formation of the di- and triphosphorylated species, the latter substance being the active one. The triester formation takes place to a much greater extent in the herpes-infected cells. Thus, acyclovir displays a high therapeutic activity against herpesvirus and very low toxicity against uninfected host cells. The selectivity of action is manifested in the fact that a 3000-fold higher concentration of acyclovir is needed to inhibit uninfected cell multiplication.

An example of pH-dependent bioactivation relates to the action of the anti-ulcer drug omeprazole (**14.69**). The drug is an effective inhibitor of gastric acid secretion by inhibiting the gastric H$^+$, K$^+$-ATPase. This enzyme is responsible for the gastric acid production and is located in the secretory membranes of the parietal cells. Omeprazole is, *per se*, inactive but requires transformation within the acidic compartment of the parietal cells into the active inhibitor, a cyclic sulfenamide (**14.70**). This intermediate reacts with thiol groups in the enzyme forming a disulphide complex (**14.71**) thereby inactivating the enzyme

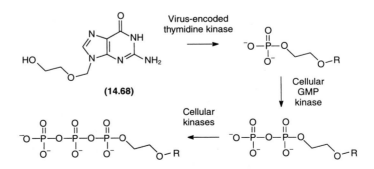

Figure 14.9 Bioconversion of antiviral agent acyclovir (**14.68**), to the pharmacologically active triphosphate ester.

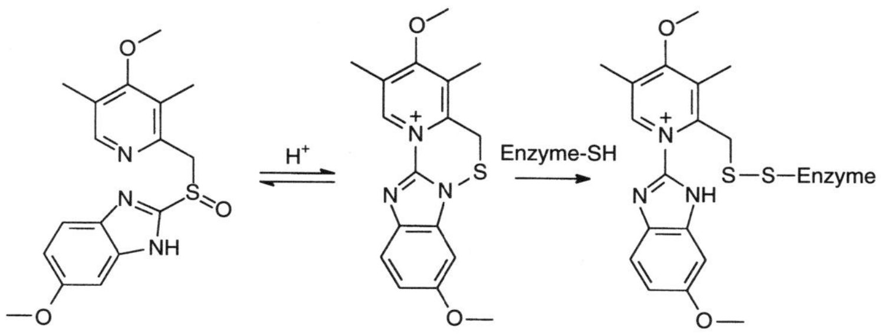

(14.69)   **(14.70)**   **(14.71)**

Scheme 14.23

(Scheme 14.23). A combination of factors, therefore, contributes to the specific action of omeprazole:

(1) Omeprazole is a weak base (pK$_a$ of the pyridine nitrogen is 4.0) and the drug concentrates in acidic compartments, i.e. in the parietal cells, which have the lowest pH of the cells in the body
(2) The low pH value of the parietal cells initiates the conversion of omeprazole into the active inhibitor in the vicinity of the target enzyme
(3) The active inhibitor is a permanent cation with limited possibilities to permeate the membranes of the parietal and other cells, and thus will be retained at its site of action
(4) At physiological pH 7.4 omeprazole has good stability and only modest conversion to the active species occurs

There are various colonic disorders warranting delivery of effective amounts of drug compounds selectively to the diseased site. The ability of the gut microflora to hydrolyze different chemical bonds has formed the basis for design of several prodrug types. The prodrug sulfasalazine (**14.72**) has long been used in the management of colon inflammatory disorders like ulcerative colitis. After passage through the small intestine the active species, 5-aminosalicylic acid (5-ASA) (**14.74**), is released from the prodrug after cleavage of the azo-bond by action of azo-reductases secreted from colonic bacteria. However, disadvantages of sulfasalazine therapy include absorption of intact prodrug from the small intestine and systemic adverse reactions. A more elegant prodrug of 5-ASA, olsalazine (**14.73**), has been developed, consisting of two 5-ASA molecules linked together by an azo-bond (Scheme 14.24). The latter twin prodrug releases two molecules of 5-ASA in the colon and due to its highly polar nature only negligible amounts are absorbed from the small intestine.

The examples cited in the last two sections illustrates the utility of the prodrug concept to achieve site-specific drug delivery. For the design of prodrugs directed

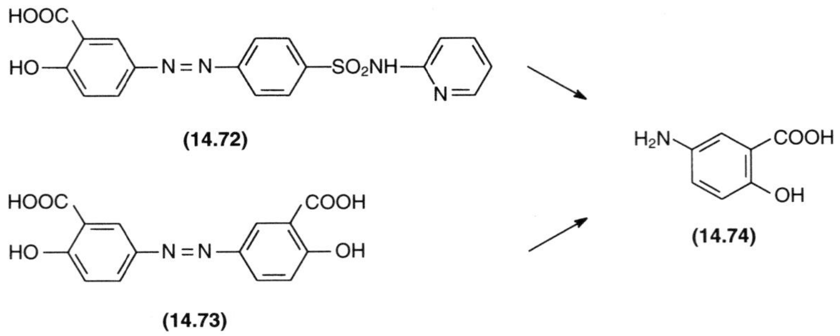

(14.72)

(14.73)

(14.74)

Scheme 14.24

selectively to their site of action, the following basal criteria must be taken into consideration:

(1) The prodrug should be able to reach the site of action
(2) The prodrug should be converted efficiently to the drug at the site of action
(3) The parent active should to some extent be retained or trapped at the target site for a sufficient period of time to exert its effect

The reason why attempts to promote site-specific drug delivery via prodrugs have failed in many cases, is that not all criteria have been met.

14.4.3   Improvement of drug formulation

Successful development of a drug candidate includes the design of dosage forms exhibiting suitable shelf-lives. Despite the fact that solid oral dosage forms are the most used types of formulations, the chemical kinetics of drug degradation in the solid state is far from fully understood. For a drug which is susceptible to hydrolysis it is primarily moisture in the dosage form that causes its instability. In this case, stability problems might be circumvented by using a poorly soluble prodrug derivative or salt. Changing the properties of a drug in the crystalline state by bioreversible derivatization may also lead to improved *in vitro* stability. Dinoprostone (prostaglandin E_2, PGE_2) (**14.75**) is a crystalline solid (mp 63 °C), stable at room temperature for only a short period of time, but liquefies and decomposes rapidly after a few months. As other β-ketols, PGE_2 is easily dehydrated under formation of prostaglandin A_2. Based on the assumption that the decomposition rate was

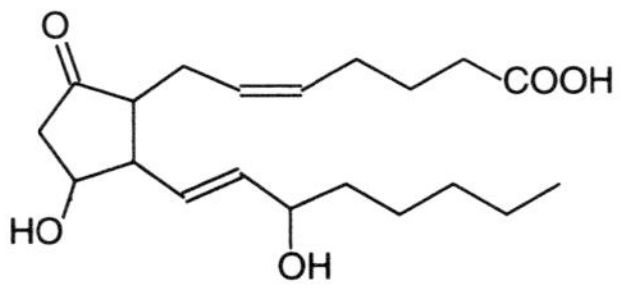

(14.75)

related to the crystalline interaction energy, a series of *para*-substituted phenyl esters of PGE$_2$ was synthesized. Storage of these higher melting esters at room temperature for up to 30 months revealed no detectable deterioration.

Intramuscular oil depot injections are available for long-term administration of antipsychotics and a number of steroids. The principal role of depot neuroleptic therapy is to ensure patient compliance. Oily injections are marketed for steroid hormones exhibiting low and variable oral bioavailability due to extensive first-pass metabolism in the gastrointestinal tract and the liver. Pharmacokinetic studies have demonstrated that the rate of release of chemical entities from oil solutions is, at least partly, related to the pH-dependent oil vehicle–water distribution coefficient. The prodrug approach has successfully been applied on a variety of drugs to design derivatives, most often in the form of ester derivatives, possessing suitable lipophilicities and thereby desired durations of action. After i.m. administration the prodrugs are slowly released from the injection site. Reconversion to the parent drug may take place in the tissue fluid at the injection site or in the blood. The rate of prodrug liberation from the oil vehicle decreases with increasing lipophilicity of the derivatives. In case of the neuroleptic agent, fluphenazine (**14.76**) duration of action is 6–8 h after intramuscular injection. In contrast, the more lipophilic enanthate ester **14.77** and decanoate ester **14.78** show a duration of action of 1–2 and 3–4 weeks, respectively, following i.m. injection in a sesame oil vehicle. Similar long-acting fatty acid ester prodrugs of various other clinically used neuroleptics such as flupenthixol, zuclopenthixol and haloperidol are available. Clinically, depot neuroleptics possess several advantages over short-acting oral forms including enhanced patient compliance, reduced relapse and rehospitalization rate, and reduced daily dose.

Several steroids are also frequently used in the form of long-acting prodrugs. Thus, for testosterone (**14.62**) the following esters have been used in oil solutions or suspensions: cypionate (**14.79**), isocaproate, valerate, phenylpropionate, enanthate and undecanoate.

The greatest utility of the prodrug approach in solving pharmaceutical formulation problems is probably to modify the aqueous solubility of drugs. Whereas poorly water-soluble bioreversible derivatives, such as the palmitate esters of

(**14.76**)	R = H
(**14.77**)	R = (C=O)C$_6$H$_{13}$
(**14.78**)	R = (C=O)C$_9$H$_{19}$

(**14.79**)

chloramphenicol and clindamycin, have been designed to mask the bitter taste of the parent antibacterial agents, the prodrug approach has mainly been used to increase the water solubility of drugs, thereby allowing convenient solution formulations for intravenous and ophthalmic use to be prepared (see also Section 14.2.2.2).

Ester formation has long been recognized as an effective way to enhance the aqueous solubility of drugs containing a hydroxy functional group (Drug-OH). Water-soluble derivatives might be obtained from dicarboxylic acid hemiesters (notably hemisuccinates), sulphate esters, phosphate esters, α-amino or related short-chained aliphatic amino acid esters, and aminomethylbenzoate esters. These types of esters should ideally provide high water solubility at the pH of optimum stability, sufficient stability in aqueous solution, i.e. shelf-lives above 2 years, combined with a rapid and quantitative conversion to the parent drug *in vivo*. Hemisuccinate esters do, however, possess limited solution stability and, in addition, they exhibit a slow and incomplete conversion *in vivo* to the parent agent. This has been reported for esters of various corticosteroids, chloramphenicol, and metronidazole. Sulphate esters are, in contrast, rather stable in solution, but an impediment to their use might be a high resistance to enzymatic hydrolysis. In general, phosphate ester sodium salts are freely soluble in water and they exhibit a reasonable stability in aqueous solution. The susceptibility of phosphate ester prodrugs to undergo enzyme-mediated hydrolysis may, however, vary dependent on the chemical nature of the parent drug. Whereas α-amino or related short-chained aliphatic amino acid esters might be cleaved by plasma hydrolases, such derivatives are prevented from being employed in ready-to-use aqueous formulations due to their limited solution stability. The major reason for the high instability of the latter ester type in aqueous solution at pH values affording their favorable water solubility (pH 3–5) is the strongly electron-withdrawing effect of the protonated amino group which activates the ester linkage towards hydroxide ion attack. In particular cases, facilitation of hydrolysis may additionally arise from intramolecular catalysis by the terminal amino group. An effective and simple means to avoid the hydrolysis facilitating effect of the amino group and yet retain a rapid rate of enzymatic ester hydrolysis is to incorporate a phenyl group between the ester moiety and the amino group. In this case intramolecular catalytic reactions of the amino group is no longer possible due to steric hindrance. Such *N*-substituted 3- or 4-aminomethyl benzoate esters have been found to be readily soluble in water at weakly acidic pH values and to possess a high stability in such solutions in combination with a feasible susceptibility towards enzymatic cleavage. Thus, the 4-(morpholinomethyl)benzoate ester (**14.80**) of metronidazole possesses a predicted shelf-life of more than 10 years in aqueous solution pH 4 and 25 °C.

(14.80)

Table 14.6 Examples of water-soluble prodrug derivatives of drugs containing a hydroxy group (Drug-OH) and their chemical and enzymatic reactivity

Prodrug derivatives		Stability in solution	Enzymatic lability
Hemisuccinates	$\text{Drug}-O-\overset{\overset{O}{\|}}{C}-CH_2CH_2-\overset{\overset{O}{\|}}{C}-O^-$	Limited	Limited
Sulphates	$\text{Drug}-O-SO_3^-$	High	Low
Phosphates	$\text{Drug}-O-PO_3^{2-}$	High	High/Limited
α-Amino acid esters	$\text{Drug}-O-\overset{\overset{O}{\|}}{C}-\overset{\overset{R}{\|}}{C}H-NH_3^+$	Limited	High
Dialkylaminoacetates	$\text{Drug}-O-\overset{\overset{O}{\|}}{C}-CH_2-\overset{\overset{R_1}{\|}}{\overset{}{N}}^+H\overset{}{\underset{R_2}{\|}}$	Limited	High
Aminomethyl benzoate esters*	$\text{Drug}-O-\overset{\overset{O}{\|}}{C}-\langle\text{ring}\rangle-CH_2-\overset{\overset{R_1}{\|}}{N}^+H\overset{}{\underset{R_2}{\|}}$	High	High

Note
*3 or 4 position.

In human plasma, the half-life of the prodrug is less than 1 min. The stability characteristics of the ester types dealt with above are summarized in Table 14.6.

A novel prodrug approach for improving the water solubility of poorly soluble drugs containing a tertiary amine group relates to the formation of N-phosphonooxymethyl derivatives which can be considered as double prodrugs since regeneration of the parent amine initially requires phosphatase catalyzed hydrolysis of the phosphate ester bond. The resulting hydroxymethyl intermediate undergoes spontaneous degradation releasing the parent amine and formaldehyde (Scheme 14.25). The prodrug derivative (14.81) obtained from N-phosphonooxymethylation of the tricyclic dibenzoxazepine antipsychotic agent loxapine (14.82) showed a more than 15 000-fold improvement in solubility at pH 7.4 relative to loxapine and the predicted shelf-life of an aqueous formulation was about 2 years.

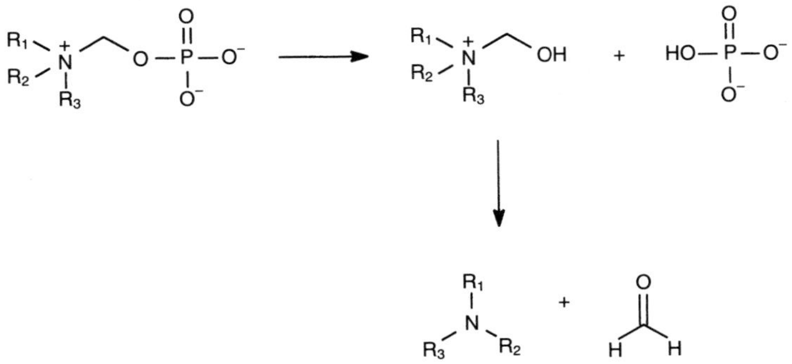

Scheme 14.25

(14.81)   (14.82)

Following i.v. administration to beagle dogs the prodrug was found to be rapidly and quantitatively converted to the parent drug.

FURTHER READING

Bagshawe, K. (Theme ed.) (1996) Enzyme-prodrug therapy. *Adv. Drug Delivery Rev.*, **22**, 265–376.

Bundgaard, H. (ed.) (1985) *Design of Prodrugs*. Amsterdam: Elsevier.

Bundgaard, H. (1989) The double prodrug concept and its applications. *Adv. Drug Delivery Rev.*, **3**, 39–65.

Larsen, C. (1989) Dextran prodrugs – structure and stability in relation to therapeutic activity. *Adv. Drug Delivery Rev.*, **3**, 103–154.

Oliyai, R. and Stella, V.J. (1993) Prodrugs of peptides and proteins for improved formulation and delivery. *Ann. Rev. Pharmacol. Toxicol.*, **32**, 521–544.

Sloan, K.B. (ed.) (1992) *Prodrugs, Topical and Ocular Drug Delivery*. New York: Marcel Dekker Inc.

Soyez, H., Schacht, E. and Vanderkerken, S. (1996) The crucial role of spacer groups in macromolecular prodrug design. *Adv. Drug Delivery Rev.*, **21**, 81–106.

Stella, V.J. (Theme ed.) (1996) Low molecular weight prodrugs. *Adv. Drug Delivery Rev.*, **19**, 1–330.

Stella, V.J., Mikkelsen, T.J. and Pipkin, J.D. (1980) Prodrugs: the control of drug delivery via bioreversible chemical modifications. In *Drug Delivery Systems, Characteristics and Biomedical Applications*, edited by R.L. Juliano, pp. 112–176. New York: Oxford University Press.

Yang, C.Y., Dantzig, A.H. and Pidgeon, C. (1999) Intestinal peptide transport systems and oral drug availability. *Pharm. Res.*, **16**, 1331–1343.

Chapter 15

Peptides and peptidomimetics

Kristina Luthman and Uli Hacksell

15.1 INTRODUCTION

A large number of endogenous peptides have been isolated and characterized (Table 15.1). These peptides are involved in a wide range of important physiological processes both centrally and peripherally. Drug intervention with the formation, breakdown or receptor interaction of peptides might provide therapeutic opportunities. The most well-known drug that interacts with peptide receptors is morphine. It was isolated from opium in 1803. However, whereas its analgesic efficacy and other CNS effects were discovered already in the nineteenth century, the fact that morphine interacts with receptors for opiate peptides was verified only relatively recently. Currently, numerous drug discovery efforts are focussed on processes involving peptides and intense research and development efforts during the past 30 years have provided important peptide interacting drugs such as captopril and losartan.

15.1.1 Peptide structure

Already in 1902, Hofmeister and Fischer independently reported that peptides consist of amino acids (Table 15.2) linked via amide bonds (peptide bonds). A peptide have a chain length between 2 and 50 amino acids whereas proteins include more than 50 amino acids. The different properties of the individual amino acids together with the amino acid sequence (the primary structure) determine the physico-chemical properties of the peptides. All amino acids except glycine are chiral (Figure 15.1). In Nature, the L-configuration is predominating but peptides from micro-organisms and some opioid peptides isolated from the skin of amphibians also contain D-amino acids.

Most peptides are flexible and frequently adopt a large number of conformations in solution. This flexibility is caused by the rotation about single bonds within each amino acid. The torsions in the backbone of particular interest for peptide over-all conformations are the ψ, ϕ and ω angles (Figure 15.2). Many combinations of ψ and ϕ angles are disallowed because of unfavorable steric interactions. The relationship between the ψ, ϕ and energy is often visualized in Ramachandran maps in which the approximate areas of allowed ψ/ϕ angles can be identified. Short peptides exist in a multitude of conformations in solution whereas longer peptides may adopt stable secondary structures such as α-helices, β-sheets and turns.

Table 15.1 Some important endogenous peptides

Peptide	Amino acid sequence
Angiotensin I (Ang I)	DRVYIHPFHL
Angiotensin II (Ang II)	DRVYIHPF
Arginine vasopressin (AVP)	CYFQNCPRG-NH$_2$
Bradykinin	RPPGFSPFR
Cholecystokinin (CCK-33)	CGNLSTCMLGTYTQDFNKFHTFPQTAIGVGAP-NH$_2$
Dynorphin B	YGGFLRRIRPKLKWDNQ
Endomorphin I	YPWF-NH$_2$
Endomorphin II	YPFF-NH$_2$
β-Endorphin	YGGFMTSEKSQTPLVTLFKNAIIKNAYKKGQ
Endothelin (ET-1)	CSCSSLMDKECVYFCHLDIIW
(Leu)Enkephalin	YGGFL
(Met)Enkephalin	YGGFM
Galanin	GWTLNSAGYLLGPHAIDNHRSFHDKYGLA-NH$_2$
Gastrin	pEGPWLEEEEEAY(SO$_3$H)GYGWMDF-NH$_2$
Gastrin releasing peptide	APVSVGGGTVLAKMYPRGNHWAVGHLM-NH$_2$
Ghrelin	GSS(OOCn-C$_7$H$_{15}$)FLSPEHQKAQQRKESKKPPAKLQPR
Gonadotropin-releasing hormone (Gn-RH)	pEHWSYGLRPG-NH$_2$
Neurokinin A (NKA)	HKTDSFVGLM-NH$_2$
Neurokinin B (NKB)	DMHDFFVGLM-NH$_2$
Neuropeptide Y (NPY)	YPSKPDNGPEDAPAEDMARYYSALRHYINLITRQRY-NH$_2$
Neurotensin (NT)	pELYQNKPRRPYIL
Oxytocin	CYIQNCPLG-NH$_2$
Somatostatin (SST)	AGCKNFFWKTFTSC
Substance P (SP)	RPKPQQFFGLM-NH$_2$
Thyrotropin-releasing hormone (TRH)	pEHP-NH$_2$
Vasoactive intestinal peptide (VIP)	HSDAVFTDNYTRLRKQMAVKKYLNSILN-NH$_2$

Table 15.2 The chemical name of the 20 common amino acids and their 3 and I letter codes

Alanine	Ala	A	Leucine	Leu	L
Arginine	Arg	R	Lysine	Lys	K
Asparagine	Asn	N	Methionine	Met	M
Aspartic acid	Asp	D	Phenylalanine	Phe	F
Cystein	Cys	C	Proline	Pro	P
Glutamic acid	Glu	E	Serine	Ser	S
Glutamine	Gln	Q	Threonine	Thr	T
Glycine	Gly	G	Tryptophan	Trp	W
Histidine	His	H	Tyrosine	Tyr	Y
Isoleucine	Ile	I	Valine	Val	V

15.1.2 Solid phase peptide synthesis

A major milestone in peptide chemistry was achieved in 1953 with the isolation, characterization and synthesis of the peptides oxytocin and vasopressin

Figure 15.1 Structures of L- and D-amino acids.

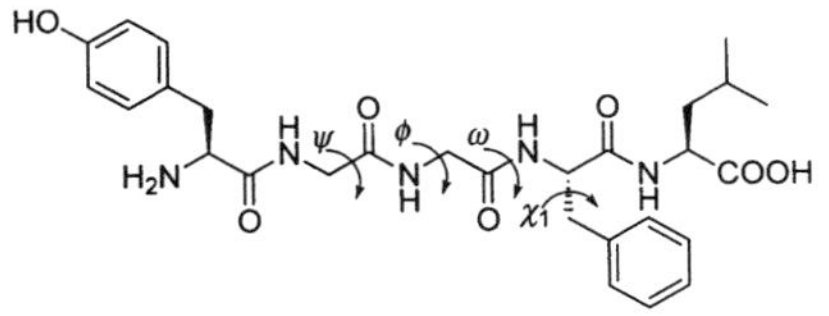

Tyrosyl-glycyl-glycyl-phenylalanyl-leucine (Leu-Enkephalin)

Tyr-Gly-Gly-Phe-Leu (YGGFL)

Figure 15.2 Structures of Leu-enkephalin. Also shown are the ψ, ϕ, ω and χ torsion angles.

(*J. Am. Chem. Soc.*, 1953, 75, 4879 and 4880). Another major step in the synthesis of biologically active peptides and peptide analogs was the introduction of the solid phase synthetic method by Merrifield in 1963 (*J. Am. Chem. Soc.*, 1963, 85, 2149). In this method, the peptide is synthesized from the C-terminal to the N-terminal end (Figure 15.3). The C-terminal amino acid is linked to an insoluble polystyrene based polymer and the peptide is then conveniently synthesized by sequential coupling of properly protected amino acids. The most commonly used N-terminal protecting groups are the base labile 9-fluorenylmethoxycarbonyl (Fmoc) and the acid labile *tert*-butoxycarbonyl (Boc) moieties. The carboxylic acid function has to be activated before coupling. Protecting groups and coupling reagents are improved continuously.

The synthesized peptide is cleaved from the polymer resin and fully deprotected by HF- or TFA-treatment. The synthesis may be performed either by using single amino acid couplings or the fragment condensation technique. The latter strategy is mainly used in the synthesis of longer peptide and small proteins, but also in the synthesis of modified peptides using non-peptidic building blocks.

The peptide synthesis of today has been automated. Although the synthesis of a peptide is trivial a considerable amount of time has to be spent on its purification, usually using reversed phase HPLC or electrophoresis techniques. Synthesized peptides are characterized by amino acid analysis, mass spectrometry, and NMR-spectroscopy. Sequence analyses can be performed by Edman degradation and mass spectrometry (FAB-MS and MS-MS). Production of endogenous peptides and proteins may also be achieved using genetic engineering techniques.

15.1.3 Biosynthesis of peptides

Peptide precursors are biosynthesized on the ribosome as higher molecular forms (prepropeptides) (Figure 15.4). During the transport through the endoplasmatic reticulum to the Golgi apparatus, an N-terminal signal peptide of 20–30 amino

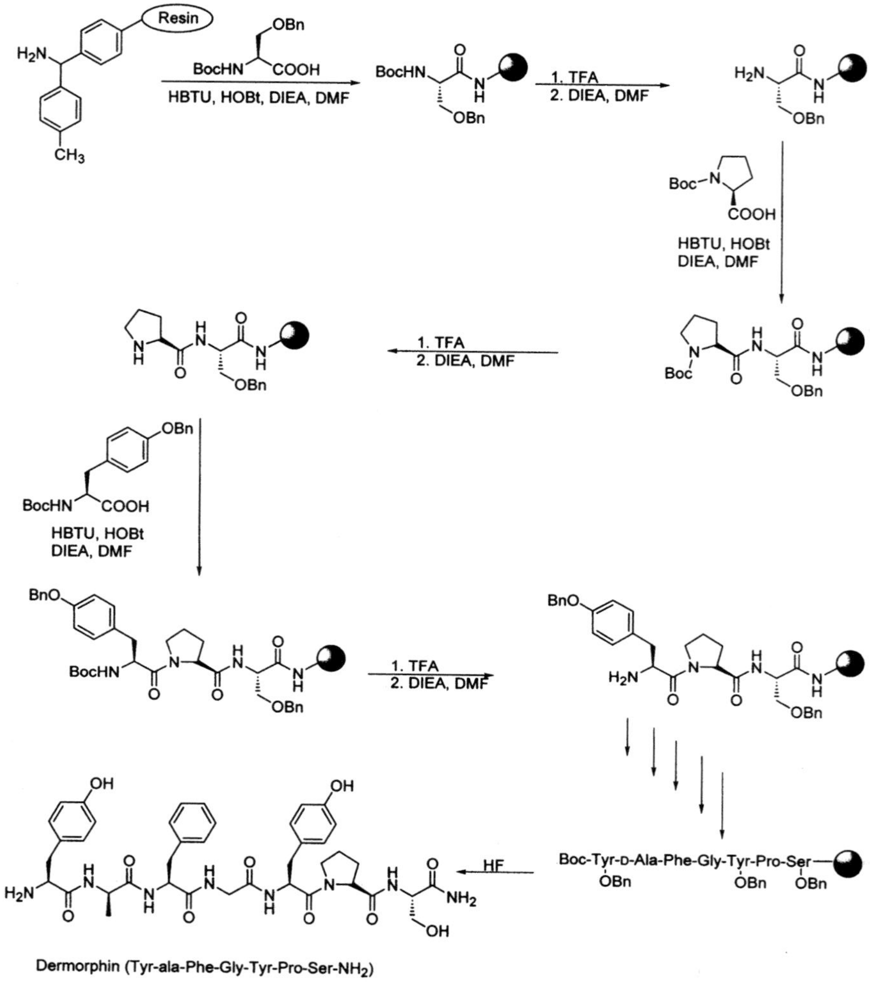

Figure 15.3 Solid phase synthesis of the amphibian heptapeptide dermorphin. HBTU: 2-(1H-benzotriazol-1-yl)-1,1,3,3-tetramethyluronium hexafluorophosphate; HOBt: 1-hydroxybenzotriazole; DIEA: diisopropylethylamine; DMF: dimethylformamide; TFA: trifluoroacetic acid; •: polystyrene resin with a specific spacer for synthesis of C-terminal amidated peptides.

acids is cleaved off to generate the propeptide. This cleavage is catalyzed by specific peptidases. The propeptides are further processed to their active forms and structural modifications like acetylation, glycosylation, sulphation, phosphorylation, or C-terminal amidation may occur. The peptides are stored in synaptic vesicles and are released into the environment by appropriate stimuli. The peptides act mainly as neurotransmitters, neuromodulators, and hormones, thus influencing a series of vital functions such as metabolism, immune defence, digestion, respiration, sens-

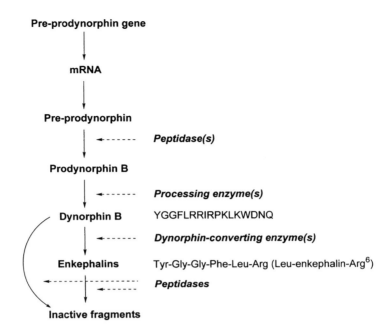

Pre-prodynorphin gene

↓

mRNA

↓

Pre-prodynorphin

  ←------ *Peptidase(s)*

↓

Prodynorphin B

  ←------ *Processing enzyme(s)*

↓

Dynorphin B   YGGFLRRIRPKLKWDNQ

  ←------ *Dynorphin-converting enzyme(s)*

↓

Enkephalins   Tyr-Gly-Gly-Phe-Leu-Arg (Leu-enkephalin-Arg[6])

  ←------ *Peptidases*

↓

Inactive fragments

Figure 15.4 Flowchart showing the biosynthesis of dynorphin B and its breakdown.

itivity to pain, reproduction, behavior and electrolyte levels. The breakdown of a peptide *in vivo* is frequently less specific than that of small molecular transmitters since it involves peptidases of low specificity. The peptide fragments formed on peptide degradation may be inactive or display biological activity; e.g. dynorphin B produces the potent hexapeptide Leu-enkephalin-Arg[6] on degradation.

Some endogenous peptides such as the amyloid precursor protein (APP) which is believed to be responsible for the neurodegeneration in Alzheimer's disease, are quite toxic. The membrane anchored APP can be cleaved by β- and γ-secretases to form a 42-amino acid peptide called amyloid β peptide (Aβ) (Figure 15.5). This peptide is quite hydrophobic and is prone to nucleation and fibril formation. The Aβ-production ultimately leads to amyloid plaque formation in the brain of Alzheimer patients. The β-secretase cleavage of APP is considered the rate-limiting step in the Aβ-synthesis and an intense search for inhibitors of this enzyme is ongoing.

15.1.4 Peptide–G-protein coupled receptor interactions

Many peptide receptors belong to the GPCR super family. Frequently only a small number of amino acids (4–8) are responsible for the recognition and activation of the GPCR (the 'message' part). These important amino acids can be identified by amino acid substitutions which lead to pronounced changes in the biological response. The part of the peptide not directly involved in the binding to the GPCR (the 'address' part) serves to fix the important amino acids in a

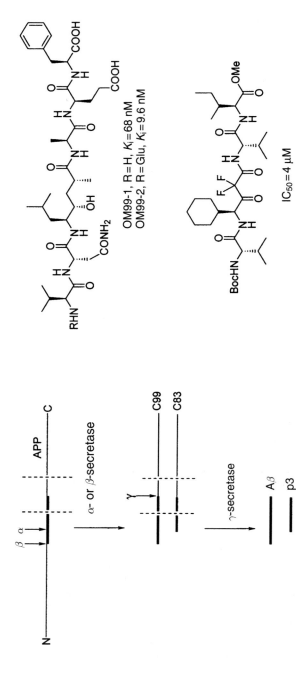

Figure 15.5 Schematic representation of the Aβ-formation from amyloid precursor protein (APP) by β- and γ-secretase cleavage (left). Dotted lines represent the lipid bilayer. Pseudopeptides with inhibitory activity towards γ-secretase (right).

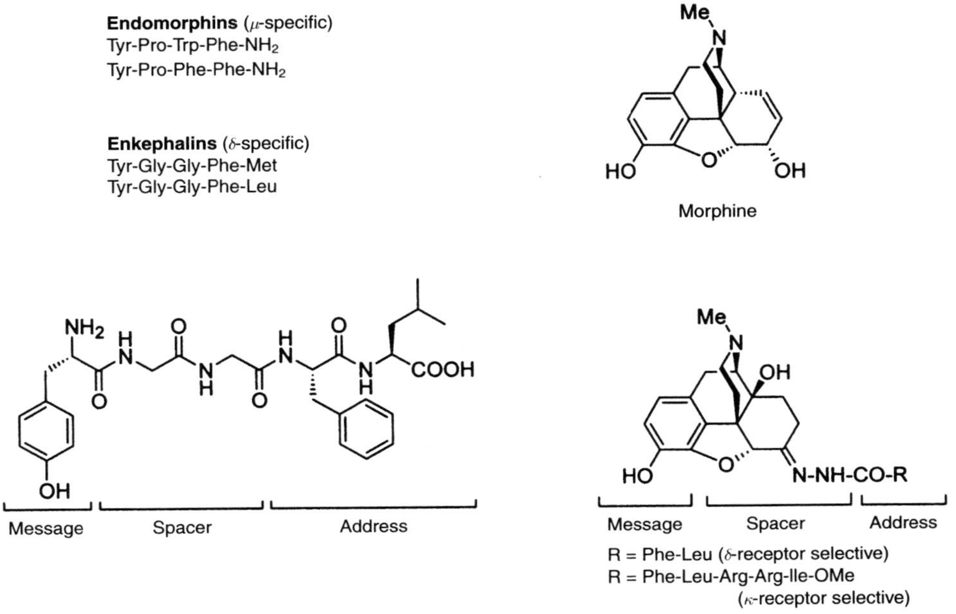
Endomorphins (μ-specific)
Tyr-Pro-Trp-Phe-NH2
Tyr-Pro-Phe-Phe-NH2
Enkephalins (δ-specific)
Tyr-Gly-Gly-Phe-Met
Tyr-Gly-Gly-Phe-Leu
Me
N
HO
O
OH
Morphine
NH2
H
N
O
N
H
COOH
OH
Message
Spacer
Address
OH
N-NH-CO-R
Message
Spacer
Address
R = Phe-Leu (δ-receptor selective)
R = Phe-Leu-Arg-Arg-Ile-OMe
(κ-receptor selective)

Figure 15.6 Structural relationship between the endomorphins, enkephalins and the peptidomimetic morphine. Also illustrated is the concept of message and address parts of peptides.

proper spatial arrangement and confers additional affinity and selectivity for the receptor. The concept of address and message parts in enkephalin is illustrated in Figure 15.6.

15.2 STRATEGIES FOR PEPTIDOMIMETIC DRUG DISCOVERY

The peptide receptors and the enzymes involved in the biosynthesis and degradation of peptides have become attractive targets in drug discovery research. Most biologically active peptides display receptor affinities (K_D) in the nM–pM range (10^{-9}–10^{-12} M). However, peptides are rarely useful as drugs due to their (i) low oral bioavailability; (ii) rapid degradation by endogenous peptidases; (iii) rapid excretion through liver and kidneys; and (iv) side effects due to their interaction with several different receptors (lack of selectivity). Hence, current research in the field mainly deals with the challenging task of circumventing these limitations; orally effective and metabolically stable analogs of peptidic hormones, neurotransmitters, and neuromodulators are needed and could lead to drugs with useful pharmacological/therapeutical profiles. These compounds are often referred to as 'peptidemimetics' or 'peptidomimetics'.

According to Morgan and Gainor, peptidomimetics can be defined as 'structures which serve as appropriate substitutes for peptides in interaction with receptors and enzymes. The mimics must possess not only affinity but also efficacy or substrate function'. The most well-known peptidomimetic is probably morphine which acts as an agonist on opiate receptors (Figure 15.6). The research on peptidomimetics deals with peptides and proteins as lead compounds for the discovery of other classes of compounds through a variety of research strategies. Since peptide–receptor antagonists/inverse agonists or enzyme inhibitors do not interact with receptors in the same way as the endogenous peptide they should not be regarded as peptidomimetics. However, all ligands for peptide receptors or peptide degrading enzymes are termed peptidomimetics in the current literature.

In general, a successfully designed peptidomimetic should be metabolically stable, have good (preferably oral) bioavailability, have high receptor affinity and selectivity, and should produce a minimum of side effects. However, today it is not known how to rationally convert (*de novo*) a peptide into a non-peptide while maintaining the biological activity. There is no strategy which guarantees the discovery of ligands with high affinity, efficacy, and specificity. In general, the discovery of novel ligands for peptide receptors has not been based on a thorough understanding of the key-intermolecular interactions. Instead, receptor-based random screening has been the most rewarding method. Below follows an outline of different strategies used in the development of peptidomimetics.

15.2.1   Design of peptidomimetics

A design process which is based on the primary structure of a peptide and on insight into its biological activity may be used for the development of peptidomimetics. Such a process requires a close collaboration between specialists from the areas of synthetic chemistry, NMR-spectroscopy, crystallography, molecular modeling, and biology. In 1980, Farmer described how to convert a peptide into a peptidomimetic. He defined a set of rules (The Farmer's rules) for this process:

1   'The design of nonpeptidic analogs of a bioactive peptide should start from the simplest conceivable structures that might possibly have a peptidomimetic activity.' Large parts of the peptide can be removed without loss of activity and determinations of the smallest active fragment can be performed by a stepwise cleavage of amino acids from both the N- and the C-terminal ends of the natural peptide. Hydrophobic residues are usually important for receptor binding but polar residues are likely to be important for intrinsic activity.

2   'A nonpeptidic analog of a bioactive peptide should not occupy space outside that believed to be occupied by the peptide itself.' In addition, the functional groups should be maintained during the first stages of the conversion of a peptide into a non-peptide.

3   'Conformational flexibility should be maximized until lead activity is discovered in a nonpeptidic structure.' At least some conformational flexibility should be retained in the first set of mimetic compounds. Potency and selectivity may then be improved by introduction of conformational constraints.

4   'The design of nonpeptidic peptidomimetics should rely heavily on mimicking the topology of backbone peptide bonds, especially where there are regular secondary structures.' Analogs of secondary structures such as α-helices or β-sheets are unlikely to exhibit selectivity. Analogs mimicking tertiary structures should be more useful.

Experimental studies of designed drugs should be performed continuously during the design process and should provide information on pharmacodynamic as well as pharmacokinetic parameters such as biological activity, absorption, first-pass metabolism, CNS-penetration (if important), and water solubility. In addition, structure–activity relationships should be deduced. Several examples are available in the literature which demonstrate that Farmer's rules can successfully be employed.

15.2.1.1   Amino acid manipulations

Following the identification of the smallest active fragment of a peptide the role of each amino acid should be determined. Initially, a systematic replacement of the side chains with methyl groups, i.e. exchange of one amino acids at the time for alanine (Ala scan), can be performed. This should allow the identification of side chains of importance either for the receptor interaction or for folding of the peptide into its bioactive conformation. Phenylalanine scans indicate the role of hydrophobicity in special parts on the peptide. A systematic replacement of L-amino acids with D-amino acids or proline scans may be informative in the initial exploration of structural requirements for receptor recognition and binding. A more elaborate strategy may also involve the systematic introduction of conformational constraints by, e.g. N- or α-methylations (the conformational flexibility of the modified peptide should change dramatically due to the limited rotation around the ψ/ϕ bonds). Several unnatural amino acids in which the physico-chemical parameters differ from the natural amino acids, have been synthesized. Selected examples are shown in Figure 15.7. The common feature of these structures is the conformationally constrained side chains. The amino acids Tic and Aib are frequently used as replacements for Phe and Ala, respectively.

15.2.1.2   Peptide backbone modifications

In large peptides, the backbone mainly serves as a structural matrix. The conformation of the backbone positions the side chains in defined spatial positions which allow optimal interactions with the enzyme or receptor protein. The amide bonds themselves may also be of importance for binding to enzymes and receptors. Several amide bond isosteres have been designed, synthesized and introduced into peptide analogs. These fragments are mainly used to enhance the stability towards protease degradation but may also be useful tools in studies of structural mimicry. An appropriate amide bond replacement should, e.g. exhibit similar geometrical, conformational, electrostatical, and hydrogen bonding properties as the amide bond itself. Although a large number of amide isosteres are known 'a convincing imitation of the amide bond in the ground state has not yet been achieved' according to Giannis and Kolter. Some examples of amide isosteres are shown in Figure 15.8.

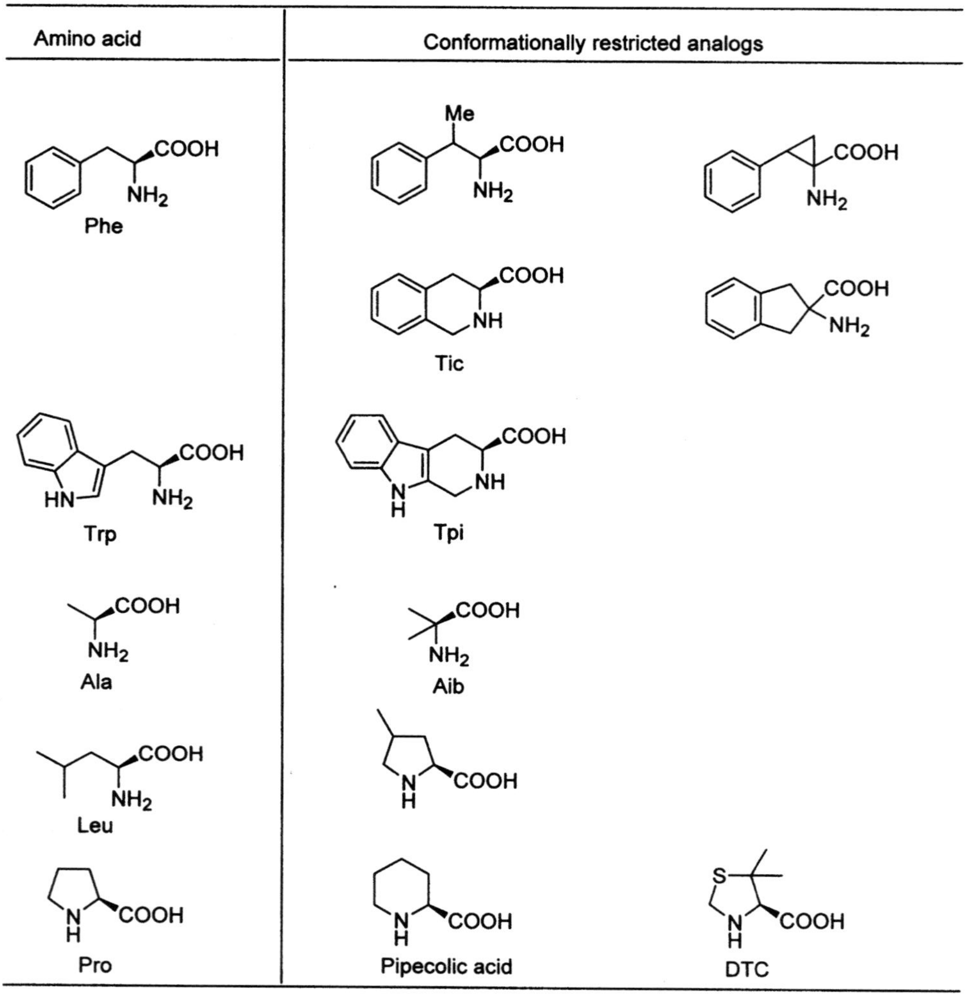

Amino acid	Conformationally restricted analogs

Figure 15.7 Some unnatural amino acids which impose conformational constraints when introduced in peptides.

Retro-inverse isosteres not only reverse the direction of the peptide but also have the L-amino acids exchanged for D-amino acids. Incorporation of a retro-inverse isostere results in a pseudopeptide with a similar topology as the native peptide, however, it is no longer sensitive to peptidase degradation.

15.2.1.3 Di(oligo)peptidomimetics

Replacement of larger structural moieties with di- or tripeptidomimetic structures are of interest since these modified peptides bridge the gap between peptide

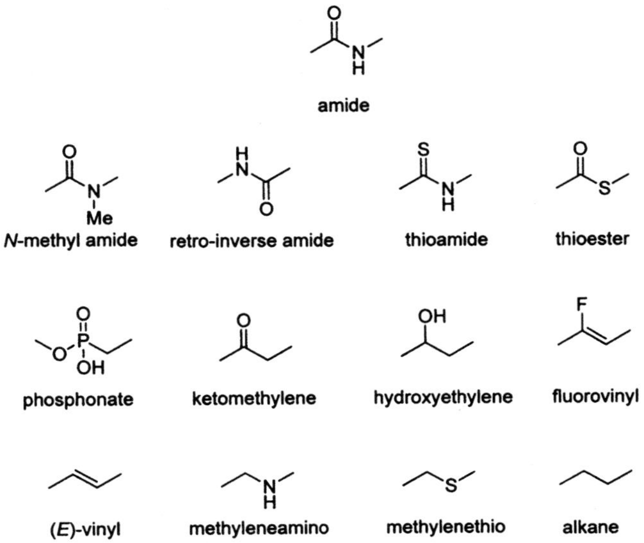

Figure 15.8 Some amide isosteres.

analogs and non-peptidic structures. Several lactams have been synthesized as bridging elements to stabilize certain backbone conformations. These mimetic structures are based on side chain to side chain, or side chain to backbone cyclizations (Figure 15.9). Mimetic moieties involving the peptide bond, such as azole-derived mimetics, have also been successfully used as dipeptide replacements. It should be noted, however, that the incorporation of a specific di(oligo)-peptidomimetic moiety into different peptides may affect the biological activity differently.

15.2.1.4 *Local or global conformational constraints*

The bioactive conformation of a peptide is the conformation recognized by and/or interacting with the binding domain(s) of a receptor or enzyme. Unfortunately, the bioactive conformation of a peptide may be poorly populated in the absence of the receptor and, consequently, it may be quite different from conformations observed by e.g. NMR-spectroscopy or X-ray crystallography. Molecular mechanics calculations and molecular dynamics studies of isolated peptides have also been performed in attempts to deduce the bioactive conformations of peptides but, in general, these studies are non-informative. Recently, computational studies have been performed in which the peptide has been allowed to interact with the receptor structure. However, bioactive conformations are probably best deduced by use of conformationally restricted mimetics.

Introduction of conformational constraints aims to stabilize either local or global conformations. Local conformational constraints could include the replacement

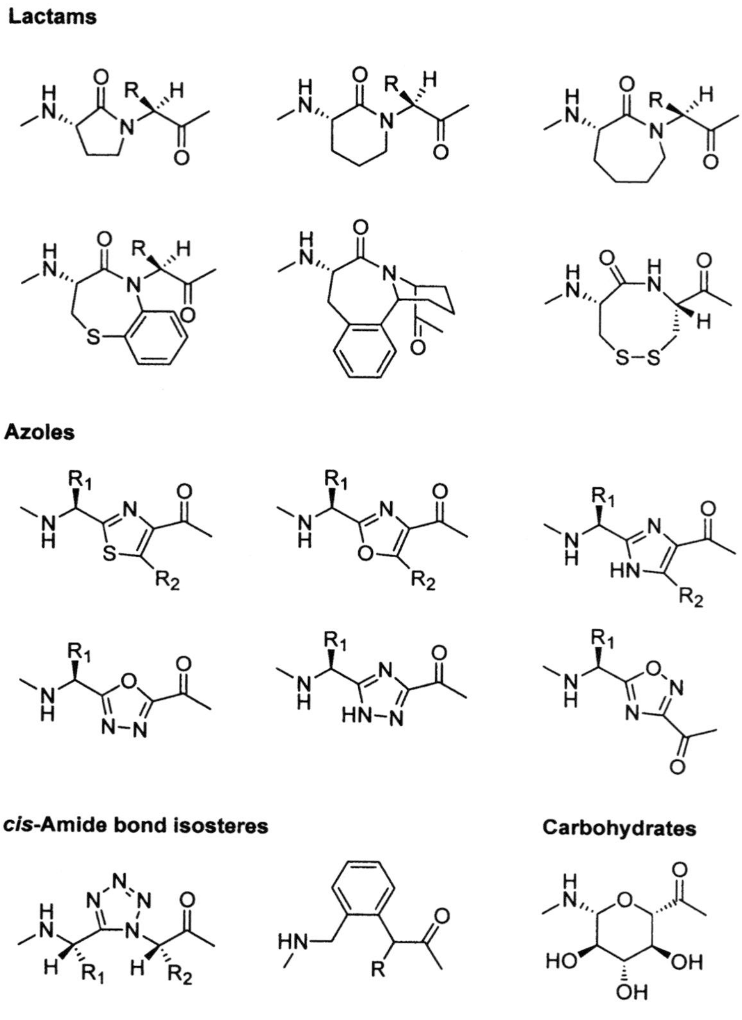

Lactams

Azoles

cis-Amide bond isosteres   **Carbohydrates**

Figure 15.9 Some dipeptidomimetics.

of the amide moiety by isosteres (methylamino, ketomethylene, inverse amide, etc.) and introduction of amino acid residues/mimics which restrict the conformational flexibility. A disadvantage with these approaches is that the introduction of local constraints may have unpredicted effects on the over-all conformational equilibrium. Global constraints may involve cyclic disulfide bridges. Alternatively, side chains not involved in the receptor recognition/interaction could be connected by cyclization. Backbone to backbone cyclizations provide another type of global conformational constraints (Figure 15.10).

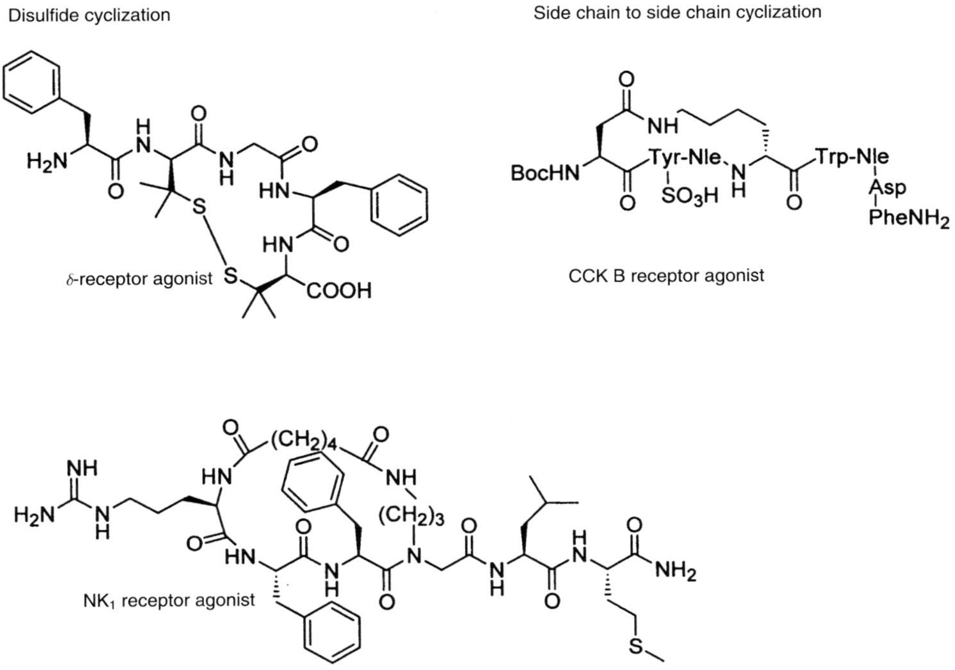
Disulfide cyclization
δ-receptor agonist
Side chain to side chain cyclization
BocHN
Tyr-Nle
SO3H
Trp-Nle
Asp
PheNH2
CCK B receptor agonist
(CH2)4
(CH2)3
NK1 receptor agonist

Figure 15.10 Some peptides which have been cyclized to restrict global conformational mobility.

15.2.1.5 *Mimics of peptide secondary structures*

There are three classes of secondary structure elements of a peptide: (1) α-helices; (2) β-sheets; and (3) turns and loops. A secondary structure mimetic is a structural moiety that, when incorporated into a peptide, forces the peptide to adopt a specific conformation.

15.2.1.6 *β- and γ-turn mimetics*

Turns and loops are important conformational characteristics of peptides and proteins. A β-turn is formed from four amino acids and is stabilized by a hydrogen bond between the first and the third amino acid. A γ-turn is formed in a similar way from three amino acids (Figure 15.11). Large numbers of turn mimetics have been designed and synthesized but most have resulted in inactivity when incorporated into peptides. A selection of turn mimetics are shown in Figure 15.11.

15.2.1.7 *α-helix and β-sheet mimetics*

α-Helix and β-sheet motifs are well characterized structural features of peptides and proteins. Some examples of α-helix initiators and β-sheet inducers are shown in Figure 15.12.

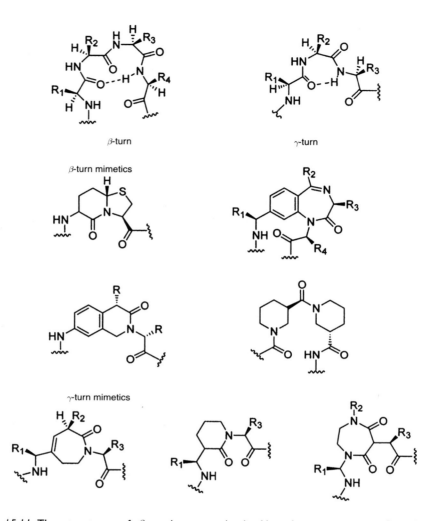

Figure 15.11 The structures of β- and γ-turns (top). Also shown are some β- and γ-turn mimetics.

15.2.1.8   Scaffold mimetics

Topological constraints may also provide information about the bioactive conformation; important amino acid side chains are positioned in proper relative positions onto a molecular template (scaffold), i.e. in agreement with the bioactive topology. The optimal molecular scaffold appears to be a highly functionalized small (5–7-membered) ring of defined stereochemistry. In Figure 15.13, some interesting scaffold mimetics are shown.

The strategies described above are empirical and time consuming. Novel combinatorial chemistry techniques that permit the controlled synthesis of peptide

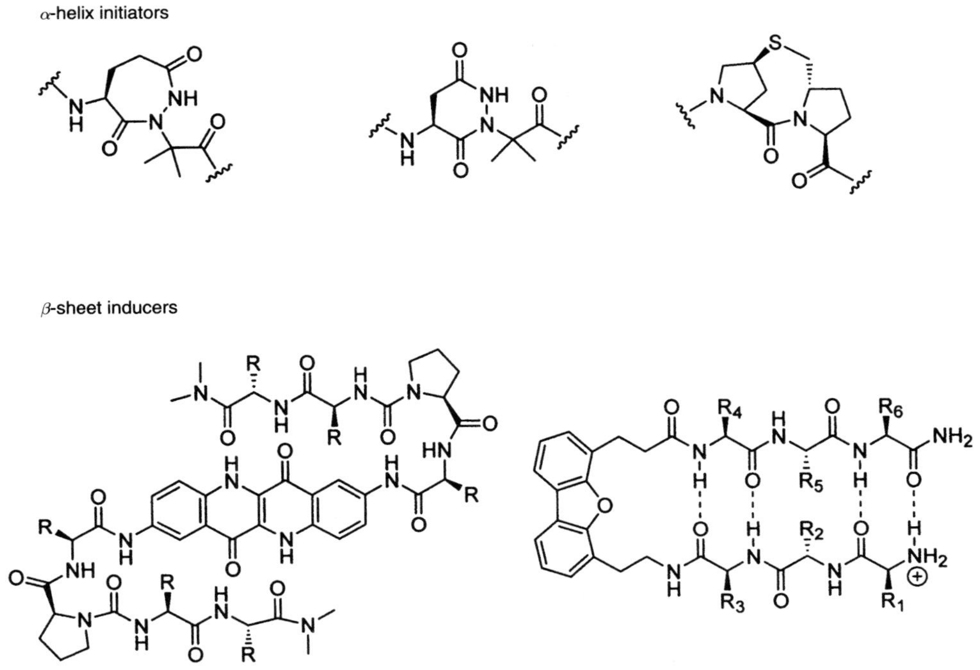

α-helix initiators

β-sheet inducers

Figure 15.12 Structures mimicking various aspects of peptide secondary structure.

libraries in which various mimetic moieties are introduced would probably lead to a more efficient research process.

15.2.2 Discovery of peptidomimetics using receptor/enzyme-based screening

Extensive efforts have been put into peptide–receptor-based screening of small molecules, natural products, or microbial broths. Although identified leads may show quite weak affinity structural optimization may improve both affinity and selectivity. Most frequently, receptor antagonists have been discovered by this approach. However, in recent years, an increased number of peptide receptor agonist have been identified. The main reason for this trend is believed to be the use of functionalized assays in high throughput screening.

Access to the detailed structure of the binding site of a peptide receptor or enzyme active site would make it possible to use structure-based design technology in attempts to generate efficient agonists/substrates or antagonists/inhibitors. Unfortunately, our knowledge about the structure of ligand binding sites on receptors is very limited. However, structures of several active sites of enzymes have been obtained. In addition, their mechanisms of action have been deduced and this information can also be used efficiently in the lead optimization process as

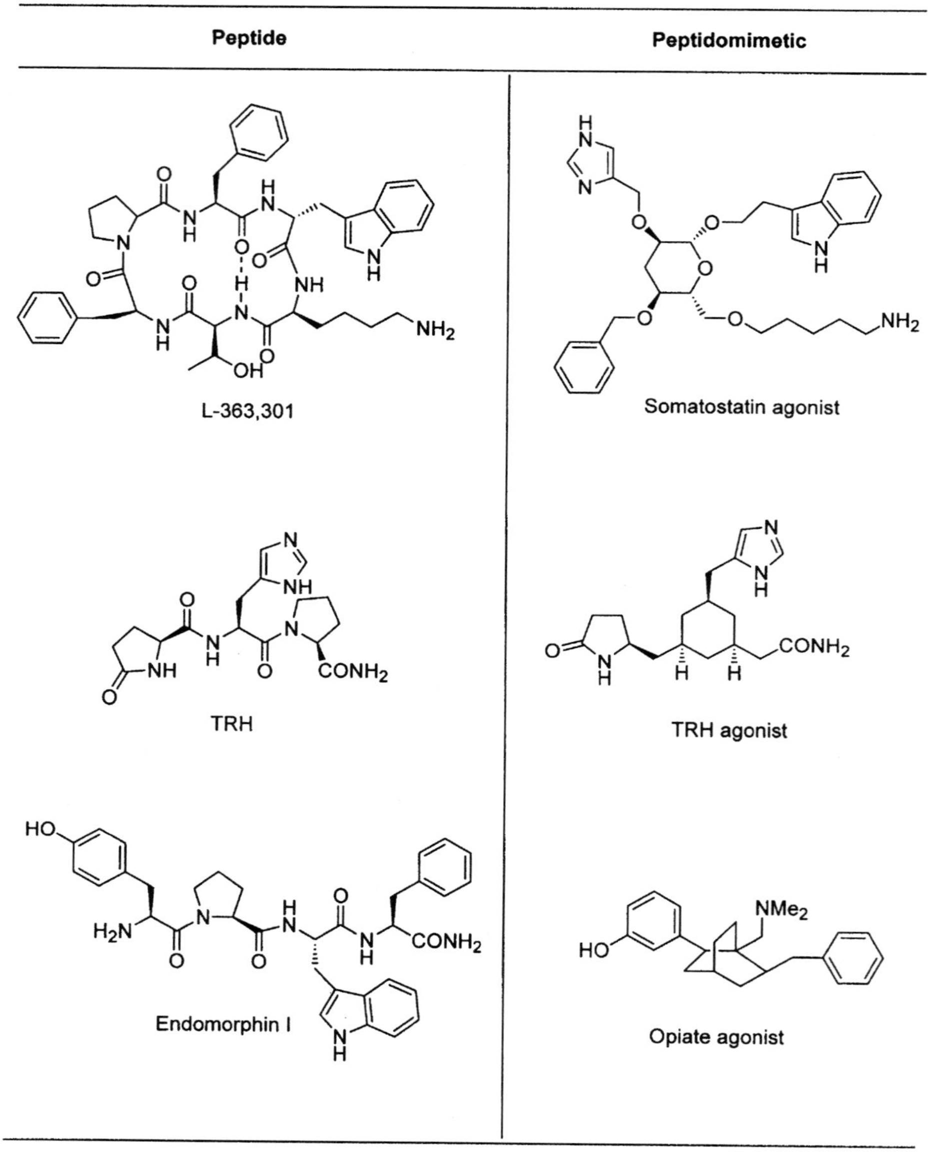
Peptide
Peptidomimetic
L-363,301
Somatostatin agonist
TRH
TRH agonist
Endomorphin I
Opiate agonist
NH2
CONH2
NMe2
HO

Figure 15.13 Some examples of scaffold-based peptidomimetics.

exemplified by the discovery of the ACE inhibitors (Figure 15.14). In the following sections several examples will be given of peptidomimetics developed after design-based optimization of lead compounds identified in screening programs. Examples of agonists developed from antagonist structures will be given, e.g. angiotensin II, cholesystokinin, bradykinin and arginine vasopressin receptor agonists.

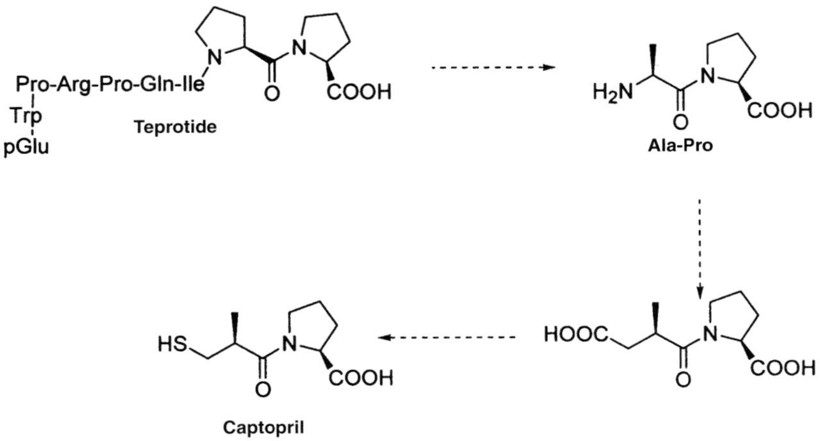

Figure 15.14 The process leading to the discovery of captopril.

15.2.2.1 *Angiotensin converting enzyme (ACE) inhibitors and angiotensin II receptor ligands*

The ACE-inhibitors were discovered using the nonapeptide teprotide, that was isolated from snake venom, as the molecular lead (Figure 15.14). The optimization of the lead started from the weak inhibitor Ala-Pro, a modified C-terminal fragment of teprotide. The ACE is known to be a metalloprotease with a Zn^{2+} ion in the active site and a carboxylic acid group was introduced to increase the co-ordination of the inhibitor to the enzyme. The successful result of this modification led to the replacement of the carboxylic acid group by a thiol function which co-ordinates even stronger to Zn. The resulting compound, captopril, has been used as an orally active antihypertensive drug for several years.

An early example of discovery of non-peptidic peptide–receptor ligands by receptor-based screening followed by design-based optimization is provided by the angiotensin II receptor (AT_1) antagonist DuP753 (Losartan, Figure 15.15) that was developed from S-8308 which also contains an imidazole moiety. The design was carried out using computer modeling and it has been suggested that the side chains of amino acids Tyr, Ile, and Phe in AngII are mimicked correctly by DuP753. Recently, also AT_1 receptor agonists e.g. L-162,313 and L-162,782 were discovered in screening programs for antagonists (Figure 15.15). Interestingly, the structural similarities between the novel agonists and antagonists are profound, L-162,782 and L-162,389 differ only in one methyl group (Figure 15.15).

15.2.2.2 *Cholecystokinin (CCK) receptor ligands*

Another early example of discovery of non-peptidic peptide–receptor ligands is provided by the cholecystokinin (CCK) receptor antagonists MK-329 and L-365,260 (Figure 15.16) that were developed from Asperlicin. The CCK-receptor affinity of Asperlicin was discovered by screening. These antagonists contain the

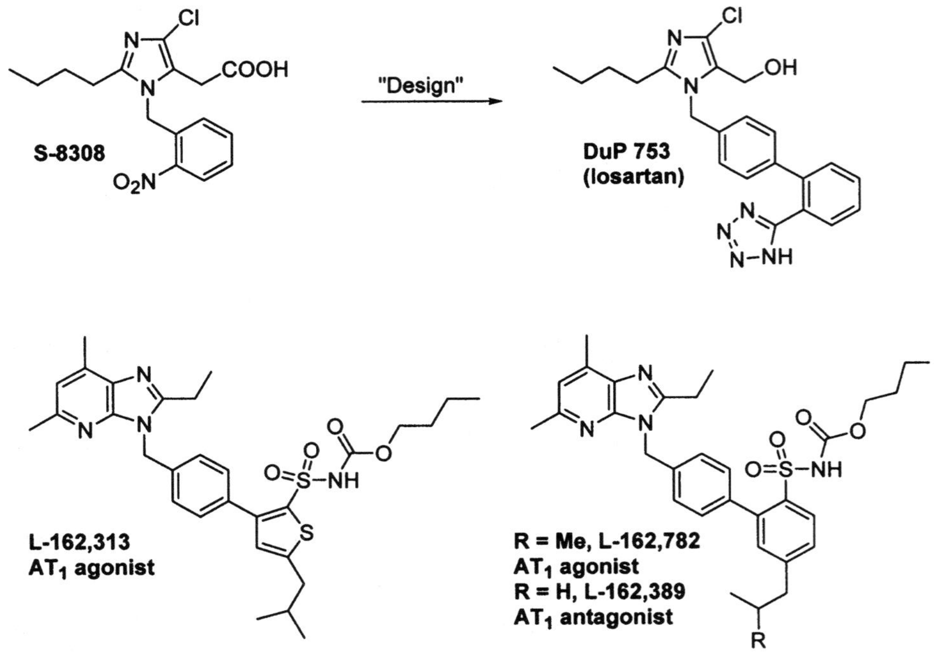

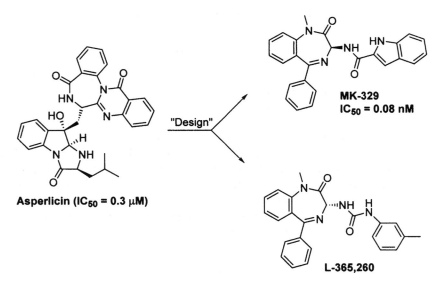

Figure 15.15 The AT_1-receptor antagonist DuP753 was developed from S-8308. Recently structurally related non-peptidic agonists were also discovered.

Figure 15.16 Peptide receptor ligands from receptor-based screening. Two CCK antagonists have been developed from asperlicin.

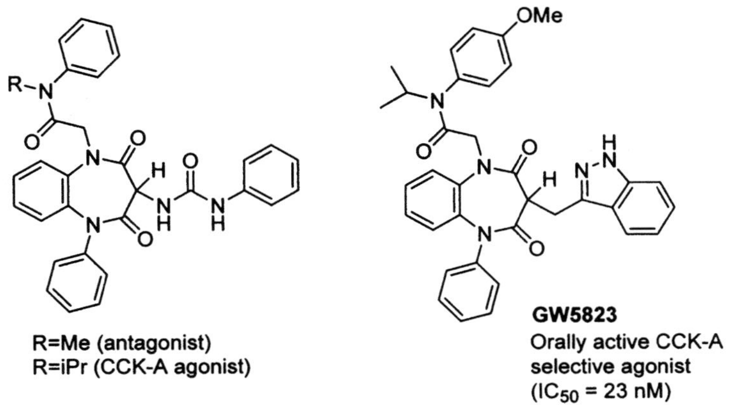

Figure 15.17 CCK-A receptor agonists based on the 1,5-benzodiazepine framework. The successful use of the 'agonist trigger' is shown.

1,4-benzodiazepine structure. The benzodiazepine moiety is also present in many other non-peptidic peptide–receptor ligands and has been termed a 'privileged structure' for peptide receptor affinity.

The term 'agonist trigger' was coined during the development of CCK receptor agonists containing a 1,5-benzodiazepin framework (Figure 15.17). The agonist/ antagonist activity could be modulated by the N^1-anilinoacetamido moiety, an N^1-methyl group gave antagonist activity whereas an isopropyl group gave agonist activity. The successful use of a combination of information obtained from Asperlicin and the agonistic effect triggered by an isopropyl group lead to the development of the first orally active CCK-A selective agonist GW5823 (Figure 15.17).

15.2.2.3 Arginine Vasopressin (AVP) receptor ligands

Recently a series of arginine vasopressin (AVP) V_2 receptor agonists based on the benzazepin skeleton was discovered. The design of agonists was based on a lead structure obtained by analysis of metabolites from antagonists, such as tolvaptan (Figure 15.18). A large series of compounds were synthesized with high affinity for the V_2 receptor but with varying functional activities. The agonist effect was determined as percentage of maximal cAMP accumulation. The V_2-receptor agonist activity is severely restricted by the size of the P1 region of the receptor and even small structural changes in this region could lead to drastic differences in agonist action. Therefore, it was hypothesized that this region contains an activation cavity. The P2 binding region seems to be important for the affinity. Some agonist structures are shown in Figure 15.18.

15.2.2.4 Bradykinin receptor ligands

The structural similarities between agonists and antagonists at peptide receptors can also be illustrated by ligands for the bradykinin B_2-receptor. Agonists at the

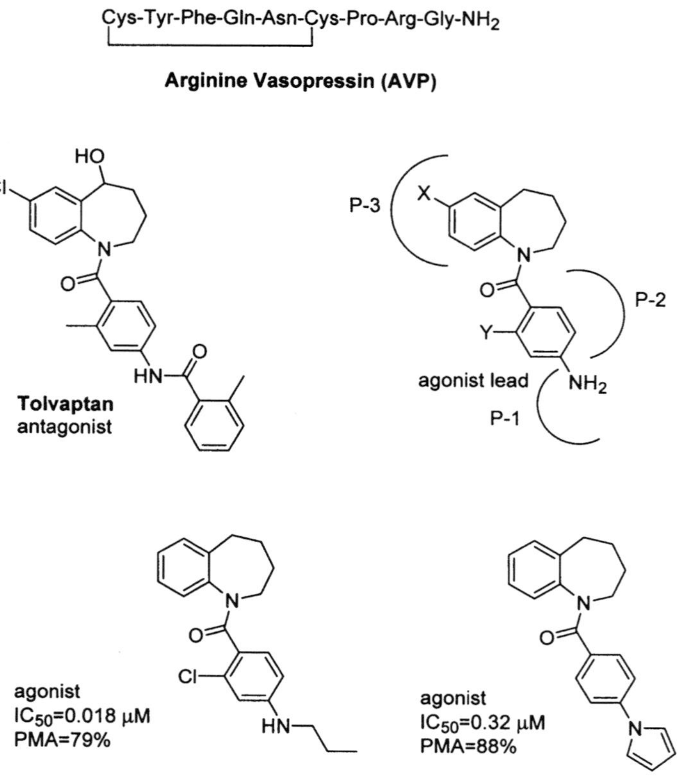

Cys-Tyr-Phe-Gln-Asn-Cys-Pro-Arg-Gly-NH$_2$

Arginine Vasopressin (AVP)

Figure 15.18 Design of novel non-peptidic AVP agonists based on the benzazepine skeleton. PMA = percentage of maximal cAMP accumulation at a concentration of 1 μM. The P-1, P-2 and P-3 binding regions are also shown.

B$_2$-receptor are expected to be important e.g. in hypertension, and several peptidic agonists are known. The first non-peptidic B$_2$-agonist FR190997 was recently identified among a large series of bradykinin-receptor antagonists (Figure 15.19).

15.2.2.5 Mimetics of growth hormone regulating peptides

Growth hormone release is regulated by different peptides such as growth hormone releasing hormone (GH-RH), growth hormone secretagogues (GHS), and somato-statin. It was not until recently the endogenous ligand for the GHS receptor was identified to be the 28 amino acid peptide ghrelin. Ghrelin is a linear peptide containing an *n*-octanoyl modification on Ser3. Several non-peptidic agonists at the GHS-receptor(s) has been identified, they exhibit a large structural diversity (Figure 15.20).

Growth hormone release is negatively regulated by somatostatin activation of the sst$_2$-receptor subtype. Somatostatin regulates also the release of other hormones such as glucagon, insulin and gastrin, the different functional activities being regulated by activation of different sst-receptor subtypes. Non-peptidic subtype

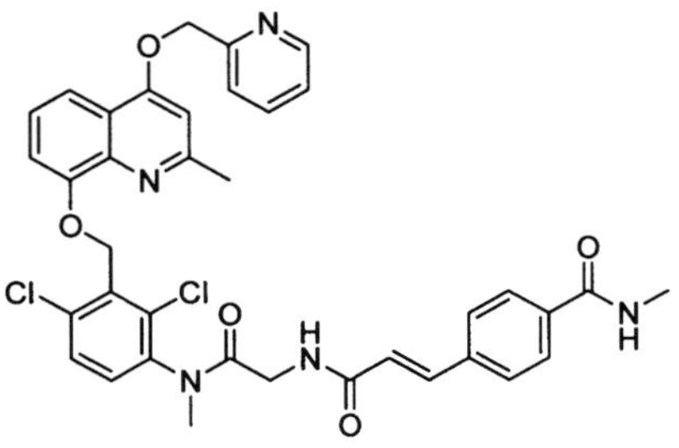

FR190997

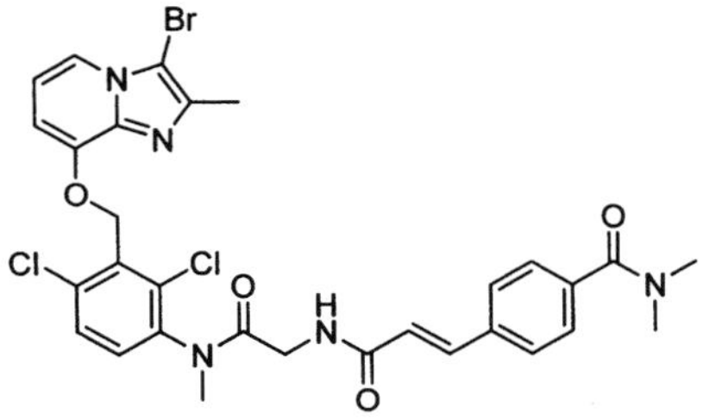

FR167344

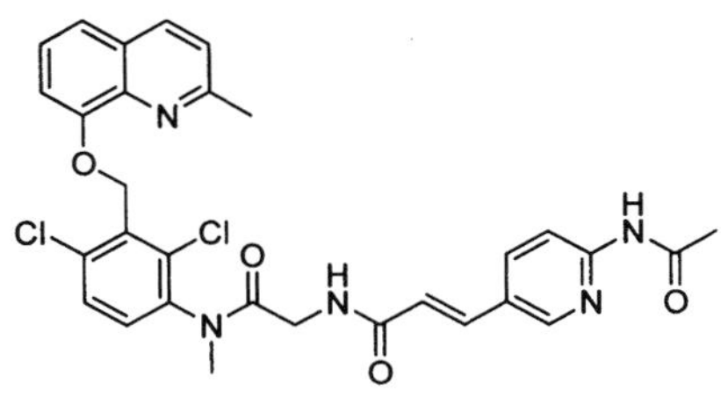

FR173657

Figure 15.19 The bradykinin B_2-receptor agonist FR190997 and some structurally related antagonists.

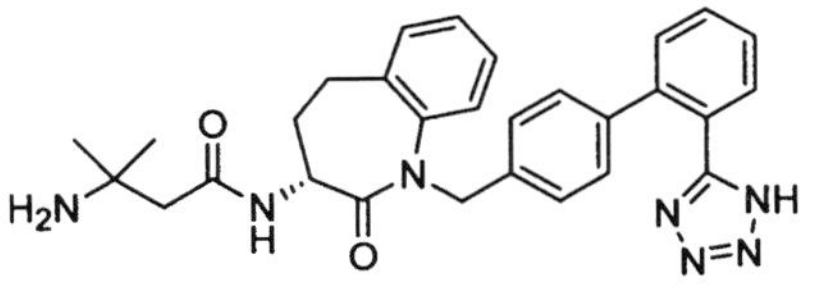

L-692,429

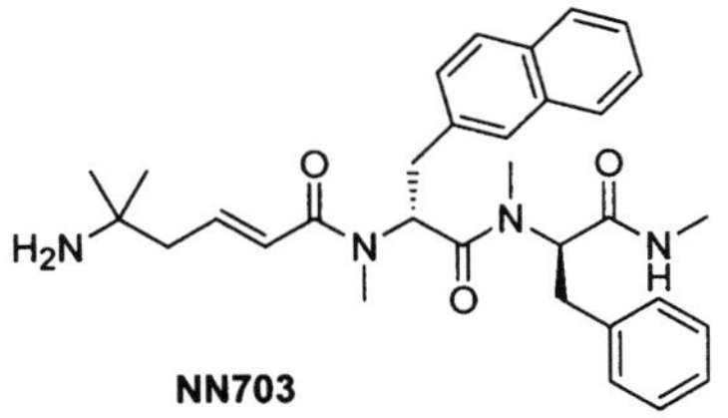

NN703

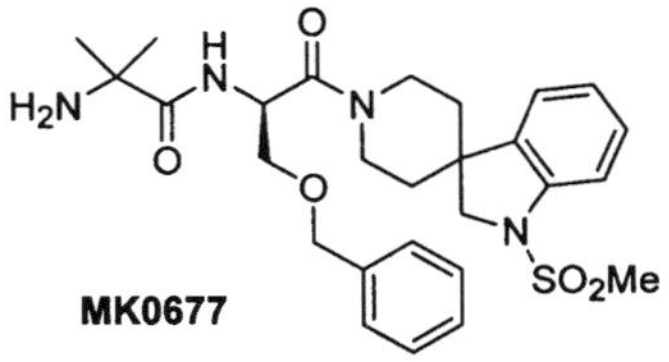

MK0677

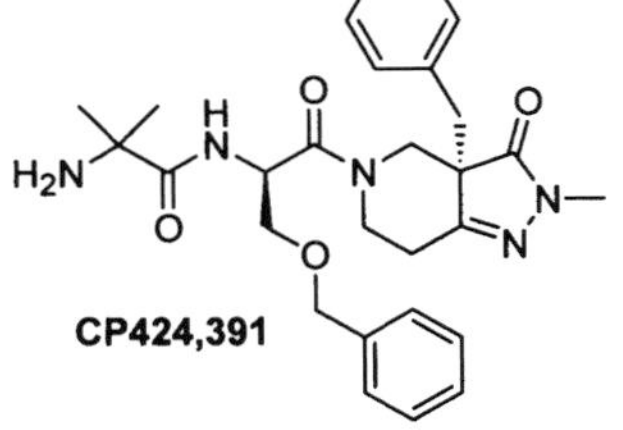

CP424,391

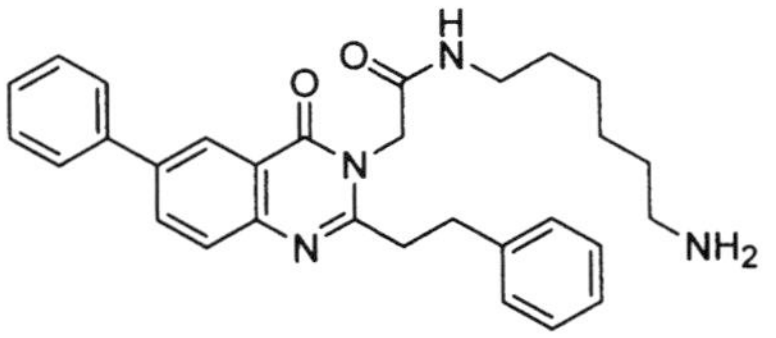

Figure 15.20 Some non-peptidic GHS-receptor agonists.

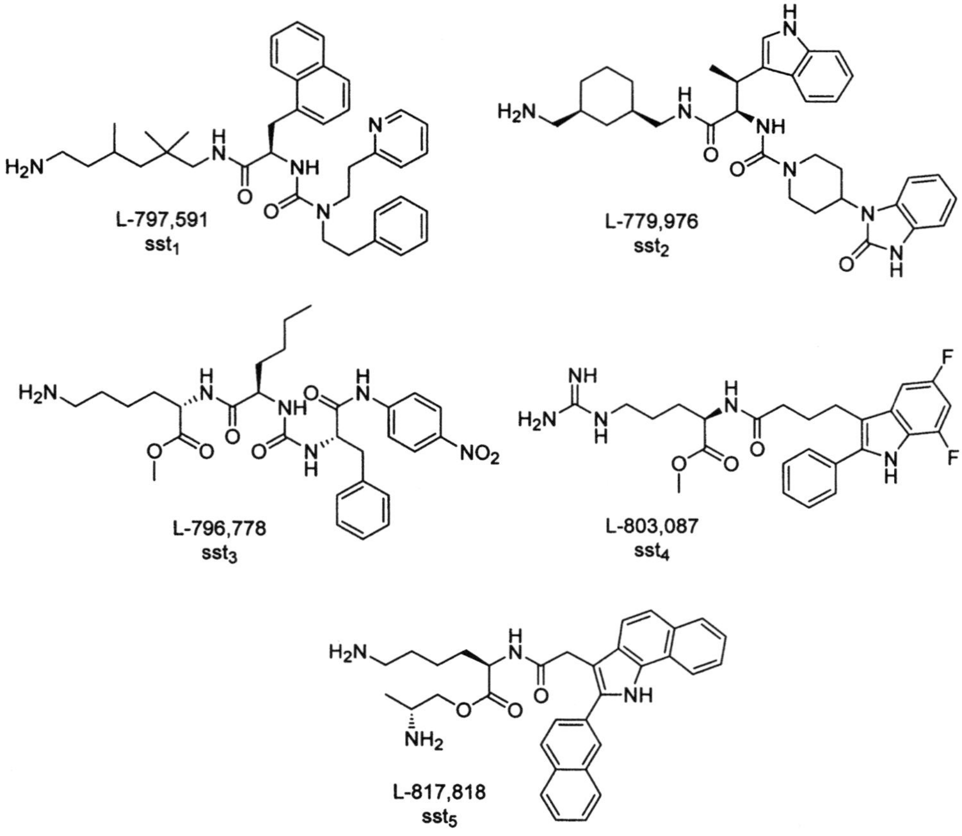

Figure 15.21 Subtype specific somatostatin receptor agonists have been identified by a combination of combinatorial chemistry and molecular modeling.

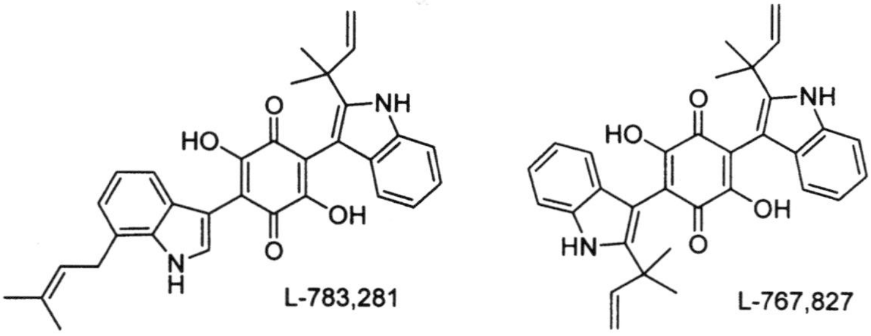

Figure 15.22 Recently discovered small molecule insulin mimetics.

receptor specific agonists have been identified by a combination of combinatorial chemistry and molecular modeling using the cyclic hexapeptide somatostatin agonist (L-363,377) as a lead (Figure 15.21).

15.2.2.6 Small molecule insulin mimetics

Recently non-peptide small molecule insulin mimetics were discovered. The quinone derivative L-783,281, isolated from a fungal extract, showed potent anti-diabetic activity. Interestingly, the mimetic has been shown to bind to a different binding site on the insulin receptor than insulin itself. The structurally related compound hinulliquinone (L-767,827) also showed activity in the antidiabetic assay, however this symmetrical molecule was a 100 times less potent than L-783,281 (Figure 15.22).

FURTHER READING

Adang, A.E.P., Hermkens, P.H.H., Linders, J.T.M., Ottenheijm, H.C.J. and van Staveren, C.J. (1994) Case histories of peptidomimetics: progression from peptide to drugs. *Recl. Trav. Chim. Pays-Bas*, **113**, 63–78.

Aquino, C.J., Armour, D.R., Berman, J.M., Birkemo, L.S., Carr, R.A.E., Croom, D.K., Dezube, M., Dougherty, Jr., R.W., Ervin, G.N., Grizzle, M.K., Head, J.E., Hirst, G.C., James, M.K., Johnson, M.F., Miller, L.J., Queen, K.L., Rimele, T.J., Smith, D.N. and Sugg, E.E. (1996) Discovery of 1,5-benzodiazepines with peripheral cholecystokinin (CCK-A) receptor agonist activity. 1. Optimization of the agonist 'trigger'. *J. Med. Chem.*, **39**, 562–569.

Aramori, I., Zenkoh, J., Morikawa, N., Asano, M., Hatori, C., Sawai, H., Kayakiri, H., Satoh, S., Inoue, T., Abe, Y., Sawada, Y., Mizutani, T., Inamura, N., Nakahara, K., Kojo, H., Oku, T. and Notsu, Y. (1997) Nonpeptide mimic of bradykinin with long-acting properties at the bradykinin B₂ receptor. *Mol. Pharmacol.*, **52**, 16–20.

Bednarek, M.A., Feighner, S.D., Pong, S.-S., Kulju McKee, K., Hreniuk, D.L., Silva, M.V., Warren, V.A., Howard, A.D., van der Ploeg, L.H.Y. and Heck, J.V. (2000) Structure–function studies on the new growth hormone-releasing peptide, ghrelin: minimal sequence of ghrelin necessary for activation of growth hormone secretagogue receptor 1a. *J. Med. Chem.*, **43**, 4370–4376.

Beeley, N.R.A. (2000) Can peptides be mimicked? *Drug Discovery Today*, **5**, 354–363.

Bélanger, P.C. and Dufresne, C. (1986) Preparation of exo-6-benzyl-exo-2-(m-hydroxy-phenyl)-1-dimethylaminomethylbicyclo[2.2.2]octane. A non-peptide mimic of enkephalins. *Can. J. Chem.*, **64**, 1514–1520.

Benz, H. (1994) The role of solid-phase fragment condensation (SPFC) in peptide synthesis. *Synthesis*, 337–358.

Berts, W. and Luthman, K. (1999) Synthesis of a complete series of C-4 fluorinated Phe-Gly mimetics. *Tetrahedron*, **55**, 13819–13830.

Borg, S., Estenne-Bouhtou, G., Luthman, K., Csöregh, I., Hesselink, W. and Hacksell, U. (1995) Synthesis of 1,2,4-oxadiazole, 1,3,4-oxadiazole, and 1,2,4-triazole-derived dipeptidomimetics. *J. Org. Chem.*, **60**, 3112–3120.

Borg, S., Vollinga, R.C., Labarre, M., Payza, K., Terenius, L. and Luthman, K. (1999) Design, synthesis, and evaluation of Phe-Gly mimetics: heterocyclic building blocks for pseudopeptides. *J. Med. Chem.*, **42**, 4331–4342.

Boyle, S., Guard, S., Higginbottom, M., Horwell, D.C., Howson, W., McKnight, A.T., Martin, K., Pritchard, M.C., O'Toole, J., Raphy, J., Rees, D.C., Roberts, E., Watling, K.J.,

Woodruff, G.N. and Hughes, J. (1994) Rational design of high affinity tachykinin NK_1 receptor antagonists. *Bioorg. Med. Chem.*, **2**, 357–370.

Chorev, M. and Goodman, M. (1993) A dozen years of retro-inverso peptidomimetics. *Acc. Chem. Res.*, **26**, 266–273.

Chung, Y.J., Christianson, L.A., Stanger, H.E., Powell, D.R. and Gellman, S.H. (1998) A β-peptide reverse turn that promotes hairpin formation. *J. Am. Chem. Soc.*, **120**, 10555–10556.

de Tullio, P., Delarge, J. and Pirotte, B. (1999) Recent advances in the chemistry of cholecystokinin receptor ligands (agonists and antagonists). *Curr. Med. Chem.*, **6**, 433–455.

Duncia, J.V., Carini, D.J., Chiu, A.T, Johnson, A.L., Price, W.A., Wong, P.C., Wexler, R.R. and Timmermans, P.B.M.W.M. (1992) The discovery of DuP753, a potent, orally active nonpeptide angiotensin II receptor antagonist. *Med. Res. Rev.*, **12**, 149–191.

Evans, B.E., Bock, M.G., Rittle, K.E., DiPardo, R.M., Whitter, W.L., Veber, D.F., Anderson, P.S. and Freidinger, R.M. (1986) Design of potent, orally effective, nonpeptidal antagonists of the peptide hormone cholecystokinin. *Proc. Natl. Acad. Sci. USA*, **83**, 4918–4922.

Farmer, P.S. (1980) Bridging the gap between bioactive peptides and nonpeptides: some perspectives in design. *Drug Design*, Vol. X, pp. 119–143.

Gallop, M.A., Barrett, R.W., Dower, W.J., Fodor, S.P.A. and Gordon, E.M. (1994) Applications of combinatorial technologies to drug discovery. 1. Background and peptide combinatorial libraries. *J. Med. Chem.*, **37**, 1233–1251.

Gante, J. (1994) Peptidomimetics – tailored enzyme inhibitors. *Angew. Chem. Int. Ed. Engl.*, **33**, 1699–1720.

Giannis, A. and Kolter, T. (1993) Peptidomimetics for receptor ligands – Discovery, development, and medical perspectives. *Angew. Chem. Int. Ed. Engl.*, **32**, 1244–1267.

Gilon, C., Halle, D., Chorev, M., Selinger, Z. and Byk, G. (1991) Backbone cyclization: a new method for conferring conformational constraint on peptides. *Biopolymers*, **31**, 745–750.

Golic Grdadolnik, S., Mierke, D.F., Byk, G., Zeltser, I., Gilon, C. and Kessler, H. (1994) Comparison of the conformation of active and nonactive backbone cyclic analogs of substance P as a tool to elucidate features of the bioactive conformation: NMR and molecular dynamics in DMSO and water. *J. Med. Chem.*, **37**, 2145–2152.

Gordon, E.M., Barrett, R.W., Dower, W.J., Fodor, S.P.A. and Gallop, M.A. (1994) Applications of combinatorial technologies to drug discovery. 2. Combinatorial organic synthesis, library screening strategies, and future directions. *J. Med. Chem.*, **37**, 1385–1401.

Ghosh, A.K., Shin, D., Downs, D., Koelsch, G., Lin, X., Ermolieff, J. and Tang J. (2000) Design of potent inhibitors for human brain memapsin 2 (β-secretase). *J. Am. Chem. Soc.*, **122**, 3522–3523.

Graf von Roedern, E. and Kessler, H. (1994) A sugar amino acid as a novel peptidomimetic. *Angew. Chem. Int. Ed. Engl.*, **33**, 687–689.

Henke, B.R., Aquino, C.J., Birkemo, L.S., Croom, D.K., Dougherty, Jr., R.W., Ervin, G.N., Grizzle, M.K., Hirst, G.C., James, M.K., Johnson, M.F., Queen, K.L., Sherrill, R.G., Sugg, E.E., Suh, E.M., Szewczyk, J.W., Unwalla, R.J., Yingling, J. and Willson, T.M. (1997) Optimization of 3-(1*H*-indazol-3-ylmethyl)-1,5-benzodiazepines as potent, orally active CCK-A agonists. *J. Med. Chem.*, **40**, 2706–2725.

Hirschmann, R. (1991) Medicinal chemistry in the golden age of biology: lessons from steroid and peptide research. *Angew. Chem. Int. Ed. Engl.*, **30**, 1278–1301.

Hirschmann, R., Nicolaou, K.C., Pietranico, S., Leahy, E.M., Salvino, J., Arison, B., Cichy, M.A., Spoors, P.G., Shakespeare, W.C., Sprengler, P.A., Hamley, P., Smith III, A.B., Reisine, T., Raynor, K., Maechler, L., Donaldson, C., Vale, W., Freidinger, R.M., Cascieri, M.R. and Strader, C.D. (1993) *De novo* design and synthesis of somatostatin non-peptide peptidomimetics utilizing β-D-glucose as a novel scaffolding. *J. Am. Chem. Soc.*, **115**, 12550–12568.

Hirschmann, R., Hynes, Jr., J., Cichy-Knight, M.A., van Rijn, R.D., Sprengeler, P.A., Spoors, P.G., Shakespeare, W.C., Pietranico-Cole, S., Barbosa, J., Liu, J., Yao, W., Rohrer, S. and Smith, A.B., III. (1998) Modulation of receptor and receptor subtype affinities using diastereomeric and enantiomeric monosaccharide scaffolds as a means to structural and biological diversity. A new route to ether synthesis. *J. Med. Chem.*, **41**, 1382–1391.

Hirst, G.C., Aquino, C., Birkemo, L., Croom, D.K., Dezube, M., Dougherty, Jr., R.W., Ervin, G.N., Grizzle, M.K., Henke, B., James, M.K., Johnson, M.F., Momtahen, T., Queen, K.L., Sherrill, R.G., Szewczyk, J., Willson, T.M. and Sugg, E.E. (1996) Discovery of 1,5-benzodiazepines with peripheral cholecystokinin (CCK-A) receptor activity (II). Optimization of the C3 amino substituent. *J. Med. Chem.*, **39**, 5236–5245.

Hong, L., Koelsch, G., Lin, X., Wu, S., Terzyan, S., Ghosh, A.K., Zhang, X.C. and Tang, J. (2000) Structure of the protease domain of memapsin 2 (β-secretase) complexed with inhibitor. *Science*, **290**, 150–153.

Houghten, R.A. (1985) General method for the rapid solid-phase synthesis of large numbers of peptides: specificity of antigen–antibody interaction at the level of individual amino acids. *Proc. Natl. Acad. Sci. USA*, **82**, 5131–5135.

Houghten, R.A., Pinilla, C., Blondelle, S.E., Appel, J.R., Dooley, C.T. and Cuervo, J.H. (1991) Generation and use of synthetic peptide combinatorial libraries for basic research and drug discovery. *Nature*, **354**, 84–86.

Howson, W. (1995) Rational design of tachykinin receptor antagonists. *Drug News Perspect.*, **8**, 97–103.

Hruby, V.J. (1982) Conformational restrictions of biologically active peptides via amino acid side chain groups. *Life Sci.*, **31**, 189–199.

Hruby, V.J., Al-Obeidi, F. and Kazmierski, W. (1990) Emerging approaches in the molecular design of receptor-selective peptide ligands: conformational, topographical and dynamic considerations. *Biochem. J.*, **268**, 249–262.

Hruby, V.J. (1993) Conformational and topographical considerations in the design of biologically active peptides. *Biopolymers*, **33**, 1073–1082.

Hruby, V.J. and Balse, P.M. (2000) Conformational and topographical considerations in designing agonist peptidomimetics from peptide leads. *Current Med. Chem.*, **7**, 945–970.

Humphrey, J.M. and Chamberlin, A.R. (1997) Chemical synthesis of natural product peptides: coupling methods for the incorporation of noncoded amino acids into peptides. *Chem. Rev.*, **97**, 2243–2266.

Höllt, V. (1986) Opioid peptide processing and receptor selectivity. *Ann. Rev. Pharmacol. Toxicol.*, **26**, 59–77.

Hölzemann, G. (1991) Peptide conformation mimetics part 1 and 2. *Kontakte (Darmstadt)*, 3–12, 55–63.

Kahn, M. (1993) Peptide secondary structure mimetics: recent advances and future challenges. *Synlett*, 821–826.

Kalindjian, S.B., Dunstone, D.J., Low, C.M.R., Pether, M.J., Roberts, S.P., Tozer, M.J., Watt, G.F. and Shankley, N.P. (2001) Nonpeptide cholecystokinin-2 receptor agonists. *J. Med. Chem.* **44**, 1125–1133.

Kazmierski, W.M. (ed.) (1999) *Methods Mol. Med.*, **23**(Peptidomimetics Protocols). Totowa, New Jersey, USA: Humana Press.

Kessler, H. (1982) Conformation and biological activity of cyclic peptides. *Angew. Chem. Int. Ed. Engl.*, **21**, 512–523.

Kim, H.-O. and Kahn, M. (2000). A merger of rational drug design and combinatorial chemistry: development and application of peptide secondary structure mimetics. *Combinatorial Chemistry & High Throughput Screening*, **3**, 167–183.

Kivlighn, S.D., Huckle, W.R., Zingaro, G.J., Rivero, R.A., Lotti, V.J., Chang, R.S.L., Schorn, T.W., Kevin, N., Johnson, Jr., R.G., Greelee, W.J. and Siegl, P.K.S (1995) Discovery of L-162,313: a nonpeptide that mimics the biological actions of angiotensin II. *Am. J. Physiol.*, R820–R823.

Kojima, M., Hosoda, H., Date, Y., Nakazato, M., Matsuo, H. and Kangawa, K. (1999) Ghrelin is a growth-hormone-releasing acylated peptide from stomach. *Nature*, **402**, 656–660.

Kondo, K., Ogawa, H., Shinohara, T., Kurimura, M., Tanada, Y., Kan, K., Yamashita, H., Nakamura, S., Hirano, T., Yamamura, Y., Mori, T., Tominaga, M. and Itai, A. (2000) Novel design of nonpeptide AVP V$_2$ receptor agonists: structural requirements for an agonist having 1-(4-aminobenzoyl)-2,3,4,5-tetrahydro-1H-1-benzazepin as a template. *J. Med. Chem.*, **43**, 4388–4397.

Kreil, G. (1994) Peptides containing a D-amino acid from frogs and molluscs. *J. Biol. Chem.*, **269**, 10967–10970.

Liao, S., Alfaro-Lopez, J., Shenderovich, M.D., Hosohata, K., Lin, J., Li, X., Stropova, D., Davis, P., Jernigan, K.A., Porreca, F., Yamamura, H.I. and Hruby, V.J. (1998) *De novo* design, synthesis, and biological activities of high-affinity and selective non-peptide agonists of the δ-opioid receptor. *J. Med. Chem.*, **41**, 4767–4776.

Liskamp, R.M.J. (1994) Conformationally restricted amino acids and dipeptides, (non)peptidomimetics and secondary structure mimetics. *Recl. Trav. Chim. Pays-Bas*, **113**, 1–19.

Moore, C.L., Leatherwood, D.D., Diehl, T.S., Selkoe, D.J. and Wolfe, M.S. (2000) Difluoro ketone peptidomimetics suggest a large S1 pocket for Alzheimer's γ-secretase: implications for inhibitor design. *J. Med. Chem.*, **43**, 3434–3442.

Morgan, B.A. and Gainor, J.A. (1989) Approaches to the discovery of non-peptide ligands for peptide receptors and peptidases. *Ann. Rep. Med. Chem.*, **24**, 243–252.

Olson, G.L., Bolin, D.R., Bonner, M.P., Bös, M., Cook, C.M., Fry, D.C., Graves, B.J., Hatada, M., Hill, D.E., Kahn, M., Madison, V.S., Rusiecki, V.K., Sarabu, R., Sepinwall, J., Vincent, G.P. and Voss, M.E. (1993) Concepts and progress in the development of peptide mimetics. *J. Med. Chem.*, **36**, 3039–3049.

Olson, G.L., Cheung, H.-C., Chiang, E., Madison, V.S., Sepinwall, J., Vincent, G.P., Winokur, A. and Gary, K.A. (1995) Peptide mimetics of thyrotropin-releasing hormone based on a cyclohexane framework: design, synthesis, and cognition-enhancing properties. *J. Med. Chem.*, **38**, 2866–2879.

Ostresh, J.M., Husar, G.M., Blondelle, S.E., Dörner, B., Weber, P.A. and Houghten, R.A. (1994) 'Libraries from libraries': Chemical transformation of combinatorial libraries to extend the range and repertoire of chemical diversity. *Proc. Natl. Acad. Sci. USA*, **91**, 11138–11142.

Ramachandran, G.N. and Sasisekharan, V. (1968) Conformation of polypeptides and proteins. *Adv. Prot. Chem.*, **23**, 283–437.

Rist, B., Entzeroth, M. and Beck-Sickinger, A.G. (1998) From micromolar to nanomolar affinity: a systematic approach to identify the binding site of CGRP at the human calcitonin gene-related peptide 1 receptor. *J. Med. Chem.*, **41**, 117–123.

Rohrer, S.P., Birzin, E.T., Mosley, R.T., Berk, S.C., Hutchins, S.M., Shen, D.-M., Xiong, Y., Hayes, E.C., Parmar, R.M., Foor, F., Mitra, S.W., Degrado, S.J., Shu, M., Klopp, J.M., Cai, S.-J., Blake, A., Chan, W.W.S., Pasternak, A., Yang, L., Patchett, A.A., Smith, R.G., Chapman, K.T. and Schaeffer, J.M. (1998) Rapid identification of subtype-selective agonists of the somatostatin receptor through combinatorial chemistry. *Science*, **282**, 737–740.

Saulitis, J., Mierke, D.F., Byk, G., Gilon, C. and Kessler, H. (1992) Conformation of cyclic analogues of substance P: NMR and molecular dynamics in dimethyl sulfoxide. *J. Am. Chem. Soc.*, **114**, 4818–4827.

Schmidhammer, H. (1998) Opioid receptor antagonists. *Prog. Med. Chem.*, **35**, 83–132.

Schulz, G.E. and Schirmer, R.H. (1979) *Principles of Protein Structure*. New York: Springer-Verlag.

Schmidt, B., Lindman, S., Tong, W., Lindeberg, G., Gogoll, A., Lai, Z., Thörnwall, M., Synnergren, B., Nilsson, A., Welch, C.J., Sohtell, M., Westerlund, C., Nyberg, F., Karlén, A. and Hallberg, A. (1997) Design, synthesis and biological activities of four angiotensin II receptor ligands with γ-turn mimetics replacing amino acid residues 3–5. *J. Med. Chem.*, **40**, 903–919.

Schmitz, R. (1985) Friedrich Wilhelm Sertürner and the discovery of morphine. *Pharmacy in History*, **27**, 61–74.

Spatola, A.F. (1983) Peptide backbone modifications: a structure–activity analysis of peptides containing amide bond surrogates, conformational constraints, and related backbone replacements. In *Chemistry and Biochemistry of Amino Acids, Peptides, and Proteins*, Vol. VII, edited by B. Weinstein, pp. 267–357, New York: Marcel Dekker.

Toniolo, C. (1990) Conformationally restricted peptides through short-range cyclizations. *Int. J. Peptide Protein Res.*, **35**, 287–300.

Wiley, R.A. and Rich, D.H. (1993) Peptidomimetics derived from natural products. *Med. Res. Rev.*, **13**, 327–384.

Zhang, B., Salituro, G., Szalkowski, D., Li, Z., Zhang, Y., Royo, I., Vilella, D., Diez, M.T., Pelaez, F., Ruby, C., Kendall, R.L., Mao, X., Griffin, P., Calaycay, J., Zierath, J.R., Heck, J.V., Smith, R.G. and Moller, D.E. (1999) Discovery of small molecule insulin mimetic with antidiabetic activity in mice. *Science*, **284**, 974–977.

Chapter 16

Classical antiviral agents and design of new antiviral agents

Piet Herdewijn and Erik de Clercq

16.1 CLASSICAL ANTIVIRAL AGENTS

16.1.1 Introduction

More than 50 years have elapsed since the discovery of the first antiviral agents, i.e. methisazone and 5-iodo-2′-deoxyuridine. In contrast to the evolution in other fields, the antiviral chemotherapy has evolved very slowly at the start. The reasons therefore are multiple:

- close association between the replicative cycle of the virus and the metabolism of the cell;
- the intracellular location of the virus;
- viruses possess considerable fewer virus-associated or -encoded enzymes than bacteria;
- effective vaccines have been developed for the prevention of some severe viral infections; and
- antiviral research is a high-risk enterprise for industry.

However, the interest in antiviral chemotherapy has been boosted considerably since the identification, now more than 15 years ago, of HIV (human immuno deficiency virus) as the causative agent of the acquired immune deficiency syndrome (AIDS).

Viral infections can vary from mild and transient to severe and irreversible, and occasionally lead to death. Viral infections can cause chronic degenerative disease and are also implicated in various forms of cancer in man. Many viral infections, even if not life-threatening, have an important socio-economic impact.

The classical antiviral agents that are, at present, used in the clinic have all evolved from random screening and serendipity. The rational design of antivirals is a relatively new approach and has mainly been used in the anti-HIV field and more recently in the anti-HCV (hepatitis C virus) field. All antiviral agents depend for their activity on interactions with the virus-encoded enzymes. Progress in the molecular biology of viral–host interaction has uncovered new targets for antiviral chemotherapy, and thus, compounds with a different chemical structure. In the first part of this chapter, an overview is given of classical antiviral agents. In the second part, more recent developments in antiviral drug design are summarized.

(16.1)
5'-Iodo-2'-deoxyuridine

(16.2)
Thymidine

(16.3)
Zidovudine

5-Iodo-2'-deoxyuridine (IdUrd, IDU) (**16.1**) has a structure that is very similar to that of the natural nucleoside thymidine (**16.2**). The van der Waals radius of an iodo group is somewhat larger than that of a methyl group, and the pKa of 5-iodouracil, the 6-membered heterocyclic unit of 16.1, is about 1.5 units lower than that of thymine, the corresponding heterocyclic unit of 16.2. This results from the inductive effect of the iodo group in the 5-position. These slight differences are apparently sufficient for IdUrd to become a rather selective antiviral agent. W.H. Prusoff synthesized IdUrd first in 1959 by iodination of 2'-deoxyuridine with iodine/nitric acid. IdUrd is active against the multiplication of *Herpes simplex* virus type 1 (HSV-1), *Herpes simplex* virus type 2 (HSV-2) and vaccinia virus (VV) *in vitro* and has proven efficacious in the treatment of herpes eye infections (i.e. herpetic keratitis). Its toxicity, however, does not allow systemic use.

Also there is a great resemblance in the structures of thymidine and 3'-azido-3'-deoxythymidine (zidovudine, AZT) (**16.3**). Here, the 3'-position is substituted with an azido group. This compound was the first to be approved by the FDA for the treatment of AIDS patients. J.P. Horwitz synthesized it first in 1964 starting from thymidine. Also, the modes of action of IdUrd and zidovudine are quite similar. They have to be metabolized intracellularly to their 5'-triphosphate derivatives and these triphosphates then interact with (viral) DNA synthesis.

These two nucleoside analogs (IDU and AZT), which resemble very well their natural counterpart, have had a tremendous impact on antiviral research. IDU has long been a model compound for the design of new and more selective antiherpes agents. The advent of AIDS, the identification of a retrovirus as the causative agent of the disease and the observation that its replication can be blocked by simple nucleosides, gave an important incentive to the search for new antiviral agents.

In this chapter, we will see how selectivity can be obtained by interference with virus-specific targets. The identification of specific, virus-encoded, enzymes has proved the key step in the design of new antiviral compounds.

In the design of new nucleoside analogs, targeted at viral DNA synthesis, the discovery of HPMPC [(S)-1-(3-hydroxy-2-phosphonylmethoxypropyl)cytosine] (**16.4**) and PMPA [(R)-9-(2-phosphonylmethoxypropyl)adenine] (**16.5**) as potent inhibitors of CMV (cytomegalo virus) and HIV, respectively, could be considered as important progress. Their antiviral activity clearly indicates that mimicking nucleoside metabolites, e.g. nucleoside monophosphates, can overcome at least

(16.4)   (16.5)

the first step of intracellular phosphorylation. It also proves that such phosphonate analogs can be taken up by the cell sufficiently well to exhibit their antiviral action. This brings us one step nearer to the target (viral DNA) site.

Nucleosides are naturally occurring molecules, which play a crucial role in cell multiplication and function. As a consequence, cells contain a whole battery of enzymes for the anabolism and catabolism of nucleosides. All of these enzymes are potential targets for the action of the modified nucleosides, and this can lead to premature death of the cell. Especially the interaction of the inhibitor with normal cellular DNA may be hazardous in that it could lead to mutagenicity, carcinogenicity or teratogenicity. Moreover, good *in vitro* antiviral activity not necessarily predicts equivalent *in vivo* activity. These considerations make the design of new nucleoside antivirals both a difficult and challenging task.

16.1.2 Base-modified pyrimidine nucleosides as antiherpes agents

The intracellular metabolism and mode of action of IdUrd (**16.1**) can be presented as follows (Scheme 16.1):

IdUrd can be phosphorylated by both cellular and virus-encoded thymidine kinases (i). However, IdUrd is phosphorylated more efficiently by the HSV-encoded thymidine kinase than by the cellular thymidine kinase, which explains its (modest) selectivity as an antiherpes agent. IdUrd 5'-monophosphate is then phosphorylated to the diphosphate (ii) and triphosphate (iii). IdUrd can be incorporated in both cellular and viral DNA. This incorporation impairs the subsequent transcription and replication processes and is believed to be the major reason for the activity and toxicity of IdUrd. As also evident from the above reaction scheme (Scheme 16.1), IdUrd (**16.1**) is a substrate for thymidine phosphorylase (iv) and for thymidylate synthase (v). Both processes lead to deactivation (of IdUrd). Together with the feedback inhibition of the phosphorylated products on the regulatory enzymes of nucleotide biosynthesis, the general biochemical reaction scheme as depicted for IdUrd also holds for most other pyrimidine nucleoside analogs, and could explain their antiviral activity and toxicity.

A crucial enzyme in the anabolism of pyrimidine 2'-deoxynucleosides is the thymidine kinase, which phosphorylates the nucleoside to its 5'-monophosphate derivative. Some herpes viruses (i.e. HSV-1, HSV-2) and also *Varicella-zoster* virus

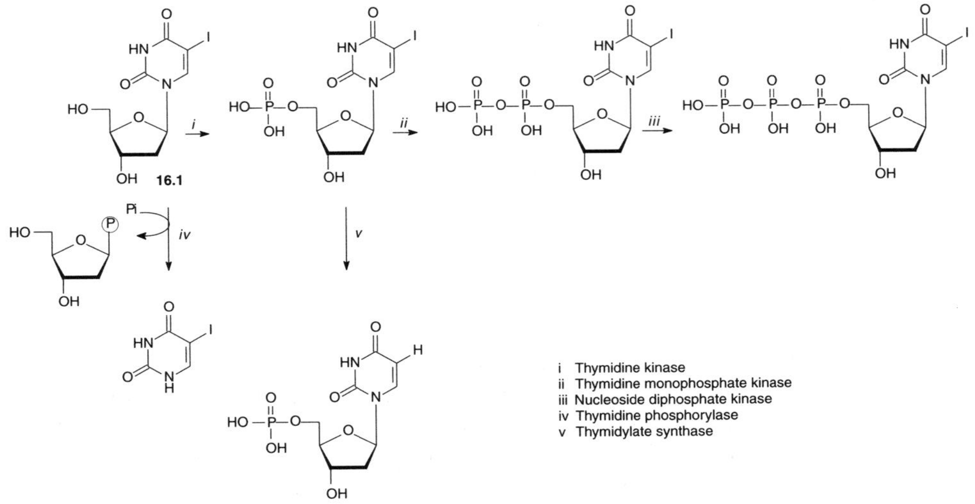

Scheme 16.1

i   Thymidine kinase
ii Thymidine monophosphate kinase
iii Nucleoside diphosphate kinase
iv Thymidine phosphorylase
v   Thymidylate synthase

(VZV) encode for their own thymidine kinase. Introduction of a substituent in the 5-position of the pyrimidine ring has led to compounds with higher affinity for the virus-encoded enzyme than for the cellular enzyme, and thus greater selectivity as antiviral agents. Pertinent examples of this 'second' generation of antiviral compounds are 5-ethyl-2′-deoxyuridine (EtdUrd) (**16.6**) and, even more so, 5-(*E*)-bromovinyl-2′-deoxyuridine (BVdUrd, BVDU) (**16.7**).

There is a marked difference in the phosphorylation capacity of the thymidine kinases of different herpes viruses. While the HSV-1-encoded thymidine kinase is capable of converting BVdUrd to its 5′-monophosphate and further onto its 5′-diphosphate, the HSV-2-encoded thymidine kinase is unable to further phosphorylate BVdUrd monophosphate onto its diphosphate. This differential behavior in phosphorylation may explain the differences found in the activity of BVdUrd against HSV-1 and HSV-2. The mode of binding of BVdUrd to the HSV-1 thymidine kinase has been determined (Figure 16.1). The 3-NH and 4-CO groups of the pyrimidine moiety interact with Gln-125. The bulky 5-substituent occupies a pocket available in the neighborhood of residues Trp-88, Tyr-132, Arg-163 and Ala-167. A change in conformation of one residue (Tyr-132) is needed for accommodation of the bromovinyl group. The binding mode of the deoxyribose moiety of BVdUrd is similar to that of dThd.

The BVdUrd and EtdUrd can also be incorporated into DNA. Because of the specific phosphorylation of EtdUrd and BVdUrd by the virus-infected cells, only the virus-infected cells that have allowed phosphorylation of the compounds will be sensitive to their eventual antiviral action (following incorporation into DNA).

The BVdUrd is superior in potency to any other antiherpes agent against both HSV-1 and VZV infections, i.e. it is 1000-fold more active *in vitro* against VZV than acyclovir, the most commonly used drug for the treatment of VZV infections. The VZV is responsible for primary (varicella or chickenpox) and recurrent (zoster and

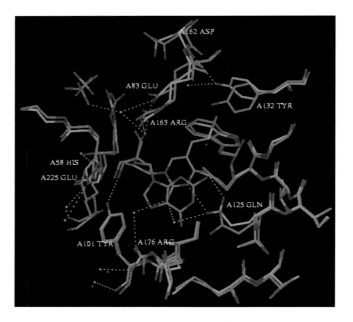

(16.6)　　　　　(16.7)　　　　　(16.8)　　　　　(16.9)

Figure 16.1 Binding of BrvdUrd and acyclovir (**16.11**) in the active site of the thymidine kinase (TK) of *Herpes simplex* virus type 1. The pyrimidine moiety of BrvdUrd has an orientation different from that of the guanine moiety of acyclovir. Intermolecular hydrogen bonding is shown for the TK/BrvdUrd complex.

shingles) infections, following reactivation of the virus. BVdUrd (brivudin) is currently the most potent antiviral agent on the market for the treatment of VZV infections.

The IdUrd monophosphate can be dehalogenated by thymidylate synthase to give dUrd monophosphate (Scheme 16.1), which is the natural substrate for the enzyme. Thymidylate synthase is responsible for the conversion of dUrd monophosphate to dThd monophosphate using N^5, N^{10}-methylenetetrahydrofolic acid as methyl donor. This is the key enzyme in the *de novo* biosynthesis of the dThd metabolites (Scheme 16.2).

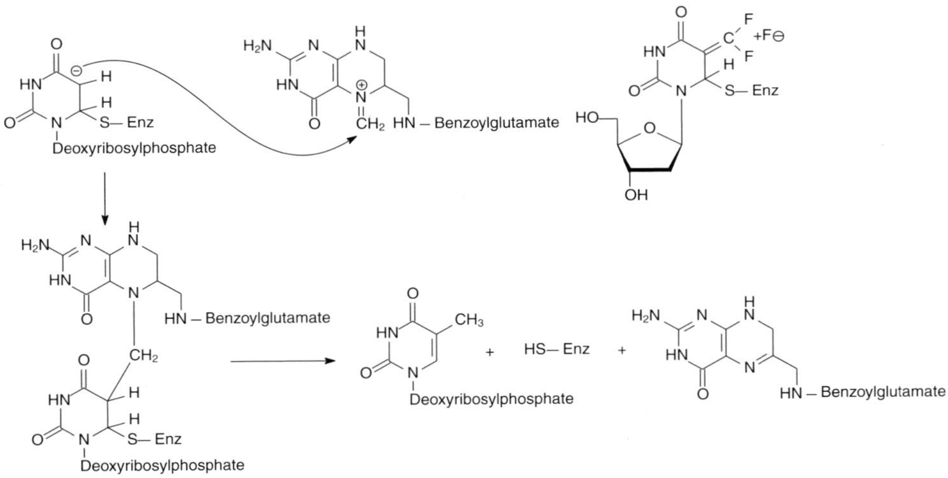

Scheme 16.2

When the iodo group of IdUrd (**16.1**) is replaced by a strong electron withdrawing substituent (X), which forms a stable C–X bond, the compound could inhibit thymidylate synthase without functioning as a substrate. This is the case for 5-fluoro-2'-deoxyuridine (**16.8**) and 5-trifluoromethyl-2'-deoxyuridine (**16.9**). The pK$_a$ of 5-fluorouracil is 8.04, as compared to 7.35 for 5-trifluoromethyluracil and 9.94 for thymine, the 6-membered heterocyclic unit containing a methyl group in the 5-position. While 5-fluorouracil is used in cancer chemotherapy, 5-trifluoromethyl-2'-deoxyuridine (F$_3$dThd, TFT) (**16.9**) is used for the topical treatment of herpetic keratitis.

F$_3$dThd (**16.9**) is phosphorylated by viral and cellular kinases to the monophosphate and further to the di- and triphosphate. Here again, phosphorylation is more efficient in HSV-infected than uninfected cells. Incorporation into DNA occurs and could contribute to the antiviral activity of F$_3$dThd. However, F$_3$dThd owes its antiviral activity mainly to the inhibition of thymidylate synthase. The mode of action of F$_3$dThd can be explained by assuming a nucleophilic attack of the enzyme at the 6-position of the heterocyclic base, which leads to the generation of a reactive difluoromethylene at the 5-position (Scheme 16.2). This enzyme is an interesting target for those viruses, which do not encode for a functional thymidine kinase. These viruses must rely on the *de novo* biosynthesis of dThd monophosphate starting from *N*-carbamoylaspartate to form the necessary quantities of dThd triphosphate that are needed for their own DNA synthesis.

16.1.3 Sugar-modified purine nucleosides

9-(β-D-Arabinofuranosyl)adenine (ara-A) (**16.10**) is a naturally occurring nucleoside, which was synthesized 8 years before it was isolated. Ara-A is an antiviral agent with a multiple mode of action. Theoretically, drugs that have multiple modes of action are most likely to avoid drug-virus resistance but, they may also have the highest risk for toxic side effects. The relative role of the different actions in the overall antiviral activity of ara-A is not well known. Ara-A is phosphorylated to its monophosphate and further to its di- and triphosphate. This triphosphate inhibits DNA polymerases, which could explain the activity of ara-A against DNA viruses. Ara-A can also be incorporated into both host cell DNA and viral DNA. Furthermore, ara-A inhibits methyltransferase reactions presumably through inhibition of S-adenosylhomocysteine hydrolase and accumulation of S-adenosylhomocysteine. The latter acts as a product inhibitor of transmethylation reactions such as those involved in the maturation of viral mRNA. Ara-A has been used for the treatment of HSV-1 encephalitis and *Herpes zoster* in immunocompromised patients, but is now surpassed by acyclovir for this purpose. A major disadvantage of ara-A is that it is promptly deaminated *in vivo* by adenosine deaminase, converting the amino group into an oxo group. The resulting hypoxanthine analog has markedly reduced antiviral activity as compared to ara-A.

The search for inhibitors of the adenosine deamination reaction has led to the discovery at the Wellcome Research Laboratories of 9-(2-hydroxyethoxymethyl) guanine (acyclovir) (**16.11**) as an antiviral agent. This compound, whose action is surprisingly similar to that of the aforementioned pyrimidine nucleoside analogs, has oriented research in the direction of the acyclic nucleoside analogs. This research has yielded a number of active congeners, i.e. 9-(1,3-dihydroxy-2-propoxymethyl)guanine (ganciclovir) (**16.12**) and penciclovir (**16.13**). As of today, acyclovir has remained the 'gold' standard for the treatment of HSV infections, whereas ganciclovir is used in the treatment of CMV infections, and both penciclovir (as its prodrug form, famciclovir) and acyclovir (as its prodrug form, valaciclovir) for the treatment of VZV infections.

All of these compounds can be considered as analogs of 2′-deoxyguanosine or carbocyclic 2′-deoxyguanosine (*vide infra*) from which the 2′-carbon (ganciclovir, penciclovir) or both the 2′- and 3′-carbons (acyclovir) have been deleted. The antiviral activity of acyclovir was discovered by accident, whereas ganciclovir (**16.12**) was the result of a structure–activity design starting from acyclovir as the model compound. From a structural viewpoint, ganciclovir is more closely related to 2′-deoxyguanosine than is acyclovir.

The antiviral activity of acyclovir (**16.11**) can be explained by the same biochemical reaction scheme as presented for IdUrd (Scheme 16.1). There are, however, subtle differences that explain the greater selectivity of acyclovir. Acyclovir is phosphorylated to its monophosphate by a virus-specific thymidine/deoxycytidine kinase, which actually recognizes acyclovir as a deoxycytidine analog. Viruses, which encode for such an enzyme (HSV-1, HSV-2, VZV, but not CMV) are susceptible to the antiviral action of acyclovir. Although the natural substrates for this enzyme are pyrimidine nucleosides, it apparently accepts purine derivatives as substrates. The structure of the complex of HSV-1 thymidine kinase with acyclovir, ganciclovir and penciclovir has been determined by X-ray crystallography. The guanine moiety of all three compounds lay in a similar location, with hydrogen bond pairing being made with Gln-125 via the 1-NH and 6-CO groups (Figure 16.1). In uninfected cells, phosphorylation occurs to a limited extent. The monophosphate of acyclovir is phosphorylated to the diphosphate by GMP kinase and further to its triphosphate by various cellular enzymes. The triphosphate of

(16.10)
Ara-A

(16.11)
Acyclovir

(16.12)
Ganciclovir

(16.13)
Penciclovir

acyclovir is a competitive inhibitor of dGTP for the viral DNA polymerase and can also function as a substrate resulting in the incorporation of acyclovir into DNA and chain termination. Acyclovir is given orally or intravenously in the treatment of HSV and VZV infections, and topically in the treatment of HSV infections (i.e. herpetic keratitis and herpes labialis). For oral use, acyclovir, because of its limited oral bioavailability is now substituted by its oral prodrug form, valaciclovir.

As compared to acyclovir, ganciclovir (**16.12**) is more easily phosphorylated in CMV-infected cells by the virus-encoded (UL 97) protein kinase and its triphosphate has a five-fold greater affinity than ACV (acyclovir) triphosphate for CMV DNA polymerase. Ganciclovir can be incorporated both internally and at the 3′-terminal end of DNA. Ganciclovir is active against HSV-1, HSV-2, VZV, CMV and EBV. It is fairly toxic for the bone marrow (neutropenia). Its clinical use is restricted to the treatment of CMV infections in immunocompromised patients.

Penciclovir (**16.13**) has the same antiviral spectrum as acyclovir. As compared to acyclovir, penciclovir leads to higher triphosphate concentrations in virus-infected cells and its antiviral activity persists for a longer time after removal of the compound. In fact, after removal of acyclovir, antiviral activity rapidly disappears. Not only penciclovir, but also BVdUrd (**16.7**) and ganciclovir (**16.12**) show persistent antiviral activity after the drugs have been removed from the medium. This is due to the greater stability of their triphosphates as compared to that of acyclovir triphosphate.

16.1.4   Ribavirin

In contrast with the preceding compounds, ribavirin (**16.14**) has a broad spectrum activity against RNA and DNA viruses both *in vitro* and *in vivo*. R.K. Robins first synthesized ribavirin. The structural requirements for the broad-spectrum antiviral activity of ribavirin are very stringent. The compound shows its greatest potency against myxo (influenza) and paramyxo (respiratory syncytial) virus infections. Ribavirin also shows activity against some hemorrhagic fever viruses such as Lassa, Machupo, Pichinde, Rift Valley and Hantaviruses. Therapeutic efficacy has been demonstrated with ribavirin, given as a small-particle aerosol, in infants suffering from respiratory syncytial virus (RSV) infection. The compound has been approved for the treatment of RSV infections, as well as human hepatitis C virus (HCV) infections, for the latter only in combination with interferons.

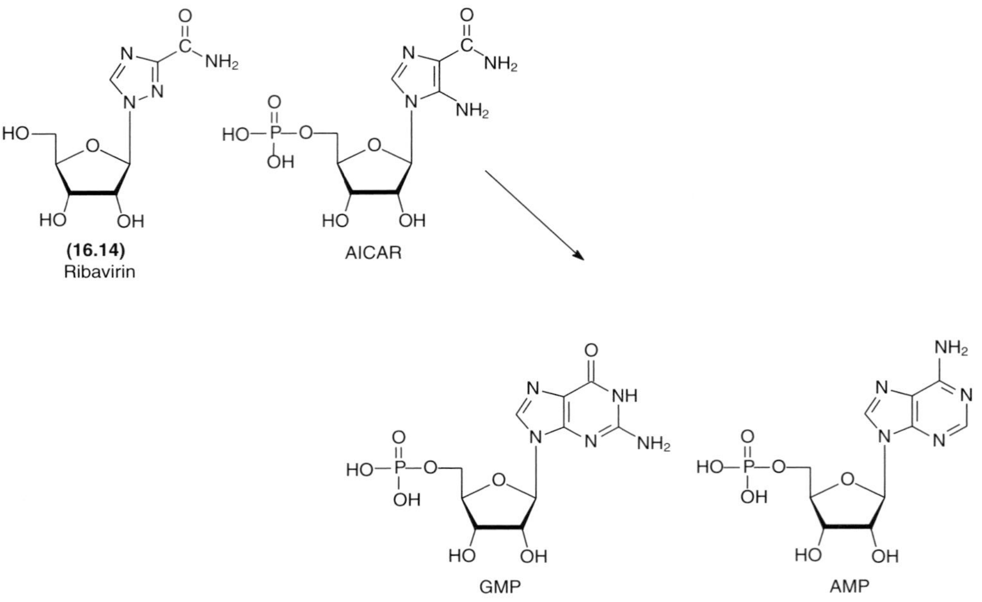

Scheme 16.3

The mode of action of ribavirin is multipronged and may also vary from one virus to another. Ribavirin (5′-monophosphate) can be considered as an analog of AICAR (Scheme 16.3) which is a precursor of both AMP and GMP.

As has been elucidated by X-ray crystallography studies, there is a nice resemblence between ribavirin and guanosine; by rotating the amide group, also good resemblence is found between ribavirin and adenosine (Scheme 16.3).

16.1.5 Compounds which inhibit the replication of the human immunodeficiency virus (HIV)

Human immunodeficiency virus is a retrovirus, which means that, once it has infected the cell, its genomic RNA is transcribed to proviral DNA by a virus-specific enzyme (the RT). This enzyme has a broader substrate specificity than cellular DNA polymerases, and has since long been recognized as a target for antiviral chemotherapy. Here, the task to design specific antiviral agents is somewhat more difficult than for herpes viruses, since HIV does not encode for a virus-specific kinase which could confine the metabolism of the nucleoside analogs to the virus-infected cells.

Fifteen compounds have now been approved for the treatment of HIV infection from which zidovudine (**16.3**) was the first one. Nine of them are targeted at the viral RT and the other six are targeted at the viral protease. Among the reverse transcriptase inhibitors, six are nucleoside analogs (zidovudine (**16.3**)) didanosine (**16.15**), zalcitabine (**16.16**), stavudine (**16.17**), lamivudine (**16.18**), abacavir (**16.19**). These dideoxynucleoside analogs must be phosphorylated through

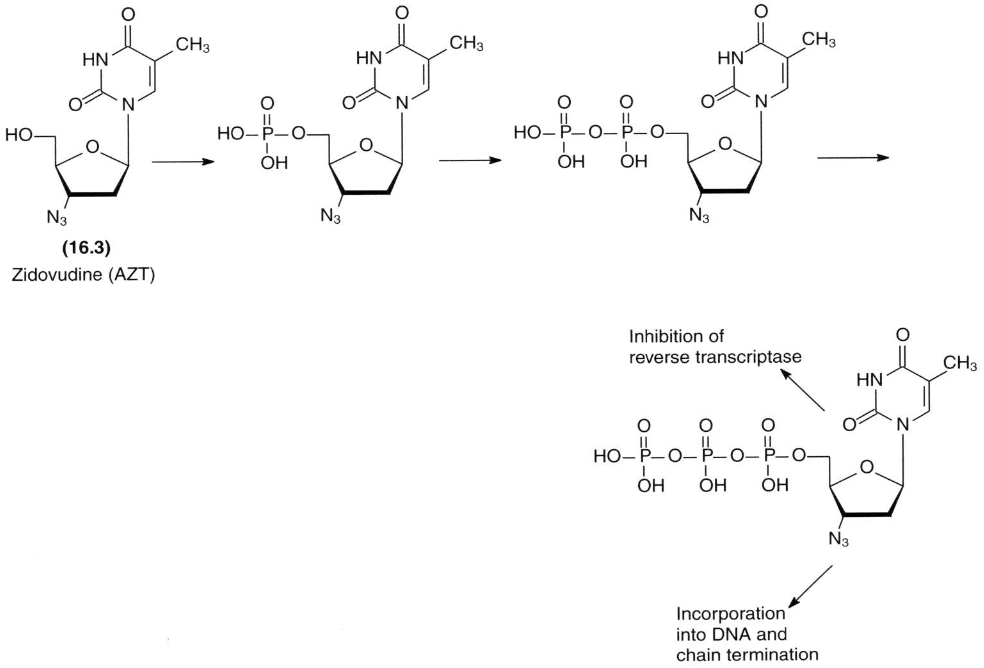

(16.3)
Zidovudine (AZT)

Inhibition of
reverse transcriptase

Incorporation
into DNA and
chain termination

Scheme 16.4

three consecutive kinase reactions to the triphosphate form before they can interact as competitive inhibitors with respect to the natural substrates at the RT. The intracellular metabolism of dideoxynucleosides is dependent on the type of compound, the type of cell and the anabolic state of the cells.

Zidovudine is phosphorylated by the cellular thymidine kinase to its 5'-mono-phosphate (Scheme 16.4). This 5'-monophosphate is then phosphorylated to the di- and triphosphate by thymidylate kinase and, subsequently, nucleoside-5'-diphosphate kinase, respectively. As the efficiency of conversion of zidovudine-5'-monophosphate to its diphosphate by thymidylate kinase is much lower than the efficiency of phosphorylation of the natural substrate, zidovudine-5'-mono-phosphate accumulates in the cells. In its triphosphate form, AZT is a more efficient inhibitor of the RT than of the cellular DNA polymerases. The AZT is incorporated into DNA and functions as a chain terminator.

The active metabolite of didanosine (**16.15**) is dideoxyadenosine-5'-triphosphate. Didanosine is first converted to dideoxyinosine-5'-monophosphate. Through a sequential action of adenylosuccinate synthetase and lyase, dideoxyadenosine-5'-monophosphate is formed which is further converted to the above mentioned triphosphate. Stavudine (**16.17**) is less efficiently phosphorylated to its 5'-mono-phosphate than zidovudine but readily proceeds from its monophosphate onto its di- and triphosphate so that equivalent levels of the active metabolites (5'-triphos-phates) are attained into the cells. Zalcitabine (**16.16**), lamivudine (**16.18**) and

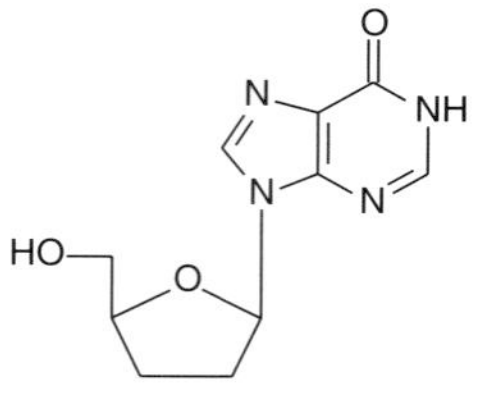

(16.15)
Didanosine

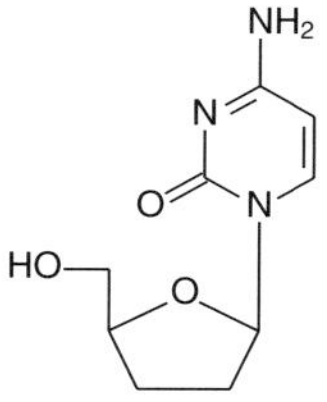

(16.16)
Zalcitabine

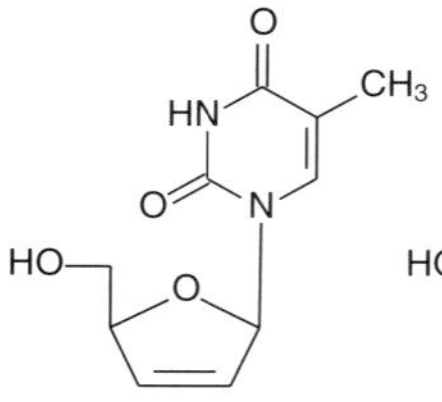

(16.17)
Stavudine

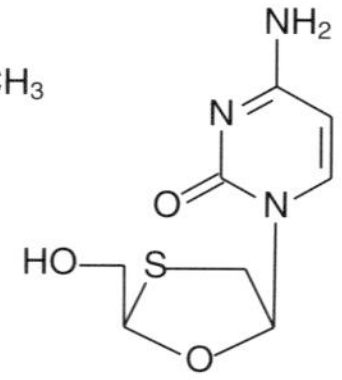

(16.18)
Lamivudine

abacavir (**16.19**) are also converted intracellularly to their active triphosphates. All these triphosphates inhibit DNA polymerase α, β and γ to a lesser extent than RT and, once incorporated, all these nucleosides function as chain terminators. As a rule, the relative ability of the dideoxynucleoside analogs to generate 5′-triphosphates intracellularly is of greater importance in determining the eventual capacity to block HIV replication than the relative abilities of the resultant triphosphates to inhibit the viral RT.

Abacavir is phosphorylated by adenosine phosphotransferase to abacavir monophosphate, which is then converted by a cytosolic deaminase to carbovir monophosphate before being further processed to the di- and triphosphate of carbovir (the guanine analog of abacavir) (scheme 16.5). This intracellular activation pathway enables abacavir to overcome the pharmacokinetic and toxicological deficiencies of carbovir while maintaining potent and selective anti-HIV activity.

The NNRTIs nevirapine (**16.20**), delavirdine (**16.21**) and efavirenz (**16.22**) block the HIV-1 RT reaction through interaction with an allosterically located, non-substrate binding 'pocket' site. This binding pocket is located at about 10 Å distance from the substrate-binding site. The binding of an NNRTI and NRTI (nucleoside reverse transcriptase inhibitor) to the RT is a co-operative process, and this might explain the synergistic effect of both types of inhibitors when used in combination.

Several studies have revealed a common mode of binding for the different NNRTIs with their target site at the HIV-1 RT. The NNRTIs cause a repositioning of the three-stranded β-sheet in the p66 subunit (containing the catalytic aspartic acid

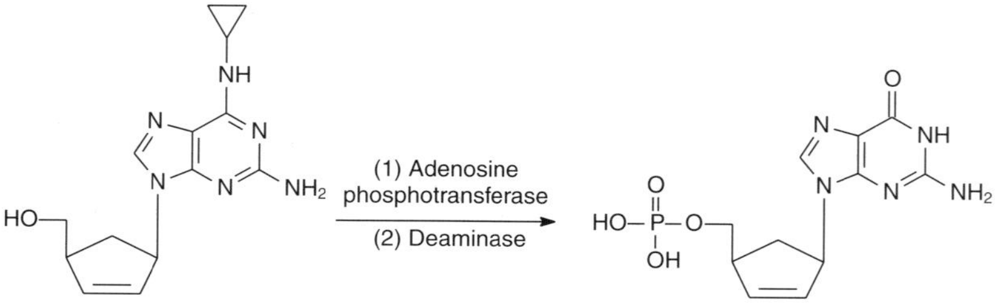

(16.19)
Abacavir

(1) Adenosine phosphotransferase

(2) Deaminase

Carbovir 5′-O-monophosphate

Scheme 16.5

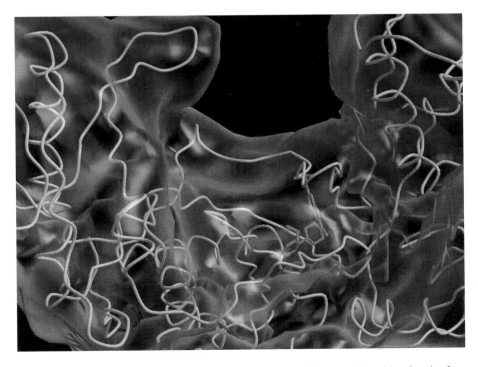

(16.20)
Nevirapine

(16.21)
Delavirdine

(16.22)
Efavirenz

residues 110, 185 and 186). This suggests that the NNRTIs inhibit HIV-1 RT by locking the active catalytic site in an inactive conformation. As an example, the binding of delavirdine to HIV-1 RT is described (Figure 16.2). Delavirdine is hydrogen-bonded to the main chain of Lys-103 and extensively interact with Pro-236 by hydrophobic contacts. Part of delavirdine protrudes into the solvent creating a channel between Pro-236 and the polypeptide segments 225–226 and 105–106.

The HIV protease inhibitors [saquinavir (**16.23**), ritonavir (**16.24**), indinavir (**16.25**) (Figure 16.3), nelfinavir (**16.26**), amprenavir (**16.27**) and lopinavir (**16.28**) prevent the cleavage of the gag and gag-pol precursor polyproteins to the functional proteins (p17, p24, p7, p6, p2, p1, protease, RT, integrase), thus arresting maturation

Figure 16.2 Mode of binding of delavirdine (**16.21**) to HIV RT. Colors used are blue for the fingers, yellow for the palm, red for the thumb domain and gray for the rest.

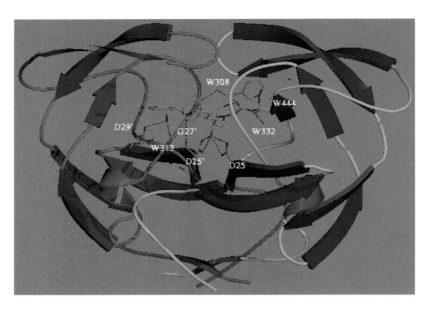

Figure 16.3 Structure of HIV-1 protease in complex with indinavir (**16.25**).

(16.23)
Saquinavir

(16.24)
Ritonavir

(16.25)
Indinavir

(16.26)
Nelfinavir

(16.27)
Amprenavir

(16.28)
Lopinavir

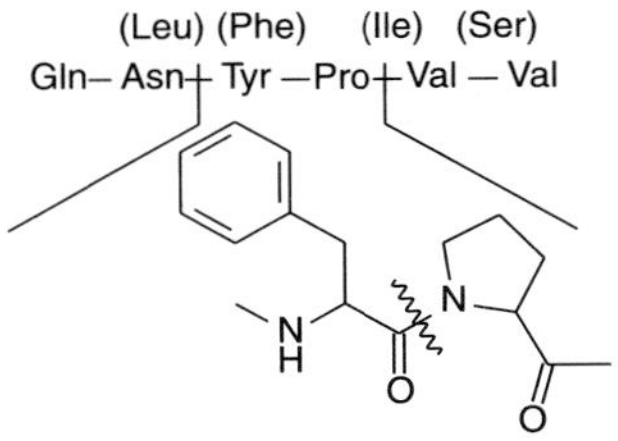

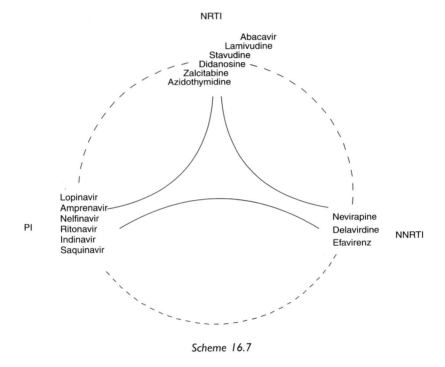

Phenylalanine-Proline cleavage site of HIV-protease
in the gag-pol polyprotein

Scheme 16.6

Scheme 16.7

and thereby blocking infectivity of the nascent virions. The HIV protease inhibitors have been tailored after the target peptidic linkage in the gag and gag-pol polyproteins that need to be cleaved by the viral protease, i.e. the phenylalanine-proline sequence at positions 167 and 168 of the gag-pol polyprotein.

All protease inhibitors that are currently licensed for the treatment of HIV infection, are peptidomimetics where the carbonyl group of the peptide bond is substituted by an hydroxyethylene group (Scheme 16.6).

Synergistic anti-HIV activity is observed when NRTIs are combined with other NRTIs or NNRTIs or with protease inhibitors (PIs). This treatment regimen allows the individual compounds to be used at lower doses and, in preventing virus break-through, they also prevent the virus from becoming resistant to the compounds.

Combination of NRTIs, NNRTIs and PIs (Scheme 16.7) have been found to decrease HIV viral load, to increase CD4 count and to decrease mortality and delay disease progression, particularly in AIDS patients with advanced immune suppression. When initiated during early asymptomatic HIV infection, highly active anti-retroviral therapy (HAART) initiates rapid reversal of disease-induced T-cell activation, while preserving pretherapy levels of immune function, suggesting that therapeutic benefit may be gained from early aggressive anti-HIV chemotherapy.

16.2 DESIGN OF NEW ANTIVIRAL AGENTS

16.2.1 Nucleoside prodrugs

The activity of a compound *in vivo* is highly dependent on the formulation in which the compound is presented. Active research is focused on developing prodrugs with optimal bioavailability. Apart from the classical approach of using esters as prodrugs, other approaches are based on the knowledge of the different enzymes involved in nucleoside metabolism. One of the oldest examples in the nucleoside field is the use of ara-A 5′-monophosphate (**16.29**) (Scheme 16.8). Ara-A has a very low solubility in water (approximately 0.5 mg/ml). Administration of ara-A by infusion requires large volumes (2 liter for an adult person). The greater solubility of ara-A monophosphate permits the use of smaller infusion volumes.

Another enzyme which has proved valuable in the prodrug design is xanthine oxidase. Guanine nucleosides are very insoluble in water because of the strong intermolecular associations through hydrogen bonds and stacking between the base moieties. As a consequence, compounds such as acyclovir (**16.11**) are quite insoluble in body fluids. The 6-deoxy analog of acyclovir (desiclovir) (**16.31**) is more soluble and is metabolized *in vivo* by xanthine oxidase to acyclovir. When administered orally, 6-deoxyacyclovir gives the same blood levels of acyclovir as those obtained with intravenous acyclovir. An analogous approach has also proved successful for ganciclovir (**16.12**). The diacetyl derivative of the 6-deoxy analog of ganciclovir (**16.30**) gives peak plasma concentrations after 1 h which are tenfold higher than those detected following an equivalent oral dose of ganciclovir. This prodrug (**16.30**) has been given the name of famciclovir, which has been launched for the systemic (i.e. oral) treatment of HSV and VZV infections.

Abacavir (**16.19**) is another example of a prodrug form of a purine nucleoside. This compound is intracellularly activated to (−)-carbovir triphosphate, as mentioned above.

The therapeutic armamentarium of acyclic anti-HSV and anti-VZV nucleosides has been extended to the L-valyl ester of acyclovir (valaciclovir) (**16.32**). This drug is a prodrug of acyclovir, and has been developed because of the low oral bioavailability of the parent compound. It is used for the systemic (i.e. oral) treatment of HSV and VZV infections. Valaciclovir is absorbed through a stereospecific transporter of the intestine cells and is rapidly hydrolyzed upon absorption, yielding acyclovir.

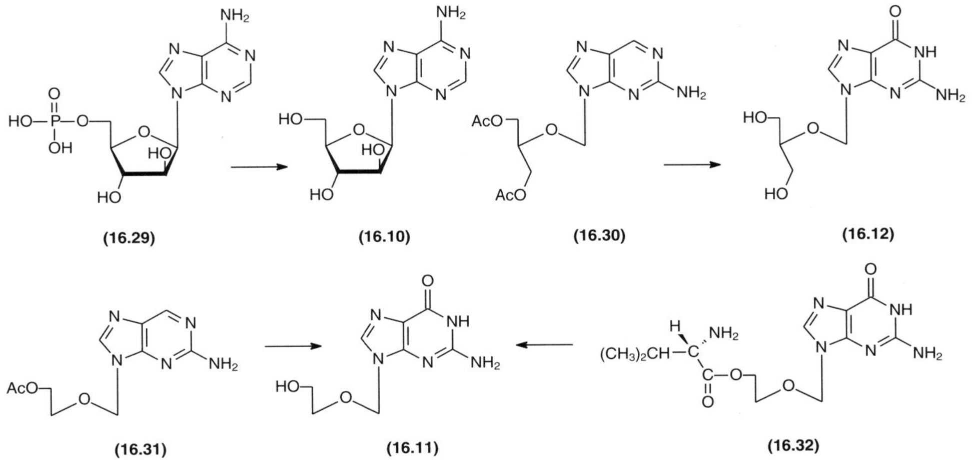

(16.29) (16.10) (16.30) (16.12)

(16.31) (16.11) (16.32)

Scheme 16.8

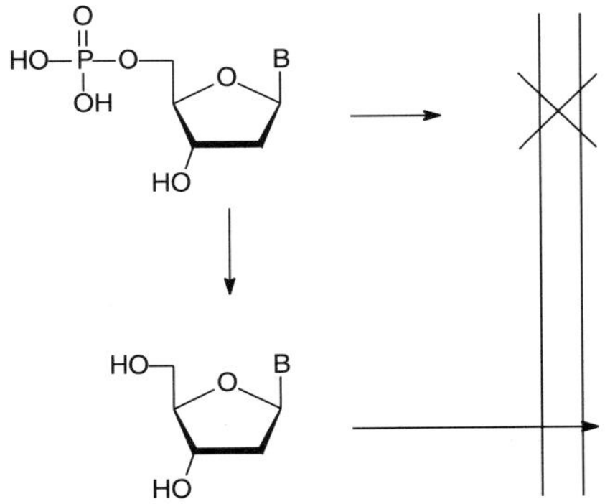

Scheme 16.9

16.2.2 Analogs of 5′-monophosphates and nucleotide prodrugs

As most, if not all, nucleosides need to be phosphorylated to exert their antiviral activity, an interesting approach would be based upon the use of the phosphorylated derivatives themselves.

The main problem associated with this approach, however, is that the phosphorylated derivatives are as such not taken up by cells (Scheme 16.9). Furthermore, 5′-*O*-phosphates of nucleosides are easily dephosphorylated by esterases which thereby release the parent nucleosides.

The cyclic monophosphate of ganciclovir (**16.33**), however, is taken up intact by the cell and opened intracellularly to the (*S*)-enantiomer of ganciclovir monophosphate (Scheme 16.10), which is then further phosphorylated to the triphosphate.

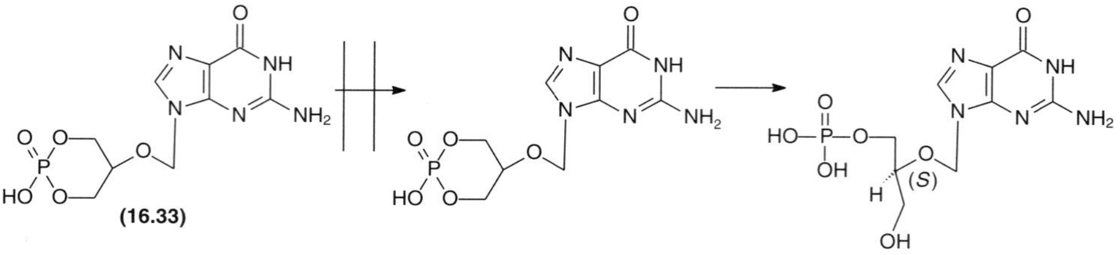

Scheme 16.10

This compound (2′-norcGMP) (**16.33**) shows a broad-spectrum activity against DNA viruses (i.e. HSV-1, HSV-2, CMV, VZV and also against TK⁻ HSV strains) *in vitro*. It is also effective orally and topically in preventing orofacial HSV-1 infection and genital HSV-2 infection in mice.

Because the first phosphorylation by nucleoside kinase is the rate-limiting step in the metabolic activation of most anti-HIV dideoxy nucleoside analogs, several prodrug strategies have been designed to bypass the nucleoside kinase step. These 'masked' nucleotides can penetrate cells and deliver the nucleoside 5′-monophosphate intracellularly. For example, the stavudine-MP prodrug (**16.34**) containing an ester at the phosphate moiety and a methyl ester of alanine linked to the phosphate through a phosphoramidate linkage, showed anti-HIV activity superior to that of stavudine (**16.17**) and, in contrast to stavudine, proved also active against HIV in thymidine kinase-deficient cells. Following intracellular uptake, the stavudine-MP triester gives rise to the formation of stavudine-MP, stavudine-DP and stavudine-TP and also to a new metabolite, alaninyl stavudine-MP, which could be considered as an intracellular depot form of stavudine and/or stavudine-MP.

A logic pursuit of this approach has led to the development of the nucleoside phosphonate derivatives. In designing such compounds, one should take into account that a glycosidic bond is *a priori* sensitive to chemical and enzymatic degradation, whereas an alkylated purine or pyrimidine base should not have this problem. Thus, a new series of purine and pyrimidine derivatives with an aliphatic side chain and a phosphonate group attached to it was developed. The first compound of this series, (*S*)-HPMPA or (*S*)-9-(3-hydroxy-2-phosphonylmethoxy-propyl)adenine (**16.35**) was conceived after another acyclic nucleoside, (*S*)-DHPA or (*S*)-9-(2,3-dihydroxypropyl)adenine (**16.36**), that had been synthesized earlier

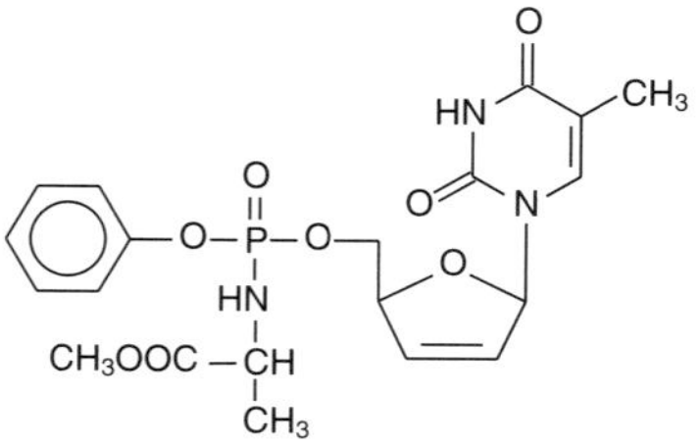

(16.34)

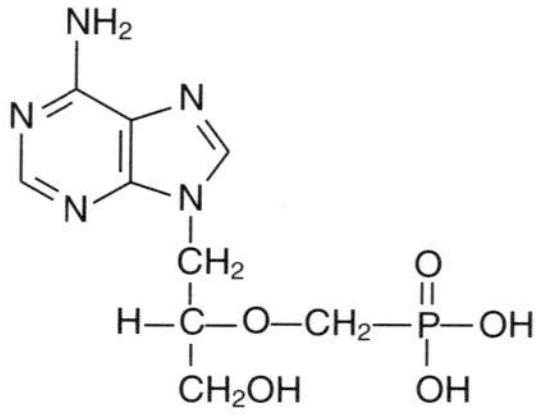

(16.35)
(*S*)-HPMPA

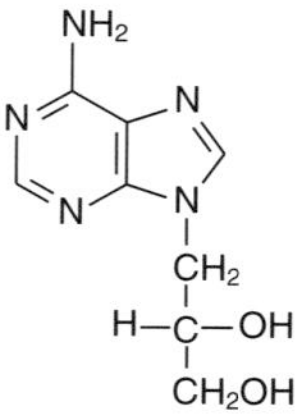

(16.36)
(*S*)-DHPA

and shown to inhibit the multiplication of several DNA viruses (i.e. vaccinia virus) and RNA viruses (i.e. vesicular stomatitis virus) *in vitro*.

(*S*)-HPMPA (**16.35**) has broad-spectrum activity against DNA viruses (i.e. HSV-1, TK⁻ HSV-1, HSV-2, VZV, TK⁻ VZV, CMV, EBV, pox- and adenoviruses). The most interesting features of this compound are, on the one hand, that it is stable against metabolic degradation but is capable of penetrating cells, thus circumventing the need for phosphorylation by dThd kinase (or other nucleoside kinases). Within the cell, (*S*)-HPMPA is further phosphorylated by cellular enzymes (i.e. AMP kinase and/or PRPP synthetase) to its diphosphoryl derivative. (*S*)-HPMPA inhibits viral DNA synthesis at a concentration which is several orders of magnitude lower than the concentration required for inhibition of cellular DNA synthesis. Three compounds, derived from (*S*)-HPMPA, show even more interesting activity: PMEA (adefovir) (**16.37**) and (*S*)-HPMPC (cidofovir) (**16.4**) and PMPA (tenofovir) (**16.5**). As PMEA (**16.37**) and PMPA (**16.5**) are not sufficiently bioavailable by the oral route, they are administered in their oral prodrug forms: *bis*(POM)PMEA (**16.38**) and *bis*(POC)PMPA (**16.39**), respectively (Scheme 16.11).

Cidofovir (HPMPC) (**16.4**) is active against herpes, adeno, polyoma, papilloma and pox viruses. Cidofovir delays progression of CMV retinitis in patients with AIDS. It has been formally licensed for this indication. Cidofovir also holds great promise for the treatment of various papilloma virus-associated lesions. The antiviral activity spectrum of adefovir is unique in that it encompasses both retroviruses and hepadnaviruses as well as herpes viruses. It could be used for the treatment of HIV and HBV infections as well as for the prophylaxis of herpes virus infections and is now primarily pursued, as its oral prodrug form (adefovir

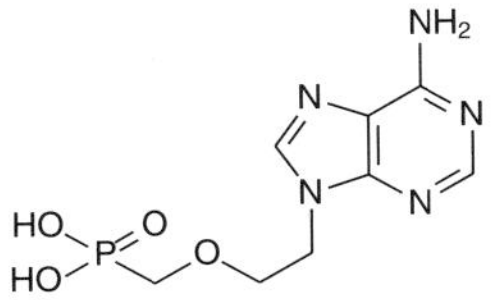

(16.37)

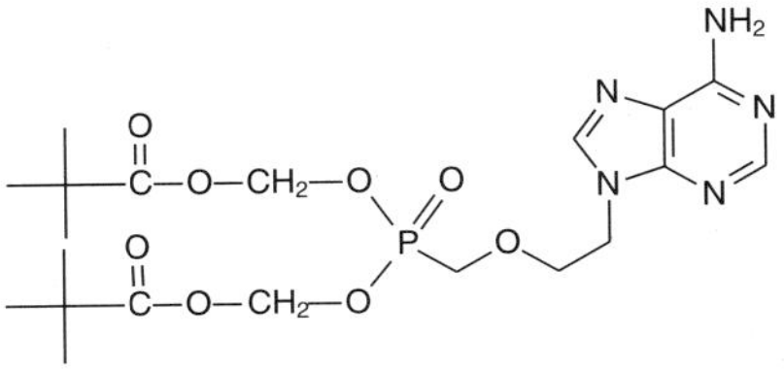

(16.38)
bis(pivaloyloxymethyl)-
9-(2-phosphonomethoxyethyl)adenine

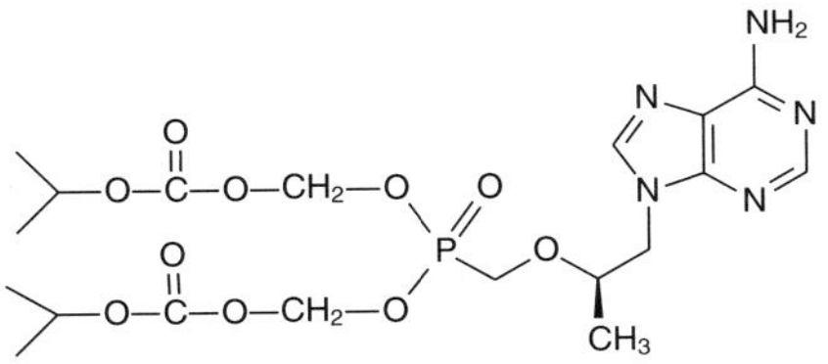

(16.39)
bis[(isopropoxycarbonyl)oxymethyl]-
(*R*)-9-(2-phosphonomethoxypropyl)adenine

Scheme 16.11

dipivoxil or bis (POM)PMEA) for the treatment of HBV infections. The activity of PMPA is confined to retroviruses and hepadnaviruses. It is pursued in its oral prodrug form (tenofovir disoxoproxil or bis(POC)PMPA), for the treatment of HIV infections.

The main advantage of the acyclic nucleoside phosphonates over the 'classical' nucleoside analogs is their prolonged antiviral action, which allows infrequent dosing, i.e. once daily for the oral formulation of adefovir and tenofovir; once weekly for intravenous or intralesional cidofovir; once daily for cidofovir if applied topically as eyedrops or gel.

16.2.3   Nucleosides with the non-natural L-configuration

All nucleosides described in the previous sections, except for **16.18** (lamivudine), possess the D-configuration. Until recently, it was generally accepted that nucleosides belonging to the L-series would not be accepted as substrates for enzymes and, thus, not active. Surprising results, however, were obtained with these 'mirror-image' nucleosides.

Dideoxycytidine (**16.16**) is very active against HIV (EC$_{50}$:0.01 µM), but is also quite toxic (CC$_{50}$:10 µM). CC$_{50}$ is defined as the concentration required to reduce cell growth by 50%. Its L-isomer (**16.40**) is slightly less active against HIV (EC$_{50}$:0.02 µM) but has markedly lower toxicity (CC$_{50}$:100 µM). This difference has also been observed with 3'-thia-2',3'-dideoxycytidine. The activity (EC$_{50}$) and toxicity (CC$_{50}$) of the compound with the 'natural' (+)-structure is 0.25 µM and 1 µM, respectively. The 'unnatural' (−)-isomer (**16.18**) is as active (0.2 µM) but less toxic (>100 µM). A striking characteristic of **16.40** and **16.18** and of their 5-fluorinated congeners (**16.41**) and (**16.42**) is that they are not only active against HIV but also HBV, which extends their potential use to the treatment of this latter disease. It has been suggested that the low toxicity of the L-series is due to the fact that these non-natural compounds are not transported into mitochondria. Part of the toxicity of the anti-HIV nucleosides zidovudine, zalcitabine and didanosine could be attributed to the inhibition of mitochondrial DNA synthesis.

16.2.4   Non-nucleoside antivirals outside the anti-HIV field

Numerous non-nucleoside compounds have been described that show *in vitro* antiviral activity against a wide variety of viruses. Some of these compounds have been marketed. Already in the fifties, methisazone (**16.43**) was mentioned for

(16.40) X = H
(16.41) X = F

(16.18) X = H
(16.42) X = F

prophylactic use against smallpox and therapeutic use against the complications of vaccinia virus vaccination.

Amantadine (**16.44**) and rimantadine (**16.45**) target the influenza A virus M2 protein, a membrane protein that is essential to virus replication. They are used in the prophylaxis and early treatment of influenza A virus infections; in this regard rimantadine is as efficacious as amantadine and less prone to toxic side effects (i.e. for the CNS). Phosphonoformic acid (PFA) (**16.46**) has been pursued for the treatment of CMV infections (particularly retinitis) in immunocompromised patients, as an alternative to ganciclovir (**16.12**) treatment, and for the treatment of TK⁻ HSV infections, also in immunocompromised patients, following resistance development to acyclovir (**16.11**).

Haemagglutinin and neuraminidase are glycoproteins that occur on the surface of influenza virus and they interact with receptors which contain terminal neuraminic acid residues. Neuraminidase destroys receptors recognized by haemagglutinin by cleaving the α-ketosidic bond linking a terminal neuraminic acid residue to the adjacent oligosaccharide moiety. One of the effects of neuraminidase inhibitors is that virions stay attached to the membrane of infected cells and to each other and virus spread is inhibited. Neuraminidase is a tetramer composed of a cytoplasmic tail, a transmembrane domain, a stalk region, and a globular head. The residues forming the active site are highly conserved among all A and B influenza viruses. Reversible competitive neuraminidase inhibitors, zanamivir (**16.47**), oseltamivir (**16.48**) and RWJ-270201 (**16.49**), inhibit replication of both influenza A and B viruses. Zanamivir is delivered by inhalation because of its low oral bioavailability whereas oseltamivir is administered orally. Early treatment with either drug reduces the severity and duration of influenza symptoms.

Interferons have been proposed for the treatment of several viral infections, i.e. due to rhinovirus, influenza virus, herpes viruses, papilloma virus, adenovirus, hepatitis B virus, hepatitis C virus and others, but their usefulness has remained

(16.43)   (16.44)   (16.45)   (16.46)

(16.47)
Zanamivir

(16.48)
Oseltamivir

(16.49)
RWJ-270201

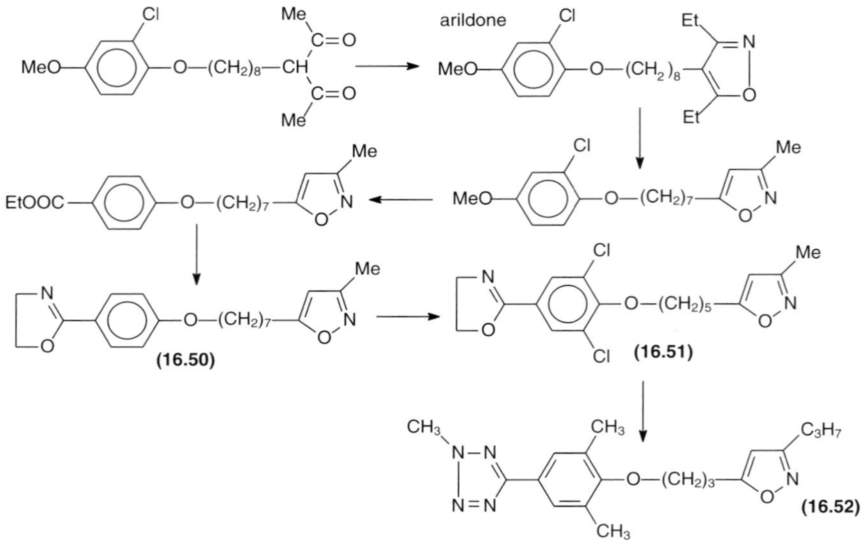

Scheme 16.12

controversial. Disoxaril (**16.50**) and its 4-methyloxazoline analog exhibit broad-spectrum activity both against rhinoviruses and enteroviruses. These compounds are derived from arildone, a compound which is quite active against poliovirus but only marginally active against rhinoviruses. Systematic variation of the substituents on the phenyl ring and introduction of different heterocyclic rings on the 'other side' has led to the discovery of disoxaril (**16.50**) as a potent antirhinovirus compound (Scheme 16.12).

These compounds specifically bind to the viral capsid and inhibit uncoating of the viral RNA. The interaction of these compounds with the viral capsid protein VP1 of rhinovirus-14 has been studied by X-ray crystallography. These compounds fit into a specific hydrophobic pocket, which corresponds to the cell receptor binding site and interacts with domains 1 and 2 of ICAM-1 (Figure 16.4). Elucidation of the mode of action of the compounds at the molecular level may lead to compounds with greater activity and selectivity. Following this lead, an analog of disoxaril, WIN 54954 (**16.51**) was shown to be more effective than disoxaril. However, due to the acid lability, the oxazoline ring, these molecules only have a short half-life. New analogs with a tetrazole ring such as **16.52** were, therefore, designed. These molecules likewise demonstrate a broad-spectrum activity against human rhinoviruses at ±0.02 μM.

A problem in the development of antirhinovirus compounds is the number of different serotypes (>100). Given the relative harmlessness of the common cold infection, any candidate drug has to be absolutely free of toxic side effects to be acceptable for clinical use. Nevertheless, a good antirhinovirus compound will be of great value because of the socio-economic impact of this disease. The problem with the above mentioned compounds is that they do not demonstrate a significant

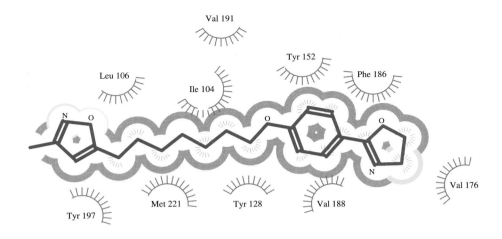

Figure 16.4 Interaction of compound **16.50** with the capsid VPI of rhinovirus-14.

16.53
Pleconaril

clinical effect against the infection if administered after the onset of symptoms. However, they are able to reduce the symptoms of the infection when used prophylactically (i.e. disoxaril (**16.50**) and WIN 54954 (**16.51**) against human Coxsackie A21 virus infection).

Pleconaril (**16.53**) is a metabolically stable capsid-function inhibitor with an oral bioavailability of 70%. It is a broad-spectrum antiviral showing potent antienterovirus and antirhinovirus activity. The integration of pleconaril into the capsid of picornaviruses prevents the virus from attaching to cellular receptors and from uncoating. Pleconaril has been shown to have clinical benefits and a favorable safety profile.

16.2.5   New developments in the anti-HIV-field

The replicative cycle of HIV-1 offers a wealth of potential targets for antiviral agents. The currently used anti-HIV agents interact with either the RT or viral protease. The most important alternative targets together with an example of an inhibitor are given in Table 16.1.

A great variety of polyanionic compounds have been described to block HIV replication through interference with virus adsorption to the cell surface. They are

Table 16.1 Targets in the replicative cycle of HIV-1 and potential inhibitory agents

Target	Potential anti-HIV agent
Viral adsorption through binding to the viral envelope glycoprotein gp120	Polysulfates or -sulfonates
Viral entry through blockade of the viral co-receptors CXCR4 or CCR5	Bicyclams
Virus-cell fusion, through binding to the viral glycoprotein gp41	T-20 peptide
Viral assembly and disassembly, through NCp7 zinc-finger-targeted agents	DIBA
Proviral DNA integration through integrase inhibitors	L-chicoric acid
Viral mRNA transcription, through inhibitors of the transcription process.	Fluoroquinolone K-12

assumed to exert their anti-HIV activity by shielding off the positively charged sites in the V3 loop of the viral envelope glycoprotein (gp120), which is necessary for virus attachment to the cell surface heparan sulphate (the primary binding site to the CD4 receptor of the $CD4^+$ cells). The major role of polysulfate or sulfonate compounds in the management of HIV infections may reside in the prevention of sexual transmission of HIV infection, as these compounds, if applied as a vaginal formulation, may successfully block HIV infection through both virus-to-cell and cell-to-cell contact.

To enter cells, following binding with the CD4 receptor, the HIV-1 particles must interact with the CXCR4 co-receptor or CCR5 co-receptor. CXCR4 is the co-receptor for X4 HIV-1 strains that infect T-cells, and CCR5 is the co-receptor for R5 HIV-1 strains that infect macrophages. These receptors normally act as receptors for chemokines. The bicyclams are highly potent and selective inhibitors of HIV-1 and HIV-2 replication. They bind to the CXCR4 receptor, which is a co-receptor for HIV entry into T-cells. The activity spectrum of bicyclam is restricted to those HIV variants (T-tropic) that use the CXCR4 receptor for entering the cells. The most potent compound is AMD 3329 (**16.54**), with an EC_{50} value against HIV-1 and HIV-2 replication of 0.8 and 1.6 nM respectively, which is about three- to five-fold lower than the EC_{50} of AMD 3100 (**16.55**). In Phase I clinical trial, **16.55** is well tolerated following single 15 min i.v. injection of doses of 10, 20, 40 and 80 µg/kg.

The interaction of the HIV-1 envelope glycoprotein gp120 with the co-receptor CXCR4 or CCR5, respectively, is followed by a spring-loaded action of the viral glycoprotein gp41, that then anchors into the target cell membrane. This initiates the fusion of the two lipid bilayers, that of the viral envelope with that of the cellular plasma membrane. T-20 is a synthetic, 36-amino acid peptide corresponding to residues 127–162 of the ectodomain of gp41. T-20 was selected after a specific domain predictive of α-helical secondary structure. T-20 afforded 100% blockade of virus-mediated cell–cell fusion at concentrations ranging from 1 to 10 ng/ml. An initial clinical trial has been carried out with T-20 in 16 HIV-infected adults. At 100 mg twice daily, T-20 achieved by 15 day a 1.5- to 2.0-fold reduction in

(16.54)

(16.55)

(16.56)

plasma HIV RNA. In a preliminary study, 1000-fold suppression of HIV-1 RNA was maintained for 20 weeks, no evidence of genotypic resistance to T-20 was observed, and no anti-T-20 antibodies were detected after 28 weeks of administration of T-20.

The two zinc fingers in the nucleocapsid (NCp7) protein comprise the proposed molecular target for zinc-releasing compounds such as the 2,2'-dithiobisbenzamide-1 (DIBA) (**16.56**). This compound can interfere with both early (uncoating, disassembly) and late phases (packing, assembly) of retrovirus replication. Its effect at the late phase (assembly) would result in abnormal processing of the gag precursor, due to the formation of intermolecular cross-links among the zinc fingers of adjacent NCp7 molecules and the release of non-infectious virus particles. The DIBA is able to enter intact virions, and the cross-linkage of NCp7 in virions correlates with loss of infectivity and decreased proviral DNA synthesis during acute infection.

Retrovirus integration requires at least two viral components, the retroviral enzyme integrase, and *cis*-acting sequences at the retroviral DNA termini U3 and U5 ends of the long terminal repeats (LTRs). Since HIV, like other retroviruses, cannot replicate without integration into a host chromosome, integrase has been considered as an attractive therapeutic target. A well documented HIV integrase inhibitor is L-chicoric acid (**16.57**). Integrase was identified as the molecular target for the action of L-chicoric acid when a single amino acid substitution in the integrase made the corresponding HIV-1 mutant resistant to L-chicoric acid.

(16.57)

(16.58)

(16.59)

However, it has been demonstrated that this diacid owes its anti-HIV activity in cell culture primarily to an interaction with the viral envelope gp120 and, consequently, inhibition of virus adsorption. Meanwhile, diketo acid (DKA) (**16.58**) derivatives have been identified as 'genuine' intergrase inhibitors that owe their anti-HIV activity in cell culture to integrase inhibition.

At the transcription level, HIV gene expression may be inhibited by compounds that interact with cellular factors that bind to the LTR promoter and that are needed for basal level transcription, such as the NF-κB inhibitors. Greater specificity, however, can be expected from those compounds that specifically inhibit the transactivation of the HIV LTR promoter by the viral Tat protein. Tat may be important, not only for translocation but also for nuclear localization and *trans*-activation, and thus targeting of the Tat basic domain may provide great scope for therapeutic intervention in HIV-1 infection. A number of compounds have been reported to inhibit HIV-1 replication through interference with the transcription process, e.g. the fluoroquinolones. The inhibitory effects of the fluoroquinolones on the HIV-1 LTR-driven gene expression may at least in part be attributed to inhibition of the Tat function. The fluoroquinolone K-12 [**16.59**] acts synergistically with RT and PIs.

FURTHER READING

Advances in Antiviral Drug Design, Vol. 1, edited by E. De Clercq, pp. 1–329. London, England: JAI Press, Inc. 1993; Vol. 2, (pp. 1–233), 1996; Vol. 3, (pp. 1–237), 1999.

Rotbart, H. (2000) Antiretroviral therapy for enteroviruses and rhinoviruses. *Antiviral Chem. and Chemother.*, **11**, 261–271.

Gubareva, L., Kaiser, L. and Hayden, F.G. (2000) Influenza virus neuraminidase inhibitors. *The Lancet*, **355**, 827–835.

Chapter 17

Anticancer agents

Ingrid Kjøller Larsen and Jette Sandholm Kastrup

17.1 DNA AS TARGET FOR ANTICANCER DRUGS

The DNA molecule is essential for the growth of all living cells and so far it has been the main target for anticancer drug action. Some of these drugs act directly on the DNA molecule, either by drug-induced DNA damage or by some kind of alteration of DNA (Section 17.1.1), whereas other drugs prevent nucleic acid synthesis by inhibiting one or more of the enzymes involved in the DNA synthesis, or by disturbing the DNA function by incorporation of 'wrong pieces' into the DNA molecule (Section 17.1.2).

The DNA interacting drugs prevent cell growth, but not only cancer cell growth. Unfortunately, the growth of normal cells is also blocked. The cytotoxic effect is most serious on rapidly dividing cells, i.e. in addition to tumor cells also the cells of normal bone marrow, gut, skin epithelium, and mucosa of the mouth.

The lack of selectivity of cancer drugs is one of the main problems in cancer chemotherapy. All the known abnormal biological phenomena of cancer cells (e.g. excessive cell proliferation, loss of tissue-specific characteristics, invasiveness, and metastasis) seem to be based on normal biological functions of the cells, e.g. by use of normal enzyme systems. The abnormality of malignant tumor growth is connected to the regulation of cell growth and caused by mutations in control genes, which are converted to oncogenes. The introduction of gene therapy might be a very important step forward in the treatment of cancer in the future. In most gene therapy approaches, full, healthy genes are introduced as substitutes for wrong versions ('mutation compensation'). Inhibition of expression of unwanted genes by using DNA or RNA binding agents might also be possible (cf. Section 17.1.1.5).

It should be noticed that most anticancer drugs interfering with DNA or DNA synthesis also exhibit a variety of actions on other targets in the cells. The classification of anticancer drugs in this chapter is based on the mode of action of the specified anticancer agents, which is generally believed to be responsible for the cytotoxic activity.

All drugs with action directly on the DNA molecule affect all fast-growing cells without preference for a special phase of the cell cycle (phase non-specific agents). They are, however, usually more effective against proliferating cells than against resting cells, where no DNA replication may occur for long periods of time. Drugs interfering with one or more of the enzymes involved in DNA synthesis are most effective in one phase of the cell cycle, i.e. the S phase of the cell cycle, which is the period of DNA synthesis (S phase specific agents).

One of the very serious problems in cancer chemotherapy is the development of drug resistance. Most drugs are initially very effective, but subsequent therapy may fail because the tumor cells have become non-sensitive to the drug. In many cases, the mechanisms of resistance to antitumor drugs are known and are mentioned later in this chapter under the individual classes of drugs.

In recent years, the existence of multidrug resistance (MDR) has been recognized. The MDR is characterized by cross-resistance to a group of structurally and mechanistically distinct antitumor agents including the anthracyclines (daunomycin and adriamycin), the vinca alkaloids (vincristine and vinblastine), colchicine and podophyllotoxins, and actinomycin D. However, this resistance does not extend to all anticancer agents, for example antimetabolites (e.g. methotrexate, cytarabine, and thioguanine) and alkylating agents (e.g. carmustine and cyclophosphamide) are not affected.

There are probably several different mechanisms by which cells can be cross-resistant to multiple drugs. However, MDR is commonly associated with high levels of a membrane-associated phosphoglucoprotein (Pgp), which is a transport protein with pertinent homology to bacterial transport proteins. The Pgp functions as an energy (ATP) dependent drug efflux pump. It has been shown that the drug efflux from cells, in which the gene for Pgp is expressed, increases with resistance. The detailed mechanism by which Pgp pumps drugs out of cells is not fully understood.

17.1.1   Drugs interacting directly with DNA

The functions of the DNA molecule can be influenced by drugs in different ways. Damage to DNA, where covalent bond formation is involved, is performed by the category of compounds usually called alkylating agents, including some anticancer antibiotics (Section 17.1.1.1). *cis*-Platinum co-ordination complexes modify the DNA structure by binding of the metal ions directly to DNA (Section 17.1.1.2). Breakdown of the DNA molecule (DNA strand scission) is caused by other antibiotic agents (Section 17.1.1.3). The intercalating agents (Section 17.1.1.4) disturb DNA function by intercalating between the base pairs, but normally without bond breakage or formation. Antisense anticancer agents (Section 17.1.1.5) are designed to perform their action on nucleic acids (blocking of specified base sequences) by a combination of intercalating and alkylating abilities, in addition to hydrogen bonding and hydrophobic interactions.

17.1.1.1   Alkylating agents

At least six major classes of alkylating agents are employed in cancer chemotherapy (cf. Scheme 17.1, where representative structures are given). All these compounds undergo a reaction in which an alkyl group becomes covalently linked to some cellular constituent, preferably the DNA molecule.

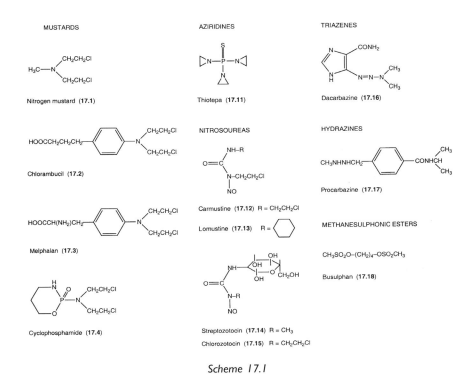

Scheme 17.1

17.1.1.1.1   Nitrogen mustards

Nitrogen mustard (**17.1**), mustine, mechlorethamine, di(2-chloroethyl)-methylamine is a volatile liquid, but it is administered clinically as the chloride. The salt is crystalline, but hygroscopic, and has to be dissolved in water immediately before use (intravenous saline infusion), because it is unstable in aqueous solution. The compound is very irritating (vesicant) to skin and mucous membranes, thus the acute side effects are severe and painful. The most serious delayed side effect is bone marrow depression, as also for all other alkylating agents. Nitrogen mustard has a very rapid alkylating effect and is therefore valuable in life-threatening situations.

Nitrogen mustard was the first drug used in cancer chemotherapy. It was discovered during the second world war that the war gas *sulphur mustard* [S(CH$_2$-CH$_2$-Cl)$_2$] and the isosterically related compound nitrogen mustard have anti-tumor activity. The sulphur mustard is too reactive and toxic for clinical use. Nitrogen mustard is also a very reactive drug with a number of toxic side effects, but it has proved to be a very useful drug and it is still in clinical use, often in combination with other drugs.

The proposed mechanism of action of nitrogen mustard is shown in Scheme 17.2. The molecule forms a reactive cyclic intermediate, an aziridinium ion, by release of a chloride ion. This aziridinium ion is an electrophile, which attacks

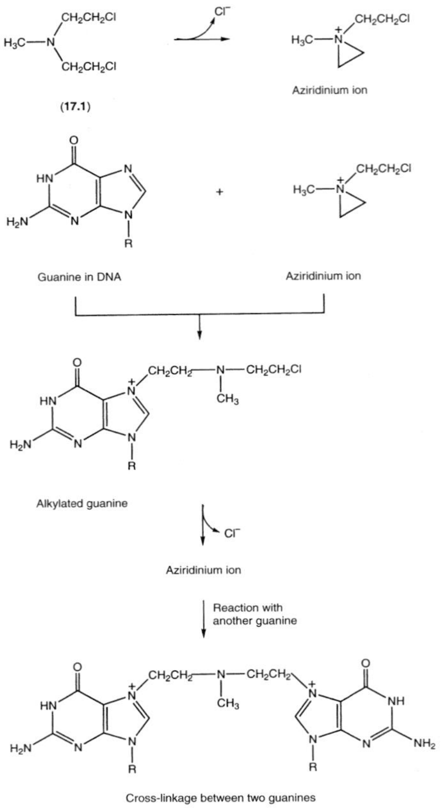

Scheme 17.2

electron-rich centers (nucleophiles) in biological macromolecules. The reaction is an S_N2 process, as the bimolecular reaction with the nucleophile is the rate controlling step, which obeys second-order kinetics. The formation of the aziridinium ion is a very fast unimolecular reaction, when CH_3 (or another alkyl group) is connected to the N-atom of the nitrogen mustard.

The nucleophilic groups, which can be attacked by the electrophile formed from nitrogen mustard, may be amino, hydroxyl, sulphhydryl or imidazole moieties in proteins and nucleic acids. The reaction of major importance in the cytotoxic effect of nitrogen mustards is the formation of a covalent bond with the N-7 atom of a guanine base of DNA. N-7 is thought to be the preferred position for purin alkylation, because it is easier accessible than N-3, and N-1 is involved in hydrogen bonding in a Watson–Crick base pair.

The other chloroethyl side chain of nitrogen mustard can undergo a similar cyclization and react with another nucleophilic group. If this second reaction involves an N-7 of a guanine base from an opposite strand of the double helix, the result is cross-linking between the DNA strands. Intra-strand cross-links can also be formed, and, in addition, reactions between monoalkylated DNA and another nucleic acid or a protein are possible. There is a good correlation between DNA cross-linking and inhibition of cell growth, and DNA cross-links are generally believed to be responsible for the antitumor activity of bifunctional alkylating agents, e.g. nitrogen mustards. However, as many cellular constituents, including membrane proteins, can be alkylated, it might be assumed that the cytotoxicity is a result of many diverse effects.

Nitrogen mustard is easily hydrolyzed. This happens when the initially formed aziridinium ion reacts with a water molecule instead of a nucleophilic group of a biomacromolecule. In this case, an inactive hydroxy form of the compound $[CH_3N(CH_2CH_2OH)_2]$ is formed. A considerable amount of the injected drug is actually inactivated before reaching the biological targets.

Evidence for the formation of cross-links between two different DNA strands of the double helix has been obtained from different experiments. Alkylation of DNA bases, and especially intra- and interstrand cross-linking, disturbs the functions of the DNA molecule in different ways. The cross linkages prevent separation of the individual strands, thereby mainly inhibiting DNA replication, but DNA transcription will also be influenced. In addition, it is now accepted that alkylating agents kill tumor cells by inducing apoptosis (programmed cell death).

All living cells are able to repair DNA damage, whether accidentally arisen or due to alkylating agents, by the DNA repair system, involving several enzymes (e.g. endonucleases, repair polymerase and ligase). Drug resistance of cells treated with nitrogen mustards (or other cross-linking agents) is due to an increased ability of the resistant cells to excise the cross-linked residues in DNA and repair the defect.

Chlorambucil (**17.2**), 4-[*bis*(2-chloroethyl)amino)benzenebutanoic acid], is a synthetically prepared, crystalline compound. This aromatic nitrogen mustard was introduced at an early stage of cancer therapy. It has a milder effect than nitrogen mustard, no serious acute side effects, and it can be given orally. The long-term toxicity is bone marrow depression.

Melphalan (**17.3**), 4-[*bis*(2-chloroethyl)amino)-L-phenylalanine], is another crystalline nitrogen mustard with an aryl group attached to the N-atom. This drug was also developed as a drug with less reactivity (see below) than nitrogen mustard. In addition, it was originally synthesized in support of the idea that attachment of a mustard group to a naturally occurring carrier (in this case phenylalanine) might increase the effectiveness, because of increased affinity for certain biological sites. Since phenylalanine is a precursor for melanin, it was hoped that melphalan would preferentially accumulate in melanomas and thereby produce a selective effect. This early attempt on site-directed mustard effect was not successful, but still melphalan is a widely used drug, because of its pharmacological properties.

The mechanism of action of chlorambucil and melphalan is similar to that of nitrogen mustard (Scheme 17.2). One of the advantages of nitrogen mustards, as compared to sulphur mustard, is that the third substituent (CH_3 in nitrogen mustard) can be varied in order to introduce some variation of the reactivity of the drug. Attachment of an aromatic ring to the nitrogen atom, as in chlorambucil and melphalan, decreases the rate of alkylation. The electron withdrawing effect of the ring, and/or delocalization of the lone pair electrons, makes the nitrogen atom less nucleophilic and the rate of cyclization much slower than for alkyl nitrogen mustards. This step (formation of aziridinium ion by first order cyclization) is probably the rate limiting step in the case of aryl nitrogen mustards, and the reaction is believed to be an S_N1 type process.

The decreased reactivity of aromatic nitrogen mustards can be advantageous for several reasons. The drug can be given orally, whereas nitrogen mustard has to be be given intravenously. The higher stability allows time for absorption and wide distribution before degradation (hydrolysis) and before extensive alkylation. Finally, the acute side effects are much less severe. The biological effects are the same.

Cyclophosphamide (**17.4**), 1-*bis*(2-chloroethyl)amino-1-oxo-2-aza-5-oxaphosphoridine, is a nitrogen mustard with an oxazaphosphorine ring attached to the N-atom. It was synthesized originally as a transport form (prodrug) for nornitrogen mustard [normustine, $HN(CH_2CH_2Cl)_2$], which is also an active alkylating agent, but too toxic and with a low therapeutic index. The biochemical rationale behind this early approach to the development of a target-directed prodrug was that the compound should be enzymatically converted into the active compound *in vivo* by phosphoramidase enzymes, which were thought to be more abundant in tumors compared with normal tissue. Later it was demonstrated, however, that simple enzymatic cleavage is not the reason for the bioactivation of cyclophosphamide.

Cyclophosphamide (CPA) is one of the most effective alkylating agents with a wide application in cancer chemotherapy against many different neoplastic diseases. It can be given either orally or intravenously and its side effects are less severe and easier to control than those of nitrogen mustard (**17.1**). Immunosuppression is a side effect, which has led to its use to prevent transplant rejection. In addition, CPA has a number of undesirable side effects, some of which are probably caused by one or more of the metabolites.

Cyclophosphamide has to be metabolically activated in the body before it can alkylate cellular constituents. The CPA by itself is not cytotoxic to cells in culture (*in vitro*), but cells are killed, when incubated with both the drug and a liver homogenate, which can convert it into the active form. The mechanism of the metabolic activation of CPA has been extensively studied. The metabolic degradation pathway is considered to be as shown in Scheme 17.3. The oxidation product 4-hydroxy-CPA (**17.5a**) either undergoes further oxidation (detoxification) into 4-keto-CPA (**17.6**) or tautomerizes into the open-chain aldehyde aldophosphamide (**17.5b**). Aldophosphamide may be oxidized into carboxy-CPA (**17.7**), a detoxification reaction, or the enol form of **17.5b** may undergo a spontaneous β-elimination (reverse Michael addition) to give acrolein (**17.8**) and phosphoramide mustard (**17.9**). In addition, nornitrogen mustard (**17.10**) is formed as a decomposition product (hydrolysis, non-enzymatic) of several of the above mentioned compounds.

Phosphoramide mustard (**17.9**) is generally believed to be the final cytotoxic agent. Due to its polar nature, phosphoramide mustard is not capable of penetrating cell membranes and therefore has to be formed intracellularly. Neither of the two major urinary metabolites (**17.6**) and (**17.7**) is significantly cytotoxic and represents inactivated excretion products. Acrolein (**17.8**) and phosphoramide

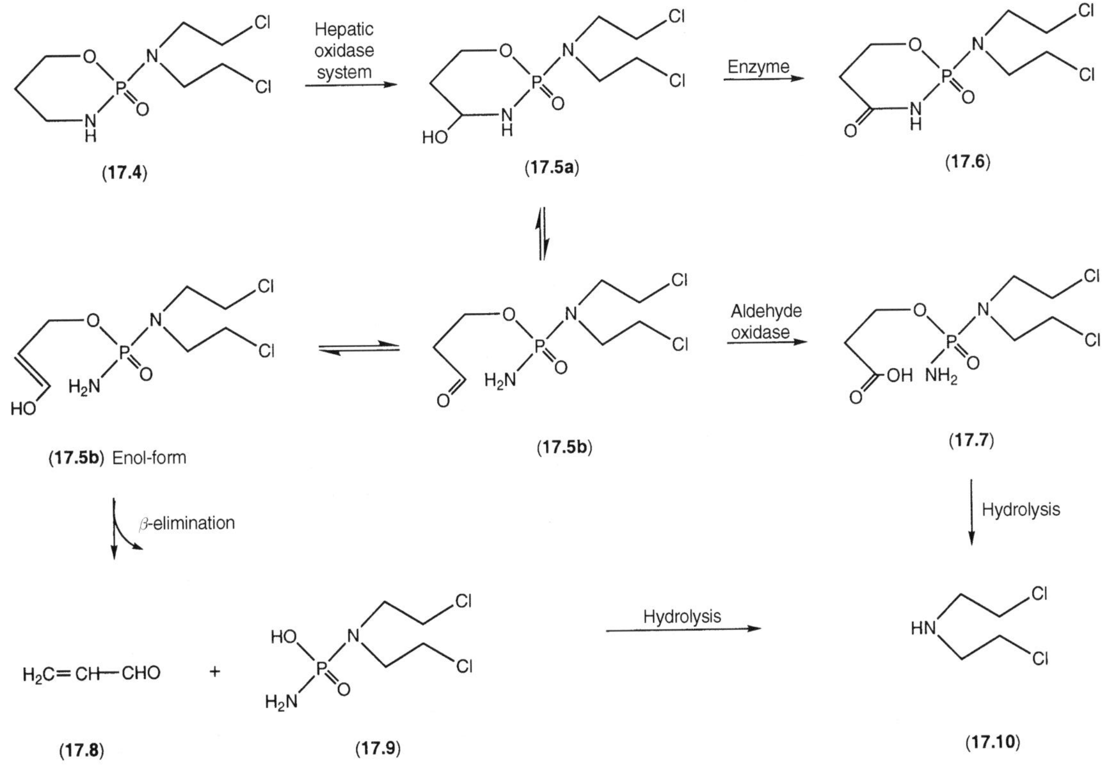

Cl
N
O
P
O
N
H
Cl
(17.4)
Hepatic
oxidase
system
(17.5a)
HO
Enzyme
(17.6)
(17.5b) Enol-form
H2N
HO
(17.5b)
Aldehyde
oxidase
OH
NH2
(17.7)
β-elimination
Hydrolysis
H2C=CH—CHO
+
(17.8)
(17.9)
HN
(17.10)

Scheme 17.3

mustard are produced in equimolar amounts during the metabolism of CPA. Because of the known toxicities of acrolein one might expect it to contribute to the final cytotoxicity of CPA. This is unlikely, however, as phosphoramide mustard is cytotoxic at levels considerably below the level of acrolein required for cytotoxicity. Some role for acrolein in the pharmacology of CPA cannot be excluded, however. Thus, the bladder toxicity observed in patients treated with CPA is caused by acrolein and can be diminished by co-administration of the drug with an alkyl sulphide (e.g. MESNA, sodium 2-mercaptoethanesulphonate), which reacts with acrolein by a Michael's reaction. The reaction product is then excreted.

Phosphoramide mustard, as well as nornitrogen mustard, are powerful cytostatic agents, also *in vitro*, and high levels of both compounds can be detected in plasma 1–10 h after CPA infusion. Phosphoramide mustard is considered to be the ultimate alkylating agent for several reasons, e.g. because it is a more powerful alkylating agent than nornitrogen mustard. In addition, nornitrogen mustard is a secondary amine and may, after formation of an aziridinium ion, deliver H^+ to solvent, thereby forming the uncharged chloroethylaziridine, which is relatively resistant to nucleophilic attack.

Phosphoramide mustard (**17.9**) is an alkylating agent because of its ability to form an aziridinium ion in contrast to CPA (**17.4**), where the withdrawing electronegative effect of the ring, and delocalization of the lone pair electrons, makes the N-atom less nucleophilic and the rate of initial cyclization very slow. In phosphoramide mustard, which is deprotonated at physiological pH (pKa of the OH group is 4.75), the nucleophilic effect of the N-atom is not decreased because of strong contributions of the resonance forms with the negative charge on the two oxygen atoms of the phosphoramide group and therefore negligible delocalization of the lone pair on the N-atom with the chloroethyl substituents.

The main biological effect of CPA is the same as that of nitrogen mustard, i.e. formation of DNA cross links by alkylation of guanine N-7. The initial phosphoramide-DNA adduct is unstable and converted to the corresponding nornitrogen mustard adduct G-nor-G. Monoalkylation also occurs. Other oxazaphosphorines used therapeutically are *ifosfamide* with one of the chloroethyl substituents positioned at the N-atom of the oxazaphosphorine ring, and *trofosfamide*, which has this substituent as a third chloroethyl group.

17.1.1.1.2 Aziridines

Thiotepa (**17.11**), triethylenethiophosphoramide, *tris*(1-aziridinyl)phosphine sulphide, is a hexasubstituted triamide of thiophosphoric acid. Thiotepa is unstable in acid and is poorly absorbed from the gastrointestinal tract. It is therefore given intravenously or used topically, e.g. to treat papillary carcinoma of the bladder. The major side effect is bone marrow depression.

Thiotepa is a trifunctional alkylating agent containing aziridine rings. It has been developed as an analog of the reactive aziridinium ion formed from nitrogen mustard, in order to obtain a deactivated alkylating agent. The aziridine ring is less attractive to nucleophiles because of the lack of a positive charge. However, if the third substituent on the N-atom of the aziridine ring is an electron-withdrawing group, some positive charge (electron deficiency) arises on the C-atoms of the aziridine ring, due to polarization of the bonds.

17.1.1.1.3 Nitrosoureas

Carmustine (**17.12**), BCNU, *N,N'-bis*(2-chloroethyl)-*N*-nitrosourea, and the structural analog *lomustine* (**17.13**), CCNU, *N*-(2-chloroethyl)-*N'*-cyclohexyl-*N*-nitrosourea, are developed as a result of the observation of promising antileukemic properties of *N*-methyl-*N*-nitrosourea in routine screening of this compound. The compounds are rather unstable in acidic and alkaline aqueous solutions. The BCNU has to be given intravenously, whereas CCNU can be administered orally.

The nitrosoureas are unionized at physiological pH and consequently they have much higher lipid solubility than the nitrogen mustards and other alkylating agents. Their ability to pass the blood–brain barrier renders them especially useful in the treatment of CNS neoplasm (e.g. brain tumors and metastases). The BCNU and CCNU both produce nausea and vomiting, and the delayed side effects are bone marrow depression, leukopenia, and thrombocytopenia. The BCNU is more toxic of the two compounds.

A number of theories on the mechanism of action of the nitrosoureas has been proposed. It is evident that these drugs are alkylating as well as carbamoylating agents and that cross-linking of DNA is a consequence of alkylation. The proposed mechanisms for the alkylation and carbamoylation outlined in Scheme 17.4 are based on the mechanism of decomposition of nitrosoureas in aqueous solution at pH 7.4. Base abstraction of the amide hydrogen atom produces an unstable intermediate, which rapidly decomposes to yield the corresponding alkylisocyanate and 2-chloroethanediazohydroxide. The isocyanate formed is capable of carbamoylating proteins, e.g. lysine and cysteine residues. By spontaneous decomposition of the diazohydroxide and reaction with a nucleophilic center, e.g. of base X, the DNA is monoalkylated. Preferably O-6 but also N-7 of guanine may be alkylated (β-chloroethylated). In a second step, an ethylene bridge is formed by reaction with the cytosine (base Y) on the complementary strand and elimination of a chloride ion. The DNA-protein cross links as well as monoalkylated nucleic acids and proteins can also occur as the result of alkylation with nitrosoureas. Resistance to nitrosoureas is caused by enzymatical removal of chloroethyl groups, thereby preventing formation of DNA interstrand cross links.

Streptozotocin (**17.14**), an anticancer antibiotic isolated from *Streptomyces achromogenes*, is a nitrosourea derivative with a glucose moiety at one N-atom and a methyl group at the other. By substitution of this methyl group with a chloroethyl group *chlorozotocin* (**17.15**) was obtained, which shows lower toxicity (myelosuppression) than streptozotocin. The drugs are retained in the β-cells of the islets of Langerhans and can be used experimentally to induce diabetes in laboratory animals. Insulin chock is a dangerous acute toxicity. Because of the β-cell effect the drugs can be used against metastatic islet cell carcinoma. The compounds probably act by alkylation of nucleophilic sites, but the precise mechanism has not been well worked out. The glucose moiety of the drugs may be of importance for the lower myelosuppression.

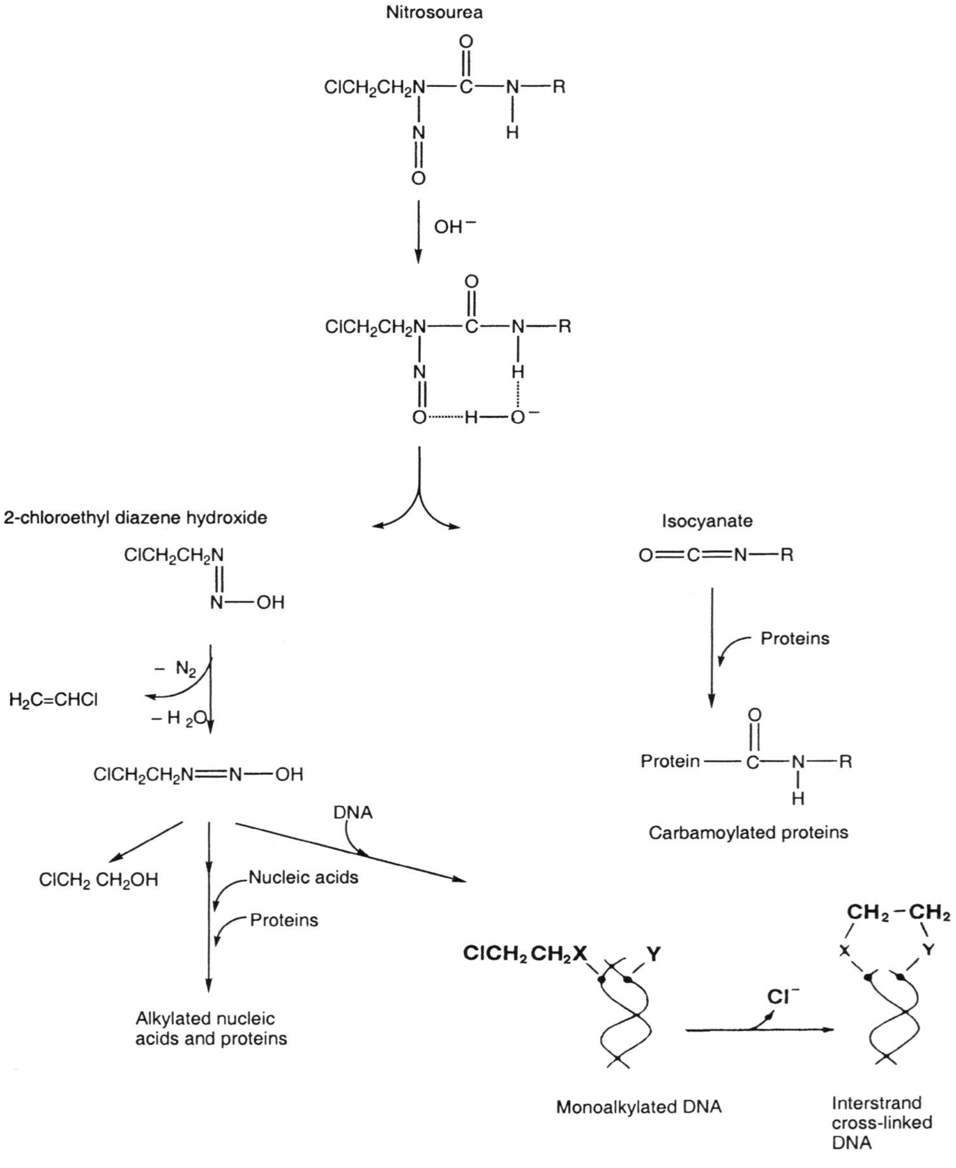

Nitrosourea

$$ClCH_2CH_2N-\overset{\overset{\displaystyle O}{\|}}{C}-\underset{\underset{\displaystyle H}{|}}{N}-R$$
$$\underset{\underset{\displaystyle O}{\|}}{N}$$

↓ OH⁻

$$ClCH_2CH_2N-\overset{\overset{\displaystyle O}{\|}}{C}-\underset{\underset{\displaystyle H}{|}}{N}-R$$

2-chloroethyl diazene hydroxide

$$ClCH_2CH_2N$$
$$\underset{\underset{\displaystyle N-OH}{\|}}{}$$

$- N_2$

$H_2C=CHCl$

$- H_2O$

$ClCH_2CH_2N{=}{=}N-OH$

DNA

Isocyanate

$$O{=}C{=}N-R$$

↓ Proteins

$$Protein-\overset{\overset{\displaystyle O}{\|}}{C}-\underset{\underset{\displaystyle H}{|}}{N}-R$$

Carbamoylated proteins

$ClCH_2\,CH_2OH$

Nucleic acids

Proteins

Alkylated nucleic
acids and proteins

ClCH₂CH₂X   **Y**

Cl⁻

Monoalkylated DNA

CH₂−CH₂
X   Y

Interstrand
cross-linked
DNA

Scheme 17.4

17.1.1.1.4   Triazenes

Dacarbazine (**17.16**), DTIC, 5-(3,3-dimethyl-1-triazenyl)-1-*H*-imidazole-4-carbox-amide, is a compound, which is stable in solution, but has to be protected against light. The drug is given intravenously and produces severe nausea and vomiting and sometimes a flu-like syndrome of fever. Dacarbazine has appeared to be particularly suitable for the treatment of malignant melanoma.

Dacarbazine was originally developed as a structural analog of 5-aminoimidazole-4-carboxamide, an intermediate in purine biosynthesis. It is, however, now known that the cytotoxicity of the drug is due to its alkylating (methylating) action, rather than to inhibition of purine biosynthesis. The generally accepted mechanism (metabolism and subsequent chemical decomposition) is shown in Scheme 17.5.

The monomethyl derivative produced via the corresponding hydroxymethyl derivative by enzymatic oxidation decomposes spontaneously (non-enzymatically) to form 5-aminoimidazole-4-carboxamide (the major metabolite excreted in the urine) and the methylating agent, which is methane diazohydroxide $CH_3-N=N-OH$. This methylating agent attacks nucleophilic groups in DNA and other cellular constituents. An important site of *in vivo* alkylation is the N-7 position of guanine, and the 7-methylguanine product has been identified in the urine of patients given ^{14}C-methyl-dacarbazine.

Many triazenes have been investigated in which the imidazole ring has been replaced by other heterocyclic systems or phenyl derivatives in a search for second-generation antitumor triazenes with enhanced selectivity and activity. The studies have shown that the nature of the aromatic moiety does not affect the activity markedly. Substitution of one of the methyl groups of the triazene moiety has no effect on antitumor activity, provided that the replacement alkyl group can undergo oxidative dealkylation (depends e.g. on chain length and bulkyness of the alkyl group). If both methyl groups of the triazene N-atom are substituted by other

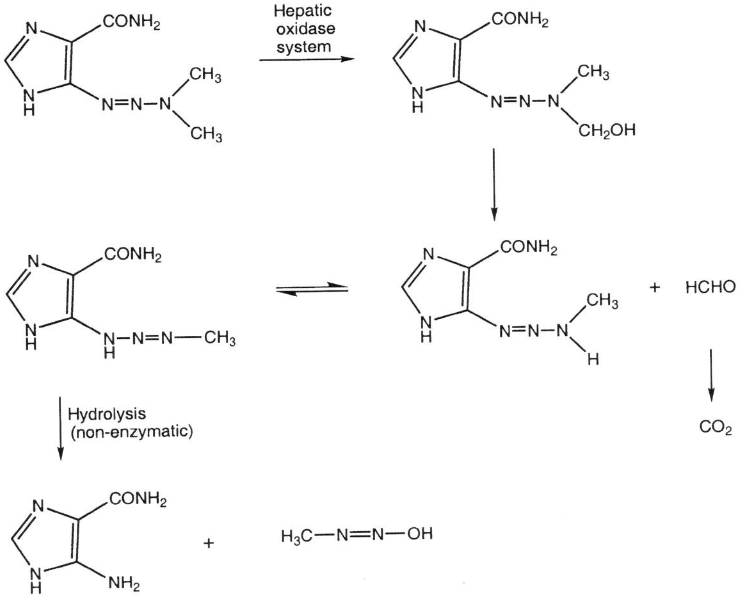

Scheme 17.5

alkyl groups, total loss of activity is observed. It is not yet fully understood why methyl substituents predispose so decisively towards the activity of the triazenes.

17.1.1.1.5 Hydrazines

Procarbazine (**17.17**), *N*-(1-methylethyl)-4-[(2-methylhydrazino)methyl]-benzamide, is used as the chloride of the hydrazine. This compound was synthesized as a potential monoamine oxidase (MAO) inhibitor, but it was later shown to have antitumor effect. It is clinically used both in combination drug therapy and in various drug protocols to treat e.g. melanoma and Hodgkin's disease. Procarbazine can penetrate into the cerebrospinal fluid and has been used to treat malignant brain tumors. Its side effects are similar to those of typical alkylating agents, but it also causes psychopharmacological effects consistent with its ability to inhibit MAO.

Procarbazine is inactive *in vitro* and requires enzymatic activation before it shows antitumor activity. *In vivo* it is rapidly converted to azo-procarbazine, $CH_3-N=N-CH_2-C_6H_4-CONHCH(CH_3)_2$, probably by hepatic microsomal enzymes. Several pathways have been proposed for the conversion of this intermediate to the major urinary metabolite *N*-isopropylterephthalamic acid, $HOOC-C_6H_4-CONHCH(CH_3)_2$. Methane is observed as a minor metabolite, and it has been suggested that methyl radicals or methyl carbocations are the biologically active methylating agent.

17.1.1.1.6 Methanesulphonate esters

Busulphan (**17.18**), myleran, 1,4-*bis*(methanesulphonyloxy)butane is unstable in aqueous solution, but can still be given orally and is well absorbed from the gastrointestinal tract. It is excreted in the urine as methanesulphonic acid and several metabolites, which are derived from the alkylating butylene moiety. It is a very mild alkylating agent with no acute side effects and it is useful mainly in the treatment of patients with chronic granulocytic leukemia. A number of long-term side effects are observed, among those bone marrow depression.

Busulphan is a bifunctional alkylating agent, which has a reactivity considerably lower than that of nitrogen mustard. The mechanism of the alkylation is believed to be similar to that of nitrogen mustards. The alkyl–oxygen bond splits with the methanesulphonate moiety as the leaving group when reacting with nucleophilic centers of the cell constituents, including N-7 of guanine bases, but also with sulphhydryl groups of cysteines in proteins. Diguanyl derivatives can be formed as a reaction product between busulfan and nucleotides, and cross-linking of DNA is believed to be the main reason for the cytotoxic activity of busulphan.

17.1.1.2 Metal complex binding to DNA

Platinum co-ordination complexes with the formula *cis*-PtA_2X_2, where X is a uninegative, readily exchangeable group, and A is ammonia or an amine, have been known for many years to exhibit antitumor properties. The initial trials were very promising, but the toxic side effects, e.g. renal toxicity, appeared to be a serious limitation of the use of the Pt-complexes as anticancer agents. Improved administration procedures have now resulted in large-scale clinical application of *cis*-Pt-complexes, especially in combination with many other anticancer drugs. It is generally believed that the antitumor properties of *cis*-Pt-complexes are mainly based on interactions of these compounds with DNA. Introduction of Pt-complexes is regarded as one of the most important acquisitions in cancer chemotherapy of the last two decades.

Cisplatin (**17.19**), *cis*-diamminedichloroplatinum(II), possesses a very broad spectrum of activity and is one of the most widely used anticancer drugs. It is routinely administered by intravenous infusion, and supplied as a lyophylized powder, because of the low solubility in water. Cisplatin is particularly used in combination therapy, e.g. with paclitaxel (taxol **17.39**), cyclophosphamide and bleomycin, in the treatment of testicular cancer, but good response in the treatment of several other cancer forms has been observed. In particular, promising results have been obtained with cisplatin in combination with paclitaxel in treatment of ovarian cancer, and there is a broad consensus that this combination represents a significant advance in the treatment of advanced ovarian cancer.

Several methods have been used in order to elucidate the mechanism of action of cisplatin and other Pt-complexes. It is known that cisplatin interacts with DNA by specific binding to the guanine N-7 sites. Binding to cytosine N-3, adenine N-1, and adenine N-7 is also possible, but is less common. A second binding interaction readily takes place on the same strand of DNA, most frequently at another guanine base being a next-neighbor. Interstrand cross-linking is also possible.

Detailed information on the nature of the binding of cisplatin to DNA has been obtained from studies of the model complexes consisting of cisplatin bound to short DNA fragments. The accurate structure in solution of the adduct *cis*-Pt(NH$_3$)$_2$-[d(GpG)] has been studied using high-resolution NMR techniques, and the solid-state structure of the very similar adduct *cis*-Pt(NH$_3$)$_2$-[d(pGpG)] was solved using X-ray diffraction (Figure 17.1). The geometry of the two adducts (in solution and in the solid-state) was shown to be substantially the same. Pt binds to the two guanine bases of the dinucleotide by co-ordination through N-7, and the conformational changes of the overall structure of the nucleotide are limited to small changes in the position of the sugar ring at the 5′ side of d(GpG) and of the dihedral angle between the guanine bases. The distortion of the DNA structure, after chelation of cisplatin to a GpG sequence, should therefore be rather small.

Molecular modeling studies suggested a helix distortion, which can best be described as a kink or a bend in the helical axis of about 40°. This has now been confirmed by the X-ray structure determination of a double-stranded DNA dodecamer containing cisplatin (Figure 17.2). The biological consequences of the

Cisplatin (**17.19**) Carboplatin (**17.20**)   Oxaliplatin (**17.21**)

A = NH$_3$ X = Cl

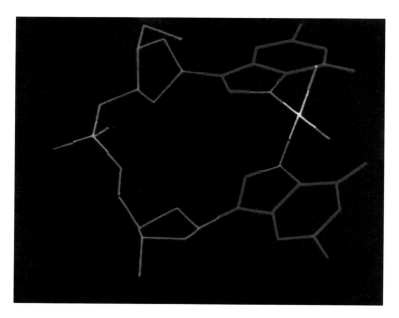

Figure 17.1 Structural model of the Pt(NH$_3$)$_2$ [d(GpG)] adduct, determined from analysis of the NMR spectra. From Reedijk, J. in *NMR Spectroscopy in Drug Research*, eds. J.W. Jaroszewski, K. Schaumburg and H. Kofod. Munksgaard, Copenhagen 1988, with permission by Munksgaard.

DNA distortion (bending and unwinding) are not quite clear, but high-mobility-group (HMG)-domain proteins seem to be involved. The ultimate result is that cell replication is hampered. The cytotoxic effects of cisplatin might, however, be considered to be due to the combined effects of various lesions.

It has been known for sometime that also *trans*-PtA$_2$X$_2$, e.g. *trans*-diamminedichloroplatinum(II), binds to DNA, but these complexes have much lower cytotoxic effect and no anticancer activity. As the binding affinities to the nucleobases are quite comparable with those of the *cis* complexes, the different activity must originate from differences related to the bifunctional binding. The NMR studies have shown that *trans*-Pt compounds can chelate to GNG sequences (N = A, T or C) through the guanine N-7 atoms, but the distortion of DNA after such *trans* binding is larger. This has prompted the hypothesis that repair enzymes recognize and remove the *trans* compound easier than the *cis* compound. It may also be possible that the distortion of DNA is of a nature that do not cause erroneous binding of HMG-domain proteins.

Several thousands of analogs of cisplatin has been synthesized and tested in order to enhance the therapeutic index and or reduce the resistance development. So far, most analogs are found to be so-called 'me too' versions of cisplatin. One of the few, which has provided definite advantage over cisplatin is *carboplatin* (**17.20**), *cis*-diammine-1,1-cyclobutanedicarboxylatoplatinum(II). Carboplatin has, however, afforded benefit in reducing some of the toxic side effects, and has now replaced cisplatin in many clinical situations. It has the same spectrum of

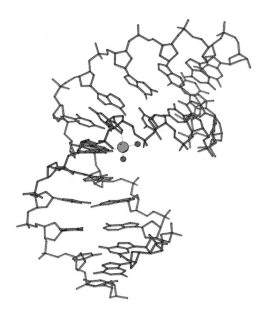

Figure 17.2 The X-ray structure of a double-stranded DNA dodecamer (shown in red) containing cisplatin (Pt ion shown in green and amine ligands in blue). The DNA structure has been modified by binding of cisplatin to two neighbouring intrastrand guanine bases. The structure is generated using the program Molscript with co-ordinates from Protein Data Bank.

anticancer activity and is not active in cisplatin-resistant cancers. Another analog of cisplatin, *oxaliplatin* (**17.21**), appears to have a somewhat different spectrum of antitumor activity. Introduction of this drug, in monotherapy as well as in combination with fluorouracil (**17.30**), represents a significant advance in the treatment of advanced colorectal cancer and is registered for this use in several European countries.

SAR studies have been performed on *cis*-platinum compounds with the following conclusions:

1   The nature of the leaving group X in PtA_2X_2 determines the rate of the substitution reactions. Strongly bound groups, such as thiocyanate, lead to inactivity in biological systems. On the other hand, very labile groups, such as H_2O or NO_3^-, give rise to very toxic compounds with little or no antitumor activity. It should be mentioned in this context that both chloride ions of e.g. cisplatin are replaced by water molecules before the binding to DNA occurs inside the cells. This does not happen outside the cells, as the concentration of chloride ions in the extracellular fluid is very high.

2   The nature of the amine group A co-ordinated to platinum also influences anticancer activity. Active compounds have at least one hydrogen atom at the N-atom of the amine ligand, which should not be too large.

3   The net-charge of the complexes has to be zero. Presumably, charged complexes are unable to cross the cell membranes.

17.1.1.3 Degradation of DNA

Anticancer agents of a wide range of structural types have been observed to produce strand breaks in DNA *in vivo* and *in vitro*. These include some of the earlier mentioned categories of compounds, e.g. nitrosoureas, but this is not the primary cytotoxic action of these compounds, as it appears to be in the case of *bleomycin*. This drug binds to DNA and causes strand scissions by an oxidative attack involving chelated iron and free radical species.

Bleomycin (**17.22**): Bleomycins are a group of related glucopeptide antibiotics isolated from *Streptomyces verticillus*. Bleomycin A_2 (Scheme 17.6) is the major component of the bleomycin employed clinically (as the sulphate). The various bleomycins differ only in their terminal amine moieties. In bleomycinic acid, which is inactive, the terminal amine moiety is replaced by a hydroxyl group.

Bleomycin (BLM) can be given by a number of parenteral routes, but it is most commonly injected intravenously. The drug is widely distributed in the tissues, except in brain tissue. Apparently BLM cannot enter the cerebrospinal fluid in any significant concentration. The highest concentrations of active drug are found in skin and lung. This is important because these two sites are very susceptible to BLM toxicity. The most common acute side effects involve the skin and mucous membranes, and the most severe, dose-limiting BLM toxicity is the pulmonary toxicity. The BLM is unique among the available antitumor antibiotics by producing very little bone marrow depression. For this reason, it is particularly useful in combination therapy with nearly all major anticancer drugs.

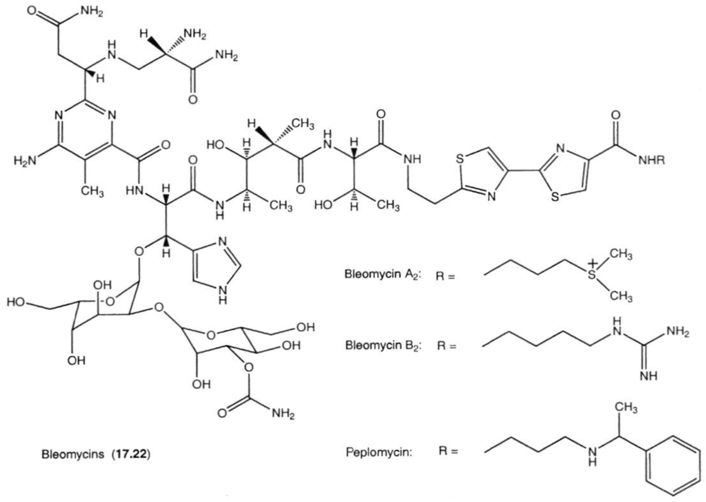

Scheme 17.6

The chemistry and biological effects and mechanism of action of BLM have been extensively studied. The glycopeptide contains several unusual amino acids and sugars, a pyrimidine ring, an imidazole ring, and a bithiazole ring system. X-ray structure determination of BLM has not been reported, and the structure shown in Scheme 17.6 is based on conventional methods and confirmed by high-resolution, 2D NMR spectroscopy.

The BLM molecule contains at least four functional domains. The left part of the molecule is the metal chelating domain, where the oxidative reaction with DNA is initiated. The bithiazole and C-terminal substituent are known to be involved in DNA binding, and the linker region (the pentapeptide) has been shown to be of importance to the efficiency of DNA cleavage by BLM. The function of the fourth domain, the carbohydrate moiety, is not well understood, but may be important for metal ion co-ordination.

The BLM binds in the minor grove of DNA with specific DNA sequences (5′GC3′ and 5′GT3′ sites) leading to sequence selectivity in DNA cleavage. Computer analysis and modeling of a DNA–BLM complex has been performed, but the structure of the complex has not yet been confirmed by X-ray analysis. The reaction by which DNA strand scission is effected by BLM has been found to require Fe(II) and O_2 as cofactors. The ultimate agent of DNA damage is an active BLM dioxygen species.

Bleomycin forms one-to-one complexes with several metals, e.g. copper, zinc, iron, and cobalt. The BLM–Cu(II) complex is the most stable complex and also the natural form produced by fermentation. It is inactive and resistant to BLM hydrolase, a BLM inactivating enzyme. The BLM hydrolase is present in cells and hydrolyses metal-free BLM, resulting in inactivation of BLM.

After injection of BLM (metal-free) it binds to Cu(II) ions in blood to form the stable BLM–Cu(II) complex. Inside the cells, the copper of the complex is removed reductively and trapped by other proteins, leaving BLM free to form the active iron complex (or to enzymatical inactivation). Thus, the Cu(II) complex of BLM protects against inactivation and provides transport and distribution of BLM in the body in an inactive form.

The structure of the Fe(II) complex of BLM is shown in Scheme 17.7. The structure of the iron complex is based on the X-ray structure of a model compound, i.e. a copper complex of a smaller part of the BLM molecule, lacking the sugar and bithiazole moieties. In the oxygenated iron complex there is strong evidence suggesting that dioxygen is the sixth ligand.

In the cells the oxygenated complex, BLM-Fe(II)-O_2, is further converted into a transient ferric species called 'activated BLM', which produces the oxidative species that initiate DNA degradation by abstraction of a H-atom at C-4′ of a backbone sugar ring. The degradation of DNA by BLM has been studied by identification of the products (DNA fragments) formed, and, while degrading the deoxyribose, BLM releases the bases undamaged. This is compatible with a site-specific generation of an oxygen radical species close to a susceptible site on the deoxyribose moiety and remote from the bases.

One of the disadvantages of BLM treatment is the development of pulmonary fibrosis. A lot of semi-synthetic BLM analogs have been prepared in order to find an active drug with lower pulmonary toxicity, e.g. *peplomycin*, a BLM with a

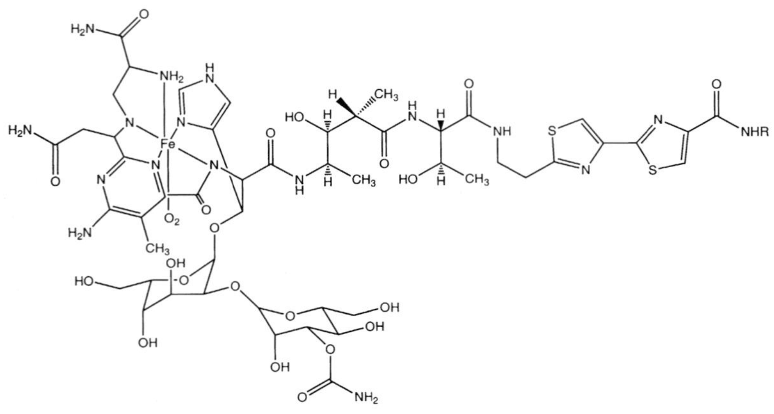

Scheme 17.7

synthetic terminal amine (Scheme 17.6). Semi-synthetic BLM analogs can be prepared by reaction of the Cu(II) complex of BLM acid with the amine in the presence of a coupling reagent for peptide synthesis. The BLM acid is prepared enzymatically from native BLM in order to avoid cleavage also of other peptide bonds in the molecule. The Cu(II) co-ordination protects the primary amino group in the α-position of the terminal β-aminoalanine moiety and prevents inter- and intramolecular coupling.

17.1.1.4 Intercalating agents

Several compounds bind reversibly to double-stranded DNA by intercalation, i.e. by squeezing in between adjacent base pairs of DNA. Such compounds have to be rather planar and are most often aromatic ring systems, which are held between the flat purine and pyrimidine rings by van der Waals' forces and charge-transfer complex formation. Some of the compounds also bind covalently, in some cases after metabolic transformation, e.g. *benzopyrene*, which is a carcinogen. Intercalating drugs can be primarily antibacterial (e.g. *aminoacridines*), antimalarial (e.g. *mepacrine*), or carcinostatic agents (e.g. *actinomycin D, daunorubicin* and *doxorubicin*). In this chapter, only the anticancer agents will be considered.

Several techniques have been used to characterize the interactions of intercalating agents with DNA. Evidence for binding to DNA can be obtained by determination of the association constant and number of binding sites. Intercalating agents give rise to increase in the length of DNA, as shown diagrammatically in Figure 17.3. This unwinding property of intercalators can be used in several ways to demonstrate that drugs bind to DNA by intercalation. One method is to investigate the effect of the drugs on the supercoiling of closed circular duplex DNA, by monitoring the rate of sedimentation, which decreases by unwinding. The anticancer antibiotic *mithramycin* is an example of a drug, which binds to DNA in a different way, as it does not change DNA supercoiling. Detailed information on the nature of the binding of intercalating agents to DNA can be obtained by studying

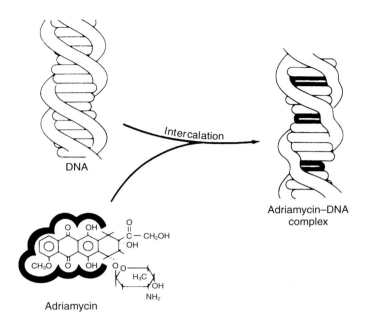

Figure 17.3 Diagrammatic model of intercalation of the flat part of the adriamycin molecule (in black) into DNA, showing local unwinding of the helical structure. From Lerman, L.S. *J. Cell. Comp. Physiol.*, **64**, Suppl. 1:1 (1964) with permission by LISS (Alan R. Liss, Inc.). New York.

model drug–DNA complexes by NMR methods or – when crystalline complexes are available – by X-ray structure determinations. In addition, molecular modeling methods have become increasingly significant in recent years.

The DNA intercalation has various biological consequences, e.g. inhibition of DNA replication and transcription, probably due to prevention of DNA/RNA polymerase activity. The cytotoxicity of intercalating agents is believed to be primarily a consequence of the DNA interaction, but DNA breakage (strand scissions), generated by some of the drugs in a reaction involving the nuclear enzyme topoisomerase II, contributes to the cytotoxicity and may play an important role in their mutagenic and carcinogenic activity.

Actinomycin D (**17.23**), d-actinomycin, AMD, is an anticancer antibiotic isolated from *Streptomyces* species. It is given by rapid flowing infusion, because injection is accompanied by severe local reaction. Additional serious side effects, both acute and delayed, have limited the clinical application, but the drug is still in use, e.g. in combined chemoradiotherapy.

The AMD molecule consists of an aminophenoxazone ring system, to which two identical cyclic pentapeptides are attached. The first and the last amino acids are linked by the formation of a lactone ring. Information on the binding of AMD to DNA was originally obtained from the X-ray structure determination of a drug–nucleoside model complex (Figure 17.4).

N-methylvaline

CH(CH₃)₂ HC(CH₃)₂

O═C CH CH C═O

NCH₃ NCH₃

Sarcosine Sarcosine

L-proline L-proline

D-valine D-valine

C═O C═O

CH₃HC—CH CH—CHCH₃

NH NH

Threonine

C═O C═O

NH₂

N

O

CH₃ CH₃

O

Actinomycin D (17.23)

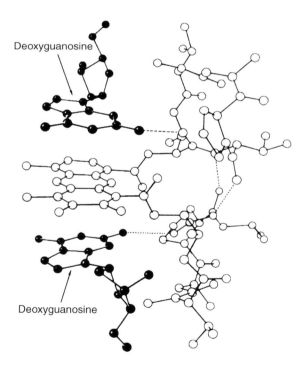

Deoxyguanosine

Deoxyguanosine

Figure 17.4 The X-ray structure of the actinomycin–deoxyguanosine complex. The two deoxy-guanosine molecules stack on alternate sides of the phenoxazone ring. Hydrogen bonds are indicated by dashed lines. (Redrawn from Sobell, H.M. *et al.* (1971), *Nature New Biol.*, **231**, 200 with permission by Macmillan Journals Ltd.).

The study showed that the planar phenoxazone ring of AMD in the model complex is squeezed in between the planar guanine bases of two deoxyguanosine molecules. Strong hydrogen bonds connect the 2-amino groups of guanine and the carbonyl oxygen of threonine residues in the cyclic peptides and contribute to the strong binding of AMD to DNA. Based on model building, the cyclic peptides were suggested to lie in the minor grove of DNA. This was confirmed by structure determination of a model complex consisting of AMD and the self-complementary double helix DNA octamer d(GAAGCTTC), Figure 17.5. The numerous van der Waals interactions between the peptide side chains and DNA contribute considerably to the tight binding of AMD.

Daunorubicin (**17.24**), daunomycin, and *doxorubicin* (**17.25**), adriamycin, are both anthracycline antibiotics isolated from various *Streptomyces* species. The compounds are unstable in alkaline and acidic aqueous solution and cannot be given orally. Although daunorubicin and doxorubicin have very similar chemical structures, doxorubicin is more cytotoxic and has a wider spectrum of antitumor activity. The reasons for these differences in activity are not quite clear. Both drugs bind tightly to DNA with comparable association constants (ca. $10^5 M^{-1}$). The differences in potency and clinical use may be due to differences in cellular pharmacokinetics, uptake, transport and distribution of the drugs.

Doxorubicin has the broadest range of clinical usefulness of the anticancer drugs in routine clinical use and has established activity against several solid tumors, which earlier were relatively unresponsive to chemotherapy. Daunorubicin is primarily used to treat acute leukemia. The side effects of the two anthracycline drugs are similar, e.g. nausea and vomiting, alopecia, myelosuppression and cardiotoxicity (cardiomyopathy). The cardiotoxicity, which is the most serious side effect limiting the doses and the duration of the treatment, is connected to the quinone moiety of the aromatic ring system, which, after reduction to a semi-quinone radical species, induces lipid peroxidation by a free radical mechanism. The involvment of iron has been suggested, and iron-chelators are considered for use as cardioprotective agents against doxorubicin-mediated cardiotoxicity. In addition, thousands of analogs have been synthesized and tested in order to find effective drugs without – or with lower – cardiotoxicity.

The anthracyclines daunorubicin and doxorubicin have a characteristic four-ring structure (rings A–D), the aglycon chromophore, which is linked, via a glycoside bond, to an amino sugar, daunosamine. The rings B–D constitute the anthracycline

Daunomycin (**17.24**) R = H
Adriamycin (**17.25**) R = OH

Mitoxantrone (**17.26**)
$R_1 = R_2 = NHCH_2CH_2NHCH_2CH_2OH$

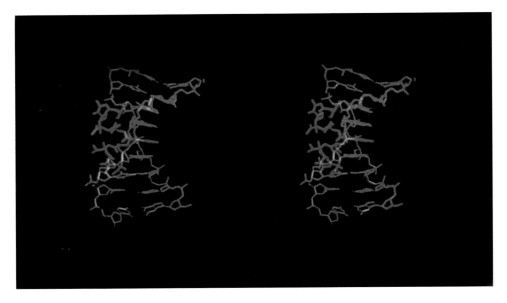

Figure 17.5 Stereoview of the AMD-d(GAAGCTTC) complex. The AMD molecule is shown in magenta, the DNA octamer in green. This side view of the complex shows the intercalation of the chromofore in the G5C5 site and the cyclic peptides of AMD in the minor groove. The structure was generated using the program SYBYL with co-ordinates from Protein Data Bank.

nucleus. The only difference between the structures of the two drugs is in the C-9 side chain of ring A, doxorubicin being the C-14 hydroxy derivative of daunorubicin.

The interaction of anthracycline drugs with DNA by intercalation has been demonstrated by several methods. Detailed information on the daunorubicin-DNA interactions has been obtained from X-ray structure determinations of several model complexes, e.g. of daunorubicin co-crystallized with the self-complementary DNA hexamer d(CGTACG). The six-base pair fragment of the double helix of DNA binds two molecules of daunorubicin (plus several water molecules and two sodium ions). The structure of part of this model compound is shown in Figure 17.6, which focuses on four base pairs of the hexamer with daunorubicin intercalated.

In the model complex, the planar anthracycline part of the daunorubicin molecule is squeezed in between the layers of C–G base pairs of the right-handed DNA double helix (B-DNA), at the CpG sites of both ends of the hexamer duplex (cf. the structure of the doxorubicin–DNA hexamer complex shown in Figure 17.7). The long axis of the anthracycline aglycon is almost perpendicular to the direction of the base pair hydrogen bonds. This is in contrast to model complexes of other drugs, e.g. *proflavine* in complex with the dinucleotide d(CpG), where the long axis is parallel to the base pairs (parallel overlap). As a result of the non-parallel intercalation of the daunorubicin aglycon, the amino sugar ring is placed in the

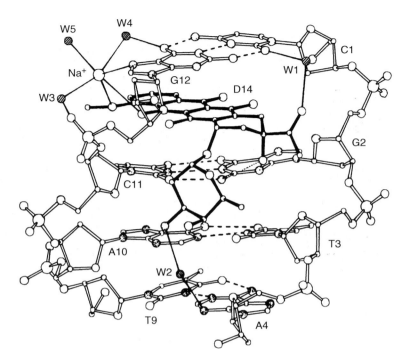

Figure 17.6 Diagram of daunomycin (D14) intercalated into the DNA hexamer. Four base pairs are shown (G12:C1, C11:G2, A10:T3, and T9:A4). Hydrogen bonds in base pairs are represented by dashed lines, other hydrogen bonds by dotted lines (those involving O-9) or thin lines (those involving bridging water molecules, W1 and W2). From Wang, H.-J. *et al.* (1987) *Biochemistry*, **26**, 1152 , with permission by The American Chemical Society.

minor groove of DNA, while the ring D of the anthracycline moiety protrudes on the major groove side. The distance between the base pairs of the intercalation site is increased from the normal 3.4 to 6.8 Å, and this can be achieved by adjusting the torsion angles of the phosphate ester backbones, resulting in a slightly distorted DNA fragment (unwinding of the DNA double helix).

The model complex shows that the cyclohexene ring A of the daunorubicin aglycon is almost planar, with the exception of C-9, which is displaced in the same direction as the amino sugar relative to the plane of the aglycon. This arrangement, in combination with the axially placed hydroxyl group at C-9, gives rise to several specific hydrogen bonding interactions, which stabilize the binding of daunorubicin. The hydroxyl oxygen atom O-9 is involved in two hydrogen bonds, both to nitrogen atoms of the guanine base G2 below the intercalator. Another hydrogen bonding system is seen on the other side of the aglycon ring system involving the C-13 oxygen atom O-13. This carbonyl oxygen is hydrogen bonded via a water molecule (W1) to a carbonyl oxygen atom of the cytosine ring C1 in the base pair above the intercalator. In this way, the OH group and the side chain at C-9 of ring A together serves as an anchor for the daunorubicin molecule and

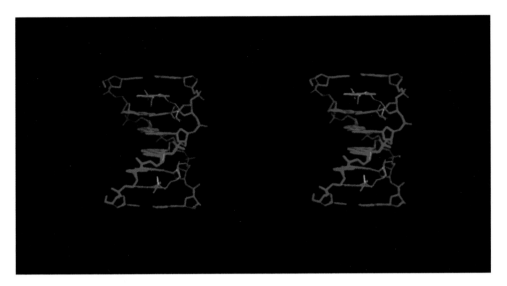

Figure 17.7 A stereoview of the adriamycin-d(CGATCG) complex. The two antibiotic molecules are shown in green, the DNA hexamer in red. The structure was generated using the program SYBYL with co-ordinates from Protein Data Bank.

contributes considerably to the stability of the binding complex, in addition to the 'stacking forces' at the intercalation site.

The amino sugar portion of daunorubicin is held in a proper orientation by the hydrogen bonding system of the C-9 substituents. It fits snugly into the minor groove, but this position excludes any interaction between the positively charged amino group of the sugar ring and the negatively charged phosphate oxygen atoms of the backbone. The X-ray results show that the sugar ring is very mobile, probably due to the lack of strong specific hydrogen bonding as well as ionic interactions. It is believed that the amino sugar is the recognition site for the enzyme topoisomerase II during the process leading to the formation of a ternay DNA–drug–enzyme complex and ultimately to enzyme-mediated DNA cleavage.

Several X-ray structures of the model complexes have now been determined. The model complexes consisting of the DNA hexamer d(CGATCG) and dauno-rubicin and doxorubicin, respectively, are almost isostructural. In both structures, the anthracycline antibiotic intercalate with d(CpG) as the intercalation site, indi-cating some sequence specificity of the drugs. Theoretical as well as experimental studies indicate that the third base pair is also of importance and should preferably be an A–T base pair (triplet recognition). In the doxorubicin complex, the O-14 hydroxyl group is hydrogen bonded to a nearby phosphate group via a water molecule.

Structure–activity studies, involving numerous synthetic, semisynthetic as well as natural anthracycline analogs, have been performed with the aim of finding structural analogs with reduced toxicity and/or a wider spectrum of activity. The testing for anticancer activity of compounds with modifications in the amino sugar moiety showed relatively low limitations for structural variations in this part of the drug molecule. The chirality of the 4'-position can be changed, *epirubicin* (4'-epidoxorubicin) has antitumor activity comparable to doxorubicin and is in clinical use. The compound has reduced cardiotoxicity when compared to doxorubicin, probably due to a more extensive metabolism (conversion to the 4'-O-beta-D-glucuronide). *Idarubicin* (4-demethoxydaunorubicin) is a highly potent antileukemic drug. A notable property of this analog is represented by its rate of cell uptake, which is distinctly higher when compared with that of the parent 4-methoxylated compound daunorubicin.

The presence of a cationic charge on the sugar ring connected to the aglycon seems to be of importance. Acylation of the amino group leads to markedly lower potency as is the case when the amino group is replaced by a hydroxy group. In all anthracycline aminoglycosides reported earlier, the amino sugar was invariably directly attached to the aglycone. However, recently a 'third generation' doxorubicin analog (MEN 10755) was reported with a disaccharide attached to the aglycone, in which the dounosamine is the second sugar ring. This compound has shown very promising antiproliferative activity when tested in a spectrum of human tumors and is undergoing clinical trials. The design of disaccharide compounds was based on the consideration that extension of the sugar moiety might increase the capacity of the topoisomerase enzyme to recognize the DNA–drug complex, and actually increased enzyme-mediated DNA cleavage was observed using MEN 10755 and enzyme preparations *in vitro*.

The anticancer agent, *mitoxanthrone* (**17.26**), is an aminoalkyl-substituted anthraquinone, i.e. a derivative in which the amino sugar, as well as ring A, are replaced by side chains with several possibilities for hydrogen bonding and protonation (hydroxy and amino functions). X-ray structure determination of a mitoxantrone–nucleotide model complex has not been published, but computer modeling and energy calculations have shown that this compound, as well as several analogs, can also bind intercalatively with DNA, and that the aminoalkyl substituents are used to anchor the molecules. Mitoxanthrone is an example of a drug designed on the basis of knowledge on drug–DNA interactions obtained from model complexes.

The methoxy group on C-4 of ring D of the anthracyclines is not required for anticancer activity, idarubicin is, as mentioned, a highly active compound. This is in accordance with the model, which shows that ring D protrudes out into the major groove without direct interaction with the DNA helix. *Carminomycin*, in which the methoxy group is replaced with an OH group, also has antitumor activity. The hydroquinone system is more sensitive to structural changes. The overlap of the rings B and C with base pairs is relatively small, but the oxygen atoms on each side of the rings may play a stabilizing role by being stacked with the bases. Methylation of the hydroxy groups results in loss of potency and lower affinity to DNA.

The geometry and substitutions of ring A are most important for the activity of anthracycline antibiotics. This is in full agreement with the model, which shows that this part anchors the molecules by hydrogen bonding to the bases on either side of the intercalator. The chirality at C-9 and C-7 cannot be changed without loss of activity. Substitution of the C-9 hydroxy group with a methyl group also leads to inactive compounds, and when the hydroxy group is removed, compounds with reduced affinity to DNA and lowered anticancer efficacy are obtained. Ring A cannot be 9,10-dehydrogenated without loss of activity, probably because the proper 'sofa'-conformation of this ring is thereby hindered. The C-9 side chain has to be of small size and with one or two oxygen atoms, which can provide for the hydrogen bonding to the base pair above the intercalator molecule.

Several drug design studies are aimed at developing sequence-specific DNA intercalators, e.g. *bis*-intercalators in which two intercalating ligands are bridged by a central linking chain, in order to obtain specific effects and stronger binding to DNA. Such compounds might become of interest in gene therapy.

17.1.1.5 *Antisense agents*

Nucleic acids are the targets for the so-called antisense agents, which are under design and development for e.g. anticancer and antivirus chemotherapy. The antisense gene-targeted therapeutic approach is a new and emerging technique, for selective manipulation of gene activity. In this technique an 'antisense' sequence (inverted piece of the gene code) complementary to the coding strand is used to specifically lock unto potentially dangerous genetic messengers, canceling their ability to do harm. The bad gene could be a cancer-causing oncogene, and this is one of the potential roles of antisense agents in cancer therapy.

Antisense agents normally target the gene's messenger RNA (mRNA), as they are designed to bind with and block the specific piece corresponding to the bad gene on DNA (Figure 17.8). Translation of the genetic information is thereby blocked, and the ribosomal production of the corresponding protein is prevented (the antisense strategy). Alternatively, it is possible to use the double-stranded DNA as target. In this case, the compounds (oligonucleotides, 'oligos') are called anti-gene agents, as they block the gene by binding directly to DNA, forming a local triple helix (the antigene approach).

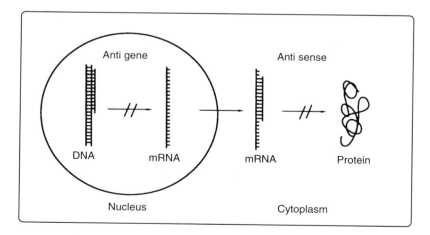

Figure 17.8 Schematic illustration of the antisense/antigene DNA principle. (The drawing was kindly provided by Professor Peter E. Nielsen, Research Center for Medical Bio-technology, University of Copenhagen, Denmark).

The major technical problems in using antisense/antigene agents as drugs are to figure out (1) how to penetrate into the cells; (2) how to prevent degradation of the oligos by nucleases; and (3) how to obtain effective binding to the target. Improvement of stability and cellular uptake of oligos have been obtained by chemical changes in the phosphodiester group. In addition, it appears that oligos with 10–15 bases are able to effectively block a gene.

Peptide nucleic acids (PNAs) are nucleic acid mimics showing a promising potential as gene-specific drugs. The PNAs are oligonucleotides in which the backbone is replaced by a peptide-like backbone of N-(2-aminoethyl)glycine units that bind with high affinity to complementary sequences of DNA and RNA. The PNAs are easy to prepare, water soluble and stable at biological conditions. The main problem is that PNAs does not readily enter the cells. The cellular uptake of PNA might be facilitated by conjugation to carrier molecules or incorporation into liposomes, and then the basis for the development of gene-specific drugs of decisive value in gene chemotherapy seems to be very good. Oligonucleotides with other modifications of the nucleotide backbone are currently being developed, e.g. phosphorothioates with a sulphur atom substituting one of the non-bridging oxygen atoms, and locked nucleic acids (LNAs) consisting of 2'-O, 4'-C methylene bicyclonucleotides, i.e. with a 'locked' normal backbone.

The new approach in anticancer, antibacterial and antivirus research, based on mRNA (or duplex DNA) as the primary drug target, is very promising and might lead to the desired goal in chemotherapy: selective cell death.

17.1.2 Drugs interfering with DNA synthesis

A number of different enzymes are involved in the synthesis of DNA and these are potential targets for anticancer (as well as antibacterial and antiviral) drug action. Inhibitors of these enzymes, which also often are called antimetabolites, block more or less crucial steps in DNA synthesis. Most of the drugs so far used in cancer chemotherapy were found by routine screening of the compounds and their mechanism of action was established later. Now, several of the structures of the enzymes involved in DNA synthesis are known from X-ray structure determinations, and new drugs are being designed and developed using this knowledge (structure-based drug design). Anticancer agents with effect as inhibitors of enzymes involved in DNA synthesis are specific for the S-phase of the cell cycle.

17.1.2.1 Inhibition of tetrahydrofolate synthesis

Folic acid analogs have for many years been used in the chemotherapy of infectious and neoplastic diseases. These drugs act by inhibiting the enzyme dihydrofolate reductase (DHFR). This enzyme, which is widely distributed in nature (from bacteria, protozoa and plants to man), converts dihydrofolic acid to tetrahydrofolic acid in the presence of NADPH as a cofactor (Scheme 17.8).

The DHFR is one of the enzymes that has been most thoroughly studied, and the 3D-structure of the protein is known from X-ray structure determinations of DHFR from many different origins (e.g. E. coli, L. casei, chicken and man). Some of the structures are known both without and with inhibitor and/or cofactor

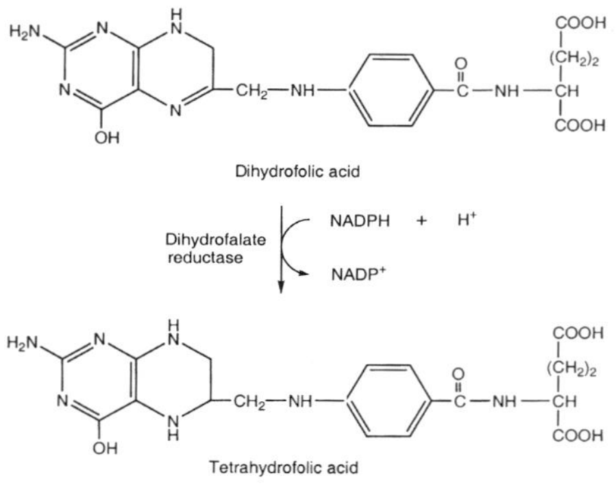

Scheme 17.8

(NADPH) bound to the enzyme in a binary or ternary complex, showing the interactions between the drug and its 'receptor' (the biomacromolecule). Some of the inhibitors of DHFR have become useful in the treatment of cancer, e.g. *methotrexate*, others as antibacterial drugs, e.g. *trimethoprim*, while *pyrimethamine* is used as an antimalarial drug. Only the anticancer drug methotrexate is discussed in more detail. The other drugs will be mentioned for comparison in an attempt to understand the differential use of the drugs.

Methotrexate (**17.27**), MTX, is closely related to folic acid (Scheme 17.9), and the compound can be prepared synthetically. The MTX has a low aqueous solubility, and the risk of nephrotoxicity can be minimized in patients on high dose therapy by alkalinizing the urine. The MTX is widely used in cancer chemotherapy, most often in combination with other drugs. It has serious side effects, both acute effects,

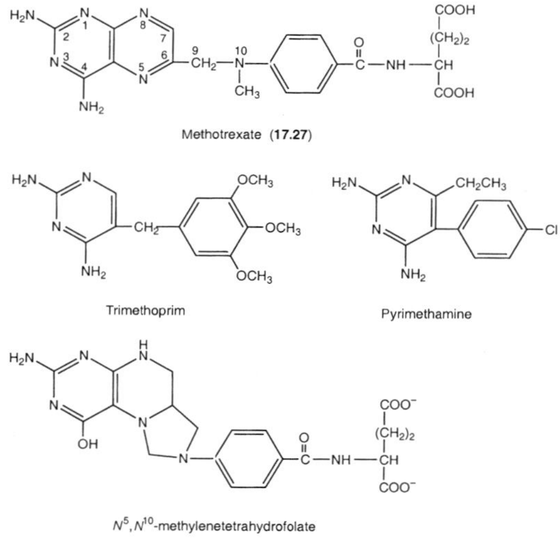

Scheme 17.9

e.g. ulceration, and delayed toxicities as bone marrow depression and – particularly with high doses – hepatic toxicity.

The MTX and other folic acid analogs are potent competitive inhibitors of DHFR ($K_i < 10^{-9}$ M). There are several consequences of inhibiting the synthesis of tetrahydrofolate, since this compound is further converted *in vivo* to N^5, N^{10}-methylenetetrahydrofolate (methylene-THF, Scheme 17.9), which functions as a cofactor for various enzymes involved in one-carbon transfer reactions, e.g. for the enzyme thymidylate synthase (cf. Figure 17.12). The most critical effect leading to cell death after exposure to MTX is probably the indirect inhibition of the action of thymidylate synthase and thereby blocking of the production of deoxythymidylate, which is required for the synthesis of DNA. The MTX is actively transported into the cells, and the ability of various tumor cells to transport MTX seems to be related to their ability to respond to the drug. Increased cellular content of DHFR due to increased rate of enzyme synthesis is probably the main reason for resistance to MTX.

The amino acid sequences for a number of DHFRs (i.e. enzymes from several different sources) have been determined, and, as expected, they have common features. The sequence identity between enzymes from different vertebrates is in the region of 75–90%, between the vertebrate enzymes and the bacterial enzymes, on the other hand, only about 20–30%. Nevertheless, X-ray crystallographic studies of the DHFRs have shown that there is a high degree of resemblance in the folding of the main chains of these enzymes. As an example of this, the tertiary structures of DHFR from chicken liver and from *E. coli* are shown in Figure 17.9.

Common to these, and other known DHFR structures, is a central 8-stranded β-sheet area with the strands denoted βA–H. In addition, the molecules contain four helical regions, αB, αC, αE and αF. The molecules have a bi-lobed appearance, as the active site forms a 15 Å deep cleft in the central part of the molecule between the B and C helices. The width of this cleft has been observed to be 1.5–2.0 Å greater in the vertebrate enzymes than that in the bacterial enzymes. In addition to that, the foldings mostly differ in the loop areas at the surface of the enzyme. Nevertheless, it seems evident that the structural differences between enzymes are responsible for the highly selective inhibition of *E. coli* DHFR exhibited by trimethoprim and the particular selectivity of pyrimethamine for DHFR of the malarial protozoan *Plasmodium berghei*. Recently, the structure of the fungal pathogen *Pneumocystis carnii* DHFR has been determined, and structure-based drug design is in progress. Development of selective drugs is important, because this infective agent is critical to AIDS patients, causing the severe pneumonia that is a major cause of death.

X-ray crystallographic studies of the enzyme–inhibitor complex of e.g. DHFR from *E. coli* and MTX show the binding interactions between drug and protein (Figure 17.10A). As it appears from the figure, there are good contacts to side chains of amino acids at the active site of the protein. The pteridine ring interacts with Asp-27 through the electrostatic interactions at N-1 and the 2-amino group (salt bridges or 'charge-assisted' hydrogen bonds). The pKa value for N-1 of MTX has been shown to be much higher in the complex than in free MTX (10 and 5.7, respectively), which implies that in the complex, the pteridine ring is protonated at physiological pH. In addition to inhibitor binding, Asp-27 appears to play an

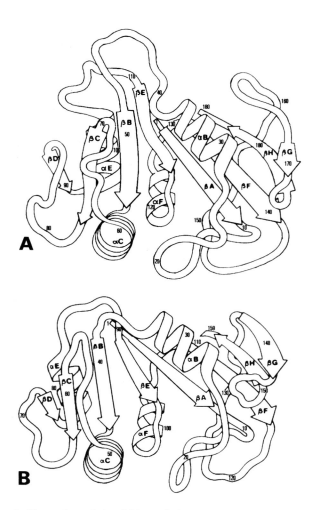

Figure 17.9 Schematic illustration of the folding of the main chain, A of chicken liver, and B of *E. coli* DHFR (From Beddell, C.R. in *X-Ray Crystallography and Drug Action*, eds. A.S. Horn and C.J. De Ranter, Oxford University Press, Oxford 1984 with permission by Oxford University Press).

important functional role in the reduction of the enzyme substrate. The 4-amino group of the pteridine ring is hydrogen bonded to backbone carbonyl groups behind the drug (not shown). The α-carboxylic group of the glutamate moiety of MTX is involved in strong hydrogen bonding (charge-assisted) with the guanidinium group of Arg-57, whereas the γ-carboxylic group is not directly bonded to the protein. The benzene moiety of MTX is sandwiched between Ile-50 and Leu-28 forming hydrophobic (or van der Waals) contacts to these residues.

In Figure 17.10B, the X-ray structure of the trimethoprim (TMP) complex with *E. coli* DHFR is illustrated. As it can be seen, there are qualitative similarities between the binding of the two drugs, MTX and TMP. The 2,4-diamino-

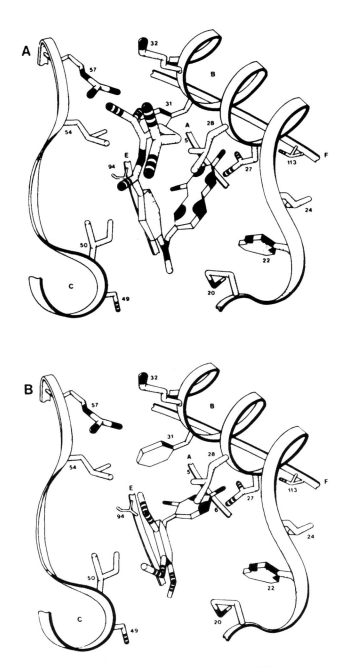

Figure 17.10 Schematic illustration of the active site of *E. coli* DHFR; A with bound methotrexate, and B with bound trimethoprim. Selected atoms of drugs and protein side chains are highlighted: oxygen by stripes, nitrogen in black, and sulphur by hatching. (From Beddell, C.R. – see legend to Figure 17.9).

pyrimidine rings bind in the same manner, the benzene rings are involved in hydrophobic interactions, and charged-assisted hydrogen bonds are formed to Asp-27 in both cases. However, TMP does not have a carboxylic group and cannot interact electrostatically with Arg-57. On the other hand, the trimethoxy-phenyl ring fits very favorably into the more narrow active site cleft of *E. coli* DHFR. The relatively subtle structural differences are apparently largely respons-ible for the 3000-fold difference in affinity of TMP for *E. coli* DHFR compared to the chicken liver enzyme.

The structure of the *E. coli* DHFR-TMP complex has been used for modeling studies with the aim of designing analogs of TMP with higher affinities for the enzyme. This study is a very early example of structure-based drug design. The TMP analogs in which one *meta*-methoxy group was replaced by carbalkoxy substituents of varying lengths were designed (Scheme 17.10). Modeling experi-ments using computer graphics indicated that the compound with five methylene groups in the chain was able to interact particularly well with Arg-57 in the same way as methotrexate.

The compounds were synthesized and tested for enzyme affinity, and the compound with five methylene groups was found to be most active. X-ray structure determination of *E. coli* DHFR complexed with this carbalkoxy analog was performed in order to determine the actual position of the analog in the active site. The study shows that the compound actually is binding as modeled (Figure 17.11). Because of unfavorable biopharmaceutical properties this analog did not become a new antibacterial drug, but similar analogs are being developed.

Other methods, e.g. classical QSAR, have been used for rational design and analysis of inhibitors of DHFR. However, the most obvious approach to the design of novel inhibitors is the utilization of the 3D-structures of the enzyme. With detailed knowledge of the structure of the enzymes of different origin (vertebrate, bacterial, fungal etc.), the opportunities for rational design of selective inhibitors are optimal.

17.1.2.2   Inhibition of purine and pyrimidine synthesis

Analogs of purine and pyrimidine block one or more steps in the purine/pyrimidine synthesis. Both categories of compounds have to be converted in the cells into the corresponding nucleotides before they become active. Several analogs of purine and pyrimidine nucleotides are important as antiviral agents and are discussed in Chapter 16.

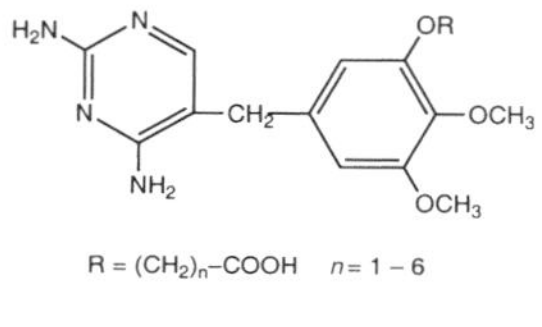

$R = (CH_2)_n-COOH$ $n = 1 - 6$

Scheme 17.10

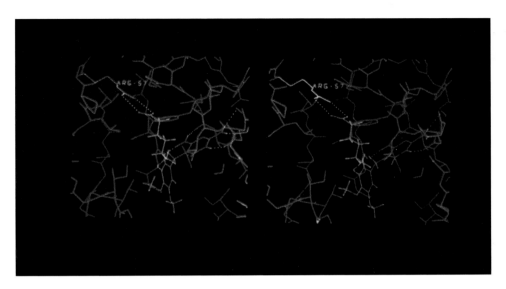

Figure 17.11 The active site of *E. coli* DHFR with an carbalkoxy analog of trimethoprim bound (C, green; H, white; N, blue; O, red). (From Hitchings, G.H. *et al.* in *Design of Enzyme Inhibitors as Drugs*, eds. M. Sandler and H.J. Smith. Oxford University Press, Oxford 1989, with permission by Oxford University Press.

6-mercaptopurine (**17.28**)   6-thioguanine (**17.29**)   5-fluorouracil (**17.30**)

6-Mercaptopurine (**17.28**), 6-MP, and *6-thioguanine* (**17.29**), 6-TG, are purine analogs, which can be given orally, and are used in the treatment of leukemias. Bone marrow depression is the principal toxic effect of both drugs. Allopurinol can be given to inhibit xanthine oxidase degradation of 6-MP into thiouric acid, thereby preventing renal damage.

The 6-MP acts as a normal substrate for the enzyme hypoxanthine–guanine phosphoribosyl transferase and is thus converted into the nucleotide 6-mercaptopurine ribose phosphate (6-MPRP). This nucleotide interferes with an early step in the purine biosynthesis by inhibiting the enzyme phosphoribosylpyrophosphate (PRPP) amidotransferase. In addition, several other enzymatic pathways are inhibited, and cell death may be the result of a combination of different events. The 6-TG is also converted *in vivo* to the nucleotide (6-TGRP), but it has a much weaker inhibitory effect on the enzymes involved in purine synthesis, e.g. the amidotransferase. The cytotoxic action of 6-TG seems to be primarily due to incorporation into DNA of the nucleotide 6-TGRP after further phosphorylation into the triphosphate.

Fluorouracil (**17.30**), 5-FU, is a synthetically prepared pyrimidine analog with a close structural relationship to the natural base uracil. The drug can be given orally, e.g. as the orally formulated drug tegafur/uracil (UFT), which is a combination of uracil and tegafur (5-FU linked to a dehydroxylated ribose sugar ring, that is hydroxylated *in vivo* by hepatic enzymes leading to a slow but sustained level of 5-FU in the cells). The 5-FU is effective against several types of solid tumors. In combination with oxaliplatin (**17.21**), 5-FU is now successfully used in the treatment of colorectal cancer. The 5-FU has severe side effects, both acute and delayed.

Like the thiopurines, 5-FU has to be converted *in vivo* into a nucleotide, 5-fluoro-2'-deoxyuridine-5'-monophosphate (FdUMP), before it becomes active as a cytotoxic drug. This conversion can be accomplished via different pathways involving various enzymes, and resistance to 5-FU might be due to decreased activity of some of these enzymes.

The FdUMP blocks DNA synthesis by inhibition of the enzyme thymidylate synthase (TS). This enzyme catalyzes the conversion of dUMP into dTMP, which subsequently is incorporated into DNA (Figure 17.12). The FdUMP inhibits the enzyme irreversibly after acting as a normal substrate through part of the catalytic cycle. First, a sulphhydryl group of the enzyme (cysteine-SH) reacts with C-6 of FdUMP (Scheme 17.11). The cofactor methylene-THF then adds to C-5, and, in the case of the substrate dUMP, a proton is removed from C-5 of the bound nucleotide. However, the C–F bond of the bound inhibitor FdUMP cannot be broken, and the catalysis is blocked at the stage where a ternary covalent complex is formed, consisting of enzyme, FdUMP and cofactor.

This mechanism has been confirmed by the X-ray structure determinations of TS from several sources, e.g. *E. coli*, *L. casei*, and human TS, both with and without

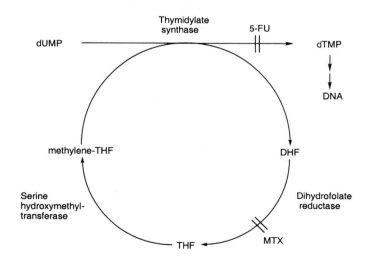

Figure 17.12 Schematic representation of the conversion of dUMP (deoxyuridine monophosphate) into dTMP (deoxythymidine monophosphate). DHF = dihydrofolate, THF = tetrahydrofolate, and methylene-THF = N^5N^{10}-methylenetetrahydrofolate. Fluorouracil (5-FU) inhibits the methylation of dUMP, and MTX blocks the regeneration of THF from DHF.

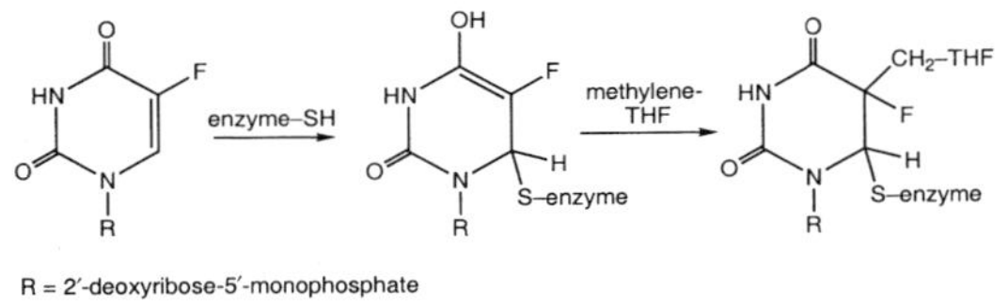

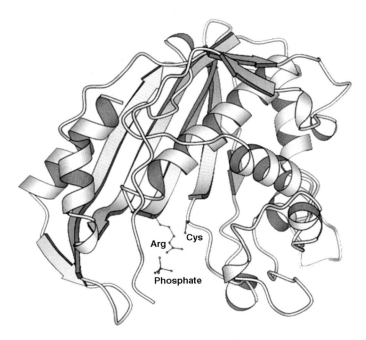

R = 2'-deoxyribose-5'-monophosphate

Scheme 17.11

inhibitor and/or cofactor or cofactor analog. In the native enzyme, the cysteine residue that reacts with C-6 of FdUMP is situated in the active site cleft with hydrogen bonding to an arginine residue (Figure 17.13) and is thereby activated (more nucleophilic). In complexes with inhibitor (or substrate) and cofactor (or cofactor analog), covalent bonds connect the inhibitor with enzyme and cofactor (short distances are observed, Figures 17.14 and 17.15).

The 5-FU has been used in cancer treatment for more than 40 years. However, TS is still an attractive target for anticancer drugs because of its central position in the pathway of DNA synthesis. Co-administration of leucovorin (5-formyl-THF) is now frequently used. Leucovorin is rapidly converted *in vivo* to 5-methyl-THF and further to methylene-THF. Excess of this cofactor ensures the tight binding of FdUMP to the enzyme, the result being optimal inhibition of TS and increased cytotoxic effect of 5-FU.

Figure 17.13 Ribbon representation of the folding of the main chain of TS. Two important residues and a bound phosphate ion in the active site cleft are shown. The figure is generated using the program Molscript with co-ordinates from Protein Data Bank.

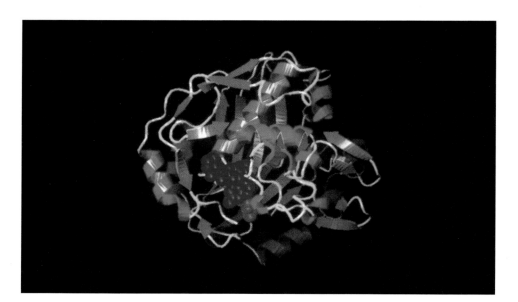

Figure 17.14 The structure of TS of *E. coli* with substrate (in magenta) and co-factor analog (in blue) bound in active site. The structure was generated using the program 'O' with co-ordinates from Protein Data Bank.

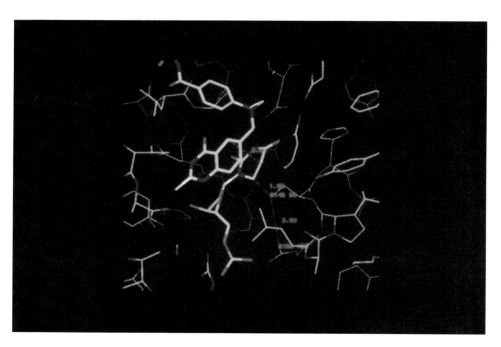

Figure 17.15 The active site of TS with substrate and co-factor analog bound (N, blue; O, red). Dashed lines indicate short distances. The structure was generated using the program 'O' with co-ordinates from Protein Data Bank.

Thymidylate synthase is extensively used for structure-based drug design. Several new cofactor analogs are being developed, some of them very promising and in clinical testing. Also other advanced computer methods are being used, e.g. screening of all compounds of a data base of commercial available compounds for molecules that fits to the active site of *L. casei* TS, using a molecular docking program (DOCK). In addition to retrieving the substrate and several known inhibitors, some previously unknown putative inhibitors were proposed, e.g. phenolphthalein analogs. These compounds, which were found to inhibit TS in the micromolar range, do not resemble the substrate dUMP. X-ray structure determinations of the TS-drug complexes showed that the compounds bind in the active site cleft at another binding region 6–9 Å displaced compared to the substrate. The phenolphthalein analogs are a novel family of tight-binding specific TS inhibitors, found by the use of the known target protein structure, which might lead to the development of new drugs in chemotherapy.

17.1.2.3   Inhibition of DNA/RNA polymerases

The DNA polymerases catalyze the step-by-step addition of deoxynucleotide units to the new DNA strand during DNA replication and are potential targets for anticancer and antiviral drug action. Very few inhibitors of DNA polymerases are in clinical use in cancer therapy, whereas several inhibitors (substrate analogs) have become useful in curing virus infections (see Chapter 16). The compounds are purine or pyrimidine analogs, and some of them are also incorporated into DNA.

Cytarabine (**17.31**), cytosine arabinoside, Ara-C, is a pyrimidine nucleoside analog with a structural change in the ribose ring. The drug is poorly absorbed orally, and it is routinely given intravenously or by continuous infusion methods because of rapid hepatic deamination by cytosine deaminase into inactive ara-U (uracil arabinoside). It is used primarily in the treatment of acute leukemias. The principal toxicities are nausea, vomiting, and bone marrow depression. Ara-C is converted *in vivo* into the active nucleotide triphosphate Ara-CTP by enzymes that treat Ara-C as a normal substrate. Ara-CTP is an analog of the deoxycytidine triphosphate substrate of DNA polymerase and inhibits this enzyme competitively. As a consequence, DNA synthesis and cell growth is inhibited. Resistance to Ara-C is probably associated with high levels of deaminase activity.

Cytarabine (**17.31**)   Vidarabine (**17.32**)

Vidarabine (**17.32**), adenine arabinoside, Ara-A, is a purine nucleoside analog with a similar mechanism of action as Ara-C, but this drug is primarily used as an antiviral agent. Structural modifications of Ara-A and Ara-C, as well as co-administration of a deaminase inhibitor, have been used in order to avoid inactivation of the drugs.

17.1.2.4 *Inhibition of ribonucleotide reductase*

The enzyme *ribonucleotide reductase* (RNR) is an essential component of all living cells. The function of the enzyme is to participate in the synthesis of DNA by catalyzing the conversion of all of the four ribonucleotides into the corresponding deoxyribonucleotides, see Scheme 17.12. This is the only pathway for the formation of deoxyribonucleotides, and the reaction is believed to be a rate limiting step in DNA synthesis. Consequently, RNR is an obvious target for anticancer as well as antibacterial and antiviral drug action. The only RNR inhibitor in clinical use is *hydroxyurea*, but other compounds are in clinical trial. Design and development of selective antiviral agents will also be possible, as some viruses (e.g. herpes simplex virus, HSV) code for their own enzyme system. Structural differences between host and virus enzymes exist and are being utilized in drug design.

Hydroxyurea (**17.33**), *N*-hydroxyurea, hydrea, is a crystalline compound, which is routinely given orally, as it is water soluble and well absorbed from the gastrointestinal tract. It is excreted very rapidly and has to be given in very high and

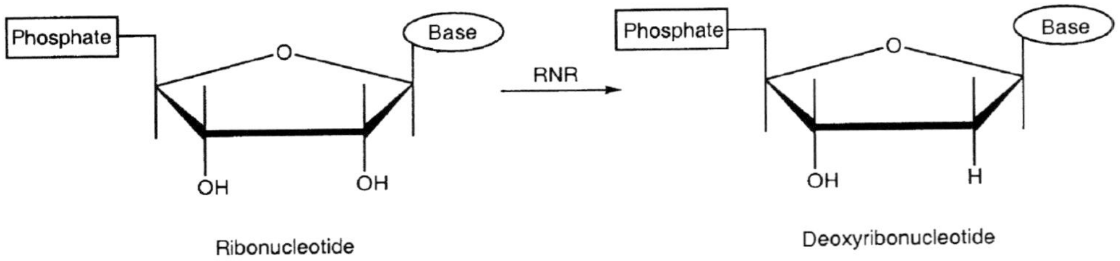

Ribonucleotide   Deoxyribonucleotide

Scheme 17.12

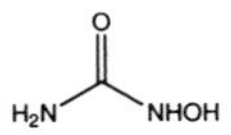

Hydroxyurea (**17.33**)

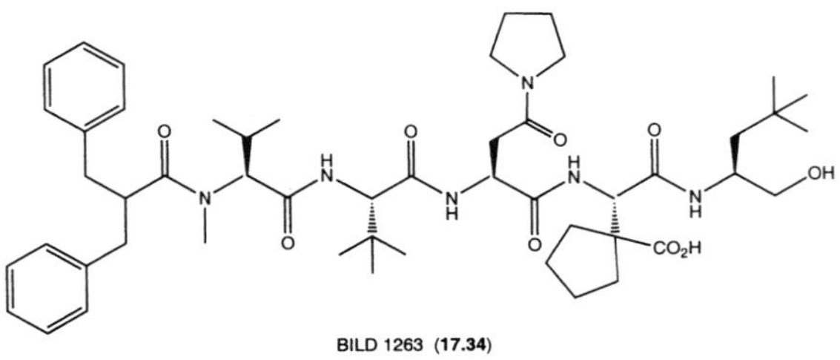

BILD 1263 (**17.34**)

frequent doses. Hydroxyurea is primarily used to treat chronic myelogenous leukemia, but has also demonstrated activity in malignant melanoma and other solid tumors. The acute side effects are mild and bone-marrow depression is the dose-limiting toxicity. Recently, hydroxyurea has been introduced in the treatment of HIV-1 infection because of its inhibitory action in viral replication and to its potentialization of the activitiy of the nucleosides, e.g. AZT (cf. Chapter 16).

Hydroxyurea inhibits RNR by interfering with the smaller of the two proteins, of which the enzyme consists (protein R2, Figure 17.16). R2 is unusual in containing a free radical group (a tyrosyl radical), which is essential for catalysis. This radical is destroyed (reduced to a normal tyrosine residue) by hydroxyurea, and the enzyme function is thereby prevented. Hydroxyurea is an iron chelator, but the iron centers of protein R2 are not affected by the drug. The function of the iron is to generate and stabilize the free radical group.

Studies on analogs of hydroxyurea have indicated that inhibitors of this type (radical scavengers) have to be rather small molecules. X-ray structure determination of protein R2 of the *E. coli* and mammalian enzymes has shown that the tyrosyl radical (and iron center) is buried in a hydrophobic pocket in R2 of *E. coli*, whereas it is more accessible in R2 of the mammalian RNR. The structure of the

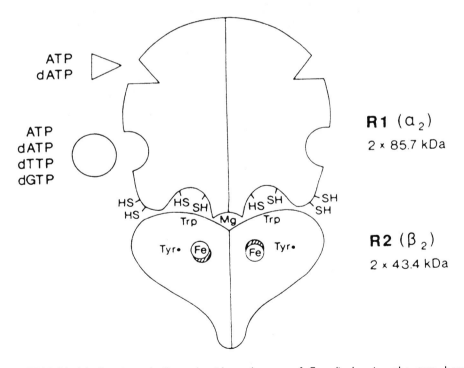

Figure 17.16 Model drawing of ribonucleotide reductase of *E. coli* showing the two homo-dimeric proteins, R1 and R2, the effector sites and the redox-active sulphhydryl groups on R1, and the iron centers and tyrosyl radicals on R2. (The drawing was kindly provided by Professor Britt-Marie Sjöberg, Department of Molecular Biology, University of Stockholm, Sweden).

R1 subunit of *E. coli* RNR has also been determined, and the R1R2 holoenzyme complex has been modeled on the basis of the two separate protein structures (Figure 17.17).

The carboxy terminal of R2 is known to be involved in the R1R2 association. Consequently, peptidomimetics, i.e. analogs of oligopeptides with amino acid sequences corresponding to the carboxy terminal of the R2 subunit of RNR of HSV, have been developed as selective antivirus agents. These compounds inhibit the enzyme by interfering with the interphase between the subunits, thereby preventing association of the subunits. BILD 1263 (**17.34**) was the first HSV R1R2 subunit association inhibitor published with antiviral activity *in vivo*. Other peptidomimetics are being developed, including cyclic peptide inhibitors, with effect on the mammalian RNR where the R2 carboxy terminal is different. Disruption of protein–protein interactions is a relatively new strategy of inhibitor design for the development of chemotherapeutic agents.

17.2 MITOTIC APPARATUS AS TARGET FOR DRUGS

The mitotic inhibitors act by interfering with the mitosis of cells and thereby inducing mitotic arrest. Mitosis takes place during the M phase of the cell cycle, and drugs that prevent cell division by interfering with mitosis are M phase specific. Mitotic arrest is induced because of damage to the spindle apparatus. Consequently, the chromatides, which are separated in the metaphase, are prevented from being pulled toward opposite poles in the following anaphase.

The separate threads of the spindle apparatus are built as a microtubule system. Microtubules are hollow, cylindrical structures built up of the protein tubulin, which consists of two subunits, α- and β-tubulin, with very similar amino acid sequences. The cylinder consists of 13 rows of tubulin heterodimers, the protofilaments. The microtubule cylinder can also be regarded as consisting of a helical array of alternating α- and β-tubulin subunits (Figure 17.18). Most of the mitotic inhibitors disrupt microtubule assembly by binding with high affinity to tubulin. Some of the drugs have a common binding site (the *vinca alkaloids*) and others a different, but probably common, binding site (*podophyllotoxin* and *colchicine*). *Taxanes*, on the other hand, promote the assembly of tubulin to microtubules and prevent depolymerization by binding to tubulin at a separate site.

Microtubules are found as a ubiquitous substituent in cells and have several other functions than being elements in mitosis. Microtubules are part of the cytoskeleton, and take part in intracellular transport and communication. Some of the toxic side effects of the mitotic inhibitors may be due to disturbance of these phenomena.

17.2.1 Drugs interfering with the Vinca alkaloid binding site of tubulin

Vinblastine (**17.35**) and *vincristine* (**17.36**) are constituents of the Madagascar periwinkle *Vinca rosea* Linn. Vinblastine (VBL) is found in much larger quantity than

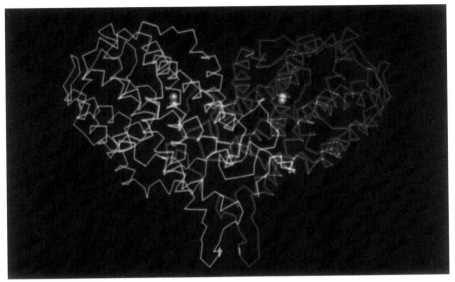

Plate (A)

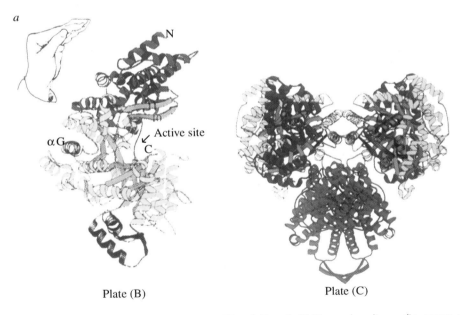

Plate (B)

Plate (C)

Figure 17.17 The structures of (A) protein R2 of *E. coli* RNR as the dimer (in green and magenta) with the iron atoms in red; (B) protein R1 of *E. coli* RNR as the monomer. The colors illustrate different domains of the protein; and (C) the R1R2 holoenzyme modeled on the basis of the separate X-ray structures of R1 and R2. The R2 dimer is colored in red. The figures were kindly provided by Professor Hans Eklund, Department of Molecular Biology, Biomedical Center, Uppsala, Sweden.

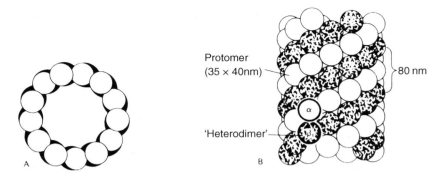

Figure 17.18 Schematic model of a microtubule, showing the pattern of tubulin subunits. A is a cross-sectional view showing the arrangement of the 13 protofilaments. B is a longitudinal view showing the surface lattice of α and β subunits. (From Bryan, J. (1974) *Fed. Proc.*, **33**, 152 with permission by the Federation of American Societies for Experimental Biology).

vincristine (VCR), but it is easily converted synthetically into the clinically more useful drug VCR (conversion of a methyl group into a formyl group). The VBL and VCR are used as the sulphates and are given intravenously because of bad and unpredictable absorption from the gastrointestinal tract. The compounds are highly irritating to tissue and great care has to be taken to avoid extravasation and contact with eyes. The dose-limiting toxicity of VBL is bone marrow depression, whereas VCR is considered to be bone marrow sparing compared to most anticancer drugs. Neurotoxicity is dose-limiting for VCR, on the other hand, while this is a less frequent and serious problem with VBL. The reasons for these differences in toxicity of the structurally very similar compounds are not fully understood.

The clinical use of the drugs is also different. The VCR is given in combination therapy to induce remission in acute lymphocytic leukemia of childhood, and it has actually revolutioned the therapy of this disease, as 90–100% of the patients are achieving complete remission. Very high percentages of remission are also achieved in the treatment of Hodgkin's disease with combinations of drugs including VCR or VBL. Both drugs are used in the treatment of several other cancer diseases.

Vinblastine **(17.35)** R = CH$_3$

Vincristine **(17.36)** R = CHO

The vinca alkaloids are known to bind to tubulin at a common binding site. As a result of this binding, the tubulin units cannot polymerize to form microtubules, a reversible reaction, which occurs in the presence of Mg^{2+} and GTP in addition to the microtubules-associated proteins (MAPs). Only when GTP is bound to tubulin the filament can grow, and only from one end (the plus end). Thus, the microtubules are in dynamic equilibrium with tubulin in cytosolic solution. When VBL (or VCR) is bound to tubulin, new GTP-tubulin units cannot be added to the filaments, and the growth is thereby prevented. Dissociation of tubulin units from the minus end can still occur, and the result is rapid disappearance of the spindle apparatus.

The binding site of the vinca alkaloids is located to the β-subunit of tubulin, but very little is known on the nature of the binding. In addition to the vinca alkaloids, compounds of other natural sources, and with quite different structures, share binding site with the vinca alkaloids. Some of these, e.g. the *dolastatin* peptides derived from a marine origin, are in clinical trials.

17.2.2 Drugs interfering with the colchicine binding site of tubulin

The two drugs mentioned below are not commonly used in cancer therapy, but are considered for comparison with the vinca alkaloids and the taxanes.

Podophyllotoxin (**17.37**) can be isolated from extracts of the roots of *Podophyllum peltatum* L. (American mandrake), and is primarily used in the treatment of condyloma. *Colchicine* (**17.38**) is the major alkaloid of the meadow saffron *Colchicum autumnale* L. It is an active antimitotic drug, but the toxicity of the compound has limited its use to the treatment of gout and related inflammatory disease states. However, analogs with lower toxicity are still being developed.

Like the vinca alkaloids, podophyllotoxin (PODO) and colchicine (COL) both inhibit mitosis by binding to tubulin and thereby preventing microtubule assembly. The two drugs share a common binding site, which is distinct from the VBL binding site. It has been proposed that, while VBL/VCR prevent longitudinal interactions between tubulin subunits, COL and PODO seem to prevent microtubule assembly by inhibiting lateral interactions between subunits in adjacent protofilaments. The binding of both COL and PODO to tubulin is tight, but, although practically irreversible, probably non-covalent in nature. Details on the nature of the bindings are not yet known.

Podophyllotoxin (**17.37**)

Colchicine (**17.38**)

17.2.3   Drugs stabilizing the assembly of tubulin into microtubules

Paclitaxel (**17.39**), taxol, is a plant product isolated from the cortex of the western yew *Taxus brevifolia*. The compound has a very low solubility in water, and this has caused serious problems related to its formulation. It is most often used as an emulsion with Cremophor EL (a polyethoxylated castor oil) as the surfactant, and taxol is now the trade-marked name of this formulation. However, the formulation is far from ideal and others are under investigation. The allergic reactions observed in some patients are probably caused by the solvent, but improved administration procedures, including premedication with glucocorticoides and antihistamines, have reduced this problem.

Another problem is the very low yield of paclitaxel from the cortex of *T. brevifolia*. However, the compound can be produced semisynthetically from a precursor that is obtained in higher yield. Paclitaxel is now in Phase III trials and in clinical use against ovarian cancer and breast cancer, but has also effect against a variety of other cancer diseases. The major side effect of paclitaxel, in addition to hypersensitivity, is neurotoxicity.

Paclitaxel is a taxane diterpenoid characterized by its ester side chain at C-13 (the *N*-benzoyl-β-phenylisoserine ester of the compound *baccatin III*) and by its oxetane ring D. The X-ray structure of paclitaxel has been determined, as well as of *docetaxel* (earlier taxotere that now is the trade-marked name for a formulation using Tween 80 as solvent). Docetaxel is a C-10 deacylated analog of paclitaxel with the *N*-benzoyl group replaced by a *tert*-butoxycarbonyl group. The structures clearly show a cup-like shape of the taxane skeleton (Figure 17.19). Docetaxel is also a promising anticancer drug and is progressing through clinical trials. Though very similar structures, there are significant differences in the pharmacology of the two agents.

Unlike other plant-derived antimitotic agents (colchicine, podophyllotoxin and the vinca alkaloids), which inhibit microtubule assembly, the taxanes actually promote the assembly of tubulin and stabilize the microtubules formed against depolymerization. The cytotoxicity is related to the microtubule-mediated interruption of mitosis, resulting from distortion of the mitotic spindle.

The drugs bind to the β-subunit of tubulin, and an understanding of the binding of taxanes to microtubules has recently been obtained by the structure determination of a tubulin-drug complex at low resolution (3.7 Å). Two-dimensional zinc-induced crystalline sheets of tubulin, stabilized by docetaxel, were obtained and studied by electron crystallography (Figure 17.20). The structure shows that the drug binds to β-tubulin in a pocket near to the lateral interaction between the

Taxol (**17.39**)

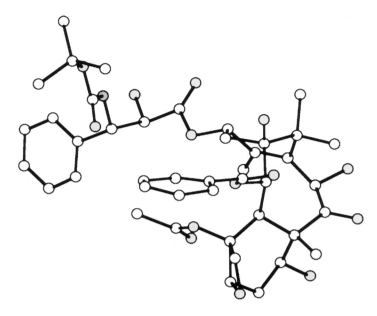

Figure 17.19 The X-ray structure of docetaxel (taxotere), generated using the program MacMimic with co-ordinates from Cambridge Structural Data Base. Oxygen atoms are light gray and nitrogen dark gray.

β-subunits. In this way, a strengthening of the lateral contacts and thereby stabilization of the protofilament adhesion may be obtained. In the α-subunit, the corresponding binding pocket is occupied by a loop, which is not present in β-tubulin. More detailed structures are still needed for the design of improved anticancer drugs.

However, some information on taxanes has been obtained indirectly by SAR studies. Beccatin III, without the ester side chain at C-13, is significantly less active than paclitaxel, indicating the importance of this side chain for the activity. An *N*-acyl group is required in the side chain (benzoyl in paclitaxel, and *tert*-butoxy-carbonyl in docetaxel). Various paclitaxel analogs that lack the 3′-phenyl group of the side chain are significantly less active than paclitaxel. A free 2′-hydroxy group (or a hydrolysable ester) is required, and a change of the chirality at 2′ and 3′ leads to less active compounds.

Structural variations along the upper part (C-6–C-12) of the taxol molecule (e.g. acylation or removal of an OH group) do not greatly affect the bioactivity, suggesting that this region is not intimately involved in binding to tubulin. The lower part, on the other hand, including C-14, C-1–C-5 and the unusual oxetane ring at C-4–C-5, appears to be a region, which is crucial to the activity of taxol, as structural changes has major effects on activity. Opening of the oxetane ring with electrophilic reagents yields products, which are less active than paclitaxel, and also the benzoyl-oxy group at C-2 is required. The oxetane ring is relatively inert chemically, and it has been suggested that its role simply may be to act as a lock to maintain the

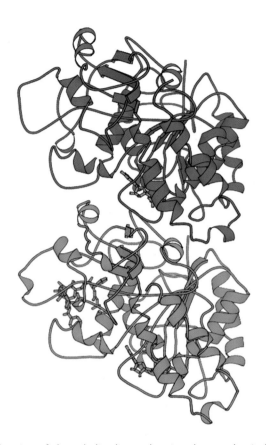

Figure 17.20 Ribbon drawing of the tubulin dimer showing the α subunit (in purple) with bound GTP (in gray) and the β subunit (in green) containing GDP (in gray) and taxotere (in red). The structure was obtained by electron crystallography and determined to 3.7 Å resolution. The figure is generated using the program Molscript with co-ordinates from Protein Data Bank.

conformation of the diterpenoid ring system of paclitaxel. The cup-like shape of the ring system is conserved in the known X-ray structures of taxanes.

FURTHER READING

Arcamone, F. (1984) Structure–activity relationships in antitumour anthracyclines. In *X-Ray Crystallography and Drug Action*, edited by A.S. Horn and C.J. De Ranter, pp. 367–388. Oxford: Clarendon Press.

Arcamone, F., Animati, F., Capranico, G., Lombardi, P., Pratesi, G., Manzini, S., Supino, R. and Zunino, F. (1997) New developments in antitumor anthracyclines. *Pharmacol. Ther.*, **76**, 117–124.

Boddy, A.V. and Yule, S.M. (2000) Metabolism and pharmacokinetics of oxazaphosphorines. *Clin. Pharmacokinet.*, **38**, 291–304.

Champness, J.N., Kuyper, L.F. and Beddell, C.R. (1986) Interaction between dihydrofolate reductase and certain inhibitors. In *Topics in Molecular Pharmacology*, Vol. 3, edited by A.S.V. Burgen, G.C.K. Roberts and M.S. Tute. Amsterdam: Elsevier.

Cody, V., Galitsky, N., Luft, J.R., Pangborn, W., Gangjee, A., Devraj, R., Queener, S.F. and Blakeley, R.L. (1997) Comparison of ternary complexes of pneumosystis carnii and wild-type human dihydrofolate reductase with coenzyme NADPH and a novel classical antitumor furo[2,3-d]pyrimidine antifolate. *Acta Cryst.*, D**53**, 638–649.

Cohen, J. (ed.) (1989) *Oligodeoxynucleotides Antisense Inhibitors of Gene Expressions*. London: The Macmillan Press.

Danenberg, P.V., Malli, H. and Swenson, S. (1999) Thymidylate synthase inhibitors. *Semin. Oncol.*, **26**, 621–631.

Dedon, P.C. and Goldberg, I.H. (1992) Free-radical mechanisms involved in the formation of sequence-dependent bistranded DNA lesions by the antitumor antibiotics bleomycin, neocarzinostatin, and calicheamicin. *Chem. Res. Toxicol.*, **5**, 311–332.

Friedman, O.M., Myles, A. and Colvin, M. (1979) Cyclophosphamide and related phosphoramide mustards. Current status and future prospects. In *Advances in Cancer Chemotherapy*, Vol. 4, edited by A. Rosowsky, pp. 143–204. New York: Marcel Dekker.

Hardy, L.W., Finer-Moore, J.S., Montfort, W.R., Jones, M.O., Santi, D.V. and Stroud, R.M. (1987) Atomic structure of thymidylate synthase. Target for rational drug design. *Science*, **235**, 448–455.

Hecht, S.M. (2000) Bleomycin: new perspectives on the mechanism of action. *J. Nat. Prod.*, **63**, 158–168.

Iwasaki, S. (1993) Antimitotic agents: chemistry and recognition of tubulin molecule. *Med. Res. Rev.*, **13**, 183–198.

Joshua-Tor, L. and Sussman, J.L. (1993) The coming age of DNA crystallography. *Curr. Opin. Struct. Biol.* **3**, 323–335.

Judson, I. and Kelland, L.R. (2000) New developments and approaches in the platinum arena. *Drugs*, **59** (Suppl. 4), 29–36.

Kingston, D.G.I. (1994) Taxol: the chemistry and structure–activity relationships of a novel anticancer agent. *TIBTECH*, **12**, 222–227.

Kingston, D.G.I. (2000) Recent advances in the chemistry of taxol. *J. Nat. Prod.* **63**, 726–734.

Knudsen, H. and Nielsen, P.E. (1997) Application of peptide nucleic acid in cancer therapy. *Anti-Cancer Drugs*, **8**, 113–118.

Kuyper, L.F. (1989) Inhibitors of dihydrofolate reductase. In *Computer-Aided Drug Design. Methods and Applications*, edited by T.J. Perun and C.L. Propst, pp. 327–364. New York: Marcel Dekker.

Larsen, I.K. (1990) Inhibition of the enzyme ribonucleotide reductase. In *Frontiers in Drug Research. Crystallographic and Computational Methods*, edited by B. Jensen, F.S. Jørgensen and H. Kofod, pp. 47–57. Copenhagen: Munksgaard.

Liehr, S., Barbosa, J., Smith, A.B. and Cooperman, B.S. (1999) Synthesis and biological activity of cyclic peptide inhibitors of ribonucleotide reductase. *Org. Lett.*, **I**, 1201–1204.

Liuzzi, M., Déziel, R., Moss, N., Beaulleu, P., Bonneau, A.-M., Bousquet, C., Chafouleas, J.G., Garneau, M., Jarmillo, J., Krogsrud, R.L., Lagacé, L., McCollum, R.S., Nawooy, S. and Guindon, Y. (1994) A potent peptidomimetic inhibitor of HSV ribonucleotide reductase with antiviral activity *in vivo*. *Nature*, **372**, 695–698.

Lown, J.W. (1983) The chemistry of DNA damage by antitumour drugs. In *Molecular Aspects of Anti-Cancer Drug Action*, edited by S. Neidle and M.J. Waring, pp. 283–314. London: The Macmillan Press.

McCormick, J.E. and McElhinney, R.S. (1990) Nitrosoureas from chemist to physician: classification and recent approaches to drug design. *Eur. J. Cancer*, **26**, 207–221.

Mirkes, P.E., Brown, N.A., Kajbaf, M., Lamb, J.H., Farmer, P.B. and Naylor, S. (1992) Identification of cyclophosphamide-DNA adducts in rat embryos exposed *in vitro* to 4-hydroperoxocyclophosphamide. *Chem. Res. Toxicol.*, **5**, 382–385.

Nielsen, P.E., Egholm, M. and Buchardt, O. (1994) A DNA mimic with a peptide backbone. *Bioconjugate Chemistry*, **5**, 3–7.

Nogales, E., Whittaker, M. Wolf, S.G. and Downing, K.H. (1998) Structure of the $\alpha\beta$-tubulin dimer by electron crystallography. *Nature*, **391**, 199–203.

Nordlund, P. and Eklund, H. (1993) Structure and function of *Escherichia coli* ribonucleotide reductase protein R2. *J. Mol. Biol.*, **232**, 123–164.

Pratt, W.B. and Ruddon, R.W. (eds.) (1979) *The Anticancer Drugs*. Oxford: Oxford University Press.

Reedijk, J. (1988) Structure determination of platinum antitumour compounds and their adducts with DNA. In *NMR Spectroscopy in Drug Research*, edited by J.W. Jaroszewski, K. Schaumburg and H. Kofod, pp. 341–357. Copenhagen: Munksgaard.

Shoichet, B.K., Stroud, R.M., Santi, D.V., Kuntz, I.D. and Perry, K.M. (1993) Structure-based discovery of inhibitors of thymidylate synthase. *Science*, **259**, 1445–1450.

Sugiura, Y., Takita, T. and Umezawa, H. (1985) Bleomycin antibiotics: metal complexes and their biological action. In *Metal Ions in Biological Systems*, Vol. 19, edited by H. Sigel, pp. 81–108, New York: Marcel Dekker.

Takahara, P.M., Rosenzweig, A.C., Frederick, C.A. and Lippard, S.J. (1995) Crystal structure of double-stranded DNA containing the major adduct of the anticancer drug cisplatin. *Nature*, **377**, 649–652.

Wang, A.H.-J. (1992) Intercalative drug binding to DNA. *Curr. Opin. Struct. Biol.*, **2**, 361–368.

Weiss, R.B. and Christian, M.C. (1993) New cisplatin analogues in development. *A review. Drugs*, **46**, 360–377.

Wilman, D.E.V. and Connors, T.A. (1983) Molecular structure and antitumour activity of alkylating agents. In *Molecular Aspects of Anti-Cancer Drug Action*, edited by S. Neidle and M.J. Waring, pp. 233–282. London: The Macmillan Press.

Index

THE RIGHTS OF REFUGEES UNDER INTERNATIONAL LAW

JAMES C. HATHAWAY

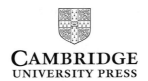

CAMBRIDGE
UNIVERSITY PRESS

CAMBRIDGE UNIVERSITY PRESS

Cambridge, New York, Melbourne, Madrid, Cape Town, Singapore, São Paulo

CAMBRIDGE UNIVERSITY PRESS

The Edinburgh Building, Cambridge, CB2 2RU, UK

Published in the United States of America by Cambridge University Press, New York

www.cambridge.org
Information on this title: www.cambridge.org/9780521542630

First published 2005

Printed in the United Kingdom at the University Press, Cambridge

A catalogue record for this book is available from the British Library

ISBN-13 978-0-521-83494-0 hardback
ISBN-10 0-521-83494-5 hardback
ISBN-13 978-0-521-54263-0 paperback
ISBN-10 0-521-54263-4 paperback

In memory of Lisa Gilad

"[D]ecisions had at times given the impression that it was a conference for the protection of helpless sovereign states against the wicked refugee. The draft Convention had at times been in danger of appearing to the refugee like the menu at an expensive restaurant, with every course crossed out except, perhaps, the soup, and a footnote to the effect that even the soup might not be served in certain circumstances."

Mr. Rees, International Council of Voluntary Agencies (Nov. 26, 1951)

"[I]t was clearly in the best interests of refugees that [the Refugee Convention] should be cast in a form which would be acceptable to governments, thus inducing them to accept at least certain commitments ... Otherwise, they would be obliged to enter reservations which would probably exclude even those minimum commitments. Liberalism which was blind to the facts of reality could only beat the air."

Mr. Rochefort, Representative of France (Nov. 30, 1951)

CONTENTS

vii

ACKNOWLEDGMENTS

This book has evolved over the course of more than a decade. It was inspired by a call from the refugee law pioneer Atle Grahl-Madsen, shortly before his death. Professor Grahl-Madsen asked me to consider preparing a comprehensive analysis of the rights of refugees, drawing freely upon notes which he had authored during the 1960s (which were subsequently published in full by UNHCR in 1997). Grahl-Madsen's prescient vision was to link an updated study of the rights derived from the Refugee Convention with analysis of relevant norms of international human rights – thus yielding a truly comprehensive understanding of the refugee rights regime. As always, Grahl-Madsen was ahead of the curve: he foresaw that the days in which recognition of refugee status would lead with relatively little debate to respect for relevant legal entitlements would not last forever, and that there was therefore an urgent need for the academy to consolidate a clear understanding of the international legal rules that define the baseline entitlements that follow from refugee status. This book is my effort to do justice to his vision.

My own sense was that the study of legal norms would be most fruitful if tested against the hard facts of refugee life on the ground. The design for a mixed legal–empirical study emerged with the generous support of colleagues at York University's interdisciplinary Centre for Refugee Studies, in particular David Dewitt, Winona Giles, Diana Lary, and Penny Van Esterik. The university supported the launch of this research by awarding me the Walter L. Gordon Research Professorship for the academic year 1994–1995; the research effort itself was generously funded by Canada's Social Sciences and Humanities Research Council. At the same time, the International Academy of Comparative Law kindly appointed me General Rapporteur for a transnational study of the implementation of refugee rights around the world: with the extraordinary support of a team of twenty-eight National Rapporteurs, the analytical framework which grounds this book emerged. As the footnotes throughout this volume make clear, I remain enormously indebted to this group of eminent scholars who shared my commitment to developing an understanding of refugee rights capable of meeting real challenges in often difficult circumstances.

xiii

Much of the book was written while I was on the faculty of Osgoode Hall Law School of York University, in Toronto. Deans Jim MacPherson and Marilyn Pilkington were unfailingly supportive of my ambitions. My talented law colleagues Bill Angus and John Evans provided regular and much-needed advice, and were consistently encouraging of my efforts. My ever-supportive best friend Jamie Cameron kept my spirits high, even when I felt impossibly weighed down by the enormity of this undertaking – a role which I am thankful she still plays for me.

During the early years of this research, I had the honor to work with an outstanding team in the Law Unit of the Centre for Refugee Studies. Leanne MacMillan and Alex Neve coordinated the legal research work, and tolerated my wholly unreasonable requests with grace and true professionalism. Enthusiastic and top-quality research assistance was provided by an able team of graduate students, in particular by Michael Barutciski and Jeanne Donald. Unique recognition is owed to John Dent, who became my true partner in this research effort. John began work on this study while a graduate student in political science, and pursued the project full time after completing his degree. Not only did he conceive and execute a truly extraordinary empirical research effort, but he worked side by side with me on development of the book's legal analysis as well. Simply put, this book would never have emerged without John's invaluable insights and contributions.

When I moved to the University of Michigan Law School in 1998, it was in large part because then-Dean Jeffrey Lehman shared my vision to develop an unparalleled curriculum in international and comparative refugee and asylum law. Jeff found the resources to support my work, and allowed me to focus my energies entirely on thinking about refugee protection concerns. His successor Evan Caminker has been similarly generous to me, and has found the time to help me shape my research agenda. Wonderful colleagues at the Law School have given freely of their knowledge and perspectives – in particular, Christine Chinkin, Rob Howse, Chris McCrudden, Catharine MacKinnon, Roberta Morris, Bruno Simma, and Eric Stein. I am grateful also for the fine research assistance of Anne Cusick and Dipen Sabharwal. Louise Moor and Larissa Wakim not only helped me fine-tune my research, but agreed to coordinate much of the Program in Refugee and Asylum Law in order to give me the time to complete my writing. And from beginning to end of this endeavor, the outstanding resources of the University of Michigan Law Library have been made available to me. Law Librarian Margaret Leary met with me on my first day at the faculty to assess my research needs; her colleague Barb Garavaglia created a system that allowed me nearly painlessly to monitor key legal and social developments; and Aimee Mangan ensured that every research request I made was answered not only promptly, but with an attention to detail that most academics can only dream of.

A special acknowledgment is owed to an amazing group of visiting faculty and senior graduate students – Michelle Foster, Rodger Haines, Seong Soo Kim, Luis Peral, Dipen Sabharwal, and Seyoum Tesfay – each of whom generously read draft chapters of the book, and met regularly over the course of the winter 2003 term to discuss them. This process significantly sharpened my thinking, and was critical in identifying for me where additional work was required. Rodger and Luis have proved the best of friends and colleagues to me, continuing to provide wise counsel from afar at a moment's notice.

Nor have I benefited only from the assistance of colleagues close to home. Christian Wolff, a graduate student at Oxford's Refugee Studies Centre, undertook a massive empirical updating project for me in 2003–2004 – spanning literally every concern, in every part of the world. His efforts were heroic, and the research unearthed of enormous value to ensuring the continuing relevance of the case studies presented here. Chris Nash of the European Council on Refugees and Exiles, as well as academics Lee Anne de la Hunt, David Turton, and Marjoleine Zieck, was key among a group of persons I prevailed upon to advise me. I also acknowledge with gratitude the comments on my research from students to whom it has been presented at the Oxford University Refugee Studies Centre, as well as from researchers at Amnesty International in London where I have had the privilege to teach refugee law for many years.

Some of the most direct assistance I have received has been from a wonderful group of support persons – Wendy Rambo and Rose della Rocca at Osgoode Hall, and Baiba Hicks, Janice Proctor, and Karen Rushlow at Michigan. They have all taken a serious interest in this project, and found creative ways to advance the flow of this research, for which I am most grateful.

I have also received extraordinary support from Cambridge University Press to bring this book into being. Finola O'Sullivan believed in this project from the start, and ensured that standard publishing procedures were tailored to meet the particular challenges of producing this book. Diane Ilott was the model of a perfectionist editor: her proposals for revision were routinely thoughtful, and of real assistance to me. And Maureen MacGlashan has created a wonderful set of tables and indices, which I am confident will enable even the most demanding reader to navigate this book with ease.

And finally, there is a cast of wonderful people who have kept me sane during the long period of research and writing. John Moreau suffered more than anyone from my dedication to this work; I owe him more than I can say. My canine pal Otis patiently watched nearly every keystroke from the beginning to end of this writing project, silently communicating his unfailing confidence that I could see the project through. And last but definitely not least, I have been blessed with the very best of friends and family who supported me during interminable bouts of anxiety and stress. To my parents, Bernice and Charles Hathaway; and to Virginia Gordan in Ann Arbor,

Paul Gravett and Mark Hand on Salt Spring Island, and Howard and Pat Frederick in Tucson: thank you for never letting me down.

This book is dedicated to my dear friend Lisa Gilad – social anthropologist, advocate for social justice, and refugee law decision-maker – who died tragically before she could see her inspired agenda to better the lot of refugees through to completion. Lisa was committed to the view that law could make a critical difference to the welfare of refugees, and worked tirelessly to inspire a humane understanding of protection principles among her colleagues, as well as in the broader community of persons working with refugees in government, academia, and on the front lines. My hope is that this study will contribute to the work of others who, like Lisa, believe that refugee protection can best be assured by a steadfast commitment to clear rules, interpreted in context, and applied with compassion.

James C. Hathaway
Ann Arbor, Michigan
December 2004

Every effort has been made to secure necessary permissions to reproduce copyright material in this work, though in some cases it has proved impossible to trace copyright holders. If any omissions are brought to our notice, we will be happy to include appropriate acknowledgments on reprinting.

TABLE OF CASES

I. International decisions

International Court of Justice

Permanent Court of International Justice

UN Committee Against Torture

UN Human Rights Committee

World Trade Organization Appellate Body

II. Regional Decisions

African Commission on Human and Peoples' Rights

European Court of Human Rights

European Court of Justice

Interamerican Commission on Human Rights

III. National Decisions

Australia

France

Germany

Hong Kong

India

Switzerland

United Kingdom

United States

TABLE OF TREATIES AND OTHER INTERNATIONAL INSTRUMENTS

---

[2] As discussion of the Refugee Convention in general permeates the whole of the text (i.e.
passim) only discussion of particular articles is included in this Table.

ABBREVIATIONS FOR COURTS
AND TRIBUNALS CITED

Au. HC	Austria, High Court
Aus. FC	Australia, Federal Court
Aus. FFC	Australia, Full Federal Court
Aus. HC	Australia, High Court
Can. FC	Canada, Federal Court
Can. FCA	Canada, Federal Court of Appeal
Can. IRB	Canada, Immigration and Refugee Board
Can. SC	Canada, Supreme Court
ECHR	European Court of Human Rights
ECJ	European Court of Justice
Eng. CA	England, Court of Appeal
Eng. HC	England, High Court
Eng. QBD	England, Queen's Bench Division
Eur Comm	European Commission on Human Rights
Fr. CE	France, Conseil d'Etat
Ger. AC	Germany, Administrative Court
Ger. FCC	Germany, Federal Constitutional Court
Ger. FASC	Germany, Federal Administrative Supreme Court
HK PC	Hong Kong, Privy Council
ICJ	International Court of Justice
India SC	India, Supreme Court
Inter-Am Comm HR	Inter-American Commission on Human Rights
Jap. SC	Japan, Supreme Court
NZ CA	New Zealand, Court of Appeal
NZ HC	New Zealand, High Court
NZ RSAA	New Zealand, Refugee Status Appeals Authority
NZ SC	New Zealand, Supreme Court
PCIJ	Permanent Court of International Justice
SA CC	South Africa, Constitutional Court
SA HC	South Africa, High Court
SA SCA	South Africa, Supreme Court of Appeal
Sw. FC	Switzerland, Federal Court
Tokyo DC	Japan, Tokyo District Court

1

Tokyo HC	Japan, Tokyo High Court
UK HL	United Kingdom, House of Lords
UK SIAC	United Kingdom, Special Immigration Appeals Commission
UNCAT	United Nations Committee Against Torture
UNHCHR	United Nations High Commissioner for Human Rights
UNHCR	United Nations High Commissioner for Refugees
UNHRC	United Nations Human Rights Committee
US AG	United States, Attorney General
US BIA	United States, Board of Immigration Appeals
US CA2	United States, 2nd Circuit Court of Appeals
US CA4	United States, 4th Circuit Court of Appeals
US CA7	United States, 7th Circuit Court of Appeals
US CA8	United States, 8th Circuit Court of Appeals
US CA9	United States, 9th Circuit Court of Appeals
US CA11	United States, 11th Circuit Court of Appeals
US DCCa	United States, District Court, California
US DCEDNY	United States, District Court, Eastern District of New York
US DCNDCa	United States, District Court, Northern District of California
US DCSDNY	United States, District Court, Southern District of New York
US IC	United States, Immigration Court
US SC	United States, Supreme Court
US SJCMass	United States, Supreme Judicial Court of Massachusetts
WTO AB	World Trade Organization Appellate Body

INTRODUCTION

The greatest challenge facing refugees arriving in the developed world has traditionally been to convince authorities that they are, in fact, entitled to recognition of their refugee status.[1] What level of risk is required by the "well-founded fear" standard? What sorts of harm are encompassed by the notion of "being persecuted"? Is there a duty to seek an internal remedy within one's own country before seeking refugee protection abroad? What is the meaning of the five grounds for protection, and what causal connection is required between those grounds and the risk of being persecuted? Most recently, significant attention has also been paid to the nature of the circumstances under which a person may be excluded from, or deemed no longer to require, protection as a refugee.

While debate continues on these and other requirements for qualification as a Convention refugee,[2] there is no denying that the decade of the 1990s gave rise to a marked increase in both the extent and depth of judicial efforts to resolve the most vexing definitional controversies. Senior appellate courts now routinely engage in an ongoing and quite extraordinary transnational judicial conversation[3] about the scope of the refugee

---

[1] The core of the international legal definition of a refugee requires that "owing to well-founded fear of being persecuted for reasons of race, religion, nationality, membership of a particular social group or political opinion, [the applicant] is outside the country of his nationality and is unable or, owing to such fear, is unwilling to avail himself of the protection of that country": Convention relating to the Status of Refugees, 189 UNTS 2545, done July 28, 1951, entered into force Apr. 22, 1954 (Refugee Convention), supplemented by the Protocol relating to the Status of Refugees, 606 UNTS 8791, done Jan. 31, 1967, entered into force Oct. 4, 1967 (Refugee Protocol).

[2] In its recent Global Consultations on International Protection, the United Nations High Commissioner for Refugees (UNHCR) identified as issues of particular salience the scope of the "membership of a particular social group" category; gender-related persecution; the nature of the duty to seek internal protection or relocation; and the cessation and exclusion clauses. See E. Feller et al. eds., *Refugee Protection in International Law* (2003) (Feller et al., *Refugee Protection*), at 263–552.

[3] See A.-M. Slaughter, "A Typology of Transjudicial Communication," (1994) 29 *University of Richmond Law Review* 99.

definition,[4] and have increasingly committed themselves to find common ground.[5] Indeed, the House of Lords has suggested that courts have a legal responsibility to interpret the Refugee Convention in a way that ensures a common understanding across states of the standard of entitlement to protection:

> [A]s in the case of other multilateral treaties, the Refugee Convention must be given an independent meaning ... without taking colour from distinctive features of the legal system of any individual contracting state. In principle therefore there can only be one true interpretation of a treaty ...
>
> In practice it is left to national courts, faced with the material disagreement on an issue of interpretation, to resolve it. But in doing so, [they] must search, untrammelled by notions of [their] national legal culture, for the true autonomous and international meaning of the treaty.[6]

In contrast to the progress achieved by courts in conceiving a shared understanding of the Convention refugee definition, there has been only minimal judicial engagement with the meaning of the various rights which follow from recognition of Convention refugee status. Although most of the Refugee Convention is in fact devoted to elaborating these entitlements, there is only a smattering of judicial guidance on a small minority of the rights set by the treaty. Even in the academic literature, only the core duty of *non-refoulement* and, to a lesser extent, the duties of non-expulsion and non-penalization, have received any serious attention.[7] This analytical gap is

---

[4] The contemporary jurisprudence of leading asylum states on the scope of Convention refugee status is collected at the University of Michigan's Refugee Caselaw Site, www.refugeecaselaw.org.

[5] The establishment in 1995 of the International Association of Refugee Law Judges (IARLJ), now comprising members from some forty asylum states, is a particularly noteworthy means of advancing this sense of refugee law as a common enterprise. In 2002, the IARLJ convened its first Advanced Workshop on Refugee Law, in which appellate judges from around the world met to seek consensus on refugee definition issues identified by them as particularly challenging. See J. Hathaway, "A Forum for the Transnational Development of Refugee Law," (2003) 15(3) *International Journal of Refugee Law* 418.

[6] *R v. Secretary of State for the Home Department, ex parte Adan and Aitseguer*, [2001] 2 WLR 143 (UK HL, Dec. 19, 2000).

[7] The only refugee rights which have received relatively extensive academic attention are Arts. 31–33. See e.g. G. Stenberg, *Non-Expulsion and Non-Refoulement* (1989); W. Kälin, *Das Prinzip des Non-Refoulement* (1982). Even in the context of its recent Global Consultations on International Protection, UNHCR drew particular attention to only three refugee rights: the rights of *non-refoulement* (Art. 33), freedom from penalization or detention for illegal entry (Art. 31), and protection of family unity: Feller et al., *Refugee Protection*, at 87–179, 185–258, and 555–608. Those academic works that do address the full range of refugee rights are all quite dated, including N. Robinson, *Convention relating to the Status of Refugees: Its History, Contents and Interpretation* (1953); A. Grahl-Madsen, *Commentary on the Refugee Convention 1951* (1963, pub'd., 1997); and P. Weis, *The Refugee Convention, 1951: The Travaux Préparatoires Analysed with a Commentary by Dr. Paul Weis* (posthumously pub'd., 1995).

no doubt largely the result of the tradition of most developed states simply to admit refugees, formally or in practice, as long-term or permanent residents. While not required by the Refugee Convention,[8] this approach has led de facto to respect for most Convention rights (and usually more). Because refugee rights were not at risk, there was little perceived need to elaborate their meaning.

In recent years, however, governments throughout the industrialized world have begun to question the logic of routinely assimilating refugees, and have therefore sought to limit their access to a variety of rights.[9] Most commonly, questions are now raised about whether refugees should be allowed to enjoy freedom of movement, to work, to access public welfare programs, or to be reunited with family members. In a minority of states, doubts have been expressed about the propriety of exempting refugees from compliance with visa and other immigration rules, and even about whether there is really a duty to admit refugees at all. There is also a marked interest in the authority of states to repatriate refugees to their countries of origin, or otherwise to divest themselves of even such duties of protection as are initially recognized.

This movement towards a less robust form of refugee protection mirrors the traditional approach in much of the less developed world. For reasons born of both pragmatism and principle, poorer countries – which host the overwhelming majority of the world's refugees[10] – have rarely contested the eligibility for refugee status of those arriving at their borders.[11] Yet this conceptual generosity has not always been matched by efforts to treat the refugees admitted in line with duties set by the Refugee Convention. In far too many cases, refugees in less developed states have been detained, socially marginalized, left physically at risk, or effectively denied the ability to meet even their most basic needs. The imperative clearly to define the rights which follow from refugee status, while of comparatively recent origin in most

---

[8] See chapters 4.1 and 7.4 below.

[9] See e.g. J. Hathaway, "The Emerging Politics of *Non-Entrée*," (1992) 91 *Refugees* 40, also published as "L'émergence d'une politique de non-entrée," in F. Julien-Laferrière ed., *Frontières du droit, Frontières des droits* (1993), at 65; and, in particular, G. Noll, *Negotiating Asylum: The EU Acquis, Extraterritorial Protection, and the Common Market of Deflection* (2000).

[10] As of Dec. 31, 2003, for example, just under 80 percent of the world's refugees were protected in Africa, the Middle East, or South and Central Asia: US Committee for Refugees, *World Refugee Survey 2004* (2004), at 4–5.

[11] In some instances, particularly in Africa, the commitment to a more expansive understanding of refugee status has been formalized in regional treaty or other standards. See J. Hathaway, *The Law of Refugee Status* (1991) (Hathaway, *Refugee Status*), at 16–21; and G. Goodwin-Gill, *The Refugee in International Law* (1996) (Goodwin-Gill, *Refugee in International Law*), at 20–21.

industrialized states, is of long-standing duration in much of the less developed world.

The goal of this book is therefore to give renewed life to a too-long neglected source of vital, internationally agreed human rights for refugees. More specifically, the analysis here seeks to elaborate an understanding of refugee law which is firmly anchored in legal obligation, and which is accordingly detached from momentary considerations of policy and preference. The essential premise is that refugees are entitled to claim the benefit of a deliberate and coherent system of rights.

It will be clear from this formulation that the Refugee Convention and its Protocol are conceived here not as accords about immigration, or even migration, but as part and parcel of international human rights law. This view is fully in line with the positions adopted by senior courts which have analyzed the object and purpose of the Refugee Convention. In perhaps the earliest formulation, the Supreme Court of Canada embraced the view that the essential purpose of the Refugee Convention is to identify persons who no longer enjoy the most basic forms of protection which a state is obliged to provide. In such circumstances, refugee law provides surrogate or substitute protection of basic human rights:

> International refugee law was formulated to serve as a back-up to the protection one expects from the State of which an individual is a national. It was meant to come into play only when that protection is unavailable, and then only in certain situations.[12]

Complementing this analysis, the House of Lords more recently affirmed that the fundamental goal of refugee law is to restore refugees to affirmative protection:

> The general purpose of the Convention is to enable the person who no longer has the benefit of protection against persecution for a convention reason in his own country to turn for protection to the international community.[13]

Justice Kirby of the High Court of Australia has moreover linked the goals of refugee law directly to the more general human rights project:

> [The Refugee Convention's] meaning should be ascertained having regard to its object, bearing in mind that the Convention is one of several

---

[12] *Canada v. Ward*, (1993) 103 DLR 4th 1 (Can. SC, June 30, 1993). More recently, Justice Bastarache of the same court affirmed that "[t]he overarching and clear human rights object and purpose is the background against which interpretation of individual provisions must take place": *Pushpanathan v. Minister of Citizenship and Immigration*, 1998 Can. Sup. Ct. Lexis 29 (Can. SC, June 4, 1998), at para. 59.

[13] *Horvath v. Secretary of State for the Home Department*, [2000] 3 All ER 577 (UK HL, July 6, 2000), per Lord Hope of Craighead.

important international treaties designed to redress "violation[s] of basic human rights, demonstrative of a failure of state protection" ... It is the recognition of the failure of state protection, so often repeated in the history of the past hundred years, that led to the exceptional involvement of international law in matters concerning individual human rights.[14]

As these formulations make clear, refugee law is a remedial or palliative branch of human rights law. Its specific purpose is to ensure that those whose basic rights are not protected (for a Convention reason) in their own country are, if able to reach an asylum state, entitled to invoke rights of substitute protection in any state party to the Refugee Convention. As such, the right of entry which is undoubtedly the most visible consequence of refugee law is, in fact, fundamentally consequential in nature, and of a duration limited by the persistence of risk in the refugee's state of origin.[15] It is no more than a necessary means to a human rights end, that being the preservation of the human dignity of an involuntary migrant when his or her country of origin cannot or will not meet that responsibility. In pith and substance, refugee law is not immigration law at all, but is rather a system for the surrogate or substitute protection of human rights.

Despite its obvious relevance and widespread ratification,[16] the Refugee Convention has only rarely been understood to be the primary point of reference when the well-being of refugees is threatened. In particular, there has too often been a tendency simply to invoke non-binding UNHCR or other institutional policy positions. When legal standards are brought to bear, there appears to have been a tacit assumption that whatever concerns refugees face can (and should) be addressed by reliance on the more recently evolved general system for the international protection of human rights.[17]

---

[14] *Minister for Immigration and Multicultural Affairs v. Khawar*, [2002] HCA 14 (Aus. HC, Apr. 11, 2002), per Kirby J. See also *Applicant "A" and Ano'r v. Minister for Immigration and Multicultural Affairs*, (1997) 190 CLR 225 (Aus. HC, Feb. 24, 1997), per Kirby J. at 296–297, holding that the term "refugee" is "to be understood as written against the background of international human rights law, including as reflected or expressed in the Universal Declaration of Human Rights (esp. Arts. 3, 5, and 16) and the International Covenant on Civil and Political Rights (esp. Arts. 7, 23)."

[15] See chapter 4.1 below.

[16] As of October 1, 2004, 145 states were a party to either the Refugee Convention or Refugee Protocol. Madagascar, Monaco, Namibia, and St. Kitts and Nevis were a party only to the Convention; Cape Verde, the United States of America, and Venezuela were a party only to the Protocol: UNHCR, www.unhcr.ch (accessed Nov. 19, 2004).

[17] "In traditional international law, the 'responsibility of States for damage done in their territory to the person or property of foreigners' frequently appears closely bound up with two great doctrines or principles: the so-called 'international standard of justice', and the principle of the equality of nationals and aliens ... What was formerly the object of these two principles – the protection of the person and his property – is now intended to be

It is, of course, true that all persons are today understood to possess legally defined human rights worthy of official validation across time and societies. States acknowledge in principle that they may not invoke raw power, sovereign political authority, or cultural diversity to rationalize failure to ensure the basic rights of persons subject to their jurisdiction – including refugees.[18] The range of international human rights instruments is moreover indisputably vast, and growing. Yet, more than half a century after inauguration of the United Nations system of international human rights law, we must concede that there are only minimal legal tools for the imposition of genuine and truly universal state accountability. The adjustment to an understanding of human rights law conceived outside the political processes of individual nation-states has required a painstaking process of reconciling divergent values and political priorities, which is far from complete. Instead of a universal and comprehensive system of human rights law, the present reality is instead a patchwork of standards of varying reach, implemented through mechanisms that range from the purely facilitative to the modestly coercive.[19] Despite all of its successes, the human rights undertaking is very much a work in progress, with real achievements in some areas, and comparatively little in others.

This fragmentary quality of international human rights law has too often been ignored by scholars and advocates. In a perhaps unconscious drive to will the universal human rights project to early completion, there has been a propensity to overstate the authentic reach of legal norms by downplaying, or even recasting, the often demanding standards which govern the recognition of principles as matters of international law. In the result, there is now a troubling disjuncture between law as declared and law recognized as a meaningful constraint on the exercise of state authority.

The view advanced here, in contrast, is that the protection of refugees is better pursued by the invocation of standards of indisputable legal authority,

---

accomplished by the international recognition of the essential rights of man. Under this new legal doctrine, the distinction between nationals and aliens no longer has any *raison d'être*, so that both in theory and in practice these two traditional principles are henceforth inapplicable. In effect, both of these principles appear to have been outgrown by contemporary international law": F. V. Garcia Amador et al., *Recent Codification of the Law of State Responsibility for Injuries to Aliens* (1974), at 1.

[18] Belgium at one point proposed incorporation in the Refugee Convention of at least Arts. 18 and 19 of the Universal Declaration of Human Rights. The proposal was defeated because of agreement with the views of the British representative "that a convention relating to refugees could not include an outline of all the articles of the Universal Declaration of Human Rights; furthermore, by its universal character, the Declaration applied to all human groups without exception, and it was pointless to specify that its provisions applied also to refugees": Statement of Sir Leslie Brass of the United Kingdom, UN Doc. E/AC.32/SR.11, Jan. 25, 1950, at 8.

[19] See generally P. Alston and J. Crawford eds., *The Future of UN Human Rights Treaty Monitoring* (2000).

and in particular by reliance on widely ratified treaty law. This study therefore seeks clearly to adumbrate, in both theoretical and applied terms, the authentic scope of the international legal rights which refugees can bring to bear in states of asylum. This approach is based on a firm belief that the creative synthesis of imperfect norms and mechanisms is the best means of pursuing meaningful state accountability in the present legal context, and that the international refugee rights regime provides an important, and thus far insufficiently exploited, opportunity to advance this goal.

In light of this purpose, this book does not address other than incidentally a variety of related issues. Most obviously, it is not a study of the refugee definition.[20] Neither does it seek to explain the work of the institutions charged with the protection of refugees at the domestic or international levels,[21] or the ways in which the refugee protection regime as a whole could be more effectively configured.[22]

Nor does this book present a detailed analysis of the full range of highly specialized human rights treaties established by the United Nations and regional bodies. This decision to avoid canvassing all potentially pertinent international human rights was not taken lightly, since it is clearly correct that particular refugees also benefit incidentally from the protection of specialized branches of international human rights law. Refugees who are members of other internationally protected groups, such as racial minorities, women, and children, may avail themselves of specialized treaty rights in most states.[23] Other refugees will be entitled to claim rights and remedies in consequence of their reasons for flight, a matter of particular importance to those who have escaped from war.[24] Still other refugees will be received in parts of the world

---

[20] The scope of the Convention refugee definition is discussed in detail in Hathaway, *Refugee Status*; in relevant portions of Goodwin-Gill, *Refugee in International Law*, at 32–79; and in A. Grahl-Madsen, *The Status of Refugees in International Law* (vol. I, 1966), at 142–304. Particularly influential analyses of the domestic interpretation of the Convention refugee definition include D. Anker, *The Law of Asylum in the United States* (1999); W. Kälin, *Grundriss des Asylverfahrens* (1990); and F. Tiberghien, *La protection des réfugiés en France* (1999).

[21] On this issue, see in particular G. Loescher, *The UNHCR and World Politics: A Perilous Path* (2001); and A. Helton, *The Price of Indifference: Refugees and Humanitarian Action in the New Century* (2002).

[22] See J. Hathaway ed., *Reconceiving International Refugee Law* (1997).

[23] Of particular importance are the International Convention on the Elimination of All Forms of Racial Discrimination, UNGA Res. 2106A(XX), adopted Dec. 21, 1965, entered into force Jan. 4, 1969; the Convention on the Elimination of All Forms of Discrimination against Women, UNGA Res. 34/180, adopted Dec. 18, 1979, entered into force Sept. 3, 1981; and the Convention on the Rights of the Child, UNGA Res. 44/25, adopted Nov. 20, 1989, entered into force Sept. 2, 1990.

[24] See e.g. T. Meron, *Human Rights and Humanitarian Norms as Customary Law* (1989), at 3–78.

that have adopted regional human rights conventions now clearly understood to embrace non-nationals, in particular the European Convention for
the Protection of Human Rights and Fundamental Freedoms,[25] or in which
there is a transnational human rights regime specifically designed to assist
refugees, as in the case of the regional refugee convention adopted in 1969 by
the Organization of African Unity.[26]

The decision not to engage in depth with the full range of regional and
specialized human rights norms in no way reflects a view that these standards
are not of real importance to refugees. They are not, however, standards that
apply universally to all refugees: only a subset of refugees are women, or
children, or members of racial minorities. An even smaller percentage of
refugees can claim the protection of any one of the regional human rights or
refugee treaties. Because of the specialized nature of these accords, they
cannot reasonably be invoked in aid of the goal of this study, that being to
define the common core of human rights entitlements that inhere in *all*
refugees, in all parts of the world, simply by virtue of being refugees. This
more foundational, and hence more limited, enterprise is designed to elaborate the common *corpus* of refugee rights which can be asserted by refugees
in any state party to the Refugee Convention or Protocol, whatever the
refugee's specific identity or circumstances. The hope is that others will
build upon this basic analysis to define the entitlements of sub-groups of
the refugee population entitled to claim additional protections.

One critical deviation from the commitment to this fairly strictly defined
analytical focus has, however, been made. The rights regime presented here is
the result of an effort to synthesize the entitlements derived from conventional refugee law with those rights codified in the two foundational treaties
of the international human rights system, the International Covenant on
Civil and Political Rights and its companion International Covenant on
Economic, Social and Cultural Rights.[27] The specificity of analysis has been
compromised in this way partly because it is clear that a treatment of refugee
law which takes no account whatever of more general human rights norms
would clearly present an artificially narrow view of the human rights of
refugees. More specifically, though, this analytical synthesis was necessary
in order to present an interpretation of the Refugee Convention which
complies with the view, set out below, that the alignment of refugee law

---

[25] 213 UNTS 221, done Nov. 4, 1950, entered into force Sept. 3, 1953.

[26] Convention governing the Specific Aspects of Refugee Problems in Africa, 10011 UNTS
14691, done Sept. 10, 1969, entered into force June 20, 1974, at Arts. II–VI.

[27] International Covenant on Civil and Political Rights, UNGA Res. 2200A(XXI), adopted
Dec. 16, 1966, entered into force Mar. 23, 1976 (Civil and Political Covenant); International
Covenant on Economic, Social and Cultural Rights, UNGA Res. 2200A(XXI), adopted
Dec. 16, 1966, entered into force Jan. 3, 1976 (Economic, Social and Cultural Covenant).

with international human rights law is required by the duty to interpret the Refugee Convention in context, and taking real account of its object and purpose.[28]

The specific decision to present a merged analysis of refugees' rights and of rights grounded in the two Human Rights Covenants is moreover defensible in view of the unique interrelationships between these particular treaties and refugee law.[29] At a formal level, more than 95 percent of the state parties to the Refugee Convention or Protocol have also signed or ratified both of the Human Rights Covenants.[30] Even more important, about 86 percent of the world's refugees reside in states which have signed or ratified the two Covenants on Human Rights, more even than the 68 percent who reside in a state party to the Refugee Convention or Protocol.[31] As such, both in principle and in practice, refugee rights will in the overwhelming majority of cases consist of an amalgam of principles drawn from both refugee law and the Covenants. Second, and of particular importance, the Covenants and the Refugee Convention aspire to comparable breadth of protection, and set consistently overlapping guarantees. As will be clear from the analysis

---

[28] See chapter 1.3.3 below.

[29] In principle, it would also have made sense to incorporate analysis of rights that are universally binding as authentic customary norms or general principles of law since, to the extent such standards inhere in all persons, refugees are clearly entitled to claim them. But because only protection from systemic racial discrimination is clearly so defined (see chapter 1.2 below) – and since that right is already included in the more general duty of non-discrimination set by the Civil and Political Covenant – the focus here is limited to the cognate rights stated in the two Human Rights Covenants.

[30] Of the 145 state parties to the Refugee Convention, only eight have not signed or ratified either of the Human Rights Covenants: Antigua and Barbuda, Bahamas, Fiji, Holy See, Mauritania, Papua New Guinea, St. Kitts and Nevis, and Tuvalu. Three have signed or ratified only the International Covenant on Civil and Political Rights: Botswana, Haiti, and Mozambique. One state party to the Refugee Convention has signed or ratified only the International Covenant on Economic, Social and Cultural Rights: Solomon Islands: United Nations High Commissioner for Human Rights (UNHCHR), www.unhchr.ch (accessed Nov. 19, 2004).

[31] Of the Dec. 31, 2003 world refugee population of 11,852,900, 86 percent (10,289,700) were residing in a state that has signed or ratified the International Covenant on Civil and Political Rights and 86 percent (10,269,200) were residing in a state that has signed or ratified the International Covenant on Economic, Social and Cultural Rights. In contrast, only 8,148,200 refugees – 68 percent of the total refugee population – resided in a state party to the Refugee Convention or Protocol. These figures are derived from statistics in US Committee for Refugees, *World Refugee Survey 2004* (2004), at 4–5; UNHCHR, www.unhchr.ch (accessed Nov. 19, 2004); and UNHCR, www.unhcr.ch (accessed Nov. 19, 2004). Most rights in the Covenants are granted to all persons physically present in the territory, including refugees, although less developed countries are afforded some latitude in deciding the extent to which economic rights will be extended to non-nationals: Civil and Political Covenant, at Art. 2(1), and Economic, Social and Cultural Covenant, at Art. 2(2)–(3).

below, even when refugee law is the source of a stronger or more contextualized form of protection on a given issue, it is usually the case that the Covenants contribute in some way to the clarification of the relevant responsibilities of states.

In conceiving this work, an effort has been made to be attentive to the central importance of facts. Because a work of scholarship on refugee law seems more likely to be of value if it does not restrict itself simply to the elucidation of legal norms in abstract terms, the treatment of each right in this book begins with an overview of relevant protection challenges in different parts of the world. Some cases present the current reality faced by refugees; others highlight important protection challenges in the recent past. An effort has also been made to include examples from all parts of the world, and impacting diverse refugee populations. The analysis that follows seeks to engage with these practical dilemmas, and to suggest how refugee law should guide their resolution. This approach reflects a strong commitment to the importance of testing the theoretical analysis of human rights standards against the hard facts of protection dilemmas on the ground. The hope is that by taking this approach, the reliability of the analysis presented here is strengthened, and the normative implications of the study are made more clear.

The opening chapter of the book presents an analysis of the fundamental background question of the sources of international law, with a focus on how principles about the sources of law should be applied to identify human rights of genuinely universal authority. This analysis is based upon a theory of modern positivism, which accepts that international law is most sensibly understood as a system of rules agreed to by states, intended to govern the conduct of states, and ultimately enforced in line with the will of states. The theory of international law embraced here is thus in a very real sense a conservative one, predicated on a rigorous construction of the sources of law. Drawing on this theoretical approach, the study identifies those universal rights of particular value to refugees, even as it explains why the rights of refugees are for the most part best defended not by reference to universal custom or general principles of law, but rather by reliance on clear duties codified in treaty law.

Because of this study's primary commitment to reliance on treaty law, chapter 1 concludes with an overview of the approach taken throughout the study to the interpretation of treaties, with specific reference to the construction of the treaties at the heart of this study, the Refugee Convention and Protocol, and the two Human Rights Covenants. It is suggested that there are powerful reasons to defer neither to literalism nor to state practice in discerning the true meaning of these accords. To the contrary, it is both legally correct and more substantively productive to construe the text of refugee and other human rights treaties in the light of their context, objects and purposes as discerned, in particular, from careful study of their drafting history. Equally important, the interpretations of cognate rights rendered by United

Nations treaty supervisory bodies should be understood to be a vital source of contemporary guidance on the content of refugee rights. This is so not only because the advancement of human rights is at the core of refugee law's object and purpose, but more generally because the resultant normative synthesis furthers the commitment to interpret treaties in good faith, and as living instruments.

Chapter 2 moves from analysis of general legal principles to address the specific content of the international refugee rights regime. It begins by tracing the origins of refugee rights in the international law on aliens, through to its codification in the present Convention and Protocol relating to the Status of Refugees. This chapter also introduces the essential approach of the foundational refugee treaties, and shows how they have been complemented both by "soft law" standards and by the evolution of contemporary treaties on human rights and the rights of aliens. Particular attention is paid to the development of general norms of non-discrimination law, and to their relevance as a protective mechanism for refugees. The chapter concludes by explaining why, despite progress in related fields of law, the specific entitlements set by refugee law remain fundamental to ensuring the human dignity of refugees.

Chapter 3 introduces the rather unique principles governing entitlement to claim the rights set by the Refugee Convention. As a fundamental principle, the acquisition of refugee rights under international law is not based on formal status recognition by a state or agency, but rather follows simply and automatically from the fact of substantive satisfaction of the refugee definition. As UNHCR has affirmed:

> A person is a refugee within the meaning of the 1951 Convention as soon as he fulfils the criteria contained in the definition. This would necessarily occur prior to the time at which his refugee status is formally determined. Recognition of his refugee status does not therefore make him a refugee, but declares him to be one. He does not become a refugee because of recognition, but is recognized because he is a refugee.[32]

Despite this critical understanding of refugee status determination as a purely declaratory process, the Refugee Convention does not grant all rights immediately and absolutely to all refugees. To the contrary, it strikes a reasonable balance between meeting the needs of refugees and respecting the legitimate concerns of state parties. In this sense, the Convention reflects the commitment of the drafters to the establishment of a treaty that is both politically realistic, and of positive benefit to refugees.[33]

---

[32] UNHCR, *Handbook on Procedures and Criteria for Determining Refugee Status* (1979, re-edited 1992), at para. 28.

[33] See generally J. Hathaway and A. Cusick, "Refugee Rights Are Not Negotiable," (2000) 14(2) *Georgetown Immigration Law Journal* 481.

While all refugees benefit from a number of core rights, additional entitlements accrue as a function of the nature and duration of the attachment to the asylum state. Some rights inhere as soon as the refugee comes under a state's authority; a second set when he or she enters its territory; others once the refugee is lawfully within the territory of a state party; a fourth group only when the refugee is lawfully staying or durably residing there; and a few rights govern the pursuit of a durable solution to refugeehood. The nature of the duty to extend rights to refugees is moreover defined through a combination of absolute and contingent criteria. A small number of rights are guaranteed absolutely to refugees, and must be respected even if the host government does not extend these rights to anyone else, including to its own citizens. More commonly, though, the standard for compliance varies in line with the relevant treatment afforded another group under the laws and practices of the receiving country. Under these contingent rights standards, the scope of entitlement is conceived as a function of the rights of aliens generally, of the nationals of most-favored states, or as equivalent to those afforded citizens of the host country itself. The Refugee Convention moreover incorporates an overarching duty of non-discrimination between and among refugees, and strictly limits the ability of states to suspend refugee rights, even for national security reasons.

Chapters 4–7 are the heart of the book. They offer a detailed analysis of the substance of refugee rights, drawing on both the norms of the Refugee Convention itself and on cognate standards set by the Covenants on Human Rights. Rather than grouping rights on the basis of traditional categories (e.g. civil, political, economic, social, or cultural), these chapters are structured around the refugee experience itself. This organizational structure reflects the Refugee Convention's commitment, described in chapter 3, to define eligibility for protection on the basis of degrees of attachment to the host state.[34]

Chapter 4 therefore addresses those rights agreed to be immediately (if provisionally) acquired upon coming under the jurisdiction of a state party, as well as those which inhere upon reaching its territory, even before any steps have been taken to verify refugee status. These initial rights speak to the extraordinary personal vulnerability of asylum-seekers, and to the importance of safeguarding their most basic interests until and unless a decision is taken formally to verify their refugee status. A second set of modestly more extensive human rights, described in chapter 5, is deemed suited to the condition of refugees who have met the host state's legal requirements for

---

[34] It is also hoped that adoption of a chapter structure which draws attention to the delays set by refugee law for the acquisition of rights will facilitate critical assessment of the Convention's implicit assumptions regarding the timing and duration of the legal commitment to protection.

lawful presence, including by having satisfied national requirements for the assessment of their refugee status. As in the case of the first set of rights, these enhanced protections inhere until and unless a decision is reached to deny recognition of refugee status.

Once a refugee is authorized to remain in the asylum country, he or she benefits from additional rights, discussed in chapter 6, understood to be necessary to ensuring that the refugee can establish a durable and fully dignified life until and unless the reasons for departure from the home state come to an end. A final group of human rights, set out in chapter 7, is associated with the movement toward the solution of refugee status, whether this is by way of return home, by resettlement in a third country, or by the residual solution of permanent integration in the host state.

An epilogue to the book seeks to open debate on the larger and more political issues of just how the rights set by refugee law should be enforced. Returning to themes introduced in chapter 2, attention is given to the failure of the international community to establish an overarching supervisory mechanism for the Refugee Convention of the kind now in place for virtually every other major United Nations human rights treaty, as well as to the viability of the alternative, national and agency-based enforcement systems upon which refugees are largely compelled to rely. This chapter also introduces the much larger question of the continuing practicality of a rights-based system for the protection of refugees, particularly given the often radical difference between the political, social, and economic circumstances known to the drafters of the Refugee Convention, and those which exist in the states where refugees are most commonly received today.

The thesis which underlies this study is that the specificity of refugee entitlements is too often ignored – not only by those governments which often treat refugees as little more than the beneficiaries of humanitarian discretion, but also by scholars and advocates who too readily assume that generic human rights law is a sufficient answer to the needs of refugees. The objective here is to correct these common misperceptions, and to affirm the importance of refugee-specific rights. While the structures by which refugee law is implemented are no doubt in need of creative reinvigoration and perhaps even of fundamental retooling, it is nonetheless vital to endorse the recognition by states of "the enduring importance of the 1951 Convention, as the primary refugee protection instrument which ... sets out rights, including human rights, and minimum standards of treatment that apply to persons falling within its scope."[35] In an era in which there is no more than selective

---

[35] "Declaration of States Parties to the 1951 Convention and/or its 1967 Protocol relating to the Status of Refugees," UN Doc. HCR/MMSP/2001/09, Dec. 13, 2001, incorporated in Executive Committee of the High Commissioner's Program, "Agenda for Protection," UN Doc. EC/52/SC/CRP.9/Rev.1, June 26, 2002, at Part II, Preamble, para. 2.

ability and inclination to put down human rights abuse abroad, and in which traditional human rights afford few immediate and self-actuating sources of relief, refugee law stands out as the single most effective, truly autonomous remedy for those who simply cannot safely remain in their own countries. The surrogate protection of human rights required by refugee law is too valuable a tool not to be widely understood, and conscientiously implemented.

International law as a source of refugee rights

A study of the rights of refugees under international law must first stake out a position on the critical question of what counts as international law. There is, of course, a simple answer to this question: refugee rights are matters of international law to the extent they derive from one of the accepted trio of international law sources: treaties, custom, or general principles of law.[1] But while technically correct, this facile response fails to do justice to real disagreements about how rules derived from custom or general principles are to be identified and, more specifically, about whether general rules of recognition can fairly be applied to the identification of human rights norms. While this book in no sense aspires to analyze these concerns in depth, it begins with a brief explanation of the reasoning which led to the adoption here of a relatively conservative understanding of the sources of both custom and general principles premised on a consent-based, modern positivist view of international law.

In the second part of this chapter, the rules of recognition are applied to determine whether there are human rights derived from custom, general principles of law or treaties of universal reach which, by virtue of the generality of those sources of law, inhere in all persons. Any protections guaranteed by all states to all persons will, of course, accrue to the benefit of refugees. Yet while in principle universal human rights law[2] should provide the common denominator of protections owed to refugees throughout the world, the analysis here suggests that in practice it delivers little by way of legal entitlement. Because the tests for recognition of a universal norm are appropriately demanding, the protective ambit of universal human rights law is, at best, exceedingly modest.

---

[1] Statute of the International Court of Justice, 59 Stat. 1055 (1945), adopted June 26, 1945, entered into force Oct. 24, 1945 (ICJ Statute), at Art. 38(1).

[2] The term "universal international law" is distinguished from the concept of "general international law," which embraces rules of law which deal with issues of general interest and which are binding on the large majority of (but not all) members of the international community. See generally G. Danilenko, *Law-Making in the International Community* (1993) (Danilenko, *Law-Making*), at 9–10.

The third part of this chapter therefore focuses squarely on treaty law, the most important contemporary source of refugee rights. It presents an understanding of the rules of treaty interpretation which requires significant deference to be afforded the context, object, and purpose of refugee and other human rights treaties. This approach draws on recognition that purely literal interpretation of text is to be avoided under international law. It further acknowledges that evidence of state practice is no more than conditionally relevant in general terms, and of considerably less value in the interpretation of human rights conventions than other treaties. The text of a refugee or other human rights treaty should instead be construed in a way that ensures its effectiveness, as conceived by reference to both the intentions of the drafters and the contemporary social and legal environment within which the treaty must function. To this end, the analysis of refugee rights presented here draws significantly on both the *travaux préparatoires* of the Refugee Convention and on the authoritative interpretations of cognate rights rendered by the United Nations treaty bodies.

1.1 A modern positivist understanding of the sources of universal rights

The simplicity of the assertion that the Charter of the United Nations has ushered in a new era of universally accepted human rights norms is attractive, but untenable as an honest description of the legal landscape. To date, and despite rhetoric to the contrary,[3] states simply have not been willing comprehensively to limit their sovereignty in favor of the essential dignity of the human person. While some see continued patterns of human rights abuse as little more than evidence of a failure to *respect* universal human rights law, this approach begs the question of the origins of those universal rights. Most obviously, because relatively consistent state practice is an essential element for the development of custom, it surely follows that significant inconsistent state practice undermines reliance on customary international law as a source of universal human rights. Yet countervailing practice seems, as discussed below, too often to be either dismissed or even ignored altogether by large parts of the scholarly community.

---

[3] See e.g. I. Cotler, "Human Rights as the Modern Tool of Revolution," in K. Mahoney and P. Mahoney eds., *Human Rights in the Twenty-First Century: A Global Challenge* 7 (1993), at 10: "[T]he post World War II explosion in international human rights law – the internationalization of human rights, and the humanization of international law – turned [the] traditional international law theory on its head. Accordingly, international human rights law would now be premised on the notion that every state has an obligation to protect not only any aliens within its midst, but its own citizens. Individuals, then, are not objects, but subjects of international law with rights and remedies that are justiciable in both domestic and international fora."

Clarity about the defining characteristics of the formal sources of universal international law has been fundamentally compromised by a blurring of the boundary between the law and the politics of human rights. This entanglement of admittedly worthy moral claims with matters of strict legal duty is not only intellectually and legally dubious, but risks stigmatizing all human rights law as no more than a matter of aspiration.[4] This study therefore begins by confronting the proclivity to exaggerate the ambit of universal human rights law. It then defines and applies more defensible criteria for the validation of universal human rights.

Because treaties normally create duties only for states that choose to adhere to them,[5] genuinely universal human rights norms are most likely to be generated through either custom or general principles of law. Both of these sources formalize as generally applicable international law those standards which states treat as binding on themselves, without the necessity of codification. Specifically, custom validates consistent and uniform interstate practices that have come to be regarded by governments as matters of obligation.[6] General principles of international law, in turn, are normally derived from domestic standards present in the legal cultures of a significant majority of states.[7] To the extent that a

---

[4] As cogently observed by Laws LJ, "[n]othing, surely, is more elementary than the certainty required for the identification of what is and is not law . . . ; and we must not be seduced by humanitarian claims to a spurious acceptance of a false source of law": *R (European Roma Rights Centre and Others) v. Immigration Officer at Prague Airport*, [2003] EWCA Civ 666 (Eng. CA, May 20, 2003, rev'd. on another ground at [2004] UKHL 55 (UK HL, Dec. 9, 2004)), at para. 100.

[5] The Charter of the United Nations may sensibly be considered to be an exception to this rule, both because of its near-universal acceptance by states and because of its foundational status within the international legal system: see chapter 1.2.3 below. Other treaties may be explicitly or impliedly declaratory of universal custom or general principles of law, this implication arising most logically when a treaty is adopted without any significant opposition. Finally, a treaty may on occasion indirectly give rise to universal norms through interaction with customary lawmaking, for example where non-adhering states consistently act and are dealt with as though bound by a treaty's terms. But these exceptions apart, treaties ordinarily apply only to those states that have opted to be bound by them.

[6] Under the "natural law" view articulated by Lauterpacht, custom is merely the way through which preexisting law is revealed. "Custom is actual practice in pursuance of or in obedience to what is *already* law [emphasis added]": E. Lauterpacht ed., *International Law: The Collected Papers of Hersch Lauterpacht* (1970) (Lauterpacht, *Collected Papers*), at 238. But this perspective really cannot be maintained in a pluralistic world in which there is no universal agreement on the source or content of moral obligation.

[7] The alternative construction of general principles of law defines them to be "no more than a modern formulation of the law of nature which played a decisive part in the formative period of international law and which underlay much of its subsequent development. For there is no warrant for the view that the law of nature was mere speculation which gave a legal form to deductive thinking on theology and ethics. It was primarily a generalization of the legal experience of mankind": Lauterpacht, *Collected Papers*, at 74–75. To the contrary, it is suggested here that "natural law" is a culturally specific normative structure, the imposition of which on universal law is untenable.

pervasive sense of obligation can be located either in the agreed structure for the conduct of international relations or across systems of domestic governance, a universally binding legal standard may be declared to exist.

As described here, the existence of clear and consistent acceptance by states is a precondition to recognition of a standard as either customary law or a general principle of law. A universally binding human right cannot be brought into existence by simple declaration. Rather, a universal norm can be established only when states concretize their commitment to a particular principle either through their actions toward each other (custom) or by pervasively granting rights within their own political communities (general principles). It is the rigor of this standard that makes it possible for what are effectively supranational standards to emerge from a purely international legal system. Because a significant pattern of inconsistent state practice can always defeat the emergence of a new universal norm, there is no substantive departure from international law's commitment to reserving to states the authority to define the limits of acceptable state conduct. This is the *realpolitik* of international human rights law: there is simply no accepted mechanism by which states may presently be forced to accept universally binding standards.[8] Once such standards are established, however, non-conforming state practice is appropriately understood to be simply a violation of the universal norm, at least until and unless a new rule emerges through the same process of general recognition among states.

These descriptions of the ways in which universal human rights law may arise are firmly rooted in a positivist validation of the will of states.[9] The international human rights law system, even with its increasing openness to injections of individuated and collective concern, remains firmly anchored in a process of state auto-determination of the acceptability of state conduct. It is simply not honest to pretend that human rights norms may somehow descend and be binding upon states that have opted only for loose collaboration within a continuing system of nation-state sovereignty. Rules should instead be said to be part of international law only if they have been explicitly or impliedly agreed to by the states thereby said to be bound. Scholars and non-state actors may influence the course of interstate agreement; but states, and only states, make international law.[10]

---

[8] Dissenting states can dissociate themselves from an emerging customary norm by timely and persistent objection to the rule in question. The question of peremptory (*jus cogens*) norms is discussed at chapter 1.1.3 below.

[9] The understanding of the sources of law set out here was first advanced in J. Hathaway, "America, Defender of Democratic Legitimacy?," (2000) 11(1) *European Journal of International Law* 121.

[10] But see e.g. M. Byers, *Custom, Power and the Power of Rules: International Relations and Customary International Law* (1999) (Byers, *Custom*), which invokes non-legal approaches in aid of a less state-centered understanding of customary international law.

Many, perhaps most, scholars – particularly those who adhere to the now-dominant, policy-oriented school of thought developed at New Haven[11] – will see the affirmation here of legal positivism as unduly conservative, perhaps even simply as old-fashioned. Yet the alternative, policy-oriented, view is most certainly not immune from criticism. In particular, it depletes international law of the certainty required for meaningful accountability. Indeed, the extraordinarily vague and potentially far-reaching nature of the policy-oriented paradigm in practice dissuades governments from treating international law as a meaningful source of real obligations at all.[12] Whatever substantive breadth is sacrificed by positivism's insistence on evidence of consent is arguably more than compensated for by gains in meaningful enforceability that accrue from an understanding of international law as a system of state-generated, consent-based rules and operations. As Kingsbury has observed in an insightful analysis of Oppenheim's positivist understanding of international law,

> [I]t is difficult to argue that a robust theory of international law has as yet accompanied . . . newer accounts of more and more inclusive and complex international society, with disaggregated states, an infinite diversity of non-state actors, private or hybrid rule-making, and an ever-expanding range of topics covered by competing systems or fragments of norms. The extensive cognitive and material reconstruction required to actualize emancipatory projects . . . is indicative of the scale of the challenge. However unappealing Oppenheim's [positivist] approach has seemed, its coherence and manageability are normative attractions that make its continuing political influence intelligible.[13]

The policy-oriented understanding of international law also suffers from a basic problem of political legitimacy. Stripping the theory of any pretense of

[11] See e.g. M. McDougal and F. Feliciano, *Law and Minimum World Public Order* (1961).

[12] The very fluid, policy-oriented account of international law may have been devised precisely because it imposes so few clear obligations on states. As a response to the traditional isolationism of the United States, a non-threatening understanding of international law may have been thought strategically necessary to induce greater American participation in international legal regimes. And as Kingsbury has observed, this fluid approach may also serve contemporary American priorities. "If no balance [of power] exists, and one state becomes preponderant, that state will pursue 'anti-formalist' approaches where these suit it better. Thus, after the decline and collapse of the USSR, a US scholarly focus on 'governance,' 'regimes,' 'managerial compliance,' 'decision process' and the like, and a US tendency to negotiate detailed multilateral rule-making treaties which it does not then ratify, may reflect in some areas of international law a US preference for anti-formal malleability that is influenced by the aura of preponderant power": B. Kingsbury, "Legal Positivism as Normative Politics: International Society, Balance of Power and Lassa Oppenheim's Positive International Law," (2002) 13(2) *European Journal of International Law* 401 (Kingsbury, "Legal Positivism"), at 421.

[13] Kingsbury, "Legal Positivism," at 416.

political neutrality, Anthony D'Amato argues that international law is comprised simply of those norms derived from state practice which facilitate systemic homeostasis or equilibrium.[14] Law is process, and is therefore essentially indistinguishable from international relations, or even from plain old international politics. As such, the inherent ambiguity of policy-oriented definitions provides extraordinary camouflage for the exercise of unilateral action in defiance of even broadly accepted norms.[15] The murky definitions of international law proposed by Myres McDougal and the generation of legal theorists who followed his lead are therefore not simply harmless efforts to take account of an increasingly complex international reality. This policy-oriented school of international law is, at its core, fundamentally anti-democratic.

Specifically, by rejecting legal positivism's concern to limit the scope of international law to those standards agreed by sovereign states to bind them, the policy-oriented perspective on international law facilitates an equation of international law with whatever norms are of value to dominant states. By deeming the process through which norms and institutions are agreed to be as much law as the resultant norms and institutions themselves, and by equating political and economic power with legitimate rule-making authority, the policy-oriented school of international law provides a ready-made justification for defiance of established international norms and procedures by powerful countries.[16] After all, if rules and institutions established by consent are no more "law" than is the process of interstate power-brokering and influence, then rules and institutions can freely be ignored when they fail to serve the interests of hegemonic states. Indeed, where rules and institutions work counter to international homeostasis (i.e. the situation in which those who dominate continue to dominate), the extreme version of the thesis as articulated by

---

[14] A. D'Amato, "On the Sources of International Law," paper presented at the University of California at Berkeley, Jan. 18, 1996, at 68: "There are no mysterious 'sources' of international law. The rules of international law derive from the behavior (or practice) of states as they interact with each other within the international system. Both the states, and the system itself, have an overarching goal: to persist through time. Rules of law, accordingly, play a role in facilitating this persistence, primarily by signaling to states a class of prohibited behaviors. If a state ignores a prohibitory rule, it risks creating friction with other states that could lead to a rupture of systemic equilibrium."

[15] As Koskenniemi has argued, those who embrace an understanding of law predicated on the enforcement of so-called underlying values "have irrevocably left formalism for hermeneutics. Law is now how it is interpreted. As the 'deep-structural' values which the interpretation is expected to reveal do not exist independently of human purposes, we are down the slippery slope of trying to identify those purposes": M. Koskenniemi, "'The Lady Doth Protest Too Much': Kosovo, and the Turn to Ethics in International Law," (2002) 65(2) *Modern Law Review* 159 (Koskenniemi, "The Lady"), at 164.

[16] See e.g. M. Reisman, "Unilateral Action and the Transformations of the World Constitutive Process: The Special Case of Humanitarian Intervention," (2000) 11(1) *European Journal of International Law* 3 (Reisman, "Unilateral Action").

D'Amato holds that an understanding of international law *must* be derived from the political process, even when it contradicts established rules and processes. The policy-oriented school of international law has thus spawned a new version of natural law thinking under which the will of powerful states is simply substituted for that of God or nature.[17]

This is not to say that a consent-based, positivist understanding of international law is without limitations of its own.[18] Most obviously, it is an error to believe that such a rule-based understanding of law will necessarily govern other than relatively routine forms of interaction among states. In the context of high

---

[17] For example, if a powerful state wants to avoid compliance with the duty to refrain from the unilateral use of force pursuant to the UN Charter, law as process serves the purpose. Simply redefine a Western-dominated unofficial network as a source of law and grant powerful states the right to interpret and act upon its prescriptions, and voilà: unilateral intervention in a foreign country is now legal. But what if that same unofficial network suggests the need to rid the world of land mines that kill and maim thousands of innocent civilians every year? Ironically, the policy-oriented school of international law as process can still serve the needs of powerful countries. Because key states remain the final arbiters of the result of the diffuse lawmaking conversation, no action need be taken if the social authenticity of the speakers is called into question. In short, the fungibility of policy-oriented views of international law can be manipulated in ways that the fairly clear requirements of legal positivism cannot. See e.g. Reisman "Unilateral Action," at 15. Even more moderate accounts of "modern custom" leave enormous room for the imposition of subjective preferences. For example, Roberts' "reflective interpretive concept" would derive customary norms from "commonly held subjective values about right and wrong that have been adopted by a majority of states in treaties and declarations": A. Roberts, "Traditional and Modern Approaches to Customary International Law: A Reconciliation," (2001) 95(4) *American Journal of International Law* 757 (Roberts, "Traditional and Modern Approaches"), at 778. In the end, however, the vagueness of this standard leaves powerful states with extraordinary interpretive space.

[18] This study does not address in any detail criticisms which are relatively easily answered, e.g. those noted in Roberts, "Traditional and Modern Approaches," at 767 ff. First, it is said that a positivist understanding of customary law "lacks democratic legitimacy": ibid. This seems an odd criticism, since the reliance on the words of scholars, select international conferences, declarations understood to be non-binding, or on views articulated by powerful states – all relied upon by the proponents of so-called "modern custom" – seem significantly more anti-democratic. Second, it is said that traditional custom is "too clumsy and slow": ibid. But if speed is of the essence, the obvious answer is to proceed by way of treaty-making. Third, it is asserted that customary law has at times been declared on the basis of less than over-whelming practice. While this is true, the need for empirically verifiable acceptance by states under traditional custom at least provides an objective basis (absent from modern custom) to challenge the declaration of a customary norm. Fourth and finally, it is said that custom inaccurately assumes that states have perfect knowledge of state practice and an awareness that failure to respond will result in the imposition of legal obligations upon them. This seems doubtful: states *are* aware that they need to respond, and unlimited resources are no longer required in the age of the Internet and widely disseminated information on state practice in order for governments to be able to participate in (or to challenge) the creation of custom that would limit their sovereignty. See e.g. R. Gaebler and M. Smolka-Day, *Sources of State Practice in International Law* (2002).

stakes, inherently political situations, formal rules are unlikely to be outcome-determinative.[19] It is nonetheless better to concede the limited ambit of meaningful international law than to sacrifice the commitment to legal certainty and enforceability that positivism affords in most spheres of relatively routine interaction.[20]

Traditional positivism is also subject to the criticism that gender, racial, and other forms of bias permeate domestic legal systems, and hence limit the extent to which a state's agreement to be bound internationally truly reflects the consent of all of its people. While there is some force in this argument, positivism may nonetheless actually be a valuable means of taking critical insights about the reality of power onboard in practical ways. Specifically, a modern understanding of positivism as conceived here is anchored in recognition of the overarching and powerful commitment of international law to the establishment of broad-ranging, substantive equality.[21] Because no rule is immune from the duty of all states to ensure equal benefit of all laws to all persons, modern positivism both compels and facilitates the challenging of domestic legal and other constraints which disfranchise women and minorities.[22] So conceived, the commitment to respect for consent-based rules is in no sense antithetical to social and political

---

[19] Writing at the beginning of the twentieth century, this point was colorfully (if somewhat depressingly) made by Baker. "No general or admiral worth the name would pause in difficult strategy, or at the moment of victory, because some effeminate Article of the Second Hague Convention or other grandmotherly Conference forbade him to do so and so. All that can be hoped for is the exercise of well known, plain and intelligent rules which do not interfere with the act of war, but cause it to be waged with more humanity. Elaborate rules prescribed by the delegates sitting at ease in the Palace of Peace, or in any other place, will never be followed when the safety of an empire or life or liberty is in serious jeopardy": G. Baker ed., *Halleck's International Law* (1908), at vi. Even in a contemporary context, "formal rules work well in a domestic normality where situations are routine and the need to honor the formal validity of the law by far outweighs incidental problems in its application. The benefits of exceptionless compliance offset the losses ... But this is otherwise in an international emergency of some gravity ... The point of the rule (that is, the need to prevent serious and large scale violations of human rights) is more important than its formal validity ... In the international situation ... and especially if the situation is defined as a 'serious violation of fundamental rights,' the need to uphold the formal validity of the law cannot be compared to the weight of the impulse to act now": Koskenniemi, "The Lady," at 168–169.

[20] Specifically, a positivist understanding of international law may be said to count among its advantages "the distinctive formulation and interpretation of legal rules as a basis for clarity and stability; their reduction in writing to increase certainty and predictability; the elaboration of distinct legal institutions; the development of ethically autonomous professional roles, such as that of international judge; and the separation of legal argument from moral arguments as a means to overcome disagreement": Kingsbury, "Legal Positivism," at 422.

[21] See chapter 2.5.5 below.

[22] "[I]t does not suffice only to provide a hearing to the claims of the political other but also to include in political contestation the question about *who* are entitled to make claims and *what kinds* of claims pass the test of validity. Without such self-reflexivity formalism will

progress. To the contrary, a rule-based approach to international law actually supports efforts to compel governments to confront historic patterns of exclusion. This compatibility of criticality with the positivist project has been recognized at least since the time of Oppenheim:

> This task of the science of international law is very important and must not be neglected if we want international law to develop progressively and to bring more and more matters under its sway ... Nothing prevents us from applying the sharp knife of criticism, from distinguishing between what is good and bad according to our individual ideas, and from proposing improvements.[23]

At the very least, a consent-based understanding of international law ensures that as more socially inclusive understandings of power and politics evolve at the domestic level in an increasing number of states, these automatically impact the international lawmaking process as well (because the consent of these more inclusive systems of governance will be required to create new international law). In this sense, positivism reinforces and entrenches domestic gains on the international plane.

A third concern is that the consent-based foundation of legal positivism is attenuated by its willingness to impose what amounts to a contract of adhesion on new states – those states that wish to be recognized must sign on to the established rules of general international law. While this is true, this violation of full-fledged consent theory is a less egregious intrusion on those states' self-determination than is the neo-natural law alternative, which effectively gives powerful states the right to define law not only at the moment of a new state's independence, but indefinitely. As Koskenniemi has observed, "the very claim that one is arguing from the position of authenticity – for example, a given notion of human rights, or self-determination – involves an objectionable attempt to score a political victory outside politics."[24] In contrast, legal positivism's insistence on the consent of states is not only a critical means of ensuring that international law is actually taken seriously by the states that it purports to bind. It is also the least illegitimate basis for a system that purports to govern in the absence of a mechanism for the direct enfranchisement of real people.[25] In Kingsbury's terms, "a formal international law based on consent has an

---

freeze into the justification of one or another substantive policy [emphasis in original]": Koskenniemi, "The Lady," at 174–175.

[23] L. Oppenheim, "The Science of International Law: Its Task and Method," (1908) 2(2) *American Journal of International Law* 313, at 318, 355, cited in Kingsbury, "Legal Positivism," at 426.

[24] Koskenniemi, "The Lady," at 173.

[25] As Kingsbury observes in relation to the work of Oppenheim, "an international society of states, a balance of power and a positivist conception of international law should all be pursued because they represented the best feasible means to attain ... higher normative goals": Kingsbury, "Legal Positivism," at 434.

increasing hold on the democratic imagination and on the growing number for whom anti-formalism is a specific or systemic threat."[26]

In sum, a positivist understanding of international law is an important means to advance both refugee rights, and the more general international human rights project. Evidence of consent by states establishes both substantive certainty and the political foundation required for meaningful accountability. It is an approach to international law which minimizes the potential for powerful states to bend the normative project to their will, and which sets a firm foundation from which to challenge exclusion of any part of a state's population from real participation in the decision about whether to consent to the establishment of new international law. Moreover, the major weakness of modern positivism – namely, that the analytical rigor of its rules of recognition results in a less extensive range of international legal norms than does the policy-oriented alternative – is, in fact, more apparent than real. As described in detail below, the current array of international norms of indisputable authority (in particular, of treaties) is a more than sufficient basis from which to advance the human rights project, including the protection of refugees.

1.1.1 Customary law

Under the modern positivist approach outlined above, any universal norm of human rights law must be the product of state consent. Thus, customary international law requires the existence of relatively constant and uniform state practice that has generated a sense of mutual obligation among states.[27] The process of striving for interstate agreement is no less real than in law-making by treaty, the key difference being simply that the medium of negotiation is action rather than words. There is customary law only where legally relevant actions coincide to such an extent that they can be said to represent an agreed standard of acceptable behavior.[28] As Simma and Alston note,

---

[26] Ibid. at 436. See also M.-E. O'Connell, "Re-Leashing the Dogs of War," (2003) 97(2) *American Journal of International Law* 446 (O'Connell, "Re-Leashing"), at 456, observing that "a return to stricter adherence to the positive sources of international law . . . is generally the right [approach]."

[27] The *opinio juris* requirement of custom is most usefully understood in modern context to require that the practice be acknowledged by states to circumscribe the range of their sovereign authority. This may be inferred from consistent de facto reference to the standard, or from explicit invocation of its authority.

[28] "[I]f absolute and universal uniformity were to be required, only very few rules could rank as general customary rules of international law. Nevertheless, it appears that, because of the underlying requirement of consent, the condition of constancy and uniformity is liable on occasion to be interpreted with some rigidity when there is a question of ascertaining a customary rule of general validity": Lauterpacht, *Collected Papers*, at 62.

customary lawmaking is a process of inductive reasoning in which retrospection on empirical reality provides a normative projection for the future.[29]

Yet some maintain that the *actions* from which custom arises can consist solely of words.[30] By construing international legal discourse to be a form of state action,[31] it is possible to reach the startling conclusion that actual interstate practice is not requisite to the development of customary law.[32] Official statements that are neither formalized through treaty nor consistent with prevailing state practice are presented as authoritative representations of the state of international law.[33] In reality, however, pronouncements at conferences and in international fora cannot be said to show any intention to be bound.[34] More fundamentally, the proponents of this exaggerated definition of state "practice" deny the most elementary distinction between treaties and

---

[29] B. Simma and P. Alston, "The Sources of Human Rights Law: Custom, *Jus Cogens*, and General Principles," (1988–1989) 12 *Australian Year Book of International Law* 82 (Simma and Alston, "Sources of Human Rights Law"), at 89.

[30] "Statements are conduct. They count as examples of state practice regardless of the *opinio juris* that they also reflect": O'Connell, "Re-Leashing," at 448.

[31] As Byers has observed, "[t]he newly independent non-industrialized States found themselves in a legal system which had been developed primarily by relatively wealthy, militarily powerful States. They consequently sought to change the system. They used their numerical majorities to adopt resolutions and declarations which advanced their interests. They also asserted, in conjunction with a significant number of legal scholars (and perhaps with the International Court of Justice), that resolutions and declarations are instances of State practice which are potentially creative, or at least indicative, of rules of customary international law ... Powerful States, for the most part, along with some scholars from powerful States, have resisted these developments. They have emphatically denied that resolutions and declarations can be State practice": Byers, *Custom*, at 41.

[32] "Approximately two centuries after the rise of the positivist view, a new theory [of customary international law (CIL)] is beginning to take hold in some quarters. The theory derives norms of CIL in a loose way from treaties (ratified or not), UN General Assembly resolutions, international commissions, and academic commentary – but all colored by a moralism reminiscent of the natural law view": J. Goldsmith and E. Posner, "Understanding the Resemblance Between Modern and Traditional Customary International Law," (2000) 40(2) *Virginia Journal of International Law* 639 (Goldsmith and Posner, "Modern and Traditional"), at 640.

[33] "The passage of norms agreed upon in international conferences into customary law through the practice, including the acquiescence, of states constitutes a common, generally accepted method of building customary international law. But an attempt to endow customary law status instantly upon norms approved by consensus or near-consensus at international conferences raises serious questions": T. Meron, *Human Rights and Humanitarian Norms as Customary Law* (1989) (Meron, *Human Rights*), at 87. This more cautious approach is helpfully elaborated by Roberts, who suggests that there is a need to "broaden our understanding of state practice to include considerations of intrastate action ... obligations being observed ... and reasons for a lack of protest over breaches": Roberts, "Traditional and Modern Approaches," at 777.

[34] "[R]esolutions and recommendations ..., however sympathetic one may be towards their motivation and purpose, cannot themselves establish a legal rule binding in

custom: custom is not simply a matter of words, wherever or by whomever uttered,[35] but is a function of what is happening in the real world.[36]

1.1.2 General principles of law

As an alternative to custom, universally applicable human rights might also be established as general principles of law. As traditionally conceived, a general principle of law is established not on the basis of uniform state practice as under custom, but by virtue of the consistency of domestic laws across a significant range of countries. International law can validly emerge in such circumstances because states have already consented to the binding authority of the standard within their own spheres of governance. As extrapolations from the laws which states have themselves chosen to enact, general principles of law are in principle consistent with the consensualist foundation of international law.

In contrast, a revisionist formulation of this source of international law would not only embrace norms common to domestic legal systems, but would also validate key declarations of the General Assembly and other

international law": *Sepet and Bulbul v. Secretary of State for the Home Department*, [2003] UKHL 15 (UK HL, Mar. 20, 2003). See also *Garza v. Lappin*, (2001) 253 F 3d 918 (US CA7, June 14, 2001), at 924–925: "The American Declaration of the Rights and Duties of Man, on which the Commission relied in reaching its conclusions in Garza's case, is an aspirational document which, as Garza admitted in his petition ... did not on its own create an enforceable obligation on the part of the OAS member nations."

[35] The resolutions of the General Assembly may, however, provide evidence of *opinio juris*, or confirm the existence of a norm of customary international law: *Legality of the Threat or Use of Nuclear Weapons*, [1996] ICJ Rep 226, at para. 70. It remains the case, however, that inconsistent state practice precludes the development of a customary norm despite strong evidence of *opinio juris*: ibid. at para. 73.

[36] For example, in rejecting the argument that a system to prevent the departure of Roma refugee claimants from the Czech Republic was in breach of a customary international legal duty not to frustrate efforts to seek asylum, the House of Lords took note of many authoritative principles adopted in international fora and otherwise that might support such a position, but ultimately concluded that those principles had not "received the assent of ... nations": *R v. Immigration Officer at Prague Airport et al., ex parte European Roma Rights Centre et al.*, [2004] UKHL 55 (UK HL, Dec. 9, 2004), at para. 27. In reaching this conclusion, Lord Bingham cited the decision of Cockburn CJ in *R v. Keyn*, (1876) 2 Ex D 63 (Eng. Exchequer Division, Nov. 11, 1876), at 202, that "even if entire unanimity had existed in respect of the important particulars ... in place of so much discrepancy of opinion, the question would still remain, how far the law as stated by the publicists had received the assent of the civilized nations of the world. For writers on international law, however valuable their labours may be in elucidating and ascertaining the principles and rules of law, cannot make the law. To be binding, the law must have received the assent of the nations who are to be bound by it. This assent may be express, as by treaty or the acknowledged concurrence of governments, or may be implied from established usage": ibid. at para. 27.

major international deliberative bodies as general principles of law.[37] While more honest than the conversion of words into actions by "instant custom,"[38] this proposal flatly contradicts the most fundamental tenet of the international legal system, namely that there is no universal legislature or executive that can create law that is binding on all states. The General Assembly is constitutionally prohibited from engaging in general lawmaking,[39] and even the authority of the Security Council is delegated by states within the limits of Chapter VII of the United Nations Charter.[40] Yet the suggested renovation of the general principles framework would allow the simple pronouncement of the General Assembly on a matter within the *jus cogens* substantive sphere to give rise to international law.[41] This would be so even though the foundational norm itself had never been accepted as a source of legal obligation.

[37] See e.g. R. Falk, *The Status of Law in International Society* (1970), at 174–184; and G. Abi-Saab, "Cours général de droit international public," (1987) 207 *Recueil de cours* 173, at 173–178. "Admittedly, the dominant view understands this concept in a narrow sense, as referring to legal principles developed *in foro domestico*. But, as many writers have pointed out in various contexts, there is no necessity to restrict the notion of 'general principles' in this way. For the drafters of the Statute [of the International Court of Justice] the decisive point was that such principles were not to be derived from mere speculation; they had rather to be made objective through some sort of general acceptance or recognition by States. Such acceptance or recognition, however, may also be effected on the *international plane*" [emphasis in original]: Simma and Alston,"Sources of Human Rights Law," at 102.

[38] As Simma observed, "this is as far as mainstream theory, based on state consent, can take this issue; if we are to go beyond this, we will have to look to legal hermeneutics and linguistic theory": B. Simma, "Book Review," (1998) 92(3) *American Journal of International Law* 577, at 578.

[39] Charter of the United Nations, 59 Stat. 1031 (1945), done June 26, 1945, entered into force October 24, 1945 (UN Charter), at Arts. 10–18. These articles authorize the General Assembly to make binding decisions only on a range of administrative matters. "Article 18 [of the Charter] deals with '*decisions*' of the General Assembly 'on important questions.' These 'decisions' do indeed include certain recommendations, but others have dispositive force and effect. Among these latter decisions, Article 18 includes suspension of rights and privileges of membership, expulsion of Members, 'and budgetary questions'": *Certain Expenses of the United Nations*, [1962] ICJ Rep 151, at 163.

[40] "The primary place ascribed to international peace and security is natural, since the fulfilment of the other purposes will be dependent upon the attainment of that basic condition. These purposes are broad indeed, but neither they nor the powers conferred to effectuate them are unlimited. Save as they have entrusted the Organization with the attainment of these common ends, the Member States retain their freedom of action": *Certain Expenses of the United Nations*, [1962] ICJ Rep 151, at 168.

[41] The International Law Commission has affirmed that the peremptory character of a norm is fundamentally "the particular nature of the subject-matter with which it deals": International Law Commission, "Draft Articles on the Law of Treaties," at 67, cited in M. Ragazzi, *The Concept of International Obligations* Erga Omnes (1997) (Ragazzi, *Erga Omnes*), at 49.

The alliance of a reconstituted general principles lawmaking with the *jus cogens* doctrine raises a second concern. Classification as a general principle of law would follow not from compliance with formal rules of recognition, but from an assessment of whether the standard's subject matter resonates within a character-defined sphere of *jus cogens*. This formulation plays into the hands of those who posit the existence of some overarching philosophical structure on those rights established through the consensual process of interstate lawmaking.

1.1.3 Jus cogens *standards*

Properly conceived, the idea of *jus cogens* or higher, peremptory law, is a helpful way of bringing order to international law without feigning the existence of supranational authority. *Jus cogens* is a general principle of law based on the near-universal commitment of national legal systems to insulating certain basic norms from derogation.[42] It sanctions the establishment of an outer limit to the range of subjects on which states may legitimately contract, enforced by the invalidation of conflicting treaties. The *jus cogens* principle is recognized in the Vienna Convention on the Law of Treaties as the basis for giving precedence to any treaty that embodies "a norm accepted and recognized by the international community of States as a whole as a norm from which no derogation is permitted."[43]

Jus cogens is not, therefore, a source of law. It is rather a hierarchical designation that attaches to laws that have come into existence by the usual modes of international lawmaking. The attribution of status as "higher law" derives from the intersection of such a freestanding law with the general principle of law prohibiting agreements that are inconsistent with the most basic values of the international community.[44] *Jus cogens* is best understood as a means of giving greater enforceability to norms that have already acquired the status of universal law by operation of general principles or

---

[42] A. Verdross, "*Jus Dispositivum* and *Jus Cogens* in International Law," (1966) 60(1) *American Journal of International Law* 55, at 61. See also M. McDougal, H. Lasswell, and L. Chen, *Human Rights and World Public Order: The Basic Policies of an International Law of Human Dignity* (1980) (McDougal et al., *World Public Order*), at 339–340: "The newly emphasized notion of *jus cogens* had its origin, in various roughly equivalent forms, in national legal systems. In most legal systems, it is a key institutional postulate that some policies are so intensely demanded, and so fundamental to the common interest of the community, that private parties cannot be permitted to deviate from such policies by agreement. In fact, this notion is so widespread and so common that it could be said to be part of the general principles of law regarded as [an] authoritative source of international law."

[43] Vienna Convention on the Law of Treaties, 1155 UNTS 331, done May 23, 1969, entered into force Jan. 27, 1980 (Vienna Convention), at Art. 53.

[44] See generally F. Domb, "Jus Cogens and Human Rights," (1976) 6 *Israeli Yearbook of Human Rights* 104.

custom (including custom interacting with treaty).[45] Human rights that are matters of *jus cogens* are therefore "super rights" that trump conflicting claims.[46] It is not possible, however, for a right to have force as *jus cogens* without first acquiring status as law through one of the recognized modes of international lawmaking.

The challenge is to ensure that *jus cogens* is defined in a way that ensures evolution away from its parochial origins in natural law and which advances respect for the consensual premise of international lawmaking. In a world of diverse values, the most useful approach would be to build upon the accepted formalities of international lawmaking. There should be evidence that the putative *jus cogens* norm occupies a privileged position in the context of accepted traditional sources of international law.[47] Thus, for example, where custom and treaty law intersect, it may be reasonable to suggest that common normative standards may be said to be fundamental to transnational community values. One might similarly attribute privileged stature to a pervasively subscribed treaty, or to customary norms or general principles that have shown their durability through application to varied circumstances over time and across cultures. The uniting principle suggested here respects state control over international law, in that "higher law" evolves as a function of the extent and degree of affirmation by states.[48] It similarly acknowledges the

---

[45] Thus, for example, the International Law Commission has recommended not only that states be prohibited from recognizing as lawful a situation created by a serious breach of a peremptory norm, but that they also undertake to cooperate in bringing such a breach to an end: "Draft Articles on Responsibility of States for Internationally Wrongful Acts," UN Doc. A/56/10, Ch. IV.E.1, adopted Nov. 2001 (International Law Commission, "Draft Articles"), at Arts. 40–41.

[46] "Third States would have the right and the duty to question the illegal act, and to refrain from recognizing it or giving it legal effect": Meron, *Human Rights*, at 200. More recently, the International Law Commission has determined that all states must take all lawful means to end human rights abuse which involves breach of a peremptory norm and are not required to recognize a situation created by such a breach: "Report of the International Law Commission," UN Doc. A/56/10 (2001), at Part II, Ch. III, Arts. 40–41.

[47] "[T]he important point about the expression 'acceptance and recognition' is not to decide in the abstract which source(s) can produce norms of *jus cogens*, but to assess whether the 'intrinsic value' of a certain rule and the fact that it is 'rooted in the international conscience' . . . are reflected in the acceptance and recognition of that rule as a rule of *jus cogens*": Ragazzi, *Erga Omnes*, at 54.

[48] The human rights suggested by the International Law Commission to be peremptory norms – namely, freedom from slavery, genocide, racial discrimination, *apartheid*, and torture; and respect for the basic rules of international humanitarian law, and the right to self-determination – would likely all qualify as *jus cogens* norms based upon the approach recommended here. See "Report of the International Law Commission," UN Doc. A/56/10 (2001), at "Commentary to Article 26," para. 5; and "Commentary to Article 40," paras. 3–5. But note that the Supreme Court of Canada has characterized the prohibition of torture merely as "an emerging peremptory norm of international law": *Suresh v. Canada*, [2002] 1 SCR 3 (Can. SC, Jan. 11, 2002).

truly exceptional nature of defining any standards to be matters of "high illegality" in an essentially coordinative body of law.[49]

At present, however, the utility of the *jus cogens* doctrine is threatened by a range of politically expedient actions. On the one hand, there is an unhealthy tendency on the part of some scholars in powerful states to equate hegemonic political or ideological traditions with universal values. This "character defined" approach to *jus cogens*, impliedly endorsed by the renovation of general principles previously outlined,[50] fails to recognize the impossibility in a pluralist world of defining peremptory norms based on particularized notions of which rights are intrinsic and undeniable.[51] Common human rights standards will be agreed to for varied reasons, and taking account of diverging world views. If there is to be a recognition of standards that trump other norms, the defining characteristic of these *jus cogens* principles must itself be accepted by all those it purports to bind.

Conversely, there are those in the less developed world who see *jus cogens* as a way to override international law established without their full participation, thereby accelerating the pace of global institutional and normative reform.[52]

---

[49] "Jurists have from time to time attempted to classify rules, or rights and duties, on the international plane by use of terms like 'fundamental' or, in respect of rights, 'inalienable' or 'inherent.' Such classifications have not had much success, but have intermittently affected the interpretation of treaties by tribunals": I. Brownlie, *Principles of Public International Law* (2003) (Brownlie, *Public International Law*), at 488. For example, the Supreme Court of Canada addressed the question whether the prohibition of torture is a peremptory norm under international law in a very cautious way. "Although the Court is not being asked to pronounce on the status of the prohibition on torture in international law, the fact that such a principle is included in numerous multilateral instruments, that it does not form part of any known domestic administrative practice, and that it is considered by many academics to be an emerging, if not established, peremptory norm, suggests that it cannot be easily derogated from": *Suresh v. Canada*, [2002] 1 SCR 3 (Can. SC, Jan. 11, 2002).

[50] See chapter 1.1.2 above.

[51] "In fact, the [International Law Commission] commentary and most authors on the subject essentially contend that peremptory rules exist because they are needed . . . The urgent need to act that the concept suggests fundamentally challenges the consensual framework of the international system by seeking to impose obligations on dissenting states that the 'international community' deems fundamental": D. Shelton, "Righting Wrongs: Reparations in the Articles on State Responsibility," (2002) 96(4) *American Journal of International Law* 833, at 843.

[52] "The numerical majority favoring far-reaching and rapid changes in the existing international legal order . . . discovered an ideal opportunity to reformulate community interests and some of its basic rules of behavior. The temptation has emerged to use *jus cogens* as a possible normative vehicle for introducing sweeping reforms dictated by the majority. While writers from developing countries display a growing interest in the non-consensual foundations of *jus cogens* [citing to T. Rao, "International Custom," (1979) 19 *Indian Journal of International Law* 515, at 520], recent practice indicates that the Third World decision makers do not hesitate to use the *jus cogens* concept for legislative purposes": Danilenko, *Law-Making*, at 239.

Recognizing the numerical strength of the less developed world in the General Assembly, there have been efforts to characterize its resolutions as constitutive of *jus cogens*. But this approach runs afoul of the principle, described above, that *jus cogens* is not a source of law, but is rather a label that attaches to an otherwise validly conceived law because of its centrality to collective consensus on basic standards. Because the General Assembly and its subordinate bodies have no general lawmaking authority,[53] their resolutions are not usually binding.[54] There is therefore no law to which the *jus cogens* designation can adhere. The only exceptions would be where the resolution is simply the codification of a preexisting custom or general principle of law, or where it has achieved such status over time since passage of the resolution.

It is, of course, perfectly legitimate to argue for the replacement of traditional modes of international lawmaking by a more parliamentary, community-based system of supranational authority. It is, however, duplicitous to pretend that there is presently agreement in favor of such a shift. It is doubly dishonest to argue that the *jus cogens* rule, designed to bring order to established forms of law, can be relied upon to assert the existence of an order of authority superior to standards devised through the three established modes of lawmaking.

1.2 The present scope of universal human rights law

The most fundamental problem with the various efforts to expand the scope of international law is that states have generally not been willing to acknowledge their force. As the gap between declared universal law and the practice of states widens, advocates of an expansive interpretation of universal human rights norms may inadvertently be contributing to the destruction of a meaningful system of general interstate obligation toward humankind. The net result of the persistent overstatement of the reach of custom, general principles, and *jus cogens* is not, as presumably hoped, the effective incorporation of new standards into a clear and practical system of enforceable duties. Instead,

---

[53] "The functions of the General Assembly for which it may establish such subsidiary organs include, for example, investigation, observation and supervision, but the way in which such subsidiary organs are utilized depends on the consent of the State or States concerned": *Certain Expenses of the United Nations*, [1962] ICJ Rep 151, at 165.

[54] "Although the decisions of the General Assembly are endowed with full legal effect in some spheres of the activity of the United Nations and with limited legal effects in other spheres, it may be said, by way of a broad generalization, that they are not legally binding upon the Members of the United Nations": *South West Africa (Voting Procedure)*, [1955] ICJ Rep 67, at 115 (Separate Opinion of Judge Lauterpacht). This is not to say, however, that they may not contribute to the evolution of customary international law, by providing relevant evidence of *opinio juris*: *Legality of the Threat or Use of Nuclear Weapons*, [1996] ICJ Rep 226, at para. 70.

wishful legal thinking sends the signal that the very notion of universal human rights law is essentially rhetorical, thereby diluting the force of whatever standards truly command (or may one day command) the respect of states. In the end, this melding of international law and politics yields little beyond politics.[55]

Some may counter that the distinction between the law and the politics of human rights is in any event artificial. At one level, this is true. International law is in general the product of power, and is a system of authority premised on the retention of power by nation-states. More profoundly, international law unquestionably entrenches rules that privilege the goals of those states that presently dominate international life, with concomitant marginalization of the aspirations of less powerful countries.[56] The conclusion might therefore be reached that the effective melding of law and politics through sweeping pronouncements on the content of universal human rights law at worst serves simply to make clear the artificial or unprincipled elevation of certain norms to the realm of binding authority.[57]

While perhaps principled, this analysis is strategically flawed. It is simply not true that the international political process is a more hospitable environment for the generation of fair-minded and equitable standards of acceptable conduct than is the international lawmaking regime.[58] International politics, no less than international law, is dominated by the strategic concerns of present-day power-holders. Moreover, even where standards evolve in arguably democratic fora such as the General Assembly of the United Nations, it is abundantly clear that the highly politicized nature of such processes provides no guarantee that the interests of the intended beneficiaries of human rights law will be well served. Most important, and in contrast to international law (and most forms of domestic politics), international politics affords no structure within which states must justify their stewardship of human rights in a public and expert forum.

---

[55] "Despite certain special characteristics, such as the types of evidence marshalled to establish customary human rights, human rights cannot but be considered a subject within the theory and discipline of public international law. Undue emphasis on the uniqueness of human rights will not advance their acceptance, on the broadest possible scale, as international law": Meron, *Human Rights*, at 101.

[56] See generally B. S. Chimni, *International Law and World Order* (1993).

[57] "Modern customary international law (CIL) does not constrain nations any more than old CIL did. When nations decline to violate CIL, this is usually because they have no reason to violate it. Nations would act no differently if CIL were not a formally recognized source of law. Modern CIL is mostly aspirational, just as old CIL was": Goldsmith and Posner, "Modern and Traditional," at 672.

[58] This is conceded even by some of those who would effectively merge international law and politics. McDougal et al. note that "[t]he procedures in the General Assembly are so crude and cumbersome that prescriptions may still be manipulated to serve special interests rather than common interests": McDougal et al., *World Public Order*, at 277.

For these reasons, the cause of human dignity is best served by the maintenance of a credible and recognizable distinction between the law and the politics of international human rights. This bifurcation does not take anything away from resort to the political process as one mechanism to promote respect for human dignity. It does, however, ensure that in at least some circumstances, a rule-based alternative can be invoked in support of human rights.

When, then, can a particular interest be said to be enforceable against all states as a matter of universal human rights law? First, some human rights may have the status of customary international law. The test is whether they can be located within a relatively constant and uniform interstate practice that has generated a sense of mutual obligation among states. There must be a coincidence of relevant *actions*, not simply official statements, sufficient to establish an agreement among states to be bound to a particular standard of conduct. Pronouncements in universal fora and elsewhere may help to establish that states view themselves as legally obligated to adhere to established patterns of conduct (*opinio juris*). There is, however, no substitute for that conduct.[59]

Second, some universal human rights may flow from general principles of law, meaning that they are pervasively recognized as binding norms across the domestic laws of states. The existence of a clear pattern of relevant domestic legislation, like practice and *opinio juris* in the case of custom, provides suitably clear evidence of the intention of states formally to be bound.

Third, universal human rights law might also be set by a treaty of genuinely universal reach. In this regard, particular attention should be paid to the Charter of the United Nations, thus far the only treaty that may establish human rights obligations that bind all members of the international community.[60]

---

[59] Thus, for example, the House of Lords declined to find a customary international right of conscientious objection to military service on the grounds that despite significant *opinio juris*, "evidence before the House does not disclose a uniformity of practice ... Of 180 states surveyed ..., some form of conscription was found to exist in 95. In 52 of those 95 states, the right of conscientious objection was found not to be recognized at all ... It could not, currently, be said that there is *de facto* observance of anything approaching a uniform rule": *Sepet and Bulbul v. Secretary of State for the Home Department*, [2003] UKHL 15 (UK HL, Mar. 20, 2003), at para. 18. The same conclusion had been reached by Laws LJ in the Court of Appeal, though he helpfully observed that "a universal practice need not be shown": *Sepet v. Secretary of State for the Home Department*, [2001] EWCA Civ 681 (Eng. CA, May 11, 2001), at para. 77.

[60] "In the event of a conflict between the obligations of the Members of the United Nations under the present Charter and their obligations under any other international agreement, their obligations under the present Charter shall prevail": UN Charter, at Art. 103. The Convention on the Rights of the Child, UNGA Res. 44/25, adopted Nov. 20, 1989, entered into force Sept. 2, 1990, enjoys comparably broad accession. Yet because of the relative power of one of the two states which are not parties – the United States of America – it is difficult to argue that this treaty can be treated as a source of universal obligation.

1.2.1 Human rights under customary international law

It must be acknowledged at the outset that the very nature of customary international law sits uncomfortably with the search for universal norms of human rights. Customary law exists to formalize interstate practice that has come to represent an agreed benchmark of acceptable relations between and among states. Custom has legitimacy as law only because interstate behavior is accepted by states as an ongoing medium of negotiation. It is clearly understood by governments that there is no customary law until there is both agreement on "terms" signaled by constant and relatively uniform interstate practice, and a sufficient expression of the willingness of states to be bound by that agreement. This structure is highly unlikely to produce universal human rights norms, as was observed by Lord Hoffmann in the House of Lords:

> I do not think it is possible to apply the rules for the development of rules of international law concerning the relations of states with each other (for example, as to how boundaries should be drawn) to the fundamental human rights of citizens against the state. There are unhappily many fundamental rights which would fail such a test of state practice, and the Refugee Convention is itself a recognition of this fact. In my opinion, a different approach is needed. Fundamental human rights are the minimum rights which a state ought to concede to its citizens. For the purpose of deciding what these minimum rights are, international instruments are important even if many states in practice disregard them ... [because they] show recognition that such rights ought to exist.[61]

The essential problem with reliance on custom is that human rights will only rarely be subject to the kind of interstate give and take that is the essence of customary lawmaking.[62] The requisite pattern of dealing may, for example, be observed in regard to the rights of aliens, where the mutual self-interest of states of nationality and the states in which aliens are located has produced observable patterns of affirmative protection and forbearance.[63] Relevant interaction between and among states regarding the rights of human beings generally, however, is rare.[64]

---

[61] *Sepet and Bulbul v. Secretary of State for the Home Department*, [2003] UKHL 15 (UK HL, Mar. 20, 2003), per Lord Hoffmann at para. 41.

[62] "The customary law of human rights is not established by a record of claims and counter-claims between the foreign ministries of countries concerned with the protection of their rights as states and the rights of their respective nationals": Meron, *Human Rights*, at 100.

[63] See chapter 2.1 below.

[64] International humanitarian law is another area where states have a comparatively clear self-interest in ensuring mutual respect for basic norms of human dignity during conflict. As such, it is not surprising that customary norms have also evolved in this field. Thus, the International Court of Justice has observed that the Regulations under the Fourth Hague

Schachter made a creative effort to overcome this problem by counting the willingness of states to condemn particular forms of human rights abuse as a relevant form of interstate dealing.[65] His argument is that consistent censure of invidious conduct is a sufficiently clear pattern of interaction to render the condemned conduct contrary to customary law. The problem with this approach, however, is that the activity consistently engaged in by states (study and condemnation) is not the subject of the putative customary norm (for example, freedom from arbitrary detention).[66] Because the basis of customary law formation is concrete performance or self-restraint *in regard to* the matter said to acquire binding force, the behavior relied upon by Schachter can at best reinforce as customary law the Charter-derived *droit de regard*.[67] But it is not authority for the existence of new substantive norms of universal human rights law.

A more compelling renovation of customary international lawmaking to accommodate the possibility of evolution in human rights law might be based on scrutiny of the actual human rights records of states. The treatment a state metes out to its own population has not usually been understood to be an ongoing process of negotiating acceptable international standards of conduct. It may, however, be possible to locate the required appreciation of legal significance in the Charter's good faith undertaking to act in support of human rights.[68] If this commitment is viewed as a sufficient "signal" to states of the potential legal relevance of their human rights conduct, the basis exists

Convention of 1907 "were prepared 'to revise the general laws and customs of war' existing at that time. Since then, however, the International Military Tribunal of Nuremberg has found that the 'rules laid down in the Convention were recognised by all civilised nations, and were regarded as being declaratory of the laws and customs of war' (Judgment of the International Military Tribunal of Nuremberg, 30 September and 1 October 1946, p. 65). The Court itself reached the same conclusion when examining the rights and duties of belligerents in their conduct of military operations (*Legality of the Threat or Use of Nuclear Weapons*, Advisory Opinion, ICJ Rep 1996 (I), p. 256, para. 75). The Court considers that the provisions of the Hague Regulations have become part of customary law": *Legal Consequences of the Construction of a Wall in the Occupied Palestinian Territory*, ICJ Gen. List No. 131, decided July 9, 2004, at para. 89.

[65] O. Schachter, *International Law in Theory and Practice* (1991) (Schachter, *International Law*), at 337–340.

[66] "The performance of most substantive human rights obligations ... lacks this element of interaction proper; it does not 'run between' States in any meaningful sense": Simma and Alston, "Sources of Human Rights Law," at 99.

[67] This duty of states to submit to scrutiny by the General Assembly and its specialized human rights bodies is discussed in chapter 1.2.3 below at pp. 46–47.

[68] State members "pledge themselves to take joint and separate action in cooperation with the Organization for the achievement of the purposes set forth in Article 55," which include "universal respect for, and observance of, human rights and fundamental freedoms for all without distinction as to race, sex, language, or religion": UN Charter, at Arts. 56 and 55(c).

to search for evidence of both constant and relatively uniform state practice and *opinio juris*.

Yet even application of this understanding of customary lawmaking could not justify the list of universally binding human rights commonly contended for. A composite list of the human rights argued by senior publicists to have acquired force as matters of customary law includes freedom from (1) systemic racial discrimination; (2) genocide; (3) slavery; (4) extrajudicial execution or enforced disappearance; (5) torture, cruel, inhuman, or degrading treatment; (6) prolonged arbitrary detention; and (7) serious unfairness in criminal prosecution.[69] Of these, only the first – freedom from systemic racial discrimination – appears to be a clear candidate for customary international legal status. While race-based discrimination remains prevalent in much of the world,[70] formally codified racial disfranchisement is now virtually unknown.[71] Coupled with the explicit and powerful *opinio juris* supplied by no less a source than the Charter of the United Nations,[72] systemic racial discrimination is sensibly understood to be a violation of customary international law.

---

[69] This list includes those rights identified as matters of customary international law by any of American Law Institute, *Restatement of the Law: The Foreign Relations Law of the United States* (1987); Brownlie, *Public International Law*; R. Jennings and A. Watts eds., *Oppenheim's International Law* (1992) (Jennings and Watts, *Oppenheim's*); Meron, *Human Rights*; Schachter, *International Law*; or P. Sieghart, *The Lawful Rights of Mankind* (1985) (Sieghart, *Rights of Mankind*).

[70] Indeed, the World Conference against Racism "recognize[d] and affirm[ed] that, at the outset of the third millennium, a global fight against racial discrimination, xenophobia and related tolerance and all their abhorrent and evolving forms and manifestations is a matter of priority for the international community": "Report of the World Conference against Racism, Racial Discrimination, Xenophobia and Related Intolerance," UN Doc. A/CONF.189/12 (2001), at para. 3.

[71] With the demise of the South African *apartheid* system, only relatively isolated cases of systemic racial discrimination remain. For example, the Roma are subject to a citizenship law in the Czech Republic that is conceived in a way that renders them de jure stateless; under Hungarian law, and throughout much of Central and Eastern Europe, the Roma are systemically denied many of the essential rights of citizenship: see e.g. A. Warnke, "Vagabonds, Tinkers, and Travelers: Statelessness Among the East European Roma," (1999) 7 *Indiana Journal of Global Legal Studies* 335, at 356, 359; and "Racism, Racial Discrimination, Xenophobia and All Forms of Discrimination," UN Doc. E/CN.4/2000/16, Feb. 10, 2000, at para. 35. Formal racial disfranchisement is also clear in Malaysia's "New Economic Policy," which – while its days may be numbered – still reserves the majority of government jobs and university places for indigenous Malays to the exclusion of the ethnic Chinese population: "The slaughter of sacred cows," 367 *The Economist* 10 (Apr. 5, 2003).

[72] "The Purposes of the United Nations are ... [t]o achieve international cooperation in solving international problems ... and in promoting and encouraging respect for human rights and for fundamental freedoms for all without distinction as to race, sex, language, or religion": UN Charter, at Art. 1(3). See chapter 1.2.3 below, at p. 44.

In contrast, however, the need to identify relatively constant state practice defeats the assertion of customary international legal status in relation to the balance of the asserted interests. While perhaps a close case,[73] even the assertion of a right to freedom from genocide is difficult to reconcile to a raft of contemporary genocides, including those in Afghanistan,[74] Bangladesh,[75] Bosnia,[76] Burundi,[77] Cambodia,[78] East Timor,[79] Guatemala,[80] Iraq,[81] Rwanda,[82] and Sudan.[83] Indeed, the pervasiveness of this phenomenon has led Kushner and Knox to characterize the present era as "an age of genocide."[84] State practice is moreover consistent, at best, with an extremely

---

[73] Most authoritatively, the International Court of Justice has suggested that freedom from genocide is a universal legal norm. "The origins of the [Genocide] Convention show that it was the intention of the United Nations to condemn and punish genocide as a 'crime under international law' involving a denial of the right of existence of entire human groups, a denial which shocks the conscience of mankind and results in great losses to humanity, and which is contrary to moral law and the spirit and aims of the United Nations ... The first consequence arising from this conception is that the principles underlying the [Genocide] Convention are principles which are recognized by civilized nations as binding on States, even without any conventional obligation": *Reservations to the Convention on the Prevention and Punishment of the Crime of Genocide*, [1951] ICJ Rep. 15, at 23.

[74] D. Bronkhoerst ed., "Genocide: Not a Natural Disaster: A Report on the National Conference on Genocide, Rotterdam, The Netherlands, 10 October 1997," Centre for Conflict Research, Amsterdam (1997).

[75] A. Jongman ed., *Contemporary Genocides: Causes, Cases, Consequences* (1996) (Jongman, *Contemporary Genocides*); P. Chakma, "The Genocide in the Chittagong Hill Tracts," (1989) 5(3) *Seeds of Peace* 4, at 4–6; A. McGregor, "Genocide in Chittagong Hill Tracts," (1991) 2 *On the Record* 11.

[76] G. Andreopoulos, *Genocide: Conceptual and Historical Dimensions* (1994) (Andreopoulos, *Genocide*).

[77] C. Sherrer, *Genocide and Crisis in Central Africa: Conflict Roots, Mass Violence and Regional War* (2002) (Sherrer, *Genocide and Crisis*); C. Jennings, *Across the Red River: Rwanda, Burundi and the Heart of Darkness* (2000) (Jennings, *Red River*); R. Lemarchand, *Burundi: Ethnic Conflict and Genocide* (1995).

[78] Jongman, *Contemporary Genocides*; Andreopoulos, *Genocide*.

[79] Andreopoulos, *Genocide*.

[80] "Genocide and Mass Murder in Guatemala, 1960–1996," (1999) 23 *ISG Newsletter* 9, at 9–12, 17.

[81] Jongman, *Contemporary Genocides*; Andreopoulos, *Genocide*.

[82] Sherrer, *Genocide and Crisis*; Jennings, *Red River*; Andreopoulos, *Genocide*.

[83] H. Fein, "Genocide by Attrition in Sudan and Elsewhere," (2002) 29 *ISG Newsletter* 7, at 7–9; R. Omaar and A. De Waal, *Facing Genocide: The Nuba of Sudan* (1995); M. Salih, D. Guha-Sapir, and T. Cannon, "Resistance and Response: Ethnocide and Genocide in the Nuba Mountains, Sudan," (1995) 36(1) *GeoJournal* 71, at 71–78.

[84] T. Kushner and K. Knox, *Refugees in an Age of Genocide: Global, National and Local Perspectives During the Twentieth Century* (1999). See also R. Falk, "The Challenge of Genocide and Genocidal Politics in an Era of Globalization," in T. Dunne and N. Wheeler eds., *Human Rights in Global Politics* (1999), at 177. A more general global, historical overview of genocide is provided in I. Charney, *Encyclopedia of Genocide* (1999).

narrowly defined right to be free from slavery;[85] a broader view suggests that there are not less than 27 million, and perhaps as many as 200 million, slaves in the world today.[86] Non-conforming state practice is also a serious impediment to recognition of the last four of the proposed list of seven putative customary human rights. In 2002 alone, there were credible reports of extrajudicial execution and of enforced disappearance in thirty-three countries; of torture, cruel, inhuman, or degrading treatment in one hundred and six states; of prolonged arbitrary detention in fifty-four countries; and of major unfairness in criminal prosecution in thirty-five states.[87] The generality and pervasiveness of abusive

[85] "The cumulative evidence contained in this report substantiates *prima facie* that, although chattel-slavery in the former traditional sense no longer persists in any significant degree, the prevalence of several forms of slavery-like practice continues unabated": B. Whitaker, "Slavery: Report prepared by the Special Rapporteur of the Sub-Commission on Prevention of Discrimination and Protection of Minorities," UN Doc. E/CN.4/Sub.2/ 1982/20/Rev.1, at 37. More than a decade later, however, continuing instances of chattel-slavery were documented in Brazil, Mauritania, Sudan, and Thailand: Anti-Slavery International, Factsheets D (1994), E (1994), and G (1994). See also B. Lance, *Of Human Bondage: An Investigation into Slavery in Present-Day Sudan* (1999) and R. Funari, "Brazil – Slaves to Misery," (April 2002) *Anti-Slavery Reporter* 8, at 8–9.

[86] "My best estimate of the number of slaves in the world today is 27 million. This number is much smaller than the estimates put forward by some activists, who give a range as high as 200 million, but it is the number I feel I can trust [based on a 'strict definition of slavery']": K. Bales, *Disposable People: New Slavery in the Global Economy* (2000), at 8–9. The higher number of as many as 200 million slaves includes persons subject to chattel-slavery, serfdom, debt bondage, servile forms of marriage, and exploitation as children: Anti-Slavery International, Factsheet G (1994). A broad definition of slavery is consistent with the approach of the Supplementary Convention on the Abolition of Slavery, the Slave Trade, and Institutions and Practices Similar to Slavery, 266 UNTS 3, done Sept. 7, 1956, entered into force Apr. 30, 1957. This broader understanding adds significantly to the complexity of calculating the actual number of slaves in the world. For example, the UN Working Group on Contemporary Forms of Slavery has appealed to "Governments concerned [to] carry out independent and comprehensive surveys, at the local level, to identify the number and location of people held in debt bondage": "Report of the Working Group on Contemporary Forms of Slavery on its Twenty-Sixth Session," UN Doc. E/ CN.4/Sub.2/2001/30, July 16, 2001.

[87] These statistics are based on Amnesty International, *Report 2003* (2003). The geographical breakdowns are as follows. Extrajudicial execution: seventeen (Africa), nine (Americas), two (Europe and Central Asia), five (Middle East and North Africa). Enforced disappearance: five (Africa), twelve (Americas), four (Asia Pacific), six (Europe and Central Asia), six (Middle East and North Africa). Torture, cruel, inhuman or degrading treatment: twenty-one (Africa), twenty (Americas), twenty (Asia Pacific), twenty-seven (Europe and Central Asia), eighteen (Middle East and North Africa). Detention without charge or trial: seventeen (Africa), seven (Americas), fourteen (Asia Pacific), four (Europe and Central Asia), twelve (Middle East and North Africa). Major unfairness in criminal prosecution includes reports of prisoners of conscience: six (Africa), two (Americas), eight (Asia Pacific), six (Europe and Central Asia), thirteen (Middle East and North Africa).

state behavior in regard to even these core interests therefore contradict any assertion of customary legal protection.

1.2.2 Human rights derived from general principles of law

An alternative approach more in keeping with the structure of international law may therefore be to search for universal human rights within the general principles of law. As argued by Simma and Alston, "the concept of a 'recognized' general principle seems to conform more closely than the concept of custom to the situation where a norm invested with strong inherent authority is widely accepted though widely violated."[88] In keeping with accepted modes of international lawmaking, the relevant test of a general principle of law is whether the proposed universal standard has been pervasively recognized in the domestic laws of states.[89] If the only evidence of "acceptance" consists of declarations and other non-binding statements at the domestic or international level, there is an insufficient basis upon which to assert the norm as binding on states. Formalization in domestic law, like constant and relatively uniform interstate practice coupled with *opinio juris*, affords concrete evidence of intention to be bound.

Perhaps because commentators usually appeal to customary international law to justify the proclamation of new universal human rights, there are no official surveys that conclusively document the extent to which human rights have been codified in the laws of states. In several important cases, this information gap could be closed by synthesis of existing country-specific data on compliance with international human rights undertakings. Because some human rights treaties explicitly require state parties both to enact domestic legislation to protect one or more human rights and to report their efforts to an international supervisory body, the information base already exists to seek out new universal human rights norms rooted in the general principles of law.

For example, states adhering to the Genocide Convention agree to enact legislation to punish all acts intended to destroy, in whole or in part, a

---

[88] Simma and Alston, "Sources of Human Rights Law," at 102.

[89] It is, of course, difficult to provide a precise quantification of the degree of support required. An indication of the strength of support that should exist before amendment of truly fundamental principles comes into force is, however, provided by the Statute of the International Criminal Court, UN Doc. A/CONF.183/9, done July 17, 1998, entered into force July 1, 2002. Art. 121 of that treaty provides that while amendments to it may be adopted by a two-thirds majority of state parties, an amendment will come into force only once seven-eighths of state parties have accepted or ratified the amendment. If that figure were extrapolated to the broader context, a general principle of law should be located in the domestic laws of some 168 countries.

national, ethnic, racial or religious group.[90] State parties to the International Covenant on Civil and Political Rights undertake to protect by domestic law the right of every human being not to be arbitrarily deprived of life.[91] The Convention against Torture requires effective legislative measures to prevent acts of torture.[92] The Slavery Convention, Supplementary Convention on the Abolition of Slavery, International Covenant on Civil and Political Rights, and the Convention on the Elimination of All Forms of Discrimination against Women all require states to enact a formal prohibition on slavery and the slave trade in all their forms.[93] The International Covenant on Civil and Political Rights, the Convention on the Elimination of All Forms of Discrimination against Women, and the International Convention on the Elimination of All Forms of Racial Discrimination go beyond the Charter's prohibition in principle of systemic discrimination to require legislation

---

[90] Convention on the Prevention and Punishment of the Crime of Genocide, UNGA Res. 260A(III), adopted Dec. 9. 1948, entered into force Jan. 12, 1951 (Genocide Convention), at Art. V. In contrast to the other instruments discussed here, there is no periodic reporting requirement under the Genocide Convention which facilitates evaluation of compliance with this obligation. An effort in the 1980s by the Sub-Commission on Human Rights to survey relevant domestic legislation yielded only twenty-three responses: B. Whitaker, "Revised and Updated Report on the Question of the Prevention and Punishment of the Crime of Genocide," UN Doc. E/CN.4/Sub.2/1985/6. Official verification of pervasive compliance with this duty to legislate is therefore presently lacking, though a recent study notes that "[a] large number of States have enacted legislation concerning the prosecution and repression of genocide, most by amending their penal or criminal codes in order to add a distinct offence": W. Schabas, *Genocide in International Law: The Crime of Crimes* (2002), at 4–5. Yet the same author urges caution in assessing the practical effect of the Genocide Convention. "Fifty years after its adoption, [the Genocide Convention] has fewer than 130 State parties, a rather unimpressive statistic when compared with the other major human rights treaties of the United Nations system which, while considerably younger, have managed to approach a more general degree of support by the nations of the world. The reason is not the existence of doubt about the universal condemnation of genocide, but unease among some States with the onerous obligations that the treaty imposes, such as prosecution or extradition of individuals, including heads of State": ibid. at 3.

[91] International Covenant on Civil and Political Rights, UNGA Res. 2200A(XXI), adopted Dec. 16, 1966, entered into force Mar. 23, 1976 (Civil and Political Covenant), at Art. 6(1).

[92] Convention against Torture and Other Cruel, Inhuman or Degrading Treatment or Punishment, UNGA Res. 39/46, adopted Dec. 10, 1984, entered into force June 26, 1987 (Torture Convention), at Arts. 2(1) and 4.

[93] Slavery Convention, 60 LNTS 253, done Sept. 25, 1926, entered into force Mar. 9, 1927, at Art. 6, as amended by Slavery Protocol, 212 UNTS 17, done Oct. 23, 1953, entered into force July 7, 1955; Supplementary Convention on the Abolition of Slavery, the Slave Trade, and Institutions and Practices Similar to Slavery, 226 UNTS 3, done Sept. 7, 1956, entered into force April 30, 1957, at Arts. 1, 5, 6, and 8(2); Civil and Political Covenant, at Art. 8(1); and Convention on the Elimination of All Forms of Discrimination against Women, UNGA Res. 34/180, adopted Dec. 18, 1979, entered into force Sept. 3, 1981 (Discrimination Against Women Convention), at Art. 6.

variously to end all forms of generalized discrimination, outlaw hate propaganda, and establish affirmative protections against discrimination.[94] Where states have reported their various laws to fulfil legislative responsibilities under these treaties, it may therefore be possible to define a general principle of law to coincide with the seminal treaty norm.

[In view of the large number of states that have formally undertaken to legislate regarding these five human rights, they seem particularly ripe for scrutiny under the rules of general principles lawmaking. There are some indications that positive results are likely. The United Nations Center for Human Rights has, for example, already declared that "[a]s a legally permitted labour system, traditional slavery has been abolished everywhere."[95] Similarly, a study issued by the Institut Henri Dunant affirmed that "[a]lmost every State has some form of legislation prohibiting detention officials, or any individual, from torturing or treating a detainee inhumanly,"[96] and that even the "few states [which] do not have specific legislative protection against torture ... have alternative protections against action such as ill treatment."[97] If fortified by careful and probing analysis of domestic legislative records, reliance on general principles of law therefore offers the possibility of expanding universal human rights law in a manner consonant with the accepted formalities of international lawmaking. To date, however, this critical groundwork remains largely undone. Much less are there legally authoritative declarations of the status of particular human rights as general principles of law.

1.2.3 Human rights set by the United Nations Charter

Because of the real challenges of asserting international human rights law grounded in either custom or general principles, the most compelling basis upon which to posit the existence of a universal law of human rights is sometimes located in the Charter of the United Nations. That accord sets unambiguous human rights obligations only for states that exercise

---

[94] Civil and Political Covenant, at Arts. 20(2) and 26; Discrimination Against Women Convention, at Art. 2(b), (c), (f), and (g); and International Convention on the Elimination of All Forms of Racial Discrimination, UNGA Res. 2106A(XX), adopted Dec. 21, 1965, entered into force Jan. 4, 1969 (Racial Discrimination Convention), at Arts. 2(1)(d) and 4(a), (b).

[95] United Nations Center for Human Rights, "Fact Sheet No. 14: Contemporary Forms of Slavery" (1991), at 4, available at www.unhchr.ch (accessed Nov. 19, 2004).

[96] P. Williams, "Treatment of Detainees: Examination of Issues Relevant to Detention by the United Nations Human Rights Committee" (1990) (Williams, "Treatment of Detainees"), at 31. The extent of state compliance with the duty to avoid torture or inhuman treatment while in detention has recently been surveyed in the context of persons seeking refugee status: Lawyers' Committee for Human Rights, "Review of States' Procedures and Practices Relating to Detention of Asylum-Seekers" (2002).

[97] Williams, "Treatment of Detainees," at 31.

trusteeship authority on behalf of the United Nations.[98] The source of a more general duty to respect human rights, in contrast, is usually located in the ambiguous pledge made by states in Arts. 55 and 56 to "take joint and separate action in cooperation with the Organization" in furtherance of human rights and fundamental freedoms.[99] It is not self-evident, however, that this "pledge" of cooperative action imports an agreement to be held accountable in law for breaches of human rights.[100] Indeed, there is force in Jennings' view that the most that can be derived from these articles is a good faith obligation to act in support of the Charter.[101] The language of Arts. 55 and 56 is too

---

[98] UN Charter, at Arts. 75–85. This view was affirmed by the International Court of Justice in its advisory opinion on *Legal Consequences for States of the Continued Presence of South Africa in Namibia*, [1971] ICJ Rep 6, at para. 131: "Under the Charter of the United Nations, the former Mandatory had pledged itself to observe and respect, in a territory having an international status, human rights and fundamental freedoms for all without distinction as to race. To establish instead, and to enforce, distinctions, exclusions and limitations exclusively based on grounds of race, color, descent or national or ethnic origin which constitute a denial of fundamental rights is a flagrant violation of the purposes and principles of the Charter."

[99] An *obiter* reference in *United States Diplomatic and Consular Staff in Teheran*, [1980] ICJ Rep 3, at para. 91 affords indirect support for viewing the Charter as a binding source of human rights obligations. In contrast, in the decision in *Military and Paramilitary Activities in and Against Nicaragua*, [1986] ICJ Rep 14, at para. 261, the Court suggests that a good faith undertaking to observe human rights should be regarded as a form of political, rather than legal, obligation.

[100] The drafting history of Arts. 55 and 56 also provides reason to doubt the intention for the Charter to give rise to general human rights obligations. "It is interesting to observe that the text of what is now article 56 originally suggested a pledge 'to take separate and joint action and to co-operate with the Organization.' This clearly suggested 'separate action' by members of the organization regardless of whether or not other members took any action. The USA found this formula unacceptable; other drafts were unacceptable to other delegations and, accordingly, the present text emerged. From the drafting history one may deduce that no obligation to take action exists unless it is in co-operation with the Organization": P. Gandhi, "The Universal Declaration of Human Rights at Fifty Years: Its Origins, Significance and Impact," (1998) 41 *German Yearbook of International Law* 206 (Gandhi, "Universal Declaration"), at 225.

[101] "There is no provision in the Charter laying down *expressis verbis* that there is a legal obligation resting upon nations to observe human rights and fundamental freedoms. However, in basic constitutional instruments such as the Charter, there is less room for reasoning that although one of the objects of the United Nations is to promote respect for human rights and fundamental freedoms, its members are not under a duty to respect and observe them; or that the pledge – the undertaking – of Art. 56 can, as a matter of good faith, have any other meaning. The members of the United Nations are under *at least a moral – and, however imperfect, a legal –* duty to use their *best efforts*, either by agreement or, whenever possible, by enlightened actions of their own judicial and other authorities, to act in support of a crucial purpose of the Charter. Nevertheless, the provisions of the Charter on the subject do not themselves signify a full and effective guarantee of human rights on the part of international society [emphasis added]": Jennings and Watts, *Oppenheim's*, at 989.

hortatory and vague to create a legal duty to adhere to a comprehensive human rights regime.

Indeed, the text of Arts. 55 and 56 would sustain the argument that whatever enforceable human rights pledge is made is strictly context-specific. The language of Arts. 55 and 56 *requires* states to honor their human rights pledge only if failure to do so might jeopardize conditions of stability and well-being between or among nations. This is because the binding commitment of states in Art. 56 is simply to take action "for the achievement of the *purposes* set forth in Article 55 [emphasis added]." Art. 55, in turn, posits human rights as one of three initiatives that should be promoted by the United Nations to realize the objective of creating "conditions of stability and well-being that are necessary for peaceful and friendly relations among nations based on respect for the equal rights and self-determination of peoples." The *purposes* of Art. 55, which Art. 56 binds states to promote, are therefore pursuit of stability and well-being among nations. Respect for human rights is an instrumentality through which the United Nations is to advance this objective, but it is not in itself a purpose of Art. 55. From this perspective, states have not committed themselves to an all-embracing human rights undertaking, but are duty-bound to respect human rights only if non-compliance would adversely affect interstate relations. This interpretation establishes reciprocity of rights and enforceability, since the Security Council is empowered to demand the compliance of states only as far as necessary "for the maintenance of international peace and security."

On this reading of the Charter, it is unclear whether there could be any such thing as an authoritative interpretation of the human rights commitment made by states in the United Nations Charter. This is because the obligations of states and the reciprocal power of the Security Council do not presume any need to define human rights. States are accountable not for failure to adhere to human rights *per se*, but for actions that are disruptive of peaceful and friendly relations among nations. It is immaterial whether the cause of the disruption is or is not a breach of human rights. Similarly, the Security Council is not restricted to intervention simply when particular norms are at risk: its authority, like the obligations of states, is defined solely by an evaluation of risk to international peace and security. In sum, because the structure of the Charter presents no need to distinguish human rights from other interests, it cannot logically be argued that its effectuation requires the reading-in of externally defined human rights norms.

The importation of a broad range of human rights standards into the Charter is difficult to justify even if one were to adopt the more liberal view of Arts. 55 and 56 as creating a legally binding duty to promote human rights in good faith. Incorporation by reference of such standards is usually justified on the grounds that because the Charter does not contain an endogenous definition of the duty to respect "human rights and fundamental freedoms," core standards subsequently adopted by the United Nations should acquire universal force as authoritative interpretations of the Charter-based obligations.[102] Yet the question arises whether there really is a substantive gap of the kind that would warrant incorporation by reference of much of the *corpus* of international human rights law.

Specifically, the Charter's commitment to non-discrimination on the grounds of race, sex, language, or religion is explicit.[103] One might moreover assume United Nations competence to address any human rights that have attained universal stature by operation of custom or general principles,[104] and most certainly any rights within the *erga omnes* sphere.[105] Given these definitive points of reference, there is no basis to assert that the pledge of states would be rendered meaningless absent the importation of human rights standards from various declarations and treaties. That is, there is nothing patently unreasonable in the suggestion that whatever human rights obligations are assumed by states under the Charter are of relatively narrow scope.

Moreover, the idea of invoking the Charter to give indirect universal legal force to either the Universal Declaration of Human Rights, or to the two

---

[102] See e.g. L. Sohn, "The Human Rights Law of the Charter," (1977) 12 *Texas International Law Journal* 129, at 133. The authorities for and against this proposition are canvassed in Gandhi, "Universal Declaration," at 228–234.

[103] "The Purposes of the United Nations are: ... (3) To achieve international co-operation ... in promoting and encouraging respect for human rights and for fundamental freedoms for all without distinction as to race, sex, language, or religion": UN Charter, at Art. 1(3). See chapter 1.2.1 above at p. 36.

[104] In *Military and Paramilitary Activities in and Against Nicaragua*, [1986] ICJ Rep 14, at para. 267, the International Court of Justice confirmed the legitimacy of scrutiny of human rights norms which exist independently of treaty: "The Court also notes that Nicaragua is accused by the 1985 finding of the United States Congress of violating human rights. This particular point requires to be studied independently of the question of the existence of a 'legal commitment' by Nicaragua towards the Organization of American States to respect these rights; *the absence of such a commitment would not mean that Nicaragua could with impunity violate human rights* [emphasis added]."

[105] "An essential distinction should be drawn between the obligations of a state towards the international community as a whole, and those arising vis à vis another state in the field of diplomatic protection. By their very nature, the former are the concerns of all states. In view of the importance of the rights involved, all states can be held to have a legal interest in their protection; they are obligations *erga omnes*. Such obligations derive ... from the outlawing of acts of aggression, and of genocide, and also from the principles and rules concerning the basic rights of the human person, including protection from slavery and racial discrimination. Some of the corresponding rights of protection have entered into the body of general international law ...; others are conferred by international instruments of a universal or quasi-universal character": *Barcelona Traction, Light and Power Company Limited (Belgium v. Spain)*, [1970] ICJ Rep 3. The notion of a norm *erga omnes* reflects the view that "international law does not only govern the reciprocal relations between states, but also involves considerations going beyond the mere sum of their individual interests": Ragazzi, *Erga Omnes*, at 218.

Human Rights Covenants, is cause for concern.[106] The Declaration was passed as a non-binding resolution of the General Assembly.[107] It was the clear intention of states that the Declaration serve as a foundational statement of principle, with legal obligations to follow from accession to what became the two Covenants.[108] Moreover, despite the clear evidence of respect generated since 1948 for the principles enshrined in the Declaration, the International Court of Justice has not yet found the Universal Declaration of Human Rights to be a source of binding obligations. In the *Nicaragua* case, for example, the Court could not "find an instrument with legal force, whether unilateral or synallagmatic, whereby Nicaragua has committed itself in respect of the principle or methods of holding elections."[109] More

[106] Justice Callinan of the High Court of Australia, for example, has observed that "the Universal Declaration of Human Rights ... [is] still in many respects an aspirational rather than an effective and enforceable instrument": *S157/2002 v. Commonwealth of Australia*, [2003] HCA 2 (Aus. HC, Feb. 4, 2003), per Callinan J. at para. 116. But see e.g. R. Higgins, *The Development of International Law Through the Political Organs of the United Nations* (1963).

[107] "The language of the Universal Declaration, the circumstances and the reasons of its adoption, and, above all, the clearly and emphatically expressed intention of the States, Members of the United Nations, who voted for the Resolution of the General Assembly, show clearly that the Declaration is not by its nature and by the intention of its parties a legal document imposing legal obligations": H. Lauterpacht, *International Law and Human Rights* (1950), at 408. Thus, "[t]he [Universal] Declaration has been of considerable value as supplying a standard of action and of moral obligation. It has been frequently referred to in official drafts and pronouncements, in national constitutions and legislation, and occasionally – with differing results – in judicial decisions. These consequences of the Declaration may be of significance so long as restraint is exercised in describing it as a legally binding instrument": Jennings and Watts, *Oppenheim's*, at 1002–1004.

[108] See Gandhi, "Universal Declaration," at 239: "The reason why the Declaration was adopted so speedily may ... be put down to the fact that most governments present at the Paris session of the General Assembly clearly believed they were not adhering to a document imposing legally binding norms. The General Assembly had already instructed the Human Rights Commission to prepare a convention (or two Covenants as they later emerged) covering the same rights: such an operation would have been completely otiose if it had been intended that the terms of the [Universal Declaration of Human Rights] should be legally binding."

[109] *Military and Paramilitary Activities in and Against Nicaragua*, [1986] ICJ Rep 14, at para. 261. In contrast, Art. 21(3) of the Universal Declaration of Human Rights provides that "[t]he will of the people shall be the basis of the authority of government; this will shall be expressed in periodic and genuine elections which shall be by universal and equal suffrage and shall be held by secret vote or by equivalent free voting procedures": UNGA Res. 217A(III), Dec. 10, 1948 (Universal Declaration). In a similar vein, the International Court of Justice declined to recognize the *erga omnes* character of the right to protection against denial of justice even though Arts. 7–11 of the Universal Declaration of Human Rights speak to this issue: *Barcelona Traction, Light and Power Company Limited (Belgium v. Spain)*, [1970] ICJ Rep 3, at para. 91.

generally, the Court has (appropriately) "rhetorically relied on the [Universal] Declaration as a touchstone of legality,"[110] but has otherwise insisted that there is no basis in law to equate a "political pledge" made in a non-binding accord to a legal obligation to respect human rights.[111] The alternative of effectively reading-in the content of the Human Rights Covenants (or other treaties) is even more problematic, since that approach amounts to giving universal force to treaties open to particularized accession, and agreed to in fact by substantially less than the whole of the international community. If the Human Rights Covenants were intended to function as universally applicable definitions of universally binding, Charter-based human rights undertakings, why would formal accession by states be made purely optional?

While not a source of legally binding obligations, a more expansive human rights jurisdiction resides with the General Assembly and the specialized human rights organs established under its authority.[112] Art. 13 of the Charter empowers the General Assembly to initiate studies and make recommendations for the purpose of "assisting in the realization of human rights and fundamental freedoms for all without distinction as to race, sex, language, or religion." Art. 10 authorizes discussion in the General Assembly of any such questions. Ultimately, however, these powers are in the nature of a *droit de regard*: the General Assembly and its subordinate bodies may scrutinize and discuss human rights, they may even recommend that states bring pressure to bear on non-compliant governments, but they have no right to require conformity

---

[110] Schachter, *International Law*, at 337. Of particular relevance is the *obiter dictum* that "[w]rongfully to deprive human beings of their freedom and to subject them to physical constraint in conditions of hardship is in itself manifestly incompatible with the *principles* of the Charter of the United Nations, as well as with the *principles* enunciated in the Universal Declaration of Human Rights [emphasis added]": *United States Diplomatic and Consular Staff in Teheran*, [1980] ICJ Rep 3, at para. 91. The fact that the breach of "principles" of both the Charter and the Universal Declaration is not characterized as a breach of *law* is noteworthy.

[111] "The Organization of American States Charter has already been mentioned, with its respect for the political independence of member States; in the field of domestic policy, it goes no further than to list the social standards to the application of which the Members 'agree to dedicate every effort' ... It is evident that provisions of this kind are far from being a commitment to the use of particular political mechanisms": *Military and Paramilitary Activities in and Against Nicaragua*, [1986] ICJ Rep 14, at para. 261. A dissenting opinion of Judge Tanaka, however, takes the opposite view. "[T]he Universal Declaration of Human Rights adopted by the General Assembly in 1948, although not binding itself, constitutes evidence of the interpretation and application of the relevant Charter provisions": *South West Africa Case (Ethiopia v. South Africa; Liberia v. South Africa), Second Phase*, [1966] ICJ Rep 6, at 293 (Dissenting Opinion of Judge Tanaka).

[112] These include the Commission and Sub-Commission on Human Rights, the Commission on the Status of Women, and the High Commissioner for Human Rights. See generally H. Steiner and P. Alston, *International Human Rights in Context* (2000) (Steiner and Alston, *International Human Rights*), at 597–602.

with any standards.[113] It is in this political sense that a broad range of international human rights have standing *erga omnes*:[114] states must submit to scrutiny by the General Assembly and specialized human rights bodies, since human rights are legitimately matters of concern to all.[115] There is, however, no reason to equate this *droit de regard* with a legally binding obligation of states to comply with human rights norms that have neither attained status as universally binding norms, nor been specifically adhered to.[116]

Taken together, the dispositions of the Charter establish only a skeletal legal regime to enforce universal human rights. There are situation-specific duties to respect human rights that flow from fiduciary duties assumed by trustee states under Chapter XII, and consequential human rights duties set by the Security Council under its Chapter VII peace and security jurisdiction. In the absence of accession to more specific treaties, however, a more broadly based duty to respect human rights is in essence a function simply of a given state's vulnerability to whatever particular forms of international political pressure may be generated by the General Assembly and its subsidiary bodies.

In sum, and despite its intuitive appeal, there is little reason to believe that the human dignity of refugees can be adequately safeguarded simply by reliance on universally applicable norms of human rights law. Customary

[113] "[I]t is the Security Council which, exclusively, may order coercive action ... The word 'action' must mean such action as is solely within the province of the Security Council. It cannot refer to recommendations which the Security Council might make ... because the General Assembly under Article 11 has a comparable power": *Certain Expenses of the United Nations*, [1962] ICJ Rep 151, at 163–165.

[114] As Ragazzi concludes in his comprehensive study of the subject of obligations *erga omnes*, the legal notion is more carefully constrained to include only a narrowly defined set of norms which set prohibitive duties, which bespeak basic instrumental principles, and which have already met the *jus cogens* standard: Ragazzi, *Erga Omnes*, at 215. But see J.-A. Carillo Salcedo, "Book Review: The Concept of International Obligations *Erga Omnes*," (1998) 92(4) *American Journal of International Law* 791, arguing for the effective merger of the legal and more broad-ranging notions of a norm *erga omnes*.

[115] "[T]he most interesting feature of this development is that the growing acceptance of the *erga omnes* character of human rights has not been limited to the basic rights of the human person only ... [T]he UN Assistant Secretary-General for Human Rights ... has emphasized that one of the accomplishments of the United Nations has been to consolidate the principle that human rights are a matter of international concern *that the international community is entitled to discuss* [emphasis added]": Meron, *Human Rights*, at 187–189.

[116] While the Court in *Barcelona Traction* affirmed that all states have a legal interest in the protection of "basic rights of the human person" (para. 34), it equally clearly denied that all rights affirmed in the Universal Declaration of Human Rights give rise to *erga omnes* enforceability. The right to protection against denial of justice (stipulated in Universal Declaration Arts. 7–11), for example, does "not confer on States the capacity to protect the victims of infringements of such rights irrespective of their nationality" (para. 91): *Barcelona Traction, Light and Power Company Limited (Belgium v. Spain)*, [1970] ICJ Rep 3, at paras. 34, 91.

international law likely protects refugees from systemic racial discrimination, as well as from subjection to genocide or the most basic forms of slavery. General principles of law likely confirm these rights, and establish in addition the right to be protected from arbitrary deprivation of life, torture, and a broader range of discriminatory practices. The UN Charter, even if viewed as a general source of human rights, adds little if anything to this list. In short, without reference to treaty-based human rights law, and most specifically to the Refugee Convention and the Covenants on Human Rights, refugees would be entitled to no more than a bare minimum of rights.

1.3 An interactive approach to treaty interpretation

Even as much of the international law academy has embraced an extraordinarily expansionist understanding of both custom and general principles of law, there has been a failure adequately to develop the potential for treaty law to play a genuinely transformative role in the international system. The better place for liberality is not in defining what amounts to law – where state resistance can both be expected, and be dispositive in practical terms – but rather in the elaboration of the approach to be taken by courts and tribunals in the interpretation of rules of undisputed authority. Without doubt, the rules of treaty interpretation formally embraced by states afford significant room to secure many of the gains presumably of interest to those who posit expansionist theories of the sources of universally applicable law. And because the process of treaty interpretation operates in more formal and rule-oriented settings, it is better positioned to generate dependable and rights-regarding results.

To this end, the discussion here seeks to explain how the Vienna Convention's codification of the rules of treaty interpretation[117] should be applied in the context of human rights treaties generally, and in relation to the Refugee

---

[117] The Vienna Convention approach has been recognized by the International Court of Justice as embodying customary norms of treaty interpretation: *Kasikili/Seduda Island (Botswana v. Namibia), Preliminary Objections*, [1996] ICJ Rep 803, at 812; *Territorial Dispute (Libyan Arab Jamahiriya v. Chad)*, [1994] ICJ Rep 6, at 21; *Arbitral Award of 31 July 1989 (Guinea-Bissau v. Senegal)*, [1991] ICJ Rep 53, at 69. Thus, for example, "[t]he WTO Panels and the Appellate Body rely on the treaty interpretation rules expressed in the Vienna Convention on the Law of Treaties as the basic rules for interpreting WTO instruments. This is because those rules are generally regarded as a codification of the public international law rules of treaty interpretation as a matter of general (or customary) international law": M. Lennard, "Navigating by the Stars: Interpreting the WTO Agreements," (2002) 5 *Journal of International Economic Law* 17 (Lennard, "Navigating by the Stars"), at 17–18. See also I. Sinclair, *The Vienna Convention and the Law of Treaties* (1984) (Sinclair, *Vienna Convention*), at 153: "There is no doubt that Articles 31 to 33 of the [Vienna] Convention constitute a general expression of the principles of customary international law relating to treaty interpretation."

Convention and Protocol in particular. There has for too long been an anachronistic fixation with literalism, with insufficient attention paid to the duty to read text in line with the context, object, and purpose of a treaty. It is suggested here that this approach misreads the authentic rules of treaty interpretation, and bespeaks a lack of creativity within the bounds expressly sanctioned by states.

While not seeking to promote a wholly teleological approach to treaty interpretation, the view advanced here is that account must be more rigorously taken of the clear duty to read the text of treaties in consonance with their fundamental purposes. To this end, courts charged with interpretation of the Refugee Convention have increasingly recognized that particular assistance is likely to be gleaned from the drafting history (largely as recorded in the *travaux préparatoires*) and by seeking to locate refugee law principles within the broader complex of general human rights obligations.

1.3.1 The perils of "ordinary meaning"

The well-known general rule of treaty interpretation, codified in Art. 31(1) of the Vienna Convention, is that "[a] treaty shall be interpreted in good faith in accordance with the ordinary meaning to be given to the terms of the treaty in their context and in the light of its object and purpose."[118] Paragraph 2 of Art. 31 defines the "context" relevant to treaty interpretation; paragraph 3 requires that this understanding of a treaty's "context" be supplemented by interpretive agreements between the parties, subsequent practice in application of the treaty, and relevant rules of international law; and paragraph 4 validates special meanings intended to be given to treaty terms by the parties.[119] As emphasized by the International Law Commission, which drafted the provision,[120] this rather complex formulation was adopted in order

> to indicate that the application of the means of interpretation in the article would be a single combined operation. All the various elements, as they were present in any given case, would be thrown into the crucible, and their interaction would give the legally relevant interpretation. Thus [Art. 31] is entitled "General *rule* of interpretation" in the singular, not "General *rules*" in the plural, because the Commission desired to emphasize that the

---

[118] Vienna Convention, at Art. 31(1).

[119] "Article 31(4) . . . was nearly deleted by the International Law Commission in a late draft of what became the Vienna Convention, on the basis that the so-called 'special' meaning would in any case be the 'ordinary' meaning in the particular context, in terms of the Article 31(1) rules. The reference to a special meaning does not seem to add much to the other provisions, probably only emphasizing the burden of proof resting on those claiming such a meaning": Lennard, "Navigating by the Stars," at 44–45.

[120] "The Commission's proposals . . . were adopted virtually without change by the Conference and are now reflected in Articles 31 and 32 of the Convention": Sinclair, *Vienna Convention*, at 115.

process of interpretation is a unity and that the provisions of the article form a single, closely integrated rule.[121]

Art. 31(1) therefore embodies what is termed here an *interactive understanding* of treaty interpretation.[122] As Aust makes clear, "[a]though at first sight paragraphs 1, 2 and 3 might appear to create a hierarchy of legal norms, this is not so: the three paragraphs represent a logical progression, nothing more."[123] More specifically, Bos affirms that the article "refers the interpreter to the *concurrent* use of no less than three methods, *viz.*, the grammatical (ordinary meaning to be given to the terms of the treaty), the systematic (in their context) and the teleological method (in the light of its object and purpose)."[124]

The guidance afforded by the International Court of Justice is similarly supportive of an interactive understanding of the basic rule of treaty interpretation.[125] The Court has determined that

> one must certainly start ... from the "ordinary meaning" of the terms used ... but not in isolation. For treaty interpretation rules there is no "ordinary meaning" in the absolute or the abstract. That is why Article 31 of the Vienna Convention refers to "good faith" and to the ordinary meaning "to be given" to the terms of the treaty "in their context and in light of its object and purpose." It is, therefore, a fully qualified "ordinary meaning" ... The elucidation of the "ordinary meaning" of terms used in the treaty to be interpreted requires ... that due account be taken of those various interpretative principles and elements, and not only of the words or expressions used in the interpreted provisions in isolation.[126]

---

[121] [1966] 2 *Yearbook of the International Law Commission*, at 219–220.

[122] This is to be distinguished from a hierarchical approach under which context, object, and purpose are to be considered only where a treaty's text cannot be relied upon to disclose its "ordinary meaning." See e.g. M. Fitzmaurice, "The Law and Procedure of the International Court of Justice 1951–4: Treaty Interpretation and Other Treaty Points," (1957) 33 *British Yearbook of International Law* 203, at 204–207; and D. O'Connell, *International Law* (1970), at 253: "In so far as [the logic inherent in the treaty] can be discovered by reference to the terms of the treaty itself, it is impermissible to depart from those terms. In so far as it cannot, it is permissible."

[123] A. Aust, *Modern Treaty Law and Practice* (2000) (Aust, *Treaty Law*), at 187.

[124] M. Bos, "Theory and Practice of Treaty Interpretation," (1980) 27 *Netherlands International Law Review* 135 (Bos, "Theory and Practice"), at 145. See also P. Reuter, *Introduction to the Law of Treaties* (1995) (Reuter, *Law of Treaties*), at 75: "These carefully and subtly graduated elements constitute, primarily and simultaneously, the basic guidelines of interpretation."

[125] To the same effect, the European Court of Human Rights has determined that "[i]n the way in which it is presented in the 'general rule' of Article 31 of the Vienna Convention on the Law of Treaties, the process of interpretation is a unity, a single combined operation; this rule, closely integrated, places on the same footing the various elements enumerated in the four paragraphs of the Article": *Golder v. United Kingdom*, [1975] 1 EHRR 524 (ECHR, Feb. 21, 1975), at para. 30.

[126] *Land, Island and Maritime Frontier Dispute (El Salvador v. Honduras)*, [1992] ICJ Rep 351, at 719 (Separate Opinion of Judge Torres Bernandez).

Thus, "[t]he word obtains its meaning from the context in which it was used";[127] indeed, "[w]ords communicate their meaning from the circumstances in which they are used. In a written instrument their meaning *primarily* is to be ascertained from the context, setting, in which they are found [emphasis added]."[128]

There is, however, no doubt that literalism continues to have real appeal, particularly to governments and courts anxious to simplify their own task, or to be seen to be making "more objective" decisions. There is an undeniable comfort in the possibility of simply looking up a disputed term in the dictionary.[129] Yet this is false objectivity at its worst,[130] since it is surely right that "[e]tymological and grammatical bases are arbitrary and unreliable; their use is of limited theoretical value and fruitless as a method of proof."[131] The risks of dictionary-shopping[132] and of serious interpretive inconsistency are moreover magnified when there is more than one authentic linguistic version of a treaty,[133] nearly always the case for refugee and other international human rights treaties.[134]

---

[127] *Constitution of the Maritime Safety Committee of the Intergovernmental Maritime Consultative Organization (IMCO)*, [1960] ICJ Rep 150, at 158.

[128] *Certain Expenses of the United Nations*, [1962] ICJ Rep 151, at 184 (Separate Opinion of Judge Spender).

[129] As Merrills has succinctly observed, "[i]nterpreting a text involves more than looking up the meanings of words in a dictionary": J. Merrills, *The Development of International Law by the European Court of Human Rights* (1993) (Merrills, *European Court*), at 76.

[130] McNair was of the view that the duty to give treaty terms their "ordinary meaning" "begs the question whether the words are, or are not clear – a subjective matter because they may be clear to one man and not clear to another, and frequently to one or more judges and not to their colleagues": Lord McNair, *The Law of Treaties* (1961) (McNair, *Treaties*), at 372.

[131] Bos, "Theory and Practice," at 149.

[132] "[I]t is an approach which lends itself to an unseemly ransacking of dictionaries for the *mot juste* appropriate to the case at hand. This does not assist in a principled analysis of the issues": *Refugee Appeal 71427/99* (NZ RSAA, Aug. 16, 2000), at 11.

[133] "When a treaty has been authenticated in two or more languages, the text is equally authoritative in each language, unless the treaty provides or the parties agree that, in case of divergence, a particular text shall prevail": Vienna Convention, at Art. 33(1).

[134] In the case of the Refugee Convention, the English and French texts are equally authoritative: Convention relating to the Status of Refugees, 189 UNTS 2545, done July 28, 1951, entered into force Apr. 22, 1954 (Refugee Convention), at Conclusion. For the Refugee Protocol, as well as for the two Human Rights Covenants, the situation is still more complex, as the Chinese, English, French, Russian, and Spanish texts are equally authentic: Protocol relating to the Status of Refugees, 606 UNTS 8791, done Jan. 31, 1967, entered into force Oct. 4, 1967 (Refugee Protocol), at Art. XI; Civil and Political Covenant, at Art. 53; International Covenant on Economic, Social and Cultural Rights, UNGA Res. 2200A(XXI), adopted Dec. 16, 1966, entered into force Jan. 3, 1976 (Economic, Social and Cultural Covenant), at Art. 31. As Steiner and Alston have observed, "[s]ometimes corresponding words in different versions may shed more light on the intended meaning; at other times, they are plainly inconsistent": Steiner and Alston, *International Human Rights*, at 109.

In such circumstances, it is difficult to imagine how a coherent, transnational understanding of a treaty can emerge from a predominant focus on text.[135]

This is not to suggest that the inherent fungibility of language means that text should not be carefully considered in the construction of a treaty,[136] but simply that the results of a perusal of text must be synthesized with other considerations before arriving at a final interpretation of the treaty.[137] As Aust has cogently concluded, "[p]lacing undue emphasis on text, without regard to what the parties intended; or on what the parties are believed to have intended, regardless of the text; or on the perceived object and purpose in order to make the treaty more 'effective,' irrespective of the intentions of the parties, is unlikely to produce a satisfactory result."[138]

Interestingly, the rejection of literalism as the core of treaty interpretation has been specifically approved in the judicial review of refugee law decisions. One of the earliest clear commitments to a broad, interactive understanding of treaty interpretation was stated by Chief Justice Brennan of the High Court of Australia:

> In interpreting a treaty, it is erroneous to adopt a rigid priority in the application of interpretative rules ... Although the text of a treaty may itself reveal its object and purpose or at least assist in ascertaining its object and purpose, assistance may also be obtained from extrinsic sources. The form in which a treaty is drafted, the subject to which it relates, the history of its negotiations and comparison with earlier or amending instruments

[135] "Choosing to rely upon nothing else but the text of the treaty, one delivers onself up to all its possible shortcomings ... For, as one might have expected, it is not immediately clear what the implications of the concept are: what, indeed, is the ordinary sense of 'ordinary meaning'?": Bos, "Theory and Practice," at 147–149.

[136] In *European Roma Rights Centre v. Immigration Officer at Prague Airport*, [2002] EWCA 1989 (Eng. QBD, Oct. 8, 2002), for example, the court sensibly relied on the plain requirement of the Refugee Convention that a refugee must be "outside the country of his nationality" in order to dismiss an argument based on the Refugee Convention's object and purpose that refugee rights inhere also in persons still seeking to leave their own country. Much the same approach was taken by the Court of Appeal in *R (Hoxha) v. Secretary of State for the Home Department*, [2002] EWCA Civ 1403 (Eng. CA, Oct. 14, 2002), at para. 48, where the Court determined that the broad humanitarian aims of the treaty could not override the "agreed limitations which are contained within the terms of the Convention itself," specifically "the particular causes of persecution which have to be shown."

[137] For this reason, the goal of interpreting a treaty according to the natural and ordinary meaning of the words employed "is not an absolute one. Where such a method of interpretation results in a meaning incompatible with the spirit, purpose and context of the clause or instrument in which the words are contained, no reliance can validly be placed on it": *South West Africa Case (Ethiopia v. South Africa; Liberia v. South Africa), Preliminary Objections*, [1962] ICJ Rep 319, at 336.

[138] Aust, *Treaty Law*, at 185.

relating to the same subject may warrant consideration in arriving at the true interpretation of its text.[139]

The focus of the interpretive exercise is therefore an understanding of the text of the treaty, but text must be interpreted in context and purposively, rather than literally.

1.3.2 Context

In the case of the Refugee Convention, the treaty's "context," as defined in Art. 31(2) and supplemented by Art. 31(3) of the Vienna Convention, provides some important (thought largely issue-specific) interpretive assistance. For example, the Final Act of the conference which adopted the Refugee Convention[140] is a clear example of an "agreement relating to the treaty, which was made between all the parties in connexion with the conclusion of the treaty."[141] As described below, its commitments on such questions as family unity may therefore be invoked to interpret the formal text of the treaty.[142]

More generally, as Judge Weeramantry has noted,

> An obvious internal source of reference is the preamble to the treaty. The preamble is a principal and natural source from which indications can be gathered of a treaty's objects and purposes even though the preamble does not contain substantive provisions. Article 31(2) of the Vienna Convention sets this out specifically ... [and] this Court ... has made substantial use of it for interpretational purposes.[143]

As such, account should be taken of the fact that the first two operative paragraphs of the Preamble to the Refugee Convention unequivocally establish the human rights purposes of the treaty:

> *The High Contracting Parties,*
>   *Considering* that the Charter of the United Nations and the Universal Declaration of Human Rights ... have affirmed the principle that human beings shall enjoy fundamental rights and freedoms without discrimination,

---

[139] *Applicant "A" and Ano'r v. Minister for Immigration and Multicultural Affairs*, (1997) 190 CLR 225 (Aus. HC, Feb. 24, 1997), per Brennan CJ.

[140] "Final Act of the United Nations Conference of Plenipotentiaries on the Status of Refugees and Stateless Persons," 189 UNTS 37.

[141] Vienna Convention, at Art. 31(2)(a).

[142] See chapter 4.6 below.

[143] *Arbitral Award of 31 July 1989 (Guinea-Bissau v. Senegal)*, [1991] ICJ Rep 53, at 142 (Dissenting Opinion [on another point] of Judge Weeramantry). The decisions cited in which the International Court of Justice has relied upon the preamble to a treaty for interpretive purposes include *Rights of Nationals of the United States in Morocco*, [1952] ICJ Rep 176, at 196; and *Asylum Case (Colombia/Peru)*, [1950] ICJ Rep 266, at 282.

Considering that the United Nations has, on various occasions, manifested its profound concern for refugees and endeavoured to assure
refugees the widest possible exercise of these fundamental rights and
freedoms, ...

Have agreed as follows.[144]

The Preamble to the Refugee Protocol similarly affirms the fundamental
human rights purpose of the regime, and expressly stipulates the intention
of state parties to ensure that "equal status should be enjoyed by all refugees,"
including those who became refugees as the result of "new refugee situations
[that] have arisen since the [1951] Convention was adopted."[145]

Beyond matters formally recognized as part of the context for purposes of
treaty interpretation, Art. 31(3) directs attention to several related sources of
understanding. For example, the UNHCR's *Handbook on Procedures and
Criteria for Determining Refugee Status*, as well as many of the Conclusions
on International Protection issued by the state members of UNHCR's
Executive Committee, are to be taken into account as evidence of "subsequent agreement between the parties" on the meaning of the treaty.[146]
Even more clearly, reliance may be placed on the recent Declaration of States
Parties, issued at the December 2001 Ministerial Meeting of States Parties

---

[144] Refugee Convention, at Preamble, paras. 1, 2, 3, and 8. In the case of *European Roma
Rights Centre v. Immigration Officer at Prague Airport*, [2002] EWCA 1989 (Eng. QBD,
Oct. 8, 2002), portions of the Preamble to the Convention were invoked to contest the
legality of efforts to prevent would-be refugees from departing their own country. On the
facts of the case, however, the court reasonably held that the Refugee Convention's
general commitment to respect for human rights could not compel an interpretation at
odds with the ordinary meaning of the treaty, which plainly grants rights only to a person
who is "outside the country of his nationality": ibid. at paras. 42–43.

[145] Refugee Protocol, at Preamble, paras. 3, 4.

[146] Clearly, however, the scope of agreement manifested should not be overstated. As the
English Court of Appeal correctly observed in relation to the *Handbook*, "[a]spirations
are to be distinguished from legal obligations. It is significant that a number of the
passages [from the *Handbook*] relied on by the appellants are expressed in terms of what
'could' or 'should' be done": *R (Hoxha) v. Secretary of State for the Home Department*,
[2002] EWCA Civ 1403 (Eng. CA, Oct. 14, 2002). More specifically, Aust treats the
Handbook as part of the context of the treaty, appropriately referenced under Art. 31(2)
of the Vienna Convention: Aust, *Treaty Law*, at 191. Conversely, a decision of the English
Court of Appeal considered the *Handbook* instead to be evidence of "international
practice within article 31(3)(b) of the Vienna Convention": *R v. Secretary of State for
the Home Department, ex parte Adan and Aitseguer*, [1999] 3 WLR 1274 (Eng. CA, July 23,
1999, appeal to the House of Lords dismissed without comment on this issue). Neither of
these positions seems entirely correct, as the *Handbook* and Conclusions on International
Protection are logically viewed as "subsequent agreement between the parties regarding
the interpretation of the treaty or the application of its provisions": Vienna Convention,
at Art. 31(3)(a). It must be acknowledged, however, that not all state parties are members
of the UNHCR Executive Committee at any given moment, and that not all members of
the Executive Committee are parties to the Convention or Protocol. However, the

to mark the fiftieth anniversary of the Refugee Convention.[147] That Declaration of all state parties recognized, *inter alia*, that the 1951 Convention was of "enduring importance"; affirmed that all persons within its scope are entitled to "rights, including human rights, and minimum standards of treatment"; and specifically acknowledged "the continuing relevance and resilience of this international regime of rights and principles."

1.3.3 Object and purpose, conceived as effectiveness

In contrast to the fairly self-evident meaning of the duty to consider a treaty's text and Art. 31's specific definition of its context and related matters, there is no express guidance in the Vienna Convention on how to apply the third part of the general rule of interpretation, respect for the treaty's "object and purpose." This inquiry is complicated by unwarranted anxiety about reliance on the preparatory work of the treaty in order to discern object and purpose. But even if that concern is overcome, a more fundamental challenge remains. Since a treaty is to be understood as presently speaking rather than forever defined by the circumstances in which it was conceived, how can its historical "object and purpose" be authoritatively renewed in a way that does not invite speculation or the introduction of unbridled subjectivity? To this end, there is real value in a merger of the inquiry into a treaty's object and purpose with advancement of the more general duty to interpret a treaty in a way that ensures its effectiveness. Specifically, an interpretation of text made "in the light of [the treaty's] object and purpose" should take account of the historical intentions of its drafters, yet temper that analysis to ensure the treaty's effectiveness within its modern social and legal setting.

overwhelming majority of the more than sixty states represented on the Executive Committee are parties to the Convention or Protocol, and all state parties are invited to observe and to comment upon draft proposals under consideration by the Executive Committee. While this process is no doubt imperfect, it is difficult to imagine in practical terms how subsequent agreement among 145 state parties to the Refugee Convention could more fairly be generated. See generally chapter 2.5.2 below for a discussion of the legal relevance of these standards. It is not suggested, however, that the various institutional policy papers issued by UNHCR should be treated as evidence of subsequent agreement among the parties to the Convention, since there is no comparable deliberative process among states in their development.

[147] "Declaration of States Parties to the 1951 Convention and/or its 1967 Protocol relating to the Status of Refugees," UN Doc. HCR/MMSP/2001/09, Dec. 13, 2001, incorporated in Executive Committee of the High Commissioner's Program, "Agenda for Protection," UN Doc. EC/52/SC/CRP.9/Rev.1, June 26, 2002. The Declaration was welcomed by the UN General Assembly in UNGA Res. A/RES/57/187, Dec. 18, 2001, at para. 4. The December 2001 Ministerial Meeting has particular significance in that it was the first occasion on which a meeting at the ministerial level of all state parties to the Refugee Convention and Protocol was convened.

The starting point for analysis of a treaty's object and purpose should ordinarily be the historical record of the treaty's drafting.[148] So long as care is taken to distinguish between statements made which merely express one state's views and those which drive or capture consensus, the published records of the interstate drafting process that resulted in a treaty[149] (generally referred to as its *travaux préparatoires*)[150] can be a rich source of information about its object and purpose.[151] There is nonetheless a frequent reluctance to rely on the *travaux*,[152] motivated at least in part by the fact that the Vienna

---

[148] As Sinclair describes the process, "[t]he would-be interpreter is ... expected, when confronted with a problem of treaty interpretation (which, *ex hypothesi*, involves an argument as to the meaning of text), to have recourse to all the materials which will furnish him with evidence as to what is the meaning to be attributed to the text; such materials will naturally include the *travaux préparatoires* of the treaty, and all the circumstances of its conclusion. It is only when he has available to him all the necessary materials that he will be in a position to assess their relative value and weight in the light of the rules laid down in the Convention": Sinclair, *Vienna Convention*, at 117.

[149] This is not to endorse strong reliance on the full range of what might be considered to be the preparatory work of a treaty. Rather, "[t]he value of the material will depend on several factors, the most important being authenticity, completeness, and availability. The summary record of a conference prepared by an independent and skilled secretariat, such as that of the United Nations, will carry more weight than an unagreed record produced by a host state or a participating state": Aust, *Treaty Law*, at 198.

[150] "[T]here may however be cases where neither the text of the treaty nor the *travaux préparatoires* gives a sufficiently comprehensive view of the historical background and where recourse may therefore be had to extrinsic evidence": Sinclair, *Vienna Convention*, at 141.

[151] But see e.g. Reuter, *Law of Treaties*, at 97–98: "[R]ecourse to preparatory work means treading uncertain ground: its content is not precisely defined nor rigorously certified, and it reveals the shortcomings or potential blunders of the negotiators as well as their reluctance to confront true difficulties. Moreover, preparatory work is not always published, and even when it is there could be some misgivings about invoking it against States, even more numerous on account of the modern methods of accession, [involving states] which did not take part in the negotiations." In some cases, however – the Refugee Convention being one – the preparatory work is carefully defined, approved by states, and published. Moreover, evidence of "shortcomings and blunders," so long as it is recognized as such, may actually help to elucidate the meaning of provisions ultimately adopted. In these circumstances, resort to the *travaux* by states which choose to accede to a treaty without having participated in its negotiation enables them more clearly to understand the duties they are contemplating undertaking than would, for example, mere reliance on ambiguous text.

[152] See e.g. E. Lauterpacht and D. Bethlehem, "The Scope and Content of the Principle of *Non-Refoulement*," in Feller et al., *Refugee Protection* 87 (Lauterpacht and Bethlehem, "*Non-Refoulement*"), at para. 47: "While reference by international courts and tribunals to the *travaux préparatoires* of a treaty is common, it is a practice that has significant shortcomings particularly in the case of treaties negotiated at a time and in circumstances far distant from the point at which the question of interpretation and application arises. The *travaux préparatoires* of the 1951 Refugee Convention must, therefore ... be approached with care." The authors rely on this general position to reject parts of the

Convention treats the preparatory work of a treaty as a "supplementary means of interpretation" listed in Art. 32, rather than as part of the "general rule of interpretation" stated in Art. 31.[153] Yet this characterization of the role of the *travaux* as supplementary to the main duty to interpret text purposively and in context has been said by Judge Jessup to be more the result of habit than derived from principle:

> In my opinion, it is not necessary – as some utterances of the two international courts might suggest – to apologize for resorting to *travaux préparatoires* as an aid to interpretation. In many instances the historical record is valuable evidence to be taken into account in interpreting a treaty. It is tradition, rather than law or logic, which has at times led to judicial statements that the evidence is used merely to confirm an interpretation which is supposed to have already been derived from the bare words of the text or even of the text in its context.[154]

Indeed, the International Court of Justice has in practice relied on the *travaux*[155] not only to confirm the meaning of text,[156] but also to fill textual voids[157] and to

Refugee Convention's drafting history inconsistent with their preferred positions (ibid. at paras. 70, 103), yet invoke the *travaux* where these appear to support their favored views (ibid. at paras. 124, 150, 171). While the concern to ensure that account is taken of the modern circumstances in which a treaty must operate is, of course, well founded, this objective can be secured by a more broadly based, interactive interpretive structure oriented to reading treaties as living instruments: see text below at pp. 62–68. This approach takes nothing away from the real interpretive value of the *travaux préparatoires*, even as it insists on considering the *travaux* together with other sources of guidance.

[153] "Recourse may be had to supplementary means of interpretation, including the preparatory work of the treaty and the circumstances of its conclusion, in order to confirm the meaning resulting from the application of article 31, or to determine the meaning when the interpretation according to article 31: (a) leaves the meaning ambiguous or obscure; or (b) leads to a result which is manifestly absurd or unreasonable": Vienna Convention, at Art. 32.

[154] *South West Africa Case (Ethiopia v. South Africa; Liberia v. South Africa), Second Phase*, [1966] ICJ Rep 6, at 352 (Dissenting Opinion of Judge Jessup).

[155] A broad range of *travaux* has been consulted by the International Court of Justice, including "negotiation records, minutes of commission proceedings, committee debates preceding the adoption of a convention, preliminary drafts of provisions, diplomatic exchanges, and government memoranda": M. Ris, "Treaty Interpretation and ICJ Recourse to *Travaux Préparatoires*: Towards a Proposed Amendment of Articles 31 and 32 of the Vienna Convention on the Law of Treaties," (1991) 14(1) *Boston College International and Comparative Law Review* 111, at 133.

[156] See e.g. *Aegean Sea Continental Shelf Case (Greece v. Turkey)*, [1978] ICJ Rep 3, at 13–14; *Border and Transborder Armed Actions (Nicaragua v. Honduras), Jurisdiction and Admissibility*, [1988] ICJ Rep 69, at 90.

[157] See e.g. *Reservations to the Convention on the Prevention and Punishment of the Crime of Genocide*, [1951] ICJ Rep 15 (interpreting the Genocide Convention to determine the permissibility of reservations).

answer interpretive issues of first impression.[158] Even where there has been an effort to characterize reliance on the *travaux* as purely confirmatory of an interpretation reached on the basis of Art. 31 sources, Rosenne suggests that this may be more a matter of form than of substance:

> [T]hat case law would be much more convincing if from the outset the court or tribunal had refused to admit consideration of *travaux préparatoires* until it had first been established whether or not the text was clear, but in fact ... on all these occasions the *travaux préparatoires* had been fully and extensively placed before the court or the arbitral tribunal by one or other of the parties, if not by both. In the circumstances, to state that the *travaux préparatoires* had been used only to confirm an opinion already arrived at on the basis of the text of the treaty was coming close to a legal fiction.[159]

Sir Humphrey Waldock has similarly opined that "the reference to confirmation and, *a fortiori*, verification tended to undermine the text of a treaty in the sense that there was an express authorisation to interpret it in the light of something else; nevertheless, that was what happened in practice."[160]

Beyond the fact that the *travaux* appear in practice to figure prominently as a primary point of reference in the actual interpretation of treaties,[161] there is reason to doubt that it was ever intended that their characterization as supplementary means of interpretation was designed to discourage interpreters from relying upon them. Sir Ian Sinclair, actively involved in the drafting of the Vienna Convention, takes the view that "no rigid sequential limitation on resort to *travaux*, by their categorization as 'supplementary means,' was intended."[162] Waldock affirms that "there had certainly been no intention of discouraging *automatic recourse* to preparatory works for the general understanding of a treaty [emphasis added]."[163] Judge Schwebel goes

---

[158] See e.g. *Military and Paramilitary Activities in and Against Nicaragua (Nicaragua v. United States), Jurisdiction*, [1984] ICJ Rep 392, at 406 (interpreting the Statute of the International Court of Justice to determine the validity of a declaration of jurisdiction by the Permanent Court of International Justice).

[159] S. Rosenne, [1964] 1 *Yearbook of the International Law Commission*, at 292, para. 17.

[160] Sir Humphrey Waldock, [1964] 1 *Yearbook of the International Law Commission*, at 283, para. 65.

[161] "The European Court of Human Rights and the European Court of Justice have made use of *travaux préparatoires* for a variety of purposes and, on the evidence considered so far, it might be thought that they should be regarded as a major component in the courts' decisions": Merrills, *European Court*, at 92.

[162] Sinclair, *Vienna Convention*, at 116. He explains further that "[t]he distinction between the general rule of interpretation and the supplementary means of interpretation is intended rather to ensure that the supplementary means do not constitute an alternative, autonomous method of interpretation divorced from the general rule": ibid.

[163] "United Nations Conference on the Law of Treaties, Official Records of the First Session," UN Doc. CONF.39/11, at 184 (33rd Meeting), cited in Lennard, "Navigating by the Stars," at 24.

farther still, contending that the duty of good faith interpretation may at times require departure from an ordinary meaning thought to be "clear" in order to do justice to the drafters' intentions as disclosed by reference to the *travaux*.[164]

In short, there appears to be neither theory nor practice to justify the view that the designation of a treaty's preparatory work as a supplementary means of interpretation requires that it be relegated to an inherently subordinate or inferior place in a comprehensive, interactive process of treaty interpretation. The more sensible understanding of the *travaux*'s status as a supplementary means of interpretation is instead that they are to be treated as a means by which to achieve the interpretive goal set by Art. 31.[165] That is, the preparatory work is supplementary in the sense that its role is to provide *evidence of* the true meaning of a treaty's text construed purposively, in context, and with a view to ensuring its effectiveness.[166]

---

[164] "If, as Article 31 itself prescribes, a treaty is to be interpreted 'in good faith,' surely the provision of Article 32 regarding recourse to preparatory work must be understood to be meaningful rather than meaningless. If preparatory work may be invoked only when it confirms the ordinary meaning otherwise deduced, the provision for its application in Article 32 approaches the meaningless. But if preparatory work may be invoked to correct the ordinary meaning otherwise deduced (if not to inform and influence the interpretation of the treaty from the outset), it and the provisions of Article 32 are accorded a meaningful place": S. Schwebel, "May Preparatory Work be Used to Correct, Rather than Confirm, the 'Clear' Meaning of a Treaty Provision?," in L. Makasczyk ed., *Theory of International Law at the Threshold of the 21st Century: Essays in Honour of Krzysztof Skubiszewski* 541 (1996) (Schwebel, "Preparatory Work"), at 546. Aust observes in this regard that "[t]his is no doubt how things work in practice; for example, the parties to a dispute will always refer the tribunal to the *travaux*, and the tribunal will inevitably consider them along with all the other material put before it. [Judge Schwebel's] suggestion is therefore a useful addition to the endless debate on the principles of interpretation": Aust, *Treaty Law*, at 197.

[165] See Sinclair, *Vienna Convention*, at 116: "The distinction between the general rule of interpretation and the supplementary means of interpretation is intended rather to ensure that the supplementary means do not constitute an alternative, autonomous method of interpretation divorced from the general rule."

[166] This understanding appears to be in line with the approach of the International Court of Justice in *Legal Consequences of the Construction of a Wall in the Occupied Palestinian Territory*, (2004) ICJ Gen. List No. 131, decided July 9, 2004. Immediately after referring to the duty to interpret a treaty in good faith and in accordance with the ordinary meaning to be given to its terms in their context and in the light of its object and purpose, the Court cited the full text of Art. 32 of the Vienna Convention: ibid. at para. 94. It then relied extensively on the *travaux* to determine that Art. 2 of the Fourth Geneva Convention is applicable even during an occupation not involving armed conflict on the grounds that "[t]his interpretation reflects the intention of the drafters of the Fourth Geneva Convention to protect civilians who find themselves, in whatever way, in the hands of the occupying Power . . . That interpretation is confirmed by the Convention's *travaux préparatoires*": ibid. at para. 95.

In line with the understanding, there is quite a low threshold for deeming the text of a treaty to be "ambiguous or obscure," thus justifying resort to its preparatory work under the terms of Art. 32.[167] Indeed, it has been argued that the mere fact of an interpretive dispute triggers the right of reliance on the *travaux*:[168]

> It is undeniable that, when [the parties'] conflicting arguments are matched together, the meaning of some of the treaty's provisions are ambiguous or obscure; indeed each of the Parties maintained that the opposing interpretation led to results which, if not manifestly absurd, were unreasonable. Thus, according to the Vienna Convention, this is a case in which recourse to the preparatory work and circumstances of the Treaty's conclusion was eminently in order.[169]

To the same effect, Judge Spender opined that "[a]lthough the cardinal rule of interpretation is that words are to be read, if they may be read, in their ordinary and natural sense ... ambiguity may be hidden in the plainest and most simple of words even in their ordinary and natural meaning."[170]

---

[167] Vienna Convention, at Art. 32(a). Thus, for example, the House of Lords looked to the drafting history of Art. 33 of the Refugee Convention, noting that the *travaux* are "a legitimate guide to interpretation if the effect of a provision is in doubt and the *travaux préparatoires* yield a clear and authoritative answer": *R v. Immigration Officer at Prague Airport et al., ex parte European Roma Rights Centre et al.*, [2004] UKHL 55 (UK HL, Dec. 9, 2004), at para. 17.

[168] "One can, almost by definition, assume that a dispute about the interpretation of a treaty provision which reaches the stage of international adjudication will have arisen because the text is ambiguous or obscure": Sinclair, *Vienna Convention*, at 142.

[169] *Elettronica Sicula (USA v. Italy)*, [1989] ICJ Rep 15, at 97 (Dissenting Opinion of Judge Schwebel). See also *Judgment No. 273 of the UN Administrative Tribunal*, [1982] ICJ Rep 325, at 463 (Dissenting Opinion of Judge Schwebel): "The Court should do exactly as it has done in prior cases in which the meaning of a treaty or legislative text has been at issue: examine the preparatory work which gave rise to it. If it is objected that resort to this supplementary means of interpretation is justified only where the text is not clear, it is submitted that the text's lack of clarity is sufficiently shown by the differences about its interpretation which are demonstrated as between the Court's opinion and dissenting opinions in this case." Judge Schwebel has developed this position in his scholarship, observing that "the terms of a treaty which come before the Court for interpretation, if not usually obscure, are often 'ambiguous.' If this were not so, that is, if they did not lend themselves to argument attaching different meaning to their terms, they would not likely be legally contested at all. Moreover, it is not infrequent that the 'ordinary meaning' of the terms of a treaty, even if found unambiguously such, leads to a result which, if not 'manifestly absurd' is 'unreasonable' – at any rate, in the view of one of the parties to the dispute": Schwebel, "Preparatory Work," at 543. To similar effect, the European Court of Human Rights determined in *James v. United Kingdom*, (1986) 8 EHRR 123 (ECHR, Feb. 21, 1986), at para. 64, that "confronted with a text whose interpretation has given rise to such disagreement, the court considers it proper to have recourse to the *travaux préparatoires* as a supplementary means of interpretation."

[170] *Northern Cameroons Case*, [1963] ICJ Rep 15, at 88 (Separate Opinion of Judge Spender).

More generally, the way in which Art. 32 is framed supports giving the *travaux* pride of place as a source of evidence regarding a treaty's purpose, context, and intended effects. In authorizing reliance on supplementary means of treaty interpretation, Art. 32 singles out only "the preparatory work of the treaty and the circumstances of its conclusion" as definitively relevant. This unique recognition of the value of the *travaux* is very much in line with the relatively routine resort by many domestic courts to them in order to assist in the process of treaty interpretation.[171] Indeed, the House of Lords recently made clear that a focus on words alone – without a serious effort to come to grips with the historical goals understood to underpin the Refugee Convention – is unlikely to yield a sound understanding of the treaty's language:

> Inevitably the final text will have been the product of a long period of negotiation and compromise . . . It follows that one is more likely to arrive at the true construction of Article 1(A)(2) by seeking a meaning which makes sense in the light of the Convention as a whole, and the purposes which the framers of the Convention were seeking to achieve, rather than by concentrating exclusively on the language. A broad approach is what is needed, rather than a narrow linguistic approach.[172]

This observation neatly brings analysis of the role of a treaty's preparatory work full circle. The goal of interpretation is to discern a "true construction" of text. Yet such an understanding will only be possible when account is taken not only of words, but also of the treaty's object and purpose. A critical part of that interactive interpretive process – one which makes it "more likely" that a treaty will be accurately construed – is the careful consideration of the deliberations of the convention's drafters.

---

[171] See e.g. *Fothergill v. Monarch Airlines*, [1981] AC 251 (UK HL, July 10, 1980), per Diplock LJ at 283, in which the view is expressed that "an English court might well be under a constitutional obligation" to consider the *travaux* of a treaty where the text is ambiguous or obscure. American courts also make extensive use of the *travaux* in the construction of treaties: see e.g. *Volkswagenwerk Aktiengesellschaft v. Schlunk*, (1988) 486 US 694 (US SC, June 15, 1988); *Eastern Airlines v. Floyd*, (1991) 499 US 530 (US SC, Apr. 17, 1991); and, in the context of refugee law, *Sale, Acting Commissioner, Immigration and Naturalization Service, et al., Petitioners v. Haitian Centers Council, Inc., et al.*, 509 US 155 (US SC, Jan. 12, 1993). As Sinclair concludes, "there is now a growing tendency, even in the municipal courts of States which do not permit recourse to *travaux préparatoires* in construing statutes or other domestic legislative instruments, to apply this supplementary means of interpretation in determining the meaning of those statutes which give the force of domestic law to the provisions of international treaties": Sinclair, *Vienna Convention*, at 144.

[172] *R v. Secretary of State for the Home Department, ex parte Adan*, [1999] 1 AC 293 (UK HL, Apr. 2, 1998). See also *INS v. Cardoza Fonseca*, (1987) 480 US 421 (US SC, Mar. 9, 1987), at 437–438, in which the United States Supreme Court took account of the *travaux préparatoires* in its analysis of the meaning of "well-founded fear" in the Convention refugee definition.

Yet not even the most careful review of a treaty's *travaux* can in and of itself accurately identify its "object and purpose." Despite the real deference owed to evidence of the objectives being pursued by the representatives of governments that drafted, negotiated, and bound themselves to the treaty,[173] a treaty's object and purpose cannot reasonably be forever locked in time. To the contrary, because treaties are living instruments, evidence of historical intent should be balanced against more contemporary evidence of the social and legal context within which original intentions are now to be implemented.[174] To quote Judge Lauterpacht, "the true intentions of the parties may on occasion be frustrated if exclusive importance is attached to the meaning of words divorced from the social and legal changes which have intervened in the long period following upon conclusion of those treaties."[175]

To this end, the obligation to interpret the text of a treaty in the light of its object and purpose should be conceived as incorporating the overarching duty to interpret a treaty in a way that ensures its effectiveness.[176] The duty to promote a treaty's effectiveness is, in turn, derived from the more general obligation of good faith treaty interpretation.[177] As framed by the International Law Commission, "[w]hen a treaty is open to two interpretations, one of which does and the other does not enable the treaty to have appropriate effects, good faith and the objects and purposes of the treaty *demand* that the former interpretation should be adopted [emphasis added]."[178] To quote Judge Lauterpacht once more,

> The preponderant practice of the Court itself has ... been based on principles of interpretation which render the treaty effective, rather than

[173] In any event, good faith treaty interpretation requires fidelity to the intentions of the parties: [1966] 2 *Yearbook of the International Law Commission* 211.

[174] "An even more dynamic variant of the teleological approach is the so-called theory of 'emergent purpose' whereby the object and purpose itself is not regarded as fixed and static": Sinclair, *Vienna Convention*, at 131.

[175] Lauterpacht, *Collected Papers*, at 133.

[176] See Bos, "Theory and Practice," at 150: "In the International Law Commission's view, the 'object and purpose' phrase in Article 31, paragraph 1, is the consecration of the maxim *ut magis valeat quam pereat.*"

[177] According to the International Law Commission, good faith implies the requirement to remain faithful to the intentions of the parties, refraining from defeating them by a literal interpretation: [1966] 2 *Yearbook of the International Law Commission* 211. The *pacta sunt servanda* principle is codified in the Vienna Convention, at Art. 26: "Every treaty in force is binding upon the parties to it and must be performed by them in good faith." As Aust observes, "[i]nterpretation is part of the performance of the treaty, and therefore the process of examining the relevant materials and assessing them must be done in good faith": Aust, *Treaty Law*, at 187. The obligation to construe treaties in good faith does not, however, amount to an independent source of substantive obligation: *R v. Immigration Officer at Prague Airport et al., ex parte European Roma Rights Centre et al.*, [2004] UKHL 55 (UK HL, Dec. 9, 2004), at paras. 19 (per Lord Bingham) and 57–62 (per Lord Hope).

[178] [1966] 2 *Yearbook of the International Law Commission* 219.

ineffective. These principles are not easily reconcilable with restrictive interpretation conceived as the governing rule of construction.[179]

Yet despite the legal logic and common sense appeal of interpreting a treaty in a way that makes it effective[180] – thereby automatically renewing the treaty's historical object and purpose to take account of modern social and legal realities – there is nonetheless a real risk that this principle may simply provide cover for the imposition of a decision-maker's policy preferences. It is therefore important to constrain the process for identification of the "appropriate effects" of a treaty by reference to two types of objective criteria.

First, there will sometimes be important factual shifts in the social reality within which a treaty must function. In the context of refugee protection, for example, the current array of *non-entrée* policies,[181] designed to prevent refugees from accessing the territory of many states, simply did not exist when the Refugee Convention was concluded in 1951. Nor was the modern social welfare state then fully developed. Yet the Refugee Convention prohibits the *refoulement* of refugees, and grants refugees access to such rights as public relief, housing, and social security.[182] If the commitment of states to the regulation of modern refugee flows within the framework of the Refugee Convention is to be honored, it follows that an effort must be made to understand the ways in which the duties in force are to be applied within host societies as presently constructed.[183] The interpretive challenge – and

---

[179] H. Lauterpacht, *The Development of International Law by the International Court* (1958), at 304.

[180] The principle of effectiveness has been relied upon, for example, in *Corfu Channel Case (United Kingdom v. Albania), Merits*, [1949] ICJ Rep 4, at 24–26; and *Free Zones of Upper Savoy and the District of Gex Case*, [1929] PCIJ Rep, Series A, No. 22, at 13. More recently, the World Trade Organization Appellate Body invoked the duty to interpret treaties so as to advance their effectiveness in *Canada – Term of Patent Protection*, Dec. No. WT/DS170/R (WTO AB, Oct. 2000), at para. 6.49. The United States Supreme Court has recognized the effectiveness principle in e.g. *Bacardi Corp. of America v. Domenech*, (1940) 311 US 150 (US SC, Dec. 9, 1940), at 163; and *Jordan v. Tashiro*, (1928) 278 US 123 (US SC, Nov. 19, 1928), at 127.

[181] See generally J. Hathaway, "The Emerging Politics of *Non-Entrée*," (1992) 91 *Refugees* 40; also published as "L'émergence d'une politique de non-entrée," in F. Julien-Laferrière ed., *Frontières du droit, Frontières des droits* 65 (1993).

[182] These concerns are addressed at chapters 4.1, 4.4, 6.1.3, 6.3, and 6.4 below.

[183] See A. North and N. Bhuta, "The Future of Protection – The Role of the Judge," (2001) 15(3) *Georgetown Immigration Law Journal* 479, at 484, in which the authors affirm the critical importance of refugee law judges being "pragmatic and responsive to new realities." Indeed, as noted above, state parties to the Refugee Convention and Protocol have formally insisted upon precisely this understanding by recognizing "the continuing relevance and resilience of [the Convention's] regime of rights and principles, including at its core the principle of non-refoulement", even as they took note of the "complex features of the evolving environment in which refugee protection has to be provided, including ... mixed population flows, [and] the high costs of hosting large numbers of

duty – is thus to translate historical understanding of refugee rights in a way that positions them to meet the protection challenges presented by altered social and political circumstances.[184]

Second and more specifically, it is important that treaties be interpreted in a way that reconciles them to their contemporary international legal context.[185] Perhaps most obviously, the Refugee Convention was only the second binding human rights treaty promulgated by the United Nations, having come into force more than two decades before the Human Rights Covenants.[186] Yet because refugees are normally entitled to claim the benefit of general human rights treaties, and specifically because the subject matter of the Covenants overlaps frequently with that of the Refugee Convention, it is important that some coherence be given to cognate concepts under these treaties. The Supreme Court of Canada has made this point clearly:

> [T]he Refugee Convention itself expresses a "profound concern for refugees," and its principal purpose is to "assure refugees the widest possible exercise of . . . fundamental rights and freedoms." This negates the suggestion that the provisions of the Refugee Convention should be used to deny rights that other legal instruments make universally available to everyone.[187]

Indeed, the fact that the Covenants are regularly interpreted by a legally authoritative process which requires engagement with real cases involving

refugees and asylum-seekers": "Declaration of States Parties to the 1951 Convention and/ or its 1967 Protocol relating to the Status of Refugees," UN Doc. HCR/MMSP/2001/09, Dec. 13, 2001, incorporated in Executive Committee of the High Commissioner's Program, "Agenda for Protection," UN Doc. EC/52/SC/CRP.9/Rev.1, June 26, 2002. The Declaration was welcomed by the UN General Assembly in Res. A/RES/57/187, Dec. 18, 2001, at para. 4. This Declaration is to be taken into account together with the context of the Refugee Convention in interpreting the provisions of the treaty: see text above, at pp. 54–55.

[184] The unambiguous text of a treaty nonetheless sets a limit to the range of possible interpretations of a treaty so as to meet contemporary challenges. For example, the fact that refugee rights are limited to persons who are outside their own country was sensibly determined by the House of Lords to foreclose the possibility of granting Art. 33 rights to persons still within their own state. "[T]here is no want of good faith if a state interprets a treaty as meaning what it says and declines to do anything significantly greater than or different from what it agreed to do. The principle . . . *pacta sunt servanda* cannot require departure from what has been agreed. This is more obviously true where a state or states very deliberately decided what they were and were not willing to undertake to do": *R v. Immigration Officer at Prague Airport et al., ex parte European Roma Rights Centre et al.*, [2004] UKHL 55 (UK HL, Dec 9, 2004), at para. 19.

[185] This understanding is analogous to the view that "it is a rule of interpretation that a text emanating from a Government must, in principle, be interpreted as producing and as intended to produce effects in accord with existing law and not in violation of it": *Rights of Passage over Indian Territory (Portugal v. India), Preliminary Objections*, [1957] ICJ Rep 125, at 142.

[186] See chapters 2.4 and 2.5 below.

[187] *Suresh v. Canada*, [2002] 1 SCR 3 (Can. SC, Jan. 11, 2002).

real people (while the Refugee Convention is not)[188] gives additional impetus to the logic of ensuring a harmonious construction of rights and duties.[189]

The duty to interpret treaties as living instruments able to function as part of a complex and evolving legal environment is now widely accepted. While its origins are in European human rights law,[190] it has been embraced more broadly in, for example, both European economic law[191] and international trade law.[192] In the latter context, appellate jurisprudence has affirmed that

[188] See Epilogue below, at pp. 992–998.

[189] In a decision challenging the detention of a non-removable failed asylum-seeker, the Full Federal Court of Australia not only drew heavily on the Civil and Political Covenant, but expressly addressed the relevance of the views of the Human Rights Committee adopted under its authority to receive complaints of breach of that treaty. "Although the views of the Committee lack precedential authority in an Australian court, it is legitimate to have regard to them as the opinions of an expert body established by the treaty to further its objectives by performing functions that include reporting, receiving reports, [and] conciliating and considering claims that a state party is not fulfilling its obligations": *Minister for Immigration and Multicultural and Indigenous Affairs v. Al Masri*, (2003) 197 ALR 241 (Aus. FFC, Apr. 15, 2003). More recently, a commitment to taking real account of the work of UN human rights supervisory bodies was expressed by Justice Kirby of the High Court of Australia, who noted that "[i]n ascertaining the meaning of the [International Covenant on Civil and Political Rights] . . . it is permissible, and appropriate, to pay regard to the views of the [UN Human Rights Committee] . . . Such views do not constitute legally binding rulings for the purposes of international law. However, they are available to municipal courts, such as this, as the opinions of independent experts in international law, to assist in the understanding of the requirements of that law for whatever weight the municipal legal system accords to it. In Australia, that is the weight of persuasive influence. No more; but no less": *Minister for Immigration and Multicultural and Indigenous Affairs v. B and B*, [2004] HCA 20 (Aus. HC, Apr. 29, 2004), per Kirby J, at para. 148.

[190] "[T]he Convention is a living instrument which, as the Commission rightly stressed, must be interpreted in the light of present day conditions. In the case now before it, the court cannot but be influenced by the developments and commonly accepted standards in the penal policy of the member states of the Council of Europe in this field": *Tyrer v. United Kingdom*, (1978) 2 EHRR 1 (ECHR, Apr. 25, 1978), at para. 31. Merrills concludes that "[t]he principle that the Convention must be interpreted as a 'living instrument' is now generally accepted": Merrills, *European Court*, at 79.

[191] The evolutionary approach is described as "particularly appropriate in Community law where . . . the treaties provide mainly a broad programme or design rather than a detailed blueprint": L. Brown and T. Kennedy eds., *Brown and Jacobs: The Court of Justice in the European Communities* (2000), at 339.

[192] "The Appellate Body has accepted in its treaty interpretations that it may be evident from a treaty that a term has an evolutionary meaning, with some built-in 'elasticity' to accommodate new shades of meaning as they develop, while respecting the bargain that has been struck": Lennard, "Navigating by the Stars," at 75. As a general matter, "[t]he WTO Panels and the Appellate Body rely on the treaty interpretation rules expressed in the *Vienna Convention* . . . as the basic rules for interpreting WTO instruments. This is because those rules are generally regarded as codification of the public international law rules of treaty interpretation": ibid. at 17.

Interpretation cannot remain unaffected by the subsequent development of law ... Moreover, an international instrument has to be interpreted and applied within the entire legal system prevailing at the time of interpretation.[193]

Members of the International Court of Justice have similarly pointed out the importance of seeking conceptual concordance among closely connected treaties. In the *North Sea Continental Shelf Cases*, for example, Judge Ammoun insisted that it was "imperative in the present case to interpret [the treaty] in the light of the formula adopted in the other three [related] conventions, in accordance with the method of integrating the four conventions by co-ordination."[194] Judge Mosler has opined that "[t]he method of interpreting a treaty by reference to another treaty, although it is sometimes contested, has rightly been admitted in the decisions of the Court."[195] Most generally, the International Court of Justice has determined that "an international instrument has to be interpreted and applied within the framework of the entire legal system *prevailing at the time of the interpretation* [emphasis added]"[196] – a principle expressly affirmed in the context of international human rights law.[197] Indeed, this approach is arguably compelled by Art. 31(3) of the Vienna Convention, which requires that treaty interpretation take account of "any relevant rules of international law applicable in the relations between the parties."[198]

---

[193] *US – Import Prohibition of Certain Shrimp and Shrimp Products*, WTO Dec. No. WT/DS58/AB/R (WTO AB, Oct. 12, 1998), at para. 130.

[194] *North Sea Continental Shelf Cases (Federal Republic of Germany/Denmark; Federal Republic of Germany/Netherlands)*, [1969] ICJ Rep 3, at 125 (Separate Opinion of Judge Ammoun).

[195] *Constitution of the Maritime Safety Committee of the Intergovernmental Maritime Consultative Organization (IMCO)*, [1960] ICJ Rep 73, at 126 (Separate Opinion of Judge Mosler).

[196] *Legal Consequences for States of the Continued Presence of South Africa in Namibia*, [1971] ICJ Rep 6. Sinclair concludes that "there is scope for the narrow and limited proposition that the evolution and development of the law can be taken into account in interpreting certain terms in a treaty which are by their very nature expressed in such general terms as to lend themselves to an evolutionary interpretation. But this must always be on condition that such an evolutionary interpretation does not conflict with the intentions and expectations of the parties as they may have been expressed during the negotiations preceding the conclusion of the treaty": Sinclair, *Vienna Convention*, at 140.

[197] "Treaties that affect human rights cannot be applied in such a manner as to constitute a denial of human rights as understood at the time of their application": *Gabcikovo–Nagymaros Project (Hungary/Slovakia)*, [1997] ICJ Rep 7, at 114–115 (Judge Weeramantry).

[198] Vienna Convention, at Art. 31(3). Sinclair explains that the paragraph as originally drafted by the International Law Commission initially referred only to "rules of international law *in force at the time of [the treaty's] conclusion* [emphasis added]." He observes

The evolutionary principle was recently applied by the House of Lords to refugee law in a way that blends it seamlessly with the duty to respect historical intentions:

> It is ... plain that the Convention must be seen as a living instrument in the sense that *while its meaning does not change over time, its application will.* I would agree with the observation [that] ... "[u]nless it is seen as a living thing, adopted by civilized countries for a humanitarian end which is constant in motive but mutable in form, the Convention will eventually become an anachronism [emphasis added]."[199]

In line with this formulation, an interpretive approach that synthesizes foundational insights from analysis of the historical intentions of a treaty's drafters with understandings derived from the normative legal context and practical landscape within which treaty duties are now to be implemented is the most objective and legally credible means of identifying how best to make the treaty effective. It is an approach fully in line with the basic obligation of *pacta sunt servanda*, since it honors the original goals which prompted elaboration of the treaty even as it refuses to allow those commitments to

that the italicized words "were intended to reflect the general principle that a juridical fact must be appreciated in the light of the law contemporary with it. During the course of second reading in the Commission, some members suggested that the text as it then stood failed to deal with the problem of the effect of an evolution of the law on the interpretation of legal terms in a treaty and was therefore inadequate. For this reason, the Commission concluded that it should omit a temporal element and transfer this element of interpretation to paragraph 3 as being an element extrinsic both to the text and to the 'context' as defined in paragraph 2": Sinclair, *Vienna Convention*, at 138–139. Aust, in contrast, takes the view that cognate treaties are appropriately referenced as supplementary means of interpretation pursuant to Art. 32 of the Vienna Convention, writing that "[o]ne may also look at other treaties on the same subject matter adopted *either before or after* the one in question which use the same or similar terms [emphasis added]": Aust, *Treaty Law*, at 200.

[199] *Sepet and Bulbul v. Secretary of State for the Home Department*, [2003] UKHL 15 (UK HL, Mar. 20, 2003), per Lord Bingham. In reaching this conclusion, Lord Bingham adopted the reasoning of Sedley J in *R v. Immigration Appeal Tribunal, ex parte Shah*, [1997] Imm AR 145 (Eng. QBD, Nov. 11, 1996), at 152. He further approved of the observation of Laws LJ in *R v. Secretary of State for the Home Department, ex parte Adan and Aitseguer*, [1999] 3 WLR 1274 (UK CA, July 23, 1999), that "[i]t is clear that the signatory states intended that the Convention should afford continuing protection for refugees in the changing circumstances of the present and future world. In our view the Convention has to be regarded as a living instrument: just as, by the Strasbourg jurisprudence, the European Convention on Human Rights is so regarded." More specifically, Lord Bingham observed that "the reach of an international human rights convention is not forever determined by the intentions of those who originally framed it. Thus ... the House was appropriately asked to consider a mass of material illustrating the movement of international opinion among those concerned with human rights and refugees in the period, now a very significant period, since the major relevant conventions were adopted": [2003] UKHL 15, at para. 11.

atrophy through passage of time.[200] It is moreover an approach to treaty interpretation that results in the marriage of the duty to advance a treaty's effectiveness with the more basic obligation to interpret text purposively, and in context.

1.3.4 But what about state practice?

One challenge to this understanding of the rules of treaty interpretation is rooted in Art. 31(3)(b) of the Vienna Convention, which provides that treaties are to be interpreted in the light of "any subsequent practice in the application of the treaty which establishes the agreement of the parties regarding its interpretation."[201] Since governments often seek to minimize the practical effect of their refugee law and other human rights commitments, it might be argued that this state practice should trump, or at least attenuate, the results of interpreting text purposively, in context, and with a view to ensuring the treaty's effectiveness. However, while state practice is often of clear value in the interpretation of bilateral treaties involving purely interstate interests, there are good reasons to read this provision narrowly as a guide to the construction of multilateral treaties in general, and of multilateral human rights treaties in particular.

The most basic concern arises from international law's commitment to the view that no grouping of states can impose obligations on a third state without the latter's express or implied consent thereto.[202] As such, reliance on less-than-unanimous practice by the parties to a treaty in order to interpret the obligations of *all* parties to that treaty raises a problem of consent to be bound by that practice-derived interpretation. As Judge Spender observed,

> In the case of multilateral treaties, the admissibility and value as evidence of subsequent conduct of one or more parties thereto encounter particular difficulties. If *all* the parties to a multilateral treaty where the parties are fixed and constant pursue a course of conduct in their attitude to the text of the treaty, and that course of conduct leads to an inference, and one

---

[200] "Given the freedoms guaranteed under the Universal Declaration of Human Rights and other international conventions, it could not have been consistent with the purpose of the Refugee Convention to require that persons claiming to be refugees be deprived of their fundamental human rights and freedoms in the country from [which] they are seeking protection": *Minister for Immigration and Multicultural Affairs v. Mohammed*, (2000) 98 FCR 405 (Aus. FFC, May 5, 2000), per French J.

[201] Vienna Convention, at Art. 31(3)(b).

[202] See Vienna Convention, at Arts. 34 ("A treaty does not create either obligations or rights for a third State without its consent") and 35 ("An obligation arises for a third State from a provision of a treaty if the parties to the treaty intend the provision to be the means of establishing the obligation and the third State expressly accepts that obligation in writing").

inference only, as to their common intention and understanding at the time they entered into the treaty as to the meaning of the text, the probative value of their conduct ... is manifest. If, however, only one or some but *not all* of them by subsequent conduct interpret the text in a certain manner, that conduct stands upon the same footing as the unilateral conduct of one party to a bilateral treaty. The conduct of such one or more could not of itself have any probative value or provide a criterion for judicial interpretation [emphasis added].[203]

While it is true that the International Law Commission did not accept a proposal to require the express consent of all parties to a treaty as a condition for the application of Art. 31(3)(b) of the Vienna Convention,[204] the International Court of Justice has thus far seemed disinclined to promote ease of reliance on Art. 31(3)(b) at the expense of overriding the views of state parties to a treaty which have not at least acquiesced in the allegedly interpretive practice.[205]

Even if the problem of reliance on non-unanimous practice to interpret the duties of all state parties to a treaty could be overcome, Art. 31(3)(b) gives less weight to state practice as an interpretive tool than is commonly assumed.

---

[203] *Certain Expenses of the United Nations*, [1962] ICJ Rep 151, at 191 (Separate Opinion of Judge Spender).

[204] [1966] 2 *Yearbook of the International Law Commission* 222. The rejection of this requirement may be read, however, as a rejection of the requirement for the *express* (rather than simply passive) assent of all parties to the interpretive practice in question. Thus, Sinclair employs rather fungible language, concluding that "paragraph 3(b) of Article 31 of the Convention does not cover subsequent practice in general, but only a specific form of subsequent practice – that is to say, *concordant subsequent practice* common to all the parties [emphasis added]": Sinclair, *Vienna Convention*, at 138. Aust similarly concludes that "[i]t is not necessary to show that each party has engaged in a practice, only that all have accepted it, albeit tacitly": Aust, *Treaty Law*, at 195.

[205] In the *Asylum Case*, for example, Judge Read indicated that the practice of all parties to a treaty should be taken into account (though in the case at hand lack of time, space and information compelled him to review only the practice of the disputing states): *Asylum Case (Colombia/Peru)*, [1950] ICJ Rep 266. Judge van Wyk observed that "[t]he weight to be attached to such conduct must necessarily depend on the circumstance of each case. Where for a relatively lengthy period after the execution of any agreement, *all* the parties by conduct accept the position that the agreement does not embody a particular obligation, then such conduct must bear considerable weight in a determination whether that obligation exists or not [emphasis added]": *South West Africa Case (Ethiopia v. South Africa; Liberia v. South Africa), Second Phase*, [1966] ICJ Rep 6, at 135–136 (Separate Opinion of Judge van Wyk). And in the *Namibia Case*, Judge Spender reiterated his view that a treaty "cannot be altered by the will of the majority of the member states, no matter how often that will is expressed or asserted against a protesting minority and no matter by how large the majority – or how small the minority": *Legal Consequences for States of the Continued Presence of South Africa in Namibia (South West Africa) Notwithstanding Security Council Resolution 276 (1970)*, [1971] ICJ Rep 16, at 31. This view was affirmed in the case by Judge Bustamante (ibid. at 291), and by Judge Winiarski in his dissenting opinion (ibid. at 234).

The provision does not validate *all* state practice as part of the general rule of interpretation; rather, it expressly sanctions reliance only on a subset of state practice, namely "subsequent practice in the application of the treaty, which establishes the agreement of the parties regarding its interpretation."[206] The purposive nature of legally relevant practice requires, in effect, that the practice in question have been motivated by a sense of legal obligation (*opinio juris*).[207] As Judge Fitzmaurice summarized the rule, evidence of state practice is a useful tool for the construction of a treaty where "it is possible and reasonable to infer from the behavior of the parties that they have regarded the interpretation they have given the instrument in question as the legally correct one, and have tacitly recognized that, in consequence, certain behavior was legally incumbent upon them."[208] Thus, in Judge Winiarski's view, "[i]t is sometimes difficult to attribute any precise legal significance to the conduct of the contracting parties, because it is not always possible to know with certainty whether they have acted in a certain manner because they consider that the law so requires or allows, or for reasons of expediency."[209] In the context of refugee and other international human rights treaties, expedient or other self-interested conduct by governments is distressingly common,[210] thus taking much state practice under such accords outside the scope of Art. 31's general rule of interpretation.[211]

It is nonetheless true that state practice which does not meet the requirements of Art. 31(3)(b) may still be considered as a (non-enumerated)

---

[206] Vienna Convention, at Art. 31(3)(b). Indeed, the approach of the Permanent Court of International Justice was to validate only state practice which shed light on the intent of the parties *at the time they concluded the treaty*: *Treaty of Lausanne Case*, [1925] PCIJ Rep, Series B, No. 13, at 24.

[207] "[I]nterpretive conduct must have been motivated by a sense of legal obligation. For example, in the *Asylum Case*, the [International Court of Justice] thought that the granting of asylum in the cases referred to it may have been the product of political expediency rather than an indication of the existence of a legal obligation. This requirement is the same as that found for the development of a customary norm through the practice of states ... [T]he strength of evidence of practice will often lie in its inadvertent nature: the agent acts on a non-politically motivated interpretation of the provision in question, rather than consciously attempting to establish a practice": G. McGinley, "Practice as a Guide to Treaty Interpretation," [Winter 1985] *Fletcher Forum* 211 (McGinley, "Practice as a Guide"), at 218.

[208] *Certain Expenses of the United Nations*, [1962] ICJ Rep 151, at 201 (Separate Opinion of Judge Fitzmaurice).

[209] Ibid. at 232 (Dissenting Opinion – on another proposition – of Judge Winiarski).

[210] See the detailed empirical analysis of failures to respect refugee rights in chapters 4–7 below.

[211] See e.g. the approach of the European Court of Human Rights, which has taken the view that state practice is not within the bounds of Art. 31(3)(b) unless motivated by *opinio juris*: *Cruz Varas v. Sweden*, (1991) 14 EHRR 1 (ECHR, Mar. 20, 1991), at para. 100; *Soering v. United Kingdom*, (1989) 11 EHRR 439 (ECHR, July 7, 1989), at para. 103.

supplementary means of interpretation under Art. 32 of the Vienna Convention.[212] It may be admitted into evidence "because practice represents the common-sense practical interpretation of the treaty under the varied contingencies of its ongoing operation."[213] Like evidence of historical intent (also admitted under Art. 32), data on state practice may be an important means by which to come to grips with the challenges of a treaty's current operational setting, thereby advancing the process of interpreting a treaty so as to promote its effectiveness.[214] Yet even while promoting this understanding of the relevance of state practice, McGinley does not recommend that evidence of state practice be treated as inherently of value:

> The practice may be so vast as to make it virtually unavailable to the court of the parties. Or, much may be unrecorded or otherwise unavailable. It may be generated at will by the parties and be highly self-serving. Moreover, because practice is amenable to subjective interpretation, it may be readily bent to particular points of view. Finally, judicial selectivity is often a problem: acts ignored by one judge may be given special significance by another.[215]

Beyond these general concerns, particular caution is warranted before relying on general evidence of practice by state parties to interpret refugee and other international human rights treaties. These treaties are unique applications of international law, in that they are expressly designed to constrain state conduct for the benefit of actual human beings. This purpose could be fundamentally frustrated if the construction of the duties assumed by states were to be determined by the very state practices sought to be constrained. Indeed, if refugee and other human rights treaties are interpreted in ways that defer to contemporary state practice, there is a very real risk that state auto-determination of the scope of obligations will trump the existence of obligations at all. As the American representative to the Ad Hoc Committee which drafted the Refugee Convention observed, "the mere fact that the provisions of a convention required a change in the existing laws of any country was not a valid argument against them. If all national laws were to remain unchanged, why should there be a convention?"[216] Thus, at least when interpreting bodies of law specifically designed by states to limit state

---

[212] Sinclair, *Vienna Convention*, at 138; McGinley, "Practice as a Guide," at 221.

[213] McGinley, "Practice as a Guide," at 227.

[214] As noted above, the fact that a treaty's preparatory work and the circumstances of its conclusion are the only listed supplementary means of interpretation may suggest that they are worthy of special consideration in the interpretive process: see chapter 1.3.3 above, at p. 61.

[215] McGinley, "Practice as a Guide," at 219.

[216] Statement of Mr. Henkin of the United States, UN Doc. E/AC.32/SR.37, Aug. 16, 1950, at 15. See also Statement of Mr. Weis of the IRO, ibid. at 16.

autonomy for the benefit of third parties, Art. 31(3)(b) should be read quite narrowly.[217]

This constrained view of the relevance of state practice to interpreting refugee and other human rights treaties is very much in line with the classic approach taken to the construction of "lawmaking treaties," that is, treaties under which

> the Contracting States do not have any interests of their own; they merely have, one and all, a common interest, namely, the accomplishment of those high purposes which are the *raison d'être* of the convention. Consequently, in a convention of this type, one cannot speak of individual advantages to States, or of the maintenance of a perfect balance between rights and duties.[218]

In the case of lawmaking treaties – of which refugee and other human rights accords are surely a paradigmatic example[219] – it is recognized that "the character of the treaty may affect the question whether the application of a particular [interpretive] principle, maxim or method is suitable in a particular case."[220] Specifically, where a treaty is "less a manifestation of free will than a calling to mind of principle obligatory for every civilized State, less a contract than universally valid regulation of objective law . . . in the matter of interpretation, validity of the convention is placed outside the sphere of the will of the Contracting Parties."[221]

This notion that the interpretation of lawmaking treaties should not be directed solely or even principally to advancing the interests of the contracting parties has some fairly clear implications.[222] For example, an interpretive

---

[217] In line with this view, it is arguably appropriate that "[g]enerally speaking, human rights treaty interpretation is characterized by the 'teleological' approach": B. Simma, "How Distinctive Are Treaties Representing Collective Interest? The Case of Human Rights Treaties," in V. Gowlland-Debbas ed., *Multilateral Treaty Making – The Current Status of and Reforms Needed in the International Legislative Process* 83 (2000), at 84.

[218] *Reservations to the Convention on the Prevention and Punishment of the Crime of Genocide*, [1951] ICJ Rep 15, at 26. Judge de Visscher defined lawmaking treaties as treaties the object of which is the laying down of common rules of conduct (*normes de conduite communes*): C. de Visscher, *Problèmes d'interpretation judiciare en droit international public* (1963) (de Visscher, *Problèmes d'interpretation*), at 128.

[219] The remarks of the International Court of Justice – see text above, at note 218 – were made in the context of construction of the Genocide Convention.

[220] Remarks of Sir Humphrey Waldock, Chief Rapporteur of the International Law Commission for the Draft Articles on the Law of Treaties, [1964] 2 *Yearbook of the International Law Commission* 55.

[221] De Visscher, *Problèmes d'interpretation*, at 38 (translation).

[222] "[N]ot all treaties contain 'law.' Some . . . instead of 'law' carry 'obligations.' The difference was said to be of importance precisely in the matter of interpretation, for treaties carrying 'obligations' may be expected to be interpreted with a very heavy emphasis on the will of the parties, in contrast with treaties containing 'law,' the construction of which to a degree may be influenced by the collective state-interest": Bos, "Theory and Practice," at 156.

principle such as *in dubio mitius*[223] is of limited value, since it is based on the assumption that governments negotiating treaties seek to secure particular benefits from other states at a minimal cost to their own sovereignty and self-interest. This background assumption is of doubtful currency in the case of a treaty designed precisely to limit state sovereignty in the interests of advancing more general goals for the international community as a whole. The pertinence of state practice as an aid in the interpretation of lawmaking treaties intended to promote refugee and other human rights is similarly suspect. Because these treaties are conceived to advance common "high purposes" by binding and constraining the autonomy of governments, their very nature compels a more particularized approach to interpretation. In the words of the European Court of Human Rights, it is necessary in such cases "to seek the interpretation that is most appropriate in order to realise the aim and achieve the objective of the treaty, not that which would restrict to the greatest possible degree the obligations undertaken by the parties."[224]

In sum, Art. 31(3)(b) is not a significant impediment to the logic of interpreting refugee and other human rights treaties on the basis of an approach committed to interpreting text in context, purposively, and with a view to ensuring the treaty's effectiveness. Less-than-unanimous state practice is at best an awkward source of guidance on the meaning of multilateral treaties. Moreover, the Vienna Convention does not require deference to all state practice, but only to such practice as derives from a sense of legal obligation, rather than – as is most common in the human rights context – from state self-interest or expediency. Even where evidence of state practice is tendered not as relevant to establishing a treaty's context but more generally

---

[223] The principle of *in dubio mitius* posits that if the wording of a treaty provision is not clear, preference should be given to the interpretation that gives rise to a minimum of obligations for the parties. For example, the WTO Appellate Body has held that "[t]he principle of *in dubio mitius* applies in interpreting treaties, in deference to the sovereignty of states. If the meaning of the term is ambiguous, that meaning is to be preferred which is less onerous to the party assuming an obligation, or which interferes less with the territorial and personal supremacy of a party, or involves less general restrictions upon the parties": *European Communities – Measures Affecting Meat and Meat Products (EC Hormones)*, WTO Dec. No. WT/DS26/AB/R (WTO AB, Jan. 16, 1998), at para. 154. While this reasoning makes clear why the principle ought not to govern the interpretation of lawmaking treaties, there are also more general reasons to be skeptical about its propriety. It has been questioned in McNair, *Treaties*, at 765, and in Jennings and Watts, *Oppenheim's*, at 1278: "[I]n applying this principle, regard must be had to the fact that the assumption of obligations constitutes the primary purpose of the treaty and that, in general, the parties must be presumed to have intended the treaty to be effective."

[224] *Wemhoff v. Germany*, (1968) 1 EHRR 55 (ECHR, June 27, 1968), at para. 23. See also *Klass v. Germany*, (1979) 2 EHRR 214 (ECHR, Sept. 6, 1978), at para. 42, where the Court determined that restrictions on human rights are to be narrowly construed in light of the fundamental human rights objectives of the European Convention on Human Rights.

as a supplementary means of interpretation, it is surely doubtful that practice which contests or limits the scope of refugee and other human rights is a helpful means of interpreting lawmaking treaties conceived in order to advance precisely those rights.

The interpretive approach adopted here can briefly be summarized. One should begin with the text of the Refugee Convention, and seek to understand it not on the basis of literal constructions but rather in a way that takes real account of its context, and which advances its object and purpose.[225] In addition to formal components of context, such as the Final Act of the conference that adopted the Convention and the Preambles to the Convention and its Protocol, the context includes subsequent interpretive agreement among the parties, in particular the relevant Conclusions issued by the state members of UNHCR's Executive Committee. The analysis here draws regularly as well on the primary indicia of the object and purpose of the refugee treaty, both historical and contemporary. The main record of the original goals of the drafters is accessible through the extensive and officially compiled *travaux* of the Convention's drafting.[226] The analysis here tests the historical understanding against evidence of contemporary factual challenges to the treaty's effectiveness, and synthesizes the interpretation so derived with analysis of the vast array of primary and secondary materials which elaborates the interpretation of cognate rights under general international human rights law. This interactive process is intended to yield a genuinely comprehensive understanding of the rights of refugees as presently conceived under international law.

---

[225] "[O]nly a broad approach to the text, and to the legal rights which the Convention affords, will fulfill its objectives": *Chen Shi Hai v. Minister for Immigration and Multicultural Affairs*, (2000) 170 ALR 553 (Aus. HC, Apr. 13, 2000), per Kirby J.

[226] The *travaux préparatoires* of the Refugee Convention are helpfully collected in a three-volume looseleaf set: A. Takkenberg and C. Tahbaz eds., *The Collected Travaux Préparatoires of the 1951 Geneva Convention relating to the Status of Refugees* (1989). The main contributions to the Convention's development were made by the Ad Hoc Committee on Statelessness and Related Problems, which met at Lake Success, New York, during January–February 1950; by a reconvened Ad Hoc Committee on Refugees and Stateless Persons, which met again at Lake Success, New York, during August 1950; and by a Conference of Plenipotentiaries, which met in Geneva during July 1951. The analysis here draws heavily on discussions in these three fora.

The evolution of the refugee rights regime

The origins of refugee rights are closely intertwined with the emergence of the general system of international human rights law. Like international human rights, the refugee rights regime is a product of the twentieth century. Its contemporary codification by the United Nations took place just after the adoption of the Universal Declaration of Human Rights, and was strongly influenced by the Declaration's normative structure.

In a more fundamental sense, though, the refugee rights regime draws heavily on the earlier precedents of the law of responsibility for injuries to aliens and international efforts to protect national minorities. This chapter highlights the conceptual contributions made by each of these bodies of international law to the emergence of specific treaties to govern the human rights of refugees. It then introduces the essential structure of the 1951 Refugee Convention,[1] still the primary source of refugee-specific rights in international law. Finally, this chapter takes up the question of the relationship between the refugee rights regime and subsequently enacted treaties, particularly those that establish binding norms of international human rights law. The view is advanced that refugee rights should be understood as a mechanism by which to answer situation-specific vulnerabilities that would otherwise deny refugees meaningful benefit of the more general system of human rights protection. Refugee rights do not exist as an alternative to, or in competition with, general human rights. Nor, however, has the evolution of a broad-ranging system of general human rights treaties rendered the notion of refugee-specific rights redundant.

2.1 International aliens law

The process of governance is normally premised on a closed system of obligation. Rules are established to support the polity's functional interdependence, without expectation that outsiders will conduct themselves by those standards. There is therefore a potential conflict when foreigners seek

---

[1] Convention relating to the Status of Refugees, 189 UNTS 2545, done July 28, 1951, entered into force Apr. 22, 1954 (Refugee Convention).

entry into a territory governed by rules of conduct different from those that prevail in their home country. While it is generally conceded that the territorial sovereign may formally insist on compliance with prevailing standards as a condition of entry, there are often practical considerations which argue against such inflexibility.[2] Governments have long understood that it is sensible to attenuate otherwise valid laws to encourage the entry of desirable outsiders.

For example, the ancient Greeks accepted that their rules denying legal capacity to foreigners posed a barrier to the attraction of foreign craftsmen able to enrich the quality of their communal life. Their answer was the establishment of a separate legal regime to govern the conduct of skilled foreigners, the standards of which were sufficiently attractive to facilitate the desired level of settlement.[3] Similar practices evolved as part of the medieval law merchant. By the thirteenth century, it had become common for associations of traveling merchants to negotiate various forms of immunity and privilege with European rulers anxious to promote economic growth through foreign trade. These merchants were ultimately allowed to govern themselves, autonomously administering their own laws within the territory of foreign sovereigns.

The emergence of nation-states in the sixteenth century provided the context within which to formalize this ad hoc pattern of special rights granted to traders by various European rulers. Governments undertook the bilateral negotiation of treaties in which safe passage and basic civil rights were mutually guaranteed to merchants and others wishing to do business or to travel in the partner state. By the late nineteenth century, a network of "friendship, commerce, and navigation" treaties consistently guaranteed certain critical aspects of human dignity to aliens admitted to most trading states.[4] Because these agreements were pervasively implemented in the domestic laws of state parties, certain human rights universally guaranteed to aliens were identified as general principles of law.[5] These included recognition of the alien's juridical personality, respect for life and physical integrity, and personal and spiritual liberty within socially bearable limits. Aliens were afforded no political rights, though resident aliens were subject to reasonable public duties. In the economic sphere, there was a duty of

[2] See generally R. Lillich, *The Human Rights of Aliens in Contemporary International Law* (1984) (Lillich, *Rights of Aliens*), at 5–40.

[3] C. Phillipson, *The International Law and Custom of Ancient Greece and Rome* (1911), at 122–209.

[4] H. Walker, "Modern Treaties of Friendship, Commerce and Navigation," (1958) 42 *Minnesota Law Review* 805 (Walker, "Treaties of Friendship"), at 823.

[5] C. Amerasinghe, *State Responsibility for Injuries to Aliens* (1967) (Amerasinghe, *State Responsibility*), at 23; A. Roth, *The Minimum Standard of International Law Applied to Aliens* (1949) (Roth, *Minimum Standard*), at 113. See generally chapter 1.1.2 above.

non-discrimination among categories of aliens where they were allowed to engage in commercial activity. There was also an obligation to provide adequate compensation for denial of property rights where aliens were allowed to acquire private property. Finally, aliens were to be granted access to a fair and non-discriminatory judicial system to enforce these basic rights.[6]

The protection of aliens was not restricted to the few rights which attained the status of general principles of law. States heavily engaged in foreign commerce and investment were understandably anxious to garner additional protections for their nationals working abroad. They pursued this objective by continuing to negotiate bilateral treaties to supplement entitlements under the general alien rights regime. These particularized agreements allowed consenting governments mutually to accord a variety of rights to each other's citizens, to a degree befitting the importance attached to the bilateral relationship. An important innovation to emerge from this process of bilateral negotiation was the definition of aliens' rights by a combination of absolute and contingent standards of protection.[7]

The definition of rights in absolute terms, traditionally used at the national level, did not translate well to the framing of bilateral accords on alien protection. First, the meaning attributed to a particular entitlement (for example, freedom of internal movement) had always to be interpreted through the often divergent cultural and juridical lenses of each state party. The national state might, for example, assume that this right allowed the legally admitted alien to choose his or her place of residence in the receiving state, while the latter state intended it to mean only freedom to travel without restrictions. The definition of broad rights in absolute terms might therefore result not in strengthened protection, but instead in a lack of clarity.

Second, unambiguous, absolute standards could work to the long-term disadvantage of aliens residing in states in which rights were in evolution. Host states were not disposed continuously to renegotiate bilateral protection agreements, and were especially unlikely to entertain requests for amendment from foreign governments of modest influence. The citizens of less important states might therefore find themselves denied the benefits of protections extended to the nationals of more-favored countries. Even for the citizens of more influential countries, the definition of aliens' rights in absolute terms could be counter-productive: a static definition of rights would mean that new protections afforded citizens of the host country would not accrue automatically to even most-favored aliens.

To respond to these concerns, bilateral negotiations tended to couple absolute protection of a limited core of clearly understood rights with a

---

[6] This carefully constructed list of rights universally held by aliens was based on an empirical survey spanning 150 years: Roth, *Minimum Standard*, at 134–185.

[7] See generally Walker, "Treaties of Friendship," at 810–812.

broader range of entitlements loosely defined in contingent terms. The standard of protection for contingent rights was not discernible simply by reference to the literal scope of the treaty. It was set instead as a function of the relevant treatment accorded another group likely to secure maximum protection under the receiving state's laws, usually either the nationals of "most-favored" states, or the citizens of the state of residence itself. The precise content of the duty was therefore not fixed, but evolved in tandem with an exterior state of law and fact presumed to be a reliable benchmark of the best treatment that could be secured from the receiving state.

Walker aptly characterizes this system of contingent rights as providing for "built-in equalization and adjustment mechanisms."[8] The definition of aliens' rights by a combination of general principles of law and bilateral agreements of varying scope and rigor resulted in different classes of foreigners enjoying protection of sometimes different rights, and to differing degrees. All aliens, however, were in theory entitled to at least the benefit of the limited set of rights established by the general principles of aliens law. At first glance, international aliens law might therefore appear to be an important source of rights for refugees. After all, refugees are by definition persons who are outside the bounds of their own state.[9]

The general principles that emerged from the network of interstate arrangements on the protection of aliens do not, however, endow aliens themselves with rights and remedies. International aliens law was conceived very much within the traditional contours of international law: the rights created are the rights of national states, enforced at their discretion under the rules of diplomatic protection and international arbitration. While injured aliens may benefit indirectly from the assertion of claims by their national state, they can neither require action to be taken to vindicate their loss, nor even compel their state to share with them whatever damages are recovered in the event of a successful claim.[10] The theory underlying international aliens law is not the need to restore the alien to a pre-injury position. As summarized by Brierly, the system reflects "the plain truth that the injurious results of a denial of justice are not, or at any rate are not necessarily, confined to the

---

[8] Ibid. at 812.

[9] "[T]he term 'refugee' shall apply to any person who ... is outside the country of his nationality and is unable or, owing to such fear, is unwilling to avail himself of the protection of that country": Refugee Convention, at Art. 1(A)(2). See generally A. Grahl-Madsen, *The Status of Refugees in International Law* (vol. I, 1966) (Grahl-Madsen, *Status of Refugees I*), at 150–154; G. Goodwin-Gill, *The Refugee in International Law* (1996) (Goodwin-Gill, *Refugee in International Law*), at 40; and J. Hathaway, *The Law of Refugee Status* (1991) (Hathaway, *Refugee Status*), at 29–63.

[10] "The fate of the individual is worse than secondary in this scheme: it is doctrinally non-existent, because the individual, in the eyes of traditional international law, like the alien of the Greek city-State regime, is a non-person": Lillich, *Rights of Aliens*, at 12.

individual sufferer or his family, but include such consequences as the mistrust and lack of safety felt by other foreigners similarly situated."[11]

In any event, refugees are unlikely to derive even indirect protection from the general principles of aliens law because they lack the relationship with a state of nationality legally empowered to advance a claim to protection.[12] Aliens law is essentially an attempt to reconcile the conflicting claims of governments that arise when persons formally under the protection of one state are physically present in the sovereign territory of another. Whatever benefit accrues to the injured alien is incidental to resolution of this potential for interstate conflict. The essential condition for application of aliens law to refugees and stateless persons is therefore absent, since they are without a national state likely to view injuries done to them as a matter of official concern.

The emergence of general principles of aliens law nonetheless signaled a critical conceptual breakthrough in international law, which laid the groundwork for the subsequent development of the refugee rights regime. First, aliens law recognizes the special vulnerabilities which attend persons outside the bounds of their national state. Aliens have no right to participate in, or to influence, a foreign state's lawmaking process, yet are subjected to its rigors. As such, the domestic laws of the foreign state might, in the absence of international law, make no or inadequate provision for the alien to access meaningful protection against harm:

> [T]he individual, when he leaves his home State, abandons certain rights and privileges, which he possessed according to the municipal law of his State and which, to a certain limited extent, especially in a modern democracy, gave him control over the organization of the State ... In a foreign State, he is at the mercy of the State and its institutions, at the mercy of the inhabitants of the territory, who in the last resort accord him those rights and privileges which they deem desirable. This is a situation which hardly corresponds to modern standards of justice.[13]

---

[11] Cited in Amerasinghe, *State Responsibility*, at 59. As Amerasinghe demonstrates, however, many of the rules governing the procedures for assertion of a claim and calculation of damages are intimately related to the position of the injured alien: ibid. at 61–65.

[12] While no longer sustainable in view of obligations assumed by adherence to the United Nations Charter and particular treaties, the classical predicament of persons without a nationality is captured by L. Oppenheim, *International Law: A Treatise* (1912), at 369: "It is through the medium of their nationality only that individuals can enjoy benefits from the existence of the Law of Nations ... Such individuals as do not possess any nationality enjoy no protection whatever, and if they are aggrieved by a State they have no way to redress, there being no State that would be competent to take their case in hand. As far as the Law of Nations is concerned, apart from morality, there is no restriction whatever to cause a State to abstain from maltreating to any extent such stateless individuals."

[13] Roth, *Minimum Standard*, at 113.

Aliens law effects a minimalist accommodation of the most basic concerns of foreigners in the interest of continued international intercourse. It is a formal acknowledgment that commercial linkages and other aspects of national self-interest require legal systems to adapt to the reasonable expectations of non-nationals.

Second, the development of aliens law brought the vindication of particularized harms within the realm of international legal relations. A state which fails to live up to the minimum standards of protection owed to aliens can be forced to answer for its failures through the formal mechanisms of diplomatic protection and international arbitration. International law was transformed from a system focused solely on resolving the conflicting corporate interests of states, to a regime in which the particularized harms experienced by at least some individual human beings are subsumed within the definition of the national interest.

Third, given that international legal accountability would mean nothing without effective action, aliens law embraced surrogacy as the conceptual bridge between particularized harms and international enforceability. Because individuals are not recognized actors in international legal relations, all wrongs against a citizen are notionally transformed into harms done to the national state, which is deemed to enjoy a surrogate right to pursue accountability in its sole discretion.[14] This is not a trustee relationship, as national states are required neither to take the needs of the injured individual into account, nor to make restitution of any proceeds derived from enforcement. As unfair as it undoubtedly is that the persons who actually experience a loss abroad have so little control over process or recovery of damages, the surrogacy relationship implemented by international aliens law nonetheless serves the objective of forcing foreign states to take respect for the human dignity of aliens more seriously. As observed by Amerasinghe,

> International society as a whole is, perhaps, content to keep the law in a fairly undeveloped state. Thus, it has become more an instrument for keeping in check the powers of States vis à vis aliens, emanating from extreme theories of State sovereignty, than a reflection of the proper aspirations of an international society seeking to reconcile the conflicting interests of State and alien with a view to ensuring ideal justice for the individual.[15]

Fourth, and most specifically, the parallel system of bilateral agreements on the protection of aliens showed how rights could be defined across cultures, and

---

[14] "Nationality is a juridical and political link that unites an individual with a State and it is that link which enables a State to afford protection against all other States": L. Sohn and T. Buergenthal, *The Movement of Persons Across Borders* (1992) (Sohn and Buergenthal, *Movement of Persons*), at 39.

[15] Amerasinghe, *State Responsibility*, at 285.

in a way that maintained its currency in changing circumstances. Only a few clearly understood and established rights were normally phrased as absolute undertakings. For the most part, the standard of protection was set in contingent terms, effectively assimilating the aliens of the state parties either to "most-favored" foreigners or even to citizens of the territorial state. The objective of protection came therefore to be understood in terms of non-discrimination, extending to whatever core interests were viewed by the negotiating states as necessary to sustain the desired level of interstate relations.

2.2 International protection of minorities

A second body of law which influenced the structure of the international refugee rights regime was the League of Nations system for the protection of national minorities. Like aliens law, the Minorities Treaties which emerged after the First World War were intended to advance the interests of states. Their specific goal was to require vanquished states to respect the human dignity of resident ethnic and religious minorities, in the hope of limiting the potential for future international conflict:

> We are trying to make a peaceful settlement, that is to say, to eliminate those elements of disturbance, so far as possible, which may interfere with the peace of the world ... The chief burden of the war fell upon the greater Powers, and if it had not been for their action, their military action, we would not be here to settle these questions. And, therefore, we must not close our eyes to the fact that, in the last analysis, the military and naval strength of the Great Powers will be the final guarantee of the peace of the world ... Nothing, I venture to say, is more likely to disturb the peace of the world than the treatment which might in certain circumstances be meted out to minorities. And, therefore, if the Great Powers are to guarantee the peace of the world in any sense, is it unjust that they should be satisfied that the proper and necessary guarantee has been given?[16]

The Minorities Treaties marked a major advance over the conceptual framework of international aliens law. Whereas the concern under aliens law had been simply to set standards for the treatment abroad of a state's own nationals, the Minorities Treaties provided for external scrutiny of the relationship between foreign citizens and their own government. Minorities were guaranteed an extensive array of basic civil and political entitlements, access to public employment, the right to distinct social, cultural, and educational institutions, language rights, and an equitable share of public funding. The duty to respect these rights was imposed on the governments of defeated states as a condition precedent to the restoration of sovereign authority over their

---

[16] Speech by United States President Wilson to the Peace Conference, May 31, 1919, cited in L. Sohn and T. Buergenthal, *International Protection of Human Rights* (1973), at 216–217.

territories. While no formal international standing was granted to minority citizens themselves, enforcement of interstate obligations relied heavily on information garnered from petitions and other information provided by concerned individuals and associations. The welfare of particular human beings was thereby formally recognized as a legitimate matter of international attention.

Beyond their conceptual importance as limitations on state sovereignty over citizens, the Minorities Treaties also broke new ground in procedural terms. After the 1878 Treaty of Berlin, complaints had been made that victorious states took advantage of their right to supervise the protection of minorities to intervene oppressively in the vanquished states' internal affairs. Rather than overseeing the conduct of the defeated states directly, the Great Powers which emerged from the First World War therefore opted to establish the first international system of collectivized responsibility for the enforcement of human rights. The Great Powers requested the Council of the just-established League of Nations to serve as guarantor of the human rights obligations set by the Minorities Treaties. Once ratified, the treaties were submitted to the Council, which then resolved formally to take action in response to any risk of violation of the stipulated duties.[17] The League of Nations went on to establish an elaborate petition system to ensure that Council members had the benefit of the views of both minorities and respondent governments before taking action in a particular case.

This system was in no sense a universal mechanism to protect human rights. It was applicable only to states forced to accept minority rights provisions as part of the terms of peace, and to a smaller number of states that made general declarations to respect minority rights as a condition of admission to the League of Nations. Nor did the Minorities Treaties system challenge the hegemony of states as the only parties able to make and enforce international law. Petitions from minorities were a source of critical information to the League's Council, but did not enfranchise individuals or collectivities as participants in the enforcement process.

The minorities system nonetheless contributed in important ways to the evolution of both international human rights law and the refugee rights regime. The Minorities Treaties firmly established the propriety of international legal attention to the human rights of at-risk persons inside sovereign states. Whereas aliens law considered harms against individuals merely as evidence in the adjudication of competing claims by states, the system of minorities protection reversed the equation. The focus of concern became the well-being of the

---

[17] The Permanent Court of International Justice could be asked to render advisory opinions on contentious legal issues. See e.g. *Greco-Bulgarian Communities*, [1930] PCIJ Rep, Ser. B, No. 17; *Access to German Minority Schools in Upper Silesia*, [1931] PCIJ Rep, Ser. A/B, No. 40; *Minority Schools in Albania*, [1935] PCIJ Rep, Ser. A/B, No. 64.

minorities themselves, albeit a concern driven by the desire to avoid consequential harm to the peace and security of the international community.

Equally important, the Minorities Treaties provided the context for collectivization of international responsibility for supervision of human rights. They showed the viability of an enforcement process vested in the community of states, yet open to the voices of particular individuals and collectivities. In contrast to aliens law, the minorities system did not condition enforcement on the initiative of a particular state, but established a direct role for the international community itself in the assertion of human rights claims. This evolution was very important to refugees and stateless persons, who are by definition not in a position to look to their national state to protect their interests.

2.3 League of Nations codifications of refugee rights

Aliens law was the first legal system to deny the absolute right of states to treat persons within their jurisdiction in whatever manner they deemed appropriate. It recognized the special vulnerabilities of persons outside their national state, and established a combination of absolute and contingent duties owed to aliens. It was enforceable by a system of *interstate accountability*, operationalized at the bilateral level. The League of Nations system for protection of national minorities built on these achievements, but strengthened enforceability by replacing pure bilateral accountability with the first system of *collectivized surrogacy*. The concern of the international community was transformed from simply the facilitation of national protective efforts, to direct engagement as the source of residual protection for those whose interests were not adequately safeguarded by national governments. States were directly accountable to the international community for actions in disregard of human rights within their own borders. The legal framework for an international refugee rights regime draws on the progressive refinements achieved under these two systems.

The early efforts of the international community to protect refugees stemmed from a series of exoduses in the years following the end of the First World War: some 2 million Russians, Armenians, and others were forced to flee their countries between 1917 and 1926. The flight of these refugees unfortunately coincided with the emergence of modern systems of social organization throughout most of Europe. Governments began to regulate large parts of economic and social life, and to safeguard critical entitlements for the benefit of their own citizens. This commitment to enhanced investment in the well-being of their own citizenry led states to reassert the importance of definite boundaries between insiders and outsiders, seen most clearly in the reinforcement of passport and visa controls at their frontiers. Equally important, access to such important social goods as the right to work and public housing was often limited to persons able to prove citizenship.

The impact of this shift in European social organization was mitigated by the network of bilateral treaties of friendship, commerce, and navigation established under the rubric of international aliens law.[18] These agreements guaranteed the nationals of contracting states access while abroad to most of the benefits normally reserved for citizens. The essential precondition was reciprocity: the citizens of one state could expect benefits in the cooperating state only if their own government in turn ensured the rights of citizens of that partner state. If reciprocity was not respected, or if there was no bilateral arrangement between an individual's home state and the foreign country into which entry was sought, access to the territory, or at least to important social benefits, would likely be denied.

This reciprocity requirement was disastrous for early groups of refugees. Most had no valid identity or travel documents to prove their nationality in a cooperating state. Worse still, the 1.5 million Russian refugees who fled the Bolshevik Revolution were formally denationalized by the new Soviet government, and therefore clearly ineligible to benefit from any bilateral arrangement. Without documentation to establish their eligibility for entry and residence, refugees were either turned away or, if able to avoid border controls, barred from work and other regulated sectors. Lacking valid travel documents, they were not able to move onward from first asylum states in search of better living conditions. The result was many truly desperate people, often destitute and ill, unable either to return to their home state or to live decent lives abroad.

The first generation of refugee accords was an attempt to respond to the legally anomalous situation of refugees.[19] As observed by the League of Nations Advisory Commission for Refugees, "the characteristic and essential feature of the problem was that persons classed as 'refugees' have no regular nationality and are therefore deprived of the normal protection accorded to the regular citizens of a State."[20] Like all aliens, refugees were essentially at the mercy of the institutions of a foreign state. In contrast to other foreigners, however, refugees clearly could not seek the traditional remedy of diplomatic protection from their country of nationality:

> The refugee is an alien in any and every country to which he may go. He does not have the last resort which is always open to the "normal alien" – return to his own country. The man who is everywhere an alien has to live in unusually difficult material and psychological conditions. In most cases

---

[18] Bilateral aliens treaties are discussed above, at pp. 76–78.

[19] See generally J. Hathaway, "The Evolution of Refugee Status in International Law: 1920–1950," (1984) 33 *International and Comparative Law Quarterly* 348 (Hathaway, "Evolution of Refugee Status"), at 350–361.

[20] "Report by the Secretary-General on the Future Organisation of Refugee Work," LN Doc. 1930.XIII.2 (1930), at 3.

he has lost his possessions, he is penniless and cannot fall back on the various forms of assistance which a State provides for its nationals. Moreover, the refugee is not only an alien wherever he goes, he is also an "unprotected alien" in the sense that he does not enjoy the protection of his country of origin. Lacking the protection of the Government of his country of origin, the refugee does not enjoy a clearly defined status based upon the principle of reciprocity, as enjoyed by those nationals of those states which maintain normal diplomatic relations. The rights which are conferred on such nationals by virtue of their status, which is dependent upon their nationality, are generally unavailable to him. A refugee is an anomaly in international law, and it is often impossible to deal with him in accordance with the legal provisions designed to apply to aliens who receive assistance from their national authorities.[21]

Confronted by largely unstoppable flows of desperate people who did not fit the assumptions of the international legal system, states agreed that it was in their mutual self-interest to enfranchise refugees within the ranks of protected aliens. To have decided otherwise would have exposed them to the continuing social chaos of unauthorized and desperate foreigners in their midst. Equally important, it was understood that the credibility of border controls and of the restriction of socioeconomic benefits to nationals was at stake: by legitimating and defining a needs-based exception to the norm of communal closure, refugee law sustained the protectionist norm. So long as the admission of refugees was understood to be formally sanctioned by states, their arrival would cease to be legally destabilizing.

The mechanisms adopted to address the plight of refugees followed from experience under predecessor systems. As under aliens law, the fundamental goal was to adapt to the reasonable expectations of non-nationals in the interest of the continued well-being of the international system. This objective was implemented through the collectivized surrogacy model developed by the Minorities Treaties regime: refugees did not become the holders of particular rights, but were entitled to benefit from actions taken for them by a succession of League of Nations high commissioners. In particular, the League of Nations was empowered by various treaties and arrangements to respond to the legal incapacity of refugees by providing them with substitute documentation, which states agreed to treat as the functional equivalent of national passports. A system of surrogate consular protection emerged as well. Representatives of the High Commissioner were authorized by states to perform tasks normally reserved to states of nationality, such as establishing identity and civil status, and certifying educational and professional qualifications.

---

[21] "Communication from the International Refugee Organization to the Economic and Social Council," UN Doc. E/1392, July 11, 1949, at App. I.

These first refugee agreements did not set specific responsibilities for states, other than cooperation in the recognition of League of Nations documentation. There was generally no need for greater precision, as most European states continued to afford relatively generous benefits to the nationals of "most-favored states" to whom refugees were effectively assimilated. The refugee problem was moreover perceived by states to be a passing phenomenon, which would resolve itself either through consensual naturalization in the state of residence or by return of the refugee to the state of origin when conditions normalized.[22] There was accordingly no need to do more than bring refugees within the ranks of admissible foreigners.

The 1928 Arrangement relating to the Legal Status of Russian and Armenian Refugees,[23] however, departed from this pattern. Increasing political and economic instability, coupled with the persistence of the "temporary" refugee problem, had led some states to refuse to assimilate refugees to most-favored foreigners. As generosity subsided, the League of Nations elected to standardize the range of rights that should be extended to refugees. While framed as a series of non-binding recommendations to states, the 1928 Arrangement set standards for the recognition of personal status, and emphasized the inappropriateness of conditioning refugee rights on respect for reciprocity by their home state. The Arrangement also addressed a number of more detailed concerns, such as access to the courts, the right to work, protection against expulsion, equality in taxation, and the nature of national responsibilities to honor League of Nations identity certificates.

Reliance on moral suasion alone to induce uniform respect for the human dignity of refugees did not, however, prove satisfactory:

> The results so far secured, however, leave something to be desired as regards both the legal status and conditions of life of refugees. The replies received [from states] to the enquiry into the application of the Arrangement ... show that there is still much to be done before the position of refugees in all countries is such as no longer to call for strong and continued international action. The striking feature of the replies and of the established known facts is the comparative inefficacity of the recommendations.[24]

---

[22] "A final solution of the refugees problem can accordingly only be furnished by naturalisation in the countries in which the refugees reside, or by restoring their original nationality to them. As neither of these alternatives is possible *at the moment*, it has been necessary to institute a *provisional system of protection* which is embodied in the Inter-Governmental Arrangements of 1922, 1924, 1926 and 1928 [emphasis added]": "Report by the Secretary-General on the Future Organisation of Refugee Work," LN Doc. 1930.XIII.2 (1930), at 3.

[23] Arrangement relating to the Legal Status of Russian and Armenian Refugees, 89 LNTS 53, done June 30, 1928.

[24] "Report by the Inter-Governmental Advisory Commission for Refugees on the Work of its Fourth Session," 12(2) LN OJ 2118 (1931), at 2119.

The Great Depression had understandably fortified the resolve of states to preserve scarce entitlements for their own citizens. Unlike other foreigners who responded by leaving, however, refugees could not return home.

The dilemma was sufficiently serious that in 1933 the League of Nations Intergovernmental Commission, charged with oversight of refugee protection, argued that "[t]he desirability of a convention aiming at securing a more stable legal status for refugees [was] unanimously recognized,"[25] and that "the stabilization of the legal status of refugees can only, owing to the very nature of the steps to be taken, be brought about by a formal agreement concluded by a certain number of States concerned."[26] The resultant 1933 Convention relating to the International Status of Refugees[27] is one of the earliest examples of states agreeing to codify human rights as matters of binding international law.[28] Equally important, it opened the door to a new way of thinking about the human rights of aliens. Aliens' rights had previously been conceived to respond to a fixed set of circumstances, namely those typically encountered by traders and other persons traveling or residing abroad in pursuit of commercial opportunities.[29] Many risks faced by refugees in foreign states were, however, different from those which typically confronted business travelers. The Refugee Convention of 1933 met this challenge by setting a rights regime for a subset of the alien population, tailored to its specific vulnerabilities.

Many rights set by the 1933 Convention simply formalized and amplified the recommendations set out in the 1928 Arrangement. An important addition was the explicit obligation of states not to expel authorized refugees, and to avoid *refoulement*, defined to include "non-admittance at the frontier."[30] Three key socioeconomic rights were also added to the 1928 list. First, the Convention granted refugees some relief from the stringency of foreign labor restrictions, and proscribed limitations of any kind after three

---

[25] "Report of the Intergovernmental Commission and Communication from the Governing Body of the Nansen International Office," LN Doc. C.311.1933 (1933), at 1.

[26] "Work of the Inter-Governmental Advisory Commission for Refugees during its Fifth Session and Communication from the International Nansen Office for Refugees," 5(1) LN OJ 854 (1933), at 855.

[27] 159 LNTS 3663, done Oct. 28, 1933, entered into force June 13, 1935 (1933 Refugee Convention).

[28] The 1933 Refugee Convention established the second voluntary system of international supervision of human rights (preceded only by the 1926 Slavery Convention, 60 LNTS 253, done Sept. 25, 1926, entered into force Mar. 9, 1927).

[29] See chapter 2.1 above, at pp. 76–77.

[30] "Each of the Contracting Parties undertakes not to remove or keep from its territory by application of police measures, such as expulsions or non-admittance at the frontier (*refoulement*), refugees who have been authorised to reside there regularly, unless the said measures are dictated by reasons of national security or public order": 1933 Refugee Convention, at Art. 3.

years' residence, where the refugee was married to or the parent of a national, or was an ex-combatant of the First World War. Second, refugees were granted access to the host state's welfare and relief system, including medical care and workers' compensation. Third, access to education was to be facilitated, including by the remission of fees. This enumeration was later said to have "confer[red] upon refugees the maximum legal advantages which it had been possible to afford them in practice."[31]

The 1933 Convention drew on the precedent of aliens law to establish a mixed absolute and contingent rights structure. Some rights, including recognition of legal status and access to the courts, were guaranteed absolutely. More commonly, one of three contingent rights formulations was used. Refugees were to have access to work, social welfare, and most other rights on the same terms as the nationals of most-favored nations. Exceptionally, as with liability to taxation, refugees were assimilated to citizens of the host state. Education rights, conversely, were mandated only to the extent provided to foreigners generally. This pattern of variant levels of obligation toward refugees continues to the present day.[32] It is noteworthy, however, that the 1933 Convention guaranteed almost all refugee rights either absolutely or on terms of equivalency with the citizens of most-favored states.

In practice, however, the 1933 Convention did not significantly expand refugee rights. Only eight states ratified the treaty, several with major reservations. The assimilation of refugees to most-favored foreigners in any event proved an inadequate guarantee of reasonable treatment, as the intensification of the unemployment crisis led states to deny critical social benefits, including the right to work, even to established foreigners:

> Some countries have found it necessary to introduce restrictions on the employment of foreign workers and, as a result, refugees who had been employed for years have been deprived of their livelihood, while in other countries, as a result of these restrictions, refugees have become vagrants, and this has been considered a sufficient reason for their expulsion. Unlike other foreigners in a similar position, these refugees could not be repatriated. Their lot has become a tragic one, since they have been obliged to enter first one country and then another illegally; many of them are thus compelled to live as outlaws.[33]

The strategy of assimilating refugees to aliens, while valuable in the earlier, more cosmopolitan era, now condemned refugees to real hardships. Yet

---

[31] "Work of the Inter-Governmental Advisory Commission for Refugees during its Eighth Session," LN Doc. C.17.1936.XII (1936), at 156.

[32] See chapters 3.2 and 3.3 below.

[33] "Report Submitted to the Sixth Committee to the Assembly of the League of Nations: Russian, Armenian, Assyrian, Assyro-Chaldean, Saar and Turkish Refugees," LN Doc. A.45.1935.XII (1935).

return home had not been possible for most refugees, and few European states had agreed to grant naturalization.[34]

One answer to this dilemma would have been to extend national treatment to refugees. The League of Nations, however, was engaged in a rearguard action intended simply to preserve the "most-favored alien" guarantees secured under the 1933 Convention. Some states were unwilling to grant refugees rights even at this level of obligation. Others declined to sign the accord for fear that the intensifying economic crisis might force them to renounce the Convention peremptorily, in breach of its one-year notice requirement. Rather than expanding rights, therefore, the international agenda was very much focused on easing the requirements of the 1933 Convention or even drafting a new, more flexible, accord to induce states to bind themselves to some standard of treatment, even if a less exigent one.[35] This was hardly the moment to make progress on a more inclusive rights regime for refugees.

The extent of the retreat from meaningful protection of refugees can be seen in the 1936 Provisional Arrangement concerning the Status of Refugees coming from Germany.[36] While continuing the approach of stipulating legally binding duties of states, no attempt was made to guarantee refugees more than identity certificates, protection from expulsion, recognition of personal status, and access to the courts. Even at that level, only seven states adhered. As it worked to establish a more definitive regime for refugees from the German Reich, the League of Nations was therefore drawn to two critical points of consensus. First, given the insecurity about economic and political circumstances, governments were likely to sign only if able quickly to renounce obligations. Second, and more profoundly, it was understood that truly adequate protection would be provided only if refugee rights were effectively assimilated to those of nationals, a proposition flatly rejected by most European states. Unlike the countries of Europe, however, most overseas countries of resettlement were "inclined to offer greater facilities for the naturalization of refugees."[37] The League of Nations therefore decided that

---

[34] "Unfortunately, for various reasons, [naturalisation] encountered considerable difficulties even before countries became reluctant, owing to their unemployment problems, to increase the number of workers ... [A] surprisingly small percentage of refugees had succeeded in obtaining naturalisation, and those modest results, combined with existing political and economic conditions, do not suggest that too much hope should be pinned to naturalisation as a general and early remedy for the refugee problem in Europe": ibid. at 2.

[35] "Work of the Inter-Governmental Advisory Commission for Refugees during its Eighth Session," LN Doc. C.17.1936.XII (1936), at 156–157.

[36] 3952 LNTS 77, done July 4, 1936.

[37] "Report Submitted by the Sixth Committee to the Assembly: Russian, Armenian, Assyrian, Assyro-Chaldean, Saar and Turkish Refugees," LN Doc. A.45.1935.XII (1935), at 2.

"[a] suitable distribution of refugees among the different countries might help to solve the problem."[38]

The resulting 1938 Convention concerning the Status of Refugees coming from Germany[39] reflected this shift. While most of the rights mirrored the comprehensive list established by the 1933 Convention, two new provisions of note were included. Art. 25 reversed the position of the predecessor 1933 Convention, allowing states to accede to the regime without committing themselves to give any notice before renouncing it. While it was hoped that this new flexibility would encourage states to adhere for as long as circumstances allowed, in fact only three states – Belgium, France, and the United Kingdom – ultimately agreed to be bound by it (none of which availed itself of the early renunciation option). The more prophetic novation of the 1938 Convention stipulated that "[w]ith a view of facilitating the emigration of refugees to oversea countries, every facility shall be granted to the refugees and to the organizations which deal with them for the establishment of schools for professional re-adaptation and technical training."[40] In light of the unwillingness of European states to grant meaningful rights to refugees, there was indeed no option other than to pursue the resettlement of refugees in states outside the region.

This adoption of what Coles has styled an "exilic bias" in refugee law[41] led to a de-emphasis on the elaboration of standards to govern refugee rights. Between 1938 and the adoption of the present Refugee Convention in 1951, the consistent emphasis of a succession of treaties and intergovernmental arrangements was to resettle overseas any refugees who could not be expected to integrate or repatriate within a reasonable time. As the countries to which refugees were relocated agreed to assimilate them to citizens, the traditional need to address the legal incapacity of refugees through the guarantee of a catalog of rights was considered no longer to exist.

The early refugee agreements, in particular the 1933 Convention, nonetheless provided the model for two conceptual transitions at the heart of the modern refugee rights regime. First, they introduced the idea of freely accepted international supervision of national compliance with human rights. This quiet revolution in thinking transformed collective supervision of human rights from a penalty to be paid by subordinate states, as under the League of Nations Minorities Treaties system, to a means of advancing the shared objectives of states through cooperation. Of equal importance, the

---

[38] "Work of the Inter-Governmental Advisory Commission for Refugees during its Eighth Session," LN Doc. C.17.1936.XII (1936), at 159.

[39] 192 LNTS 4461, done Feb. 10, 1938 (1938 Refugee Convention).

[40] Ibid. at Art. 15.

[41] G. Coles, "Approaching the Refugee Problem Today," in G. Loescher and L. Monahan eds., *Refugees and International Relations* 373 (1990).

1928 and subsequent accords reshaped the substance of the human rights guaranteed to aliens. Rather than simply enfranchising refugees within the traditional aliens law regime, states tailored and expanded those general principles to meet the real needs of refugees. The consequential decisions to waive reciprocity, and to guarantee basic civil and economic rights in law, served as a direct precedent for a variety of international human rights projects, including the modern refugee rights regime.

2.4 The Convention relating to the Status of Refugees

In the years immediately following the Second World War, the international community pursued the repatriation of European refugees when possible, failing which an effort was made to arrange for overseas resettlement. There was a fortuitous coalescence of interests, as the postwar economic boom in states of the New World had opened doors to new sources of labor. The scale of the resettlement project was massive: between 1947 and 1951, the International Refugee Organization (IRO) relocated more than 1 million Europeans to the Americas, Israel, Southern Africa, and Oceania. The IRO had its own specialized staff, a fleet of more than forty ships, and, most important, enjoyed the political and economic support of the developed world.[42]

As the June 1950 date for termination of the mandate of the IRO neared, it was clear that not all Second World War refugees could be either repatriated or resettled. A strategy was moreover needed to address impending refugee flows from the Communist states of the East Bloc. In this context, the United Nations proposed the effective assimilation of all stateless persons, including refugees, under a new international regime.[43] While political antagonism undermined realization of this holistic vision,[44] a process was initiated which led ultimately both to the establishment of the United Nations High Commissioner for Refugees (UNHCR), and to the preparation of the 1951 Refugee Convention. This Convention, which remains the cornerstone of modern international refugee law, resurrected the earlier commitment to codification of legally binding refugee rights.

---

[42] See generally L. Holborn, *The International Refugee Organization: A Specialized Agency of the United Nations* (1956); Independent Commission on International Humanitarian Issues, *Refugees: The Dynamics of Displacement* (1986), at 32–38.

[43] United Nations Department of Social Affairs, "A Study of Statelessness," UN Doc. E/1112, Feb. 1, 1949 (United Nations, "Statelessness").

[44] See J. Hathaway, "A Reconsideration of the Underlying Premise of Refugee Law," (1990) 31(1) *Harvard International Law Journal* 129, at 144–151.

In part, the desire of states to reach international agreement on the human rights of refugees was simply a return to pre-Depression traditions.[45] States had always understood that it was in their self-interest to ensure that the arrival and presence of refugees did not become a socially destabilizing force.[46] While desperate circumstances at the end of the Second World War had led to massive intergovernmental efforts to resettle refugees overseas, the restoration of relative normalcy now prompted states to demand a return to greater individuated control over the process of refugee protection.[47] It was argued that the appropriate level of interstate coordination of refugee protection could be secured through the moral suasion of a high commissioner armed with agreed common standards of conduct.[48] In most cases, however, states could again be counted on to facilitate the integration of those refugees who were unable to return home.[49]

This return to particularized responsibility would be feasible, however, only if it were possible simultaneously to consolidate the commitment of other states to accept a share of responsibility for the European refugee burden.[50] Born of political and strategic solidarity, and nourished by economic advantage, the postwar resettlement effort had proved extremely

[45] "If the General Council accepts the recommendation ... with regard to the termination of the [International Refugee] Organization's care and maintenance programme, the Director-General [of IRO] assumes that Governments will wish to revert to their traditional pre-war policy in granting material assistance to refugees. Thus individual Governments would undertake to provide for any necessary care and maintenance of refugees living on their territories": "Communication from the International Refugee Organization to the Economic and Social Council," UN Doc. E/1392, July 11, 1949, at 8.

[46] "The stateless person in the country he is able to reach and which is ready to admit him usually finds no encouragement to settle there. And yet, if he is not to remain beyond the pale of society and to become an 'international vagabond' he must be integrated in the economic life of the country and settle down": United Nations, "Statelessness," at 23. See generally chapter 2.3 above, at pp. 84–85.

[47] "[T]he proposal to set up a high commissioner's office would give that institution the functions of coordination and liaison, and would leave to States the political responsibility which should properly be theirs. The time had come to impose that responsibility on States. The principal States concerned in the refugee problem, in fact, were claiming it": Statement of Mr. Fenaux of Belgium, 9 UNESCOR (326th mtg.), at 618 (1949).

[48] "The French and Belgian Governments considered that an international convention was essential to settle the details of the measures which national authorities would have to put into effect": Statement of Mr. Rochefort of France, ibid.

[49] "Existing conventions which were limited in scope needed to be brought up-to-date and a new consolidated draft convention prepared ... The 1933 Convention could be used as a basis for the new convention": Statement of Mr. Rundall of the United Kingdom, ibid. at 623.

[50] "In effect, an appeal was made to all governments to accord the same treatment to all refugees, in order to reduce the burden on contracting governments whose geographical situation meant that the greater part of the responsibility fell on them": Statement of Mr. Desai of India, UN Doc. E/AC.7/SR.166, at 18 (1950). See also Statement of Mr. Rochefort

important to recovery efforts in Western Europe. Europeans were therefore anxious to enlist external support to insure against the prospect of purely European responsibility for refugee flows from Eastern and Central Europe. The experience of the IRO had shown that the willingness of refugees to resettle outside Europe was contingent on the establishment of a common denominator of basic entitlements in overseas states. The IRO had thus regularly negotiated bilateral agreements with resettlement states to ensure the protection of refugees, particularly during the period before they were naturalized. With the impending termination of the IRO's mandate, the establishment of a guaranteed core of refugee rights was therefore a critical element in maintaining the viability of overseas resettlement as a residual answer to refugee protection needs. Access by refugees to work and social security were especially crucial.[51]

The modern system of refugee rights was therefore conceived out of enlightened self-interest. To the prewar understanding of assimilation as a source of internal stability were added concerns to promote burden-sharing and to set the conditions within which states could independently control a problem of interstate dimensions:

> This phase, which will begin after the dissolution of the International Refugee Organization, will be characterized by the fact that the refugees will lead an independent life in the countries which have given them shelter. With the exception of the "hard core" cases, the refugees will no longer be maintained by an international organization as they are at present. They will be integrated in the economic system of the countries of asylum and will themselves provide for their own needs and for those of their families. This will be a phase of the settlement and assimilation of the refugees. Unless the refugee consents to repatriation, the final result of that phase will be his integration in the national community which has given him shelter. It is essential for the refugee to enjoy an equitable and stable status, if he is to lead a normal existence and become assimilated rapidly.[52]

2.4.1 Substantive rights

The substantive rights set by the Convention have their origins in two main sources. Most of the entitlements are derived from the 1933 Refugee

of France, 9 UNESCOR (326th mtg.), at 616 (1949): "Not the least of the merits of the International Refugee Organization was that it had enlisted many distant countries in the work of providing asylum for refugees, the burden of which had for long been supported by the countries of Europe alone."

[51] Communication from the International Refugee Organization to the Economic and Social Council, UN Doc. E/1392, July 11, 1949, at paras. 35–37.

[52] "Memorandum by the Secretary-General to the Ad Hoc Committee on Statelessness and Related Problems," UN Doc. E/AC.32/2, Jan. 3, 1950, at 6–7.

Convention, explicitly acknowledged to be the model for the 1951 agreement. A key secondary source, however, was the 1948 Universal Declaration of Human Rights.[53] It influenced the redrafting of the content of several rights found in the 1933 Refugee Convention, and accounted for six additions to the earlier formulation of refugee rights.[54] Of the four rights with no obvious predecessor, the cryptically named right to "administrative assistance" essentially codifies the assumption by state parties of the consular role previously played by the high commissioners for refugees of the League of Nations.[55] Three provisions, namely protection against penalization for illegal entry, exemption from exceptional measures applied against co-nationals, and the right to transfer externally acquired assets to a country of resettlement,[56] represent net additions to the conceptualization of refugee rights.

The rights set by the Refugee Convention include several critical protections which speak to the most basic aspects of the refugee experience, including the need to escape, to be accepted, and to be sheltered. Under the Convention, refugees are not to be penalized for seeking protection, nor exposed to the risk of return to their state of origin. They are entitled to a number of basic survival and dignity rights, as well as to documentation of their status and access to national courts for the enforcement of their rights.

Beyond these basic rights, refugees are also guaranteed a more expansive range of civil and socioeconomic rights. While falling short of the comprehensive list of civil rights promoted by the Universal Declaration of Human Rights, the Refugee Convention nonetheless pays significantly more attention to the definition of a sphere of personal freedom for refugees than did any of the earlier refugee agreements. The inability of states to make any reservations

---

[53] Universal Declaration of Human Rights, UNGA Res. 217A(III), Dec. 10, 1948 (Universal Declaration).

[54] These include the rights to non-discrimination, housing, naturalization, property, freedom of internal movement, and religious freedom. As a general matter, there was an assumption that rights declared in the Universal Declaration of Human Rights formed the clear backdrop to the Refugee Convention. In the words of the British delegate, "a Convention relating to refugees could not include an outline of all the articles of the Universal Declaration of Human Rights; furthermore, by its universal character, the Declaration applied to all human groups without exception and it was pointless to specify that its provisions applied also to refugees": Statement of Sir Leslie Brass of the United Kingdom, UN Doc. E/AC.32/SR.11, Jan. 25, 1950, at 8. Yet it is equally clear that there was no appetite on the part of all delegates to codify in binding form all of the rights recognized in the Declaration. France, for example, was of the view that the Refugee Convention ought not to render binding the full notion of freedom of opinion and expression codified in Art. 19 of the Universal Declaration of Human Rights: Statement of Mr. Rain of France, ibid. at 9.

[55] Refugee Convention, at Art. 25. See chapter 2.3 above, at pp. 85–86.

[56] Refugee Convention, at Arts. 31 ("refugees unlawfully in the country of refuge"), 8 ("exemption from exceptional measures"), and 30 ("transfer of assets").

to their obligation to guarantee protection against discrimination, religious freedom, and access to the courts entrenches a universal minimum guarantee of basic liberties for refugees.[57]

Of particular importance are the guarantees of key socioeconomic rights that integrate refugees in the economic system of the country of asylum or settlement, enabling them to provide for their own needs. Basic rights to property and work are supplemented by a guarantee of access to the asylum country's social safety net. Refugees are also to be treated as citizens under labor and tax legislation. There are important parallels between these key socioeconomic rights and those negotiated under the 1939 and 1949 migrant labor conventions of the International Labor Organization (ILO).[58] The ILO pioneered international legal protections against economic vulnerability, challenging the assumption of aliens law that persons outside their own country require only guarantees of basic civil rights.[59] Recognizing that refugees, like migrant workers, face the risk of economic marginalization and exploitation, the 1951 Refugee Convention goes a substantial distance toward enfranchising refugees within the structures of the social welfare state.

Finally, the Convention establishes rights of solution, intended to assist refugees to bring their refugee status to an end. The promotion of repatriation is not addressed, consistent with the position of the drafters that return should result only from the voluntary decision of a particular refugee,[60] or in consequence of a determination by the asylum state that the basis for the individual's claim to protection has ceased to exist.[61] In contrast, provision is made for the issuance of travel documents and transfer of assets that would be necessary upon resettlement, and also for the alternative of naturalization in the asylum state.

2.4.2 Reservations

Refugee Convention, Art. 42   Reservations
    1. At the time of signature, ratification or accession, any State may make reservations to articles of the Convention other than to articles 1, 3, 4, 16(1), 33, 36–46 inclusive.
    2. Any State making a reservation in accordance with paragraph 1 of this article may at any time withdraw the reservation

---

[57] Ibid. at Art. 42(1). Protection against *refoulement* is similarly insulated from reservations by state parties.

[58] See chapter 2.5.4 below, at pp. 152–153.   [59] See chapter 2.1 above, at pp. 76–77.

[60] See chapter 2.4 above, at p. 93; and generally chapter 7.2 below.

[61] Refugee Convention, at Art. 1(C). See generally Grahl-Madsen, *Status of Refugees I*, at 367–411; Hathaway, *Refugee Status*, at 189–214; and chapter 7.1 below.

by a communication to that effect addressed to the Secretary-General of the United Nations.

All substantive rights other than to non-discrimination, freedom of religion, access to the courts, and protection against *refoulement* may be excluded or modified by a state through reservation upon signature, ratification, or accession to the Convention.[62] An evaluation of refugee rights in any particular state therefore requires that account be taken of the terms of participation consented to by the state in question.[63] The requirement that refugees lawfully staying in an asylum state benefit from the same right to access wage-earning employment as most-favored foreigners has attracted the largest number of reservations.[64] There has also been a noticeable reluctance fully to embrace the rights of refugees to enrol in public schools, benefit from labor and social security legislation, and enjoy freedom of movement within the territory of the asylum state.[65]

2.4.3 Temporal and geographical restrictions

Refugee Convention, Art. 1   Definition of the term "refugee"
A. For the purposes of the present Convention, the term "refugee" shall apply to any person who: . . . (2) [a]s a result of events occurring before 1 January 1951 and owing to well-founded fear of being persecuted for reasons of race, religion, nationality, membership of a particular social group or political opinion, is outside the country of his nationality and is unable, or owing to

---

[62] The Executive Committee of the High Commissioner's Program has, however, voted to endorse an Agenda for Protection which stipulates that "States Parties [are] to give consideration to withdrawing reservations lodged at the time of accession and, where appropriate, to work towards lifting the geographical reservation": "Declaration of States Parties to the 1951 Convention and/or its 1967 Protocol relating to the Status of Refugees," UN Doc. HCR/MMSP/2001/09, Dec. 13, 2001, incorporated in Executive Committee of the High Commissioner's Program, "Agenda for Protection," UN Doc. EC/52/SC/CRP.9/Rev.1, June 26, 2002, at Part III, Goal 1, Point 1. More generally, the International Law Commission is presently preparing a Guide to Practice on the question of reservations to treaties, including recommendations with respect to the withdrawal or modification of reservations and interpretive declarations: "Report of the International Law Commission on the Work of its 55th Session," UN Doc. A/CN.4/537, Jan. 21, 2004, at paras. 170–200.

[63] See generally S. Blay and M. Tsamenyi, "Reservations and Declarations under the 1951 Convention and the 1967 Protocol relating to the Status of Refugees," (1990) 2(4) *International Journal of Refugee Law* 527.

[64] Twenty-one governments have qualified their acceptance of at least some part of Art. 17 (wage-earning employment) of the Refugee Convention: UNHCR, "Declarations under section B of Article 1 of the Convention," available at www.unhcr.ch (accessed Apr. 13, 2004).

[65] Arts. 22 (public education), 24 (labor legislation and social security) and 26 (freedom of movement) have each attracted nine or more reservations: ibid.

such fear, is unwilling to avail himself of the protection of that country; or who, not having a nationality and being outside the country of his former habitual residence as a result of such events, is unable or, owing to such fear, is unwilling to return to it …

> B. (1) for the purposes of this Convention, the words "events occurring before 1 January 1951" in article 1, section A, shall be understood to mean either
>
> (a) "events occurring in Europe before 1 January 1951"; or
>
> (b) "events occurring in Europe or elsewhere before 1 January 1951";
>
> and each Contracting State shall make a declaration at the time of signature, ratification or accession, specifying which of these meanings it applies for the purpose of its obligations under this Convention.

It is moreover possible for a government to restrict its obligations on temporal or geographical grounds. As initially conceived, a state party to the 1951 Refugee Convention could elect to limit its obligations to persons whose fear of being persecuted was the result of events which occurred before January 1, 1951. The 1967 Protocol relating to the Status of Refugees[66] abolishes this temporal limitation for the overwhelming majority of states that have agreed also to be bound by its terms. However, four governments acceded to the Refugee Convention, but have not gone on to adopt the Protocol. Madagascar, Monaco, Namibia, and St. Kitts and Nevis are therefore under no legal duty to honor the Refugee Convention in respect to the claims of contemporary refugees.

Art. 1(B) of the Refugee Convention also allows a government to restrict its obligations on a geographical basis, specifically to protect only European refugees. In addition to availing themselves of the temporal limitation discussed in the preceding paragraph, Madagascar and Monaco have also chosen to invoke this prerogative to avoid legal responsibility toward non-European refugees. The terms of the Refugee Protocol also allow the governments of Congo, Malta, and Turkey to maintain in force a previously declared geographical restriction to European refugees, even while acceding to the Protocol. This option, however, is available only to states which had entered a geographical reservation under the Refugee Convention before the adoption of the Refugee Protocol in 1967.[67] Because Hungary acceded to the

---

[66] Protocol relating to the Status of Refugees, 606 UNTS 8791, done Jan. 31, 1967, entered into force Oct. 4, 1967 (Refugee Protocol).

[67] "The present Protocol shall be applied by the States Parties hereto without any geographic limitation, save that *existing declarations* made by States already Parties to the Convention in accordance with article 1B(1)(a) of the Convention, shall, unless extended under article 1B(2) thereof, apply also under the present Protocol [emphasis added]": Refugee Protocol, at Art. I(3).

Refugee Convention and Protocol only in 1989, it did not meet this requirement. Its attempt to sustain a geographical limitation upon accession to the
Protocol was therefore legally invalid, perhaps explaining the withdrawal of
the same in 1998.

2.4.4 Duties of refugees

Governments may legitimately expect refugees to comply with general laws,
regulations, and public order measures. Such obligations may not, however,
treat refugees less favorably than other resident aliens. Most important, there
is no reciprocity of rights and obligations under the Refugee Convention.
While refugees who breach valid laws of the host country are clearly subject to
the usual range of penalties, states are prohibited from invoking the failure of
refugees to comply with generally applicable duties as grounds for the withdrawal of rights established under the Convention.

> **Refugee Convention, Art. 2   General obligations**
> **Every refugee has duties to the country in which he finds himself,**
> **which require in particular that he conform to its laws and regula-**
> **tions as well as to measures taken for the maintenance of public**
> **order.**

The original draft of the Refugee Convention contained a chapter that
imposed three kinds of obligation on refugees: to obey laws, pay taxes, and
perform military and other kinds of civic service.[68] The duty to respect the
law was simply "a reminder of the essential duties common to nationals as
well as to foreigners in general."[69] Liability to taxation and military conscription on the same terms as citizens was viewed as a fair contribution to expect
from a refugee "residing in the country of asylum, enjoying a satisfactory
status, and earning his living there."[70] Just as refugees should benefit from
most of the advantages that accrue to nationals, so too should they assume
reasonable duties toward the state that afforded them protection.

There were two quite different reactions to the proposal to codify the
duties owed by refugees to an asylum state. A number of governments felt
that such a provision was superfluous in view of the general duty of foreigners
to obey the laws of their country of residence.[71] Moreover, as the American

---

[68] United Nations, "Memorandum by the Secretary-General to the Ad Hoc Committee on
Statelessness and Related Problems," UN Doc. E/AC.32/2, Jan. 3, 1950, at 31–33. Chapter IV
was entitled "Responsibilities of Refugees and Obligations Incumbent upon Them."
[69] Ibid. at 31.   [70] Ibid. at 32.
[71] "[T]he article was unnecessary, as it contained nothing which was not obvious. Indeed, it
was generally known that the laws of a country applied not only to its nationals but also to
the foreigners residing in its territory, whether they were refugees or not": Statement of

representative argued, "refugees themselves would not be signing the Convention and would not be asked to do any more than anyone else in the country in which they took refuge."[72] In legal terms, "[i]t was impossible to write into a convention an obligation resting on persons who were not parties thereto."[73] It was therefore suggested that there was no need to include specific mention of the obligations of refugees.

However, France and several other states were adamant that

> such a provision [was] indispensable. It would have a moral application in all countries where there was no obligation on the immigrant alien to take an oath of loyalty or allegiance or to renounce [one's] former nationality. The purpose ... was not to bring about the forcible absorption of refugees into the community, but to ensure that their conduct and behavior was in keeping with the advantages granted them by the country of asylum.[74]

These countries had little patience for the argument that refugees were already obliged to respect the laws of their host states:

> [I]t should not be forgotten that what to some seemed obvious did not, unfortunately, square with the facts. That was proved by France's experience. The obligations of refugees should therefore be stressed and an appropriate clause inserted. Too often the refugee was far from conforming to the rules of the community ... Often, too, the refugee exploited the community.[75]

Largely out of respect for the significant refugee protection contributions made by France,[76] it was decided to include a specific reference in the Convention to the duties of refugees. The compromise was that while

Mr. Larsen of Denmark, UN Doc. E/AC.32/SR.11, Jan. 25, 1950, at 10. See also Statement of Mr. Guerreiro of Brazil, ibid., and Statement of Mr. Kural of Turkey, ibid. at 11. "Since an alien is subject to the territorial supremacy of the local state, it may apply its laws to aliens in its territory, and they must comply with and respect those laws": R. Jennings and A. Watts eds., *Oppenheim's International Law* (1992), at 905. See also chapter 2.1 above, at p. 76.

[72] Statement of Mr. Henkin of the United States, UN Doc. E/AC.32/SR.34, Aug. 14, 1950, at 7.

[73] Statement of Mr. Herment of Belgium, UN Doc. A/CONF.2/SR.3, July 3, 1951, at 22.

[74] Statement of Mr. Rochefort of France, UN Doc. E/AC.32/SR.34, Aug. 14, 1950, at 4. See also Statements of Mr. Perez Perozo of Venezuela and Mr. Herment of Belgium, ibid. at 5. A similarly exigent understanding of the duties owed by refugees is clear in remarks made by Mr. Robinson of Israel, UN Doc. E/AC.32/SR.12, Jan. 25, 1950, at 7: "[A] refugee was a foreigner *sui generis* to whom the draft convention accorded special status and in certain cases even equality with the nationals of the recipient country. The refugee thus obtained certain privileges and it was only fair to balance those by conferring upon him *greater* responsibilities [emphasis added]."

[75] Statement of Mr. Rochefort of France, UN Doc. E/AC.32/SR.34, Aug. 14, 1950, at 7–8.

[76] See e.g. Statements of Mr. Henkin of the United States, UN Doc. E/AC.32/SR.23, Feb. 3, 1950, at 8 and UN Doc. E/AC.32/SR.34, Aug. 14, 1950, at 6–7; and Statement of Mr. Robinson of Israel, UN Doc. A/CONF.2/SR.4, July 3, 1951, at 8.

refugees would not be subject to any particularized duties, the Convention would make clear that refugee status may not be invoked to avoid whatever general responsibilities are imposed upon other residents of the host country.[77] The notion of a specific enumeration of refugee duties was dropped.[78]

The unwillingness of the drafters to subject refugees to special duties can most clearly be seen in the debate about regulation of the political activities of refugees. It was argued that refugees tend to be more politically active than other immigrants,[79] and that their militancy could threaten the security interests of an asylum state.[80] The French government therefore proposed to allow governments "to restrict or prohibit political activity on the part of refugees."[81] Strong exception was taken to this proposal, both on grounds of general principle and because it suggested a right to treat refugees less favorably than other resident foreigners.[82] The result was agreement that while "laws prohibiting or restricting political activity for foreigners generally

---

[77] The essence of the French plea could be satisfied by the inclusion of "a moral *per contra*" falling short of an enforceable legal duty: Statement of Mr. Rochefort of France, UN Doc. E/AC.32/SR.34, Aug. 14, 1950, at 4.

[78] "[T]he Committee had altered the structure of the draft convention, which was meant to cover the liabilities as well as the rights of refugees": Statement of Mr. Weis of the International Refugee Organization, UN Doc. E/AC.32/SR.12, Jan. 25, 1950, at 10.

[79] "It was not too difficult to ask a foreign national to leave the country but it was often virtually impossible to expel a refugee. Different measures had to be taken for the two groups. Moreover, it had been the experience of some States that foreign nationals rarely engaged in political activity, while refugees frequently did so": Statement of Mr. Cuvelier of Belgium, UN Doc. E/AC.32/SR.23, Feb. 3, 1950, at 10–11.

[80] A restriction of the political rights of refugees "should not be regarded as a discriminatory measure against refugees but rather as a security measure. While it was embarrassing to favour the withdrawal of rights from a group of people, it would be better to do that than to expose that group of people – refugees – to the more drastic alternative of deportation": Statement of Mr. Devinat of France, ibid. at 9. See also Statement of Mr. Larsen of Denmark, UN Doc. E/AC.32/SR.10, Jan. 24, 1950, at 10: "[R]efugees who had found freedom and security in another country should not be permitted to engage in political activity which might endanger that country."

[81] France, "Proposal for a Draft Convention," UN Doc. E/AC.32/L.3, Jan. 17, 1950 (France, "Draft Convention"), at Art. 8, General Obligations. See also Statement of Mr. Kural of Turkey, UN Doc. E/AC.32/SR.23, Feb. 3, 1950, at 11: "[S]ince the draft convention was to be a definitive document governing the status of refugees, it might conveniently be invoked by the latter in order to sanction undesirable political activity."

[82] "[H]e regarded it as undesirable to include in a United Nations document a clause prohibiting political activities – a very broad and vague concept indeed . . . In the absence of a specific clause on the subject, [governments] would still have the right to restrict political activities of refugees as of any other foreigners. On the other hand, the inclusion of the clause might imply international sanction of such a restriction. The possibility of such an interpretation was undesirable": Statement of Mr. Henkin of the United States, UN Doc. E/AC.32/SR.23, Feb. 3, 1950, at 8. See also Statements of Mr. Chance of Canada and Mr. Larsen of Denmark, ibid. at 9.

would be equally applicable to refugees,"[83] the Convention would not authorize states to impose any additional restrictions on refugees.[84]

With the elimination of a specific chapter on the duties of refugees, the question of the liability of refugees to taxation was transferred to the "administrative measures" section of the Convention.[85] The reference to a duty of refugees to perform military or other service was deleted altogether, leaving this issue to the discretion of particular states.[86] This left only a general obligation to respect the laws and regulations of the host state, included in the draft Convention as a symbolic recognition of the basic responsibility of refugees:

---

[83] Statement of Mr. Perez Perozo of Venezuela, ibid. at 11. See also Statements by each of the representatives of the United States, Canada, Denmark, and China affirming a state's sovereign authority to limit the political rights of foreigners: ibid. at 8–9. This view is, of course, consonant with the traditional view under international aliens law, discussed in chapter 2.1 above, at p. 76. In view of the general applicability of Art. 19 of the subsequently enacted International Covenant on Civil and Political Rights, UNGA Res. 2200A(XXI), adopted Dec. 16, 1966, entered into force Mar. 23, 1976 (Civil and Political Covenant), however, it is questionable whether governments continue to enjoy a comparable discretion to limit the expression of political opinions by non-citizens. As observed by the Human Rights Committee, "the general rule is that each one of the rights must be guaranteed without discrimination between citizens and aliens. Aliens receive the benefit of the general requirement of non-discrimination in respect of the rights guaranteed in the Covenant, as provided for in article 2 thereof. This guarantee applies to aliens and citizens alike": UN Human Rights Committee, "General Comment No. 15: The position of aliens under the Covenant" (1986), UN Doc. HRI/GEN/1/Rev.7, May 12, 2004, at 140, para. 2. See generally chapter 2.5.5 below.

[84] Robinson's comment that "Article 2 must be construed to mean that refugees not only must conform with the laws and general regulations of the country of their residence but are also subject to whatever curbs their reception country may consider necessary to impose *on their political activity* in the interest of the country's 'public order'[emphasis added]" is therefore not an accurate summary of the drafting history. See N. Robinson, *Convention relating to the Status of Refugees: Its History, Contents and Interpretation* (1953) (Robinson, *History*), at 72; and P. Weis, *The Refugee Convention, 1951: The Travaux Préparatoires Analysed with a Commentary by Dr. Paul Weis* (posthumously pub'd., 1995) (Weis, *Travaux*), at 38. To be valid under Article 2, curbs on political activity cannot be directed solely at refugees or a subset of the refugee population, but must apply generally, for example to aliens or all residents of the asylum state. The duty of non-discrimination must, of course, also be respected in the designation of the group to be denied political rights (see generally chapters 2.5.5 and 3.4 below). The interpretation of the duty to conform to "public order" measures, upon which Robinson and Weis base their arguments, is discussed below at pp. 102–103.

[85] See chapter 4.5.2 below.

[86] The vote to reject this provision was 4–3 (4 abstentions): UN Doc. A/AC.32/SR.12, Jan 25, 1950, at 9. "The Committee was not, however, the appropriate body to legislate on the very difficult question of military service. No provision regarding that question should be included in the convention; it should be solved by the operation of national legislation within the general framework of international law": Statement of Mr. Larsen of Denmark, ibid. at 8.

> [W]hen article 2 had been drafted, many representatives had felt that there
> was no need for it. It had been maintained that the laws of a given country
> obviously applied to refugees and aliens as well as to nationals of the
> country. Article 2 had been introduced for psychological reasons, and
> to maintain a balance, because the draft Convention tended to over-
> emphasize the rights and privileges of refugees. It was psychologically
> advantageous for a refugee, on consulting the Convention, to note his
> obligations towards his host country.[87]

This general obligation was subsequently strengthened in only one respect.
The original formulation of Art. 2 imposed a duty on refugees "to conform to
the [host state's] laws and regulations, *including* measures taken for the
maintenance of public order [emphasis added]."[88] This wording suggested
that only public order[89] measures codified in laws or regulations could
legitimately be applied against refugees. Without any substantive discussion
in the drafting committee, however, Art. 2 was amended to authorize a state
to require refugees to "conform to its laws and regulations *as well as* to
measures taken for the maintenance of public order [emphasis added]."[90]
On the basis of the literal meaning of Art. 2, refugees are therefore *prima facie*
bound by any general measures taken in the interest of public order, whether
or not formalized by law or regulation.[91]

Importantly, Art. 2 cannot be relied upon to legitimate an otherwise
invalid measure. Because it merely recognizes the duty of refugees to comply
with valid laws, regulations, and public order measures established apart
from the Refugee Convention, the legality of a particular constraint must
be independently established, including by reference to any relevant requirements of the Refugee Convention itself or general international human rights
law. For example, a domestic law or public order measure that purported to
prevent refugees from practicing their religion would not be saved by Art. 2,

---

[87] Statement of Mr. Robinson of Israel, UN Doc. A/CONF.2/SR.3, July 3, 1951, at 21.

[88] UN Doc. E/AC.32/L.32, Feb. 9, 1950, at 3.

[89] The term "public order" was selected to convey the meaning of the civil law concept of
"*ordre public*": Robinson, *History*, at 72; Weis, *Travaux*, at 38.

[90] UN Doc. E/1850, Aug. 25, 1950, at 15. This language is identical to that included in the
Convention as finally adopted.

[91] It is doubtful, however, that "public order" encompasses all measures viewed as necessary
in the interest of public morality. The Egyptian delegation proposed a specific provision to
this effect. "In any case, whether the Belgian amendment was adopted or not, the Egyptian
delegation considered it necessary to add to the end of article 2 the words 'and of
morality,' for morality was inseparable from public order": Statement of Mr. Mostafa of
Egypt, UN Doc. A/CONF.2/SR.3, July 3, 1951, at 23. This suggestion attracted no interest,
and was not proceeded with. But see Weis, *Travaux*, at 38: "Although this is not explicitly
stated, refugees may be expected to behave in such a manner, for example, in their habits
and dress, as not to create offence in the population of the country in which they find
themselves."

as it would be contrary to the explicit requirements of Art. 4 of the Refugee Convention.[92] Similarly, while governments are free to impose conditions of admission on refugees by regulation or contract, these must be in compliance with the rights otherwise guaranteed to refugees under the Convention.[93] Particular care is called for to ensure that the *ordre public* provision is not invoked in defense of a clearly invidious distinction.[94] Nowak argues in the context of the Civil and Political Covenant that "the purpose for interference does not relate to the specific *ordre public* of the State concerned but rather to an international standard of the democratic society."[95] A comparable benchmark should govern resort to the public order authority under Art. 2 of the Refugee Convention, thereby ensuring that the common purpose of advancing refugee rights is not undermined.[96]

---

[92] See generally chapter 4.7 below.

[93] A proposal that would have required refugees, for example, to remain in the employment found for them by the host government was advanced by Australia: UN Doc. A/CONF.2/10. "The Australian Government was put to considerable expense in selecting migrants, in contributing to the cost of their journey to Australia, in arranging for their reception, and generally in helping them to adapt to their new place in the community. It had therefore been regarded as reasonable that migrants should recognize their obligations to their new country, and continue to do work for which they were most needed for a limited period": Statement of Mr. Shaw of Australia, UN Doc. A/CONF.2/SR.3, July 3, 1951, at 20. The United Nations High Commissioner replied that the Australian objective could best be met by enforcing the obligations against the refugee on the basis of domestic regulation or contract, rather than by a specific duty in the Refugee Convention itself: Statement of Mr. van Heuven Goedhart, UNHCR, UN Doc. A/CONF.2/SR.4, July 3, 1951, at 4. More specifically, the British delegate observed that "[h]e believed that the Australian delegation was not so much concerned with the failure of a refugee to comply with conditions, as with the need for ensuring that the specific conditions imposed on entry to Australia conformed with the provisions of the draft Convention ... [I]t seemed to him that the question of whether the Australian practice was permissible must be considered in the light of other articles of the draft Convention which imposed certain conditions upon States. He would therefore suggest that the Australian representative should withdraw his amendment [to Art. 2]": Statement of Mr. Hoare of the United Kingdom, ibid. at 6. The Australian amendment to Art. 2 was subsequently withdrawn: ibid. at 7.

[94] *Ordre public* is a "highly dangerous civil law concept ... [which] covers at least as much ground as public policy in English-American law and perhaps much more": J. Humphrey, "Political and Related Rights," in T. Meron ed., *Human Rights in International Law: Legal and Policy Issues* 171 (1984) (Meron, *Human Rights in International Law*), at 185. The contentious nature of the notion of *ordre public* is discussed below in chapter 5.1, at pp. 679–690; in chapter 5.2, at pp. 715–716; and in chapter 6.7, at pp. 900–901.

[95] M. Nowak, *UN Covenant on Civil and Political Rights* (1993) (Nowak, *ICCPR Commentary*), at 213. Nowak makes specific reference to an attempt by South Africa to justify *apartheid*-era restrictions as necessary to its own particular *ordre public*.

[96] "Since *ordre public* may otherwise lead to a complete undermining of freedom of expression and information – or to a reversal of rule and exception – particularly strict requirements must be placed on the necessity (proportionality) of a given statutory restriction. Furthermore, the *minimum requirements* flowing from a common

Most important, there is no basis whatever to assert that Art. 2 authorizes a decision either to withdraw refugee status or to withhold rights from refugees on the grounds of the refugee's failure to respect laws, regulations, or public order measures. The Conference of Plenipotentiaries considered this question in the context of a Belgian proposal that would have transformed Art. 2 from a statement of principle to a condition of eligibility for continuing protection:

> Only such refugees as fulfil their duties toward the country in which they find themselves and in particular conform to its laws and regulations as well as to measures taken for the maintenance of public order, may claim the benefit of this Convention.[97]

This proposal met with serious disapproval. The representative of Israel asserted that the proposal "was a revolutionary departure from the original intention of article 2,"[98] which posed very serious dangers:

> If it were to be adopted, refugees who were guilty, for example, of minor infractions of the law would be deprived of all their rights and privileges. To try to make saints out of refugees would be to set the Convention at naught. Again, while he believed in the good faith of the countries that would sign the Convention, it could not be denied that xenophobia existed in certain countries, and junior officials who disliked refugees might seek pretexts to deprive them of their rights.[99]

The British delegate agreed that "[t]he Belgian amendment would confer on States full power to abolish refugee status for any infractions of the laws of the country concerned, which ... would, in fact, nullify all the rights conferred by the Convention."[100]

In an attempt to preserve the essence of the Belgian initiative, France suggested that refugee rights should be forfeited only consequent to a breach of the most serious duties owed to a host state, and on the basis of a fair procedure:

international standard for this human right, which is so essential for the maintenance of democracy, may not be set too low": ibid. at 357.

[97] UN Doc. A/CONF.2/10. The Belgian delegate insisted that his amendment raised no issue of substance, but was instead "mainly a question of form": Statement of Mr. Herment of Belgium, UN Doc. A/CONF.2/SR.3, July 3, 1951, at 18. Later, however, he conceded that "[h]is amendment would permit Contracting States to withdraw the benefit of the provisions of the Convention from refugees contravening the laws and regulations of the receiving country, or failing to fulfil their duties towards that country or guilty of disturbing public order": ibid. at 22.

[98] Statement of Mr. Robinson of Israel, UN Doc. A/CONF.2/SR.3, July 3, 1951, at 21.

[99] Ibid.

[100] Statement of Mr. Hoare of the United Kingdom, ibid. at 22. See also Statement of Mr. Chance of Canada, ibid. at 23: "[T]he inclusion of [the] clause might frustrate the purposes of the Convention"; and Statement of Baron van Boetzelaer of the Netherlands, ibid. at 24.

> Any refugee guilty of grave dereliction of duty and who constitutes a danger
> to the internal or external security of the receiving country may, by appro-
> priate procedure assuring maximum safeguards for the person concerned,
> be declared to have forfeited the rights pertaining to the status of refugees,
> as defined in this Convention.[101]

As the President of the Conference observed, this more carefully framed
amendment allowed the delegates to address the fundamental question of
"whether a refugee who failed to fulfil certain conditions should forfeit the
rights proclaimed in the draft Convention, even if his country of refuge did
not expel him."[102] The proponents of the French amendment argued that this
approach to Art. 2 was actually of benefit to refugees, since it would allow a
host state to protect its vital interests without resorting to the more extreme
alternatives of either withdrawing refugee status or expulsion.[103] Refugees
would be deprived of the special benefits of the Refugee Convention, but
would be subjected to no particular disabilities. Most important, the incorporation of a forfeiture provision in Art. 2 was said to be an important source
of protection for the majority of refugees who might otherwise be stigmatized
by the actions of a troublesome minority:

> It was actually a matter of fundamental interest to refugees generally that
> the measures advocated by the French delegation should be taken against
> such refugees as carried on activities constituting a danger to the security of
> the countries receiving them. If certain disturbances provoked by orga-
> nized bands were allowed to increase in France, the final outcome would be
> a wave of xenophobia, and public opinion would demand not merely the

---

[101] UN Doc. A/CONF.2/18. "[T]he word 'duty' in the French amendment referred to the duties
mentioned in the first line of article 2 itself, which were incumbent on the refugee as
a resident in the receiving country ... [T]he concept of 'receiving country' ... covered ...
both the 'receiving country' and what was meant by the 'country of selective immigration.' With regard to the procedure to be adopted in respect of the forfeiture by the
refugee of the rights pertaining to his status, it should be noted that the measures in
question related to extremely serious – and, incidentally, rare – cases, and came within
the category of counter-espionage operations. No country could possibly be expected
to expatiate in an international forum on the measures which it proposed to adopt in
that connexion. 'Forfeiture' of his rights by the refugee would transfer him from the
jurisdiction of the international convention to that of the legislation currently in force
in the countries concerned": Statement of Mr. Rochefort of France, UN Doc. A/
CONF.2/SR.4, July 3, 1951, at 9.

[102] Statement of the President, Mr. Larsen, UN Doc. A/CONF.2/SR.4, July 3, 1951, at 5. See
also Statement of Mr. Hoare of the United Kingdom, ibid. at 6.

[103] "[T]he person subjected to [the measures contemplated] would preserve his status as [a]
refugee; the pronouncement of his forfeiture of rights would in no way withdraw that
status from him, but would simply have the effect of depriving him of all or some of the
benefits granted by the Convention": Statement of Mr. Herment of Belgium, ibid. at 10.

application of the measures laid down in the French proposal, but the expulsion of a great many innocent refugees.[104]

On the other side of the argument, UNHCR and the United Kingdom preferred that no restrictions on refugee rights be possible. Unless the risk posed was serious enough to meet the requirements for exclusion from refugee status[105] or expulsion from the country,[106] the host country should continue to respect all rights guaranteed by the Convention. It would be inappropriate to include in the Convention "a provision by virtue of which a State would be able to treat a refugee as a pariah."[107] This view prevailed, and the French amendment was withdrawn.[108]

The legal position is therefore clear: Art. 2 does not authorize the withdrawal of refugee rights for even the most serious breaches of a refugee's duty to the host state.[109] Because there is no reciprocity of rights and obligations under the Refugee Convention, refugees must be dealt with in the same ways as any other persons who violate a generally applicable law, regulation, or public order measure.[110] Refugees are subject only to the same penalties as

---

[104] Statement of Mr. Rochefort of France, ibid. at 11.

[105] "[W]hile some provision such as that proposed by the French delegation was desirable, it would more appropriately be placed in article 1, among the provisions relating to the exclusion from the benefits of the Convention of certain categories of refugees ... [A] refugee dealt with as proposed in the French amendment ... would cease to be a refugee for the purposes of the Convention": Statement of Mr. van Heuven Goedhart, UNHCR, ibid. at 9–10. The requirements for exclusion from refugee status are discussed in Grahl-Madsen, *Status of Refugees I*, at 262–304; Hathaway, *Refugee Status*, at 214–229; and Goodwin-Gill, *Refugee in International Law*, at 95–114.

[106] "In his view, it should be recognized that in the last resort a country might be obliged to return the offender to the country from which he came ... [but] [i]t would be wrong to exclude any such person from the benefits of the Convention while he still remained as a refugee in a particular country": Statement of Mr. Hoare of the United Kingdom, UN Doc. A/CONF.2/SR.4, July 3, 1951, at 10. See generally chapter 5.1 below.

[107] Statement of Mr. Hoare of the United Kingdom, UN Doc. A/CONF.2/SR.4, July 3, 1951, at 11.

[108] Statement of Mr. Rochefort of France, UN Doc. A/CONF.2/SR.24, July 17, 1951, at 19.

[109] "[N]on-observance [by a refugee] of his 'duties' according to Article 2 has no effect in international law": Grahl-Madsen, *Status of Refugees I*, at 58.

[110] "What was important was that the refugee should not constitute a problem, and that he should conform to the laws and regulations to which he was subject. When he failed to do so, appropriate sanctions should be applied, and repeated violations of the regulations might reasonably warrant expulsion. Until he was expelled, however, he should be treated in accordance with the provisions of the Convention and be subject only to such sanctions as were applicable to other law-breakers": Statement of Mr. Hoeg of Denmark, UN Doc. A/CONF.2/SR.4, July 3, 1951, at 4–5. The only exception is the right of refugees to receive travel documents, which may be suspended under the explicit terms of the Convention where required by "compelling reasons of national security or public order": Refugee Convention, at Art. 28. See generally chapter 6.6 below.

others, and may not be threatened with withdrawal of the particular benefits of refugee status.[111] All rights under the Convention are to be respected in full until and unless refugee status is either validly withdrawn under Art. 1, or the strict requirements for expulsion or *refoulement* are met.[112]

The decision to reject a "middle ground" position that would have authorized the forfeiture of specific rights as an alternative to the withdrawal of refugee status or expulsion is conceptually important. The ability of the host state to enforce its laws and regulations in the usual ways, for example by incarceration, is in no sense compromised by the Refugee Convention. The argument that failure to allow states to withdraw Convention rights from refugees would compel them to resort to the withdrawal of status or expulsion is therefore fallacious. Even the specific concern of the French drafter to be in a position to deal with spies who might infiltrate the refugee population[113] can readily be addressed by generic counter-espionage legislation to which refugees would clearly be subject in common with the population at large.

The proposed right of forfeiture would have transformed Art. 2 from an affirmation of the duty of refugees to respect laws of general application to a mechanism for the differential treatment of refugees on the basis of their heightened vulnerability. Yet refugee rights are not rewards or bonuses; they are rather the means by which the international community has agreed to restore to refugees the basic ability to function within a new national community. The rights set by the Convention are the core minimum judged necessary to compensate refugees for the situation-specific disabilities to which involuntary migration has subjected them. To have sanctioned the withdrawal from refugees of some part of this restitutionary package of rights would therefore have injected a distinctively punitive dimension into the Refugee Convention. The position ultimately adopted, in contrast, requires refugees to comply with all general legal requirements of the host state and to pay the usual penalties for any breach of the law, but ensures that they are not denied the rights deemed necessary to offset the specific hardships of forced migration.

---

[111] Thus, for example, the threat of the Thai government in July 2003 to revoke the registration of any refugee who "break[s] any Thai laws" was clearly inconsistent with the requirements of the Refugee Convention: "Thais to intern 1,500 Burmese," *International Herald Tribune*, July 3, 2003, at 1. Swaziland also acted contrary to international law when it withdrew refugee status from thirty-seven refugees and ordered their "provisional isolation" because they had embarrassed Prince Sobandla by protesting during a visit to a refugee camp. The Prince justified the decision on the grounds of "gross misconduct and breach of refugee ethics": *Times of Swaziland*, July 19, 2002.

[112] Refugee Convention, at Arts. 32 and 33, discussed below at chapters 5.1 and 4.1 respectively.

[113] See text above, at p. 105, n. 101.

2.4.5 Non-impairment of other rights

Refugee Convention, Art. 5   Rights granted apart from this Convention
Nothing in this Convention shall be deemed to impair any rights and benefits granted by a Contracting State to refugees apart from this Convention.

The original purpose of Art. 5 was to safeguard the privileges of particular refugee classes that existed at the time the Convention came into force.[114] The provision as first adopted at the Second Session of the Ad Hoc Committee provided that "[n]othing in this Convention shall be deemed to impair any rights and benefits granted by a Contracting State to refugees *prior to or apart from* this Convention [emphasis added]."[115] At the Conference of Plenipotentiaries, however, the President declared that the words "prior to or" were "redundant," resulting in the decision to safeguard simply rights and benefits granted refugees "apart from" the Convention.[116] While there was no discussion on point, the literal meaning of the provision as adopted therefore requires states to honor not only preexisting obligations, but also whatever duties might accrue to refugees in the future.[117]

The basic goal of affirming preexisting rights is consistent with other parts of the Convention, for example the recognition of refugee status granted under earlier agreements, as well as the decision to insulate previously recognized refugees from the new rules for cessation of status due to change of circumstances.[118] The International Refugee Organization had sometimes negotiated agreements with particular states that provided for stronger rights than those codified in the Convention, which the drafters wished to ensure were not challenged on the basis of an assertion that the earlier rights were superseded by the provisions of the Refugee Convention.[119] The validity of

---

[114] "The committee also thought it advisable to make it clear that the adoption of the present Convention should not impair any greater rights which refugees might enjoy prior to or apart from this Convention": "Report of the Ad Hoc Committee on Refugees and Stateless Persons, Second Session," UN Doc. E/1850, Aug. 25, 1950 (Ad Hoc Committee, "Second Session Report"), at 11.

[115] UN Doc. E/AC.32/L.42/Add.1, at 8, adopted by the Committee as Art. 3(a): UN Doc. E/AC.32/SR.43, Aug. 25, 1950, at 14.

[116] Statement of the President, Mr. Larsen, UN Doc. A/CONF.2/SR.5, Nov. 19, 1951, at 18.

[117] See also Weis, *Travaux*, at 44: "It resulted from the history of the Article that both rights and benefits granted prior to the Convention and subsequently to its entry into force are meant."

[118] Refugee Convention, at Arts. 1(A)(1) and 1(C)(5). See generally Grahl-Madsen, *Status of Refugees I*, at 108–119, 307–309, and 367–369; and Hathaway, *Refugee Status*, at 6 and 203–204.

[119] Robinson, *History*, at 79. See chapter 2.4.1 above, at p. 93.

rights granted by free-standing international agreement was instead to be determined by the terms of those agreements.

Second, refugees sometimes benefited from social legislation adopted in particular countries that was quite progressive relative to the "lowest common denominator" of rights guaranteed in the Refugee Convention. Art. 5 was intended to provide balance by signaling that the sometimes minimal rights it had been possible to secure for refugees in the cut and thrust of negotiation did not require the withdrawal from refugees of more generous protections granted under domestic law.[120] The Refugee Convention could not, of course, require governments to safeguard superior rights, but neither should it serve as a pretext to diminish the quality of protection already enjoyed by refugees.[121]

The express provision validating free-standing duties owed to refugees adds nothing to the legal enforceability of such duties. Nonetheless, it is a valuable affirmation of the concern of the drafters "to grant refugees as many rights as possible, not to restrict them."[122] As originally conceived, Art. 5 may even have been intended to authorize discrimination in favor of particular sub-groups of the refugee population, a matter now generally proscribed by general international human rights law.[123] The continuing importance of Art. 5, while largely symbolic, lies both in its encouragement to states to legislate domestically beyond the standards of the Refugee Convention and, particularly, in its insistence that state parties continue to accord refugees all advantages that accrue to them by virtue of other international agreements,[124] including under bilateral treaties with the refugee's country of origin.[125]

Most important, Art. 5 should be read as requiring governments to respect the array of important international human rights accords negotiated in recent

---

[120] Art. 5 is stated in peremptory terms ("*[n]othing* in this Convention shall be deemed to impair [emphasis added]"): Refugee Convention, at Art. 5.

[121] Weis, *Travaux*, at 44.   [122] Robinson, *History*, at 79.

[123] To the extent that the discrimination is both systematic and based on race, sex, language, or religion, it contravenes a universally binding human right established by the Charter of the United Nations: see chapter 1.2.3 above, at p. 44. More generally, there is now a pervasive norm of non-discrimination established by the Civil and Political Covenant that binds those states that have adhered to it: see chapter 2.5.5 below, at p. 125 ff. Differential treatment designed and carefully tailored to achieve substantive equality ("affirmative action") is not, however, discriminatory under international law: see chapter 2.5.5 below, at pp. 124–125.

[124] In relation to the comparable provision of the Civil and Political Covenant, Nowak argues that "the *savings clause* ... gives expression to the principle that the rights of the Covenant merely represent *a minimum standard* and that the cumulation of various human rights conventions, domestic norms and customary international law may not be interpreted to the detriment of the individual": Nowak, *ICCPR Commentary*, at 95.

[125] See generally chapter 3.2.2 below.

years. These international human rights conventions generally regulate the treatment of all persons subject to a state's jurisdiction, and are therefore critical sources of enhanced protection for refugees. Art. 5 of the Refugee Convention makes clear that the drafters were aware that refugees would be protected by additional rights acquired under the terms of other international agreements, and that they specifically intended that this should be so. The next section examines the most important of these complementary sources of refugee rights that have come into existence since the drafting of the Refugee Convention.

2.5 Post-Convention sources of refugee rights

Apart from the minority of refugees who continued to benefit from special arrangements negotiated by the International Refugee Organization or codified in earlier treaties, the internationally defined rights of most refugees in 1951 were essentially limited to those set by the Refugee Convention. As shown above, international aliens law was of no real benefit to refugees, since refugees have no national state likely to view injuries done to them as a matter of official concern.[126] A general system of conventional international human rights law had yet to emerge. The scope of universal norms of human rights law, then as now, was decidedly minimalist.[127]

Since 1951, authoritative interpretations of rights set by the Refugee Convention have been issued, and some binding enhancements to refugee-specific rights secured at the regional level. Advances in refugee rights since 1951 have, however, largely occurred outside of refugee law itself. While aliens law has yet to evolve as a meaningful source of protection, the development of a pervasive treaty-based system of international human rights law has filled many critical gaps in the Refugee Convention's rights regime. Because treaty-based human rights are framed in generic terms, however, there is a continuing role for the Refugee Convention in responding to the particular disabilities that derive from involuntary migration. It is nonetheless clear that the evolution of human rights conventions that include refugees within their scope has resulted in a net level of legal protections significantly greater than envisaged by the Refugee Convention. By synthesizing refugee-specific and general human rights, it is now possible to respond to most critical threats to the human dignity of refugees.

2.5.1 Protocol relating to the Status of Refugees

There have been few formal changes to the refugee rights regime since the entry into force of the Refugee Convention. The 1967 Refugee Protocol is a

---

[126] See chapter 2.1 above, at p. 79.   [127] See chapter 1.2 above.

treaty which incorporates the Refugee Convention's rights regime by reference,[128] and extends those protections to all refugees by prospectively eliminating the Convention's temporal and geographical limitations for those
countries which choose to be bound by it. The Protocol is not, as is commonly believed, an amendment to the 1951 Convention: as Weis has
observed, "[w]ith the entry into force of the Protocol there exist, in fact,
two treaties dealing with the same subject matter."[129] The Full Federal Court
of Australia has reached the same conclusion, noting that states may accede to
the Protocol without first becoming a party to the Convention, and that those
which do so are immediately bound to grant the rights described in the
Convention to a broader class of persons – that is, to modern refugees from
all parts of the world – than would have been the case by accession to the
Convention itself.[130]

More ominously, and in contrast to the provisions of the Refugee
Convention, countries which are bound only by the Protocol have the
option at the time of accession to deny other state parties the right to refer
a dispute regarding their interpretation or application of the Protocol to the
International Court of Justice.[131] One of the two countries eligible to have
made this election, Venezuela, has in fact excluded the Court's

---

[128] Refugee Protocol, Art. I(1).

[129] P. Weis, "The 1967 Protocol relating to the Status of Refugees and Some Questions
relating to the Law of Treaties," (1967) *British Yearbook of International Law* 39, at 60.
More specifically, "[t]he procedure for revision of the 1951 Convention, as provided for
in its terms, was not resorted to in view of the urgency of extending its personal scope to
new groups of refugees and of the fact that the amended treaty would have required fresh
consent by the states parties to the Convention. Instead, a new instrument, the 1967
Protocol relating to the Status of Refugees, was established, which does not amend the
1951 Convention and modifies it only in the sense that States acceding to the Protocol
accept the material obligations of the Convention in respect of a wider group of persons.
As between the state parties to the Convention, it constitutes an *inter se* agreement by
which they undertake obligations identical *ratione materiae* with those provided for in
the Convention for additional groups of refugees not covered by the Convention on
account of the dateline of 1 January 1951. As regards states not parties to the Convention,
it constitutes a separate treaty under which they assume the material obligations laid
down in the Convention in respect of refugees defined in Art. 1 of the Protocol, namely
those covered by Art. 1 of the Convention and those not covered by reason of the
dateline": ibid. at 59.

[130] *Minister for Immigration and Multicultural Affairs v. Savvin*, (2000) 171 ALR 483 (Aus.
FFC, Apr. 12, 2000), per Katz J. Justice Katz thus concludes that "for parliament to
describe the 1951 Convention as having been 'amended' by the 1967 Protocol is inaccurate. At the same time, however, for a state like Australia, which was already bound by the
1951 Convention before acceding to the 1967 Protocol, the error is one of no practical
significance": ibid.

[131] Under Art. VII(1) of the Refugee Protocol, a state may enter a reservation regarding Art.
IV of the Protocol, which establishes the right of other state parties to refer a dispute to
the International Court of Justice. In contrast, Art. 42 of the Refugee Convention, which

jurisdiction.[132] Several other states which have acceded to the Protocol, but which are also parties to the Convention, have purported to make a similar election. Yet because of the mandatory provisions regarding the Court's jurisdiction contained in the Convention, a dispute involving one of these states – Angola, Botswana, China, Congo, El Salvador, Ghana, Jamaica, Rwanda, and Tanzania – may still be referred to the International Court of Justice so long as it involves the interpretation or application of the Convention, rather than of the Protocol. As the substantive content of the two treaties is largely identical, it would seem open to a state party to the Convention to refer a dispute involving interpretation of the refugee definition or of refugee rights, so long as the subject matter is not uniquely relevant to post-1951 refugees.

A decade after the advent of the Protocol, the United Nations Conference on Territorial Asylum considered, but ultimately rejected, the codification of a new treaty which would set a clear right to enduring protection for refugees. It reached agreement in principle to require states to facilitate the admission of a refugee's spouse and minor or dependent children, and explicitly to interpret the duty of *non-refoulement* to include "rejection at the frontier."[133] The Conference was also of the view that the enjoyment of refugee rights could legitimately be made contingent on compliance with the laws of the state of asylum. No effort has been made, however, either to resuscitate the asylum convention project, or to formalize as matters of law the consensus achieved on either family reunification or the scope of the duty of *non-refoulement*.

2.5.2 Conclusions and guidelines on international protection

Rather than formulate new refugee rights, the focus of effort since 1975 has been to elaborate the content of existing standards in non-binding resolutions adopted by the state members of the agency's governing body, the Executive Committee of the High Commissioner's Program. These "Conclusions on the International Protection of Refugees"[134] have addressed

addresses the scope of permissible reservations to that treaty, does not allow states to enter a reservation to Art. 38, the equivalent of Art. IV of the Protocol. "While the Convention provides for obligatory jurisdiction of the International Court of Justice in any dispute relating to its interpretation or application, one reason for the Protocol was for some States to be able to make reservations to this jurisdictional clause": Sohn and Buergenthal, *Movement of Persons*, at 113.

[132] The other eligible country, the United States of America, did not elect to exclude the jurisdiction of the International Court of Justice. Because the option is available only at the time of accession, the United States cannot make such an election in the future.

[133] UN Doc. A/CONF.78/12, Feb. 4, 1977. See generally A. Grahl-Madsen, *Territorial Asylum* (1980).

[134] These are periodically published in looseleaf form in UN Doc. HCR/IP/2, and are collected at www.unhcr.ch (accessed Nov. 20, 2004). UNHCR has also issued "A Thematic Compilation of Executive Committee Conclusions" (March 2001), which organizes relevant Executive Committee Conclusions under sixty major chapters.

such matters as non-rejection and *non-refoulement*,[135] exemption from penalties for illegal entry,[136] conditions of detention,[137] limits on expulsion and extradition,[138] family unity,[139] the provision of identification documents,[140] physical security,[141] and the rights to education[142] and to undertake employment.[143] An effort has also been made to interpret rights to respond to the special vulnerabilities of refugees who are children,[144] women,[145] elderly,[146] or caught up in a large-scale influx.[147] While not matters of law, these standards have strong political authority as consensus resolutions of a formal body of government representatives expressly responsible for "providing guidance and forging consensus on vital protection policies and practices."[148] The Canadian Federal Court of Appeal has thus appropriately recognized that Executive Committee Conclusions are deserving of real deference:

> [I]n Article 35 of the [Refugee] Convention the signatory states undertake to cooperate with the Office of the United Nations High Commissioner for Refugees (UNHCR) in the performance of its functions and, in particular, to facilitate the discharge of its duty of supervising the application of the Convention. Accordingly, considerable weight should be given to recommendations of the Executive Committee of the High Commissioner's Program on issues relating to refugee determination

[135] See UNHCR Executive Committee Conclusions Nos. 1 (1975), 5 (1977), 6 (1977), 17 (1990), 22 (1981), 29 (1983), 50 (1988), 52 (1988), 55 (1989), 62 (1990), 65 (1991), 68 (1992), 71 (1993), 74 (1994), 77 (1995), 81 (1997), 82 (1997), and 85 (1998), available at www.unhcr.ch (accessed Nov. 20, 2004).

[136] Ibid. at Nos. 44 (1986), 55 (1989), and 85 (1998).

[137] Ibid. at Nos. 3 (1977), 7 (1977), 36 (1985), 44 (1986), 46 (1987), 47 (1987), 50 (1988), 55 (1989), 65 (1991), 68 (1992), 71 (1993), 85 (1998), and 89 (2000).

[138] Ibid. at Nos. 7 (1977), 9 (1977), 17 (1980), 21 (1981), 44 (1986), 50 (1988), 55 (1989), 61 (1990), 68 (1992), 71 (1993), 79 (1996), and 85 (1998).

[139] Ibid. at Nos. 1 (1975), 9 (1977), 15 (1979), 22 (1989), 24 (1989), 47 (1987), 74 (1994), 84 (1997), 85 (1998), and 88 (1999).

[140] Ibid. at Nos. 8 (1977), 18 (1980), 24 (1981), 35 (1984), 64 (1990), 65 (1991), 72 (1993), 73 (1993), and 91 (2001).

[141] Ibid. at Nos. 20 (1980), 25 (1982), 29 (1983), 44 (1986), 45 (1986), 46 (1987), 48 (1987), 54 (1988), 55 (1989), 58 (1989), 72 (1993), 74 (1994), 77 (1995), 87 (1999), and 98 (2003).

[142] Ibid. at Nos. 47 (1987), 58 (1989), 59 (1989), 74 (1994), 77 (1995), 80 (1996), 84 (1997), and 85 (1998).

[143] Ibid. at Nos. 50 (1988), 58 (1989), 64 (1990), and 88 (1999).

[144] Ibid. at Nos. 47 (1987), 59 (1989), 72 (1993), 73 (1993), 74 (1994), 79 (1996), 85 (1998), 87 (1999), and 89 (2000).

[145] Ibid. at Nos. 32 (1983), 39 (1985), 46 (1987), 54 (1988), 60 (1989), 64 (1990), 68 (1992), 71 (1993), 73 (1993), 74 (1994), 77 (1995), 79 (1996), 81 (1997), 85 (1998), 87 (1999), and 89 (2000).

[146] Ibid. at Nos. 32 (1983), 85 (1998), 87 (1999), and 89 (2000).

[147] Ibid. at Nos. 19 (1980), 22 (1981), 25 (1982), 44 (1986), 81 (1997), 85 (1998), and 100 (2004).

[148] Ibid. at No. 81 (1997).

and protection that are designed to go some way to fill the procedural void in the Convention itself.[149]

Specifically, UNHCR's authority under Article 35 of the Refugee Convention[150] is a sufficient basis for the agency to require state parties to explain treatment of refugees that does not conform to the Conclusions on Protection adopted by the agency's governing body. This authority to require the international community to engage in a dialogue of justification is comparable to the human rights *droit de regard* enjoyed by the General Assembly:[151] UNHCR may legitimately expect states to respond to concerns about the adequacy of refugee protection as measured by reference to Conclusions adopted by the state members of its Executive Committee, though it has no power to require compliance with those or any other standards.[152]

It is less clear, however, to what extent standards recommended by UNHCR, but which have not been adopted as a Conclusion of its Executive Committee, are to be afforded comparable deference. There is a traditional practice of giving particular weight to the UNHCR's *Handbook on Procedures and Criteria for Determining Refugee Status*,[153] a comprehensive analysis of the basic precepts of refugee law prepared at the behest of the Executive Committee more than a quarter of a century ago.[154] The Supreme Court of

---

[149] *Rahaman v. Minister of Citizenship and Immigration*, 2002 ACWSJ Lexis 1026 (Can. FCA, Mar. 1, 2002), per Evans JA. To similar effect see *Attorney General v. E*, [2000] 3 NZLR 257 (NZ CA, July 11, 2000), at 269.

[150] "The Contracting States undertake to co-operate with the Office of the United Nations High Commissioner for Refugees . . . in the exercise of its functions, and shall in particular facilitate its duty of supervising the application of the provisions of this Convention": Refugee Convention, at Art. 35(1).

[151] See chapter 1.2.3 above, at pp. 46–47.

[152] States recently affirmed "the fundamental importance of UNHCR as the multilateral institution with the mandate to provide international protection to refugees . . . and recall[ed] [their] obligations as States Parties to cooperate with UNHCR in the exercise of its functions; [and] [u]rge[d] all states to consider ways that may be required to strengthen the implementation of the 1951 Convention and/or 1967 Protocol and to ensure closer cooperation between States Parties and UNHCR to facilitate UNHCR's duty of supervising the application of the provisions of these instruments": "Declaration of States Parties to the 1951 Convention and/or its 1967 Protocol relating to the Status of Refugees," UN Doc. HCR/MMSP/2001/09, Dec. 13, 2001, incorporated in Executive Committee of the High Commissioner's Program, "Agenda for Protection," UN Doc. EC/52/SC/CRP.9/Rev.1, June 26, 2002, at Part I, paras. 8–9. The challenge of ensuring meaningful supervision and enforcement of the Refugee Convention is briefly taken up in the Epilogue below, at pp. 992–998.

[153] UNHCR, *Handbook on Procedures and Criteria for Determining Refugee Status* (1979, reedited 1992) (UNHCR, *Handbook*).

[154] In 1977, the Executive Committee "[r]equested the Office to consider the possibility of issuing – for the guidance of Governments – a handbook relating to procedures and criteria for determining refugee status": UNHCR Executive Committee Conclusion

the United States, for example, determined that "the Handbook provides significant guidance" on the interpretation of refugee law;[155] the British House of Lords has gone farther, acknowledging that by virtue of UNHCR's statutory authority, "[i]t is not surprising ... that the UNHCR Handbook, although not binding on states, has high persuasive authority, and is much relied on by domestic courts and tribunals."[156] Yet not even the *Handbook* is treated as a source of legal obligation. The House of Lords has warned that the *Handbook* "is of no binding force either in municipal or international law,"[157] while the New Zealand Court of Appeal has similarly insisted that the *Handbook* "cannot override the function of [the decision-maker] in determining the meaning of the words of [the Refugee] Convention."[158] Indeed, courts have recently become increasingly guarded in their appraisal of the *Handbook*'s authority,[159] finding, for example, that it is "more [of] a practical guide ... than ... a document purporting to interpret the meaning of relevant parts of the Convention."[160] In its most recent statement on point, the House of Lords observed only that the *Handbook* "is recognized as an important source of guidance on matters to which it relates"[161] – a significantly less enthusiastic endorsement than the same court issued just two years earlier.[162]

The decline in the deference afforded the *Handbook* is no doubt largely attributable to the increasing dissonance between some of its positions and

---

No. 8, "Determination of Refugee Status" (1977), at para. (g), available at www.unhcr.ch (accessed Nov. 20, 2004).

[155] *Immigration and Naturalization Service v. Cardoza Fonseca*, (1987) 480 US 421 (US SC, Mar. 9, 1987), at 439, n. 22.

[156] *R v. Secretary of State for the Home Department, ex parte Adan and Aitseguer*, [2001] 2 WLR 143 (UK HL, Dec. 19, 2000), per Lord Steyn. The *Handbook* has been treated as solid evidence of the current state of international practice on interpretation of refugee law: *R (Hoxha) v. Secretary of State for the Home Department*, [2002] EWCA Civ 1403 (Eng. CA, Oct. 14, 2002), at para. 36.

[157] *R v. Secretary of State for the Home Department, ex parte Bugdaycay*, [1987] AC 514 (UK HL, Feb. 19, 1987), per Lord Bridge of Harwich at 525; cited with approval in *M v. Attorney General*, [2003] NZAR 614 (NZ HC, Feb. 19, 2003).

[158] *S v. Refugee Status Appeals Authority*, [1998] 2 NZLR 291 (NZ CA, Apr. 2, 1998), at 300. See also *M v. Attorney General*, [2003] NZAR 614 (NZ HC, Feb. 19, 2003).

[159] In *WAGO of 2002 v. Minister for Immigration and Multicultural and Indigenous Affairs*, 194 ALR 676 (Aus. FFC, Dec. 20, 2002), the Australian Full Federal Court declined to find any error in the determination that the provisions in the UNHCR *Handbook* "were not part of the law of Australia and did not provide grounds for legal review of the Tribunal's decision."

[160] *NADB of 2001 v. Minister for Immigration and Multicultural Affairs*, [2002] FCAFC 326 (Aus. FFC, Oct. 31, 2002). See also *Todea v. MIEA*, (1994) 20 AAR 470 (Aus. FC, Dec. 22, 1994), at 484.

[161] *Sepet and Bulbul v. Secretary of State for the Home Department*, [2003] UKHL 15 (UK HL, Mar. 20, 2003), at para. 12.

[162] See text above, at n. 156.

those which have resulted from the intensive period of judicial activism in refugee law, which began in the early 1990s. In contrast to earlier times when there were few authoritative decisions on the content of refugee law, many state parties today have developed their own, often quite comprehensive, judicial understandings of many aspects of international refugee law. Where no domestic precedent exists, courts are increasingly (and appropriately) inclined to seek guidance from the jurisprudence of other state parties to the Convention.[163] In this more mature legal environment, UNHCR's views on the substance of refugee law – at least where these are not formally codified through the authoritative process of Executive Committee decision-making – will inevitably not be treated as uniquely pertinent, but will instead be considered and weighed as part of a more holistic assessment of the current state of refugee law obligations.

Indeed, the recent proliferation of various forms of UNHCR position papers on the interpretation of refugee law has made it increasingly difficult for even state parties committed to a strong UNHCR voice to discern the precise agency position on many key protection issues. Of greatest concern, the agency's Department of International Protection has commenced release of "Guidelines on International Protection"[164] under a process approved in only the most general terms by its Executive Committee.[165] While explicitly intended to be "complementary" to the standards set out in the *Handbook*,[166] the standards at times appear to conflict with the advice of the *Handbook*.[167] Such conflicts have not gone unnoticed by courts: in a recent decision, for

---

[163] See J. Hathaway, "A Forum for the Transnational Development of Refugee Law: The IARLJ's Advanced Refugee Law Workshop," (2003) 15(3) *International Journal of Refugee Law* 418.

[164] As of September 2004, six sets of Guidelines had been issued by UNHCR: UN Docs. HCR/GIP/02/01 (gender-related persecution); HCR/GIP/02/02 (membership of a particular social group); HCR/GIP/03/03 (cessation); HCR/GIP/03/04 (internal relocation alternative); HCR/GIP/03/05 (exclusion); and HCR/GIP/04/06 (religion-based claims).

[165] At its fifty-third session, the UNHCR's Executive Committee requested UNHCR "to produce complementary guidelines to its *Handbook on Procedures and Criteria for Determining Refugee Status*, drawing on applicable international legal standards, on State practice, on jurisprudence and using, as appropriate, the inputs from the debates in the Global Consultations' expert roundtable discussions": Executive Committee of the High Commissioner's Program, "Agenda for Protection," UN Doc. EC/52/SC/CRP.9/Rev.1, June 26, 2002, at Part III, Goal 1, Point 6. The Executive Committee clearly did not intend that these guidelines should be the sole, or even the primary, means of advancing the development of refugee law, since it simultaneously agreed that the agency should "explore areas that would benefit from further standard-setting, such as [Executive Committee] Conclusions or other instruments to be identified at a later stage": ibid. at Goal 1, Point 7.

[166] Executive Committee of the High Commissioner's Program, "Agenda for Protection," UN Doc. EC/52/SC/CRP.9/Rev.1, June 26, 2002, at Part III, Goal 1, Point 6.

[167] For example, on the question of what has traditionally been referred to as the "internal flight alternative," the *Handbook* directs attention to the retrospective question of

example, the Full Federal Court of Australia declined to follow the approach to criminal law exclusion recommended in the *Handbook*, preferring to adopt the tack endorsed in the UNHCR's Global Consultations process and subsequently codified in a Guideline on International Protection.[168] Similarly, the Canadian Federal Court of Appeal relied upon the "less categorical" approach taken to the definition of a "manifestly unfounded claim" in UNHCR's Global Consultations process to conclude that there is no international consensus on the meaning of this term – even though the judgment acknowledged the existence of a formally adopted Executive Committee conclusion directly on point, characterized by the Court as providing for a "restricted meaning" to be given to the notion.[169] In contrast, the New Zealand Court of Appeal declined to give significant weight to the new wave of UNHCR institutional positions because of their questionable legal pedigree:

> The Guidelines do not, however, have a status in relation to interpretation of the Refugee Convention that is equal to that of the resolutions of the UNHCR Executive Committee ... I have focussed ... on the Executive Committee's views which in any event I regard as the most valuable guide for the Court.[170]

whether the applicant "could have sought refuge in another part of the same country": UNHCR, *Handbook*, at para. 91. Yet in its "Guideline on International Protection: Internal Flight or Relocation Alternative," UN Doc. HCR/GIP/03/04 – expressly said to be a "supplement" to the *Handbook* – UNHCR suggests that assessment should instead focus on "whether the proposed area provides a meaningful alternative in the future. The forward-looking assessment is all the more important": ibid. at para. 8. The point is not that the new standard is less appropriate than that set by the *Handbook*, but simply that the effort to promote inconsistent approaches will only engender confusion and lack of respect for UNHCR standard-setting. Adding to this concern, while the new Guidelines are in principle intended to "draw on" the expert advice received during the agency's Global Consultations process (Executive Committee of the High Commissioner's Program, "Agenda for Protection," UN Doc. EC/52/SC/CRP.9/Rev.1, June 26, 2002, at Part III, Goal 1, Point 6), the Guidelines at times diverge from even the formal conclusions reached through that process. See e.g. J. Hathaway and M. Foster, "Membership of a Particular Social Group," (2003) 15(3) *International Journal of Refugee Law* 477, at para. 44. Yet in at least one case, an appellate court gave weight to the new Guidelines on the express grounds that "[t]hey ... result from the Second Track of the Global Consultations on International Protection Process": *Minister for Immigration and Multicultural Affairs v. Applicant S*, [2002] FCAFC 244 (Aus. FFC, Aug. 21, 2002).

[168] "By consensus, it was agreed [at the Lisbon Expert Roundtable of the Global Consultations] on the question of balancing [the risks of return against the seriousness of the crime committed] ... [that] state practice indicates that the balancing test is no longer being used in common law and in some civil law jurisdictions": *NADB of 2001 v. Minister for Immigration and Multicultural Affairs*, [2002] FCAFC 326 (Aus. FFC, Oct. 31, 2002).

[169] *Rahaman v. Minister of Citizenship and Immigration*, 2002 ACWSJ Lexis 1026 (Can. FCA, Mar. 1, 2002).

[170] *Attorney General v. Refugee Council of New Zealand Inc.*, [2003] 2 NZLR 577 (NZ CA, Apr. 16, 2003), per McGrath J. at para. 111. Justice Glazebrook gave the Guidelines somewhat greater weight, noting that "it is also appropriate to have regard to ... the

We thus find ourselves at a moment of significant normative confusion on the appropriate source of UNHCR institutional advice on the substance of international refugee law. The critical role of UNHCR in providing Art. 35 guidance to state parties is compromised not only by the sheer volume of less-than-fully-consistent advice now emanating from a multiplicity of UNHCR sources, but more fundamentally by recent efforts to draft institutional positions at such a highly detailed level that they simply cannot be reconciled with the binding jurisprudence of state parties. It would therefore be in the best interest of all that general principles of refugee law interpretation intended to be taken seriously by state parties be codified in formal, and clearly authoritative, resolutions of the UNHCR's Executive Committee. More detailed guidance may sensibly be gleaned from a compendium of norms prepared by the agency itself, but that advice should rather be presented in a unified form that does not risk the confusion or conflicts of the present array of the *Handbook*, Guidelines, and various other UNHCR position papers. More preliminary thinking is best presented as such, with any effort at codification by the agency delayed until there is truly a clear and principled consensus achieved in the jurisprudence of state parties.

2.5.3 Regional refugee rights regimes

Regional refugee law in Africa establishes auxiliary rights for refugees in that region. The Convention governing the Specific Aspects of Refugee Problems in Africa[171] requires participating states of the African Union (formerly the Organization of African Unity) to "use their best endeavors consistent with their respective legislation[ ] to receive refugees and to secure [their] settlement" until and unless voluntary repatriation is possible.[172] The duty of *non-refoulement* is explicitly recognized within the region to prohibit rejection at the frontier, and to apply whenever there is a risk to the refugee's "life, physical integrity, or liberty."[173] Equally important, states bind themselves to take account of the security needs of refugees, settling them away from the frontier with their country of origin.[174] In return, refugees are to respect the asylum state's laws and comply with public order measures. They are also prohibited from engaging in "subversive activities against any Member State of the OAU," and even from expressing political or other views if "likely to

---

Guidelines ... because the Immigration Service refers to them ... and cannot be seen to 'pick and choose' the parts it wishes to comply with. It is also relevant that New Zealand will be judged in the light of those Guidelines by the Office of UNHCR in its monitoring role": ibid. at para. 271.

[171] Convention governing the Specific Aspects of Refugee Problems in Africa, 10011 UNTS 14691, done Sept. 10, 1969, entered into force June 20, 1974 (OAU Convention).

[172] Ibid. at Arts. II(1) and V.   [173] Ibid. at Art. II(3).   [174] Ibid. at Art. II(6).

cause tension between Member States."[175] The African Convention therefore goes beyond the basic indifference of the Refugee Convention to the political rights of refugees,[176] and purports to deny some forms of political free speech as the cost of enhanced basic protection rights.[177]

The Cartagena Declaration of 1984[178] has been recommended to states in the Americas by the General Assembly of the Organization of American States.[179] Although it is not a binding agreement akin to the African Union's treaty, the Cartagena Declaration provides a clear statement of the region's optic on desirable protections for refugees. The inclusive African reading of the duty of *non-refoulement* and that region's undertaking to ensure the physical protection of refugees are adopted by the OAS.[180] There are moreover commitments to refugee integration, self-sufficiency, employment, and family reunification.[181] The Cartagena Declaration explicitly affirms the continuing value of the Refugee Convention's rights regime,[182] and does not condition its expanded definition of refugee rights on the renunciation of political or other activity. To date, however, it has not been formalized as a matter of binding law.

2.5.4 International human rights law

While there has been only modest evolution of the refugee rights regime since 1951, the broader field of international human rights law has undergone exponential change. The Refugee Convention was only the second major human rights convention adopted by the United Nations.[183] The only contemporaneous formulation of international human rights was the Universal Declaration of Human Rights, an unenforceable General Assembly resolution.[184] Today, on the other hand, binding international human rights law has been established by the 1966 Human Rights Covenants, specialized universal accords, and regional human rights regimes in Europe, Africa, and the Americas. As the UNHCR's Executive Committee has observed, the modern duty of protection therefore

---

[175] Ibid. at Art. III.   [176] See chapter 2.4.4 above, at pp. 100–101.

[177] While the African treaty's failure to guarantee political rights to refugees is likely not in contravention of the Refugee Convention itself (see chapter 6.7 below, at pp. 882–885), its sweeping prohibition on political activities cannot be reconciled to duties under the Covenant on Civil and Political Rights: see chapter 6.7 below at pp. 897–905.

[178] OAS Doc. OEA/Ser.L/II.66, Doc.10, Rev.1, at 190–193 (OAS Cartagena Declaration).

[179] See UNHCR, "OAS General Assembly: an Inter-American Initiative on Refugees," (1986) 27 *Refugees* 5.

[180] OAS Cartagena Declaration, at Part III(5), (6), and (7).

[181] Ibid. at Part III(6), (11), and (13).   [182] Ibid. at Part III(8).

[183] The Refugee Convention was preceded by the Convention on the Prevention and Punishment of the Crime of Genocide, UNGA Res. 260A(III), adopted Dec. 9, 1948, entered into force Jan. 12, 1951.

[184] See chapter 1.2.3 above, at p. 45.

goes beyond simply respecting the norms of refugee law; it includes also the obligation "to take all necessary measures to ensure that refugees are effectively protected, including through national legislation, and in compliance with their obligations under international human rights and humanitarian law instruments bearing directly on refugee protection."[185]

Indeed, the maturation of human rights law over the past half-century has to a certain extent filled the vacuum of protection that required the development of a refugee-specific rights regime in 1951. As a preliminary matter, it might therefore be asked whether the rights regime set by the Refugee Convention retains any independent value in the modern era of general guarantees of human rights.

It is certainly true that refugees will sometimes find it in their interests to rely on generally applicable norms of international human rights law, rather than on refugee-specific standards.[186] Of greatest significance to refugees, nearly all internationally recognized *civil rights* are declared to be universal and not subject to requirements of nationality.[187] The International Covenant on Civil and Political Rights generally extends its broad-ranging protection to "everyone" or to "all persons."[188] Each contracting state undertakes in Art. 2(1) to ensure the rights in the Covenant "to all individuals within its territory and subject to its jurisdiction ... without distinction of any kind, such as race, colour, sex, language, religion, political or other opinion, national or social origin, property, birth or other status." While nationality is not included in this illustrative list, it has been determined to be embraced by the residual category of "other status."[189] Thus, the Human Rights Committee has explicitly affirmed that "the general rule is that each one of the rights of the Covenant must be guaranteed without discrimination between citizens and aliens. Aliens must receive the benefit of the general requirement of non-discrimination in respect of the rights guaranteed by the Covenant."[190] More recently, the Committee has held that rights may not be

---

[185] UNHCR Executive Committee Conclusion No. 81, "General Conclusion on International Protection" (1997), at para. (e), available at www.unhcr.ch (accessed Nov. 20, 2004).

[186] The UNHCR Executive Committee has, for example, affirmed "that States must continue to be guided, in their treatment of refugees, by existing international law and humanitarian principles and practice bearing in mind the moral dimension of providing refugee protection": UNHCR Executive Committee Conclusion No. 50, "General Conclusion on International Protection" (1988), at para. (c), available at www.unhcr.ch (accessed Nov. 20, 2004).

[187] The exceptions are that only citizens are granted the rights to vote, to run for office, and to enter the public service: Civil and Political Covenant, at Art. 25.

[188] See chapter 2.5.5 below, at pp. 127–128.

[189] One commentator prefers to ground his analysis in the notion of nationality as a "distinction of any kind": Lillich, *Rights of Aliens*, at 46.

[190] UN Human Rights Committee, "General Comment No. 15: The position of aliens under the Covenant" (1986), UN Doc. HRI/GEN/1/Rev.7, May 12, 2004, at 140, para. 2.

limited to citizens of a state, but "must also be available to all individuals, regardless of nationality or statelessness, such as asylum-seekers [and] refugees."[191] The Civil and Political Covenant is therefore a critical source of rights for refugees, mandating attention to matters not addressed in the Refugee Convention, such as the rights to life and family, freedoms of opinion and expression, and protection from torture, inhuman or degrading treatment, and slavery.

On the other hand, because the Covenant on Civil and Political Rights is addressed primarily to persons who reside in their state of citizenship, it does not deal with refugee-specific concerns, including recognition of personal status, access to naturalization, immunity from penalization for illegal entry, the need for travel and other identity documents, and especially protection from *refoulement*. Moreover, even where the subject matter of the Civil and Political Covenant is relevant to refugees, the Covenant often formulates rights on the basis of inappropriate assumptions. For example, the Civil and Political Covenant sets guarantees of fairness in judicial proceedings, but does not deal with the more basic issue of access to a court system.[192] Yet refugees and other aliens, unlike citizens, are not always able freely to invoke judicial remedies. Perhaps most ominously, governments faced with genuine public emergencies are authorized to withdraw all but a few core civil rights from non-citizens,[193] even if the measures taken would ordinarily amount to impermissible discrimination on grounds of national origin, birth, or other status.[194] In the result, though the Covenant on Civil and Political Rights in

[191] UN Human Rights Committee, "General Comment No. 31: The nature of the general legal obligations of states parties to the Covenant" (2004), UN Doc. HRI/GEN/1/Rev.7, May 12, 2004, at 192, para. 10.

[192] Compare Civil and Political Covenant, at Arts. 14–16, with the Refugee Convention, at Art. 16.

[193] The rights which cannot be suspended are the rights to life; freedom from torture, cruel, inhuman, or degrading treatment or punishment; freedom from slavery; freedom from imprisonment for contractual breach; freedom from *ex post facto* criminal law; recognition as a person; and freedom of thought, conscience, and religion: Civil and Political Covenant, at Art. 4(2).

[194] Ordinarily, emergency derogation must not be imposed in a discriminatory way. However, the grounds of impermissible discrimination for emergency derogation purposes explicitly omit reference to several of the general grounds on which discrimination is prohibited under the Civil and Political Covenant. The omissions include discrimination on the grounds of political or other opinion; national origin; property; birth or other status. Compare Civil and Political Covenant, at Arts. 2(1) and 4(1). The UN Special Rapporteur on the Rights of Non-Citizens has suggested that "[t]his omission, according to the *travaux préparatoires*, was intentional because the drafters of the Covenant understood that States may, in time of national emergency, have to discriminate against non-citizens within their territory": UN Commission on Human Rights, "Preliminary Report of the Special Rapporteur on the Rights of Non-Citizens," UN Doc. E/CN.4/Sub.2/2001/20, June 6, 2001, at para. 37.

principle extends its protections to refugees, it does not dependably provide for all basic civil rights needed to address their predicament.

The continuing value of refugee-specific rights despite the advent of broad-ranging international human rights law is even more apparent in the field of *socioeconomic rights*. While the basic non-discrimination obligation under the International Covenant on Economic, Social and Cultural Rights[195] is essentially indistinguishable from that set by the Civil and Political Covenant,[196] developing countries are authorized to decide, considering their economic situation, the extent to which they will guarantee the economic rights of the Convention to non-nationals.[197] If subjected to this fundamental limitation, the vast majority of the world's refugees (who are located in the less developed world) might be denied employment or subsistence rights. The Refugee Convention, in contrast, sets absolute, if less exigent, expectations of states in the field of economic rights.

Second, as with the Civil and Political Covenant, the substantive formulation of general socioeconomic rights in the Economic, Social and Cultural Covenant does not always provide sufficient contextual specificity to ensure respect for the most critical interests of refugees. For example, while the Economic, Social and Cultural Covenant establishes a general right to an

[195] International Covenant on Economic, Social and Cultural Rights, UNGA Res. 2200A(XXI), adopted Dec. 16, 1966, entered into force Jan. 3, 1976 (Economic, Social and Cultural Covenant).

[196] Two kinds of distinction are sometimes asserted. First, while state parties to the Civil and Political Covenant agree to *grant* rights to all without discrimination, the contemporaneously drafted Economic, Social and Cultural Covenant requires only an undertaking that whatever rights are granted may be *exercised* without discrimination: compare Civil and Political Covenant, at Art. 2(1) and Economic, Social and Cultural Covenant, at Art. 2(2). Superficially, this would suggest that whereas the Civil and Political Covenant prohibits limitation of the category of rights holders, the formulation in the Economic, Social and Cultural Covenant does not. In fact, however, the various rights in the Economic, Social and Cultural Covenant are granted to "everyone" or "all," nullifying any practical distinction between the non-discrimination clauses in the two Covenants. Second, the non-discrimination provision in the Civil and Political Covenant seems to be more inclusively framed than its counterpart in the Economic, Social and Cultural Covenant. Whereas the former prohibits "distinction of any kind, such as" a distinction based on the listed forms of status, the Economic, Social and Cultural Covenant prohibits "discrimination of any kind as to" the enumerated types of status. But unless it is suggested that no differentiation, even on patently reasonable grounds, can ever be permissible in relation to rights under the Civil and Political Covenant, no concrete consequences flow from use of the word "distinction" rather than "discrimination." Nor does it matter that one Covenant prohibits discrimination "such as" that based on certain grounds, while the other proscribes discrimination "as to" those same grounds. Because the list under both Covenants includes the generic term "other status," the net result in each case is an inclusive duty of non-discrimination, including, for example, non-discrimination in relation to refugees and other aliens.

[197] Economic, Social and Cultural Covenant, at Art. 2(3).

adequate standard of living, it does not explicitly guarantee equal access to rationing systems, a matter of frequent immediate concern to involuntary migrants in war zones and other areas of crisis.[198]

Most critically, generally applicable socioeconomic rights are normally conceived simply as duties of progressive implementation.[199] Under the Economic, Social and Cultural Covenant, for example, states are required simply to "take steps" progressively to realize Economic, Social and Cultural rights to the extent possible within the limits of their resources.[200] The Refugee Convention, on the other hand, treats socioeconomic rights on par with civil and political rights. They are duties of result, and may not be avoided because of competition within the host state for scarce resources.

2.5.5 Duty of equal protection of non-citizens

As among the various protections now guaranteed by international human rights law, the duty of non-discrimination clearly has the potential to be of greatest value to refugees. Because it is an overarching principle governing the allocation of a wide array of, in particular, public goods, the legal duty of non-discrimination can be an effective means by which to address the need to enfranchise refugees on a multiplicity of fronts. To the extent that the main concern of refugees is to be accepted by a host community, a guarantee of non-discrimination might in fact be virtually the only legal guarantee that many refugees require.

The value of protection against discrimination is, of course, a function of how that duty is framed. As McCrudden has observed,

> There is no one legal meaning of equality or discrimination applicable in the different circumstances; the meanings of equality and discrimination are diverse. There is no consistency in the circumstances in which stronger or weaker concepts of equality and discrimination currently apply. There is no one organizing principle or purpose underlying the principles of equality and non-discrimination currently applicable; the justifications offered for the legal principles of equality and non-discrimination are diverse.[201]

---

[198] Compare Economic, Social and Cultural Covenant, at Art. 11, with Refugee Convention, at Art. 20.

[199] In the case of the Civil and Political Covenant, the Human Rights Committee has observed that "[t]he requirement under article 2, paragraph 2, to take steps to give effect to the Covenant rights is unqualified and of immediate effect. A failure to comply with this obligation cannot be justified by reference to political, social, cultural or economic considerations within the State": UN Human Rights Committee, "General Comment No. 31: The nature of the general legal obligations imposed on states parties to the Covenant" (2004), UN Doc. HRI/GEN/1/Rev.7, May 12, 2004, at 192, para. 14.

[200] Economic, Social and Cultural Covenant, at Art. 2(1).

[201] C. McCrudden, "Equality and Discrimination," in D. Feldman ed., *English Public Law* (vol. XI, 2004) (McCrudden, "Equality"), at para. 11.02.

Despite the breadth of possible applications, Fredman helpfully suggests that the common core of non-discrimination law is to ensure "that individuals should be judged according to their personal qualities. This basic tenet is contravened if individuals are subjected to detriment on the basis only of their status, their group membership, or irrelevant physical characteristics."[202]

The core understanding of non-discrimination thus requires simply that irrelevant criteria not be taken into account in making allocations: it is essentially a fairly formal prohibition of arbitrariness, which requires that any unequal treatment be "properly justified, according to consistently applied, persuasive, and acceptable criteria."[203] It follows, of course, that not every differential allocation is discriminatory: the concern is to draw a line between invidious (discriminatory) and socially acceptable (non-discriminatory) distinctions. While this can be a vexed question, international human rights law normally stipulates grounds on which distinctions are presumptively arbitrary, including where allocations are based on forms of status or personal characteristics which are either immutable or fundamental to one's identity. Because decisions predicated on such criteria are clearly prone to stereotypical and hence arbitrary assumptions, they undermine the duty to consider individuals on their own merits.

Non-discrimination law's insistence on non-arbitrariness is often more rigorously conceived where "prized public goods"[204] – including human rights – are at stake. This may, for example, take the form of heightened scrutiny or insistence on a proportionality test in the assessment of the rationality of the differential allocation under scrutiny. Critically, non-discrimination may also be conceived in a way that moves the principle beyond simply a prohibition of allocations shown to be based on irrelevant or otherwise arbitrary criteria (which requires often difficult, if not impossible, comparative assessments) to include also a prohibition of conduct which *in effect*, even if not by design, results in an arbitrary allocation at odds with the duty to ensure that individuals are treated in accordance with their particular merits. Indeed, formal equality of treatment may itself result in discrimination. As Fredman writes, "treating people in the same way regardless of their differing backgrounds frequently entrenches difference."[205] Most important of all, non-discrimination may also be understood to be not only a prohibition of arbitrary allocations – whether by design, or as measured by effects – but also an affirmative guarantee of equal opportunity. Under such an understanding, non-discrimination requires public authorities "to do more than ensure the absence of discrimination ... but also to act positively to promote equality of opportunity between different groups

---

[202] S. Fredman, *Discrimination Law* (2001) (Fredman, *Discrimination*), at 66.
[203] McCrudden, "Equality," at para. 11.71.   [204] Ibid. at para. 11.76.
[205] Fredman, *Discrimination*, at 106.

throughout all policy making and in carrying out all those activities to which the duty applies."[206]

The core guarantee of non-discrimination in international human rights law is that found in Art. 26 of the Civil and Political Covenant. This unique and broadly applicable guarantee of non-discrimination provides that:

> All persons are equal before the law and are entitled without any discrimination to the equal protection of the law. In this respect, the law shall prohibit any discrimination and guarantee to all persons equal and effective protection against discrimination on any ground such as race, colour, sex, language, religion, political or other opinion, national or social origin, property, birth or other status.[207]

While there are many other guarantees of non-discrimination – for example, Art. 2 in each of the Human Rights Covenants, and Art. 3 of the Refugee Convention – Art. 26 is unique in that its ambit is not limited to the allocation of simply the rights found in any one instrument. Art. 26 rather governs the allocation of all public goods, including rights not stipulated by the Covenant itself. As summarized in General Comment 18 of the Human Rights Committee,

> [A]rticle 26 does not merely duplicate the guarantee already provided for in article 2 [of the Civil and Political Covenant] but provides in itself an autonomous right. It prohibits discrimination in law or in fact in any field regulated and protected by public authorities. Article 26 is therefore concerned with the obligations imposed on States parties in regard to their legislation and the application thereof. Thus, when legislation is adopted by a State party, it must comply with the requirement of article 26 that its content should not be discriminatory. In other words, the application of the principle of non-discrimination contained in article 26 is not limited to those rights which are provided for in the Covenant.[208]

---

[206] McCrudden, "Equality," at para. 11.187.   [207] Civil and Political Covenant, at Art. 26.

[208] UN Human Rights Committee, "General Comment No. 18: Non-discrimination" (1989), UN Doc. HRI/GEN/1/Rev.7, May 12, 2004, at 146, para. 12. This principle has been affirmed in the jurisprudence of the Human Rights Committee, including, for example, in *Pepels v. Netherlands*, UNHRC Comm. No. 484/1991, UN Doc. CCPR/C/51/D/484/1991, decided July 15, 1994, at para. 7.2; and *Pons v. Spain*, UNHRC Comm. No. 454/1991, UN Doc. CCPR/C/55/D/454/1991, decided Oct. 30, 1995, at para. 9.3. In *Teesdale v. Trinidad and Tobago*, UNHRC Comm. No. 677/1996, UN Doc. CCPR/C/74/D/677/1996, decided Apr. 1, 2002, for example, the Committee "recall[ed] its established jurisprudence that article 26 of the Covenant prohibits discrimination in law and in fact in any field regulated and protected by public authorities": ibid. at para. 9.8. It thus determined that it had the authority to determine whether the discretionary decision of the President regarding whether to commute a death sentence was exercised in a discriminatory way.

The first branch of Art. 26, equality before the law, is a relatively formal prohibition of negative conduct: it requires simply that there be no discrimination in the enforcement of existing laws. Several delegates to the Third Committee of the General Assembly argued that this guarantee of procedural non-discrimination, standing alone, was insufficient. For example, the representative of the Philippines observed that the obligation to ensure equality before the law would not preclude states from "providing for separate but equal facilities such as housing, schools and restaurants for different groups."[209] The Polish delegate agreed, pointing out that even much South African *apartheid*-era legislation could be reconciled to a guarantee of equality before the law.[210] These concerns suggested the need for a duty of non-discrimination addressed not just to the process of law enforcement, but to the *substance* of laws themselves.

The precedent drawn upon by the drafters of the Civil and Political Covenant was the principle advanced in the Universal Declaration of Human Rights of a right to *equal protection of the law*.[211] As reframed in the Covenant, the equal protection component of Art. 26 is an extraordinarily inclusive obligation, requiring that "the legislature must refrain from any discrimination when enacting laws ... [and] is also obligated to prohibit discrimination by enacting special laws and to afford effective protection against discrimination."[212] While commentators are not unanimous in their interpretation of Art. 26,[213] both the literal text of this article and an appreciation of its drafting history suggest that this provision was designed to be an extraordinarily robust guarantee of non-discrimination including, in particular, an affirmative duty to prohibit discrimination and effectively to protect all persons from discrimination.[214]

It is true that the provision was originally drafted as no more than a guarantee of "equality before the law," and that the second sentence's prohibition of discrimination was amended to reinforce this purpose by linking the duty of non-discrimination to the goal of equality before the

---

[209] UN Doc. A/C.3/SR.1098, at para. 25.   [210] UN Doc. A/C.3/SR.1101, at para. 21.

[211] "All are equal before the law and are entitled without any discrimination to equal protection of the law. All are entitled to equal protection against any discrimination in violation of this Declaration and against any incitement to such discrimination": Universal Declaration, at Art. 7.

[212] Nowak, *ICCPR Commentary*, at 468.

[213] A narrow view of the scope of Art. 26 is argued by Vierdag, who concludes that "[t]he starting point was, and remained, to provide a guarantee of 'equality before the law.' All later additions were proposed and adopted with the strengthening of this principle in mind": E. Vierdag, *The Concept of Discrimination in International Law, with a Special Reference to Human Rights* (1973), at 126.

[214] See Nowak, *ICCPR Commentary*, at 462–465.

law through insertion of the words "[i]n this respect." As Nowak correctly observes, however, an intervening amendment expanded the scope of the first sentence's guarantee to include also the sweeping notion of "equal protection of the law." In the result, the correlative phrase "[i]n this respect" is logically read to require the prohibition of discrimination and the effective protection against discrimination in *both* senses stipulated in the first sentence, namely equality before the law *and* equal protection of the law.[215]

Refugees and other non-citizens are entitled to invoke Art. 26's duty to avoid arbitrary allocations and its affirmative duty to bring about non-arbitrary allocations since the Human Rights Committee has determined "that each one of the rights of the Covenant must be guaranteed without discrimination between citizens and aliens,"[216] a principle explicitly determined to extend to refugees and asylum-seekers.[217] Because the second branch of Art. 26 – the duty to ensure "equal protection of the law" – may reasonably be read to set an obligation to take the steps needed to offset the disadvantages which involuntary alienage creates for the enjoyment of rights,[218] it might even be thought that Art. 26 would be a sufficient basis

---

[215] "[S]ince the adoption of the Indian amendment, the passage 'in this respect' no longer relates only to equality before the law but also to equal protection of the law. That this involves two completely different aspects of the principle of equality was made unmistakably clear by the Indian delegate": ibid. at 464–465.

[216] UN Human Rights Committee, "General Comment No. 15: The position of aliens under the Covenant" (1986), UN Doc. HRI/GEN/1/Rev.7, May 12, 2004, at 140, para. 2. In the Committee's decision of *Karakurt v. Austria*, UNHRC Comm. No. 965/2000, UN Doc. CCPR/C/74/D/965/2000, decided Apr. 4, 2002, two members of the Committee took the opportunity to affirm that "[i]n [their] view distinctions based on citizenship fall under the notion of 'other status' in article 26": ibid. at Individual Opinion of Members Rodley and Scheinen. While General Comment No. 15 interprets only the Civil and Political Covenant, it is reasonable to assume that the virtually identical prohibition of discrimination on the basis of "other status" in the Economic, Social and Cultural Covenant will be similarly interpreted to protect the entitlement of aliens to national treatment in relation to its catalog of rights.

[217] UN Human Rights Committee, "General Comment No. 31: The nature of the general legal obligation imposed on states parties to the Covenant" (2004), UN Doc. HRI/GEN/1/Rev.7, May 12, 2004, 192, at para. 10.

[218] In *Nahlik v. Austria*, UNHRC Comm. No. 608/1995, UN Doc. CCPR/C/57/D/608/1995, decided July 22, 1996, the Committee was faced with an objection by Austria that "the communication [was] inadmissible … since it relates to alleged discrimination within a private agreement, over which the State party has no influence. The Committee observes that under articles 2 and 26 of the Covenant the State party is under an obligation to ensure that all individuals within its territory and subject to its jurisdiction are free from discrimination, and consequently the courts of States parties are under an obligation to protect individuals against discrimination, whether this occurs within the public sphere or among private parties in the quasi-public sector of, for example, employment": ibid. at

to require asylum states to bring an end to any laws or practices that set refugees apart from the rest of their community.[219]

Despite the apparent extraordinary potential of Art. 26, however, it is unlikely in practice to prove a sufficient mechanism for the full enfranchisement of refugees. This is because Art. 26, like common Art. 2 of the Covenants,

para. 8.2. In *Waldman v. Canada*, UNHRC Comm. No. 694/1996, UN Doc. CCPR/C/67/ D/694/1996, decided Nov. 3, 1999, the Human Rights Committee observed that "[t]he material before the Committee does not show that members of the Roman Catholic community or any identifiable section of that community are now in a disadvantaged position compared to those members of the Jewish community that wish to secure the education of their children in religious schools. Accordingly, the Committee rejects the State party's argument that the preferential treatment of Roman Catholic schools is nondiscriminatory because of its Constitutional obligation": ibid. at para. 10.4 – implying that differentiation which *was* directed to combating disadvantage would not likely be found to be discriminatory. Such a construction is in line with the jurisprudence of many developed states with respect to comparably framed domestic guarantees of non-discrimination. "What is required by Congress is the removal of artificial, arbitrary, unnecessary barriers to employment when the barriers operate invidiously to discriminate on the basis of racial or other impermissible classification": *Griggs v. Duke Power Co.*, 401 US 424 (US SC, Mar. 8, 1971), at 430–431. "At the heart of the prohibition of unfair discrimination lies a recognition that the purpose of our new constitutional and democratic order is the establishment of a society in which all human beings will be accorded equal dignity and respect regardless of their membership of particular groups": *President of the Republic of South Africa v. Hug CCT*, (1997) 4 SA 1 (SA CC, Apr. 8, 1997).

[219] But in *Sahak v. Minister for Immigration and Multicultural Affairs*, [2002] FCAFC 215 (Aus. FFC, July 18, 2002), the Full Federal Court of Australia was called upon to consider whether there was a breach of the duty of non-discrimination contained in Art. 5 of the International Convention on the Elimination of All Forms of Racial Discrimination, UNGA Res. 2106A(XX), adopted Dec. 21, 1965, entered into force Jan. 4, 1969 (Racial Discrimination Convention). Under Art. 5, states "undertake to prohibit and to eliminate racial discrimination in all its forms and to guarantee the right of everyone, without distinction as to race, color, or national or ethnic origin, to equality before the law, notably in the enjoyment of . . . [t]he right to equal treatment before the tribunals and all other organs administering justice": ibid. at Art. 5(a). The claim involved persons seeking recognition of their refugee status who did not speak English, and who were detained in a facility with only limited availability of interpreters. They had done everything in their power to meet the twenty-eight-day deadline for applying for judicial review of the rejection of their refugee claims but could not comply because of lack of documentation, interpreters, and lawyers in the detention facility. Their argument that the judicial review rules amounted, in effect, to race-based discrimination was, however, rejected on the formal grounds that "the Act does not deprive persons of one race of a right [to judicial review] that is enjoyed by another race, nor does it provide for differential operation depending on the race, color, or national or ethnic origin of the relevant applicant. For example, persons whose national origin is Afghani or Syrian are able to take advantage of the relevant right if their comprehension of the English language is sufficient, or if they have access to friends or professional interpreters so as to overcome the language barrier . . . Any differential effect . . . is not based on race, color, descent or national or ethnic origin, but rather on the individual personal circumstances of each applicant." North J, in dissent, opted for an effects-based understanding of the duty of non-

does not establish a simple guarantee of equal protection of the law for refugees or any other group.[220] While initially proposed as such, the right as ultimately adopted is in fact an entitlement "*without any discrimination* to the equal protection of the law [emphasis added]."[221] To give effect to this formulation, the Human Rights Committee inquires whether a differential allocation of rights is "reasonable and objective."[222] If the differentiation is found to meet this test, it is not discriminatory and there is accordingly no duty either to desist from differentiation or to take positive steps to equalize opportunity under Art. 26.

Three particular trends in the application of the "reasonable and objective" standard may work against the interests of refugees and other non-citizens. First, the Committee has too frequently been prepared to recognize

discrimination, writing that "to say that any differential impact is suffered not because of national origin, but rather as a result of individual personal circumstances, appears to me to adopt a verbal formula which avoids the real and practical discrimination." Invoking the decision of the US Supreme Court in *Griggs v. Duke Power Co.*, 401 US 424 (US SC, 1971), at 430–431, he concluded that "[t]o approach anti-discrimination provisions in [a formal, intent-based] way would rob them of much of their intended force."

[220] But see T. Clark and J. Niessen, "Equality Rights and Non-Citizens in Europe and America: The Promise, the Practice, and Some Remaining Issues," (1996) 14(3) *Netherlands Quarterly of Human Rights* 245, in which it is argued that the duty of non-discrimination requires the minimization of distinctions between aliens and nationals.

[221] The original amendment of India to add to the first sentence the words "and are entitled to equal protection of the law" (UN Doc. A/C.3/L.945) was sub-amended by a proposal of Argentina and Chile (UN Doc. A/C.3/L.948) to insert between the words "are entitled" and "to equal protection of the law" the words "without any discrimination": UN Doc. A/5000, at para. 103 (1961).

[222] For example, the Committee determined in *Broeks v. Netherlands*, UNHRC Comm. No. 172/1984, decided Apr. 9, 1987, at para. 13, that "[t]he right to equality before the law and to equal protection of the law without any discrimination does not make all differences of treatment discriminatory. A differentiation based on reasonable and objective criteria does not amount to prohibited discrimination within the meaning of article 26." See also *Danning v. Netherlands*, UNHRC Comm. No. 180/1984, decided Apr. 9, 1987; and *Zwaan-de Vries v. Netherlands*, UNHRC Comm. No. 182/1984, decided Apr. 9, 1987. At one point, the test appeared to have been watered down to a simple assessment of "reasonableness." In *Simunek et al. v. Czech Republic*, UNHRC Comm. No. 516/1992, UN Doc. CCPR/C/54/D/516/1992, decided July 19, 1995, the Committee held that "[a] differentiation which is compatible with the provisions of the Covenant and is based on reasonable grounds does not amount to prohibited discrimination within the meaning of article 26": ibid. at para. 11.5. But the traditional "reasonable and objective" formulation has been affirmed in more recent jurisprudence: see e.g. *Oord v. Netherlands*, UNHRC Comm. No. 658/1995, UN Doc. CCPR/C/60/D/658/1995, decided July 23, 1997, at para. 8.5; *Foin v. France*, UNHRC Comm. No. 666/1995, UN Doc. CCPR/C/67/D/666/1995, decided Nov. 3, 1999, at para. 10.3; *Waldman v. Canada*, UNHRC Comm. No. 694/1996, UN Doc. CCPR/C/67/D/694/1996, decided Nov. 3, 1999, at para. 10.4; and *Wackenheim v. France*, UNHRC Comm. No. 854/1999, UN Doc. CCPR/C/67/D/854/1999, decided July 15, 2002, at para. 7.4.

differentiation on the basis of certain categories, including non-citizenship, as presumptively reasonable. Second and related, the Committee has paid insufficient attention to evidence that generally applicable standards may impact differently on differently situated groups, thereby failing to do justice to a substantive understanding of the right to equal protection of the law.[223] And third and most generally, the Human Rights Committee routinely affords governments an extraordinarily broad margin of appreciation rather than engaging in careful analysis of both the logic and extent of the differential treatment.

Turning to the first concern, some kinds of differentiation seem simply to be assumed to be reasonable by the Human Rights Committee. The Committee, for example, apparently feels that it is self-evidently reasonable to deny unmarried spouses the social welfare rights granted to married spouses,[224] or to withhold general guarantees of legal due process from

---

[223] "Fair equality of opportunity differs from the simple non-discrimination principle ... in being positive as well as negative in its requirements and in taking into account some of the prior existing disadvantages ... The two principles differ also in the conception of the social processes of inequality on which they tend to be grounded. A demand for fair equality of opportunity is more often than not based on a recognition of the structural sources of unequal opportunity and in particular on an acceptance of what has become known as 'institutional discrimination.' Finally, fair equality of opportunity, again unlike the simple non-discrimination principle, requires questions to be asked not only about the precise basis on which the good being distributed is deserved but also about the nature of the good being distributed": C. McCrudden, "Institutional Discrimination," (1982) 2(3) *Oxford Journal of Legal Studies* 303, at 344–345.

[224] "[T]he decision to enter into a legal status by marriage, which provides, in Netherlands law, both for certain benefits and for certain duties and responsibilities, lies entirely with the cohabiting persons. By choosing not to enter into marriage, Mr. Danning and his cohabitant have not, in law, assumed the full extent of the duties and responsibilities incumbent on married couples. *Consequently*, Mr. Danning does not receive the full benefits provided for in Netherlands law for married couples [emphasis added]": *Danning v. Netherlands*, UNHRC Comm. No. 180/1984, decided Apr. 9, 1987, at para. 14. See also *Sprenger v. Netherlands*, UNHRC Comm. No. 395/1990, UN Doc. CCPR/C/44/D/395/1990, decided Mar. 31, 1992. The use of the conjunction "consequently" erroneously suggests a logical nexus between the absence of the legal duties and responsibilities of married spouses and ineligibility for social welfare benefits. Whatever reasonable differentiation may be made between married and unmarried cohabitants, the needs of couples of both classes for income support consequent to the disability of one partner are not obviously distinct. The Human Rights Committee did not, however, even consider this question. The Committee has recently affirmed this approach in its decision of *Derksen v. Netherlands*, UNHRC Comm. No. 976/2001, UN Doc. CCPR/C/80/D/1976/2001, decided Apr. 1, 2004, at para. 9.2: "The Committee reiterates that not every distinction amounts to prohibited discrimination under the Covenant, as long as it is based on reasonable and objective criteria. The Committee recalls that it has earlier found that a differentiation between married and unmarried couples does not amount to a violation of article 26 of the Covenant, since married and unmarried couples are subject to different legal regimes and the decision whether or not to enter into a legal status by marriage lies entirely with the [cohabiting] persons."

military conscripts.[225] On the basis of the drafting history of the Covenant, there is a clear risk that differentiation based on lack of citizenship may similarly be assumed to be reasonable, in at least some circumstances.

Specifically, several delegations, including the Indian representative who spearheaded the drive to include the guarantee of equality before the law, made it clear that they were not suggesting that all distinctions between nationals and aliens should be eradicated.[226] The non-discrimination clause was said not to prohibit measures to control aliens and their enterprises, particularly since Art. 1 of the Covenant guarantees the right of peoples to permanent sovereignty over their natural wealth and resources.[227] An effort to confine Art. 26's protection against discrimination to "citizens" rather than to "all persons" was not adopted,[228] but this decision was predicated on a general agreement that it is sometimes reasonable to distinguish between citizens and aliens.[229] The critical point is that the drafters of the Civil and Political Covenant recognized that states enjoy latitude to allocate some rights differentially on the basis of citizenship, without thereby running the risk of engaging in discriminatory conduct of the kind prohibited by Art. 26, or by common Art. 2 of the Covenants.

The extent to which the Human Rights Committee will deem differentiation based on citizenship to be the basis for objective and reasonable categorical differentiation remains unclear. On the one hand, the Committee has adopted the view that where particular categories of non-citizens are treated differently (both from each other, and from citizens) by virtue of the terms of a bilateral treaty based on reciprocity, the treaty-based origin of the distinction can justify a general finding that it is based on objective and reasonable

[225] "He merely alleges that he is being subjected to different treatment during the period of his military service because he cannot appeal against a summons like a civilian. The Committee observes that the Covenant does not preclude the institution of compulsory military service by States parties, even though this *means* that the rights of individuals may be restricted during military service, within the exigencies of such service [empahsis added]": *RTZ v. Netherlands*, UNHRC Comm. No. 245/1987, decided Nov. 5, 1987, at para. 3.2. See also *MJG v. Netherlands*, UNHRC Comm. No. 267/1987, decided Mar. 24, 1988; and *Brinkhof v. Netherlands*, UNHRC Comm. No. 402/1990, UN Doc. CCPR/C/48/D/402/1990, decided July 27, 1993, at para. 6.2. While the Committee suggests that military status "means" that due process rights may be restricted, it is incredible that the Human Rights Committee would not even ask *why* it was necessary to deprive all conscripts of their general legal right to contest a summons.

[226] See UN Docs. E/CN.4/SR.122, at 5–7; E/CN.4/SR.173, at paras. 46, 67, and 76; and E/CN.4/SR.327, at 7.

[227] Statement of the Representative of France, UN Doc. E/CN.4/SR.173, at para. 19.

[228] This oral proposal by the Representative of Indonesia (UN Doc. A/C.3/SR.1102, at para. 48) was ultimately withdrawn.

[229] See UN Docs. A/C.3/SR.1098, at paras. 10 and 55; A/C.3/SR.1099, at paras. 18, 26, 31, and 36; A/C.3/1100, at para. 10; A/C.3/SR.1101, at paras. 40, 43, and 53; A/C.3/SR.1102, at paras. 17, 24, 27, 29, and 51.

grounds, and is therefore non-discriminatory.[230] More recently, though, the Committee has insisted that a categorical approach to deeming differentiation based upon citizenship to be reasonable cannot always be justified:

> Although the Committee had found in one case ... that an international agreement that confers preferential treatment to nationals of a State party to that agreement might constitute an objective and reasonable ground for differentiation, no general rule can be drawn therefrom to the effect that such an agreement in itself constitutes a sufficient ground with regard to the requirements of article 26 of the Covenant.[231]

This second case involved a challenge to Austria's assertion that the applicant's status as a non-citizen of Austria or the European Economic Area barred him from holding a post on a work council to which he had been elected. In addressing the complaint of discrimination based on citizenship, the Committee helpfully determined that

> it is necessary to judge every case on its own facts. With regard to the case at hand, the Committee has to take into account the function of a member of a work council, i.e., to promote staff interests and to supervise compliance with work conditions ... In view of this, it is not reasonable to base a distinction between aliens concerning their capacity to stand for election for a work council solely on their different nationality. Accordingly, the Committee finds that the author has been the subject of discrimination in violation of article 26.[232]

In the result, the Committee's position seems to be that while in some circumstances it will be reasonable to exclude non-citizens as a category from

---

[230] "The Committee observes ... that the categories of persons being compared are distinguishable and that the privileges at issue respond to separately negotiated bilateral treaties which necessarily reflect agreements based on reciprocity. The Committee recalls its jurisprudence that a differentiation based on reasonable and objective criteria does not amount to prohibited discrimination within the meaning of article 26": *Oord v. Netherlands*, UNHRC Comm. No. 658/1995, UN Doc. CCPR/C/60/D/658/1995, decided July 23, 1997, at para. 8.5.

[231] *Karakurt v. Austria*, UNHRC Comm. No. 965/2000, UN Doc. CCPR/C/74/D/965/2000, decided Apr. 4, 2002, at para. 8.4.

[232] Ibid. The unwillingness to assume nationality to be a valid ground for differential treatment is clear also from an earlier decision of the Committee in response to a complaint brought by 743 Senegalese nationals who had served in the French army prior to independence in 1960. The Committee found that French legislation that froze their military pensions on the grounds of nationality (while simultaneously allowing for increases to the pensions of comparably situated retired soldiers of French citizenship) was not based on objective and reasonable criteria, and was therefore discriminatory. It observed that "[t]here has been a differentiation by reference to nationality acquired upon independence. In the Committee's opinion, this falls within the reference to 'other status' in the second sentence of article 26": *Gueye v. France*, UNHRC Comm. No. 196/1985, decided Apr. 3, 1989, at para. 9.4.

the enjoyment of rights, there are other situations in which citizenship (or lack thereof) cannot be deemed a valid ground of categorical differentiation. The present moment can thus be most accurately described as one of legal uncertainty on this point: until and unless the jurisprudence of the Human Rights Committee assesses the propriety of categorical differentiation based on citizenship across a broader range of issues, it will be difficult to know which forms of exclusion are likely to be found valid, and which are in breach of Art. 26.

A second and related concern is that the Human Rights Committee has traditionally shown only modest willingness to act on the principle that a rule that applies to everyone can nonetheless be discriminatory where the rule's application impacts differently on different groups of people. In *PPC v. Netherlands*,[233] for example, the issue was whether an income support law that determined eligibility for assistance on the basis of revenue during the month of September alone was discriminatory. The applicant had received an income in excess of the minimum wage during only two months of the year, of which September was one. On the basis of consideration of nothing other than his September income, PPC was denied access to the income support program. In considering his complaint, the Human Rights Committee, however, did not even consider the fact that the applicant was clearly in no different need than a person who had received identical income during a month other than September, and who would consequently have been granted benefits under the law:

> [T]he scope of article 26 does not extend to differences of results in the application of common rules in the allocation of benefits ... Such determination is ... uniform for all persons with a minimum income in the Netherlands. Thus, the Committee finds that the law in question is not *prima facie* discriminatory.[234]

The Committee's highly formalistic understanding of equality is also clear in its response to a challenge to the legality of a Quebec language law that denied merchants the right to advertise in other than the French language. The Committee found no evidence of discrimination against the English-speaking minority in that province on the grounds that the legislation

---

[233] UNHRC Comm. No. 212/1986, decided Mar. 24, 1988.

[234] *PPC v. Netherlands*, ibid. at para. 6.2. Like the Swedish school benefits cases, discussed below, at pp. 140–141, the facts in this case may not amount to discrimination, since the differential rights allocation was not the result of stigmatization on the grounds of actual or imputed group identity. This does not, however, make the differentiation "reasonable." As discussed below, the Committee's unwillingness to scrutinize the application of facially neutral rules on the basis of this skewed understanding of "reasonableness" has resulted in the failure to recognize discrimination against linguistic minorities, women, and immigrants.

contained only "general measures applicable to all those engaged in trade, regardless of their language."[235] The views of the Committee take no account of the fact that the impact of the language law on French and English speakers was in fact quite different. Whereas most French language merchants could continue to communicate with their majority clientele in their preferred language (French), the law prohibited most English language merchants from advertising to their principal customer base in its preferred language (English). The Human Rights Committee did not even inquire into whether there was *in fact* a difference in the impact of the law on English and French language merchants, noting simply that "[t]his prohibition applies to French speakers as well as to English speakers, so that a French speaking person wishing to advertise in English, in order to reach those of his or her clientele who are English speaking, may not do so. Accordingly the Committee finds that the [English-speaking merchant] authors have not been discriminated against on the ground of their language."[236]

The Human Rights Committee's reluctance to engage with the discriminatory ramifications of facially neutral laws has ironically led it to countenance real discrimination even against groups, such as women and minorities, whose equality rights it has otherwise insisted upon. For example, after the Committee declared discriminatory a Dutch unemployment benefits system that imposed tougher eligibility criteria for women than for men, the Netherlands government abolished the facially discriminatory requirement. Women who would have received benefits but for the subsequently abolished criterion were, however, prevented from making a retroactive claim on the grounds that they were not in fact unemployed on the date they made their claims for retroactive benefits. Finding that both men and

---

[235] *Ballantyne and Davidson v. Canada* and *McIntyre v. Canada*, UNHRC Comm. Nos. 359/1989 and 385/1989 (joined on Oct. 18, 1990), UN Docs. CCPR/C/40/D/359/1989 and CCPR/C/40/D/385/1989, decided Mar. 31, 1993, at para. 11.5. See also *Singer v. Canada*, UNHRC Comm. No. 455/1991, UN Doc. CCPR/C/51/D/455/1991, decided July 26, 1994.

[236] *Ballantyne and Davidson v. Canada* and *McIntyre v. Canada*, UNHRC Comm. Nos. 359/1989 and 385/1989 (joined on Oct. 18, 1990), UN Docs. CCPR/C/40/D/359/1989 and CCPR/C/40/D/385/1989, decided Mar. 31, 1993, at para. 11.5. This is a case that cried out for nuanced analysis under the affirmative action rubric. There are some important social reasons that suggest the need to reinforce the place of the French language in Quebec society, but the Committee ought logically to have given careful consideration to whether the particular approach adopted was reasonable in the sense of adequately taking account of the individuated capabilities and potentialities of persons outside the beneficiary group. Relevant issues would include whether the legislation impairs the rights of members of the non-beneficiary class more than is necessary to accomplish its objectives, and whether the negative impact of the affirmative action program on members of the non-beneficiary group is disproportionate to the good thereby sought to be achieved for those within the target group. See text below, at p. 139, n. 252.

women were allowed to claim retroactive benefits only if unemployed, the Human Rights Committee dismissed the allegation of discrimination.[237]

This result completely misses the salient point that limiting the ability to make a retroactive claim *in practice* had radically different consequences for men and women. Whereas men could have claimed the benefits at the time they were unemployed (because they were eligible to do so), women were legally prevented from receiving benefits because of the then-prevailing discriminatory eligibility requirement. The apparently neutral demand that all applicants be unemployed at the time of requesting retroactive benefits – when the state itself stood in the way of women complying with that facially neutral requirement – was most certainly discriminatory in its effect. A genuinely non-discriminatory retroactivity rule ought to have accommodated the legal disability formerly imposed on women.

Of greatest concern to refugees, a similar superficiality of analysis has unfortunately informed the Committee's consideration of cases involving allegations of discrimination against non-citizens. For example, restrictions on the right to family unity imposed by immigration controls have received short shrift. In *AS v. Canada*, the Committee ruled that the refusal to allow the applicant's daughter and grandson to join her in Canada because of their economic and professional status did not even raise an issue potentially cognizable as discrimination.[238] Yet surely it is clear that the family reunification rules impact disproportionately on recent immigrants and other non-citizens, and can – if not objective and reasonable – discriminate against them in relation to their human right to live with their families.

Similarly, in *Oulajin and Kaiss v. Netherlands*,[239] the Human Rights Committee upheld a Dutch law that paid child support in respect of the natural children of Dutch residents wherever the children might live, but which denied support for foster children who were not resident in the Netherlands. Dutch authorities argued that this distinction was reasonable because whereas a "close, exclusive relationship . . . is presumed to exist in respect of one's own children . . . it must be made plausible in respect of foster children."[240] In fact, however, the bar on payment to foster children

---

[237] *VdM v. Netherlands*, UNHRC Comm. No. 478/1991, UN Doc. CCPR/C/48/D/478/1991, decided July 26, 1993; *Araujo-Jongen v. Netherlands*, UNHRC Comm. No. 418/1990, UN Doc. CCPR/C/49/D/418/1990, decided Oct. 22, 1993; *JAMB-R v. Netherlands*, UNHRC Comm. No. 477/1991, UN Doc. CCPR/C/50/D/477/1991, decided Apr. 7, 1994.

[238] UNHRC Comm. No. 68/1980, decided Mar. 31, 1981. It was held that the negative resettlement assessment was "in conformity with the provisions of existing Canadian law, the application of which did not in the circumstances of the present case give rise to any question of discrimination": ibid. at para. 8.2(c).

[239] *Oulajin and Kaiss v. Netherlands*, UNHRC Comm. Nos. 406/1990 and 426/1990, UN Docs. CCPR/C/46/D/406/1990 and CCPR/C/46/D/426/1990, decided Oct. 23, 1992.

[240] Ibid. at para. 2.5.

resident abroad was absolute, and could not be dislodged by evidence of a de facto close and exclusive relationship. The migrant workers who appealed to the Committee pointed out that both their natural and foster children were being raised under precisely the same conditions in Morocco, and that the presumption of a weaker bond between parents and foster children that gave rise to the statutory prohibition of payments to non-resident foster children was rooted in a stereotypical Western understanding of family obligations. The separation of the migrant workers from their children, both natural and foster, was moreover a function of their limited rights as non-citizens. They had not wished to leave their children in Morocco, but were required to do so under the terms of their immigration authorizations.

Taking absolutely no account of the fundamentally different circumstances of migrant workers and Dutch citizens, the Committee found the support scheme to be non-discriminatory, as "applicants of Dutch nationality, residing in the Netherlands, are also deemed ineligible for child benefits for their foster children who are resident abroad."[241] More generally, four members appended an individual opinion in which they suggested that states should be free in all but the most egregious cases to allocate social benefits as they see fit, without fear of running afoul of Art. 26:

> With regard to the application of article 26 of the Covenant in the field of economic and social rights, it is evident that social security legislation, which is intended to achieve aims of social justice, necessarily must make distinctions. It is for the legislature of each country, which best knows the socio-economic needs of the society concerned, to try to achieve social justice in the concrete context. Unless the distinctions made *are manifestly discriminatory or arbitrary*, it is not for the Committee to reevaluate the complex socio-economic data and substitute its judgment for that of the legislatures of States parties [emphasis added].[242]

This unwillingness to consider the ways in which foreign citizenship or residence abroad may give rise to the need for special accommodation in order to achieve substantive equality is also apparent from the decision in *SB v. New Zealand*.[243] Entitlement to a New Zealand government pension was reduced by the amount of any other government pension, but not by any sums payable under a private pension. The complainant, an immigrant to New Zealand, argued that he stood at a disadvantage relative to native New Zealanders since all pensions in his country of origin were accumulated in a state-administered fund. Because all of his pension benefits therefore derived

---

[241] Ibid. at para. 5.4.

[242] Ibid. at para. 3 of the Individual Opinion of Messrs. Kurt Herndl, Rein Müllerson, Birame N'Diaye, and Waleed Sadi.

[243] UNHRC Comm. No. 475/1991, UN Doc. CCPR/C/50/D/475/1991, decided Mar. 31, 1994.

from a government-administered plan, they were counted against his entitlement to a New Zealand pension. A New Zealand national, on the other hand, who was allowed to contribute the same monies to a private pension scheme, would see no reduction in his entitlement to a New Zealand government pension. The Human Rights Committee saw no arguable claim of discrimination, invoking its standard reasoning that the law was not explicitly discriminatory in relation to non-citizens.[244] As in the case of the migrant workers' application for benefits in respect of their foster children, the Committee showed no sensitivity to the different way in which a facially neutral law can impact on persons who are not, or who have not always been, citizens of the country in question.

There is, however, cause for optimism in a series of cases contesting the validity of laws designed to effect restitution to persons deprived of property by Communist regimes.[245] These cases did not actually involve an allegation of discriminatory impact in the application of facially neutral laws: to the contrary, the laws being contested explicitly denied compensation to persons able to meet citizenship and other criteria.[246] Yet because the governments argued that despite the language of the relevant laws there had been no intention to discriminate against non-citizens, the Committee felt compelled to take up the question of discriminatory effects. It did so most clearly in its decision of *Adam v. Czech Republic*, where it specifically determined that there is no need to find an intention to discriminate in order to establish a breach of Art. 26:

> The State party contends that there is no violation of the Covenant because the Czech and Slovak legislators had no discriminatory intent at the time of the adoption of Act 87/1991. The Committee is of the view, however, that the intent of the legislature is not dispositive in determining a breach of article 26 of the Covenant, but rather the consequences of the enacted legislation. Whatever the motivation or intent of the legislature, a law may still contravene article 26 of the Covenant if its effects are discriminatory.[247]

---

[244] "[T]he Act does not distinguish between New Zealand citizens and foreigners ... [A] deduction takes place in all cases where a beneficiary also receives a similar [government-administered] benefit ... from abroad": *SB v. New Zealand*, UNHRC Comm. No. 475/1991, UN Doc. CCPR/C/50/D/475/1991, decided Mar. 31, 1994, at para. 6.2.

[245] The seminal case was *Simunek et al. v. Czech Republic*, UNHRC Comm. No. 516/1992, UN Doc. CCPR/C/54/D/516/1992, decided July 19, 1995.

[246] For example, the issue in *Simunek et al. v. Czech Republic*, ibid., was whether the Czech government had discriminated by passing a law which granted restitution for property confiscated during the Communist era, but only to those who were citizens and permanent residents of the Czech Republic on September 30, 1991.

[247] *Adam v. Czech Republic*, UNHRC Comm. No. 586/1994, UN Doc. CCPR/C/57/D/586/1994, decided July 23, 1996.

This position has been affirmed in subsequent decisions dealing with laws that were similarly explicit in their denial of rights to non-citizens.[248]

The Committee's most direct affirmation that discrimination contrary to Art. 26 can be discerned on the basis of effects without proof of intent came in a decision which found a Dutch law to be discriminatory because it provided survivorship benefits for the children of unmarried parents, but only if they were born after a particular date. In that context, the Committee unambiguously affirmed that "article 26 prohibits both direct and indirect discrimination, the latter notion being related to a rule or measure that may be neutral on its face without any intent to discriminate but which nevertheless results in discrimination because of its exclusive or disproportionate adverse effect on a certain category of persons."[249] It remains to be seen whether the Committee will adopt the same approach when called upon to assess the reasonableness of rules which discriminate in fact against non-citizens despite their complete facial neutrality[250] – including, for example, rules on

[248] See e.g. *Blazek v. Czech Republic*, UNHRC Comm. No. 857/1999, UN Doc. CCPR/C/72/D/857/1999, decided July 12, 2001, at para. 5.8; and *Brok v. Czech Republic*, UNHRC Comm. No. 774/1997, UN Doc. CCPR/C/73/D/774/1997, decided Oct. 31, 2001, at para. 7.2.

[249] *Derksen v. Netherlands*, UNHRC Comm. No. 976/2001, UN Doc. CCPR/C/80/D/1976/2001, decided Apr. 1, 2004, at para. 9.3. See also *Althammer v. Austria*, UNHRC Comm. No. 998/2001, UN Doc. CCPR/C/78/D/1998/2001, decided Aug. 8, 2003, at para. 10.2, which noted that "a violation of article 26 can also result from the discriminatory effect of a rule or measure that is neutral at face value or without intent to discriminate. However, such indirect discrimination can only be said to be based on the grounds enumerated in Article 26 of the Covenant if the detrimental effects of a rule or decision exclusively or disproportionally affect persons having a particular race, color, sex, language, religion, political or other opinion, national or social origin, property, birth or other status. Furthermore, rules or decisions with such an impact do not amount to discrimination if they are based on objective and reasonable grounds." Specifically as regards sex discrimination, the Human Rights Committee has taken the view that "[t]he State party must not only adopt measures of protection, but also positive measures in all areas so as to achieve the effective and equal empowerment of women. States parties must provide information regarding the actual role of women in society so that the Committee may ascertain what measures, in addition to legislative provisions, have been or should be taken to give effect to these obligations, what progress has been made, what difficulties are encountered and what steps are being taken to overcome them": UN Human Rights Committee, "General Comment No. 28: The equality of rights between men and women" (2000), UN Doc. HRI/GEN/1/Rev.7, May 12, 2004, at 178, para. 3.

[250] There is some cause for optimism in the Committee's recently expressed view that "an indirect discrimination may result from a failure to treat different situations differently, if the negative results of such failure exclusively or [disproportionately] affect persons of a particular race, colour, sex, language, religion, political or other opinion, national or social origin, property, birth or other status": *Godfried and Pohl v. Austria*, UNHRC Comm. No. 1160/2003, UN Doc. CCPR/C/81/D/1160/2003, decided July 9, 2004.

immigration, child support, and pension entitlement adjudicated in earlier cases without the benefit of an effects-based analysis.[251]

The third and most fundamental concern about the Human Rights Committee's non-discrimination analysis is its tendency to assume the reasonableness of many state-sanctioned forms of differentiation, rather than to condition a finding of reasonableness on careful analysis. There has, in particular, been a reluctance to delve into the facts of particular cases in order to ensure that the differential treatment is actually proportionate to the social good thereby being advanced.[252] For example, the case of *Debreczeny v.*

[251] The specificity of the approach in the property restitution cases is clear from the views of the Committee that it has determined only that "a requirement in the law for citizenship as a necessary condition for restitution of property previously confiscated by the authorities makes an arbitrary, and, consequently, a discriminatory distinction between individuals who are equally victims of prior state confiscations, and constitutes a violation of article 26 of the Covenant": *Des Fours v. Czech Republic*, UNHRC Comm. No. 747/1997, UN Doc. CCPR/C/73/D/747/1997, decided Oct. 30, 2001, at para. 8.4. It is also important to note that in both the property restitution cases and even in the decision of *Derksen v. Netherlands*, UNHRC Comm. No. 976/2001, UN Doc. CCPR/C/80/D/1976/2001, decided Apr. 1, 2004, the impugned legislation was, in fact, explicit about the category of persons to whom benefits would be denied (non-citizens in the former cases, children born before a particular date in the latter decision). The Committee has yet to apply the indirect discrimination doctrine to a situation in which there is no such explicit limitation in the law or practice being scrutinized. Moreover, the Committee in *Derksen*, ibid., seemed at pains to make clear that the government's recent decision to extend survivorship benefits to the children of unmarried parents was critical to the finding of discrimination. "In the circumstances of the present case, the Committee observes that under the earlier [law] the children's benefits depended on the status of the parents, so that if the parents were unmarried, the children were not eligible for the benefits. However, under the new [law], benefits are being denied to children born to unmarried parents before 1 July 1996 while granted in respect of similarly situated children born after that date": ibid. at para. 9.3. Yet if the Committee is truly committed to an effects-based approach to the identification of indirect discrimination, it is unclear why a law designed along the lines of the former law – which provided benefits for the children of married parents, but not for the children of unmarried parents – would not amount to discrimination in fact against the children of unmarried parents. Indeed, the rejection in this same case of a claim by the child's mother for benefits on the grounds that she and her (now deceased) partner failed to be married and hence to establish entitlement under the survivorship regime applicable to spouses suggests the extraordinarily fragile nature of the Committee's new-found commitment to the eradication of indirect discrimination.

[252] For example, to determine whether a law that infringes a protected right may nonetheless be adjudged a "reasonable limitation" for Canadian constitutional law purposes, the Supreme Court of Canada has determined that the government's objective must be pressing and substantial, and that there is proportionality between means and end. To determine the latter question of proportionality, consideration should be given to whether the limitation on the right is carefully designed to achieve its objective; whether it constrains the right to the minimum extent truly necessary; and whether the benefit of the limitation outweighs the harm occasioned by infringement of the right: *R v. Oakes*,

Netherlands[253] involved a police officer who was excluded from membership on a municipal council by reason of a law deeming membership of the council to be incompatible with the subordinated position of a police officer to local authorities. While the Committee logically noted the "objective and reasonable" goal of avoiding conflicts of interest, it failed to explain why the *complete exclusion* of the police officer from holding local political office was a proportionate means to achieve that goal.[254]

Deference to state assertions of reasonableness is also evident in two cases against Sweden involving the denial of financial assistance for school meals and textbooks to children attending private schools. The Human Rights Committee found no reason to uphold the claims of discrimination on the grounds that the government might "reasonably and objectively" choose to treat public and private schools (not students) differently.[255] The Committee observed that students who wish to receive the benefits should exercise their option to attend a public school. Yet surely if "reasonableness" has any significance in the context of discrimination analysis, it should be to direct

[1986] 1 SCR 103 (Can. SC, Feb. 28, 1986). The importance of a law's objective cannot compensate for its patent over-breadth. As such, the Supreme Court of Canada has struck down legislation advancing critical objectives when the means adopted are not proportional to the objective, e.g. involving the protection of children from sexual offenders (*R v. Heywood*, [1994] 3 SCR 761 (Can. SC, Nov. 10, 1994)), the protection of female children from the harm caused to them by premature intercourse (*R v. Hess*, [1990] 2 SCR 906 (Can. SC, Oct. 4, 1990)) and the protection of persons from the health risks of tobacco use (*RJR-Macdonald Inc. v. Canada*, [1995] 3 SCR 199 (Can. SC, Sept. 25, 1995)).

[253] UNHRC Comm. No. 500/1992, UN Doc. CCPR/C/53/D/500/1992, decided Apr. 3, 1995.

[254] Similarly, the Committee upheld the reasonableness of the retroactive reclassification of a member of the Polish civic militia as a member of the prior regime's security forces, thereby making him ineligible for reappointment in the post-Communist government: *Kall v. Poland*, UNHRC Comm. No. 552/1993, UN Doc. CCPR/C/60/D/552/1993, decided July 14, 1997. In a dissenting opinion, Members Evatt and Medina Quiroga wrote that "it has to be examined whether the classification of the author's position as part of the Security Police was both a necessary and proportionate means for securing a legitimate objective, namely the re-establishment of internal law enforcement services free of the influence of the former regime, as the State party claims, or whether it was unlawful or arbitrary and or discriminatory, as the author claims": ibid.

[255] In *Blom v. Sweden*, UNHRC Comm. No. 191/1985, decided Apr. 4, 1988, the Committee declared that "[i]n deciding whether or not the State party violated article 26 by refusing to grant *the author, as a pupil* of a private school, an education allowance for the school year 1981/82, whereas *pupils* of public schools were entitled to education allowances for that period, the Committee bases its findings on the following observations. The State party's educational system provides for both private and public education. The State party cannot be deemed to act in a discriminatory fashion if it does not provide the same level of subsidy *for the two types of establishment*, when the private system is not subject to State supervision [emphasis added]": ibid. at paras. 10.2–10.3. That the Committee failed to grapple with the issue of whether there was truly a difference in the needs of the two classes of student is readily apparent from its reference to the legitimacy of withholding funds from one of two kinds of *establishment*.

attention to whether or not the differential rights allocation is made on the basis of real differences of need between the persons affected – here, the students attending the private schools and those in public schools. There is, however, no evidence that the Committee even canvassed this issue, much less that it found some reason implicitly to declare that *all students* in attendance at a private school are by virtue of that status in no need of personal financial assistance. In these cases reliance on a "reasonableness" test rather than on serious analysis of the real needs and interests of the persons involved served simply to legitimate state discretion.[256]

This extraordinary deference to state perceptions of reasonableness has even led the Committee to condone clear unfairness in the purported pursuit of justice. While some form of restitution was clearly called for in the case of Uruguayan civil servants dismissed by the former military government for their political affiliations, the Human Rights Committee in *Stalla Costa v. Uruguay*[257] did not even consider whether the particular affirmative action program adopted – which effectively blocked access to civil service recruitment for a whole generation of younger Uruguayans – was unduly intrusive on the rights of the non-beneficiary class. Instead, the Committee was content to find the program to be "reasonable and objective," observing simply that "[t]aking into account the social and political situation in Uruguay during the years of military rule, in particular the dismissal of many public servants . . . the Committee *understands* the enactment . . . by the new democratic Government of Uruguay as a measure of redress [emphasis added]."[258]

Indeed, it is "understandable" that the new government would wish to afford redress to the improperly fired civil servants. This general legitimation is precisely the result compelled by scrutiny of a differential rights allocation in relation to no more than a "reasonableness" test. That the program is "understandable" does not, however, make it non-discriminatory. A decision on this latter issue should have led the Committee to consider, for example, whether there were other means of redress open to the Uruguayan government that would not have had such a devastating impact on persons not previously employed by the state.

There are many other examples in which state-sanctioned differentiation is simply assumed to be reasonable without meaningful analysis. The Committee has rejected claims of discrimination based on an assumption of reasonable differentiation where social welfare benefits were calculated

---

[256] The Swedish school benefits cases could, however, legitimately be rejected on the basis that they do not involve differentiation on the grounds of actual or imputed group identity. They may, in other words, be examples of arbitrariness in rights allocation, rather than discrimination as such. See generally text above, at p. 124.

[257] UNHRC Comm. No. 198/1985, decided July 9, 1987.

[258] *Stalla Costa v. Uruguay*, ibid. at para. 10.

based on a presumption of greater support from cohabiting family members than from non-related cohabitants;[259] where active and retired employees who were similarly situated economically were treated differently for purposes of pension calculation;[260] where compensation was paid to military personnel, but not to civilians, who were detained by enemy soldiers during wartime;[261] where a legal aid system funded counsel for the civil defendant in a criminal case at nearly three times the rate paid to counsel for the plaintiff;[262] where the government elected to bar only one of several forms of employment understood to be inconsistent with respect for human dignity, with severe economic consequences for the former employees;[263] and where a

[259] "In the light of the explanations given by the State party, the Committee finds that the different treatment of parents and children and of other relatives respectively, contained in the regulations under the Social Security Act, is not unreasonable nor arbitrary, and its application in the author's case does not amount to a violation of article 26 of the Covenant": *Neefs v. Netherlands*, UNHRC Comm. No. 425/1990, UN Doc. CCPR/C/51/D/425/1990, decided July 15, 1994, at para. 7.4.

[260] "In the instant case, the contested differentiation is based only superficially on a distinction between employees who retired before 1 January 1992 and those who retired after that date. Actually, this distinction is based on a different treatment of active and retired employees at the time. With regard to this distinction, the Committee considers that the author has failed to substantiate, for purposes of admissibility, that the distinction was not objective or how it was arbitrary or unreasonable. Therefore, the Committee concludes that the communication is inadmissible": *Nahlik v. Austria*, UNHRC Comm. No. 608/1995, UN Doc. CCPR/C/57/D/608/1995, decided July 22, 1996, at para. 8.4.

[261] "As regards the claim that the exclusion of civilian detainees from entitlements under the War Pensions Act is discriminatory, the Committee notes from the information before it that the purpose of the Act is specifically to provide pension entitlements for disability and death of those who were in the service of New Zealand in wartime overseas, not to provide compensation for incarceration or for human rights violations. In other words if disability arises from war service it is irrelevant to the entitlement to a pension whether the person suffered imprisonment or cruel treatment by captors. Keeping in mind the Committee's prior jurisprudence according to which a distinction based on objective and reasonable criteria does not constitute discrimination within the meaning of article 26 of the Covenant, the Committee considers that the authors' claim is incompatible with the provisions of the Covenant and thus inadmissible": *Drake v. New Zealand*, UNHRC Comm. No. 601/1994, UN Doc. CCPR/C/59/D/601/1994, decided Apr. 3, 1997, at para. 8.5.

[262] "The Committee recalls that differences in treatment do not constitute discrimination, when they are based on objective and reasonable criteria. In the present case, the Committee considers that representation of a person presenting a civil claim in a criminal case cannot be equalled to representing the accused. The arguments advanced by the author and the material he provided do not substantiate, for purposes of admissibility, the author's claim that he is a victim of discrimination": *Lestourneaud v. France*, UNHRC Comm. No. 861/1999, UN Doc. CCPR/C/67/D/861/1999, decided Nov. 3, 1999, at para. 4.2.

[263] "The Committee is aware of the fact that there are other activities which are not banned but which might possibly be banned on the basis of grounds similar to those which justify the ban on dwarf tossing. However, the Committee is of the opinion that, given that the

state's law codified a presumption that military officers of a predecessor state presented a risk to national security and were therefore ineligible for citizenship.[264] In a recent and particularly clear example of the Committee's abdication of its role seriously to examine the merits of a state's assertion of the reasonableness of differentiation, a twenty-year residence requirement for purposes of voting on self-determination for New Caledonia was upheld as non-discriminatory:

> [T]he Committee considers that, in the present case, the cut-off points set for the ... referendums from 2014 onwards are not excessive inasmuch as they are in keeping with the nature and purpose of these ballots, namely a self-determination process involving the participation of persons able to prove sufficiently strong ties to the territory whose future is being decided. This being the case, these cut-off points do not appear to be disproportionate with respect to a decolonization process involving the participation of residents who, over and above their ethnic origin or political affiliation, have helped, and continue to help, build New Caledonia through their sufficiently strong ties to the territory.[265]

ban on dwarf tossing is based on objective and reasonable criteria and the author has not established that this measure was discriminatory in purpose, the mere fact that there may be other activities liable to be banned is not in itself sufficient to confer a discriminatory character on the ban on dwarf tossing. For these reasons, the Committee considers that, in ordering the above-mentioned ban, the State party has not, in the present case, violated the rights of the author as contained in article 26 of the Covenant": *Wackenheim v. France*, UNHRC Comm. No. 854/1999, UN Doc. CCPR/C/67/D/854/1999, decided July 15, 2002, at para. 7.5.

[264] The law in question presumes that foreigners who have served in the armed forces of another country pose a threat to Estonian national security. In this case, "the Tallinn Administrative Court ... found that the author had not been refused citizenship because he had actually acted against the Estonian state and its security in view of his personal circumstances. Rather, for the reasons cited, the author was in a position where he could act against Estonian national security ... It observed that there was no need to make out a case of a specific individual threat posed by the author, as he had not been accused of engaging in actual activities against the Estonian state and its security": *Borzov v. Estonia*, UNHRC Comm. No. 1136/2002, UN Doc. CCPR/C/81/D/1136/2002, decided Aug. 25, 2004, at para. 2.5. The Committee nonetheless determined that "the State party concluded that a grant of citizenship to the author would raise national security issues generally on account of the duration and level of the author's military training, his rank and background in the armed forces of the then USSR ... [T]he author did enjoy a right to have the denial of his citizenship application reviewed by the courts of the State party. Noting, furthermore, that the role of the State party's courts in reviewing administrative decisions, including those decided with reference to national security, appears to entail genuine substantive review, the Committee concludes that the author has not made out his case that the decision taken by the State party with respect to the author was not based on reasonable and objective grounds": ibid. at para. 7.4.

[265] *Gillot v. France*, UNHRC Comm. No. 932/2000, UN Doc.CCPR/C/75/D/932/2000, decided July 15, 2002, at para. 14.7.

The Committee did not even examine the question whether "sufficiently strong ties" might be demonstrated by a period of residence significantly less than twenty years, much less the allegation that the goal of the requirement was to disfranchise an ethnic minority of the population.[266]

The critical difference that careful analysis of the reasonableness of differentiation can make is evident from examination of a pair of cases which alleged that the automatic prolongation of alternative military service was discriminatory in relation to genuine conscientious objectors. In *Järvinen v. Finland*,[267] the Human Rights Committee considered Finland's rule requiring conscientious objectors to military service to undertake alternative service for double the period of military service. The doubling of service time for conscientious objectors was said by the state to be justified on the grounds that it was necessary in order to discourage abuse of the non-combatant option. The Committee agreed, finding that the scheme was "reasonable" based on the importance of administrative workability, and because there was no intention to discriminate. No effort was made to assess whether the risk of abuse under the new system truly required such a significant disparity between the duration of military and alternative service, much less whether it was necessary to impose the prolonged service on persons willing to submit to careful scrutiny of their reasons for refusal to engage in military service.

In contrast, the Human Rights Committee more recently arrived at the opposite conclusion when it refused simply to accept the state party's assertion of reasonableness. In a series of decisions rendered against France on facts essentially indistinguishable from those considered in *Järvinen*, the Committee rejected the reasonableness of a double-time civilian service alternative imposed in the interests of ensuring that only true conscientious objectors would avoid military service:

> Any differentiation, as the Committee has had the opportunity to state repeatedly, must ... be based on reasonable and objective criteria. In this context, the Committee recognizes that the law and practice may establish differences between military and national alternative service and that such differences may, in a particular case, justify a longer period of service, provided that the differentiation is based on reasonable and objective criteria, *such as the nature of the specific service concerned or the need for a special training in order to accomplish that service*. In the present case,

---

[266] "The authors also consider the period of residence determining the right to vote in referendums from 2014 onwards, namely 20 years, to be excessive. They again assert that the French authorities are seeking to establish an electorate of Kanaks and Caldoches for whom, moreover, the right to vote is maintained even in the event of lengthy absences from New Caledonia": *Gillot v. France*, ibid. at para. 3.10.

[267] UNHRC Comm. No. 295/1988, decided July 25, 1990.

however, the reasons forwarded by the State party do not refer to such criteria or refer to criteria in general terms without specific reference to the author's case, *and are rather based on the argument that doubling the length of service was the only way to test the sincerity of an individual's convictions.* In the Committee's view, such argument does not satisfy the requirement that the difference in treatment involved in the present case was based on reasonable and objective criteria. In the circumstances, the Committee finds that a violation of article 26 occurred, since the author was discriminated against on the basis of his conviction of conscience [emphasis added].[268]

There could surely be no more compelling example of why a real injustice can be done when the assessment of reasonableness fails to scrutinize the reasons advanced by states for practices which raise *prima facie* claims of discrimination.[269] Regrettably, only a minority of the jurisprudence under Art. 26 takes up this question,[270] and none of it has thus far engaged in more sophisticated proportionality analysis.

---

[268] *Foin v. France*, UNHRC Comm. No. 666/1995, UN Doc. CCPR/C/67/D/666/1995, decided Nov. 3, 1999, at para. 10.3. See also *Maille v. France*, UNHRC Comm. No. 689/1996, UN Doc. CCPR/C/69/D/689/1996, decided July 10, 2000; and *Venier and Nicolas v. France*, UNHRC Comm. Nos. 690/1996 and 691/1996, UN Docs. CCPR/C/69/D/690/1996 and CCPR/C/69/D/691/1996, decided July 10, 2000.

[269] See also *Young v. Australia*, UNHRC Comm. No. 941/2000, UN Doc. CCPR/C/78/D/941/2000, decided Aug. 6, 2003, in which the refusal of the Committee to defer to the government's assertion that it was "reasonable" to distinguish between same-sex and opposite-sex couples for purposes of entitlement to veterans' benefits led to a finding of discrimination contrary to Art. 26. In contrast to the usual pattern of deference, the Committee here noted that "[t]he State party provides no arguments on how this distinction between same-sex partners, who are excluded from pension benefits under law, and unmarried heterosexual partners, who are granted such benefits, is reasonable and objective, and no evidence which would point to the existence of factors justifying such a distinction has been advanced": ibid. at para. 10.4.

[270] A somewhat unstructured analysis underpins some of the Committee's decisions. For example, in one case the Committee explicitly articulated the view that the disfranchisement of past property owners in favor of current tenants was rendered reasonable by virtue of the existence of a system to compensate the former owners. "The State party has justified the (exclusionary) requirement that current tenants of former State-owned residential property have a 'buy first option' even vis-à-vis the former owner of the property with the argument that tenants contribute to the maintenance of the property through improvements of their own. The Committee does not consider that the fact of giving the current tenants of former State-owned property priority in the privatization sale of such property is in itself unreasonable; the interests of the 'current tenants', who may have been occupying the property for years, are deserving of protection. If the former owners are, moreover, compensated on equal and non-discriminatory terms ... the interplay between Act XXV of 1991 and of Act LXVIII of 1993 can be deemed compatible with article 26 of the Covenant": *Somers v. Hungary*, UNHRC Comm. No. 566/1993, UN Doc. CCPR/C/53/D/566/1993, decided July 23, 1996, at para. 9.8. More recently, in *Love v. Australia*, UNHRC Comm. No. 983/2001, UN Doc.

The point is not that the Human Rights Covenants' guarantees of non-discrimination – in particular, Art. 26 of the Civil and Political Covenant – will never be of value to refugees and other non-citizens. To the contrary, non-discrimination law will be a critically important remedy for refugees if recent, positive developments continue and take hold – specifically, if there is clear rejection of the view that categorical distinctions based on citizenship are to be assumed to be reasonable; if there is a genuine preparedness to take account of the discriminatory effects of superficially neutral laws and practices; and if the nascent preparedness to begin real interrogation of state assertions of reasonableness continues. The Human Rights Committee has moreover shown an awareness that refugee rights should follow from their unique predicament as involuntary expatriates,[271] and has indicated a particular disinclination to find restrictions to be reasonable insofar as individuals are unable to comply by virtue of having been forced to seek refugee status abroad.[272] But all of these developments must be seen for what they are: modest and recent shifts away from what has traditionally been a rather

CCPR/C/77/D/983/2001, decided Mar. 25, 2003, a case involving an allegation of age discrimination in the context of a mandatory retirement requirement for commercial airline pilots, the Committee observed that "it is by no means clear that mandatory retirement age would generally constitute age discrimination. The Committee takes note of the fact that systems of mandatory retirement age may include a dimension of workers' protection by limiting the life-long working time, in particular when there are comprehensive social security schemes that secure the subsistence of persons who have reached such an age. Furthermore, reasons related to employment policy may be behind legislation or policy on mandatory retirement age . . . [T]he Committee's task [is to assess] whether any particular arrangement for mandatory retirement age is discriminatory. In the present case, as the State party notes, the aim of maximising safety to passengers, crew and persons otherwise affected by flight travel was a legitimate aim under the Covenant. As to the reasonable and objective nature of the distinction made on the basis of age, the Committee takes into account the widespread national and international practice, at the time of the author's dismissals, of imposing a mandatory retirement age of 60. In order to justify the practice of dismissals maintained at the relevant time, the State party has referred to the ICAO regime which was aimed at, and understood as, maximising flight safety. In the circumstances, the Committee cannot conclude that the distinction made was not, at the time of Mr Love's dismissal, based on objective and reasonable considerations": ibid. at paras. 8.2–8.3.

[271] "These victims of political persecution sought residence and citizenship in other countries. Taking into account that the State party itself is responsible for the departure of the authors, it would be incompatible with the Covenant to require them permanently to return to the country as a prerequisite for the restitution of their property or for the payment of appropriate compensation": *Simunek et al. v. Czech Republic*, UNHRC Comm. No. 516/1992, UN Doc. CCPR/C/54/D/516/1992, decided July 19, 1995, at para. 11.6.

[272] In *Blazek v. Czech Republic*, UNHRC Comm. No. 857/1999, UN Doc. CCPR/C/72/D/857/1999, decided July 12, 2001, the Committee observed "that it cannot conceive that the distinction on grounds of citizenship can be considered reasonable in the light of the fact that the loss of Czech citizenship was a function of their presence in a State in which they

superficial and deferential jurisprudence on the meaning of non-discrimina-tion. Until the recent evolution is solidified and enhanced by, for example, incorporation of an analytically rigorous proportionality test,[273] refugees and other non-citizens are still not positioned dependably to benefit from most of the rights guaranteed to citizens.

2.5.6 International aliens law

As the preceding discussion makes clear, the inadequacy of international human rights law as a response to the vulnerabilities of refugees is in part a function of its inattention to the concerns of aliens generally. Inapplicable assumptions and outright exclusions reflect the orientation of international human rights law to meeting the needs of most of the world's population, who are citizens of their state of residence. At least until a more inclusive understanding of non-discrimination law evolves on the international plane, refugees, like other non-citizens, cannot depend on the general system of human rights protection adequately to address those of their concerns that are specifically a function of non-citizenship.

The early response of the United Nations to this dilemma was essentially to deny it. The Special Rapporteur of the International Law Commission, F. V. Garcia-Amador, confidently proclaimed that there was no need for a special legal regime to benefit aliens. His draft codification of the rights of aliens provides that "aliens enjoy the same rights and the same legal guarantees as nationals," these being "the 'universal respect for, and observance of, human rights and fundamental freedoms' referred to in the Charter of the United Nations and in other general, regional and bilateral instruments."[274] As

were able to obtain refuge": ibid. at para. 5.8. This is consistent with Art. 6 of the Refugee Convention, which requires that refugees be exempted from requirements "which by virtue of their nature a refugee is incapable of fulfilling": Refugee Convention, at Art. 6. See generally chapter 3.2.3 below.

[273] As the International Court of Justice has recently observed, the Human Rights Committee has appropriately insisted in other contexts of consideration on the propor-tionality of restrictions of rights before finding them to be lawful. "The Court would observe that the restrictions provided for under Article 12, paragraph 3, of the International Covenant on Civil and Political Rights [dealing with freedom of move-ment] are, by the very terms of that provision, exceptions to the right of freedom of movement contained in paragraph 1. In addition, it is not sufficient that such restrictions be directed to the ends authorized; they must also be necessary for the attainment of those ends. As the Human Rights Committee put it, they 'must conform to the principle of proportionality' and 'must be the least intrusive instrument amongst those which might achieve the desired result' (CCPR/C/21/Rev.1/Add.9, General Comment No. 27, para. 14)": *Legal Consequences of the Construction of a Wall in the Occupied Palestinian Territory*, (2004) ICJ Gen. List No. 131, decided July 9, 2004, at para. 136.

[274] F. V. Garcia Amador et al., *Recent Codification of the Law of State Responsibility for Injuries to Aliens* (1974), at 5, 129.

previously shown, however, the Charter establishes only a limited duty of non-discrimination,[275] and the two Human Rights Covenants are not sufficiently attentive to the concerns and disabilities of aliens.[276] Because bilateral treaties do not enable aliens themselves to take action, but rather create rights between governments, they provide no effective recourse for refugees.[277] The upshot of Garcia-Amador's proposal, therefore, would have been to leave refugees with a fragmentary combination of rights derived from some treaties and general principles of law.[278]

A more forthright assessment of the problem was offered by the Special Rapporteur of the Sub-Commission on Prevention of Discrimination and Protection of Minorities, Baroness Diana Elles. She argued that the Universal Declaration of Human Rights was not a binding instrument, and could not therefore confer legal rights on aliens; that the Covenants on Human Rights offered at best patchwork protection to non-citizens; and that the many exclusions and permissible limitations in international instruments provided a substantively inadequate response to the vulnerabilities of persons outside their own country.[279] Although the Special Rapporteur's efforts were therefore clearly premised on the need to establish legally enforceable rights for aliens,[280] it is ironic that the product of her efforts within the Sub-Commission was itself completely unenforceable. The General Assembly adopted the Declaration on the Human Rights of Individuals Who are not

---

[275] See chapter 1.2.3 above, at p. 44.   [276] See chapter 2.5.4 above, at pp. 121–123.

[277] See chapter 2.1 above, at pp. 78–79.

[278] "Admittedly, there is a body of opinion that may regard [codification of aliens' rights] as surplusage. Although the law governing the Responsibility of States for Injuries to Aliens was one of international law's first attempts to protect human rights, according to some authorities it has been preempted, in whole or in part, by the generation by the United Nations of new international human rights norms applicable to nationals and aliens alike. The fact that not all states subscribe to such norms and that, in any event, the machinery to implement them generally is non-existent or inadequate, is overlooked or ignored in such quarters. Thus, if one accepts the preemption argument, aliens actually may have less protection now than in years past": R. Lillich, "Editorial Comment: The Problem of the Applicability of Existing International Provisions for the Protection of Human Rights to Individuals Who are not Citizens of the Country in Which They Live," (1976) 70(3) *American Journal of International Law* 507, at 509.

[279] D. Elles, "Aliens and Activities of the United Nations in the Field of Human Rights," (1974) 7 *Human Rights Journal* 291, at 314–315.

[280] "What the Charter does not say is that there should be no distinction between alien and nationals ... [T]he alien, although his human rights and fundamental freedoms must be respected, may not necessarily expect equal treatment with nationals ... Continued violations of the rights of aliens in many parts of the world give grounds for doubting whether there are sufficient sanctions available against a host state without some judicial body of the highest quality and esteem, with the power to enforce judgements": "International Provisions Protecting the Human Rights of Non-Citizens," UN Doc. E/CN.4/Sub.2/393/Rev.1 (1979), at 5–7.

Nationals of the Country in which They Live,[281] but has yet to consider the codification of a binding catalog of rights for non-citizens.

Most recently, in August 2000 the Sub-Commission appointed Prof. David Weissbrodt as Special Rapporteur on the Rights of Non-Citizens, and charged him to prepare "a comprehensive study of the rights of non-citizens," which would "take into account the different categories of citizens regarding different categories of rights in countries of different levels of development with different rationales to be offered for such distinctions."[282] Weissbrodt's final report, delivered in May 2003,[283] takes a position between those of his two predecessors. Like Baroness Elles, he forthrightly catalogs the numerous ways in which non-citizens are explicitly excluded from many core treaty-based guarantees of human rights. His report acknowledges that political rights and freedom of internal movement are not clearly extended to non-citizens under the Civil and Political Covenant; that Art. 2(3) of the Economic Covenant allows poorer states to withhold economic rights from non-citizens; and that the International Convention on the Elimination of All Forms of Racial Discrimination does not preclude distinctions, exclusions, restrictions, or preferences between citizens and non-citizens.[284] He even alludes to possible reasons to question the value of non-discrimination law.[285]

Despite his recognition of the limitations of international human rights law, the thrust of Prof. Weissbrodt's report – like that of Garcia-Amador – is nonetheless that the human rights of non-citizens can be satisfactorily regulated under existing norms of international law.[286] This is, of course, a much more credible position today than it was when taken by Garcia-Amador in 1974.[287] To back up his position, the Special Rapporteur includes a summary

---

[281] UNGA Res. 40/144, adopted Dec. 13, 1985.

[282] "The rights of non-citizens: Preliminary report of the Special Rapporteur," UN Doc. E/CN.4/Sub.2/2001.20, June 6, 2001, at paras. 4–5.

[283] "The rights of non-citizens: Final report of the Special Rapporteur," UN Doc. E/CN.4/Sub.2/2003/23, May 26, 2003.

[284] Ibid. at paras. 18–22. Importantly, "[t]he Committee [on the Elimination of Racial Discrimination] . . . affirms that article 1, paragraph 2, must not be interpreted to detract in any way from the rights and freedoms recognized and enunciated in other instruments, especially the Universal Declaration of Human Rights, the International Covenant on Economic, Social and Cultural Rights and the International Covenant on Civil and Political Rights": UN Committee on the Elimination of Racial Discrimination, "General Recommendation XI: Non-citizens" (1993), UN Doc. HRI/GEN/1/Rev.7, May 12, 2004, at 205, para. 3.

[285] "The rights of non-citizens: Final report of the Special Rapporteur," UN Doc. E/CN.4/Sub.2/2003/23, May 26, 2003, at para. 23.

[286] "In general, international human rights law requires the equal treatment of citizens and non-citizens": ibid. at para. 1.

[287] See text above, at pp. 147–148.

of state practice in a number of countries,[288] and draws together the jurisprudence and concluding observations of the UN and regional human rights treaty bodies.[289] To the extent that work remains to be done – Weissbrodt pointed in a draft of his report, in particular, to the increasing number of distinctions among non-citizens *inter se*,[290] as well as barriers on access to citizenship,[291] and also provided a more broad-ranging (if somewhat eclectic) addendum of state practice which fails to respect the human rights of non-citizens[292] – the approach recommended is greater clarity and coordination among the standards applied by the existing human rights supervisory bodies,[293] not the establishment of new norms. For example, he suggests that there may indeed be particular value in vindicating the rights of non-citizens via scrutiny under the widely ratified Racial Discrimination Convention,[294] since most non-citizens are, in fact, racial minorities (remembering that "race" is defined therein to include *inter alia* national or ethnic origin[295]).

In essence, Weissbrodt provides a road map of how the existing legal norms of human rights law can more effectively be brought to bear on many of the problems faced by non-citizens around the world. Despite the obvious value to advocates and decision-makers of a report oriented in this way, the weakness of this approach is that it is prone to downplay the gaps in international human rights law. In particular, the report fails to grapple with the limited value of non-discrimination law as presently interpreted, including the problems for non-citizens that arise from the Human Rights Committee's often categorical approach to the definition of a "reasonable"

---

[288] In a very interesting self-reporting exercise, twenty-two governments submitted responses to a questionnaire prepared by the Special Rapporteur regarding their own standards and practice in relation to the rights of non-citizens: "The rights of non-citizens: Final report of the Special Rapporteur," UN Doc. E/CN.4/Sub.2/2003/23/Add.4, May 26, 2003.

[289] See "The rights of non-citizens: Final report of the Special Rapporteur," UN Doc. E/CN.4/Sub.2/2003/23/Add.1. While not directly relevant to the international standard of non-citizens' rights, Weissbrodt also cataloged relevant regional standards and jurisprudence: see "The rights of non-citizens: Final report of the Special Rapporteur," UN Doc. E/CN.4/Sub.2/2003/23/Add.2, May 26, 2003.

[290] "The rights of non-citizens: Progress report of the Special Rapporteur," UN Doc. E/CN.4/Sub.2/2002/25, June 5, 2002, at paras. 25–42.

[291] Ibid. at paras. 43–49.

[292] "The rights of non-citizens: Progress report of the Special Rapporteur," UN Doc. E/CN.4/Sub.2/2002/25/Add.3, June 5, 2002. Weissbrodt's final report contains a more methodically organized (if still highly selective) indication of officially validated concerns: "The rights of non-citizens: Final report of the Special Rapporteur," UN Doc. E/CN.4/Sub.2/2003/23/Add.3, Add.4, May 26, 2003.

[293] "The rights of non-citizens: Final report of the Special Rapporteur," UN Doc. E/CN.4/Sub.2/2003/23, May 26, 2003, at paras. 31–33, 39–40.

[294] Ibid. at para. 34.   [295] Racial Discrimination Convention, at Art. 1(1).

justification for differentiation; the breadth of the margin of appreciation it extends to governments; and its traditional disinclination to implement in practice its commitment in principle to an effects-based approach to the analysis of discrimination.[296] Indeed, the final report (optimistically) mis-states the actual status of the Human Rights Committee's jurisprudence on non-discrimination, suggesting that justifications will be found to be reasonable only if "they serve a legitimate State objective *and are proportional to the achievement of that objective* [emphasis added]."[297]

More generally, the report simply does not aspire to provide solid answers to the underlying challenge of the exclusion of non-citizens from key parts of human rights law, including by the legal prerogative of less developed states to deny economic rights to non-citizens,[298] and by the general inability of non-citizens to claim some civil and political rights,[299] most especially when an emergency is proclaimed.[300] While the decision to defer consideration of these issues may derive from a politically realistic calculus, it remains that the Sub-Commission's most recent effort does not move us concretely towards a

[296] See chapter 2.5.5 above, at pp. 129–147.

[297] "The rights of non-citizens: Final report of the Special Rapporteur," UN Doc. E/CN.4/Sub.2/2003/23, May 26, 2003, at paras. 1, 6, and 17. But see chapter 2.5.5 above, at pp. 139–145. Only one academic and one regional (not UN) decision are offered as support for this proposition: ibid. at n. 13. It is noteworthy that the (unwarranted) reference to "proportionality" did not feature in earlier drafts of the report, e.g. "The rights of non-citizens: Progress report of the Special Rapporteur," UN Doc. E/CN.4/Sub.2/2002/25, June 5, 2002, at para. 28: "The Human Rights Committee has similarly observed in General Comment 18 that differences in treatment may be permissible under the Covenant 'if the criteria for such differentiation are reasonable and objective and if the aim is to achieve a purpose which is legitimate under the Covenant' (para. 13)."

[298] The report observes only that "[a]s an exception to the general rule of equality, it should be noted that article 2(3) must be narrowly construed, may be relied upon only by developing countries, and only with respect to economic rights": "The rights of non-citizens: Final report of the Special Rapporteur," UN Doc. E/CN.4/Sub.2/2003/23, May 26, 2003, at para. 19.

[299] The report simply acknowledges that non-citizens do not enjoy full rights under Arts. 25 (political rights), 12(1) (internal freedom of movement), and 12(4) (freedom from deprivation of the right to enter one's own country), and notes the constraints on these limits set by the Human Rights Committee: ibid. at para. 18.

[300] This concern was given substantial attention in a draft version of Weissbrodt's report: see "The rights of non-citizens: Progress report of the Special Rapporteur," UN Doc. E/CN.4/Sub.2/2002/25, June 5, 2002, at paras. 13, 19–20. Specifically, it was observed that "[u]nlike the general anti-discrimination clause found in article 2(1), the derogation clause does not include 'national origin' among the impermissible grounds for discrimination. This omission, according to the *travaux préparatoires*, reflects the drafters' recognition that States often find it necessary to discriminate against non-citizens in time of national emergency": ibid. at para. 20. Interestingly, no comparable acknowledgment of this restriction is included in the final report of the Special Rapporteur.

strategy for engaging – even incrementally – with these foundational concerns.

Despite the absence of broadly based progress, some concrete normative progress has been achieved in the establishment of binding rights for at least a subset of non-citizens. The International Convention on the Protection of the Rights of All Migrant Workers and Members of their Families entered into force on July 1, 2003, though only a small minority of states has thus far ratified it.[301] To the extent that refugees may avail themselves of this treaty's provisions, it helpfully imposes obligations to provide, for example, emergency healthcare, children's education, fair conditions and employment, and the right to be protected against abuse and attacks. More generally, non-citizens may invoke rights under the various conventions established by the International Labor Organization to regulate migration for employment purposes.[302] Governed by an amalgam of state, employer, and worker representatives, the ILO has produced several treaties on international labor standards which, when ratified by states, are legally binding. Additional guidance is often provided by more detailed recommendations, which do not have the force of law.[303] The ILO's progressive codification of migrant worker rights is an important source of enforceable socioeconomic rights for

---

[301] UNGA Res. 45/158, adopted Dec. 18, 1990, entered into force July 1, 2003. Only twenty-five states have both signed and ratified the treaty: www.unhchr.ch (accessed Nov. 19, 2004).

[302] In 1939, the ILO adopted Convention No. 66, the Convention concerning the Recruitment, Placing and Conditions of Labor of Migrants for Employment, together with the accompanying Recommendation No. 61, Recommendation concerning the Recruitment, Placing and Conditions of Labor of Migrants for Employment. Convention No. 66 never secured sufficient ratifications to enter into force. It was updated in 1949 by Convention No. 97, the Convention concerning Migration for Employment (Revised) and its Recommendation No. 86, Recommendation concerning Migration for Employment (Revised). Convention No. 97 came into force shortly after the adoption of the Refugee Convention, and is a parallel source of rights for refugees lawfully admitted to residence in a state party. The ILO has since produced Convention No. 143, the Migrant Workers (Supplementary Provisions) Convention, 1975 and the companion Recommendation No. 151, Migrant Workers Recommendation, 1975. The 1975 accord deals with migration in abusive conditions and provides for equality of opportunity and treatment of migrant workers. See generally International Labor Conference et al., *Conventions and Recommendations Adopted by the International Labor Conference, 1919–1966* (1966) (International Labor Conference et al., *Conventions and Recommendations*) and Lillich, *Rights of Aliens*, at 73–74.

[303] Of particular note is Recommendation No. 86 (1949) which proposes a model agreement for the regulation of labor migration. Several of these non-binding standards speak explicitly to the needs of refugees, regarded as a subset of persons who seek employment outside their own country. First, some additional rights are added to the binding list of matters to be guaranteed on terms of equality with nationals. These include rights to recognition of travel documents, adaptation assistance, naturalization, participation in collective labor agreements, private property, and of access to food and suitable housing.

resident aliens, including those refugees who are lawfully admitted as immigrants to an asylum state. This is particularly so because ILO procedures allow enforcement action to be initiated not just by states, but equally by worker and employer organizations.[304] The critical limitation of the ILO standards is, however, that they apply only in states that voluntarily adhere to them, and generally regulate the treatment only of refugees lawfully admitted as immigrants to the state in question.

Overall, there is little doubt that non-citizens have benefited in important ways from the post-Convention evolution of international human rights law, particularly as regards their entitlement to claim most civil and political rights. On the other hand, a conservative approach has generally been taken to interpretation of broadly applicable guarantees of non-discrimination; emergency derogation can erode practical access to many civil and political rights; and poorer states remain legally entitled to exclude non-citizens from the enjoyment of most generally applicable economic rights. In these circumstances, the Refugee Convention remains a critical source of protection. In particular, it sets economic rights which must be honored in all countries; it insulates many key civil and political rights from derogation; and more generally, the Refugee Convention entrenches a broad range of entitlements which are fundamental to avoiding the specific predicaments of involuntary alienage. As such, refugee law must be understood still to be the cornerstone of the refugee rights regime, even as it has been buttressed in important ways by more general norms of human rights law.

Second, equal access to trades and occupations is established, but only "to the extent permitted under national laws and regulations." Third, migrant workers who are "lawfully within" the territory are entitled to equality of treatment with respect to hygiene, safety, and medical assistance; and, as far as the state regulates such matters, to weekly rest days, admission to educational institutions, recreation, and welfare. Fourth, the model agreement extends most of these equality rights to refugees' family members, an entitlement not proposed for the families of other alien workers. See International Labor Conference et al., *Conventions and Recommendations*.

[304] See generally F. Wolf, "Human Rights and the International Labour Organization," in Meron, *Human Rights in International Law*, at 273.

The structure of entitlement under the Refugee Convention

The universal rights of refugees are today derived from two primary sources – general standards of international human rights law, and the Refugee Convention itself. As the analysis in chapter 2 makes clear, the obligations derived from the Refugee Convention remain highly relevant, despite the development since 1951 of a broad-ranging system of international human rights law. In particular, general human rights norms do not address many refugee-specific concerns; general economic rights are defined as duties of progressive implementation and may legitimately be denied to non-citizens by less developed countries; not all civil rights are guaranteed to non-citizens, and most of those which do apply to them can be withheld on grounds of their lack of nationality during national emergencies; and the duty of non-discrimination under international law has not always been interpreted in a way that guarantees refugees the substantive benefit of relevant protections.

On the other hand, general human rights law adds a significant number of rights to the list codified in the Refugee Convention, and is regularly interpreted and applied by supervisory bodies able to refine the application of standards to respond to contemporary realities. Because both refugee law and general human rights law are therefore of real value, the analysis in chapters 4–7 synthesizes these sources of law to define a unified standard of treatment owed to refugees.

This chapter examines the fairly intricate way in which rights are attributed and defined under the Refugee Convention. Most fundamentally, the refugee rights regime is not simply a list of duties owed by state parties equally to all refugees. An attempt is instead made to grant enhanced rights as the bond strengthens between a particular refugee and the state party in which he or she is present. While all refugees benefit from a number of core rights, additional entitlements accrue as a function of the nature and duration of the attachment to the asylum state. The most basic set of rights inheres as soon as a refugee comes under a state's de jure or de facto jurisdiction; a second set applies when he or she enters a state party's territory; other rights inhere only when the refugee is lawfully within the state's territory; some when the refugee is lawfully staying there; and a few rights accrue only upon satisfaction of a durable residency requirement.[1] Before any given right can be claimed by a particular refugee, the nature of his or her attachment to the host state must therefore be defined. The structure of the attachment system is incremental: because the levels build on one another (a refugee in a state's territory is also under its jurisdiction; a refugee lawfully present is also present; a refugee lawfully residing is also lawfully present; and a refugee durably residing is also lawfully residing), rights once acquired are retained for the duration of refugee status.[2]

Second, as under the 1933 Convention and the predecessor regime of aliens law, the standard of treatment owed to refugees is defined through a combination of absolute and contingent criteria. A few rights are guaranteed absolutely to refugees, and must be respected even if the host government does not extend these rights to anyone else, including its own citizens.[3] More commonly, the standard for compliance varies as a function of the relevant treatment afforded another group under the laws and practices of the receiving country. Under these contingent rights standards, refugees are entitled to be assimilated either to nationals of a most-favored state, or to citizens of the asylum state itself.[4] If no absolute or contingent standard is specified for a given right, refugees benefit from the usual standard of treatment applied to non-citizens present in the asylum state.[5] In applying this general residual standard, however, refugees must be exempted from any criteria which a refugee is inherently unable to fulfill,[6] and may not be subjected to any exceptional measures applied against the citizens of their state of origin.[7]

Third, an asylum state may not grant preferred treatment to any subset of the refugee population. The interaction of the Refugee Convention's endogenous rule of non-discrimination and the general duty of non-discrimination requires that all refugees benefit from equal access to rights in the host country.

Fourth and finally, states enjoy a limited discretion to withhold some rights from particular refugees on the grounds of national security.[8] In contrast to treaties such as the Civil and Political Covenant,[9] however, the

---

[1] See chapter 3.1 below.
[2] "The structure of the 1951 Convention reflects [a] 'layering' of rights": "Letter from R. Andrew Painter, UNHCR Senior Protection Officer, to Robert Pauw," (2003) 80 *Interpreter Releases* 423, at 427.
[3] See chapter 3.3.3 below.
[4] See chapters 3.3.1 and 3.3.2 below. It will be recalled that this approach establishes a built-in equalization and adjustment mechanism, since contingent rights vary as a function of the relevant treatment afforded another group under the laws and practice of the state party. See chapter 2.1 above, at pp. 77–78.
[5] See chapter 3.2 below.   [6] See chapter 3.2.3 below.
[7] See chapter 3.5.2 below.   [8] See chapter 3.5.1 below.
[9] "In time of public emergency which threatens the life of the nation and the existence of which is officially proclaimed, the States Parties to the present Covenant may take measures

Refugee Convention does not allow states to derogate from their obligations on a generalized basis, even in time of war or other serious national emergency.

The enforcement of these rights is to be accomplished by the attribution to UNHCR of a surrogate protector role comparable to that played by the various High Commissioners during the League of Nations era,[10] supplemented by the non-derogable agreement of state parties to submit any dispute regarding interpretation or application of the Refugee Convention to the International Court of Justice.[11] There is moreover potential for the national courts and tribunals of many state parties to enforce refugee rights directly, and for United Nations and other human rights bodies to take account of refugee-specific obligations in the interpretation of generally applicable human rights obligations.

3.1 Attachment to the asylum state

Refugees are entitled to an expanding array of rights as their relationship with the asylum state deepens. At the lowest level of attachment, some refugees are simply subject to a state's *jurisdiction*, in the sense of being under its control or authority. A greater attachment is manifest when the refugee is physically present *within a state's territory*. A still more significant attachment is inherent when the refugee is deemed to be *lawfully present* within the state. The attachment is greater still when the refugee is *lawfully staying* in the country. Finally, a small number of rights are reserved for refugees who can demonstrate *durable residence* in the asylum state. As the refugee's relationship to the asylum state is solidified over the course of this five-part assimilative path, the Convention requires that a more inclusive range of needs and aspirations be met.

---

derogating from their obligations under the present Covenant to the extent strictly required by the exigencies of the situation, *provided that such measures are not inconsistent with their other obligations under international law* and do not involve discrimination solely on the ground of race, color, sex, language, religion or social origin. No derogation from articles 6, 7, 8 (paragraphs 1 and 2), 11, 15, 16 and 18 may be made under this provision [emphasis added]": International Covenant on Civil and Political Rights, UNGA Res. 2200A(XXI), adopted Dec. 16, 1966, entered into force Mar. 23, 1976 (Civil and Political Covenant), at Art. 4(1)–(2). The provision requiring continuing respect for "other obligations under international law" clearly imports the duty of state parties to the Refugee Convention to implement their duties under that treaty even when derogation from Covenant rights is allowed. With regard to the right of derogation under the Civil and Political Covenant, see UN Human Rights Committee, "General Comment No. 29: Derogations during a state of emergency" (2001), UN Doc. HRI/GEN/1/Rev.7, May 12, 2004, at 184.

[10] See chapter 2.3 above, at p. 85.
[11] Convention relating to the Status of Refugees, 189 UNTS 2545, done July 28, 1951, entered into force Apr. 22, 1954 (Refugee Convention), at Art. 38.

The drafters' decision to grant refugee rights on an incremental basis reflected the experience of states confronted with the unplanned arrival of refugees at their frontiers. While overseas asylum states continued mainly to receive refugees preselected for resettlement,[12] several European countries were already faced with what has today become the dominant pattern of refugee flows, namely the unplanned and unauthorized arrival of refugees at a state's borders. The drafters of the Convention explicitly considered how best to align the refugee rights regime with this transition from an essentially managed system of refugee migration, to a mixed system in which at least some refugees would move independently:

> [T]he initial reception countries were obliged to give shelter to refugees who had not, in fact, been properly admitted but who had, so to speak, imposed themselves upon the hospitality of those countries. As the definition of refugee made no distinction between those who had been properly admitted and the others, however, the question arose whether the initial reception countries would be required under the convention to grant the same protection to refugees who had entered the country legally and those who had done so without prior authorization.[13]

The compromise reached was that any unauthorized refugee, whether already inside or seeking entry into a state party's territory, would benefit from the protections of the Refugee Convention.[14] Such refugees would not, however, immediately acquire all the rights of "regularly admitted" refugees, that is, those pre-authorized to enter and to reside in an asylum state. Instead, as under then-prevailing French law, basic rights would be granted to all refugees, with additional rights following as the legal status of the refugee was consolidated.[15] The Refugee Convention implements this commitment by defining a continuum of legal attachment to the asylum state.

---

[12] "The Chairman, speaking as the representative of Canada, observed that the question raised by the initial reception countries did not apply to his country, which was separated by an ocean from the refugee zones. Thanks to that situation, all refugees immigrating to Canada were *ipso facto* legally admitted and enjoyed the recognized rights granted to foreigners admitted for residence": Statement of Mr. Chance of Canada, UN Doc. E/AC/32/SR.7, Jan. 23, 1950, at 12.

[13] Statement of Mr. Cuvelier of Belgium, ibid.

[14] "It did not, however, follow that the convention would not apply to persons fleeing from persecution who asked to enter the territory of the contracting parties ... [W]hether or not the refugee was in a *regular position*, he must not be turned back to a country where his life or freedom could be threatened [emphasis added]": Statement of Mr. Henkin of the United States, UN Doc. E/AC.32/SR.20, Feb. 1, 1950, at 11–12.

[15] "[T]he problem would be seen more clearly if it were divided into three different aspects: the first concerned the treatment of refugees before they had reached an understanding with the authorities of the recipient countries; the second referred to their right to have their situation regularized and the conditions in which that was to be done; the third dealt with their rights after they had been lawfully authorized to reside in the country, which meant, in the case of France, after they were in possession of a residence card and a work card": Statement of Mr. Rain of France, UN Doc. E/AC/32/SR.15, Jan. 27, 1950, at 15.

N.B.

In practice, however, some or all refugee rights are at times withheld by states pending the affirmative validation of entitlement to Convention refugee status.[16] It is, of course, true that the rights set by the Refugee Convention are those only of genuine Convention refugees, not of every person who seeks recognition of refugee status. But because it is one's de facto circumstances, not the official validation of those circumstances, that gives rise to Convention refugee status,[17] genuine refugees may be fundamentally disadvantaged by the withholding of rights pending status assessment.[18] They are rights holders under international law, but are precluded from exercising

[16] See e.g. *Krishnapillai v. Minister of Citizenship and Immigration*, [2002] 3(1) FC 74 (Can. FCA, Dec. 6, 2001), in which the court expressed the view that "in a case involving a Convention refugee claimant and not, as in this case, a Convention refugee . . . [t]he Convention . . . did not apply": ibid. at para. 25. Thus, for example, the court was of the view that Art. 16's guarantee of access to the courts – which actually inheres in all persons who are in fact refugees as soon as they come under a state's jurisdiction – could be claimed only "once their refugee status had been determined": ibid. at para. 27.

[17] "A person is a refugee within the meaning of the 1951 Convention as soon as he fulfils the criteria contained in the definition. This would necessarily occur prior to the time at which his refugee status is formally determined. Recognition of his refugee status does not therefore make him a refugee but declares him to be one. He does not become a refugee because of recognition, but is recognized because he is a refugee": UNHCR, *Handbook on Procedures and Criteria for Determining Refugee Status* (1979, reedited 1992) (UNHCR, *Handbook*), at para. 28. This reasoning was approved in *R (Hoxha) v. Secretary of State for the Home Department*, [2002] EWCA Civ 1403 (Eng. CA, Oct. 14, 2002). But see the earlier decision of the same court in *R v. Secretary of State for the Home Department, ex parte Jammeh*, [1998] INLR 701 (Eng. CA, July 30, 1998), at 710–711, which suggested that "[i]t is . . . a reasonable policy in accordance with the Convention not to confer upon would-be immigrants refugee status and rights that go with that until the entitlement to that status has been established." But this approach does not accord with the text of the Refugee Convention. "Article 1(A)(2) of the 1951 Convention does not define a 'refugee' as being a person who has been *formally recognized* as having a well-founded fear of persecution, etc. . . . [A] person who satisfies the conditions of Article 1(A)(2) is a refugee regardless of whether he or she has been formally recognized as such pursuant to a municipal law process": E. Lauterpacht and D. Bethlehem, "The Scope and Content of the Principle of *Non-Refoulement*," in E. Feller et al. eds., *Refugee Protection in International Law* 87 (Lauterpacht and Bethlehem, "*Non-Refoulement*"), at para. 90.

[18] This point was recognized by the English Court of Appeal in *Khaboka v. Secretary of State for the Home Department*, [1993] Imm AR 484 (Eng. CA, Mar. 25, 1993), holding "that a refugee is a refugee both before and after his claim for asylum as such may have been considered and accepted . . . It is common sense and a natural reading of article 31(1). The term 'refugee' means what it says. It will include someone who is subsequently established as being a refugee": ibid. at 489. In a subsequent decision of the Queen's Bench Division, this point was affirmed, though with the appropriate qualification that whether a refugee is entitled to particular rights is a function of the level of attachment which governs access to that right. The court was clearly anxious that an interpretation that withheld refugee rights until after status recognition could work a serious injustice, particularly as regards the right in Art. 16(1) of the Refugee Convention to access the courts. "[T]he use of the word 'refugee' [in Art. 16(1)] is apt to include the aspirant, for

their legal rights during the often protracted domestic processes by which their entitlement to protection is verified by officials. Unless status assessment is virtually immediate, the adjudicating state may therefore be unable to meet its duty to implement the Refugee Convention in good faith.[19]

This dilemma can only be resolved by granting any person who claims to be a Convention refugee the provisional benefit of those rights which are not predicated on regularization of status, in line with the Convention's own attachment requirements.[20] As UNHCR has observed,

> Every refugee is, initially, also an asylum-seeker; therefore, to protect refugees, asylum-seekers must be treated on the assumption that they may be refugees until their status has been determined. Otherwise, the principle of *non-refoulement* would not provide effective protection for refugees, because applicants might be rejected at borders or otherwise returned to persecution on the grounds that their claim had not been established.[21]

Governments that wish to be relieved of the presumptive (if minimalist) responsibility towards asylum-seekers have the legal authority to take steps to expedite formal determination of refugee status, including by resort to a

---

were that not so, if in fact it had to be established that he did fall within the definition of 'refugee' in article 1, he might find that he could have no right of audience before the court because the means of establishing his status would not be available to him so that he could not have access to the courts of this country on judicial review": *R v. Secretary of State for the Home Department, ex parte Jahangeer*, [1993] Imm. AR 564 (Eng. QBD, June 11, 1993), at 566.

[19] "The principle of good faith underlies the most fundamental of all norms of treaty law – namely, the rule *pacta sunt servanda* ... Where a third party is called upon to interpret the treaty, his obligation is to draw inspiration from the good faith that should animate the parties if they were themselves called upon to seek the meaning of the text which they have drawn up": I. Sinclair, *The Vienna Convention and the Law of Treaties* (1984), at 119–120. An example of the clear risk of failure to adopt this approach is provided by the decision of the government of Venezuela to adopt a policy of "excluded tolerance" of Colombian asylum-seekers on their territory. While there is little doubt that many Colombians in flight from the conflict in their state are Convention refugees, the Venezuelan decision not to consider the merits of their claims has, in practice, denied them access to services and assistance to which they are, in fact, legally entitled: (2003) 128 *JRS Dispatches* (Mar. 17, 2003).

[20] These include rights which are subject to no level of attachment, rights which inhere in refugees simply physically present, and – once the requirements for status verification have been met – rights which are afforded to refugees who are lawfully present: see chapters 3.1.1, 3.1.2, and 3.1.3 below. More sophisticated rights (those that require lawful stay, or durable residence: see chapters 3.1.4 and 3.1.5 below) need be granted only after affirmative verification of refugee status. Importantly, all rights provisionally respected can be immediately withdrawn in the event an applicant is found not to be a Convention refugee.

[21] UNHCR, "Note on International Protection," UN Doc. A/AC.96/815 (1993), at para. 11.

fairly constructed procedure for "manifestly unfounded claims" if necessary.[22] Convention rights may be summarily withdrawn from persons found through a fair inquiry not to be Convention refugees. Such an approach enables a state to meet its obligations towards genuine refugees who seek its protection, consistent with the duty to ensure that at least certain basic rights accrue even before regularization of status.[23]

3.1.1 Subject to a state's jurisdiction

While most rights in the Refugee Convention inhere only once a refugee is either in, lawfully in, lawfully staying in, or durably residing in an asylum country, a small number of core rights are defined to apply with no qualification based upon level of attachment.[24] While as a practical matter these rights will in most cases accrue to a refugee simultaneously with those that apply once the refugee arrives at a state party's territory, there are some circumstances in which a refugee will be under the control and authority of a state party even though he or she is not physically present in, or at the border of, its territory.

For example, what of a situation in which a state exercises de facto control in territory over which it has no valid claim to lawful jurisdiction? A state

---

[22] Manifestly unfounded claims are "those which are clearly fraudulent or not related to the criteria for the granting of refugee status laid down in the 1951 United Nations Convention relating to the Status of Refugees nor to any other criteria justifying the granting of asylum": UNHCR Executive Committee Conclusion No. 30, "The Problem of Manifestly Unfounded or Abusive Applications for Refugee Status or Asylum" (1983), at para. (d), available at www.unhcr.ch (accessed Nov. 20, 2004).

[23] In a decision addressing exclusion from refugee status under Art. 1(F)(b), the High Court of Australia impliedly endorsed the view that refugee status is to be provisionally presumed pending the outcome of a status inquiry. Chief Justice Gleeson in a majority judgment observed that "[w]hatever the operation of the expression 'admission ... as a refugee' in other systems of municipal law, in Australia there would be nothing to which the language could apply. It would be necessary to read the words 'prior to his admission to that country as a refugee' as meaning no more than 'prior to his entry into that country.' The preferable solution is to read the reference to 'admission ... as a refugee' as a reference to putative admission as a refugee": *Minister for Immigration and Multicultural Affairs v. Singh*, (2002) 186 ALR 393 (Aus. HC, Mar. 7, 2002). Justice Callinan, in dissent, similarly observed that "[c]ontrary to a submission made in this court ... I am of the opinion that the words 'prior to his admission to that country as a refugee' should be understood to mean 'prior to his entry into the country in which he seeks or claims the status of a refugee.' Otherwise the purpose of the Convention would be subverted in that the nature of the applicant's prior criminal conduct could only be explored after he had been accorded refugee status": ibid.

[24] See Refugee Convention, at Arts. 3 ("non-discrimination"), 13 ("movable and immovable property"), 16(1) ("access to courts"), 20 ("rationing"), 22 ("education"), 29 ("fiscal charges"), 33 ("prohibition of expulsion or return – 'refoulement'"), and 34 ("naturalization").

might invade and take authority over the territory of another country; or it might appropriate authority over part of the *res communis*, such as the high seas. While it is not possible in such circumstances to argue that the state must respect refugee rights in such a place as the natural corollary of the state's de jure jurisdiction (because there is no right to control the territory), there is no denying that the state is exercising de facto jurisdiction over the territory in question. From the perspective of the refugee, moreover, the state's control and authority over him or her – whether legally justified or not – is just as capable of either inflicting harm or providing assistance as would be the case if the state's formal jurisdiction were fully established there.

As a general matter, of course, states do not assume international legal duties in the world at large, but only as constraints on the exercise of their sovereign authority – thus, normally applicable within the territory over which they are entitled to exercise jurisdiction. As the European Court of Human Rights has recently affirmed, "the jurisdictional competence of a State is primarily territorial."[25] In the particular context of refugee law, moreover, governments were emphatic in their rejection of a duty to reach out to refugees located beyond their borders, accepting only the more constrained obligation not to force refugees back to countries in which they might be persecuted.[26] The small set of core refugee rights subject to no attachment requirement nonetheless applies to state parties which exercise de facto jurisdiction over refugees not physically present in their territory. This is not only a natural conclusion from the way in which the text of the Refugee Convention is framed, but is an understanding that is consistent with basic principles of public international law.

The starting point for analysis is the plain language of the Refugee Convention, in which all but a very small number of core refugee rights *are* reserved for those who reach a state's territory, or who meet the requirements of a higher level of attachment. The decision generally to constrain the application of rights on a territorial or other basis creates a presumption that no such limitation was intended to govern the applicability of the rights not subject to such textual limitations. To assert that the few rights which are explicitly subject to no level of territorial attachment should nonetheless be treated as though they were so constrained would run afoul of the basic principle of interpretation that a good faith effort should be made to construe the text of a treaty in the light of its context – which clearly includes the balance of the provisions of the treaty itself.[27]

This textual reading is in several cases directly confirmed by the drafting history of the Convention. As regards property rights,[28] for example, the

---

[25] *Bankovic et al. v. Belgium et al.*, 11 BHRC 435 (ECHR, Dec. 12, 2001), at para. 59.
[26] See chapter 4.1 below, at pp. 300–301.   [27] See chapter 1.3.2 above.
[28] Refugee Convention, at Art. 13.

drafters debated, but ultimately rejected, higher levels of attachment because they wished to ensure that refugees could claim property rights even in a state party where they were not physically present (on the same basis as other non-resident aliens).[29] Similarly, the absence of a level of attachment for purposes of the right to tax equity[30] was driven by the goal of ensuring that state parties would limit any effort to tax refugees not present on their territory by reference to the rules applied to non-resident citizens.[31] The right of access to the courts[32] was also broadly framed specifically to ensure that refugees had access to the courts of all state parties, not just those of a country where they might be physically present.[33] In each of these cases, the failure to stipulate a level of attachment was intentional, designed to grant refugees rights in places where they might never be physically present.[34]

The same explanation does not apply, however, to the decision not to stipulate any level of attachment for purposes of access to elementary education.[35] The generality of the way in which this obligation was framed followed from the drafters' determination to honor the "urgent need" for, and compulsory nature of, access by all to the most basic forms of education in line with the formula of the Universal Declaration of Human Rights – and specifically to ensure that even non-resident refugee children had access to schooling.[36] Because this particular goal might have been achieved by adoption of the next-lowest level of attachment (physical presence in the asylum state), it is arguable that the absence of any attachment requirement for this right is more the product of modest over-exuberance than of clear design. Yet there seems little doubt that had the drafters been aware that states might (as is increasingly the case) detain refugees extraterritorially, the fervor of their convictions about the fundamental importance of access to basic education would almost certainly have led them to opt for the present unqualified formulation.[37]

---

[29] See chapter 4.5.1 below, at pp. 526–527.   [30] Refugee Convention, at Art. 29.
[31] See chapter 4.5.2 below, at p. 532.   [32] Refugee Convention, at Art. 16(1).
[33] See chapter 4.10 below, at p. 645. Taking account of interaction with relevant provisions of the Civil and Political Covenant, Art. 16(1) may in some circumstances have relevance also to enabling refugees to access courts to enforce refugee rights violated extraterritorially: see chapter 4.10 below, at p. 650.
[34] "[S]everal provisions of the 1951 Convention enable a refugee residing in one Contracting State to exercise certain rights – as a refugee – in another Contracting State ... [T]he exercise of such rights is not subject to a new determination of his refugee status": UNHCR Executive Committee Conclusion No. 12, "Extraterritorial Effect of the Determination of Refugee Status" (1978), at para. (c), available at www.unhcr.ch (accessed Nov. 20, 2004).
[35] Refugee Convention, at Art. 22.   [36] See chapter 4.8 below, at p. 597.
[37] This approach is not rendered unworkable by virtue of practical concerns, for example the viability of delivering elementary education immediately, or while onboard a ship. Even those rights which inhere immediately clearly do so only on their own terms. As regards

The right of access to systems which ration consumer goods[38] could also technically apply extraterritorially in line with its textual formulation, but only if the state in question operates a general rationing system in the place where it purports to exercise control over the refugee.[39] Since this duty pertains only to systems which distribute essential goods (e.g. foodstuffs), there is a clear logic to the requirement that in such circumstances refugees under a state's extraterritorial control should have access to rationed goods. No real significance should be given to the fact that the Convention's provision on naturalization[40] is not constrained by a level of attachment since, as elaborated below, this provision really is not the basis for any rights at all, but is more in the nature of non-binding advice to states.[41]

This then leaves us with only two core refugee rights that would, under the understanding of the plain meaning of the text advanced here, be of general practical relevance to state parties which choose to exercise extraterritorial jurisdiction over refugees: a duty of non-discrimination (between and among refugees);[42] and the obligation not to return them, directly or indirectly, to a place where they risk being persecuted for a Convention reason (*non-refoulement*).[43] Beyond these duties, the state party would be obligated only to act in accordance with the general standard of treatment[44] – that is, treating the refugees under its authority at least as well as it treats aliens generally,[45] exempting them from reciprocity or insurmountable requirements,[46] respecting their personal status (e.g. family and matrimonial rights),[47] and honoring rights acquired apart from the Refugee Convention itself.[48] This is certainly a modest set of expectations, and not one which could credibly be argued to render the plain meaning of the Convention's text in any sense unworkable. Much less is it an approach at odds with the treaty's object and purpose. To the contrary, if states were able with impunity to reach out beyond their borders to force refugees back to the risk of being persecuted, whether as a general matter or in relation to only particular groups of refugees, the entire Refugee Convention – which is predicated on the ability

---

public education, for example, refugees need only receive "the same treatment as is accorded to nationals." Thus, there is no breach of refugee law if refugees are subject only to the same delays or constraints in establishing educational facilities that might apply, for example, to citizens living in a comparably remote area. But such considerations must be addressed with the same promptness and effectiveness that would apply in the case of citizens of the state party.

[38] Refugee Convention, at Art. 20.   [39] See chapter 4.4.1 below, at p. 467, n. 861.
[40] Refugee Convention, at Art. 34.   [41] See chapter 7.4 below, at pp. 982–983.
[42] Refugee Convention, at Art. 3. See chapter 3.4 below.
[43] Refugee Convention, at Art. 33. See chapter 4.1 below.   [44] See chapter 3.2 below.
[45] See chapter 3.2.1 below.   [46] See chapters 3.2.2 and 3.2.3 below.
[47] See chapter 3.2.4 below.   [48] See chapter 2.4.5 above.

of refugees to invoke rights of protection in state parties – could, as a practical matter, be rendered nugatory.

Assuming, then, that the plain meaning of the Convention's textual framing of a small number of core rights does not – in contrast to the treaty's general approach – stipulate a territorial or other required level of attachment, does it follow that these rights bind state parties wherever they act?

This is an increasingly debated question in international human rights law generally. The present range of approaches among courts and treaty supervisory bodies is, to some extent, attributable to the fact that the scope of duties under various relevant treaties is differently conceived. As the International Court of Justice has recently observed, the starting point for analysis of the scope of a treaty's obligations is clearly the language of the relevant treaty, interpreted in a manner that advances its object and purpose.[49] Thus, the four Geneva Conventions, dealing with the protection of the victims of war, are exceptional in obligating state parties "to respect and to ensure respect for the present Convention *in all circumstances* [emphasis added]."[50] Other treaties are more constrained, usually imposing obligations on state parties only where they exercise jurisdiction, which is presumptively the case in their own territory.[51] For example, the Convention against Torture imposes a duty to protect persons "in any territory under its jurisdiction,"[52] while the Civil and Political Covenant applies to persons "within [a state party's] territory and subject to its jurisdiction."[53] In most cases, human rights treaties tend either to be silent on the question,[54] or to bind states to

---

[49] *Legal Consequences of the Construction of a Wall in the Occupied Palestinian Territory*, (2004) ICJ Gen. List No. 131, decided July 9, 2004, at paras. 108–109. The Court gave particular attention to relevant jurisprudence under the Civil and Political Covenant, as well as to its *travaux préparatoires* in identifying the object and purpose. This is very much in line with the interactive approach to treaty interpretation advocated here: see chapter 1.3.3 above.

[50] Geneva Convention relative to the Protection of Civilian Persons in Time of War, 75 UNTS 287, done Aug. 12, 1949, entered into force Oct. 21, 1950, at Art. 1.

[51] "The Court would observe that, while the jurisdiction of States is primarily territorial, it may sometimes be exercised outside the national territory. Considering the object and purpose of the International Covenant on Civil and Political Rights, it would seem natural that, even when such is the case, States parties to the Covenant should be bound to comply with its provisions": *Legal Consequences of the Construction of a Wall in the Occupied Palestinian Territory*, (2004) ICJ Gen. List No. 131, decided July 9, 2004, at para. 109.

[52] Convention against Torture and Other Cruel, Inhuman or Degrading Treatment or Punishment, UNGA Res. 39/46, adopted Dec. 10, 1984, entered into force June 26, 1987, at Art. 2(1).

[53] Civil and Political Covenant, at Art. 2(1).

[54] For example, International Covenant on Economic, Social and Cultural Rights, UNGA Res. 2200A(XXI), adopted Dec. 16, 1966, entered into force Jan. 3, 1976 (Economic, Social and Cultural Covenant); International Convention on the Elimination of All Forms of

protect the rights of persons either "subject to"[55] or "within"[56] their jurisdiction.

Yet there is in fact a surprising commonality of approach in the interpretation of most treaties. For example, the Interamerican Commission on Human Rights, deriving its authority from the American Declaration on the Rights and Duties of Man (which is silent on the question of the ambit of obligations) has determined that "no person under the authority and control of a state, regardless of his or her circumstances, is devoid of legal protection for his or her fundamental and non-derogable human rights."[57] To similar effect, the UN Human Rights Committee has read Art. 2(1) of the Civil and Political Covenant disjunctively, thus finding that the obligation to respect rights "within [a state's] territory and subject to its jurisdiction" means that "a State party must respect and ensure the rights laid down in the Covenant to anyone within the power or effective control of that State Party, even if not situated within the territory of the State Party."[58]

In a recent case, however, the European Court of Human Rights was called upon to consider the more vexing question of whether a state may also be

Racial Discrimination, UNGA Res. 2106A(XX), done Dec. 21, 1965, entered into force Jan. 4, 1969; Convention on the Elimination of All Forms of Discrimination Against Women, UNGA Res. 34/180, adopted Dec. 18, 1979, entered into force Sept. 3, 1981; and the American Declaration of the Rights and Duties of Man, OAS Res. XXX (1948).

[55] Optional Protocol No. 1 to the Civil and Political Covenant, 999 UNTS 172, adopted Dec. 16, 1966, entered into force Mar. 23, 1976, at Art. 1; American Convention on Human Rights, 1144 UNTS 123, adopted Nov. 22, 1969, entered into force July 18, 1978, at Art. 1.

[56] Optional Protocol No. 2 to the Civil and Political Covenant, 1648 UNTS 414, adopted Dec. 15, 1989, entered into force July 11, 1991, at Art. 1; European Convention for the Protection of Human Rights and Fundamental Freedoms, 213 UNTS 221, done Nov. 4, 1950, entered into force Sept. 3, 1953, at Art. 1.

[57] Interamerican Commission on Human Rights, "Request for Precautionary Measures Concerning the Detainees at Guantanamo Bay, Cuba," Mar. 12, 2002; "Request for Precautionary Measures Concerning Detainees Ordered Deported or Granted Voluntary Departure," Sept. 26, 2002.

[58] UN Committee on Human Rights, "General Comment No. 31: The nature of the general legal obligation imposed on states parties to the Covenant" (2004), UN Doc. HRI/GEN/1/Rev.7, May 12, 2004, at 192, para. 10. This reading was affirmed as accurate by the International Court of Justice in *Legal Consequences of the Construction of a Wall in the Occupied Palestinian Territory*, (2004) ICJ Gen. List No. 131, decided July 9, 2004, at para. 109: "The *travaux préparatoires* of the Covenant confirm the Committee's interpretation of Article 2 of that instrument. These show that, in adopting the wording chosen, the drafters of the Covenant did not intend to allow States to escape from their obligations when they exercise jurisdiction outside their national territory. They only intended to prevent persons residing abroad from asserting, vis-à-vis their State of origin, rights that do not fall within the competence of that State, but of that of the State of residence (see the discussion of the preliminary draft in the Commission on Human Rights, E/CN.4/SR.194, para. 46; and United Nations, Official Records of the General Assembly, Tenth Session, Annexes, A/2929, Part II, Chap. V, para. 4 (1955))."

held to account for breach of its obligations when its actions *impact* on the exercise of human rights abroad, even if it does not exercise *jurisdiction* there.[59] In a thorough and wide-ranging discussion, the Court determined in *Bankovic* that NATO state parties to the European Convention did not violate that treaty when they authorized the bombing of Yugoslavia, resulting in civilian deaths in that country.[60] It reached this conclusion on the grounds that the victims of the attacks were not under the jurisdiction of the NATO countries:

> Article 1 of the Convention must be considered to reflect [the] ordinary and essentially territorial notion of jurisdiction, other bases of jurisdiction being exceptional and requiring special justification in the particular circumstances of each case.[61]

The Court helpfully spelled out the circumstances in which public international law recognizes a state's extraterritorial jurisdiction. First,

> recognised instances of the extra-territorial exercise of jurisdiction by a State include cases involving the activities of its diplomatic or consular agents abroad and on board craft and vessels registered in, or flying the flag of, that State. In these specific situations, customary international law and treaty provisions have recognised the extra-territorial exercise of jurisdiction by the relevant State.[62]

And second, in line with the Court's own holdings in *Loizidou v. Turkey*[63] and *Cyprus v. Turkey*,[64] jurisdiction is also established where a state exercises "effective control of an area outside its national territory":[65]

> [R]ecognition of extra-territorial jurisdiction by a Contracting State is exceptional: it [is appropriate] when the respondent State, through the effective control of the relevant territory and its inhabitants abroad as a consequence of military occupation or through the consent, invitation or

---

[59] This question should be distinguished from more general issues of state responsibility, which focus on secondary rules (what follows from breach of an international legal obligation), not on primary rules (when has an international legal obligation been breached). That is, there must first be a determination of fault under a primary rule (the question being addressed here); only then does the question of the nature of state responsibility arise: see generally J. Crawford, "The ILC's State Responsibility Articles," (2002) 96(4) *American Journal of International Law* 773, at 874.

[60] *Bankovic et al. v. Belgium et al.*, 11 BHRC 435 (ECHR, Dec. 12, 2001).

[61] Ibid. at para. 61.   [62] Ibid. at para. 73.

[63] *Loizidou v. Turkey*, 23 EHRR 513 (ECHR, Dec. 18, 1996).

[64] "Having effective overall control over Northern Cyprus, [Turkey's] responsibility cannot be confined to the acts of its own soldiers or officials in Northern Cyprus but must also be engaged by virtue of the acts of the local administration which survives by virtue of Turkish military and other support": *Cyprus v. Turkey*, 35 EHRR 30 (ECHR, May 10, 2001), at para. 77.

[65] *Bankovic et al. v. Belgium et al.*, 11 BHRC 435 (ECHR, Dec. 12, 2001), at para. 70.

acquiescence of the Government of that territory, exercises all or some of the public powers normally to be exercised by that Government.[66]

The Court expressly rejected that "cause-and-effect notion of jurisdiction" contended for by the applicants,[67] limiting this second exceptional basis for a finding of jurisdiction to circumstances where there is evidence of "control [by a state party], whether it [is] exercised directly, through the . . . armed forces, or through a subordinate local administration."[68]

In considering the relevance of this decision to refugee law, it must certainly be acknowledged that the silence of the Refugee Convention on the general ambit of the obligations it imposes – and most certainly on the ambit of the small group of rights subject to no level of attachment – is less constraining than the "within [a state party's] jurisdiction" clause in the European Convention.[69] It is also true that the *Bankovic* decision has been criticized for having failed to recognize the logic of an understanding of jurisdiction for purposes of human rights law that is more broadly construed than that under public international law generally.[70] Yet the International

---

[66] Ibid. at para. 71. Similarly, the US Supreme Court recently noted that under the agreement between the United States and Cuba, the Guantanamo Base is – while under Cuban sovereignty – nonetheless under the "complete jurisdiction" of the United States for the duration of its lease with Cuba. On this basis, Justice Kennedy sensibly concluded that Guantanamo Bay "is in every practical respect a United States territory": *Rasul v. Bush*, Dec. No. 03–334, June 28, 2004.

[67] *Bankovic et al. v. Belgium et al.*, 11 BHRC 435 (ECHR, Dec. 12, 2001), at para. 75. "[T]he applicants' submission is tantamount to arguing that anyone adversely affected by an act imputable to a Contracting State, wherever in the world that act may have been committed or its consequences felt, is thereby brought within the jurisdiction of that State": ibid.

[68] Ibid. at para. 70. See also *Military and Paramilitary Activities in and Against Nicaragua*, [1986] ICJ Rep 14, at para. 115, in which the International Court of Justice determined that the relevant issue to establish responsibility is the "level of control exercised by the state to whom the acts might be attributed."

[69] The authors of a recent opinion commissioned by UNHCR on the scope of the Refugee Convention's duty of *non-refoulement* assert what amounts to an effects-based jurisdiction: "[P]ersons will come within the jurisdiction of a State in circumstances in which they can be said to be under the effective control of that State or are affected by those acting on behalf of the State more generally, wherever this occurs": Lauterpacht and Bethlehem, "*Non-Refoulement*," at para. 67.

[70] See e.g. A. Trilsch, "*Bankovic v. Belgium*," (2003) 97(1) *American Journal of International Law* 168: "[A]s the Court itself pointed out in *Loizidou* and *Cyprus v. Turkey*, and confirmed in the present decision, the applicability of the Convention does not depend on whether the extraterritorial act in question was lawful or unlawful – a distinction that is, in contrast, decisive in determining a state's jurisdiction under public international law. Having regard to the object and purpose of the Convention, these conceptual differences invite us to consider whether, instead of having the recognition of jurisdiction . . . depend on the exercise of effective (territorial) control, the point of reference should lie in the exercise of state authority as such."

Court of Justice has recently taken much the same tack as did the European Court of Human Rights.

In its *Advisory Opinion on the Legal Consequences of the Construction of a Wall in the Occupied Palestinian Territory*,[71] the Court was required to determine the reach of Israel's obligations under international law. It determined that while the primary point of reference is the specific provisions of a given treaty interpreted in light of the accord's object and purpose, obligations must normally be held to apply in any territory over which a state party exercises "effective jurisdiction."[72] Indeed, even when a treaty's terms might incline towards a more purely territorial sense of obligation, "it is not to be excluded that it applies both to territories over which a State party has sovereignty and to those over which that State exercises territorial jurisdiction."[73] Strikingly, however, despite the breadth of the Court's analysis of the scope of application of both human rights and humanitarian law obligations, it did not take the view that liability might ever follow on the basis simply that a state party's actions had an impact over persons in a foreign country – suggesting that it might well be inclined to take a position on the notion of "cause-and-effect jurisdiction" akin to that embraced in *Bankovic.*

The reasoning of the International Court of Justice may, however, helpfully illustrate the application of the second basis for extraterritorial jurisdiction identified by the European Court of Human Rights, that being where a state through effective control "exercises all or some of the public powers normally to be exercised by that Government." In finding that Israel exercises jurisdiction in the Occupied Palestinian Territory, the ICJ noted with approval the practice of the Human Rights Committee to deem de facto jurisdiction to be established when the official agents of a state act in the territory of another country.[74] Applying this approach, the Court recognized "the exercise of effective jurisdiction by Israeli security forces [in the

---

[71] *Legal Consequences of the Construction of a Wall in the Occupied Palestinian Territory*, (2004) ICJ Gen. List No. 131, decided July 9, 2004.

[72] Ibid. at paras. 109–110.   [73] Ibid. at para. 112.

[74] "The Court would observe that, while the jurisdiction of States is primarily territorial, it may sometimes be exercised outside the national territory. Considering the object and purpose of the International Covenant on Civil and Political Rights, it would seem natural that, even when such is the case, States parties to the Covenant should be bound to comply with its provisions. The constant practice of the Human Rights Committee is consistent with this. Thus, the Committee has found the Covenant applicable where the State exercises its jurisdiction on foreign territory. It has ruled on the legality of acts by Uruguay in cases of arrests carried out by Uruguayan agents in Brazil or Argentina (case No. 52/79, *López Burgos v. Uruguay*; case No. 56/79, *Lilian Celiberti de Casariego v. Uruguay*). It decided to the same effect in the case of the confiscation of a passport by a Uruguayan consulate in Germany (case No. 106/81, *Montero v. Uruguay*)": *Legal Consequences of the Construction of a Wall in the Occupied Palestinian Territory*, (2004) ICJ Gen. List No. 131, decided July 9, 2004, at para. 109.

Occupied Territory]."[75] In other words, the Court understands effective jurisdiction to be established abroad where a state's agents exercise an important aspect of public power (in this case, police powers); having established that exercise of public power, the Court did not feel the need to inquire further into whether Israel also exercises a broader array of public powers in the Occupied Territory. While falling short of a pure effects-based approach to jurisdiction, the Court's holding makes clear that effective jurisdiction – and hence liability for breach of human rights – can be established even where the territorial government (here, the Palestinian Authority) continues to exercise many or even most of the public powers usually associated with governance.

For present purposes, the real importance of these decisions is that they make clear that it is not permissible to limit the underlying jurisdictional basis for state accountability on a narrowly territorial basis. To the contrary, the recognized circumstances in which jurisdiction extends beyond territory are sufficient to define a "legal space (*espace juridique*)"[76] within which those Refugee Convention rights not subject to a territorial or other level of attachment are, at a minimum, applicable.[77]

Assuming, then, that rights under the Refugee Convention not subject to an express level of attachment apply on the basis of the default position regarding jurisdiction in public international law, it may be concluded that the governments of state parties are bound to honor these rights not only in territory over which they have formal, de jure jurisdiction, but equally in places where they exercise effective or de facto jurisdiction outside their own territory.[78] At a minimum, this includes both situations

---

[75] Ibid. at para. 110.

[76] Ibid. at para. 80. Indeed, the Court's determination was largely in line with the perspective advanced by the defendant states (Belgium, Czech Republic, Denmark, France, Germany, Greece, Hungary, Iceland, Italy, Luxembourg, Netherlands, Norway, Poland, Portugal, Spain, Turkey, and the United Kingdom) that "[t]he exercise of 'jurisdiction' ... involves the assertion or exercise of legal authority, actual or purported, over persons owing some form of allegiance to that State or who have been brought within that State's control ... [It] generally entails some form of structured relationship normally existing over a period of time": ibid. at para. 36.

[77] In the context of refugee law, the English Court of Appeal has affirmed the link between control and jurisdiction. "There was no doubt that Mr. D was within the 'jurisdiction' of the United Kingdom, however that expression might be interpreted, because the United Kingdom was asserting rights over him, in particular the right to expel him to the country from whence he had come": *Kaya v. Haringey London Borough Council*, [2001] EWCA Civ 677 (Eng. CA, May 1, 2001).

[78] "In view of the purposes and objects of human rights treaties, there is no a priori reason to limit a state's obligation to respect human rights to its national territory. Where agents of the state, whether military or civilian, exercise power and authority (jurisdiction, or de facto jurisdiction) over persons outside national territory, the presumption should be that

in which a state's consular or other agents take control of persons abroad,[79] and where the state exercises some significant public power in territory which it has occupied, or in which it is present by consent, invitation, or acquiescence.

A helpful example of the latter circumstance derives from the right of states to extend their jurisdiction into what would otherwise be the *res communis* of the high seas by claiming a contiguous zone extending up to twelve miles beyond the external perimeter of their territorial sea. A contiguous zone, unlike the territorial sea or another part of a state's territory, is not an area of sovereign authority. It is, however, a zone in which specialized jurisdiction may be exercised including, for example, enforcement of the state's customs or immigration laws.[80] To the extent that a state party opts to establish a contiguous zone – and most obviously where the claim to extended jurisdiction includes the right to regulate the movement of persons within the zone – refugees present within the area of expanded territorial jurisdiction are thus

---

the state's obligation to respect the pertinent human rights continues. That presumption could be rebutted only when the nature and content of a particular right or treaty language suggest otherwise": T. Meron, "Extraterritoriality of Human Rights Treaties," (1995) 89(1) *American Journal of International Law* 78, at 80–81.

[79] This view was adopted not only by the International Court of Justice, but also by the European Court of Human Rights, which noted that the respondent governments accepted the view set out in its earlier decision of *Öcalan v. Turkey*, Dec. No. 46221/99 (unreported) (ECHR, Dec. 14, 2000) that jurisdiction was established by an official act of arrest and detention outside a state's territory, said by the respondent states to be "a classic exercise of such legal authority or jurisdiction over those persons by military forces on foreign soil": *Bankovic et al. v. Belgium et al.*, 11 BHRC 435 (ECHR, Dec. 12, 2001), at para. 37. The House of Lords recently affirmed the logic of this basic principle, finding that "a member state could, through the actions of its agents outside its territory, assume jurisdiction over others in a way that could engage the operation of the [European Convention on Human Rights]": *R v. Immigration Officer at Prague Airport et al., ex parte European Roma Rights Centre et al.*, [2004] UKHL 55 (UK HL, Dec. 9, 2004), at para. 21. Inexplicably, the decision nonetheless concluded that the actions of British immigration officers stationed at Prague Airport did not meet the relevant standard. Lord Bingham observed simply that he had "the greatest doubt whether the functions performed by the immigration officers at Prague, even if they were formally treated as consular officials, could possibly be said to be an exercise of jurisdiction in any relevant sense over non-UK nationals": ibid. This conclusion does not seem to accord with the broad approach adopted by both the European Court of Human Rights and, in particular, the International Court of Justice.

[80] Convention on the Territorial Sea and Contiguous Zone, 516 UNTS 205, done Apr. 29, 1958, entered into force Sept. 10, 1964, at Art. 24; and United Nations Convention on the Law of the Sea, UN Doc. A/CONF.62/122, done Dec. 10, 1982, entered into force Nov. 16, 1994, at Art. 33. Similarly, a state may claim an exclusive economic zone of up to 200 miles from the baseline of the territorial sea in which it may, *inter alia*, construct artificial islands and regulate immigration to and from any such artificial islands: ibid. at Arts. 55–75, in particular Art. 60(2).

entitled to claim the benefit of those rights which apply without qualifications based upon level of attachment.[81]

3.1.2 Physical presence

Several additional rights – to freedom of religion, to receive identity papers, to freedom from penalization for illegal entry, and to be subject to only necessary and justifiable constraints on freedom of movement – accrue to all refugees who are simply "in" or "within" a contracting state's territory.[82] Any refugee physically present, lawfully or unlawfully, in territory under a state's jurisdiction may invoke these rights.[83] This conclusion follows not only from the plain meaning of the language of "in" or "within,"[84] but also from the express intention of the drafters,[85] who insisted that these rights must be granted even to "refugees who had not yet been regularly admitted into a country."[86] This position is also consistent with the context of the

---

[81] But see *Sale, Acting Commissioner, Immigration and Naturalization Service, et al., Petitioners v. Haitian Centers Council, Inc., et al.*, 509 US 155 (US SC, Jan. 12, 1993) in which the majority of the United States Supreme Court determined that Art. 33 of the Refugee Convention was not intended to apply extraterritorially, in particular on the high seas. A contrary position is elaborated in chapter 4.1.3 below, at pp. 336–339.

[82] See Refugee Convention, at Arts. 4 ("religion"), 27 ("identity papers"), 31(1) ("non-penalization for illegal entry or presence") and 31(2) ("movements of refugees unlawfully in the country of refuge").

[83] But see *Minister for Immigration and Multicultural Affairs v. Khawar*, [2002] HCA 14 (Aus. HC, Apr. 11, 2002), per Justices McHugh and Gummow: "Nor does the Convention specify what constitutes entry into the territory of a contracting state so as then to be in a position to have the benefits conferred by the Convention. Rather, the protection obligations imposed by the Convention upon contracting states concern the status and civil rights to be afforded refugees who are within the contracting states." While somewhat unclear, the passage might be read to suggest that rights which inhere upon mere presence in a state may be withheld on the basis that, as a matter of law, the state has determined the person not to have formally entered its territory. Such an approach would confuse mere physical presence with lawful presence (see chapter 3.1.3 below). The fact that the drafters did not elaborate the meaning of "in" or "within" a state's territory simply confirms the self-evident plain meaning of those terms, i.e. physical presence in the territory of the state in question.

[84] See G. Stenberg, *Non-Expulsion and Non-Refoulement* (1989) (Stenberg, *Non-Expulsion*), at 87: "The statement that a person is present in the territory of a State indicates that he is physically within its borders."

[85] Mr. Larsen of Denmark persuaded the Ad Hoc Committee to draw up "a number of fairly simple rules for the treatment of refugees not yet authorized to reside in a country": Statement of Mr. Larsen of Denmark, UN Doc. E/AC.32/SR.15, Jan. 27, 1950, at 22. To similar effect, the representative of the International Refugee Organization stressed the importance of including in the Convention "provisions concerning refugees who had not yet been regularly admitted": ibid. at 18.

[86] Statement of Mr. Henkin of the United States, ibid. at 18. The Danish representative similarly distinguished between "refugees regularly resident" and "those . . . who had just

Convention as a whole, most notably with the approach taken to the provisional suspension of rights in the context of a national emergency.[87]

Under general principles of territorial jurisdiction, this level of attachment enfranchises, for example, not only refugees within a state's land territory, but also those on its inland waterways or territorial sea,[88] including on islands, islets, rocks, and reefs; it includes also those in the airspace above each of these.[89] The Australian Senate was therefore acting very much in line with international law when it rejected a government proposal to "excise" some 3,500 islands from the portion of the national territory in which refugee protection obligations would have been deemed applicable.[90] A state's territory moreover includes both its ports of entry,[91] and so-called "international zones" within a state's territory.[92] To the extent that a state acquires additional territory by accretion, cession, conquest, occupation, or prescription,[93] it is bound to honor rights that apply at this second level of attachment in such territory.

arrived in the initial reception country": Statement of Mr. Larsen of Denmark, UN Doc. E/AC.32/SR.16, Jan. 30, 1950, at 11.

[87] The interpretation of the Refugee Convention as granting rights even prior to formal verification of status is buttressed by the specific incorporation of Art. 9 in the Refugee Convention, which allows governments provisionally to suspend the rights of persons not yet confirmed to be refugees *if* the asylum state is faced with war or other exceptional circumstances. It follows from the inclusion of this provision in the Convention that, absent such extreme circumstances, states cannot suspend rights pending verification of status. See generally chapter 3.5.1 below.

[88] See e.g. UNHCR Executive Committee Conclusion No. 97, "Conclusion on Protection Safeguards in Interception Measures" (2003), available at www.unhcr.ch (accessed Nov. 20, 2004), at para. (a)(i): "The State within whose sovereign territory, or territorial waters, interception takes place has the primary responsibility for addressing any protection needs of intercepted persons."

[89] I. Brownlie, *Principles of Public International Law* (2003) (Brownlie, *Public International Law*), at 105.

[90] "Island excision thrown out: hunt for new plan," *Sydney Morning Herald*, Nov. 25, 2003, available at www.smh.com.au (accessed Nov. 25, 2003). In defending the excision, the Defence Minister said that the government had excised Christmas Island "because that was seen as an easy route to get the protections under Australian law": "Plan to excise islands doomed: Hill," *Canberra Times*, June 17, 2002, at A-10. Indeed, the Immigration Minister was reported to have said that "he could not rule out placing Tasmania outside Australia's immigration borders": "Refugee boats will 'aim for mainland,'" *Canberra Times*, June 11, 2002, at A-1. Such notions led one commentator to observe, in line with rules of international law, that "if the whole of Australia were excised from the migration zone, maybe it could be excised from all the rest of the law that gives people rights to access the courts ... The islands today; the rest of Australia tomorrow. There is no difference": C. Hull, "Excising islands: where will it all end?," *Canberra Times*, June 21, 2002, at A-13.

[91] G. Goodwin-Gill, *The Refugee in International Law* (1996) (Goodwin-Gill, *Refugee in International Law*), at 123.

[92] *Amuur v. France*, [1996] ECHR 25 (ECHR, June 25, 1996).

[93] See generally M. Shaw, *International Law* (2003), at 417–441.

A state is not, however, required to grant rights defined by this level of attachment to refugees with which it may come into contact in territory under the full sovereign authority of another state, including in particular refugees who arrive at a state's embassy or other diplomatic post abroad. While such premises are immune from intrusion,[94] they are neither assimilated to the territory of the state that established the diplomatic mission, nor otherwise free from the legal control of the territorial state.[95] Because a diplomatic post is not a part of the territory of the state whose interests it represents, the primary responsibility to honor the rights of any refugees physically present there falls to the country in which the post is located.[96]

3.1.3 Lawful presence

Refugees who are not simply physically present, but who are also *lawfully in* the territory of a state party, are further entitled to claim the rights that apply at the third level of attachment. Lawful presence entitles refugees to be protected against expulsion, enjoy a more generous guarantee of internal freedom of movement, and engage in self-employment.[97] Lawful

---

[94] Vienna Convention on Diplomatic Relations, 500 UNTS 95, done Apr. 18, 1961, entered into force Apr. 24, 1964, at Art. 22.

[95] *Asylum Case (Colombia v. Peru)*, [1950] ICJ Rep 266. Brownlie, however, suggests that the reference to "special arrangements" in the Vienna Convention on Diplomatic Relations, at Art. 41, "makes room for bilateral recognition of the right to give asylum to political refugees within the mission": Brownlie, *Public International Law*, at 348. The traditional practice of Latin American states to honor a grant of diplomatic asylum is codified in the Caracas Convention on Diplomatic Asylum, OAS Doc. OEA/Ser.X/1, entered into force Dec. 29, 1954.

[96] If the "refugees" in question are nationals of the territorial state, they have no entitlement to refugee rights as they will not have satisfied the alienage requirement of the Convention refugee definition. See generally A. Grahl-Madsen, *The Status of Refugees in International Law* (vol. I, 1966) (Grahl-Madsen, *Status of Refugees I*), at 150–154; J. Hathaway, *The Law of Refugee Status* (1991) (Hathaway, *Refugee Status*), at 29–33; and Goodwin-Gill, *Refugee in International Law*, at 40. A more interesting question arises with regard to third-country nationals who arrive at a consulate or embassy, however. To the extent that consular or embassy officials have jurisdiction over such persons in line with norms of customary international law (see chapter 3.1.1 above, at pp. 169–170), the state in whose consulate or embassy the refugee is located is logically bound to respect those rights not subject to territorial or a higher level of attachment (including, for example, the duty of *non-refoulement*). It would, in this sense, exercise jurisdiction concurrently with the territorial state. Yet only the territorial state would be bound to honor those rights which require physical presence in a state's territory, or a higher level of attachment.

[97] See Refugee Convention, at Arts. 18 ("self-employment"), 26 ("freedom of movement"), and 32 ("expulsion"). Goodwin-Gill, however, asserts that Art. 32 rights need be granted only to refugees who are "in the State on a more or less indefinite basis": Goodwin-Gill, *Refugee in International Law*, at 308. He offers no legal argument to justify this clear deviation from the express provisions of the Convention, relying instead on a bald appeal

presence was broadly conceived,[98] including refugees in any of three situations.

First, a refugee is lawfully present if admitted to a state party's territory for a fixed period of time, even if only for a few hours. Whether the refugee resides elsewhere and is merely transiting through the second state[99] or is sojourning there for a limited time,[100] his or her presence is lawful so long as it is officially sanctioned.[101] This clarification was particularly important to representatives concerned to grant a limited range of supplementary rights to refugees living near a frontier, who might wish to pursue commercial interests in a neighboring state.[102] As the French delegate remarked, "it could not be argued that where there was no residence, the situation was irregular."[103]

> to the importance of achieving consistency with relevant state practice. State practice may, of course, assist in establishing the *interpretation* of a treaty provision: Vienna Convention on the Law of Treaties, 1155 UNTS 331, done May 23, 1969, entered into force Jan. 27, 1980 (Vienna Convention), at Art. 31(3)(b). However, state practice standing alone cannot give rise to a legal norm which may be relied upon to challenge the applicability of a conflicting treaty stipulation: see generally chapters 1.1.1 and 1.3.4 above.
>
> [98] The French representative described this level of attachment as "a very wide term applicable to any refugee, whatever his origin or situation. It was therefore a term having a very broad meaning": Statement of Mr. Juvigny of France, UN Doc. E/AC.32/SR.42, Aug. 24, 1950, at 12.
>
> [99] "Mr. Guerreiro (Brazil) asked whether the phrase 'refugees lawfully in their territory' was intended to cover refugees in transit through a territory . . . Mr. Henkin (United States of America) explained that the provisions . . . were really intended to apply to all refugees lawfully in the country, even those who were not permanent residents. There was no harm in the provision even if it theoretically applied to refugees who were in a country for a brief sojourn, since the individuals would hardly seek the benefit of the rights contemplated": Statements of Mr. Guerreiro of Brazil and Mr. Henkin of the United States, UN Doc. E/AC.32/SR.25, Feb. 10, 1950, at 5. See also Statement of Mr. Herment of Belgium, UN Doc. E/AC.32/SR.42, Aug. 24, 1950, at 17, that rights allocated at this second level of attachment would accrue to refugees "merely passing through a territory."
>
> [100] "The expression 'lawfully in their territory' included persons entering a territory even for a few hours, provided that they had been duly authorized to enter": Statement of Mr. Henkin of the United States, UN Doc. E/AC.32/SR.41, Aug. 23, 1950, at 14; see also Statements of Mr. Henkin of the United States at UN Doc. E/AC.32/SR.42, Aug. 24, 1950, at 20 and 32.
>
> [101] "[T]he mere fact of lawfully being in the territory, even without any intention of permanence, must suffice": N. Robinson, *Convention relating to the Status of Refugees: Its History, Contents and Interpretation* (1953) (Robinson, *History*), at 117.
>
> [102] "The difficulties raised were . . . not academic, at least in the case of refugees living near a frontier": Statement of the Chairman, Mr. Larsen of Denmark, UN Doc. E/AC.32/SR.41, Aug. 23, 1950, at 18. For example, it was suggested that the rights granted to refugees lawfully present in a state would accrue even to "a [refugee] musician [who] was staying for one or two nights in a country": Statement of the Chairman, Mr. Larsen of Denmark, UN Doc. E/AC.32/SR.42, Aug. 24, 1950, at 16–17.
>
> [103] Statement of Mr. Juvigny of France, UN Doc. E/AC.32/SR.42, Aug. 24, 1950, at 20. "For example, there were aliens lawfully in France without being resident. As evidence of that

Second and of greater contemporary importance, the stage between "irregular" presence and the recognition or denial of refugee status, including the time required for exhaustion of any appeals or reviews, is also a form of "lawful presence."[104] Presence is lawful in the case of "a person ... not yet in possession of a residence permit but who had applied for it and had the receipt for that application. *Only those persons who had not applied, or whose applications had been refused, were in an irregular position* [emphasis added]."[105] The drafters recognized that refugees who travel without pre-authorization to a state party, but who are admitted to a process intended to assess their suitability for admission to that or another state, should "be considered, for purposes of the future convention, to have been regularly admitted."[106] Thus, for example, the Full Federal Court of Australia determined in *Rajendran* that a Sri Lankan applicant whose refugee case had yet to be determined was nonetheless "lawfully in" Australia by virtue of his provisional admission under domestic regulations for purposes of pursuing his claim.[107]

Yet because the full contours of "lawful presence" are not settled, there is a body of British jurisprudence which suggests that where a state party's domestic laws – in contrast to those considered by the Australian court – do not authorize presence for purposes of pursuing a claim to refugee status, asylum-seekers are not lawfully present, and hence cannot claim rights defined by the third level of attachment.[108] This approach is said to be based on the decision of the House of Lords in 1987 in *Bugdaycay*,[109] which

---

he mentioned the case of Belgian nationals, who needed only an identity card to spend a few hours in France. They would be in France lawfully, even though not resident": ibid.

[104] The French description of the three phases through which a refugee passes distinguished the second step of "regularization" of status from the third and final stage at which "they had been lawfully authorized to reside in the country": Statement of Mr. Rain of France, UN Doc. E/AC.32/SR.15, Jan. 27, 1950, at 15.

[105] Ibid. at 20.

[106] Statement of Mr. Henkin of the United States, ibid. at 20.

[107] "In the present case, Mr. Rajendran entered the country on a visitor's visa. He now holds a bridging visa. If his application for a [refugee status-based] protection visa is ultimately unsuccessful ... that visa will cease to have effect at the time stipulated in the relevant Migration Regulations ... whereupon he will cease both to be lawfully in Australia and to be able to invoke Article 32": *Rajendran v. Minister for Immigration and Multicultural Affairs*, (1998) 166 ALR 619 (Aus. FFC, Sept. 4, 1998). The same reasoning was impliedly adopted by the South African Supreme Court of Appeal, which determined that the child of a person seeking recognition of refugee status is "a child who is lawfully in this country": *Minister of Home Affairs v. Watchenuka*, (2004) 1 All SA 21 (SA SCA, Nov. 28, 2003), at para. 36, per Nugent JA.

[108] A comparable position was taken in the United States prior to the establishment of a domestic procedure for the determination of refugee status, enacted by the Refugee Act 1980: see *Chim Ming v. Marks*, (1974) 505 F 2d 1170, at 1172 (US CA2, Nov. 8, 1974).

[109] *R v. Secretary of State for the Home Department, ex parte Bugdaycay*, [1987] AC 514 (UK HL, Feb. 19, 1987).

determined that not even temporary admission to the UK gave rise to lawful presence under British law.[110] Insisting that it could not revisit the issue determined in *Bugdaycay*, the English Court of Appeal upheld the denial of public housing to a Kurdish husband and wife on the grounds that they were not lawfully present in the United Kingdom while they awaited a decision on their refugee claims:

> There is no settled international meaning of the term "lawfully," not merely in international but national law. The word is a notoriously slippery expression, that can mean a wide range of things in different contexts. One has to ask oneself why that expression is used in the [Refugee Convention] at all. By far the most obvious explanation [for the choice of this phrase] . . . is that the contracting parties to the Convention wished to reserve to themselves the right to determine conditions of entry, at least in cases not covered by the Refugee Convention.[111]

The Court therefore found that the immigration regulation which denied the lawful presence of a person temporarily admitted "does go to the lawfulness of the person's presence and is directly relevant to the question of whether,

[110] Ibid. at 526. There is no indication that relevant portions of the Convention's drafting history – e.g. those speaking to both temporary admission, and to presence before status was regularized as examples of lawful presence (see text above, at pp. 174–175) – were drawn to the attention of the House of Lords. With the benefit of these insights, at least a core international understanding of "lawful presence" for refugee law purposes might well have been identified. In any event, Lord Bridge was clearly led to conclude against finding temporarily present persons to be "lawfully in" the country because of a mistaken belief that "if [this] argument is right, it must apply equally to any person arriving in this country . . . whether he is detained or temporarily admitted pending a decision on his application for leave to enter. It follows that the effect of the submission, if it is well-founded, is to confer on any person who can establish that he has the status of a refugee . . . but who arrives in the United Kingdom from a third country, an indefeasible right to remain here, since to refuse him leave to enter and direct his return to the third country will involve the United Kingdom in the expulsion of a 'refugee lawfully in their territory' contrary to article 32(1)": ibid. at 526. But states may lawfully (and often do) interpose an eligibility determination procedure to determine whether some other state may be said to have primary responsibility to determine the claim to refugee status. If it is determined that the initial responsibility lies with another country and instructions for removal to that country are issued, the initial lawful presence of the refugee comes to an end, and Art. 32 no longer governs his or her removal (though Art. 33 remains applicable). See chapter 5.1 below, at pp. 663–664.

[111] *Kaya v. Haringey London Borough Council*, [2001] EWCA Civ 677 (Eng. CA, May 1, 2001), at para. 31. The constraint perceived to flow from the decision of the House of Lords in *Bugdaycay* is clear. "An international treaty has only one meaning. That is the teaching of the House of Lords in *Adan* . . . It was not open to [counsel for the applicant] to argue in this Court, as he at one time sought to do, that Lord Bridge had taken an approach incorrect in international law as to the construction of the Refugee Convention. In my judgment, Lord Bridge's exposition is a binding exposition of the meaning and implications of virtually the same phrase with which we are concerned": ibid.

under national rules, the seeker for asylum is 'unlawfully present' in this country."[112]

As a starting point, the logic of deference to national legal understandings of lawful presence is clearly sensible. Not only is it correct that there is no uniform and comprehensive international standard by reference to which lawful presence can be determined but, as the debates cited above regarding temporary admission confirm,[113] the drafters did generally intend for the third level of attachment to be determined by reference to national standards. Yet there is no indication that this deference was intended to be absolute, a proposition which – if carried to its logical conclusion – could result in refugees never being in a position to secure more than rights defined by the first two of the five levels of attachment agreed to by state parties.[114] Indeed, as much as was recognized by the English Court of Appeal when it determined that "the contracting parties to the Convention wished to reserve to themselves the right to determine conditions of entry, *at least in cases not covered by the Refugee Convention* [emphasis added]."[115] That is, a state's general right to define lawful presence is constrained by the impermissibility of deeming presence to be unlawful in circumstances when the Refugee Convention – and by logical extension, other binding norms of international law – deem presence to be lawful.[116] While this is in most cases a minimalist constraint on the scope of domestic discretion, it is nonetheless one that is important to ensuring the workability of a treaty intended to set a common international standard.[117]

Interpretation of the notion of "lawful presence" should therefore look primarily to domestic legal requirements, interpreted in the light of the small number of international legal understandings on point, in particular those

---

[112] Ibid. at para. 33. The provision in question was s. 11 of the Immigration Act 1971, which provided that "[a] person arriving in the United Kingdom by ship or aircraft shall for the purposes of this Act be deemed not to enter the United Kingdom unless he disembarks, and on disembarkation at a port shall further be deemed not to enter the United Kingdom so long as he remains in such area (if any) at the port as may be approved for this purpose by an immigration officer ... and a person who has not otherwise entered the United Kingdom shall be deemed not to do so as long as he is detained, or temporarily admitted or released while liable to detention."

[113] See text above, at p. 174.

[114] This result would only be precluded by the ability to establish lawful stay on the basis of de facto toleration of ongoing presence. See chapter 3.1.4 below, at pp. 186–187.

[115] *Kaya v. Haringey London Borough Council*, [2001] EWCA Civ 677 (Eng. CA, May 1, 2001), at para. 31.

[116] "The question whether an alien is 'lawfully' within the territory of a State is a matter governed by domestic law, which may subject the entry of an alien to the territory of a State to restrictions, *provided they are in compliance with the State's international obligations* [emphasis added]": UN Human Rights Committee, "General Comment No. 27: Freedom of movement" (1999), UN Doc. HRI/GEN/1/Rev.7, May 12, 2004, at 173, para. 4.

[117] See Introduction above, at p. 2.

reached by the drafters of the Refugee Convention.[118] Deference to domestic law cannot therefore be absolute. At a minimum, the domestic meaning of lawful presence should not be adopted for refugee law purposes where to do so would be at odds with the normative requirements of the Refugee Convention. For example, current British law purports to treat only persons who seek refugee status at a port or airport as lawfully present.[119] Yet as a matter of international law, all persons who seek recognition of refugee status within a reasonable period of time after their arrival in a state are entitled to the same rights as those who seek protection immediately upon arrival.[120] Because "lawful presence" is being construed not in the abstract, but as an integral part of the Refugee Convention, it would be contrary to the duty to interpret a treaty's terms in their context to defer to a domestic understanding of lawful presence which conflicts with the requirements of the Refugee Convention itself. In the result, where persons seeking recognition of refugee status meet the requirements of Art. 31 – that is, they "present themselves without delay to the authorities and show good cause for their illegal entry or presence"[121] – their presence must be deemed lawful, even if they fail to claim refugee status immediately, or to meet some other domestic requirement at odds with Art. 31.

An even more worrisome position is that a refugee is not lawfully present until permanent residence is granted,[122] or at least until refugee status has

---

[118] See text above, at pp. 174–175; and below, at pp. 183–185.

[119] In *O v. London Borough of Wandsworth*, [2000] EWCA Civ 201 (Eng. CA, June 22, 2000), the Court of Appeal observed that its "first difficulty is understanding [the argument that] all asylum-seekers are said to be here lawfully. As [counsel] acknowledged, only those who claim asylum at the port of entry and are granted temporary admission, or who claim asylum during an extant leave, are here lawfully; the rest are here unlawfully albeit, of course, they are irremovable until their claims have been determined (or they can be returned to a safe third country)." See also *R (Saadi) v. Secretary of State for the Home Department*, [2002] UKHL 41 (UK HL, Oct. 31, 2002), in which the House of Lords held that even a person who "complied with reporting conditions" immediately upon entry into the United Kingdom was still not lawfully present. As the judgment observed, "until the state has 'authorized' entry, the entry is unauthorized." Regrettably, the latter case appears to have been argued on the grounds of the importance of recognizing a "restriction on liberty" in such circumstances, rather than on the basis of the need not to contravene Art. 31 or other provisions of the Refugee Convention.

[120] The Convention provides that states "shall not impose penalties, on account of their illegal entry or presence, on refugees who, coming directly from a territory where their life or freedom was threatened ... enter *or are present* in their territory without authorization, *provided they present themselves without delay* to the authorities and show good cause for their illegal entry or presence [emphasis added]": Refugee Convention, at Art. 31(1). See chapter 4.2 below.

[121] Refugee Convention, at Art. 31(1). This provision does not require immediate presentation of a claim upon arrival in a state party: see chapter 4.2.1 below, at pp. 391–392.

[122] There is rather dated German authority for the view that Art. 32 rights, which require lawful presence, accrue only once a refugee who has entered the state unlawfully secures lawful residence in the state party: *Yugoslav Refugee (Germany) Case*, 26 ILR 496 (Ger.

been formally verified.[123] This position contradicts the plain meaning of "lawful presence." In line with the approach taken in *Rajendran*,[124] it cannot sensibly be argued that persons who avail themselves of domestic laws which authorize entry into a refugee status determination or comparable procedure are not lawfully present.[125] So long as a refugee has provided authorities with the information that will enable them to consider his or her entitlement to refugee status – in particular, details of personal and national

FASC, Nov. 25, 1958), at 498 (reporting German Federal Administrative Supreme Court Dec. BverGE 7 (1959), at 333). A comparable, though somewhat less demanding, standard has been suggested by the New Zealand Court of Appeal, which determined that a person positively determined to be a Convention refugee was not lawfully present because he had "not been granted a permit to enter New Zealand": *Attorney General v. Zaoui*, Dec. No. CA20/04 (NZ CA, Sept. 30, 2004), at paras. 32–33.

[123] Grahl-Madsen, for example, equivocates in his analysis of the status of refugees awaiting verification of their claims by authorities. He suggests that "a refugee may be 'lawfully' in a country for some purposes while 'unlawfully' there for other purposes ... Furthermore, a refugee's presence may, on the face of it, be 'illegal' according to some set of rules (e.g. aliens legislation), yet 'legal' within a wider frame of reference (e.g. international refugee law)": A. Grahl-Madsen, *The Status of Refugees in International Law* (vol. II, 1972) (Grahl-Madsen, *Status of Refugees II*), at 363. He ultimately adopts the definition of "regularization" stated by the British delegate to the Conference of Plenipotentiaries, namely "the acceptance by a country of a refugee for permanent settlement, not the mere issue of documents prior to the duration of his stay": Statement of Mr. Hoare of the United Kingdom, UN Doc. E/CONF.2/SR.14, July 10, 1951, at 16. While this approach was endorsed by the representatives of some states not then experiencing the direct arrival of refugees, it was rejected as insufficiently attentive to the situation of those countries, such as France, that were obliged to process refugees arriving directly through a process of regularization involving successive stages (see the description of the French system provided by the Belgian delegate to the Ad Hoc Committee at UN Doc. E/AC.32/SR.15, Jan. 27, 1950, at 22). The equation of lawful presence with formal recognition of refugee status is nonetheless still advocated by some: see e.g. M. Pellonpää, *Expulsion in International Law: A Study in International Aliens Law and Human Rights with Special Reference to Finland* (1984), at 292.

[124] See text above, at p. 175.

[125] The inappropriateness of the equation of a "lawful presence" with admission to permanent residence was explicitly brought to the attention of the Conference of Plenipotentiaries by its President, who expressed the view that "such a suggestion would probably cover the situation in the United States of America, where there were [only] two categories of entrants, those legally admitted and those who had entered clandestinely. But it might not cover the situation in other countries where there were a number of intermediate stages; for example, certain countries allowed refugees to remain in their territory for a limited time": Statement of the President, Mr. Larsen of Denmark, UN Doc. A/CONF.2/SR.14, July 10, 1951, at 17. The only response to this clarification was an assertion by the representative of the United States that his country's system was not quite as simple as the President had implied. No delegate, however, challenged the accuracy of the President's understanding of "lawful presence" as including refugees subject to the various "intermediate stages" which a country might establish for refugees coming directly to its territory.

identity, and the facts relied upon in support of the claim for admission – there is clearly a legal basis for the refugee's presence.[126] The once irregularly present refugee is now lawfully present,[127] as he or she has satisfied the administrative requirements established by the state to consider which persons who arrive without authorization should nonetheless be allowed to remain there.[128]

This understanding of "lawful presence" is moreover consistent with the general approach of the Refugee Convention in at least two ways. First, an interpretation of "lawful presence" predicated on official recognition erroneously presupposes that states are necessarily under an obligation formally to verify refugee status. While there clearly is an implied duty to proceed to the assessment of refugee status if a state party elects to condition access to refugee rights on the results of such verification,[129] governments are otherwise free to dispense with a formal procedure of any kind: they must simply

---

[126] Consistent with the duty of states to implement their international legal obligations in good faith (see chapter 1.3.3 above, at p. 62), it must be possible for all Convention refugees to fulfill any such requirements. Excluded, therefore, are any requirements that are directed to matters unrelated to refugee status, including suitability for immigration on economic, cultural, personal, or other grounds. Account must also be taken of any genuine disabilities faced by particular refugees, for example by reason of language, education, mistrust, or the residual effects of stress or trauma, which may make it difficult for them to provide authorities with the information required to verify their refugee status. Because refugee status assessment involves a *shared* responsibility between the refugee and national authorities (see UNHCR, *Handbook*, at para. 196), it is the responsibility of the receiving state to take all reasonable steps to assist refugees to state their claims to protection with clarity. See generally W. Kälin, "Troubled Communication: Cross-Cultural Misunderstandings in the Asylum Hearing," (1986) 20 *International Migration Review* 230; J. Hathaway, *Rebuilding Trust* (1993); A. Leiss and R. Boesjes, *Female Asylum Seekers* (1994); UNHCR, "Refugee Children: Guidelines on Protection and Care" (1994); R. Barsky, *Constructing a Productive Other: Discourse Theory and the Convention Refugee Hearing* (1994); UNHCR, "Guidelines on Policies and Procedures in Dealing with Unaccompanied Children Seeking Asylum" (1997).

[127] Grahl-Madsen suggests one potentially important exception to this general principle. He argues that a refugee who is detained pending verification of his claim to Convention refugee status (presumably on grounds that meet the justification test of Art. 31(2) of the Convention) can no longer be considered to be "lawfully" present: Grahl-Madsen, *Status of Refugees II*, at 361–362. This conclusion is clearly tenable, though not based on decisions reached during the drafting process. A detained refugee claimant would still be entitled to those rights which are not restricted to refugees whose presence is lawful, i.e. the rights defined by the first level of attachment.

[128] UNHCR has similarly opined that "[a]t a minimum, the 1951 Convention provisions that are not linked to lawful stay or residence would apply to asylum-seekers in so far as they relate to humane treatment and respect for basic rights": UNHCR, "Reception of Asylum-Seekers, Including Standards of Treatment, in the Context of Individual Asylum Systems," UN Doc. EC/GC/01/17, Sept. 4, 2001, at para. 3.

[129] In considering a comparable issue – whether it was lawful to deny an appeal of a refusal of refugee status to a person granted the alternative status of "exceptional leave to

respect the rights of persons who are, in fact, refugees.[130] Indeed, most less developed states – which host the majority of the world's refugees – do not operate formal refugee status assessment procedures. In these circumstances, the conditioning of "lawful presence" on formal verification of refugee status would allow a genuine refugee to be held hostage to a decision never to undertake the processing of his or her claim to Convention refugee status. He or she would be effectively barred from access to rights defined by the third level of attachment – a proposition which is difficult to reconcile to the duty to implement treaty obligations in good faith.[131]

Second, the understanding of lawful presence as conditioned on formal acceptance as a refugee conflates the categories of "lawful presence" and "lawful stay."[132] Even as the drafters varied the level of attachment applicable

remain" – the Master of the Rolls, Lord Phillips, eloquently captured the nature of this dilemma. "Refugees who arrive in this country are anxious to have their status as refugees established. This is not merely because recognition of their refugee status will carry with it the entitlement to remain here, but because it will ensure that they are accorded Convention rights while they are here ... There is no doubt that this country is under an obligation under international law to enable those who are in truth refugees to exercise their Convention rights ... Although Convention rights accrue to a refugee by virtue of his being a refugee, unless a refugee claimant can have access to a decision-maker who can determine whether or not he is a refugee, his access to Convention rights is impeded": *Saad v. Secretary of State for the Home Department*, [2001] EWCA Civ 2008 (Eng. CA, Dec. 19, 2001). In a much earlier decision, the German Federal Administrative Supreme Court observed that "the Federal Republic, when ratifying the Convention, assumed an obligation to grant to a foreign refugee requesting the same the requisite recognition of his status. This is not expressly provided for in the Convention, but it follows from the legal duty to carry out the terms of the Convention in the municipal sphere": *Yugoslav Refugee (Germany) Case*, 26 ILR 496 (Ger. FASC, Nov. 25, 1958), at 497 (reporting German Administrative Supreme Court Dec. BverGE 7 (1959), at 333).

[130] Thus, for example, the Australian Full Federal Court has determined that the "obligations imposed by Article 33 fall short of creating a right in a refugee to seek asylum, or a duty on [the] part of the Contracting State to whom a request for asylum is made, to grant it, even if the refugee's status as such has not been recognized in any other country": *Rajendran v. Minister for Immigration and Multicultural Affairs*, (1998) 166 ALR 619 (Aus. FFC, Sept. 4, 1998). But see W. Kälin, "Towards a Concept of Temporary Protection: A Study Commissioned by the UNHCR Department of International Protection" (1996), at 32: "Although the 1951 Convention does not contain any provisions relating to national status determination procedures, the principle of good faith in fulfilling treaty obligations requires, as has been recently stressed by the German Constitutional Court, that states parties to the Convention institute a procedure which allows for determination of who is entitled to the guarantees of the 1951 Convention." Yet since many less developed countries do not in fact have any such procedure, this assertion begs the question whether all such governments are thereby in breach of the (implied) duty to institute such a procedure. More generally, on what basis could it be argued that a state which in fact grants all Convention rights to persons who claim refugee status is somehow in breach of its treaty obligations?

[131] Vienna Convention, at Art. 31(1). See chapter 1.3.3 above, at p. 62.

[132] See chapter 3.1.4 below.

to specific rights, they expressly opted to grant some rights at an intermediate point between "physical presence" and "lawful stay" – namely, "lawful presence."[133] Yet under the alternative interpretation, there is no such intermediate point. Refugees would move directly from being merely physically (but "irregularly") present, to securing simultaneously all the rights associated with both "lawful presence" and "lawful stay" when and if permission to remain is granted.[134] Such an approach clearly does not comport with the explicit structure of the Convention.

The view that persons present with a form of authorization that falls significantly short of ongoing permission to remain are nonetheless to be deemed lawfully present follows also from relevant determinations of the United Nations Human Rights Committee, interpreting the right to freedom of internal movement under the Civil and Political Covenant (which inheres in all persons "lawfully within the territory of a State").[135] In *Celepli v. Sweden*,[136] the Committee considered the case of a rejected refugee claimant formally ordered to be expelled to Turkey, but not in fact removed on humanitarian grounds. Despite the issuance of the expulsion order, the Committee determined the applicant to be "lawfully present" in Sweden:

---

[133] A detailed analysis of the notion of "lawful presence" is provided in Stenberg, *Non-Expulsion*, at 87–130. Stenberg ultimately concludes that "[t]here is . . . a lack of *opinio juris* on the part of States to include refugees whose status has not been recognized [within] the scope of [lawful presence for purposes of] Article 32": ibid. at 130. This conclusion seems to be based upon an overly deferential understanding of the role of state practice in the interpretation of treaties, as contrasted with its role in the formation of customary law: see chapter 1.3.4 above. On the other hand, Stenberg's examination of both the internal structure of the Convention and its drafting history leads her to essentially the same conclusion as reached here regarding the meaning of "lawful presence." As a general matter, she observes that "the drafters of the 1951 Convention intended the term 'lawfully' in Article 32(1) to signify lawful presence in the territory of a contracting State in the sense that the term has in general national immigration law . . . [T]aking into account the declaratory character of the determination of the alien's refugee status, it also seems clear that Article 32 was intended to protect not only those whose refugee status already had been recognized by the expelling State but also those whose status had not yet been recognized when the expulsion measures were initiated": ibid. at 121. Stenberg's analysis is that "for the purposes of national immigration law, an alien is 'lawfully' in the territory of the State in question if he has entered the territory in accordance with the conditions laid down in national immigration law, or his sojourn has afterwards been regularized. If, however, his entry and stay were subject to certain conditions – which for instance is the case when he has been admitted for a fixed period of time – and he no longer complies with these conditions, he cannot be considered to be lawfully in the territory": ibid. at 88.

[134] See Robinson, *History*, at 117.   [135] Civil and Political Covenant, at Art. 12(1).

[136] *Celepli v. Sweden*, UNHRC Comm. No. 456/1991, UN Doc. CCPR/C/51/D/456/1991, decided Mar. 19, 1993.

The Committee notes that the author's expulsion was ordered on 10 December 1984, but that this order was not enforced and that the author was allowed to stay in Sweden, subject to restrictions on his freedom of movement. The Committee is of the view that, following the expulsion order, the author was lawfully in the territory of Sweden, for purposes of article 12, paragraph 1, of the Covenant, only under the restrictions placed upon him by the State party.[137]

Clearly, if a *rejected* refugee claimant not removed on humanitarian grounds is "lawfully present" by virtue of the host government's decision not to enforce the removal order, there can be little doubt that a refugee claimant admitted to a status determination procedure and authorized to remain pending assessment of his or her case is similarly lawfully present. Indeed, the Human Rights Committee recently affirmed its position on the meaning of "lawful presence," expressly citing its findings in *Celepli* as authority for the proposition that:

> [t]he question whether an alien is "lawfully" within the territory of a State is a matter governed by domestic law, which may subject the entry of an alien to the territory of a State to restrictions, provided they are in compliance with the State's international obligations. In that connection, the Committee has held that an alien who entered the State illegally, but whose status *has been regularized*, must be considered to be lawfully within the territory [emphasis added].[138]

This analysis blends neatly with the understanding of the Refugee Convention advanced above. A rejected refugee claimant ordered expelled but whom the state has determined not to remove on humanitarian grounds is, in the view of the Human Rights Committee, a person whose status has "been regularized" and hence one who must be considered to be – at least for the duration of that permission to remain – "lawfully present." This conclusion makes sense because such a person – like a person seeking recognition of his or her refugee status – has satisfied the administrative requirements established by the state to determine which non-citizens should be allowed to remain, at least provisionally, in its territory. It makes clear that lawful presence is an intermediate category which occupies the ground between illegal presence on the one hand, and a right to stay on the other.

In addition to authorized short-term presence and presence while undergoing refugee status verification, the Refugee Convention foresees a third form of lawful presence. In many asylum countries, particularly in the less developed world, there is no mechanism in place to assess the refugee status

---

[137] Ibid. at para. 9.2.
[138] UN Human Rights Committee, "General Comment No. 27: Freedom of movement" (1999), UN Doc. HRI/GEN/1/Rev.7, May 12, 2004, at 173, para. 4.

of persons who arrive to seek protection.[139] Other states may on occasion opt to suspend formal status determination procedures for some or all asylum-seekers, who are thereupon assigned to an alternative (formal or informal) protection regime.[140] In either of these situations – including where governments divert refugees into so-called "temporary protection" regimes[141] – a refugee's presence should be deemed lawful.[142] This is because the decision not to authenticate refugee status, whether generally or as an exceptional measure, must be considered in the context of the government's legal duty to grant Convention rights to all persons in its territory who are *in fact* refugees, whether or not their status has been assessed.[143]

This understanding of "lawful presence" draws upon the *prima facie* legal right of individuals seeking protection to present themselves in the territory of a state which has chosen to adhere to the Refugee Convention. By choosing to become a party to the Convention, a state party signals its preparedness to grant rights to refugees who reach its jurisdiction. A state that wishes to protect itself against the possibility of receiving non-genuine claims is free to establish a procedure to verify the refugee status of those who seek its protection. But if a state opts not to adjudicate the status of persons who claim to be Convention refugees, it must be taken to have acquiesced in the asylum-seekers' assertion of entitlement to refugee rights, and must immediately

---

[139] See e.g. Lawyers' Committee for Human Rights, *African Exodus: Refugee Crisis, Human Rights and the 1969 OAU Convention* (1995), at 29–30.

[140] For example, the temporary protection policies adopted by some European states in response to the arrival of refugees from Bosnia-Herzegovina actually diverted asylum-seekers away from formal processes to adjudicate refugee status, or at least suspended assessment of status for a substantial period of time: Intergovernmental Consultations on Asylum, Refugee and Migration Policies in Europe, North America and Australia, *Report on Temporary Protection in States in Europe, North America and Australia* (1995) (IGC, *Temporary Protection*), at 79, 118.

[141] Kälin writes that "lawful presence" "refers to presence authorized by law which ... may be of a temporary nature. Thus, these provisions may be invoked by those among the temporarily protected who are Convention refugees": W. Kälin, "Temporary Protection in the EC: Refugee Law, Human Rights, and the Temptations of Pragmatism," (2001) 44 *German Yearbook of International Law* 221 (Kälin, "Temporary Protection"), at 221.

[142] "Generally, an alien is considered to be 'lawfully' in a territory if he possesses proper documentation ... has observed the frontier control formalities, and has not overstayed the period for which he has been allowed to stay by operation of law or by virtue of 'landing conditions.' He may also be 'lawfully' in the territory even if he does not fulfil all the said requirements, *provided that the territorial authorities have dispensed with any or all of them* and allowed him to stay in the territory anyway [emphasis added]": Grahl-Madsen, *Status of Refugees II*, at 357.

[143] The critical point is that refugee status determination is merely a declaratory, not a constitutive, process. Convention rights inhere in a person who is in fact a Convention refugee, whether or not any government has recognized that status: UNHCR, *Handbook*, at para. 28.

grant them those Convention rights defined by the first three levels of attachment. This is because while the Convention does not require states formally to determine refugee status,[144] neither does it authorize governments to withhold rights from persons who are in fact refugees because status assessment has not taken place. A general or situation-specific decision by a state party not to verify refugee status therefore amounts to an implied authorization for Convention refugees to seek protection without the necessity of undergoing a formal examination of their claims. In such circumstances, lawful presence is presumptively coextensive with physical presence.

Lawful presence can come to an end in a number of ways. For refugees resident in another state who were authorized to enter on a strictly temporary basis, lawful presence normally concludes with the refugee's departure from the territory. The lawful presence of a sojourning refugee may also be terminated by the issuance of a deportation or other removal order[145] issued under a procedure that meets the requirements of the Refugee Convention, in particular Art. 33. The same is true of a refugee admitted upon arrival into a procedure designed to identify the country which is to examine his or her claim under the terms of a responsibility-sharing agreement: his or her lawful presence in the state conducting the inquiry comes to an end when and if an order is made for removal to a partner state.[146]

In the case of refugees whose presence has been regularized by admission to a refugee status verification procedure, or who have sought protection in the territory of a state that has established no such mechanism, lawful presence terminates only if and when a final determination is made either not to recognize, or to revoke, protection in a particular case. A final decision that an individual does not qualify for refugee status, including a determination made under a fairly administered process to identify manifestly unfounded claims to refugee status,[147] renders an unauthorized entrant's continued presence unlawful, and results in the forfeiture of all Convention rights provisionally guaranteed during the status assessment process.[148] Similarly, a determination that an individual has ceased to be a refugee on the grounds

---

[144] The decision on whether or not to establish such a system is within the discretion of each state party: ibid., at para. 189.

[145] "The expression 'lawfully within their territory' throughout this draft convention would exclude a refugee who, while lawfully admitted, has over-stayed the period for which he was admitted or was authorized to stay or who has violated any other condition attached to his admission or stay": "Report of the Ad Hoc Committee on Statelessness and Related Problems," UN Doc. E/1618, Feb. 17, 1950, at Annex II (Art. 10).

[146] Critically, however, so long as the refugee remains in the territory or otherwise under the jurisdiction of the removing country, the duty of *non-refoulement* (Art. 33) continues to apply.

[147] See text above, at p. 175.   [148] Ibid.

set out in Article 1(C) of the Convention eliminates the legal basis for the former refugee's presence in the state.[149]

3.1.4 Lawful stay

Those refugees who are not simply lawfully in a country's territory, but who are lawfully staying there, benefit from additional rights: freedom of association, the right to engage in wage-earning employment and to practice a profession, access to public housing and welfare, protection of labor and social security legislation, intellectual property rights, and entitlement to travel documentation.[150] There was extraordinary linguistic confusion in deciding how best to label this third level of attachment.[151] The term "lawfully staying" was ultimately incorporated in the Convention as the most accurate rendering of the French language concept of "résidant régulièrement," the meaning of which was agreed to be controlling.[152]

Most fundamentally, "résidence régulière" is not synonymous with such legal notions as domicile or permanent resident status.[153] Instead, the

---

[149] See generally Grahl-Madsen, *Status of Refugees I*, at 367–412; Hathaway, *Refugee Status*, at 189–205; and Goodwin-Gill, *Refugee in International Law*, at 80–87.

[150] Refugee Convention, at Arts. 14 ("artistic and industrial property"), 15 ("right of association"), 17 ("wage-earning employment"), 19 ("liberal professions"), 21 ("housing"), 23 ("public relief"), 24 ("labour legislation and social security"), and 28 ("travel documents"). In specific circumstances, the benefit of Arts. 7(2) ("exemption from reciprocity") and 17(2) (exemption from restrictive measures imposed on aliens in the context of "wage-earning employment") may also be claimed: see chapters 3.2.2 and 6.1.1 below.

[151] "The Chairman emphasized that the Committee was not writing Anglo-American law or French law, but international law in two languages. The trouble was that both the English-speaking and the French-speaking groups were trying to produce drafts which would automatically accord with their respective legal systems and accepted legal terminology": Statement of the Chairman, Mr. Larsen of Denmark, UN Doc. E/AC.32/SR.42, Aug. 24, 1950, at 25.

[152] "The Committee experienced some difficulty with the phrases 'lawfully in the territory' in English and 'résidant régulièrement' in French. It decided however that the latter phrase in French should be rendered in English by 'lawfully staying in the territory'": "Report of the Style Committee," UN Doc. A/CONF.2/102, July 24, 1951.

[153] "He could not accept 'résidant régulièrement' if it was to be translated by 'lawfully resident,' which would not cover persons who were not legally resident in the English sense. It would not, for example, cover persons staying in the United States on a visitor's visa, and perhaps it might not even cover persons who had worked for the United Nations for five years in Geneva. The word 'residence' in English, though not exactly equivalent to 'domicile,' since it was possible to have more than one residence, had much of the same flavour": Statement of Mr. Henkin of the United States, UN Doc. E/AC.32/SR.42, Aug. 24, 1950, at 24. But see the contrary interpretation of the Canadian government implicit in its reservation to the Refugee Convention, available at www.unhcr.ch (accessed Nov. 19, 2004): "Canada interprets the phrase 'lawfully staying' as referring only to refugees admitted for permanent residence; refugees admitted for temporary residence will be

drafters emphasized that it was the refugee's de facto circumstances which determine whether or not the fourth level of attachment is satisfied.[154] The notion of "résidance régulière" is "very wide in meaning ... [and] implie[s] a settling down and, consequently, a certain length of residence."[155] While neither a prolonged stay[156] nor the establishment of habitual residence[157] is required, the refugee's presence in the state party must be ongoing in practical terms.[158] Grahl-Madsen, for example, argues that lawful stay may be implied from an officially tolerated stay beyond the last date that an individual is allowed to remain in a country without securing a residence permit (usually three to six months).[159]

    accorded the same treatment with respect to the matters dealt with in Articles 23 and 24 as is accorded visitors generally."

[154] "[T]here were two alternatives: either to say 'résidant régulièrement' and 'lawfully resident,' or to say 'lawfully' in which case 'résidant' must be omitted, otherwise, there would be too many complications in the translation of the various articles ... [I]t would be better to say 'régulièrement,' since 'légalement' seemed too decidedly legal": Statement of Mr. Juvigny of France, UN Doc. E/AC.32/SR.42, Aug. 24, 1950, at 33–34. In the context of a judgment interpreting the distinct, but related, notion of "habitual residence," the House of Lords insisted upon comparable flexibility and sensitivity to specific facts. "It is a question of fact ... Bringing possessions, doing everything necessary to establish residence before coming, having a right of abode, seeking to bring family, 'durable ties' with the country of residence or intended residence, and many other facts have to be taken into account. The requisite period is not a fixed period. It may be longer where there are doubts. It may be short": *Nessa v. Chief Adjudication Officer*, Times Law Rep, Oct. 27, 1999 (UK HL, Oct. 21, 1999).

[155] Statement of Mr. Juvigny of France, UN Doc. E/AC.32/SR.42, Aug. 24, 1950, at 12.

[156] "[T]he expression 'résidant régulièrement' did not imply a lengthy stay, otherwise the expression 'résidence continue' ... would have been employed": Statement of Mr. Juvigny of France, UN Doc. E/AC.32/SR.41, Aug. 23, 1950, at 17.

[157] "In the articles in question, the term used in the French text had been 'résidence habituelle' which implied some considerable length of residence. As a concession, the French delegation had agreed to substitute the words 'résidance régulière' which were far less restrictive in meaning": Statement of Mr. Juvigny of France, UN Doc. E/AC.32/SR.42, Aug. 24, 1950, at 12.

[158] The French representative suggested that the refugee's presence would have to be "more or less permanent" to satisfy the third level of attachment: Statement of Mr. Juvigny of France, ibid.

[159] "Considering that three months seems to be almost universally accepted as the period for which an alien may remain in a country without needing a residence permit ... it would seem that once a refugee, having filed the requisite application, has remained for more than three months, he should be considered 'lawfully staying,' even though the authority for his continued sojourn merely is a 'provisional receipt' or its equivalent ... This leads us to the more general observation, that a refugee is 'résidant régulièrement' ('lawfully staying') ... if he is in possession of a residence permit (or its equivalent) entitling him to remain there for more than three months, or if he actually is lawfully present in a territory beyond a period of three months after his entry (or after his reporting himself to the authorities, as the case may be)": Grahl-Madsen, *Status of Refugees II*, at 353–354.

Perhaps of greatest contemporary importance, it is clear that refugees in receipt of "temporary protection" who have become de facto settled in the host state[160] are to be considered to be "résidant régulièrement":

> [I]n all those articles the only concrete cases that could arise were cases implying some degree of residence, if only temporary residence; and temporary residence would be covered by the present wording, at least as far as France was concerned ... That was why he also considered, for reasons of principle, that having abandoned the idea of *"résidence habituelle"* and accepted the concept of *"résidence régulière,"* the French delegation had conceded as much as it could.[161]

Indeed, the British representative, in attempting to translate the French concept to English, proposed the phrase "lawfully resident (temporarily or otherwise)."[162] The American representative, however, argued that *any* English language formulation that included the word "resident" would fail accurately to capture the broad meaning conveyed by the French understanding of "résidant." In English, he suggested, the word "resident" would not encompass a temporary stay.[163] It was therefore important to draft an English language text that would not be open to misinterpretation, for example, by denying rights to refugees staying "for a number of months."[164] The result of the Ad Hoc Committee's deliberations was therefore a decision to translate "résidant régulièrement" into English as "lawfully living in their territory."[165]

---

[160] "[T]hese guarantees [can] be invoked by the Convention refugees who are among the temporarily protected persons only after a certain period when it becomes clear that return is not imminent and that the country of refuge has become 'home' for the persons concerned, at least for the time being": Kälin, "Temporary Protection," at 222.

[161] Statement of Mr. Juvigny of France, UN Doc. E/AC.32/SR.42, Aug. 24, 1950, at 15.

[162] Statement of Sir Leslie Brass of the United Kingdom, ibid. at 29.

[163] "[I]n the light of the exposition given by the representative of France there might prove to be a distinction of substance between the English and French texts ... It appeared that 'résidant régulièrement' covered persons temporarily resident, except for a very short period, whereas according to English law he understood the word 'resident' could not apply to a temporary stay": Statement of Mr. Henkin of the United States, ibid. at 14. It was for this reason that the American representative objected to the British proposal, ibid. at 29, which he referred to as "a contradiction in terms": Statement of Mr. Henkin of the United States, ibid. at 29.

[164] "[H]e did not understand the exact connotation of the French word 'résidant,' but apparently it could be applied to persons who did not make their home in a certain place but stayed there for a number of months. Such persons would apparently be 'résidant régulièrement' but they would not, in the United States of America at least, be lawfully resident. To be lawfully resident in a place, a man must make his home there; it need not be his only home but it must be a substantial home": Statement of Mr. Henkin of the United States, ibid. at 26.

[165] "The English text referred to refugees 'lawfully in the territory' while the French referred to a refugee 'régulièrement résidant,' the literal English equivalent of the latter phrase

The Conference of Plenipotentiaries maintained the French language formulation of the fourth level of attachment as "résidant régulièrement," but
reframed it in English as "lawfully staying in their territory."[166] This minor
terminological shift brought the English language phrasing even more closely
into line with the broadly inclusive meaning of "résidant régulièrement." In
any event, the Conference resolved any linguistic ambiguity once and for all
by explicitly agreeing that the French concept of "résidant régulièrement" is
to be regarded as the authoritative definition of the fourth level of
attachment.[167]

The fourth level of attachment set by the Refugee Convention is therefore
characterized by officially sanctioned, ongoing presence in a state party,
whether or not there has been a formal declaration of refugee status, grant
of the right of permanent residence, or establishment of domicile there.[168]
This understanding is consistent with the basic structure of the Refugee
Convention, which does not require states formally to adjudicate status or
assign any particular immigration status to refugees,[169] and which is content

havingamorerestrictiveapplication.Re-examiningtheindividualarticles,itwasdecided
in most instances that the provision in question should apply to all refugees whose
presence in the territory was lawful ... In one case [the right to engage in wage-earning
employment] the Committee agreed that the provision should apply only to a refugee
'régulièrement résidant' on the territory of a Contracting State. The English text adopted
is intended to approximate as closely as possible the scope of the French term": "Report of
the Ad Hoc Committee on Refugees and Stateless Persons, Second Session," UN Doc. E/
1850, Aug. 25, 1950 (Ad Hoc Committee, "Second Session Report"), at 12.

[166] At the Conference of Plenipotentiaries, the decision was reached to reserve a number of
rights allocated by the Ad Hoc Committee to refugees who were simply lawfully present
(public assistance, social security, housing, freedom of association, and access to liberal
professions) for refugees who were lawfully staying in the state party. This agreement to
transfer these rights to persons able to satisfy the higher level of attachment seems to have
been facilitated by the agreement to adopt a generous understanding of "résidant
régulièrement" not tied to formal legal categories. The final attribution of rights between
the second and third levels of attachment was apparently agreed to in the Style
Committee of the Conference of Plenipotentiaries: "Report of the Style Committee,"
UN Doc. A/CONF.2/102, July 24, 1951.

[167] Ibid. at para. 5. See also Grahl-Madsen, *Status of Refugees II*, at 351–352: "Against this
background it seems justified to give precedence to the French term and not to ponder
too much over the difference between the expressions 'lawfully staying' and 'lawfully
resident' ... Both expressions apparently mean the same thing."

[168] As a practical matter, "evidence of permanent, indefinite, unrestricted or other residence
status, recognition as a refugee, issue of a travel document, [or] grant of a re-entry visa
will raise a strong presumption that the refugee should be considered as lawfully staying
in the territory of a Contracting State. It would then fall to that State to rebut the
presumption by showing, for example, that the refugee was admitted for a limited time
and purpose, or that he or she is in fact the responsibility of another State": Goodwin-
Gill, *Refugee in International Law*, at 309.

[169] See chapter 3.1.3 above, at pp. 180–181.

to encourage, rather than to require, access to naturalization or other forms of permanent status.[170]

3.1.5 Durable residence

Only a few rights are reserved for refugees who are habitually resident in an asylum state: in addition to rights defined by the first four levels of attachment, such refugees are entitled to benefit from legal aid systems, and to receive national treatment in regard to the posting of security for costs in a court proceeding.[171] After a period of three years' residence, refugees are also to be exempted from both requirements of legislative reciprocity,[172] and any restrictive measures imposed on the employment of aliens.[173] As can be seen from the short list of rights subject to the fifth level of attachment, there was little enthusiasm among the drafters for the conditioning of access to refugee rights on the satisfaction of a durable residence requirement.

> **Refugee Convention, Art. 10   Continuity of residence**
> 1. Where a refugee has been forcibly displaced during the Second World War and removed to the territory of a Contracting State, and is resident there, the period of such enforced sojourn shall be considered to have been lawful residence within that territory.
> 2. Where a refugee has been forcibly displaced during the Second World War from the territory of a Contracting State and has, prior to the date of entry into force of this Convention, returned there for the purpose of taking up residence, the period of residence before and after such enforced displacement shall be regarded as one uninterrupted period for any purposes for which uninterrupted residence is required.

In deciding whether or not a refugee meets a particular residence requirement, "[t]he point at issue [is] ... continuous residence, not legal residence."[174] Thus, the drafters made specific provision to accommodate the predicament of persons forcibly deported during the Second World War. Those refugees who elected to remain in the territory of the state to which they had been deported would be considered to have been resident in that country during the period of enforced presence.[175] Even though the state to

---

[170] Refugee Convention, at Art. 34.   [171] Ibid. at Art. 16(2).   [172] Ibid. at Art. 7(2).

[173] An earlier exemption from alien employment restrictions is required in the case of a refugee who was already exempt from such requirements at the time the Convention entered into force for the state party; or where the refugee is married to, or the parent of, a national of the state party: ibid. at Art. 17(2).

[174] Statement of Mr. Cuvelier of Belgium, UN Doc. E/AC.32/SR.22, Feb. 2, 1950, at 5. See also Statement of Mr. Weis of the IRO, ibid.

[175] Refugee Convention, at Art. 10(1).

which deportation had been effected may not have legally consented to their entry, the focus on de facto residence led to an agreement that "the country to which a person had been deported would accept the period spent there as a period of regular residence."[176]

Recognizing that other refugees would prefer to have the time spent in enforced sojourn abroad credited toward the calculation of their period of residence in the state from which they had been removed, the drafters agreed that a victim of deportation[177] could elect to be treated as continually resident in the country from which the deportation was effected.[178] Even though such a refugee had not actually been resident in the contracting state during the time he or she was subject to deportation, "[t]he authors of the Convention sought to mitigate the results of interruption of residence not due to the free will of the refugee, and to provide a remedy for a stay without *animus* and without permission, which are usually required to transform one's 'being' in a certain place into 'residence.'"[179]

The resultant Art. 10 of the Convention is today only of hortatory value,[180] as it governs the treatment only of Second World War deportees.[181] Nonetheless, the debates on Art. 10 make two points of continuing relevance. First, the calculation of a period of residence is not a matter simply of ascertaining how long a refugee has resided outside his or her own country, but rather how much time the refugee has spent in the particular state party in which fourth level of attachment rights are to be invoked. Periods of residence in an intermediate country are not to be credited to the satisfaction of a

[176] Statement of the Chairman, Mr. Chance of Canada, UN Doc. E/AC.32/SR.22, Feb. 2, 1950, at 7.

[177] "It presumably was not intended to refer to persons displaced by the Government of the country on account of their suspicious or criminal activities, but only to persons forcibly displaced by enemy or occupying authorities": Statement of Mr. Perez Perozo of Venezuela, UN Doc. E/AC.32/SR.35, Aug. 15, 1950, at 12.

[178] Refugee Convention, at Art. 10(2).   [179] Robinson, *History*, at 96.

[180] The restrictive language was adopted notwithstanding a plea to extend the benefit of Art. 10 to all refugees. "[I]t was an important matter . . . to be credited, as constituting residence, with the time spent . . . in enforced displacement, or with the period before or after such displacement, in cases where the refugee had returned to his receiving country to re-establish his residence there. The latter provision was all the more useful in view of the fact that, under certain national legislation, the period of residence normally had to be extended if residence was interrupted. Nevertheless, the provisions of article [10(2)] merely remedied an occasional situation caused by the second world war, without providing any [general] solution": Statement of Mr. Rollin of the Inter-Parliamentary Union, UN Doc. A/CONF.2/SR.10, July 6, 1951, at 7.

[181] The article was arguably obsolete even at the time the Refugee Convention came into force, as nearly a decade had elapsed since the end of the Second World War and few, if any, rights were conditioned on continuous residence of more than five years.

durable residence requirement.[182] The calculation of a period of residence should, however, be carried out with due regard to the particular disabilities faced by refugees.[183] In keeping with the spirit of Art. 10 of the Convention, this may include either a period of enforced presence in the state party, or the time during which continuous residence was interrupted by forces beyond the refugee's control.

In sum, the general language of the five levels of attachment facilitates application of the Refugee Convention across the full range of states, despite their often widely divergent approaches to the legal reception of refugees. It moreover allows governments a reasonable measure of flexibility in deciding for themselves how best to operationalize refugee law within their jurisdictions.

Yet because access to rights is defined by practical circumstances rather than by any official decision or status, the Refugee Convention prevents states from invoking their own legalistic categories as the grounds for withholding rights from refugees. Some rights apply simply once a state has jurisdiction over a refugee; others by virtue of physical presence in a state's territory, even if illegal; a third set when that presence is either officially sanctioned or tolerated; further rights accrue once the refugee has established more than a transient or interim presence in the asylum state; and even the most demanding level of attachment requires only a period of de facto continuous and legally sanctioned residence. In no case may refugee rights be legally denied or withheld simply because of the delay or failure of a state party to process a claim, assign a status, or issue a confirmation of entitlement.

3.2 The general standard of treatment

Once the rights to which a particular refugee are entitled have been identified on the basis of the level of attachment test outlined above, the next step is to define the required standard of compliance. Many rights in the Convention are expressly defined to require implementation on the basis of either a contingent or an absolute standard of achievement. These are referred to here as "exceptional standards of treatment," the interpretation of which is addressed below.[184] Absent express provision of this kind, however, refugees are to be treated at least as well as "aliens generally."

---

[182] It was agreed that the time spent in the state of deportation could not be credited toward the satisfaction of a durable residence requirement in a third state, since the deportation had not resulted in any kind of attachment to the third state. "[T]he principle of the transfer from one State to another of acquired rights with respect to residence should be rejected": Statement of the Chairman, Mr. Chance of Canada, UN Doc. E/AC.32/SR.22, Feb. 2, 1950, at 8.

[183] See chapter 3.2.3 below, at p. 208.   [184] See chapter 3.3 below.

Under traditional norms of international aliens law, the assimilation of refugees to "aliens generally" would provide little assurance of meaningful protection.[185] This is because the primary responsibility to protect the interests of aliens lies with their state of nationality, which is expected to engage in diplomatic intervention to secure respect for the human rights of its citizens abroad. Because refugees are by definition persons whose country of nationality either cannot or will not protect them, traditional aliens law could be expected to provide them with few benefits.[186] For this reason, an essential aspect of international refugee protection has always been to provide surrogate international protection under the auspices of an international agency – presently UNHCR – which is to undertake the equivalent of diplomatic intervention on behalf of refugees.[187]

More fundamentally, the very existence of relevant rights for aliens can also depend on the efforts of the refugee's state of nationality.[188] Absent consideration of the Refugee Convention and other treaties, each state determines for itself whether any rights will be granted to non-citizens beyond the limited range of rights guaranteed to all aliens under general principles of law.[189] Some countries have routinely granted aliens most of the rights extended to their own citizens.[190] A second group of states applies a

---

[185] See chapter 2.1 above, at pp. 78–79.   [186] See generally chapters 2.1 and 2.5.6 above.

[187] See chapter 2.3 above, at p. 85; and Epilogue below, at pp. 992–993.

[188] "At the root of the idea of the juridical status of foreigners is the idea of reciprocity. The law considers a foreigner as a being in normal circumstances, that is to say, a foreigner in possession of a nationality. The requirement of reciprocity of treatment places the national of a foreign country in the same position as that in which his own country places foreigners": United Nations, "Memorandum by the Secretary-General to the Ad Hoc Committee on Statelessness and Related Problems," UN Doc. E/AC.32/2, Jan. 3, 1950 (Secretary-General, "Memorandum"), at 28. "Reciprocity refers to the interdependence of obligations assumed by participants within the legal schemes created by human rights law . . . In other words, obligations are reciprocal if their creation, execution and termination depend on the imposition of connected obligations on others. International law, being a system based on the formal equality and sovereignty of States, has arisen largely out of the exchange of reciprocal rights and duties between States": R. Provost, "Reciprocity in Human Rights and Humanitarian Law," (1994) 65 *British Yearbook of International Law* 383 (Provost, "Reciprocity"), at 383.

[189] See chapter 2.1 above, at pp. 76–77.

[190] The definition of recognized approaches to reciprocity is not without confusion. Borchard, for example, identifies only two systems, namely diplomatic and legislative reciprocity: E. Borchard, *The Diplomatic Protection of Citizens Abroad* (1915) (Borchard, *Diplomatic Protection*), at 71–72. In contrast, the document prepared by the United Nations Department of Social Affairs, "A Study of Statelessness," UN Doc. E/1112, Feb. 1, 1949 (United Nations, "Statelessness"), at 17–18, which served as the basis for drafting of the Refugee Convention, argues that there are two approaches to reciprocity, namely diplomatic and de facto. While de facto reciprocity as defined by the UN Study and legislative reciprocity as defined by Borchard are comparable in that the referent for duties owed to aliens is a domestic, rather than an international standard, it is clear that a

presumption in favor of the equivalent treatment of aliens and nationals, but reserves the right to withdraw particular rights from those refugees and other aliens whose national state fails to extend comparable protections to foreign citizens, whether by its domestic laws (legislative reciprocity) or practices (de facto reciprocity). A third approach denies the logic of routine assimilation of aliens to nationals for the purpose of rights allocation. In states that rely on the theory of diplomatic reciprocity, a fundamental distinction is made between privileged aliens, who are automatically treated largely on par with nationals, and other aliens. Foreigners within the residual category receive rights beyond those required by the general principles of law only if their state of citizenship agrees by treaty to guarantee analogous rights to foreigners under its jurisdiction.[191]

There is, of course, no reason to expect the states from which refugees flee to agree to reciprocity as a means of assisting their citizens who seek refuge abroad. Before the advent of refugee law, the severing of the bond between refugees and their state of citizenship often left refugees with no more than bare minimum rights in those states that grounded their treatment of foreigners in the existence of reciprocity. This dilemma led the League of Nations to stress the humanitarian tragedy that would ensue if refugees were subjected to the usual rules. The League also urged that there was no practical purpose served by the application of rules of reciprocity to refugees:

> [R]efusal to accord national treatment to foreigners in the absence of reciprocity is merely an act of mild retaliation. The object [of reciprocity] is to reach, through the person of the nationals concerned, those countries which decline to adopt an equally liberal regime ... But what country or which Government can be reached through the person of a refugee? Can the refugee be held responsible for the legislation of his country of origin? Clearly, the rule of reciprocity, if applied to refugees, is pointless and therefore unjust. The injury caused to refugees by the application of this rule is substantial since the rule constantly recurs in texts governing the status of foreigners. Since the condition of reciprocity cannot be satisfied, refugees are denied the enjoyment of a whole series of rights which are accorded in principle to all foreigners.[192]

---

number of the Refugee Convention's drafters insisted upon the relevance of the dichotomy between reciprocity systems based on domestic legislation, as contrasted with those based on domestic practice, in the partner state. See in particular comments of Mr. Perez Perozo of Venezuela, UN Doc. E/AC.32/SR.11, Jan. 25, 1950, at 3; and the exchange between the representatives of the Netherlands and Belgium at the Conference of Plenipotentiaries, UN Doc. A/CONF.2/SR.24, July 17, 1951, at 22.

[191] See generally Borchard, *Diplomatic Protection*, at 71–73.

[192] Secretary-General, "Memorandum," at 29, citing statement of the French government when submitting the 1933 Refugee Convention for legislative approval.

The predecessor 1933 Refugee Convention therefore exempted refugees from all requirements of reciprocity,[193] meaning that the baseline standard of treatment for refugees included all rights that might ordinarily have been secured by interstate negotiation. This clause had no impact on the first category of states which did not condition the treatment of refugees on reciprocity in any event. Importantly, its implications for states of the third category (those which relied on diplomatic reciprocity) were also relatively modest. Because diplomatic reciprocity does not work from an underlying presumption that aliens should receive full rights, exemption from reciprocity in diplomatic reciprocity states brought refugees only within the ranks of the residual category of foreigners. In diplomatic reciprocity states, many critical rights were simply not "on offer" to other than partner countries. Exemption from reciprocity therefore merely required diplomatic reciprocity states to assimilate refugees to second-tier resident aliens, not to enfranchise them within the ranks of preferred aliens.

The ramifications of exemption from reciprocity had, however, been significant for countries of the second category, which conditioned alien rights on legislative or de facto reciprocity. In these states, exemption from reciprocity revived the presumption that aliens should be assimilated to nationals, thereby effectively guaranteeing national treatment for refugees. In contrast to states that relied on diplomatic reciprocity, countries that embraced legislative or de facto reciprocity "usually grant[ed] foreigners the same rights as their subjects, reserving however the power to apply retorsion to the nationals of countries where aliens generally or their subjects alone [were] handicapped by the particular disability in question."[194]

This historical background is important for understanding the approach taken in the current Refugee Convention. It was initially proposed that, as under the 1933 Convention, refugees protected by the 1951 Convention should simply be assimilated to the citizens of states with which the asylum country had reciprocity arrangements.[195] While some states supported this position, including Denmark[196] and the United

---

[193] "The enjoyment of certain rights and the benefit of certain favours accorded to foreigners subject to reciprocity shall not be refused to refugees in the absence of reciprocity": Convention relating to the International Status of Refugees, 159 LNTS 3663, done Oct. 28, 1933, entered into force June 13, 1935 (1933 Refugee Convention), at Art. 14.

[194] Borchard, *Diplomatic Protection*, at 72.

[195] "The enjoyment of the rights and favours accorded to foreigners subject to reciprocity shall not be refused to refugees (and stateless persons) in the absence of reciprocity": Secretary-General, "Memorandum," at 28.

[196] "Denmark used reciprocity simply as a means to ensure that Danes in foreign countries received the privileges that were granted to nationals of those countries in Denmark. In such cases he felt that refugees should be granted the same privileges although there could

States,[197] France pointed to the fact that only three of the eight state parties to the 1933 Convention had actually accepted the duty to exempt refugees from reciprocity.[198] Arguing the importance of pragmatism, it tabled an alternative formulation premised on the denial to refugees of all rights conditioned on diplomatic reciprocity, and stipulating that rights conditioned on legislative or de facto reciprocity would accrue to refugees only after the passage of a number of years in the asylum country.[199] States that relied on legislative or de facto reciprocity would thereby find themselves on a similar footing with countries that embraced diplomatic reciprocity.[200]

3.2.1 Assimilation to aliens

Refugee Convention, Art. 7(1)
Except where this Convention contains more favourable provisions, a Contracting State shall accord to refugees the same treatment as is accorded to aliens generally.

The drafters conceived the general standard of treatment in Art. 7(1) in fairly broad terms. While it is clearly less comprehensive than the complete exemption from reciprocity endorsed in the 1933 Refugee Convention, the purpose

be no question of reciprocity": Statement of Mr. Larsen of Denmark, UN Doc. E/AC.32/SR.36, Aug. 15, 1950, at 18–19.

[197] "[I]n the United States of America as in the United Kingdom, problems of reciprocity did not arise but . . . he, too, had no objection to the inclusion of the article for the sake of countries differently situated . . . The main object was to ensure that aliens should not be penalised because they had no nationality and that where privileges were generally enjoyed by aliens, through treaties or in any other way, refugees should have the same privileges": Statement of Mr. Henkin of the United States, UN Doc. E/AC.32/SR.34, Aug. 14, 1950, at 15–16.

[198] Only Bulgaria, France, and Italy did not enter a reservation or qualification to Art. 14 of the 1933 Convention: United Nations, "Statelessness," at 93–97. It is noteworthy that Bulgaria and Italy routinely assimilated aliens to foreigners in any event, and France relied on diplomatic reciprocity (thereby allowing it to reserve a category of privileged aliens, exemption from reciprocity notwithstanding). The article was not in force for any legislative or de facto reciprocity state where it would clearly have had the greatest impact.

[199] "The enjoyment of certain rights and the benefit of certain privileges accorded to aliens subject to reciprocity shall not be refused to refugees in the absence of reciprocity in the case of those enjoying them at the date of signature of the present Convention. As regards other refugees, the High Contracting Parties undertake to give them the benefit of these provisions upon completion of [a certain period of] residence": France, "Proposal for a Draft Convention," UN Doc. E/AC.32/L.3, Jan. 17, 1950 (France, "Draft Convention"), at 4.

[200] Only refugees who enjoyed exemption from reciprocity under the 1933 Convention or another pre-1951 instrument are entitled immediately to be assimilated to the ranks of privileged foreigners: Refugee Convention, at Art. 7(3). See chapter 3.2.2 below, at p. 203.

of Art. 7(1) is to ensure that refugees receive the benefit of all laws and policies which normally apply to aliens.

The primary value of Art. 7(1) is to incorporate by reference all general sources of rights for non-citizens. Urged by the American delegate to ensure that the general standard "should cover all rights to be granted to refugees and not only those which were actually specified in the draft convention,"[201] the report of the First Session of the Ad Hoc Committee succinctly notes that "[t]he exemption from reciprocity relates not only to rights and benefits specifically covered by the draft convention, but also to such rights and benefits not explicitly mentioned in the draft Convention."[202] Even as the attitude of states towards the timing and scope of exemption from reciprocity hardened over the course of the drafting process, there was no weakening of this basic commitment to comprehensive application of the general standard of treatment.[203] Simply put, refugees cannot be excluded from any rights which the asylum state ordinarily grants to other foreigners. Thus, the general standard of Art. 7(1) ensures that refugees may claim the narrow range of rights set by international aliens law,[204] as well as the benefit of any international legal obligations (for example, those set by the Human Rights Covenants[205]) which govern the treatment of aliens in general.

The "aliens generally" standard was also a useful means by which to meet the concerns of diplomatic reciprocity states. France and Belgium were particularly adamant that the Refugee Convention should not compel them to treat refugees on par with the citizens of special partner states.[206] The adoption of the "aliens generally" baseline standard was intended to avoid any assertion that the general duty includes the obligation to grant refugees special rights reserved for preferred aliens, for example the citizens of countries affiliated in an economic or political union.[207] Because exceptional

---

[201] Statement of Mr. Henkin of the United States, UN Doc. E/AC.32/SR.23, Feb. 3, 1950, at 4.

[202] "Report of the Ad Hoc Committee on Statelessness and Related Problems," UN Doc. E/1618, Feb. 17, 1950 (Ad Hoc Committee, "First Session Report"), at Annex II.

[203] See Refugee Convention, at Art. 7(5): "The provisions of paragraphs 2 and 3 apply both to the rights and benefits referred to in articles 13, 18, 19, 21, and 22 of this Convention *and to rights and benefits for which this Convention does not provide* [emphasis added]."

[204] See chapter 2.1 above, at pp. 76–77. [205] See chapter 2.5.4 above.

[206] "[C]ountries such as Belgium, which were linked to certain other countries by special economic and customs agreements, did not accord the same treatment to all foreigners. Belgium, for example, placed nationals of the Benelux countries for certain periods on a quasi-equal footing with Belgian citizens": Statement of Mr. Cuvelier of Belgium, UN Doc. E/AC.32/SR.10, Jan. 24, 1950, at 5. See chapter 3.2 above, at p. 195.

[207] Mr. Cuvelier subsequently repeated "that refugees could not benefit from reciprocal treatment in cases where the right or privilege in question was granted solely as a result of an international agreement between two countries": Statement of Mr. Cuvelier of Belgium, UN Doc. E/AC.32/SR.23, Feb. 3, 1950, at 4. The Israeli delegate thereupon

rights of this kind do not ordinarily inhere in "aliens generally,"[208] the new general standard allows them to be withheld from refugees.[209]

Yet even as the drafters recognized the importance of enabling states to maintain special relationships by means of diplomatic reciprocity, there was a determination to limit the exclusion of refugees to situations in which the attribution of particular rights to non-citizens was truly part of a special regime. Thus, all but one of the substantive Convention rights that require implementation only at the baseline "aliens generally" standard[210] – rights to property, self-employment, professional practice, housing, and secondary

suggested, and the Committee agreed, that "that interpretation should be placed on the record": Statement of Mr. Robinson of Israel, ibid. As helpfully clarified by the British delegate, refugees cannot automatically claim the benefit of "a special treaty between two countries": Statement of Sir Leslie Brass of the United Kingdom, ibid.

[208] See e.g. Statement of Mr. Cuvelier of Belgium, UN Doc. E/AC.32/SR.10, Jan. 24, 1950, at 5; Statement of Mr. Larsen of Denmark, ibid.; and Statement of the International Refugee Organization, in United Nations, "Compilation of the Comments of Governments and Specialized Agencies on the Report of the Ad Hoc Committee on Statelessness and Related Problems," UN Doc. E/AC.32/L.40, Aug. 10, 1950 (United Nations, "Compilation of Comments"), at 34–35: "The main reason why the Ad Hoc Committee decided to change the wording of the Articles relating to reciprocity . . . was that it did not wish the Article to relate to treaty provisions conferring preferential treatment on aliens of a particular nationality. It is certain that since 1933 there has been a general development in the granting of preferential treatment to aliens of a particular nationality on the basis of customs, political and economic associations founded on geographical or historical connections. It may be held that some qualification should be made to the original formula concerning reciprocity, as included in the Conventions of 1933 and 1938, in order to overcome any misinterpretation which may lead to the belief that an article concerning the exemption from reciprocity might have as a consequence the legal entitlement for refugees to the benefits of preferential treatment."

[209] Special guarantees of reciprocal treatment, such as those negotiated by partner states in an economic or customs union, do not automatically accrue to refugees. The benefits of such forms of diplomatic reciprocity are normally extended to refugees only where the Refugee Convention stipulates that refugees are to be treated either as "most-favored foreigners," or on par with the nationals of the asylum state. "[A] distinction should be drawn between the clause relating to exemption from reciprocity and the provisions of some articles which specified whether refugees should be accorded the most favorable treatment or be subject to the ordinary law. Where such provisions were set forth in an article there was no need to invoke the clause on exemption from reciprocity. It was obvious, in fact, that where refugees were accorded the most favorable treatment there would be no point in invoking the clause respecting exemption from reciprocity . . . The paragraph on exemption from reciprocity would apply only where articles failed to define the treatment accorded to refugees": Statement of Mr. Giraud of the Secretariat, UN Doc. E/AC.32/SR.11, Jan. 25, 1950, at 6. See generally chapter 3.3.1 below.

[210] The exception is the right to freedom of movement set by Art. 26, which requires only that refugees be allowed to "choose their place of residence and to move freely within [the state party's] territory, subject to any regulations applicable to aliens generally in the same circumstances": Refugee Convention, at Art. 26. While there is no textual requirement to grant refugees internal mobility rights on terms "as favorable as possible," whatever

and higher education – are actually phrased to require "treatment as favourable as possible and, in any event, not less favourable than that accorded to aliens generally."[211] As the Belgian delegate insisted, this form of words requires more than simply adherence to the principle of non-discrimination.[212]

First and most specifically, the phrase was agreed to circumscribe the ability of governments to refuse refugees the benefits of rights only formally subject to diplomatic reciprocity. The Report of the First Session of the Ad Hoc Committee explains this precise choice of language:

> The formula used in [Art. 13, on movable and immovable property] and in several others – i.e., "treatment as favorable as possible and, in any event, not less favorable than that accorded to aliens generally in the same circumstances" – is intended to assure that refugees will, *regardless of reciprocity*, be treated at least as well as other aliens and to encourage countries to give them better treatment where this is possible [emphasis added].[213]

As such, while it was understood that refugees would not benefit from special rights genuinely associated with unique bilateral or similar arrangements,[214] it was agreed that there is no good reason to deny refugees rights that are in fact available to most non-citizens. This was in keeping with the reason given by governments for refusal immediately to exempt refugees from all reciprocity requirements. Their concern was the importance of not undermining their special political and economic relationships; there is no such risk once the rights in question are no longer reserved for only the citizens of select partner states, but are in fact extended to the nationals of most foreign

---

constraints are to be imposed on freedom of movement must derive from "regulations," not simply from the exercise of bureaucratic or other discretion or directive.

[211] Refugee Convention, at Arts. 13, 18, 19, 21, and 22.

[212] The matter arose in the context of a French criticism that an American proposal to grant refugees "the most favorable treatment possible and, in any event, not less favorable than that given to foreigners generally as regards housing accommodations" was unnecessary in view of the duty of non-discrimination. In response, the Belgian delegate "pointed out that the United States text was not redundant, inasmuch as it required the High Contracting Parties not merely not to discriminate against refugees, but to ensure them 'the most favorable treatment possible'": Statement of Mr. Cuvelier of Belgium, UN Doc. E/AC.32/SR.24, Feb. 3, 1950, at 13.

[213] Ad Hoc Committee, "First Session Report," at Annex II.

[214] "This article [on exemption from reciprocity] is intended to meet the situation in various countries where certain rights are accorded to aliens subject to reciprocity. In such cases there is no objection on the part of the State to aliens enjoying these rights, and the purpose of conferring them subject to reciprocity is merely to obtain similar rights for its nationals in foreign countries. The Article will confer these rights on refugees; they would otherwise be prevented from having them in view of their lack of nationality. The Article is not intended to relate to rights specifically conferred by bilateral treaty and which are not intended to be enjoyed by aliens generally": "Comments of the Committee on the Draft Convention," UN Doc. E/AC.32/L.32/Add.1, Feb. 10, 1950, at 2–3.

states.[215] Thus, where there is truly generality of access to a given set of rights – as evinced by, for example, relevant domestic laws or practices, a pervasive pattern of bilateral or multilateral agreements, or de facto enjoyment of the right by most aliens – the right in question automatically accrues to refugees as well.

Second and more generally, the duty to grant refugees "treatment as favorable as possible" requires a state party to give consideration in good faith to the non-application to refugees of limits generally applied to aliens. It was proposed in order to ensure that "refugees would be granted not the most favorable treatment, but a treatment more favorable than that given to foreigners generally."[216] The spirit of this responsibility is nicely captured by the comments of the British government that it would be prepared to "consider sympathetically the possibility of relaxing the conditions upon which refugees have been admitted."[217]

3.2.2 Exemption from reciprocity

Refugee Convention, Art. 7   Exemption from reciprocity

. . .

2. After a period of three years' residence, all refugees shall enjoy exemption from legislative reciprocity in the territory of the Contracting States.

---

[215] "If the French Government and a small State concluded a treaty providing for certain rights to be granted to Frenchmen, and the same rights to be granted to nationals of that State in France, was the advantage granted to the citizens of a single country to be accorded by France to all refugees? As he interpreted it, article [7] did not mean that it was necessary to accord that treatment to all refugees. He had observed from the summary records of the Committee that the United Kingdom representative had accepted that article because it contained the word 'generally.' But where did the general treatment of aliens begin? Was it when there was reciprocal treatment with one or two other States or when there was such treatment with a very large number of other States? . . . France was prepared to give refugees the treatment given to aliens generally, but did not intend to give better treatment to refugees than that given to the majority of aliens": Statement of Mr. Juvigny of France, UN Doc. E/AC.32/SR.34, Aug. 14, 1950, at 11–12. See also Statement of Mr. Henkin of the United States, ibid. at 16: "It was also necessary to cover cases where reciprocity treaties existed with many countries and were hence equivalent to legislative reciprocity. The representative of France had raised the question of how many such treaties must exist, whether 5 or 50. He could not himself suggest a draft but the Drafting Committee would have to, so long as it was clear what was desired." Notwithstanding this assurance, the quantitative issue was resolved neither by the Drafting Committee, nor by any subsequent body that participated in the preparation of the Refugee Convention.

[216] Statement of Mr. Henkin of the United States, UN Doc. E/AC.32/SR.13, Jan. 26, 1950, at 14. Under this intermediate standard, a government should at least consider providing preferential treatment for refugees. See also Statement of Mr. Kural of Turkey, ibid. at 15.

[217] United Nations, "Compilation of Comments," at 40.

> 3. Each Contracting State shall continue to accord to refugees the rights and benefits to which they were already entitled, in the absence of reciprocity, at the date of entry into force of this Convention for that State.
>
> 4. The Contracting States shall consider favourably the possibility of according to refugees, in the absence of reciprocity, rights and benefits beyond those to which they are entitled according to paragraphs 2 and 3, and to extending exemption from reciprocity to refugees who do not fulfil the conditions provided for in paragraphs 2 and 3.
>
> 5. The provisions of paragraphs 2 and 3 apply both to the rights and benefits referred to in articles 13, 18, 19, 21 and 22 of this Convention and to rights and benefits for which this Convention does not provide.

The general standard of treatment under the Refugee Convention is, for reasons described above, premised on the continued existence of preferred aliens regimes in states that rely on diplomatic reciprocity. In such states, refugees may not insist that they be afforded rights reserved by treaty for the citizens of countries with which the asylum state has a special relationship.[218] In an effort to avoid the imposition of radically different obligations on state parties that embrace distinct understandings of reciprocity, a decision was taken to delay the assimilation of refugees to citizens in states that rely on either of the two remaining forms of reciprocity, legislative and de facto reciprocity.[219]

The need for a special approach to legislative and de facto reciprocity states arises from the quite different impact of a "general standards" baseline duty of protection in such countries. Because states that rely on legislative and de facto reciprocity acknowledge an underlying *presumption* in favor of the assimilation of aliens to citizens,[220] implementation of the "general standards" requirement would effectively have required the immediate assimilation of all refugees to citizens. Because Art. 7(1) requires that refugees receive the benefit of rights routinely granted to non-preferred foreigners on the basis of reciprocity,[221] all rights "on offer" under a legislative or de facto reciprocity system would presumptively accrue to them. Application of this

---

[218] See chapter 3.2.1 above, at pp. 197–198.

[219] While the text of the articles speaks only to "legislative reciprocity," it is clear from the drafting history that this term was used in contradistinction to "diplomatic reciprocity." As observed by its Belgian co-sponsor, the term "legislative reciprocity" "was emphatically not designed to exclude *de facto* reciprocity": Statement of Mr. Herment of Belgium, UN Doc. A/CONF.2/SR.24, July 17, 1951, at 22. There is a logical basis for this assertion, grounded in differing ways of categorizing approaches to reciprocity. See chapter 3.2 above, at pp. 193–194, n. 190.

[220] See chapter 3.2 above, at pp. 193–194.   [221] Ibid.

general standard of treatment would therefore have imposed a significantly more onerous obligation on states that rely on legislative or de facto reciprocity.

This result was attenuated by delaying the time at which refugees are granted the benefit of rights ordinarily subject to legislative or de facto reciprocity.[222] The Ad Hoc Committee's recommendation that "a legal obligation in this sense would be acceptable only in regard to refugees who had resided in the country for a given period"[223] led to the decision to defer exemption from legislative reciprocity until a refugee has resided in an asylum state for three years.[224]

The net result is that the general standard of treatment under the modern Refugee Convention endorses a significant, though not complete, retrenchment from the requirement of the 1933 Refugee Convention that refugees should be exempted from all reciprocity requirements. By virtue of Art. 7(1)'s limited duty to accord to refugees all rights that inhere in "aliens generally," refugees may legitimately be refused any diplomatic reciprocity rights which accrue only to preferred nationals, such as those of partner states in an economic or political union. In reliance on Art. 7(2), states may also withhold for up to three years any rights that are reserved for the nationals of states which have met the requirements of legislative or de facto reciprocity. It is only when Convention rights formally subject to reciprocity are in fact generally enjoyed by aliens that refugees too may claim these rights by virtue of the phrasing of the specific articles of the Convention which require implementation only at the baseline level.[225] Because refugees are never to be treated less well than the average foreigner, the prerogative of asylum states

---

[222] Austria was one of the few states present that relied primarily on legislative reciprocity. Because it was a country of first asylum for large numbers of refugees who would ultimately be granted resettlement elsewhere, the three-year delay in according exemption from reciprocity effectively met its most pressing concerns. See Comments of the Government of Austria, in United Nations, "Compilation of Comments," at 5, 32: "Considering the great number of refugees, however, who are in the country and are still coming, Austria cannot be expected to grant a permanent refuge to all who are now on Austrian territory. The Federal Government of Austria rather expects States which are much larger and economically much stronger to adopt the same generous attitude towards immigration and naturalization of refugees as that shown by Austria ... Rights which can be granted generally to a small number of aliens on the basis of reciprocity could not be extended, especially in matters of welfare and labor, to the several hundreds of thousands of refugees in Austria."

[223] Ad Hoc Committee, "Second Session Report," at 12.

[224] The determination of when the requirement of "three years' residence" has been satisfied should be made in accordance with the spirit of Art. 10 ("continuity of residence"). See chapter 3.1.5 above, at pp. 191–192.

[225] See chapter 3.2.1 above, at pp. 199–200.

to withhold rights on the basis of any form of reciprocity comes to an end once the rights in question are enjoyed by most aliens.[226]

Some drafters clearly recognized the inappropriateness of subjecting refugees to the harshness of reciprocity.[227] While unable to overcome the protectionist views of the majority of states, they nonetheless secured an amendment that shields many pre-1951 refugees from any attempt to reduce rights based on reciprocity principles.[228] Of greater contemporary relevance, Art. 7 was also amended to oblige states to give consideration to the waiver of legislative and de facto reciprocity requirements before the elapse of the three-year residency requirement.[229] As Robinson[230] and Weis[231] affirm, Art. 7(4) is not merely hortatory, but requires governments to give real

---

[226] See Statement of Sir Leslie Brass of the United Kingdom, UN Doc. E/AC.32/SR.41, Aug. 23, 1950, at 7: "[P]aragraph 2 of article [7] must be interpreted in the light of paragraph 1."

[227] "According to [the draft of Art. 7(3)] . . . certain refugees would continue to enjoy the reciprocity which they had previously enjoyed; that included the legislative reciprocity mentioned in the second paragraph, as well as diplomatic and *de facto* reciprocity. On the other hand, new refugees would . . . enjoy exemption from reciprocity only after a period of three years' residence in the receiving country. He appreciated the reasons for which certain States felt obliged to limit the rights of new refugees in that way, but pointed out that there were other States which visualized the possibility of extending the idea of reciprocity even to non-statutory refugees": Statement of Baron van Boetzelaer of the Netherlands, UN Doc. A/CONF.2/SR.24, July 17, 1951, at 21–22.

[228] "Each Contracting State shall continue to accord to refugees the rights and benefits to which they were already entitled, in the absence of reciprocity, at the date of entry into force of this Convention for that State": Refugee Convention, at Art. 7(3).

[229] "The Contracting States shall consider favourably the possibility of according to refugees, in the absence of reciprocity, rights and benefits beyond those to which they are entitled according to paragraphs 2 and 3, and to extending exemption from reciprocity to refugees who do not fulfil the conditions provided for in paragraphs 2 and 3": Refugee Convention, at Art. 7(4). The Ad Hoc Committee had "expressed the hope that States would give sympathetic consideration to extending rights, as far as possible, to all refugees without regard to reciprocity, particularly where the rights have no relation to the requirements of residence, as for example, compensation for war damages and persecution": Ad Hoc Committee, "Second Session Report," at 11–12.

[230] "[T]he [Ad Hoc] Committee expressed the hope that states would give sympathetic consideration to extending rights, as far as possible, to all refugees without regard to reciprocity, particularly where the rights have no relation to the requirements of residence. This 'hope' was transformed by the Conference [of Plenipotentiaries] into a special clause which must have more meaning than 'hope.' It is a recommendation to the Contracting States . . . In other words, a state cannot be forced to accord these rights, but there must be a well-founded reason for refusing their accordance": Robinson, *History*, at 88–89.

[231] "It is only a recommendation, but imposes nevertheless a mandatory obligation to consider favourably the granting of wider rights and benefits": P. Weis, *The Refugee Convention, 1951: The Travaux Préparatoires Analysed with a Commentary by Dr. Paul Weis* (posthumously pub'd., 1995) (Weis, *Travaux*), at 57.

attention to the logic of continued application of reciprocity requirements to refugees. While not formally obliged to grant rights subject to legislative or de facto reciprocity during the first three years a refugee resides in its territory, Art. 7(4) "uses the word 'shall' to indicate that it *requires* the states to consider favorably the possibility of according such rights."[232]

In any event, it is today legally dubious that states also bound by the International Covenant on Civil and Political Rights may validly withhold refugee rights on the grounds of an absence of reciprocity.[233] The Covenant's general guarantee of non-discrimination requires that rights allocated by a state to any group presumptively be extended to all persons under its jurisdiction.[234] Legislative and de facto reciprocity are particularly vulnerable, as the decision to deny rights to only those aliens whose national states have not agreed to reciprocal treatment is explicitly a means of pressuring other *states* to grant protection to foreign citizens.[235] As observed by the American representative to the Ad Hoc Committee, "[t]he purpose of making . . . rights subject to reciprocity was to encourage other countries to adopt an equally liberal regime towards foreigners in their territory. Naturally there was nothing to be gained by making the rights subject to reciprocity where a refugee was concerned."[236] In view of the impossibility of advancing the explicitly instrumentalist goals of most reciprocity regimes through the

---

[232] Robinson, *History*, at 89.

[233] This is certainly the case where the rights in question are themselves guaranteed by international law. For example, the UN Human Rights Committee has expressed the view that "the provisions in [Azerbaijan's] legislation providing for the principle of reciprocity in guaranteeing Covenant rights to aliens are contrary to articles 2 and 26 of the Covenant": "Concluding Observations of the Human Rights Committee: Azerbaijan," UN Doc. CCPR/CO/73/AZE, Nov. 12, 2001, at para. 20. A recent analysis of the role of reciprocity in international human rights law asserts the potential value of reciprocity in the context of a system which still lacks a centralized enforcement mechanism. It none-theless insists that countermeasures must be carefully targeted, lest the goals of human rights law be undermined. "At a general level, the notion of enforcing human rights law through disregard for its norms seems incompatible with this rationale, indeed, the *raison d'être*, of that body of law . . . [A] mechanism that would permit infringements of human rights to be echoed by further infringements of human rights would undoubtedly under-mine the structure of human rights as a body of compulsory norms limiting the actions of the State": Provost, "Reciprocity", at 444–445.

[234] See chapter 2.5.5 above, at pp. 126–128.

[235] Whether preferred rights secured by special forms of diplomatic reciprocity are equally vulnerable to attack on the basis of the duty of non-discrimination is less clear. Where enhanced rights are granted only to citizens of those states with which the asylum country is linked in a form of political or economic union, for example, this may be said to reflect an effective assimilation of those aliens to the political or economic community of the partner state. The non-discrimination analysis ought therefore to focus on whether the rights in question can be said to reflect the unique abilities and potentialities of members of a shared political and economic community. See chapter 2.5.5 above, at p. 128 ff.

[236] Statement of Mr. Henkin of the United States, UN Doc. E/AC.32/SR.23, Feb. 3, 1950, at 2.

person of refugees,[237] an attempt to rely on the restrictive portions of Art. 7 is unlikely to meet modern understandings of the duty of non-discrimination, the broad margin of appreciation afforded state parties notwithstanding.[238]

3.2.3 Exemption from insurmountable requirements

Refugee Convention, Art. 6   The term "in the same circumstances"
For the purpose of this Convention, the term "in the same circumstances" implies that any requirements (including requirements as to length and conditions of sojourn or residence) which the particular individual would have to fulfil for the enjoyment of the right in question, if he were not a refugee, must be fulfilled by him, with the exception of requirements which by their nature a refugee is incapable of fulfilling.

As previously noted, most Convention rights that require implementation only at the baseline standard – rights to property, self-employment, professional practice, housing, and post-primary education[239] – are textually framed to require "treatment as favourable as possible and, in any event, not less favourable than that accorded to aliens generally in the same circumstances." Governments are also allowed to restrict the internal mobility of refugees lawfully present in their territory "subject to any regulations applicable to aliens generally in the same circumstances."[240] The same phrase is used to modify the duty to assimilate refugees to the nationals of most-favored states in relation to the rights to association and to wage-earning employment: "the most favourable treatment accorded to nationals of a foreign country, in the same circumstances."[241]

This language reflects the view of the drafters that where refugee rights are defined to require only the baseline standard of treatment – that is, assimilation to aliens generally – refugees should have to qualify in essentially the same way as other aliens. The initial approach of the Ad Hoc Committee was quite strict, suggesting that refugees should have to meet "the same requirements, including the same length and conditions of sojourn or residence, which are prescribed for the national of a foreign state for the enjoyment of the right in question."[242] The Committee rejected proposals that would have

---

[237] See chapter 3.2 above, at p. 194.   [238] See chapter 2.5.5 above, at pp. 129–145.
[239] Refugee Convention, at Arts. 13, 18, 19, 21, and 22.   [240] Ibid. at Art. 26.
[241] Ibid. at Arts. 15, 17. Comparable phrasing is employed to define the duty of tax equity in Art. 29 ("[no] taxes ... other or higher than those which are ... levied on their nationals in similar situations").
[242] Ad Hoc Committee, "Second Session Report," at 15.

required states to judge comparability solely on the basis of terms and conditions of stay in the asylum state.[243] The Belgian and American representatives argued that such an approach was too restrictive, but were able to persuade the Committee only that governments should be entitled to consider a wide variety of criteria in determining whether a refugee is truly similarly situated to other aliens granted particular rights.[244]

At the Conference of Plenipotentiaries, the Australian delegate lobbied unsuccessfully to grant states even more discretion to withhold rights from refugees. Mr. Shaw proposed "[t]hat nothing in this Convention shall be deemed to confer upon a refugee any right greater than those enjoyed by other aliens."[245] This position was soundly denounced, and ultimately withdrawn.[246] As the Austrian representative observed, "[i]f it were to be posited that refugees should not have rights greater than those enjoyed by other aliens, the Convention seemed pointless, since its object was precisely to provide for specially favourable treatment to be accorded to refugees."[247] The Conference nonetheless agreed that where rights are defined at the baseline "aliens generally" standard, governments could legitimately deny access to particular rights on the grounds that a given refugee is not truly "in the same circumstances" as other aliens enjoying the right in question.

In line with the thinking of the Ad Hoc Committee, representatives to the Conference were not persuaded that states should have to judge the comparability of a refugee's situation on the basis solely of the conditions of his or her sojourn or residence.[248] As Grahl-Madsen has observed, "[i]n most countries certain rights are only granted to persons satisfying certain criteria, for example with regard to age, sex, health, nationality, education, training, experience, personal integrity, financial solvency, marital status, membership of a professional association or trade union, or residence, even length of residence within the country or in a particular place. There may also be strict

---

[243] Proposal of the Chairman, Mr. Larsen of Denmark, UN Doc. E/AC.32/SR.36, Aug. 15, 1950, at 9; and Proposal of Mr. Robinson of Israel, UN Doc. E/AC.32/SR.42, Aug. 24, 1950, at 23.

[244] Statements of Mr. Herment of Belgium and Mr. Henkin of the United States, UN Doc. E/AC.32/SR.42, Aug. 24, 1950, at 24.

[245] Proposal of Australia, UN Doc. A/CONF.2/19, July 3, 1951.

[246] See e.g. criticisms voiced by Mr. Herment of Belgium and Mr. von Trutzschler of the Federal Republic of Germany, UN Doc. A/CONF.2/SR.6, July 4, 1951, at 5–6.

[247] Statement of Mr. Fritzler of Austria, ibid. at 6.

[248] The United Kingdom representative sought to restrict the comparison to only "requirements as to length and conditions of sojourn or residence," but withdrew his proposal in the face of substantial disagreement. See Statements of Mr. Hoare of the United Kingdom, UN Doc. A/CONF.2/SR.34, July 25, 1951, at 16; and UN Doc. A/CONF.2/SR.35, July 25, 1951, at 36.

rules for proving that one possesses the required qualifications, e.g. by way of specified diplomas or certificates."[249]

Broader concerns of this kind were likely of importance to the drafters. The Belgian delegate, for example, expressly suggested that evidence of occupational or professional qualification might be a legitimate ground upon which to condition access to certain rights.[250] The British representative insisted that the notion of "in the same circumstances" was "defined in its implications, not in its meaning."[251] While conditions of residence or sojourn were obviously the primary concerns,[252] it would be undesirable to particularize all possible grounds for defining similarity of circumstances "since that might result in the vigorous application of all possible requirements applicable to foreigners in the country of asylum."[253] Thus, Art. 6 is framed in open-ended language,[254] allowing governments "some latitude ... to decide within the general conception that refugees were not to have more privileged treatment than aliens generally as to the conditions which must be fulfilled."[255]

This discretion is not, however, absolute. Apart from the requirements now imposed by general principles of non-discrimination law,[256] the major caveat to the prerogative granted states to define the basis upon which the comparability of a refugee's situation is to be assessed is the duty to exempt refugees from insurmountable requirements. Even as governments insisted on the authority to require refugees to qualify for rights and benefits on the same terms as other aliens, they recognized that the very nature of refugeehood – for example, the urgency of flight, the severing of ties with the home state, and the inability to plan for relocation – may sometimes make compliance with the usual criteria a near-impossibility:

---

[249] A. Grahl-Madsen, *Commentary on the Refugee Convention 1951* (1963, pub'd. 1997) (Grahl-Madsen, *Commentary*), at 23.

[250] "To give an example, it might be that a refugee would wish to procure a document allowing him to exercise a profession or ply a trade. The element of sojourn or residence would count, of course, but other considerations might also come into play, such as the kind of trade or profession the refugee wished to engage in": Statement of Mr. Herment of Belgium, UN Doc. A/CONF.2/SR.34, July 25, 1951, at 17.

[251] Statement of Mr. Hoare of the United Kingdom, ibid. at 17.   [252] Ibid. at 16.

[253] Statement of Mr. Hoare of the United Kingdom, UN Doc. A/CONF.2/SR.35, July 25, 1951, at 35.

[254] "[T]he treatment of foreigners was not necessarily uniform, but would depend in many instances upon the individual's circumstances and claims to consideration": Statement of Mr. Hoare of the United Kingdom, UN Doc. A/CONF.2/SR.3, July 3, 1951, at 22.

[255] Statement of Mr. Hoare of the United Kingdom, UN Doc. A/CONF.2/SR.35, July 25, 1951, at 35.

[256] See chapter 2.5.5 above.

For example, in some eastern European countries a person had to fulfil certain qualifications relating to residence in order to be eligible for social security. The definition . . . was too rigid, and would weaken the Convention . . . The special circumstances of refugees must be recognized.[257]

The validity of this concern was endorsed without opposition, leading the Conference of Plenipotentiaries to adopt a joint British–Israeli amendment to require governments to exempt refugees from requirements "which by their nature a refugee is incapable of fulfilling."[258]

As suggested by the concerns of the Israeli representative that led to the redrafting of Art. 6,[259] general criteria based on length of sojourn or residence may be relied on to assess the entitlement of refugees, but may not be mechanistically applied. Some flexibility to take account of difficulties faced by refugees in meeting the usual standard is clearly called for. For example, Grahl-Madsen suggests that requirements to produce certificates of nationality, or documentation of educational or professional qualification or experience acquired in the refugee's country of origin may sometimes fall within the insurmountable requirements exception.[260] This does not mean that refugees should be admitted to jobs for which they are truly unqualified, but simply that if "the refugee is unable to produce a certificate from the university in the country of origin where he graduated, he must be allowed to prove his possession of the required academic degree by other means than the normally required diploma."[261] This is because the very nature of the refugee experience may have denied the individual the time to amass or to carry all relevant documentation when leaving his or her country, and there may be no present means to compel authorities there to issue the requisite certification from abroad.[262]

The net result is a fair balance between a general principle of assimilating refugees to other aliens – both in the positive sense of granting them access to particular benefits, and in the negative sense of requiring compliance with the usual rules for entitlement to those benefits – and the equally obvious need to render substantive justice to refugees in the application of those principles. Even when rights require implementation only to the same extent granted aliens generally, whatever impediments an individual refugee faces by virtue of the uprooting and dislocation associated with refugeehood should not be relied upon to deny access to rights.

---

[257] Statement of Mr. Robinson of Israel, UN Doc. A/CONF.2/SR.5, July 4, 1951, at 19.

[258] The proposal was adopted on a 22–0 (2 abstentions) vote: UN Doc. A/CONF.2/SR.26, July 18, 1951, at 10.

[259] See text above, at note 257.   [260] Grahl-Madsen, *Commentary*, at 23.

[261] Ibid. at 23.   [262] See Weis, *Travaux*, at 46–47.

3.2.4 Rights governed by personal status

Refugee Convention, Art. 12   Personal status

1. The personal status of a refugee shall be governed by the law of the country of his domicile or, if he has no domicile, by the law of the country of his residence.

2. Rights previously acquired by a refugee and dependent on personal status, more particularly rights attaching to marriage, shall be respected by a Contracting State, subject to compliance, if this be necessary, with the formalities required by the law of that State, provided that the right in question is one which would have been recognized by the law of that State had he not become a refugee.

Under the dominant civil law understanding, the personal status of a non-citizen – including, for example, his or her legal capacity, family and matrimonial rights, and entitlement to benefit under rules of succession and inheritance – is ordinarily to be determined by the law of the country of which the individual is a national.[263] Thus, to determine whether a non-citizen child has been validly adopted, whether an alien is entitled to an interest in his or her spouse's property by virtue of marriage, or whether a will made by a non-citizen abroad is legally valid, reference should be made to the legal standards prevailing in the alien's country of citizenship.

There are some good reasons for this legal point of departure. For example, if the validity of a marriage were to be determined by reference to the age of consent wherever a couple happened to reside or even to visit, it is clear that international travel could pose a major risk to the stability of some fundamental personal relationships. In order to avoid such disruptions without

---

[263] The traditional civil law approach is to look to the law of nationality to determine an alien's personal status, a heritage of late nineteenth- and early twentieth-century nationalism. This approach was codified in the Hague Conventions on Private International Law of 1902, and is still the rule in most civilian systems. Yet there are important exceptions (such as Switzerland). The basic common law rule (prevailing in the UK, the US, etc.) has always been to look to the law of domicile. On the whole, reference to domicile or habitual residence seems to be the path of the future: see E. Scoles et al., *Conflict of Laws* (2000) (Scoles et al., *Conflict*), at 242–245. This is especially so as the result of invocation of the non-discrimination principles in EU law, leading to a focus on domicile or, more precisely, "habitual residence." "The European Court of Justice appears to be inclined to establish a 'Community concept' of residence for benefit purposes which is based on the facts of a person's living arrangements rather than the legal rules prevailing in each member state": D. Mabbett and H. Bolderson, "Non-Discrimination, Free Movement, and Social Citizenship in Europe: Contrasting Positions for EU Nationals and Asylum-Seekers," paper presented at the ISSA Research Conference on Social Security, Helsinki, Sept. 25–27, 2000, at 2, available at www.issa.int/pdf/helsinki2000/topic1/2mabbett.pdf (accessed Apr. 30, 2005).

denying courts in a country of residence or transit the ability to determine with certainty the personal status of a non-citizen within their territory, most civil law states have traditionally chosen to anchor analysis in the rules governing personal status in the non-citizen's own country. Adoption of this approach is a pragmatic means by which to enable persons to move between countries without thereby jeopardizing basic entitlements. It is also arguably a principled standard, since the rules which determine an individual's fundamental personal status are those which govern in the country to which that person owes his or her primary political allegiance.

Yet in the case of a refugee, by definition a person who no longer enjoys the assumed bond between citizen and state, the drafters of the Refugee Convention were of the view that there is no principled basis for application of the usual civil law approach to the determination of personal status. To the contrary, some representatives felt that it was ethically wrong to hold refugees hostage to personal status rules which prevailed in the countries which they had fled. The Danish representative advanced the argument that "[r]efugees should not be treated by the host country in accordance with the very laws – such as the Nürnberg Laws – that might have caused them to become refugees."[264] As summarized by Mr. Giraud of the Committee Secretariat,

> A refugee was characteristically a person who had broken with his home country and who no longer liked its laws. That fact constituted a strong reason for not applying to him the laws of his home country. Furthermore, it would make for more harmonious relations if the laws of the country in which the refugee had established domicile or residence were applied to him.[265]

The logic of not binding refugees to personal status rules in force in their country of origin thus has much in common with the basic premise of the duty to exempt refugees from exceptional measures. As discussed below, it would make little sense to stigmatize a refugee as an enemy alien on the basis of his or her formal possession of the nationality of a state the protection of which the refugee does not enjoy.[266] Similarly, it is difficult to understand why rights should be withheld from a refugee by the application of principles governing his or her personal status in the country of origin, but which are

---

[264] Statement of Mr. Larsen of Denmark, UN Doc. E/AC.32/SR.8, Jan. 23, 1950, at 2. See also Statement of Mr. Robinson of Israel, ibid.: "It would hardly be fair to say that a man who had fled from his country with the intention of never going back retained his nationality ... [N]o refugee should be forced to accept the laws of the country of which he was a national." Mr. Cha of China insisted that "refugees should be treated in accordance with the laws of the country which had given them asylum," invoking his country's aversion to the extraterritorial application of national laws: ibid.

[265] Statement of Mr. Giraud of the Secretariat, ibid. at 4.

[266] See chapter 3.5.2 below, at p. 272.

inconsistent with the rules which determine personal status in the asylum state. Yet this would have been precisely the result – at least in most civil law states – of a strict application of the general rule under Art. 7(1) that refugees should, without a provision to the contrary, receive "the same treatment as is accorded to aliens generally."

Principled concerns were not, however, solely responsible for the decision to reverse the precedent of most earlier refugee treaties, under which the rules of the refugee's country of citizenship generally determined his or her personal status.[267] To the contrary, the driving force for reform appears to have been the practical experience of the International Refugee Organization, which was concerned that the traditional nationality rule had caused real problems for refugees in the field of family rights, particularly in regard to the capacity to enter into marriage, and the ability to dissolve a marriage.[268] Reliance on the status rules of the refugee's country of citizenship was moreover said to be fraught with administrative difficulty.[269] An example offered by the Israeli delegate to the Conference of Plenipotentiaries gives some sense of this concern:

---

[267] The primary exception related to refugees who had no citizenship; the personal status of such refugees was determined by reference to their country of domicile or habitual residence. On the other hand, the 1933 Refugee Convention determined personal status by reference to domicile or residence for all refugees. While most refugees covered by this treaty were stateless, some were not. See Weis, *Travaux*, at 106. The reformist character of Art. 12 was new to the drafters. "[P]aragraph 1 introduces an innovation. It makes no distinction between refugees who are stateless *de jure* and those who are stateless only *de facto*. In point of fact persons in either category no longer enjoy the protection of their countries of origin": Secretary-General, "Memorandum," at 25.

[268] "The IRO had experienced great difficulties in cases where the principle of domicile and residence had not been applied": Statement of Mr. Weis of the International Refugee Organization, UN Doc. E/AC.32/SR.8, Jan. 23, 1950, at 5. More specifically, "the question of the right to contract marriage raised difficulties: countries which had so far applied the national law did so only in so far as it did not conflict with their public policy. It might therefore happen that the same consideration of domestic public policy might be raised in deciding the capacity of the refugee to contract marriage under the law of his country of domicile or residence. Moreover, the dissolution of marriages raised a question of competence: the courts of many countries refused to decree a dissolution of marriage if the national law of the person concerned was not obliged to recognize the validity of their ruling": Statement of Mr. Weis of the International Refugee Organization, UN Doc. E/AC.32/SR.9, Jan. 24, 1950, at 3–4.

[269] "In practice, the application of their own national law to refugees would involve great difficulties. Even if they had kept their own nationality, the authorities of their country of origin were unfavourably disposed towards them, and if a court of a reception country were to apply to those authorities for information needed to establish their personal status, it would presumably have difficulty obtaining such data": Statement of Mr. Kural of Turkey, UN Doc. E/AC.32/SR.7, Jan. 23, 1950, at 13. See also Statement of Mr. von Trutzschler of the Federal Republic of Germany, UN Doc. A/CONF.2/SR.7, July 5, 1951, at 11: "There were grave technical objections to applying the law of the country of origin."

Taking, by way of example, the case of a person whose place of origin was Vilna, and who had sought asylum in a country where in matters of international private law the courts applied the law of the country of origin, the courts would have to establish whether they should apply the Polish Civil Code, that of Lithuania before its annexation by the Soviet Union, or the Soviet Civil Code for the constituent republics of the Union. Such a decision would involve political considerations, and courts in some countries might be unwilling to go into such matters.[270]

The alternative recommended by the Secretariat was to allow refugees to benefit from the traditional common law position, under which a non-citizen's personal status is determined by the rules which prevail in his or her country of domicile. Because a refugee's state of domicile is ordinarily the country of asylum,[271] this approach was thought to facilitate the work of domestic courts involved in the adjudication of refugee rights:[272]

Such a solution would be to the advantage of the refugees, and would be welcomed also by other inhabitants of the country who may have legal proceedings with refugees, and by the courts of the country. Courts will be freed from the very difficult task of deciding which law is applicable and of discovering what are the provisions of foreign laws in a particular regard. Moreover, in some countries, courts may exercise jurisdiction with regard to aliens only if their decisions are recognized by the courts of the country of nationality of the alien. The present provisions would, by applying the law of domicile or of residence, eliminate this limitation with regard to refugees.[273]

In the end, even the French representative – who had tabled an opposing draft, under which personal status would have continued to be decided by reference to the rules of the refugee's country of nationality[274] – was persuaded that a refugee's personal status should instead be governed by the standards applicable in his or her country of domicile.[275] As summarized by the Danish representative,

---

[270] Statement of Mr. Robinson of Israel, UN Doc. A/CONF.2/SR.7, July 5, 1951, at 11–12.

[271] "[T]he principle applied in this article is the most simple because in the majority of cases a refugee adopts the country of asylum as his domicile and thus the personal status will easily be established and reference to foreign law will be avoided": Robinson, *History*, at 102.

[272] "Whereas during normal times, when there were few foreigners in a country, the application of the national law would not cause insurmountable difficulties, the courts would be inundated with work if, at a time when the number of refugees amounted to hundreds of thousands, they had to refer in each case to a national law with which they were unfamiliar": Statement of Mr. Kural of Turkey, UN Doc. E/AC.32/SR.7, Jan. 23, 1950, at 14.

[273] Ad Hoc Committee, "First Session Report," at Annex II.

[274] France, "Draft Convention," at 3–4.

[275] Statement of Mr. Rain of France, UN Doc. E/AC.32/SR.8, Jan. 23, 1950, at 5. "The Committee was, in fact, trying to bring about the application of a new rule in countries

With regard to refugees, the Committee had decided that their personal status would be governed by the law of their country of domicile ... That being the case, all other criteria had been abandoned. Consequently, in those states where the law of the country of domicile ... was applied, refugees would receive the same treatment as other aliens; in other countries, they would be granted a special status.[276]

In truth, however, it is not entirely clear that the approach adopted in Art. 12 of the Refugee Convention answers either the ethical or practical concerns which arise in determining a refugee's personal status. As a matter of principle, there is some force to the original assertion of the French representative that reliance on the rules of a refugee's country of nationality was often more consistent with "the national traditions of the refugees" themselves.[277] Indeed, the only non-governmental intervention on this issue opposed the shift to the determination of personal status based on the rules of domicile on the grounds that it failed to recognize the desire of many refugees ultimately to return to their country of origin:

> That a political refugee who had a horror of his country of origin, and had no intention whatsoever of returning to it, should find himself given the personal status provided by the legislation of the host government seemed reasonable. But would it be reasonable, it might still be asked, to impose on refugees who were still attached to their country of origin and lived only in the hope of returning to it (as formerly the German anti-fascists had done and as the Spanish Republicans were doing at present), a personal status which might vary considerably according to their country of residence, and to adopt that measure, according to changes in circumstances in the country of domicile, without the person affected having an opportunity of expressing his own desires on the matter?[278]

More generally, the Egyptian representative to the Conference of Plenipotentiaries provided an example which shows clearly the potential ethical difficulty of assigning personal status on the basis of the rules applying in the country of domicile:

> The majority of the Egyptian population was Mohammedan, its personal status being governed by Koranic law, whereas the personal status of other sections of the population was governed by the law of their respective religions or faiths ... [E]ach of these legal systems conceived of the

having a French legal tradition. The French idea had not met with a favorable reception so far, either on questions of principle or on those of application; in every case, it had had to yield to other ideas": Statement of Mr. Rain of France, UN Doc. E/AC.32/SR.9, Jan. 24, 1950, at 12.

[276] Statement of Mr. Larsen of Denmark, UN Doc. E/AC.32/SR.9, Jan. 24, 1950, at 11.

[277] Statement of Mr. Rain of France, UN Doc. E/AC.32/SR.8, Jan. 23, 1950, at 3.

[278] Statement of Mr. Rollin of the Inter-Parliamentary Union, UN Doc. A/CONF.2/SR.10, July 6, 1951, at 8.

> principle of personal status in a different way ... [T]he status of aliens (other than Mohammedan aliens) in Egypt was governed by their personal status under the law of their own country, reference to that law being made by Egyptian law. If the personal status of a refugee was governed by the law of his country of domicile, or, if he had no domicile, by the law of his country of residence, and if that refugee was established in Egypt, there would be difficulty deciding which among the various types of personal status of domicile or residence should be granted to him.[279]

The result of Art. 12's deference to the rules of the domicile state in the case posited by the Egyptian representative would be that the refugee's personal status would be determined on the basis of the rules advocated by his or her religion, even if the refugee's personal preference (and prior experience in the country of origin) were to have his or her personal status determined on a secular basis.

At the level of practicality, objection may also be taken to the shift to a primary reliance on the rules of the country of "domicile" on the grounds of the inherent ambiguity of that notion. Scoles et al., for example, cite Justice Holmes' famous quotation in *Bergner and Engel Brewing Co. v. Dreyfus*[280] that

> what the law means by domicile is the one technically pre-eminent headquarters, which as a result either of fact or fiction every person is compelled to have in order that by aid of it, certain rights and duties which have attached to it by law may be determined.[281]

Because the notion of domicile places a premium on the place which an individual considers to be "home," it clearly presents a particular difficulty for refugees:

> If a political refugee intends to return to the country from which he fled as soon as the political situation changes, he retains his domicile there unless the desired political change is so improbable that his intention is discounted as merely an exile's longing for his native land; but if his intention is not to return to that country even when the political situation has changed, he can acquire a domicile of choice in the country to which he has fled.[282]

This confusion was evident in the comments of even the experts from the common law countries which had traditionally relied on domicile to determine the personal status of non-citizens. Sir Leslie Brass, for example, asserted that an individual's domicile in English law was "the country in which the refugee had established his permanent residence."[283] But as the

---

[279] Statement of Mr. Mostafa of Egypt, UN Doc. A/CONF.2/SR.7, July 5, 1951, at 10.
[280] 172 Mass 154, at 157; 51 NE 531, at 532 (US SJC Mass, Oct. 29, 1898).
[281] Scoles et al., *Conflict*, at 245.
[282] L. Collins, *Dicey and Morris on the Conflict of Laws* (2000) (Collins, *Dicey*), at 129.
[283] Statement of Sir Leslie Brass of the United Kingdom, UN Doc. E/AC.32/SR.9, Jan. 24, 1950, at 2.

American representative later noted, "a refugee might in some instances have his domicile in another country to the one in which he was living."[284] The representative of the IRO thought that a refugee's country of domicile was his or her "centre of existence."[285] The most helpful explanation, offered at the Conference of Plenipotentiaries by the British representative, was that

> [i]n Anglo-Saxon law there were two concepts: the domicile of origin, and the domicile of choice. The former might or might not be the place of birth; the latter was acquired by the personal choice of the person concerned . . . It would be very exceptional if a refugee, fleeing from his country of origin, did not adopt the country of asylum as his domicile of choice.[286]

In view of the fungibility of the concept of "domicile" even in the common law states accustomed to its use, it is little wonder that so many representatives of civil law countries expressed confusion about how to apply it in practice. France observed that "it seemed . . . that the word 'domicile' bore a different meaning in English from that generally accepted by those taking part in the present Conference."[287] Israel "drew attention to the ambiguity of the term 'domicile,' which was interpreted differently by different legal systems. In any case, it was quite possible for a person to have his residence in one country and his domicile in another."[288] The Chinese representative offered a practical example to illustrate his discomfort with the vagueness of the notion of domicile:

> [I]t should be specified how long a refugee was required to reside in a country in order to be considered as domiciled there. Otherwise it would be difficult to know whether he was really domiciled in a reception country, as had been the case with certain Jews who had taken refuge in Shanghai before the war and had been considered at the time to be domiciled there but who had lost that right later under the Japanese occupation and had finally been repatriated to Poland or directed to Israel. The application of the law of domicile seemed therefore to raise serious difficulties.[289]

This led the Chinese representative to conclude that "the term 'domicile' . . . mean[s] the place where a person desired to live and carry out his business,"[290] a view not corrected by any other delegate.

---

[284] Statement of Mr. Henkin of the United States, UN Doc. E/AC.32/SR.36, Aug. 15, 1950, at 6.

[285] Statement of Mr. Weis of the International Refugee Organization, ibid. at 7.

[286] Statement of Mr. Hoare of the United Kingdom, UN Doc. A/CONF.2/SR.7, July 5, 1951, at 9.

[287] Statement of Mr. Rochefort of France, ibid. at 14.

[288] Statement of Mr. Robinson of Israel, UN Doc. E/AC.32/SR.8, Jan. 23, 1950, at 4.

[289] Statement of Mr. Cha of China, UN Doc. E/AC.32/SR.9, Jan. 24, 1950, at 2.

[290] Statement of Mr. Cha of China, UN Doc. E/AC.32/SR.36, Aug. 15, 1950, at 5.

In the end, no clear definition of domicile was ever agreed to.[291] It was pragmatically, if perhaps unhelpfully, decided that "the courts of the reception country would determine the domicile ... of [refugees]."[292] While the unwillingness of the majority to accede to strong pleas in favor of reference instead to the rules on personal status prevailing in the refugee's country of "residence" or "habitual residence"[293] must surely be taken as evidence that domicile – at least as understood in the mid-twentieth century – was not simply synonymous with those notions, this dichotomy is, in practice, increasingly anachronistic. Because the present trend is for common law states to reform their law of "domicile" to bring it into line with the civil law concept of "habitual residence,"[294] the distinction between these notions may not long survive.

[291] As Robinson observes, "[t]he difference between the various concepts of domicile may provoke certain conflicts, especially when a refugee moves from the area of one concept to that of another or when the personal status of a refugee residing in one area is to be established in another. In doubtful cases, the law of the country of habitual residence of the refugee must be decisive": Robinson, *History*, at 102.

[292] Statement of Mr. Guerreiro of Brazil, UN Doc. E/AC.32/SR.8, Jan. 23, 1950, at 6. See also Statement of Sir Leslie Brass of the United Kingdom, ibid.

[293] In the Ad Hoc Committee, the French representative expressed his preference for reliance on the rules prevailing in a refugee's country of residence. He "considered it advisable, in view of the complicated procedure which might be required to establish the distinction between domicile and residence, and in the interests of the refugees, to retain only the reference to the law of the country of residence in paragraph 1": Statement of Mr. Rain of France, UN Doc. E/AC.32/SR.8, Jan. 23, 1950, at 7. This view was voiced as well at the Conference of Plenipotentiaries. The representative of the Netherlands argued that "it would be better to replace the word ['domicile'] by the expression 'habitual residence,' which left no room for misinterpretation": Statement of Baron van Boetzelaer of the Netherlands, UN Doc. A/CONF.2/SR.7, July 5, 1951, at 5. See also Statement of Mr. Fritzer of Austria, ibid. at 6. On the other hand, the Colombian representative preferred the notion of domicile because it "implied a legal relation between a person and his domicile, whereas that of residence implied simply a stay in a place, without any legal relation between the person and the place in question": Statement of Mr. Giraldo-Jaramillo of Colombia, ibid. at 8. And, seemingly oblivious to the views and concerns of most civil law delegates, the British representative asserted simply that "if the concept of 'habitual residence' was introduced, certain countries might find themselves in difficulties, because the concept had not formally existed in their legal system and would require interpretation by the courts. The concept of domicile, on the other hand, was well-known": Statement of Mr. Hoare of the United Kingdom, ibid. at 9. It is noteworthy, however, that even the idea of "residence" may also be prone to imprecision. For example, the Belgian representative expressed his concern about how to deal with the case of "a refugee domiciled in China, where he had his family and his business, [but] who might visit Belgium on a business trip. If he should happen to die in Belgium, it would be ludicrous to determine his status on the basis of the law of the *country of residence*. He would normally be subject to the law of China, his country of domicile [emphasis added]": Statement of Mr. Cuvelier of Belgium, UN Doc. E/AC.32/SR.8, Jan. 23, 1950, at 7.

[294] "The notion of habitual residence appears to be emerging as a concept acceptable to lawyers from both common law and civil law traditions, as representing a compromise between domicile and nationality, or at least as a more acceptable connecting factor than

If a refugee does not have a country of domicile,[295] Art. 12 as adopted does allow for reference to the rules on personal status of the refugee's country of "residence."[296] Yet even with this back-up rule,[297] it may sometimes be difficult to know precisely how to define a refugee's personal status. As candidly observed by the American representative, "[t]he article ... raise[d] certain issues because a refugee might be in a transit camp with neither domicile nor residence."[298] Indeed, a refugee who seeks recognition of his or her status, but who has not yet been admitted to a status determination procedure, may also be a person with neither a domicile nor a residence. In keeping with the underlying spirit of Art. 12, however, it would be best to refrain from defining personal status on the basis of the rules existing in the individual's state of origin.[299] Unless the refugee applicant has a stronger attachment to some other state, the logical default position would be to refer to the usual rules which define personal status in the transit or asylum country confronted with the need to determine the individual's personal status.

Which forms of personal status, then, are to be determined by reference to the rules of the refugee's domicile state? While the Chairman of the Ad Hoc Committee was insistent that the Convention provide a clear definition of

domicile to be used as an alternative to nationality. The reform of the law of domicile in England is taking the concept closer to that of habitual residence, which is also not far removed from the understanding of domicile prevalent in United States jurisdictions": Collins, *Dicey*, at 154.

[295] The British representative to the Ad Hoc Committee suggested that everyone should be understood to have a country of domicile. "If it meant, in the case of his own country, that the personal status of refugees would be determined in accordance with the law of domicile, he could accept the paragraph, since everyone had a domicile under English law": Statement of Sir Leslie Brass of the United Kingdom, UN Doc. E/AC.32/SR.8, Jan. 23, 1950, at 6.

[296] "[T]he two criteria – domicile and residence – were not simply juxtaposed in the paragraph under consideration: it was to be noted that the law of the country of domicile was to be applied in the first instance, the law of the country of residence to be applied only if the country of the refugee's domicile was unknown or in doubt. While preference was thus given to the criterion of domicile, the notion of residence had been introduced because it was often easier to establish residence than domicile": Statement of Mr. Giraud of the Secretariat, UN Doc. E/AC.32/SR.8, Jan. 23, 1950, at 4–5.

[297] "Decisions should ... be based wherever possible on 'domicile,' and only exceptionally on 'residence'": Statement of Mr. Robinson of Israel, UN Doc. E/AC.32/SR.36, Aug. 15, 1950, at 6.

[298] Statement of Mr. Henkin of the United States, ibid. at 7.

[299] See text above, at p. 210. "[T]he types of personal status obtaining in some countries might be incompatible with human dignity, and it could be argued that they were one of the reasons which had led to a person's fleeing his country. It would not be just for Contracting States to apply them": Statement of Mr. Rochefort of France, UN Doc. A/CONF.2/SR.7, July 5, 1951, at 9.

relevant forms of personal status,[300] the majority of Committee members successfully resisted his plea.[301] The French and British delegates argued that it was unlikely that any agreement was possible on this subject, given its extraordinary legal complexity.[302] As in the case of the definition of "domicile," it was therefore decided that "it would be for each State which signed the convention to interpret the expressions within it within the framework of its own legislation and in the light of the concepts that were most akin to its own juridical system."[303] But this domestic discretion should be informed by "the Secretariat study … [which] was an adequate exposé of the concept of personal status. It was for the contracting states to decide finally upon the elements of that status, in the light of the interpretation given by the Secretariat and of the records of the Committee meetings, without, however, being bound by those texts."[304]

The Secretariat's Study refers to three types of personal status governed by Art. 12.[305] The first, "[a] person's capacity (age of attaining majority, capacity of the married woman, etc.)"[306] elicited no debate during the drafting of the Convention. While the primary concern of the Study involved the preservation of the property rights of married women (discussed below[307]), comparable dilemmas might arise for a woman coming from a state in which women were not allowed to have independent legal or economic status. Such a

---

[300] Statements of the Chairman, Mr. Chance of Canada, UN Doc. E/AC.32/SR.9, Jan. 24, 1950, at 3, 11. The same concern was expressed by the Egyptian representative to the Conference of Plenipotentiaries, Mr. Mostafa, UN Doc. A/CONF.2/SR.7, July 5, 1951, at 10: "It would … be desirable for the Convention to define what was meant by personal status. The question was undoubtedly a very complex one, and might involve lengthy discussion."

[301] The Israeli delegate argued that the Committee "would have to choose between an ideal convention, which would obtain only a few signatures, and a less satisfactory document which would be ratified by a greater number of States. If the Committee did not want the convention to become a dead letter, it must place a limit upon its ambitions": Statement of Mr. Robinson of Israel, UN Doc. E/AC.32/SR.9, Jan. 24, 1950, at 6.

[302] "[I]t would be dangerous for the Ad Hoc Committee to follow the course advocated by the Chairman … Indeed, it was unlikely that such a definition would be in harmony with the various legislations of the States signatories … Such a notion should not … be defined in a convention dealing solely with refugees, but rather in an instrument dealing with private international law in general": Statement of Mr. Rain of France, ibid. at 4. See also Statement of Sir Leslie Brass of the United Kingdom, ibid. at 5: "He did not consider that the members of the Committee were competent to work out definitions of that kind."

[303] Statement of Mr. Larsen of Denmark, ibid. at 4.

[304] Statement of Mr. Robinson of Israel, ibid. at 8. See also Statements of Sir Leslie Brass of the United Kingdom, ibid.; Mr. Kural of Turkey, ibid.; and Mr. Rain of France, ibid. at 9.

[305] United Nations, "Statelessness," at 24.   [306] Ibid.

[307] See text below, at pp. 221–222.

woman might find – if reference were made by the reception state to the rules on status in the country of origin – that "[s]he [could] neither sign a lease, acquire property nor open a bank account. Her economic activity [would be] hampered and her chances of settling down and becoming assimilated [would be] jeopardized."[308] By virtue of Art. 12, however, the refugee woman is entitled to have her personal status assessed by reference to the norms prevailing in her new country of domicile (or residence, if domicile had yet to be acquired). Similarly, a refugee coming from a country in which the age of majority is, for example, twenty-one years old to an asylum state in which an individual is deemed an adult at eighteen years old, is entitled to the benefit of that lower age of majority.

The second head of personal status identified in the Study is status relevant to "family rights (marriage, divorce, recognition and adoption of children, etc.) . . . [and] [t]he matrimonial regime in so far as this is not considered a part of the law of contracts."[309] It seems clear that these forms of status were uppermost in the minds of the drafters,[310] in particular because some states had taken the view that the non-citizen status of refugees meant that authorities in the asylum country could not apply their own rules to decide on eligibility for entry into or dissolution of a marriage.[311] But by virtue of Art. 12's stipulation that the personal status of refugees is to be governed by the rules of the domicile state, "[t]he authorities of the country of [domicile] will therefore be competent to celebrate marriages in accordance with the rules regarding form and substance of the place where the marriage is celebrated. Similarly courts will be competent to decree divorces in accordance with the *lex fori* establishing the conditions for divorce."[312] The breadth of relevant forms of status is clear from the explanatory notes to the paragraph of the draft article originally specifically devoted to family law matters, which observed "that personal status includes family law (that is to say filiation, adoption, legitimation, parental authority, guardianship and curatorship, marriage and divorce) and the law concerning successions."[313] While this paragraph was later deleted as a superfluous elaboration of the basic rule set out in paragraph 1, it is clear that there was agreement that a broad-ranging set of refugee family law status concerns is to be governed

---

[308] United Nations, "Statelessness," at 25.   [309] Ibid. at 24.

[310] See text above, at pp. 211–212.

[311] Among the specific concerns identified in the Study were requirements to produce identity or other documents available only from the authorities of the country of origin, the production of civil registration documents, and possession of particular kinds of residence permits: United Nations, "Statelessness," at 25–26.

[312] Ibid. at 25.   [313] Secretary-General, "Memorandum," at 25.

by the law of the domicile state,[314] whatever the rules generally applicable to other non-citizens.[315]

Third and finally, the Study suggests that Art. 12 governs personal status relevant to issues of "[s]uccession and inheritance in regard to movable and in some cases to immovable property."[316] Specific reference was required because of the ambiguity about whether such concerns were squarely matters of family law status.[317] The ambivalent phrasing ("and in some cases to immovable property") follows from the fact that inheritance of real property is not in all jurisdictions a matter regulated by personal status.[318] Clearly, the duty to assess a refugee's personal status by reference to the rules of the domicile state gives the refugee no practical advantage where personal status is not relevant (for citizens or others) to particular forms of succession or inheritance.

[314] Some substantive concerns were raised in relation to the details of the proposed Art. 12(2) (see e.g. the comments of Mr. Guerreiro of Brazil, UN Doc. E/AC/32/SR.9, Jan. 24, 1950, at 5). But in the end, no objection was taken to the request of the representative of the International Refugee Organization "to include in the Committee's report a paragraph explaining that paragraph 2 had been deleted because, in the opinion of the Committee, paragraph 1 fully covered the points raised in paragraph 2 and also because the law differed considerably in various States, particularly with regard to the questions referred to in paragraph 2. The report might then state that the Committee had unanimously agreed that the questions dealt with in paragraph 2 ought not to be governed by the rules concerning the substance, form and competence of the national law, even in the countries in which such questions were usually governed by that law": Statement of Mr. Weis of the IRO, ibid. at 13–14. The actual text of the relevant passage in the Committee's report is significantly more succinct. It notes simply that "[t]he Committee decided that it was not necessary to include a specific reference to family law, as this was covered by paragraph 1": Ad Hoc Committee, "First Session Report," at Annex II.

[315] "[T]he main purpose was to regulate the position of those countries where aliens were subject to their own national law": Statement of Sir Leslie Brass of the United Kingdom, UN Doc. E/AC.32/SR.9, Jan. 24, 1950, at 9. This was unequivocally accepted by, for example, the French delegate, who agreed that "there could be no further question of applying national law to the personal status of refugees and there was no distinction to be made between the various countries": Statement of Mr. Rain of France, ibid.

[316] United Nations, "Statelessness," at 24.

[317] The French delegate posed a question (which was never answered on the record) to the Secretariat, namely "whether it considered that the law of succession was part of family law and whether it should therefore be understood that the rules of substance of the country of domicile ... applied both to family law, particularly to the celebration and dissolution of marriage, and to the law of succession": Statement of Mr. Rain of France, UN Doc. E/AC.32/SR.9, Jan. 24, 1950, at 6.

[318] "In matters of succession ... the transfer of real estate [in Brazil] was carried out in accordance with the legislation of the country where the real estate was, and not in accordance with that of the refugee's country of domicile": Statement of Mr. Guerreiro of Brazil, ibid. at 5.

It should be emphasized that these three forms of personal status – namely, status relevant to personal capacity, family rights and the matrimonial regime, and succession and inheritance – were agreed to simply as general points of reference.[319] They neither bind states as a matter of formal law, nor restrict the forms of personal status potentially governed by Art. 12.[320]

The final concern of Art. 12, addressed by para. 2, is to avoid situations in which the determination of a refugee's personal status by reference to the rules of the domicile country would result in the impairment of rights acquired by the refugee in his or her country of origin.[321] Under this provision, "[r]ights previously acquired by a refugee and dependent on personal status, more particularly rights attaching to marriage, shall be respected by a Contracting State." Two matters were of particular concern.

First, it was felt "undesirable to modify without reason the capacity of married women or the matrimonial regime."[322] To the extent that the position of women in the country of origin was superior to that which prevailed in the asylum state, application of the general rule of Art. 12 (that is, determination of personal status on the basis of the rules of the country of domicile) might result in a deprivation of acquired rights:

> At the time of their marriage these women may have been residing in their country of origin and have possessed the nationality of that country. In many cases, under their national law, marriage did not diminish their capacity but required the complete separation of the property of each spouse. Having become [a refugee] and being resident in a reception country the law of which restricts the capacity of married women and, where there is no marriage contract, requires the married couple to observe a matrimonial regime differing from that of separate estate, a woman in this position often finds her rights actually disputed.[323]

---

[319] See text above, at p. 218.

[320] Indeed, the British representative observed "that the definition given in the Secretariat study gave only a very vague idea of the concept of personal status": Statement of Sir Leslie Brass of the United Kingdom, UN Doc. E/AC.32/SR.9, Jan. 24, 1950, at 8. The Turkish delegate concurred, noting that "[i]n point of fact, the concept of personal status would be determined by the laws and customs of each country, with due regard to the preparatory work of the convention": Statement of Mr. Kural of Turkey, ibid.

[321] "Paragraph 2 is the result of the generally accepted validity of 'acquired (or vested) rights' which ought not be disturbed": Robinson, *History*, at 103.

[322] Secretary-General, "Memorandum," at 26. See also Statement of Mr. Weis of the International Refugee Organization, UN Doc. E/AC.32/SR.36, Aug. 15, 1950, at 8: "[P]aragraph 2 provided for exceptional treatment for refugees in a very narrow field ... The paragraph as a whole mainly concerned property rights connected with marriage, in respect of which it would be difficult for refugees to comply with the law of their country of domicile."

[323] United Nations, "Statelessness," at 25.

Second, the French representative voiced his desire to ensure respect for spousal rights resulting from "the acts of religious authorities to whom refugees were amenable, if performed in countries admitting the competence of such authorities."[324] If only secular marriage were authorized in the asylum state, a refugee couple might find that its union was not recognized there.

In each case, there was agreement that it would be inappropriate to allow the operation of the general rule in Art. 12 to deprive the refugee of his or her status-based acquired rights.[325] In a fundamental sense, then, Art. 12(2) goes a substantial distance towards meeting the non-governmental concern expressed at the Conference of Plenipotentiaries that greater deference should be paid to the preferences of the refugees themselves about how their personal status should be determined.[326] While not allowing refugees to elect the basis upon which their personal status is decided, Art. 12 read as a whole will often give refugees the best of both worlds. For example, a woman who comes from a country where the separate legal identity of women is not recognized is entitled under Art. 12(1) to claim the benefit of a more progressive status regime in her new country of domicile. But if the status of women is inferior in the domicile state to that which prevailed in her state of origin, she may nonetheless invoke Art. 12(2) to insist on respect for rights previously acquired under the more favorable regime.

In its original form, Art. 12(2) would have safeguarded "[r]ights acquired under a law other than the law of the country of domicile."[327] On the suggestion

---

[324] Statement of Mr. Rain of France, UN Doc. E/AC.32/SR.9, Jan. 23, 1950, at 14.

[325] Paragraph 2 of Art. 12 expressly exempts "[r]ights previously acquired by a refugee and dependent on personal status, *more particularly rights attaching to marriage* [emphasis added]." While less explicit than the Secretary-General's original draft (which set out that "rights attaching to marriage" included "matrimonial system, legal capacity of married women, etc.": Secretary-General, "Memorandum," at 24), the deletion of the explanatory language was without any evident substantive effect: Statement of Mr. Robinson of Israel, UN Doc. E/AC.32/SR.9, Jan. 24, 1950, at 15. Moreover, when the American representative suggested the deletion of the explicit reference to marital rights altogether, the Chairman successfully argued "that those rights were indeed of particular importance and that special reference should be made to them": Statement of the Chairman, Mr. Chance of Canada, ibid. On the question of marital rights acquired by virtue of a religious ceremony, the drafting history records that "[t]he Chairman explained, after consultation with the representative of the Assistant Secretary-General, that the Secretariat had considered that the provisions of [paragraph 2] covered all acquired rights including those resulting from the acts of religious authorities to whom the refugees were amenable, if performed in countries admitting the competence of such authorities": Statement of the Chairman, Mr. Chance of Canada, ibid. at 14. The French representative thereupon withdrew his amendment that would have explicitly made this point, "not because there was any intention to rescind those provisions but because they were covered by the general terms of . . . the Secretariat draft": Statement of Mr. Rain of France, ibid. at 15.

[326] See text above, p. 213.   [327] Secretary-General, "Memorandum," at 24.

of the Belgian representative,[328] and taking account of the British delegate's insistence that the goal of Art. 12(2) was to ensure that "an individual's personal status and acquired rights before he became a refugee should be respected,"[329] the Second Session of the Ad Hoc Committee amended the text to refer to rights "previously acquired."[330] The essential concern was that while refugees should not forfeit status-based rights acquired prior to their admission to their new state of domicile, asylum states should not be obligated to respect any rights acquired by a refugee who might choose to leave his or her new domicile state temporarily in order to acquire rights not available in that country.

This point was expressly canvassed during debate on a (subsequently deleted) paragraph which stipulated that "[w]ills made by refugees ... in countries other than the reception country, in accordance with the laws of such countries, shall be recognized as valid."[331] While the explanatory comment on the paragraph made clear that its purpose was to preserve the legal force of wills made by the refugee pre-departure, but which had not been amended to conform to the specific requirements of the state of reception,[332] the Belgian delegate observed that there might well be a conflict between the text itself and its principled objective:

> Thus in the case of a Polish refugee who had spent some time in Germany and had then taken up permanent residence in Belgium, a will made in Poland would, according to the comment, be valid in Belgium, whereas according to [the text] it would be valid if it had been made either in Poland or in Germany.[333]

In the discussion that followed, the essence of the Belgian delegate's concern was recognized. But it was made clear that the key question was temporal, not jurisdictional. Mr. Larsen of Denmark, for example,

> considered that it was reasonable to include in the article relating to the personal status of refugees a provision guaranteeing the validity of wills made by them *before their arrival in the countries which became their country of domicile or residence*. On the other hand, he did not see why that provision should be drafted so as to grant the refugees, after their arrival

---

[328] Statement of Mr. Herment of Belgium, UN Doc. E/AC.32/SR.36, Aug. 15, 1950, at 4.

[329] Statement of Sir Leslie Brass of the United Kingdom, ibid. at 8.

[330] Ad Hoc Committee, "Second Session Report," at 17.

[331] Secretary-General, "Memorandum," at 24.

[332] "It frequently happens that refugees have made a will in their country of origin in accordance with the provisions of the law of that country and are convinced that the will they brought away with them remains valid. The will may not however conform to the rules as regards form and substance of the country of residence. As a result, persons who believe they have taken the necessary steps to protect the interests of their next of kin die intestate": ibid. at 26.

[333] Statement of Mr. Cuvelier of Belgium, UN Doc. E/AC.32/SR.9, Jan. 24, 1950, at 17.

in the country of domicile or of residence, the privilege of making wills in other countries in accordance with the laws of those countries and of having those wills recognized as valid in the reception countries; privileges of that nature were never granted to aliens and there was consequently no reason why they should be given to refugees [emphasis added].[334]

Similarly, the Chairman and the French representative affirmed that the focus should be on whether the will had been drawn up prior to arrival in the asylum country, whether in the state of origin or elsewhere.[335] A purposive interpretation of Art. 12(2) would thus safeguard status-based rights acquired prior to arrival in the asylum country, whether in the refugee's state of origin or in any intermediate country.

The decision to delete a specific textual reference to the continuing validity of wills made by refugees before arrival in the asylum state was reached for two reasons.[336] On the one hand, it was felt that there was no need to affirm the legality of wills simply because the formalities of their execution abroad did not correspond with those of the domicile state.[337] As the Belgian representative observed, "if the only purpose of [the provision] was to recall the principle *locus regit actum*, the paragraph was wholly unnecessary, inasmuch as the principle was generally recognized and respected."[338] Conversely, there was no agreement to honor refugee wills executed prior

---

[334] Statement of Mr. Larsen of Denmark, ibid. at 17. See also Statement of Mr. Rain of France, ibid. at 19: "A refugee who had made a will in his country of origin *or in transit* thought that his will was valid ... That was what the text said; that was, in fact, what should be said. The only amendment necessary was to make it clear that the provision applied to wills made before arrival in the country of reception [emphasis added]."

[335] "[I]f the provision were made only for wills drawn up in the country of origin, [the paragraph] would be of academic interest only; there was every reason to believe that the country of origin would not be prepared to allow the heirs to take possession of the property left to them, even if it was still in existence": Statement of the Chairman, Mr. Chance of Canada, ibid. at 19.

[336] It is important to note, however, that "the vote in favour of the deletion of the reference to wills should not be interpreted as weakening in any way the force of the paragraph ... dealing with acquired rights": Statement of Mr. Rain of France, UN Doc. E/AC.32/SR.10, Jan. 24, 1950, at 4. In response, "[t]he Chairman confirmed Mr. Rain's interpretation of the vote. The reference to wills had been deleted because it would entail conflict with domestic law. The courts of reception countries could be relied upon to deal fairly with refugees in the matter": Statement of the Chairman, Mr. Chance of Canada, ibid.

[337] "[T]here seemed to be general agreement regarding the validity of wills made by refugees in their country of origin in so far as the form was concerned": Statement of Mr. Cuvelier of Belgium, ibid. at 3.

[338] Statement of Mr. Cuvelier of Belgium, UN Doc. E/AC.32/SR.9, Jan. 24, 1950, at 18. The Secretariat had, in fact, suggested that this was the sole purpose of the paragraph. "[T]he Secretariat had intended to refer to the form of a will rather than to its provisions. For example, the will of a Russian refugee in France would be recognized as valid with respect to form; the validity of its provisions, however, would have to be determined according to local law or, in the case of landed property, according to the law of the country in which the property was situated": Statement of Mr. Giraud of the Secretariat, ibid. In fact, however, the explanatory notes to the draft under consideration make clear that the

to arrival to the extent that they contained substantive provisions contrary to the laws of the asylum state.[339] The British representative

> feared that the proposal would actually permit the refugee, by his will, to alter the law of the reception country. For example . . . a refugee residing in England could, by means of a will made in his country of origin, tie up property in England in perpetuity.[340]

The example provided by the Danish delegate was perhaps more poignant:

> Some countries, such as Denmark, did not allow the testator to disinherit his children; the children must be assured of their rightful share, and the testator could dispose freely of the remaining portion only. Other countries, such as the United Kingdom, allowed the testator to dispose of the whole of his estate as he pleased.[341]

In the end, the drafters acknowledged only a commitment in principle to encourage courts in asylum countries "wherever possible, [to] give effect to the wishes of the [refugee] testator."[342] On matters of substance, however, most states felt that the substantive validity of refugee wills should be subject to the usual legal and public policy concerns pertaining in the asylum country.[343]

Indeed, the drafters agreed to a public policy limitation on the duty to honor the previously acquired status-based rights of refugees. Following from the debate about refugee wills, it was agreed by the Ad Hoc Committee "that the article did not require rights previously acquired by a refugee to be recognized by a country if its law did not recognize them on grounds of public policy or otherwise. It had been decided that the provisions of the article were in any case subject to that general reservation, which was implied and need not therefore be written into it."[344] The Conference of Plenipotentiaries, however, decided to make the public policy limitation

---

paragraph was intended to safeguard refugee wills "as regards form and substance": Secretary-General, "Memorandum," at 26.

[339] "A will drawn up in the country of origin might contain clauses which were not in conformity with the laws of the country of residence, particularly those dealing with public order": Statement of Mr. Henkin of the United States, UN Doc. E/AC.32/SR.10, Jan. 24, 1950, at 2.

[340] Statement of Sir Leslie Brass of the United Kingdom, ibid. at 3.

[341] Statement of Mr. Larsen of Denmark, UN Doc. E/AC.32/SR.9, Jan. 24, 1950, at 17.

[342] Ad Hoc Committee, "First Session Report," at Annex II.

[343] "The Chairman, speaking as the representative of Canada, acknowledged that the Government of the reception country would have to make some derogation to domestic law, thus placing the refugee in a favoured position. It might therefore be wiser to delete [the specific reference to refugee wills]": Statement of Mr. Chance of Canada, UN Doc. E/AC.32/SR.10, Jan. 24, 1950, at 3. The provision was thereupon deleted by a vote of 7–2 (2 abstentions): ibid.

[344] Statement of Sir Leslie Brass of the United Kingdom, UN Doc. E/AC.32/SR.41, Aug. 23, 1950, at 8. See also Statement of Mr. Weis of the International Refugee Organization, UN Doc. E/AC.32/SR.36, Aug. 15, 1950, at 9: "He wondered whether . . . rights [should be

explicit. Mr. Hoare of the United Kingdom proposed that the phrase, "provided the right is one which would have been recognized by the law of that State had he not become a refugee,"[345] be added to Art. 12(2). This amendment would meet his concern

> that States should not be required to respect rights previously acquired by a refugee when they were contrary to their own legislation. A State could not protect a right which was contrary to its own public policy.[346]

The specific example considered by the Conference was "the position of a divorced refugee who had obtained his divorce in a country the national legislation of which recognized divorce, but [who] was resident in a country, like Italy, where divorce was not recognized."[347] It was agreed that the asylum country could not reasonably be asked to issue documentation certifying the divorce, since "if a particular country did not recognize divorce, it could not possibly issue a certificate authenticating such a status ... [T]he right [must be] one which would have been recognized by the law of the particular State had the person in question [not] become a refugee."[348] This may be technically right, since Art. 12(2) requires only respect for previously acquired, status-based rights, not an affirmative duty to certify such entitlements.

Of more concern, however, the Belgian and French representatives opined that "[t]he purpose of the United Kingdom amendment was to place refugees on the same footing as aliens in respect of rights dependent on personal status ... [I]n the case cited by the French representative the courts of the receiving country would have to decide whether they would have recognized a divorce granted in the same circumstances to two aliens who were not refugees."[349] While the context of the remark suggests a more limited purport,[350] the comment as stated cannot be reconciled to the text of Art. 12, read as a whole.

made] dependent not only on compliance with the formalities prescribed by the law of the country of domicile but also on the [exigencies] of public order."

[345] Statement of Mr. Hoare of the United Kingdom, UN Doc. A/CONF.2/SR.25, July 17, 1951, at 4.

[346] Statement of Mr. Hoare of the United Kingdom, UN Doc. A/CONF.2/SR.7, July 5, 1951, at 13. See also Statements of Mr. Schurch of Switzerland, ibid. at 12: "Swiss law recognized acquired rights, but only subject to provisions concerning public order"; and the President, Mr. Larsen of Denmark, ibid. at 15: "It was essential to make some provision ensuring that such rights did not conflict with the legislation of the country in which the refugee became domiciled."

[347] Statement of Mr. Rochefort of France, UN Doc. A/CONF.2/SR.25, July 17, 1951, at 4–5.

[348] Statement of Mr. Hoare of the United Kingdom, ibid. at 5.

[349] Statement of Mr. Herment of Belgium, ibid. at 5–6. See also Statement of Mr. Rochefort of France, ibid. at 6.

[350] "[I]n principle States which forbad divorce did so only to their own nationals. It was solely for reasons of public order that a State might decide not to recognize divorces

The essential reason for Art. 12 is precisely to exempt refugees from the rules ordinarily applying to (non-refugee) aliens,[351] not to assimilate them to aliens. And while the British amendment – which was unfortunately not discussed further before being approved by the Conference[352] – was clearly intended to authorize state parties to refrain from the recognition of forms of previously acquired status which "was contrary to its own public policy,"[353] there is absolutely no basis to assert that its goal was to undermine the already agreed, essential goals of Art. 12. Thus, a reception state which does not recognize divorce as a matter of public law or policy cannot be compelled by virtue of Art. 12(2) to recognize a refugee's rights flowing from divorce.[354] If, on the other hand, the reception state has no domestic impediment to divorce, but refrains for policy reasons from recognizing the rights following from the divorce abroad of non-citizens, it would nonetheless be required by Art. 12(2) to recognize the rights of refugees accruing from divorce. In essence, the only legal or public policy concerns which are relevant to Art. 12(2) are those which apply generally in the reception state, not those which apply to non-citizens or a subset thereof. Robinson, for example, suggests that "rights resulting from polygamy in a country where it is prohibited"[355] could legitimately be resisted under the public policy exception to Art. 12(2).

The final requirement for availment by a refugee of Art. 12(2) is that he or she comply, "if this be necessary, with the formalities required by the law of [the contracting] State." This requirement was in the original draft of the Convention, and mirrors the precedents of the 1933 and 1938 Refugee Conventions.[356] The essential purpose of this requirement is "to protect the interests of third parties."[357]

---

between foreigners or not to authorize them to divorce in its territory": Statement of Mr. Herment of Belgium, ibid. at 5.

[351] See text above, at pp. 210–211. See also Weis, *Travaux*, at 107: "The main intent of the provision is, indeed, to subtract the refugee from the application of the law of the country of his nationality, considering that they have left that country and that that law may have undergone changes with which the refugees do not agree."

[352] See UN Doc. A/CONF.2/SR.25, July 17, 1951, at 9.

[353] Statement of Mr. Hoare of the United Kingdom, UN Doc. A/CONF.2/SR.7, July 5, 1951, at 13.

[354] It may be, however, that a general prohibition of divorce is no longer permitted under international law. "A special problem . . . results from the question of the permissibility of prohibitions of divorce, as continue to exist in some States influenced by Canon law . . . The systematic analysis of Art. 23 [of the Civil and Political Covenant] in light of its wording as compared with similar provisions under international law and its historical background . . . leads to the result that an *absolute divorce prohibition* in conjunction with the precept of monogamy – i.e., when persons who are in agreement that their marriage is ruined are compelled by the State to lead a new family life without the statutory protection of a 'legal family' – not only constitutes interference with private and family life pursuant to Art. 17, but also *violates their right to marry* pursuant to Art. 23(2) [emphasis in original]": M. Nowak, *UN Covenant on Civil and Political Rights* (1993) (Nowak, *ICCPR Commentary*), at 412.

[355] Robinson, *History*, at 103.   [356] Secretary-General, "Memorandum," at 26.   [357] Ibid.

Robinson suggests, for example, that "the law of the country in which recognition is sought may prescribe that foreign adoptions have to be confirmed by [a] local court or that the special matrimonial regime (separation of property or the right of the husband to administer the property of his wife) be registered in certain records."[358] This requirement is thus not a substantive limitation on the scope of Art. 12(2) rights, but merely an acknowledgment that a refugee's previously acquired rights are not immune from the asylum state's usual requirements to register or otherwise give general notice of the existence of rights as a condition precedent to their invocation.

3.3 Exceptional standards of treatment

Where refugee rights are guaranteed in the Convention only at the baseline level of assimilation to aliens generally – rights to internal freedom of movement, property, self-employment, professional practice, housing, and post-primary education[359] – the net value of the Refugee Convention may indeed be minimal. For the most part, states are required to grant these rights to refugees only to the extent they have freely chosen to extend comparable entitlements to other admitted aliens. Conversely, if only citizens or most-favored foreigners (or no non-citizens at all) are entitled to these rights, they may legitimately be denied to refugees. As the American representative to the Ad Hoc Committee succinctly observed, "when the Convention gave refugees the same privileges as aliens in general, it was not giving them very much."[360]

The major caveat to this conclusion follows from the fact that the general standard of treatment under Art. 7(1) incorporates by reference all general norms of international law. As noted above, this means that general principles both of international aliens law and of international human rights law accrue automatically to the benefit of refugees.[361] International aliens law adds to the baseline standard of treatment at least in a negative sense: while refugees need not be granted the right to acquire private property, their legitimately acquired property may not be taken from them without adequate compensation.[362] As there is still no agreement on the codification of an affirmative right to own private property as a matter of international human rights law, even this modest protection is of some value.[363]

In most cases, general norms of international human rights law are of the greatest value in supplementing the content of refugee rights defined at the

---

[358] Robinson, *History*, at 104.   [359] See chapter 3.2.1 above, at pp. 198–199.
[360] Statement of Mr. Henkin of the United States, UN Doc. E/AC.32/SR.37, Aug. 16, 1950, at 7.
[361] See chapter 3.2.1 above, at p. 197.   [362] See chapter 2.1 above, at p. 77.
[363] The right of refugees to protection of property is discussed below, at chapter 4.5.1.

"aliens generally" standard of treatment.[364] For example, the Civil and Political Covenant guarantees freedom of internal movement to "everyone" lawfully within a state's territory, subject only to specific types of limits applied on a non-discriminatory basis.[365] By virtue of Art. 7(1) of the Refugee Convention, once refugees are lawfully present – that is, once they have been admitted to a status verification procedure, temporary protection regime, or authorized de facto to remain without investigation of their need for protection[366] – any continuing constraints on internal freedom of movement must thereafter be justified by reference to the standards of the Civil and Political Covenant.[367]

Similarly, the other four refugee rights defined at the "aliens generally" baseline standard of treatment – rights to self-employment, professional practice, housing, and secondary and higher education – are the subject of cognate rights in the Economic, Social and Cultural Covenant.[368] At least in developed states, the incorporation by reference of these norms under Art. 7(1) of the Refugee Convention means that the rights must be guaranteed on the terms set by the Covenant to refugees without discrimination.[369] But as previously noted, because the Economic, Social and Cultural Covenant authorizes less developed states to withhold economic rights from non-citizens,[370] the dilemma for the majority of refugees who are protected in such states may be acute.

Happily, most rights in the 1951 Convention are to be extended to refugees not at the baseline standard, but at a higher standard: on par with the rights extended to most-favored foreigners, to the same extent granted citizens of the asylum state, or simply in absolute terms. Where a right is defined to require treatment at any of these higher levels, protections beyond the general standard accrue to refugees.[371] By explicitly requiring states to meet an

---

[364] See chapters 1.2 and 2.5.4 above.

[365] Civil and Political Covenant, at Arts. 12 and 2(1). As previously noted, aliens have been held by the Human Rights Committee to benefit from protection against discrimination on the grounds of "other status": see chapter 2.5.5 above, at p. 127.

[366] See chapter 3.1.3 above.

[367] The right of refugees to enjoy internal freedom of movement is discussed below, at chapters 4.2.4 and 5.2.

[368] Economic, Social and Cultural Covenant, at Arts. 6(1), 11(1), and 13(2)(b).

[369] The broad margin of appreciation afforded states under prevailing notions of non-discrimination law remains problematic, however. See chapter 2.5.5 above, at pp. 129–145.

[370] See chapter 2.5.4 above, at p. 122.

[371] "[A] distinction should be made between the clause relating to exemption from reciprocity and the provisions of some articles which specified whether refugees should be accorded the most favorable treatment or be subject to the ordinary law. Where such provisions were set forth in an article there was no need to invoke the clause on exemption from reciprocity. It was obvious, in fact, that where refugees were accorded the most favorable treatment there would be no point in invoking the clause respecting exemption from reciprocity": Statement of Mr. Giraud of the Secretariat,

exceptional standard of treatment, the Convention requires that refugees benefit from treatment superior to that enjoyed by aliens generally.[372] Indeed, the pervasive incorporation of these exceptional standards of treatment means that the Refugee Convention is in many ways at least as generous – and in some cases, more generous – than earlier refugee conventions which relied simply on a waiver of requirements of reciprocity for refugees.

3.3.1 Most-favored-national treatment

Two rights in the Refugee Convention – the rights to freedom of non-political association[373] and to engage in wage-earning employment[374] – are guaranteed to refugees to the same extent enjoyed by most-favored foreigners.[375] This means that refugees may automatically claim the benefit of all guarantees of associative freedom and to engage in employment extended to the nationals of any foreign state. Refugees may nonetheless still be granted less favorable treatment in relation to these rights than that enjoyed by citizens of the host country, subject to the requirements of general non-discrimination law.[376]

As earlier observed, governments were not prepared routinely to assimilate refugees to the citizens of states with which they had special economic or political relationships.[377] There was a general belief, however, that the right to work (and the related right to freedom of association, particularly to join trade unions) warranted treatment at this standard. In proposing that

UN Doc. E/AC.32/SR.11, Jan. 25, 1950, at 5–6. The representative of the United Kingdom took the lead on this issue, noting that he "did not see how there could be any question of a reciprocity provision applying except in cases where the treatment of the refugee was to be the same as that accorded to foreigners generally": Statement of Sir Leslie Brass of the United Kingdom, UN Doc. E/AC.32/SR.23, Feb. 3, 1950, at 4–5. This led the Chairman to observe that "the draft proposed by the United Kingdom representative accurately stated what was in the minds of the Committee members and he would therefore invite them to accept it": Statement of the Chairman, Mr. Chance of Canada, ibid. at 6.

[372] See e.g. Statement of Mr. Henkin of the United States, UN Doc. E/AC.32/SR.36, Aug. 15, 1950, at 11: "His delegation believed that refugees should be treated better than other aliens in some respects, and that the provisions in the draft Convention which accorded better treatment to refugees than to aliens were not of such major importance as to create grave problems for many countries. Therefore, if it could be agreed that in general a minimum treatment should be accorded to refugees and that that treatment should be no worse that that given to aliens in general, and that in some respects the refugees should even have certain advantages, the articles could safely be left to the Drafting Committee."

[373] The rights of refugees to freedom of expression and association are discussed below, at chapter 6.7.

[374] The right of refugees to engage in wage-earning employment is discussed below, at chapter 6.1.

[375] Refugee Convention, at Arts. 15, 17(1).   [376] See chapter 2.5.5 above.

[377] See chapter 3.2.1 above, at pp. 197–199.

refugees enjoy preferred access to the right to work, the French representative observed that

> it was legitimate and desirable to accord the most favourable treatment to refugees to engage in wage-earning employment, and not only the treatment accorded to foreigners generally, because refugees by their very nature were denied the support of their Governments and could not hope for governmental intervention in their favour in obtaining exceptions to the general rule by means of conventions. France was thus merely being faithful to the spirit which had heretofore guided United Nations action in favour of refugees: the purpose of that action was to obtain for refugees the advantages which Governments sought to have granted to their own subjects.[378]

As the American representative to the Ad Hoc Committee put it, "without the right to work, all other rights were meaningless."[379]

The Committee therefore agreed to break with precedent,[380] and based the Convention's right to work on a French proposal that refugees be granted "the most favourable treatment given to nationals of a foreign country."[381] Governments accepted this exceptional standard of treatment with clear awareness of the impact of their decision. In its comments on the Ad Hoc Committee's draft, for example, Austria recognized that the standard amounted to a "most favoured nation clause" that would require that "hundreds of thousands of refugees" be assimilated to the "relatively small" number of foreigners traditionally granted most-favored-national access to employment.[382] The United Kingdom commented that this standard would mean that refugees would be allowed to work as steamship pilots, a job traditionally reserved for British and French citizens.[383] Belgium insisted that it would be forced to enter a reservation to the article "in view of the economic and customs agreements existing between Belgium and certain neighbouring countries."[384] Norway indicated that it, too, would have to

---

[378] Statement of Mr. Rain of France, UN Doc. E/AC.32/SR.13, Jan. 26, 1950, at 2.

[379] Statement of Mr. Henkin of the United States, UN Doc. E/AC.32/SR.37, Aug. 16, 1950, at 12.

[380] "[T]he text proposed by the French delegation represented an advance upon the provisions of previous conventions ... While it was understandable that some delegations should hesitate to accept the innovation ... it would be surprising if the Committee should wish to retreat from the results obtained by the previous Conventions, and to end with a text which would contribute nothing towards the improvement of the conditions of the refugee": Statement of Mr. Cuvelier of Belgium, UN Doc. E/AC.32/SR.13, Jan. 26, 1950, at 8–9.

[381] France, "Draft Convention," at 6.

[382] United Nations, "Compilation of Comments," at 43.

[383] Ibid. at 44; Statement of Sir Leslie Brass of the United Kingdom, UN Doc. E/AC.32/SR.13, Jan. 26, 1950, at 14.

[384] Statement of Mr. Herment of Belgium, UN Doc. A/CONF.2/SR.9, July 6, 1951, at 8.

reserve on the exceptional standard of treatment because of "the regional policy of the Scandinavian countries in respect of the labor market."[385]

The inevitability of reservations notwithstanding,[386] the President of the Conference of Plenipotentiaries appealed to states to "seek the golden mean, and, if possible, by precept and example, to encourage others to withdraw their reservations at a later stage. If the Conference worked along those lines he believed it might be possible to arrive at a just and effective instrument."[387] In the end, the Conference rejected the two extremes – assimilation of refugees to nationals,[388] and treatment at the residual standard of the rights of aliens generally[389] – and agreed that refugees would be entitled to engage in

---

[385] Statement of Mr. Anker of Norway, ibid. at 14.

[386] As observed by the Chairman of the Ad Hoc Committee, "[i]t had, of course, been realised that the inclusion of provisions which, without representing ideals to strive for, were too generous for some Governments to accept, would lead to their making reservations, but it had been thought that such a course might in the long run have a good effect even on Governments which felt themselves unable to accord the treatment prescribed in the Convention immediately upon signing it. Other such cases had arisen in the past where refugees and those who had the interests of refugees at heart had addressed appeals to Governments applying low standards, pointing to the higher standards applied by other Governments, and so had gradually produced an improvement in their policies": Statement of the Chairman, Mr. Larsen of Denmark, UN Doc. E/AC.32/SR.37, Aug. 16, 1950, at 11–12. In fact, a large number of states have entered either sweeping reservations or other major qualifications to the duty to treat refugees as most-favored nationals for purposes of either or both of Arts. 15 and 17. These include Austria, Bahamas, Belgium, Botswana, Ethiopia, Iran, Ireland, Latvia, Liechtenstein, Malawi, Mexico, Monaco, Papua New Guinea, Sierra Leone, Uganda, Zambia, and Zimbabwe. More modest qualifications have been entered by Angola, Chile, Denmark, Ecuador, Finland, France, Honduras, Jamaica, Madagascar, Mozambique, Norway, Sweden, and the United Kingdom. Yet Mr. Larsen's optimism has been partly borne out. The reservations to Art. 17 entered by Brazil, Greece, Italy, and Switzerland have been revoked: UNHCR, Declarations and Reservations to the 1951 Convention relating to the Status of Refugees, www.unhcr.ch (accessed July 15, 2003).

[387] Statement of the President, Mr. Larsen of Denmark, UN Doc. A/CONF.2/SR.9, July 6, 1951, at 14. As the American representative stated, it was best to "incorporate in the convention a clause providing for a real improvement in the refugees' [right to work], even if that clause were to result in reservations which, it might be hoped, would not be very numerous or extensive": Statement of Mr. Henkin of the United States, UN Doc. E/AC.32/SR.13, Jan. 26, 1950, at 8.

[388] This approach was strongly promoted by Yugoslavia, with the support of Germany. See UN Doc. A/CONF.2/SR.9, July 6, 1951, at 4–5.

[389] "A country such as Italy ... could definitely not consider assuring commitments regarding the employment or naturalization of foreign refugees, which could only add to the difficulties already confronting the Italian economy ... [T]he Italian Government could do no more than allow refugees to benefit by the laws and regulations concerning work, employment, salaried professions, insurance and so on, which at the moment applied to all aliens resident in Italy": Statement of Mr. Del Drago of Italy, ibid. at 9.

employment on the basis of "the most favourable treatment accorded to nationals of a foreign country in the same circumstances."[390]

In addition to the relevant references made by the drafters of the Convention,[391] a helpful sense of the breadth of this exceptional standard of treatment can be distilled from the text of the reservations and declarations entered by state parties which have not agreed to grant most-favored-national treatment to refugees. Most obviously, most-favored-national treatment includes the benefits of bilateral and multilateral arrangements with special partner states. The "preferential treatment" which the nationals of Brazil and Portugal enjoy in each other's territory;[392] the "privileges" of Danish, Finnish, Icelandic, Norwegian, and Swedish citizens in each of those countries;[393] and the "rights which, by law or by treaty" are granted by Spain to the nationals of Andorra, the Philippines, Portugal, and Latin America are examples.[394] The benefits of special regional and sub-regional arrangements are included[395] – for example, the privileges enjoyed by Central Americans in states of that area,[396] and nationals of states belonging to the East African Community and the African Union.[397] More generally, most-favored-national treatment includes any privileges accorded to foreign citizens under "special co-operation agreements,"[398] "commonwealth-type" arrangements,[399] "agreements . . . for the purpose of establishing special conditions for the transfer of labor,"[400] "establishment" treaties,[401] and by virtue of any "customs, economic or political agreements."[402] Perhaps most important, the very nature of the most-favored-national standard means that it is inherently subject to evolution. As observed by Robinson,

> the "most favorable treatment accorded to nationals of a foreign country" is a dynamic concept: it varies from country to country, and from time to time. Every new agreement with a foreign country may create a new basis

---

[390] Refugee Convention, at Art. 17(1). The language in Art. 15 (right of association) is the same.

[391] See text above, at pp. 231–232.

[392] See reservations of Brazil and Portugal: UNHCR, Declarations and Reservations to the 1951 Convention relating to the Status of Refugees, www.unhcr.ch (accessed July 15, 2003).

[393] See reservations of Denmark, Finland, Norway, and Sweden: ibid.

[394] See reservation of Spain: ibid.

[395] See reservations of Belgium, Guatemala, Iran, Luxembourg, Netherlands, Spain, and Uganda: ibid.

[396] See reservation of Guatemala: ibid.   [397] See reservation of Uganda: ibid.

[398] See reservation of Angola: ibid.

[399] See reservation of Portugal upon acceding to the Protocol: ibid. See also reservation of Spain, safeguarding special rights with the nationals of "the Latin American countries": ibid.

[400] See reservation of Norway: ibid.   [401] See reservation of Iran: ibid.

[402] See reservations of Belgium, Iran, Luxembourg, Netherlands: ibid.

for the treatment, and the expiration of existing conventions may reduce the scope of the treatment.[403]

3.3.2 National treatment

Refugees are to be assimilated to citizens of the asylum state for purposes of religious freedom,[404] the protection of artistic and industrial property rights,[405] entitlement to assistance to access the courts (including legal aid),[406] participation in rationing schemes,[407] enrolment in primary education,[408] inclusion in public welfare systems,[409] entitlement to the benefits of labor legislation and social security,[410] and for purposes of tax liability.[411] This exceptional standard of treatment explicitly proscribes any attempt to justify distinctions between the treatment of refugees and citizens, as these articles usually require that the rights afforded refugees be "the same" as those enjoyed by nationals.[412] Taxes imposed on refugees may not be "other or higher than those which are or may be levied on [the host state's] nationals in similar situations."[413] And perhaps most interesting, refugees enjoy "treatment at least as favorable as that accorded to … nationals"[414] to practice their religion and to ensure the religious education of their children. As elaborated below, this is the only provision in the Convention premised on an explicit commitment to substantive equality between refugees and citizens.[415]

With the exception of the right to religious freedom, each of these rights was defined to require assimilation to citizens in the first draft of the treaty proposed by the Secretary-General in January 1950.[416] The explanations provided there for requiring national treatment are instructive. In some

---

[403] Robinson, *History*, at 110.

[404] The right of refugees to freedom of religion is discussed below, at chapter 4.7.

[405] The right of refugees to the protection of intellectual property rights is discussed below, at chapter 6.5.

[406] The right of refugees to assistance to access the courts is discussed below, at chapter 6.8.

[407] The right of refugees to benefit from rationing systems is discussed below, at chapter 4.4.

[408] The right of refugees to education is discussed below, at chapter 4.8.

[409] The right of refugees to benefit from public welfare systems is discussed below, at chapter 6.3.

[410] The right of refugees to fair working conditions is discussed below, at chapter 6.1.2; the right to social security is discussed below, at chapter 6.1.3.

[411] The right of refugees to equity in taxation is discussed below, at chapter 4.5.2.

[412] Refugee Convention, at Arts. 14, 16(2), 20, 22(1), 23, and 24(1).

[413] Ibid. at Art. 29.   [414] Ibid. at Art. 4.

[415] Substantive equality may, however, be more generally required by virtue of the interaction of the Refugee Convention with Art. 26 of the Civil and Political Covenant. See chapter 2.5.5 above, at pp. 127–128.

[416] Secretary-General, "Memorandum."

cases, the goal was consistency with prior or cognate international law. Equality in regard to taxation had already been required by the 1933 Refugee Convention,[417] and there was a pattern of bilateral and multilateral treaties, including those negotiated under the auspices of the ILO, that assimilated aliens to nationals for purposes of social security.[418] There were practical reasons to grant refugees national treatment under labor legislation, namely that "it was in the interests of national wage-earners who might have been afraid [that] foreign labor, being cheaper than their own, would have been preferred."[419] Similarly, while the right of refugees to sue and be sued "in principle ... is not challenged, in practice there are insurmountable difficulties to the exercise of this right by needy refugees: the obligation to furnish *cautio judicatum solvi* and the refusal to grant refugees the benefit of legal assistance make this right illusory."[420]

In two cases, the importance of assimilation was cited to justify national treatment. Primary education should be available on terms of equality with nationals "because schools are the most rapid and most effective instrument of assimilation."[421] An appeal to principle was relied on to justify national treatment with regard to artistic and industrial property rights, "since intellectual and industrial property is the creation of the human mind and recognition is not a favour."[422] And finally, simple fairness was said to require the equal treatment of refugees and nationals with regard to both access to rationing and systems for public relief. Rationing regulated the distribution of items "of prime necessity,"[423] and "[p]ublic relief can hardly be refused to refugees who are destitute because of infirmity, illness or age."[424]

The one national treatment right added to the Secretary-General's list is the right to religious freedom. A non-governmental representative to the Conference of Plenipotentiaries noted that "the negative principle of non-discrimination as expressed in article 3" did not "ensure the development of the refugee's personality."[425] It was important, he suggested, that the Convention contain a "positive definition of the spiritual and religious freedom of the refugee."[426] The delegates to the Conference agreed, noting that religious freedom conceived in affirmative terms is an "inalienable"[427] right.

---

[417] Ibid. at 31.   [418] Ibid. at 38.   [419] Ibid. at 37.   [420] Ibid. at 30.

[421] Ibid. at 38. It was also noted that primary education "satisfies an urgent need," in consequence of which it was already compulsory in most states: ibid.

[422] Ibid. at 27.   [423] Ibid. at 38.   [424] Ibid. at 39.

[425] Statement of Mr. Buensod of Pax Romana, UN Doc. A/CONF.2/SR.11, July 9, 1951, at 9–10.

[426] Ibid. at 10.

[427] Statements of Msgr. Comte of the Holy See and Mr. Montoya of Venezuela, UN Doc. A/CONF.2/SR.30, July 20, 1951, at 11–12.

There were nonetheless concerns that the first working draft, in which what became Art. 4 was framed as an absolute right,[428] imposed too stringent an obligation on states.[429] Yet it was recognized that the alternative of authorizing states to invoke regulatory or public order limits on religious freedom had, in practice, resulted in hardship for refugees. As the Canadian representative commented, "[i]t was well known that certain sects often committed in the name of their religion acts contrary to *l'ordre public et les bonnes moeurs.*"[430] The compromise position suggested by the President of the Conference was that refugees should benefit from "the same treatment in respect of religion and religious education . . . as . . . nationals."[431]

This approach was, however, rejected by the Conference. The Holy See argued that assimilation to nationals was insufficient because "in countries where religious liberty was circumscribed, refugees would suffer."[432] It was important, he said, "to guarantee refugees a minimum of religious liberty in such countries."[433] His point was not that refugees benefit from "preferential treatment" vis-à-vis citizens.[434] Nonetheless, purely formal parity with nationals was not sufficient:

> His sole concern was that [refugees] should be given equal treatment with nationals. It was known that, precisely on account of their position as refugees, they are frequently handicapped in the practice of their religion. It was with that consideration in mind that he had put forward his amendment.[435]

This argument for substantive equality led the representative of the Holy See to propose a unique standard of treatment, namely that refugees should enjoy

---

[428] "The Contracting States shall grant refugees within their territories complete freedom to practice their religion both in public and in private and to ensure that their children are taught the religion they profess": UN Doc. A/CONF.2/94.

[429] Egypt, Luxembourg, and the Netherlands all felt that an affirmative right to religious freedom should be subject to the requirements of "national law": Statements of Mr. Sturm of Luxembourg, Mr. Mostafa of Egypt, and Baron van Boetzelaer of the Netherlands, UN Doc. A/CONF.2/SR.30, July 20, 1951, at 11–14. Belgium and even the Holy See felt a "public order" limitation would be acceptable: Statements of Mr. Herment of Belgium and Msgr. Comte of the Holy See, ibid. at 14.

[430] Statement of Mr. Chance of Canada, ibid. at 17.

[431] Statement of the President, Mr. Larsen of Denmark, ibid. at 17.

[432] Statement of Msgr. Comte of the Holy See, UN Doc. A/CONF.2/SR.33, July 24, 1951, at 7.

[433] Ibid. The French representative agreed, but noted that such a position "had been rejected [in the Style Committee] on the grounds that Contracting States could not undertake to accord to refugees treatment more favorable than that they accorded to their own nationals": Statement of Mr. Rochefort of France, ibid. at 7–8. The British representative bluntly observed that the Holy See's approach might "be open to interpretation as an innuendo to the effect that the treatment of nationals in respect of religious freedom was not as liberal as it might be": Statement of Mr. Hoare of the United Kingdom, ibid. at 8.

[434] Statement of Msgr. Comte of the Holy See, ibid. at 8.   [435] Ibid.

"treatment at least as favorable as that accorded ... nationals."[436] Governments are thus obliged not to deny refugees any religious freedom enjoyed by citizens, and moreover commit themselves in principle to take measures going beyond strict formal equality in order to recognize "that religious freedom as an abstract principle might be of little value if divorced from the practical means of ensuring it."[437]

3.3.3 Absolute rights

The balance of the Refugee Convention's substantive rights[438] – that is, those defined to require treatment neither at the "aliens generally" baseline standard, nor at one of the two exceptional standards (assimilation to most-favored foreigners, or to the citizens of the asylum country) – are absolute obligations. For the most part, the decision not to set a contingent standard of treatment follows logically from the fact that there is no logical comparator group for these rights.[439] Refugees are, for example, entitled to turn to the host country for administrative assistance, identity papers, and travel documents (because, unlike both citizens and most aliens, refugees have no national state willing to provide them with such facilities).[440] Other rights follow from the unique nature of refugeehood: the right to avoid penalties for unauthorized entry, to avoid expulsion or *refoulement*, to the recognition of preexisting rights based on personal status, and to take assets abroad in the event of resettlement.[441]

The absolute nature of the right of refugees to access the courts of state parties[442] (though entitlement to legal aid and to waiver of technical requirements for access inheres in refugees only to the extent granted to citizens of the refugee's place of residence[443]) follows the precedents of international aliens law[444] and the 1933 Convention, and elicited no debate.[445] While Art. 34's provisions on the assimilation and naturalization of refugees are likewise subject to no contingency, there is really no substantive right contained in

---

[436] The Conference approved this revised language 20–0(1 abstention): ibid. at 9.

[437] Statement of Mr. Petren of Sweden, ibid. at 9. It is clear, however, that Art. 4 does not oblige governments to take specific affirmative measures to advance the religious freedom of refugees. See chapter 4.7 below, at pp. 582–583.

[438] A number of the Convention's articles do not establish free-standing rights, but define the context within which enumerated rights must be implemented. See Refugee Convention, at Arts. 2, 3, 5–12(1), and 35–46.

[439] See generally the discussion of absolute and contingent rights developed under international aliens law in chapter 2.1 above, at pp. 77–78.

[440] Refugee Convention, at Arts. 25, 27, and 28.   [441] Ibid. at Arts. 12(2), 30–33.

[442] Ibid. at Art. 16(1).   [443] Ibid. at Art. 16(2). See chapter 6.8 below.

[444] See chapter 2.1 above, at p. 77.

[445] "[I]n principle the right of a refugee to sue and be sued is not challenged": Secretary-General, "Memorandum" at 30.

this provision. State parties are encouraged to facilitate the integration of refugees, but are under no binding duty to do so.

3.4 Prohibition of discrimination between and among refugees

As previously described, the general purpose of the legal duty of non-discrimination is defined by Fredman as being to ensure "that individuals should be judged according to their personal qualities."[446] Consideration has already been given to such key questions as the differences between formal equality ("equality before the law") and substantive equality ("equal protection of the law"); the relative importance of intention and effects in assessing whether discrimination of either kind is demonstrated; and the extent to which international law requires positive efforts to remedy unjustifiable distinctions, rather than just a duty to desist from discriminatory conduct.[447] The earlier focus was on whether the broad duty of non-discrimination – in particular, that set by Art. 26 of the Civil and Political Covenant – might actually be sufficient in and of itself to require the equal protection of refugees and other non-citizens, in which case specific norms of aliens and refugee law might be rendered essentially superfluous. Based on a close examination of the jurisprudence of the Human Rights Committee, however, the conclusion was reached that despite its textual breadth, Art. 26 could not yet be relied upon dependably to enfranchise non-citizens. In particular, account was taken of the Committee's tendency simply to accept some categorical distinctions (often including non-citizenship) as an inherently reasonable basis upon which to treat people differently; a pattern of unjustifiably broad deference to national perceptions of reasonable justification; and, in particular, only a nascent preparedness to take seriously the discriminatory effects of facially neutral laws. The conclusion was therefore reached that despite its value to counter some types of differential treatment, non-discrimination law has not yet evolved to the point that refugees and other non-citizens can safely assume that it will provide a sufficient answer to the failure to grant them rights on par with citizens.

The analysis here draws on some of these same principles, but to investigate a different question. Even if many distinctions in the ways that non-citizens, including refugees, are treated relative to citizens are deemed reasonable, does the legal duty of non-discrimination nonetheless provide a meaningful response to more specific types of disfranchisement which may be experienced by subsets of the refugee population?

To a real extent, the inappropriateness of differential allocations of refugee rights is clear from the fact that the language of the Refugee Convention

---

[446] S. Fredman, *Discrimination Law* (2001) (Fredman, *Discrimination*), at 66.
[447] See chapter 2.5.5 above.

presupposes that whatever entitlements are held by virtue of refugee status should inhere in *all* refugees. In setting the refugee definition, the drafters of the Convention were at pains carefully to limit the beneficiary class. They excluded, for example, persons who have yet to leave their own country, who cannot link their predicament to civil or political status, who already benefit from surrogate national or international protection, or who are found not to deserve protection.[448] Beyond these explicit strictures, however, refugees are conceived as a generic class, all members of which are equally worthy of protection.

Yet there are in fact often significant differences in the way that particular subsets of Convention refugees are treated by states. Perhaps most commonly, differentiation is based upon nationality. Saudi Arabia recognized Iraqis displaced as a result of the Gulf War as refugees even as it left thousands of refugees from other countries within its borders without status, and summarily deported at-risk Somalis.[449] India has allowed Tibetan refugees full access to employment, but limited – in some cases severely – the opportunities to earn a livelihood for refugees from Sri Lanka and, in particular, those from Bangladesh.[450] The United States has a long-standing practice of dealing much more harshly with refugees arriving from Haiti than with those who come from Cuba. Most fundamentally, it pursues a formal policy of interdiction and routine detention of Haitian refugees at Guantanamo Bay, while simultaneously allowing Cuban refugees free access to its territory.[451]

---

[448] See generally Grahl-Madsen, *Status of Refugees I*; and Hathaway, *Refugee Status*.

[449] "The Saudi Arabian government contends that 'Islamic principles rather than international law' are the basis for its extension of haven to Iraqi refugees. The government has failed to sign the international treaties and instruments that protect refugees from forced repatriation. It has not articulated an official policy regarding refugees or asylum": Lawyers' Committee for Human Rights, *Asylum Under Attack: A Report on the Protection of Iraqi Refugees and Displaced Persons One Year After the Humanitarian Emergency in Iraq* (1992), at 64. More generally, a Canadian government report observed that "Saudi Arabia is ... known for its policies of discrimination against refugees in general, regardless of whether or not they are Muslims ... In March 1991, for example, shortly after the downfall of Mohamed Siad Barre and when fighting was fierce in both northern and southern Somalia, Saudi Arabia deported some 950 immigrant workers to Somalia": Immigration and Refugee Board Documentation, Information, and Research Branch, "Kenya, Djibouti, Yemen and Saudi Arabia: The Situation of Somali Refugees" (1992), at 5.

[450] Tibetan refugees have been issued certificates of identity which enable them to undertake gainful employment, and even to travel abroad and return to India. Sri Lankan refugees, in contrast, have been allowed to engage only in self-employment, while Bangladeshi refugees have not been allowed to undertake employment of any kind: B. Chimni, "The Legal Condition of Refugees in India," (1994) 7(4) *Journal of Refugee Studies* 378, at 393–394.

[451] As Naomi and Norman Zucker conclude, "the United States has singled out Cubans and Haitians for diametrically opposite treatment. Cubans who quit their island are assisted

Even when Haitian refugees manage to reach US territory, they are ineligible to seek release on bond and must have their claims assessed under the abbreviated "expedited removal" procedure, rather than under the usual refugee status assessment rules.[452] In another example of differential treatment based on nationality, the British government announced in 2002 that the citizens of three countries – Liberia, Libya, and Somalia – would no longer benefit from its usual practice of granting a right of permanent residence to recognized refugees.[453] The United Kingdom also ended in-country appeal rights for persons seeking refugee status from a list

in coming to the US, are called political refugees, and are given asylum, while Haitians who leave their island are labeled economic migrants, interdicted at sea, and returned to Haiti": N. and N. Zucker, "United States Admission Policies Toward Cuban and Haitian Migrants," paper presented at the Fourth International Research and Advisory Panel Conference, Oxford, Jan. 5–9, 1994, at 1. "After it was accused of discrimination, the Carter administration granted Haitians the status of 'entrants,' on par with Cubans; however, in mid-1981 the Reagan administration reinstated differential treatment and began incarcerating apprehended Haitians . . . [President Clinton] pledged to change the policy . . . [but he] reversed himself immediately after taking office to prevent a flood of refugees that would weaken his political base in Florida": A. Zolberg, "From Invitation to Interdiction: US Foreign Policy and Immigration since 1945," in M. Teitelbaum and M. Weiner eds., *Threatened Peoples, Threatened Borders: World Migration and US Policy* 144 (1995), at 145–146. The failure of the American judiciary to end the double standard is described in T. James, "A Human Tragedy: The Cuban and Haitian Refugee Crises Revisited," (1995) 9(3) *Georgetown Immigration Law Journal* 479. "If an interdicted Haitian does manage to communicate a fear of return, the Coast Guard notifies the INS, which transports an asylum officer to the ship in order to conduct a preliminary credible fear interview. If the asylum officer determines that the individual does have a credible fear of return, then the person is transferred to Guantanamo Bay, Cuba . . . The treatment afforded interdicted Haitians starkly contrasts with the enhanced procedures applied to interdicted Cubans and Chinese, both nationalities that have strong political allies in Washington, D. C.": Women's Commission for Refugee Women and Children, "Refugee Policy Adrift: The United States and Dominican Republic Deny Haitians Protection" (2003), at 18.

[452] Lawyers' Committee for Human Rights, *Imbalance of Powers: How Changes to US Law and Policies Since 9/11 Erode Human Rights and Civil Liberties* (2003), at 30. While the routine denial of access to full asylum procedures in theory applies to all refugees who arrive by sea, Cubans are expressly exempted from its provisions: US Department of Justice, "Notice Designating Aliens Subject to Expedited Removal Under Section 235(b)(1)(A)(iii) of the Immigration and Naturalization Act," Order No. 2243–0, Nov. 13, 2002. Because boat arrivals in the United States are mainly either Haitian or Cuban, the policy is effectively aimed at Haitian refugees. Amnesty International reported that the US government overtly defended this policy on the grounds that "it is longstanding US policy to treat Cubans differently from other aliens": Letter from Bill Frelick, Director, Refugee Program, Amnesty International USA, to Director, Regulations and Forms Services Division, Immigration and Naturalization Service, Dec. 13, 2002, at 2.

[453] A. Travis, "Blunkett plans to end asylum-seekers' automatic right to claim benefits," *Guardian*, Oct. 8, 2002, at 9.

of ten countries (those subsequently admitted to the European Union in 2004).[454]

Nationality-based exclusion may even be directed at all refugees coming from an entire region. For example, Uganda has granted protection to refugees coming from Ethiopia, Iraq, Sri Lanka, and Eritrea, but has shown indifference to the needs of refugees arriving from countries with which it shares a land border.[455] Sudan has recognized the refugee status of persons arriving from neighboring countries (except Chad), but has expected refugees from Arab states "to stay on an informal and unofficial basis."[456] The European Union has gone farther still, agreeing by treaty that member states may ordinarily declare any refugee claim from a citizen of an EU country to be inadmissible.[457] Conversely, Southern African states have often refused to grant protection to refugees from outside that region, earning them a public rebuke from UNHCR.[458]

---

[454] United Kingdom, "Certification Under Sections 94 and 115 of the Nationality and Immigration Act 2002: List of Safe Countries," Nov. 15, 2002. Claims by nationals of listed states are to be presumed to be "clearly unfounded," with the result that appeals must ordinarily be pursued after removal back to the country of origin.

[455] D. Kaiza, "Uganda: Kampala Refugee Policy is 'Bad,'" available at www.unhcr.ch (accessed July 12, 2003). Ugandan refugee policy seems to be largely ad hoc, with some ethnic groups – for example, ethnic Banyarwandans from neighboring Rwanda – suffering disproportionately: J. Kabrera, "Potential for Naturalization of Refugees in Africa: The Case of Uganda," paper presented at the Silver Jubilee Conference of the African Studies Association of the United Kingdom, Cambridge, Sept. 14–16, 1988, at 9.

[456] UN Committee on the Elimination of Racial Discrimination, "Concluding Observations of the Committee on the Elimination of Racial Discrimination: Sudan," UN Doc. CERD/C/304/Add.116, Apr. 27, 2001, at para. 15.

[457] "Given the level of protection of fundamental rights and freedoms by the Member States of the European Union, Member States shall be regarded as constituting safe countries of origin in respect of each other for all legal and practical purposes in relation to asylum matters. Accordingly, any application for asylum made by a national of a Member State may be taken into consideration or declared admissible for processing by another Member State only in [exceptional] cases": Protocol on Asylum for Nationals of Member States of the European Union, annexed to the Treaty establishing the European Community, OJ 97/340/01, at 103 (Nov. 10, 1997). By virtue of this provision, "the right of EU citizens to claim asylum in a neighbouring EU State has been effectively removed, unless a Member State chooses to reinstate such a right ... One striking anomaly of this situation is that third country nationals resident in a Member State may still apply for asylum within the Union: the only way in which they have more rights than nationals. But of course the main threat of the Protocol is one of principle, as it sets a very bad precedent for other regions of the world, linking the legal right of asylum to the political and economic alliance of neighbouring countries": European Council on Refugees and Exiles, "Analysis of the Treaty of Amsterdam in so far as it relates to asylum policy" (Nov. 10, 1997), at 8–9.

[458] "The United Nations refugee agency ... lambasted the 14 members of the Southern African Development Community (SADC) for rejecting refugees from outside the region. 'There is a tendency within SADC of not accepting refugees from outside the region. This is unacceptable,' UNHCR Southern Africa Director Nicolas Bwakira told a

Protection may also be skewed for purely political reasons: for example, long-standing political ties with North Korea have led China to refuse recognition to any refugee arriving from that country.[459] Sex can play an important role in limiting access to refugee rights, as was the case for women refugees from Somalia who were denied access to adequate health facilities, food, or educational opportunities while in receipt of asylum in Ethiopia.[460] The same sort of disfranchisement occurred when Nepal distributed critical supplies to Bhutanese refugees, including even food and shelter, only to male heads of household. This practice made it nearly impossible for female refugees estranged from their husbands to survive.[461]

Nor is the pattern of differentiation among refugees limited to actions grounded in nationality, politics, or sex. Since the arrival of the "boat people," Australia has routinely detained refugees who present themselves without a valid entry visa, even as it has in most cases allowed refugees arriving on a tourist or student visa to remain at liberty while their claims

---

news conference ... Most SADC countries [except Zambia] bar refugees from West Africa and the Horn of Africa": *Reuters*, Jan. 27, 2000.

[459] "China, North Korea's principal ally, claims it is bound by its treaty obligations to Pyongyang": "Inside the Gulag," *Guardian*, July 19, 2002, at 23. "[T]he underlying reason Beijing does not welcome them, Chinese analysts say, is that it believes the fall of Communism in Eastern Europe was precipitated when Hungary allowed tens of thousands of East German refugees to pass through on their way to the West in 1989. 'If we gave them refugee status, millions would pour over our doorstep,' said a Chinese scholar who advises the North Korean and Chinese governments. 'That would cause a humanitarian crisis here and a collapse of the North. We can't afford either'": J. Pomfret, "China cracks down on North Korean refugees," *Washington Post*, Jan. 22, 2003, at A-01. The UN High Commissioner for Refugees announced that "[i]n China, the plight of North Koreans who leave their country illegally remains a serious concern. For a number of years UNHCR has been making efforts to obtain access to them, but this has consistently been denied. An analysis of currently available information recently carried out by our Department of International Protection concludes that many North Koreans may well be considered refugees. In view of their protection needs, the group is of concern to UNHCR ... [T]he principle of *non-refoulement* must be respected": "UNHCR Designates North Korean Refugees as a Group of Concern," Opening Statement by Mr. Ruud Lubbers, United Nations High Commissioner for Refugees, at the Fifty-fourth Session of the Executive Committee of the High Commissioner's Program, Geneva, Sept. 29, 2003.

[460] In response, UNHCR announced that in the context of its assistance programs in Ethiopia, "[r]efugee women will be encouraged to take the lead role in the supervision of food": UNHCR, "Global Appeal 2002: Ethiopia" (2002), at 79. See also US Committee for Refugees, *World Refugee Survey 2002* (2002), at 74.

[461] "This policy ... imposes particular hardship on women trying to escape abusive marriages. Either these women must stay in violent relationships, leave their relationships (and thus relinquish their full share of aid packages), or marry another man, in which cases they lose legal custody of their children": Human Rights Watch, "Nepal/Bhutan: Refugee Women Face Abuses," Sept. 24, 2003. See generally Human Rights Watch, "Trapped by Inequality: Bhutanese Refugee Women in Nepal" (2003).

to refugee status are assessed.[462] Even once recognized as refugees, those who initially arrive without authorization are granted only a renewable, three-year temporary protection visa (as contrasted with the permanent status granted those who arrive with a visa), and are moreover not entitled to reunification with their family members.[463] Pakistan provided inferior material assistance to the less educated, rural Afghan refugees in Baluchistan than to their urban co-nationals in the North West Frontier Province.[464] Some countries, at one point including the United States,[465] have refused to admit refugees who are HIV-positive.[466] In sum, refugees are frequently subjected to differences in treatment based on factors extraneous to their need for protection. The net result is a critical challenge to the notion that a universal common denominator of rights can be said to follow from refugee status.

[462] P. Mares, *Borderline: Australia's Treatment of Refugees and Asylum Seekers* (2002), at 6. See also C. Steven, "Asylum-Seeking in Australia," (2002) 36(3) *International Migration Review* 864, at 889: "Less favorable treatment has been given to unauthorized arrivals claiming asylum than those who arrive legally. Mandatory detention in prison-like conditions has been introduced to ensure that asylum-seekers are not permitted to enter nor disappear into the community before their cases have been determined, and to ensure that rejected asylum-seekers can be removed from Australia without difficulty."

[463] P. Mathew, "Australian Refugee Protection in the Wake of the *Tampa*," (2002) 96(3) *American Journal of International Law* 661, at 673.

[464] K. Connor, "Geographical Bias in Refugee Treatment Within Host Countries," paper prepared for the RSP/QEH Refugee Participation Network, 1988, at 1–5. See also S. Khattak, "Refugee Policy Politics: Afghans in Pakistan," paper presented at the Conference of Scholars and Other Professionals Working on Refugees and Displaced Persons in South Asia, Dhaka, Bangladesh, Feb. 9–11, 1998, at 6–7.

[465] In *Haitian Centers Council Inc. v. Sale*, (1993) 823 F Supp 1028 (US DCEDNY, June 8, 1993) it was determined that the indefinite detention in Guantanamo by the United States of HIV-positive Haitian refugees was not lawful. "The Clinton Administration, through the Department of Justice, did not appeal the order and admitted the infected Haitians": L. Macko, "Acquiring a Better Global Vision: An Argument Against the United States' Current Exclusion of HIV-Infected Immigrants," (1995) 9(3) *Georgetown Immigration Law Journal* 545, at 546, n. 14. At present, an HIV test is required of all persons seeking permanent residence in the United States, excepting only those who apply through cancellation of removal. Refugees who apply through the legalization program may secure a waiver of ineligibility based on HIV status where concerns of family unity, humanitarianism, or public interest are demonstrated: San Francisco AIDS Foundation, "Gaining Legal Immigrant Status," available at www.sfaf.org (accessed Dec. 16, 2003).

[466] "UNHCR and IOM have issued a joint policy which opposes the use of mandatory HIV screening and restrictions based on a refugee's HIV status. Nevertheless, some States have adopted mandatory HIV testing for refugees, and exclude those who test positive": UNHCR, "Refugee Resettlement: An International Handbook to Guide Reception and Integration" (2002), at 155.

Refugee Convention, Art. 3   Non-discrimination
The Contracting States shall apply the provisions of this
Convention to refugees without discrimination as to race, religion
or country of origin.

Economic, Social and Cultural Covenant, Art. 2

. . .

2. The States Parties to the present Covenant undertake to
guarantee that the rights enunciated in the present Covenant will
be exercised without discrimination of any kind as to race, colour,
sex, language, religion, political or other opinion, national or
social origin, property, birth or other status.

3. Developing countries, with due regard to human rights and
their national economy, may determine to what extent they would
guarantee the economic rights recognized in the present Covenant
to non-nationals.

Civil and Political Covenant, Art. 2(1)
Each State Party to the present Covenant undertakes to respect
and to ensure to all individuals within its territory and subject to
its jurisdiction the rights recognized in the present Covenant,
without distinction of any kind, such as race, colour, sex, language,
religion, political or other opinion, national or social origin, property, birth or other status.

Civil and Political Covenant, Art. 26
All persons are equal before the law and are entitled without any
discrimination to the equal protection of the law. In this respect, the
law shall prohibit any discrimination and guarantee to all persons
equal and effective protection against discrimination on any ground
such as race, colour, sex, language, religion, political or other opinion, national or social origin, property, birth or other status.

The drafting history of the Refugee Convention provides little guidance
on the substantive reach of Art. 3's duty of non-discrimination. The Swiss
delegate, for example, acknowledged only "measures of a humiliating
character" to be discriminatory.[467] Egypt tried unsuccessfully to exclude
action necessary for the maintenance of public order from the scope of
discrimination.[468] No interest was shown in a Greek effort to ensure that

---

[467] Statement of Mr. Schurch of Switzerland, UN Doc. A/CONF.2/SR.4, July 3, 1951, at 15.
[468] Statement of Mr. Mostafa of Egypt, UN Doc. A/CONF.2/SR.5, July 4, 1951, at 12. The
British delegate thought that "the acknowledged right of any State to safeguard the
requirements of public order and morality was extraneous to the subject-matter of

actions necessary for "public safety" were immune from scrutiny under Art. 3.[469] The most precise comment on the meaning of non-discrimination was offered by the American representative, who thought that discrimination meant "denying to one category of persons certain rights and privileges enjoyed by others in identical circumstances."[470] In line with principles of treaty interpretation earlier described,[471] this conceptual uncertainty should be remedied by taking account of the parameters of the duty of non-discrimination elaborated under the terms of cognate treaties – including, for example, under the Human Rights Covenants, described above.[472] Most fundamentally, this means that even a differential allocation of rights on the basis of a prohibited ground will not amount to discrimination if demonstrated to meet international standards of "reasonableness."[473]

In drafting Art. 3, consensus was reached on the critical point that the duty of non-discrimination is not restricted to actions taken within a state's territory, but governs as well a state's actions towards persons seeking to enter its territory. While the English language draft of Art. 3 produced by the Second Session of the Ad Hoc Committee appeared to prohibit only discrimination by a state "against a refugee within its territory,"[474] the French language formulation was not predicated on successful entry into a state's territory.[475] At the Conference of Plenipotentiaries, the French delegate successfully argued against the narrowness of the duty proposed in the English text:

> [T]he statement that the State should not discriminate against a refugee within its territory on account of his race, religion or country of origin seemed to suggest that the State was perfectly entitled to discriminate against persons *wishing* to enter its territory, that was to say, against persons not yet resident in its territory. He therefore proposed that the words "within its territory" be deleted.[476]

Article 3", while the Dutch representative argued that "[i]t would be dangerous to add a provision to Article 3 which would to some extent emasculate it": Statements of Mr. Hoare of the United Kingdom and Baron van Boetzelaer of the Netherlands, ibid. at 14.

[469] Statement of Mr. Philon of Greece, ibid. at 12–13.

[470] Statement of Mr. Warren of the United States of America, ibid. at 4.

[471] See chapter 1.3.3 above, at pp. 64–68.

[472] The practice of the Human Rights Committee in interpreting the duty of non-discrimination is described in chapter 2.5.5 above.

[473] See chapter 2.5.5 above, at pp. 129–145.   [474] UN Doc. E/1850, Aug. 25, 1950, at 15.

[475] "Aucun Etat contractant ne prendra de mesures discriminatoires sur son territoire, contre un réfugié en raison de sa race, de sa religion ou de son pays d'origine": UN Doc. A/CONF.2/72, July 11, 1951, at 1. See also Statement of the President, UN Doc. A/CONF.2/SR.4, July 3, 1951, at 19.

[476] Statement of Mr. Rochefort of France, UN Doc. A/CONF.2/SR.4, July 3, 1951, at 18–19.

The rationale for the territorial limitation captured in the draft English language text had, in fact, been simply to ensure that states were left complete freedom to administer their own systems of immigration law.[477] Once it was recognized that the admission of refugees to durable asylum or permanent residency is not in any event governed by the Refugee Convention,[478] it proved possible to secure the consent of states to a duty of non-discrimination with extraterritorial application.[479] In line with the fact that Art. 3 governs all rights in the Refugee Convention, including Art. 33's duty of *non-refoulement*, the American interdiction and detention of black Haitian asylum-seekers on the high seas, while simultaneously allowing predominantly white Cuban asylum-seekers to proceed to Florida, is (unless determined to be reasonable by reference to international standards) in breach of Art. 3's duty of non-discrimination.

In contrast to the agreement on this point, there was real debate about the substantive breadth of Art. 3. As initially conceived, the provision was intended to prohibit discrimination not only against particular subsets of the refugee population, but against refugees in general. The Belgian draft of Art. 3 submitted to the Ad Hoc Committee provided that:

> The High Contracting Parties shall not discriminate against refugees on account of race, religion or country of origin, *nor because they are refugees* [emphasis added].[480]

The latter part of the duty – imposing a duty not to discriminate on the basis of refugee status itself – did not survive the Conference of Plenipotentiaries.

---

[477] "The history of the drafting of Article 3 showed that if the words 'within its territory' were deleted, the Convention would affect the whole field of immigration policy . . . There was no subject on which Governments were more sensitive or jealous regarding their freedom of action than on the determination of immigration policies . . . If the proposed deletion were made, certain Governments might feel that their policy of selection was affected by the Convention, and they might accordingly be hesitant about acceding to it": Statement of Mr. Warren of the United States of America, UN Doc. A/CONF.2/SR.5, July 4, 1951, at 5.

[478] "It was noted during the discussion that . . . the Convention does not deal either with the admission of refugees (in countries of first or second asylum) or with their resettlement (in countries of immigration)": "Report of the Committee Appointed to Study Article 3," UN Doc. A/CONF.2/72, July 11, 1951, at 3.

[479] "It was thought that the words 'within its territory' in the place where they occurred in the English text could be interpreted *a contrario* as permitting such discrimination outside the territory of the Contracting State. *A document drawn up under the auspices of the United Nations ought not to be susceptible to such an interpretation* [emphasis added]": ibid. at 2. The consensus definition of this Committee – which deleted the limitation "within its territory" – was the basis for the version of Art. 3 finally adopted: UN Doc. A/CONF.2/SR.18, July 12, 1951, at 18, and UN Doc. A/CONF.2/SR.24, July 17, 1951, at 19–21.

[480] Statement of Mr. Cuvelier of Belgium, UN Doc. E/AC.32/SR.24, Feb. 3, 1950, at 11.

Even there, some delegates clearly believed it should be retained. For example, the French representative insisted that equality between groups of refugees was an insufficiently inclusive goal, as "if all refugees received equally bad treatment, the State concerned could claim to have observed the provisions of Article 3."[481] Particularly where all refugees in a given asylum state belong to the same race or religion, or come from the same country, skewed rights allocations that are in substance racially, religiously, or nationally motivated might not be caught by a simple prohibition of discrimination *between classes of refugees* (since all refugees would be equally harmed). Some representatives therefore identified the need for a stronger commitment to prohibit the kinds of discriminatory actions that generate refugee flows in the first place.[482]

Despite these concerns, the Israeli delegate successfully moved the deletion of Art. 3's prohibition of discrimination against refugees in general on the grounds that this issue was already regulated by the Convention's provisions on required standards of treatment.[483] This position was in line with the view he had earlier expressed in the Ad Hoc Committee that priority should be given to the express language which defined the various levels of obligation:

> It was important to clear up the exact place of Article 3 in the Convention and its relation to the other articles. It proclaimed a principle, but the exact conditions under which refugees might enjoy the benefits conferred by it were enumerated in later articles. There was nothing abnormal about that. The United Nations Charter itself began by speaking of the "sovereign equality" of all members of the United Nations and then proceeded to divide those members into great Powers and small Powers, permanent and non-permanent members of the Security Council, members with the right of veto and members without. There would be no objection to retaining Article 3 as formulated, on the understanding that its function was to establish a principle to which the exceptions would be specified in later articles, as was usual practice in any legal instrument.[484]

---

[481] Statement of Mr. Rochefort of France, UN Doc. A/CONF.2/SR.4, July 3, 1951, at 18.

[482] "Such a provision was all the more necessary because most refugees had left their countries of origin in order to escape discrimination on grounds of race, religion, or political opinion": Statement of Mr. Cuvelier of Belgium, UN Doc. E/AC.32/SR.24, Feb. 3, 1950, at 11.

[483] Statement of Mr. Robinson of Israel, UN Doc. A/CONF.2/SR.4, July 3, 1951, at 17–19. While the textual modification to Art. 3, in which the words "nor because they are refugees" were deleted, arguably determines this issue, it should be noted that even after the adoption of the Israeli motion, remarks of the Australian, French, and American delegates during the final substantive discussion of this article support a broader reading: UN Doc. A/CONF.2/SR.5, July 4, 1951, at 7–9. Moreover, the final language proposed by the Style Committee was said to be primarily designed to restrict the substantive ambit of this duty of non-discrimination to actions of a kind regulated by the Refugee Convention: UN Doc. A/CONF.2/72, July 11, 1951, at 3.

[484] Statement of Mr. Robinson of Israel, UN Doc. E/AC.32/SR.34, Aug. 14, 1950, at 9.

It is, of course, true that the extent of permissible differentiation between refugees and citizens in the delivery of rights is explicitly set out in the Refugee Convention's mixed contingent and absolute rights structure.[485] Many of the rights in regard to which the issue of discrimination vis-à-vis nationals might arise are required to be implemented only insofar as they are guaranteed to some other category of non-citizens.[486] To this extent, the Refugee Convention clearly presumes the legitimacy of treating refugees less favorably than citizens with respect to any of the rights defined by a contingent standard less than nationality. For example, Art. 17 requires only that refugees benefit from "the most favorable treatment accorded to nationals of a foreign country in the same circumstances" as regards the right to work. In view of this clear language, the structure of the Refugee Convention argues against a finding of discrimination simply because refugees enjoy access to work on terms less favorable than those extended to citizens.

Conversely, a duty of non-discrimination between citizens and refugees would add nothing to the force of those rights that are already defined to mandate implementation on terms of parity with citizens. All refugees must be assimilated to nationals in terms of the rights to rationing, primary education, and fair taxation.[487] Where the relevant degree of attachment is satisfied, refugees are also entitled to national treatment in regard to religion and religious education, artistic rights and industrial property, public relief, labor legislation, social security, and legal assistance and security for costs before the courts.[488] The duty to implement these rights on terms of parity with nationals is actually more powerful than a duty of non-discrimination relative to nationals would be, since the issue of reasonable differentiation inherent in non-discrimination analysis simply does not arise.

As discussed earlier,[489] the prohibition of generalized discrimination against refugees is in any event now largely achieved by the binding duty of non-discrimination subsequently codified in the Human Rights Covenants. Art. 2 of each of the Covenant on Civil and Political Rights and the Covenant on Economic, Social and Cultural Rights prohibits discrimination on the

---

[485] See chapters 3.2 and 3.3 above.

[486] Freedom of association and the right to engage in employment are guaranteed at the level of most-favored-national treatment; the rights to private property, internal freedom of movement, housing, and to engage in self- and professional employment are granted to refugees only to the extent afforded aliens generally.

[487] Refugee Convention, at Arts. 20, 22, and 29.

[488] See chapter 3.3.2 above. Equality of treatment with regard to religion and religious education are guaranteed to all refugees "within the territory"; rights to public relief, and to benefit from labor and social security legislation to all refugees who are "lawfully staying"; and the protection of artistic rights and industrial property and access to legal assistance and avoidance of security for costs to refugees who are "habitually resident."

[489] See chapter 2.5.5 above, at pp. 127–128.

basis of a list of grounds, including "other status."[490] Relying on this open-ended formulation, the duty of non-discrimination has been authoritatively interpreted to establish the general rule "that each one of the rights of the Covenant must be guaranteed without discrimination between citizens and aliens,"[491] and specifically to require that rights not be limited to citizens of a state, but that they "must also be available to all individuals, regardless of nationality or statelessness, such as asylum-seekers [and] refugees."[492] Unlike Art. 3 of the Refugee Convention (which prohibits only discrimination of particular kinds against refugees – namely on the basis of race, religion, or country of origin), the duty set by the Covenants is thus fully inclusive, prohibiting every kind of status-based discrimination (including on the basis of refugee status) in relation to a right established by the Covenants. This guarantee of non-discrimination found in Art. 2 of each of the Human Rights Covenants therefore partly fills the gap left by the limited prohibition of discrimination *against refugees in general* in the Refugee Convention.

First, where a given right is found in both the Refugee Convention and one of the Covenants, Art. 2 of the Covenants disallows discrimination relative to nationals. In such circumstances, it is simply not necessary to rely on the relevant refugee right in order to contest treatment below national treatment. Since virtually all rights in the Covenants must be implemented without discrimination between nationals and non-citizens,[493] refugees who invoke the cognate Covenant protection can effectively avoid the lower standard of treatment prescribed by the Refugee Convention.

For example, Art. 15 of the Refugee Convention guarantees freedom of association to refugees only to the extent of "the most favourable treatment accorded to nationals of a foreign country, in the same circumstances." The failure to grant refugees the same associational rights as citizens would therefore not contravene the terms of the Refugee Convention. On the other hand, because the right to freedom of association is also established by Art. 22 of the Civil and Political Covenant and by Art. 8 of the Economic, Social and

---

[490] See chapter 2.5.5 above, at p. 125.

[491] UN Human Rights Committee, "General Comment No. 15: The position of aliens under the Covenant" (1986), UN Doc. HRI/GEN/1/Rev.7, May 12, 2004, at 140, para. 2. While this General Comment interprets only the Civil and Political Covenant, it is reasonable to assume that the virtually identical prohibition of discrimination on the basis of "other status" in the Economic, Social and Cultural Covenant will be similarly interpreted to protect the entitlement of aliens to national treatment in relation to its catalog of rights. The relevance of the minor differences in the language of the prohibition of discrimination in the two Human Rights Covenants is discussed in chapter 2.5.5 above, at note 130.

[492] UN Human Rights Committee, "General Comment No. 31: The nature of the general legal obligation imposed on states parties to the Covenant" (2004), UN Doc. HRI/GEN/1/Rev.7, May 12, 2004, at 192, para. 10.

[493] Civil and Political Covenant, at Art. 2(1).

Cultural Covenant, refugees can invoke Art. 2 of the Covenants as the basis for asserting the same *prima facie* entitlement to associational rights as nationals. It would then fall to the state party denying equal treatment to advance the case that the distinction between refugees and citizens should be adjudged reasonable.[494] In addition to freedom of association, refugees may rely on parallel provisions in the Covenants (which are subject to a general duty of non-discrimination) to assert a right to national treatment in access to employment, housing, and internal freedom of movement,[495] each of which is guaranteed by the Refugee Convention only at a lower contingency level.[496]

Second, reliance on the Covenants to assert a duty of non-discrimination relative to nationals may actually allow refugees to contest a broader range of substantive disfranchisement. This is because the Covenants guarantee a significant number of rights not provided for at all in the Refugee Convention. In particular, the Civil and Political Covenant establishes the rights to life, to freedom from slavery, against torture, cruel, inhuman, and degrading treatment, to liberty and security of the person, freedom of thought, conscience, and religion, to leave the country, to equality before courts and tribunals,[497] against retrospective application of criminal law, to recognition as a person, to protection of family, children, and privacy, against advocacy of hatred or discrimination, to freedom of opinion, expression, and assembly, and to the protection of minority rights.[498] Additional rights derived from the Economic, Social and Cultural Covenant include guarantees of just and favorable working conditions, adequate food and clothing, protection of the family (including of mothers and of children), secondary and

---

[494] See chapter 2.5.5 above, at pp. 128–145.

[495] Only refugees who are "lawfully in the territory of a State Party" may claim the right to non-discrimination relative to nationals in regard to internal freedom of movement and choice of place of residence: Civil and Political Covenant, at Art. 12(1).

[496] Under the Refugee Convention, the rights to self-employment, professional employment, housing, and internal freedom of movement are granted to refugees only to the extent afforded to aliens generally (Articles 18, 19, 21, and 26). Access to wage-earning employment is guaranteed to refugees at the most-favored-national level (Article 17). The comparable provisions in the Human Rights Covenants make no differentiation between the entitlement of nationals and aliens (Economic, Social and Cultural Covenant, at Arts. 6 and 11; Civil and Political Covenant, at Art. 12, which does, however, require lawful presence in the state's territory).

[497] International aliens law also prohibits discrimination by courts against aliens (including refugees) in the adjudication of claims involving core rights, such as legal status, physical security, personal and spiritual liberty, and some economic and property rights. While not enforceable by refugees themselves, this customary norm of international aliens law can nonetheless be invoked as evidence of a principled, legally defined limitation on discrimination. See chapter 2.1 above, at pp. 76–77.

[498] Civil and Political Covenant, at Arts. 6–11, 12(2), 14–21, 23–24, and 27.

higher education, social security, access to healthcare, and participation in cultural life.[499] Each of these rights must in principle be guaranteed to non-citizens, including refugees, without discrimination relative to nationals.

Beyond the context-specific duty of non-discrimination derived from Art. 2 of the Covenants, additional value may also be secured from Art. 26 of the Civil and Political Covenant. As elaborated earlier, Art. 26 establishes a general duty to guarantee everyone equality before the law and the equal protection of the law without discrimination.[500] As a matter of principle, this overarching duty should be understood to compel states not only to avoid any intentional disfranchisement of refugees, but also affirmatively to adopt measures which provide refugees with the substantive benefit of all public goods.[501] In theory, even the levels of attachment set by the Refugee Convention are themselves subject to scrutiny under Art. 26 to ensure that the withholding of benefits from some refugees is justifiable.

The major challenge to the efficacy of the various non-discrimination rights set by the Human Rights Covenants is that, as previously described, the contemporary practice of the Human Rights Committee has been to defer to state perceptions of "reasonableness" in determining whether a given form of differentiation amounts to discrimination.[502] Whether the assessment occurs under one of the endogenous Art. 2 guarantees or in relation to the more generally applicable Art. 26, a refugee arguing that inequality of treatment is discriminatory must make the case that certain kinds of differential allocation should be understood to be impermissible as a general matter, or at least in particular circumstances. Given the mixed success in advancing this argument on behalf of non-citizens generally,[503] it is by no means clear that general norms of non-discrimination law will, in practice, make up for the decision to exclude discrimination against refugees in general from the scope of Art. 3 of the Refugee Convention. On the other hand, reliance on the Human Rights Covenants can at least compel states to justify differential treatment of refugees as a class, in contrast to Art. 3 of the Refugee Convention.

Stripped of its role in prohibiting discrimination against refugees as a group, the purpose of Art. 3 of the Refugee Convention as finally adopted is instead to disallow any discrimination in the allocation of Convention rights between and among refugees on the basis of race, religion, or country of origin. While not requiring that all groups of refugees who arrive in an asylum country be treated identically, Art. 3 establishes a presumption that differential treatment based on any of the enumerated grounds is illegitimate.

---

[499] Economic, Social and Cultural Covenant, at Arts. 7, 9–13, and 15.
[500] See chapter 2.5.5 above, at pp. 125–129.   [501] See chapter 2.5.5 above, at pp. 126–128.
[502] See chapter 2.5.5 above, at pp. 128–145.
[503] See chapter 2.5.5 above, at pp. 131–133 and 135–138.

This presumption would apply, for example, in the case of India's decision to grant permission to work to Tibetan refugees, even as Sri Lankan refugees were restricted to self-employment and Bangladeshi refugees afforded no right to earn a livelihood.

As is clear from its text, however, Art. 3 (in contrast, for example, to Art. 26 of the Civil and Political Covenant) applies only to matters that are regulated by the Refugee Convention. Those who drafted the provision emphasized that "[t]he members of the Committee were in full agreement in their adherence to the principle of non-discrimination, in their desire to reach an acceptable (preferably a unanimous) solution *which should cover the whole Convention*, and in their determination *not to 'legislate' beyond the Convention* [emphasis added]."[504] Their particular concern was to avoid any implication that states are subject to a duty to administer their immigration laws in a non-discriminatory way.[505] Art. 3 is not therefore a generalized prohibition of discrimination, but speaks only to invidious differentiation in the implementation of rights set by the Refugee Convention.[506]

In considering the question of whether a Convention right is engaged, it is important to take real account of the breadth of the protected interest. For example, states are not under a legal obligation to grant any form of durable or permanent status to even recognized refugees. Yet Art. 34 of the Refugee Convention, while setting a weak obligation, is nonetheless not purely hortatory: as the analysis below makes clear, Art. 34 is breached where a state party simply does not allow refugees to secure its citizenship, and refuses to provide a cogent explanation for that inaccessibility.[507] As such, the complete bar imposed by Australia on access to even durable residence in the case of recognized refugees who arrive without authorization, and even more clearly the British decision to exclude the nationals of three countries from the usual right to secure permanent residence, may well amount to discrimination unless found to be reasonable by reference to international standards. Similarly, the right of access to the courts under Art. 16(1) of the Refugee Convention requires that all refugees be able to pursue any remedies that are within the usual subject-matter jurisdiction of the courts.[508] The United Kingdom's decision substantively to withdraw the right to appeal a negative refugee status assessment from the citizens of certain countries – since an

---

[504] "Report of the Committee Appointed to Study Article 3," UN Doc. A/CONF.2/72, July 11, 1951, at 3.

[505] See text above, at p. 246.

[506] "The non-discrimination provision in article 3 is limited to the application of 'the provisions of this convention.' Article 3 does not contain a freestanding non-discrimination provision. It resembles the weak provision in article 14 of the European Convention on Human Rights (1950)": *R v. Immigration Officer at Prague Airport et al., ex parte European Roma Rights Centre et al.*, [2004] UKHL 55 (UK HL, Dec. 9, 2004), at para. 43.

[507] See chapter 7.4 below, at pp. 988–989.   [508] See chapter 4.10 below, at pp. 646–649.

appeal that can be pursued only once a refugee is returned to the place in which persecution is feared is not in substance an appeal that is capable of ensuring protection against that risk – should thus be understood *prima facie* to raise an issue of discrimination contrary to Art. 3.[509]

Importantly, the implementation of a Convention right may be implicated even in actions or policies which are not on their face linked to an interest protected by the Convention. For example, the nature of the refugee status determination procedure is not specifically regulated by the Refugee Convention, thus suggesting that discrimination in relation to such procedural matters would be unlikely to infringe Art. 3. But to the extent that it can be shown that a heightened risk of rejection is the foreseeable consequence of the American decision to require all Haitians to make their claims to refugee status in the truncated "expedited removal" system (rather than under the more elaborate procedures applicable to the citizens of other states),[510] an issue of compliance with Art. 33's duty of *non-refoulement* arises. Because the duty of *non-refoulement* is set by the Convention itself, the discriminatory nature of the American policy of requiring Haitians to establish their claims under inferior procedures can be challenged by reference to Art. 3's duty of non-discrimination.

---

[509] In considering whether this system was fair, the English Court of Appeal relied upon the fact that the listed countries – which include, for example, both the Czech Republic and Slovakia, each of which has in fact produced genuine (Roma) refugees recognized as such by many state parties – had been determined by the government to be countries from which applications for protection are to be deemed "clearly unfounded." The Court reasoned that so long as individuals had an opportunity nonetheless to demonstrate that they had an arguable claim, there was no inherent unfairness in a general policy of denying in-country appeal rights to refugee claimants from the listed states: *R (ZL) v. Secretary of State for the Home Department*, [2003] 1 WLR 1230 (Eng. CA, Jan. 24, 2003). In view of the way in which this challenge was framed, the Court was not called upon explicitly to consider the requirements of either Art. 16(1) or Art. 3 of the Refugee Convention. Had it done so, it is likely that the real challenge to a discrimination claim under Art. 3 would have been to decide whether the existence of an individuated "escape valve" was sufficient to render the system as a whole a "reasonable" enterprise. In this regard, it is noteworthy that an American court determined that Art. 16 of the Refugee Convention should be considered in the adjudication of a comparable claim of discrimination. In assessing the legitimacy of a US rule that required stowaways to have their refugee claims determined solely by an official rather than having the usual access to an immigration judge, the US Court of Appeals (4th Cir.) cited Art. 16(1) of the Refugee Convention, noting that it was indirectly incorporated into US law. It went on to determine that the relevant domestic statute should be understood to require the Attorney General "to establish a single procedure for asylum claims that appl[ies] to all applicants without distinction": *Selgeka v. INS*, 184 F 3d 337 (US CA4, June 7, 1999).

[510] See University of California Hastings College of the Law, "Annual Reports on Implementation of Expedited Removal" (1998, 1999, and 2000), available at www.uchastings.edu (accessed Aug. 24, 2004).

In contrast, because the Convention does not establish a right to family reunification, Australia's policy of withholding this right from some refugees, even if that exclusion were implemented on the basis of a prohibited ground, cannot be successfully contested under Art. 3. As in the case of claims of discrimination against refugees generally, however, the Human Rights Covenants provide at least a partial answer to the fact that Art. 3 addresses only discrimination in relation to rights that are specifically provided for in the Refugee Convention. This is because the guarantee of equal benefit of the law without discrimination set by Art. 26 of the Civil and Political Covenant applies not only to matters regulated by that Covenant; rather, "[i]t prohibits discrimination in law or in fact in any field regulated and protected by public authorities."[511] As such, a state bound by both Art. 3 of the Refugee Convention and Art. 26 of the Civil and Political Covenant must now abide by a duty of non-discrimination in the allocation of any legal rights.

A second concern is that the Refugee Convention's duty of non-discrimination is strictly limited to the three listed grounds of race, religion, and country of origin. The protection against discrimination on grounds of "country of origin" is of particular value, given the prevalence of discrimination against refugees based upon their citizenship. There can be little doubt that this ground is sufficient, for example, to contest the nationality-based Saudi refusal to recognize the refugee status of other than Iraqis. A purposive reading of prohibition of discrimination on grounds of "country of origin" would moreover extend also to practices and policies which are aimed at refugees from a given category of states. Thus, the refusals of Uganda, Sudan, and some Southern African states to recognize the refugee status of persons coming from particular groups of states or regions is also inconsistent with the Convention's duty of non-discrimination. Even more clearly, any attempt to implement the European Union treaty sanctioning formal inadmissibility bars on refugees originating inside the Union would contravene Art. 3.[512]

It remains, however, that Art. 3's restriction to only three grounds is oddly conceived. It does not, for example, replicate the United Nations Charter's prohibition of discrimination on the grounds of race, sex, language, or

---

[511] UN Human Rights Committee, "General Comment No. 18: Non-discrimination" (1989), UN Doc. HRI/GEN/1/Rev.7, May 12, 2004, at 146, para. 12. See generally chapter 2.5.5 above, at pp. 126–128.

[512] G. Goodwin-Gill, "The Individual Refugee, the 1951 Convention and the Treaty of Amsterdam," in E. Guild and C. Harlow eds., *Implementing Amsterdam: Immigration and Asylum Rights in EC Law* 141 (2001), at 158–159. Nor is it an answer to this concern to assert the right of European Union citizens simply to move to another member state, as "free movement within the European Union is to be withheld by most EU states from the union's new members for between five and ten years": R. Prasad, "No place of refuge: What EU enlargement means for the much-persecuted Roma population is that they may have no escape from ethnic violence and abuse," *Guardian*, Oct. 24, 2002, at 21.

religion.[513] Even though the drafters expressed a desire to conform to the Universal Declaration of Human Rights,[514] they refused to sanction an open-ended duty of non-discrimination of the kind contained in the Universal Declaration.[515] Nor does it include the Universal Declaration's explicit references to color, sex, language, political or other opinion, social origin, property, or birth as prohibited bases of discrimination.[516] While some of the drafters defended the scope of Art. 3 on the basis of its symmetry with the usual grounds on which refugees were persecuted, the failure to make reference to political opinion as a prohibited ground of discrimination was acknowledged to be at odds with this understanding of the purpose of Art. 3.[517] Thus, for example, Art. 3 cannot be relied upon to challenge the political bias of China's refusal to protect refugees from North Korea.

A particularly disturbing discussion occurred in response to a proposal that sex be included as a prohibited ground of discrimination. Some states

---

[513] See chapter 2.4.1 above, at p. 94. In a dissenting opinion in the Full Federal Court of Australia, the view was taken that where differential treatment of certain refugees resulted largely from their inability to communicate in English, this was – if examined on the basis of effects – discrimination on grounds of national origin. "[T]o say that any differential impact is suffered not because of national origin, but rather as a result of individual personal circumstances, appears to me to adopt a verbal formula which avoids the real and practical discrimination which flows as a result of the operation of the [twenty-eight-day limit to seek review]": *Sahak v. Minister for Immigration and Multicultural Affairs*, [2002] FCAFC 215 (Aus. FFC, July 18, 2002), per North J. The majority of the Court, however, was of the view that "such discrimination or disadvantage as arose from the practical operation of ... the Act ... does not deprive persons of one race of a right that is enjoyed by another race, nor does it provide for differential operation depending upon the race, color, or national or ethnic origin of the relevant applicant. For example, persons whose national origin is Afghani or Syrian are able to take advantage of the relevant right if their comprehension of the English language is sufficient, or if they have access to friends or professional interpreters so as to overcome the language barrier": ibid.

[514] Statement of Mr. Cuvelier of Belgium, UN Doc. E/AC.32/SR.24, Feb. 3, 1950, at 11.

[515] The Yugoslavian delegate, Mr. Makiedo, unsuccessfully proposed that the list be made open-ended by the addition of the words "or for other reasons": UN Doc. A/CONF.2/SR.4, July 3, 1951, at 13.

[516] Universal Declaration of Human Rights, UNGA Res. 217A(III), Dec. 10, 1948, at Art. 2.

[517] "Political opinion," together with race and religion, was acknowledged to be one of the three traditional grounds that led persons to seek protection as refugees: Statement of Mr. Cuvelier of Belgium, UN Doc. E/AC.32/SR.24, Feb. 3, 1950, at 11. Yet it was omitted in the statement of the President of the Conference of Plenipotentiaries that "the original idea underlying Article 3 [was] that persons who had been persecuted on account of their race or religion, for example, should not be exposed to the same danger in their country of asylum": UN Doc. A/CONF.2/SR.5, July 4, 1951, at 10. The Yugoslavian delegate later sought (unsuccessfully) to justify an open-ended list of prohibited grounds of discrimination on the basis that "[t]he President had suggested that the text was satisfactory because it in fact enumerated all the reasons for which refugees were generally persecuted. There were, however, others, such as the holding of certain political opinions": Statement of Mr. Makiedo of Yugoslavia, ibid. at 12.

took umbrage at the mere suggestion that any government might be guilty of sex discrimination,[518] while others clearly acknowledged that sex discrimination was common, but ought not to be challenged.[519] One state actually defended its opposition to including sex as a prohibited basis of discrimination on the grounds that to prohibit discrimination on the basis of sex might interfere with cigarette distribution quotas.[520] The lack of serious and principled intellectual engagement in this discussion confirms the essentially arbitrary approach to the decision on which substantive grounds to include in Art. 3. The final 17–1 (5 abstentions) vote in opposition to any expansion of the scope of Art. 3 makes clear, however, that there is no basis upon which to argue that the Refugee Convention was intended to grant refugees the benefit of a comprehensive duty of non-discrimination.[521] The women refugees denied equal access to health facilities, food, and educational opportunities by Ethiopia and Nepal cannot therefore claim protection under Art. 3's duty of non-discrimination.

Here again, however, the interaction between the Refugee Convention and the guarantee of equal benefit of the law without discrimination set by Art. 26

---

[518] "He would ... oppose the insertion of the words 'and sex' which would imply that certain countries at present practised discrimination on grounds of sex. Such was not the case": Statement of Mr. Rochefort of France, UN Doc. A/CONF.2/SR.5, July 4, 1951, at 9. It is interesting to consider whether this position should be taken as an acknowledgment that reception countries *were* engaged in discrimination on the enumerated grounds of race, religion, and country of origin.

[519] "If that were done ... States whose legislation provided for different hours of work for men and women, for instance, might be hesitant to accede to the Convention": Statement of Mr. Warren of the United States, ibid. at 10. "The President added that ... married women might be prevented by national legislation from establishing their own domiciles. The inclusion of a reference to sex in Article 3 might therefore present legislative difficulties for the State in question": Statement of the President, ibid.

[520] "[T]he inclusion of a reference to sex might well conflict with national legislation, and he was therefore opposed to it as well. To quote one example, during a tobacco shortage in Austria the ration for women had been smaller than that for men. It had been alleged in the constitutional courts that that was a violation of the equality of the sexes, but the finding of the courts had been that women needed less tobacco than men. Thus, to include the reference to sex might bring the Convention into conflict with national legislation, because a woman refugee might not obtain as many cigarettes as a male refugee": Statement of Mr. Fritzer of Austria, ibid. at 11. The trivialization of the importance of sex discrimination – not to mention the fact that cigarette distribution is clearly not within the substantive ambit of the Refugee Convention – attest to a shockingly weak grasp of the issues at hand.

[521] Ibid. at 12. Interestingly, the observer from the Confederation of Free Trade Unions resurrected the issue of amending Art. 3 to embrace sex discrimination during final reading of the Convention. There is no reported discussion of her proposal, the present text of Art. 3 being adopted without amendment by a vote of 21–0(1 abstention): UN Doc. A/CONF.2/SR.33, July 24, 1951, at 7.

of the Civil and Political Covenant now establishes an expanded breadth of protection. Art. 3 of the Refugee Convention clearly establishes that there was an explicit intention to insulate refugee rights from discrimination (albeit then on the basis of only the three enumerated grounds). Art. 26 of the Civil and Political Covenant, in turn, today requires that any rights (including to non-discrimination) allocated to one group be presumptively extended to all. Taken together, the protections of Art. 3 of the Refugee Convention must now be read to apply generally, that is without discrimination based upon *any of the grounds* set by Art. 26, namely race, color, sex, language, religion, political or other opinion, national or social origin, property, birth or other status.[522]

On the basis of this analysis, the refusal by some states (once including the United States) to protect HIV-positive refugees, and the Pakistani decision to deny certain material assistance rights to less educated, rural refugees – both immune from challenge under Art. 3 of the Refugee Convention standing alone – are nonetheless appropriately subject to scrutiny under Art. 26 of the Civil and Political Covenant (the discrimination against HIV-positive refugees being on the basis of immutable health status, while that against less educated, rural refugees being for reasons of social origin or property). In contrast, even this combination of legal duties may not suffice to find Australia in breach of the duty of non-discrimination when it routinely detains refugees arriving unlawfully, but not those who arrive with some form of legal status. Because the Human Rights Committee has yet clearly to embrace an effects-based approach to analysis of whether actions amount to discrimination for a relevant reason,[523] the fact that the detention policy as written is directed to persons simply on the basis of a

---

[522] Civil and Political Covenant, at Art. 26.

[523] See chapter 2.5.5 above, at pp. 133–139. It has been argued by some that the impact of Australia's detention policy, and the circumstances in which it was implemented, suggest that it is essentially driven by considerations of race. "Boat people are predominantly South-East Asian asylum-seekers who come to Australia by sea without authority ... They are all unlawful non-citizens ... Although Australia had a detention policy, it had been used only for specific cases and only for individuals until the arrival of the boat people. It was activated to incarcerate this particular group. This discriminatory response arose out of the fear of Australia's 'significant other': Asia": D. McMaster, *Asylum Seekers: Australia's Response to Refugees* (2001), at 2–3. Alternatively, Fonteyne suggests that the underlying basis for discrimination might be the region (or countries) of origin. "[T]he policy in effect violate[d] the non-discrimination standard mandated by Article 3 of the Refugee Convention (as only boat people, and not on-shore applicants are routinely detained, and boat people in reality predominantly come from particular geographic regions)": J.-P. Fonteyne, "Illegal Refugees or Illegal Policy?," in Australian National University Department of International Relations ed., *Refugees and the Myth of the Borderless World* (2002), at 16.

failure to comply with immigration laws may well defeat the discrimination claim.[524]

Even where it is necessary to rely on the non-discrimination duty set by Art. 26 of the Covenant, Art. 3 of the Refugee Convention may be of real value in addressing the central question in non-discrimination analysis of whether a differential allocation of refugee rights may be found to be "reasonable." In answering this question, reliance should be placed on the fact that Art. 3 of the Refugee Convention defines a series of entitlements that are presumptively to follow from refugee status. These include not only rights which mirror those found in the Covenants and elsewhere (e.g. freedom of movement, right to work), but also other rights uniquely relevant to the situation of refugees (e.g. non-penalization for illegal entry, *non-refoulement*, and access to identity documents). A state party seeking to justify differential protection of some part of the refugee population on any status-based ground therefore faces a particular hurdle when the subject matter of the differentiation is a right expressly guaranteed in the Refugee Convention itself: because these are rights that are explicitly intended to inhere in persons who are refugees *simply because* they are refugees, the government withholding these rights should be expected to overcome that presumption in seeking to demonstrate the reasonableness of its failure to treat all refugees equally.

Despite both its direct and indirect value to contesting discrimination against subsets of the refugee population, the efficacy of Art. 3 is nonetheless sometimes questioned on the grounds that it appears to be overridden by Art. 5 of the Refugee Convention, which provides that "[n]othing in this Convention shall be deemed to impair any rights and benefits granted by a Contracting State to refugees apart from this Convention."[525] Because Art. 3 is subordinate to conflicting provisions of the Convention,[526] it is arguable that Art. 5 authorizes states to grant superior rights to preferred categories of refugees, so long as no class receives treatment below the minimum standard

---

[524] The issue of whether discrimination against "boat people" was a violation of the duty of non-discrimination on the basis of "other status" was not adjudicated by the Human Rights Committee in *A v. Australia*, UNHRC Comm. No. 560/1993, UN Doc. CCPR/C/59/D/560/1993, decided April 30, 1997. Australia's detention of the "boat people" was, however, found to violate Arts. 9(1), 9(4), and 2(3) of the Civil and Political Covenant. The question of Australia's breach of the duty to avoid arbitrary detention is examined in chapter 4.2.4 below, at p. 430; the only point being made here is that the approach to detention is unlikely to be determined to be *discriminatory*, not that it is lawful. Even if the status of "unlawful entrant" is deemed a form of "other status" for purposes of non-discrimination analysis, the deference traditionally afforded states to engage in differential treatment based upon non-citizen status would likely result in a finding of reasonable justification, thereby defeating the claim of discrimination: see chapter 2.5.5 above, at pp. 129–133.

[525] See generally chapter 2.4.5 above, at pp. 128–145.   [526] See text above, at p. 248.

of treatment required by the Convention.[527] Particularly because Art. 5 was originally incorporated in the Convention immediately after the duty of non-discrimination,[528] it may therefore be read to authorize governments to depart from the principle of Art. 3 if a subset of the refugee population is thereby benefited.[529]

The better view, however, is that Art. 5 should be given a narrow reading.[530] As previously argued, the drafting history suggests that it was addressed to the maintenance of certain historical advantages accorded refugees at the time the Refugee Convention was drafted.[531] In any event, there is nothing in Art. 5 that *requires* a reading that abrogates Art. 3's duty of non-discrimination. If understood as an interpretive provision that encourages governments to uphold standards higher than those mandated by the Refugee Convention,[532] Art. 5 and Art. 3 can clearly be read in harmony. This means, however, that Art. 5 cannot be relied upon to countenance privileges granted to only a select subset of refugees subsequent to the entry into force of the Refugee Convention. Rights and benefits may be granted to refugees apart from the Convention, but they may not be differentially allocated on the grounds of race, religion, or country of origin. Thus, for example, if access to the labor market on terms of parity with nationals is granted immediately to any part of the refugee population, it must be extended to all absent a showing of differing capabilities and potentialities sufficient to justify the preferred treatment of only a subset of the refugee population.

In sum, Art. 3 of the Refugee Convention and cognate provisions of the Human Rights Covenants combine to provide a solid guarantee of non-discrimination between and among refugee sub-populations. While to a real extent the Covenants provide the greatest value, Art. 3 of the Refugee Convention plays an important role by defining a core sphere of interests in regard to which the allocation of differential rights to refugees should be presumed not to be justifiable. Art. 3 of the Refugee Convention, in other words, acts as an important check on the possibility of an overly broad interpretation of "reasonableness" that could undermine the scope of the

---

[527] See e.g. S. Blay and M. Tsamenyi, "Reservations and Declarations under the 1951 Convention and the 1967 Protocol relating to the Status of Refugees," (1990) 2(4) *International Journal of Refugee Law* 527 (Blay and Tsamenyi, "Reservations"), at 556–557.

[528] UN Doc. E/AC.32/SR.43, Sept. 28, 1950, at 14.

[529] See Weis, *Travaux*, at 44; and Robinson, *History*, at 76.

[530] See chapter 2.4.5 above, at pp. 109–110.   [531] See chapter 2.4.5 above, at pp. 108–109.

[532] There was clearly interest in encouraging states to grant protections that exceed those stipulated by the Refugee Convention. See e.g. the exchange between Mr. Warren of the United States and Mr. Herment of Belgium: UN Doc. A/CONF.2/SR.5, July 4, 1951, at 8; and generally, chapter 2.4.5 above.

general duty of non-discrimination. While it remains unclear whether Art. 26 of the Civil and Political Covenant will force states increasingly to equate refugees to nationals for the purpose of rights allocation, Art. 26 has considerable value as a complementary prohibition of *discrimination between classes of refugees* in the allocation of a wide-ranging set of rights, and on the basis of any type of actual or imputed group identity.

Equally important, the drafting history of the Refugee Convention makes it clear that refugees are owed a duty of non-discrimination wherever they are encountered, not just once admitted to an asylum country. And because Art. 26 of the Civil and Political Covenant requires that all laws must extend protection without discrimination "on any ground," governments that are bound by both treaties must now extend this broad-ranging protection against discrimination to claims grounded in any form of status, not just in relation to the three grounds set out in Art. 3 of the Refugee Convention.

3.5 Restrictions on refugee rights

A state that makes no reservation to the terms of the Convention, and which does not avail itself of the formal option to limit its obligations temporally[533] or geographically,[534] may validly restrict refugee rights under only one of two very narrow circumstances. First, a small number of Convention rights may be withdrawn for reasons of security or criminality, in accordance with the express terms of the relevant articles of the Convention.[535] Second, the rights of persons whose refugee status has yet to be confirmed may be provisionally suspended on national security grounds during a war or other grave emergency.

---

[533] This can be achieved by acceding to the Refugee Convention, without also acceding to the Refugee Protocol. See chapter 2.4.3 above, at pp. 97–98.

[534] A state may restrict its obligations to persons who became refugees as the result of events occurring in Europe by acceding to the Refugee Convention, but not to the Refugee Protocol, and making a declaration at the time of signature, ratification, or accession specifying that it is governed by the interpretation of the refugee definition set out in Art. 1(B)(1)(a) of the Refugee Convention. Those states which became parties to the Refugee Convention and which elected to adopt the interpretation set out in Art. 1(B)(1)(a) prior to 1967 may also validly retain that geographical limitation, even while broadening the temporal scope of their obligations by accession to the Refugee Protocol. Other governments that opt to bind themselves to refugees without temporal limitation by accession to the Refugee Protocol must, however, also accept obligations without geographical limitation. See chapter 2.4.3 above, at pp. 97–98.

[535] These include Art. 33 (*non-refoulement*: "may not, however, be claimed . . . [if] danger to the security of the country . . . or who, having been convicted by a final judgment of a particularly serious crime, constitutes a danger to the community of that country"); Art. 32 (freedom from expulsion: "save on grounds of national security or public order"); and Art. 28 (travel documents: "unless compelling reasons of national security or public order otherwise require"). See generally chapters 4.1.4, 5.1, and 6.6 below.

The provisional measures taken for security reasons during a grave emergency must, however, come to an end once refugee status is verified. Refugees must also be exempted from any peacetime measures of retaliation or retorsion imposed on the grounds of their formal nationality. And most fundamentally, the Refugee Convention – in contrast, for example, to the Civil and Political Covenant – does not grant governments a general right to suspend or withhold Convention rights, even under emergency situations.

3.5.1 Suspension of rights for reasons of national security

Refugee Convention, Art. 9   Provisional measures
Nothing in this Convention shall prevent a Contracting State, in time of war or other grave and exceptional circumstances, from taking provisionally measures which it considers to be essential to the national security in the case of a particular person, pending a determination by the Contracting State that that person is in fact a refugee and that the continuance of such measures is necessary in his case in the interests of national security.

The drafters of the Convention considered, but rejected, an all-embracing power of derogation in time of national crisis.[536] The British proponent of the derogation clause wanted governments to be in a position to withhold rights from refugees if faced with a mass influx during wartime or other crisis. Because it would be impossible immediately to verify whether each person should be excluded from refugee status on security grounds,[537] governments might otherwise be effectively compelled to grant rights to persons who represented a danger to the host state.[538] His concern was valid, since a significant number of rights accrue to refugees even before their status has

---

[536] "A contracting State may at a time of national crisis derogate from any particular provision of this Convention to such extent only as is necessary in the interests of national security": Proposal of the United Kingdom, UN Doc. E/AC/32/L.41, Aug. 15, 1950.

[537] Refugee Convention, at Art. 1(F). The exclusion clauses which form an integral part of the definition of refugee status also provide critical safeguards for governments. On this topic, see generally Grahl-Madsen, *Status of Refugees I*, at 262–304; and Hathaway, *Refugee Status*, at 214–233.

[538] "He recalled the critical days of May and June 1940, when the United Kingdom had found itself in a most hazardous position; any of the refugees within its borders might have been fifth columnists, masquerading as refugees, and it could not afford to take chances with them. It was not impossible that such a situation could be reproduced in the future": Statement of Sir Leslie Brass of the United Kingdom, UN Doc. E/AC.32/SR.21, Feb. 2, 1950, at 8. See also the comments of Mr. Theodoli of Italy, UN Doc. E/AC.32/SR.34, Aug. 14, 1950, at 20: "[T]he main concern was to know whether at a time of crisis the Contracting States could resort to exceptional measures. He referred to the situation of Italy at the outset of the war when thousands of refugees had flocked to the frontiers of Italy."

been formally determined.[539] Yet, as the American delegate insisted, it was equally important that any exception to the duties owed refugees be limited to "very special cases."[540] The focus of attention therefore became how to ensure that states faced with a critical emergency could protect vital national security interests during the time required to investigate particular claims to refugee status.[541]

The resultant Art. 9 grants state parties the discretion to withhold rights from refugees "in time of war or other grave and exceptional circumstances." Serious economic difficulties do not warrant a suspension of rights.[542] Nor is it sufficient for a government to invoke "public order" concerns,[543] or even "national security" interests.[544] While the original formulation, in which governments could suspend rights only during a "national emergency," was

---

[539] See generally chapters 3.1.1, 3.1.2, and 3.1.3 above. The assurance of the representative of the United States that "the doubts of the United Kingdom representative might be resolved by the fact that any Government would be free to hold that any individual was not a *bona fide* refugee, in which case none of the provisions of the convention would apply to him" failed to recognize this critical point: Statement of Mr. Henkin of the United States, UN Doc. E/AC.32/SR.21, Feb. 2, 1950, at 8. See also UN Doc. E/AC.32/SR.34, Aug. 14, 1950, at 19.

[540] Statement of Mr. Henkin of the United States, UN Doc. E/AC.32/SR.34, Aug. 14, 1950, at 21. In particular, Mr. Henkin agreed that the Convention "ought not to prevent Governments in time of war from screening refugees to weed out those who were posing as such for subversive purposes." His concern was simply that "any limitation . . . ought to be defined more precisely than had been proposed, rather than leaving it open to countries to make far-reaching reservations. He would like the limitation to be as narrow as was possible": Statement of Mr. Henkin of the United States, UN Doc. E/AC.32/SR.35, Aug. 15, 1950, at 6.

[541] "The President recalled that . . . there had been no doubt that dangerous persons, such as spies, had to be dealt with under national laws. The question had then been raised as to the action to be taken in respect of refugees on the declaration of a state of war between two countries, which would make it impossible for a particular State to make an immediate distinction between enemy nationals, in the country, supporting the enemy government, and those persons who had fled from the territory of that enemy country. The Ad Hoc Committee had come to the conclusion that, while a government should not be in a position to treat persons in the latter category as enemies, it would need time to screen them": Statement of the President, Mr. Larsen, UN Doc. A/CONF.2/SR.6, July 4, 1951, at 15.

[542] Statement of Mr. Robinson of Israel, UN Doc. E/AC.32/SR.34, Aug. 14, 1950, at 21.

[543] A suggestion to adopt this traditional formulation made by Mr. Perez Perozo of Venezuela was not taken up by the drafters: UN Doc. E/AC.32/SR.35, Aug. 15, 1950, at 10. Thus, for example, the suggestion by Zimbabwe that it would "round up" urban refugees not employed or attending school in urban centers and remove them to refugee camps because "[s]ome of the refugees could end up being destitute or getting involved in illegal activities or prostitution for survival" would not be justified under Art. 9: see *Daily News* (Harare), May 20, 2002.

[544] This language was suggested by Mr. Shaw of Australia: UN Doc. A/CONF.2/SR.6, July 4, 1951, at 13. It was, however, "felt that there might be reasonable grounds for objecting to the Australian proposal that the phrase 'or in the interests of national security' should be

ultimately softened,[545] more than just "grave tension"[546] is clearly required. The circumstances must truly be "exceptional."[547]

Assuming relevant exceptional circumstances to exist, officials may take only "measures which [the state] considers to be *essential* to the national security in the case of a particular person [emphasis added]." The specific steps must therefore follow from a good faith assessment of the risk to national security that would follow from a failure to act.[548] Historically, the purpose of Art. 9 was to allow for flexibility where the government of the asylum state is faced with the risk of overthrow by illegal means.[549] This is in line with Grahl-Madsen's classic understanding of national security:

inserted, since it would enable a State to take exceptional measures at any time, and not only in time of war or a national emergency": Statement of Mr. Hoare of the United Kingdom, ibid. at 14. See also Statements of Mr. Chance of Canada and Baron van Boetzelaer of the Netherlands, ibid. In the result, only a subset of national security concerns, namely those that arise during war or other grave and exceptional circumstances, were deemed sufficient to justify provisional measures.

[545] This standard was adopted by the Ad Hoc Committee on Refugees and Stateless Persons at its Second Session: UN Doc. E/AC.32/8, Aug. 25, 1950, at 16. It was, however, dropped at the Conference of Plenipotentiaries, at which it was noted that "the expression 'national emergency' seemed unduly restrictive": Statement of Mr. Rochefort of France, UN Doc. A/CONF.2/SR.6, July 4, 1951, at 14.

[546] The Australian delegate proposed the language "time of grave tension, national or international," which was explicitly rejected by the Conference of Plenipotentiaries: UN Doc. A/CONF.2/SR.6, July 4, 1951, at 16. The French view that derogation should be allowed in the event of "cold war, approximating to a state of war, tension, a state of emergency or an international crisis calling for certain precautions" must therefore also be taken to have been impliedly rejected: ibid. at 14.

[547] This language was proposed by the representative of the Netherlands, and adopted by the British delegate in the motion which ultimately was approved at the Conference of Plenipotentiaries: ibid. at 16. It remains that this is a more fluid standard than, for example, that subsequently adopted in the Civil and Political Covenant, which allows a suspension of rights only if there is a "public emergency which threatens the life of the nation": Civil and Political Covenant, at Art. 4(1).

[548] "It had therefore been decided that there should be a blanket provision whereby, *in strictly defined* circumstances of emergency, derogation from any of the provisions of the Convention would be permitted in the interests of national security [emphasis added]": Statement of Mr. Hoare of the United Kingdom, UN Doc. A/CONF.2/SR.28, July 19, 1951, at 6.

[549] "It must be borne in mind that … each government had become more keenly aware of the current dangers to its national security. Among the great mass of refugees it was inevitable that some persons should be tempted to engage in activities on behalf of a foreign Power against the country of their asylum, and it would be unreasonable to expect the latter not to safeguard itself against such a contingency": Statement of Mr. Hoare of the United Kingdom, UN Doc. A/CONF.2/SR.16, July 11, 1951, at 8. See also Statement of Mr. Chance of Canada, ibid.: "In drafting [Art. 33], members of [the Ad Hoc] Committee had kept their eyes on the stars but their feet on the ground. Since that time, however, the international situation had deteriorated, and it must be recognized,

> If a refugee is spying against his country of residence, he is threatening the national security of that country ... The same applies if he is engaged in activities directed at the overthrow by force or other illegal means of the government of his country of residence, or in activities which are directed against a foreign government, which as a result threatens the government of the country of residence with intervention of a serious nature.[550]

There is also little doubt that national security may be at risk where there is a fundamental threat to a state's citizens, wherever they may be located.[551] But as Lord Slynn observed for the House of Lords in *Rehman*, "I do not accept that these are the only examples of action which makes it in the interests of national security to deport a person."[552]

In line with greater contemporary concern about the risks of terrorism,[553] senior courts have come to embrace a more ample understanding of national security. They have expressed concern that the traditional definition of national security, under which there is a requirement to show the risk of a direct impact on the host state,

> limits too tightly the discretion of the executive in deciding how the interests of the state, including not merely military defense but democracy, the legal and constitutional systems of the state, need to be protected. I accept that there must be a real possibility of an adverse effect on the [host state] for what is done by the individual under inquiry, but I do not accept that it has to be direct or immediate.[554]

---

albeit with reluctance, that at present many governments would find difficulty in accepting unconditionally the principle [of *non-refoulement*]."

[550] A. Grahl-Madsen, "Expulsion of Refugees," in P. Macalister-Smith and G. Alfredsson eds., *The Land Beyond: Collected Essays on Refugee Law and Policy by Atle Grahl-Madsen* 7 (2001), at 8.

[551] This was accepted even at the initial hearing level: *Rehman v. Secretary of State for the Home Department*, [1999] INLR 517 (UK SIAC, Sept. 7, 1999) per Potts J, at 528. This decision was subsequent considered in *Secretary of State for the Home Department v. Rehman*, [2000] 3 WLR 1240 (Eng. CA, May 23, 2000); and in *Secretary of State for the Home Department v. Rehman*, [2001] UKHL 47 (UK HL, Oct. 11, 2001), discussed below.

[552] *Secretary of State for the Home Department v. Rehman*, [2001] UKHL 47 (UK HL, Oct. 11, 2001), per Lord Slynn of Hadley at para. 16.

[553] "It seems to me that, in contemporary world conditions, action against a foreign state may be capable indirectly of affecting the security of the United Kingdom. The means open to terrorists both in attacking another state and attacking international or global activity by the community of nations, whatever the objectives of the terrorist, may be capable of reflecting on the safety and well-being of the United Kingdom or its citizens. The sophistication of means available, the speed of movement of persons and goods, the speed of modern communication, are all factors which may have to be taken into account in deciding whether there is a real possibility that the national security of the United Kingdom may immediately or subsequently be put at risk by the action of others": ibid.

[554] Ibid. See also *Attorney General v. Zaoui*, Dec. No. CA20/04 (NZ CA, Sept. 30, 2004), at para. 135: "It is clear from the *travaux préparatoires* for the Refugee Convention that there

Thus, the House of Lords in *Rehman* expressly authorized the executive to adopt a "preventative or precautionary" approach to the assessment of risks to national security,[555] finding that "[t]he United Kingdom is not obliged to harbour a terrorist who is currently taking action against some other state (or even in relation to a contested area of land claimed by another state) if that other state could realistically be seen by the [executive] as likely to take action against the United Kingdom and its citizens."[556]

The Supreme Court of Canada not only endorsed the logic of the *Rehman* decision, but defined a relatively liberal evidentiary framework for meeting the broadened test of a risk to national security. In *Suresh*, the Court first acknowledged that not every danger to the public of a host state rises to the level of a threat to national security,[557] and that it was generally accepted that "under international law the state must prove a connection between the terrorist activity and the security of the deporting country."[558] In line with the House of Lords, it held that "possible future risks must be considered,"[559] and that the risk to national security "may be grounded in distant events that indirectly have a real possibility of harming Canadian security."[560] But in defining how the ultimate question of a "real and serious possibility of adverse effect [on] Canada"[561] should be proved, the Supreme Court of Canada went beyond the approach of the House of Lords to endorse what appears to be an evidentiary presumption grounded in modern global interdependence, namely that proof of a risk to the security of another country is generally probative of a threat to Canadian national security:

> International conventions must be interpreted in the light of current conditions. It may once have made sense to suggest that terrorism in one country *did not necessarily implicate* other countries. But after the year 2001, that approach is no longer valid [emphasis added].[562]

---

was intended to be a margin of appreciation for States in the interpretation of that phrase ... Indeed, one would expect that views on security could well differ between States, depending on the particular circumstances of those States ... Views as to what would constitute a danger to national security can also legitimately change over time."

[555] *Secretary of State for the Home Department v. Rehman*, [2001] UKHL 47 (UK HL, Oct. 11, 2001), per Lord Slynn of Hadley at para. 17.

[556] Ibid. at para. 19.

[557] *Suresh v. Canada*, [2002] 1 SCR 3 (Can. SC, Jan. 11, 2002), at para. 84.

[558] Ibid. at para. 85, citing J. Hathaway and C. Harvey, "Framing Refugee Protection in the New World Disorder," (2001) 34(2) *Cornell International Law Journal* 257, at 289–290.

[559] *Suresh v. Canada*, [2002] 1 SCR 3 (Can. SC, Jan. 11, 2002), at para. 88.

[560] Ibid. The views of the House of Lords and Supreme Court of Canada on this point were adopted by the New Zealand Court of Appeal in *Attorney General v. Zaoui*, Dec. No. CA20/04 (NZ CA, Sept. 30, 2004), at para. 147.

[561] *Suresh v. Canada*, [2002] 1 SCR 3 (Can. SC, Jan. 11, 2002), at para. 88.

[562] Ibid. at para. 87.

The implied assertion that terrorism in one country necessarily implicates the security of other countries is surely an empirical overstatement. But if understood to suggest instead that a connection is more likely than not, there are good grounds to accept the notion of a (rebuttable) presumption, namely that proof of risk to the most basic interests of one state by reason of the refugee's actions justifies a *prima facie* belief that the refugee poses a risk to the national security of his or her host state. This more moderate notion seems to infuse the Court's summary of the meaning of national security:

> [A] person constitutes a "danger to the security of Canada" if he or she poses a serious threat to the security of Canada, whether direct or indirect, and bearing in mind the fact that the security of one country *is often dependent* on the security of other nations. The threat must be "serious," in the sense that it must be grounded on objectively reasonable suspicion based on evidence and in the sense that the threatened harm must be substantial rather than negligible [emphasis added].[563]

In sum, a refugee poses a risk to the host state's national security if his or her presence or actions give rise to an objectively reasonable, real possibility of directly or indirectly inflicted substantial harm to the host state's most basic interests, including the risk of an armed attack on its territory or its citizens, or the destruction of its democratic institutions.

In an appropriate case, provisional measures necessary to counter a threat to national security may involve suspension of any of the rights set by the Refugee Convention,[564] even authorizing states to mandate generalized internment pending status determination.[565] As such, the recent decision of the United States that critical national security interests require the detention of persons applying for recognition of refugee status from any of more than thirty Arab and Muslim countries could potentially be justifiable within the

---

[563] Ibid. at para. 90.

[564] See Mr. Hoare's intervention to this effect at UN Doc. A/CONF.2/SR.6, July 4, 1951, at 13. Because Art. 9 explicitly takes precedence over any contrary requirement in the Refugee Convention ("Nothing in this Convention shall prevent a Contracting State . . . from taking provisionally measures which it considers to be essential"), a government is not required to respect even the limitations on security-based resort to expulsion and *refoulement* set out in Art. 32 and 33 so long as the criteria of Art. 9 are satisfied. But see the discussion of the requirement that the provisional measures be "essential," at p. 267 below.

[565] "Everyone would agree that a Government in time of crisis might be forced to intern refugees in order to investigate whether they were genuine or not and therefore a possible danger to the security of the country": Statement of Mr. Bienenfeld of the World Jewish Congress, UN Doc. E/AC.32/SR.34, Aug. 14, 1950, at 18. See also Statement of Mr. Hoare of the United Kingdom, UN Doc. A/CONF.2/SR.28, July 19, 1951, at 6: "The kind of action which he envisaged States might take under the provisions of [Art. 9] would be, for example, the wholesale immediate internment of refugees in time of war, followed by a screening process, after which many could be released."

parameters of what Art. 9 allows.[566] But because only "essential" restrictions are authorized, the state is limited to taking measures that are logically connected to avoidance of the threat to national security.[567] While provisional measures may be taken collectively against all refugees, or in relation to a national or other subset of the refugee population,[568] this kind of wholesale suspension of rights will be justifiable as "essential" only in response to an extremely compelling threat to national security.[569] Thus, for example, there can be no presumption that the existence of a "mass influx" of refugees necessarily grants states the authority provisionally to suspend rights.[570]

---

[566] "The Department of Homeland Security announced... 'Asylum applications from nations where al-Qa'ida, al-Qa'ida sympathisers and other terrorist groups are known to have operated will be detained for the duration of their processing period'... It described the initiative as temporary, 'reasonable and prudent'": A. Gumbel, "On the brink of war: US to round up all Muslim and Arab asylum-seekers: Security," *Independent*, Mar. 19, 2003, at 10.

[567] In his description of the scope of "exceptional measures," the British representative to the Ad Hoc Committee made clear that actions taken must be directly related to the threat perceived. "He wished to explain that the term 'exceptional measures' covered not only internment but such measures as restrictions on the possession of wireless apparatus, in order to prevent the reception of code messages and the conversion of receiving into transmitting apparatus": Statement of Sir Leslie Brass of the United Kingdom, UN Doc. E/AC.32/SR.35, Aug. 15, 1950, at 8.

[568] The reference to measures "in the case of a particular person" was agreed to without any substantive discussion, apparently on the grounds that the original reference to "any person" was unduly general relative to the usual reference in the Convention to "refugees": UN Doc. A/CONF.2/SR.6, July 4, 1951, at 13. Taking account of the purpose of the article as a whole, Grahl-Madsen's view that this reference is intended to "restrict the applicability of provisional measures to individual persons, thus ruling out large scale measures against groups of refugees" should not be adopted: Grahl-Madsen, *Commentary*, at 45. Measures are taken in the case of a particular person whether they are *directed against* a particular person, or simply *define the treatment* of a particular person on the basis of a generalized assessment. This clause may therefore be read to allow provisional measures to be taken in particular cases so long as those measures derive from a (specific or general) assessment that national security would be jeopardized but for the actions in question.

[569] The requirement that the provisional "measures... *be essential*... in the case of a particular person [emphasis added]" can be read to mean that the government in question should satisfy itself that the consequential violation of the human rights of particular refugees is an unavoidable necessity to avert the security risks occasioned by war or other exceptional circumstances. A refusal to sanction resort to "avoidable" provisional measures is consistent with the insistence of the drafters that this authority be "exceptional" and reserved for "very special cases": see text above, at pp. 261–262.

[570] Some scholars nonetheless erroneously suggest that it is permissible to deliver less than full respect for refugee rights in the case of a "mass influx." B. S. Chimni, for example, has written that "[i]t is often the complaint of states in the [South Asian] region that the rights regime embodied in the 1951 Convention is unsuited to the conditions of the poor world as they do not have the resources to fulfill their obligations. In this respect there is a

Perhaps most important, Art. 9 does not authorize generalized derogation on an ongoing basis, but only as a provisional measure.[571] A state that wishes to avail itself of the provisional measures authority must proceed in good faith to verify the claims to refugee status of all persons whose rights are thereby suspended.[572] If a particular person is found not to be a Convention refugee, including on the basis of criminal or other exclusion under Art. 1(F), no rights under the Refugee Convention accrue, and removal from the territory or the imposition of other restrictions is allowed.[573] If, on the other hand, an individual is found to satisfy the Convention refugee definition, Art. 9 establishes a presumption that the provisional measures shall come to an end.[574]

Provisional measures may be maintained in force in a particular case only if security concerns remain to be investigated even at the time a determination of refugee status is made. War or other exceptional circumstances might deny a government the resources routinely to investigate each applicant for refugee status. Inquiries would instead be instigated only in response to a particular concern which might or might not surface in time to be thoroughly canvassed before a determination of refugee status was made. If the authorities of an asylum state were denied the ability to investigate even late-

---

need for research to determine a minimal core of assistance and the bundle of rights to be applicable in situations of mass influx": B. Chimni, "The Law and Politics of Regional Solution of the Refugee Problem: The Case of South Asia," RCSS Policy Studies 4, Regional Centre for Strategic Studies, Colombo (1998), at 13.

[571] This is, of course, clear from the literal text of the article, which explicitly sanctions a state "taking provisionally measures which it considers to be essential to the national security ... pending a [refugee status] determination." Indeed, while the Australian representative argued perhaps most strenuously for a wide-ranging power of derogation, even he made clear "that it was never his delegation's intention to open the way to an indefinite extension of the circumstances in which states could take exceptional measures": Statement of Mr. Shaw of Australia, UN Doc. A/CONF.2/SR.6, July 4, 1951, at 14.

[572] "During the war . . . [i]t was impossible to give all persons entering the country as refugees a thorough security examination, which had to be deferred till exceptional circumstances made it necessary": Statement of Sir Leslie Brass of the United Kingdom, UN Doc. E/AC.32/SR.35, Aug. 15, 1950, at 8. As Robinson observes, "[t]he purpose of Art. 9 is to permit the wholesale provisional internment of refugees in time of war, followed by a screening process": Robinson, *History*, at 95.

[573] Countervailing domestic or international legal obligations, for example duties to avoid removal under the Convention against Torture and Other Cruel, Inhuman or Degrading Treatment or Punishment, UNGA Res. 39/46, adopted Dec. 10, 1984, entered into force June 26, 1987, may operate independently to prevent removal from the asylum country.

[574] Robinson argues that the provisional measures "have to be suspended if the person involved can prove conclusively his status as a refugee": Robinson, *History*, at 95. The literal meaning of Art. 9 cannot, however, sustain this interpretation. The requirement that in the case of a refugee "the continuance of such measures [must be] necessary in his case in the interests of national security" is, however, a sufficient basis to argue that absent such a finding, provisional measures must be terminated.

breaking security risks in a specific case, they might take a less generous attitude toward the admission of refugees.[575]

The drafting Committee therefore approved an exception to the presumption that a positive determination of refugee status ends the application of provisional measures. If there is a specific finding in regard to a particular refugee "that such measures are still necessary in his case in the interests of national security,"[576] the Committee agreed that it should be possible to continue provisional measures for the time it takes to investigate the concerns. As an exception to the general purpose of Art. 9, however, this authority must be restrictively construed. In particular, it authorizes only the continuance of provisional measures, not the establishment of indefinite restrictions in the interests of national security.[577] Nor does it provide any general authority to limit the rights of persons already recognized to be Convention refugees.[578]

The duty to terminate provisional measures does not mean, however, that the government of the asylum country is prevented from protecting itself against risks to its national security posed by a person recognized as a genuine refugee. It must, however, ground its actions in the authority of a particular article of the Convention, rather than relying on the generic authority of Art. 9.[579] There is therefore no logical inconsistency between the strictly temporary and situation-specific nature of provisional measures and the understandable concern of governments to be in a position to safeguard their basic interests.

In sum, provisional measures may be taken only in time of war or comparable exceptional circumstances, and on the basis of a good faith assessment that they are essential to protection of the receiving state's most vital national interests. The specific actions authorized are broad-ranging, though they must be logically connected to eradication of the security concern and be justifiable as essential, taking full account of the particularized harms

---

[575] "In his country refugees were granted legal status after a previous examination on their entering the country; later information obtained sometimes threw new light on their possible danger to the community. If the State were not permitted to take measures against refugees in the light of such later information, it would be less willing to accord them citizen status": Statement of Mr. Winter of Canada, UN Doc. E/AC.32/SR.35, Aug. 15, 1950, at 10.

[576] UN Doc. E/1850, Aug. 25, 1950, at 16. There is no indication that the rephrasing of the provision ("that the continuance of such measures is necessary in his case") was intended to effect a substantive change of any kind.

[577] This is clear both from the reference to the continuance of "such measures," and from the inclusion of the provision as part of an article expressly dedicated to provisional measures.

[578] Art. 9 authorizes the "continuance" of provisional measures in exceptional cases, but not their initiation or reestablishment.

[579] See p. 260 above, at n. 535.

consequentially occasioned. Provisional measures may not be of indefinite duration, but instead normally come to an end if and when an individual's refugee status is formally verified. While they may exceptionally be continued where case-specific national security concerns have not been resolved by the time refugee status is formally determined, provisional measures may not otherwise be applied against persons already recognized as Convention refugees.

3.5.2 Exemption from exceptional measures

Refugee Convention, Art. 8   Exemption from exceptional measures
With regard to exceptional measures which may be taken against the person, property or interests of nationals of a foreign State, the Contracting States shall not apply such measures to a refugee who is formally a national of the said State solely on account of such nationality. Contracting States which, under their legislation, are prevented from applying the general principle expressed in this article, shall, in appropriate cases, grant exemptions in favour of such refugees.

Outside the context of war or comparable crisis, the drafters of the Refugee Convention opposed any general right of states to suspend refugee rights.[580] Of particular concern was the practice following the Second World War of subjecting refugees to confiscatory and other penalties imposed on enemy aliens:

> After the Second World War, many refugees who had been persecuted by the Governments of the Axis countries were subjected to exceptional measures taken against the nationals of enemy countries (internment, sequestration of property, blocking of assets, etc.) because of the fact that formally they were still *de jure* nationals of those countries. The injustice of such treatment was finally recognized and many administrative measures (screening boards, special tribunals, creation of a special category of "non-enemy" refugees, etc.) were used to mitigate the practice.[581]

To ensure that refugees would not be stigmatized by the fact of their formal nationality,[582] the International Refugee Organization played an instrumental

---

[580] See text above, at p. 261.
[581] Secretary-General, "Memorandum," at 48.
[582] The nature of the dilemma is neatly summarized in Ad Hoc Committee, "First Session Report," at 42: "Unless a refugee has been deprived of the nationality of his country of origin he retains that nationality. Since his nationality is retained, exceptional measures applied . . . to such nationals would be applied to him. The article provides therefore that exceptional measures shall not be applied only on the grounds of his nationality." The French delegate to the Ad Hoc Committee indicated that "the word 'formally' meant

role in persuading governments to adopt Art. 44 of the 1949 Geneva Convention relative to the Protection of Civilian Persons in Time of War:

> [T]he Detaining Power shall not treat as enemy aliens exclusively on the basis of their nationality *de jure* of an enemy State, refugees who do not, in fact, enjoy the protection of any Government.[583]

As the Secretary-General convincingly argued, "[i]f this rule is to be applied in time of war, a similar rule must *a fortiori* be applied in time of peace. The object of Art. [8] is to remove both the person and property and interest of refugees from the scope of exceptional measures."[584]

Nor was the concern of the drafters restricted to the particular measures that had been taken at the end of the Second World War. The French representative to the Ad Hoc Committee observed that refugees were sometimes penalized during peacetime on the grounds of their formal nationality by subjection to both retaliatory measures and restrictions resulting from economic or financial crisis.[585] While states required a margin of discretion to withhold rights from persons claiming refugee status during wartime, Mr. Juvigny insisted that there was no basis to assert a comparable prerogative during peacetime.[586] The decision was therefore taken to separate the rules relating to exceptional measures applicable only during war or comparable emergencies (Art. 9) from those governing measures which might be taken at any time (Art. 8).[587]

'legally'": Statement of Mr. Juvigny, UN Doc. E/AC.32/SR.35, Aug. 15, 1950, at 7. Grahl-Madsen concludes that "[t]he word 'formally' means 'legally' or *de jure*, that is to say, according to the municipal law of the State concerned": Grahl-Madsen, *Commentary*, at 40.

[583] Geneva Convention relative to the Protection of Civilian Persons in Time of War, 75 UNTS 287, done Aug. 12, 1949, entered into force Oct. 21, 1950, at Art. 44. The Red Cross recently affirmed that Art. 8 of the Refugee Convention "clearly reflects Article 44 of the Fourth Geneva Convention": "Humanitarian Debate: Law, Policy, Action," in (2001) 83(843) *International Review of the Red Cross* 633.

[584] Secretary-General, "Memorandum," at 48.

[585] Statement of Mr. Juvigny of France, UN Doc. E/AC.32/SR.35, Aug. 15, 1950, at 5.

[586] The French representative noted the importance of "making a distinction between two types of exceptional measures . . . namely: on the one hand, measures taken in peacetime or during crises of a non-military type . . . and, on the other hand, measures taken in exceptional circumstances which affected peace or national security. The provisions relating to the latter type of measures would naturally be more severe than the former": ibid.

[587] "The measures referred to in article [8] were not designed only for times of emergency. A second paragraph should be added to cover the particular case of emergency in which the rights of refugees could be restricted, but only as little as was absolutely necessary": Statement of Mr. Robinson of Israel, UN Doc. E/AC.32/SR.34, Aug. 14, 1950, at 22. In the Report of the Ad Hoc Committee, the two concerns were therefore addressed in different paragraphs of the same article. The Report notes simply that "the Committee thought it advisable to add a paragraph in order to clarify the application of this article in regard to

The logic of exempting refugees from measures of retaliation or retorsion is fairly straightforward. The sorts of penalties sometimes applied against the citizens of a particular nationality during peacetime – for example, freezing or blocking of assets, the denial of visas, or curbing of civil liberties – are intended to punish or pressure the state of nationality to act or refrain from acting in a particular way. As observed above in the discussion of reciprocity,[588] there is little reason to believe that a state which is the target of acts of retaliation or retorsion would be influenced by the suffering of persons who have rejected its protection by the act of seeking refugee status. The injustice of including refugees in the scope of exceptional measures is therefore clear.[589]

The context governed by Art. 8 is quite broad.[590] It is applicable during time of war or other critical national emergency, though the more specific provisions of Art. 9 grant states expanded authority over refugees still seeking recognition of their status in such extreme circumstances. In addition, Art. 8 governs resort to exceptional measures during a "cold war, approximating a state of war, tension, a state of emergency or an international crisis calling for certain internal precautions."[591] There could also be a temporary dispute between states, for example in consequence of trade concerns or the failure to pay damages.[592] Diplomatic relations may have been suspended or broken off completely. In all such circumstances, whatever measures may be taken *en bloc* against the citizens of the offending state may not be applied against refugees, irrespective of the duration and character of a particular refugee's presence.[593]

---

measures related to national security in time of war and national emergency": Ad Hoc Committee, "Second Session Report," at 12. The Conference of Plenipotentiaries adopted a British proposal (UN Doc. A/CONF.2/26) to separate the two paragraphs into distinct articles of the Convention: UN Doc. A/CONF.2/SR.6, July 4, 1951, at 16.

[588] See chapter 3.2.2 above, at pp. 204–205.

[589] The over-breadth of such measures may also violate the duty of non-discrimination. See chapter 2.5.5 above, at pp. 144–145.

[590] "[I]t was impossible to legislate for future possible contingencies . . . It was, therefore, important that [Art. 8] should be made as flexible as possible": Statement of Mr. Petren of Sweden, UN Doc. A/CONF.2/SR.26, July 19, 1951, at 9.

[591] Statement of Mr. Rochefort of France, UN Doc. A/CONF.2/SR.6, July 4, 1951, at 14.

[592] In the Ad Hoc Committee, the Israeli representative "inquired whether the article was broad enough to include possible retaliation and retorsion by countries against subjects of States with which they had a temporary disagreement. He did not think that exceptional measures of that kind should apply to refugees from countries against whose subjects such measures were directed": Statement of Mr. Robinson of Israel, UN Doc. E/AC.32/SR.21, Feb. 2, 1950, at 7. The Chairman, Mr. Chance of Canada, confirmed that such measures would be precluded by Art. 8: ibid. at 8.

[593] Indeed, Grahl-Madsen suggests that "[t]here can be no doubt that the Article applies to all Convention refugees, irrespective of whether they are present in the territory of the Contracting State concerned": Grahl-Madsen, *Commentary*, at 40.

There are two important qualifications to this general rule. First, the duty to exempt refugees from exceptional measures governs only measures taken solely on the grounds of nationality.[594] Because the objective of Art. 8 is to avoid unfairly stigmatizing refugees on the basis of their possession of a formal, but de facto ineffective, nationality,[595] only "wholesale measures"[596] defined by nationality contravene Art. 8. Robinson observes that

> a state is free to apply to a refugee exceptional measures if they are taken on grounds other than his [formal] nationality. Thus Art. 8 ... would not hinder the application of exceptional measures on account of the economic or political activity or special unwanted contacts of a refugee, if such activity or contacts are, in general, a reason for applying all or some of the exceptional measures.[597]

As this analysis suggests, the critical issue is the generality of the measure in question.[598] So long as the exceptional measure is not aimed simply at persons of a particular nationality, but is instead applicable to all persons who meet the contingent standard that governs the right suspended, then refugees cannot complain that they too are subject to its impact.[599] For

---

[594] "[T]he word 'solely' ... indicated that, while exceptional measures could be taken against refugees, they could not be taken on the grounds of nationality alone": Statement of Mr. Henkin of the United States, UN Doc. E/AC.32/SR.21, Feb. 2, 1950, at 7. This understanding was affirmed by both the Turkish representative, ibid., and by the Chairman, Mr. Chance of Canada, ibid. at 8: "[T]he article would prevent exceptional measures of retaliation or retorsion from being applied to refugees solely on the grounds of their nationality."

[595] "Article 8 does not mention former nationals of a foreign State. If, however, measures are taken against persons solely because they are, or have been (at any time) or are suspected of being, nationals of a certain State, it goes without saying that the case will fall within the scope of Article 8": Grahl-Madsen, *Commentary*, at 40. See also Statement of the President, Mr. Larsen of Denmark, UN Doc. E/AC.32/SR.35, Aug. 15, 1950, at 6; and Robinson, *History*, at 93–94: "[I]n practice denaturalized citizens of an enemy state or persons whose origin was in such a state were frequently subjected to all or some of the measures taken against nationals. A proper interpretation of Art. 8 would lead us to the conclusion that mere former citizenship or origin in such a state cannot *a fortiori* be a reason for the application of exceptional measures to a refugee."

[596] Weis, *Travaux*, at 75.   [597] Robinson, *History*, at 91.

[598] See Grahl-Madsen, *Commentary*, at 39: "The reference to 'nationals of a foreign State' considerably restricts the applicability of the Article. It does not apply to measures which may be taken against stateless persons as such, or against aliens generally, not to speak of measures which are directed at one's nationals and aliens without discrimination."

[599] "The Belgian representative appeared to be opposed to any possibility of interning refugees; the text however only prohibited such internment if it were effected simply on account of the refugees' nationality. In 1939–40, and at later periods, the French authorities had interned not only aliens, but also a few French nationals suspected of fifth-column activities. Such a measure, which only conditions of crisis could justify, could not be prohibited under article [8]": Statement of Mr. Juvigny of France, UN Doc. E/AC.32/SR.35, Aug. 15, 1950, at 7.

example, refugees are entitled to property rights on terms "not less favourable than [those] accorded to aliens generally in the same circumstances."[600] Confiscatory exceptional measures applied to all aliens (whatever their nationality) would thus not contravene Art. 8. On the other hand, refugees are entitled to access rationing systems on terms of equality with nationals of the asylum state.[601] Exceptional measures directed to aliens generally cannot therefore lawfully be applied against refugees, since refugees are outside the scope of the group legally subject to the measures. Importantly, exceptional measures that do not contravene Art. 8 may nonetheless be challenged on the basis of the general duty of non-discrimination,[602] though the margin of appreciation usually accorded states may undercut the utility of that remedy.[603]

Second, the goal of Art. 8 is to ensure that exceptional measures defined by nationality do not, in practice, result in the denial of rights to refugees. The Swedish government waged a determined battle at the Conference of Plenipotentiaries to ensure that Art. 8 was not understood to require governments to rewrite domestic laws that fail to codify an exemption from exceptional measures in the case of refugees. Originally, the Swedish objective seemed to be to grant states a near-complete right to decide for themselves when refugees should benefit from an exemption from exceptional measures.[604] But as the Belgian representative noted, the validation of state discretion to define the circumstances in which exemption is warranted "would considerably reduce the rights accorded to refugees by the Convention."[605] More specifically:

> It was . . . to be feared that [the Swedish approach] would result in a regime
> of arbitrary decisions, since countries of residence would be at liberty either

---

[600] Refugee Convention, at Art. 13.   [601] Ibid. at Art. 20.   [602] See chapter 2.5.5 above.
[603] See chapter 2.5.5 above, at pp. 128–145.
[604] Sweden asserted that "[o]ne could easily imagine cases in which it would appear fully justified to maintain the confiscation of the property of a refugee even if that property, in his hands, did not constitute a menace to national security. A person might for instance have fled from Nazi Germany at a very late stage of the Second World War after having been a militant Nazi up to then. Should States decide to take certain measures against the nationals of another State, it would have to be left to their administrations to decide whether refugees from the country in question could be exempted from them": Statement of Mr. Petren of Sweden, UN Doc. A.CONF.2/SR.27, July 18, 1951, at 28–29. Yet, as the British representative subsequently observed (UN Doc. A/CONF.2/SR.28, July 19, 1951, at 8), each state party would first have to determine whether or not the individual in question even qualified as a refugee. In the case cited by the Swedish delegate, there is good reason to believe that exclusion from refugee status under Art. 1(F)(a) is a real possibility. In any event, it is unclear that a militant Nazi fleeing Nazi Germany would in any sense have a well-founded fear of being persecuted in Nazi Germany.
[605] Statement of Mr. Herment of Belgium, UN Doc. A/CONF.2/SR.27, July 18, 1951, at 31.

not to apply to a refugee the exceptional measures which they might be obliged to take against the person, property or interests of other nationals of his country of origin, or to grant certain exemptions in the case of such refugees. Refugees would therefore have no absolute right to exemption from the application of those measures, and decisions as to the cases in which exemption was appropriate would be left to Governments.[606]

Even more emphatically, the Canadian representative asserted that the Swedish initiative resulted in an approach to Art. 8 that was "guilty of the unhappy fault of, so to speak, taking away with one hand what it gave with the other. In its original form, and before an attempt had been made to take into account the circumstances and laws of a certain country, the article had consisted of a simple and straightforward statement."[607]

Confronted with such direct attacks, the Swedish government sought to downplay the significance of the amendment it had sponsored to the text of Art. 8. It insisted that the addition of the words "or shall provide for appropriate exemptions in respect of such refugees"[608] was simply intended to allow governments the option of meeting their Art. 8 obligation either by way of a generic exemption for refugees from exceptional measures, or by extending case-specific exemptions to all refugees.[609] Whichever option was taken, the result would be the same, namely, a mandatory duty to exempt refugees from exceptional measures.[610] As the President of the Conference concluded, "the problem turned on the question of whether the application of certain measures should be ensured by means of automatic legislation or by means of exemptions. *In either case the obligations of the State would be the same* [emphasis added]."[611]

---

[606] Statement of Mr. Herment of Belgium, UN Doc. A/CONF.2/SR.28, July 19, 1951, at 8.

[607] Statement of Mr. Chance of Canada, UN Doc. A/CONF.2/SR.34, July 25, 1951, at 18.

[608] UN Doc. A/CONF.2/37.

[609] The French representative's view of the Swedish approach was that it "was very far from suggesting measures of an illiberal nature. It laid upon states the obligation to grant certain exemptions at the time when they were unable to observe the general principle enunciated in the article. If that principle was not acceptable to States, they would enter a general reservation to the article. He would interpret the words 'ou accorderont' as imposing an obligation to grant exemptions": Statement of Mr. Rochefort of France, UN Doc. A/CONF.2/SR.34, July 25, 1951, at 20.

[610] "Either legislation could be passed exempting certain categories of aliens from the application of the enemy property act, or some arrangement could be made to enable such persons to claim the return of their property provided they could substantiate their right to restoration. Those two possibilities must both be allowed for, or administrative difficulties would arise": Statement of Mr. Petren of Sweden, UN Doc. A/CONF.2/SR.28, July 19, 1951, at 8.

[611] Statement of the President, Mr. Larsen of Denmark, UN Doc. A/CONF.2/SR.34, July 25, 1951, at 19.

In a last-minute effort to capture the essence of this consensus,[612] the Canadian representative persuaded delegates to accept an oral amendment to the previously accepted Swedish phrasing of Art. 8. Sadly, the precise language chosen can be construed so as to give rise to the very concern that both the Canadian delegate and the Conference as a whole appeared determined to avoid.[613] Instead of the Swedish language "or shall provide for appropriate exemptions in respect of such refugees,"[614] the Canadian amendment adopted by the Conference provides that state parties whose domestic legislation prevents the granting of *en bloc* exemption from exceptional measures to refugees "shall, *in appropriate cases*, grant [exemptions] in favour of such refugees [emphasis added]."[615] Thus, even though the Swedish government had been content with language that appeared quite clearly to impose a mandatory duty to exempt all refugees (albeit via a process of particularized exemptions), the literal text of the Canadian amendment – which includes the qualifying phrase "in appropriate cases" – may be read to suggest that there will be some cases in which exemption will not be appropriate, and hence not necessary.[616]

This is clearly a case in which reliance simply on the plain language of the treaty would result in an interpretation that is inconsistent not only with the general purpose of the Refugee Convention,[617] but moreover with the express

[612] "[H]e believed that the meeting was on the brink of agreement. There was no objection to the general principle that no exceptional measures should be applied to a refugee solely on account of his nationality": Statement of Mr. Chance of Canada, ibid. at 22.

[613] "The Conference posed the question whether the word 'shall' should be interpreted as being mandatory or permissive and came out firmly in favor of the first interpretation[ ]. With regard to substance if not to form, the obligations of the Contracting States would be the same whether they based themselves on the first or the second sentence": Grahl-Madsen, *Commentary*, at 41. Robinson, however, takes the view that "the second sentence (included by the Conference) considerably restricts the import of this article ... It is obvious that the sentence was included in order to 'appease' states which are not or would not be willing to accept the general rule as expressed in the first sentence": Robinson, *History*, at 90–91.

[614] UN Doc. A/CONF.2/37.

[615] The oral amendment proposed by Canada referred to "exceptions" rather than "exemptions": Statement of Mr. Chance of Canada, UN Doc. A/CONF.2/SR.34, July 25, 1951, at 22.

[616] See e.g. Robinson, *History*, at 93: "What these cases are depends on what the law provides; in other words, by domestic legislation the state can fix the instances in which exemption is granted but the limits cannot be such as to refuse exemption when it would not threaten the proper application of the measures and their contemplated effects."

[617] "By entering reservations to Article 8, a State reserves the right, for instance, in time of war to intern refugees considered to be enemy aliens. While conceding that the fact of internment may not necessarily undermine the humanitarian basis of the Convention in every case, the very fact of internment or other related restrictions defeat[s] the ideal of the Convention as the vehicle for providing a safe haven for the refugee in the State of

intention of every state that addressed the desirable scope of Art. 8 at the Conference of Plenipotentiaries. This unhappy result can be avoided, however, by seeing the reference to "appropriate cases" not as an invitation to exercise discretion, but as a shorthand reference to any effort to impose exceptional measures solely on account of nationality. It is clear, however, that states need not formally enact exemptions from exceptional measures that accrue to the benefit of refugees, so long as they are prepared in practice dependably to grant refugees exemption from such measures.[618]

refuge where he or she may enjoy basic civil liberties": Blay and Tsamenyi, "Reservations," at 554.

[618] Robinson argues that "[i]f, as seems to be the case, 'legislation' refers not only to past but also to future laws, the second sentence is an 'invitation' to enact [legislation prohibiting *en bloc* exemption from exceptional measures for refugees], wherever it does not yet exist. From the viewpoint of a state it is undoubtedly more prudent not to be bound by a general rule of exemption": Robinson, *History*, at 93. It is unclear that this is so. Given the consensus in favor of a duty to exercise discretion in favor of refugees, the net result may simply be increased processing costs for the asylum country.

Rights of refugees physically present

This chapter addresses those rights which follow automatically and immediately from the simple fact of being a Convention refugee within the effective jurisdiction of a state party. These primary protection rights must continue to be respected throughout the duration of refugee status, with additional rights accruing once the asylum-seeker's presence is regularized, and again when a refugee is allowed to stay or reside in the asylum country.

Convention rights can obviously not be claimed until all the requirements of the Convention refugee definition are satisfied, including departure from one's own state.[1] But since refugee rights are defined to inhere by virtue of refugee status alone, they must be respected by state parties until and unless a negative determination of the refugee's claim to protection is rendered. This is because refugee status under the Convention arises from the nature of one's predicament rather than from a formal determination of status.[2] Refugee rights, however, remain inchoate until and unless the refugee comes under the de jure or de facto jurisdiction of a state party to the Convention. This is because the Convention binds particular state parties, each of which is required to meet obligations only within its own sphere of authority.[3]

Assuming that these two conditions are met, what rights ought refugees to be able to invoke as matters of basic entitlement, whether or not their status has been formally assessed? While the extension of some rights can logically

---

[1] "For the purposes of the present Convention, the term 'refugee' shall apply to any person who ... *is outside the country of his nationality* and is unable or ... is unwilling to avail himself of the protection of that country; or who, not having a nationality and *being outside the country of his former habitual residence* ... is unable or ... unwilling to return to it [emphasis added]": Convention relating to the Status of Refugees, 189 UNTS 2545, done July 28, 1951, entered into force Apr. 22, 1954 (Refugee Convention), at Art. 1(A)(2).

[2] "A person is a refugee within the meaning of the 1951 Convention as soon as he fulfils the criteria contained in the definition. This would necessarily occur prior to the time at which his refugee status is formally determined. Recognition of his refugee status does not therefore make him a refugee but declares him to be one. He does not become a refugee because of recognition, but is recognized because he is a refugee": UNHCR, *Handbook on Procedures and Criteria for Determining Refugee Status* (1979, reedited 1992) (UNHCR, *Handbook*), at 9. See chapter 3.1 above, at pp. 157–160.

[3] See chapter 3.1.1 above, at pp. 160–161.

be delayed until a refugee's status has been regularized, for example by admission to a procedure for verification of refugee status, which refugee interests should be immediately and unconditionally recognized?

There are six categories of vital concern. First, persons who claim to be refugees are generally entitled to enter and remain in the territory of a state party until and unless they are found not to be Convention refugees. Second, they should not be arbitrarily detained or otherwise penalized for seeking protection. Third, it should be possible to meet essential security and economic subsistence needs while the host state takes whatever measures it deems necessary to verify the claim to Convention refugee status. Fourth, basic human dignity ought to be respected, including by respect for property and related rights, preservation of family unity, honoring freedom of thought, conscience, and religion, and by the provision of primary education to refugee children. Fifth, authoritative documentation of identity and status in the host state should be made available. Sixth, asylum-seekers must have access to a meaningful remedy to enforce their rights, including to seek a remedy for breach of any of these primary protection rights.

4.1 Right to enter and remain in an asylum state (*non-refoulement*)

The most urgent need of refugees is to secure entry into a territory in which they are sheltered from the risk of being persecuted. This fundamental concern must somehow be reconciled to the fact that all of the earth's territory is controlled or claimed by governments which, to a greater or lesser extent, restrict access by non-citizens. This clash of priorities has led to proposals to lease land from states on which to shelter refugees,[4] and even to attempts to establish internationally supervised sanctuaries for would-be refugees within the territory of their own states.[5] To date, however, limited international authority and resources have prevented these options from replacing entry into a foreign state as the most logical means to access safety. The stakes are high: refugees denied admission to a foreign country are likely either to be returned to the risk of persecution in their home state, or to be thrown into perpetual "orbit" in search of a state willing to authorize entry.

There are many historical cases which illustrate the potentially grave consequences of a failure to recognize this need of refugees to be able to enter another state. A particularly notorious example involved 907 German Jews who

---

[4] E. Burton, "Leasing Rights: A New International Instrument for Protecting Refugees and Compensating Host Countries," (1987) 19(1) *Columbia Human Rights Law Review* 307.

[5] These regimes are effectively critiqued in B. Frelick, "Preventive Protection and the Right to Seek Asylum: A Preliminary Look at Bosnia and Croatia," (1992) 4(4) *International Journal of Refugee Law* 439; and A. Shacknove, "From Asylum to Containment," (1993) 5(4) *International Journal of Refugee Law* 516.

fled persecution in their homeland aboard the ocean liner *St. Louis*. After the Cuban government refused to recognize their entrance visas, these refugees were denied permission to land by every country in Latin America. The United States dispatched a gunboat to ensure that the *St. Louis* remained at a distance which prevented its passengers from swimming ashore. Canada argued that the passengers of the *St. Louis* were not a Canadian problem. As Abella and Troper observe, "the Jews of the *St. Louis* returned to Europe, where many would die in the gas chambers and crematoria of the Third Reich."[6]

Similarly blunt denials of access continue to face modern refugees. One of the most notorious cases was the "pushback" order issued by the Thai Ministry of the Interior in 1988. The government deputized fishermen in Khlong Yai to prevent entry of any boats which might be carrying Vietnamese refugees, an order interpreted by fishermen "as a mandate to abuse defenceless boat people. Smugglers, fearing prosecution or vigilante attack, dumped their human cargo into the gulf."[7] Nepal has often refused entry to Tibetan asylum-seekers, including Buddhist monks and nuns, who have thereupon been returned to, and jailed by, Chinese authorities.[8] Hundreds of refugees fleeing conflict in Sierra Leone were summarily sent back by Guinea.[9] Namibia imposed a dusk-to-dawn curfew – with soldiers being ordered to shoot violators – along a 450 km stretch of the Kavango river in late 2001. This effectively prevented Angolan refugees seeking to escape violence in that country's Cuando Cuban Province from being able to seek asylum, since Angolan government and UNITA patrols could be safely avoided only at night.[10] In the wake of the flight of ethnic Albanians from Kosovo, Greek officials simply turned away twenty busloads of refugees at the Macedonian border on the grounds that because they had "not been informed of the influx," they were not prepared to admit the refugees.[11] And Jordan admitted only about 150 of more than 1,000 Iranian, Palestinian, Sudanese, Somali, and

---

[6] I. Abella and H. Troper, *None is Too Many: Canada and the Jews in Europe 1933–1948* (1992), at 64.

[7] A. Helton, "Asylum and Refugee Protection in Thailand," (1989) 1(1) *International Journal of Refugee Law* 20 (Helton, "Thailand"), at 28.

[8] In 1990, Nepalese border guards refused entry to forty-three Tibetan asylum-seekers, including twenty-seven monks and six nuns, who were thereupon jailed by Chinese authorities in Gutsa Prison: US Committee for Refugees, "Tibetan Refugees: Still At Risk" (1990), at 2. There are also efforts to remove the Tibetans after they have entered Nepal. In a recent operation carried out jointly by Nepalese and Chinese authorities, the Tibetans were "carried crying and screaming into vehicles before being driven in the direction of the border": Amnesty International, "Nepal: Forcible Return of Tibetans to China Unacceptable," June 2, 2003.

[9] "Refugee influx concerns President," (1999) 41 *JRS Dispatches* (Jan. 15, 1999).

[10] "Curfew could trap Angolan refugees, says UNHCR," *UN Integrated Regional Information Networks*, Oct. 30, 2001.

[11] J. Hooper, "They vanished in the night: 10,000 refugees unaccounted for after camp cleared," *Guardian*, Apr. 8, 1999, at 1.

Syrian refugees who had received asylum in Iraq, but who were forced to flee that country when threatened by armed Iraqis after the collapse of Saddam Hussein's government.[12]

Turn-back policies can also be implemented by the complete closure of borders. Both Zaïre and Tanzania at times simply closed their borders to refugees attempting to flee the brutal conflict for dominance between Hutus and Tutsis in Northeastern Africa.[13] Tanzania's Foreign Minister reportedly told his Parliament that "[e]nough is enough. Let us tell the refugees that the time has come for them to return home, and no more should come."[14] In 1999, Macedonia cited the failure of Greece, Turkey, Bulgaria, and the European Union to do enough for Kosovo Albanian refugees as justification for its decision to close its borders to all but the most frail refugees, as well as those destined for another country.[15] After providing a haven for more than 2 million Afghan refugees, the Pakistani government closed its borders to most new arrivals in November 2000,[16] arguing that it had not received the support

---

[12] "The refugees told UNHCR that groups of armed Iraqis forced them from their homes and threatened that, if they refused to leave Iraq, the men would be killed and the women raped. Others said that they fled because of the lack of food and water in the places where they normally reside, including the Bijii and Balediyat neighborhoods in Baghdad, and the al-Hurriya and al-Tash refugee camps outside of Baghdad": Human Rights Watch, "US and Allies Must Protect Refugees; Jordan Should Not Block Trapped Refugees," Apr. 23, 2003.

[13] On August 19, 1994, Deputy Prime Minister Malumba Mbangula of Zaïre declared that no refugees would be allowed to cross from Rwanda into Zaïre. Immediately prior to his announcement, 120 refugees per minute had been crossing into Zaïre at the frontier post of Bakavu: "Le Zaïre ferme ses frontières aux réfugiés," *Le Monde*, Aug. 22, 1994, at 4. As some 50,000 refugees attempted to flee ethnic clashes in Burundi, the Tanzanian government officially closed its border with Burundi on March 31, 1995: US Agency for International Development, "Rwanda: Civil Strife/Displaced Persons Situation Report No. 4," Apr. 5, 1995, at 4. The Tanzanian Prime Minister told Parliament that "[t]he gravity of the situation, especially for those coming from Burundi and Rwanda, has made it inevitable for Tanzania to take appropriate security measures by closing her border with Burundi and Rwanda": Speech by the Prime Minister to the Parliament of Tanzania, June 15, 1999, at 5, on file at the library of the Oxford University Refugee Studies Centre.

[14] "Border closure triggers debate," *Guardian*, July 19, 1995.

[15] "Macedonia today effectively closed its borders to tens of thousands of ethnic Albanian refugees caught in no-man's land at the Kosovo frontier, saying the numbers had driven it to the breaking point ... The Interior Minister ... said it was time for its neighbors ... to take up their share of the burden ... Macedonia has become increasingly bitter in recent days about what it sees as the slow response of its neighbors and Western nations to provide help": "Beleaguered Macedonia tries to staunch flood from Kosovo," *New York Times*, Apr. 4, 1999, at A-10.

[16] "Tens of thousands [of refugees] have been camped in the open since January [2001] ... The UNHCR said that more than 80,000 were squatting in squalid conditions on a strip of land at Jalozai, and more were arriving each day": E. MacAskill, "Pakistan keeps Annan from 'world's worst' camp," *Guardian*, Mar. 13, 2001, at 14.

it required from the international community.[17] Its policy was adopted by the other five countries bordering Afghanistan after the September 11, 2001 attack on the World Trade Center.[18]

Blunt barriers can serve much the same end as border closures. During the *apartheid* era, South Africa erected a 3,000 volt electrified, razor wire fence to prevent the entry of refugees from Mozambique.[19] In the summer of 2002, France and the United Kingdom cooperated to build a double fence around the French railway terminal near Calais in order to "close the last loophole" for refugees wishing to travel to Britain in order to seek asylum.[20] A year later, the British immigration minister reported that "the French port was proving impenetrable, without any noticeable shift of asylum-seekers to other ports in northern France or Belgium."[21]

---

[17] "Pakistan rightly complains about the economic burden of supporting such a large influx of people. More than 30,000 crossed in the weeks before the border was closed. The UNHCR appealed for $7.5 million for its Afghan programme this year. It received just $2 million. For every $200 donated for each refugee in the Balkans, just $20 is given for each Afghan refugee. That's a quarter of the cost of one ticket for the Khyber steam train": R. McCarthy, "Comment," *Guardian*, Nov. 27, 2000, at 20.

[18] K. Kenna, "Pakistan closes border to desperate Afghans," *Toronto Star*, Nov. 3, 2001, at A-14. "'If we open the gates freely, we will have to be ready for another 2 million refugees,' Pakistan's president, Gen. Pervez Musharraf, said recently. 'There will be social and economic problems. Do we want another 2 million refugees?'": R. Chandrasekaran, "Predicted outpouring of Afghan refugees is more like trickle," *Washington Post*, Nov. 1, 2001, at A-21. "Many refugees said they tried to enter Pakistan, only to be turned away. Although the United Nations estimates that more than 130,000 refugees have crossed into Pakistan since Sept. 11 [2001], most either have Pakistani identification cards, family members willing to sponsor them, or the money to hire smugglers to take them across unmanned sections of the border": J. Pomfret, "Refugees endure lives of squalor in Taliban camp," *Washington Post*, Nov. 21, 2001, at A-01. By November 2001, "[a]n estimated 100,000 asylum-seekers [were] stranded in the Afghanistan desert": K. Kenna, "Pakistan closes its border to Afghani males," *Hamilton Spectator*, Nov. 28, 2001, at C-05. See generally Human Rights Watch, "Closed Door Policy: Afghan Refugees in Pakistan and Iran" (2001).

[19] As of 1990, official statistics reported that ninety-four refugees had been killed trying to get through the fence: C. Nettleton, "Across the Fence of Fire," (1990) 78 *Refugees* 27, at 27–28. But observers report that the toll was likely much higher. "On the 9th of July 1988, while on a visit to the fence . . . a soldier on the border assured me that while patrolling the fence he used to find between 4–5 bodies per week (in the fence) which, if true, would then mean an average of 200 casualties per year on the southern section of the fence": South African Bishops' Conference, Bureau for Refugees, "The Snake of Fire: Memorandum on the Electric Fence Between Mozambique and South Africa" (1989), at 2–3.

[20] A. Travis, "French to close 'last' way for refugees to use tunnel," *Guardian*, June 26, 2002, at 8.

[21] A. Travis, "New asylum centres open by end of year," *Guardian*, May 9, 2003, at 6, quoting remarks by immigration minister Beverley Hughes to the House of Commons on May 8, 2003.

Even refugees who manage to cross an asylum state's border may still face summary ejection by officials. Cambodia forcibly arrested Montagnard refugees living in Koh Nheak, and forcibly returned them to Vietnamese border police;[22] it has also deported Chinese refugees under the formal protection of UNHCR.[23] Despite the continuation of conflict between the Sri Lankan army and LTTE rebels, Tamil refugees from Sri Lanka were returned by India to Talaimannar in northern Sri Lanka.[24] Pakistani police have randomly stopped Afghan men to check their identification, and driven those without papers to the Afghan border for immediate expulsion.[25] Many Colombians crossing the Rio de Oro to seek protection in Venezuela from paramilitary violence have been intercepted by army patrols, and forced back to Colombia.[26] Australia came under attack from UNHCR in 2003 when it ordered that a boat carrying asylum-seekers be towed back to Indonesia, despite the fact that the boat was already inside Australian territory near Melville Island.[27] The United States has acted similarly. In January 2000, for example, "an overloaded fishing boat with more than 400 Haitians aboard was turned away from the south Florida coast, its passengers transferred to Coast Guard cutters and quickly sent back to Haiti – apparently with no questions asked."[28]

At times, the ejection of refugees can be both a matter of formal policy, and truly massive in scope. In July 1999, Zambia ordered the immediate deportation without court review of all nationals of the Democratic Republic of Congo (clearly including many refugees), noting that "it is necessary that

---

[22] "Subsequently, around the third week of January 2003, another group of 30 Montagnards ... was again arrested by the Cambodian police near Koh Nheak. But the men in this second group were reportedly beaten up by the Cambodian police before they were handed over to the Vietnamese border guards": (2002) 126 *JRS Dispatches* (Feb. 13, 2002).

[23] "Two Chinese asylum-seekers ... were deported by the Cambodian authorities on 9 August 2002 and are now being held in detention in China's Hunan Province ... The Chinese couple are Falun Gong practitioners and were persons of concern under the protection of the UNHCR in Cambodia": (2002) 117 *JRS Dispatches* (Aug. 29, 2002).

[24] (2000) 74 *JRS Dispatches* (July 5, 2000).

[25] P. Constable, "Afghan refugees facing eviction," *Washington Post*, June 16, 2001, at A-14.

[26] S. Wilson, "Influx burdens Venezuela," *Washington Post*, Oct. 1, 2000, at A-28. Venezuelan President Hugo Chavez reportedly gave Colombians an eight-day ultimatum to leave the country or face repatriation: (2000) 78 *JRS Dispatches* (Sept. 15, 2000).

[27] "UNHCR's spokesman Kris Jankowski ... said that by sending them to Indonesia, which has not signed the [Refugee Convention], Australia ... had shirked its obligations under international law ... 'These people had already entered Australian territory and should have been given access to a fair asylum procedure ... Instead they were sent back to a country which has no asylum procedure in place and where there is no possibility of being granted durable asylum'": UNHCR, "UN refugee agency says Australia has shirked its international obligations," Nov. 11, 2003.

[28] S. Pressley, "In Little Haiti, the Elian fight sheds a painful light," *Washington Post*, Jan. 15, 2000, at A-03.

these people are cleared because they are not budgeted for."[29] In 2001, the Iranian government ordered the removal of several thousand refugees into western Afghanistan against their will. According to UN sources, the Afghans were "randomly rounded up in neighborhoods in the capital city or villages and towns around the border area, then taken to a detention center and put back on trucks without any recourse."[30] More recently, Thailand rebuked UNHCR for seeking to delay its plan to repatriate more than 100,000 ethnic Burmese refugees.[31] Indeed, the Thai National Security Council announced in January 2003 that it would no longer welcome any refugees from neighboring countries, and "would force them back home as soon as the authorities found them."[32]

Ejection is at times carried out by non-state agents with the encouragement or toleration of authorities. For example, immediately after Kenyan President Moi decreed that Ugandan and other refugees would have to leave his country, "police and members of the youth wing of the ruling Kenya African National Union (KANU) began seizing refugees from their homes, bars and lodges ... Despite urgent appeals to the [UNHCR], refugees [were] being persecuted by the security forces and at least one thousand [were] deported across the Ugandan border."[33] Similarly, Liberian and Sierra Leonean refugees fled Guinea in late 2000 after a wave of xenophobic violence was unleashed when President Lansana Conte encouraged citizens to form militia groups[34] with a view to forcing refugees to "go home."[35]

Beyond rejection at the border or being physically forced back to their country of origin, refugees may be subject to removal when refused access to a procedure

---

[29] *Xinhua News Agency* (Lusaka), July 19, 1999, quoting Zambian Deputy Minister for Home Affairs Edwin Hatembo.

[30] P. Baker and A. Sipress, "Concern grows over refugees," *Washington Post*, Dec. 1, 2001, at A-16, quoting Yusuf Hassan, spokesman for UNHCR in Kabul.

[31] "General Khajadpai says the government's policy is to close the camps and send the people back home. But non-governmental border relief agencies say they do not want to send the Burmese back, citing the country's uncertain political and economic outlook, and reports of clashes and violence by pro-Burmese government groups opposing greater Karen autonomy": *Voice of America News*, Aug. 19, 2000.

[32] (2003) 125 *JRS Dispatches* (Jan. 27, 2003).

[33] Africa Watch, "Kenya: Illegal Expulsion of More Than 1000 Refugees" (1990), at 1. Somali refugees were also pushed back from border camps within Kenya: Africa Watch, "Kenya: Forcible Return of Somali Refugees; Government Repression of Kenyan Somalis" (1989); and F. del Mundo, "The Future of Asylum in Africa," (1994) 96 *Refugees* 3, at 7. When in 1997 Moi referred to refugees as "foreign spies and criminals," the police responded with enthusiasm, including a pattern of arbitrary arrests, detention without charge, and forcible removal: G. Verdirame, "Refugees in Kenya: Between a Rock and a Hard Place," unpublished paper on file at the library of the Oxford University Refugee Studies Centre, 1998, at 2–3.

[34] D. Farah, "For refugees, hazardous haven in Guinea," *Washington Post*, Nov. 6, 2000, at A-24.

[35] "Over 400 refugees arrived in Monrovia on 12 October following a two-day sea voyage. Many complained of being beaten and raped by Guineans": (2000) 80 *JRS Dispatches* (Oct. 16, 2000).

to verify their refugee status. For example, Japan declined to consider the refugee claims of Chinese pro-democracy dissidents in the immediate post-Tiananmen era, and forced many of them back to China.[36] China refuses to consider the claims of refugees from North Korea, insisting on its right forcibly to return refugees to that country under the terms of a bilateral agreement.[37] Malaysian police waiting outside the local UNHCR office have arrested and deported Indonesians seeking to make appointments to have their refugee status claims processed.[38] Namibia has summarily classified Angolan refugees as "illegal immigrants" subject to removal without affording them any opportunity to apply for asylum;[39] Zimbabwe treated Rwandan refugees in much the same way.[40] UN workers trying to verify the refugee claims of persons who had arrived from Afghanistan were ordered by the Pakistani government to cease their efforts when it became clear that the majority qualified for protection.[41] Thailand bluntly refused UNHCR's request to recognize the status of ethnic Karen refugees who had arrived from Burma, arguing that "[i]f we toe the agency's line, thousands of Shan people may flood into Thailand."[42]

---

[36] Asia Watch, "Japan: Harassment of Chinese Dissidents" (1990), at 1. "In a number of cases, the authorities refused to renew visas which were about to expire and individual Chinese students were told to return home, including some who had played a prominent part in the pro-democracy movement and who were clearly at risk of serious human rights violations in China": Amnesty International, "Japan: Inadequate Protection for Refugees and Asylum Seekers" (1993), at 8.

[37] "Asylum in China," *Washington Post*, May 12, 2002, at B-06. "[P]osters had appeared along the border between China and North Korea exhorting Chinese to turn in North Korean refugees and warning of steep fines for harboring a refugee": J. Pomfret, "China steps up repatriation of North Korean refugees," *Washington Post*, July 23, 2001, at A-16. Moreover, when a small number of North Korean refugees managed to enter foreign embassies prepared to resettle them, China bluntly ordered the foreign governments concerned to turn over North Korean refugees to China for purposes of immediate removal to North Korea: Human Rights Watch, "China: Protect Rights of North Korean Asylum Seekers," Nov. 19, 2002. After a number of refugees entered the South Korean embassy, Foreign Ministry spokesperson Kong Quan is quoted as having stated, "We require the South Korean Embassy to hand these people over to the Chinese side to be dealt with": J. Pomfret, "China presses Seoul to turn over four North Korean refugees," *Washington Post*, May 29, 2002, at A-13. The Chinese government has even stopped the departure of a group of North Korean refugees from China to South Korea and Japan: "Back to the gulag," *Washington Post*, Jan. 27, 2003, at A-18.

[38] "The UNHCR office has now closed its operations because of the continued police presence outside its office. Although police arrested some Burmese and Bangladeshi asylum-seekers, most of those arrested are Achenese": Human Rights Watch, "Malaysia: Don't Return Indonesian Asylum Seekers," Aug. 29, 2003.

[39] *Mail & Guardian* (Johannesburg), Mar. 27, 2000.

[40] *Daily News* (Harare), Feb. 21, 2003.   [41] "Nowhere to turn," *Toronto Star*, Apr. 8, 2001.

[42] "UNHCR . . . said last week that 4,300 illegal immigrants had been turned away from the Mae La refugee camp in Thailand's western Tak province despite UNHCR requests to let them stay": *Agence France Presse*, Aug. 19, 2001.

The refusal to process claims to refugee status may also be more specifically focused. Some European states have traditionally been unwilling to assess the refugee status of unaccompanied persons less than eighteen years old;[43] the Australian immigration minister urged states to adopt much the same position as a general rule.[44] During the 1991 Gulf War, New Zealand enacted legislation which effectively precluded authorities from fully considering the claims of refugees – in practice, mostly Muslims – presumed to present a risk to national security.[45] Thus, Pakistanis provisionally classified as refugees by immigration authorities – but who "the police say . . . fit the general 'profile' of terrorists, although there was no positive evidence pointing to that"[46] – were removed before their claims to protection were considered on the merits. The New Zealand Court of Appeal conceded that "because of the security risk . . . Government officers may have at times to send away, and perhaps back to persecution, persons who *may* have genuine reasons to fear persecution for their political beliefs"; but that "such persons as the appellants may be seen as, in a sense, casualties of war."[47] The United States has similarly asserted the right to deny asylum to refugees on security and related grounds without the need fully and fairly to investigate entitlement to refugee status.[48]

---

[43] (2000) 76 *JRS Dispatches* (Aug. 3, 2000).

[44] K. Lawson, "Send minors back home immediately: Ruddock," *Canberra Times*, Oct. 2, 2002, at A-7.

[45] The "Provisional Procedures for Determining Refugee Status Applications During the Gulf War Where There is a Security Risk" were in effect between January 28, 1991 and April 30, 1991: R. Haines, *International Academy of Comparative Law National Report for New Zealand* (1994), at 57. Their operation was explained by authorities as being that "[d]uring the course of the Gulf War, a person disembarks in New Zealand and before having been granted a permit applies for refugee status. At that point, a preliminary security screening is performed by the police to determine whether the person can be given a security clearance. If the result of that security screening is negative, then the provisional procedures apply": W. F. Birch, Minister of Labour of New Zealand, "Provisional Procedures for Determining Refugee Status Applications During the Gulf War Where There is a Security Risk," paper on file at the library of the Oxford University Refugee Studies Centre.

[46] *D v. Minister of Immigration*, [1991] 2 NZLR 673 (NZ CA, Feb. 13, 1991), at 675.

[47] Ibid. at 676. The Court did observe, however, that "[i]t would appear . . . that the Gulf War may have brought to light a deficiency in the New Zealand legislation for dealing with persons arriving in this country and claiming refugee status . . . Where security clearance is available, such persons can be allowed to remain here while the refugee question is fully investigated . . . But in practice they cannot be fully used within 28 days . . . Yet if security clearance cannot be given, there is no statutory provision for detaining such people for more than 28 days and there is no way in which the Court could invent such a provision": Ibid.

[48] "'We don't do investigations,' the general counsel of the immigration agency, Paul Virtue, said. 'There is a low evidentiary threshold for finding whether someone is eligible for

Refugees may also face removal because of practical weaknesses in the operation of domestic asylum systems. The system itself may simply be unsound, as is the case in Austria where inexpert border guards play an often decisive role in the registration and adjudication of asylum claims,[49] or in South Africa where officers in repatriation centers have little awareness of refugee law.[50] The risk may also follow from failure of even a carefully designed procedure to take notice of the most accurate human rights data. For example, in January 2002, the United Kingdom summarily deported members of opposition parties to Zimbabwe, basing its decision on dated Home Office risk assessments rather than on updated Foreign Office warnings of a serious deterioration of conditions there.[51]

Initiatives to promote voluntary repatriation are sometimes used as the pretext to engage in the disguised withdrawal of protection from refugees. For example, Turkey allowed Iraqi officials to "visit" Kurdish refugees in Turkey

asylum here. It is wholly unlike a criminal case . . . ' The immigration service says it has the right to deny the Iraqis [who worked with the CIA against then-President Saddam Hussein] asylum without the normal due process required under law because they arrived without visas and have never been officially allowed to enter the United States": J. Risen, "Evidence to deny 6 Iraqis asylum may be weak, files show," *New York Times*, Oct. 13, 1998, at A-9.

[49] A report of two fact-finding missions to interview rejected asylum-seekers in Hungary concluded that "almost all [refugees] were handed over to Hungarian authorities after only one day of arrest in Austria, and in only two cases was an asylum procedure conducted in Austria . . . Both conversations with refugees and reports from the two representatives of Hungarian NGOs show that the interviews conducted by the foreigners police or the border authorities are not aimed at documenting possible reasons for fleeing. The inquiries concentrate on the route of flight and escape agents. Only well-informed refugees who explicitly request asylum manage to access the asylum procedure": Asylkoordination Österreich, "Bericht über die Fact-finding-mission in Ungarn am 20 Mai 1998 und 15 Juni 1998" (1998), at 1 (unofficial translation). This is a long-standing concern: see E. Wiederin, *International Academy of Comparative Law National Report for Austria* (1994), at 7–8.

[50] The South African Human Rights Commission found that "most officers [at the Lindela Repatriation Centre] were not trained to make decisions about asylum . . . and referred all those cases to a few, overloaded senior immigration officers. People at Lindela who claimed they were asylum-seekers were not given the opportunity to apply for asylum as was the policy. The commission heard that immigration officers at Lindela had repeatedly asked for training": "Home Affairs ignores SAHRC recommendations," *Business Day*, Dec. 13, 2000.

[51] "They were waiting for him at the airport, just as he feared. Gerald Mukwetiwa was still recovering from the eight-hour flight to Harare when British immigration officers handed him over to their Zimbabwean counterparts. But the airport officials were not what they seemed. They were members of Zimbabwe's feared Central Intelligence Organisation . . . [A]n *Observer* investigation has discovered that scores of members of opposition parties in Zimbabwe face being sent back to President Mugabe's regime with little regard for their safety": P. Harris and M. Bright, "Crisis in Zimbabwe: Special Investigation: They flee here for safety but are sent back to face death," *Observer* (London), Jan. 13, 2002, at 8.

to promote their repatriation. This encouragement was reinforced by ill-treatment at the hands of their Turkish hosts, including reductions in food and water supplies for those who did not return to Iraq.[52] In August 2002, Rwanda not only allowed members of a Congolese rebel group backed by it to meet with refugees from the Democratic Republic of Congo in order to promote their return home, but advised the refugees that both camp services and the offer of transportation home would soon be withdrawn from those who did not choose to repatriate.[53] India coerced Sri Lankans to repatriate through a combination of arbitrary arrests, withholding stipends and food rations, blocking information about conditions in Sri Lanka, and pressuring the refugees to sign consent forms they could not read.[54] Roma refugees from Kosovo felt compelled to leave Macedonia after being denied basic sanitary facilities and services there.[55] Hundreds of Burundian refugees reported to be voluntarily repatriating from Tanzania were actually leaving because of dramatic reductions in their food rations, coupled with denial of the right to earn a living through economic activity.[56] Nearly 1,000

---

[52] "Amnesty International's concern is intensified by reports received in the past eighteen months that hundreds of Iraqi Kurds ... have 'disappeared' in custody, were tortured or executed in Iraq, after surrendering to the authorities under official amnesties or after receiving assurances that they would come to no harm": Amnesty International, "Iraqi Kurds: At Risk of Forcible Repatriation from Turkey and Human Rights Violations in Iraq" (1990), at 1, 7. "Even those asylum-seekers recognized by UNHCR as refugees are not safe in Turkey. Amnesty International knows of numerous cases where non-Europeans recognized by the Ankara office of the UNHCR as refugees were detained by the Turkish authorities and sent back to their country of origin, despite protests by UNHCR": Amnesty International, "Turkey: *Refoulement* of Non-European Refugees – A Protection Crisis" (1997).

[53] US Committee for Refugees, "The Forced Repatriation of Congolese Refugees Living in Rwanda," Nov. 13, 2002. See also "Opening Statement by Mr. Ruud Lubbers, United Nations High Commissioner for Refugees, at the Fifty-Third Session of the Executive Committee of the High Commissioner's Programme," Sept. 30, 2002, at 4: "In Rwanda I remain concerned about the imposed return of Congolese refugees, and I have taken this up with the Rwandan government."

[54] "We felt compelled to go back because the conditions in the camp were so bad. We came [back to Sri Lanka] with the impression that we would be taken back to our villages. The Indian police at the camp assured us that the Sri Lankan army and police could protect us. We had no radio, no letters, no direct contact with Sri Lanka": Asia Watch, "Halt Repatriation of Sri Lankan Tamils" (1993), at 18, quoting an interview with a Sri Lankan refugee. "[A] leaflet distributed by the Tamil Nadu government officers in camps refers to the refugees as cowards, and poses the question, 'Are only your lives dear?' The leaflet also urged the refugees to shed their cowardice and return to Sri Lanka": Tamil Information Centre, "Tamils Concerned Over Safety of Refugee Returnees to Sri Lanka," Nov. 18, 1992.

[55] (2003) 133 *JRS Dispatches* (May 30, 2003).

[56] (2000) 76 *JRS Dispatches* (Aug. 3, 2000). A coalition of non-governmental groups noted that Tanzania was also "placing political and psychological pressure" on the refugees to return: *UN Integrated Regional Information Networks*, May 15, 2002. More recently, a leading humanitarian organization working with Burundian refugees in Tanzania reported that "[a]mong the reasons for departure mentioned by the refugees were bad

refugees returned to Sudan because they were starving in camps in Uganda.[57] As part of its strategy to force Afghan refugees to return home, Pakistan barred foreign aid agencies from providing material assistance to refugees in the Jalozai camp.[58] Refugees International determined that Bangladesh, working in concert with UNHCR, was promoting the repatriation of Rohingya refugees from Burma by "creat[ing] an environment in which protection for the Rohingya is virtually untenable ... Methods of coercion ... include a reduction in certain basic entitlements, including food, withholding of medical services or pharmaceuticals, forced relocation within camps to poorer housing, beatings, and, most commonly, threats of and actual jail sentences."[59] The government of the United States engaged in threats, subterfuge, and other forms of coercion to persuade Salvadorans to agree "voluntarily" to depart.[60] Australia offered Afghan families a twenty-eight-day option to abandon their asylum claims and return home in exchange for a payment of up to A$10,000[61] – with the warning that those who did not accept "at some point down the track ... will be going home."[62] Tanzania relied on an agreement with Rwanda and UNHCR to impose an arbitrary deadline by which all refugees from Rwanda were required "voluntarily" to repatriate.[63]

conditions in the refugee camps in western Tanzania, where food rations had been cut by 50 percent since February, and only recently increased to 72 percent": "Limitations in refugee camps forcing hundreds to leave," *UN Integrated Regional Information Networks*, May 15, 2003, quoting a statement issued by the Tanganyika Christian Refugee Service.

[57] "[T]he refugees accused UNHCR and the World Food Program of abandoning them": (2000) 75 *JRS Dispatches* (July 20, 2000).

[58] R. McCarthy, "Wrapped in plastic, the rejected wait to die," *Guardian*, Mar. 16, 2001, at 15.

[59] Refugees International, "Lack of Protection Plagues Burma's Rohingya Refugees in Bangladesh," May 30, 2003.

[60] *Orantes-Hernandez v. Meese*, (1988) 685 F Supp 1488 (US DCCa, Apr. 29, 1988), affirmed as *Orantes-Hernandez v. Thornburgh*, (1990) 919 F 2d 549 (US CA9, Nov. 29, 1990).

[61] "Refugee groups criticised the measures. 'It's bribery on the one hand and blackmail on the other,' Simon O'Neill, a spokesman for Refugee Action Collective, told the ABC": P. Barkham, "Australia offers Afghan asylum-seekers £3,800 to go home," *Guardian*, May 24, 2002, at 6.

[62] K. Lawson, "Afghan detainees to be offered $2000 each to go home," *Canberra Times*, May 24, 2002, at A-3, quoting a spokesman for immigration minister Philip Ruddock. It was reported that "[t]he UNHCR welcomed the scheme being voluntary and people being given 28 days to respond": ibid.

[63] "[T]he message was clear. The Tanzanian Government had decided that national security concerns had the highest priority and that these concerns would prevail. Although it did agree to individual screening of those who did not return as of [Dec. 31, 1996], this option was not in any systematic way made known to the refugees. In addition, the whole set-up of this mass return certainly did not suggest that it would be feasible for a refugee to receive special treatment and an evaluation of the merits of his or her claim. Correspondingly, no formal mechanism was provided or established for identifying individuals who risked persecution if they were to be sent back": A. Eggli, *Mass Refugee Influx and the Limits of Public International Law* (2001) (Eggli, *Mass Influx*), at 247. A

Beyond the refusal of protection at or within its borders, a state can also use arm's-length legal maneuvers to repel asylum-seekers in areas of arrogated jurisdiction beyond its formal frontiers. Most notoriously, the United States not only interdicted Haitians fleeing the murderous Cedrás dictatorship on the high seas, but forced the asylum-seekers to board its Coast Guard vessels, destroyed their boats, and delivered the refugee claimants directly into the arms of their persecutors.[64] The United States continues to engage in interdiction and forcible repatriation of Haitian and some other refugees in international waters. While current practice is to conduct a cursory review of protection needs onboard the interdicting ship,[65] the United States nonetheless maintains that it has no legal obligations to interdicted refugees, even if they manage to reach its territorial sea.[66] Australia similarly seeks to turn away refugees in international waters before they can reach its territory, though it does not return them directly

similar absolutism was clear in the subsequent repatriation effort by Tanzania. "The repatriation program was launched in November 2002 rooted in a tripartite agreement signed in Geneva by UNHCR and the Tanzanian and Rwandan governments. The agreement provides that every effort will be made to complete the operation 'by the end of December 2002' . . . Refugees said that public statements by Tanzanian authorities declaring that all Rwandans must repatriate by December 31 completely eroded their sense of safety": Lawyers' Committee for Human Rights, "Rwandans May Be Forced to Leave Tanzanian Refugee Camps," Dec. 27, 2002.

[64] Tang Thanh Trai Le, *International Academy of Comparative Law National Report for the United States* (1994), at 11. This was not the first attempt by the United States to exercise authority over asylum-seekers in international waters. In 1993, three boats carrying 659 Chinese asylum-seekers were intercepted by the United States in international waters off the coast of Mexico. Based on cursory Immigration and Naturalization Service and UNHCR screening, one person was accepted for protection in the United States, while the rest were handed over to Mexico for return to China: ibid. at 13.

[65] President Clinton ordered US authorities to "attempt to ensure that smuggled aliens detained as a result of US enforcement actions, whether in the US or abroad, are fairly assessed and/or screened by appropriate authorities to ensure protection of *bona fide* refugees": US President William Clinton, "Alien Smuggling," Doc. PDD-9, June 18, 1993, at 1–2. But in practice, "it appears that Haitians and Dominicans received very minimal or no procedural protections while the Chinese received some degree of screening . . . ": K. Musalo, "Report of the Expedited Removal Study" (2000), at n. 44. In the case of interdicted Haitians, access to protection amounted to the reading of the following declaration at least once to those onboard: "This is (interpreter name) speaking for the captain of the Coast Guard Cutter *Valiant*. We would like to remind you again that you can speak to the interpreters or any Coast Guard person on board about specific problems, issues, or medical concerns that you may wish to tell us about": ibid. at note 48.

[66] "Aliens interdicted within United States territorial waters do not have a right to exclusion proceedings . . . [T]he [Immigration and Nationalization Act's] sections relating to asylum and withholding do not require that an exclusion hearing be provided for aliens interdicted within territorial waters": US Department of Justice, Office of Legal Counsel, "Memorandum for the Attorney General: Immigration Consequences of Undocumented Aliens' Arrival in United States Territorial Waters," Oct. 13, 1993, at 9, 14.

to their country of origin. For example, the Australian troop ship *HMAS Manoora* paused on its well-publicized journey to ferry refugees taken from the *Tampa* to be processed in Nauru in order to intercept an Indonesian fishing boat, the *Aceng*, carrying 237 (largely Iraqi) asylum-seekers believed to have been bound for Australia.[67] More recently, British Home Secretary Blunkett confirmed that Royal Navy ships might be used to intercept unauthorized migrants being smuggled in the eastern Mediterranean Sea.[68] The UK has, however, already extended control efforts beyond its borders under a land-based system of stationing its immigration officers at foreign airports to screen out passengers bound for Britain deemed likely to seek refugee protection there – effectively trapping such persons inside their own country.[69]

Rather than relying on physical interdiction, it is more common for states to seek to avoid the arrival of refugees by the adoption of relatively invisible *non-entrée* policies.[70] In essence, the goal of these mechanisms is to implement legal norms which have the effect of preventing refugees from even reaching the point of being able to present their case for protection to asylum state authorities.

The classic mechanism of *non-entrée* is to impose a visa requirement on the nationals of genuine refugee-producing countries, enforced by sanctions against any carrier that agrees to transport a person without a visa. Canada, for example, has long required the nationals of countries likely to produce refugees to obtain a visa before boarding a plane or otherwise coming to

---

[67] P. Barkham, "Migrants step ashore to flowers and fences," *Guardian*, Sept. 20, 2001, at 17. These refugees were similarly taken to Nauru.

[68] A. Travis, "French to close 'last' way for refugees to use tunnel," *Guardian*, June 26, 2002, at 8. One commentator observed that "[t]his would be a new departure for Britain indeed – though already a staple of Australian political theatre – and gives a literal twist to Blair's war on asylum": S. Milne, "Declaration of war on asylum," *Guardian*, May 23, 2002, at 18.

[69] "In the first 10 days British officials were at the [Prague] airport, 90 people – mostly Roma – were refused entry to the UK": R. Prasad, "Airport colour bar," *Guardian*, July 30, 2001, at 15. Officials operated under an instruction that particular national groups could be targeted for enhanced scrutiny where "there is statistical evidence showing a pattern or trend of breach of the immigration laws by persons of that nationality": H. Young, "Ministerial double-talk simply masks a racist law," *Guardian*, Apr. 24, 2001, at 16. The likelihood of "breach of immigration laws" was taken to include unauthorized arrival for purposes of making a refugee claim; indeed, the Home Office resumed the scheme after it had been adjudged to have served its original deterrent purpose because of "a renewed increase in claims for asylum by Czech citizens": S. Hall, "Protests as Prague airport screening resumes," *Guardian*, Aug. 28, 2001, at 2. It is reported that senior UK immigration officials are also stationed as "airline liaison officers" in Accra, Dhaka, Delhi, Colombo, and Nairobi: P. Field, "Breaching the fortress," *Guardian*, June 24, 2002, at 19.

[70] *Non-entrée* is a term coined to describe the array of legalized policies adopted by states to stymie access by refugees to their territories. See J. Hathaway, "The Emerging Politics of *Non-Entrée*," (1992) 91 *Refugees* 40.

Canada.[71] Because a visa will not be issued for the purpose of seeking refugee protection, only those who lie about their intentions or secure forged documentation are able successfully to satisfy the inquiries of the transportation company employees who effectively administer Canadian law abroad.[72] Most persons in these states, however, are simply barred from traveling to Canada altogether. Much the same approach is taken by New Zealand. When introducing a visa requirement for Indonesian nationals in 1998, the Immigration Minister justified his actions on the grounds that "[t]here have been over 300 refugee applications received in the last four months alone from Indonesian nationals ... By suspending the visa-free status for Indonesian nationals we are better placed to manage the risk of people seeking refugee status once they arrive here."[73] Britain was equally candid when it imposed a visa requirement on Zimbabweans in 2003: the High Commissioner to Zimbabwe indicated that the visa requirements "were intended to reduce the rising number of Zimbabweans seeking asylum in the UK."[74] The European Union has adopted an even more sweeping visa control policy. Building upon earlier arrangements

[71] "Canada is buffered from large scale [refugee] flows by the United States and, to a lesser extent, by Europe. What the government does to reinforce or counteract those buffers affects how accessible Canada is to people who do not submit to selection abroad, or who are in such circumstances that they cannot do so. The record of successive governments in imposing visa requirements on sources of refugee claims emphasizes the policy choice": R. Girard, "Speaking Notes for an Address to the Conference on Refuge or Asylum – A Choice for Canada," unpublished paper, 1986, on file at the library of the Centre for Refugee Studies, York University, at 4. "There is a correlation between the imposition of a visa requirement by Canada and the kinds of human rights abuses that cause refugees to flee. The worse the human rights abuses, the more likely the country is to have a visa requirement imposed on it": Canadian Council for Refugees, "Interdicting Refugees" (1998), at 23.

[72] See generally E. Feller, "Carrier Sanctions and International Law," (1989) 1(1) *International Journal of Refugee Law* 48 (Feller, "Sanctions"); and Danish Refugee Council and Danish Center of Human Rights, "The Effect of Carrier Sanctions on the Asylum System" (1991).

[73] "Indonesian nationals require visas to enter New Zealand," New Zealand Executive Government News Release, Oct. 21, 1998, quoting Minister of Immigration Hon. Tuariki Delamere.

[74] "UK tries to stop entry of Zimbabweans," *Daily News* (Harare), Nov. 8, 2002, referring to comments made by High Commissioner Brian Donnelly. Interestingly, even the British government conceded that in 2001 (that is, even before the onset of the most serious human rights abuse in Zimbabwe) 115 of 2,115 asylum applications in the UK by Zimbabweans had been found to be genuine: ibid. In the decision of *European Roma Rights Centre v. Immigration Officer at Prague Airport*, [2002] EWCA 1989 (Eng. QBD, Oct. 8, 2002), the court noted that "[o]ne of the objectives of imposing new visa regimes ... is to address the questions of asylum overload. When, for example, Colombia and Ecuador were included as visa states, this was directly in response to an increase in the number of those nationals coming to the United Kingdom in order to apply for asylum."

agreed to by core EU members,[75] the European Council now requires all member states to impose visas on the nationals of some 131 countries – including, for example, such refugee-producing countries as Afghanistan, Iraq, Somalia, and Sudan.[76] The effectiveness of visa controls as a means of barring genuine refugees from securing protection is clear. When Sweden imposed a visa requirement on Bosnians in 1992, for example, asylum requests by Bosnians dropped immediately from 2,000 to less than 200 per week.[77] More generally, Kjaerum suggests that much of the nearly 50 percent drop in the number of refugees seeking asylum in Europe from 1992 to 1998 was due to the impact of visa and related policies.[78]

A second mechanism of *non-entrée* is the deportation chain that can be set in motion by "first country of arrival" and "safe third country" rules. Taken together, "first country of arrival" and "safe third country" rules have traditionally posed a legal barrier to the entry into Europe of very large numbers of refugees.[79] For example, during the early 1990s invocation of these rules resulted in the return of refugees by Greece to Turkey, Libya, and the Sudan, from where some were then returned to their countries of origin.[80] Similarly, Norway returned Kosovo Albanian asylum-seekers to Sweden (where their claims had already been rejected), with the knowledge that they would be returned by Sweden to Serbia.[81]

The "first country of arrival" principle purports to collectivize responsibility to protect refugees among a select group of participating states. The two formal

---

[75] See generally J. Hathaway, "Harmonizing for Whom? The Devaluation of Refugee Protection in the Era of European Economic Integration," (1993) 26(3) *Cornell International Law Journal* 719, at 722–728.

[76] EC Reg. No. 539/2001 (Mar. 15, 2001). Exemptions are possible for persons admitted to a temporary protection regime, but not more generally: Council Directive 2001/55/EC (July 20, 2001), at Art. 8.3.

[77] M. Eriksson, *International Academy of Comparative Law National Report for Sweden* (1994), at 19.

[78] M. Kjaerum, "Refugee Protection Between State Interests and Human Rights: Where is Europe Heading?," (2002) 24 *Human Rights Quarterly* 513, at 515.

[79] "There is now a latent danger of a deportation chain – in breach of international law – at the end of which refugees will find themselves dumped back in the country from which they fled. Far from mutually clarifying responsibilities for examining refugee status, the concept of safe third countries serves merely to justify refusing access to the asylum process": S. Teloken, "The Domino Effect," (1993) 94 *Refugees* 38, at 40.

[80] Z. Papassiopi-Passia, *International Academy of Comparative Law National Report for Greece* (1994), at 59. The new Law 2452/1996, however, "abolished the conditions of admissibility and laid down that 'an alien who is in any way on Greek territory shall be recognized as a refugee and shall be granted asylum if the conditions of Article 1(A) of the Geneva Convention . . . are fulfilled'": A. Skordas, "The New Refugee Legislation in Greece," (1999) 11(4) *International Journal of Refugee Law* 678, at 681.

[81] T. Einarsen, *International Academy of Comparative Law National Report for Norway* (1994), at 23. See also G. Tjore, "Norwegian Refugee Policy," (2002) 35 *Migration* 193, at 203.

harmonization regimes thus far established – that predicated on the Dublin Convention and Dublin Regulation in Europe,[82] and the more embryonic arrangement between Canada and the United States[83] – assign protective responsibility to the first partner state in which a given refugee arrives (at least where there are no issues of prior authorization to travel or family unity[84]). Other participating states are authorized summarily to remove the refugee to that single designated state, without conducting any examination of the merits of the claim to protection.

The "first country of arrival" principle is also increasingly applied in the domestic laws of states in many parts of the world. A variant of the principle is implicit in United States law which denies asylum to persons it deems to have been "firmly resettled" in another asylum state even if there is no reason to believe that the refugee can, in fact, return there.[85] At an informal level, the "first country of arrival" principle is often relied upon even in the less developed world. For example, persons seeking asylum in Kenya have been told by UNHCR to go back to Uganda or Tanzania through which they may already have passed.[86] Ugandan officials, in turn, have refused to consider the claims of Rwandan refugees previously present in Tanzania, even as Tanzania was threatening the refugees with forced repatriation to Rwanda.[87] South Africa ordered its border officials to turn back or detain refugees who traveled to that country via safe

[82] Convention Determining the State Responsible for Examining Applications for Asylum Lodged in One of the Member States of the European Communities, June 15, 1990, 30 ILM 425 (1991) (Dublin Convention), at Arts. 4–8; European Council Reg. EC 343/2003, Feb. 18, 2003 (Dublin Regulation).

[83] Agreement between the Government of Canada and the Government of the United States Regarding Asylum Claims Made at Land Borders, Aug. 30, 2002, (2002) 79(37) *Interpreter Releases* 1446, at Art. 4.

[84] Priority in the determination of the state responsible for assessing refugee status is given to the member state in which an applicant's family members live, or are already being assessed for refugee status; and secondly, to the state, if any, which is responsible for a person's entry and presence within the European Union: Dublin Regulation.

[85] "Whether Germany will re-admit the Nasirs is not . . . a question which is now before us. Although the Nasirs may have trouble re-entering Germany, 'the pertinent regulations [8 CFR §208.13(c)(2)(i)(B)] specifically focus on resettlement status prior to the alien's entry into this country; they preclude a deportable alien from bootstrapping an asylum claim simply by unilaterally severing these existing ties to a third country after arriving in the United States'": *Nasir v. Immigration and Naturalization Service*, 30 Fed. Appx 812 (US CA9, Feb. 7, 2002).

[86] (1999) 53 *JRS Dispatches* (July 16, 1999).

[87] "Ethnic Rwandese asylum-seekers entering [Uganda] from Tanzania are no longer recognised by this government, Minister for Disaster Preparedness Brg. Moses Ali has said. 'On advice of UNHCR, the government stopped recognising Rwandese asylum-seekers from Tanzania since they were already accessing international protection,' Ali said": "Government no longer recognises Rwanda asylum-seekers," *Monitor* (Kampala), Oct. 7, 2002. See also *UN Integrated Regional Information Networks*, Dec. 21, 2002.

neighboring countries – though that policy was ordered withdrawn when challenged in the High Court.[88]

The "first county of arrival" rule is in essence a specific application of what have come to be known as "safe third country" rules, which authorize a person claiming refugee status to be sent to any "safe" state through which he or she may have passed en route to the country in which he or she is now present. Indeed, European law allows even the state designated to consider a refugee claim to send the refugee applicant onward to a "safe third country," including even to a non-European state, and whether or not that country is bound by refugee law. To qualify as a "safe third country" there must simply be a determination that the destination country is prepared to consider the applicant's refugee claim, and will not expose the claimant to persecution, (generalized) risk of torture or related ill-treatment, or *refoulement*.[89] Indeed, the European Union has recently sanctioned what has come to be known as the "super safe third country" notion, allowing refugees to be sent with no risk assessment whatever to states that are bound by both the Refugee Convention and the European Convention on Human Rights, which are adjudged to observe their provisions, and which operate a formal asylum procedure.[90]

Nor is application of the "safe third country" rule limited to states which participate in formal harmonization regimes. Some governments not party to any such agreement have unilaterally opted not to consider the claims of persons for whom a "safe third country" can be identified. In Australia, for example, this means that refugee claims are not addressed on the merits if the person seeking protection can be sent to another state to which he or she will be admitted; where there is no real chance of being persecuted for a Convention reason; and from which there is no real chance of *refoulement* to the country of origin.[91] Notably, the Australian version of the "safe third country" rule, in contrast to that adopted by the European Union, does not require that the applicant be granted access to a refugee status determination

---

[88] "Department of Home Affairs Backs Down on Asylum Policy," *Business Day*, May 10, 2001. See e.g. *Katambayi and Lawyers for Human Rights v. Minister of Home Affairs et al.*, Dec. No. 02/5312 (SA HC, Witwatersrand Local Division, Mar. 24, 2002), in which the court intervened to stop the removal of a refugee claimant in transit at Johannesburg Airport, ordering the government "to allow [the applicant] to apply for asylum in South Africa."

[89] Council Directive on minimum standards of procedures in Member States for granting and withdrawing refugee status, Doc. 8771/04, Asile 33 (Apr. 29, 2004) (EU Procedures Directive), at Art. 27.1.

[90] Ibid. at Art. 35A(2).

[91] *V872/00A v. Minister for Immigration and Multicultural Affairs*, [2002] FCAFC 185 (Aus. FFC, June 18, 2002).

procedure in the destination country. Nor is the destination country limited to a state through which the applicant passed en route to Australia.

A third variant of *non-entrée* is the designation of entire countries or populations as manifestly not at risk, and hence unworthy of serious consideration for refugee status. Since being sanctioned by European immigration ministers in the early 1990s,[92] this concept has been a tool of *en bloc* exclusion of nationally defined groups. For example, the "safe country of origin" designation has been applied by Switzerland to all of India,[93] and by Germany to Romania and Senegal.[94] France treats some thirteen countries as presumptively safe, including Mali and Ghana.[95] Britain began applying the "safe country of origin" principle more recently, but has included a particularly wide range of states on its "white list" – for example, Bangladesh, Serbia, Sri Lanka, and Ukraine.[96] Applications for asylum made by persons from listed states are examined in the UK in a "fast-track" procedure designed to reach a result within ten days.[97]

The safe country of origin principle has recently been codified in European Union law, albeit with an explicit safeguard provision:[98] asylum states are entitled to assume that all nationals of listed countries are not refugees, though applicants must be allowed to attempt to rebut the presumption that their claims

---

[92] "Resolution on Manifestly Unfounded Applications for Asylum," Ad Hoc Group on Immigration Doc. SN4822/1/92 (WG1 1282), 1992.

[93] W. Kälin, *International Academy of Comparative Law National Report for Switzerland* (1994), at 22. By the late 1990s, this list included also Albania, Bulgaria, the Czech Republic, Gambia, Hungary, Poland, Romania, Senegal, and Slovakia: R. Boed, "Human Rights Postscript: Comments on the Concept of 'Safe Country of Origin,'" (1997) 7 *Human Rights Interest Group Newsletter* 15 (Boed, "Safe Country"), at 16.

[94] R. Hofmann, *International Academy of Comparative Law National Report for Germany* (1994), at 5. Other countries deemed safe by German law have included Bulgaria, the Czech Republic, Ghana, Hungary, Poland, and Slovakia: Boed, "Safe Country," at 16.

[95] M. Toumit, "Les associations refusent que le droit d'asile soit a la botte de l'interieur," *Le Monde*, Feb. 20, 2003.

[96] A. Travis, "Outcry as asylum 'white list' extended," *Guardian*, June 18, 2003, at 7.

[97] "The Home Office ... said the introduction of a 'white list' of countries – from which applications were presumed to be unfounded – had halved the number of applications from those countries": A. Travis, "Tough asylum policy hits genuine refugees," *Guardian*, Aug. 29, 2003, at 11.

[98] A high-profile decision by Sweden in 2001 to refuse protection to a US citizen on the grounds that the US was a "safe country" may have accounted for some of the pressure to constrain the applicability of the principle. The applicant was a justice of the peace who had campaigned to make US law enforcement officials more accountable, leading to vicious reprisals which authorities were apparently powerless either to prevent or redress. The Swedish decision that the claim was "manifestly unfounded" because the United States is "an internationally recognized democracy" was criticized by Members of the European Parliament, who observed "that his case raises serious questions about the EU's proposed common asylum policy": J. Henley, "Swedes face call for asylum u-turn," *Guardian*, June 21, 2001, at 14.

are unfounded in the context of an accelerated procedure.[99] The safe country of origin rule moreover applies as among European Union states in a tacit if significantly more aggressive way, since European Union law now significantly constrains the recognition of refugee status to EU citizens.[100] Thus, for example, at-risk members of the Roma community in EU states have no effective means of securing refugee status within Europe, even though free movement within the Union is being withheld from the citizens of most of the states recently admitted for a period of years.[101] The UN High Commissioner for Refugees has nonetheless recommended a more aggressive and collectivized application of the "safe country of origin" notion by European countries.[102]

[99] EU Procedures Directive, at Art. 30.
[100] "'Refugee' means a *third country national* who, owing to a well-founded fear of being persecuted for reasons of race, religion, nationality, political opinion or membership of a particular social group, is outside the country of nationality [emphasis added]": EU Procedures Directive, at Art. 2(c). Moreover, "[t]his Directive is without prejudice to the Protocol on asylum for nationals of Member States of the European Union as annexed to the Treaty Establishing the European Community": ibid. at Preamble, para. 13. Under the Protocol on Asylum for Nationals of Member States of the European Union, annexed to the Treaty establishing the European Community, OJ 97/340/01, at 103 (Nov. 10, 1997), it is agreed that "Member States shall be regarded as constituting safe countries of origin in respect of each other for all legal and practical purposes in relation to asylum matters." It is further agreed that asylum applications are only receivable from a European national where the European Council is engaged in action against the country of origin, where the country of origin has derogated from the European Convention on Human Rights, or with the exceptional consent of the destination country – though the European Council must be informed of such a decision, and the claim must in any event be treated as "manifestly unfounded."
[101] "'It is frankly absurd that people can routinely claim that they are in fear of their lives in Poland or the Czech Republic,' [UK Home Secretary David Blunkett] wrote. 'These are democratic countries which live under the rule of law.' The UN, the European Commission, and even the Foreign Office disagree. A report by the UN's Human Rights Committee last year said it was 'deeply concerned about the discrimination against the Roma and the persistent allegations of police harassment.' This year's Foreign Office human rights report acknowledges that new anti-discrimination laws in the 10 [newly admitted EU] countries have not banished 'ingrained attitudes' towards minorities": R. Prasad, "No place of refuge," *Guardian*, Oct. 24, 2002, at 21.
[102] "Since the time that you collectively declared ten EU candidate countries to be 'safe countries of origin,' it is interesting to note that the number of applications from these countries has dropped. My Office is ready to consider more such situations, wherever there is a clear indication that flows are composed, overwhelmingly, of persons without a valid claim for international protection. For these groups, why not pool your processing and reception resources, with the aim of reaching decisions more quickly and disencumbering domestic systems ... Such an approach could have a dynamic impact on your harmonization process. Is it not time to move ahead with this?": UNHCR, "Statement by Mr. Ruud Lubbers, UN High Commissioner for Refugees, at Informal Meeting of the European Union Justice and Home Affairs Council, Veria, March 28, 2003."

The determination of many states to rely on *non-entrée* policies has reached new heights in recent years, with states apparently prepared even to deem parts of their own territory to be outside their own territory, with the hope of thereby avoiding protection responsibilities to persons present therein. A particularly insidious mechanism of *non-entrée* is the designation by some states of part of their airports as a so-called "international zone," in which neither domestic nor international law is said to apply.[103] Invoking this mechanism, France and other states have summarily expelled persons seeking recognition of their refugee status without any examination of their need for protection.[104] Even more creatively, the Australian government has sought to "excise" more than 3,500 of its islands from Australia's self-declared "migration zone."[105] In essence, the result would be that refugees arriving at one of the excised islands – including not only main destinations for those arriving by boat from Southeast Asia, such as Christmas Island, but even an island only 2 km from the coast of the Australian mainland[106] – would not be entitled to have their claims assessed under Australia's refugee status determination system. Rather, they would be treated as though they were in an overseas refugee camp and considered for discretionary admission either immediately or after having their circumstances considered in the territory of a partner state, such as Nauru, to which they might be removed.[107] While the Australian Senate has consistently disallowed regulations and defeated

---

[103] Z. Papassiopi-Passia, *International Academy of Comparative Law National Report for Greece* (1994), at 15–17.

[104] See D. Lochak, "L'accès au territoire français: la réglementation," in F. Julien-Laferrière ed., *Frontières du droit, Frontières des droits* (1993), at 179.

[105] Australia's "migration zone" includes land above the low water mark and sea within the limits of a port in a State or Territory but does not include the sea within a State or Territory or the "territorial sea" of Australia: Migration Act 1958, as amended, ss. 5(1) and 7. While Australia has attempted to escape much legal responsibility in its territorial seas, such efforts are of no value as matters of international law. "The provision in the Migration Act which in effect excludes territorial waters from Australia's domestically created 'Migration Zone' is internationally incapable of excluding [the duty of *non-refoulement*] ... As the 1969 Vienna Convention on the Law of Treaties (Article 27) expressly indicates, domestic legislation cannot be used to escape treaty obligations": Jean Pierre Fonteyne, "Skulduggery on the high seas," *Canberra Times*, Sept. 11, 2001, at A-9.

[106] K. Lawson, "Ruddock flags alternative plan," *Canberra Times*, June 18, 2002, at 3, referring to Milingimbi Island, said to be 1–2 km from the mainland at low tide.

[107] "A person who enters ... an 'excised offshore place' now becomes an 'offshore entry person.' The Law empowers the arrest and detention of an offshore entry person (or those who would become so should they enter an excised offshore place ...) and removal from Australian territory to a designated place outside Australia ... Furthermore the law prohibits judicial proceedings relating to offshore entry by an 'offshore entry person' ... [including the] right to apply for a [protection or other] visa. The exception relates to proceedings brought under the original jurisdiction of the High Court under Section 75 of the Constitution, which of course cannot be utilized once the individual concerned has been removed from Australian territory": F. Motta, "Between a Rock and a Hard Place: Australia's Mandatory Detention of Asylum Seekers," (2002) 20(3) *Refuge* 12 (Motta, "Rock"), at 17.

legislation authorizing the excision of the islands,[108] the government refuses to abandon the strategy.[109]

Beyond all of the strategies deployed to date to avoid the admission of refugees, an even more assertive form of collectivized action may still emerge. The UNHCR, for example, has declared itself committed to the negotiation of a "Convention Plus" regime under which the secondary movement of refugees beyond their regions of origin would be discouraged in exchange for the agreement of developed countries to provide resettlement opportunities and development assistance.[110] The British government has proposed the establishment of "regional protection areas" to which persons claiming refugee status outside their own region would be sent for processing in an internationally funded and administered center. Only those "most in need" would be resettled to a (developed) state outside the region of origin.[111] In line with this general goal, the Intergovernmental Consultations on Refugees, Asylum and Migration Policies – an informal grouping of core members of the EU in addition to Australia, Canada, New Zealand, Norway, Switzerland, and the United States – is developing what it describes as a proposal for "effective protection" predicated on reducing demand for secondary and tertiary movement out of regions of origin, and on enhancing the capacity of countries in regions of origin to protect genuine refugees.

In sum, refugees face a broad array of practices and policies which may prevent them from entering and remaining in an asylum state. They may face blunt pushbacks from a state's territory, whether in particular instances, as part of a generalized border closure, or by the erection of physical barriers to access. Even if able to enter an asylum state, they may be summarily ejected by specific official action, under mass removal policies, or by non-state agents acting with the encouragement or toleration of the state. Refugees may also be sent away because they are denied access to a system to verify their refugee status, or because whatever system is in place fails accurately to identify them as refugees. Refugees are also frequently forced back to their country of origin under the pretext of "voluntary" repatriation efforts. Governments at times even reach out into international areas, particularly the high seas, to repel

[108] "Mr. Ruddock was given the power to excise islands by regulation in laws passed by Parliament late [in 2001]. Regulations are disallowable by Parliament . . . and when Mr. Ruddock tried in May to excise the thousands of northern islands, the Senate blocked the move. Mr. Ruddock tried again with legislation instead, but last week the Senate threw out the legislation": K. Lawson, "Ruddock puts excising ploy to the test," *Canberra Times*, Dec. 19, 2002, at A-4.
[109] "Mr. Ruddock's spokesman did not rule out . . . excising individual islands off the northern coast if suspicious boats appeared, despite the Senate's position, saying the 'principle of excision' remained on the agenda": ibid.
[110] "Lubbers Proposes 'Convention Plus' Approach," UNHCR Press Release, Sept. 13, 2002.
[111] United Kingdom (Home Office), "A New Vision for Refugees," Mar. 7, 2003.

refugees heading for their territory. There is an ever-expanding array of *non-entrée* policies which rely on law to deny entry to refugees. These include the classic approach of imposing visa controls on refugee-producing states, enforced by carrier sanctions; deportation chains set in motion by "first country of arrival" and "safe third country" rules; the *en bloc* denial of access to persons from states deemed to be safe for all their citizens; and even the designation of parts of a state's territory as an "international zone" or as "excised" for purposes of access to refugee protection systems. In the future, there is reason to believe that refugees may be routinely sent back to their regions of origin for status assessment, with only a minority selected there for resettlement to extra-regional countries.

Refugee Convention, Art. 33   Prohibition of expulsion or return ("refoulement")

1. No Contracting State shall expel or return ("refouler") a refugee in any manner whatsoever to the frontiers of territories where his life or freedom would be threatened on account of his race, religion, nationality, membership of a particular social group or political opinion.

2. The benefit of the present provision may not, however, be claimed by a refugee whom there are reasonable grounds for regarding as a danger to the security of the country in which he is, or who, having been convicted by a final judgment of a particularly serious crime, constitutes a danger to the community of that country.

Art. 33 of the Refugee Convention is the primary response of the international community to the need of refugees to enter and remain in an asylum state.[112] The duty of *non-refoulement* is not, however, the same as a right to asylum from persecution,[113] in at least two ways. First and most critically, the

---

[112] The ambiguous relationship between *non-refoulement* and a right of entry is clear from the remark of Justices McHugh and Gummow of the High Court of Australia that "[a]lthough none of the provisions in Chapter V [of the Refugee Convention] gives to refugees a right to enter the territory of a contracting state, in conjunction they provide some measure of protection": *Minister for Immigration and Multicultural Affairs v. Khawar*, [2002] HCA 14 (Aus. HC, Apr. 11, 2002), per McHugh and Gummow JJ.

[113] Interestingly, even the (non-binding) Universal Declaration of Human Rights provides only that "[e]veryone has the right to seek and to enjoy in other countries asylum from persecution" – a formulation which stops distinctly short of requiring states to grant asylum: Universal Declaration of Human Rights, UNGA Res. 217A(III), Dec. 10, 1948 (Universal Declaration), at Art. 14(1). Perhaps most tellingly, not even a vague formulation of this kind made its way into the (binding) Covenant on Civil and Political Rights. This treaty provides only that "[e]veryone shall be free to leave any country, including his own": International Covenant on Civil and Political Rights, UNGA Res. 2200A(XXI), adopted Dec. 16, 1966, entered into force Mar. 23, 1976 (Civil and Political Covenant), at Art. 12(2).

duty of *non-refoulement* only prohibits measures that cause refugees to "be pushed back into the arms of their persecutors";[114] it does not affirmatively establish a duty on the part of states to receive refugees.[115] As an obligation "couched in negative terms,"[116] it constrains, but does not fundamentally challenge, the usual prerogative of states to regulate the entry into their territory of non-citizens.[117] State parties may therefore deny entry to refugees so long as there is no real chance that their refusal will result in the return of the refugee to face the risk of being persecuted.[118] This is so even if the refugee has not previously been recognized as a refugee by any other country.[119] But where there is a real risk that rejection will expose the refugee "in any manner whatsoever" to the risk of being persecuted for a Convention ground, Art. 33 amounts to a de facto duty to admit the refugee, since admission is normally the only means of avoiding the alternative, impermissible consequence of exposure to risk.

---

[114] Statement of Mr. Chance of Canada, UN Doc. E/AC.32/SR.21, Feb. 2, 1950, at 7.

[115] Art. 33 was said to be "a negative duty forbidding the expulsion of any refugee to certain territories but [which] did not impose the obligation to allow a refugee to take up residence": Statement of Mr. Weis of the International Refugee Organization, UN Doc. E/AC.32/SR.40, Aug. 22, 1950, at 33. See E. Lauterpacht and D. Bethlehem, "The Scope and Content of the Principle of *Non-Refoulement*," in E. Feller et al. eds., *Refugee Protection in International Law* 87 (Lauterpacht and Bethlehem, "*Non-Refoulement*"), at para. 76: "[T]he 1951 Convention and international law generally do not contain a right to asylum ... [W]here States are not prepared to grant asylum to persons who have a well-founded fear of persecution, they must adopt a course of action which does not amount to *refoulement*. This may involve removal to a safe third country or some other solution such as temporary protection or refuge."

[116] *M38/2002 v. Minister for Immigration and Multicultural and Indigenous Affairs*, [2003] FCAFC 131 (Aus. FFC, June 13, 2003).

[117] "Apart from any limitations which may be imposed by specific treaties, states have been adamant in maintaining that the question of whether or not a right of entry should be afforded an individual, or to a group of individuals, is something which falls to each nation to resolve for itself": *Minister for Immigration and Multicultural Affairs v. Khawar*, [2002] HCA 14 (Aus. HC, Apr. 11, 2002), per McHugh and Gummow JJ. This formulation was endorsed in *R v. Immigration Officer at Prague Airport et al., ex parte European Roma Rights Centre et al.*, [2004] UKHL 55 (UK HL, Dec. 9, 2004), at para. 19.

[118] In defining the relevant evidentiary standard for sending a refugee to another state in line with Art. 33, the Full Federal Court of Australia has helpfully insisted that the destination country must be one in which "the applicant will not face a *real chance* of persecution for a Convention reason," and that there is not "a *real chance* that the person might be refouled [from the state of immediate destination] to a country where there will be a *real risk* of persecution [emphasis added]": *V872/00A v. Minister for Immigration and Multicultural Affairs*, [2002] FCAFC 185 (Aus. FFC, June 18, 2002).

[119] *Rajendran v. Minister for Immigration and Multicultural Affairs*, (1998) 166 ALR 619 (Aus. FFC, Sept. 4, 1998).

The second critical distinction between *non-refoulement* and a right of asylum follows directly from the purely consequential nature of the implied duty to admit refugees under Art. 33. Because the right of entry that flows from the duty of *non-refoulement* is entirely a function of the existence of a risk of being persecuted, it does not compel a state to allow a refugee to remain in its territory if and when that risk has ended. Thus, "[r]efugee status is a temporary status for as long as the risk of persecution remains."[120] Indeed, as the High Court of Australia has observed,

> The term "asylum" does not appear in the main body of the text of the [Refugee] Convention; the Convention does not impose an obligation upon contracting states to grant asylum or a right to settle in those states to refugees arriving at their borders.[121]

4.1.1 Beneficiaries of protection

The original prohibition of *refoulement*, contained in the 1933 Convention, could be claimed only by "refugees who have been authorized to reside [in the state party] regularly."[122] In line with this precedent, the original drafts of the duty of *non-refoulement* in the 1951 Refugee Convention seemed also to advocate this restriction:[123] the explicit prohibition of *refoulement* applied only to refugees whose arrival was sanctioned by the asylum state. Yet both the Secretary-General's and French drafts of the Convention also contained an additional sub-paragraph not conditioned on authorized entry, providing for a duty "in any case not to turn back refugees to the frontiers of their country of origin, or to territories where their life or freedom would be threatened."[124]

---

[120] *R v. Secretary of State for the Home Department, ex parte Yogathas*, [2002] UKHL 36 (UK HL, Oct. 17, 2002), per Lord Scott.

[121] *Minister for Immigration and Multicultural Affairs v. Khawar*, [2002] HCA 14 (Aus. HC, Apr. 11, 2002), per McHugh and Gummow JJ. See also *Ruddock v. Vadarlis*, (2001) 110 FCR 491 (Aus. FFC, Sept. 18, 2001), at 521: "By Art. 33, a person who has established refugee status may not be expelled to a territory where his life and freedom would be threatened for a Convention reason. Again, there is no obligation on the coastal state to resettle in its own territory."

[122] Convention relating to the International Status of Refugees, 159 LNTS 3663, done Oct. 28, 1933, entered into force June 13, 1935 (1933 Refugee Convention), at Art. 3.

[123] The drafts prepared by both the Secretary-General and France that were before the Ad Hoc Committee on Statelessness and Related Problems in February 1950 accorded protection against *refoulement* only to refugees "who have been authorized to reside [in the state party] regularly": United Nations, "Proposal for a Draft Convention," UN Doc. E/AC.32/2, Jan. 17, 1950 (United Nations, "Draft Convention"), at 45 (draft Art. 24(1)); and France, "Proposal for a Draft Convention," UN Doc. E/AC.32/L.3, Jan. 17, 1950 (France, "Draft Convention"), at 9 (draft Art. 19(1)).

[124] United Nations, "Draft Convention," at 45 (draft Art. 24(3)); and France, "Draft Convention," at 9 (draft Art. 19(3)).

A non-governmental text submitted by the Agudas Israel World Organization was, however, selected over the two official drafts as the basis for this part of the work of the Ad Hoc Committee on Statelessness and Related Problems.[125] Under the Agudas approach as modified by the delegates, the distinct provisions addressing *non-refoulement* and non-return to the risk of persecution were collapsed into a single provision applicable to all refugees, with no mention of the need for authorized arrival.[126] This critical conceptual shift attracted no comment.[127] The drafting process thereafter proceeded on the assumption that prior permission to reside in the asylum state was not a relevant issue.[128] This decision to protect all refugees from the risk of *refoulement* is clearly of huge importance to most contemporary refugees, since they have generally not been authorized to travel to, much less to reside in, the state from which they request protection. Because of this shift, for example, the Greek turn-back of busloads of Kosovar refugees because their entry had not been previously authorized was in breach of Art. 33.

On a related point, it has previously been explained why the duty of *non-refoulement* inheres on a provisional basis even before refugee status has been formally assessed by a state party.[129] In brief, because it is one's de facto

---

[125] UN Doc. E/AC.32/SR.20, Feb. 1, 1950, at 3. The representative of the United Kingdom argued that this text "presented the question of expulsion and non-admittance in a more logical form than did the others": ibid.

[126] "Each of the High Contracting Parties undertakes not to expel or to turn back refugees to the frontiers of territories where their life or freedom would be threatened on account of their race, religion, nationality or political opinions": UN Doc. E/AC.32/L.22, Feb. 1, 1950.

[127] Indeed, an exchange between the Venezuelan, French, and Canadian representatives makes clear that the provision was not to be limited to refugees lawfully admitted to residency. "The Chairman, speaking as the representative of Canada, said that his country was in a similar situation to that of Venezuela in that shiploads of emigrants were often landed far away from any port control authorities. The difficulties entailed by such practices were, however, very small compared with those facing European countries. That was why he wanted to achieve unanimity on article [33], which gave refugees the minimum guarantees to which they were entitled": Statement of Mr. Chance of Canada, UN Doc. E/AC.32/SR.22, Feb. 2, 1950, at 22.

[128] A Swiss protest that the article "concerned only refugees lawfully resident in a country and not those who applied for admission or entered the country without authorization" evoked an immediate answer from the Israeli representative that in fact "[t]he Swiss observer was apparently under a misapprehension with regard to the application of article [33]. In the discussions at the first session it had been agreed that article [33] referred both to refugees legally resident in a country and those who were granted asylum for humanitarian reasons. Apparently the Swiss Government was prepared to accept the provisions of the article with regard to lawfully resident refugees but not to those entering illegally and granted asylum. He feared that the Swiss Government might find its interpretation in conflict with the general feeling which had prevailed in the Committee when it had drafted the article": Statements of Mr. Schurch and Mr. Robinson, UN Doc. E/AC.32/SR.40, Aug. 22, 1950, at 32–33.

[129] See chapter 3.1 above, at pp. 158–160.

circumstances, not the official validation of those circumstances, that gives rise to Convention refugee status, genuine refugees may be fundamentally disadvantaged by the withholding of rights pending status assessment. They are rights holders under international law, but could be precluded from exercising their legal rights during the often protracted domestic processes by which their entitlement to protection is verified by officials. Unless status assessment is virtually immediate, the adjudicating state may therefore be unable to meet its duty to implement the Refugee Convention in good faith. While Convention rights clearly inhere (even provisionally) only on the basis of satisfaction of the relevant attachment requirement, the duty of *non-refoulement* is one of a small number of rights that is not contingent even on arrival at a state's territory, much less on the formal adjudication of status.[130] The duty therefore applies whether or not refugee status has been formally recognized.

A somewhat more contentious question is whether the beneficiary class for protection against *refoulement* under the terms of Art. 33 is the same as the class of refugees defined by Art. 1 of the Refugee Convention. On the one hand, a narrow textual analysis might lead one to believe that not all refugees are guaranteed Art. 33 rights, since the text of the provision prohibits only the return of refugees to places where their "life or freedom would be threatened" for a Convention reason.[131] As Weis affirms, however, the drafting history of the Convention makes it quite clear that there was no intention to grant protection against *refoulement* to only a subset of refugees.[132] Rather, the reference to "life or

---

[130] See chapter 3.1.1 above, at pp. 161–164.

[131] In a misguided effort to reconcile domestic US law (which does not grant protection against *refoulement* to all persons who meet the Convention refugee definition, but rather entitles them only to seek discretionary relief from the Attorney General) to the requirements of international law, the US Supreme Court seized on the "life or freedom" language in Art. 33 to validate the more limited American approach. It was therefore led to determine that "those who can only show a well-founded fear of persecution are not entitled to anything, but are eligible for the discretionary relief of asylum": *Immigration and Naturalization Service v. Cardoza Fonseca*, (1987) 480 US 421 (US SC, Mar. 9, 1987). But see generally J. Hathaway and A. Cusick, "Refugee Rights Are Not Negotiable," (2000) 14(2) *Georgetown Immigration Law Journal* 481.

[132] "The words 'where their life or freedom was threatened' may give the impression that another standard is required than for refugee status in Article 1. This is, however, not the case. The Secretariat draft referred to refugees 'escaping from persecution' and to the obligation not to turn back refugees 'to the frontier of their country of origin, or to territories where their life or freedom would be threatened on account of their race, religion, nationality, or political opinions.' In the course of drafting the words 'country of origin,' 'territories where their life or freedom was threatened' and 'country in which he is persecuted' were used interchangeably. The reference to Article 1 of the Convention was introduced mainly to refer to the dateline of 1 January 1951 but it also indicated that there was no intention to introduce more restrictive criteria than that of 'well-founded fear of persecution' used in Article 1(A)(ii)": P. Weis, *The Refugee Convention, 1951: The Travaux Préparatoires Analysed with a Commentary by Dr. Paul Weis* (posthumously pub'd., 1995) (Weis, *Travaux*), at 303, 341.

freedom" was intended to function as a shorthand for the risks that give rise to refugee status under the terms of Art. 1.[133] The drafting history not only supports this view, but affords no evidence whatever for the contrary thesis that this choice of language was intended fundamentally to limit the ability to claim the Convention's most basic right.[134]

Lauterpacht and Bethlehem have more recently advanced the extreme opposite thesis, namely that "the threat contemplated in Article 33(1) [may be] broader than simply the risk of persecution .... [including] a threat to life or freedom [that] may arise other than in consequence of persecution."[135] In support of this thesis, they rely on the broadening of UNHCR's competence as an agency, on the humanitarian objectives of the Refugee Convention, and on the fact that various regional human rights instruments are now understood to provide for more broadly applicable forms of protection against *refoulement*. This leads them to conclude that "a broad reading of the threat *contemplated by Article 33(1)* is warranted [emphasis added],"[136] and specifically that:

> [T]he words "where his life or freedom would be threatened" must be construed to encompass circumstances in which a refugee or asylum-seeker (a) has a well-founded fear of being persecuted, (b) faces a real risk of torture or cruel, inhuman or degrading treatment or punishment, or (c) faces other threats to life, physical integrity, or liberty.[137]

Putting to one side the question of whether there is today a broader duty of *non-refoulement* under customary international law,[138] and recognizing that the threats noted in (b) and (c) are in any event likely to fall within modern understandings of a risk of "being persecuted,"[139] the analysis presented is

---

[133] See chapter 4.2.1 below, at pp. 399–401, for discussion of the choice of comparable language for Art. 31(1).

[134] As Grahl-Madsen observes, "it was quite unwittingly that the concept of 'life [or] freedom' was introduced [into] Article 31, and it seems that the widening of [the] scope of the provision ... must not lead us to restrict its meaning with regard to the kinds of persecution which warrant exemption from penalties. It is likewise inadmissible to use the language of Articles 31 and 33 to restrict the meaning of 'persecution' in Article 1. The word 'freedom' must be understood in its widest sense": A. Grahl-Madsen, *Commentary on the Refugee Convention 1951* (1963, pub'd. 1997) (Grahl-Madsen, *Commentary*), at 175.

[135] Lauterpacht and Bethlehem, "*Non-Refoulement*," at para. 127.

[136] Ibid. at paras. 128–132.   [137] Ibid. at para. 133.   [138] See chapter 4.1.6 below.

[139] Justice Kirby of the High Court of Australia has observed that "decision-makers in several other jurisdictions [have approached] the meaning of the word 'persecuted' by reference to the purpose for which, and the context in which, it appears rather than strictly by reference to local dictionaries ... [The Refugee Convention's] meaning should be ascertained having regard to its object, bearing in mind that the Convention is one of several important international treaties designed to redress 'violation[s] of basic human rights, demonstrative of a failure of state protection'": *Minister for Immigration and Multicultural Affairs v. Khawar*, [2002] HCA 14 (Aus. HC, Apr. 11, 2002), per Kirby J. For example, the Canadian Supreme Court has held that "[u]nderlying the Convention is the international community's commitment to the assurance of basic human rights without discrimination .... Persecution, for

simply unsustainable as a matter of law. The fact that there has been an expansion of UNHCR's agency mandate and of the duty of non-return under international human rights law more generally cannot be invoked to determine the meaning of Art. 33(1) of the Refugee Convention. While reference can, of course, be made to understandings of these more general developments in order to interpret cognate ambiguous language,[140] evolution outside of refugee law cannot be relied upon to override the linkage between the risks described in Art. 33(1) and entitlement to recognition of refugee status under Art. 1.[141]

The middle-ground position – namely, that Art. 33's guarantee against *refoulement* where "life or freedom would be threatened" for a Convention ground extends to situations where there is a risk of "being persecuted" for a Convention ground – was adopted by Lord Goff in the decision of the House of Lords in *Sivakumaran*:

> It is, I consider, plain, as indeed was reinforced in argument by counsel for the High Commissioner with reference to the *travaux préparatoires*, that the *non-refoulement* provision in Article 33 was intended to apply to all persons determined to be refugees under Article 1 of the Convention.[142]

The approach has also been routinely endorsed in the Australian jurisprudence,[143] is affirmed in the more recent English caselaw,[144] and has been

example, undefined in the Convention, has been ascribed the meaning of sustained or systemic violation of basic human rights demonstrative of a failure of state protection": *Canada v. Ward*, (1993) 103 DLR 4th 1 (Can. SC, June 30, 1993). "[C]ore entitlements [relevant to the meaning of 'being persecuted'] … may be found by reference either to obligations under international law (obligations between states), or by reference to the human rights of individuals, for example pursuant to the conventions on human rights, or as recognized by the international community at large": *Sepet v. Secretary of State for the Home Department*, [2001] EWCA Civ 681 (Eng. CA, May 11, 2001), per Waller LJ, appeal to the House of Lords rejected in *Sepet and Bulbul v. Secretary of State for the Home Department*, [2003] UKHL 15 (UK HL, Mar. 20, 2003).

[140] See chapter 1.3.3 above, at pp. 64–68.   [141] See chapter 1.3.2 above, at p. 52.

[142] *R v. Secretary of State for the Home Department, ex parte Sivakumaran*, [1988] 1 All ER 193 (UK HL, Dec. 16, 1987), per Lord Goff at 202–203.

[143] "Article 33 states the principle of *non-refoulement*, which applies to persons who are refugees within the meaning of Article 1. Although the definition of 'refugee' in Article 1 and the identification of persons subject to the *non-refoulement* obligation in Article 33 differ, it is clear that the obligation against [*refoulement*] applies to persons who are determined to be refugees under Article 1": *M38/2002 v. Minister for Immigration and Multicultural and Indigenous Affairs*, [2003] FCAFC 131 (Aus. FFC, June 13, 2003). See also *Minister for Immigration and Multicultural Affairs v. Savvin*, (2000) 171 ALR 483 (Aus. FFC, Apr. 12, 2000).

[144] "In my judgment it is Art. 1 … which must govern the scope of Art. 33 rather than the other way round": *Adan v. Secretary of State for the Home Department*, [1997] 1 WLR 1107 (Eng. CA, Feb. 13, 1997), per Simon Brown, LJ. While the House of Lords reversed the result reached in the Court of Appeal, four members of the House of Lords (Lord Lloyd of Berwick, Lord Goff of Chieveley, Lord Nolan, and Lord Hope of Craighead) nonetheless specifically endorsed the views of Simon Browne LJ on this point: *R v. Secretary of State for the Home Department, ex parte Adan*, [1999] 1 AC 293 (UK HL, Apr. 2, 1998), at 306, 301, 312, and 312.

adopted in New Zealand.[145] Not only is it a position that is firmly rooted in the actual intentions of the drafters, but it most effectively meshes with the internal structure of the Convention itself. In contrast, the conservative view championed by the American Supreme Court[146] implies that at least some persons with a well-founded fear of being persecuted may nonetheless be forced back to persecution unless the risk they face is particularly egregious – surely an interpretation at odds with the Convention's basic purpose of ensuring that refugees are granted the Convention's protections.[147] Equally of concern, the liberal optic seems designed effectively to require state parties to the Refugee Convention to implement duties that in fact follow from other human rights conventions – even if states are not actually parties to those other accords. The middle-ground position on Art. 33 contended for here, in contrast, ensures that all persons who are refugees are protected from return to the risks which gave rise to that status: no more, and no less.

4.1.2 Nature of the duty of non-refoulement

It follows from the endorsement of a coordinated understanding of Arts. 1 and 33 described above[148] that there is at least one, quite fundamental limitation on the scope of Art. 33's duty of *non-refoulement*. If the duty of *non-refoulement* under Art. 33 of the Refugee Convention can be claimed only by persons who are, in fact, refugees, then it is not a right that inheres in persons who have yet to leave their own country. This is because Art. 1 of the Convention defines a refugee as a person who "is outside the country of his nationality."[149] Art. 33 is not therefore a constraint on actions which deny would-be refugees the ability to leave their own state.

---

[145] The New Zealand Court of Appeal has determined that the scope of prohibited return under Art. 33(1) "is usually interpreted as covering all situations where the refugee risks any type of persecution for a Convention reason": *Attorney General v. Zaoui*, Dec. No. CA20/04 (NZ CA, Sept. 30, 2004), at para. 36.

[146] As previously noted, the United States Supreme Court takes the view that a risk to "life or freedom" is a more demanding notion than a risk "of being persecuted": see text above at p. 304, n. 131.

[147] "*The High Contracting Parties* . . . [c]onsidering that it is desirable to revise and consolidate previous international agreements . . . and to extend the scope of and the protection accorded by such instruments by means of a new agreement . . . [h]ave agreed as follows": Refugee Convention, at Preamble. The Convention then provides a definition of refugee status in Art. 1, and defines the rights that follow from refugee status in Arts. 2–34.

[148] See chapter 4.1.1 above, at pp. 306–307.

[149] Refugee Convention, at Art. 1(A)(2). In the case of persons who are stateless, Art. 1 requires that they be "outside the country of [their] former habitual residence": ibid.

This issue was thoroughly considered in the English *European Roma Rights Centre* case.[150] One of the arguments advanced was that the pre-entry clearance procedure operated by British authorities at Prague Airport was in breach of Art. 33. It was agreed that the system was "aimed principally at stemming the flow of asylum-seekers from the Czech Republic, the vast majority of these being of Romani ethnic origin (Roma), and that in this it has plainly had some considerable success."[151] Moreover, it was also understood that "[t]he object of these controls . . . so far as asylum countries are concerned, is to prevent [refugees] from reaching [British] shores."[152] The key issue was therefore "whether a scheme designed to prevent any such asylum claims (whether genuine or otherwise) being made in the United Kingdom is inconsistent with the United Kingdom's obligations in international law, in particular under the Convention."[153] The Court of Appeal determined that it was not:

> That Article 33 of the Convention has no direct application to the Prague operation is plain . . . [I]t applies in terms only to refugees, and a refugee is defined . . . as someone necessarily "outside the country of his nationality" . . . For good measure, Article 33 forbids "*refoulement*" to "frontiers" and, whatever precise meaning is given to the former term, it cannot comprehend action which causes someone to remain on the same side of the frontier as they began; nor indeed could such a person be said to have been returned to any frontier.[154]

This conclusion is legally sound, even as it clearly points to a serious protection risk that arises by virtue of the gap between the duty of *non-refoulement* and a broader notion of access to asylum.[155] In truth, in-country interdiction schemes would be more effectively challenged as violations by the home state

---

[150] *R (European Roma Rights Centre and Others) v. Immigration Officer at Prague Airport*, [2003] EWCA Civ 666 (Eng. CA, May 20, 2003), rev'd on other grounds at [2004] UKHL 55 (UK HL, Dec. 9, 2004).

[151] *R (European Roma Rights Centre and Others) v. Immigration Officer at Prague Airport*, [2003] EWCA Civ 666 (Eng. CA, May 20, 2003), at para. 3.

[152] Ibid. at para. 1.   [153] Ibid. at para. 18.

[154] Ibid. at para. 31. The House of Lords agreed, noting succinctly that "[t]he requirement that a foreign national applying for refugee status must, to qualify as a refugee, be outside his country of nationality is unambiguously expressed in the Convention definition of refugee": *R v. Immigration Officer at Prague Airport et al., ex parte European Roma Rights Centre et al.*, [2004] UKHL 55 (UK HL, Dec. 9, 2004), at para. 16.

[155] In the High Court decision, it is recorded that counsel advanced the argument that the Prague pre-screening system is "if not in breach of an express term or obligation under the Convention, yet a breach of the obligation of good faith owed by a signatory state, in that it would be preventing those seeking asylum from gaining international protection": *European Roma Rights Centre v. Immigration Officer at Prague Airport*, [2002] EWCA 1989 (Eng. HC, Oct. 8, 2002), at para. 34. In response, the court noted that "[t]he UNHCR has, it seems, reservations about a pre-clearance system, but it does not explain

of Art. 12(2) of the Civil and Political Covenant, which provides that "[e]veryone shall be free to leave any country, including his own."[156] The Human Rights Committee has determined that

> Freedom to leave the territory of a State may not be made dependent on any specific purpose or on the period of time the individual chooses to stay outside the country. Thus traveling abroad is covered, as well as departure for permanent emigration. Likewise, the right of the individual to determine the State of destination is part of the legal guarantee.[157]

This right may only be limited for a reason deemed legitimate under the Covenant,[158] and may in any event not be limited on a discriminatory basis.[159] Thus, at least in a situation akin to the Prague Airport case – where the prohibition of seeking protection abroad is unlikely to be deemed a legitimate reason for denial of the right to leave one's country, and where the prohibition was, at least in practice, implemented on a race-specific basis[160] – the home state should be found in breach of the Covenant. Indeed, both the home state and any

---

either how in practice it is to be distinguished from a visa system, and whether that system too is to be regarded as objectionable, and if so on what basis, or how the position it takes ... is consistent with its own Handbook": ibid. at para. 49. The House of Lords emphatically rejected the notion that the duty of good faith treaty interpretation could effectively result in the imposition of duties at odds with the text of the treaty, finding that "there is no want of good faith if a state interprets a treaty as meaning what it says and declines to do anything significantly greater than or different from what it has agreed to do": R. v. Immigration Officer at Prague Airport et al., ex parte European Roma Rights Centre et al., [2004] UKHL 55 (UK HL, Dec. 9, 2004), per Lord Bingham at para. 19. See generally the discussion of the implications of the duty of good faith interpretation in the opinion of Lord Hope, ibid. at paras. 57–64, leading to the conclusion that "[w]hat the Convention does is assure refugees of the rights and freedoms set out in chapters I to V when they are in countries that are not their own. It does not require the state to abstain from controlling the movements of people outside its border who wish to travel to it in order to claim asylum": ibid. at para. 64.

[156] Civil and Political Covenant, at Art. 12(2).

[157] UN Human Rights Committee, "General Comment No. 27: Freedom of movement" (1999), UN Doc. HRI/GEN/1/Rev.7, May 12, 2004, at 173, para. 8.

[158] This right is subject only to "restrictions ... provided by law, [and which] are necessary to protect national security, public order (ordre public), public health or morals or the rights and freedoms of others, and are consistent with the other rights recognized in the present Covenant": Civil and Political Covenant, at Art. 12(3). The scope of these permissible limitations is discussed at chapter 6.7 below, at pp. 897–902.

[159] Art. 12(3) requires that restrictions be "consistent with the other rights recognized in the present Covenant"; if discriminatory, e.g. on grounds of race, there would be a breach of both Arts. 2(1) and 26 of the Covenant, thus disqualifying them from meeting the requirements of Art. 12(3): Civil and Political Covenant, at Art. 12.

[160] Indeed, the House of Lords struck down the British pre-screening system at Prague Airport precisely on the grounds that "[a]ll the evidence before us, other than that of the intentions of those in charge of the operation, which intentions were not conveyed to the officers on the ground, supports the inference that Roma were, simply because they were Roma, routinely treated with more suspicion and subjected to more intensive and

foreign countries with which it chooses to share jurisdiction over departure from its territory should be held jointly liable for a breach of Art. 12(2).[161] But this does not change the fact that prohibitions on departure operated from within the territory of one's own state, and which preclude exit altogether, cannot breach rights under the Refugee Convention, including to protection against *refoulement*:

> Article 33 . . . is concerned only with where a person must not be sent, not with where he is trying to escape from. The Convention could have, but chose not to, concern itself also with enabling people to escape their country by providing for a right of admission to another country to allow them to do so . . .
>
> In an ideal world there would no doubt be provision for states to facilitate the escape of persecuted minorities . . . I am satisfied, however, that on no view of the Convention is this within its scope. The distinction between, on the one hand, a state preventing an aspiring asylum-seeker from gaining access from his own country to its territory, and on the other hand returning such a person to his own country . . . can be made to seem a narrow and unsatisfactory one. In my judgment, however, it is a crucial distinction to make and it is supported by both the text of the Convention and by the authorities dictating its scope.[162]

Art. 33 is similarly incapable of invalidating the classic tool of *non-entrée*: visa controls imposed on the nationals of refugee-producing states,[163]

---

intrusive questioning than non-Roma . . . [S]etting up an operation like this, prompted by an influx of asylum seekers who are overwhelmingly from one comparatively easily identifiable racial or ethnic group, requires enormous care if it is to be done without discrimination. That did not happen. The inevitable conclusion was that the operation was inherently and systematically discriminatory and unlawful": *R v. Immigration Officer at Prague Airport et al., ex parte European Roma Rights Centre et al.*, [2004] UKHL 55 (UK HL, Dec. 9, 2004), per Baroness Hale at para. 97.

[161] The UN Human Rights Committee has read Art. 2(1) of the Civil and Political Covenant disjunctively, finding that the obligation to respect rights "within [a state's] territory and to all persons subject to [its] jurisdiction" means that "a State party must respect and ensure the rights laid down in the Covenant to anyone within the power or effective control of that State Party, even if not situated within the territory of the State Party": UN Human Rights Committee, "General Comment No. 31: The nature of the general legal obligation imposed on states parties to the Covenant" (2004), UN Doc. HRI/GEN/1/Rev.7, May 12, 2004, at 192, para. 10. See generally chapter 3.1.1 above, at pp. 165–169.

[162] *R (European Roma Rights Centre and Others) v. Immigration Officer at Prague Airport*, [2003] EWCA Civ 666 (Eng. CA, May 20, 2003), at paras. 37, 43, affirmed in this regard in *R v. Immigration Officer at Prague Airport et al., ex parte European Roma Rights Centre et al.*, [2004] UKHL 55 (UK HL, Dec. 9, 2004), at paras. 13–17.

[163] In many cases, of course, visa requirements are imposed for general migration control reasons, with no intent to stop the departure of refugees. Yet it remains that visa controls are unquestionably crude mechanisms that fail to distinguish between persons at risk of persecution and others, or between those at-risk persons who can safely access protection in other countries, and those who have no options.

enforced by carrier sanctions.[164] Visa control policies are generally enforced in countries of origin by airline and other common carriers, aware that failure to do so could result in penalties or prosecution by the destination country. Because no country issues visas for the purpose of entering its asylum system, any traveler who honestly states that he or she intends to claim refugee status upon arrival will in practice be turned back at the port of departure. Countries of origin are normally aware of such practices, or could readily inform themselves with minimal effort.[165]

In contrast to in-country interception of the kind implemented by the United Kingdom at Prague Airport, most visa controls – including, for example, those routinely imposed by Canada, New Zealand, and now required by European Union law – operate passively, with no need for the state imposing the controls to establish a physical presence in the would-be refugee's country of origin. UNHCR argued before the English courts that reliance could be placed on this distinction in order to strike down the Prague system without simultaneously invalidating visa control systems that operate to keep refugees inside their own countries. It suggested "that there is a distinction to be made between 'the active interdiction or interception of persons seeking refuge from persecution' on the one hand and 'passive regimes, such as visa controls and carrier sanctions' on the other." The Court of Appeal sensibly found this distinction to be without merit:[166]

---

[164] UNHCR has traditionally seemed unwilling to confront the fact that the denial of access to refugees by the imposition of visa controls is not simply the inadvertent consequence of a general policy of migration control, but can actually be a policy targeted at those who wish to claim protection. For example, the only mention of visa controls in UNHCR's position paper on interception notes that "[s]tates have a legitimate interest in controlling irregular migration. Unfortunately, existing controls, such as visa requirements and the imposition of carrier sanctions . . . often do not differentiate between genuine asylum-seekers and economic migrants. National authorities, including immigration and airline officials posted abroad, are frequently not aware of the paramount distinction between refugees, who are entitled to international protection, and other migrants, who are able to rely on national protection": UNHCR, "Interception of Asylum-Seekers and Refugees: The International Framework and Recommendations for a Comprehensive Approach," UN Doc. EC/50/SC/CRP.17, June 9, 2000 (UNHCR, "Interception"), at para. 17.

[165] See Feller, "Sanctions"; and J. Hathaway and J. Dent, *Refugee Rights: Report on a Comparative Survey* (1995), at 13–14.

[166] *R (European Roma Rights Centre and Others) v. Immigration Officer at Prague Airport*, [2003] EWCA Civ 666 (Eng. CA, May 20, 2003), at para. 48. In another context, though, UNHCR seemed to argue that visa controls *can* breach Art. 33. "Immigration control measures, although aimed principally at combatting irregular migration, can seriously jeopardize the ability of persons at risk of persecution to gain access to safety and asylum. As pointed out by UNHCR in the past, the exclusive resort to measures to combat abuse, without balancing them by adequate means to identify genuine cases, *may result in the refoulement of refugees* [emphasis added]": UNHCR, "Interception," at para. 18.

In my judgment, there is nothing in these criticisms and indeed the Prague scheme seems to me to constitute if anything a less, rather than more, serious problem for would-be asylum-seekers than visa control . . .

. . . [Objections] to visa controls . . . do not sound in international law. Rather one must hope that when in truth acute humanitarian concerns arise states will respond beyond the strict call of their international obligations. This, I believe, is the only answer the Court is entitled to give when [counsel] conjures up the spectre of a fresh holocaust. Visa controls are, in short, clearly not outlawed under the Convention or under international law generally.[167]

The Court is quite right that visa controls, which operate routinely and in many places, actually pose a greater risk to refugees than do in-country interception schemes, which tend to be more selective and less routinely operationalized.[168] Yet the Court is equally correct that "[o]n the basis of the [Refugee] Convention as it stands at present, there is no obligation on a signatory state not to introduce or continue a system of immigration control, whether by way of a requirement for visas or by the operation of a pre-clearance system."[169]

As in the case of in-country interdiction schemes described above, the most effective legal avenue to challenge visa control systems of this sort is to invoke Art. 12 of the Civil and Political Covenant, in this case in order to hold the home state liable for its complicity in efforts conducted under its jurisdiction to stymie the departure of at-risk persons who wish to claim refugee status abroad.[170] The UN Human Rights Committee has indicated its view

---

[167] *R (European Roma Rights Centre and Others) v. Immigration Officer at Prague Airport*, [2003] EWCA Civ 666 (Eng. CA, May 20, 2003), at paras. 49–50. The House of Lords was in full agreement on this point, noting that "[h]ad a visa regime been imposed, the effect on the appellants, so far as concerned their applications for asylum, would have been no different. But it could not plausibly be argued that a visa regime would have been contrary to the practice of nations": *R v. Immigration Officer at Prague Airport et al., ex parte European Roma Rights Centre et al.*, [2004] UKHL 55 (UK HL, Dec. 9, 2004), at para. 28.

[168] See also *R v. Uxbridge Magistrates Court, ex parte Adimi*, [1999] 4 All ER 520 (Eng. HC, July 29, 1999), per Simon Brown L J: "Although under the Convention subscribing states must give sanctuary to any refugee who seeks asylum (subject only to removal to a safe third country), they are by no means bound to facilitate his arrival. Rather they strive increasingly to prevent it. The combined effect of visa requirements and carrier's liability has made it well nigh impossible for refugees to travel to countries of refuge without false documents."

[169] *R (European Roma Rights Centre and Others) v. Immigration Officer at Prague Airport*, [2003] EWCA Civ 666 (Eng. CA, May 20, 2003), at para. 49, affirmed in this regard in *R v. Immigration Officer at Prague Airport et al., ex parte European Roma Rights Centre et al.*, [2004] UKHL 55 (UK HL, Dec. 9, 2004), at para. 34.

[170] See text above, at pp. 308–310. In addition to reliance on Art. 12(2) of the Civil and Political Covenant, it has also been contended that where visa controls are applied after a refugee's departure from his or her own country – for example, in a transit country – this

that, in at least some cases, the operation of a system of visa controls and carrier sanctions will put a state party in breach of the duty to respect the right of persons to leave their own country, and more generally to enjoy freedom of international movement:

> The practice of States often shows that legal rules and administrative measures adversely affect the right to leave, in particular, a person's own country. It is therefore of the utmost importance that States parties report on all legal and practical restrictions on the right to leave which they apply both to nationals and to foreigners, in order to enable the Committee to assess the conformity of these rules and practices with article 12, paragraph 3 [which defines permissible limitations on this right]. States parties should also include information in their reports on measures that impose sanctions on international carriers which bring to their territory persons without required documents, where those measures affect the right to leave another country.[171]

The case for finding a breach of Art. 12 would seem particularly strong where the visa requirement is set explicitly to avoid the departure of at-risk persons; but there is more generally a real question about the legitimacy of even visas set to regulate non-coerced migration, but which are known in practice also to preclude the freedom of movement of would-be refugees.

It may, however, be more difficult to find a breach of Art. 12(2) of the Covenant by the country which imposed the visa controls since, in contrast to situations in which that country actually operates an in-country interdiction

---

may amount to a breach of the Refugee Convention's Art. 31, which prohibits the imposition of penalties on refugees for illegal entry or presence: see chapter 4.2 below. This possibility was raised by the English High Court in relation to refugees interdicted in the United Kingdom because they did not have the required Canadian visas for onward travel. In *R v. Uxbridge Magistrates Court, ex parte Adimi*, [1999] 4 All ER 520 (Eng. HC, July 29, 1999), Simon Brown LJ observed, "If I am right in saying that refugees are ordinarily entitled to choose where to claim asylum and that a short stopover en route in a country where a traveller's status is in no way regularized will not break the requisite directness of flight, then it must follow that these applicants would have been entitled to the benefit of Article 31 had they reached Canada and made their asylum claims there. If Article 31 would have availed them in Canada, then logically its protection cannot be denied to them [in the United Kingdom] merely because they have been apprehended en route." Indeed, on the basis of this argument, it might even be possible to find the state which established the visa controls to be liable for breach of Art. 31 where it exercises shared jurisdiction with the transit state – for example, by staffing or overseeing the personnel who enforce the visa controls. The real difficulty in relying on Art. 31 as an alternative to the (substantively inadequate) Art. 33, however, is that it does not prohibit the classic result of a visa control, namely return to the country of origin. As is detailed below, the drafters were clear that expulsion or return are not to be considered "penalties" for the purposes of Art. 31 protection: see chapter 4.2.3 below, at pp. 412–413.

[171] UN Human Rights Committee, "General Comment No. 27: Freedom of movement" (1999), UN Doc. HRI/GEN/1/Rev.7, May 12, 2004, at 173, para. 10.

scheme, it is not clear that the state which sets the visa controls is in any sense exercising (even shared) jurisdiction over the place of departure. While the Human Rights Committee has a long-standing practice of holding states liable for the extraterritorial actions of their agents,[172] the International Court of Justice has recently affirmed the jurisdictional foundation of such liability, noting that "the International Covenant on Civil and Political Rights is applicable in respect of acts done by a State in the exercise of its jurisdiction outside its own territory":[173]

> The *travaux préparatoires* of the Covenant confirm the [UN Human Rights] Committee's interpretation of Article 2 of that instrument. These show that, in adopting the wording chosen, the drafters of the Covenant did not intend to allow States to escape from their obligations when they exercise jurisdiction outside their national territory. They only intended to prevent persons residing abroad from asserting, vis-à-vis their State of origin, rights that do not fall within the competence of that State, but of that of the State of residence.[174]

In essence, liability for extraterritorial actions follows where a state party exercises "effective jurisdiction."[175] While this will be a question of fact in each case, it is far from clear that a state can be said to exercise jurisdiction by the simple issuance of policies intended to apply extraterritorially, but which are wholly implemented by third parties operating inside the sovereign territory of another state.[176]

---

[172] See e.g. *Casariego v. Uruguay*, UNHRC Comm. No. 56/1979, decided July 29, 1981, at paras. 10.1–10.3: "Article 2(1) of the Covenant places an obligation upon a state party to respect and to ensure rights 'to all individuals within its territory and subject to its jurisdiction,' but it does not imply that the state party concerned cannot be held accountable for violation of rights under the Covenant which its agents commit upon the territory of another state, whether with the acquiescence of the government of that state or in opposition to it ... [I]t would be unconscionable to so interpret the responsibility under Article 2 of the Covenant, as to permit a state party to perpetrate violations of the Covenant on the territory of another state, which violations it could not perpetrate on its own territory."

[173] *Legal Consequences of the Construction of a Wall in the Occupied Palestinian Territory*, (2004) ICJ Gen. List No. 131, decided July 9, 2004, at para. 111.

[174] Ibid. at para. 109.   [175] Ibid. at para. 110.

[176] In *Legal Consequences of the Construction of a Wall in the Occupied Palestinian Territory*, ibid., for example, the analysis of the International Court of Justice seems to have given real weight to the Israeli physical presence in the Occupied Territories. "The [Human Rights] Committee, in its concluding observations after examination of the report, expressed concern at Israel's attitude and pointed 'to the long-standing presence of Israel in [the occupied] territories, Israel's ambiguous attitude towards their future status, as well as the exercise of effective jurisdiction by Israeli security forces therein' (CCPR/C/79/Add.93, para. 10). In 2003 in face of Israel's consistent position, to the effect that 'the Covenant does not apply beyond its own territory, notably in the West Bank and

The weakness of the duty of *non-refoulement* as an answer to measures that trap would-be refugees inside their own countries aside, Art. 33 is otherwise quite a robust form of protection. In particular, the duty of *non-refoulement* has ordinarily been understood to constrain not simply ejection from within a state's territory, but also non-admittance at its frontiers.[177] Indeed, the 1933 Convention – from which the present duty of *non-refoulement* was derived – explicitly codified non-admittance as an aspect of *refoulement*.[178] This comprehensive definition corresponds to the authority enjoyed by police in some states summarily to remove aliens or to refuse them entry (*refoulement*) under a process distinct from expulsion authorized by judicial authority.[179] It was clear to the drafters that summary refusals (*refoulement*) and formally sanctioned removals (expulsion or deportation) could equally undermine the sheltering of refugees from forcible return.

The original purpose of the prohibition of *refoulement* was therefore to ensure that those states in which summary removal or denial of access was authorized by law not be allowed to rely on such provisions to subvert the

---

Gaza . . .', the Committee reached the following conclusion: 'in the current circumstances, the provisions of the Covenant apply to the benefit of the population of the Occupied Territories, for all conduct by the State party's authorities or agents in those territories that affect the enjoyment of rights enshrined in the Covenant and fall within the ambit of State responsibility of Israel under the principles of public international law' (CCPR/CO/78/ISR, para. 11). In conclusion, the Court considers that the International Covenant on Civil and Political Rights is applicable in respect of acts done by a State in the exercise of its jurisdiction outside its own territory": ibid. at paras. 110–111.

[177] See e.g. UNHCR Executive Committee Conclusion No. 6, "Non-Refoulement" (1977), at para. (c), available at www.unhcr.ch (accessed Nov. 20, 2004), acknowledging "the fundamental importance of the observance of the principle of *non-refoulement* – both at the border and within the territory of a State." "Today, there appears to be ample support for the conclusion that Article 33(1) of the Refugee Convention is applicable to rejection at the frontier of a potential host state": G. Noll et al., "Study on the Feasibility of Processing Asylum Claims Outside the EU Against the Background of the Common European Asylum System and the Goal of a Common Asylum Procedure" (2002), at 36. See generally P. Mathew, "Australian Refugee Protection in the Wake of the *Tampa*," (2002) 96(3) *American Journal of International Law* 661 (Mathew, "*Tampa*"), at 667, drawing support for this proposition from the General Assembly's Declaration on Territorial Asylum; and Lauterpacht and Bethlehem, "*Non-Refoulement*," at paras. 76–86.

[178] 1933 Refugee Convention, at Art. 3.

[179] "[T]he term 'expulsion' was used when the refugee concerned had committed some criminal offence, whereas the term '*refoulement*' was used in cases when the refugee was deported or refused admittance because his presence in the country was considered undesirable": Statement of Mr. Cuvelier of Belgium, UN Doc. E/AC.32/SR.21, Feb. 2, 1950, at 5. See also G. Goodwin-Gill, *The Refugee in International Law* (1996) (Goodwin-Gill, *Refugee in International Law*), at 117: "In the context of immigration control in continental Europe, *refoulement* is a term of art covering, in particular, summary reconduction to the frontier of those discovered to have entered illegally, and summary refusal of admission to those without valid papers."

general limitations on the expulsion of refugees.[180] If the minority of countries that practiced *refoulement* were required to temper the application of such systems in relation to refugees, all governments would face comparable obligations: refugees would be able to access the state's territory, and their removal could only be effected in accordance with the general rules governing the expulsion or deportation of refugees.[181]

The debates of the Ad Hoc Committee on Statelessness and Related Problems show a clear commitment to this basic understanding that peremptory non-admittance or ejection is normally impermissible. The United States vigorously argued that

> [w]hether it was a question of closing the frontier to a refugee who asked admittance, or of turning him back after he had crossed the frontier, or even of expelling him after he had been admitted to residence in the territory, the problem was more or less the same. Whatever the case might be, whether or not the refugee was in a regular position, he must not be turned back to a country where his life or freedom could be threatened.[182]

While the English translation of *non-refoulement* varied from "undertakes not to turn back" to "undertakes not to expel or turn back,"[183] and ultimately to "undertakes not to expel or return," the intention to proscribe both non-admittance and ejection from within a state's territory was constant.[184] Indeed,

---

[180] "Sir Leslie Brass (United Kingdom) concluded from the discussion that the notion of *refoulement* could apply to (a) refugees seeking admission, (b) refugees illegally present in a country, and (c) refugees admitted temporarily or conditionally. Referring to the practice followed in his own country, Sir Leslie stated that refugees who had been allowed to enter the United Kingdom could be sent out of the country only by expulsion or deportation. There was no concept in these cases corresponding to that of *refoulement* ... Mr. Ordonneau (France) considered that the inclusion in the draft convention of a reference to the concept of *refoulement* would not in any way interfere with the administrative practices of countries such as the United Kingdom, which did not employ it, but that its exclusion from the draft convention would place countries like France and Belgium in a very difficult position": UN Doc. E/AC.32/SR.21, Feb. 2, 1950, at 5.

[181] "The Chairman suspended the discussion, observing that it had indicated agreement on the principle that refugees fleeing from persecution ... should not be pushed back to the arms of their persecutors": Statement of Mr. Chance of Canada, ibid. at 7. See generally chapter 5.1 below on the question of the prohibition of formal expulsion or deportation of refugees.

[182] Statement of Mr. Henkin of the United States, UN Doc. E/AC.32/SR.20, Feb. 1, 1950, at 11–12. See also Statement of Mr. Robinson of Israel, ibid. at 12–13: "The article must, in fact, apply to all refugees, whether or not they were admitted to residence; it must deal with both expulsion and non-admittance."

[183] Ibid. at 12.

[184] The substitution of "return" for "turn back" was intended to be a matter of style only: Statement of Mr. Henkin of the United States, UN Doc. E/AC.32/SR.22, Feb. 2, 1950, at 20.

the Belgian co-sponsor of the text adopted by the Committee emphasized that the duty had been expanded to an undertaking "not to expel *or in any way* [return] refugees [emphasis added]"[185] precisely to ensure that it was understood that the article "referred to various methods by which refugees could be expelled, refused admittance or removed."[186] Because of the comprehensive nature of the duty of *non-refoulement*, Nepal's refusal of entry to Tibetans, Guinea's blocking of access to refugees from Sierra Leone, Namibia's order indiscriminately to shoot anyone using the only escape route open to Angolan refugees from Cuando Cuban Province, and Jordan's denial of entry to most refugees who could no longer safely remain in Iraq were no less rights-violative than the ejection of a refugee from within their territory.

Perhaps most clearly, the duty of *non-refoulement* is infringed by the actions of government officials intended to force refugees back to their country of origin. The enforced removal of refugees may occur under formally sanctioned programs of the kind implemented by Zambia against refugees from the Democratic Republic of Congo, by Iran against Afghan refugees, and by Thailand in relation to ethnic Burmese refugees. It may also be implemented with less publicity, as when Cambodia returned the Montagnard refugees to Vietnam; when India sent Tamil refugees back to Sri Lanka despite the persistence of conflict there; when Pakistani police summarily expelled undocumented Afghan refugees across the border; and when Venezuelan army patrols forced Colombian refugees home. In all of these cases, the duty of *non-refoulement* was directly and unambiguously breached.

Nor is a government insulated from liability when, rather than taking action through its own officials, it encourages non-state actors to drive refugees back to their countries of origin. Because governments are liable for the actions they promote and support, Art. 33 was clearly infringed by Kenyan President Moi's incitement to remove Ugandan and other refugees, as well as by Guinean President Conte's encouragement of his citizens to form militia groups to force refugees from Liberia and Sierra Leone to go home. More generally, as the Supreme Court of India has affirmed, governments have an affirmative duty to take such action as is necessary to avoid the *refoulement* of refugees instigated and carried out by third parties. Faced with a complaint that Chakma refugees were being subjected to an economic blockade by a student vigilante group intended to drive them out, the Court issued an unambiguous and comprehensive order to both state and

---

[185] UN Doc. E/AC.32/L.25, Feb. 2, 1950, at 1. In the draft convention finalized by the Working Group, the undertaking was rephrased to require states not to "expel or return, *in any manner whatsoever*, a refugee to the frontiers of territories where his life or freedom would be threatened [emphasis added]": UN Doc. E/AC.32/L.32, Feb. 9, 1950, at 12.

[186] Statement of Mr. Cuvelier of Belgium, UN Doc. E/AC.32/SR.22, Feb. 2, 1950, at 20.

national authorities to take whatever action was required to bring the student actions to an end.[187]

To this point, consideration has been given to the ways in which the duty of *non-refoulement* may be infringed by actions specifically intended either to block the arrival, or to bring about the return, of refugees. *Refoulement* may also be effected by a very wide range of actions taken by, or with the acquiescence of, a state party. This point was made during the drafting of the Convention by the American representative, who emphasized that "[Art. 33's] sole purpose was to preclude the forcible return of a refugee to a country in which he feared both the persecution from which he had fled and reprisals for his attempted escape."[188] This makes clear that the duty under Art. 33 is to avoid certain *consequences* (namely, return to the risk of being persecuted), whatever the nature of the actions which lead to that result.[189]

Of particular concern, *refoulement* in practice frequently arises when refugees are coerced to accept "voluntary" repatriation. At least where refugees are left with no real option but to leave, de facto enforced departure is a form of *refoulement*. For example, Art. 33 was not respected when Turkey, Rwanda, Uganda, and India withheld food, water, and other essentials from refugees in order to induce them "voluntarily" to repatriate. Pakistan's refusal to allow foreign aid agencies to provide essentials to refugees in the Jalozai camp was simply a less direct means of achieving the same rights-violative end. Macedonia's denial to refugees of sanitary facilities may have been a less egregious effort to force refugees to leave, but it still proved sufficient in practice to drive refugees back to Kosovo. The fact that Tanzania's efforts to force Rwandan refugees to return home were implemented by means of a deadline to accept "voluntary" repatriation, and even that they were implemented under an

---

[187] While India is not a party to the Refugee Convention or Protocol, the Court relied on Art. 21 of the Indian Constitution which establishes a guarantee of life and personal liberty for all. Its order was that "the State of Arunachal Pradesh shall ensure that the life and personal liberty of each and every Chakma residing within the State shall be protected and any attempt to forcibly evict or drive them out of the State by organised groups, such as the [student vigilante group], shall be repelled, if necessary by requisitioning the service of paramilitary or police force, and if additional forces are considered necessary to carry out this direction, the [State] will request the . . . Union of India to provide such additional force, and [the national government] shall provide such additional force as is necessary to protect the lives and liberty of the Chakmas": *National Human Rights Commission v. State of Arunachal Pradesh*, (1996) 83 AIR 1234 (India SC, Jan. 9, 1996), at para. 21.

[188] Statement of Mr. Henkin of the United States, UN Doc. E/AC.32/SR.22, Feb. 2, 1950, at 20.

[189] See *R v. Secretary of State for the Home Department, ex parte Yogathas*, [2002] UKHL 36 (UK HL, Oct. 17, 2002), per Lord Hope at para. 47. Thus, for example, the right of a state to effect the extradition of a refugee is subject to compliance with the duty of *non-refoulement*: Lauterpacht and Bethlehem, "*Non-Refoulement*," at paras. 71–75.

agreement with UNHCR, takes nothing away from their fundamentally rights-violative character. As courts in the United States held in enjoining American threats and subterfuge undertaken to force Salvadoran refugees to go home, the formal and legalized nature of acts which are in substance coercive does not in any sense render them lawful.[190] On the other hand, Australia was, at least initially, not acting contrary to Art. 33 when it offered Afghan families the option to abandon their refugee claims in exchange for substantial cash payments. Despite the resemblance to blackmail, the voluntary character of the program was really only clearly compromised when authorities made clear that the refugees would inevitably be forced to return home, whether or not they accepted the cash payment.

Art. 33 may be infringed by fairly blunt measures of the kind considered to this point, but may also be breached by "any measure, whether judicial or administrative, which secures the departure of an alien."[191] Most obviously, this will be the case where, as in Austria and South Africa, responsibility to protect refugees is entrusted to officials such as border guards or detention center officers who do not reliably carry out those responsibilities.[192] The duty of *non-refoulement* can also be infringed by the refusal to consider a claim to refugee status, knowing that such a refusal leaves the refugee exposed to removal on general immigration grounds.[193] As such, when countries such as China, Japan,

---

[190] In *Orantes-Hernandez v. Meese*, (1988) 685 F Supp 1488 (US DCCa, Apr. 29, 1988), affirmed as *Orantes-Hernandez v. Thornburgh*, (1990) 919 F 2d 549 (US CA9, Nov. 29, 1990), the Immigration and Naturalization Service was found to have engaged in a persistent pattern of illegal conduct and enjoined from further harassment of Salvadoran refugees.

[191] Goodwin-Gill, *Refugee in International Law*, at 122, adopted in *Re S*, [2002] EWCA Civ 843 (Eng. CA, May 28, 2002).

[192] The risk of *refoulement* in such circumstances will continue to exist under recently proposed EU rules which authorize the continuation of existing procedures at borders which do not meet all procedural requirements ordinarily governing the assessment of claims to refugee protection. "Member States may provide for procedures, in accordance with the basic principles and guarantees of chapter II, in order to decide, at the border or transit zones of the Member State, on the applications made at such locations . . . However, when procedures as set out in paragraph 1 do not exist, Member States may maintain, subject to the provisions of this Article and in accordance with the laws or regulations in force at the time of the adoption of this Directive, procedures derogating from the basic principles and guarantees described in chapter II, in order to decide, at the border or in transit zones, on the permission to enter their territory of applicants for asylum who have arrived and made an application for asylum at such locations": EU Procedures Directive, at Art. 35.

[193] See e.g. UNHCR Executive Committee Conclusion No. 6, "Non-Refoulement" (1977), available at www.unhcr.ch (accessed Nov. 20, 2004), at para. (c): "The Executive Committee . . . [r]eaffirms the fundamental importance of the observance of the principle of *non-refoulement* . . . of persons who may be subjected to persecution if returned to their country of origin irrespective of whether or not they have been formally recognized

Malaysia, Namibia, Pakistan, Thailand, and Zimbabwe denied persons claiming to be refugees access to any procedure to verify their status – and then removed them from their territory on the grounds of their illegal presence – they acted in breach of the duty of *non-refoulement*.[194] There is also no basis for a bar on considering the refugee claims made by children of the kind often applied in Europe, and advocated as a general standard by Australia. To the contrary, as the English Court of Appeal has observed, the duty to protect refugees – including children who are refugees – may well trump other considerations, including the enforcement of child custody orders.[195] And while the failure to establish an appeal or review of a negative refugee status determination does not necessarily infringe Art. 33, the fact that the duty of *non-refoulement* is binding right up to the actual moment of return[196] requires that the system have the capacity to take

as refugees." See also UNHCR Executive Committee Conclusions Nos. 79, "General Conclusion on International Protection" (1996), at para. (j), and 81, "General Conclusion on International Protection" (1997), at para. (i), both available at www.unhcr.ch (accessed Nov. 20, 2004), insisting that the duty of *non-refoulement* inheres "whether or not they have been formally granted refugee status." The notion that access to Art. 33 could be limited to persons formally recognized as refugees has been described simply as "devoid of merit": Lauterpacht and Bethlehem, "*Non-Refoulement*," at para. 89.

[194] In response to China's refusal to address the refugee claims of North Koreans, the United States Senate passed a resolution in which it called upon China to make "genuine efforts to identify and protect the refugees among the North Korean migrants encountered by Chinese authorities, including providing the refugees with a reasonable opportunity to petition for asylum": S. Con. Res. 114, 107th Congress (2002), at para. 1(A), cited in S. Murphy, "Contemporary Practice of the United States relating to International Law," (2002) 96(3) *American Journal of International Law* 706.

[195] "Having regard to the rule as to the paramountcy of the child's interests ... I would respectfully suppose that a family judge would at the very least pay very careful attention to any credible suggestion that a child might be persecuted if he were returned to his country of origin or habitual residence before making any order that such a return should be effected": *Re S*, [2002] EWCA Civ 843 (Eng. CA, May 28, 2002). To similar effect, UNHCR is of the view that "[t]he child should not be refused entry or returned at the point of entry ... As soon as a separated child is identified, a suitably qualified guardian or adviser should be appointed to assist him/her at all stages. Interviews should be carried out by specially trained personnel": UNHCR, "Asylum Processes," UN Doc. EC/GC/01/12, May 31, 2001 (UNHCR, "Asylum Processes"), at para. 46. See generally Convention on the Rights of the Child, UNGA Res. 44/25, adopted Nov. 20, 1989, entered into force Sept. 2, 1990, at Art. 22(1): "States Parties shall take appropriate measures to ensure that a child who is seeking refugee status or who is considered a refugee in accordance with applicable international or domestic law and procedures shall, whether unaccompanied or accompanied by his or her parents or by any other person, receive appropriate protection and humanitarian assistance in the enjoyment of applicable rights."

[196] The duty of *non-refoulement* "continues so long as a refugee (defined by reference to a well-founded fear of being persecuted for a reason specified in the Convention) is in the United Kingdom. If a claim for asylum is made by a person, that is to say a claim that it would be contrary to the United Kingdom's obligations for him to be removed from or required to

account of new or previously unrecognized facts[197] before return is effected.[198] It was thus inappropriate for the United Kingdom to persist in the removal of refugee claimants from Zimbabwe, even as its own Foreign Office warned of emerging risks there.

Art. 33 may also be breached when a state creates a legal ruse in order to avoid formal acknowledgment of the arrival of a refugee.[199] For example, the designation by France of part of its territory as an "international zone" in which it exercised authority but assumed no protection responsibility was legally untenable, as was affirmed by the European Court of Human Rights.[200] The same is clearly true of Australia's refusal to consider the refugee status of persons present in islands or other parts of its territory, even if that country's domestic law deems that territory to have been "excised" or otherwise rendered "foreign." All such places – and indeed the

leave the United Kingdom, that person cannot be removed from or required to leave the United Kingdom pending a decision on his claim, and, even if his asylum claim is refused, so long as an appeal is being pursued": *R (Senkoy) v. Secretary of State for the Home Department*, [2001] EWCA Civ 328 (Eng. CA, Mar. 2, 2001), at para. 15.

[197] "The obligation of the United Kingdom under the Convention is not to return a refugee ... to a country where his life or freedom would be threatened for any reason specified in the Convention. That obligation remains binding until the moment of return ... It would in my judgment undermine the beneficial object of the Convention and the measures giving effect to it in this country if the making of an unsuccessful application for asylum were to be treated as modifying the obligation of the United Kingdom or depriving a person of the right to make a fresh claim for asylum ... Any other consideration would in my view be offensive to common sense. However rarely they may arise in practice, it is not hard to imagine cases in which an initial claim for asylum might be made on insubstantial, or even bogus, grounds, and be rightly rejected, but in which circumstances would arise or come to light showing a clear and serious threat of a kind recognised by the Convention ... A scheme of legal protection which could not accommodate that possibility would in my view be seriously defective": *R v. Secretary of State for the Home Department, ex parte Onibiyo*, [1996] QB 768 (Eng. QBD, Mar. 5, 1996), cited with approval in *R v. Secretary of State for the Home Department, ex parte Nassir, The Times* (Dec. 11, 1998) (Eng. CA, Nov. 23, 1998).

[198] In considering a change of rules pursuant to which persons assigned to the UK's "fast track" system would be able to pursue an appeal from outside the country, the Court of Appeal noted that "[i]t is the prospect of removal that is [the refugees'] principal concern. If their fears are well-founded, the fact that they can appeal after they have been returned to the country where they fear persecution is scant consolation": *R (L) v. Secretary of State for the Home Department*, [2003] EWCA Civ 25 (Eng. CA, Jan. 24, 2003), at para. 54.

[199] "As a matter of fact, anyone presenting themselves at a frontier post, port, or airport will already be within State territory and jurisdiction; for this reason, and the better to retain sovereign control, States have devised fictions to keep even the physically present alien technically, legally, unadmitted": Goodwin-Gill, *Refugee in International Law*, at 123.

[200] "The Court notes that even though the applicants were not in France within the meaning of the Ordinance of 2 November 1945, holding them in the international zone of Paris-Orly Airport made them subject to French law. Despite its name, the international zone does not have extraterritorial status": *Amuur v. France*, 1996 ECHR 25 (ECHR, June 25, 1996), at para. 52.

state's territorial sea – are clearly part of its territory.[201] No form of words, and no domestic law, can change that fact. There is thus no international legal difference between opting not to consider the refugee status of persons present in "international zones" or "excised territory" and refusing to consider the refugee status of persons clearly acknowledged to be on the state's territory. Where the refusal to process a refugee claim results, directly or indirectly, in the refugee's removal to face the risk of being persecuted, Art. 33 has been contravened.

Beyond such blunt notions as "excision" and the proclamation of "international zones," *refoulement* may also result from the application of the "first country of arrival" and related rules relied upon by many states to implement the evolving network of so-called "harmonization agreements." These accords constrain the traditional prerogative of refugees to decide where they wish to seek protection.[202] A single state within a group of contracting states is designated as the sole government to which a request for recognition of refugee status may be addressed, whatever the particular circumstances or preferences of the refugee.

Interestingly, the risk inherent in such measures was explicitly considered by the drafters of the Convention. At the Conference of Plenipotentiaries, the Swedish representative introduced a proposal to frame the duty of *non-refoulement* in a way that would "cover cases where refugees were expelled to a country where their life would not be directly threatened, but where they would be threatened by further expulsion to a country where they would be in danger."[203] A consensus evolved in opposition to the proposal, for two basic reasons.

First, states rejected the Swedish initiative because they wanted to remain free to expel refugees to countries in which there was no danger of being persecuted,[204] at least insofar as the state to which removal would be effected

---

[201] See chapter 3.1.2 above, at p. 172.

[202] See e.g. UNHCR Executive Committee Conclusions Nos. 15, "Refugees Without an Asylum Country" (1979), and 58, "Problem of Refugees and Asylum-Seekers Who Move in an Irregular Manner from a Country in Which They Had Already Found Protection" (1989), both available at www.unhcr.ch (accessed Nov. 20, 2004).

[203] Statement of Mr. Petren of Sweden, UN Doc. A/CONF.2/SR.16, July 11, 1951, at 4. Specifically, the proposal was that "[n]o Contracting States shall expel or return a refugee in any manner whatsoever to the frontiers of territories where his life or freedom would be threatened on account of his race, religion, nationality, membership of a particular social group, or political opinion, *or where he would be exposed to the risk of being sent to a territory where his life or freedom would thereby be endangered* [emphasis added]": UN Doc. A/CONF.2/70, July 11, 1951.

[204] "It should, however, be pointed out that the paragraph was concerned with a special case, namely the expulsion or turning back into a territory where the refugee's life or liberty was in danger. The general case was that of expulsion to any country other than that in which the refugee would be threatened": Statement of Mr. Ordonneau of France, UN Doc. E/AC.32/SR.20, Feb. 1, 1950, at 13.

had adhered to the Convention.[205] But second, they felt that the Swedish amendment was not necessary, since "if such expulsion presented a threat of subsequent forcible return to the country of origin, the life and liberty of the refugee in question were endangered" by the removal to the intermediate state. The relevant issue was said to be the *foreseeability* of the ultimate consequences of the initial expulsion.[206] This clear prohibition of indirect *refoulement* has been neatly explained by the House of Lords:

> Suppose it is well-known that country A, although a signatory to the Convention, regularly sends back to its totalitarian and oppressive neighbour, country B, those opponents of the regime in country B who are apprehended in country A following the escape across the border. Against that background, if a person arriving in [a state party] from country A sought asylum as a refugee from country B, assuming he could establish his well-founded fear of persecution there, it would, it seems to me, be as much a breach of Article 33 of the Convention to return him to country A as to country B. The one course would effect indirectly, the other directly, the prohibited result, i.e. his return "to the frontiers of territories where his life or freedom would be threatened."[207]

Taking account of these understandings, application of the so-called "first country of arrival" principle, while not anchored in the requirements of the Refugee Convention,[208] is also not necessarily in breach of it.[209] States declined to assume particularized responsibility for all who arrive at their borders, and insisted that they retain the liberty to send refugees onward to a

---

[205] "The Swedish amendment did not state that it related to countries which did not grant the right of asylum. Such countries were not necessarily those in which persecution occurred. If the States in question were signatories to the Convention, the question would not arise, because refugees would not be returned to countries where they risked being persecuted": Statement of Mr. Rochefort of France, UN Doc. A/CONF.2/SR.16, July 11, 1951, at 10.

[206] Statement of Mr. Larsen of Denmark, ibid. at 9–10. This is consistent with the concern of the French delegation to avoid the imposition of an unduly subjective duty on states: ibid. at 4.

[207] *R v. Secretary of State for the Home Department, ex parte Bugdaycay*, [1987] AC 514 (UK HL, Feb. 19, 1987), per Lord Bridge of Harwich at 532D. This approach has been affirmed in *R v. Secretary of State for the Home Department, ex parte Yogathas*, [2002] UKHL 36 (UK HL, Oct. 17, 2002).

[208] UNHCR, "Summary Conclusions on the Concept of 'Effective Protection' in the Context of Secondary Movements of Refugees and Asylum-Seekers," Lisbon, Dec. 9–10, 2002, at para. 11, available at www.unhcr.ch (accessed Nov. 19, 2004).

[209] As observed in the House of Lords, the Refugee Convention "did not lay down any rules as to which State ought to provide protection": *R v. Secretary of State for the Home Department, ex parte Yogathas*, [2002] UKHL 36 (UK HL, Oct. 17, 2002), per Lord Hope at para. 22.

country in which there is no threat of being persecuted.[210] While UNHCR once took the view that "[t]he intentions of the asylum-seeker as regards the country in which he wishes to request asylum should as far as possible be taken into account,"[211] and most specifically "that asylum should not be refused solely on the ground that it could be sought from another State,"[212] even this institutional position has been softened over the years.[213] Indeed, UNHCR now actively encourages governments to give "consideration ... to the possibility of concluding other multilateral or bilateral Dublin-type agreements," arguing that "[s]uch agreements would serve to enhance predictability, and address concerns regarding unilateral returns."[214]

---

[210] "Article 33(1) cannot ... be read as precluding removal to a 'safe' third country, i.e. one in which there is no danger ... The prohibition of *refoulement* applies only in respect of territories where the refugee or asylum-seeker would be at risk, not more generally. It does, however, require that a State proposing to remove a refugee or asylum-seeker undertake a proper assessment as to whether the third country concerned is indeed safe": Lauterpacht and Bethlehem, "*Non-Refoulement*," at para. 116.

[211] UNHCR Executive Committee Conclusion No. 15, "Refugees Without an Asylum Country" (1979), at para. (h)(iii), available at www.unhcr.ch (accessed Nov. 20, 2004).

[212] Ibid. at para. (h)(iv).

[213] See UNHCR Executive Committee Conclusion No. 58, "Problem of Refugees and Asylum-Seekers Who Move in an Irregular Manner from a Country in Which They Have Already Found Protection" (1989), available at www.unhcr.ch (accessed Nov. 20, 2004), making an exception to the general right of refugees to choose where to seek protection where they have already found protection in some other state; UNHCR Executive Committee Conclusion No. 71, "General Conclusion on International Protection" (1993), available at www.unhcr.ch (accessed Nov. 20, 2004), acknowledging the value of designated states of protection where needed to avoid "refugee in orbit" situations; and, in particular, UNHCR Executive Committee Conclusion No. 74, "General Conclusion on International Protection" (1994), at para. (p), available at www.unhcr.ch (accessed Nov. 20, 2004), which "[a]cknowledges the value of regional harmonization of national policies to ensure that persons who are in need of international protection actually receive it."

[214] UNHCR, "Asylum Processes," at para. 18. There is reason to believe, however, that there is a less-than-unanimous consensus favoring this shift. The conclusions of one of UNHCR's Global Consultations expert roundtables, for example, posit that "[t]here is no obligation under international law for a person to seek international protection at the first effective opportunity. On the other hand, asylum-seekers and refugees do not have an unfettered right to choose the country that will determine their asylum claim in substance and provide asylum. Their intentions, however, ought to be taken into account": UNHCR, "Summary Conclusions on the Concept of 'Effective Protection' in the Context of Secondary Movements of Refugees and Asylum-Seekers," Dec. 10, 2002, at para. 11. This Conclusion cites UNHCR Executive Committee Conclusion No. 15, ibid., in support; it makes no reference to UNHCR Executive Committee Conclusions Nos. 58, "Problem of Refugees and Asylum-Seekers Who Move in an Irregular Manner from a Country in Which They Have Already Found Protection" (1989); 71, "General Conclusion on International Protection" (1993); or 74, "General Conclusion on International Protection" (1994), all available at www.unhcr.ch (accessed Nov. 20, 2004).

The concern, however, is that the consonance of collectivized protection regimes and the duty of *non-refoulement* set by Art. 33 can too easily be compromised by risks arising from the relatively mechanical way in which shared responsibility tends to be implemented.[215] Since the accords drafted to date authorize the removal of a refugee simply because he or she is admissible to a partner state, governments tend not to inquire whether indirect *refoulement* is a foreseeable risk of sending the refugee to the designated state (as the drafters assumed they would). While Art. 33 does not require a state to guarantee a refugee's well-being before expelling him to a non-persecutory country, neither does it authorize wilful blindness in the face of a readily ascertainable risk of subsequent *refoulement*. As the Supreme Court of Canada has affirmed,

> At least where Canada's participation is a necessary precondition for the deprivation, and where the deprivation is an entirely foreseeable consequence of Canada's participation, the government does not avoid [responsibility] because the deprivation in question would be effected by someone else's hand ... [W]e cannot pretend that Canada is merely a passive participant.[216]

Courts have become increasingly attentive to the risks inherent in shared responsibility systems predicated on the "first country of arrival" rule. While they have taken the view that governments may legitimately begin from the position that partner states will carry out their responsibilities in good faith,[217] this prerogative is balanced against the clear duty of the sending state to refuse removal where there is a "real risk"[218] that the partner state will not itself grant protection where warranted. This might be because there is a risk of being persecuted in the partner state itself. More commonly, the sending state would breach Art. 33 if there is a real chance that the partner state may remove the refugee claimant to another state in which the risk of *refoulement* exists. In these circumstances, there can be no question of the first state avoiding responsibility for a breach of Art. 33 simply because it does not itself directly effect the removal to the place of risk:

[215] See e.g. E. Guild, "Asylum and refugees in the EU: A practitioner's view of developments," *European Information Service* (Dec. 2000), at 215, cited with approval by Lord Hope in *R v. Secretary of State for the Home Department, ex parte Yogathas*, [2002] UKHL 36 (UK HL, Oct. 17, 2002).

[216] *Suresh v. Canada*, [2002] 1 SCR 3 (Can. SC, Jan. 11, 2002). While the focus of the court's analysis here was the indirect breach of the domestic duty to guarantee fundamental justice, the analysis is helpful in understanding a broader range of indirect risks initiated by the sending away of an individual from a state's territory.

[217] "[T]he Home Secretary and the courts should not readily infer that a friendly sovereign state which is a party to the Geneva Convention will not perform the obligations it has solemnly undertaken": *R v. Secretary of State for the Home Department, ex parte Yogathas*, [2002] UKHL 36 (UK HL, Oct. 17, 2002).

[218] Ibid.

[F]or a country to return a refugee to a state from which he will then be returned by the government of that state to a territory where his life or freedom will be threatened will be as much a breach of Article 33 as if the first country had itself returned him there direct. This is the effect of Article 33.[219]

Third, there is also a risk of *refoulement* arising from application of the "first country of arrival" rule where there is reason to believe that the laws or practices of the partner state cannot be relied upon accurately to recognize the refugee status of persons who are in fact Convention refugees. Thus, the House of Lords disallowed automatic reliance on the Dublin Convention's "first country of arrival" rule to remove refugees fleeing non-state agents of persecution to France and Germany, reasoning that the understanding of the refugee definition then embraced in those two states (which excluded such cases) did not meet the requirements of international law.[220] While minor differences of interpretation are not such as to give rise to the risk of indirect *refoulement*,[221] state parties are bound – precisely in line with the intentions of the Convention's drafters – to engage in a "rigorous examination" of the laws and practices of the proposed destination state, with "anxious scrutiny" of their duty of *non-refoulement*.[222] If it is known (or could reasonably become known) that the status determination procedure or understanding of the Convention refugee definition in the "country of first arrival" or other designated state is deficient – in consequence of which there is a real chance of eventual *refoulement* – it follows that sending a refugee to that country is a breach of the duty to avoid the *refoulement* of a refugee "in any manner whatsoever." This duty cannot be avoided simply by asserting the existence of a responsibility-sharing agreement or the fact that the destination state is itself bound to honor duties under the Refugee Convention, as was made clear by the European Court of Human Rights:

Nor can [a state] rely automatically ... on the arrangement made in the Dublin Convention concerning attribution of responsibility between

---

[219] *R v. Secretary of State for the Home Department, ex parte Adan and Aitseguer*, [2001] 2 WLR 143 (UK HL, Dec. 19, 2000), per Lord Hobhouse.

[220] "[T]he enquiry must be into the meaning of the Refugee Convention approached as an international instrument created by the agreement of contracting states as opposed to regulatory regimes established by national institutions. It is necessary to determine the autonomous meaning of the relevant treaty provision": ibid., per Lord Steyn.

[221] Lord Bingham noted that only "significant differences" of interpretation would make removal unlawful because of the importance of what he defined as "the humane objective of the Convention ... to establish an orderly and internationally agreed regime for handling asylum applications": *R v. Secretary of State for the Home Department, ex parte Yogathas*, [2002] UKHL 36 (UK HL, Oct. 17, 2002).

[222] Ibid., per Lord Hutton at para. 74; and at para. 58 per Lord Hope, citing to the holding of Lord Bridge of Harwich in *R v. Secretary of State for the Home Department, ex parte Bugdaycay*, [1987] AC 514 (UK HL, Feb. 19, 1987).

European countries for deciding asylum claims. Where states establish international organizations, or *mutatis mutandis* international agreements, to pursue cooperation in certain fields of activities, there may be implications for the protection of fundamental rights. It would be incompatible with the purpose and object of the Convention if contracting states were thereby absolved from their responsibility under the Convention . . .

The Court notes the comments of the UNHCR that, while the Dublin Convention may pursue laudable objectives, its effectiveness may be undermined in practice by the differing approaches adopted by Contracting States to the scope of protection offered.[223]

Thus, for example, Canada may not lawfully force all refugees back to the United States under its harmonization agreement with that country. At least in the cases of refugees who will not be protected from *refoulement* under US law because they are deemed "only" to satisfy the refugee definition set by Art. 1, and not the "higher standard" of Art. 33; of refugees who will be excluded from protection under American laws that do not comport with Art. 1(F) or Art. 33(2) of the Convention; or of refugees who face the risk of being persecuted for a Convention reason, even if not motivated by explicit intent (which cases are rejected under US law), return to the United States would be an act of indirect *refoulement* by Canada.[224]

Even more caution is required, however, when one moves beyond simple "first country of arrival" rules to consider the broader range of returns to a "safe third country." This includes, for example, the European Union regime which allows even the "first country of arrival" or other designated state to send the applicant away to any country through which he or she has passed, so long as that country will consider the applicant's refugee claim and avoid persecution, torture or related treatment, and *refoulement*. The Australian unilateral variant is even more aggressive, since it allows an applicant to be removed whether or not the destination country will actually consider the claim to refugee protection.

The "safe third country" notion thus raises at least three important questions. First, can return be lawfully effected to a state party which is not itself a party to the Refugee Convention? Neither the European Union nor Australian approach makes this a condition precedent to application of the norm. Second and related,

---

[223] *TI v. United Kingdom*, [2000] INLR 211 (ECHR, Mar. 7, 2000). See also *R v. Secretary of State for the Home Department, ex parte Yogathas*, [2002] UKHL 36 (UK HL, Oct. 17, 2002), per Lord Hutton, observing that the duty under Art. 33 to avoid the risk of indirect return to the risk of being persecuted "is applicable . . . notwithstanding that the person is removed from the United Kingdom to another country pursuant to the arrangements made in the Dublin Convention concerning the attribution of responsibility between European countries for deciding asylum claims."

[224] The risks inherent in this collectivized system are described in J. Hathaway and A. Neve, "Fundamental Justice and the Deflection of Refugees from Canada," (1997) 34(2) *Osgoode Hall Law Journal* 213.

is it enough that the destination state will not itself persecute the refugee (or subject him or her to related ill-treatment) or engage in *refoulement*? None of the "safe third country" rules now in place requires the destination state to respect even the rights of all refugees as established by the Convention itself, including for example to freedom of internal movement, to freedom of thought and conscience, or even to have access to the necessities of life. Third, can governments make blanket determinations of safety without examination of individuated circumstances, as is the case under the European Union's "super safe third country" notion and its rule excluding nearly all nationals of member states from eligibility for refugee status?

On the first question, it will be recalled that one of the reasons the drafters rejected the Swedish proposal expressly to address the question of indirect *refoulement* in the text of Art. 33 was a belief that *state parties to the Convention* should be free to share out the duty to protect refugees. For example, the French representative observed that "[t]he Swedish amendment did not state that it related to countries which did not grant the right of asylum ... If the States in question were signatories to the Convention, the question would not arise, because refugees would not be returned to countries where they risked being persecuted."[225] The assumption, then, was that whatever allocation of responsibility might occur would be as among countries all bound by international refugee law, and would lead to full protection of refugee rights in the destination country.

Despite the contrary assumptions of the Convention's drafters, courts have not found fault with rules (such as those applied in Australia and the European Union) that transfer responsibility for protection to countries which are outside the international refugee law regime. The Australian Full Federal Court has, for example, flatly stated that "it is not necessary to show that ... the third country is a party to the Convention."[226] Indeed, courts have at times suggested that little weight should be placed on whether a country is bound by international refugee law or not:

> [T]here can be a real chance of lack of effective protection notwithstanding that the third country in question is also a party to the Convention ... It is a sad reality of modern times that countries do not always honour human rights, whether enshrined in domestic constitutions or in international treaties to which they are parties. To treat the fact of a country being party to the Convention as conclusive would be a distortion of the Convention's language and subversive of its underlying purpose ...
> As a matter of fact, [refugees] may have better effective protection in

---

[225] Statement of Mr. Rochefort of France, UN Doc. A/CONF.2/SR.16, July 11, 1951, at 10. See text above, at pp. 322–323.

[226] *S115/00A v. Minister for Immigration and Multicultural Affairs*, [2001] FCA 540 (Aus. FFC, May 10, 2001).

some countries which are not parties to the Convention ... than in many which are.[227]

This understanding is closely connected to the approach taken by courts to the second question of just what is meant by "effective protection" in the destination state. Despite the fact that refugees under the Convention are entitled immediately to receive a small number of core rights,[228] and to benefit over time from the full range of rights set by Arts. 2–34 of the Refugee Convention,[229] judicial commentary on qualification as a "safe third country" has thus far been fairly strictly limited to determining whether the "safe third country" will respect the duty of *non-refoulement*, referred to by one court as "the engine room of the Convention."[230] The House of Lords, for example, has observed that

> [T]he Convention is directed to a very important but very simple and very practical end, preventing the return of applicants to places where they will or may suffer persecution. Legal niceties and refinements should not be allowed to obstruct that purpose. It can never, save in extreme circumstances, be appropriate to compare an applicant's living conditions in different countries if, in each of them, he will be safe from persecution or the risk of it.[231]

Because of the narrowness of the inquiry as presently conceived, it is perhaps unsurprising that courts do not insist on an inquiry into an individual's refugee status before he or she is returned to a "safe third country": where there is no risk of being persecuted there, or forced out of that state, "the question of whether a person has refugee status is simply irrelevant."[232]

---

[227] *Minister for Immigration and Multicultural Affairs v. Al-Sallal*, Dec. No. BC9907140 (Aus. FFC, Oct. 29, 1999). Yet the court ultimately concludes that "[t]he question whether [the destination state] is a party to the Convention is relevant, but not determinative either way": ibid. See *Rajendran v. Minister for Immigration and Multicultural Affairs*, (1998) 166 ALR 619 (Aus. FFC, Sept. 4, 1998), in which the court approved of the fact that the trial judge "advert[ed] to the responsibility [the destination state] had as a signatory to the Convention, and to assume that it would honour its obligations thereunder including its Article 33 obligation."

[228] See chapters 3.1.1 and 3.1.2 above.   [229] See chapter 3.1 above, at pp. 156–157.

[230] *Minister for Immigration and Multicultural Affairs v. Al-Sallal*, Dec. No. BC9907140 (Aus. FFC, Oct. 29, 1999).

[231] *R v. Secretary of State for the Home Department, ex parte Yogathas*, [2002] UKHL 36 (UK HL, Oct. 17, 2002).

[232] *Nguyen Tuan Cuong v. Director of Immigration*, [1997] 1 WLR 68 (HK PC, Nov. 21, 1996), cited with approval in *Odhiambo v. Minister for Immigration and Multicultural Affairs*, [2002] FCAFC 194 (Aus. FFC, June 20, 2002). See also *Minister for Immigration and Multicultural Affairs v. Applicant "C,"* [2001] FCA 1332 (Aus. FFC, Sept. 18, 2001): "The decision maker is not required ... to decide if the applicant is a refugee before addressing the question of effective protection in a third country."

The nature of the inquiry into the risk of *refoulement* is moreover routinely said to be fundamentally pragmatic:

> [T]he focus ... is on the end result rather than the precise procedures by which the result was achieved. The question is whether the government of the third country "would not" send the person to another country or territory otherwise than in accordance with the Geneva Convention. The concern is essentially a practical one rather than one which is theoretical.[233]

In line with this purely practical orientation, courts have insisted that there be a clear ability lawfully to enter the destination state[234] – not just "a practical capacity to bring about a lawful permission to enter and reside legally in the relevant country."[235] But there is generally no inquiry into the quality of protection available there.[236]

---

[233] *R v. Secretary of State for the Home Department, ex parte Yogathas*, [2002] UKHL 36 (UK HL, Oct. 17, 2002), per Lord Hope.

[234] This requirement may be satisfied "if the person has a legally enforceable right to enter that territory ... Likewise, if the person in fact is permitted to enter, then the principle of international comity, whether or not actually infringed, is not material and could be taken to be waived at least once entry is permitted. When these matters are put together with Article 33, it can be concluded that Australia would have no protection obligations where the safe third country consents to admit the refugee, where the refugee has a legally enforceable right to enter the safe third country, or where as a matter of fact the safe third country ... admits the refugee": *V872/00A v. Minister for Immigration and Multicultural Affairs*, [2002] FCAFC 185 (Aus. FFC, June 18, 2002). But "the Tribunal must consider whether it is satisfied that the third country will permit entry so that the applicant will not be left at the border and denied admission. In deciding whether it is satisfied the Tribunal will take into account the important matters of international obligation and comity ... as well as the significance of the decision to the individual whose life or liberty may be at risk. Where there is doubt, that doubt should be resolved in favour of the applicant": ibid. For example, the court observed in *Tharmalingam v. Minister for Immigration and Multicultural Affairs*, Dec. No. BC9905456 (Aus. FFC, Aug. 26, 1999) that "the material in the present case does indicate that the appellant now faces a risk of *refoulement* to Sri Lanka because he can apparently no longer return to France as of right."

[235] *Minister for Immigration and Multicultural Affairs v. Applicant "C,"* [2001] FCA 1332 (Aus. FFC, Sept. 18, 2001).

[236] There is even a lack of clarity regarding just how durable the right to remain in the destination state must be. In early decisions, Australian courts treated a right of residence as a requirement: *Tharmalingam v. Minister for Immigration and Multicultural Affairs*, Dec. No. BC9905456 (Aus. FFC, Aug. 26, 1999), citing to the leading precedent of *Minister for Immigration and Multicultural Affairs v. Thiyagarajah*, (1997) 80 FCR 543 (Aus. FFC, Dec. 19, 1997). But in *S115/00A v. Minister for Immigration and Multicultural Affairs*, [2001] FCA 540 (Aus. FFC, May 10, 2001), the court rejected the notion that a right of residence was required. Indeed, the Australian Full Federal Court determined that not even the risk of summary ejection from Syria for commission of a minor criminal offence would compromise that country's status as a "safe third country" for Iraqi refugees. "[A]ny chance that he would commit a criminal offense or become a security risk on return [to Syria] was both remote and insubstantial. There was therefore no real

Assuming the same concerns previously identified with regard to application of the "first country of arrival" principle – that is, that account is taken of the real risk of direct persecution and of *refoulement*, whether by intent or as the result of laws or practices which are insufficient accurately to identify genuine refugees[237] – there is little doubt that the very practical way in which "safe third country" inquiries are conceived by courts can adequately guard against the breach of Art. 33 itself, even if the refugee applicants are being sent to a state which is not formally bound by international refugee law. But the narrowness of the inquiry posited nonetheless raises a fundamental concern. Even if the state of destination will neither persecute a refugee nor send him or her elsewhere, it may nonetheless be the case that sending a refugee to a "safe third country" will result in a divestiture of Convention rights.

Under Australia's "Pacific Solution," for example, refugees removed from Australia to Nauru – which is not a party to the Refugee Convention – effectively lost the rights which they had acquired by virtue of their former presence in areas under the jurisdiction of (and subsequently, within the territory of) Australia,[238] a state party to the Convention.[239] This is a very practical concern, as the *Tampa* refugees admitted to Nauru were in fact denied the right to engage in any constructive work, remunerated or not, and were forced to live in a fenced compound under constant guard.[240] More generally, whatever protection they enjoyed de facto in Nauru was entirely vulnerable to the exercise of political discretion in a way that would not be true in a state party to the Convention.

The concern may be succinctly framed as focused on the deprivation of acquired rights. First, because the decision about whether a destination country is "safe" generally takes account of no refugee rights other than Art. 33, reliance on the "safe third country" rule as now adumbrated can

---

chance that the appellant would face deportation for either reason": *Al Toubi v. Minister for Immigration and Multicultural Affairs*, [2001] FCA 1381 (Aus. FFC, Sept. 28, 2001).

[237] See text above, at pp. 325–327.

[238] These refugees were entitled to protection against discrimination (Art. 3); to religious freedom (Art. 4); to respect for their property rights (Art. 13); to access to the courts (Art. 16(1)); to the benefit of rationing systems (Art. 20); to basic education (Art. 22); to receive identity papers (Art. 27); to equal treatment under tax laws (Art. 29); to protection against penalization for illegal entry or presence (Art. 31(1)); to be subject only to such restrictions on internal movement as are shown to be necessary, and only pending regularization of their status in the host state (Art. 31(2)); to protection against *refoulement* (Art. 33); and to be considered by the state for naturalization (Art. 34): Refugee Convention. See chapters 3.1.1 and 3.1.2 above.

[239] Moreover, if rather than being sent to Nauru the refugees had been allowed to remain in Australia for a period of "temporary" protection (even if denied access to the formal status determination procedure), they would thereby have gone on to acquire additional rights under the Refugee Convention, namely to engage in self-employment, to enjoy a broader right of internal freedom of movement, and to be protected against expulsion. See chapter 3.1.3 above.

[240] P. Barkham, "Paradise lost awaits asylum-seekers," *Guardian*, Sept. 11, 2001, at 3.

lead to a situation where refugees are routinely denied access to the very rights which the Convention was designed to ensure. Second, because the "safe third country" designation is not limited to countries which are parties to the Convention or Protocol, forcing refugees to go to such a state may amount, in practice, to a deprivation of a remedy for denial of whatever rights are in fact provided there. Rather than being treated as rights holders in line with Convention norms, refugees become little more than the objects of discretion. Yet because most refugees subject to "safe third country" removal have, in fact, already come under the jurisdiction of a state party and hence acquired at least a number of core rights, including to access a remedy for breach of their rights,[241] the deprivation is both real and important.

One answer is that the flexibility which inheres in states by virtue of the limited applicability of Art. 32 of the Convention[242] suggests that there is no clear legal basis to contest this deprivation of rights. At least when refugees are removed under "safe third country" rules *before* they become lawfully present on a state's territory (including in its territorial waters), sending them onward to a non-state party is within the bounds of the Refugee Convention so long as there is no foreseeable risk of direct or indirect *refoulement*. On the other hand, this technically plausible approach is extremely difficult to reconcile to the context, object, and purpose of the Refugee Convention itself – clearly a critical consideration in arriving at an authentic understanding of the duty of *non-refoulement*.[243] Specifically, while the drafters did not conceive Art. 33 as tantamount to a duty to grant asylum, they did opt to extend the personal scope of Art. 33 to include refugees not pre-authorized to come to their territory[244] and more generally to grant a number of basic Convention rights even before an individual is admitted to a refugee status determination procedure.[245] Perhaps most fundamentally, the Refugee Convention is not simply a treaty by which states obligate themselves to avoid *refoulement*: its scope is much broader than that, in line with the purpose set out in its Preamble of "revis[ing] and consolidat[ing] previous international agreements relating to the status of refugees and to extend the scope of and the protection accorded by such instruments by means of a new agreement" in order to "assure refugees the widest possible exercise of [their] fundamental rights and freedoms."[246] Could an interpretation of Art. 33 which effectively nullifies the ability of refugees to claim all but one of their Convention rights possibly be consistent with these clear intentions?

On balance, it is suggested here that a fair interpretation of Art. 33 would condition the right of states to remove refugees on a determination that "effective protection" worthy of the name is in fact available in the destination

---

[241] See chapter 4.10 below.   [242] See chapter 5.1 below.   [243] See chapter 1.3.3 above.
[244] See chapter 4.1.1 above, at pp. 302–303.   [245] See chapters 3.1.1 and 3.1.2 above.
[246] Refugee Convention, at Preamble, paras. 2–3.

country. Ideally, this would mean that the refugee is being sent to a state that is a party to the Refugee Convention or Protocol, and which would in fact assess his or her status and honor all relevant Convention and other rights. But not even a carefully contextualized reading of the Convention can honestly be said to require this much. On the other hand, it seems reasonable to insist that, at a minimum, a country be deemed a "safe third country" only if it will respect in practice whatever Convention rights the refugee has already acquired by virtue of having come under the jurisdiction[247] or entered the territory[248] of a state party to the Refugee Convention, as well as any other international legal rights thereby acquired; and further that there be a judicial or comparable mechanism in place to enable the refugee to insist upon real accountability by the host state to implement those rights.[249]

Under such an understanding of the "safe third country" principle, states would continue to enjoy the freedom to share out responsibility for refugee protection, including with countries that are not yet formally bound by refugee law. But they would not be able to do so in ways that are less a sharing of the responsibility to protect than an effort to deter the search for the protection to which refugees are entitled. Refugees would not be stripped of the rights which they have already acquired, even though they may have to be exercised in a country not of their choosing. This approach respects the admonition of courts that the focus of analysis should be practical and result-oriented, yet does not allow refugees to be warehoused in conditions at odds with the basic standards agreed to in the Convention. Not only is it an appropriate litmus test for particularized application of "safe third country" rules, but it sets a principled, yet practical, baseline standard for the lawful implementation of a more collectivized protection system along the general lines of those proposed by the United Kingdom, UNHCR, and the Intergovernmental Consultations.

A final *non-entrée* mechanism which must be considered is the designation of whole countries as "safe countries of origin" – essentially signaling that persons from such states are to be assumed not to be Convention refugees. In principle, this approach conflicts with the highly individuated focus required by the Convention: even if nearly all persons from a given country cannot qualify for refugee status, this fact ought not to impede recognition of refugee status to the small minority who are in fact Convention refugees. An

---

[247] See chapter 3.1.1 above.   [248] See chapter 3.1.2 above.

[249] The UN Human Rights Committee has insisted that a state party must "maintain its practice and tradition of observance of the principle of non-refoulement. When a State party expels a person to another State on the basis of assurances as to that person's treatment by the receiving State, it must institute credible mechanisms for ensuring compliance by the receiving State with these assurances from the moment of expulsion": UN Human Rights Committee, "Concluding Observations: Sweden," UN Doc. A/57/40, vol. I (2002) 57, at para. 79(12)(b).

assessment of the legality of designating "safe countries of origin" therefore hinges on whether it can dependably ensure the protection of genuine refugees coming from those states.

Most clearly, there can be no question of automatically refusing all claims from any country: an approach of this kind will inevitably force away at least some refugees.[250] Nor is it an answer to this concern to suggest that only countries which adhere to the Refugee Convention or other human rights instruments will be designated as "safe countries of origin." Sadly, even countries considered model democracies and defenders of human rights have generated – at some times, and in some circumstances – persons who are in fact Convention refugees.[251] At least where the "safe country of origin" notion is treated as a firm bar to substantive consideration of a claim to refugee status – as is effectively the case under the European Union's "super safe country" rules, and its bar on the reception of refugee claims from European Union citizens – states will not be in a position to honor their duties under Art. 33.

More commonly, however, designation of a country of origin as "safe" operates not as a bar on seeking protection as such, but rather as a procedural device which requires an applicant to establish his or her refugee status under an accelerated or otherwise truncated procedure, often with the requirement to rebut a presumption against recognition of refugee status.[252] In a particularly helpful judgment, the English Court of Appeal has insisted that such a procedure can be operated without breach of the duty of *non-refoulement* so long as it delivers a "fair hearing," including access to legal counsel.[253] The procedure may begin from a presumption of safety in the country of origin,

---

[250] UNHCR takes an equivocal position on the legality of designating whole countries of origin as presumptively safe, noting without comment that "[s]ome states have drawn up extensive lists of such countries, sometimes applying them as an automatic bar to access to the asylum procedures": UNHCR, "Asylum Processes," at para. 38. The agency seems to be willing to tolerate such an approach so long as care is taken in drawing up the list of "safe countries of origin." UNHCR refers to the need to give attention to individuated concerns as "best state practice," rather than a clear duty: ibid. at para. 39.

[251] For example, in *Roszkowski v. Special Adjudicator*, [2001] EWCA Civ 650 (Eng. CA, May 9, 2001), the court did not question the designation of Poland as a safe country of origin despite the fact that the Special Adjudicator had accepted that the Polish Roma applicants had experienced not only demands for money and beatings, but had been subjected to attacks by anti-Roma vigilantes on their apartment – including physical assaults – on three separate occasions.

[252] UNHCR offers some support for this approach, suggesting that "a proper designation of a country as a 'safe country of origin' does not, by that fact alone, serve as a declaration of cessation of refugee status in regard to refugees from that country. It should serve merely as a procedural tool to expedite processing of refugee claims": UNHCR, "Note on the Cessation Clauses," UN Doc. EC/47/SC/CRP.30 (1997) (UNHCR, "Cessation"), at para. 7.

[253] *R (L) v. Secretary of State for the Home Department*, [2003] EWCA Civ 25 (Eng. CA, Jan. 24, 2003), at paras. 30, 38.

but must give "careful consideration to the facts of the individual case."[254] Thus, it must be possible, for example, for an applicant to adduce expert medical evidence where relevant.[255] Perhaps most critically, where it becomes clear that credibility is at the heart of the case, refugee status should not ordinarily be refused without access to a more traditional refugee status inquiry.[256]

Yet even if procedural safeguards of this kind avert most risks of a breach of the duty of *non-refoulement*, there is surely still a principled objection to deeming countries in which real risks of persecution exist to be "safe countries of origin." For example, the decision of the United Kingdom to designate Pakistan as presumptively safe was characterized by a reviewing court as simply "irrational" in view of the continuing recognition of significant numbers of Pakistanis as genuine refugees and, particularly, taking account of that country's fundamental disfranchisement of its Ahmadi minority.[257] As UNHCR has suggested, account needs to be taken "not simply of international instruments ratified and relevant legislation enacted there, but also of the actual degree of respect for human rights and the rule of law, of the country's record of not producing refugees, of its compliance with human rights instruments, and of its accessibility to national or international organizations for the purpose of verifying human rights issues."[258]

4.1.3 *Extraterritorial* refoulement

Analysis to this point has focused on the implications of *non-refoulement* for refugees at a state's borders or within its territory. Increasingly, however, states are inclined to take action in areas beyond their own territory (including beyond their territorial sea) with a view to forcing refugees back to their place of origin, or at least towards some other state. The operation of interception and related strategies may in fact result in refugees being denied protection. But because these deterrent measures are premised on denial to the refugee of any direct contact with a receiving state, the question arises whether a state party which engages in arms-length actions that lead ultimately to refugees being forced back to their country of origin has breached the duty of *non-refoulement*.

---

[254] Ibid. at para. 45.   [255] Ibid. at para. 49.

[256] "Where an applicant's case does turn on an issue of credibility, the fact that the interviewer does not believe the applicant will not, of itself, justify a finding that the claim is clearly unfounded. In many immigration cases, findings on credibility have been reversed on appeal. Only where the interviewing officer is satisfied that nobody could believe the applicant's story will it be appropriate to certify the claim as clearly unfounded on the ground of lack of credibility alone": ibid. at para. 60.

[257] *R v. Secretary of State for the Home Department, ex parte Javed*, [2001] EWCA Civ 789 (Eng. CA, May 17, 2001).

[258] UNHCR, "Asylum Processes," at para. 39.

The arguments against seeing such actions as contrary to Art. 33 were accepted by the majority of the Supreme Court of the United States in the decision of *Sale v. Haitian Centers Council*,[259] a challenge to the American policy of interdicting Haitians in search of protection in international waters, and returning them to Haiti. The Court observed that "the text and negotiating history of Article 33 . . . are both completely silent with respect to the Article's possible application to actions taken by a country outside its own borders."[260] Moreover, it was noted that the original continental European understanding of *refoulement* – which spoke to rejections which occurred at, or from within, a state's borders – was in line with the textual reference in Art. 33 to the duty to avoid "return," said by the Court to denote "a defensive act of resistance or exclusion at a border rather than an act of transporting someone to [their home state, or some other country] . . . In the context of the Convention, to 'return' means to 'repulse' rather than to 'reinstate.'"[261] Indeed, it was determined by the Court that only a territory-based understanding would allow the primary duty set by Art. 33(1) to be read in consonance with the right of states under Art. 33(2) to deny protection against *refoulement* to persons who pose a danger to the security "of the country *in which he is* [emphasis added]." In the view of the American Supreme Court, reading Art. 33(1) to apply to extraterritorial deterrence "would create an absurd anomaly: dangerous aliens on the high seas would be entitled to the benefits of Art. 33(1) while those residing in the country that sought to expel them would not. It seems more reasonable to assume that the coverage of Art. 33(2) was limited to those already in the country because it was understood that Art. 33(1) obligated the signatory states only with respect to aliens within its territory."[262] Thus, the prohibition against *refoulement* was determined to accrue to the benefit only of persons "on the threshold of initial entry."[263]

These arguments have little substance. Perhaps most spurious is the construction of Art. 33(1) based on the need for consistency with Art. 33(2). Since a refugee can be ejected on national security grounds only where his or her presence or actions give rise to an objectively reasonable, real possibility of directly or indirectly inflicted substantial harm to the host state's most basic interests, including the risk of an armed attack on its territory or its citizens, or the destruction of its democratic institutions,[264] it is difficult to conceive of a situation in which a refugee not yet at or within a state's territory could be subject to such exclusion. It is thus perfectly logical that this very limited prerogative to avoid the fundamental duty of *non-refoulement* would be textually constrained

---

[259] *Sale, Acting Commissioner, Immigration and Naturalization Service, et al., Petitioners v. Haitian Centers Council, Inc., et al.*, 509 US 155 (US SC, Jan. 12, 1993).
[260] Ibid. at 178.   [261] Ibid. at 182.   [262] Ibid. at 180.   [263] Ibid. at 187.
[264] See chapter 4.1.4 below, at pp. 345–346.

to situations in which a clear and critical risk could, in fact, arise. As Justice Blackmun noted in his dissenting opinion in *Sale*, "[t]he tautological observation that only a refugee already in a country can pose a danger to the country 'in which he is' proves nothing."[265]

Second, the fact that the drafters assumed that *refoulement* was likely to occur at, or from within, a state's borders – and therefore did not expressly proscribe extraterritorial acts which lead to a refugee's return to be persecuted – simply reflects the empirical reality that when the Convention was drafted, no country had ever attempted to deter refugees other than from within, or at, its own borders. As the American representative to the Ad Hoc Committee that prepared the Refugee Convention observed in the aftermath of the *Sale* decision, "[i]t is incredible that states that had agreed not to force any human being back into the hands of his/her oppressors intended to leave themselves – and each other – free to reach out beyond their territory to seize a refugee and to return him/her to the country from which he sought to escape."[266] There is simply no basis whatever to maintain that the drafters envisaged, let alone would have sanctioned, interdiction and return as practiced on the high seas by the United States. There was certainly no historical precedent of a policy of proactive deterrence, encompassing affirmative actions intended specifically to take jurisdiction over refugees (such as forcing them onto US ships and destroying their boats), without a concomitant assumption of responsibility.

This leaves us with the Court's fairly basic literal proposition that because a state cannot "expel or return" someone who has yet to arrive at its territory, the duty to avoid "return" speaks only to "a defensive act of resistance or exclusion at a border," and not to the act of actually sending them home. Of all of the Court's arguments, this is perhaps the most disingenuous. Not only does the word "return" not have the plain meaning attributed to it,[267] but a construction which excludes actions that would actually deliver a refugee back to his or her persecutors – rather than simply resisting or excluding

---

[265] *Sale, Acting Commissioner, Immigration and Naturalization Service, et al., Petitioners v. Haitian Centers Council, Inc., et al.*, 509 US 155 (US SC, Jan. 12, 1993), at 194.

[266] L. Henkin, "Notes from the President," [1993] 5 *American Society of International Law Newsletter* 1.

[267] The definition of "return" is to "come or go back ... [to] bring, put, or send back to the ... place ... where originally belonging": *Concise Oxford Dictionary*, 9th edn (1995), at 1178. Moreover, as UNHCR argued before the Supreme Court, "the definition of '*refouler*' upon which the government relies to render the term 'return' ambiguous simultaneously renders it redundant. Under [the US government's] reading, the phrase 'expel or return' is transformed into 'expel or expel'": UNHCR, "Brief as *Amicus Curiae*," filed Dec. 21, 1992 in *McNary v. Haitian Centers Council Inc.*, Case No. 92–344, at 10 (*Sale v. Haitian Centers Council*, 509 US 155 (US SC, June 21, 1993)), reprinted in (1994) 6(1) *International Journal of Refugee Law* 85.

them – is in fact the plainest and most obvious breach of the duty conceived by the drafters, namely to prohibit measures which would cause refugees to be "pushed back into the arms of their persecutors."[268]

More generally, the US Supreme Court's approach takes no account of the previously noted decision of the drafters to amend Art. 33 in order to stipulate that the duty of *non-refoulement* prohibits return to the risk of being persecuted "in any manner whatsoever,"[269] said to "refer to various methods by which refugees could be expelled, refused admittance or removed."[270] Much less does it give any consideration to the fact that the essential purpose of the Refugee Convention is to provide rights to seriously at-risk persons able to escape from their own countries – a goal which would clearly be fundamentally undermined by an approach to Art. 33 which effectively authorized governments to deny them all rights by forcing them back home, so long as the repulsion occurred before the refugees reached a state party's territory.[271] Equally important is the policy concern expressed by the UNHCR in its *amicus curiae* brief filed in the *Sale* case:

> [The US government's] interpretation of Article 33 ... extinguishes the most basic right enshrined in the treaty – the right of non-return – for an entire class of refugees, those who have fled their own countries but have not yet entered the territory of another State. Under [the US government's] reading, the availability of the most fundamental protection afforded refugees turns not on the refugee's need for protection, but on his or her own ability to enter clandestinely the territory of another country.[272]

---

[268] Statement of the Chairman, Mr. Chance of Canada, UN Doc. E/AC.32/SR.21, Feb. 2, 1950, at 7. It is also an interpretation fundamentally at odds with the most central goal of the Refugee Convention itself, namely "to assure refugees the widest possible exercise of ... fundamental rights and freedoms": Refugee Convention, at Preamble, para. 2.

[269] See chapter 4.1.2 above, at pp. 316–317.

[270] Statement of Mr. Cuvelier of Belgium, UN Doc. E/AC.32/SR.22, Feb. 2, 1950, at 20.

[271] See UNHCR, "Interception," at para. 23: "The principle of *non-refoulement* does not imply any geographical limitation. In UNHCR's understanding, the resulting obligations extend to all government agents acting in an official capacity, within or outside national territory. Given the practice of States to intercept persons at great distance from their own territory, the international refugee protection regime would be rendered ineffective if States' agents abroad were free to act at variance with obligations under international refugee law and human rights law."

[272] UNHCR, "Brief as *Amicus Curiae*," filed Dec. 21, 1992 in *McNary v. Haitian Centers Council Inc.*, Case No. 92–344 (US SC), at 18, reprinted in (1994) 6(1) *International Journal of Refugee Law* 85. The US Supreme Court invoked arguments by both Robinson and Grahl-Madsen in support of its conclusion that Art. 33 only applies once persons reach a state party's territory. Yet both writers impliedly acknowledge the illogical policy implications of distinguishing between refugees located on either side of a border. Robinson commented that "if a refugee has succeeded in eluding the frontier guards, he is safe; if he has not, it is his hard luck": N. Robinson, *Convention relating to the Status*

Perhaps most fundamentally, the American Supreme Court's analysis seems erroneously to assume that international rights can apply only in a state's territory: no account whatever was taken of the fact that some Convention rights are explicitly not subject to a territorial or other level of attachment – including, of course, Art. 33's duty of *non-refoulement*. In line with the views of both the European Court of Human Rights and the International Court of Justice, the duty to respect these rights inheres wherever a state exercises effective or de facto jurisdiction outside its own territory, including at a minimum both situations in which a state's consular or other agents take control of persons abroad; and where the state exercises some significant public power in foreign territory which it has occupied, or in which it is present by consent, invitation, or acquiescence. There can therefore be little doubt that interception by United States military vessels in international waters easily qualifies as an exercise of de facto jurisdiction abroad.

Much the same conclusion has recently been reached by the English Court of Appeal. Noting that the Interamerican Commission on Human Rights[273] was "fiercely critical of the majority decision of the Supreme Court,"[274] the Court treated the *Sale* decision as "wrongly decided; it certainly offends one's sense of fairness."[275] It concluded that "it is impermissible to return refugees from the high seas to their country of origin."[276] All in all, the textual and historical arguments for reading Art. 33 in the narrow way posited by the

---

of Refugees: Its History, Contents and Interpretation (1953) (Robinson, *History*), at 163. Grahl-Madsen posited the scenario of a refugee approaching a frontier post some distance inside the actual frontier, who may be refused permission to proceed farther inland, but must be allowed to stay in the bit of territory situated between the actual frontier line and the control post, because any other course of action would violate Art. 33: Grahl-Madsen, *Commentary*, at 229–230.

[273] *Haitian Centre for Human Rights et al. v. United States*, Case No. 10.675, Report No. 51/96, Inter-AmCHR Doc. OEA/Ser.L/V/II.95 Doc. 7 rev., at 550 (Inter-Am Comm HR, Mar. 13, 1997).

[274] *R (European Roma Rights Centre and Others) v. Immigration Officer at Prague Airport*, [2003] EWCA Civ 666 (Eng. CA, May 20, 2003), at para. 34.

[275] Ibid. In the House of Lords, however, Lord Hope expressed some measure of support for the *Sale* decision, noting that he did "not, with respect, think that the *Sale* case was wrongly decided" since it was based on a determination that "both the text and the negotiating history of article 33 affirmatively indicated that it was not intended to have extraterritorial effect": *R v. Immigration Officer at Prague Airport et al., ex parte European Roma Rights Centre et al.*, [2004] UKHL 55 (UK HL, Dec. 9, 2004), at para. 68. Despite the clear logic of reliance on a provision's text and drafting history, the relevant analysis of the United States Supreme Court on these points was in error for reasons discussed above, at pp. 336–339.

[276] *R (European Roma Rights Centre and Others) v. Immigration Officer at Prague Airport*, [2003] EWCA Civ 666 (Eng. CA, May 20, 2003), at para. 35.

Supreme Court of the United States are simply not compelling. As Justice Blackmun concluded in his dissent,

> Today's majority ... decides that the forced repatriation of the Haitian refugees is perfectly legal because the word "return" does not mean return [and] because the opposite of "within the United States" is not outside the United States ...
>
> The Convention ... was enacted largely in response to the experience of Jewish refugees in Europe during the period of World War II. The tragic consequences of the world's indifference at that time are well known. The resulting ban on *refoulement*, as broad as the humanitarian purpose that inspired it, is easily applicable here, the Court's protestations of impotence and regret notwithstanding.[277]

It is important to signal that the notions of taking control and exercise of public power – that is, the basis for finding an exercise of de facto extra-territorial jurisdiction – should be construed in consonance with accepted principles of state responsibility. Under these rules, governments are responsible *inter alia* for "the conduct of a person or group of persons in fact acting on the instruction of, or under the direction or control of, the State,"[278] as well as for "conduct which is ... acknowledged and adopted by the State as its own."[279] Where these requirements are met, an act which would amount to an exercise of extraterritorial jurisdiction is no less so because it is committed by an entity (for example, a private corporation) under contract with a government than if committed directly by officials of the state party itself.

Perhaps of greatest contemporary relevance, state responsibility may be established by "the conduct of an organ placed at the disposal of a State by another State if the organ is acting in the exercise of elements of the governmental authority of the State at whose disposal it is placed."[280] Thus, to the extent that officials of a transit country exercise visa control or other authority on behalf of a destination state which results in the (direct or indirect) return of a refugee to his or her country of origin, this is a vicarious exercise of de facto jurisdiction by the destination state which amounts to a breach of the duty of *non-refoulement*.[281] Indeed,

---

[277] *Sale, Acting Commissioner, Immigration and Naturalization Service, et al., Petitioners v. Haitian Centers Council, Inc., et al.*, 509 US 155 (US SC, Jan. 12, 1993), at 207–208.

[278] "Draft Articles on Responsibility of States for Internationally Wrongful Acts," UN Doc. A/56/10, Ch. IV.E.1, adopted Nov. 2001 (International Law Commission, "Draft Articles"), at Art. 8.

[279] Ibid. at Art. 11.   [280] Ibid. at Art. 6.

[281] The concerns canvassed earlier where visa controls have effect within the country of origin itself – and hence necessarily impact before the person subject to them has satisfied the alienage criterion of the refugee definition – clearly do not apply once the person has successfully left his or her own country.

where both the transit state and destination state are parties to the Refugee Convention, they may in such circumstances be held jointly liable for the act of *refoulement*.[282]

None of this is to say, of course, that governments may not have legitimate cause to intercept non-citizens in areas beyond their territorial jurisdiction. For example, state parties to the Smuggling Protocol[283] may rely on that treaty to assert this authority in some circumstances:

> A State Party that has reasonable grounds to suspect that a vessel is engaged in the smuggling of migrants by sea and is without nationality or may be assimilated to a vessel without nationality may board and search the vessel. If evidence confirming the suspicion is found, that State Party shall take appropriate measures in accordance with relevant domestic and international law.[284]

Thus, at least when the vessel in question does not have a flag state,[285] state parties to the Smuggling Protocol enjoy a presumptive right to board and search vessels reasonably suspected of smuggling migrants. But this authority is in no sense at odds with the ability simultaneously to respect obligations under the Refugee Convention, including the duty of *non-refoulement*.[286] To the extent that the actions of the intercepting country are such as to amount to an exercise of de facto jurisdiction over the vessel or those onboard, it must respect Art. 33 of the Refugee Convention (and the other rights which inhere prior to arrival at a state party's territory[287]). This does not mean that all refugees onboard must be

---

[282] See G. Noll, "Visions of the Exceptional: Legal and Theoretical Issues Raised by Transit Processing Centers and Protection Zones," (2003) 5(3) *European Journal of Migration Law* 303 (Noll, "Transit Processing"), at 326: "The precise allocation of responsibility cannot be assessed in the abstract, as it would depend on the facts of the case, any agreements concluded, and the degree of control *de facto* and *de jure* of the different states involved in the operation of the scheme."

[283] Protocol against the Smuggling of Migrants by Land, Sea and Air, supplementing the United Nations Convention against Transnational Organized Crime, UNGA Res. 55/25, Annex III, 55 UNGAOR Supp. (No. 49) at 65, UN Doc. A/45/49, vol. I (2001), adopted Nov. 15, 2000, entered into force Jan. 28, 2004 (Smuggling Protocol).

[284] Ibid. at Art. 8(7).

[285] Where the vessel suspected of engaging in people smuggling has a flag state, that country's cooperation is normally to be sought before boarding or searching the vessel: ibid. at Art. 8(2).

[286] "States have a legitimate interest in controlling irregular migration. Unfortunately, existing control tools, such as visa requirements and the imposition of carrier sanctions, as well as interception measures, often do not differentiate between genuine asylum-seekers and economic migrants. National authorities, including immigration and airlines officials posted abroad, are frequently not aware of the paramount distinction between refugees, who are entitled to international protection, and other migrants, who are able to rely on national protection": UNHCR, "Interception," at para. 17.

[287] See chapter 3.1.1 above.

admitted to the territory of the state which undertakes the interception; but it does mean that having opted to take jurisdiction, the state party must not act in contravention of its freely assumed international responsibilities to protect refugees.[288]

4.1.4 Individuated exceptions

States are not bound to honor the duty of *non-refoulement* in the case of persons who are individually determined to pose a fundamental threat to the receiving state.[289] Specifically, particularized *refoulement* is legal on the grounds of compelling reasons of national security, or where a refugee convicted of a particularly serious crime is shown to be a danger to the host community.[290]

There is frequently confusion between the right of a state to expel or return dangerous refugees pursuant to Art. 33(2) and the exclusion of fugitives from justice under Art. 1(F)(b) of the Convention.[291] Art. 1(F)(b), inserted at the insistence of countries which perceived themselves to be vulnerable to large

---

[288] "Interception measures should not result in asylum-seekers and refugees being denied access to international protection, or result in those in need of international protection being returned, directly or indirectly, to the frontiers of territories where their life or freedom would be threatened on account of a Convention ground, or where the person has other grounds for protection based on international law. Intercepted persons found to be in need of international protection should have access to durable solutions": UNHCR Executive Committee Conclusion No. 97, "Conclusion on Protection Safeguards in Interception Measures" (2003), at para. (a)(iv), available at www.unhcr.ch (accessed Nov. 20, 2004).

[289] "The benefit of the present provision may not, however, be claimed by *a refugee* whom there are reasonable grounds for regarding as *a danger* to the security of the country in which *he* is, or who, having been convicted by *a final judgment* of *a particularly serious crime*, constitutes *a danger* to the community of that country [emphasis added]": Refugee Convention, at Art. 33(2).

[290] Lauterpacht and Bethlehem suggest that – the clear language of Art. 33(2) notwithstand-ing – there is today a basis for understanding the duty of *non-refoulement* to include no exceptions whatever: Lauterpacht and Bethlehem, "*Non-Refoulement*," at paras. 151–158. The argument is based on an unsound construction of Art. 33(2) which draws on a mix of regional norms, norms derived from other instruments, and policy positions of inter-national agencies. While the authors "are not ultimately persuaded that there is a sufficiently clear consensus opposed to exceptions to *non-refoulement* to warrant reading the 1951 Convention without them," they nonetheless insist that the exceptions "must be read subject to very clear limitations": ibid. at para. 158.

[291] See e.g. Immigration and Refugee Board of Canada Decision No. T89–0245, Sept. 12, 1989, in which the Board inappropriately employed the exclusion clause in Art. 1(F)(b) to bar a claimant on the basis of a combination of pre-entry and Canadian criminality for which sentence had been served. This case ought reasonably to have been assessed against the standards of Art. 33(2); if met, the claimant would retain refugee status, but lose the benefit of protection against *refoulement*.

flows of refugees,[292] is designed to afford the possibility of pre-admission exclusion on the basis of a relatively low standard of proof ("serious reasons for considering"),[293] and without recourse to a formal trial to assess the criminal charge. The expediency of this recourse is balanced against its very narrow scope: it applies only to persons believed to have committed serious, pre-entry crimes which remain justiciable. The distinctiveness of Art 1(F)(b) and Art. 33(2) must be recognized, as was pointedly observed by Mr. Justice Bastarache of the Supreme Court of Canada:

> [P]ersons falling within Art. 1(F) of the Convention are automatically excluded from the protections of the [Convention]. Not only may they be returned to the country from which they have sought refuge without any determination ... that they pose a threat to public safety or national security, but their substantive claim to refugee status will not be considered. The practical implications of such an automatic exclusion, relative to the safeguards of the [Art. 33(2)] procedure, are profound.[294]

Art. 33(2) codifies the original[295] and more broadly applicable criminality provision. It provides the means for states to expel or return two categories of refugees. First, it authorizes the *refoulement* of any refugee with respect to whom there are reasonable grounds for regarding him or her as a danger to the security of the asylum country, whether or not there is an allegation of criminality. Second, Art. 33(2) sanctions the removal of refugees adjudged to endanger the safety of the community of the asylum country because of particularly serious crimes committed in the state of refuge or elsewhere, whether or not those crimes remain justiciable.[296]

---

[292] "France's reason for taking such a firm stand on the subject lay in the fact that she had to administer the right of asylum under much more difficult conditions than did countries which were in a position to screen immigrants carefully at their frontiers": Statement of Mr. Rochefort of France, UN Doc. A/CONF.2/SR.24, July 17, 1951, at 13. See also Statement of Mr. Makiedo of Yugoslavia, ibid. at 18. These states were concerned not to undermine the possibilities for resettlement of the refugees admitted: "If refugee status was to be granted to criminals, immigration countries could not fail to question its value": Statement of Mr. Rochefort of France, UN Doc. A/CONF.2/SR.19, July 13, 1951, at 7.

[293] A. Grahl-Madsen, *The Status of Refugees in International Law* (vol. I, 1966) (Grahl-Madsen, *Status of Refugees I*), at 289.

[294] *Pushpanathan v. Minister of Citizenship and Immigration*, 1998 Can. Sup. Ct. Lexis 29 (Can. SC, June 4, 1998), at para. 13.

[295] Indeed, it was argued by the United Kingdom that there was no need for a criminality exclusion clause in Art. 1(F) in view of Art. 33(2): Statement of Mr. Hoare of the United Kingdom, UN Doc. A/CONF.2/SR.24, July 17, 1951, at 4. See also Statement of Baron van Boetzelaer of the Netherlands, UN Doc. A/CONF.2/SR.29, July 19, 1951, at 12: "Common criminals should not enjoy the right of asylum; but that consideration had already been taken care of in article [33] of the draft Convention."

[296] See e.g. *I v. Belgium* (Feb. 13, 1987), (1987) 46 *Revue du droit des étrangers* 200, summarized at (1989) 1(3) *International Journal of Refugee Law* 392, in which Belgium

In cases that fall under Art. 33(2), the asylum country is authorized to expel or return even refugees who face the risk of extremely serious forms of persecution.[297] Its standard of proof, however, is more exacting than that set by Art. 1(F)(b). As described in more detail below, the criminality branch of Art. 33(2) requires conviction by a final judgment of a particularly serious crime, rather than simply "serious reasons for considering" that a person may be a criminal.[298] Also, it is not enough that the crime committed has been "serious," but it must rather be "particularly serious." Beyond this, there must also be a determination that the offender "constitutes a danger to the community."

So construed, Art. 1(F)(b) and Art. 33(2) form a coherent and logical system. A person is denied refugee status under Art. 1(F)(b) if admission as a refugee would result in the protection of an individual who has not expiated serious criminal acts. While this may appear harsh, it is the only means available to ensure that refugee law does not benefit fugitives from justice.[299] Because ordinary crimes cannot normally be prosecuted in other than the country where they were committed, any response short of the exclusion of common law criminals from the refugee protection system (and consequential amenability to deportation) would undermine international comity in the fight against crime.

If, in contrast, the concern is not complicity in the avoidance of criminal responsibility, but instead protection of the core interests of the host state or of its citizenry, there is no need to deny refugee status. Thus, Art. 33(2) does not annul refugee status, but simply authorizes a host government to divest itself of its particularized protective responsibilities.[300] The individual in question remains a refugee, and is therefore entitled both to UNHCR institutional assistance and to the protection of any other state party the safety and security of

---

relied on Art. 33(2) to expel a refugee sentenced to three years' imprisonment in respect of a major theft in Belgium. It is, however, open to serious question whether theft is appropriately considered to be a "particularly serious crime," since it would not qualify as even a "serious crime" for purposes of exclusion under Art. 1(F)(b).

[297] "The exclusion clause now refers to crimes committed 'prior to his (the refugee's) admission to that country (i.e. the country of asylum) as a refugee' while persons who have committed a serious crime in the country of residence remain refugees, but may in certain conditions be denied asylum and returned to their country of origin (Article 33(2) of the Convention)": P. Weis, "The Concept of the Refugee in International Law," (1960) 87 *Journal du droit international* 928, at 984.

[298] See text below, at pp. 349–352.

[299] Despite the prerogative afforded by Art. 33(2), state parties to other human rights treaties – for example, to the European Convention on Human Rights, to the Convention against Torture, and to the International Covenant on Civil and Political Rights – will be subject to additional constraints on removal as a result of these other treaty obligations: see chapter 4.1.6 below, at pp. 368–370.

[300] See e.g. *Moses Allueke*, Dec. No. 188981 (Fr. CE, Nov. 3, 1999), confirming that while criminal convictions registered in France would allow the applicant to be excluded from the benefit of protection against *refoulement*, they were not a basis for the withdrawal of refugee status as such.

which is not infringed by the refugee's presence within its territory. This distinction was clearly understood by the Supreme Court of Canada:

> The purpose of Article 1 is to define who is a refugee. Article 1(F) then establishes categories of persons who are specifically excluded from that definition. The purpose of Article 33 of the Convention, by contrast, is not to define who is and who is not a refugee, but rather to allow for the *refoulement* of a *bona fide* refugee to his or her native country where he or she poses a danger to the security of the country of refuge, or to the safety of the community . . . Thus, the general purpose of Article 1(F) is not the protection of the society of refuge from dangerous refugees, whether because of acts committed before or after the presentation of a refugee claim; that purpose is served by Article 33 of the Convention.[301]

The first category of persons legitimately subject to *refoulement* comprises those "whom there are reasonable grounds for regarding as a danger to the security of the [reception] country." The notion of "reasonable grounds" has been helpfully defined by Madame Justice Glazebrook of the New Zealand Court of Appeal to require "that the State concerned cannot act either arbitrarily or capriciously and that it must specifically address the question of whether there is a future risk and the conclusion on the matter must be supported by evidence."[302] While national security was not precisely defined in the drafting debates, there are indications that delegates to the Conference of Plenipotentiaries were particularly concerned about the possibility of Communist infiltration.[303] Under the modern

---

[301] *Pushpanathan v. Minister of Citizenship and Immigration*, 1998 Can. Sup. Ct. Lexis 29 (Can. SC, June 4, 1998), at para. 58. To similar effect, the New Zealand Court of Appeal has determined that "Art. 1(F) is concerned with past acts. Art. 33(2) is only concerned with past acts to the extent that they may serve as an indication of the behaviour one may expect from the refugee in the future. The danger that the refugee constitutes must be a present or future danger": *Attorney General v. Zaoui*, Dec. No. CA20/04 (NZ CA, Sept. 30, 2004), at para. 166.

[302] *Attorney General v. Zaoui*, Dec. No. CA20/04 (NZ CA, Sept. 30, 2004), at para. 133. In his concurring opinion, Mr. Justice William Young observed that "these words must be interpreted so as to ensure that [the state party] conforms to its obligations under the Refugee Convention and thus in light of the international understanding of what they mean (or imply)": ibid. at para. 198.

[303] "It must be borne in mind that . . . each government had become more keenly aware of the current dangers to its national security. Among the great mass of refugees it was inevitable that some persons should be tempted to engage in activities on behalf of a foreign Power against the country of their asylum, and it would be unreasonable to expect the latter not to safeguard itself against such a contingency": Statement of Mr. Hoare of the United Kingdom, UN Doc. A/CONF.2/SR.16, July 11, 1951, at 8. See also Statement of Mr. Chance of Canada, ibid.: "In drafting [Art. 33], members of [the Ad Hoc] Committee had kept their eyes on the stars but their feet on the ground. Since that time, however, the international situation had deteriorated, and it must be recognized, albeit with reluctance, that at present many governments would find difficulty in accepting unconditionally the principle [of *non-refoulement*]."

jurisprudential views analyzed earlier, however, invocation of a national security argument is appropriate where a refugee's presence or actions give rise to an objectively reasonable, real possibility of directly or indirectly inflicted substantial harm to the host state's most basic interests, including the risk of an armed attack on its territory or its citizens, or the destruction of its democratic institutions.[304]

Despite the breadth of this modern understanding of national security, it may still be misapplied in practice. It is not appropriate, for example, to assert the importance of safeguarding international relations as the basis for excluding refugees on national security grounds.[305] Nor is there any basis in international law for deeming a refugee to pose a threat to national security because property or economic interests might be adversely impacted by his or her presence.[306] Much less can national security be said to justify the denial of protection in order to discourage the departure of other persons from the refugee's country of origin.[307]

[304] See chapter 3.5.1 above, at pp. 264–266. In contrast, Lauterpacht and Bethlehem assert that an interpretation of this kind would be "inconsistent with the nature of [the] compromise [between state and individual interests], and with the humanitarian and fundamental character of the prohibition of *refoulement*," in consequence of which the national security exemption set by Art. 33(2) "does not address circumstances in which there is a possibility of danger to the security of other countries or to the international community more generally": Lauterpacht and Bethlehem, "*Non-Refoulement*," at para. 165.

[305] "Concerns about New Zealand's reputation can be taken into account [under Art. 33(2)] only if they impinge to such a serious extent on national security that they could fairly be said to constitute a danger to national security": *Attorney General v. Zaoui*, Dec. No. CA20/04 (NZ CA, Sept. 30, 2004), at para. 141. But see *Suresh v. Minister of Citizenship and Immigration*, 2000 DLR Lexis 49 (Can. FCA, Jan. 18, 2000), reversed on appeal in *Suresh v. Canada*, [2002] 1 SCR 3 (Can. SC, Jan. 11, 2002). "[T] he 'security of Canada' . . . logically extends to situations where the integrity of Canada's international relations and obligations are affected."

[306] Contrary to this understanding, the court in *Cheema v. Immigration and Naturalization Service*, 183 DLR (4th) 629 (US CA9, Dec. 1, 2003), simply adopted without any analysis a nearly unbounded test of "national security" posited by the Board of Appeals, namely that there is a risk to national security where the individual concerned "(1) endangers the lives, *property* or *welfare* of United States citizens; (2) *compromises* the national defense of the United States; or (3) materially damages the *foreign relations or economic interests* of the United States [emphasis added]."

[307] In overruling a decision of the Board of Immigration Appeals that no national security threat had been shown in the case of an unauthorized entrant from Haiti, the Attorney General took the unusual step of issuing a "binding determination," specifically said to be treated as a precedent in future cases, that national security would be compromised by the release on bail of Haitian entrants because this "would tend to encourage further surges of mass migrations from Haiti by sea, with attendant strains on national and homeland security resources": *In re DJ*, 2003 BIA Lexis 3 (US AG, Apr. 17, 2003). Incredibly, the Attorney General explicitly advanced a deterrent rationale for his decision, asserting that "surges in such illegal migration by sea injure national security by diverting valuable Coast Guard and DOD resources from counter-terrorism and homeland security responsibilities": ibid.

A more difficult question is whether the national security exception to the duty of *non-refoulement* can be invoked in order to avoid the risk of retaliation by those who would persecute a refugee. The US Board of Immigration Appeals has emphatically asserted that such exclusion is not lawful:

> The immigration judge did not find that the applicant himself would seek to undermine the security of the United States. Instead, she found that the decision of the United States to offer [asylum to] the applicant, a high profile person involved in a violent political crisis . . . might involve the United States in that crisis or cause this country to become the target of violent conflict. If our country shelters him, foreign violent opponents of his may well consider our territory an appropriate battleground . . .
>
> We conclude that the immigration judge's interpretation . . . is flawed. The case law establishes that an alien would properly be considered a danger to the security of the United States when the alien himself poses the danger . . . We have found no authority to support the immigration judge's interpretation . . . that an alien would properly be considered a danger to the security of the United States when the decision of the United States to grant the alien asylum might encourage others to commit violence against the United States in retaliation for that decision. The purpose of asylum is to protect an individual who is in danger based on, among other things, his political opinion. This purpose would be severely undermined if we denied asylum because some third party who opposed the alien's political opinion contemplated violence against the United States (or the alien himself) in retaliation for granting him the protective relief of asylum.[308]

While clearly a highly principled position, this view takes an overly narrow view of the notion of national security. For purposes of Art. 33(2), the question ought to be whether there genuinely is a real chance of retaliation; and if so, whether the nature of the retaliation poses a risk of substantial harm to the host state's most basic interests – such as an armed attack on its territory or its citizens, or the destruction of its democratic institutions. If these strict criteria are satisfied, the national security exception to the duty of *non-refoulement* may legitimately be invoked, and the refugee required to leave the host state. Art. 33 should, however, be read in consonance with Arts. 31 and 32 to allow dangerous refugees the opportunity to seek entry into a non-persecutory state, as an alternative to being returned to their home country.[309]

Even where vital interests of this kind are involved, a state seeking to rely on the national security exception to the duty of *non-refoulement* must, of course, undertake a careful assessment of the security threat actually posed by

---

[308] *In re Anwar Haddam*, 2000 BIA Lexis 20 (US BIA, Dec. 1, 2000).
[309] See Weis, *Travaux*, at 343.

the particular refugee whose *refoulement* is being contemplated.[310] The Art. 33(2) inquiry "requires the person him or herself to constitute a danger to national security. This clearly implies that there must be some element of causation."[311] Thus, as the Supreme Court of Canada has insisted, it cannot be assumed that a person poses a risk to national security based on the fact of group membership, or other affiliation alone – the risk must rather be proved on the basis of fair procedures.[312] This was, in fact, the key problem with New Zealand's peremptory denial of protection to Muslim asylum-seekers during the first Gulf War. By requiring each refugee claimant to rebut a presumption that he or she *was* a security risk legitimately subject to *refoulement*, the government skewed what is intended to be a particularized and highly exceptional form of protection for states. A restrictive approach is clearly called for,[313] with the state asserting the danger posed by the refugee logically expected to establish a case for the refugee to answer.[314]

[310] "Following the events of September 11 . . . a number of States have strengthened measures to combat illegal migration and the misuse of asylum systems. While UNHCR supports measures to combat misuse of asylum systems, I am concerned that in some cases indiscriminate measures have led to non-admission, denial of access to asylum procedures, and even incidents of *refoulement*": UNHCR, "Opening Statement of the UN High Commissioner for Refugees, Ruud Lubbers, at the 53rd Session of the Executive Committee of the High Commissioner's Program," Sept. 30, 2002.

[311] *Attorney General v. Zaoui*, Dec. No. CA20/04 (NZ CA, Sept. 30, 2004), at para. 148.

[312] In line with the approach of the Supreme Court of Canada, the permissibility of *refoulement* based upon the fact of group membership might be better considered not on the basis of the national security leg of Art. 33(2), but rather on the basis of the other branch of Art. 33(2), which authorizes *refoulement* in the case of persons who are shown to pose a danger to the community of their intended host state, but only after final conviction of a particularly serious crime. "[C]ontrary to the government's submission, [we would] distinguish 'danger to the security of Canada' from 'danger to the public,' although we recognize that the two phrases may overlap. The latter phrase clearly is intended to address threats to individuals in Canada, but its application is restricted by requiring that any individual who is declared to be a 'danger to the public' have been convicted of a serious offence . . . The government's suggested reading of 'danger to the security of Canada' effectively does an end-run around the requirements of Article 33(2) of the Refugee Convention that no one may be refouled as a danger to the community of the country unless he has first been convicted by a final judgment of a particularly serious crime": *Suresh v. Canada*, [2002] 1 SCR 3 (Can. SC, Jan. 11, 2002), at para. 84. It would seem to follow that if a state wishes to exclude a refugee from protection against *refoulement* on the basis of his or her membership of a terrorist or other organization, the host state should criminalize that membership, successfully prosecute and convict the alleged member, and show that he or she poses a danger to the security of the country.

[313] See *Attorney General v. Zaoui*, Dec. No. CA20/04 (NZ CA, Sept. 30, 2004), at para. 136: "[I]t is clear that the Art. 33(2) exception must be interpreted restrictively. In my view, this means that the danger to security must be serious enough to justify frustrating the whole purpose of the Refugee Convention by sending a person back to persecution."

[314] In *NSH v. Secretary of State for the Home Department*, [1988] Imm AR 410 (Eng. CA, Mar. 23, 1988), the English Court of Appeal held that the grounds for determining an applicant

Beyond concerns of national security, *refoulement* is also allowed in the case of a refugee who has been "convicted by a final judgment of a particularly serious crime," and who is determined to constitute "a danger to the community" of the asylum state. In contrast to Art. 1(F)(b) of the Refugee Convention, the purpose of which is simply to ensure that extraditable criminals cannot avoid prosecution and punishment abroad by claiming refugee status, the criminality exclusion set by Art. 33(2) exists to enable host states to protect the safety of their own communities from criminal refugees who are shown to be dangerous.[315] This right to engage in the *refoulement* of dangerous criminals is, however, carefully constrained.

First, the gravity of criminality which justifies *refoulement* under Art. 33(2) is higher than that which justifies the exclusion of fugitives from justice under Art. 1(F)(b) of the Convention. Art. 1 denies protection to an extraditable criminal who has committed a "serious non-political crime outside the country of refuge prior to his admission to that country as a refugee."[316] "Serious" criminality in this context is normally understood to mean acts that involve violence against persons, such as homicide, rape, child molesting, wounding, arson, drugs trafficking, and armed robbery.[317] The gravity of

---

to be a risk to the national security of a country must in fact be reasonable before protection against *refoulement* may validly be denied. While the courts cannot expect all evidence to be placed before them, the assertion of risk must be "sufficiently particularized" to substantiate the reasonableness of exclusion. In the view of the New Zealand Court of Appeal, "it is incumbent upon the [state party] to provide as much information as is possible, without risking the disclosure of the classified security information itself": *Attorney General v. Zaoui*, Dec. No. CA20/04 (NZ CA, Sept. 30, 2004), at para. 72. In general terms, "[t]he relevant authorities must specifically address the question of whether there is a future risk [to national security]; and their conclusion on the matter must be supported by evidence": Lauterpacht and Bethlehem, "*Non-Refoulement*," at para. 168.

[315] See J. Hathaway and C. Harvey, "Framing Refugee Protection in the New World Disorder," (2001) 34(2) *Cornell International Law Journal* 257. In describing the different functions of Art. 1(F)(b) and Art. 33(2) of the Refugee Convention, Lord Mustill observed that the argument that Art. 1(F)(b) should be used to exclude dangerous refugees "overlooks Article 33(2) of the 1951 Convention ... The state of refuge has sufficient means to protect itself against harbouring dangerous criminals without forcing on an offence, which either is or is not a political crime when and where committed, a different character according to the opinions of those in the receiving state about whether the refugee is an undesirable alien": *T v. Secretary of State for the Home Department*, [1996] 2 All ER 865 (UK HL, May 22, 1996), per Lord Mustill. See also *Pushpanathan v. Minister of Citizenship and Immigration*, 1998 Can. Sup. Ct. Lexis 29 (Can. SC, June 4, 1998), at para. 73.

[316] Refugee Convention, at Art. 1(F)(b). See generally Grahl-Madsen, *Status of Refugees I*, at 289–304; J. Hathaway, *The Law of Refugee Status* (1991) (Hathaway, *Refugee Status*), at 221–226; and Goodwin-Gill, *Refugee in International Law*, at 101–108.

[317] Grahl-Madsen, *Status of Refugees I*, at 297; Hathaway, *Refugee Status*, at 224; Goodwin-Gill, *Refugee in International Law*, at 104–106.

harm necessary to justify the *refoulement* of a person who qualifies for refugee status – expressly framed as a "particularly" serious crime – is clearly higher still, and has been interpreted to require that even when the refugee has committed a serious crime, *refoulement* is only warranted when account has been taken of all mitigating and other circumstances surrounding commission of the offence.[318]

For example, the Australian Full Federal Court was called upon to consider whether Art. 33(2) was appropriately applied in the case of a person who had been detained by Australia for more than two years before his Convention refugee status was confirmed. By reason of his protracted detention, he began to experience severe paranoid delusions. After his release, and while in a delusional state, he went to an acquaintance's home armed with a knife and threatened to kill her. He subsequently made further threats against the woman's life, ultimately resulting in his arrest on one count of aggravated burglary and five counts of threats to kill. He was convicted of those charges, and sentenced to a term of three-and-a-half years' imprisonment. The Court reviewing the decision that *refoulement* was justified held that the offences ought not to have been deemed "particularly serious" without consideration of "the fact that it was the appellant's psychological illness that led to the commission of the offenses. It should have taken into account that the appellant's conduct was directed to a person whom he believed, as a consequence of his psychological illness, had been conspiring to cause him harm. The Tribunal should have considered the extent to which the psychological illness reduced the moral culpability of the appellant in much the same way as his psychological illness was taken into account in sentencing the appellant for having committed those offenses." As a general principle, the Court concluded:

> On its proper construction, Article 33(2) does not contemplate that a crime will be characterized as particularly serious or not particularly serious merely by reference to the nature of the crime that has been committed, although this may suffice in some cases. The reason is that there are very many crimes where it is just not possible to determine whether they are particularly serious without regard to the circumstances surrounding their commission.[319]

Second, while refugee status is to be withheld from persons reasonably suspected of criminal conduct under Art. 1(F)(b), the *refoulement* of refugees is permissible only when there has actually been conviction by a final

---

[318] *Betkoshabeh v. Minister for Immigration and Multicultural Affairs*, (1998) 157 ALR 95 (Aus. FC, July 29, 1998), at 102, reversed on grounds of mootness at (1999) 55 ALD 609 (Aus. FFC, July 20, 1999).
[319] Ibid.

judgment. Appeal rights should therefore have expired or been exhausted,[320] limiting the risk of *refoulement* strictly to those whose criminality has been definitively established in accordance with accepted, general legal norms.

Third and most important, the nature of the conviction and other circumstances must justify the conclusion that the refugee in fact constitutes a danger to the community[321] from which protection is sought.[322] Because danger follows from the refugee's criminal character, it does not matter whether the crime was committed in the state of origin, an intermediate state, or the asylum state.[323] Nor is it relevant whether the claimant has or has not served a penal sentence or otherwise been punished. In contrast to exclusion from refugee status under Article 1(F)(b) of the Convention, however, particularized *refoulement* cannot be based on the refugee's criminal record *per se* – as seems increasingly to be the practice in the United States, for example.[324]

---

[320] Statement of Mr. Hoare of the United Kingdom, UN Doc. A/CONF.2/SR.16, July 11, 1951, at 14. See also Lauterpacht and Bethlehem, "*Non-Refoulement*," at para. 188: "'Final judgment' must be construed as meaning a judgment from which there remains no possibility of appeal. It goes without saying that the procedure leading to the conviction must have complied with minimum international standards."

[321] "[I]t is evident that [the word 'community'] is intended as a reference to the safety and well-being of the population in general, in contrast to the national security exception which is focused on the larger interests of the State": Lauterpacht and Bethlehem, "*Non-Refoulement*," at para. 192.

[322] For example, a proposal to authorize the *refoulement* of habitual offenders convicted of a series of less serious crimes was not accepted: Statements of Mr. Theodoli of Italy and Mr. Hoare of the United Kingdom, UN Doc. A/CONF.2/SR.16, July 11, 1951, at 16–17.

[323] "Moreover, the possibility of a refugee committing a crime in a country other than his country of origin or his country of asylum could not be ignored. No matter where a crime was committed, it reflected upon the personality of the guilty individual, and the perpetrator was always a criminal ... The President pointed out that paragraph 2 [of Article 33] afforded a safeguard for States, by means of which they could rid themselves of common criminals or persons who had been convicted of particularly serious crimes in other countries": Statements of Mr. Rochefort of France and Mr. Larsen of Denmark, UN Doc. A/CONF.2/SR.35, July 25, 1951, at 24. But see Lauterpacht and Bethlehem, "*Non-Refoulement*," at para. 149. Because the authors do not recognize Art. 1(F)(b) as restricted to justiciable criminality, they argue that the need to avoid overlap between Arts. 1(F)(b) and 33(2) compels the conclusion that the latter speaks only to crimes committed *after* admission to a state party as a refugee.

[324] See decision of the US Attorney General overruling the US Board of Immigration Appeals in *In re YL*, 2002 BIA Lexis 4 (US AG, Mar. 5, 2002), in which the Board had found that an aggravated drug trafficking felony did not amount to a "particularly serious crime" based on evidence of cooperation with authorities, a limited criminal record, and the fact that the applicant had been sentenced at the low end of the applicable sentencing guideline range. The Attorney General reversed the decision, and imposed a nearly absolute understanding of a "particularly serious crime": "It is my considered judgment that aggravated felonies involving unlawful trafficking in controlled substances presumptively constitute particularly serious crimes ... Only under the most extenuating circumstances that are both extraordinary and compelling would departure from this

Refoulement is instead authorized only as a "last resort"[325] where there is no alternative mechanism to protect the community in the country of asylum from an unacceptably high risk of harm.[326] The practice of some states to give dangerous refugees the option of indefinite incarceration in the asylum state as an alternative to *refoulement* is therefore one mechanism to be considered, since it protects the host community, yet averts the risk of being persecuted.[327] In the end, however, the Refugee Convention accepts that in extreme and genuinely exceptional cases, the usual considerations of humanity must yield to the critical security interests of the receiving state.[328] Thus, if the demanding criteria of Art. 33(2) are satisfied, an asylum state may, assuming there is no other option, remove a refugee convicted of a particularly serious crime who poses a danger to the host community's safety – even if the only option is to send the refugee to his or her country of origin.[329]

interpretation be warranted or permissible ... We find that the crime of trafficking of drugs is inherently a particularly serious crime ... As we find trafficking in drugs to inherently be a particularly serious crime, no further inquiry is required into the nature and circumstances of the respondent's convictions": ibid. The inappropriateness of this approach is clear from the decision of *In re Mengisteab Bahta*, 2000 BIA Lexis 16 (US BIA, Oct. 4, 2000) in which a refugee from Ethiopia was ordered to be removed back to his country on the grounds that he had been convicted (under a plea bargain) of the offense of attempted possession of stolen property. Despite the nature of the offense and the fact that he had received only a thirty-six-month suspended sentence, the classification of his crime as an aggravated felony under US law was deemed by the majority sufficient to justify his removal.

[325] *Attorney General v. Zaoui*, Dec. No. CA20/04 (NZ CA, Sept. 30, 2004), at para. 139.

[326] Thus, "the danger involved is not a present or future danger that a person may commit a crime as that can be dealt with by the ordinary criminal law": ibid. at para. 167. This is in line with the view of the drafters of the Refugee Convention. For example, "the Swiss Government wished to reserve the right in quite exceptional circumstances to expel an undesirable alien, even if he was unable to proceed to a country other than the one from which he had fled, since the Federal Government might easily find itself so placed that there was no other means of getting rid of an alien who had seriously compromised himself": Statement of Mr. Schurch of Switzerland, UN Doc. E/AC.32/SR.40, Aug. 22, 1950, at 32.

[327] The drafters of the Convention, however, assumed this option to be no better than *refoulement*. "To condemn such persons to lifelong imprisonment, even if that were a practicable course, would be no better solution": Statement of Mr. Hoare of the United Kingdom, UN Doc. A/CONF.2/SR.16, July 11, 1951, at 8. In line with this concern, it has been determined in the United States – based not only on domestic law, but also on its understanding of international law – that indefinite detention is not a lawful option: *Kim Ho Ma v. Attorney General*, 208 F 3d 951 (US CA9, Apr. 10, 2000).

[328] "A State would always be in a position to protect itself against refugees who constituted a danger to national security or public order": Statement of Msgr. Comte of the Holy See, UN Doc. E/CONF.2/SR.16, July 11, 1951, at 5.

[329] There must, however, be "the necessity for an appreciable alleviation of the danger to be effected by deportation": *Attorney General v. Zaoui*, Dec. No. CA20/04 (NZ CA, Sept. 30, 2004), at para. 25, per Anderson J.

By allowing states to contemplate *refoulement* in only these clear and extreme cases,[330] the drafters conceived a threshold test for permissible *refoulement* which takes real account of both refugee and communal rights. If it is shown either that a refugee is a danger to national security, or that a refugee who is a serious criminal poses a danger to the safety of the community of that country, there is therefore no additional proportionality requirement to be met: by definition, no purely individuated risk of persecution can offset a real threat to such critical security interests of the receiving state. Because the objective of Art. 33(2) is protection of the most fundamental interests of the host state and its community, a clear risk to such collective interests defeats the refugee's right to invoke the duty of *non-refoulement*.

Most writers have taken a contrary position,[331] relying largely on a single comment of the British co-sponsor of the particularized *refoulement* provision.[332] Yet the British reference to the importance of letting states weigh relative risks was actually an answer to a proposal to restrict states' margin of appreciation,[333] not an argument for a super-added proportionality test. Indeed, the British representative associated himself with his French co-sponsor's explanation of the rationale for the particularized *refoulement* clause:

> The French and United Kingdom delegations had submitted their amendment in order to make it possible for states to punish activities ... directed against national security or constituting a danger to the community ... The right of asylum rested on moral and humanitarian considerations which were freely recognised by receiving countries, but it had certain essential limitations. A country could not contract an unconditional obligation towards persons over whom it was difficult to exercise any control, and into the ranks of whom undesirable elements might well infiltrate. The problem was a moral and psychological one, and in order to solve it, it would be necessary to take into account the possible reactions of public opinion.[334]

---

[330] "The Chairman realized that the presence of particularly intractable refugees might cause certain difficulties in certain reception countries. Nevertheless, it was for the governments of those countries to find the means of making reservations to meet special cases, while accepting the principle, which applied to all civilized nations, of not expelling refugees to territories where they would meet certain death": Statement of the Chairman, Mr. Chance of Canada, UN Doc. E/AC.32/SR.20, Feb. 1, 1950, at 15.

[331] See Robinson, *History*, at 164 and Weis, *Travaux*, at 342.

[332] "It must be left to States to decide whether the danger entailed to refugees by expulsion outweighed the menace to public security that would arise if they were permitted to stay": Statement of Mr. Hoare of the United Kingdom, UN Doc. A/CONF.2/SR.16, July 11, 1951, at 8.

[333] "What was meant for example by the words 'reasonable grounds'? He considered that the wording: 'may not, however, be claimed by a refugee *who constitutes* a danger to the security of the country' would be preferable [emphasis in original]": Statement of Msgr. Comte of the Holy See, ibid. at 7–8.

[334] Statement of Mr. Rochefort of France, ibid. at 7.

This conviction that the establishment and maintenance of a relatively open refugee protection system requires a strong safeguard of the basic security interests of receiving states was precisely the reason that the Conference of Plenipotentiaries rejected the Ad Hoc Committee's unconditional insistence on strict observance of the duty of *non-refoulement*.[335]

Appearances notwithstanding, insistence that risks to national security or dangers to the host community be "balanced" against the consequences of returning a refugee has in any event actually worked against the interests of many refugees concerned. This is because, in practice, the suggestion that there are some individuated forms of harm that could be more compelling than national security or danger to the community of reception has trivialized the significance of the latter two concepts and justified an unacceptably broad reading of the scope of Art. 33(2). In holding a "balancing test" to be mandated by Art. 33(2), the English Court of Appeal, for example, authorized the government to construe relatively minor concerns as matters of national security or communal danger:

> [T]he Secretary of State argues that on the plain wording of the Article a refugee may be expelled or returned even to a country where his life or freedom would be threatened, and that no balancing exercise is necessary; expulsion or return is permitted even where the threat to life or freedom *is much more serious than* the danger to the security of the country ... Despite the literal meaning of Article 33, it would seem to me quite wrong that *some trivial danger* to national security should allow expulsion or return in a case where there was a present threat to the life of the refugee if that took place [emphasis added].[336]

The very notion that there could be any such thing as a "trivial danger to national security" to be balanced against purely individuated interests is

---

[335] "The President thought that the Ad Hoc Committee, in drafting article [33], had, perhaps, established a standard which could not be accepted. That Committee, as could be seen from its report on its second session, had felt that the principle inherent in article [33] was fundamental, and that it could not consider any exceptions to the article": Statement of the President, Mr. Larsen of Denmark, ibid. at 13.

[336] *Secretary of State for the Home Department, ex parte Chahal*, [1994] Imm AR 107 (Eng CA, Oct. 22, 1993), per Straughton LJ, violation found in *Chahal v. United Kingdom*, (1996) 23 EHRR 413 (ECHR, Nov. 15, 1996). The decision of the Court of Appeal unfortunately rejected the earlier reasoning of the same court in *NSH v. Secretary of State for the Home Department*, [1988] Imm AR 410 (Eng. CA, Mar. 23, 1988): "It may be that in many cases, particularly where a case is near the borderline, the Secretary of State will weigh in the balance all the compassionate circumstances, including the fact that the person is a refugee. But where national security is concerned I do not see that there is any legal requirement to take this course. Indeed Article 33(2) of the Convention provides that a refugee cannot claim the benefit of Article 33(1) where there are reasonable grounds for regarding him 'as a danger to the security of the country in which he is.'"

disturbing. This decision shows how assertion of the importance of a "balancing test" inadvertently legitimates an unwarranted extension of the scope of the security-based exception to the duty of *non-refoulement*. If, in contrast, national security and danger to the community are more carefully constrained as described here, it is readily apparent that they would always trump purely individuated risks, in consequence of which no super-added balancing test is required or appropriate.[337]

4.1.5 Qualified duty in the case of mass influx

Beyond the possibility of particularized exclusion under Art. 33(2), the intention to establish a broadly applicable duty of *non-refoulement* was qualified during the final phase of the drafting process[338] in order to

---

[337] These arguments were considered by the New Zealand Court of Appeal, but rejected on the twin grounds that "it is built into the concept of danger to the security of the country that the danger posed by the individual must be serious enough to warrant sending a hypothetical person back to persecution" and that "[t]he weight of authority seems to favour an additional balancing of the consequences for the particular individual if removed or deported against the danger to security": *Attorney General v. Zaoui*, Dec. No. CA20/04 (NZ CA, Sept. 30, 2004), at para. 157. The second point is not, of course, substantively persuasive in and of itself. The first point, in contrast, is clearly correct, but is answered by the duty described above to constrain the scope of "national security" grounds to circumstances in which there is an objectively reasonable, real possibility of directly or indirectly inflicted substantial harm to the host state's most basic interests: see text above, at pp. 345–346. Nor does the Court address why there is a need for a "balancing requirement" also where *refoulement* is to be authorized for reasons of particular serious criminality, since removal on this basis can in any event only be ordered once mitigating and other surrounding circumstances have been taken into account, and as a true "last resort": see text above, at pp. 349–353.

[338] The Swiss and French delegations to the Conference of Plenipotentiaries appear initially to have argued that *non-refoulement* proscribes the expulsion of refugees from within a state's territory, but not the refusal of admission: Statement of Mr. Zutter of Switzerland, UN Doc. A/CONF.2/SR.16, July 11, 1951, at 6; and Statement of Mr. Rochefort of France, ibid. On closer examination, however, it is clear that their intention was not to endorse the routine *refoulement* of refugees, but rather only to authorize states to defend their frontiers in the event of a threat to their national security engendered by a mass migration of refugees: "The Swiss Government considered that in the present instance the word ['return'] applied solely to refugees who had already entered a country, but were not yet resident there. According to that interpretation, States were not compelled to allow *large groups of persons* claiming refugee status to cross [their] frontiers [emphasis added]": Statement of Mr. Zutter of Switzerland, ibid. See also Statement of Baron van Boetzelaer of the Netherlands, ibid. at 11: "He appreciated the importance of the basic principles underlying article [33] but, as a country bordering on others, was somewhat diffident about assuming unconditional obligations *so far as mass influxes of refugees were concerned* [emphasis added]."

accommodate critical public order and national security concerns which may arise during a "mass influx."[339] The President of the Conference observed that the work of the preparatory Ad Hoc Committee had set perhaps too absolute a standard of respect for *non-refoulement*.[340] The British[341] and Swiss[342] delegates to the Ad Hoc Committee argued that the Convention should recognize the traditional prerogative of states to engage in *refoulement* where required by vital national security interests. In contrast, France[343] and the United States asserted that "it would be highly undesirable to suggest in the text . . . that there might be cases, even highly exceptional cases, where a [refugee] might be sent to death or persecution."[344] The latter view prevailed in the Ad Hoc Committee, resulting in a draft article that made no mention of any right to engage in *refoulement* under any circumstances.[345]

At the Conference of Plenipotentiaries, Switzerland and the Netherlands reasserted the customary understanding that a comprehensive and absolute

---

[339] "[M]ass influx is a phenomenon that has not been defined, but . . . , for the purposes of this Conclusion, mass influx situations may, inter alia, have some or all of the following characteristics: (i) considerable numbers of people arriving over an international border; (ii) a rapid rate of arrival; (iii) inadequate absorption or response capacity in host States, particularly during the emergency; (iv) individual asylum procedures, where they exist, which are unable to deal with the assessment of such large numbers": UNHCR Executive Committee Conclusion No. 100, "Conclusion on International Cooperation and Burden and Responsibility Sharing in Mass Influx Situations" (2004), at para. (a), available at www.unhcr.ch (accessed Nov. 20, 2004).

[340] "The President thought that the Ad Hoc Committee, in drafting article [33], had, perhaps, established a standard that could not be accepted. That Committee, as could be seen from its report on its second session, had felt that the principle inherent in article [33] was fundamental, *and that it could not consider any exceptions to the article* [emphasis added]": Statement of Mr. Larsen of Denmark, UN Doc. A/CONF.2/SR.16, July 11, 1951, at 13. As is clear from this statement, however, the absolutism of concern to the President was the unwillingness to *consider exceptions* to the duty of *non-refoulement*, as for example were argued to be necessary in the event of mass influx. The President did not take issue with the general scope of the prohibition of *refoulement* as elaborated by the Ad Hoc Committee as including both ejection and non-admittance at the frontier.

[341] "National security was a consideration which should take precedence over all others": Statement of Sir Leslie Brass of the United Kingdom, UN Doc. E/AC.32/SR.20, Feb. 1, 1950, at 4. "The United Kingdom Government had no thought of acting harshly in such cases and hoped indeed that the mere existence of the power to expel a man making trouble might serve to keep his behaviour within reasonable bounds": Statement of Sir Leslie Brass, UN Doc. E/AC.32/SR.40, Aug. 22, 1950, at 30.

[342] Statement of Mr. Schurch of Switzerland, UN Doc. E/AC.32/SR.40, Aug. 22, 1950, at 32.

[343] "[A]ny possibility, even in exceptional circumstances, of a genuine refugee . . . being returned to his country of origin would not only be absolutely inhuman, but was contrary to the very purposes of the Convention": Statement of Mr. Juvigny of France, UN Doc. E/AC.32/SR.40, Aug. 22, 1950, at 33.

[344] Statement of Mr. Henkin of the United States, ibid. at 31.

[345] UN Doc. E/1850, Aug. 25, 1950, at 25.

duty of *non-refoulement* was untenable in the face of a mass influx.[346] The President agreed, ruling that "the possibility of mass migrations across frontiers or of attempted mass migrations was not covered by article 33."[347] The French term *refoulement* was added to the English text of the article following the word "return" to ensure that the duty of non-return was understood to have "no wider meaning"[348] than the French expression, which was agreed not to apply in the event that national security or public order was genuinely threatened by a mass influx.

There is a logic to this position. In the context of individuated applications for protection, it is feasible for states scrupulously to avoid peremptory acts of *refoulement*. The applicant can be admitted to the state's territory and removed if ultimately adjudged to constitute a serious risk to either national security or the safety of the community.[349] In contrast, it is not usually practical for a country overwhelmed by a mass influx of refugees to engage in this kind of detailed, case-by-case analysis of risks to its own well-being. Governments therefore wanted the assurance that in truly exceptional circumstances, they could engage in peremptory *refoulement* to the extent truly necessary to protect their most critical national interests.

The view that there is an implied limitation on the scope of the duty of *non-refoulement* where a state is at grave risk owing to a mass influx is, however, often resisted.[350] Indeed, Lauterpacht and Bethlehem dismiss this position out of hand:

> Although by reference to passing comments in the *travaux préparatoires* of the 1951 Convention, it has on occasion been argued that the principle does not apply to [mass influx] situations, this is not a view that has any merit. It is neither supported by the text as adopted nor by subsequent practice.[351]

---

[346] "According to [the Swiss] interpretation, article [33] would not have involved any obligations *in the possible case of mass migrations* across frontiers or of attempted *mass migrations* . . . The Netherlands could not accept any legal obligation *in respect of large groups of refugees* seeking access to its territory [emphasis added]": Statement of Baron van Boetzelaer of the Netherlands, UN Doc. A/CONF.2/SR.35, July 25, 1951, at 21.

[347] Statement of Mr. Larsen of Denmark, ibid.

[348] Statement of Mr. Hoare of the United Kingdom, ibid.

[349] Refugee Convention, at Art. 1(F).

[350] Goodwin-Gill does not take a firm position on this question, though he seems inclined to the view taken here that there is no more than a conditional duty of *non-refoulement* in the context of a genuine and truly threatening mass influx. He writes that "[i]t can be argued that a mass influx is not itself sufficient to justify *refoulement*, given the likelihood of an international response to offset any potential threat to national security . . . [I]t must be admitted that the prospect of a massive influx of refugees and asylum-seekers exposes the limits of the State's obligation otherwise not to return or refuse admission to refugees": Goodwin-Gill, *Refugee in International Law*, at 141.

[351] Lauterpacht and Bethlehem, "*Non-Refoulement*," at para. 103.

At the level of text, this position ignores the explicit decision to add the French language word "*refoulement*" to the English language version of Art. 33 in order to ensure that the traditional civil law understanding of that term (which did not govern in a mass influx) would be formally recognized.[352] Moreover, most of the "state practice" invoked by these writers against the mass influx exception is not properly considered to be state practice at all.[353]

It is true, though, that relevant conclusions of UNHCR's Executive Committee may appear to argue against recognition of the mass influx exception. Most importantly, Conclusion No. 22 provides that even in situations of mass influx, "the fundamental principle of *non-refoulement* – including non-rejection at the frontier – must be scrupulously observed."[354] As evidence of the subsequent agreement of the parties regarding interpretation of the Refugee Convention,[355] Conclusion No. 22 is an appropriate source of interpretive guidance. But if the Conclusion is read as a whole, it is clear that it argues for a much less one-sided responsibility than is often suggested.[356] The duty of state parties to respect the principle of *non-refoulement* ("at least on a temporary basis") is in fact balanced against a duty of international solidarity owed by other state parties to the receiving country:

> A mass influx may place unduly heavy burdens on certain countries; a satisfactory solution of a problem, international in scope and nature, cannot be achieved without international cooperation. States *shall*, within the framework of international solidarity and burden-sharing, *take all*

---

[352] See text above, at p. 357.

[353] Various memoranda and position papers authored by regional and international agencies are cobbled together as evidence of state practice in Lauterpacht and Bethlehem, "*Non-Refoulement*," at paras. 108–110. Kälin similarly opines that "[i]t is sometimes argued that the prohibition of *refoulement*, at least regarding rejection at the frontier, does not apply in situations of mass influx. Support for this position can be found, to a certain extent, in the drafting history. *Subsequent and uniform practice . . .* however, prevails over any drafting history, [and] evidences . . . that states regularly admit large numbers of refugees to cross international borders in that in the relatively few cases of push-backs at the border, other states have protested such behaviour [emphasis added]": W. Kälin, "Towards a Concept of 'Temporary Protection': A Study Commissioned by the UNHRC Division of International Protection," unpublished paper, Nov. 12, 1996, at 13–14. But see chapter 1.1.1 above, at pp. 25–26; and, in particular, chapter 1.3.4 above, at pp. 69–72.

[354] UNHCR Executive Committee Conclusion No. 22, "Protection of Asylum-Seekers in Situations of Large-Scale Influx" (1981), at para. II(A)(2), available at www.unhcr.ch (accessed Nov. 20, 2004).

[355] See chapter 1.3.2 above, at pp. 54–55.

[356] See Lauterpacht and Bethlehem, "*Non-Refoulement*," at para. 105, suggesting that by virtue of UNHCR Executive Committee Conclusion No. 22 "[t]he applicability of the principle [of *non-refoulement*] to [mass influx] situations has . . . been affirmed unambiguously by the Executive Committee."

necessary measures to assist, at their request, States which have admitted asylum-seekers in large-scale influx situations [emphasis added].[357]

This approach draws directly on the language of the Preamble to the Refugee Convention, itself a part of the context of the treaty for interpretive purposes.[358] In the result, Executive Committee Conclusion No. 22 actually suggests an understanding of the duty of *non-refoulement* which disallows state parties any prerogative to deny entry to refugees in a mass influx situation *so long as* there is reason to believe that the risk to their critical national interests occasioned by the mass influx will be countered by timely assistance from other states.[359] Much the same conclusion flows from the limited scope of the mass influx exception as conceived by the drafters of the Convention: states are allowed to deny entry to refugees only in truly exceptional circumstances, and only to the extent truly necessary to protect their most critical national interests.[360]

---

[357] UNHCR Executive Committee Conclusion No. 22, "Protection of Asylum-Seekers in Situations of Large-Scale Influx" (1981), at para. IV(1), available at www.unhcr.ch (accessed Nov. 20, 2004).

[358] "Considering that the grant of asylum may place unduly heavy burdens on certain countries, and that a satisfactory solution of a problem of which the United Nations has recognized the international scope and nature cannot therefore be achieved without international co-operation": Refugee Convention, at Preamble. See generally chapter 1.3.2 above, at p. 53, regarding the importance of a treaty's preamble as a reference point for interpretation.

[359] On the other hand, in a general conclusion not addressed to the context of mass influx, the Executive Committee has affirmed the view that "international solidarity and burden-sharing are of direct importance to the satisfactory implementation of refugee protection principles; [but that] . . . access to asylum and the meeting by States of their protection obligations should not be dependent on burden-sharing arrangements first being in place, particularly because respect for fundamental human rights and humanitarian principles is an obligation for all members of the international community": UNHCR Executive Committee Conclusion No. 85, "Conclusion on International Protection" (1998), at para. (p), available at www.unhcr.ch (accessed Nov. 20, 2004). Not only is this conclusion not clearly oriented to the mass influx situation, but it also begs the question since – if the duty of *non-refoulement* does not extend to circumstances where fundamental interests are threatened by a genuine mass influx – a call to respect protection obligations even without burden-sharing is not infringed by recognition of the implied exception to the duty of *non-refoulement*. But see Eggli, *Mass Influx*, at 229 in which this Conclusion is said to "underscore[ ] that states should always admit these asylum-seekers, at least on a temporary basis . . . in even more explicit and unequivocal terms" than did Conclusion No. 22.

[360] A more recent Conclusion of the Executive Committee which is oriented to the understanding of duties in a mass influx situation seems, however, to take a more absolutist approach, albeit without explicit reference to the duty of *non-refoulement*. "[A]ccess to asylum and the meeting by all States of their international protection obligations should not be dependent on burden and responsibility sharing arrangements first being in place,

Most fundamentally, there can be no question of avoiding the duty of *non-refoulement* under this implied exception where the numbers arriving and the resources of the receiving state are such that security concerns can be addressed under the individuated exceptions set by Art. 33(2).[361] Thus, for example, the American interdiction of the boats of fleeing Haitians was an infringement of the rule against *refoulement*: it simply could not reasonably be said that the circumstances in the country of destination were so fragile, or the number of asylum-seekers so massive in relation to adjudicative and reception resources, that the orderly assessment of claims would have exposed the receiving state to an unacceptable risk. While Nepal's fear of Chinese retaliation may have given it greater reason to fear the security consequences of admitting refugees from Tibet, the number of arrivals was too small to warrant resort to peremptory refusal at the border. Security concerns should rather have been taken into account as part of a post-admission assessment of the threat posed by the refugee.

Even where numbers are significant and the situation of the destination state difficult, the exceptional nature of permissible *refoulement* requires good faith action by the intended state of destination. Derogation from respect for *non-refoulement* is justified in the case of mass influx only where it is the sole realistic option for a state that might otherwise be overwhelmed and unable to protect its most basic national interests.[362] Because it is such an exceptional measure, suspension of protection from *refoulement* must be carried out in a way that is minimally invasive of the human dignity of refugees. While the acute risk to states inherent in particular circumstances will sometimes justify blunt refusals of protection, the limited right of states to engage in *refoulement* should not be interpreted as a form of carte blanche to practice unnecessary harshness. Indeed, the European Union has taken the lead by enacting a Directive on Temporary Protection which eases the procedural expectations of states faced with a mass

---

particularly because respect for human rights and humanitarian principles is a responsibility for all members of the international community": UNHCR Executive Committee Conclusion No. 100, "Conclusion on International Cooperation and Burden and Responsibility Sharing in Mass Influx Situations" (2004), at Preamble. The same Conclusion moreover "[r]eaffirm[s], in regard to mass influx, the guidance on reinforcing burden and responsibility sharing, including in particular that set out in Conclusion No. 22 (XXXII) of 1981 on the protection of asylum-seekers in situations of large-scale influx": ibid. at Preamble.

[361] See chapter 4.1.4 above.

[362] "Venezuela had experienced disturbances, accompanied by violence, in which refugees from various countries had taken part; the people of Venezuela had suffered a great deal during and following those upheavals and they would not accept a convention for refugees which contained any provisions that would prevent them from defending their own institutions. It should be possible to expel all aliens, whether refugees or not, from the territory of a State [if] public order in that State was threatened": Statement of Mr. Perez Perozo of Venezuela, UN Doc. E/AC.32/SR.20, Feb. 1, 1950, at 8.

influx, even as it ensures that *refoulement* is scrupulously avoided and basic rights respected.[363]

Because of the duty to protect the state of arrival's basic interests in the least intrusive way possible, the Thai pushback policy of Vietnamese asylum-seekers was not warranted. Even though more than 500 asylum-seekers were arriving every week, Thailand effectively put itself in a position of admin-istrative incapacity by refusing an offer from the United States to build new facilities to provide for the refugees.[364] The *refoulement* of often desperately dehydrated and starving refugees back to sea was moreover unnecessarily brutal, and appears to have resulted less from specific security concerns than from a simple determination to avoid responsibility for refugees.[365] Nor can there be any excuse for the vigilante-style ejection of Rwandese and Ugandans from Kenya, or for the violent "chasing back" of refugees from Guinea. Objection may also be taken to both the South African electrified fence along its border, and the British–French double fence near Calais: these barriers effected the rejection of refugees in a way that was both too per-manent and absolutely unselective, thus failing to meet security concerns in the least rights-intrusive means possible. While no doubt a closer case,[366] Macedonia's 1999 closure of its border to Kosovo Albanian refugees appears to have been less a truly unavoidable act premised on necessity than a bargaining chip to garner increased support from other countries to cope with the refugee flow. As Eggli has concluded, Macedonia was "playing politics with refugees,"[367] making it difficult to see its actions as limited to strictly what was required in order to avoid fundamental risk to its own most basic interests.

---

[363] Council Directive on minimum standards for giving protection in the event of a mass influx of displaced persons and on the measures promoting a balance of efforts between Member States in receiving such persons and bearing the consequences thereof, Doc. 2001/55/EC (July 20, 2001) (EU Temporary Protection Directive). See generally W. Kälin, "Temporary Protection in the EC: Refugee Law, Human Rights, and the Temptations of Pragmatism," (2001) 44 *German Yearbook of International Law* 221; and J. Hathaway, "What's in a Label?," (2003) 5 *European Journal of Migration and Law* 1 (Hathaway, "Label").

[364] Helton, "Thailand," at 27.

[365] Deputy Interior Minister Somphon Klinphongsa is quoted as having stated that "the Government's policy is ... [w]e don't want our country regarded as a country of first acceptance because refugees could remain for 10 or even 20 years": ibid.

[366] There is no doubt that the security situation for Macedonia was grave: the number of refugees seeking entry was nearly 20 percent of the host country's population, and would – if admitted more than strictly temporarily – seriously exacerbate an already volatile political situation by fundamentally changing Macedonia's ethnic balance. See M. Barutciski and A. Suhrke, "Lessons from the Kosovo Refugee Crisis: Innovations in Protection and Burden-Sharing," (2001) 14(2) *Journal of Refugee Studies* 95.

[367] Eggli, *Mass Influx*, at 225.

A more compelling case can, however, be made for the legality of the border closings by Zaïre and Tanzania in the face of refugee flows from Rwanda and Burundi. Both states had been overwhelmed by hundreds of thousands of refugees, and were faced by the imminent prospect of additional flows at the time of the border closures. At least in the case of Zaïre, there was also good reason to believe that internal security could be threatened by the entry of refugees, many of whom were suspected of having committed serious criminal offenses. The decisions to suspend border crossings were moreover of limited duration, while efforts to secure international resources to protect refugees were being pursued. The desperate circumstances in Zaïre and Tanzania, and their good faith approach to a context-specific practice of *refoulement*, does not make the results any less tragic for the refugees who were denied access to safety. This situation does, however, provide an example of states confronted by the sort of "prisoner's dilemma" that the drafters of the Convention intended to be resolved in favor of the populations of states of destination.

Clearly, however, reliance on an implied exception to limit the duty of *non-refoulement* where critical interests are at stake in a mass influx is not a happy solution. It is unsatisfactory not only because it leaves refugees without protection, but also because it leaves states with only a very blunt tool to respond to difficult circumstances. UNHCR is moreover right that "[t]he need for greater clarity concerning the scope of international protection in mass influx situations is apparent, not least in view of the varying responses that have been used to address mass displacement."[368] While the agency coyly suggests that "there is nothing inherent in *the provisions of* the 1951 Convention and 1967 Protocol to preclude [them] being applied in mass influx situations [emphasis added],"[369] there is nonetheless value in UNHCR's call to explore the possibility of "another authoritative text, in addition to the 1951 Convention" to address the ways in which refugee law in general – and the duty of *non-refoulement* in particular – should be applied when the arrival of refugees genuinely imperils the most fundamental interests of receiving states.[370] Fairly conceived, an optional protocol or other agreement should bind all state parties to come to the aid of a country experiencing a mass influx by way of both burden *and* responsibility sharing; in return, it should

---

[368] UNHCR, "Protection of Refugees in Mass Influx Situations: Overall Protection Framework," UN Doc. EC/GC/01/4, Feb. 19, 2001 (UNHCR, "Mass Influx"), at para. 1.

[369] Ibid. at para. 17.

[370] Executive Committee of the High Commissioner's Program, "Agenda for Protection," UN Doc. EC/52/SC/CRP.9/Rev.1, June 26, 2002, at Part III, Goal 1, Point 10. Some general guidance on this point is now afforded by UNHCR Executive Committee Conclusion No. 100, "Conclusion on International Cooperation and Burden and Responsibility Sharing in Mass Influx Situations" (2004), available at www.unhcr.ch (accessed Nov. 20, 2004).

commit the receiving state so aided to respect all applicable refugee and other international human rights.[371] With the benefit of such a system, no state could legitimately invoke the mass influx exception to the duty of *non-refoulement* implicit in Art. 33, since the support received would negate the *in extremis* argument which is an essential condition for its application.

4.1.6 An expanded concept of non-refoulement?

There is insufficient evidence to justify the claim that the duty to avoid the *refoulement* of refugees has evolved at the universal level beyond the scope of Art. 33 of the Refugee Convention. The variants of this position that are relevant to this discussion are the assertion that *non-refoulement* has come to encompass non-rejection at the frontier, and that the principle as a whole is now properly viewed as a matter of universally binding customary international law.[372] There is, of course, no need to assess the first aspect of this alleged evolution, since *non-refoulement* as defined in Art. 33 has always included both ejection from a state and non-admission at the frontier.[373] In contrast, the claim that *non-refoulement* is no longer strictly a matter of conventional law, but is now automatically binding on all states as a matter of custom, is clearly deserving of attention.

In chapter 1 consideration was given to the tendency of some scholars to overlook the requirements of customary international lawmaking when validating the existence of new principles of universal human rights law.[374] The position taken there is that a universally binding norm cannot be brought into existence by simple declaration. Rather, a large and representative part of the community of states must concretize its commitment to a particular principle through its actions. Customary law is not simply a matter of words, wherever spoken and however frequently recited: custom can evolve only through interstate practice in which governments effectively agree to be bound through the medium of their conduct. This standard simply is not yet met in the case of the duty of *non-refoulement*.

---

[371] See UNHCR, "Mass Influx," at para. 8: "In its Conclusion No. 22 adopted in 1981, the Executive Committee defined minimum standards of immediate treatment in situations of large-scale influx. For UNHCR as well as for affected States, this Conclusion remains an important yardstick against which to measure such treatment in a mass influx of refugees. It is important to note, however, that the Conclusion was never intended as a substitute for standards of protection under the 1951 Convention."

[372] These arguments are advanced in G. Goodwin-Gill, "*Nonrefoulement* and the New Asylum Seekers," in D. Martin ed., *The New Asylum Seekers: Refugee Law in the 1980s* (1986), at 103. The author also advances a third claim, namely that some persons outside the scope of the Convention refugee definition are the beneficiaries of protection against *refoulement*. This last claim is answered in Hathaway, *Refugee Status*, at 24–27.

[373] See chapter 4.1.2 above, at pp. 315–317.

[374] See in particular chapter 1.1 above, at pp. 16–17; and chapter 1.1.1 above, at pp. 25–26.

It is of course true that there are many official pronouncements by UNHCR and others to the effect that *non-refoulement* is part of customary international law.[375] Of perhaps greatest significance, in 2001 the state parties to the Refugee Convention formally acknowledged "the principle of *non-refoulement*, whose applicability is imbedded in customary international law."[376] Yet even the *opinio juris* component of the test for customary status is not clearly satisfied, as most states of Asia and the Near East have routinely refused to be formally bound to avoid *refoulement*.[377] The Chief Justice of India, for example, has affirmed that while courts in his country "have stepped in" on occasion to prevent refugee deportations, "most often these are *ad hoc* orders. And an *ad hoc* order certainly does not advance the law. It does not form part of the law, and it certainly does not make the area clear."[378]

Most fundamentally, however, it is absolutely untenable to suggest that there is anything approaching near-universal respect among states for the principle of *non-refoulement*. To the contrary, as the recounting of state practice at the beginning of this chapter makes depressingly clear, *refoulement* still remains part of the reality for significant numbers of refugees, in most parts of the world. Indeed, the United Nations Commission on Human Rights has formally expressed its "distress" at the "widespread violation of

---

[375] A typical example is the "San Remo Declaration on the Principle of *Non-Refoulement*," issued by the International Institute of Humanitarian Law in San Remo, Italy. The San Remo Declaration is succinct: "The principle of *non-refoulement* of refugees incorporated in Article 33 of the Convention relating to the Status of Refugees of 28 July 1951 is an integral part of customary international law": ibid. In the accompanying explanatory note, the authors invoke the fact that "in the last half-century, no State has expelled or returned a refugee to the frontiers of a country where his life or freedom would be in danger ... using the argument that *refoulement* is permissible under contemporary international law": ibid. But the absence of an assertion that acts of *refoulement* are justified by legal norms is clearly not the same thing as the existence of state practice which affirms a duty not to send refugees back. The Declaration also invokes the view of the International Court of Justice that a customary norm is not defeated by subsequent inconsistent practice so long as that practice is defended as consistent with the customary norm itself. But this understanding applies only to conduct which occurs after the customary norm comes into existence – the Court did not suggest (as the San Remo Declaration impliedly does) that a customary international norm can be established (rather than not undermined) by inconsistent practice justified by reference to the putative norm.

[376] "Declaration of States Parties to the 1951 Convention and/or its 1967 Protocol relating to the Status of Refugees," UN Doc. HCR/MMSP/2001/09, Dec. 13, 2001, at para. 4, incorporated in Executive Committee of the High Commissioner's Program, "Agenda for Protection," UN Doc. EC/52/SC/CRP.9/Rev.1, June 26, 2002.

[377] See K. Hailbronner, "*Nonrefoulement* and 'Humanitarian' Refugees: Customary International Law or Wishful Legal Thinking?," in D. Martin ed., *The New Asylum Seekers: Refugee Law in the 1980s* (1986), at 128–129.

[378] J. S. Verma, "Inaugural Address," in UNHCR and SAARCLAW, *Seminar Report: Refugees in the SAARC Region: Building a Legal Framework* (1997), at 13–18.

the principle of *non-refoulement* and of the rights of refugees."[379] The effort to disguise this fact by reference to the institutional positions and practices of UNHCR mistakenly assumes that the work of international agencies can *per se* give rise to international law binding on states.

The most recent effort to assert the customary international legal status of the duty of *non-refoulement* suggests that because all but nineteen UN member states "participat[e] in some or other conventional arrangement embodying *non-refoulement*"[380] – that is, they have all agreed to be bound by at least *one of* Art. 33 of the Refugee Convention, Art. 3 of the Torture Convention, Arts. 6 and 7 of the Civil and Political Covenant, or by a comparable provision under a relevant regional treaty – it is now possible to conclude that "*non-refoulement* must be regarded as a principle of customary international law."[381] It is of course true that when a treaty-based norm stimulates a broadly embraced sense of obligation and general practice among states in general (in particular, among non-party states), a cognate customary international legal obligation emerges.[382] But there is no basis to assert that just because most countries have accepted some kind of *non-refoulement* obligation, applying to at least some kinds of cases, and in at least some contexts (many not involving refugees at all), it can now be concluded that there is a universally applicable duty of *non-refoulement* owed to refugees by all states – including the forty-five or so which have opted not to accede to either the Refugee Convention or Protocol.

Moreover, the nature of the various duties of *non-refoulement* relied upon is highly variable, and therefore does not afford the basis for even a common *opinio juris*, much less for general respect of that norm in practice. As such, even if some form of a duty of *non-refoulement* is owed by nearly all states to at least some people, there is no basis to conclude that "[t]he content of the customary principle of *non-refoulement* in a refugee context corresponds largely to ... the interpretation of Article 33 of the Refugee Convention."[383]

The net result of the persistent overstatement of the reach of custom is not, as presumably hoped, the effective incorporation of new standards into a clear and practical system of enforceable duties.[384] For example, the English courts were recently invited by UNHCR to find that the duty of *non-refoulement* should be deemed to have evolved beyond the text of Art. 33 in order to prohibit efforts to stymie the departure from their own countries of would-be refugees. UNHCR frankly acknowledged that its submissions to this

---

[379] UN Commission on Human Rights, Res. 1997/75.
[380] Lauterpacht and Bethlehem, "Non-Refoulement," at para. 210.   [381] Ibid. at para. 216.
[382] *North Sea Continental Shelf Cases (Federal Republic of Germany/Denmark; Federal Republic of Germany/Netherlands)*, [1969] ICJ Rep 3, at para. 74.
[383] Lauterpacht and Bethlehem, "Non-Refoulement," at para. 218.
[384] See chapter 1.1 above, at p. 18.

end did "not turn on the text of the Refugee Convention. Rather, they turn on understanding the international protection regime as a complex of international practice and precepts drawn from refugee law, human rights law, and general principles of international law ... Where, as in the present case, issues arise that strictly do not fall within the Convention's textual scope, its objectives and purposes should act as a reliable guide."[385]

Both the Court of Appeal and House of Lords rejected this argument in clear terms. The Court of Appeal cited with approval the view of the International Court of Justice that "although the principle of good faith is 'one of the most basic principles concerning the creation and performance of legal obligations ... it is not in itself a source of obligation where none would otherwise exist'."[386] The House of Lords was insistent that despite the obvious benefit to at-risk persons of expanding the scope of the duty of non-refoulement beyond what Art. 33 requires, there simply was not sufficient evidence of relatively consistent state practice to substantiate a relevant customary norm.[387] In the words of the High Court of Australia in a decision endorsed by both the English Court of Appeal and House of Lords,

> the Convention, like many international and municipal instruments, does not necessarily pursue its primary purpose at all costs. The purpose of an instrument may instead be pursued in a limited way, reflecting the accommodation of the differing viewpoints, the desire for limited achievement of objectives, or the constraints imposed by limited resources ...
> It would therefore be wrong to depart from the demands of language and context by invoking the humanitarian objectives of the Convention

---

[385] *R (European Roma Rights Centre and Others) v. Immigration Officer at Prague Airport*, [2003] EWCA Civ 666 (Eng. CA, May 20, 2003), at para. 28; and *R v. Immigration Officer at Prague Airport et al., ex parte European Roma Rights Centre et al.*, [2004] UKHL 55 (UK HL, Dec. 9, 2004), at paras. 22–23. Importantly, the House of Lords acknowledged the general view that "[t]he existence of the convention is no obstacle in principle to the development of an ancillary or supplementary body of law, more generous than the Convention in its application to those seeking asylum as refugees": ibid. at para. 23.

[386] *R (European Roma Rights Centre and Others) v. Immigration Officer at Prague Airport*, [2003] EWCA Civ 666 (Eng. CA, May 20, 2003), at para. 45, citing the decision on preliminary objections in *Cameroon v. Nigeria*, [1998] ICJ Rep 2, at para. 39. The House of Lords reached the same conclusion: *R v. Immigration Officer at Prague Airport et al., ex parte European Roma Rights Centre et al.*, [2004] UKHL 55 (UK HL, Dec. 9, 2004), at paras. 19, 57–62.

[387] "In considering whether the rule contended for has received the assent of the nations, it is pertinent to recall that the states parties to the 1951 Convention have not, despite much international discussion, agreed to revise its terms or extend its scope at any time since 1967 ... The House was referred to no judicial decision supporting the rule contended for ... Have the states in practice observed such a rule? It seems to me clear that they have not": *R v. Immigration Officer at Prague Airport et al., ex parte European Roma Rights Centre et al.*, [2004] UKHL 55 (UK HL Dec. 9, 2004), at para. 28.

without appreciating the limits which the Convention itself places on the achievement of them.[388]

Not only are courts disinclined to accept policy claims simply because they are advanced as customary legal claims,[389] but there is a real risk that wishful legal thinking about the scope of the duty of *non-refoulement* may send the signal that customary law as a whole is essentially rhetorical, with a resultant dilution of emphasis on the real value of those norms which really have been accepted as binding by a substantial majority of states. There is no doubt that many refugees will benefit from at least one of the various treaty-based duties of *non-refoulement*; it may also be the case that the increasing propensity of states to embrace *non-refoulement* of some kind in their domestic laws[390] may at some point give rise to at least a lowest common denominator claim based on a new general principle of law.[391] But it is simply disingenuous to assert that there is presently a universal duty of *non-refoulement* that is substantively in line with the provisions of Art. 33 and which is owed to all refugees, by all states.

In sum, most threats to the ability of refugees to enter and remain in an asylum state are in fact answered by a good faith interpretation of the Refugee Convention's prohibition of *refoulement*. There are, however, three significant gaps in the protective ambit of Art. 33. First and most fundamentally, the duty of *non-refoulement* does not constrain policies such as visa controls implemented in countries of origin, or interstate agreements to deter migration. Until and unless refugees actually leave their own state, they are not legally entitled to protection against *refoulement*, or to any other refugee rights. Second, individuals who are refugees, but who pose a risk to the national security of the state of reception, or who are particularly serious criminals who endanger its community, cannot claim protection against *refoulement* by virtue of the express exceptions set by Art. 33(2). Third, the duty of *non-refoulement* does not bind a state faced with a mass influx of refugees insofar as the arrival of refugees truly threatens its ability to protect its most basic national interests.

---

[388] *Applicant "A" and Ano'r v. Minister for Immigration and Multicultural Affairs*, (1997) 190 CLR 225 (Aus. HC, Feb. 24, 1997), per Dawson J, adopted in *R (European Roma Rights Centre and Others) v. Immigration Officer at Prague Airport*, [2003] EWCA Civ 666 (Eng. CA, May 20, 2003), at para. 36.

[389] A notable exception appears to be the New Zealand Court of Appeal, which adopted without independent analysis the view that "[t]he prohibition on refoulement, contained in art. 33(1) of the Refugee Convention, is generally thought to be part of customary international law": *Attorney General v. Zaoui*, Dec. No. CA20/04 (NZ CA, Sept. 30, 2004), at paras. 34–36.

[390] See Lauterpacht and Bethlehem, "*Non-Refoulement*," at Annex 2.2, indicating that some 125 states have thus far incorporated some aspect of a duty of *non-refoulement* in their domestic law.

[391] See chapter 1.2.2 above.

The last of these gaps – the implied exception to the duty of *non-refoulement* for refugees arriving as part of a mass influx – could be answered by more effective international burden- and responsibility-sharing arrangements.[392] The alternative of simply expanding the notion of *non-refoulement* to mass influx situations would, in contrast, exact an inappropriately high cost to the collective survival of states of destination that happen to be in the refugees' path of flight. The second concern might similarly be answered by a combination of responsibility sharing to relocate refugees to states in which they do not constitute a security risk, and burden sharing to finance the cost of allowing criminal refugees the option of incarceration or other appropriate custodial arrangements as an alternative to *refoulement*. The first dilemma is, however, the most intractable. So long as states remain adamant that there is no binding duty to allow at-risk persons to seek asylum in other countries,[393] it may be difficult to conceive an adequate international legal response to modes of *non-entrée* that effectively imprison would-be refugees within their own states. Reliance on the right of "everyone to leave any country" set by Art. 12(2) of the Civil and Political Covenant certainly has real potential value. But with the dissipation of the political and economic concerns that once sustained the commitment to refugee protection in the industrialized world, we can unfortunately expect to see an exacerbation of the tendency to endorse visa controls, carrier sanctions, and migration control agreements as exclusionary mechanisms. As a practical matter, only a fundamental recasting of the objectives and modalities of refugee protection has any realistic chance of persuading states to relinquish their tools of refugee deterrence.[394]

While beyond the scope of this book, it should be noted that evolution in treaties outside of international refugee law provides important support to the Refugee Convention's duty of *non-refoulement* as a means of facilitating entry of at least those at-risk persons able to exit their own state.[395] Art. 3(1) of the United Nations Convention against Torture, for example, explicitly prohibits the return of a person to another state where there are substantial

---

[392] See Epilogue below, at pp. 998–1002.

[393] The continued unwillingness of the community of nations to override sovereign discretion over immigration control even in situations of compelling humanitarian concern is reflected in the purely permissive nature of the "right to seek and enjoy asylum" in the Universal Declaration of Human Rights, in the absence of a duty to grant asylum in the Declaration on Territorial Asylum, and in the complete failure of the 1977 United Nations Conference on Territorial Asylum. See A. Grahl-Madsen, *Territorial Asylum* (1980).

[394] See J. Hathaway and A. Neve, "Making International Refugee Law Relevant Again: A Proposal for Collectivized and Solution-Oriented Protection," (1997) 10 *Harvard Human Rights Journal* 115; and J. Hathaway ed., *Reconceiving International Refugee Law* (1997).

[395] See Lauterpacht and Bethlehem, "*Non-Refoulement*," at paras. 5–9, 220–253.

grounds to perceive a risk of subjection to torture.[396] Arts. 6 and 7 of the International Covenant on Civil and Political Rights, which respectively require state parties to avert the arbitrary deprivation of life and to ensure that nobody is subject to cruel, inhuman or degrading treatment or punishment, have similarly been interpreted by the Human Rights Committee to prohibit removal of individuals from a state's territory to face a relevant risk:

> [T]he article 2 obligation requiring that States Parties respect and ensure the Covenant rights for all persons in their territory and all persons under their control entails an obligation not to extradite, deport, expel or otherwise remove a person from their territory, where there are substantial grounds for believing that there is a real risk of irreparable harm, such as that contemplated by articles 6 and 7 of the Covenant, either in the country to which removal is to be effected or in any country to which the person may subsequently be removed. The relevant judicial and administrative authorities should be made aware of the need to ensure compliance with the Covenant obligations in such matters.[397]

In addition to a clear duty not to return anyone to face grave risks to their physical security, there is nascent support for the view that state parties to the European Convention on Human Rights and Fundamental Freedoms will not be allowed to remove persons who face the risk of a particularly serious violation of a fairly wide range of human rights.[398] Beyond norms of non-return derived from human rights law, there is tentative judicial authority for the view that international humanitarian law should be construed to preclude the forcible repatriation of aliens who have fled generalized violence or other threats to their security arising out of internal armed conflict in their state of nationality.[399]

For at least some refugees, therefore, the insufficiency of the *non-refoulement* guarantee set by Art. 33 of the Refugee Convention is effectively

---

[396] "The Committee must decide, pursuant to paragraph 1 of article 3, whether there are substantial grounds for believing that Mr. Khan would be in danger of being subject to torture. In reaching this conclusion, the Committee must take into account all relevant considerations, pursuant to paragraph 2 of article 3, including the existence of a consistent pattern of gross, flagrant or mass violations of human rights. The aim of the determination, however, is to establish whether the individual concerned would be personally at risk of being subjected to torture in the country to which he would return ... additional grounds must exist to indicate that the individual concerned would be personally at risk": *Khan v. Canada*, UNCAT Comm. No. 15, UN Doc. CAT/C/13/D/15/1994, decided July 4, 1994, at 10.

[397] UN Human Rights Committee, "General Comment No. 31: The nature of the general legal obligation imposed on states parties to the Covenant" (2004), UN Doc. HRI/GEN/1/Rev.7, May 12, 2004, at 192, para. 12.

[398] See *R (Ullah) v. Special Adjudicator; Do v. Secretary of State for the Home Department*, [2004] UKHL 26 (UK HL, June 17, 2004).

[399] See e.g. *Orelien v. Canada*, [1992] 1 FC 592 (Can. FCA, Nov. 22, 1991); and *In re Santos*, Dec. No. A29–564–781 (US IC, Aug. 24, 1990).

remedied by the ability to invoke other standards of international law. Courts have moreover appropriately held that where a state is bound by a duty of non-return external to the Refugee Convention, the state concerned may not invoke the flexibility afforded by Art. 33 in order to counter its other legal responsibilities.[400]

4.2 Freedom from arbitrary detention and penalization for illegal entry

The ability simply to enter and remain in an asylum state is cold comfort for many refugees. As UNHCR observes, "it frequently occurs that the necessary distinction is not made either in law or in administrative practice between asylum-seekers and ordinary aliens seeking to enter the territory. The absence of such a distinction may, and in many cases does, lead to asylum-seekers being punished and detained for illegal entry in the same manner as illegal aliens."[401]

---

[400] See *Chahal v. United Kingdom*, (1996) 23 EHRR 413 (ECHR, Nov. 15, 1996), in which the court rejected the state party's argument that account should be taken of considerations of international security of the kind recognized as valid constraints on *refoulement* under Art. 33 of the Refugee Convention in order to determine obligations under Art. 3 of the European Convention. The argument was also rejected by the Supreme Court of Canada in *Suresh v. Canada*, [2002] 1 SCR 3 (Can. SC, Jan. 11, 2002): "In our view, the prohibition in the Civil and Political Covenant and the [Convention Against Torture] on returning a refugee to face the risk of torture reflects the prevailing international norm. Article 33 of the Refugee Convention protects, in a limited way, refugees from threats to life and freedom from all sources. By contrast, the CAT protects everyone, without derogation, from state-sponsored torture. Moreover, the Refugee Convention itself expresses a 'profound concern for refugees' and its principal purpose is to 'assure refugees the widest possible exercise of ... fundamental rights and freedoms.' This negates the suggestion that the provisions of the Refugee Convention should be used to deny rights that other legal instruments make universally available to everyone." The UN Human Rights Committee has moreover found even the minimal discretion to remove a person at risk of torture identified by the Supreme Court of Canada in *Suresh* to be viable under Canadian domestic law to be of doubtful legality. "The Committee does however refer, in conclusion, to the Supreme Court's holding in *Suresh* that deportation of an individual where a substantial risk of torture had been found to exist was not necessarily precluded in all circumstances. While it has neither been determined by the State party's domestic courts nor by the Committee that a substantial risk of torture did exist in the author's case, the Committee expresses no further view on this issue other than to note that the prohibition on torture, including as expressed in article 7 of the Covenant, is an absolute one that is not subject to countervailing considerations": *Ahani v. Canada*, UNHRC Comm. No. 1051/2002, UN Doc. CCPR/C/80/D/1051/2002, decided Mar. 29, 2004, at para. 10.10.

[401] UNHCR, "Note on Accession to International Instruments and the Detention of Refugees and Asylum Seekers," UN Doc. EC/SCP/44, Aug. 19, 1986 (UNHCR, "Detention Note"), at para. 33.

In some cases, there has simply been no effort to enact specific protections for refugees. In Thailand, for example, refugees without valid passports and visas are not distinguished from other illegal immigrants under the Immigration Act, and are therefore subject to arrest and deportation absent an exercise of ministerial discretion.[402] Gambia has charged asylum-seekers from Senegal with the offense of entering the country without a residence permit, and expelled them without trial.[403] The UNHCR intervened in 2001 to prevent Malawi from refusing to protect refugees from the Democratic Republic of Congo on the grounds that they did not have the required documentation to enter the country.[404] In Kenya, even refugees who had been issued UNHCR documentation were arrested and detained unless able to pay a bribe to officials.[405] Zambian officials have arrested and detained refugees as "illegal immigrants."[406] Zimbabwe arrested refugees from Rwanda for "flouting immigration laws," specifically because they crossed the border at illegal entry points.[407]

Even in states with refugee-specific legislation, the laws may not clearly preempt inconsistent immigration laws. Thus, many asylum-seekers are in practice subject to the same penalties for illegal entry as other aliens in

---

[402] "The declared policy of the Thai government since 1993 has been to force a 'crackdown' on 'illegal immigrants' within the country. Thailand does have large numbers of 'illegal immigrants,' many of whom come to the Kingdom in search of work. However, a proportion of people who enter the country 'illegally,' without documentation, are asylum-seekers and refugees, fleeing from human rights violations in their own countries. The current policy of the Thai government does not make any allowance for the special situation of those who are asylum-seekers or refugees, and the majority of those arrested without adequate documentation are prosecuted and detained for 'illegal immigration' regardless of their reason for being in the country. Once an asylum-seeker or refugee is arrested and found not to be in possession of appropriate documentation, the prosecution and detention for 'illegal immigration' follows automatically, even if this person is a UNHCR-registered 'person of concern'": Amnesty International, "Thailand: Burmese and Other Asylum-Seekers at Risk" (1994), at 3. This policy is of long-standing duration: see Lawyers' Committee for Human Rights, *Uncertain Haven* (1991), at 32–39; and T. Banbury, "Kampuchean Displaced Persons in Thailand: Between the Devil and the Deep Blue Sea," unpublished manuscript authored for the Harvard Law School Human Rights Program (1988) (Banbury, "Kampuchean Displaced Persons in Thailand").

[403] Amnesty International, "The Gambia: Forcible Expulsion (*Refoulement*) of Senegalese Asylum Seekers" (1990), at 1.

[404] "[T]he UNHCR chief in Malawi, Michael Owor, accused the government of flouting international conventions on refugees ... 'Refugees don't need papers. What sort of papers do they want?,' he said": *SAPA-SFP* (Blantyre), Apr. 17, 2001.

[405] G. Verdirame, "Human Rights and Refugees: The Case of Kenya," (1999) 12(1) *Journal of Refugee Studies* 54 (Verdirame, "Kenya"), at 59–61.

[406] In May 2000, UNHCR was able successfully to secure the release of refugees arrested for illegal presence in Zambia: *Post of Zambia*, May 29, 2000.

[407] *Daily News* (Harare), Feb. 21, 2003.

Bulgaria[408] and in Russia.[409] South African police have rounded up and detained asylum-seekers – including many with valid documents – as part of general operations to catch illegal immigrants and suspected criminals.[410] New Zealand law authorizes the prosecution of refugee claimants who seek protection there in reliance on false identity documents;[411] in the United Kingdom, even refugees in transit to a third state may be subject to criminal penalties for producing a non-genuine travel document.[412]

Illegal entry may also entail negative consequences for refugees short of prosecution under criminal or immigration laws. For example, the Illegal

---

[408] "Routinely confused with illegal migrants, asylum-seekers are frequently subject to measures restricting their freedom of movement, which amount to detention. This is particularly true at Sofia international airport, where there are numerous cases of foreigners being held (detained) in the transit zone until deportation is feasible, without any opportunity to submit an asylum application, without the length of their detention being regulated, and under inappropriate conditions – nowhere to sleep, or wash, no privacy, etc.": F. Liebaut, *Legal and Social Conditions for Asylum Seekers and Refugees in Central and Eastern European Countries* (1999) (Liebaut, *Conditions 1999*), at 9, available at www.flygtning.dk (accessed Dec. 12, 2003).

[409] "Because most far-abroad asylum-seekers, including those registered with UNHCR, never receive refugee status, Russian authorities consider them to be illegal migrants. Without legal status, they are denied most rights, including the right to work, receive social services and non-emergency medical care, and even to register marriages and births. Many schools do not accept the children of far-abroad asylum-seekers because of their illegal status": US Committee for Refugees, *World Refugee Survey 2002* (2002), at 238. To make matters worse, "[t]here continues to be widespread ignorance of refugee law ... on the part of [Russian] officials": UK Home Office, Immigration and Nationality Directorate, "Russian Federation Country Assessment" (2002), at para. 6.58.

[410] "In March 2000, during a highly publicized crackdown on crime, many refugees and asylum-seekers were illegally arrested, and [Jesuit Refugee Service] staff worked long hours each day to get some detainees out of Lindela [Repatriation Centre]": (2000) 84 *JRS Dispatches* (Dec. 18, 2000); see also (2000) 68 *JRS Dispatches* (Apr. 1, 2000) and Human Rights Watch, "South Africa Immigration Crackdown – Human Rights Groups Condemn Abuse of Refugees, Asylum-Seekers, and South Africans," May 11, 2000.

[411] In New Zealand, persons who present false documents when they arrive to seek protection, and who assume the fraudulent identity in order to secure an entry permit, may be prosecuted under s. 142(1) of the Immigration Act 1987, s. 31 of the Passports Act 1997, and/or ss. 233 and 266(1)(a) of the Crimes Act 1961. In practice, however, where prosecution occurs the case is normally adjourned pending the determination of refugee status; if refugee status is recognized, the charge is likely to be withdrawn: R. Haines, *International Academy of Comparative Law National Report for New Zealand* (1994), at 49; and R. Haines, personal communication, Sept. 9. 2003.

[412] The United Kingdom has prosecuted even asylum-seekers transiting through that country en route to North America: Amnesty International, "Cell Culture: The Detention and Imprisonment of Asylum Seekers in the United Kingdom" (1996), at 26–37; and Amnesty International, "Dead Starlings: An Update to the Amnesty International UK Report 'Cell Culture: The Detention and Imprisonment of Asylum Seekers in the United Kingdom'" (1997), at 8.

Immigration Reform and Immigrant Responsibility Act of 1996[413] provides that persons arriving in the United States without proper and valid immigration documentation are to be summarily removed from the country.[414] While not exempted from the general rule requiring summary expulsion for entry without valid documentation, refugee claimants are referred to a summary hearing to determine whether they have a "credible fear" of persecution in their country of origin.[415] If successful at this inquiry, asylum-seekers are allowed to remain in the country pending the assessment of their claims to protection and are not prosecuted for their illegal entry.[416] But unlike refugees who arrive with valid documentation, undocumented asylum-seekers are denied the right to appeal a negative assessment reached under the expedited removal process.[417] A proposal advanced by the United Kingdom in 2003 would have gone farther still: refugees arriving without documentation in a European Union state would have been required to make their case for protection under a rudimentary procedure conducted in an external processing center, rather than being admitted to a domestic asylum system.[418]

Even more seriously, some countries impose deadlines for the receipt of an application for protection as a refugee. Immediately after acceding to the Refugee Convention in 2000, for example, Mexico passed regulations under which it generally refuses to consider claims lodged more than fifteen days after the refugee's arrival in the country.[419] Poland implemented a similar regime, giving refugees only fourteen days within which to seek protection absent extenuating circumstances based on risks to life or health, or because the claim is based on facts which arose after entry.[420] Turkey imposed a five-day filing deadline (subsequently extended to ten days) – but these rules were later struck down by courts.[421]

---

[413] Pub. L. No. 104–208, 110 Stat. 3009 (1996), enacted as Division C of the Omnibus Appropriations Act of 1996, now codified in the Immigration and Nationality Act, 8 USCA § 1225.

[414] Immigration and Nationality Act, 8 USCA § 1225(b)(1)(A)(I).

[415] Ibid. at § 1225(b)(1)(B)(v).   [416] Ibid. at § 1225(b)(1)(A)(ii), b(1)(C).

[417] See generally K. Musalo, "Report on the First Three Years of Implementation of Expedited Removal," (2000) 15 *Notre Dame Journal of Law, Ethics & Public Policy* 1.

[418] "The lack of proper documentation is unrelated to protection need – a person arriving without passport and visa can obviously have valid reasons for seeking asylum. Channelling such persons into [transit processing centers] providing decreased procedural and material protection for deterrent reasons might raise issues under Article 31 of the 1951 Refugee Convention, prohibiting the imposition of penalties": Noll, "Transit Processing," at 330.

[419] Under Art. 166(VII)(a) of the Regulations of the General Law on Population, a waiver of the deadline is possible in the case of persons who become refugees *sur place*: G. Kuhner, "Detention of Asylum Seekers in Mexico," (2002) 20(3) *Refuge* 58, at 59.

[420] (1998) 5/6 *ECRE Documentation Service*.

[421] K. Kirisci, "UNHCR and Turkey: Nudging towards a Better Implementation of the 1951 Convention on the Status of Refugees" (2001), at 11–12.

By far the most common consequence of a refugee's unauthorized arrival in an asylum country is that he or she will be detained or otherwise denied internal freedom of movement.[422] In January 2001, India began detaining refugees coming from Sri Lanka in order to deter further arrivals.[423] Refugees from Pakistan arriving in Swaziland have been taken to Sidwashini Prison for having "trespassed" on Swazi territory.[424] Namibian immigration officials threatened to prosecute any citizen who failed to report an Angolan refugee in the country without authorization; once located, the refugees were forcibly transported to camps hundreds of kilometers away from the towns and villages where they had taken shelter.[425] Burmese refugees allowed to remain in Thailand after recognition of their status by UNHCR were told by the government that they would have to live in camps on the Thai–Burmese border – but were provided no assistance to travel there, and were not even guaranteed admission upon arrival at the camps.[426]

The detention of refugees is often the result of the application of general laws which authorize the detention without charge of any unauthorized migrant. In Belgium, this automatic right of detention may last for two months,[427] in

---

[422] "Although State Members of the Executive Committee adopted [Conclusion No. 44 (XXXVII)] by consensus, the recommendations contained therein appear to have had very little impact on the practice of a number of states as regards detention of refugees and asylum-seekers. On the contrary, detention under harsh conditions, for long periods and without justifiable cause has recently increased": UNHCR, "Note on International Protection," UN Doc. A/AC.96/713, Aug. 15, 1988, at para. 21. See also UNHCR, "Opening Statement by Mr. Ruud Lubbers, United Nations High Commissioner for Refugees," Sept. 30, 2002: "I am particularly concerned about the problem of detention of asylum-seekers. While many States have been able to manage their asylum systems without detentions, a more general trend towards increased use of detention – often on a discriminatory basis – is worrying."

[423] "In another attempt to deter refugees coming from the island's war zones in the north, the Indian government is detaining new arrivals in an area in the transit camp, which has been converted into a mini-jail. Conditions are appalling, as men, women and children are holed up in this overcrowded space": (2001) 85 *JRS Dispatches* (Jan. 17. 2001).

[424] "Over 12 Pakistani refugees kept at Sidwashini Prison," *Times of Swaziland*, Oct. 16, 2002.

[425] "Namibia Citizens Who Help Non-Citizens to be Dealt with Severely," *Nampa/MFAIB*, Apr. 18, 2001.

[426] (2000) 67 *JRS Dispatches* (Mar. 15, 2000).

[427] "[B]order asylum-seekers who are undocumented or whose identity cannot be estab-lished can be detained . . . during the processing of their claim under the admissibility procedure. In-country applicants who entered the country illegally may also be detained during this period, but this is rather exceptional. The detention lasts until a decision on admissibility is made, though no longer than two months . . . However, the two-month detention period can be renewed by the Minister . . . The maximum period of detention – including the detention which occurred during the processing of the claim – was initially eight months, but this was reduced to five months in 1998": F. Liebaut ed., *Legal and Social Conditions for Asylum Seekers in Western European Countries* (2000) (Liebaut, *Conditions 2000*), at 31–32.

Switzerland for three months,[428] and in Austria for six months.[429] In Malta, African refugees have been detained in miserable conditions for several months with no information about when they would be released, or their asylum applications considered.[430] Under Australian law, refugees are subject to general rules providing for the indefinite detention of non-citizens arriving without authorization:[431] discretionary release from detention is possible (though not guaranteed) only for the very young and very old, for victims of torture and others with special health needs, and for those who have remained in custody for more than six months.[432] The routine resort to the detention of persons seeking refugee status is officially justified in order "to ensure that they do not enter the Australian community until their claims to do so have been properly assessed and found to justify entry."[433] Others, however, suggest that the real motive is to

---

[428] "The detention period is limited to a maximum of three months during the asylum determination process, and for an additional maximum period of nine months if the asylum-seeker has already received a negative first instance decision and deportation proceedings have started": European Council on Refugees and Exiles, *Legal and Social Conditions for Asylum Seekers in Western European Countries, 2003* (2003) (ECRE, *Conditions 2003*).

[429] "Those applying at the airport can be held in the airport's transit zone whilst awaiting the decision of the Federal Asylum Office on whether their application is inadmissible or manifestly unfounded ... In addition, asylum-seekers may also be subject to detention measures during the asylum procedure – in particular if they have entered the country illegally and/or do not have any provisional right of residence ... Such detention must not exceed a total period of six months": ibid. at 15.

[430] (2003) 132 *JRS Dispatches* (May 15, 2003). "Migrants in detention are held in conditions which are an affront to human dignity ... People have been sleeping for months in tents, in bitter cold and flooding when it rains. Most of those with a roof over their head are severely overcrowded, like 35 people in one room. Some are not even allowed in the open air for one hour each day": (2003) 125 *JRS Dispatches* (Jan. 17, 2003).

[431] "According to the Migration Act, Division 7, Section 189, an officer must detain a person in the 'migration zone' if the officer knows or reasonably suspects that the person is an 'unlawful non-citizen' ... Detention is also mandated for a person who is unable to supply proper documentation or tries to avoid showing proper documentation that they are a lawful non-citizen ... Under the law, the period of detention is indeterminate": Motta, "Rock", at 16.

[432] "Under Australia's Migration Act, all non-citizens who unlawfully enter Australia, including those seeking asylum, are placed in detention. In rare circumstances, they may be released from detention if they meet certain criteria, such as old age, ill health, or having suffered torture or other trauma. However, the majority of asylum-seekers are detained for the duration of the asylum adjudication process, which often takes months or even years": US Committee for Refugees, *World Refugee Survey 2002* (2002), at 114. See also Motta, "Rock," at 16: "In reality ... bridging visas are rarely granted. [The Human Rights and Equal Opportunity Commission] reported in 1998 that only 2 children arriving as boat people or born in detention have been released out of a possible 581 since 1 September 1994."

[433] "Response of the Australian Government to the Views of the [UN Human Rights] Committee in Communication No. 560/1993, *A v. Australia*," June 25, 1998, at para. 5,

deter refugees and others from traveling to Australia, and to win favor with an increasingly xenophobic electorate.[434]

Even in countries where the detention of refugees is in principle more selective, it may in practice be quite routine. For example, unauthorized asylum-seekers have commonly been detained in the United States since the early 1980s.[435] Despite provision to release refugees who pass the "credible fear" pre-screening process, there is nonetheless a strong regulatory and administrative bias towards continued detention while awaiting a final adjudication of the protection claim.[436] More recently, the United States invoked

accessed at www.aph.gov.au/library (visited Nov. 19, 2004). The Immigration Minister stated that he was committed to a policy of detaining persons seeking refugee status "because no-one had invented an alternative monitoring system that worked . . . 'From our point of view, our system ensures that people are available for processing and removal if required,' he said": *Canberra Times*, Jan. 26, 2002, at C-1, quoting Immigration Minister Philip Ruddock.

[434] The Prime Minister suggested a deterrent motive, observing that "[m]andatory detention is part of the process of sending a signal to the world that you cannot come to this country illegally": P. Barkham, "PM calls asylum protest blackmail," *Guardian*, Jan. 26, 2002, at 18, quoting Prime Minister John Howard. More generally, "[i]t is said that one of the reasons why the minister is attempting to make Australia a fresh hell for those who have fled from intolerable oppression in Iraq and Afghanistan is so as to send a message to people huddling in appalling conditions in countries neighboring them that it is not worthwhile to 'jump the queue' and come to Australia by boat . . . Indeed, some suspect that the tough talk, and a sequence of mean-spirited actions, is designed as much for domestic consumption as it is to send a message abroad . . . '[I]nvasions' by boat people raise a host of . . . worries among Australians, not least about the inviolability of our borders. Add in some resentments about the activities of lawyers, and about the multi-cultural industry, and one might think that [the Immigration Minister] could not more perfectly construct a policy calculated to appeal to rednecks": "Shame of Ruddock's gulags," *Canberra Times*, June 12, 2000, at A-10.

[435] While historically refugee claimants were not detained, the practice of the Immigration and Naturalization Service from 1982 has been to detain all asylum-seekers arriving without proper documentation pending status verification. Release or "parole" is granted only in exceptional cases, such as medical emergencies or where detention is not deemed to be in the public interest: see M. Taylor, "The 1996 Immigration Act: The Detention Provisions," (1997) 74(5) *Interpreter Releases* 209. In the result, "[a]n average of 20,000 individuals were in Immigration and Naturalization Service custody each day . . . including 3,000 asylum-seekers": US Committee for Refugees, *World Refugee Survey 2002* (2002), at 279. See generally A. Helton, "Reforming Alien Detention Policy in the United States," in M. Crock ed., *Protection or Punishment: The Detention of Asylum Seekers in Australia* (1993), at 104; P. Morante, "Detention of Asylum Seekers: The United States Perspective," in J. Hughes and F. Liebaut eds., *Detention of Asylum Seekers in Europe: Analysis and Perspectives* (1998), at 85–87; and E. Acer, "Living up to America's Values: Reforming the US Detention System for Asylum Seekers," (2002) 20(3) *Refuge* 44.

[436] An asylum-seeker who is not "clearly and beyond a doubt entitled to be admitted shall be detained for a [removal] proceeding": Immigration and Nationality Act, s. 235(b)(2)(A). Undocumented aliens who apply for asylum may be released from detention only "to

national security concerns to justify the routine detention of all persons seeking protection arriving from any of thirty-three countries and two territories, most of them predominantly Muslim.[437]

At least until and unless provisions of the 2002 immigration law reform are implemented,[438] the detention of asylum-seekers in the United Kingdom remains in principle exceptional, based on a showing of good cause. Yet detention may be ordered on the basis of disregard for immigration laws, including clandestine entry, the presentation of false identity documents, or even because the refugee claimant has no personal ties to the United Kingdom.[439] There is no maximum period of detention in the United Kingdom, which may continue until a decision is made to give or to refuse leave to enter the country.[440] Short-term detention may moreover be required in the case of persons adjudged to present a "straightforward asylum claim," defined as a case which appears "to be one in which a quick decision can be reached."[441] The reason for detention in

meet a medical emergency or [when release] is necessary for a legitimate law enforcement activity": ibid. at s. 235.3(b)(4). Asylum-seekers who have passed the credible fear screening interview are eligible for release from detention "only on a case-by-case basis for urgent humanitarian reasons or significant public benefit": ibid. at s. 212(d)(5). Moreover, "[t]he decision to keep an asylum-seeker in detention is now entrusted to the Department of Homeland Security and cannot be appealed to an independent judge": Human Rights First, *In Liberty's Shadow: US Detention of Asylum Seekers in the Era of Homeland Security* (2004) (Human Rights First, *Liberty's Shadow*), at 2.

[437] "The new policy [is] part of 'Operation Liberty Shield' announced by Homeland Security Secretary Tom Ridge on March 18 ... Many of these countries have well-documented records of human rights abuse that prompt men, women and children to seek refuge in the United States ... Under the new policy, asylum-seekers could face months and even years behind bars before the immigration bureaucracy finally makes a decision on their claim. Mr. Ridge has stated that asylum-seekers will be detained throughout the time that their cases are processed": Human Rights Watch, "US 'Operation Liberty Shield' Undermines Asylum Seekers' Rights," Mar. 27, 2003.

[438] Persons subject to entrance controls may, under these reforms, be required to reside in an "accommodation center" as a condition of release from detention: Nationality, Immigration and Asylum Act 2002, c. 41 (2002), at Part 2. "The Home Office says the new accommodation centres, which will not be locked, will provide full health care and legal and education facilities, including interpreters": M. White and A. Travis, "Immigration debate," *Guardian*, Apr. 25, 2002, at 4.

[439] UNHCR, *Detention of Asylum Seekers in Europe* (1995) (UNHCR, *Detention in Europe*), at 208–209.

[440] "During the substantive consideration of a claim for asylum, a port applicant may be detained pending an interview with an immigration officer or pending a decision by the Home Office on the asylum application ... There is no limit in law to the length of time a person may be held in these circumstances, except that if someone is held for the purpose of removal, the courts may order release if there is little or no prospect of removal being carried out soon": Liebaut, *Conditions 2000*, at 311.

[441] UK Home Office Operational Enforcement Manual, Dec. 21, 2000, at para. 38.1, cited in *R (Saadi) v. Secretary of State for the Home Department*, [2002] UKHL 41 (UK HL, Oct. 31, 2002), at para. 15.

such cases is not fear of absconding or to protect the safety of the host
community, but rather that "it is in the interests of speedily and effectively
dealing with asylum claims, to facilitate the entry into the United Kingdom of
those who were entitled to do so and the removal from the United Kingdom of
those who are not."[442]

In contrast, detention in other states is both substantively and procedurally
more circumscribed. Under Italy's 2002 immigration reform, for example,
undocumented non-citizens are detained only until their identity is established – normally for hours or days, but subject to a maximum period of
twenty to thirty days.[443] In Canada, refugees and other unauthorized entrants
may be detained only if their identity cannot be established, they are judged
likely to abscond or to pose a danger to the public, they are suspected of
having violated fundamental human rights, or where necessary for an examination to be completed. An initial detention decision must be reviewed by an
immigration adjudicator within forty-eight hours and, if a decision is made
to continue the detention, that determination is reviewed seven days later,
and every thirty days thereafter.[444]

Other countries avoid the generalized detention of refugees in jails or prisons,
but routinely assign unauthorized refugees to live in reception centers, where
housing and other basic needs are met. In Denmark, for example, stay in a
reception center can be compulsory.[445] Under German law, all refugee applicants
are assigned to live in one of thirty-four federal reception centers based upon a
distribution quota agreed to by the federal and *Länder* governments. Even if the

---

[442] *R (Saadi) v. Secretary of State for the Home Department*, [2002] UKHL 41 (UK HL,
Oct. 31, 2002), at para. 18, citing testimony of Mr. Ian Martin, Oakington Detention
Centre Project Manager.

[443] Lawyers' Committee for Human Rights, "Review of States' Procedures and Practices
relating to Detention of Asylum Seekers," Sept. 2002 (LCHR, "Detention Practices"), at
55–56.

[444] Immigration and Refugee Protection Act 2001, at ss. 55–57. These new provisions, which
entered into force in 2002, have nonetheless been criticized *inter alia* on the grounds that
"it is no longer left to the adjudicator to decide whether identity has been satisfactorily
established or whether it can be. There is ... no independent oversight of an immigration officer's decision that the person's identity has not been established": Canadian
Council for Refugees, "Bill C-11 Brief" (2001), at 43. More generally, there has been a
long-standing concern that because few asylum-seekers in detention have access to legal
advice, the periodic reviews are substantively inadequate. See Canadian Council for
Refugees, "Refugee Detention in Canada" (1994), and L. Sarick, "Refugee groups,
detainees rap Canada," *Globe and Mail* (Toronto), Oct. 23, 1997, at A5.

[445] "Immediately after entry, the asylum-seeker will be taken to a registration centre at
Sandholm or Avnstrup ... If the person can establish his/her identity and travel route,
he/she will be transferred to the Red Cross reception camp. If there is insufficient
information ... the asylum-seeker can be detained in the prison section of Sandholm
Camp (under the responsibility of the Ministry of Justice) until the information can be
satisfactorily established": Liebaut, *Conditions 2000*, at 46.

refugee already has family living in Germany, he or she must stay in the assigned reception center – in principle for up to three months – before being assigned to a regional asylum center, where he or she must remain for the duration of the status verification procedure.[446] Since April 2000, persons seeking recognition of refugee status in Ireland no longer have the option to choose independent living arrangements, but are rather dispersed to hostels across the country.[447] In Switzerland, stay in a "registration center" is compulsory for all but lawfully resident minors during the time it takes to assess their application for protection.[448] Other countries, such as Norway, do not require refugee claimants to reside in a reception center, but deny state welfare benefits to asylum-seekers who choose to live elsewhere.[449] Similarly, Austria denies federal care to any refugee who abandons his or her designated accommodation for more than three days.[450] In contrast, most refugees who arrive in Sweden are housed for a few days in one of three transit centers while their claim is registered and practical needs met; but they are immediately free to arrange their own accommodation outside the centers, with no penalty in terms of their access to public support.[451]

Even in states where there is no general commitment to the detention of all asylum-seekers, detention may be routine for a subset of refugees, defined by the place or manner of entry into the asylum country. Asylum-seekers who arrive at Russian airports are prevented from submitting an application for refugee status, and are held in detention indefinitely until deportation to the country of origin can be arranged.[452] In France, asylum-seekers who apply at ports, airports, or railway stations in *zones d'attente* are also routinely

---

[446] European Council on Refugees and Exiles, "Setting Limits" (2002) (ECRE, "Limits"), at 12–13.

[447] ECRE, *Conditions 2003*.   [448] Ibid.

[449] "Accommodation in . . . transit centres is compulsory for all asylum-seekers until [police interviews and health screening] can take place, although in practice exceptions are made for asylum-seekers who already have other housing and who wish to stay there. As long as the applicant stays outside of the designated transit reception centres, he/she does not enjoy the right to any financial benefits": Liebaut, *Conditions 2000*, at 232.

[450] ECRE, *Conditions 2003*, at 19.

[451] ECRE, "Limits," at 28; LCHR, "Detention Practices," at 106–107.

[452] UNHCR, *Detention in Europe*, at 177. "Under Russian law, the government's 'Points of Immigration Control' (PIC) offices handle asylum requests at ports of entry and along Russia's vast borders, although in practice no PIC has ever accepted an asylum applicant. One of the most active of the country's 114 PIC offices is housed at Moscow's Sheremetevo-II Airport, which receives a large number of African and Asian asylum-seekers. No effective refugee screening exists at the airport": US Committee for Refugees, *World Refugee Survey 2002* (2002), at 239. While the asylum-seeker is held in the transit zone, the airline is responsible for providing him or her with food. As a result, deportations often occur at the behest of the airline itself in order to avoid this liability. It is reported that Aeroflot allows asylum-seekers to remain "for one week, but not longer; it is expensive to feed them": Amnesty International, "Russian Federation: Failure to Protect Asylum Seekers" (1997), at 12.

detained, though only pending a decision on whether their claim to be a refugee is manifestly unfounded.[453] The United States has established a new class of persons subject to its expedited removal process (and hence to routine detention[454]) consisting of persons who entered the country without authorization by sea – a rule unabashedly aimed at Haitian "boat people."[455]

The most common situation-specific reason for ordering the detention of refugees, particularly in the less developed world, is the existence of a "mass influx" of asylum-seekers.[456] Uganda confined Rwandan and Sudanese refugee populations in closed camps in Kyaka and the Masindi District respectively, and persists in a general policy of isolating larger refugee populations.[457] Kenya responded to the arrival of Ethiopian and Somali refugees by establishing closed camps, to which asylum-seekers were forcibly

---

[453] "[A]sylum seekers may be detained in waiting zones in ports, airports, and railway stations for the time 'necessary to determine whether the application is manifestly unfounded or not,' but with a maximum period of 20 days": Liebaut, *Conditions 2000*, at 85. See also US Committee for Refugees, *World Refugee Survey 2002* (2002), at 212.

[454] See text above, at pp. 372–373.

[455] Notice Designating Aliens Subject to Expedited Removal Under Section 235(b)(1)(A)(iii) of the Immigration and Nationality Act, INS Order No. 2243–02, Nov. 13, 2002, published as 67 FR 68924. As published in the Federal Register, ibid., the Notice states it was issued "in direct response to the recent arrival of hundreds of Haitian refugees off of the coast of South Florida." Moreover, the discriminatory nature of the Notice is clear from clause 5, which provides that "[e]xpedited removal proceedings will not be initiated against Cuban citizens or nationals who arrive by sea." A year prior to the issuance of the Notice, Acting Deputy Immigration and Naturalization Service Commissioner Michael Beycraft issued instructions for the routine detention of Haitians arriving in the United States, even though most had been able to demonstrate a credible fear of being persecuted: Lutheran Immigration and Refugee Service, "Detained Asylum Seekers in Miami – Urgent Action," May 16, 2002.

[456] "Problems relating to detention have also arisen in large-scale influx situations where States frequently find it necessary to place asylum-seekers in camps or reception centres due to concerns for community welfare, national security and the need to provide accommodation to large numbers of persons. In certain instances, however, asylum-seekers have been placed in 'closed camps' for unduly long periods under harsh conditions as part of a policy of 'humane deterrence' adopted as a result of a decline in resettlement prospects. In such cases refugees are required to remain in closed camps indefinitely without any immediate prospect of a solution": UNHCR, "Detention Note," at para. 39.

[457] E. Khiddu-Makubuya, *International Academy of Comparative Law National Report for Uganda* (1994), at 12. "The [Government of Uganda]/UNHCR policy is to confine refugees in camps and settlements until such a time when they can finally return home. The argument put forward is that this is the explicitly preferred 'durable' solution [because it promotes] ... economic self-sufficiency through agricultural production. On the contrary, the location of refugee camps is on waterlogged, infertile and barren land": D. Lwanga, "Refugees in Detention: A Critique of the Limitations to Justice in Uganda," paper presented at the 7th International Association for the Study of Forced Migration Conference, Johannesburg, South Africa, Jan. 8–11, 2001.

and sometimes violently transported.[458] Thailand imposed a strict policy on Cambodian refugees of detention in closed camps, reportedly enforced by the extrajudicial execution of persons discovered outside the camp boundaries.[459] UNHCR has regularly assisted in the establishment and administration of temporary holding areas for refugees arriving in a mass influx situation,[460] including for example those for Rwandan and Burundian refugees in Tanzania in 1996.[461] Perhaps most notoriously, it collaborated in the detention of Vietnamese asylum-seekers arriving in Hong Kong after 1982. Persons seeking protection were held in prison-like conditions, most for more than two years, pending a determination of their claims to refugee status under UNHCR auspices. Hong Kong's Secretary of State proclaimed that "[t]his move should make Hong Kong less attractive for refugees. When the message gets back to Vietnam, it should help to deter people from setting out ... It is urgent that word gets back to Vietnam at once that those who come will be greeted by closed camps."[462]

The conditions in which refugees are detained are often appalling. For example, in Hong Kong's Whitehead Detention Center, which held up to 25,000 people,

> each section of 2,500 people is locked 24 hours a day so that residents are confined in their own small cement section. Each hut contains at least 100 people, each of whom is allotted a space just large enough in which to lie

---

[458] African Rights, *The Nightmare Continues ... Abuses Against Somali Refugees in Kenya* (1993), at 7. More recently, it was reported that "[r]efugees living in Nairobi ... suffered from human rights abuses, many of which were linked to the Kenyan government's insistence that they reside in camps and not in urban areas": Human Rights Watch, *World Report 2003* (2003).

[459] Amnesty International, "Thailand: Extrajudicial Execution of Kampuchean Refugees" (1988). More generally, "[a]sylum seekers outside of refugee camps are considered by the Thai government to be illegal immigrants and are at risk of arrest and detention": Amnesty International, "Thailand: Widespread Abuses in the Administration of Justice" (2002), at 2.

[460] "There is a trend towards camp-like solutions on the part of UNHCR in the Horn of Africa ... The increasing permanence of UNHCR's camp operations in locations like Dadaab, however, where UNHCR protects over 100,000 mostly Somali refugees, is problematic. UNHCR tends to maintain refugees in camps, at the Kenyan government's insistence, at the expense of basic human rights including freedom of movement and the right to employment": J. Hyndman and B. Nylund, "UNHCR and the Status of Prima Facie Refugees in Kenya," (1998) 10(3) *International Journal of Refugee Law* 21, at 45–46.

[461] Information provided by UNHCR Ngara, Feb. 6, 1996; personal interview with Mr. Jean-Marc Mangin of CARE USA, Sept. 12, 1996. Even at the end of 2000, "approximately 490,000 refugees ... remained under the responsibility of UNHCR": S. van Hoyweghen, "Mobility, Territoriality and Sovereignty in Post-Colonial Tanzania," (2002) 21(1–2) *Refugee Survey Quarterly* 300, at 300.

[462] Cited in Amnesty International, "Hong Kong: Arbitrary Detention of Vietnamese Asylum Seekers" (1994), at 1.

down. Bunks are stacked three high and families are separated from other families by a sheet. The ratio of people to toilets is 50 to 1 (UNHCR recommended 20 to 1). Uniformed guards patrol the facility. The sound of unlocking and locking of gates resonates through the camp.[463]

While perhaps an extreme example, the bleak conditions faced by refugees detained in Hong Kong are not unique.[464] Detention facilities for refugees in South Korea, for example, were reported to lack heat and other necessities; conditions of detention there were moreover not subject to independent judicial or administrative review.[465] Spain came under attack from human rights groups in 2002 for detaining asylum-seekers arriving in the Canary Islands "in two extremely overcrowded old airport facilities ... At times, more than 500 migrants [were] kept in a space that the Spanish Red Cross [had] determined to be fit for fifty people."[466] The refugee detention facility in Mexico City similarly held two to three times its capacity during 2001.[467] Human rights investigators visiting a detention center in Athens in November 2000 found "150 detainees in a space ... designed for half that number. Most detainees had been held at the centre, which was filthy and roach-infested, for months; one man had been there for a full year."[468] In the United States, refugees may be detained in jails and in facilities contracted through private security firms, including in institutions built to house criminals.[469] Conditions in Australia's remote refugee detention camps are so dismal that they have been condemned by a bipartisan parliamentary

---

[463] Lawyers' Committee for Human Rights, *Uncertain Haven: Refugee Protection on the Fortieth Anniversary of the 1951 United Nations Refugee Convention* (1991), at 13–14.

[464] In general, the UN Special Rapporteur on the Rights of Non-Citizens has observed that "[a]sylum seekers, including children, pregnant women, and elderly people, have been held in detention centers without adequate health and mental health care, education, and recreation facilities": "Final Report of the Special Rapporteur of the Rights of Non-Citizens: Addendum: Examples of Practice in Regard to Non-Citizens," UN Doc. E/CN.4/Sub.2/2003/23/Add.3, May 26, 2003, at para. 14.

[465] US Committee for Refugees, *World Refugee Survey 2002* (2002), at 137.

[466] Human Rights Watch, "Spain: Migrants' Rights Violated on Canary Islands," Feb. 21, 2002.

[467] US Committee for Refugees, *World Refugee Survey 2002* (2002), at 273.

[468] Human Rights Watch, "Appalling Detention Conditions for Foreigners in Greece Says Rights Group," press release issued Dec. 20, 2000, available at www.hrw.org (accessed Dec. 13, 2003).

[469] "The Department of Homeland Security ... also rents space in state prisons and local jails around the country in order to detain asylum-seekers ... While some of these facilities are euphemistically referred to as 'detention facilities,' for those being held there, they are essentially prisons. Asylum seekers are stripped of their clothing, requiring to wear prison uniforms, transported in handcuffs and shackles, not allowed to have contact visits with family, and treated like prisoners. In some detention facilities ... detainees live in warehouse buildings and their 'outdoor' time consists of a visit to a room in the building that has a chain mesh ceiling which allows some fresh

committee, by the national ombudsman, and by United Nations inspectors.[470] As the Jesuit Refugee Service reported,

> The asylum-seekers are treated far worse than prisoners are in the prison system. Communication has been stymied, clothing provided is inadequate, and food provided is below standard. Medical and dental treatment at Woomera is also below standard. People with tooth problems have only two choices, pull the tooth or leave it. For medical complaints, water is the usual cure offered. Hunger strikes and suicide attempts are all too common at Woomera. Asylum-seekers suffer depression and anxiety. All mirrors have been removed to prevent suicide and self-mutilation ... Woomera is a miserable place to be.[471]

Of particular concern, children – both the dependants of adults seeking protection, and child refugees themselves – may not be exempted from detention regimes. At the beginning of 2003, for example, more than 300 refugee children were being detained by Australia, with some having been in custody for more than three years.[472] It was discovered in 2002 that Belgian authorities were

air to come in the room. For activity, detainees in some facilities are allowed to work in facility upkeep and paid one dollar per day for their labor": Human Rights First, *Liberty's Shadow*, at 35. "In 2001, more than half of all Immigration and Naturalization Service detainees were held in prisons or local jails intended for criminal inmates, exposing them to treatment and conditions inappropriate to their administrative detainee status": Human Rights Watch, *World Report 2002* (2002).

[470] "Detention is the first stop for those seeking asylum," *Toronto Star*, May 27, 2001; K. Lawson, "MPs 'shocked' by detention centres," *Canberra Times*, June 19, 2001, at A-3; "Centres 'like Nazi Germany,'" *Canberra Times*, May 9, 2002. Relying only on information provided by government sources, Human Rights Commissioner Chris Sidoti determined that at least one detainee "had been handcuffed for 8 hours, shackled for 7 hours, and kept in a windowless and constantly lit room for six days ... ": G. Lombard, "Setting it all to rights," *Canberra Times*, July 22, 2000. Indeed, even a study commissioned by the Immigration Minister himself found that "staff at Woomera intimidated and verbally abused detainees": P. Barkham, "Aussie rules bring despair to refugees," *Guardian*, July 27, 2001, at 16. The Western Australia Prisons Ombudsman observed, "We do not have riots in our detention centres because we have a riotous group of refugees. We have them because we run appalling systems": (2001) 103 *JRS Dispatches* (Dec. 3, 2001), quoting Western Australia Prisons Ombudsman Richard Harding.

[471] (2001) 86 *JRS Dispatches* (Feb. 3, 2001). It was reported in 2003 that detainees in some facilities could not visit friends without permission, and only then after a full-body search; that closed circuit cameras are ever-present to monitor movements; that timely medical care is not provided; and that some persons have been stripped, blindfolded, and put into solitary confinement as punishment for protesting their conditions: P. Griffiths, "The detainees have good cause to rebel," *Canberra Times*, Jan. 3, 2003, at A-11. The Woomera detention center was closed down by the government in 2003: (2003) 132 *JRS Dispatches* (May 15, 2003).

[472] These included 33 children detained at Villawood; 49 in Baxter; 3 in Maribyrnong, 20 in Port Hedland, 6 at Woomera, 169 on Nauru, and 38 on Manus: (2003) 126 *JRS Dispatches* (Feb. 13, 2003). The Immigration Minister is reported to have stated that "detaining children did not put Australia in breach of its international obligations ... [Persons

holding unaccompanied minor refugee claimants in closed "transit centers" at airports for months on end while their claims were being considered.[473] The United Kingdom even entered a reservation to the Convention on the Rights of the Child to safeguard its authority to detain refugee children[474] – an approach markedly in contrast to its general instructions to local authorities to impose secure detention on even criminal children only as a "last resort."[475]

Beyond penalties imposed directly on refugees themselves, many countries also impose criminal or other sanctions on persons or organizations responsible for assisting them to seek protection. It is now common practice for destination countries to impose sanctions against airlines and other common carriers that transport undocumented refugees to asylum states.[476] In Australia, the cost of detaining refugee claimants may be passed on to the owner of the vessel on which they arrived.[477] Under Canadian law, any person or organization transporting a non-citizen contrary to visa requirements is liable to prosecution under the Immigration and Refugee Protection Act (though in practice the government rarely prosecutes those who assist the arrival of refugees).[478] Some European countries have formalized the relaxation of such rules, to at least some extent, where refugees are involved. In

---

seeking protection as refugees] should not bring their children to Australia, he said": R. Peake, "Pressure on to free children from detention," *Canberra Times*, Aug. 2, 2002, at A-3.

[473] (2002) 121 *JRS Dispatches* (Nov. 4, 2002).

[474] L. Back et al., "Letter: Repellent views swamp the system," *Guardian*, Apr. 25, 2002, at 21.

[475] "The decision to detain children flies in the face of the government's own guidance to local authorities about the detention in secure units of children who have committed a crime or are beyond parental control. In that context, it must be a 'last resort,' with all possible alternatives having first been comprehensively considered and rejected": R. Scannell, "Letter: Plight of asylum children," *Guardian*, Aug. 2, 2002, at 21. See also R. Prasad, "Toddlers behind the razor wire," *Guardian*, July 30, 2002, at 14: "Whitehall now incarcerates children seeking asylum for unprecedented lengths of time in numbers hitherto unthought of. By expanding the use of detention, ministers shrink the rights of the child. This runs counter to Labour's social justice message: it is prepared to use the language of social inclusion for British kids, but systematically excludes foreign children seeking asylum here . . . How can the government justify imprisoning minors who have not committed any offence? Seeking asylum in Britain is not a crime, even if false papers are sometimes the only way of getting here."

[476] A detailed account of the ways in which carrier sanctions operate to prevent access to asylum is found in Amnesty International, "Cell Culture: The Detention and Imprisonment of Asylum-Seekers in the United Kingdom" (1996), at 26–37.

[477] Migration Act, s. 213. This general provision does not appear to exempt those persons who are later found to be genuine refugees or who are granted a substantive visa: see A. North and P. Decle, "Courts and Immigration Detention: 'Once a Jolly Swagman Camped by a Billabong,'" (2002) 10(1) *Australian Journal of Administrative Law* 5.

[478] "No person shall knowingly organize, induce, aid or abet the coming to Canada of one or more persons who are not in possession of a visa, passport or other document required by this Act": Immigration and Refugee Protection Act 2001, at s. 117(1). Fines of up to $1,000,000 and/or life imprisonment are possible for breach of the law: ibid. at s. 117(3). There is no exemption from this provision if the persons transported are genuine

Belgium, France, and Luxembourg, carriers are exempted from penalties if an asylum claim is deemed admissible. In Finland and Germany, on the other hand, no relief from penalization is available unless the asylum claim is ultimately determined to be well founded.[479] In 2003, the Irish Justice Minister refused to consider an exemption from fines of up to €3,000 per immigrant in the case of persons seeking refugee protection.[480] But under recent reforms, European Union countries – while obliged to impose fines on common carriers that bring inadequately documented aliens to Europe – are nonetheless encouraged not to penalize carriers where the person transported makes an application for protection in Europe.[481]

> **Refugee Convention, Art. 31   Refugees unlawfully in the country of refuge**
>
> 1. The Contracting States shall not impose penalties, on account of their illegal entry or presence, on refugees who, coming directly from a territory where their life or freedom was threatened in the sense of article 1, enter or are present in their territory without authorization, provided they present themselves without delay to the authorities and show good cause for their illegal entry or presence.
>
> 2. The Contracting States shall not apply to the movements of such refugees restrictions other than those which are necessary and such restrictions shall only be applied until their status in the country is regularized or they obtain admission into another country. The Contracting States shall allow such refugees a reasonable period and all the necessary facilities to obtain admission into another country.

refugees; such factors as motive and profit are relevant only to the penalty to be imposed: ibid. at s. 121. The refugees themselves, however, may claim the benefit of s. 133 of the Act, which provides that "[a] person who has claimed refugee protection, and who came to Canada directly or indirectly from the country in respect of which the claim is made, may not be charged with an offence ... in relation to the coming into Canada of the person, pending disposition of their claim for refugee protection or if refugee protection is conferred."

[479] European Council on Refugees and Exiles, "Legislation on carriers' liability," ECRE Information Service Bulletin No. 2, June 1999.

[480] "He said that the UNHCR's suggestion to exempt carriers from fines where the person brought to the State without proper documentation is an asylum-seeker would 'make the proposed controls unworkable and encourage the making of false asylum claims at an even higher rate than, sadly, exists in Ireland at present'": *Irish Times*, Mar. 31, 2003, quoting Justice Minister McDowell.

[481] EU Council Directive 2001/51/EC (June 28, 2001), supplementing the provisions of Art. 26 of the Convention implementing the Schengen Agreement of June 14, 1985, at Arts. 4(2) and 3. The expectation of exemption from prosecution where the person transported applies for asylum is set by the Preamble, rather than codified in an express requirement.

Civil and Political Covenant, Art. 9(1)
Everyone has the right to liberty and security of person. No one shall be subjected to arbitrary arrest or detention. No one shall be deprived of his liberty except on such grounds and in accordance with such procedure as are established by law.

Civil and Political Covenant, Art. 10(1)
All persons deprived of their liberty shall be treated with humanity and with respect for the inherent dignity of the human person.

Perhaps the most important innovation of the 1951 Refugee Convention is its commitment to the protection of refugees who travel to a state party without authorization. For the first time, the duty of *non-refoulement* was conceived as the entitlement of all refugees, including those who arrive without permission to enter the territory of an asylum country.[482] This decision to grant protection against *refoulement* to all refugees, whether authorized or unauthorized, closed the most critical protection gap that had initially prompted the drafting of a specific duty of non-penalization.[483] Because even "irregular" refugees are now shielded from return in any manner whatsoever to a place in which they are at risk, Art. 33 can be relied upon to counter penalties which raise this prospect.[484]

---

[482] See chapter 4.1.1 above, at pp. 302–303.

[483] The initial drafts of the Refugee Convention were unclear in their commitment to grant protection against *refoulement* to refugees who arrived without authorization. The Secretary-General's draft Art. 24(1) would have guaranteed that refugees "who have been authorized to reside [in the asylum country] regularly" would benefit from a guarantee that states would "not ... remove or keep [them] from [their] territory, by application of police measures, such as expulsions or non-admittance at the frontier (refoulement)": United Nations, "Draft Convention", at 46. Draft Art. 19(1) of the French draft was essentially the same, though an exception was included to protect the right to take measures "dictated by reasons of national security": France, "Draft Convention," at 9. The language of the more general obligation, not textually restricted to authorized refugees, was less explicit. Draft Art. 24(3) provided that "[e]ach of the High Contracting Parties undertakes in any case not to turn back refugees to the frontiers of their country of origin, or to territories where their life or freedom would be threatened on account of their race, religion, nationality or political opinion": United Nations, "Draft Convention," at 45 (draft Art. 24(3)). The French draft was identical, but added a qualification regarding the permissible scope of relevant political opinions ("provided these opinions are not contrary to the principles of the United Nations as set forth in the Preamble to the United Nations Charter"): France, "Draft Convention," at 9 (draft Art. 19(3)).

[484] See UNHCR Executive Committee Conclusion No. 15, "Refugees Without an Asylum Country" (1979), available at www.unhcr.ch (accessed Nov. 20, 2004), at para. (i): "While asylum-seekers may be required to submit their asylum request within a certain time limit, failure to do so, or the non-fulfilment of other formal requirements, should not lead to an asylum request being excluded from consideration."

Thus, for example, the decisions by Gambia, Malawi, and Thailand simply to arrest and deport refugees on the same terms as other illegal entrants raise the spectre of *refoulement*. The same is true of Russia's practice of expelling refugees who enter its territory at airports, and of the efforts by such countries as Mexico, Poland, and Turkey to refuse even to consider claims to refugee status which are not lodged within a fixed timeframe after arrival. Laws that subject refugees who arrive without valid documents or by passage through non-persecutory states to truncated status assessment procedures – including those in both Europe and the United States – may also result in the failure to identify and protect genuine refugees. To the extent such practices expose persons who are in fact refugees (whether or not recognized as such) to the risk of return to persecution, they violate the duty of *non-refoulement*.[485]

Yet if only penalties that force refugees back to the risk of persecution were prohibited, there would still be a risk of unfairness since refugees often have few options but to enter an asylum country without valid documentation or otherwise in breach of its migration laws.[486] As Lord Justice Simon Brown observed in the *Adimi* case,

> The need for Article 31 has not diminished. Quite the contrary. Although under the Convention subscribing states must give sanctuary to any refugee who seeks asylum (subject only to removal to a safe third country), they are by no means bound to facilitate his arrival. Rather they strive increasingly to prevent it. The combined effect of visa requirements and carrier's liability has made it well nigh impossible for refugees to travel to countries of refuge without false documents ...

---

[485] Persons are refugees when they meet the requirements of the refugee definition in fact, not simply when they are recognized as such: UNHCR, *Handbook*, at para. 28. See chapter 3.1 above, at pp. 158–160.

[486] Courts have taken the view that Art. 31 is a response to "the difficulty of gaining access to a friendly shore. Escapes from persecution have long been characterized by subterfuge and false papers ... Thus it was that Article 31(1) found its way into the 1951 UN Convention": *R v. Uxbridge Magistrates Court, ex parte Adimi*, [1999] 4 All ER 520 (Eng. HC, July 29, 1999), per Simon Brown LJ, at 523. See also *Attorney General v. Refugee Council of New Zealand Inc.*, [2003] 2 NZLR 577 (NZ CA, Apr. 16, 2003), at para. 6: "In practice, refugee status claimants often arrive at a border without appropriate documentation or with documentation which appears to be false. This may be because they have fled without papers, or are travelling on forged documents, or have destroyed their travel documents when approaching the border in order to impede their being removed on arrival"; and *Akinmade v. Immigration and Naturalization Service*, 196 F 3d 951 (US CA9, Nov. 5, 1999), finding that "we recognize that a genuine refugee escaping persecution may lie about his citizenship to immigration officials in order to flee his place of persecution or secure entry into the United States." The court adopted a helpful distinction between the (inappropriate and illegal) use of false documents falsely to secure recognition of refugee status, and the (understandable and lawful) use of false documents to escape danger or enter an asylum country: ibid.

> Self-evidently, [the purpose of Art. 31] was to provide immunity for genuine refugees whose quest for asylum reasonably involved them in breaching the law.[487]

It must, however, be acknowledged that the principled concern not to penalize refugees for explicable and often necessary breaches of migration control laws was implemented in a highly instrumentalist way. The drafters were keenly aware that without protection against penalization for unlawful entry, many refugees would opt for an "illegal existence" rather than make themselves known to authorities. They valued an orderly system for the processing of refugee claims, and realized that the threat of prosecution and punishment for the breach of general immigration laws would undoubtedly deter many unauthorized refugees from seeking to regularize their status. As observed in the Secretary-General's background study,

> In actual fact, the [refugee], since he cannot enter the territory of a State lawfully, often does so clandestinely. He will then lead an illegal existence, avoiding all contact with the authorities and living under the constant threat of discovery and expulsion. The disadvantages of this state of affairs, both for himself and for the country on whose territory he happens to be, are obvious.[488]

The drafters were of the view that "[i]t would be in keeping with the notion of asylum to exempt from penalties a refugee, escaping from persecution, who after crossing the border clandestinely, presents himself as soon as possible to the authorities of the country and is recognized as a *bona fide* refugee."[489] The underlying principled concern of Art. 31 to exempt refugees from being penalized for having entered an asylum state without authorization is therefore tempered in a critical way: only refugees who come forward to regularize their status with authorities of the host country are entitled to this immunity.

4.2.1 Beneficiaries of protection

Art. 31 does not prohibit the imposition of immigration penalties on all refugees. Because of the drafters' instrumentalist orientation, protection against penalization for illegal entry or presence is only granted to those refugees who take affirmative steps to make themselves known to officials of

---

[487] *R v. Uxbridge Magistrates Court, ex parte Adimi*, [1999] 4 All ER 520 (Eng. HC, July 29, 1999), per Simon Brown LJ at 523, 527.

[488] United Nations Department of Social Affairs, "A Study of Statelessness," UN Doc. E/1112, Feb. 1, 1949 (United Nations, "Statelessness"), at 20.

[489] United Nations, "Memorandum by the Secretary-General to the Ad Hoc Committee on Statelessness and Related Problems," UN Doc. E/AC.32/2, Jan. 3, 1950 (Secretary-General, "Memorandum"), at 46.

the asylum country, who do so within a reasonable period of time, and who satisfy authorities that their breach of immigration laws was necessitated by their search for protection. If any of these three requirements is not met, there is no exemption from forms of penalization that fall short of *refoulement*.[490]

Because no more than physical presence is required to invoke Art. 31, the provisional benefit of this right must be granted to all persons who claim refugee status, until and unless they are finally determined not to be Convention refugees:[491]

> That Article 31 extends not merely to those ultimately accorded refugee status but also to those claiming asylum in good faith (presumptive refugees) is not in doubt.[492]

---

[490] Even permissible penalization must not cause refugees to be "pushed back into the arms of their persecutors": see chapter 4.1.2 above, at pp. 318–322. The three provisos stipulated in Art. 31(1) also govern entitlement to freedom from general norms of detention for unauthorized entry, set by Art. 31(2). This is clear from the literal meaning of the reference to "such refugees" found twice in Art. 31(2). While it is true that Art. 31(2) achieved its final form before the Conference of Plenipotentiaries adopted the references in Art. 31(1) to refugees "coming directly from a territory where their life or freedom was threatened in the sense of Article 1," it is clear that the Ad Hoc Committee intended a comparable restriction of entitlement to Art. 31(2) rights. Under the joint Belgian–American redrafting of Art. 31 considered by the Ad Hoc Committee, UN Doc. E/AC.32/L.25, Feb. 2, 1950, the relevant text read: "Provided that such refugees present themselves without delay to the authorities and show good cause for their entry, the High Contracting Parties shall not impose penalties on them on account of their illegal entry or presence. The High Contracting Parties nonetheless reserve the right to apply *to such refugees* necessary police measures regarding their accommodation, residence, and movement in the territory until such time as it is possible to take a decision regarding their legal admission to the country of reception or their admission to another country [emphasis added]." The draft adopted by the Ad Hoc Committee on the same day (UN Doc. E/AC.32/L.26, Feb. 2, 1950) split this formulation into two paragraphs, retaining the reference in the second paragraph (governing restrictions on movement) to "such refugees." In the result, only refugees who satisfy the three provisos set by Art. 31(1) are entitled to invoke Art. 31(2) to contest detention which is not strictly provisional and "necessary."

[491] "Admittedly there may be an interim period between the claim to refugee status and recognition as a refugee when it may beg the question to say that the claimant is entitled to be treated as a refugee. Equally, however, it will not be possible during this period to say that the claimant is not entitled to be treated as a refugee. In those circumstances the risk of an undeserved penalty cannot be disregarded": *Attorney General v. E*, [2000] 3 NZLR 257 (NZ CA, July 11, 2000, appeal to PC refused at [2000] 3 NZLR 637). There was clearly confusion during debate regarding the moment at which refugees would be entitled to freedom of movement under Art. 31(2), but not as regards the timing of immunity from immigration penalties. See generally chapter 3.1.2 above, and text below, at pp. 390–391.

[492] *R v. Uxbridge Magistrates Court, ex parte Adimi*, [1999] 4 All ER 520 (Eng. HC, July 29, 1999), per Simon Brown LJ at 527. See also *Khaboka v. Secretary of State for the Home Department*, [1993] Imm AR 484 (Eng. CA, Mar. 25, 1993), at 489.

Indeed, the English High Court of Justice has determined that states must put in place procedures to ensure that Art. 31 protection is afforded even to "travellers recognizable as refugees, whether or not they have actually claimed asylum."[493] Only those ultimately found not to be refugees may be prosecuted for illegal entry or presence in the usual way.[494]

The first requirement to benefit from Art. 31 is that the asylum-seeker must "present [herself or himself] . . . to the authorities." As suggested above, the goal of this clause is to provide an incentive for unauthorized entrants to regularize their status with officials of the asylum state. Only refugees who come forward of their own initiative, thereby demonstrating their good faith, are immune from penalization for breach of immigration laws. Exemption from penalization should not, of course, be denied to a refugee who mistakenly reports to officials of the wrong level or branch of government. For example, an asylum-seeker who advises officials of the city where he is staying of his situation has discharged his duty to present himself to "the authorities," even if only national authorities have jurisdiction to regulate immigration or refugee protection.[495]

On the other hand, the duty to present oneself to authorities in order to claim Art. 31 protection is not usually met by an individual who claims refugee status only after being apprehended or detained by authorities,[496] as there would

---

[493] *R v. Uxbridge Magistrates Court, ex parte Adimi*, [1999] 4 All ER 520 (Eng. HC, July 29, 1999), per Simon Brown LJ at 533.

[494] Not only does a non-refugee have no right to the benefit of Art. 31, but it has also been suggested once refugee status is denied, the individual may no longer be able to show "good cause" for his or her illegal entry or presence. "[T]his condition has only a limited role in the Article. It would be satisfied by *a genuine refugee* showing that he was reasonably travelling on false papers [emphasis added]": ibid., per Simon Brown LJ at 529. The "good cause" requirement was more explicitly invoked by the New Zealand High Court to find that the benefit of Art. 31(1) accrues only to refugees who are ultimately able to prove their claim to Convention refugee status: *Jiao v. Refugee Status Appeals Authority*, [2002] NZAR 845 (NZ HC, July 29, 2002).

[495] Indeed, the Belgian representative clearly considered that local authorities were the officials who ought logically to be approached by refugees who had entered without authorization: Statement of Mr. Herment of Belgium, UN Doc. E/AC.32/SR.40, Aug. 22, 1950, at 6.

[496] At the second session of the Ad Hoc Committee, the Belgian representative voiced his concern about the logic of exemption from immigration penalties in the case of a refugee who "[t]he moment he was discovered . . . could present himself to the local authorities, explaining the reasons he had taken refuge in that territory": Statement of Mr. Herment of Belgium, ibid. The French representative replied that "in the case mentioned by the Belgian representative, the act was no longer voluntary, since the refugee who had entered illegally had been brought before the authorities by the police who discovered him. The refugee could therefore no longer benefit by the provisions of article [31]": Statement of Mr. Juvigny of France, ibid. at 7. See also Statement of Mr. Henkin of the United States, ibid.

in such a case be no genuine exercise of free will on the part of the refugee.[497] An exception to this rule is required in circumstances where a refugee is arrested or detained before he or she could reasonably have been expected to seek regularization of status. The benefit of Art. 31 should not be denied in such cases, at least so long as there is no evidence of bad faith on the part of the refugee.[498] Because refugees are only required to present themselves "without delay" in order to benefit from Art. 31, it would make no sense to deny that protection simply because apprehension by authorities was nearly immediate.

The second obligation under Art. 31 is that the voluntary reporting to authorities must occur "without delay." While it is clear that refugees who have "been in the territory a long time"[499] before presenting themselves to authorities fail this requirement, there is no duty to claim refugee status immediately upon arrival in order to benefit from Art. 31.[500] Most critically, the language of the Convention requires a non-mechanistic assessment of *bona fides*.[501] The standard will necessarily vary from person to person. A more generous interpretation is appropriate in the case of, for example, refugees who face linguistic or cultural barriers, who are uncertain about how best to seek protection, or who are traumatized or otherwise not in a position

---

[497] Exemption from penalties was said to be contingent upon "a voluntary act. A person who presented himself to the authorities of a country after crossing its frontiers without authorization was performing a voluntary act": Statement of Mr. Juvigny of France, ibid. at 7. See also Statement of Mr. Winter of Canada, ibid.: "If a refugee presented himself to the authorities involuntarily, namely, only when he had been detained, he would naturally come under the law of the country."

[498] See *R v. Uxbridge Magistrates Court, ex parte Adimi*, [1999] 4 All ER 520 (Eng. HC, July 29, 1999), per Simon Brown LJ at 528–529, indicating that the requirement of a "voluntary exonerating act" ought not to be applied in order to deny the protection of Art. 31 to a person whose "intention was to claim asylum within a short time of his arrival," but who was detained by authorities virtually as soon as he arrived in the asylum state. As Grahl-Madsen suggests, there is logically a certain interrelationship between the temporal and volitional requirements of Article 31: Grahl-Madsen, *Commentary*, at 176.

[499] Statement of Mr. Juvigny of France, UN Doc. E/AC.32/SR.40, Aug. 22, 1950, at 5.

[500] It has been suggested that there is simply a duty to present onself "within a short time of [one's] arrival" in order to benefit from Art. 31 protection: see *R v. Uxbridge Magistrates Court, ex parte Adimi*, [1999] 4 All ER 520 (Eng. HC, July 29, 1999), at 529. This test has specifically been determined not to require a refugee to claim protection "while clearing immigration controls at the port of entry": UK Soc. Sec. Comm. Dec. No. CIS/4439/1998 (Nov. 25, 1999).

[501] While the Belgian representative initially suggested that this clause contemplated "an unauthorized stay of three or four days," even he subsequently agreed that only situations of "prolonged illegal presence" were clearly excluded: Statements of Mr. Herment of Belgium, UN Doc. E/AC.32/SR.40, Aug. 22, 1950, at 4–6. The American delegate was the only representative who took the view that the "without delay" requirement imposes a duty to seek protection "immediately on entry into a country": Statement of Mr. Henkin, ibid. at 7.

immediately to make their need for protection known.[502] Because the objective of this clause is simply to ensure that asylum-seekers regularize their status "as soon as possible,"[503] it cannot be relied upon to impose arbitrary deadlines for an asylum claim to be lodged.[504] The firm deadlines to seek refugee status set by Mexico and Poland are therefore not in compliance with Art. 31; indeed, the comparable rule imposed by Turkey was found to breach the European Convention on Human Rights, precisely because of its inflexibility.[505] While the short deadlines (five to fifteen days) set by these states made their practices particularly problematic, even a less exigent deadline within which to seek protection without being subjected to migration penalties will breach Art. 31, if it is mechanistically applied. Any deadline for reporting must be administered with flexibility to take account of relevant claimant-specific circumstances.[506]

Third, the duty of non-penalization is owed only to refugees who are "coming directly from a territory where their life or freedom was threatened in the sense of Article 1" and who are able to "show good cause for their illegal entry or presence." The underlying premise of the "good cause" requirement is that exemption from immigration penalties should be reserved for refugees

---

[502] "No strict time limit can be applied to the concept 'coming directly' and each case must be judged on its merits. Similarly, given the special situation of asylum-seekers, in particular the effects of trauma, language problems, lack of information, previous experiences which often result in a suspicion of those in authority, feelings of insecurity, and the fact that these and other circumstances may vary enormously from one asylum-seeker to another, there is no time limit which can be mechanically applied or associated with the expression 'without delay'": UNHCR, "Revised Guidelines on Applicable Criteria and Standards Relating to the Detention of Asylum Seekers," Feb. 1999 (UNHCR, "Detention Guidelines"), at para. 4.

[503] Secretary-General, "Memorandum," at 46.

[504] See UNHCR Executive Committee Conclusion No. 15, "Refugees Without an Asylum Country" (1979), at para. (i), available at www.unhcr.ch (accessed Nov. 20, 2004): "While asylum-seekers may be required to submit their asylum request within a certain time limit, failure to do so, or the non-fulfilment of other formal requirements, should not lead to an asylum request being excluded from consideration."

[505] "In the Court's opinion, the automatic and mechanical application of such a short time-limit for submitting an asylum application must be considered at variance with the protection of the fundamental values embodied in Article 3 of the [European] Convention": *Jabari v. Turkey*, [2000] ECHR 368 (ECHR, July 11, 2000). Two Turkish administrative courts (*idari mahkeme*) issued rulings calling for consideration of the actual circumstances of cases before relying on the deadline for filing of a claim; the Council of State refused an appeal by the government against one of these decisions in 2000: K. Kirisci, "UNHCR and Turkey: Nudging towards a Better Implementation of the 1951 Convention on the Status of Refugees" (2001), at 11–12.

[506] The Swiss Federal Court has, however, determined that a refugee who waited only three days before reporting to the aliens police had failed to present himself "without delay" to authorities: Decision No. ASYL 1989/1, at 13 (Sw. FC, Dec. 14, 1988).

whose illegal entry is the result of some form of compulsion.[507] The drafters expected refugees to present evidence that "owing to outside pressure, [they] had been obliged to enter or re-enter particular countries illegally."[508] Clearly, "[t]he fact that a refugee was fleeing from persecution was [in and of itself] good cause,"[509] as refugees seeking to escape the risk of persecution[510] cannot be expected to satisfy immigration formalities before fleeing to safety.[511] But good cause is not limited to flight from persecution. For example, the Swiss Federal Court has determined that fear of summary rejection at the Swiss border also constitutes good cause for illegal entry into that country, entitling the asylum-seeker to benefit from Art. 31.[512]

The more contentious aspect of this clause is the "coming directly" requirement, which might be thought to pose a barrier to the eligibility for exemption from penalization of refugees who move onward after failing to secure asylum in their initial state of refuge, or who have spent some period of time in a third state before arriving to seek protection. As regards secondary movement, consideration was given to two situations: refugees might move

---

[507] While the requirement to show "good cause" was at one stage omitted from the draft of Art. 31 (see UN Doc. E/AC.32/L.26, Feb. 2, 1950), its importance was repeatedly asserted by delegates. See Statement of the Chairman, Mr. Larsen of Denmark, UN Doc. E/AC.32/SR.22, Feb. 2, 1950, at 25; Statement of Mr. Weis of the IRO, UN Doc. E/AC.32/SR.24, Feb. 3, 1950, at 7 (proposing the language "and producing valid reasons to justify their illegal entry"); and Statement of Mr. Winter of Canada, UN Doc. E/AC.32/SR.40, Aug. 22, 1950, at 5.

[508] Statement of Mr. Juvigny of France, UN Doc. E/AC.32/SR.40, Aug. 22, 1950, at 6.

[509] Statement of Mr. Hoare of the United Kingdom, UN Doc. A/CONF.2/SR.14, July 10, 1951, at 7. See also Statement of Mr. van Heuven Goedhart of UNHCR, ibid. at 5. In contrast, the representative of the Netherlands suggested that the "good cause" language would deny exemption from penalization to a refugee who entered without authorization to visit a sick relative: Statement of Baron van Boetzelaer of the Netherlands, ibid. at 8.

[510] The French representative to the Conference of Plenipotentiaries proposed at one point that Art. 31 protection be restricted to persons in flight from a "country in which he *is* persecuted [emphasis added]": Statement of Mr. Rochefort of France, UN Doc. A/CONF.2/SR.35, July 25, 1951, at 18. The British delegate successfully opposed this language, arguing that "[h]e could not vote for the French amendment, because the Conference had already accepted the definition of the term 'refugee' given in article 1. There might, too, be cases where a refugee left a country after narrowly escaping persecution but without having actually been persecuted. Such a case would not be covered by the new French amendment": Statement of Mr. Hoare of the United Kingdom, ibid. at 19. The language as adopted therefore referred to persons "coming directly from a territory where their life or freedom was *threatened* [emphasis added]": ibid. at 19.

[511] "Nor is it said that they had committed unlawful activities in other countries, even though they had arrived in this country concealed in the back of a lorry, a course understandable in view of the conditions and the risk of persecution under which some would-be asylum-seekers lived": *R (Saadi) v. Secretary of State for the Home Department*, [2002] UKHL 41 (UK HL, Oct. 31, 2002), at para. 21.

[512] Dec. *6S.737/1998/bue*, ASYL 99/2, at 21 (Sw. FC, Mar. 17, 1999).

onward because they had been refused the right to settle in their original country of refuge, or because a risk of being persecuted had emerged there.[513] The consensus reached was that the first category of secondary movers – refugees who fail to find a permanent home in their country of first refuge – must comply with immigration laws if they wish to enter another asylum country without penalization. Those whose onward movement is compelled by the risk of being persecuted, in contrast, are entitled to the benefit of Art. 31. On the more general question of the eligibility for Art. 31 protection of refugees who travel through other countries, there was agreement that the "coming directly" language does not authorize penalization on the basis of relatively brief periods of time spent in other safe countries before arrival in a state party.[514]

By way of explanation, it is important to appreciate that the "coming directly" requirement was included in Art. 31 to respond to France's view that because a right to asylum is implicit in the Refugee Convention,[515] refugees not assimilated in their first asylum country might assert the right to enter another state without authorization. France felt that only refugees in flight from the risk of being persecuted should be exempt from immigration penalties,[516] and therefore proposed an amendment that would restrict Art. 31 protection to refugees "coming direct[ly] from their country of origin."[517] While other countries did not share France's understanding that the Refugee Convention implied a right to asylum,[518] they were persuaded

---

[513] Statement of Mr. van Heuven Goedhart of UNHCR, UN Doc. A.CONF.2/SR.14, July 10, 1951, at 4–5.

[514] "The expression 'coming directly' in Article 31(1), covers the situation of a person who enters the country in which asylum is sought directly from the country of origin, or from another country where his protection, safety and security could not be assured. It is understood that this term also covers a person who transits an intermediate country for a short period of time without having applied for, or received, asylum there": UNHCR, "Detention Guidelines," at para. 4.

[515] Statement of Mr. Colemar of France, UN Doc. A/CONF.2/SR.13, July 10, 1951, at 13.

[516] "[W]hile his delegation felt that it was right to exempt from any penalties imposed for illegal crossing of the frontier refugees coming directly from their countries of origin, it did not see any justification for granting them similar exemption in respect of their subsequent movements. The initial exemption was the direct corollary of the right of asylum, but once a refugee had found asylum, article [31] in its present form would allow him to move freely from one country to another without having to comply with frontier formalities. Actually, however, there was no major reason why a refugee should not comply with those formalities": Statement of Mr. Colemar of France, ibid.

[517] UN Doc. A/CONF.2/62.

[518] "The right to asylum ... was only a right, belonging to the State, to grant or refuse asylum, not a right belonging to the individual and entitling him to insist on its being extended to him. Article [31] therefore had nothing to do with the question of the right to asylum": Statement of Mr. Hoare of the United Kingdom, UN Doc. A/CONF.2/SR.13, July 10, 1951, at 14. See also Statements of Mr. Herment of Belgium and Mr. Giraldo-Jaramillo of Colombia, ibid.

that Art. 31 protection should ordinarily obtain only in the country of first refuge.[519]

A proposal from the UNHCR that would also have granted exemption from penalization to refugees unable to find a permanent home in their first country of refuge was therefore not taken up.[520] Instead, the version of Art. 31 approved at first reading by the Conference of Plenipotentiaries explicitly limited the beneficiary class to refugees who were "unable to find asylum even temporarily."[521] This decision is consistent with the general approach of the Refugee Convention, which does not guarantee a right to permanent admission to any asylum country, but only to protection for the duration of risk.[522] Refugees granted temporary protection cannot therefore invoke a breach of legal obligation by the state of first refuge as grounds for entering another country. It is also a logical limitation on Art. 31 protection, since exemption from penalization is granted because of the urgency of the refugee's need to flee. A refugee denied assimilation in the country of first asylum, but who faces no real risk of persecution there, is not imminently at risk.[523] He or she therefore can and should comply with immigration formalities before relocating.[524] If the refugee opts simply to enter another country without authorization, there is no good reason not to impose immigration penalties on him or her, so long as the penalties do not result in *refoulement* directly or indirectly to the country in which persecution is feared.[525]

---

[519] "[A]n exception from the consequences of irregular entry should only be considered in the case of the first receiving country": Statement of Mr. Del Drago of Italy, UN Doc. A/CONF.2/SR.13, July 10, 1951, at 13. See also Statement of Mr. von Trutzschler of the Federal Republic of Germany, UN Doc. A/CONF.2/SR.14, July 10, 1951, at 7.

[520] "Such refugees might possibly be covered if the words 'and shows good cause' were amended to read 'or shows other good causes'": Statement of Mr. van Heuven Goedhart of UNHCR, UN Doc. A/CONF.2/SR.14, July 10, 1951, at 5.

[521] Ibid. at 13.

[522] J. Hathaway, "The Meaning of Repatriation," (1997) 9(4) *International Journal of Refugee Law* 551. See generally chapter 7.1 below.

[523] A contrary view was taken by the representative of Greece, who "thought that there could be no doubt that the case where a country prescribed temporary residence for a refugee and thus deprived him of his freedom of residence did constitute a case where no penalty could be imposed on him by another country into whose territory he had illegally entered or in which he was illegally present": Statement of Mr. Philon of Greece, UN Doc. A/CONF.2/SR.14, July 10, 1951, at 12.

[524] "To admit without any reservation that a refugee who had settled temporarily in a receiving country was free to enter another, would be to grant him a right of immigration which might be exercised for reasons of mere personal convenience. It was normal in such cases that he should apply for a visa to the authorities of the country in question": Statement of Mr. Colemar of France, ibid. at 10.

[525] "In order to illustrate his own point, [the French representative] would give a concrete example – that of a refugee who, having found asylum in France, tried to make his way unlawfully into Belgium. It was obviously impossible for the Belgian government to

Despite the exclusion from Art. 31 protection of refugees who enter a state unlawfully simply because they have been unable to find a permanent home in the country of first asylum, the "coming directly" language does not disfranchise two other categories of refugee. First, representatives agreed that a refugee could be said to be "coming directly" to a country of asylum even if he or she had passed through, or even been provisionally admitted to, another country. Second, it was decided that immunity from immigration penalization would be granted to the second category of secondary movers – that is, to those compelled to leave a country of asylum due to a risk of being persecuted there.

Debate on the issue of whether Art. 31 could be claimed by persons who had spent time in an intermediate country was provoked by a Belgian observation that the "coming directly" language might be inappropriately relied upon to impose penalties against "a refugee who had stayed in another country for a week or a fortnight, and had then been obliged to seek asylum in the territory of the Contracting State in question."[526] He convinced his colleagues[527] that it was important not to "exclude from the benefit of [Art. 31] any refugee who had managed to find a few days' asylum in any country through which he had passed."[528] In the result, the French proposed wording "having been unable to find" temporary asylum was replaced by a formulation in the present tense, "*being* unable to find asylum even temporarily [emphasis added]."[529] Refugees therefore "come directly" so long as they have spent no more than reasonably short periods of time in one or more other countries. The Swiss Federal Court has held, for example, that an Afghan asylum-seeker who spent one month in Pakistan and two days in Italy before arriving in Switzerland had nonetheless come "directly" to Switzerland.[530]

While the Belgian amendment ensured that refugees who had spent short periods of time in other countries without being admitted to durable protection there would not be subject to immigration penalties, it was recognized that the revised wording might inadvertently give rise to a different problem. As noted by the British representative, the new phrase "being unable to find

---

acquiesce in that illegal entry, since the life and liberty of the refugee would be in no way in danger at the time": Statement of Mr. Colemar of France, UN Doc. A/CONF.2/SR.13, July 10, 1951, at 14–15.

[526] Statement of Mr. Herment of Belgium, UN Doc. A/CONF.2/SR.14, July 10, 1951, at 12.

[527] See e.g. Statement of Mr. Philon of Greece, ibid.; and report of consensus reached, ibid. at 13.

[528] Statement of Mr. Herment of Belgium, ibid. at 12.   [529] Ibid. at 13.

[530] Dec. *6S.737/1998/bue*, ASYL 99/2 (Sw. FC, Mar. 17, 1999). In contrast, Art. 31 does not generally inhere where the stays en route are prolonged. Absent evidence of extenuating circumstances, there is no reason to question the decision of the New Zealand High Court that a refugee from Ghana was not "coming directly" to New Zealand because she had spent two weeks in Swaziland, and ten months in South Africa: *Abu v. Superintendent of Mount Eden Women's Prison*, 199 NZAR Lexis 58 (NZ HC, Dec. 24, 1999).

asylum even temporarily" might be taken to mean that "a refugee would have to establish not merely his refugee status, but also that he was unable to find asylum in any country other than the one in which he applied to settle. Thus the onus of proving a negative would be placed on the refugee himself."[531] The United Kingdom sponsored a UNHCR proposal to delete the reference to inability to find even temporary asylum[532] in order to "relieve the refugee of the onus of proving that he was unable to enter any other country where he would not be persecuted. The refugee would still have to show good cause to justify his illegal entry or presence."[533] But there could be no question of insisting that refugees demonstrate their inability to secure asylum elsewhere as a condition of immunity from immigration penalties.[534]

It follows that even though prior presence in third countries does not mean that a refugee is not "coming directly" to the asylum state, authorities in the asylum state may nonetheless take account of the circumstances of the refugee's presence in third countries in order to assess whether he or she is able to "show good cause" for illegal entry or presence.[535] In earlier debates,

---

[531] UN Doc. A/CONF.2/SR.14, July 10, 1951, at 11.

[532] The language proposed by UNHCR was: "The Contracting States shall not impose penalties, on account of his illegal entry or presence, on a refugee who enters or who is present in their territory without authorization, provided he presents himself without delay to the authorities and shows good cause for believing that his illegal entry or presence is due to the fact that his life or freedom would otherwise be threatened": UN Doc. A/CONF.2/SR.35, July 25, 1951, at 11–12.

[533] Statement of Mr. van Heuven Goedhart of UNHCR, ibid. at 12. According to Grahl-Madsen, "the main objective of the 'good cause' proviso [is] to prevent ... the obligation to exempt refugees from penalties [from being] extended to such 'refugees who wished to change their country of asylum for purely personal reasons.' However, the requirement to 'show good cause for their illegal entry or presence' cannot wholly be ignored. It seems that in view of the wording chosen, a refugee may be obliged to explain – not why he has chosen any particular country – but why his entry or presence was illegal and not regularized beforehand. Thus the requirement to show 'good cause' in the present text is closely related to the requirement of presenting oneself without delay": Grahl-Madsen, *Commentary*, at 178–179.

[534] UNHCR convinced representatives that Article 31 should not be framed in a way that "would place on refugees the very unfair onus of proving that [they] were unable to find even temporary asylum anywhere outside the country or countries in which [their] life or freedom was threatened. As there were some eighty States in the world, the difficulty of such a task required no emphasis": Statement of Mr. van Heuven Goedhart of UNHCR, UN Doc. A/CONF.2/SR.35, July 25, 1951, at 10–11.

[535] "The term 'coming directly' refers, of course, to persons who have come directly from their country of origin or a country where their life or freedom was threatened, but also to persons who have been in an intermediary country for a short time without having received asylum there": Weis, *Travaux*, at 302. A misreading of the drafting history of the Refugee Convention led an American court to precisely the opposite conclusion. The case involved the claims of Afghan Mujahedin or "freedom fighters," who initially fled Afghanistan to Pakistan and India, where they were threatened and attacked by agents

the duty to show good cause was said to "oblige the refugee to show why he had failed to secure asylum in a country adjacent to his country of origin."[536] Thus, asylum-seekers who have spent time in safe states before arriving at the asylum country have an obligation to explain their inability or reluctance to seek recognition of their refugee status in those intermediate countries.[537] Courts have, for example, accepted as reasonable the decision not to seek asylum in intermediate states which were not clearly secure, where basic human rights were not respected, which were culturally or linguistically foreign to the refugee, or in which the individual had few or no social or family connections.[538] Absent plausible reasons of this kind, however, refugees who fail to take advantage of opportunities for real protection en route

of the Afghan government and Pakistani Communists. The Afghans then traveled to the United States; some came directly from India and Pakistan, others traveled via England, Holland, and Romania. Rather than inquiring into the reasons that prompted the asylum-seekers to continue onward to the United States, and indeed with no concern for the purely transitory presence of the Afghans in countries where they were not clearly at risk, the court asserted that "petitioners may not invoke Article 31 of the Protocol because it applies only to 'refugees who come directly from a territory where their life or freedom was threatened.' In this case, all petitioners came to the United States from various countries. Not one came directly from Afghanistan ... The debates at the United Nations General Assembly Conference on the Status of Refugees and Stateless Persons that drafted the Convention indicate that exemption from the consequences of an illegal entry should be considered only in the case of the first receiving country": *Singh v. Nelson*, 623 F Supp 545 (US DCSDNY, Dec. 12, 1985), at 42. Austrian jurisprudence is equally inattentive to the contextualized meaning of "coming directly." The Austrian High Court has ruled Art. 31 inapplicable to any refugee who has even transited through another country en route to Austria. "The argument put forward in the complaint is that 'direct' entry should be interpreted as meaning that mere transit through another country, even if that country is a contracting state of the Geneva Convention, should not prevent direct entry. This does not correspond to the clearly defined provisions of Article 31 of the Convention": *VwGH 91/19/0187* (Au. HC, Nov. 25, 1991), unofficial translation by E. Wiederin, *International Academy of Comparative Law National Report for Austria* (1994), at 5.

[536] Statement of the President, Mr. Larsen of Denmark, UN Doc. A/CONF.2/SR.14, July 10, 1951, at 11. See also Statement of Mr. Zutter of Switzerland, ibid. The other concerns initially understood by the Ad Hoc Committee to be within the scope of "showing good cause," including flight from the risk of persecution, were made textually explicit by the Conference of Plenipotentiaries.

[537] See comments of the representatives of the United Kingdom, Switzerland, Australia, and Belgium at UN Doc. A/CONF.2/SR.14, July 10, 1951, at 7–10.

[538] Hathaway, *Refugee Status*, at 46–50. Such an approach is consonant with UNHCR Executive Committee Conclusion No. 15 which provides that "[t]he intentions of the asylum-seeker as regards the country in which he wishes to request asylum should as far as possible be taken into account. Regard should be had to the concept that asylum should not be refused solely on the ground that it could be sought from another state": UNHCR Executive Committee Conclusion No. 15, "Refugees Without an Asylum Country" (1979), at para. h(iii), available at www.unhcr.ch (accessed Nov. 20, 2004).

to the asylum country may validly be subjected to immigration penalties, so long as these do not give rise to the risk of *refoulement*.[539]

Beyond clarifying that Art. 31 could be invoked by refugees arriving after having spent brief periods in safe third countries, the drafters also determined that immunity from immigration penalties should not be limited to refugees coming directly "from their country of origin." A refugee who confronts a risk of persecution in a country of asylum would, like a refugee coming from his or her state of origin, not be able safely to delay departure until immigration formalities had been completed. Just as in the case of refugees coming directly from their country of origin, the need to escape logically trumps the usual duty to respect immigration laws. The President of the Conference of Plenipotentiaries therefore suggested that the Convention should exempt from penalties any refugee "coming direct[ly] from a territory where his life or freedom was threatened,"[540] an approach initially embraced as a friendly amendment by France.[541] No state opposed the extension of Art. 31 protection to refugees in secondary flight from the risk of persecution.[542] On reflection, however, the French delegate expressed concern that the precise language proposed by the President ("coming direct[ly] from a country

---

[539] See also Statement of Mr. Herment of Belgium, UN Doc. A/CONF.2/SR.13, July 10, 1951, at 14: "The purpose ... was to exempt refugees from the application of the penalties imposable for the unlawful crossing of a frontier, provided they presented themselves of their own free will to the authorities *and explained their case to them* [emphasis added]." In *R v. Uxbridge Magistrates Court, ex parte Adimi*, [1999] 4 All ER 520 (Eng. HC, July 29, 1999), at 528, the court opined that to determine whether a stay in an intermediate state was a basis for denying eligibility for Art. 31 protection, account should be taken of duration of stay, reasons for delay in departing the intermediate country, and whether or not protection had been sought or found. For reasons described above such matters should not (as the court assumed) determine whether the refugee was "coming directly" to the asylum state; these factors are nonetheless sensibly understood to be part of the inquiry into whether the refugee has "good cause" for illegal entry or presence.

[540] "A refugee in a particular country of asylum, for example, a Hungarian refugee living in Germany, might, without actually being persecuted, feel obliged to seek refuge in another country; if he then entered Denmark illegally, it was reasonable to expect that the Danish authorities would not inflict penalties on him for such illegal entry, provided he could show good cause for it": Statement of the President, Mr. Larsen of Denmark, UN Doc. A/CONF.2/SR.13, July 10, 1951, at 15.

[541] Statement of Mr. Colemar of France, ibid. See also Statement of Mr. van Heuven Goedhart of UNHCR, UN Doc. A/CONF.2/SR.14, July 10, 1951, at 5.

[542] "[H]e thought there had been no objection to the High Commissioner's interpretation, namely, that the refugee's illegal entry or presence must be proved to be due to the fact that his life or freedom would otherwise have been threatened. He (the President) considered that the French point of view should be acceptable to the other delegations, and that there need be no difference of opinion on that question": Statement of the President, Mr. Larsen of Denmark, UN Doc. A/CONF.2/SR.35, July 25, 1951, at 13. No special significance should be attributed to the language requiring a threat to "life or freedom," instead of to a "well-founded fear of being persecuted."

where his life or freedom was threatened") might undermine the finite obligation of states originally secured by the Convention's January 1, 1951 cut-off date.[543] While a refugee whose initial flight was due to post-1951 causes would not be entitled to protection, there would be no way to predict how many refugees would need to move due to risks of persecution in asylum states that might arise only after 1951.[544]

The goal of the ensuing discussion at the Conference of Plenipotentiaries was therefore to find a means to grant exemption from penalization to refugees in secondary flight from persecution that would respect the Convention's temporal limitation. The French representative felt that this goal could be achieved by "wording, which would be in accordance with Article 1."[545] His favored formulation, "coming directly from a territory in which his life or freedom would be threatened within the meaning of article 1, paragraph A, of this Convention"[546] derived from a determination to limit Art. 31 protection to persons in flight from a pre-1951 phenomenon.[547] The text as finally adopted was intended to achieve precisely this goal.[548] But with the Refugee Protocol's prospective abolition of the

---

[543] This dateline has been prospectively eliminated by the adoption of the 1967 Protocol relating to the Status of Refugees: see chapter 2.5.1 above, at pp. 110–111. The French concern therefore has no contemporary relevance for the overwhelming majority of state parties to the Convention, which are also parties to the Protocol.

[544] "As he understood the present text, a person who was the victim of events occurring in a neighbouring country after [January 1, 1951] would not come within the terms of the Convention if he crossed the border into France, whereas those who had already been authorized to take refuge in the neighbouring country as a result of events occurring before 1 January 1951 would be able to claim the benefit of the present provision. Thus there might easily be an influx of refugees who had been authorized to stay in a neighbouring country, but who, because their lives were threatened as a result of events occurring *in that country* after 1 January 1951, would be entitled to avail themselves of the clause to move into France. Thus the ceiling on commitments provided by the date of 1 January 1951 would be largely nullified [emphasis added]": Statement of Mr. Rochefort of France, UN Doc. A/CONF.2/SR.35, July 25, 1951, at 14.

[545] Ibid. at 15–16.   [546] Ibid. at 17.

[547] The British representative "felt that the time factor was already covered by the definition of the term 'refugee' in article 1. Article 31 could not therefore relate to any refugee fleeing from a country as a result of events occurring after 1 January, 1951": Statement of Mr. Hoare of the United Kingdom, ibid. at 17. The French representative insisted on the need for an additional qualification in Art. 31 "since a refugee might be a refugee under the terms of the Statute of the High Commissioner's Office [and also that] [t]he definition in article 1 did not cover conditions of admission, but only the rights to be accorded refugees": Statement of Mr. Rochefort of France, ibid.

[548] A competing British amendment was withdrawn because "the French representative found it unacceptable": Statement of Mr. Hoare of the United Kingdom, ibid. at 19. Immediately prior to the 20–0 (2 abstentions) vote to approve the final text, the French representative reiterated that the reason for the reference to Art. 1 of the Convention in the text of Art. 31 was that France, "[a]s a country of second reception . . . could not bind itself to accept refugees from all other European countries of first reception. There had to

January 1, 1951 cut-off date for refugee status,[549] the original basis for inserting the reference to persons whose life or freedom was threatened "in the sense of Article 1" has now been rendered largely moot. Because state parties to the Protocol are required to apply the Convention refugee definition without reference to the temporal limitation,[550] all refugees whose illegal entry or presence is due to the risk of being persecuted in a country of asylum are today entitled to exemption from immigration penalties.[551]

The argument has, however, been advanced that the comments of two delegates to the Conference of Plenipotentiaries suggest that the phrase "in the sense of Article 1" may also restrict access to Art. 31 protection on the grounds that it requires a refugee in secondary flight to show that the risk of persecution in the country from which secondary flight originated is on account of "race, religion, nationality, membership of a particular social group, or political opinion," meaning that Art. 31 protection would not inhere where departure is the result of a generalized risk of being persecuted there.[552] Taken in context,

---

be some limit, such as that of events occurring before 1 January 1951": Statement of Mr. Rochefort of France, ibid. at 19.

[549] See chapter 2.5.1 above, at pp. 110–111.

[550] Protocol relating to the Status of Refugees, 606 UNTS 8791, done Jan. 31, 1967, entered into force Oct. 4, 1967 (Refugee Protocol), at Art. I(2).

[551] There is no basis for an argument that the risk faced must be other than a risk of being persecuted. "The words 'where their life or freedom was threatened' may give the impression that another standard is required than for refugee status in Article 1. This is, however, not the case. The Secretariat draft referred to refugees 'escaping from persecution' and to the obligation not to turn back refugees 'to the frontier of their country of origin, or to territories where their life or freedom would be threatened on account of their race, religion, nationality, or political opinions.' In the course of drafting the words 'country of origin,' 'territories where their life or freedom was threatened' and 'country in which he is persecuted' were used interchangeably. The reference to Article 1 of the Convention was introduced mainly to refer to the dateline of 1 January 1951 but it also indicated that there was no intention to introduce more restrictive criteria than that of 'well-founded fear of persecution' used in Article 1(A)(ii)": Weis, *Travaux*, at 303.

[552] Statements of Mr. Petren of Sweden, UN Doc. A/CONF.2/SR.35, July 25, 1951, at 14–15; and of the President, Mr. Larsen of Denmark, ibid. at 18: "It might also happen, as the Swedish representative had indicated, that a refugee, as defined in article 1, escaped to a second country where his life or liberty was again in danger, but not for the reasons specified in article 1, and that for those irrelevant reasons he fled to a third country. The French representative was, presumably, concerned with the possibility of such cases coming within the terms of Article 31." In fact, as described above, this was not the concern of the French delegate. Yet the language adopted ("in the sense of Article 1") is certainly broad enough to encompass this requirement. It was also likely in the minds of the drafters, given this statement by the President just prior to the final vote on the text of Art. 31. The implications of this requirement are, however, unclear. Since the original recognition of refugee status was premised on a nexus to one of the five Convention grounds, it might reasonably be said that "but for" that initial, nexus-defined flight the refugee would not have been compelled to seek secondary protection. That is, he or she is only exposed to the risk of persecution in the asylum country because of an initial flight prompted by race, religion, nationality, membership of a particular social group, or political opinion.

however, the better view is that these interventions at the Conference were intended simply to ensure that Art. 31 protection is limited to persons whose secondary movement is motivated by a need for protection.[553] Nor should any special significance be attached to the reference to refugees coming from a "territory" (as opposed to a "country") in which they face a risk of being persecuted. The French delegate did not explain his choice of language, though it is likely that it was simply intended to track the formulation of Art. 33's duty of *non-refoulement*.[554]

A final question is whether Art. 31 can be invoked by persons or organizations that assist refugees in flight from the risk of persecution to enter an asylum country without authorization. The importance of such protection was voiced by the Swiss representative to the Ad Hoc Committee:

> Swiss federal law did not regard any person assisting [a refugee] as liable to punishment, provided his motives were above board. The provision was of some importance for voluntary organizations for aid to refugees. Article [31] did not include any such provision, and he thought the omission should be made good. It was quite possible that in domestic law, assistance to a foreigner crossing a frontier illegally might be regarded as a separate offence punishable even if the refugee was not.[555]

There was general agreement that "a refugee organization should not be penalized for having helped a refugee applying to it. That was an obvious humanitarian duty."[556] Yet no state endorsed the Swiss proposal to amend the Convention to provide for such an exemption. Concern was expressed that any such amendment might encourage organizations actually to organize or promote the illegal entry of refugees (rather than simply to respond to

---

[553] The basis for the Swedish representative's allusion to the importance of restricting the benefit of Art. 31 to persons able to show the risk of persecution for an enumerated ground was that "otherwise a refugee who had committed a theft might maintain that his freedom was in danger": Statement of Mr. Petren of Sweden, ibid. at 14–15. In other words, Art. 31 ought not to apply to persons whose illegal entry or presence was unconnected to their refugee status. This broader reading is in keeping with the more general concern to limit Art. 31 protection to refugees whose secondary movement was prompted by the need for protection. "What France wished to avoid was having to accept any refugee from a neighbouring country who *voluntarily* decided to move into France, perhaps *on the pretext* that the neighbouring country would no longer give him permission to reside there [emphasis added]": Statement of Mr. Rochefort of France, ibid. at 11.

[554] UNHCR had earlier suggested that the language of Art. 31 should mirror the duty of *non-refoulement*, which refers to "territories" where life or freedom would be threatened: Statement of Mr. van Heuven Goedhart of UNHCR, UN Doc. A/CONF.2/SR.14, July 10, 1951, at 5.

[555] Statement of Mr. Schurch of Switzerland, UN Doc. E/AC.32/SR.40, Aug. 22, 1950, at 8.

[556] Statement of Mr. Juvigny of France, ibid. at 9. See also Statements of Mr. Henkin of the United States, Mr. Perez-Perozo of Venezuela, and the Chairman, Mr. Larsen of Denmark, ibid. at 8–9.

requests for assistance). Indeed, the French representative successfully urged his colleagues to leave states the freedom to penalize "corporate bodies" that might exploit asylum-seekers.[557] The final consensus was that "it would be sufficient to make mention of the problem in the summary record of the meeting, in the hope that Governments would take note of the very liberal outlook embodied in the Swiss federal laws and follow that example."[558]

This discussion confirms that there is no legal obligation to exempt even individuals or organizations with purely humanitarian motives from penalties for assisting refugees to cross frontiers without authorization. As the text of Art. 31 makes clear, the duty of states is simply to avoid the imposition of penalties "on refugees." Yet the conceptual incongruity of penalizing individuals, organizations, or corporations for facilitating precisely the irregular entry that Art. 31 allows is surely self-evident. Recognizing that the drafters' reluctance to amend the text of Art. 31 stemmed from concern to avoid the exploitation of refugees, asylum countries should be slow to impose immigration-related penalties on innocent agents of entry.[559]

---

[557] "But assistance to refugees might go beyond the national territory, and in certain circumstances refugee organizations might literally become organizations for the illegal crossing of frontiers. He wondered whether it would be in the interests of refugees themselves that organizations of this kind, whose activities were likely to come under very much more general laws, should exist inside national territories": Statement of Mr. Juvigny of France, ibid. at 9.

[558] Statement of Mr. Juvigny of France, ibid. at 9. See also Statement of Mr. Henkin of the United States, ibid. at 8; and Statement of the Chairman, Mr. Larsen of Denmark, ibid. at 9.

[559] The English Court of Appeal found that rules which imposed a mandatory £2,000 fine on truck drivers and others for each unauthorized entrant brought to the United Kingdom by them as the result of either intent or negligence were in breach of the requirements of the European Convention on Human Rights. "[E]ven assuming, as I do, that the scheme is directed towards punishing carriers for some fault, it cannot to my mind be right to impose so high a fixed penalty without possibility of mitigation. The hallowed principle that the punishment must fit the crime is irreconcilable with the notion of a substantial fixed penalty. It is essentially, therefore, on this account rather than because of the reversed burden of proof that I would regard the scheme as incompatible with Article 6. What in particular it offends is the carrier's right to have his penalty determined by an independent tribunal. To my mind there surely is such a right . . . if . . . contrary to my belief, the scale and inflexibility of the penalty, taken in conjunction with the other features of this scheme, are not such as to deprive the carriers of a fair trial under Article 6, then I would hold them instead to impose an excessive burden on the carriers such as to violate Article 1. Even acknowledging, as I do, the great importance of the social goal which the scheme seeks to promote, there are nevertheless limits to how far the state is entitled to go in imposing obligations of vigilance on drivers (and vicarious liability on employers and hirers) to achieve it and in penalising any breach. Obviously, were the penalty heavier still and the discouragement of carelessness correspondingly greater, the scheme would be yet more effective and the policy objective fulfilled to an even higher

Thus, despite the risk that policies such as Australia's assignment of detention costs to carriers and Ireland's refusal to exempt carriers transporting refugees from sanctions will have a chilling effect on the willingness of airlines and others to allow refugees to travel, such penalties cannot be said to breach Art. 31. The same is true of the Canadian laws which authorize the criminal prosecution of persons who assist unauthorized entrants (including refugee claimants) to arrive at its territory. Importantly, however, Canada's reluctance to impose those penalties in practice against persons transporting refugee claimants in other than egregious cases is very much in line with the expectations of the Convention's drafters. Perhaps ironically, the more formalized dispensations from penalties applied in some European countries – for example, in Belgium, Finland, France, Germany, and Luxembourg – may actually be less in keeping with the goals of the drafters. Because the real basis for the drafters' reluctance to vary the text of Art. 31 was concern to punish those who are effectively "trafficking" in asylum-seekers,[560] it makes little sense to refrain from imposing carrier sanctions only where an asylum claim is ultimately found to be legally admissible, or to be substantively well founded.[561] This approach implies a duty on the part of transportation companies accurately to assess the refugee status of their passengers, and imposes liability in circumstances that are in no sense indicative of any intention to exploit. The recent move of the European Union to promote a policy of not pursuing carrier sanctions when the person transported makes a claim to refugee protection is, like the Canadian practice, more clearly in keeping with the goals of Art. 31.

---

degree. There comes a point, however, when what is achieved is achieved only at the cost of basic fairness. The price in Convention terms becomes just too high. That in my judgment is the position here": *Secretary of State for the Home Department v. International Transport Roth GmbH*, [2002] 1 CMLR 52 (Eng. CA, Feb. 22, 2002), at paras. 47, 53, per Simon Brown LJ. Interestingly, neither the issue of the impact on refugees nor the possible relevance of Art. 31 of the Refugee Convention seems to have been argued.

[560] Trafficking is defined as "the recruitment, transportation, transfer, harboring or receipt of persons, by means of threat or use of force or other forms of coercion, of abduction, of fraud, of deception, of the abuse of power or of a position of vulnerability or of the giving or receiving of payments or benefits to achieve the consent of a person having control over another person, for the purpose of exploitation": Protocol to Prevent, Suppress and Punish Trafficking in Persons, especially Women and Children, supplementing the United Nations Convention against Transnational Organized Crime, UNGA Res. 55/25, Annex II, 55 UNGAOR Supp. (No. 49) at 65, UN Doc. A/45/49, vol. I (2001), adopted Nov. 15, 2000, entered into force Dec. 25, 2003, at Art. 3.

[561] But see G. Goodwin-Gill, "Article 31 of the 1951 Convention relating to the Status of Refugees: Non-Penalization, Detention, and Protection," in E. Feller et al. eds., *Refugee Protection in International Law* 185 (2003) (Goodwin-Gill, "Article 31"), at 219: "As a matter of principle ... a carrier should not be penalized for bringing in an 'undocumented' passenger, *where that person is subsequently determined to be in need of international protection* [emphasis added]."

To summarize, a refugee in flight from the risk of being persecuted may invoke Art. 31 to avoid penalties for illegal entry or presence so long as he or she voluntarily reports to asylum state authorities within a reasonable time after crossing the frontier. The refugee must show "good cause" for illegal entry or presence, a requirement which will always be met where the breach of migration control laws is the result of flight from a risk of being persecuted. The risk of persecution may exist, however, either in the refugee's country of origin, or in a state in which protection was previously afforded. If the refugee has passed through, or spent time in, one or more non-persecutory states, he or she may be expected to provide a plausible explanation for the failure to seek protection in the intermediate states as a condition for exemption from immigration penalties, though such presence does not automatically exclude the refugee from entitlement to Art. 31 protection. Because the Convention provides protection from penalization only for refugees themselves, those who transport or otherwise assist refugees to enter asylum states without authorization are not protected from amenability to the usual regulatory or criminal penalties for such actions. The drafters assumed, however, that governments would not exercise their authority to penalize those assisting refugees to enter an asylum country absent evidence that they had acted in an exploitative way, or otherwise in bad faith.

4.2.2 Non-penalization

The substance of the duty of non-penalization was not extensively discussed by the drafters of the Refugee Convention. The core concern is to exempt refugees fleeing persecution from sanctions that might ordinarily be imposed[562] for breach of the asylum state's general migration control laws.[563] The Secretary-General's background study, for example, observed

---

[562] "The Belgian representative had urged that the penalties mentioned in the article ... should be confined to judicial penalties only. Surely that was precisely what the article stated. A judicial penalty, at least as interpreted in the code law of the Latin countries, was a penalty pronounced by the courts, not an administrative penalty": Statement of Mr. Juvigny of France, UN Doc. E/AC.32/SR.40, Aug. 22, 1950, at 5. Because the goal of the French position was to ensure that purely administrative actions were not subject to Art. 31, Grahl-Madsen logically suggests that "[t]he term 'penalties' includes imprisonment and fines, meted out as punishment by a judicial or semi-judicial body": Grahl-Madsen, *Commentary*, at 169.

[563] "The meaning of 'illegal entry or presence' has not generally raised any difficult issue of interpretation. The former would include arriving or securing entry through the use of false or falsified documents, the use of other methods of deception, clandestine entry (for example, as a stowaway), and entry into State territory with the assistance of smugglers or traffickers ... 'Illegal presence' would cover unlawful arriving and remaining, for instance, after the elapse of a short, permitted period of stay": Goodwin-Gill, "Article 31," at 196.

that while countries commonly require non-citizens to present a valid passport and visa to be legally admitted, a refugee "is rarely in a position to comply with the requirements for legal entry."[564] Equally apparent is the need of many refugees to cross borders clandestinely in order to access protection. So long as a refugee's failure to present valid travel documents or to comply with the usual immigration formalities is purely incidental to his or her flight from the risk of being persecuted, he or she should not be sanctioned "on a charge of illegal entry."[565] There is therefore no basis in international law for the practice in Russia and Bulgaria of subjecting refugees to the usual penalties for illegal entry, nor for the arrest by Zambia and Zimbabwe of refugee claimants for having entered their territory illegally. Nor may South Africa rely on its right to arrest illegal entrants to penalize refugees caught up in its more general efforts. Where efforts to penalize refugees for illegal entry are more informal, as in Kenya, the government has a duty to ensure that its officials do not take action against refugees in the hope of extracting bribes or other benefits. Nor does international law sanction the United Kingdom's policy of pursuing criminal charges against refugees found to have used false documents to pass through its territory. As an English court has observed, the right of refugees to breach migration control laws in search of protection means that the propriety of prosecution for such matters by a transit state is particularly doubtful.[566]

Interestingly, Art. 31 does not require state parties formally to incorporate an exemption for refugees from general immigration penalties. Indeed, there is not even a duty to refrain from launching a prosecution against refugees for

---

[564] Secretary-General, "Memorandum," at 46.

[565] Statement of Mr. Hoare of the United Kingdom, UN Doc. A/CONF.2/SR.13, July 10, 1951, at 14. See also Statements of Mr. Colemar of France, ibid. at 13 ("any penalties imposed for illegal crossing of the frontier"); Mr. Del Drago of Italy, ibid. at 13 ("from the consequences of irregular entry"); Mr. Herment of Belgium, ibid. at 14 ("penalties imposable for the unlawful crossing of a frontier"); the President, Mr. Larsen of Denmark, ibid. at 15 ("penalties . . . for such illegal entry"); and Mr. van Heuven Goedhart of UNHCR, UN Doc. A/CONF.2/SR.35, July 25, 1951, at 12 ("punished for such illegal entry").

[566] "[T]he [government] will surely wish to reflect upon the wisdom of prosecuting and imprisoning refugees for the use of false travel documents. Is this really a just and sensible policy? . . . In any event, the [government's] argument provides no justification whatever for prosecuting refugees in transit": *R v. Uxbridge Magistrates Court, ex parte Adimi*, [1999] 4 All ER 520 (Eng. HC, July 29, 1999), at 534. See also Goodwin-Gill, "Article 31," at 216–217: "If a State initiates action within its territory, for example, to deal with the use of false travel documents, then that State, rather than the State of intended destination, assumes the responsibility of ensuring that the refugee/asylum seeker benefits at least from those provisions of the 1951 Convention, such as Articles 31 and 33 . . . which are not dependent upon lawful presence or residence."

breach of immigration laws.[567] As much was arguably evident even in the original formulation of Art. 31, which would have required states not to "apply" penalties against refugees.[568] But the final language, in which the only obligation is not to "impose" such penalties,[569] makes this point quite clearly. Indeed, the Belgian representative to the Ad Hoc Committee observed that the immunity of a particular refugee from immigration penalties is a question to be submitted to the courts, implying the ability to lay charges in the first place.[570] It is therefore lawful for a government to charge an asylum-seeker with an immigration offense, and even to commence a prosecution, so long as no conviction is entered until and unless a determination is made that the individual is not in fact a Convention refugee.[571] The practice in New Zealand of allowing prosecutions against asylum-seekers for reliance on false travel documents to proceed pending completion of the usual refugee status verification procedures is not therefore a breach of Art. 31, so long as a verdict is not rendered pending results of the refugee inquiry.[572]

[567] See *R v. Uxbridge Magistrates Court, ex parte Adimi*, [1999] 4 All ER 520 (Eng. HC, July 29, 1999), at 533: "[I]t would seem to me clearly preferable if possible to avoid any prosecution at all rather merely than look to the remedy of a stay once it appears that immunity may arise under art. 31. I do not go so far as to say that the very fact of prosecution must itself be regarded as a penalty under art. 31 . . . But there is not the least doubt that a conviction constitutes a penalty and that art. 31 impunity is not afforded . . . by granting an absolute discharge . . . Provided that the [government] henceforth recognizes the true reach of art. 31 as we are declaring it to be, and puts in place procedures that those entitled to its protection . . . are not prosecuted, *at any rate to conviction*, . . . I am inclined to conclude that . . . the abuse of due process jurisdiction is able to provide a sufficient safety net for those wrongly prosecuted [emphasis added]."

[568] Secretary-General, "Memorandum," at 45.

[569] This shift of language can be traced to a joint proposal of Belgium and the United States, UN Doc. E/AC.32/L.25, Feb. 2, 1950. To "impose" is to "enforce compliance with": *Concise Oxford Dictionary* 682 (9th edn, 1995).

[570] Statement of Mr. Herment of Belgium, UN Doc. A/CONF.2/SR.14, July 10, 1951, at 10.

[571] "If proceedings should have been instituted against a refugee, and it becomes clear that his case [falls] under the provisions of Article 31(1), the public prosecutor will be duty bound to withdraw the case or else see to it that the refugee is acquitted. In no case may a judgment be executed, if the offence is one to which Article 31(1) applies": Grahl-Madsen, *Commentary*, at 170. See also Weis, *Travaux*, at 303: "In the case of asylum-seekers, proceedings on account of illegal entry or presence should be suspended pending examination of their request."

[572] In considering the circumstances of an Iranian refugee claimant who was charged with possession of a fraudulent French passport, the New Zealand High Court observed "[i]f it is, indeed, the case that he is found to be a true refugee then the probabilities are that the charge will be withdrawn. In any event, his *claim to refugee status* may well result in a reasonable excuse defence being successful if the case proceeds to trial [emphasis added]": *AHK v. Police*, [2002] NZAR 531 (NZ HC, Dec. 11, 2001), at para. 12. The French Conseil d'Etat has held that immigration penalties may only be applied to an asylum-seeker if and when his request for recognition of refugee status is denied: *AJDA 1977.515, Revue de droit administratif* 1977.481 (Fr. CE, May 22, 1977).

Increasingly, the penalty imposed on account of unlawful entry or presence may consist of the denial of procedural rights in the context of the refugee status determination procedure. In the United States, for example, refugees and others arriving without proper documents are diverted into an "expedited removal" process in which they enjoy significantly reduced due process rights, and no appeal rights. While persons able to show a "credible fear" of being persecuted are in principle exempted from the expedited removal system, in practice the procedure to assess exemption from this penalty is subject to myriad deficiencies.[573] In the result, refugees arriving without valid documents are not dependably safeguarded from the severe truncation of their due process rights.[574] The proposal advanced by the United Kingdom in 2003 to subject all refugees arriving without valid travel documents to an abbreviated, offshore procedure raises the same concerns in an even more obvious way: in contrast to even the American system, it was specifically and directly targeted at refugees arriving *inter alia* without valid documentation.

The case is strong that the assignment of refugees who arrive without proper documentation to abbreviated procedures is in essence a penalty inflicted for irregular entry. When a summary procedure is resorted to not on the grounds of the substantive insufficiency of a claim,[575] but rather to sanction a refugee for his or her mode of entry, such procedures take on a decidedly punitive character. Because the essential purpose of Art. 31 is to insulate refugees from penalties for the act of crossing a border without authorization, a refugee may not lawfully be denied access to ordinary legal entitlements to a complete refugee status inquiry simply because he or she has used false documents to enter the country, or otherwise contravened migration control laws. In contrast to the highly problematic American approach, however, a breach of Art. 31 may be avoided where, as under new European Union rules, the nature of the abbreviated procedure to which persons using false documents are subjected[576] is required to meet all of the usual procedural

---

[573] "Difficulties were experienced in the process with translation, with access to detainees, and with notification of material developments in the cases. These cases suggest that such problems can impact the substantive determinations made during the credible fear process": Hastings College of the Law Center for Human Rights and International Justice, "Report on the Second Year of Implementation of Expedited Removal" (1999), at 120.

[574] Ironically, if the nature of the penalty imposed by the United States for illegal entry is defined by reference to the result of the denial of due process rights – that is, expulsion – it would follow that the American law does not contravene Art. 31: see chapter 4.2.3 below, at pp. 412–413.

[575] Summary procedures are allowable under international law in the case of persons who, for example, make no arguable claim to refugee status: UNHCR Executive Committee Conclusion No. 30, "The Problem of Manifestly Unfounded or Abusive Applications for Refugee Status or Asylum" (1983), at para. (d), available at www.unhcr.ch (accessed Nov. 20, 2004).

[576] EU Procedures Directive, at Art. 23(4)(d), (f).

requirements for the fair assessment of a claim to refugee status.[577] Indeed, even under earlier European practice only refugee claimants who continued to insist on the validity of the false documentation used to secure entry, and who actually based their claims on the false identity, could be assigned to an abbreviated procedure.[578] As such, the penalty was in essence imposed for deliberate and calculated deception after arrival, not on account of illegal entry or presence.[579]

It might, however, be objected that the notion of "penalties" in Art. 31 ought to be confined to the usual sanctions imposed on persons who cross a border without permission, and not encompass, for example, the truncation of due process rights as implemented by the United States or proposed by the United Kingdom. But despite the fact that at the time of the Convention's drafting the only penalties which refugees faced on account of unauthorized entry or presence were traditional migration penalties that applied to all irregular entrants, there are nonetheless good reasons to argue that a broader range of penalties (including those imposed specifically on refugees) is in fact proscribed by Art. 31.

It is true that the original draft of Art. 31 would have supported a narrow construction of the notion of relevant "penalties." The Secretary-General's proposed wording called on states not to apply to refugees "[t]he penalties enacted against foreigners entering the territory of the Contracting Party without permission."[580] Clearly only one kind of penalty was contemplated, namely general sanctions for having entered the territory unlawfully.[581] Simultaneously on the table at the first session of the Ad Hoc Committee, however, was a joint Belgian–American proposal for Art. 31. It prefaced its requirement that states "shall not impose penalties on [refugees] on account of their illegal entry or residence" with the affirmation of a duty to afford irregularly entering refugees "treatment compatible, from both the moral and material point of view, with human dignity."[582] While the language that would have ensured that refugees could "lead as normal a life as possible"[583]

---

[577] "Member States may prioritise or accelerate any examination in accordance with the basic principles and guarantees of chapter II including where the application is likely to be well-founded or where the applicant has special needs": ibid. at Art. 23(3).

[578] *Resolution on Manifestly Unfounded Applications for Asylum*, Doc. COM(2002) 326, at para. 9(a).

[579] Ibid. at para. 9(b) and (f). This conclusion is reinforced by the fact that refugees who arrived legally could also be relegated to a truncated procedure if they deliberately made false representations, or otherwise failed to comply with their substantive legal obligations.

[580] Secretary-General, "Memorandum," at 45.

[581] See chapter 4.2 above, at pp. 382–388; and text above at pp. 405–406.

[582] UN Doc. E/AC.32/L.25, Feb. 2, 1950, at 1.

[583] Statement of Mr. Weis of the International Refugee Organization, UN Doc. E/AC.32/SR.22, Feb. 2, 1950, at 25.

was dropped because it was deemed "too ambitious,"[584] the Belgian–American approach nonetheless inspired a subtle, but important, reframing of Art. 31.

Specifically, the Chairman of the Ad Hoc Committee recommended that "the article should be re-drafted to read: 'The High Contracting Parties undertake not to impose penalties on refugees who enter or are present in their territory without prior or legal authorization.'"[585] That is, instead of prohibiting the imposition of a particular *kind of penalty* as had earlier formulations ("the penalties applied against foreigners entering the territory ... without prior permission"), Art. 31 would instead prohibit simply "penalties" *imposed on a particular group of persons*, namely "refugees who enter or are present in their territory without prior or legal authorization." As adopted by the Ad Hoc Committee, the text provided that:

> The Contracting States shall not impose penalties, on account of his illegal entry or presence, on a refugee.[586]

By moving the reference to "illegal entry or presence" into a subordinate clause, the spirit of the Chairman's proposal was maintained, and the textual meaning of Art. 31 changed from that first proposed by the Secretary-General. Instead of immunizing refugees from a particular kind of penalty, the purport of Art. 31 is that penalties (in general) are prohibited if imposed *in a particular context*, namely as the result of unlawful entry or presence. In the French language formulation as well, the reference to irregular entry or presence defines the reason or context for the imposition of penalties, not their substance.[587] Taking into account the plain meaning[588] of a "penalty" as a loss inflicted for violation of a law,[589] Art. 31 denies governments the right to subject refugees to any detriment for reasons of their unauthorized entry or

---

584 Statement of the Chairman, Mr. Chance of Canada, ibid. The general spirit of the Belgian–American amendment was adopted in what became Art. 31(2), expressly addressing the circumstances in which freedom of movement may be lawfully denied to irregularly entering refugees.

585 Statement of the Chairman, Mr. Chance of Canada, ibid.

586 "Report of the Ad Hoc Committee on Statelessness and Related Problems," UN Doc. E/1618, Feb. 17, 1950 (Ad Hoc Committee, "First Session Report"), at 7.

587 "Les Etats contractants n'appliqueront pas de sanctions pénales, *du fait de* leur entrée ou de leur séjour irréguliers, aux réfugiés qui, arrivant directement du territoire où leur vie ou leur liberté était menacée au sens prévu par l'article premier, entrent ou se trouvent sur leur territoire sans autorisation, sous la réserve qu'ils se présentent sans délai aux autorités et leur exposent des raisons reconnues valables de leur entrée ou présence irrégulières [emphasis added]": Refugee Convention, at Art. 31(1).

588 See Vienna Convention on the Law of Treaties, 1155 UNTS 331, done May 23, 1969, entered into force Jan. 27, 1980 (Vienna Convention), at Art. 31(1).

589 A penalty is "a punishment ... for a breach of a law, contract, etc." Punishment, in turn, is "the loss or suffering inflicted in the act or an instance of punishing": *Concise Oxford Dictionary* 1010, 1111 (9th edn, 1995).

presence in the asylum country. This approach is in line with the tenor of a recent administrative decision in the United Kingdom:

> In *Adimi*, it was unsurprisingly held that convictions by criminal courts were penalties under Article 31. [Counsel for the government] did not dispute that civil penalties would also fall within Article 31, but he submitted that a penalty involved a removal of a right that a person previously had. [Counsel for the claimant], on the other hand, submitted that any treatment that was less favourable than that accorded to others and was imposed on account of illegal entry was a penalty within Article 31 unless objectively justifiable on administrative grounds. I prefer [the claimant's] submission. It seems to me that [the government's] approach puts form above substance and would enable contracting states to evade Article 31 by the use of one form of words in domestic legislation rather than another.[590]

On the facts of the case, it was determined that unless the statutory requirement to seek protection "on his arrival" was construed to include applications made subsequent to the initial clearing of immigration control, the denial of income support benefits on that ground would amount to a penalty imposed for reasons of illegal entry, contrary to Art. 31 of the Refugee Convention.[591]

Despite the logic of seeing a reasonably broad range of practices resulting in a loss as "penalties" as that term is commonly understood, objection may be taken to such a broad reading on the grounds that it is at odds with the equally authoritative French language text of Art. 31 which provides for immunity only from "sanctions pénales" – thus seeming to restrict the ambit of Art. 31 to penalties understood in the narrower, criminal law sense. To counter this interpretation, Goodwin-Gill rightly points to the fact that the Human Rights Committee has refused to restrict the notion of a "penalty" in the Civil and Political Covenant's prohibition of *ex post facto* criminality in such a narrow way – even though this is a provision with a decidedly criminal law orientation.[592] Instead, the Committee has

---

[590] UK Soc. Sec. Comm. Dec. No. CIS/4439/1998 (Nov. 25, 1999), at para. 16.

[591] "Article 31 does not prohibit the imposition of such a penalty on a refugee who enters the United Kingdom illegally and then fails to present himself to authorities 'without delay.' If, therefore, the phrase 'on his arrival' in regulation 70(3A)(a) is construed in a manner which gives it the same effect as the phrase 'without delay' in Article 31, there is no conflict between the provisions. Construing the former phrase as meaning 'while clearing immigration control at the port of entry' is clearly not consistent with the construction of the latter phrase ... I therefore accept ... that Article 31 provides an additional reason for not construing 'on ... arrival' ... narrowly": ibid. at para. 18.

[592] "In seeking the most appropriate interpretation, the deliberations of the Human Rights Committee or scholars relating to the interpretation of the term 'penalty' in Article 15(1) of the Civil and Political Covenant can be of assistance": Goodwin-Gill, "Article 31," at 194. The propriety of referencing the authoritative interpretation of similar terms under cognate treaties is discussed in chapter 1.3.3 above, at pp. 64–68.

determined that "[w]hether the word 'penalty' ... should be interpreted narrowly or widely, and whether it applies to different kinds of penalties, 'criminal' and 'administrative,' ... must depend on other factors. Apart from the text ... regard must be had, *inter alia*, to its object and purpose."[593] Taking account of the decision recounted above explicitly to conceive Art. 31 not as a prohibition of a particular *kind of penalty*, but instead as a prohibition of penalties *imposed on a particular group of persons*, namely "refugees who enter or are present in their territory without prior or legal authorization," there is no sound basis to interpret the notion of a "penalty" narrowly.

4.2.3 Expulsion

There are two exceptions to the general rule that Art. 31 bars the imposition of penalties on refugees for illegal entry or presence. First, Art. 31 in no way constrains a state's prerogative to expel an unauthorized refugee from its territory. And second, as discussed below,[594] some restrictions on the freedom of movement of irregularly entering asylum-seekers are allowed pending regularization of status.

It may seem ironic that an asylum country which is generally prohibited from imposing penalties on refugees may nonetheless expel them. The drafters were, however, unambiguous on this point,[595] with Colombia going so far as to suggest an amendment that would have formally disavowed any duty to grant territorial asylum to refugees.[596] The Canadian representative successfully argued that no modification of the text was required, since "the consensus of opinion was that the right [to expel refugees who illegally enter a state's territory] would not be prejudiced by adoption of Article [31]."[597] His suggestion that "he would even regard silence on the part of the Conference as endorsement of his point of view"[598] led Colombia to withdraw its amendment.[599] Indeed, the Netherlands

---

[593] *Van Duzen v. Canada*, UNHRC Comm. No. 50/1979, decided Apr. 7, 1982, at para. 10.2. See also M. Nowak, *UN Covenant on Civil and Political Rights* (1993) (Nowak, *ICCPR Commentary*), at 278: "[E]very sanction that has not only a preventive but also a retributive and/or deterrent character is ... to be termed a penalty, regardless of its severity or the formal qualification by law and by the organ imposing it."

[594] See chapter 4.2.4 below, at pp. 420–424.

[595] See e.g. Statement of Mr. Fritzler of Austria, UN Doc. A/CONF.2/SR.13, July 10, 1951, at 12; and Statement of Mr. Herment of Belgium, ibid. at 14.

[596] UN Doc. A/CONF.2/55. "[T]erritorial asylum could not be regarded as a duty incumbent on states": Statement of Mr. Giraldo-Jaramillo of Colombia, UN Doc. A/CONF.2/SR.13, July 10, 1951, at 12.

[597] Statement of Mr. Chance of Canada, UN Doc. A/CONF.2/SR.13, July 10, 1951, at 12–13.

[598] Ibid. at 13.

[599] "[I]n the light of the foregoing discussion, the Colombian delegation would not oppose paragraph 1 of Article [31] ... Since it seemed to be the general feeling of all delegations that the granting of asylum remained a matter for the discretion of individual States, the

representative remarked that "in view of the Canadian representative's state-ment . . . that he would interpret the silence of representatives as tacit approval of the Canadian Government's interpretation of article [31], he would remain silent."[600] Thus, even the mechanistic application of a "first country of arrival" rule cannot be successfully attacked under Art. 31, as the sanction imposed under such systems is precisely expulsion to another state.

The potentially devastating impact of the clear decision not to preclude expulsion under Art. 31 is mitigated by two key factors. First, whatever right governments have to expel refugees is constrained by Art. 33's duty of *non-refoulement*.[601] Any expulsion of a refugee must therefore not expose the refugee, directly or indirectly, to a risk of being persecuted.

Second, in contrast to the situation in 1951, the laws of many countries today explicitly or implicitly authorize refugees in flight from persecution to enter their territory in search of protection. Asylum-seekers present in such states are "lawfully in" their territory,[602] and accordingly benefit from Art. 32's constraints on expulsion. As described below,[603] this means that states must invoke national security or public order grounds to expel a refugee, and that any decision to expel must be reached on the basis of a fair determination process. Thus, even expulsion practices immune from scrutiny under Art. 31 will often contravene Art. 32 where domestic law authorizes refugees arriving at its territory to seek protection.

4.2.4 *Provisional detention and other restrictions on freedom of movement*

Because the right of expulsion under Art. 31 is constrained by the additional guarantees of Art. 33 and, in many cases, of Art. 32, it is a prerogative that is only rarely a viable option for states.[604] The second and more frequently invoked exception to the duty of non-penalization is therefore the right to detain refugees who arrive unlawfully, pursuant to Art. 31(2).[605]

Art. 31(2) is one of two provisions of the Convention that defines the nature of a refugee's freedom of movement within an asylum country. The more generally applicable rule is set by Art. 26, which disallows restrictions on

---

Colombian delegation, which shared that view, would not press its amendment": Statement of Mr. Giraldo-Jaramillo of Colombia, ibid. at 14.

[600] Statement of Baron van Boetzelaer of the Netherlands, UN Doc. A/CONF.2/SR.14, July 10, 1951, at 8.

[601] See chapter 4.1 above, at pp. 300–301.

[602] See chapter 3.1.3 above, at pp. 175–183.   [603] See chapter 5.1 below.

[604] See chapter 4.2.3 above, at p. 413.

[605] UNHCR defines detention as "confinement within a narrowly bounded or restricted loca-tion, including prisons, closed camps, detention facilities or airport transit zones, where freedom of movement is substantially curtailed, and where the only opportunity to leave this limited area is to leave the territory": UNHCR, "Detention Guidelines," at Guideline 1.

refugees other than those enforced against aliens in general.[606] The Art. 26 right to freedom of movement accrues once a refugee is "lawfully in" the territory of a state party. As discussed in chapter 3, a refugee is lawfully present once formally admitted to the asylum state's refugee status verification procedure, or otherwise expressly or impliedly authorized to remain at least temporarily in that state's territory.[607] The drafters of the Convention recognized, however, that governments might require a more ample freedom to detain unauthorized refugees "before they had reached an understanding with the authorities of the recipient countries."[608] This right is, however, strictly provisional. The explicit language of Art. 31(2) requires an end to special restrictions on the movement of unauthorized refugees at such time as the refugee's status is "regularized" or he or she "obtain[s] admission into another country."

In the case of refugees not being considered for a more durable status in the asylum country, but who have instead applied to travel to some other state, Art. 31(2) authorizes detention up to the time of departure for that other state. At the urging of the Danish representative, the Ad Hoc Committee amended the applicable part of Art. 31(2) to allow detention to continue until refugees "obtain admission into another country." It was felt that the phrasing in an earlier draft, "until such time as it is possible to make a decision regarding their legal admission to . . . another country,"[609] could have been misinterpreted to require release once formal permission to travel onward had been received. The concern was that release pending removal to the other state might have allowed refugees the opportunity to abscond.[610] In principle, then, the initial decision to detain Vietnamese refugees in Hong Kong pending their relocation to other states under the Comprehensive Plan of Action was justified by Art. 31(2). But when it became clear that Hong Kong was using detention not simply as a practical means to implement the overseas relocation of refugees, but rather as an explicit mechanism of deterrence, the legality of detention came to an end. This is because the right to detain refugees under Art. 31(2) is situation specific. In this context, it authorizes only those restrictions on freedom of movement "necessary" to achieve the goal of external relocation.[611]

---

[606] See generally chapter 5.2 below.   [607] See generally chapter 3.1.3 above.

[608] Statement of Mr. Rain of France, UN Doc. E/AC.32/SR.15, Jan. 27, 1950, at 15.

[609] UN Doc. E/AC.32/L.26, Feb. 2, 1950, at 2.

[610] "He wondered whether . . . a country would be obliged to release the refugees as soon as they had obtained entry visas to another country. Some refugees might possibly use such an opportunity to remain in the country illegally": Statement of Mr. Larsen of Denmark, UN Doc. E/AC.32/SR.24, Feb. 3, 1950, at 6.

[611] The meaning of "necessary" restrictions is discussed below, at pp. 423–431. The question of the *prima facie* lawfulness of detention should not, however, be confused with the lawfulness of the conditions of detention. Where, for example, the circumstances of detention amount to a form of cruel, inhuman, or degrading treatment, continued detention is rights-violative under general norms of international human rights law.

The more controversial question is when the power of detention under Art. 31(2) ceases in relation to refugees who wish to remain in the asylum country, but whose claims to refugee status have not yet been verified. On the basis of only the record of the Conference of Plenipotentiaries, the conclusion could be reached that the termination point for special detention rules, "regularization," occurs when "after examining the appropriate files, [the government] recognize[s] him as a *bona fide* refugee."[612] Under this understanding, particularized detention measures could continue until and unless the irregular entrant is accepted "for permanent settlement."[613] Read in context, however, such a restrictive approach is not consistent with either the real intentions of the drafters or the object and purpose of the provision.

The relevant exchange at the Conference of Plenipotentiaries occurred in response to an effort by Sweden to amend Art. 31(2) to prolong the right to impose refugee-specific detention rules beyond "regularization" where needed to meet national security interests.[614] The Swedish representative was concerned that it might sometimes be necessary to detain asylum-seekers being processed for refugee status, and that the proposed cut-off point for refugee-specific detention of "regularization" would prohibit this.[615] The President, however, responded that Art. 31(2) as proposed already authorized the maintenance of security-based restrictions on movement *until a decision was reached* on the asylum-seeker's claim to refugee status.[616] More explicitly, the British representative assured the Conference that "[t]he Swedish representative had understood something different to what had been intended by the Ad Hoc Committee by the use of the words 'until his status in the country is *regularized*.' Surely, for the Ad Hoc Committee that phrase had meant the acceptance by a country of refuge for permanent settlement, and not the mere issue of documents prior to a final decision as to the duration of his stay."[617] On the basis of this interpretation, Sweden withdrew its proposed amendment.

---

[612] Statement of the President, Mr. Larsen of Denmark, UN Doc. A/CONF.2/SR.14, July 10, 1951, at 15.

[613] Statement of Mr. Hoare of the United Kingdom, ibid. at 16.

[614] "The Contracting States shall not apply to such refugees restrictions on movement other than those which are necessary and, except for reasons of national security, such restrictions shall only be applied until his status in the country is regularized": Proposal of Sweden, UN Doc. A/CONF.2/65.

[615] "[T]here was a category of refugee intermediate between those lawfully resident and those unlawfully resident in the territory of a State. The category of refugee could be tolerated by a State in its territory. There was a definite contradiction between the wording of articles [26] and [31] of the draft Convention, and the discrepancy should be brought to the notice of the Style Committee": Statement of Mr. Petren of Sweden, UN Doc. A/CONF.2/SR.14, July 10, 1951, at 16.

[616] Statement of the President, Mr. Larsen of Denmark, ibid. at 15.

[617] Statement of Mr. Hoare of the United Kingdom, ibid. at 16.

Contrary to the assumptions at the Conference, however, the Ad Hoc Committee had actually endorsed an interpretation of "regularization" which requires only that the asylum-seeker make an application to authorities for recognition of refugee status. In response to a French proposal to regulate the freedom of movement of refugees "authorized to reside within a territory"[618] (which became Art. 26), the American representative proposed that the Refugee Convention also include a specific provision to regulate the right to detain refugees "who had not yet been regularly admitted into a country"[619] (which became Art. 31(2)). This led the British representative to inquire how "regularly admitted" should be interpreted.[620] The French delegate answered him by giving a detailed description of the French asylum system, under which an immediate but provisional (and sometimes geographically limited) right to remain in France was granted to asylum-seekers.[621] Clearly concerned to maximize the protection of refugees admitted to systems of this kind that bestow rights on refugees only incrementally, the representative of the United States asserted "that persons subject to these restrictions should nevertheless be considered, for purposes of the future convention, to have been regularly admitted."[622] Critically, the French delegate agreed, noting that "[a]ny person in possession of a residence permit was in a regular position. In fact, the same was true of a person who was not yet in possession of a residence permit but who had applied for it and had the receipt for that application. *Only those persons who had not applied, or whose applications had been refused, were in an irregular position* [emphasis added]."[623]

In the view of the Ad Hoc Committee, then, "regularization" under Art. 31(2) was *not* predicated on formal recognition as a refugee. At one point, the Committee provisionally adopted language for Art. 31(2) that would have allowed refugee-specific detention to continue until a decision was reached on refugee status.[624] But the very next day, the Chairman successfully proposed a version of Art. 31(2) that restored the original reference to "regularization."[625] Even the British representative, who had earlier voiced concern

---

[618] Statement of Mr. Rain of France, UN Doc. E/AC.32/SR.15, Jan. 27, 1950, at 17.
[619] Statement of Mr. Henkin of the United States, ibid. at 18.
[620] Statement of Sir Leslie Brass of the United Kingdom, ibid. at 18.
[621] Statement of Mr. Rain of France, ibid. at 18.
[622] Statement of Mr. Henkin of the United States, ibid. at 20.
[623] Statement of Mr. Rain of France, ibid. at 20.
[624] "The High Contracting Parties nevertheless reserve the right to apply to such refugees necessary police measures ... until such time as it is possible to take a decision regarding their legal admission to the country of reception": UN Doc. E/AC.32/L.25, Feb. 2, 1950, at 2. This language was proposed jointly by Belgium and the United States. It was provisionally adopted on February 2, 1950: UN Doc. E/AC.32/L.26, Feb. 2, 1950, at 2.
[625] Statement of the Chairman, Mr. Chance of Canada, UN Doc. E/AC.32/SR.24, Feb. 3, 1950, at 6.

about this language, expressly "accepted that form of words."[626] All in all, the historical record is simply too ambiguous to justify the conclusion that "regularization" must be equated with formal recognition of refugee status.

To the contrary, a focus on the purpose and context of Art. 31(2) suggests that "regularization" of status occurs when a refugee has met the host state's requirements to have his or her entitlement to protection evaluated.[627] As previously discussed, the basic goal of Art. 31 is to provide refugees with an incentive to comply with the asylum laws of host states, rather than avoid contact with authorities.[628] That critical objective is achieved when the asylum-seeker submits to the laws of the host state, not simply when his or her claim is finally adjudicated. Equally important, an effort should be made to read Art. 31(2) in a way that avoids conflict with the other Convention rule on freedom of movement, Art. 26.[629] The general right to freedom of movement under Art. 26 inheres in refugees "lawfully in" an asylum state. It has earlier been explained why a refugee is "lawfully in" a state (as opposed to "lawfully staying" there) *inter alia* once admitted to an asylum procedure.[630] Thus, there is a general right to freedom of movement in the host state once the asylum claim is formally lodged. An interpretation that equates "regularization" with a decision on refugee status would bring the two articles into conflict, as the termination point for Art. 31(2) restrictions would be set at a higher level than that established for access to Art. 26 rights. Art. 26 would set

[626] Statement of Sir Leslie Brass of the United Kingdom, ibid.

[627] But see *R (Saadi) v. Secretary of State for the Home Department*, [2002] UKHL 41 (UK HL, Oct. 31, 2002), at para. 34, in which the House of Lords – apparently without the benefit of argument based on the requirements of the Refugee Convention – determined that "until the state has 'authorized' entry, the entry is unauthorized. The state has the power to detain ... until the application has been considered and the entry 'authorized.'" But see chapter 3.1.3 above, at pp. 175–183.

[628] See chapter 4.2 above, at p. 388.   [629] See Vienna Convention, at Art. 31(3)(c).

[630] See chapter 3.1.3 above, at pp. 175–183. This interpretation follows not only from plain language and context, but is necessitated if "lawfully in" is to be meaningfully distinguished from the higher level of attachment, "lawfully staying." The drafters agreed that a refugee is "lawfully staying" in a country when he or she benefits from officially sanctioned, ongoing presence there, whether or not there has been a formal declaration of refugee status, grant of the right of permanent residence, or establishment of domicile: see chapter 3.1.4 above, at pp. 189–190. The phrase "lawfully staying" was selected as the most accurate rendering of the French language concept of "résidant régulièrement." The original French language notion was, however, agreed to be controlling. "The Committee experienced some difficulty with the phrases 'lawfully in the territory' in English and 'résidant régulièrement' in French. It decided however that the latter phrase in French should be rendered in English by 'lawfully staying in the territory'": "Report of the Style Committee," UN Doc. A/CONF.2/102, July 24, 1951. This decision was reached *after* the discussion of "regularization" in the context of Art. 31(2), and should therefore be seen more accurately to reflect the final interpretation reached at the Conference of Plenipotentiaries.

a presumption against detention once the asylum procedure is underway, yet Art. 31(2) would authorize refugee-specific detention until the claim is adjudicated.

This conflict is readily avoided by adopting the understanding of "regularization" embraced by the Ad Hoc Committee and which advances the general purpose of Art. 31, namely that "regularization" occurs when the asylum-seeker satisfies all legal formalities requisite to refugee-status verification.[631] Under this approach, Art. 31(2) and Art. 26 play complementary, but distinct, roles in regulating the right to detain refugees. There is a clear and workable delineation of the kind intended by the drafters between situations in which freedom of movement is governed by Art. 31(2), and those in which Art. 26 applies.[632]

Thus, a refugee who enters an asylum country unlawfully, and who does not meet the requirements of Art. 31, is entitled to no immediate exemption from detention under international refugee law.[633] Once the refugee voluntarily and without delay reports to authorities, and demonstrates that his or her unauthorized entry or presence was on account of a search for

---

[631] This approach to interpretation of "regularization" would moreover be in consonance with the approach of the United Nations Human Rights Committee in interpretation of the Civil and Political Covenant. In determining that "an alien who entered the State illegally, but whose status *has been regularized*, must be considered to be lawfully within the territory [emphasis added]," the Committee cited as authority its finding that a rejected refugee claimant against whom an expulsion order had been issued but who was allowed to remain in a state party's territory on humanitarian grounds met the definition of "lawful presence": UN Human Rights Committee, "General Comment No. 27: Freedom of movement" (1999), UN Doc. HRI/GEN/1/Rev.7, May 12, 2004, at 173, para. 4, citing the decision in *Celepli v. Sweden*, UNHRC Comm. No. 456/1991, UN Doc. CCPR/C/51/D/456/1991, decided Mar. 19, 1993. If a state's decision to authorize continued presence despite the issuance of a valid expulsion order amounts to regularization of status, there can surely be little doubt that authorization to remain in a state's territory for the duration of a refugee status verification procedure also amounts to a form of regularization of status giving rise to lawful, if provisional, presence in that country.

[632] The decision to draft what became Art. 31(2) derived from the conviction that "certain provisions should also be included for refugees who had not yet been regularly admitted into a country": Statement of Mr. Henkin of the United States, UN Doc. E/AC.32/SR.15, Jan. 27, 1950, at 18.

[633] Even a purely unauthorized entrant is, however, entitled to the protection against arbitrary detention established under international human rights law. Because of the evolution of this body of law since adoption of the Refugee Convention in 1951, less significance presently follows from eligibility for Art. 31 protection against restrictions on freedom of movement. Whether or not the criteria of Art. 31 are met (voluntary reporting within a reasonable time, demonstration that breach of immigration laws was attributable to flight from a risk of persecution), the right of the asylum country to detain is subject to significant limitations. See text below, at pp. 424–425.

protection,[634] Art. 31(2) governs. The refugee is now subject only to restrictions "which are necessary." As described below,[635] this interim authority was intended to allow authorities to detain refugees while satisfying themselves of such matters as the asylum-seeker's identity, and whether or not he or she presents a security risk to the asylum state.

If the asylum country elects not to expel the refugee, but instead provisionally to allow him or her to remain in its territory (for example, while undergoing refugee-status determination), Art. 26 becomes the applicable standard for restrictions on internal movement. The refugee must, of course, submit to all necessary investigations of his or her claim to protection, and file whatever documentation or statements are reasonably required to verify the claim to refugee status. But once any such prerequisite obligations have been discharged, the refugee's presence has been regularized in the receiving state, and refugee-specific restrictions on freedom of movement must come to an end. In the result, neither the prolonged detention by Malta of African refugees nor Swaziland's imprisonment of Pakistani refugee claimants for having "trespassed" was in accordance with Art. 31(2). Much less was there any lawful basis for the decisions of Namibia and Thailand to force refugees to live on an ongoing basis only in designated camps.

Importantly, neither of the key reasons advanced to justify the drafting of Art. 31(2) can logically be invoked in support of ongoing detention while awaiting a final decision on status verification. The primary concern of the drafters was to have some means, short of expulsion, to respond to the arrival of a mass influx of refugees. As stated by the Danish representative,

> A country which was receiving large numbers of refugees could not contemplate making them re-cross the frontier or handing them over to the authorities which had persecuted them. Such refugees were often placed in camps, but it would be desirable to ensure them more normal and humane living conditions, for which purpose a certain number of fairly simple rules for the treatment of refugees not yet authorized to reside in a country should be drawn up.[636]

Art. 31(2) is therefore addressed to the rights of "refugees admitted provisionally as an emergency measure."[637] In recognition of the "real danger, on

---

[634] The nature of each of these provisos for entitlement to Art. 31 protection is discussed at chapter 4.2.1 above, at pp. 390–400.

[635] See text below, at pp. 420–421.

[636] Statement of Mr. Larsen of Denmark, UN Doc. E/AC.32/SR.15, Jan. 27, 1950, at 22. Mr. Larsen's reference to refugees not yet authorized to "reside" in the asylum country should be understood in the context of his earlier remarks, in which persons admitted provisionally to Denmark were nonetheless said to "reside" in that country: ibid. at 16–17.

[637] Statement of Mr. Weis of the IRO, UN Doc. E/AC.32.SR.21, Feb. 2, 1950, at 3.

both economic and security grounds,"[638] posed by "a great and sudden influx of refugees,"[639] Art. 31(2) affords governments some breathing space to determine how best to minimize the risks associated with their arrival.[640] As the French representative to the Ad Hoc Committee explained,

> The Secretariat had in mind the case of the Spanish refugees who had presented themselves in large numbers at the French frontier towards the end of the Spanish Civil War and for whom it had been necessary to set up reception camps to meet their immediate needs before regularizing their position and arranging for their dispersal throughout the country. The obligation to remain in those camps was clearly a considerable limitation of the right of movement . . . Such a practice might, however, prove essential in certain circumstances.[641]

Thus, objection cannot ordinarily be taken to the provisional detention of refugees arriving in the context of a mass influx until more durable arrangements can be made. On the other hand, detention even in the context of a mass influx cannot continue once the refugees' presence has been rendered lawful by passage of time.[642] This was the problem with justification for Uganda's long-term detention of Rwandan and Sudanese refugees. Where a country, like Uganda, opts neither to expel refugees nor to authenticate their Convention refugee status, it must be taken to have acquiesced in the asylum-seekers' assertion of entitlement to refugee rights after a reasonable period of time has passed, in consequence of which they enjoy the presumptive right to freedom of internal movement under Art. 26 of the Convention.[643] Nor can Art. 31(2) be looked to as legal support for Kenyan or Thai use of violence to enforce detention in response to a mass influx of refugees. As discussed below,[644] restrictions on freedom of movement, even in the context of a mass influx, must be "necessary," and may not infringe other norms of international human rights law. Brutality to impose or to enforce detention fails both tests.

Beyond enabling governments to cope with a mass influx, the second and more general objective of Art. 31(2) is to allow host states time to complete a basic inquiry into the identity and circumstances of unauthorized asylum-

---

[638] Statement of Mr. Herment of Belgium, UN Doc. E/AC.32/SR.40, Aug. 22, 1950, at 4.

[639] Statement of the President, Mr. Larsen of Denmark, UN Doc. A/CONF.2/SR.14, July 10, 1951, at 16.

[640] "If there are few illegal entrants, strict measures such as detention will be less easily justified than in the case of a mass influx, in which case the task of authorities may become overwhelming and necessitate a special *ad hoc* screening procedure": A. Grahl-Madsen, *The Status of Refugees in International Law* (vol. II, 1972) (Grahl-Madsen, *Status of Refugees II*), at 419.

[641] Statement of Mr. Rain of France, UN Doc. E/AC.32/SR.15, Jan. 27, 1950, at 14.

[642] See chapter 3.1.3 above, at pp. 183–185.   [643] See chapter 3.1.3 above, at pp. 183–184.

[644] See text below, at pp. 423–431.

seekers before releasing them into the community. At the Conference of Plenipotentiaries, Sweden and Greece asserted the importance of allowing governments to satisfy themselves that an unauthorized entrant does not pose a threat to their national security.[645] France expressed a more general concern to be in a position to investigate the identity of irregularly arriving refugees. It argued that governments should be allowed to detain asylum-seekers "for a few days, to obtain information on them. The French Government's aim in the question under discussion was that their authorities should be able to detain for a few days completely unknown persons unattached to any territory."[646] Britain also thought that Art. 31(2) should be understood to authorize "provisional detention that might be necessary to investigate the circumstances in which a refugee had entered a country."[647] This led the President of the Conference to conclude that "there was general agreement with the French representative's point of view that every State was fully entitled to investigate the case of each refugee who clandestinely crossed its frontier, and to ascertain whether he met the necessary entry requirements."[648]

This exchange makes clear that Art. 31(2) establishes only a "provisional" right of detention "for a few days," while the government of the asylum country completes a basic investigation of the asylum-seeker's identity and circumstances.[649] After that point, any ongoing detention will have to meet

---

[645] Statements of Mr. Petren of Sweden and of Mr. Philon of Greece, UN Doc. A/CONF.2/SR.14, July 10, 1951, at 15–16. The Swedish delegate had earlier tabled an amendment that would expressly authorize refugee-specific detention on national security grounds pending a formal decision on refugee status: UN Doc. A/CONF.2/65. See also Statement of Mr. van Heuven Goedhart of UNHCR, UN Doc. A/CONF.2/SR.35, July 25, 1951, at 13: "Each State was, of course, entitled to make the investigations necessary to safeguard its security."

[646] Statement of Mr. Rochefort of France, UN Doc. A/CONF.2/SR.35, July 25, 1951, at 11.

[647] Statement of Mr. Hoare of the United Kingdom, ibid. at 12.

[648] Statement of the President, Mr. Larsen of Denmark, ibid. at 13.

[649] "The detention of asylum-seekers who come 'directly' in an irregular manner should . . . not be automatic, or unduly prolonged": UNHCR, "Detention Guidelines." In *Singh v. Nelson*, 623 F Supp 545 (US DCSDNY, Dec. 12, 1985), the US District Court failed to recognize the need strictly to limit the duration of the right to detain refugees under Art. 31(2). Noting simply that "[i]t was also contemplated that in aid of its efforts to investigate the circumstances in which a refugee had entered a country, the government could detain and keep him in custody," the Court refused to deem the incarceration of Afghan claimants for more than a year to be outside the scope of Art. 31(2). In contrast, the finding of the English Court of Appeal that objection to the UK policy from 1998 to 2000 of detaining refugee claimants for the time needed to clarify their identity and the nature of their claim would have given rise to "an unanswerable claim" is curious: *R (Saadi) v. Secretary of State for the Home Department*, [2001] EWCA Civ 1512 (Eng. CA, Oct. 19, 2001), at para. 17; appeal to the House of Lords dismissed at *R (Saadi) v. Secretary of State for the Home Department*, [2002] UKHL 41 (UK HL, Oct. 31, 2002).

the requirements of Art. 26, which authorizes the detention of refugees only on the same grounds as are applied to aliens generally.[650] Because Art. 31(2) authorizes provisional detention as a necessary complement to preliminary investigation of identity and circumstances of entry, it cannot be relied upon to justify punitive detention designed to deter the arrival of other refugees of the kind that was engaged in by India against Sri Lankan refugees in 2001.[651] This prohibition of detention as a deterrent mechanism seems clearly to have been overlooked by the Attorney General of the United States who advanced precisely this ground as one of his reasons for routinely detaining Haitian claimants arriving by boat:

> [T]here is a concern that the release of aliens ... would tend to encourage further surges of mass migrations from Haiti by sea, with attendant strains on national and homeland security resources ...
>
> Encouraging such unlawful mass migrations is inconsistent with immigration policy ... While the expedited removal policy may reduce the incidence of sea-going Haitian migrants being released on bond pending removal, it hardly provides airtight assurances against future successful migrants through legal and extra-legal maneuvers, or the encouragement of additional maritime migrations likely to arise from such entries.[652]

---

[650] "[A]sylum-seekers may be detained exclusively for the purposes of a preliminary interview to identify the basis of the asylum claim. This would involve obtaining essential facts from the asylum-seeker as to why asylum is being sought and would not extend to a determination of the merits or otherwise of the claim": UNHCR, "Detention Guidelines," at Guideline 3(ii). The only situation in which provisional detention may continue is that set by Art. 9 of the Convention. Where the asylum country faces a "war or other grave and exceptional circumstances," provisional detention may be continued right up to the point of status verification in the case of an asylum-seeker found to present a risk to national security: see chapter 3.5.1 above. Any generally applicable rules on the detention of aliens who pose a threat to national security may, of course, be applied in relation to refugees in conformity with Art. 26.

[651] "Detention should not have the 'punitive' character associated with detention or imprisonment in connection with criminal offences": UNHCR, "Detention Note," at para. 47. See also UNHCR, "Detention Guidelines," at Guideline 3(iv): "Detention of asylum-seekers ... as part of a policy to deter future asylum-seekers, or to dissuade those who have commenced their claims from pursuing them, is contrary to the norms of refugee law."

[652] *In re DJ*, 2003 BIA Lexis 3 (US AG, Apr. 17, 2003). Almost as a footnote, the Attorney General observed that because the Refugee Protocol "is not self-executing," it "does not afford respondent any rights beyond what he is afforded under the federal immigration laws": ibid. Yet the Attorney General failed to acknowledge that the government of the United States is bound by Art. 31 of the Refugee Convention. His decision here to deem the reversal of the Board of Immigration Appeals' decision a "precedent binding in all future cases" therefore amounts to a clear refusal of the United States to abide by its international legal obligations.

A different problem arises in states, such as Austria, Belgium, and Switzerland, which subject unauthorized refugees to automatic periods of detention for two to six months on the basis of laws applicable to all unauthorized entrants. Because the basis for detention is not a refugee-specific law, it might be argued that automatically detaining refugees for a period of months meets the requirements of Art. 26, in that refugees are detained only in the same circumstances as other aliens. The better view, however, is that the combination of Arts. 31(2) and 26 requires governments to justify a decision to detain an asylum-seeker who arrives without authorization.[653] After all, the basic purpose of Art. 31 is to ensure that refugees are not exposed to the same penalties for unauthorized arrival as are applied to other unauthorized aliens. Read together with Art. 26, it cannot have been the intention of the drafters to authorize more stringent constraints on freedom of movement once a refugee becomes lawfully present in the host country. Thus, while restrictions on the movement of aliens that are not related to unauthorized entry or presence may validly be applied to refugees as well, the prohibition of other than minimalist detention to verify identity and circumstances of arrival for irregularly arriving refugees under Art. 31(2) should be read to enjoin governments from detaining refugees on the basis of general rules that authorize prolonged detention as a response to unauthorized entry.

In any event, the automatic prerogative to detain unauthorized entrants exemplified by the Austrian, Belgian, and Swiss rules may also run afoul of the stipulation in Art. 31(2) that the exercise of the right of provisional detention must be demonstrably "necessary." In the original draft submitted by the Secretary-General, a state was authorized to apply such measures "as *it may deem* necessary [emphasis added]."[654] The final language, which authorizes only restrictions on freedom movement "which *are* necessary [emphasis added]" was adopted to embrace the spirit of a joint Belgian–American proposal to allow states provisionally to take only "necessary police measures regarding their accommodation, residence and movement in their territory."[655] The importance of a broad but purposive understanding of the right of provisional detention was emphasized by the President of the Conference of Plenipotentiaries, who asserted that "by inserting the words 'other than those which are necessary' . . . the Ad Hoc Committee had

---

[653] As described below, the detention of aliens in general without a clear reason is today contrary to international human rights law. See text below, at pp. 424–425.

[654] Secretary-General, "Memorandum," at 45. The French proposal used the same expression: France, "Draft Convention," at 9.

[655] UN Doc. E/AC.32/L.25, Feb. 2, 1950, at 2. The American representative observed that "although the substance of the . . . article was satisfactory, its form left much to be desired": Statement of Mr. Henkin of the United States, UN Doc. E/AC.32/SR.22, Feb. 2, 1950, at 25. This led the Danish delegate, Mr. Larsen, to propose the language upon which the present formulation of Art. 31(2) is based: ibid.

intended to cover considerations of security, special circumstances, such as a great and sudden influx of refugees, or any other reasons which might necessitate restrictions of their movement."[656] Thus, UNHCR's Executive Committee has determined that

> in view of the hardship which it involves, detention should normally be avoided. If necessary, detention may be resorted to only on grounds prescribed by law to verify identity; to determine the elements on which the claim to refugee status or asylum is based; to deal with cases where refugees or asylum-seekers have destroyed their travel and/or identity documents or have used fraudulent documents in order to mislead the authorities of the State in which they intend to claim asylum;[657] or to protect national security or public order.[658]

The notion that any form of detention requires justification is, in any event, now firmly established in international human rights law. Under Art. 9(1) of the Civil and Political Covenant, no person – including an individual subject to immigration control[659] – may be deprived of his or her liberty "except on such grounds and in accordance with such procedures as are established by law."[660] The Full Federal Court of Australia has interpreted the Covenant's obligations in the context of the detention of refugee claimants to mean that not only must detention be authorized by law, but it must

---

[656] Statement of the President, Mr. Larsen of Denmark, UN Doc. A/CONF.2/SR.14, July 10, 1951, at 16.

[657] "What must be established is the absence of good faith on the part of the applicant to comply with the verification of identity process. As regards asylum-seekers using fraudulent documents or travelling with no documents at all, detention is only permissible when there is an intention to mislead, or a refusal to cooperate with the authorities": UNHCR, "Detention Guidelines," at Guideline 3(iii).

[658] UNHCR Executive Committee Conclusion No. 44, "Detention of Refugees and Asylum-Seekers" (1986), at para. (b), available at www.unhcr.ch (accessed Nov. 20, 2004).

[659] "The Committee points out that paragraph 1 is applicable to all deprivations of liberty, whether in criminal cases or in other cases such as, for example, . . . immigration control": UN Human Rights Committee, "General Comment No. 8: Right to liberty and security of persons" (1982), UN Doc. HRI/GEN/1/Rev.7, May 12, 2004, at 130, para. 1. See "Report of the Special Rapporteur, submitted pursuant to Commission on Human Rights resolution 2002/62," UN Doc. E/CN.4/2003/85 (Dec. 30, 2002) for a detailed examination of the various ways in which non-citizens are subjected to detention.

[660] Civil and Political Covenant, at Art. 9(1). See also UNHCR, "Detention Guidelines," at Guideline 3: "The permissible exceptions to the general rule that detention should normally be avoided must be prescribed by law." In the opinion of a respected commentator, "the formulation 'established by law' . . . requires[s] that the national legislature itself set down in statute all permissible restrictions. The term 'law' is to be understood here in the strict sense of a general-abstract, parliamentary statute or an equivalent, unwritten norm of common law accessible to all individuals subject to the relevant jurisdiction. Administrative provisions are thus not sufficient": Nowak, *ICCPR Commentary*, at 171.

also be subject to the claimant's right "not to be detained in circumstances which, in the individual case, are 'unproportional' or unjust."[661] More specifically, the United Nations Human Rights Committee has determined that persons who claim refugee status may not be detained "beyond the period for which the State can provide appropriate justification. For example, the fact of illegal entry may indicate a need for investigation and there may be other factors particular to the individual such as the likelihood of absconding and lack of cooperation which may justify detention for a period."[662] Where such grounds exist,[663] the detained person must nonetheless have the ability "to take proceedings before a court, in order that that court may decide without delay on the lawfulness of his detention and order his release if the detention is not lawful."[664]

---

[661] *Minister for Immigration and Multicultural and Indigenous Affairs v. Al Masri*, (2003) 197 ALR 241 (Aus. FFC, Apr. 15, 2003).

[662] *A v. Australia*, UNHRC Comm. No. 560/1993, UN Doc. CCPR/C/59/D/560/1993, decided April 30, 1997, at para. 9.4. The government of Australia did not, however, accept the Committee's findings, arguing that the lawfulness of detention was to be determined by reference to domestic, not international standards: "Response of the Australian Government to the Views of the Human Rights Committee," (1997) 9(4) *International Journal of Refugee Law* 674. The Human Rights Committee's reference to the propriety of detention to prevent a refugee from absconding is, of course, based upon the requirements of the Civil and Political Covenant rather than the Refugee Convention. A similar approach has been taken under the European Convention on Human Rights. In *Amuur v. France*, [1996] ECHR 25 (ECHR, June 25, 1996), the European Court of Human Rights determined that "[h]olding aliens in the international zone does indeed involve a restriction upon liberty ... Such confinement, accompanied by suitable safe-guards for the persons concerned, is acceptable only to enable States to prevent unlawful immigration while complying with their international obligations, particularly under the 1951 Geneva Convention relating to the Status of Refugees and the European Convention on Human Rights. States' legitimate immigration restrictions must not deprive asylum-seekers of the protection afforded by these conventions": ibid. at para. 43.

[663] The range of reasons which the Committee is prepared to consider in the assessment of reasonableness is, however, apparently open-ended. In *Bakhtiyari v. Australia*, UNHRC Comm. No. 1069/2002, UN Doc. CCPR/C/79/D/1069/2002, decided Oct. 29, 2003, the Committee determined that "in order to avoid any characterization of arbitrariness, detention should not continue beyond the period for which a State party can provide appropriate justification. In the present case, Mr Bakhtiyari arrived by boat, without dependents, with his identity in doubt and claiming to be from a State suffering serious internal disorder. In light of these factors and the fact that he was granted a protection visa and released two months after he had filed an application (some seven months after his arrival), the Committee is unable to conclude that, while the length of his first detention may have been undesirable, it was also arbitrary and in breach of article 9, paragraph 1": ibid. at para. 9.2.

[664] Civil and Political Covenant, at Art. 9(4). As the Human Rights Committee determined in the context of a review of the detention of asylum-seekers, this requirement is only met where the court review "is, in its effects, real and not merely formal." In particular, the court's authority "must include the possibility of ordering release, [and not be] limited to

The requirement that provisional detention be shown to be "necessary" in the sense that the state party is able to provide "appropriate justification" for it provides a particularly useful bulwark against overly broad assertions of a right to detain for national security reasons.[665] In addition to his determination to use detention as a means of deterring the arrival of Haitians, the US Attorney General invoked national security concerns to justify his policy of routinely detaining Haitians seeking protection in the United States:

> The Department of Defense, which is also involved in efforts to contain such overseas migrations, also asserts that the demands of mass migrations from Haiti "would create a drain on scarce assets that are being used in or supporting operations elsewhere" . . .
>
> The declarations submitted by the Immigration and Naturalization Service also substantiate a national security concern raised by the prospect of undocumented aliens from Haiti being released within the United States without adequate verification of their background, associations, and objectives.[666]

Yet the first concern expressed is so vaguely related to any meaningful understanding of a risk to national security that it could not possibly meet the test of necessity set by Art. 31(2) or international human rights law; indeed, the United States did not even attempt to demonstrate the proportionality of routine detention of all Haitians to the national security concern invoked. The second argument – the need to investigate risks presented by refugee claimants – is, of course, well within the usual ambit of reasons to undertake provisional detention under Art. 31(2). While it could therefore readily justify detention required to complete the requisite investigations of particular persons, it is difficult to imagine how it could be said to require the

---

[consideration of] mere compliance with domestic law": *A v. Australia*, UNHRC Comm. No. 560/1993, UN Doc. CCPR/C/59/D/560/1993, decided April 30, 1997, at para. 9.5. More recently, the Human Rights Committee has noted that in the case of Australia's detention system, "[j]udicial review of detention would have been restricted to an assessment of whether the author was a non-citizen without valid entry documentation, and, by direct operation of the relevant legislation, the relevant courts would not have been able to consider arguments that the individual detention was unlawful in terms of the Covenant. Judicial review of the lawfulness of detention under article 9, paragraph 4, is not limited to mere compliance of the detention with domestic law but must include the possibility to order release if the detention is incompatible with the requirements of the Covenant, in particular those of article 9, paragraph 1": *Baban v. Australia*, UNHRC Comm. No. 1014/2001, UN Doc. CCPR/C/78/D/1014/2001, decided Aug. 6, 2003, at para. 7.2.

[665] "Detention as a mechanism which seeks to address the particular concerns of States related to illegal entry requires the exercise of great caution in its use to ensure that it does not serve to undermine the fundamental principles upon which the regime of international protection is based": UNHCR, "Detention Guidelines."

[666] *In re DJ*, 2003 BIA Lexis 3 (US AG, Apr. 17, 2003).

routine detention of all persons arriving from a given country.[667] The more recent US decision to require the detention of all persons seeking refugee status from a list of mainly Muslim countries and territories on grounds of national security is not only grossly over-broad, but is likely in breach of the duty of non-discrimination.[668] The recent admonition of the Supreme Court of New Zealand is clearly appropriate:

> Article 31(2) of the Refugee Convention requires Contracting States not to apply to the movement of certain refugees restrictions other than those which are necessary. That provision ... plainly contemplates that individuals who are detained should be entitled to challenge their detention. The Solicitor-General said that national security reasons could be one reason for detention. No doubt that is so, but such reasons have to be tested in the particular case. Security cannot provide a basis for a blanket exclusion of such cases.[669]

Even assuming recognition of the importance of a particularized inquiry, the meaning of "necessary" restrictions on freedom of movement can still be difficult to discern. As noted above, the traditional approach of UNHCR has been to deem only certain *reasons* for detention to meet the necessity criterion – specifically, to deal with issues of identity, elements of the claim, document destruction, national security, or public order.[670] This was essentially the approach endorsed by the High Court of New Zealand in a thorough and broad-ranging analysis of the requirements of Art. 31 in the decision of *Refugee Council of New Zealand and D v. Attorney General*.[671] In the Court of Appeal, however, two opinions suggest the need for a more open-ended and flexible approach to assessing whether detention is necessary.[672] The

---

[667] "In assessing whether detention of asylum-seekers is necessary, account should be taken of whether it is reasonable to do so and whether it is proportional to the objectives to be achieved. If judged necessary it should only be imposed in a non-discriminatory manner for a minimal period": UNHCR, "Detention Guidelines," at Guideline 3.

[668] See chapters 2.5.5 and 3.4 above.

[669] *Zaoui v. Attorney General*, Dec. SC CIV 13/2004 (NZ SC, Nov. 25, 2004), at para. 44.

[670] See UNHCR, "Detention Guidelines," at Guideline 3. A similar reason-based approach to the interpretation of "necessary" detention seems to be preferred as well by the Human Rights Committee. In assessing whether the UK "fast track" processing system for refugees was in compliance with the Civil and Political Covenant, the Committee observed that it "is concerned that asylum-seekers have been detained in various facilities on grounds other than those legitimate under the Covenant, including reasons of administrative convenience": "Concluding Observations of the Human Rights Committee: United Kingdom," UN Doc. CCPR/CO/73, Dec. 6, 2001, at para. 16.

[671] In the High Court, Mr. Justice Baragwanath determined that provisional detention could only be ordered for reasons of administrative functionality, to preclude criminal activity, or to avoid real risk of absconding: *Refugee Council of New Zealand et al. and "D" v. Attorney General*, [2002] NZAR 717 (NZ HC, May 31, 2002).

[672] The lead judgment, authored by Mr. Justice Tipping on behalf of himself and Justices Blanchard and Anderson, does not move beyond a rather general understanding of this

reasons of Justice McGrath affirm that automatic detention clearly cannot be justified under Art. 31(2);[673] he is equally clear that "detention for the purposes of deterrence is impermissible."[674] But he is insistent that the grounds for provisional detention must not be treated as finite, but should rather "reflect the margin of appreciation that the parties to the Convention had in mind could properly be exercised."[675] Agreeing that some flexibility of this kind is required, the reasons of Justice Glazebrook suggest an approach to the determination of a "necessary" provisional constraint on a refugee's freedom of movement that takes account of both "the extent of any restrictions imposed and the reasons for such restrictions":[676]

> It is implicit ... that restrictions on freedom of movement that are less restrictive than detention should be able to be imposed more freely ... [T]he necessity standard is variable depending on the nature of the restriction on freedom of movement to be applied ...
>
> ... [T]he greater restriction there is to be on a claimant's freedom of movement, the more scrutiny should be given to the reasons for detention ... Where there is to be a major restriction on the freedom of movement through detention ... the factors discussed in [UNHCR] Guideline 3 that can point to detention being necessary [e.g. unwillingness of the claimant to cooperate in verification of identity; existence of criminal antecedents likely to jeopardize national security or public order] appear to require an element of "fault" on the part of the claimant.[677]

This is a very helpful framework within which to determine whether detention or other limits on freedom of movement are appropriately adjudged necessary. It effectively compels states to give primary consideration to constraints on freedom of movement short of detention, since such less intrusive measures will be much more readily deemed justified.[678] While there can be no question of even routine resort to such measures as residence

question: *Attorney General v. Refugee Council of New Zealand Inc.*, [2003] 2 NZLR 577 (NZ CA, Apr. 16, 2003), at para. 28.

[673] "The starting point is that New Zealand's obligations under the Refugee Convention ... include a duty to ensure that detention is not automatic for arriving persons claiming the status of refugees [citing the court's earlier decision in *Attorney General v. E*, [2000] 3 NZLR 257 (NZ CA, July 11, 2000, appeal to PC refused at [2000] 3 NZLR 637)": *Attorney General v. Refugee Council of New Zealand Inc.*, [2003] 2 NZLR 577 (NZ CA, Apr. 16, 2003), at para. 97.

[674] *Attorney General v. Refugee Council of New Zealand Inc.*, [2003] 2 NZLR 577 (NZ CA, Apr. 16, 2003), at para. 101.

[675] Ibid. at para. 102. A comparably flexible approach has recently been taken by the UN Human Rights Committee.

[676] Ibid. at para. 257.   [677] Ibid. at paras. 265, 275.

[678] In a decision successfully appealed to the Court of Appeal, the New Zealand High Court determined that "[d]etention is warranted only where 'necessary.' I would have thought that the possibility of lesser forms of control would need to be addressed before the more drastic steps of full detention could be justified ... Open centers may or may not be

restrictions or reporting requirements,[679] the view that detention should ordinarily be contemplated as a last resort[680] and normally where there is some evidence of *mala fides* or risk associated with the liberty of the refugee claimant is a sound point of departure.[681] It drives governments meaningfully to honor the presumptive right of refugees to enjoy freedom of movement, even as it affords them a flexible framework within which to justify a potentially broad range of restrictions for an open-ended set of reasons.[682]

The duty to rely on less intrusive restrictions on freedom of movement unless detention is clearly required[683] is very much in line with the intentions of the Convention's drafters. For example, the representative of the International Refugee Organization observed that the reference to

---

available in New Zealand at present. However, it is certainly commonplace in the analogous system of criminal prosecutions that persons on remand are granted bail subject to stringent conditions including daily reporting requirements, residence at a nominated address, geographical limitations upon movement, surrender of passports, curfews, and other restrictions of that nature": *E v. Attorney General*, [2000] NZAR 354 (NZ HC, Nov. 29, 1999), appeal allowed in *Attorney General v. E*, [2000] 3 NZLR 257 (NZ CA, July 11, 2000, appeal to PC refused at [2000] 3 NZLR 637).

[679] "It is significant that Article 31(2) applies to restrictions on freedom of movement generally, and not just to detention": *Attorney General v. Refugee Council of New Zealand Inc.*, [2003] 2 NZLR 577 (NZ CA, Apr. 16, 2003), at para. 259.

[680] "[T]here should be a strong, although rebuttable, presumption in favor of granting temporary permits to refugee claimants pending the determination of their refugee status": *E v. Attorney General*, [2000] NZAR 354 (NZ HC, Nov. 29, 1999), appeal allowed in *Attorney General v. E*, [2000] 3 NZLR 257 (NZ CA, July 11, 2000, appeal to PC refused at [2000] 3 NZLR 637).

[681] See e.g. *Jalloh v. Netherlands*, UNHRC Comm. No. 794/1998, UN Doc. CCPR/C/74/D/794/1998, decided Mar. 26, 2002, at para. 8.2: "[T]he author had his detention reviewed by the courts on two occasions, once twelve days after the beginning of his detention, and again two months later. On both occasions, the Court found that the author's continued detention was lawful, because he had evaded expulsion before, because there were doubts as to his identity, and because there were reasonable prospects for expulsion, as an identity investigation was still ongoing. The question remains therefore as to whether his detention was arbitrary. Recalling its previous jurisprudence the Committee notes that 'arbitrariness' must be interpreted more broadly than 'against the law' to include elements of unreasonableness. *Considering the author's flight from the open facility at which he was accommodated from the time of his arrival for around 11 months, the Committee considers that it was not unreasonable* to have detained the author for a limited time until the administrative procedure relating to his case was completed [emphasis added]."

[682] "The word 'necessary' limits both the extent of any restrictions imposed and the reasons for such restrictions": *Attorney General v. Refugee Council of New Zealand Inc.*, [2003] 2 NZLR 577 (NZ CA, Apr. 16, 2003), at para. 259.

[683] "If a less severe restriction, such as ordering the person in question to stay in a particular town or within a limited area, can be considered sufficient, the authorities are [prohibited] from applying more severe measures, such as [requiring] the refugee to stay in a certain house or in a camp, or outright detaining him": Grahl-Madsen, *Commentary*, at 182.

"necessary" measures "implied that the refugee should not be subjected to irksome restrictions, that he should be permitted to move outside the reception camp to the greatest extent possible, and that he should lead as normal a life as possible."[684] UNHCR's detention guidelines amplify this view, suggesting that "[w]here there are monitoring mechanisms which can be employed as viable alternatives to detention . . . these should be applied *first* unless there is evidence to suggest that such an alternative will not be effective in the individual case."[685] Among the alternative approaches suggested are monitoring requirements, the provision of a guarantor or surety, release on bail, and requiring refugees to reside in particular regions, or in open reception centers.[686] Neither a presumption in favor of detaining refugees of the kind employed (formally) by Australia and (de facto) by the United States, nor the relegation of refugees to closed camps in Hong Kong, Thailand, Uganda, and Kenya can be reconciled to this duty minimally to impair freedom of movement in pursuit of even legitimate investigatory goals. This duty of minimal impairment has been clearly endorsed by the Human Rights Committee in the context of a complaint of arbitrary detention made by an Afghan refugee woman and her five young children:

> Concerning Mrs Bakhtiyari and her children, the Committee observes that Mrs Bakhtiyari has been detained in immigration detention for two years and ten months, and continues to be detained, while the children remained in immigration detention for two years and eight months until their release on interim orders of the Family Court. Whatever justification there may have been for an initial detention for the purposes of ascertaining identity and other issues, the State party has not, in the Committee's view, demonstrated that their detention was justified for such an extended period.
>
> Taking into account in particular the composition of the Bakhtiyari family, the State party has not demonstrated that other, less intrusive, measures could not have achieved the same end of compliance with the State party's immigration policies by, for example, imposition of reporting obligations, sureties or other conditions which would take into account the family's particular circumstances. As a result, the continuation of immigration detention for Mrs Bakhtiyari and her children for the length of time described above, without appropriate justification, was arbitrary and contrary to article 9, paragraph 1, of the Covenant.[687]

---

[684] Statement of Mr. Weis of the IRO, UN Doc. E/AC.32/SR.22, Feb. 2, 1950, at 24–25.

[685] UNHCR, "Detention Guidelines," at Guideline 3. See also Executive Committee of the High Commissioner's Program, "Agenda for Protection," UN Doc. EC/52/SC/CRP.9/Rev.1, June 26, 2002, at Part III, Goal 1, Point 9: "States more concertedly to explore alternatives to the detention of asylum-seekers and refugees."

[686] UNHCR, "Detention Guidelines," at Guideline 4.

[687] *Bakhtiyari v. Australia*, UNHRC Comm. No. 1069/2002, UN Doc. CCPR/C/79/D/1069/2002, decided Oct. 29, 2003, at para. 9.3. See also *C v. Australia*, UNHRC Comm. No. 900/1999, UN Doc. CCPR/C/76/D/900/1999, decided Oct. 28, 2002, at para. 8.2.

A note of caution is warranted, however, before rushing to endorse various constraints on freedom of movement as alternatives to the detention of persons seeking recognition of refugee status.[688] Art. 31(2) is not only a limitation on detention, but on all measures which infringe a refugee's freedom of movement. Thus, not even a limitation on freedom of movement short of detention may be imposed without a valid justification of the kind contemplated by Art. 31(2). Equally important, no refugee-specific limitation on freedom of movement may be more than strictly provisional. The restrictions must come to an end once reasons which make it necessary come to an end – for example, when the response to the mass influx has been organized, or the preliminary assessment of identity and circumstances of entry is completed.[689] Any other or continuing constraints must be generally applicable to non-citizens in the host country, and not be imposed on account of irregular entry or presence.[690] Thus, when asylum-seekers are required to live on an ongoing basis in a reception center or hostel, as may be the case, for example, in Denmark, Germany, and Ireland, Art. 31(2) is contravened.

But what of practices such as those of Austria and Norway which allow refugee claimants to live outside the reception center only if they are prepared to give up state welfare benefits? In pith and substance, such policies seem less a constraint on freedom of movement which might raise a concern under Art. 31(2) than a restriction on access to public benefits. This restriction is in most cases lawful since, at least until and unless an issue of denial of access to the

---

[688] UNHCR clearly feels that it is waging an uphill battle against the detention of refugees. After states agreed in 1986 that detention should normally be avoided, and may legally be resorted to only for the reasons contemplated by Art. 31(2) (see UNHCR Executive Committee Conclusion No. 44, "Detention of Refugees and Asylum-Seekers" (1979)), UNHCR bluntly announced just two years later that "[a]lthough States Members of the Executive Committee adopted the Conclusion by consensus, the recommendations contained therein appear to have had very little impact on the practice of a number of states as regards detention of refugees and asylum-seekers. On the contrary, detention under harsh conditions, for long periods and without justifiable cause has recently increased": UNHCR, "Note on International Protection," UN Doc. A/AC.96/713, Aug. 15, 1988, at para. 21. The unfortunate result of this struggle to hold states to their freely assumed obligations has been a nearly exclusive concern to constrain resort to detention, even at the cost of an expansion of other restrictions on the freedom of movement of refugees. Thus, the UNHCR detention guidelines expressly posit that "[t]here is a qualitative difference between detention and other restrictions on freedom of movement. Persons who are subjected to limitations on domicile and residency are not generally considered to be in detention." Indeed, the guidelines seem almost to advocate lesser restrictions, suggesting that these constraints on freedom of movement are "options which provide State authorities with a degree of control over the whereabouts of asylum-seekers while allowing asylum-seekers basic freedom of movement": UNHCR, "Detention Guidelines," at Guidelines 1 and 4.

[689] See text above, at pp. 419–422.   [690] See text above, at pp. 421–422.

necessities of life arises,[691] states are under a duty to grant refugees access to public relief systems only once the refugee establishes an ongoing presence in the asylum country (whether or not there has been a formal declaration of refugee status, grant of the right of permanent residence, or establishment of domicile there).[692] As such, a decision to condition earlier access to welfare benefits on residence in a reception center is effectively a constraint on access to a privilege, which a refugee may choose to accept or not. The issue of whether the policy amounts to a necessary constraint on freedom of internal movement therefore does not arise.

However, once a refugee is in an asylum country on an ongoing basis, including once admitted to a temporary protection regime in the asylum state, there is a duty to assimilate him or her to nationals for the purpose of access to public relief.[693] If in such circumstances a state party persists in a policy of denying welfare benefits to refugees who refuse to reside in a reception center, its actions more clearly amount to a denial of freedom of internal movement (since the choice being offered amounts to losing one right, or losing another). The state would then be required to justify its policy by reference to Art. 26 of the Refugee Convention and, more generally, to meet the requirements of Art. 9 of the Civil and Political Covenant.[694]

Another issue of real contemporary concern is whether provisional detention can be adjudged "necessary" where it is imposed in order to ensure the efficient assessment of claims to refugee status. While not included in UNHCR's "list" of approved reasons for provisional detention,[695] courts have taken the view that short-term detention dictated by important administrative reasons may be allowed under the terms of Art. 31.[696] For example, the House of Lords gave consideration in *Saadi*[697] to the legality of the detention of refugee claimants adjudged to have "straightforward asylum claims" for seven to ten days, allowing their claims quickly to be adjudicated. Their Lordships took real account of both the practical need to deal expeditiously with a mounting volume of claims,[698] and of the quality of the

---

[691] States are obliged under international human rights law to ensure the necessities of life to persons under their jurisdiction: see chapter 4.4 below.

[692] See chapter 6.3 below.   [693] See chapter 3.1.4 above.

[694] See chapter 5.2 below.   [695] UNHCR, "Detention Guidelines," at Guideline 3.

[696] The New Zealand High Court, for example, determined that detention might be necessary "to allow the [government] to be able to perform their functions": *Refugee Council of New Zealand et al. and "D" v. Attorney General*, [2002] NZAR 717 (NZ HC, May 31, 2002).

[697] *R (Saadi) v. Secretary of State for the Home Department*, [2002] UKHL 41 (UK HL, Oct. 31, 2002).

[698] "The number of persons arriving in the United Kingdom and seeking asylum has grown considerably in recent years. Thus your Lordships were told that from July to September

detention (which included, for example, access to legal advice)[699] to arrive at the decision that detention for a few days could be ruled necessary:

> There is obviously force in the argument ... that if there is no suggestion that [the claimants] might run away, then it cannot be strictly necessary to detain them as opposed to requiring them to comply with the fixed regime enabling detailed examinations to take place. This, however, ignores the reality – large numbers of applications have to be considered intensively in a short period. If people failed to arrive on time or at all the Programme would be disrupted and delays caused not only to the individual case, but to dealing with the whole problem. If conditions in the centre were less acceptable than they are taken to be, there might be more room for doubt, but it seems to me that the need for speed justifies detention for a short period in acceptable physical conditions as being reasonably necessary.[700]

Thus, very much in line with the approach of Justice Glazebrook in the New Zealand Court of Appeal, the House of Lords adopted a flexible approach to the question of necessity, with a focus on the questions of both the reasons for detention, and the nature of the restrictions imposed. The clear implication of the judgment is that the restriction on freedom of movement would not have been deemed necessary if its duration were not so short and finite, or if the conditions of detention were less clearly rights-regarding. On balance, this seems a fair construction of the notion of "necessary" constraints, very much in line with the intention of the drafters to afford host states time to complete a basic inquiry into the identity and circumstances of unauthorized asylum-seekers before releasing them into the community.

Despite the value of a flexible approach to the assessment of whether constraints on freedom of movement are necessary, there are clearly some situations in which detention will be extraordinarily difficult to justify. In particular, it is clear that children may be lawfully detained only as a "measure of last resort."[701] A heavy onus should also rest on states that intend to detain

---

1999 the average number of applications was 7,000 a month, a 60% increase on the previous year ... This obviously placed a considerable strain on the immigration services": ibid. at para. 10.

[699] "There is obviously a deprivation of liberty in detaining people at Oakington. They cannot leave the centre, they must conform to the rules as to meal times and to being in their rooms at night. On the other hand, it is not suggested that the physical conditions – the state of the rooms, sanitation, meals – are in themselves open to criticism. Moreover, there are provisions not only for legal advice, but for medical advice, for recreation and for religious practice": ibid. at para. 17.

[700] Ibid. at para. 24.

[701] "No child shall be deprived of his or her liberty unlawfully or arbitrarily. The arrest, detention or imprisonment of a child shall be in conformity with the law and shall be

other vulnerable persons, including unaccompanied elderly persons, torture or trauma victims, and persons with a mental or physical disability.[702] The Australian and Belgian practices of detaining refugee children on a fairly routine basis are therefore unlikely to meet the requirements of Art. 31(2), or the Civil and Political Covenant. The Swiss exception for children who are "lawfully resident" is half-hearted, since international human rights law requires that the right to freedom from deprivation of liberty be implemented without discrimination of any kind.[703] And while the United Kingdom's reservation to the Convention on the Rights of the Child insulates it from responsibility under that treaty for the detention of refugee children, it remains independently accountable under the Refugee Convention and Civil and Political Covenant to overcome the presumption against the necessity of such measures.[704]

used only as a measure of last resort and for the shortest appropriate period of time": Convention on the Rights of the Child, UNGA Res. 44/25, adopted Nov. 20, 1989, entered into force Sept. 2, 1990 (Rights of the Child Convention), at Art. 37(b). "Unaccompanied minors should not, as a general rule, be detained. Where possible they should be released into the care of family members who already have residency within the asylum country. Where this is not possible, alternative care arrangements should be made by the competent child care authorities for unaccompanied minors to receive adequate accommodation and appropriate supervision. Residential homes or foster care placements may provide the necessary facilities to ensure their proper development (both physical and mental) is catered for while longer term solutions are being considered. All appropriate alternatives to detention should be considered in the case of children accompanying their parents. Children and their primary caregivers should not be detained unless this is the only means of maintaining family unity. If none of the alternatives can be applied and States do detain children, this should, in accordance with Article 37 of the Convention on the Rights of the Child, be as a measure of last resort, and for the shortest period of time": UNHCR, "Detention Guidelines," at Guideline 6. See also Executive Committee of the High Commissioner's Program, "Agenda for Protection," UN Doc. EC/52/SC/CRP.9/Rev.1, June 26, 2002, at Part III, Goal 1, Point 9: "States ... to abstain, in principle, from detaining children."

[702] "In the event that individuals falling within these categories are detained, it is advisable that this should only be on the certification of a qualified medical practitioner that detention will not adversely affect their health and well being. In addition there must be regular follow up and support by a relevant skilled professional. They must also have access to services, hospitalisation, medication counselling etc. should it become necessary": UNHCR, "Detention Guidelines," at Guideline 7.

[703] Rights of the Child Convention, at Art. 2(1). It is, of course, true that the margin of appreciation afforded states on the question of "reasonable" differences of treatment is a problematic aspect of contemporary non-discrimination jurisprudence: see chapter 2.5.5 above, at pp. 139–145.

[704] While strongly insisting on the duty to consider alternatives to detention of children, the UN Human Rights Committee has not taken the view that their detention is in all cases rights-violative. "The Committee considers that the ability for a court to order a child's release if considered in its best interests ... is sufficient review of the substantive

More generally, because generic detention regimes – such as those of Austria, Belgium, and Switzerland – are routinely applied to all unauthorized non-citizens (without requiring the state to advance specific justifications for detention), they fail even to engage with the requirement of the Refugee Convention's Art. 31(2) and of Art. 9(1) of the Civil and Political Covenant that provisional detention be demonstrably "necessary." The detention regime in the United Kingdom, in contrast, is appropriately predicated on the government adducing evidence of a need for investigation of identity or circumstances of entry; its weakness is that detention is not conceived as a strictly provisional measure.[705] The Italian detention system, on the other hand, appears more closely to conform to the requirements of both Article 31(2) and the Civil and Political Covenant, in that it is substantively circumscribed, and clearly provisional; yet even this relatively good regime fails to incorporate a requirement for routine review by an adjudicator, a critical safeguard which exists, for example, in the Canadian and French systems.[706]

While the Refugee Convention does not set standards for the conditions of detention, Art. 10 of the Civil and Political Covenant requires that all detained persons "be treated with humanity and with respect for the inherent dignity of the human person." This duty extends to any person "deprived of liberty under the laws and authority of the State."[707] Art. 10 requires states to meet a higher standard than simply the avoidance of the "cruel and inhuman" treatment prohibited by Art. 7 of the Civil and Political Covenant.[708] The Human Rights Committee has determined, for example, that Art. 10 was breached when an individual was returned to immigration detention contrary to expert medical advice.[709] It has also found a violation where a detained person was forced to sleep on the floor of a small cell without

---

justification of detention to satisfy the requirements of article 9, paragraph 4, of the Covenant ... Concerning the claim under article 24, the Committee considers that the principle that in all decisions affecting a child, its best interests shall be a primary consideration, forms an integral part of every child's right to such measures of protection": *Bakhtiyari v. Australia*, UNHRC Comm. No. 1069/2002, UN Doc. CCPR/C/79/D/ 1069/2002, decided Oct. 29, 2003, at paras. 9.5, 9.7.

[705] Similar concerns have been expressed by the United Nations Working Group on Arbitrary Detention: UN Doc. E/CN.4/1999/63/Add.4.

[706] Moreover, as the Canadian Federal Court of Appeal has observed, "[t]he onus is always on the Minister to demonstrate that there are reasons which warrant detention or continued detention ... [O]nce the Minister has made out a prima facie case for continued detention, the individual must lead some evidence or risk continued detention": *Canada v. Thanabalasingham*, [2004] FCA 4 (Can. FCA, Jan. 9, 2004), at para. 16.

[707] UN Human Rights Committee, "General Comment No. 21: Humane treatment of persons deprived of their liberty" (1992), UN Doc. HRI/GEN/1/Rev.7, May 12, 2004, at 153, para. 2.

[708] Nowak, *ICCPR Commentary*, at 186–187.

[709] "[T]his form of detention was contrary to the advice of various doctors and psychiatrists, consulted by the State party, who all advised that a further period of placement in an

medical attention or family contact,[710] as well as in the case of a detainee given only five minutes per day for personal hygiene and five minutes per day of outside exercise.[711] The severe and prolonged overcrowding experienced by refugees detained in, for example, Greece, Hong Kong, Mexico, and the Spanish Canary Islands is clearly at odds with this obligation. The relatively detailed attention to specific conditions of detention follows logically from the fact that persons detained by a government are essentially at the complete mercy of the state. Because their vulnerability to harm results specifically from an official decision to detain them, the state responsible for the detention owes detainees a "positive obligation" of care.[712] In particular, a state that elects to detain an individual may not invoke resource insufficiency as a reason for failure to meet the standards of Art. 10.[713] If, for whatever reason, a government is not in a position to ensure that persons denied their liberty are treated with humanity and respect for their inherent dignity, then it may not lawfully order their detention.

In keeping with this affirmative obligation to ensure the protection of detainees, UNHCR's Executive Committee has determined that "refugees and asylum-seekers shall, whenever possible, not be accommodated with persons detained as common criminals, and shall not be located in areas where their physical safety is endangered"[714] – a standard that calls into question the American practice of detaining refugees in ordinary jails in

---

immigration detention centre would risk further deterioration of Mr. Madafferi's mental health. Against the backdrop of such advice and given the eventual involuntary admission of Mr. Madafferi to a psychiatric hospital, the Committee finds that the State party's decision to return Mr. Madafferi to Maribyrnong and the manner in which that transfer was [e]ffected was not based on a proper assessment of the circumstances of the case but was, as such, disproportionate. Consequently, the Committee finds that this decision and the resulting detention was in violation of article 10, paragraph 1, of the Covenant": *Madafferi v. Australia*, UNHRC Comm. No. 1011/2001, UN Doc. CCPR/C/81/D/1011/2001, decided July 26, 2004, at para. 9.3.

[710] *Luyeye v. Zaïre*, UNHRC Comm. No. 90/1981, decided July 21, 1983.

[711] *Párkányi v. Hungary*, UNHRC Comm. No. 410/1990, UN Doc. CCPR/C/41/D/410/1990, decided Mar. 22, 1991.

[712] UN Human Rights Committee, "General Comment No. 21: Humane treatment of persons deprived of their liberty" (1992), UN Doc. HRI/GEN/1/Rev.7, May 12, 2004, at 153, para. 3.

[713] Art. 10 is "a fundamental and universally applicable rule . . . [T]he application of this rule, as a minimum, cannot be dependent on the material resources available in the State party": ibid. at 153, para. 4.

[714] UNHCR Executive Committee Conclusion No. 44, "Detention of Refugees and Asylum-Seekers" (1986), at para. (f), available at www.unhcr.ch (accessed Nov. 20, 2004). See also UNHCR Executive Committee Conclusion No. 85, "Conclusion on International Protection" (1998), at para. (ee), available at www.unhcr.ch (accessed Nov. 20, 2004), in which the Executive Committee "[n]ote[d] with concern that asylum-seekers detained only because of their illegal entry or presence are often held together with persons

which some facilities are shared by refugees and criminals.[715] More generally, the Executive Committee has concluded that "conditions of detention of refugees and asylum-seekers must be humane."[716] UNHCR's guidelines on the detention of asylum-seekers posit a number of specific standards to govern provisional detention,[717] largely derived from the jurisprudence under Art. 10(1) of the Civil and Political Covenant,[718] and from the United Nations' Body of Principles for the Protection of All Persons under Any Form of Detention or Imprisonment.[719] Taken together, these standards require that detained refugees have the right to be in regular contact with

---

detained as common criminals, and reiterate[d] that this is undesirable and must be avoided whenever possible, and that asylum-seekers shall not be located in areas where their physical safety is in danger"; and UNHCR, "Detention Guidelines," at Guideline 10(iii): "Separate detention facilities should be used to accommodate asylum-seekers. The use of prisons should be avoided. If separate detention facilities are not used, asylum-seekers should be accommodated separately from convicted criminals or prisoners on remand. There should be no co-mingling of the two groups."

[715] Indeed, under the Civil and Political Covenant, not even accused criminals may lawfully be detained together with convicted criminals: Civil and Political Covenant, at Art. 10(2)(a). See also Report of the United Nations Working Group on Arbitrary Detention, UN Doc. E/CN.4/1999/63, Dec. 18, 1998: "Custody of [refugees and asylum-seekers shall be] effected in public premises intended for this purpose; otherwise, the individual in custody shall be separated from persons imprisoned under criminal law."

[716] UNHCR Executive Committee Conclusion No. 44, "Detention of Refugees and Asylum-Seekers" (1986), at para. (f), available at www.unhcr.ch (accessed Nov. 20, 2004).

[717] UNHCR, "Detention Guidelines," at Guideline 10.

[718] "All persons deprived of their liberty shall be treated with humanity and with respect for the inherent dignity of the human person": Civil and Political Covenant, at Art. 10(1). As affirmed by the Human Rights Committee, "Article 10, paragraph 1 ... applies to anyone deprived of liberty under the laws and authority of the State who is held in prisons, hospitals – particularly psychiatric hospitals – detention camps or correctional institutions or elsewhere. State parties should ensure that the principle stipulated therein is observed in all institutions and establishments within their jurisdiction where persons are being held": UN Human Rights Committee, "General Comment No. 21: Humane treatment of persons deprived of their liberty" (1992), UN Doc. HRI/GEN/1/Rev.7, May 12, 2004, at 153, para. 2. Nowak summarizes the Human Rights Committee's jurisprudence on Art. 10(1) as establishing *positive State duties to ensure* certain conduct. Regardless of economic difficulties, the State must establish a minimum standard for humane conditions or detention ... In other words, it must provide detainees and prisoners with a minimum of services to satisfy their basic needs (food, clothing, medical care, sanitary facilities, communication, light, opportunity to move about, privacy, etc.)": Nowak, *ICCPR Commentary*, at 188–189.

[719] UNGA Res. 47/173, Dec. 9, 1988, Annex (UN Detention Principles). In 1997, the UN Commission on Human Rights specifically enlarged the mandate of its Working Group on Arbitrary Detention to direct it to report on "the situation of immigrants and asylum-seekers who are allegedly being held in prolonged administrative custody without the possibility of administrative or judicial remedy": "Question of arbitrary detention," UNCHR Res. 1997/50, UN Doc. E/CN.4/1997/50 (1997), at para. 4.

persons outside the detention facility;[720] to consult with legal counsel;[721] to receive basic medical care and other necessities of life (a standard not respected when, for example, South Korea failed to provide heating in refugee detention facilities);[722] to benefit from opportunities for exercise and recreation;[723] to enjoy religious freedom;[724] to access education, culture, and information;[725] and to be assured of assistance to dependent family

---

[720] "A detained or imprisoned person shall have the right to be visited by and to correspond with, in particular, members of his family and shall be given adequate opportunity to communicate with the outside world, subject to reasonable conditions and restrictions as specified by law or lawful regulations": UN Detention Principles, at Principle No. 19. See also Principles Nos. 15 and 16, ibid. The UNHCR elaborates that "[f]acilities should be made available to enable such visits. Where possible such visits should take place in private unless there are compelling reasons to warrant the contrary": UNHCR, "Detention Guidelines," at Guideline 10(iv).

[721] "A detained person shall be entitled to have the assistance of a legal counsel. He shall be informed of his right by the competent authority promptly after arrest and shall be provided with reasonable facilities for exercising it . . . If a detained person does not have a legal counsel of his own choice, he shall be entitled to have a legal counsel assigned to him by a judicial or other authority in all cases where the interests of justice so require and without payment by him if he does not have sufficient means to pay": UN Detention Principles, at Principle No. 17. Furthermore, "[a] detained or imprisoned person shall be entitled to communicate and consult with his legal counsel . . . A detained or imprisoned person shall be allowed adequate time and facilities for consultations with his legal counsel . . . The right of a detained or imprisoned person to be visited by and to consult and communicate, without delay or censorship and in full confidentiality, with his legal counsel may not be suspended or restricted save in exceptional circumstances, to be specified by law or lawful regulations, when it is considered indispensable by a judicial or other authority in order to maintain security and good order": UN Detention Principles, at Principle No. 18. See also UNHCR, "Detention Guidelines," at Guideline 10(iv).

[722] "A proper medical examination shall be offered to a detained or imprisoned person as promptly as possible after his admission to the place of detention or imprisonment, and thereafter medical care and treatment shall be provided whenever necessary. This care and treatment shall be provided free of charge": UN Detention Principles, at Principle No. 24. See also Principles Nos. 25 and 26: ibid. In addition, "[a]sylum-seekers should have the opportunity to have access to basic necessities, i.e., beds, shower facilities, basic toiletries, etc.": UNHCR, "Detention Guidelines," at Guideline 10(ix).

[723] "Asylum seekers should have the opportunity to conduct some form of physical exercise through daily indoor and outdoor recreational activities": UNHCR, "Detention Guidelines," at Guideline 10(vi).

[724] "Asylum seekers should have the opportunity to exercise their religion in practice, worship, and observance, and to receive a diet in keeping with their religion": ibid. at Guideline 10(viii).

[725] "A detained or imprisoned person shall have the right to obtain within the limits of available resources, if from public sources, reasonable quantities of educational, cultural and informational material, subject to reasonable conditions to ensure security and good order in the place of detention or imprisonment": UN Detention Principles, at Principle No. 28.

members.[726] These basic qualitative standards must, of course, be interpreted with due regard to the particular needs of children, women, and others who may be particularly vulnerable to harm while in detention.[727]

4.3 Physical security

Those who enjoyed relative privilege and safety before becoming refugees usually find their security diminished as a result of the refugee experience itself. This being said, persons who were already vulnerable – typically women, children, older persons, the disabled, and the poor – may on occasion find that becoming a refugee is a source of enhanced protection, particularly where they are received in a society that is more socially inclusive.[728] More commonly, however, refugeehood simply exposes the already disfranchised to even greater risks of physical harm. As Human Rights Watch observed, "[w]omen refugees are raped because they are refugees, because of their actual or perceived political or ethnic affiliations, and because they are women."[729]

Physical security is frequently jeopardized during the process of flight to an asylum country. The Sudanese government, for example, ordered bombing attacks on refugees attempting to flee to Ethiopia.[730] Rohingya women and girls were gang-raped by Burmese security forces as they fled the country.[731]

---

[726] "The appropriate authorities shall endeavour to ensure, according to domestic law, assistance when needed to dependent and, in particular, minor members of the families of detained or imprisoned persons and shall devote a particular measure of care to the appropriate custody of children left without supervision": ibid. at Principle No. 31.

[727] UNHCR, "Detention Guidelines," at Guidelines 6, 7, and 8.

[728] It may also be the case that the actual conditions of life for asylum-seekers may result in a revaluation of the relative importance of the skills and abilities of traditionally marginalized groups. For example, success in coping with camp life frequently puts a premium on activities within the traditional realm of "women's work," such as food-gathering, cooking, and the establishment and maintenance of living quarters. In such circumstances, women refugees have reported that the relative insecurity of life as an asylumseeker has, perhaps ironically, been a source of personal empowerment for them. See e.g. G. Garcia Hernandez and N. Garcia, "Mama Maquin Refugee Women: Participation and Organization," in W. Giles et al. eds., *Development and Diaspora: Gender and the Refugee Experience* 258 (1996), at 262.

[729] Human Rights Watch, *Human Rights Watch Global Report on Women's Human Rights* (1995), at 101. The same report notes that "[s]trong cultural stigma attached to rape further intensifies the rape victims' physical and psychological trauma. Women in refugee and displaced persons camps who acknowledge being raped may be ostracized, or even punished, by their families": ibid. at 103.

[730] D. Baligh, "International Relief Operation Saves Victims of Famine, Drought," *Associated Press*, June 9, 1991.

[731] T. Khandker and Z. Haider, "Protection [of] Refugees: Case of Rohingya Women," paper presented at the National Seminar on Refugees, Migrants, and Stateless Persons: In Search of a National Consensus, Dhaka, Dec. 29, 1997, at 5.

Many Central American refugees traveling overland to North America were subjected to extortion, kidnaping, and physical abuse in transit countries, particularly in Honduras.[732] An especially notorious case was the series of attacks between 1980 and 1984 perpetrated by Thai pirates on Vietnamese "boat people" attempting to pass through the Gulf of Thailand and South China Sea en route to Hong Kong, the Philippines, and other asylum countries. In the words of one eyewitness,

> While all the men were confined to the hold of the refugee boat . . . some, if not all of the approximately 15–20 women and young girls who were kept in the cabin of the boat were raped. The youngest of these girls was around 12 years old. Soon afterwards, the pirates set the boat on fire with all the Vietnamese on board. In the ensuing panic, the Vietnamese grabbed buoys, cans and floats, and plunged into the sea. The crews of the pirate boats then used sticks to prevent them from clinging to floating objects.[733]

Because refugees often cannot plan their escapes, travel routes and methods may be simply the most accessible, rather than the safest, way of leaving.

Even refugees who manage to reach the border of an asylum country are not immune from physical abuse.[734] Sometimes border guards take advantage of the refugees' predicament and vulnerability.[735] For example, Rwandan refugees were robbed by the predatory Zaïrian army as they entered the country in 1994,[736] and continued to be subject to attacks and looting in the camps.[737] In South Africa, refugees waiting to register at the

---

[732] See e.g. Immigration and Refugee Board of Canada, "Honduras: Persecution by Contras in Honduras, particularly in the areas bordering Nicaragua and in the city of La Ceiba, Dec. 1987 – Nov. 1988," May 1, 1989.

[733] "A Tale of Horror," (1989) 65 *Refugees* 25.

[734] The United Nations Special Rapporteur on the Rights of Non-Citizens has determined that "[t]here are reliable reports of . . . police violence, intimidation, and bullying of asylum-seekers": "Final Report of the Special Rapporteur of the Rights of Non-Citizens: Addendum: Examples of Practice in Regard to Non-Citizens," UN Doc. E/CN.4/Sub.2/2003/23/Add.3, May 26, 2003, at para. 10.

[735] As UNHCR has observed, women and girls are particularly at risk in these circumstances. "Border guards in some countries have detained refugee women or girls for weeks for their sexual use. Women have been raped by soldiers while crossing a border, and in some cases abducted and prostituted by them . . . Unaccompanied women asylum-seekers arriving by air in a country of asylum, forced to spend extended periods of time in the holding area of an airport before being transferred to a hotel where they were guarded around the clock, have been raped by their guards while the authorities were deciding to which country to expel them": UNHCR, "Note on Certain Aspects of Violence Against Women," UN Doc. A/AC.96/822, Oct. 12, 1993, at 7.

[736] African Rights, *Rwanda: Death, Despair and Defiance* (1994) (African Rights, *Rwanda*), at 661.

[737] In November 1994, for example, "Zaïrian soldiers searching for Rwandans accused of stealing opened fire on some refugees, killing and wounding more than a hundred in and

Braamfontein refugee office were reported to have been whipped and beaten by officials.[738] Malawi officials shot and killed a refugee from Eritrea while trying to force him onto a flight bound for Ethiopia,[739] while Austrian officials bound and gagged a Nigerian refugee claimant in an effort to deport him to Bulgaria, where he was pronounced dead on arrival.[740] To avoid detection by Chinese authorities intent on removing them without consideration of their protection needs, North Korean refugees are often forced to secure private protection by becoming slave laborers or prostitutes.[741]

Yet the evidence suggests that the greatest risk of physical abuse arises once refugees actually reach the camps where they are in principle to be protected. Sometimes camp officials or employees are directly responsible. For example, Iraqi refugees admitted to "temporary shelter" in Saudi Arabia during and after the Gulf War were arbitrarily detained, tortured, and even extrajudicially executed.[742] Dozens of refugees were killed by Kenyan security forces or "forcibly disappeared."[743] Many Cambodian refugees in camps along the Thai–Cambodian border were tortured and killed with impunity by Thai military officers or the Khmer Rouge officials to whom the Thais entrusted responsibility for running some camps.[744] In five extrajudicial killings of

near Katale camp, about 30 miles northeast of Goma": D. Lorch, "Pressed by Zairian troops, Rwandans flee camps," *New York Times*, Dec. 2, 1994, at A6.

[738] "On Thursday officials at the Braamfontein refugee office in Johannesburg allegedly beat approximately a thousand refugees with chains and sjamboks. A woman whose leg was fractured has been sent to hospital. Abeda Bhamjee of the Wits Law Clinic says: 'On several occasions we have noted sjambokkings as a form of crowd control, including within Home Affairs buildings'": "No place for refugees fleeing Africa's tyrants," *Sunday Independent*, Oct. 27, 2002.

[739] *Agence France Presse*, Sept. 1, 1999.

[740] "Rampant racism in Austrian police exposed," *Guardian*, Mar. 25, 2000.

[741] "There are between 10,000 and 300,000 refugees hiding in China, and monitors for Human Rights Watch found those they spoke to were resigned to a sub-human existence in China. Many fear they will be captured and sent home to serve a life sentence in one of North Korea's notorious prison camps, where inmates are reportedly experimented on with chemicals, starved or shot": J. Palmer, "Starving refugees sold as sex slaves to Chinese men," *Independent*, Nov. 19, 2002, at 13.

[742] Amnesty International, "Saudi Arabia: Unwelcome 'Guests': The Plight of Iraqi Refugees" (1994), at 1.

[743] "Police and army patrols routinely pick up refugee men, and either beat them to death or shoot them. In many cases, the bodies are then burned. Sometimes, they are demanding bribes for release, sometimes the killings are in the course of sweeps ostensibly directed against bandits ... Innumerable refugees, both women and men, have been beaten or tortured by security forces. This is common in Nairobi as well as the camps. Some have died as a consequence": African Rights, "The Nightmare Continues ... Abuses Against Somali Refugees in Kenya" (1993), at ii.

[744] "Many of the human rights abuses that characterized the population removals appear to be regular occurrences inside the refugee camps administered by the Khmer Rouge: forced labor, denial of medical care, denial of food as a means of coercion, use of civilians against their will for military purposes, and harsh penalties, including execution, for

refugees reported by Amnesty International in 1988, "the victims were apparently executed ... simply because they were found outside the camp boundaries where they had gone to collect food, firewood or building materials, or to engage in barter with Thai farmers or merchants for needed commodities."[745] Kosovar refugees taking shelter in Sarajevo were attacked by Bosnian police, who rushed into their camp at midnight and beat them indiscriminately.[746] And in Australia, an expert reported that "coercive management strategies" were employed by the officials administering refugee camps, including "teargas, room-trashings, [and] children being put into solitary confinement."[747]

Perhaps the most prevalent form of abuse by officials administering refugee camps is rape and sexual assault. For example,

> Thousands of refugee women have been raped in Kenya. While the majority of rapes are committed by shifta (armed bandits), many are also committed by policemen and soldiers, in both the camps and Nairobi ... Most are gang rapes. Some of the women have had to endure the added trauma and indignity of being raped along with their daughters, including girls as young as thirteen ... A Somali woman who has been raped is the victim of the attack itself and a victim of a set of social values that condemn a raped woman to lifelong shame and ostracism.[748]

Similarly, the United Nations has reported the rape of Tibetan refugee women by Nepalese police.[749] Sexual abuse has also occurred at the hands of relief workers. For example, two senior officials of a Catholic church agency working at the Tongogara refugee camp in Zimbabwe were fired for demanding sexual favors from refugees in return for items such as sanitary towels and blankets.[750] At the Osire refugee camp in Namibia, as many as sixty teachers

those who disobey orders": Asia Watch, "Khmer Rouge Abuses Along the Thai–Cambodian Border" (1989), at 23.

[745] Amnesty International, "Thailand: Extrajudicial Executions of Kampuchean Refugees" (1988), at 1. See also Banbury, "Kampuchean Displaced Persons in Thailand," at 27, in which the author details murders, rapes, robberies, and beatings carried out by both the Khmer Rouge forces in charge of some of the refugee camps, and by the Thai military forces.

[746] (1999) 44 *JRS Dispatches* (Mar. 1, 1999).

[747] K. Lawson, "Ruddock warns rights officials," *Canberra Times*, Jan. 23, 2002, at A-1, quoting the report of Dr. Michael Dudley, chairman of Suicide Prevention Australia and Head of Faculty of Child and Adolescent Psychiatry at the Royal Australian College of Psychiatry. The government "strongly refuted the claims": ibid.

[748] African Rights, "The Nightmare Continues ... Abuses Against Somali Refugees in Kenya" (1993), at 13.

[749] (1988) 41/42 *Human Rights Monitor* 68, reporting the observations of the Special Rapporteur on Violence Against Women, Mrs. Coomaraswamy.

[750] "Catholic refugee camp officials sacked for sex abuses," *Mail and Guardian* (Harare), July 11, 2002; "Steps taken to protect women refugees against abuse," *UN Integrated Regional Information Networks*, Dec. 2, 2002.

in the employ of the Ministry of Basic Education forced students as young as fourteen years old to have sex with them.[751] In February 2002, UNHCR and Save the Children (UK) released a report documenting patterns of sexual exploitation of refugee women and children throughout Western Africa by humanitarian workers. The workers were able to abuse their power in large measure because of the endemic scarcity of food and other resources that characterizes life in so many refugee camps.[752]

Yet much of the danger within refugee camps emanates not from authorities, but from fellow camp residents. One of the most horrifying examples was the reign of terror that persisted for Rwandan refugees inside Zaïre (now the Democratic Republic of Congo), where armed refugees continued their violence and extermination of Tutsis and moderate Hutus from within the borders of the camps themselves.[753] More recently, violence broke out among Burundian refugees at a camp in northern Mozambique based on the same ethnic tensions.[754] Risks to physical security can also be the by-product of conditions of confinement. Frequent overcrowding, failure to treat refugees with dignity, and the absence of meaningful opportunities to work, study, or otherwise occupy time set the stage for violence. For example, refugee gang violence was endemic in Hong Kong detention centers, with police failing adequately to protect refugees from the violent minority.[755]

Faulty design and management of the camps can exacerbate protection problems. There is increased likelihood of attack where communal latrines

---

[751] "Teen pregnancies soar at Osire Refugee Camp," *Namibian*, June 25, 2001; "Sexual abuse reported at Osire Refugee Camp," *Namibian*, July 5, 2001.

[752] UNHCR and Save the Children (UK), "Note for Implementing and Operational Partners on Sexual Violence and Exploitation: The Experience of Refugee Children in Guinea, Liberia and Sierra Leone based on Initial Findings and Recommendations from Assessment Mission, 22 October – 30 November 2001," Feb. 2002.

[753] African Rights, *Rwanda*, at 656–657.

[754] "One refugee from Burundi's civil war ... said his hut was burned down by another Burundian because he is a Tutsi. 'I was beaten up and my hut burned down because they hate me'": "Burundian refugees clash at camp in Mozambique," *SAPA-AFP*, Sept. 25, 2002. Hatred between Hutus and Tutsis was also responsible for violence in a refugee camp in Zimbabwe: "Refugees clash at camp," *Daily News*, Apr. 12, 2003.

[755] Weil, Gothal, and Manges, "Submission to the United Nations Working Group on Arbitrary Detention by the Lawyers Committee for Human Rights and the Women's Commission for Refugee Women and Children on behalf of approximately 40,000 Vietnamese detainees, including the families of Pham Ngoc Lam, Vuong Son Bach, and Cam Gia Ninh" (1989), at 12. "The Hong Kong Government have not done much to prevent the stress, anxiety, and fear of sexual attack and gang fights Vietnamese women and children suffer from": Hong Kong Human Rights Commission, "Report to the United Nations Committee Against Torture on the Initial Report by Hong Kong under Article 19 of the Convention Against Torture and Other Cruel, Inhuman or Degrading Treatment or Punishment" (Nov. 1995), available at www.hkhrc.org.hk (accessed Aug. 9, 2003).

are sited far from living quarters, where there is poor lighting, and where night patrols are inadequate.[756] The decision of Indian camp authorities to require Chakma refugee women to search for firewood in nearby forests "exposed them to sexual assaults – seven to eight cases are said to be reported each year. The culprits have rarely been apprehended."[757] Somali refugee women in search of firewood near three UN refugee camps in Kenya were also routinely raped, resulting in a sexual assault rate seventy-five times higher than would be expected in a community of comparable population.[758] Closed detention facilities are particularly likely to give rise to risks to physical security, with women and children the least protected and most vulnerable portion of the population.[759] As Susan Forbes Martin explains, "[t]here is evidence that psychological strains for husbands unable to assume normal cultural, social and economic roles can result in aggressive behavior towards wives and children. The enforced idleness, boredom and despair that permeate many camps are natural breeding grounds for such violence."[760] In Tanzania, for example, 95 percent of the cases of refugees seeking protection inside the Ngara camp related to domestic violence.[761]

Beyond physical security risks from officials and fellow refugees, refugees living in camps are frequently "sitting ducks" for attacks. The risk of attack may come from bandits or armed bands, particularly where refugees are located in remote areas.[762] The Ugandan rebel group "Lord's Resistance Army" has massacred Sudanese refugees in northern Uganda.[763] Bandits

---

[756] S. Forbes Martin, *Refugee Women* (1991) (Forbes Martin, *Refugee Women*), at 21.

[757] B. S. Chimni, *International Academy of Comparative Law National Report for India* (1994), at 27.

[758] K. Vick, "For Somali refugees, no safe haven: fear of rape grips women in camps," *Washington Post*, June 3, 1999, at A-19.

[759] Lawyers' Committee for Human Rights, *Inhumane Deterrence: The Treatment of Vietnamese Boat People in Hong Kong* (1989), at 14–18.

[760] Forbes Martin, *Refugee Women*, at 21. See also Helton, "Thailand," at 33: "Overcrowding, shortages of food and water, stress and the constant fear of harassment of resistance elements within the camp, have created a deteriorating social situation. Incidents of domestic violence and suicide attempts have risen dramatically."

[761] "Due to the situation in the camps, husbands are not able to afford food for their families, or clothing. They are also idle all day, and drink local brews. And their poor economic status leads to lots of violence": "Focus on sexual violence among refugees," *UN Integrated Regional Information Networks*, May 7, 2002.

[762] UNHCR, "Note on Certain Aspects of Violence Against Refugee Women," UN Doc. A/AC.96/822, Oct. 12, 1993, at 8.

[763] "At Achol Pii, home to more than 16,000 people fleeing the war zones of southern Sudan, refugees were shot at point-blank range or cruelly hacked to death with machetes. Food was looted and more than 300 huts burned down": Amnesty International, "Sudan: Amnesty International Condemns 'Callous and Calculated' Killings by Ugandan Rebels," July 18, 1996. Such attacks continue; for example "[i]n early July [2003], LRA forces

attacked Burundian refugees at the Mtabila refugee camp in Tanzania. They targeted both the Tanzanian police working there and the refugees responsible for security, as well as their family members.[764]

Armed attacks by agents of the refugees' country of origin are also frequent, and occur most commonly when refugee camps are located near insecure border areas.[765] Perhaps most notoriously, refugee camps and settlements across Southern Africa were often attacked by agents of the *apartheid*-era South African government. Between 1974 and 1986, more than 5,000 refugees from South Africa were systematically killed in camps inside Mozambique and Zambia, as well as in their homes in Botswana, Lesotho, Swaziland, and Zimbabwe.[766] Guatemalan refugees in Mexican camps in the Lacandón area, and at the Las Vétices, La Sombra, La Hamaca, and El Chupadero camps were repeatedly attacked by Guatemalan armed forces during the 1980s. The Guatemalan military government accused the refugees of being rebel sympathizers, and continued the attacks until Mexico agreed to move the camps away from the border area.[767] An Anotov plane from Sudan bombed the Olua refugee settlement camp in northern Uganda.[768] Somali refugees forced to live at a camp just 500 meters from Kenya's border with Somalia were often killed in cross-border fighting.[769] Rebels fighting the Liberian government attacked Liberian refugees left unprotected just inside

---

attacked a refugee camp in Adjumani, killing six refugees, and causing over half of the twelve thousand inhabitants to flee. On August 5, an LRA raid on the Achol Pii settlement in Pader district resulted in the deaths of about sixty people. The rebels looted all the recently-delivered food, and burned what they could not carry. They forced the camp's twenty-four thousand refugees and relief staff to flee the site": Human Rights Watch, *World Report 2003* (2003), at 89.

[764] "Curfew continues at refugee camps," *UN Integrated Regional Information Networks*, Apr. 3, 2003. Similar concerns arose at refugee camps in the Kakuma area: (2003) 127 *JRS Dispatches* (Feb. 28, 2003).

[765] R. Gorman, *Mitigating Misery* (1993), at 173–174.

[766] E. Mtango, "Military and Armed Attacks on Refugee Camps," in G. Loescher and L. Monahan eds., *Refugees and International Relations* 92 (1990) (Mtango, "Armed Attacks"), at 93.

[767] J. Simon and B. Manz, "Representation, Organization, and Human Rights Among Guatemalan Refugees in Mexico – 1980–1992," (1992) 5 *Harvard Human Rights Journal* 95, at 108–109. Sadly, however, when Mexico decided to move the Guatemalan refugees from self-settled camps near the border to interior locations in order to avoid attacks on the refugees by the Guatemalan military, authorities resorted to flagrant human rights violations, including the burning of settlements, cutting off of food supplies, and forced evictions to achieve their goal: ibid. at 109–110.

[768] (2001) 88 *JRS Dispatches* (Mar. 7, 2001).

[769] "These refugees fled inter-claim fighting in Bulo Hawa just across the border in Somalia in April and have since been living in a temporary location called Border Point 1 ... A UNHCR statement issued in May said that the proximity of Border Point 1 to the border exposed it to danger": (2002) 114 *JRS Dispatches* (June 28, 2002).

the border of Côte d'Ivoire.[770] Hundreds of thousands of refugees from Sierra Leone were required to live in isolated camps in Guinea near the border with their country of origin. Beginning in March 1999, those camps frequently came under attack in cross-border excursions by rebels and government-sponsored militias,[771] forcing the UN drastically to cut back the delivery of vital supplies. As one refugee remarked, "It is better to die at home than die in Guinea ... We are caught in a death trap here. Both sides use us as human shields. We are surrounded by guns."[772]

While refugee camps, particularly those located near insecure borders, present the greatest risk to the physical security of refugees, even refugees allowed to move freely within asylum countries often remain at risk of physical attack. Refugees in Russia, particularly those with non-Slavic features, have been regularly beaten by police.[773] There have been numerous reports of the rape of Somali refugee women in Kenya by local police and military.[774] Egyptian police beat and jailed refugees and other non-citizens in "Operation Track Down Blacks" during 2002 and 2003; disregarding even official UNHCR refugee status documentation, the police held the refugees at

---

[770] "In June 1995, the worst single cross-border attack took place at Guiglo, where 32 people died ... UNHCR appears to have made no effort to persuade the Ivoirian authorities that border settlements are unsafe for refugees, and apparently supports the policy that they should not receive assistance outside the border *zone d'accueil*": Lawyers' Committee for Human Rights, *African Exodus* (1995), at 75. Renewed fighting has since led to comparable concerns. "Liberian refugees are being indiscriminately associated with the armed opposition in Côte d'Ivoire ... They are being killed both by Ivorian security forces and groups of civilians, some of them armed by the government ...": Amnesty International, "Côte d'Ivoire: Liberian refugees at imminent risk," Feb. 20, 2003, available at http://web.amnesty.org/library (accessed Aug. 9, 2003).

[771] (1999) 50 *JRS Dispatches* (May 31, 1999).

[772] D. Farah, "For refugees, hazardous haven in Guinea," *Washington Post*, Nov. 6, 2000, quoting Ibrahim Suri Jollah, who had lived at Kaliah II camp for three years.

[773] More than 400 incidents of police harassment of refugees were recorded during the first half of 1994, with some refugees reporting several beatings in a single day: Lawyers' Committee for Human Rights, "Commitments without Compliance: Refugees in the Russian Federation" (1996), at 16. "Xenophobia and racism in Russia are increasing rapidly. In many cases, the police are more sympathetic to extremist youth groups (skinheads) which commit crimes against Chechens or Africans than to the victims. Often, the authorities do not want to prosecute these cases at all. If a case does go to court, the authorities do their best to get reduced sentences and decrease the time of imprisonment or the level of punishment": ACCORD/UNHCR, "Eighth European Country of Origin Information Seminar, Vienna, 28–29 June 2002 – Final Report: Russian Federation" (2002), at 216.

[774] Africa Watch Women's Rights Project, "Seeking Refuge, Finding Terror: The Widespread Rape of Somali Women in North Eastern Kenya," Oct. 4, 1993, at 3; F. Musse, "Women Victims of Violence: Rape in Kenya's Refugee Camps," (1994) 16 *Refugee Participation Network* 17, at 17–20.

al-Maadi and Bassatin police stations in inhumane and crowded conditions, and refused to accept food for the prisoners.[775]

Even where authorities are not directly responsible for the violence faced by refugees, they frequently create the conditions which make refugees vulnerable to attack. For example, Pakistani authorities cut off food and shelter to force Afghan refugees to move to camps near the Afghan border, even though it was well known that pro-Taliban, pro-Pushtan, and anti-foreigner sentiment in the area was high, raising serious concerns in particular for ethnic minority refugees including the Hazaras, Uzbeks, and Tajiks.[776] Because of the Kenyan and Ugandan policy of requiring refugees to live in camps, those who manage to escape to urban areas are left with few options but to sleep on the streets or in unsafe shelters where they are vulnerable to violence.[777] In September 2000, Guinean President Lansana Conte made a speech blaming refugees for border instability – leading police, soldiers, and civilian militias to launch attacks on refugee camps and against refugees in the capital city.[778]

Increasingly, anti-refugee vigilantes in asylum countries have engaged in attacks on refugees. Gangs of neo-Nazis "hunted" foreigners in the German town of Magdeburg in 1994, stabbing asylum-seekers from Africa, and beating them with iron bars. Police failed to intervene until the attacks had taken place, and then proceeded to arrest the victims.[779] The British government's policy of dispersing refugee claimants across the country also gave rise to vigilante violence, especially in areas not accustomed to the presence of racial and other minorities. Refugees in Liverpool had stones and bricks thrown through their windows;[780] Kurdish refugee claimants in Glasgow were stabbed to death.[781]

Finally, physical abuse is at times employed as part of a strategy to force refugees "voluntarily" to repatriate. Rohingya refugees were coerced to return to Burma by physical and sexual abuse at the hands of the Bangladeshi military and paramilitary forces in charge of reception camps.[782] And in

---

[775] Human Rights Watch, "Egypt: Mass Arrest of Foreigners," Feb. 10, 2003.

[776] Human Rights Watch, "Pakistan: Refugees Not Moving Voluntarily," Dec. 5, 2001.

[777] Human Rights Watch, *Hidden in Plain View* (2002).

[778] Human Rights Watch, "Guinea: Refugees Still at Risk," July 5, 2001.

[779] Human Rights Watch, "Germany for Germans: Xenophobia and Racist Violence in Germany" (1995), at 32–37; see also Amnesty International, "A Summary of Concerns in the Period May–October 1994," Doc. EUR/23/08/94 (Nov. 1, 1994).

[780] M. O'Kane, "Christmas charity appeal: Vulnerable given a cold welcome to Britain," *Guardian*, Dec. 3, 2001, at 12.

[781] V. Dodd and K. Scott, "UN body blames press for hatred of refugees," *Guardian*, Aug. 11, 2001, at 10.

[782] Human Rights Watch, *Human Rights Watch Global Report on Women's Human Rights* (1995), at 115–118. "[O]n July 20 [1997], the Bangladeshi security forces forcibly returned 187 refugees from Nayapara camp across the Naaf River to Myanmar. Apparently no one volunteered for repatriation, so the authorities picked mostly

late 1996, after most Rwandese refugees had repatriated, troops of the Democratic Republic of Congo under the command of Laurent Kabila massacred thousands of refugees who were reluctant to go back.[783]

> **Civil and Political Covenant, Art. 6(1)**
> Every human being has the inherent right to life. This right shall be protected by law. No one shall be arbitrarily deprived of his life.

> **Civil and Political Covenant, Art. 7**
> No one shall be subjected to torture or to cruel, inhuman or degrading treatment or punishment . . .

> **Civil and Political Covenant, Art. 9(1)**
> Everyone has the right to liberty and security of person . . .

Even though physical security is clearly fundamental to any notion of refugee protection, the Refugee Convention is silent on this issue. At one point, Belgium and the United States tabled a proposal that would have required states to grant refugees arriving without pre-authorization "treatment compatible, from both the moral and material view, with human dignity."[784] The Belgian co-sponsor explained that this clause would "grant the refugee the means of livelihood and . . . prevent his ill-treatment."[785] This language was not approved on the grounds that it was "too ambitious,"[786] the drafters opting instead to define with greater precision precisely which rights refugees would receive. No right to physical security was proposed or adopted.

Mtango suggests that this omission may follow from the primary concern of the drafters to ensure the economic and social well-being of refugees, the assumption being that physical safety would follow from the enforcement of norms derived from the international law of armed conflict and national asylum laws.[787] An alternative explanation is that refugee law, like the

---

women and children to be sent back": Amnesty International, "Rohingyas: The Search for Safety," Doc. ASA/13/07/97 (Sept. 1, 1997).

[783] "Killings of refugees which began in October 1996 in the camps along the DRC [Democratic Republic of Congo] border with Rwanda and Burundi continued as the AFDL [Alliance des forces démocratiques pour la libération du Congo] and its allies captured more territory, through to the DRC's western border with the Republic of Congo. The refugees who had managed to escape westwards from the camps walked hundreds of kilometres and frequently set up make-shift camps . . . Settlement in camps subsequently enabled the AFDL and its allies to locate the refugees and on occasions kill hundreds of them at a time": Amnesty International, "Deadly Alliances in Congolese Forests" (1997), at 6.

[784] UN Doc. E/AC.32/L.25, Feb. 2, 1950, at Art. 3(1).

[785] Statement of Mr. Cuvelier of Belgium, UN Doc. E/AC.32/SR.22, Feb. 2, 1950, at 24.

[786] Statement of the Chairman, Mr. Chance of Canada, ibid. at 25.

[787] Mtango, "Armed Attacks," at 97.

international human rights standards being contemporaneously developed, reflects a masculinist assumption that protection from physical attack need not be codified as a human right. Because the standards of both refugee law and international human rights law were nearly exclusively drafted by men, and because men presumed themselves to be independently able to ensure their own physical security (except, for example, during a war or while incarcerated), there was no need to draft a general right to physical security.[788]

Whatever the historical reason, we are today required to ground a right to physical security for refugees not in the Refugee Convention itself, but instead in what has been described as "a criss-cross of rules which have some bearing on the subject."[789] For example, child refugees may rely on Arts. 19, 20, 22, 34, 35, 36, and 37 of the Convention on the Rights of the Child.[790] Refugees who are threatened by armed conflict may invoke the protections of the Geneva Conventions on the Law of Armed Conflict and their Protocols, in particular Common Article 3, which prohibits acts of violence directed against persons not taking active part in hostilities.[791] But unless a refugee is able to invoke a specialized obligation of this kind, he or she must rely on the guarantee set by Art. 7(1) of the Refugee Convention, which confirms that refugees are to enjoy at least the same treatment as is afforded aliens in general.

---

[788] See generally H. Charlesworth and C. Chinkin, *Boundaries of International Law: A Feminist Analysis* (2000), at 280–287; V. Peterson, "Security and Sovereign States: What is at Stake in Taking Feminism Seriously?," in V. Peterson ed., *Gendered States: Feminist (Re)visions of International Relations Theory* (1992), at 31. Belated recognition of the importance of the right to physical security, including in a gender-specific context, has been forthcoming. At the fifty-seventh session of the Commission on Human Rights, for example, a Canadian resolution condemning violence against women as a "violation of the rights and fundamental freedoms of women" was adopted by consensus, with seventy-five co-sponsors: M. Dennis, "The Fifty-Seventh Session of the UN Commission on Human Rights," (2002) 96(1) *American Journal of International Law* 181.

[789] M. Othman-Chande, "International Law and Armed Attacks in Refugee Camps," [1990] *Nordic Journal of International Law* 153, at 153.

[790] These provisions address protection from physical or mental violence (Art. 19); special protection for children deprived of their family (Art. 20); special protection for children seeking refugee status (Art. 22); protection from sexual exploitation (Art. 34); protection from abduction or trafficking (Art. 35); protection against any form of exploitation (Art. 36); and protection against cruel, inhuman, or degrading treatment (Art. 37): Rights of the Child Convention.

[791] "In the case of armed conflict not of an international character occurring in the territory of one of the High Contracting Parties, each Party to the conflict shall be bound to apply, at a minimum, the following provisions: (1) Persons taking no active part in the hostilities ... shall in all circumstances be treated humanely, without any adverse distinction, founded on race, colour, religion or faith, sex, birth or wealth, or any other similar criteria": Geneva Convention relative to the Protection of Civilian Persons in Time of War, 75 UNTS 287, done Aug, 12, 1949, entered into force Oct. 21, 1950, at Art. 3. See Mtango, "Armed Attacks," at 103–106.

Thus, all refugees are entitled to the benefit of the narrow range of rights set by international aliens law, including the duty of every state to respect the life and physical integrity of all aliens in their territory, including refugees.[792] Yet because international aliens law unfortunately grants no directly enforceable rights to aliens themselves, this obligation will in most cases provide no practical value to refugees.[793] Of greater real importance, the ability of refugees to claim the benefit of any international legal obligations which inhere in all persons under the jurisdiction of a state party means that they are able to claim the guarantees of physical security set by the Human Rights Covenants.[794] The Human Rights Committee has made clear that the benefit of Arts. 6, 7, and 9 of the Civil and Political Covenant may be directly invoked by non-citizens under the effective jurisdiction of a state party.[795]

4.3.1 Right to life

The right to life is defined by Art. 6 of the Civil and Political Covenant to be an "inherent right," meaning that "one's right to life cannot be taken away by the state or waived, surrendered or renounced by [the individual concerned], since a human being cannot be divested, nor can he divest himself, of his humanity."[796] The right to life has been said by the International Court of Justice to be part of "the irreducible core of human rights."[797] The Human

---

[792] See chapter 2.1 above, at p. 76.

[793] See chapter 2.1 above, at pp. 78–79.

[794] "In general, the rights set forth in the Covenant apply to everyone, irrespective of reciprocity, and irrespective of his or her nationality or statelessness. Thus, the general rule is that each one of the rights of the Covenant must be guaranteed without discrimination between citizens and aliens": UN Human Rights Committee, "General Comment No. 15: The position of aliens under the Covenant" (1986), UN Doc. HRI/GEN/1/Rev.7, May 12, 2004, at 140, paras. 1–2. More specifically, state parties are required to ensure that the protection of the Covenant is "available to all individuals, regardless of nationality or statelessness, such as asylum-seekers [and] refugees": UN Human Rights Committee, "General Comment No. 31: The nature of the general legal obligation imposed on states parties to the Covenant" (2004), UN Doc. HRI/GEN/1/Rev.7, May 12, 2004, at 192, para. 10. See chapter 2.5.4 above, at pp. 120–121.

[795] "Aliens thus have an inherent right to life, protected by law, and may not be arbitrarily deprived of life. They must not be subjected to torture or to cruel, inhuman or degrading treatment or punishment ... Aliens have the full right to liberty and security of the person": UN Human Rights Committee, "General Comment No. 15: The position of aliens under the Covenant" (1986), UN Doc. HRI/GEN/1/Rev.7, May 12, 2004, at 140, para. 7.

[796] N. Jayawickrama, *The Judicial Application of Human Rights Law* (2002) (Jayawickrama, *Judicial Application*), at 256.

[797] *Legality of the Threat or Use of Nuclear Weapons*, [1996] ICJ Rep 226, at 506, per Judge Weeramantry.

Rights Committee refers to it as "the supreme right," and insists that it "is basic to all human rights"[798] and "should not be interpreted narrowly."[799]

Most obviously, the right to life prohibits acts of intentional killing by state authorities other than under the strictest controls, and in carefully limited circumstances required by law. As the Human Rights Committee has affirmed,

> States parties should take measures not only to prevent and punish depri-vation of life by criminal acts, but also to prevent arbitrary killing by their own security forces. The deprivation of life by the authorities of the State is a matter of the utmost gravity. Therefore, the law must strictly control and limit the circumstances in which a person may be deprived of his life by such authorities.[800]

The bombing of refugees in flight from Sudan, the execution of Iraqi refugees by Saudi camp officials, the murder of Rwandese refugees by troops of the Democratic Republic of Congo, and the enforced disappearance of Somali refugees by Kenyan security guards were all clearly violations of this most fundamental of all human rights.[801] Liability also inheres where a government puts unofficial agents in a position of control over refugees, and then turns a blind eye to murders committed by those to whom it has entrusted authority. Because a government may not do indirectly what Art. 6 prohibits it from doing directly, the killing of Cambodian refugees by Khmer Rouge officials who operated camps inside Thailand was an arbitrary depri-vation of life by Thailand. And as the General Comment of the Human Rights Committee makes clear, an intention to kill is not requisite to finding a breach of the right to life. Thus, for example, the disregard for the life of refugees evident in the methods of deportation employed by Malawi and Austria amounts to an infringement of the duty of affirmative protection required by Art. 6.

More generally, the right to life "is not to be understood as a negative right directed solely at the State, but rather [as a right] that calls for positive measures to ensure it."[802] Where killings are not the result of direct or indirect official acts, they nonetheless infringe Art. 6 if the state fails to take

---

[798] UN Human Rights Committee, "General Comment No. 14: Right to life" (1984), UN Doc. HRI/GEN/1/Rev.7, May 12, 2004, at 139, para. 1.

[799] UN Human Rights Committee, "General Comment No. 6: Right to life" (1982), UN Doc. HRI/GEN/1/Rev.7, May 12, 2004, at 128, para. 1.

[800] Ibid. at 128, para. 3.

[801] "The Human Rights Committee has required states to take specific and effective mea-sures to prevent the disappearance of individuals. They should establish effective facilities and procedures to investigate thoroughly cases of missing and disappeared persons in circumstances which may involve a violation of the right to life": Jayawickrama, *Judicial Application*, at 280.

[802] Nowak, *ICCPR Commentary*, at 105.

appropriate, positive steps to protect persons whose lives are known to be at risk from non-state actors.[803] When Uganda left Sudanese refugees exposed to killings by Lord's Resistance Army rebels whose objectives were clear, and when no serious effort was made by Zaïre or the UN to ensure that violent *genocidaires* and weapons were kept out of the Rwandan refugee camps, the resultant slaughter inside the camps was in breach of the right to life.

Perhaps most serious of all, decisions to force refugees to remain in areas adjacent to the frontier with their country of origin frequently expose them to cross-border raids and killings by their enemies. Especially in view of the high duty of care owed to persons detained by the state,[804] Mexico's initial insistence that Guatemalan refugees remain in camps near the border with Guatemala, and Côte d'Ivoire's comparable refusal to relocate Liberian refugees away from the Liberian frontier, were both contrary to the duty to protect life under Art. 6. UNHCR's Executive Committee has affirmed the duty of governments to mitigate the possibility of non-combatant refugees becoming the objects of armed attack.[805] Protection of physical security normally entails ensuring that refugees not be required to remain in an area which may be affected by the conflict they have fled, or by any other conflict in the country of asylum.

The state of refuge is also liable under Art. 6 where its fails to establish "effective facilities and procedures to investigate thoroughly"[806] either unofficial killings or disappearances in territory under its jurisdiction. When Hong Kong officials took no credible action to apprehend those responsible for pervasive gang killings in the refugee camps, for example, there was clearly a failure to comply with the right to life. As Nowak observes, the Human Rights Committee has generally found violations of Art. 6 on the basis of "well-documented accusations of the authors and the lack of willingness on the part of the governments to assist in resolving these deaths."[807]

---

[803] "It is the duty of the state to protect human life against unwarranted actions by public authorities as well as by private persons. This is usually done by enacting appropriate laws to criminalize the intentional taking of life and by ensuring that such laws are enforced. But the obligation to protect the right to life also implies other positive preventive measures appropriate to the general situation": Jayawickrama, *Judicial Application*, at 260.

[804] Civil and Political Covenant, at Art. 10(1).

[805] UNHCR Executive Committee Conclusion No. 48, "Military or Armed Attacks on Refugee Camps and Settlements" (1987), available at www.unhcr.ch (accessed Nov. 20, 2004). See also UNHCR Executive Committee Conclusions Nos. 27, "Military Attacks on Refugee Camps and Settlements in Southern Africa and Elsewhere" (1982), 32, "Military Attacks on Refugee Camps and Settlements in Southern Africa and Elsewhere" (1983), and 45, "Military and Armed Attacks on Refugee Camps and Settlements" (1986), all available at www.unhcr.ch (accessed Nov. 20, 2004).

[806] UN Human Rights Committee, "General Comment No. 6: Right to life" (1982), UN Doc. HRI/GEN/1/Rev.7, May 12, 2004, at 128, para. 4.

[807] Nowak, *ICCPR Commentary*, at 112.

The right to life is not, however, infringed simply because refugees die. Most Southern African states, for example, allowed refugees from the South African *apartheid* regime to move away from border areas, and took serious efforts to protect them from killings at the hands of extremely sophisticated covert incursions by the military and other agents of South Africa. Nor can Uganda be held responsible for the bombing of refugee camps in its territory by Sudan. Where loss of life results neither from intention nor a failure seriously to combat risks to life, there is no breach by the host country of Art. 6. The relevant inquiry is instead whether the authorities of the asylum state intend to kill the refugee – either directly, or indirectly, as by starvation, or exposure to illness or violence – or whether they show a lack of determination effectively to respond to known risks to life, or to pursue and prosecute those responsible for risk to, or loss of, life. Because the right to life can be infringed by either act or omission, and because it focuses broadly on whether death results from a situation characterized by "elements of unlawfulness and injustice, as well as those of capriciousness and unreasonableness,"[808] it is an important means of holding governments accountable for intentional or foreseeable threats to the lives of refugees.

4.3.2 Freedom from torture, cruel, inhuman, or degrading treatment

Many of the risks to the physical security of refugees, of course, fall short of a risk to life. Art. 7 of the Civil and Political Covenant, however, also prohibits actions which amount to torture, or to cruel, inhuman, or degrading treatment. Like the guarantee of the right to life, Art. 7 not only prohibits negative state conduct, but requires governments to take affirmative steps to protect everyone under their authority from relevant risks.[809] Equally important, a state may never justify its failure to protect all persons from torture, cruel, inhuman, or degrading treatment on the grounds of an exceptional or emergency situation:

> The text of article 7 allows of no limitation ... [E]ven in situations of public emergency ... no derogation from the provisions of article 7 is allowed and its provisions must remain in force ... [N]o justification or extenuating circumstances may be invoked to excuse a violation of article 7

---

[808] Ibid. at 111, citing comments of the Chilean representative to the Commission on Human Rights during the drafting of the Civil and Political Covenant.

[809] "It is the duty of the State party to afford everyone protection through legislative and other measures as may be necessary against the acts prohibited by article 7, whether inflicted by people acting in their official capacity, outside their official capacity or in a private capacity": UN Human Rights Committee, "General Comment No. 20: Prohibition of torture, or other cruel, inhuman or degrading treatment or punishment" (1992), UN Doc. HRI/GEN/1/Rev.7, May 12, 2004, at 150, para. 2.

for any reasons, including those based on an order from a superior officer or public authority.[810]

The definition of "torture" is relatively demanding.[811] An act may be described as torture only if four criteria are satisfied. First, the act in question must result in severe physical or mental pain or suffering. Second, the act which causes the pain or suffering must be intentional. Third, there must be a specific motivation for the intentional infliction of harm, such as the extraction of a confession, intimidation, punishment, or discrimination (but not including lawful punishment). Fourth, the act must be committed by or under the authority of a public official. By way of example, all of these criteria were met when Bangladeshi camp officials raped Rohingya refugee women with a view to terrorizing them to such a point that they would feel compelled to go back to Burma. The suffering was severe, the act of rape was intentionally inflicted by public officials, and its goal was to punish and intimidate refugees who refused to return to the risk of persecution in their own country.

While refugees are sometimes the victims of torture, they more commonly face the risk of either inhuman or cruel treatment. The prohibition of "inhuman or cruel treatment or punishment" is treated as a unified concept. That is, a clear distinction is not generally drawn between actions which are cruel, and those which are inhuman. In general, actions are "inhuman or cruel" if they meet most, but not all, of the criteria for torture.[812] Thus, acts of rape committed by state officials even if not accompanied by the specific intent required to establish torture – for example, those committed by Burmese, Kenyan, and Nepali officials – are appropriately deemed to be forms of cruel and inhuman treatment. Similarly, the intentional act of a public official intended to punish a refugee may not be "torture" if the consequent harm does not rise to the level of "severe" pain or suffering. Lesser pain or suffering, in the context of such an intentional, official, and punitive action would still

---

[810] Ibid. at 150, para. 3.

[811] While not defined in the Civil and Political Covenant, a helpful definition of "torture" may be derived from the subsequently enacted Convention against Torture and Other Cruel, Inhuman or Degrading Treatment or Punishment, UNGA Res. 39/46, adopted Dec. 10, 1984, entered into force June 26, 1987 (Torture Convention), at Art. 1(1): "For the purposes of this Convention, the term 'torture' means any act by which severe pain or suffering, whether physical or mental, is intentionally inflicted on a person for such purposes as obtaining from him or a third person information or a confession, punishing him for an act he or a third person has committed or is suspected of having committed, or intimidating or coercing him or a third person, or for any reason based on discrimination of any kind, when such pain or suffering is inflicted by or at the instigation of or with the consent or acquiescence of a public official or other person acting in an official capacity. It does not include pain or suffering arising only from, inherent in or incidental to lawful sanctions."

[812] Nowak, *ICCPR Commentary*, at 131.

amount to inhuman or cruel punishment.[813] Thus, for example, the prohibition of cruel and inhuman treatment was breached when Russian police beat non-Slavic refugees; when South African officials whipped refugees waiting to register in South Africa; when Kosovar refugees were beaten by police in Sarajevo; and when Egyptian police hunted down black refugees in order to detain them in crowded and inhumane conditions, and without access to food. And because an action is no less official when implemented by private parties encouraged by the state, the unleashing of violent attacks by Guinean citizens against refugees consequent to a speech by that country's president also amounted to a form of cruel and inhuman treatment or punishment.

A state may moreover be found to have engaged in cruel or inhuman treatment where it fails to respond appropriately to known risks of a grave quality. For example, the Human Rights Committee found a breach of Art. 7 of the Covenant where Australia continued to detain an Iranian refugee claimant even after it was clear that the prolonged detention would result in irreversible psychiatric illness:

> As to the author's allegations that his first period of detention amounted to a breach of article 7, the Committee notes that the psychiatric evidence emerging from examinations of the author over an extended period, which was accepted by the State party's courts and tribunals, was essentially unanimous that the author's psychiatric illness developed as a result of the protracted period of immigration detention. The Committee notes that the State party was aware, at least from August 1992 when he was prescribed tranquillizers, of psychiatric difficulties the author faced. Indeed, by August 1993, it was evident that there was a conflict between the author's continued detention and his sanity.
>
> Despite increasingly serious assessments of the author's conditions in February and June 1994 (and a suicide attempt), it was only in August 1994 that the Minister exercised his exceptional power to release him from immigration detention on medical grounds (while legally he remained in detention). As subsequent events showed, by that point the author's illness had reached such a level of severity that irreversible consequences were to follow. In the Committee's view, the continued detention of the author when the State party was aware of the author's mental condition and failed to take the steps necessary to ameliorate the author's mental deterioration constituted a violation of his rights under article 7 of the Covenant.[814]

In line with this focus on failure to take the steps necessary to respond to clear risks, it follows that India and Kenya were responsible for the cruel and inhuman treatment of refugee women when their camp officials refused to

[813] Jayawickrama, *Judicial Application*, at 308–311.
[814] *C v. Australia*, UNHRC Comm. No. 900/1999, UN Doc. CCPR/C/76/D/900/1999, decided Oct. 28, 2002, at para. 8.4.

provide materials for cooking fires even after learning of the rapes of women in the adjacent forests where they were compelled to forage for wood. While there may have been no specific, invidious motivation behind these governments' actions, the failure to make alternative arrangements for the provision of fuel exhibited a willful disregard for what authorities knew was the exposure of refugee women to the severe pain and suffering of rape. Similarly, China may be held liable for cruel and inhuman treatment in view of its awareness that refusal to protect North Korean refugees left them no option but to seek informal "protection" purchased by submission to sexual or other exploitation.

The known risk of serious harm at the heart of the notion of cruel and inhuman treatment need not emanate from state officials themselves, so long as the official actions contribute in a material way to the exposure to harm. Thus, Mozambique's refusal to take measures to protect minority Burundian refugees against the known risk of race-based violence at the hands of other refugees housed in the same camp; the decisions of Kenya and Guinea to force refugees from Somalia and Sierra Leone respectively to live in border camps where it was clear they would be subject to cross-border violence committed by armies from their country of origin; Pakistan's forced relocation of even minority Afghan refugees to border regions where it was clear they would be at risk of assault; as well as Tanzania's decision to require refugees to live in the remote Mtabila camp where they could not be meaningfully protected against banditry and other attacks are all examples of cruel and inhuman treatment.

Beyond acts which are torture or cruel and inhuman, Art. 7 also prohibits treatment or punishment which is "degrading." Viewed as "the weakest level of a violation of Article 7,"[815] an act is considered degrading when it is intended to humiliate the victim, or when it shows an egregious disregard for his or her humanity. As the European Court of Human Rights opined, "degrading" treatment

> humiliates or debases an individual showing a lack of respect for, or diminishing, his or her human dignity or arouses feelings of fear, anguish or inferiority capable of breaking an individual's moral and physical resistance.[816]

Australia's resort to tear gas, room-trashings, and the punitive solitary confinement of children under the guise of "management practices" shows the requisite disregard for the humanity of the refugees against whom they were directed. So too does the robbing of desperate and defenseless Rwandan refugees arriving in Zaïre by members of that country's army. Jayawickrama

---

[815] Nowak, *ICCPR Commentary*, at 133.
[816] *Pretty v. United Kingdom*, (2002) 35 EHRR 1 (ECHR, Apr. 29, 2002), at para. 52.

suggests as well that an act is also to be considered degrading where it "drives [an individual] to act against his will or conscience."[817] As such, the sexual exploitation of refugees by Zimbabwean camp workers, by Namibian teachers, and by relief workers throughout much of Western Africa – effectively forcing individuals to submit to sex as a condition of access to basic necessities or other rights – are appropriately understood to be forms of degrading treatment.

4.3.3 Security of person

The third article of the Civil and Political Covenant with a bearing on the physical security of refugees is Art. 9(1). It provides that "[e]veryone has the right to liberty and security of person." While subsequent paragraphs of Art. 9 define the ways in which the right to "liberty" informs the treatment of detained persons, Sieghart sensibly argues that independent meaning should be given to the guarantee of "security of person,"[818] even though its content is not textually elaborated. This approach conforms to the principle of treaty interpretation requiring a good faith effort to give meaning to all parts of a treaty as codified.[819]

The drafting history confirms that these words are not mere surplusage. Reference to "security of person" was added to the text of Art. 9(1) on the basis of a British proposal to the eighth session of the Commission on Human Rights,[820] apparently motivated by a desire to conform to the formulation of the predecessor Art. 3 of the Universal Declaration of Human Rights.[821] During the drafting of Art. 3 of the Universal Declaration, a Cuban proposal expressly to add a guarantee of physical integrity was turned down after discussion suggesting that the right to "security of person" already encompassed this concern.[822] Specifically, Chairperson Eleanor Roosevelt concluded that "the words 'security of person' had been chosen after lengthy discussion because they were more comprehensive than any other expression. The French representative had especially noted that they included the idea of

---

[817] Jayawickrama, *Judicial Application*, at 311.

[818] P. Sieghart, *The International Law of Human Rights* (1983), at 139.

[819] Vienna Convention, at Art. 31(1). See chapter 1.3.3 above, at p. 62.

[820] UN Doc. E/CN.4/L.137 (1952). A Polish proposal to reframe this guarantee (UN Doc. E/CN.4/L.183) was adopted by a vote of 7–5 (5 abstentions): UN Doc. E/CN.4/SR.314, at 10. See M. Bossuyt, *Guide to the "Travaux Préparatoires" of the International Covenant on Civil and Political Rights* (1987), at 196–197.

[821] Nowak, *ICCPR Commentary*, at 162. Art. 3 of the Universal Declaration of Human Rights provides that: "[e]veryone has the right to life, liberty and security of person."

[822] L. Rehof, "Article 3," in A. Eide et al. eds., *The Universal Declaration of Human Rights: A Commentary* 73 (1992) (Rehof, "Article 3"), at 77.

physical integrity."[823] As Nowak affirms, "[i]n the French Revolution, the civic right of security was accorded high priority: it granted the citizen State protection against impairment of his personal rights and his property through interference at the horizontal level."[824]

There is therefore a textual and historical basis to argue that state parties have an independent duty under Art. 9(1) of the Civil and Political Covenant to take affirmative measures to protect all persons under their authority from attacks against their personal integrity, and perhaps also their property:

> The "right to security" ... is the right to protection of the law in the exercise of the right to liberty. "Liberty and security are the two sides of the same coin." The right to security may, therefore, be applicable to situations other than the formal deprivation of liberty. For instance, a state may not ignore a known threat to the life of a person under their jurisdiction simply because he or she is not arrested or otherwise detained. There is an obligation to take reasonable and appropriate measures to protect such a person.[825]

This view has been adopted by the Human Rights Committee, which held that Art. 9(1) was infringed when the Colombian government failed to respond in a meaningful way to death threats made against a teacher who was ultimately forced to flee the country:

> Although in the Covenant the only reference to the right to security of person is to be found in article 9, there is no evidence that it was intended to narrow the concept of the right to security only to situations of formal deprivation of liberty ... States are under an obligation to take reasonable and appropriate measures to protect [persons under their jurisdiction]. An interpretation of article 9 which would allow a State party to ignore threats to the personal security of non-detained persons within its jurisdiction would render totally ineffective the guarantees of the Covenant.[826]

Under this interpretation, Germany infringed Art. 9(1) when it responded to neo-Nazi attacks on asylum-seekers in the town of Magdeburg with no more than "incredibly sloppy" police work that led to the arrest of numerous victims, but not of the German citizens who initiated the attacks.[827] And because the duty under Art. 9(1) is owed to all persons under a state's

---

[823] UNGAOR (1948), Part I (Third Committee), at 189–190, cited in Rehof, "Article 3," at 77.

[824] Nowak, *ICCPR Commentary*, at 162.

[825] Jayawickrama, *Judicial Application*, at 375–376, quoting from J. Fawcett, *The Application of the European Convention on Human Rights* (1987), at 70.

[826] *Delgado Paéz v. Colombia*, UNHRC Comm. No. 195/1985, decided July 12, 1990, at paras. 5.5–5.6.

[827] See UNHCR Executive Committee Conclusion No. 72, "Personal Security of Refugees" (1993), available at www.unhcr.ch (accessed Nov. 20, 2004), at para. (c): "The Executive

jurisdiction, the governments of Honduras and Mexico were required to take reasonable measures to protect Central American refugees traveling to North America through their territory from the known risk of abuse and extortion at the hands of smugglers.

More generally, the duty to take "reasonable and appropriate measures" to guard against risks to the physical security of refugees calls into question the general policy of closed refugee camps, clearly proven to be breeding grounds for violence, in particular against refugee women and children. It most certainly requires attention to such concerns as the location of communal latrines far from refugee living quarters and inadequate lighting and patrols, all of which give rise to known risks of rape and other forms of serious harm. The duty to avoid known risks to physical security is also grounds for contesting the legality of the British dispersal policy, under which refugees were required to live in areas where the risk of private violence was clear; as well as the refusal of Kenya and Uganda to authorize refugees to live outside of camps, thereby exposing refugees living in urban areas to vigilante and other attacks known not to elicit any protective response from the government.

Art. 9(1) would not, however, be a sufficient source of protection for the Vietnamese asylum-seekers attacked by Thai pirates. While Art. 9(1) would require Thailand to protect refugees passing through its territorial waters, and arguably through any contiguous zone declared by it,[828] human rights law does not impose an obligation to reach out to refugees attacked in adjacent portions of the high seas. Because no state is bound to afford protection of human rights in parts of the *res communis* unless it has appropriated jurisdiction over that international territory, even the broad-ranging protection of Art. 9(1) cannot establish state responsibility for all threats to the physical security of refugees in search of asylum.[829]

Committee ... [c]alls upon States vigorously to investigate violations of the personal security of refugees and asylum-seekers, and where possible to institute criminal prosecution, and where applicable strict disciplinary measures, against all perpetrators of such violations." There may indeed be evidence that the problem was not simply the unwillingness of German authorities meaningfully to intervene against private violence. The UN Committee on the Elimination of Racial Discrimination reported its concern regarding "repeated reports of racist incidents in police stations, as well as ill-treatment inflicted by law enforcement officials on foreigners, including asylum-seekers": "Concluding Observations of the Committee on the Elimination of Racial Discrimination: Germany," UN Doc. CERD/C/304/Add.115, Apr. 27, 2001, at para. 19.

[828] See generally discussion of jurisdiction over adjacent seas in chapter 3.1.1 above, at pp. 160–161.

[829] Thus, for example, UNHCR's response to the attacks on Vietnamese refugees was to address "an urgent call to all interested Governments to take appropriate action to prevent such criminal attacks whether occurring on the high seas or in their territorial waters" by, for example, undertaking increased sea and air patrols, identifying and

With the exception of this critical territorial gap, Arts. 6, 7, and 9 of the Civil and Political Covenant taken together provide a relatively sound foundation for protection of the physical security of refugees. While these duties do not, of course, insulate refugees from risks to their physical security, they can be invoked by refugees to require governments of transit and asylum countries both to avoid negative acts, and to take affirmative steps to counter unofficial risks to their well-being.

4.4 Necessities of life

Most refugees are not able immediately to meet their own needs for food, water, shelter, and healthcare. Because the flight to safety cannot always be planned, and because the logistics of travel often make it impossible for refugees to bring significant resources or provisions with them, even refugees who were self-sufficient in their homeland typically depend for survival on the generosity of the asylum country.

Frequently, the basic needs of refugees are met by the local people they first encounter in the state of reception. For instance, when refugees fleeing state-sponsored terror in Guatemala arrived in Mexico's southern states in 1981, "[t]he host population received them well, provided them with food, exchanged food for work, and bought whatever the refugees had to sell (albeit at very low prices)."[830] Similarly, when more than 50,000 Mauritanian refugees fled across the river into Senegal in 1989, they were received by the local population with offers of food and shelter before international aid agencies had time to react.[831] And when Kosovar Albanian refugees arrived in Europe during the spring of 1999, "it was as if [the] river of hostility [towards the reception of refugees in Europe] began to flow backwards ... A substantial number of people offered to take Kosovans into their own homes."[832]

Circumstances permitting, refugees may achieve a measure of self-sufficiency fairly quickly through farming, small-scale business, or wage-labor. The case of Mozambican refugees who went to Swaziland shows the ability of refugees to

prosecuting those responsible, and implementing fully the rules of general international law relating to the suppression of piracy: UNHCR Executive Committee Conclusion No. 20, "Protection of Asylum-Seekers at Sea" (1980), at paras. (c)–(e), available at www.unhcr.ch (accessed Nov. 20, 2004).

[830] F. Stepputat, *Self-Sufficiency and Exile in Mexico* (1989), at 10.

[831] "As is so often the case with boundaries drawn up by colonial powers, this one divided the peoples of the river region, so that officially they are citizens of two separate states ... These traditional links between the two peoples ensured a warm welcome for the refugees who came across from Mauritania": T. Williams, "Getting on with the Business of Living," (1991) 82 *Refugees* 7, at 8.

[832] M. Gibney, "Kosovo and Beyond: Popular and Unpopular Refugees," (1999) 5 *Forced Migration Review* 28, at 28.

meet their own basic needs when provided with opportunities for self-sufficiency by the host community:

> These refugees began to arrive in Swaziland in late 1984. The majority did not receive any international aid, relying instead on their own economic activities and on assistance from local villagers ... While the refugees did not own land, some received the use of small plots from Swazi farmers who played host to them. In order to meet all their needs, refugees undertook a variety of work. They worked for small farmers, or on large commercial farms, or set themselves up as artisans or traders.[833]

Particularly where start-up assistance is made available, initiatives of this kind can generate an extraordinarily vibrant economy. For example, the international humanitarian agency AfriCare responded to a breakdown in international aid by assisting refugees from Angola and the Democratic Republic of Congo to run their own successful enterprises in a Namibian refugee camp:

> The refugees, mostly women, work as volunteers in an agro-forestry project in the camp, planting trees and growing vegetables ... [T]he project was developed to educate refugees and also to help them grow their own food to supplement their diet. The refugees have planted fruit trees, mostly papayas ... Although it is a refugee camp for more than 20,000 refugees ... there is an open market ... Items sold at the market are fish, baked cakes, cooking oil, vegetables and various other consumables. Besides the open market, the camp features a "guesthouse" and a number of restaurants and shops owned and run by the refugees themselves.[834]

4.4.1 Freedom from deprivation

Economic, legal, and other constraints may, however, impede refugees from meeting their own needs in the short term. Where this is the case, refugees are in an extremely vulnerable position. In one of the worst examples, in November 2000 the Pakistani government decided that it would refuse international aid for its massive Afghan refugee population as part of its strategy to drive the refugees back home. It even denied the UN Secretary-General access to one of the main refugee camps, where conditions had become predictably horrific:

> Tens of thousands have been camped in the open since January [2001] and the government has refused to let the UN High Commissioner for Refugees provide basic amenities for the new arrivals. The UNHCR said that more than 80,000 were squatting in squalid conditions on a strip of land in

---

[833] D. Keen, *Refugees: Rationing the Right to Life* (1992) (Keen, *Right to Life*), at 60–61.
[834] "Self-help initiative at Osire Refugee Camp," *Namibian Economist*, June 7, 2002.

Jalozai, and more were arriving each day. The camp is known to aid workers as "Plastic City," because of the cheap plastic bags being used as tents. Faced with overflowing latrines and limited drinking water, the refugees, particularly the children, are dying almost daily.[835]

Sadly, the actions of the Pakistani government are not unique. Other governments have also denied refugees the necessities of life in order to force them home or to deter other refugees from arriving. For example, the UN Committee on Economic, Social and Cultural Rights inquired into allegations that Hong Kong had denied medical and dental treatment to asylum-seekers from Vietnam in order to force them to leave.[836] In an effort to make life unbearable for them, Vietnamese refugees in Malaysia were confined to longhouses in which refugees had only two square meters of living space per person. Of the sixty-one longhouses used to shelter refugees, ten were moreover declared structurally unsound by the Malaysian Red Crescent Society.[837] When refugees from the Democratic Republic of Congo, Rwanda, and Somalia protested the decision of Swaziland to stop paying them support allowances – their only means of supporting themselves – the government responded by arresting them and ordering their expulsion from the country.[838]

Essentials may also be withheld from refugees out of ethnic, religious, or other antagonism. For example, Iraqi Kurds in Turkey were forced to live in camps which had open privies infested by swarms of flies and insects.[839] Antipathy towards Somali refugees initially led the government of Kenya to refuse to register them as refugees, which prevented the Somalis from

---

[835] E. MacAskill, "Pakistan keeps Annan from 'world's worst' camp," *Guardian*, Mar. 13, 2001, at 14. "Although refugees continued to slip in, at year's end the border remained officially closed to them. The Pakistan government was labeling all new arrivals 'illegal immigrants.' It continued to refuse UNHCR permission to create new camps to accommodate arriving refugees, and insisted that Afghanistan is now peaceful and that Afghan refugees must return home": US Committee for Refugees, *World Refugee Survey 2001* (2001), at 163.

[836] Committee on Economic, Social and Cultural Rights, "Concluding Observations on Report of the United Kingdom," UN Doc. E/C.12/Add.10 (1996).

[837] US Government Accounting Office, "Refugees: Living Conditions are Marginal," Doc. No. UNGAO/NSIA-91-258 (1991) (US, "Living Conditions"), at 42–43.

[838] "Swaziland deports 65 refugees," *Mail & Guardian*, Sept. 4, 2002.

[839] "Privies are situated in full sunlight, without any possibility of flushing them with water . . . In the privies, faeces and other filth are piled up in the open air, covered with countless flies and other insects . . . The drainage of the camp runs off in small ditches that have been dug provisionally between the tents and along the paths. The stench is ferocious, and here too there are countless swarms of flies": German *Bundestag* Member Angelika Beer, June 12, 1989, cited in Initiative for Human Rights in Kurdistan, "Silence is Killing Them: A Report on the Situation of the Kurdish Refugees in Turkey" (1990) (IHRK, "Kurdish Refugees"), at 15.

receiving food and other general rations.[840] The necessities of life may also be denied to refugees as part of a strategy to punish them for actual or perceived misdeeds. Refugees from Sudan and Somalia, living in Kakuma camp in Kenya, were denied food for several weeks in both 1994 and 1996 as part of a strategy of collective punishment.[841] Similarly, following a dispute with Burmese refugees over the death of the driver of a logging truck, the Thai government cut all food deliveries to more than 10,000 Mon refugees.[842]

Even where there are few if any surplus resources available to meet the needs of refugees, many host countries have struggled to treat refugees fairly. In 1984, for example, acute food shortages forced Nicaragua to introduce a national rationing system for its own citizens. Each household was allowed to buy only a fixed quantity of sugar, cooking oil, rice, laundry soap, beans, and salt, at prices fixed by the government.[843] When 20,000 largely destitute Salvadoran refugees arrived to seek protection in Nicaragua, they were assimilated to nationals for purposes of participation in the rationing scheme.

On the other hand, some governments, also facing desperate circumstances, have reacted less generously. During the late 1980s, extreme drought and widespread fighting between government forces and Tigrayan and Eritrean insurgents meant that Ethiopia was unable to feed its own population. Yet it was home to some 200,000 mostly Somali and Sudanese refugees in 1987, with the refugee population rising to 740,000 by 1989. There was a critical shortfall in donor aid, with the result that the refugees' cereal rations had to be reduced from 500 grams to 375 grams per day.[844] But the situation was made much worse when international agencies, attempting to feed both

---

[840] African Rights, *The Nightmare Continues: Abuses Against Somali Refugees in Kenya* (1993) (African Rights, *Nightmare*), at 6. Human Rights Watch noted that in May 2003, "police conducted raids against 'foreigners,' arresting approximately 800 individuals who were held for several days in dismal conditions in an outdoor pen next to the Kasarani police station. At least 145 of the detainees were documented refugees who were charged with failing to register with the government – a statutory provision that was enforced for the first time, and with which no refugee could comply since government registration stopped in 1991": Human Rights Watch, *World Report 2003* (2003), at 43.

[841] Verdirame, "Kenya," at 64–66. Earlier reports suggest that because of antipathy towards ethnic Somalis, the Kenyan government initially would not allow Somali refugees to receive a general ration: African Rights, *Nightmare* at 6.

[842] Asia Watch, "Abuses Against Burmese Refugees in Thailand" (1992), at 3–4.

[843] J. Collins et al., *Nicaragua: What Difference Could a Revolution Make?* (1985) (Collins et al., *Nicaragua*), at 228–229.

[844] "Feeding the Hungry," (1996) 105 *Refugees* 16. International relief programs have generally been plagued by budget reductions since the early 1980s, even as the size of the world refugee population was increasing. "A smaller pie divided into an ever larger number of pieces has meant that, on average, each refugee receives fewer resources": Keen, *Right to Life*, at 36–37.

the domestic and refugee populations, were prohibited by the Ethiopian government from delivering food aid to areas under rebel control.[845]

> **Refugee Convention, Art. 20   Rationing**
> Where a rationing system exists, which applies to the population at large and regulates the general distribution of products in short supply, refugees shall be accorded the same treatment as nationals.
>
> **Civil and Political Covenant, Art. 6(1)**
> Every human being has the inherent right to life. This right shall be protected by law. No one shall be arbitrarily deprived of his life.
>
> **Civil and Political Covenant, Art. 7**
> No one shall be subjected to torture or to cruel, inhuman or degrading treatment or punishment . . .
>
> **Civil and Political Covenant, Art. 9(1)**
> Everyone has the right to liberty and security of person . . .
>
> **Civil and Political Covenant, Art. 10(1)**
> All persons deprived of their liberty shall be treated with humanity and with respect for the inherent dignity of the human person.

In some cases, depriving refugees of the necessities of life may give rise to a breach of the duty of *non-refoulement*. Repatriation under coercion, including situations in which refugees are left with no real option but to leave, is in breach of Art. 33 of the Refugee Convention.[846] As such, Swaziland's decision to deny refugees any means of support, then to arrest and remove them when they protested their situation, was in substance an act of *refoulement*. Even when repatriation does not in fact result, core norms of the Civil and Political Covenant already examined may be contravened by such deprivations.[847] Because the right to life set by Art. 6(1) of the Civil and Political Covenant "is the supreme right . . . [and] should not be interpreted narrowly,"[848] it

---

[845] US Committee for Refugees, *World Refugee Survey 1991* (1991), at 41. Some food aid nonetheless managed to reach rebel-held areas when donor governments re-routed their assistance to NGOs, which organized a cross-border operation to reach starving persons in Eritrea and Tigray, coordinated by Norwegian Church Aid and the Relief Society of Tigray: D. Turton, personal communication to the author, Aug. 25, 1999.

[846] See chapter 4.1.2 above, at pp. 318–319.

[847] The implications of Arts. 6 (life), 7 (torture, cruel, inhuman, degrading treatment or punishment), 9 (physical security), and 10 (rights of detainees) of the Civil and Political Covenant are discussed in detail in chapter 4.3 above, at p. 450 ff.

[848] UN Human Rights Committee, "General Comment No. 6: Right to life" (1982), UN Doc. HRI/GEN/1/Rev.7, May 12, 2004, at 128, para. 1.

prohibits threats to human life brought about not just by intentional killing, but also by planned or foreseeable malnutrition and life-threatening illness.[849] Thus, when the Thai and Kenyan governments expressly cut off all food deliveries to refugees held in their camps as a form of punishment, they contravened the duty in Art. 6(1) to protect the right to life, as well as Art. 10(1)'s duty to treat all detained persons with humanity and respect.[850] As previously described, Art. 6(1) is not simply a prohibition of negative conduct, but requires states to ensure a minimal standard of positive action to protect the right to life.[851] While governments enjoy broad discretion to decide how to implement Art. 6(1), they fail to meet their obligation if whatever measures taken are manifestly insufficient relative to known risks to life.[852]

Where the known risk is less clearly linked to immediate survival, actions to deprive refugees of the necessities of life may still violate the duty to respect physical security under Art. 9 of the Civil and Political Covenant.[853] For example, the determined effort of Pakistan to create near-complete misery in Afghan refugee camps by refusing foreign aid, as well as Hong Kong's denial of even basic medical care to asylum-seekers, should be seen as breaches of Art. 9. More generally, Art. 9's guarantee of security of person requires governments to take reasonable and appropriate measures to respond to known threats to basic personal well-being. A situation in which food rations provided to refugees are known to be so qualitatively deficient in terms of providing essential vitamins and nutrients that life-threatening illness is the predictable result would therefore also logically run afoul of the duty to ensure the physical security of refugees.

Denial to refugees of the necessities of life may moreover contravene Art. 7's prohibition of cruel, inhuman, or degrading treatment or punishment.[854] For example, the Human Rights Committee determined that imprisonment in a tiny space of virtually the exact size allocated to each Vietnamese refugee in Malaysian longhouses was a form of inhuman treatment.[855] Even less egregious denials of adequate accommodation may violate the Civil and Political Covenant. Because of the special duty of care owed to detainees under Art. 10(1), the extraordinarily unhygienic conditions to which Iraqi Kurds were subjected in Turkish camps would likely be seen as a form of

---

[849] Nowak, *ICCPR Commentary*, at 107.

[850] See discussion of Art. 10(1) in chapter 4.2.4 above, at pp. 435–439.

[851] See chapter 4.3.1 above, at pp. 451–452.   [852] Nowak, *ICCPR Commentary*, at 106.

[853] See chapter 4.3.3 above, at p. 458.

[854] See generally chapter 4.3.2 above, at pp. 454–457.

[855] Exacerbating factors in the cases considered by the Human Rights Committee included the absence of light and *incommunicado* detention: *Marais v. Madagascar*, UNHRC Comm. No. 49/1979, decided Mar. 24, 1983; *Wight v. Madagascar*, UNHRC Comm. No. 115/1982, decided Apr. 1, 1985.

inhuman treatment.[856] And because Art. 7 also prohibits degrading treatment, it is contravened by conduct outside the context of enforced detention which shows a fundamental disregard for the refugee as a person.[857] For example, where food is withheld from refugees in order to extort sexual favors, officials demonstrate the willingness to demean and objectify their victim that is the essence of degrading treatment. As Eide has observed,

> The essential point is that everyone should be able, without shame and without unreasonable obstacles, to be a full participant in ordinary, every-day interaction with other people. This means, *inter alia*, that they should be able to enjoy their basic needs under conditions of dignity. No one shall have to live under conditions whereby the only way to satisfy their needs is by degrading or depriving themselves of their basic freedoms, such as through begging, prostitution or bonded labour.[858]

The drafters of the Refugee Convention, however, paid surprisingly little attention to the importance of meeting the basic needs of refugees who arrive to seek protection. While they gave detailed attention to a variety of relatively sophisticated socioeconomic rights (for example, access to social security, fair treatment under tax laws, and even the protection of refugees' intellectual property), the Convention does not address rights to food, water, or health-care, and only regulates access to public housing for refugees once they are lawfully staying in a given country.

A variety of explanations may be offered. Most of the European states that drafted the Convention were accustomed to receiving refugees under orderly entry arrangements. Such refugees, who were immediately authorized to enter either permanently or for an extended stay, would automatically enjoy the right to engage in wage-earning or professional work. As refugees were almost always fellow Europeans, they normally possessed compatible skills, and could therefore be expected to meet basic needs from their own income. Even when refugees arrived without pre-authorization, governments in the 1940s and 1950s were still able to process these irregular entrants fairly quickly. The refugees' own assets could therefore usually see them through until their claims were recognized and work authorization granted.

More generally, the Refugee Convention predates the advent of the Western social welfare state. So long as refugees could earn their own living

---

[856] For example, in *Párkányi v. Hungary*, UNHRC Comm. No. 410/1990, UN Doc. CCPR/C/41/D/410/1990, decided Mar. 22, 1991, the allocation of only five minutes' time each day to meet personal hygiene needs (and an equally short time for outdoor exercise) was ruled a violation of Art. 10.

[857] See chapter 4.3.2 above, at pp. 456–457.

[858] A. Eide, "The Right to an Adequate Standard of Living, Including the Right to Food," in A. Eide et al. eds., *Economic, Social and Cultural Rights: A Textbook* 89 (1995) (Eide, "Standard of Living"), at 89–90.

and benefit from basic property rights, they enjoyed essentially as much protection as did most nationals. And in any event, it was assumed that UNHCR would take the lead on such issues given its institutional responsibility to administer public and private funds for material assistance to refugees.[859]

The one relevant concern addressed, however, was access by refugees to essential goods not distributed on the open market.[860] Because so many key goods had been rationed during the just-concluded Second World War, the drafters were concerned to ensure that all refugees, whether arriving with or without authorization,[861] and whether present only temporarily or indefinitely,[862] be included in any state-managed distribution systems that might be set up by asylum countries. While far from a guarantee that even basic necessities will in fact be provided to refugees, Art. 20 of the Convention ensures that refugees are assimilated to citizens for purposes of receiving allocations under rationing systems. If the rationing system provides that citizens receive vital goods free of charge, then so too must similarly situated refugees. But if the rationing system merely allocates quantities of goods that may be purchased, then the only right of refugees is to purchase goods through that allocation scheme.

There was discussion in the Ad Hoc Committee regarding the type of rationing systems in which refugees should have a right to participate. The Secretary-General's draft spoke only of systems to distribute items "of prime necessity."[863] There was agreement among the drafters that any system for the rationing of accommodation would be exempt from Art. 20, since housing is separately addressed by Art. 21 of the Convention.[864] It was also agreed

---

[859] Statute of the Office of the United Nations High Commissioner for Refugees, UNGA Res. 428(V), adopted Dec. 14, 1950, at para. 10. The United Nations had agreed to establish UNHCR in December 1949: UNGA Res. 319(IV).

[860] Robinson suggests that the value of Art. 20 is really quite modest. "It is rather unusual to treat aliens in the matter of rationing differently than nationals. Thus, the Convention only sanctions the general usage but, at the same time, strives to prevent a less favorable trend in any Contracting State": Robinson, *History*, at 119.

[861] In a critical exchange, the American representative observed "that some of the articles did not specifically indicate to which refugees they applied. He presumed that the mention of 'refugees' without any qualifying phrase was intended to include all refugees, whether lawfully or unlawfully in a territory": Statement of Mr. Henkin of the United States, UN Doc. E/AC.32/SR.41, Aug. 23, 1950, at 18. The immediate and unchallenged response of the Chairman was "that the United States representative's presumption was correct": Statement of the Chairman, Mr. Larsen of Denmark, ibid.

[862] "If a national were passing through a town for a day and received a day's rations, so would a refugee": Statement of Sir Leslie Brass of the United Kingdom, ibid. at 19.

[863] Secretary-General, "Memorandum," at 38 (draft Art. 18).

[864] While the American representative voiced concern that the housing needs of refugees be addressed (Statement of Mr. Henkin of the United States, UN Doc. E/AC.32/SR.15, Jan. 27, 1950, at 4), the notion that housing allocation schemes should be deemed "rationing

that refugees were only to have equal access to systems for the rationing of consumer goods, not products of all kinds. An American proposal that Art. 20 should apply to all "commodities in short supply"[865] was criticized by the French representative as "too far-reaching. Governments might be encouraged to ration commodities in short supply, such as common or precious metals, because they were of particular use to the country. The text of the article should make it clear that it concerned essential goods for individual use."[866] The Ad Hoc Committee's recommendation therefore referred to the rationing of "products" (rather than commodities).[867]

Suggestions were made to circumscribe the scope of Art. 20 further by limiting its scope to rationing systems for "foodstuffs" and related items,[868] or to exclude gasoline rationing systems.[869] But the comments forwarded to the Conference of Plenipotentiaries endorsed neither of these proposed limitations.[870] In order to bring the text of Art. 20 into alignment with the explanatory comments,[871] the Conference determined that refugees would be entitled to benefit as equals from rationing systems established for all "products in short supply."[872] The absence of any qualification suggests that refugees are entitled fully to participate in any system for the rationing of any consumer good.[873]

Nicaragua's decision fully to enfranchise refugees for purposes of access to its national rationing program is therefore a stellar example of compliance with Art. 20. Even though Nicaragua experienced extraordinary difficulty in

---

systems" was successfully opposed by the French representative (Statement of Mr. Rain of France, ibid. at 3). The Chairman concluded from the debate "that provisions regarding housing should not be included in the article on rationing; it would be better to state these in a separate article": Statement of the Chairman, Mr. Chance of Canada, ibid. at 4.

[865] Statement of Mr. Henkin of the United States, ibid. at 5.

[866] Statement of Mr. Rain of France, ibid. at 5.

[867] "This article applies to the generally recognized systems of rationing, which apply to the population at large and regulate the general distribution of products in short supply": "Comments of the Committee on the Draft Convention relating to the Status of Refugees," Annex II to Ad Hoc Committee, "First Session Report," at 4.

[868] Statement of Mr. Cuvelier of Belgium, UN Doc. E/AC.32/SR.15, Jan. 27, 1950, at 5.

[869] Statement of Sir Leslie Brass of the United Kingdom, ibid.

[870] But see Weis, *Travaux*, at 160: "It follows from the debate that it refers to consumer goods in short supply, not to commodities for commercial or industrial use. Petrol was also mentioned as not being included."

[871] Statement of Mr. Robinson of Israel, UN Doc. E/AC.32/SR.37, Aug. 16, 1950, at 21.

[872] This language was drafted by the Style Committee (UN Doc. A/CONF.2/102, July 24, 1951, at 11), and adopted by the Conference without discussion: UN Doc. A/CONF.2/SR.35, July 25, 1951, at 5.

[873] The French representative observed that "[I]n practice, rationing did apply principally to foodstuffs; that, however, was a question of usage which could not affect the etymological meaning of the word 'rationing.' He pointed out that, during the Second World War, products other than foodstuffs – textiles, soap, petrol and so forth – had been rationed in France": Statement of Mr. Rain of France, UN Doc. E/AC.32/SR.15, Jan. 27, 1950, at 3.

meeting the basic needs of its own population (due to a combination of absolute shortages, production and transportation difficulties, and the American government's policy of economic destabilization),[874] refugee households were given access to its rationing system on terms of equality with nationals. On the other hand, Kenya's racially motivated unwillingness to register Somali refugees, thereby denying them access to food rations, was clearly in breach of Art. 20's duty to equal access to rationing systems.[875]

One concern expressed was that Art. 20 might inadvertently require the abolition of preferential rationing systems for refugees. As the Chinese representative explained, his government had treated refugees and Chinese citizens differently under rationing systems in force during the Second World War. China had provided the Jewish and other European refugees with food rations more appropriate to their own dietary requirements and preferences. These refugees received more flour and sugar than did Chinese citizens, while the Chinese received more rice than the refugees.[876] The Chairman replied that the original language of Art. 20, requiring that refugees be dealt with under rationing systems "on the same footing as nationals,"[877] meant only that refugees "would not be treated less favorably than nationals."[878] Without any discussion, however, the Conference of Plenipotentiaries opted to delete the reference to treatment "on the same footing" as nationals in favor of a recommendation from its Style Committee that refugees receive "the same treatment" as nationals under rationing systems.[879]

It is possible that the drafters intended to insist on formal equality of rations between refugees and nationals to avert the possibility of abuse under the guise of recognition of cultural or other differences. The more likely scenario, however, is that the phrase "on the same footing as nationals" was simply viewed as out of keeping with the ways in which standards of treatment are defined elsewhere in the Convention.[880] In view of the general international legal preference to define equality as meaning substantive

---

[874] Collins et al., *Nicaragua*, at 218–219.

[875] The discriminatory refusal of Kenyan authorities to register desperate Somali refugees, knowing that they would in the result be denied access to food and other essentials, was also likely in breach of the right to life: see text above, at pp. 464–465.

[876] Statement of Mr. Cha of China, UN Doc. E/AC.32/SR.15, Jan. 27, 1950, at 3. See also Statement of Mr. Cha of China, UN Doc. E/AC.32/SR.41, Aug. 23, 1950, at 19: "He hoped that the use of the words adopted would not mean that Governments would not give rations to refugees in accordance with their needs, even if such rations were larger than those given to nationals."

[877] Secretary-General, "Memorandum," at 38.

[878] Statement of the Chairman, Mr. Chance of Canada, UN Doc. E/AC.32/SR.15, Jan. 27, 1950, at 3.

[879] UN Doc. A/CONF.2/SR.35, July 25, 1951, at 5.

[880] Even the American representative to the Ad Hoc Committee, who had championed the logic of the phrase "on the same footing as nationals," conceded that "[h]e had no

equality,[881] Art. 20 should therefore be understood to authorize some measure of operational flexibility to ensure that refugees are in fact dealt with no less favorably than nationals.

While Art. 20 governs access only to a rationing system "which applies to the population at large," this does not exclude comparably situated refugees from accessing domestic rationing systems set up for particular sub-populations. The intention of the drafters was that refugee status (or non-citizenship) not be a basis for withholding rations from refugees. Thus, the American representative noted that Art. 20 applies to systems under which "different rations [are established] for different categories of people, for example, for children."[882] A rationing system that provides goods only for children is a system which applies to a designated part of "the population at large," in consequence of which refugee children should receive the same rations as citizen children. But if the rationing program is designed only to benefit children, adult refugees have no claim to entitlement under it.[883]

Art. 20 of the Refugee Convention governs only access to rationing systems, that is, schemes established to distribute goods *because* those goods are in short supply. It is therefore not a basis for refugees to assert a right of access to public welfare or comparable systems which allocate basic necessities (or the funds to acquire them) on the basis of economic need, rather than because of the scarcity of the products themselves.[884] Most fundamentally, Art. 20 does not require the establishment of any kind of rationing system for refugees, no matter how extreme their needs. The only obligation is to ensure that refugees benefit on terms of equality with nationals under any rationing system that is established. If neither refugees nor citizens are provided with access to a rationing system – as was the case for those in rebel-held areas of Ethiopia, to which the government denied aid agencies access – then Art. 20 of the Refugee Convention is not breached.[885] The more broadly applicable duty to provide refugees with the basic necessities of life must therefore be

---

particular brief for the use of such a wording": Statement of Mr. Henkin of the United States, UN Doc. E/AC.32/SR.41, Aug. 23, 1950, at 19. See generally chapter 3.3.2 above.

[881] See chapter 2.5.5 above, at pp. 126–128.

[882] Statement of Mr. Henkin of the United States, UN Doc. E/AC.32/SR.41, Aug. 23, 1950, at 19.

[883] Robinson reaches the same result, but on the basis of a different analysis. He suggests that "Art. 20 is not applicable to allocation of certain items in favor of restricted groups or to products which are generally available in sufficient quantities but are allocated to certain groups, for instance, indigent persons, large families, at or on more favorable prices or conditions. In such circumstances, Art. 7(1) would apply": Robinson, *History*, at 119–120. This result is, in any event, compelled by the duty of non-discrimination under Art. 26 of the Civil and Political Covenant: see chapter 2.5.5 above, at pp. 126–128.

[884] The right of refugees to access public welfare systems is discussed at chapter 6.3 below.

[885] The denial of aid to these areas likely violated Art. 11 of the Economic Covenant, however. See chapter 4.4.2 below, at pp. 489–490.

established under general norms of international human rights law, rather than by reliance on any specific requirement of the Refugee Convention itself.[886]

4.4.2 Access to food and shelter

Even where there is a willingness to help refugees meet their most basic needs, it is often impossible for local economies already faced with shortages of land and jobs simply to absorb all refugees who arrive. The problem is most critical in poorer countries of the South, where there tend to be larger refugee movements and fewer indigenous resources to provide for refugees.[887] India is one of the few less developed countries that has traditionally been unwilling to accept external support for its refugee relief operations.[888] In most poorer countries, the survival of refugees has depended on international agencies providing a substantial supplement to local efforts.[889] In one particularly extreme case, the Ethiopian government was critically dependent on international aid to provide for nearly all the needs of both its large refugee population and its own nationals, during the famine of the late 1980s and early 1990s.[890] Similarly, the general impact of the drought in Zambia during 2002 meant that both refugees and their hosts were at risk of starvation.[891] As UNHCR has acknowledged,

---

[886] See chapters 4.4.2 and 4.4.3 below.

[887] As Castles has observed, in order to assess "the weight of the 'refugee burden,' [it is most] instructive ... to relate refugee populations to the wealth of the receiving country ... Refugees are overwhelmingly concentrated in the poorest countries. This puts the frequent Northern claims of being unfairly burdened by refugees in perspective": S. Castles, "The International Politics of Forced Migration," in L. Panitch and C. Leys eds., *Fighting Identities: Race, Religion, and Ethno-Nationalism* 172 (2002), at 174.

[888] B. S. Chimni, *International Academy of Comparative Law National Report for India* (1994), at 37–39.

[889] "Almost half of the world's refugees are totally dependent on international assistance for the basic needs of food, shelter, water, and health care": Forbes Martin, *Refugee Women*, at 33.

[890] Ethiopia hosted more than 700,000 refugees in the late 1980s, even as the drought created critical shortages for millions of its own nationals in northern regions: US Committee for Refugees, *World Refugee Survey 1989* (1989), at 37–38.

[891] "Food insecurity in the region will have a tremendous effect on refugee supplies, UNHCR representative Ahmed Gubartalla has said ... Gubartalla said the drought situation in the region will not spare the refugees ... 'Since October last year we have been giving half rations to the refugees and with the food situation in Zambia, rations in our camps will be complicated ... If nationals are suffering due to the drought, by extension the refugees are affected too'": "Food insecurity will affect refugee supplies, says UNHCR," *Zamnet*, June 14, 2002. In this case, Denmark responded by funding an innovative program under which critical support was provided to both refugees and the communities that received

The heavy price that major refugee hosting countries, which are among the least developed, have to pay in granting asylum is now widely recognized. Yet, the rhetoric on international solidarity and burden-sharing rarely translates into tangible support to refugee-affected areas. The international response has been uneven and often driven by political and economic considerations on the part of many donors.[892]

Because international refugee relief efforts are funded by voluntary state contributions, there is no guarantee that aid will be adequate to meet needs. For example, the funding shortfall for the 20,000 Angolan refugees in the Osire refugee camp in Namibia during 2001 resulted in severe food reductions:

> The funds available are only enough to buy 30% of the food needed . . . Food rations have already been reduced to 80% of the recommended basic monthly diet of 2,100 (17 kg) kilocalories. Due to the cut in rations, refugees now get only 8–10 kg of maize, their staple food.[893]

Beyond inadequate food, the camp was home to more than ten times the number of refugees for which it had been constructed, resulting in shortages of all kinds:

> [T]he refugee camp . . . urgently needs at least 500 more family pit latrines because existing facilities have clogged up. And although . . . there are adequate water points at present . . . the rate at which refugees are arriving in the country makes it impossible to guarantee a steady supply [of water] . . . Apart from the scarcity of tents and kerosene for cooking food, the clinic at Osire has been strenuously overstretched and more medical equipment and drugs are needed to combat possible disease outbreaks.[894]

True disaster was thankfully averted at Osire because of a last-minute response from the Swedish and American governments.[895] But similarly perilous conditions remain common. For example, UNHCR was forced to

them. "The Danish government has given UNHCR $2.6 million for refugees and their host communities in Zambia's Western Province . . . The projects formed part of the Zambia Initiative, which aims to uplift communities hosting refugees from neighboring countries living in Zambia, after it was found that many of the host communities themselves were extremely poor and battling to cope with the increased demands. Zambia is home to more than 270,000 refugees, some 225,000 of which are Angolans": "Danish government aids refugee communities," *UN Integrated Regional Information Networks*, Nov. 1, 2002.

[892] UNHCR Executive Committee, "Social and Economic Impact of Massive Refugee Populations on Host Developing Countries, as well as Other Countries: Addressing the Gaps," UN Doc. EC/49/SC/CRP.24, Sept. 3, 1999, at para. 2.

[893] *Namibian*, May 2, 2001.   [894] Ibid., Dec. 1, 2000.

[895] Ibid., May 17, 2001; US Committee for Refugees, *World Refugee Survey 2002* (2002), at 87.

put refugees in Zambia on half-rations in 2002 because of an insufficiency of aid donations.[896] In the same year, UNHCR cited financial constraints as the reason for discontinuing food and related assistance to refugees from Haiti in the Dominican Republic.[897] Funding shortfalls resulted in refugees in Kenyan camps receiving less than the World Health Organization's minimum caloric intake during most of 2002 and 2003.[898] The World Food Program was forced in 2003 to reduce food rations to refugees in Tanzania by 50 percent on top of an earlier reduction of 28 percent, leading the host government to threaten the repatriation of all refugees living in the country if the international community failed to take immediate action to stave off a violent reaction by the refugees.[899]

Shortfalls in relief funding may be the result of the political or other priorities of donor countries. For example, once a peace process was under-way in Burundi, UNHCR's budget to operate refugee camps for Burundians in Tanzania was cut by 55 percent.[900] UNHCR was unable to persuade donors to make funds available to meet even basic needs in the camps of Tanzania's Kibondo district, which continued to receive more than 100 Burundian refugees each day.[901] As the local UNICEF chief observed, "[w]hen things fizzle out in terms of CNN coverage, the funding starts to disappear."[902] Indeed, even as a massive refugee effort was underway to assist refugees in flight from Kosovo, UNHCR reported that donations to existing operations

---

[896] "Refugees on half-ration as food stocks drop," *UN Integrated Regional Information Networks*, Jan. 18, 2002.

[897] (2003) 125 *JRS Dispatches* (Jan. 27, 2003).

[898] P. Browne, "Where refugee camps are becoming a way of life," *Guardian*, June 12, 2003, at 25.

[899] "Lack of funding to feed the 500,000 refugees in Tanzania's refugee camps is leading to a 'dire' situation ... [UNHCR and WFP] have described the situation as the 'worst ever,' and said it had led to repeated calls for donor action. Furthermore, the Tanzanian authorities have reacted by warning that they might expel the refugees if the situation were to get out of hand ... 'We have said that we would not be prepared to be put into such a situation, and the alarm has been sounded. Should things deteriorate to this extent, we may have to consider the possibility of repatriating the refugees forcefully,' [the Minister of Home Affairs, Omar Ramadhani Mapuri] said": "Food situation in refugee camp 'dire,'" *UN Integrated Regional Information Networks*, Feb. 19, 2003.

[900] "The Burundi peace talks in Tanzania last year, brokered by Nelson Mandela and visited by Bill Clinton, have done the refugees more harm than good. Most of the Hutu rebel groups were excluded and the initiative has come to nothing. But it was enough to send many donors elsewhere": J. Astill, "UN refugee work in crisis as world ignores Burundi," *Guardian*, Feb. 14, 2001, at 18.

[901] "Several operations in the refugee camps ... have been severely curtailed or suspended altogether as a result of UNHCR's funding problems ... Fuel has been cut by 50%, soap distribution to refugees has been suspended, and all construction and training programs have been cancelled": (2001) 85 *JRS Dispatches* (Jan. 17, 2001).

[902] Ibid., quoting Mr. Bjorn Lungqvist of UNICEF.

had "stagnated," meaning, for example, that funds were not available even to provide Somali refugees in Kenya with firewood for cooking.[903] A reporter wrote,

> Far from safe havens, the camps [in Kenya] are so dangerous that aid workers venture into them only with armed escorts. And if the plight of ethnic Albanians has reintroduced the word "refugee" to discourse around the world, no overflow of compassion has reached the dusty Somali settlements here.[904]

The impact of such donor selectivity often falls squarely on impoverished host communities. For example, when inadequate funding led to a cut of food rations to refugees in the Kala camp of northern Zambia, riots broke out, and refugees invaded nearby villages to steal crops belonging to the local community.[905]

Even when adequate resources are in principle provided to meet refugee needs, refugees may nonetheless face food and other shortages because agencies encounter logistical barriers to the delivery of aid, for example when refugee camps are situated in remote regions. Half of the 900 km road to refugee camps in Guinea was unpaved, making it "impassable at times in the rainy season."[906] Food deliveries to the indigenous Nicaraguan refugees living in Honduras had to be suspended during the rainy season, as their settlements could only be reached by canoe.[907] It may also be impossible to reach refugees located in areas surrounded by hostile forces. For example, rebel Mozambican forces blocked the main transportation corridor used to reach refugees in Malawi in 1990.[908]

Occasionally, malnutrition stems from the rigid application by host states of general rules. While shortfalls in international assistance accounted for

---

[903] "'I cannot tell you for a fact that the contributions to Kosovo have affected the contributions to the rest,' said Michel Gabaudon, chief fund-raiser for the UN High Commissioner for Refugees ... But donations to existing operations have 'stagnated' since the outpouring for the Balkans, Gabaudon reported, and 'I have had donors say, "Where can you make cuts?"' 'If funds are cut,' he added, 'your bottom line is water and food'": K. Vick, "For Somali refugees, no safe haven," *Washington Post*, June 3, 1999, at A19.

[904] Ibid. The cuts were particularly tragic because the firewood program had obviated the need for women to scavenge for firewood in the bush, where they had been subjected to rape at a rate seventy-five times higher than would be expected in a community of that size: ibid.

[905] *SAPA-AFP*, April 15, 2001. The regional director for UNHCR characterized the situation in Zambia as a "time bomb": ibid.

[906] US, "Living Conditions," at 28.

[907] US Government Accounting Office, "Central America: Conditions of Refugees and Displaced Persons," Doc. No. UNGAO/NSIAD-89-54 (1989) (US, "Central America"), at 22.

[908] US, "Living Conditions," at 35.

much suffering at the Osire refugee camp in Namibia, the problems there were compounded by the host state's initial refusal to waive its long-standing ban on importing the refugees' staple food, maize meal.[909] Similarly, and despite the critical need for food supplies in 2002, the Zambian government initially refused to allow the World Food Program to feed more than 130,000 refugees in that country with genetically modified food provided by donors.[910] In other circumstances, food shortages result from the failure of camp or other administrators to make provision for foreseeable needs.[911] In particular, even when food reaches refugees, malnutrition may result from inadequate distribution systems. In Ethiopia, for example, the diversion of food to both Sudanese and Somali rebel movements was considered widespread.[912] Budget cuts had reduced the number of UNHCR staff assigned to monitor food distribution, in consequence of which "there was no assurance that needy refugees actually received their food allotments."[913]

In some camps where food supplies are limited, women and children are inadequately fed because cultural norms dictate that they should not eat until men have had all they wish to eat.[914] Even more egregiously, some Bhutanese

---

[909] *Namibian*, May 2, 2001. Because local maize prices were nearly double those of maize on the international market, the WFP objected to the requirement. Yet again in 2003, "[a] request to the Namibian Agronomic Board to be excused from the import restrictions has been refused. The WFP has now requested the intervention of the Home Affairs Ministry to plead for this decision to be reconsidered": "Food shortage looms for Osire refugees," *Namibian*, July 18, 2003. "The government imposed the ban to encourage the buying of maize from local farmers during the harvest period": *Namibian Economist*, Aug. 1, 2003.

[910] "Scramble for non-genetically modified food for refugees," *UN Integrated Regional Information Networks*, Jan. 12, 2002. A change of policy resulted in the food supplies being admitted later in the year: *Post* (Lusaka), Sept. 9, 2002.

[911] "Pressing food shortages are looming at Kakuma camp in Northern Kenya ... The medical coordinator claims that many children will die if food is not rushed to the camp. It seems that the authorities have known about the looming shortage for a long time but they took no measures to prevent it": (2000) 76 *JRS Dispatches* (Aug. 31, 2000).

[912] "Looting and diversion of food continued to be a problem in several SPLA zones. Action Against Hunger, a French non-governmental agency, claimed that it was expelled by the SPLA because it was about to investigate why a high rate of malnutrition existed in Labone despite adequate supplies of relief food for the civilian population. It was suspected that the SPLA deliberately kept some children in a thin and sickly state to justify continued high levels of relief food the SPLA could divert": Human Rights Watch, *World Report 1998* (1998), at 76.

[913] US, "Living Conditions," at 11.

[914] Forbes Martin, *Refugee Women*, at 35. See also G. Camus-Jacques, "Refugee Women: The Forgotten Majority," in G. Loescher and L. Monahan eds., *Refugees and International Relations* (1990) (Camus-Jacques, "Forgotten Majority"), at 148: "This [type of discriminatory practice] vividly demonstrates how refugee policies for the administration of material assistance are insufficient when such biased practices against women are allowed to develop and persist." See also UNHCR, "Note on Refugee Women and International Protection," UN Doc. EC/SCP/59, Aug. 28, 1990, at para. 30.

refugee women in Nepal have been unable to secure access to food and other aid because Nepal's system of registration required all rations to be distributed through male heads of household. In the result, women in abusive relationships "must stay in violent relationships, leave their relationships (and thus relinquish their full share of aid packages), or marry another man, in which case they lose legal custody of their children."[915]

For all these reasons, inadequate access to food is the leading cause of death among refugees.[916] As UNHCR has observed,

> Malnutrition is both a primary and secondary cause of death. There is a direct causal relationship between malnutrition and mortality in refugee sites, and this is most pronounced among children under five years of age.[917]

Sadly, the death rate for Somalis fleeing civil war actually peaked a year after reaching the "safety" of the Hartisheik camp in Ethiopia. Because of inadequate food, 46 of every 1,000 adults died, with the death rate for children reaching a staggering 150 per 1,000.[918] Refugees from the Democratic Republic of Congo arriving in Zimbabwe during the latter months of 2000 were so desperate to eat that they were selling their blankets to buy food.[919] In some circumstances, refugees will be forced to steal in order to meet their needs.[920] Afghan refugees in Pakistan were "faced with a no-win situation ... They can either move to the camps nearer the border with Afghanistan, where their security cannot be guaranteed, or they can stay in Peshawar, where their food supply and winter shelter cannot be guaranteed."[921] Conditions may even be so bad that refugees return home to face the risk of being persecuted, rather than starving in an asylum country. Starvation-induced repatriation was documented, for example, in the cases of Sudanese refugees struggling to survive in the Adjumani district of Uganda,[922] and Burundian refugees confronted with the misery of life in the Tanzanian Karago camp.[923]

Even where inadequate food rations do not lead directly to death or forced return, they may cause serious illness. Rations for some Iraqi Kurds in Turkey

---

[915] Human Rights Watch, "Nepal/Bhutan: Refugee Women Face Abuses," Sept. 24, 2003.

[916] Forbes Martin, *Refugee Women*, at 33.

[917] UNHCR Executive Committee, "Refugee Health," UN Doc. EC/1995/SC.2/CRP.29, Sept. 11, 1995.

[918] Keen, *Right to Life*, at 7–8.   [919] (2000) 80 *JRS Dispatches* (Oct. 16, 2000).

[920] "Commercial farmers involved in game and livestock farming close to the Osire Refugee Camp have accused the refugees of poaching and stock theft. Tension between the farmers and the refugees, numbering over 20,000, has occasionally resulted in some refugees being shot for trespassing": "Tension escalates near Osire Refugee Camp," *Namibian*, Jan. 30, 2002.

[921] Human Rights Watch, "Pakistan: Refugees Not Moving Voluntarily," Dec. 5, 2001.

[922] (2000) 75 *JRS Dispatches* (July 20, 2000).

[923] (2000) 76 *JRS Dispatches* (Aug. 31, 2000); (2000) 84 *JRS Dispatches* (Dec. 18, 2000).

included no milk or milk products, fruit, or vegetables,[924] and refugees from the Democratic Republic of Congo were refused any fish or meat at the Dukwe refugee camp in Botswana.[925] Potentially fatal diseases long eradicated in the North, such as scurvy, xerophthalmia, anemia, and beriberi, have made comebacks in the refugee camps of the South because of acute vitamin deficiencies.[926] For example, a shortage of niacin in food baskets led to an outbreak of pellagra among Mozambican refugees in Malawi.[927] In other situations, the only food provided may be culturally foreign or simply bad. After major food cuts to refugees in the Kigoma and Kagera regions of Tanzania in 2000, it was reported that refugees received little more than "beans which were so hard that no amount of boiling will make [them] . . . palatable."[928] One refugee mother of four children told an NGO worker that her family "eat[s] the same food day after day. It is different to the food we used to eat in Burundi, and it is not enough. But we cannot grow food so we cannot supplement our rations."[929]

Access to clean drinking water is also a frequent concern for refugees.[930] Even though UNHCR guidelines recommend 15–20 liters of water per day for each person, refugees in one camp in western Ethiopia were reported to receive less than 1 liter of water.[931] At the Maheba camp in Zambia, the death rate among Angolan refugees tripled in less than three months because

---

[924] IHRK, "Kurdish Refugees," at 11.

[925] It is reported that the UNHCR regional representative viewed the refugees' request as "unreasonable . . . If we are looking at the kilo-calories content of the food, it is in accordance with international standards": *Namibian*, Feb. 7, 2001, quoting Mangesha Kebede of the UNHCR's Regional Office in Pretoria.

[926] Keen, *Right to Life*, at 17–19; United States, "Outbreak of Beriberi Among Illegal Mainland Chinese Immigrants at a Detention Center in Taiwan," (2003) 118 *Public Health Reports* 59.

[927] US, "Living Conditions," at 41–42. See also Center for Disease Control, "International Notes: Outbreak of Pellagra Among Mozambican Refugees – Malawi, 1990," (1991) 40(13) *Morbidity and Mortality Weekly Report* 209.

[928] (2000) 75 *JRS Dispatches* (July 20, 2000).   [929] Ibid.

[930] Access to clean water may indeed be the single most important means of saving refugee lives: Keen, *Right to Life*, at 21. Keen reports that when clean water was provided to refugees in eastern Sudan, "there was a 1% death rate among those who contracted cholera in refugee camps, whereas in nearby Sudanese villages the proportion reached 20%. Non-governmental organizations realized what was happening and began to give assistance to Sudanese health centres, though this effort was impeded by lack of resources": ibid.

[931] US, "Living Conditions," at 12. The same problem occurred, though to a less drastic extent, at the Lugufu camp in Tanzania, where a water supply designed for a maximum of 40,000 persons was in fact used by more than 55,000 refugees, resulting in access to no more than 13.5 liters of water per day per person: L. Talley et al., "An Investigation of Increasing Mortality Among Congolese Refugees in Lugufu Camp, Tanzania, May–June 1999," (2001) 14(4) *Journal of Refugee Studies* 412, at 423–424.

the camp had only one functioning water borehole, rather than the twenty required for its population.[932] When refugees are not given access to safe water, they may turn in desperation to contaminated sources, a major cause of disease. For example, Iraqi refugees in Iran who were forced to use a polluted stream for drinking, washing, and bathing experienced outbreaks of cholera and typhoid.[933] Milk powder from international donors has had to be mixed with unclean water, causing severe diarrhea and even death among infants and young children.[934] And refugees given responsibility to collect water (typically women) are vulnerable to sleeping sickness, malaria, yellow fever, and river blindness.[935]

Beyond food and water, refugee survival may also depend on access to adequate shelter. Even though shelter is a crucial determinant of refugee health,[936] particularly in extreme climatic conditions, it is frequently treated as the "poor cousin" to other necessities of life. For example, more than 60,000 Kosovar refugees arriving in northern Albania were forced to sleep outside in what UNHCR described as "unsanitary, open-air ... massive sick bays."[937] Citing concerns of "perceived permanency" and cost, governments sometimes insist on the right to negotiate with international agencies about whether or not refugees should be given access to housing.[938] Thus, Iraqi Kurds arriving in Turkey were initially forced to remain in open-air camps, with no shelter of any kind.[939] Some of these refugees were eventually moved into concrete flats, while 16,000 others had to endure two years of harsh

---

[932] (2000) 82 *JRS Dispatches* (Nov. 10, 2000).

[933] M. Elkoury, "Islamic Republic of Iran: A Million Lives in the Balance," (1991) 86 *Refugees* 30, at 30.

[934] Forbes Martin, *Refugee Women*, at 37–38. "The distribution of milk powder in refugee camps constitutes an additional problem in so far as milk powder is not an acceptable substitute for breast-feeding ... When mixed with non-sterile water, milk powder can lead to severe diarrhoea with fatal results": UNHCR, "Note on Refugee Women and International Protection," UN Doc. EC/SCP/59, Aug. 28, 1990, at para. 32.

[935] Forbes Martin, *Refugee Women*, at 38.

[936] J. Rivers and G. Brown, "Physiological Aspects of Shelter Deprivation," in I. Davis ed., *Disasters and the Small Dwelling* (1981).

[937] "The deep, chest-heaving cough can be heard all throughout the night ... [A]s the flow of refugees has slowed, medical personnel have turned their attention from life-threatening trauma to the respiratory and gastrointestinal ailments": UNHCR, *Refugees Daily*, May 6, 1999.

[938] P. Goovaerts, paper prepared for the First International Workshop on Improved Shelter Response and Environment for Refugees, June 1993, at 4–7. See also R. Zetter, "Shelter Provision and Settlement Policies for Refugees: A State of the Art Review," Nordiska Afrikainstitutet Studies on Emergencies and Disaster Relief Paper No. 2 (1995), at 78.

[939] "The men are trying to make small oases of shade out of the foliage and a few blankets in the burning heat, yet these shelters are no help against the ice-cold nights in the high mountains. A sudden storm on the night of August 4 surprised tens of thousands of people who were totally without protection. After this rain, many people, especially

winters and brutal summer heat in uninsulated tents, each holding up to sixteen people.[940] Ethiopian refugees arriving in the Sudan lived for more than a year under tarpaulins because promised UNHCR tents did not materialize. When the registration of incoming Ethiopian refugees was suspended for three months in 1990, not even this shelter was available. New arrivals were forced to build makeshift shelters out of blankets and mats.[941] Sahrawi refugees in Algeria received tents, but they were destroyed in severe sandstorms because they were of the wrong shape and too weakly constructed.[942]

Even when refugees receive housing, overcrowding is a frequent problem. Nicaraguan refugees in Honduran camps squeezed up to ten family members into each of their single-room shelters.[943] Refugee claimants in the Bahamas were reported to be "living in squalor as they awaited the outcome of status determination procedures ... The Carmichael Road facility is so overcrowded that some detainees must sleep on the floors of trailer-like structures."[944] Refugee housing also frequently lacks adequate sanitation. Because Sudanese refugees in Ethiopia had no access to facilities for bathing or dishwashing in camps, they used contaminated rivers and standing pools of water for this purpose.[945] Roma refugees from Kosovo were reportedly left without even access to basic sanitary facilities at the UNHCR-run Skopje Suto Orizare camp in Macedonia.[946] The overcrowding and lack of sanitation at Spanish detention facilities in the Canary Islands were so bad that the volunteer doctors working there suspended their service in protest over the conditions.[947]

In general, the minority of refugees who seek protection in the developed world are much less likely to be denied access to the basic necessities of life. Some countries, including Canada and Norway, have opted to allow refugees

---

children, came down with fever": *Frankfurter Rundschau*, Sept. 12, 1988, cited in IHRK, "Kurdish Refugees," at 5.

[940] "The people are totally exposed to extreme climatic conditions in their tents without any protection: to severe frost in the winter and burning heat in the summer. Moreover, there are neither trees nor bushes in the camp, there is neither shade nor protection from the wind": German *Bundestag* Member Angelika Beer, June 12, 1989, cited in IHRK, "Kurdish Refugees," at 13.

[941] US, "Living Conditions," at 22–24.

[942] T. Corsellis, "The Sahrawi Refugee Camps of Western Algeria," paper presented at the Seminar on Civil Strife and Relief within the Context of the Continuum from Relief to Development, The Hague, July 1994, at 2.

[943] US, "Central America," at 17.

[944] "The Bahamas Struggle to Fulfill Refugee Obligations," (1998) 24 *Forced Migration Monitor* 8, reporting on the results of an Open Society Institute mission to the Bahamas.

[945] US, "Living Conditions," at 14.

[946] (2003) 133 *JRS Dispatches* (May 30, 2003).

[947] Human Rights Watch, "Spain: Migrants' Rights Violated on Canary Islands," Feb. 21, 2002.

subject to status verification to engage in wage-earning employment.[948] In contrast, most European countries either deny asylum-seekers the right to seek employment altogether or do so for a period of time. For example, refugees undergoing status verification may not work at all in Denmark, France, Germany, or Italy.[949] In contrast, Finland allows refugees to work after a three-month waiting period; in Sweden, the waiting period is four months.[950] Since 1998, the Netherlands has allowed a more general right of refugee claimants to work, though the duration of the work permit is a maximum of twelve weeks per annum.[951]

In most cases, refugees allowed to work in industrialized countries can meet basic needs from their own income. This is less likely to be the case, however, in states which impose real bureaucratic obstacles to receipt of a work permit, or where the nature of the authorization issued arouses the suspicion of potential employers. In Argentina, for example, refugee claimants are issued only a "certificate of precarious stay" which is not readily accepted by most businesses.[952] In addition, many refugees face language difficulties, educational differences, certification requirements, cultural barriers, and xenophobic or racist barriers to work.[953] Thus, even in asylum countries that allow refugees to work, refugees may be either channeled into low-paying, insecure jobs, or simply unable to find work at all.

Refugees in the developed world who are either prevented from working or who cannot find work must therefore turn to public or private assistance to meet their basic needs. Many countries in Western Europe have established specialized reception centers to accommodate asylum-seekers which provide residents with not only shelter, but also food or cooking facilities, as well as on-site medical assistance. Some states, including Germany and Switzerland, have traditionally met the needs of refugees only by way of a mandatory stay in a reception center.[954] Belgium has more recently adopted this policy, announcing in October 2000 that it would end the provision of financial assistance to asylum-seekers upon arrival. Food and other assistance would

---

[948] F. Crépeau and M. Barutciski, "The Legal Condition of Refugees in Canada," (1994) 7(2/3) *Journal of Refugee Studies* 239 (Crépeau and Barutciski, "Canada"), at 239–243; Liebaut, *Conditions 2000*, at 233.

[949] Liebaut, *Conditions 2000*, at 55, 96, 116–117, and 172.

[950] Ibid. at 75, 282.   [951] Ibid. at 215.

[952] S. Fraidenraij, *International Academy of Comparative Law National Report for Argentina* (1994), at 9. See generally D. Joly, *Refugees: Asylum in Europe?* (1992) (Joly, *Asylum*), at 59, who argues that uncertainty of status acts as a disincentive to offer employment to refugees.

[953] See e.g. M. Addo, *International Academy of Comparative Law National Report for the United Kingdom* (1994), at 11; J. Vedsted-Hansen, *International Academy of Comparative Law National Report for Denmark* (1994), at 2; Forbes Martin, *Refugee Women*, at 78–88.

[954] Liebaut, *Conditions 2000*, at 115, 297.

be provided only in privately run reception centers pending a decision on admissibility of the claim to refugee status.[955] In other countries, access to reception centers is voluntary, and may even be restricted. Because demand outstrips reception center capacity in France, for example, priority in admission is given to women and families.[956]

Alternatively, refugees awaiting status verification may be granted access to social assistance schemes that provide them with the funds needed to meet their own basic needs. In Canada, persons seeking recognition of their refugee status are assimilated to nationals for the purpose of access to most benefit programs.[957] Refugee claimants in Finland may also access social welfare, but have the usual social benefit amount reduced by 20 percent to account for the value of accommodation provided in reception centers – a reduction which is imposed even on refugees who live outside the centers.[958] The United Kingdom provides asylum applicants with only 70 percent of the income support paid to citizens,[959] and since 2003 has sought to bar refugees from receiving public assistance unless they make their claim to be a refugee forthwith upon arrival in the United Kingdom.[960] This provision has operated to deprive many refugee claimants of income supplements, housing benefits, and disability allowances.[961] Combined with Britain's ban on the employment of persons seeking recognition of refugee status, claimants

---

[955] (2000) 81 *JRS Dispatches* (Oct. 31, 2000).

[956] Personal communication with Antoine Decourcelle of CIMADE, Dec. 4, 2003.

[957] Crépeau and Barutciski, "Canada," at 243.

[958] Personal communication with Reetta Helander, Information Officer, Refugee Advice Center, Helsinki, Sept. 25, 2003.

[959] Refugee claimants receive a number of other in-kind benefits, which one commentator estimates bring their overall welfare benefit to about 80 percent of that provided to citizens: J. Hardy, "Tough on toys, tough on the causes of toys: How we ensure that asylum-seekers stick to life's bare essentials," *Guardian*, Dec. 20, 2000, at 18.

[960] These changes were brought in by the Social Security (Persons from Abroad) Miscellaneous Amendment Regulations 1996 (Feb. 5, 1996), and were incorporated in the Asylum and Immigration Act on July 24, 1996. They are, in essence, a penalty on account of illegal entry or presence: see chapter 4.2.2 above. This approach appears to have been the model for the European Union's Council Directive laying down minimum standards for the reception of asylum-seekers, Doc. 2003/9/EC (Jan. 27, 2003) (EU Reception Directive), at Art. 16(2), which authorizes states to "refuse reception conditions" where a claim is not made as soon as reasonably practicable after arrival: Immigration Law Practitioners' Association, [June 2004] *European Update* 10.

[961] It was estimated that about 65 percent of refugees do not apply for recognition of refugee status to an immigration officer immediately upon arrival: A. Travis, "Thousands of asylum-seekers face 'destitution,'" *Guardian*, Dec. 27, 2002, at 1. In October 1996, however, the High Court held in *R v. London Borough of Hammersmith*, [1996] EWHC Admin 90 (Eng. HC, Oct. 8, 1996) that local authorities have a duty under the 1948 National Assistance Act to provide basic services to asylum-seekers with no other means of support. The Court found it "impossible to believe that Parliament intended that an asylum-seeker, who was lawfully here and could not lawfully be removed from the

without private means can find themselves in an extraordinarily difficult position,[962] as recent evidence before the English Court of Appeal makes clear:

> Many [asylum-seekers] sleep outside [the Refugee Council] offices, in doorways, in the gardens of a local church and sometimes in telephone boxes (the only place where they are able to keep dry). They do not have enough blankets and clothing to keep them warm. They are often lonely, frightened and feel humiliated and distressed ... Staff have seen the condition of asylum-seekers visibly deteriorating after periods of rough sleeping ... On one occasion I had to tell a group of three homeless asylum-seekers to leave the building on a Friday evening during a torrential downpour with nothing more than a blanket each, a food parcel ... and a list of day centres. When I saw them the following Monday their condition had deteriorated considerably, their clothes were filthy, they had started to smell, and they had been unable to find any of the centres listed. Other clients have become depressed and have threatened suicide; one was sectioned after she was found lying across a railway track. Their story is not exceptional – we see people in this situation on a daily basis.[963]

country, should be left destitute, starving and at risk of grave illness and even death because he could find no one to provide him with the bare necessities of life": ibid. If this was the government's intention, said the Court, "it would almost certainly put itself in breach of the European Convention on Human Rights and of the Geneva Convention": ibid. More recently, the English Court of Appeal has insisted that the application of this policy must not infringe the prohibition of cruel or inhuman treatment under Art. 3 of the European Convention on Human Rights: *R (Q) v. Secretary of State for the Home Department*, [2003] EWCA Civ 364 (Eng. CA, Mar. 18, 2003); *R (S) v. Secretary of State for the Home Department*, [2003] EWCA Civ 1285 (Eng. CA, Sept. 24, 2003); *R (Limbuela) v. Secretary of State for the Home Department*, [2004] EWCA Civ 540 (Eng. CA, May 21, 2004). Shortly after issuance of the latter judgment, the government indicated that it would desist from a rigid application of s. 55 *of the Nationality, Immigration and Asylum Act 2002*, and specifically that it would no longer be applied against persons who apply for refugee status within a few days of arrival in the United Kingdom: www.refugeecouncil.org.uk (accessed June 4, 2004).

[962] Amnesty International United Kingdom, "Slamming the Door: The Demolition of the Right to Asylum in the UK" (1996), at 15; Refugee Council, "Welcome to the UK: The Impact of the Removal of Benefits from Asylum Seekers" (1996); M. Carter, Commission for Racial Equality, and the Refugee Council, "Poverty and Prejudice: A Preliminary Report on the Withdrawal of Benefit Entitlement and Impact of the Asylum and Immigration Bill" (1996). The United Kingdom previously allowed refugees who had not received an adjudication of their claim within six months to secure work authorization at that time; that policy was rescinded in July 2002. At present, permission to work is granted only if and when a positive decision on refugee status is made: British Refugee Council, "Training, Education and Employment," available at www.refugeecouncil.org.uk (accessed Dec. 13, 2003).

[963] *R (Limbuela) v. Secretary of State for the Home Department*, [2004] EWCA Civ 540 (Eng. CA, May 21, 2004), at para. 92, quoting from the evidence of Hugh Tristram of the Refugee Council.

The situation in some other countries is comparably problematic. In Italy, for example, social benefit payments to asylum-seekers end forty-five days after arrival.[964]

Generalized shortages of affordable housing in Western Europe have led to congestion in refugee reception centers.[965] Thus, the Committee on Economic, Social and Cultural Rights had noted its "concern [regarding] the living conditions of asylum-seekers in some reception centres" in the Netherlands.[966] Those refugees not admitted to centers often end up in boarding houses, or sharing dwellings with strangers. The situation for asylum-seekers in countries which provide little or no support is characterized as desperate, with homelessness among refugees a not uncommon phenomenon.[967] In Italy, Roma refugees from the former Yugoslavia have been forced by circumstances to congregate on the outskirts of Italian cities, "where living conditions are very poor."[968] Under the British government's controversial dispersal policy, asylum-seekers have been given free access to public housing. But the assigned destinations are often arbitrarily selected, remote from critical services,[969] of a poor standard,[970] and sometimes in

---

[964] "In the absence of other solutions, most ex-Yugoslavs belonging to the Roma minority have spontaneously set up unofficial camps, located on the outskirts of some Italian cities, where living conditions are extremely poor": Liebaut, *Conditions 2000*, at 172.

[965] M. Brink et al., "Reception Policies for Persons in Need of Protection in Western European States" (1993), Center for Migration Research, University of Amsterdam (Brink et al., "Reception Policies"), at 51.

[966] Committee on Economic, Social and Cultural Rights, "Concluding Observations of the Committee on the Report of the Netherlands," UN Doc. E/C.12/1/Add.25 (1998), at para. 18.

[967] The UN has, for example, recommended that Belgium take steps "to fully ensure that persons belonging to ethnic minorities, refugees and asylum-seekers are fully protected from any acts or laws which in any way result in discriminatory treatment within the housing sector": Committee on Economic, Social and Cultural Rights, "Concluding Observations on the Report of Belgium," UN Doc. E/C.12/1994/7, at para. 14.

[968] Brink et al., "Reception Policies," at 135. See also Committee on the Elimination of Racial Discrimination, "Concluding Observations on the Report of Italy," UN Doc. CERD/C/54/Misc.32/Rev. 3, Mar. 18, 1999.

[969] "One year after the passing of the 1999 *Immigration and Asylum Act*, there are evident flaws in the asylum policies brought into force. A recent report by the Audit Commission ... [revealed that] inadequate support systems outside London present a real barrier to dispersal; there is no evidence of efforts to connect people from similar backgrounds together; [and that] asylum-seekers face difficulties in obtaining food vouchers and their paltry food allowance": (2000) 82 *JRS Dispatches* (Nov. 10, 2000).

[970] The government often contracted the housing of refugee claimants to private agencies. One such contractor, Landmark Liverpool, housed 600 refugees in Merseyside in "two 15-storey tower blocks ... sold to the company by Liverpool council after they were deemed unfit for its tenants." Upon disclosure of the circumstances, the immigration minister declared this to be "completely unacceptable" and discontinued dispersals to this company: R. Prasad, "Tower block turmoil," *Guardian*, Apr. 9, 2003, at 5.

neighborhoods where there was a known risk to the physical security of refugees and other foreigners.[971] The system has had a punitive dimension, since asylum-seekers have not been allowed to spend more than seven days away from their assigned accommodation without permission.[972] Indeed, the government imposed a "one strike" rule under which refugee claimants who failed to travel to their assigned residence within forty-eight hours without reasonable excuse would be evicted from their emergency accommodation, and permanently denied access to income support.[973]

- **Economic, Social and Cultural Covenant, Article 11**
  1. The States Parties to the present Covenant recognize the right of everyone to an adequate standard of living for himself and his family, including adequate food, clothing and housing, and to the continuous improvement of living conditions. The States Parties will take appropriate steps to ensure the realization of this right, recognizing to this effect the essential importance of international co-operation based on free consent.

  2. The States Parties to the present Covenant ... recogniz[e] the fundamental right of everyone to be free from hunger ...

  Economic, Social and Cultural Covenant, Article 2(1)
  Each State Party to the present Covenant undertakes to take steps, individually and through international assistance and co-operation, especially economic and technical ... with a view to achieving progressively the full realization of the rights recognized in the present Covenant by all appropriate means ...

The most broadly framed guarantee of access to the necessities of life is Art. 11 of the Economic Covenant. Art. 11 establishes what is now understood to be an immediate obligation to alleviate hunger, as well as a duty progressively

---

[971] For example, "Mr. Justice Moses in the High Court in London heard that the Gezer family of Turkish Kurds had been spat at, threatened with dogs, and had their home attacked by a group of men ... Mr. Gezer, his wife and four children were sent to the Toryglen estate [in Scotland] in September 2001 ... Their son was bullied at school. On one occasion, the husband tried to throw himself out of a window. On October 27, their home was attacked by a group of men, and their son Ibrahim was threatened with a knife. The family was offered emergency accommodation in Glasgow, but they returned to London to live with relatives a day after the attack. The Home Office, however, insisted that they return to Glasgow and reduced their state support to the most basic level when they refused to go": A. Travis, "Shame of violence to asylum family," *Guardian*, Apr. 17, 2003, at 13.

[972] A. Travis, "Rules leave asylum-seekers with no cash for claims," *Guardian*, Nov. 26, 1999, at 5.

[973] R. Prasad, "'One strike' rule: Asylum seekers face tough new code," *Guardian*, July 25, 2001, at 4.

to implement the right to an adequate standard of living. Art. 12, addressed below,[974] focuses more specifically on the intimately related right to physical and mental healthcare.

The rights in the Economic Covenant, including those established by Arts. 11 and 12, explicitly inhere in "everyone."[975] They are also to be implemented without discrimination "of any kind as to . . . national or social origin . . . or other status."[976] The Committee on Economic, Social and Cultural Rights has therefore "extended its scrutiny of differential treatment to grounds other than those specifically enumerated," including on grounds of being either a non-citizen or a refugee.[977] As Craven concludes,

> the clear purpose of the Covenant is to protect the fundamental rights of every person without exception. That human rights are seen to adhere to every human being by virtue of their humanity means that they are possessed by every person to an equal extent. As the Preamble stresses,

[974] See chapter 4.4.3 below.

[975] For example, the Committee on Economic, Social and Cultural Rights has made clear that "[t]he right to adequate housing applies to everyone. While the reference to 'himself and his family' reflects assumptions as to gender roles and economic activity patterns commonly accepted in 1966 when the Covenant was adopted, the phrase cannot be read today as implying any limitations upon the applicability of the right to individuals or to female-headed households or other such groups": UN Committee on Economic, Social and Cultural Rights, "General Comment No. 4: The right to adequate housing" (1991), UN Doc. HRI/GEN/1/Rev.7, May 12, 2004, at 19, para. 6. See also UN Committee on Economic, Social and Cultural Rights, "General Comment No. 12: The right to adequate food" (1999), UN Doc. HRI/GEN/1/Rev.7, May 12, 2004, at 63, para. 1: "The human right to adequate food is of crucial importance for the enjoyment of all rights. It applies to everyone; thus the reference in article 11.1 to 'himself and his family' does not imply any limitation upon the applicability of this right to individuals or to female-headed households."

[976] International Covenant on Economic, Social and Cultural Rights, UNGA Res. 2200A(XXI), adopted Dec. 16, 1966, entered into force Jan. 3, 1976 (Economic, Social and Cultural Covenant), at Art. 2(2). One commentator has argued that the enumerated grounds on which discrimination is prohibited are exhaustive: A. Bayefsky, "The Principle of Equality or Non-Discrimination in International Law," (1990) *Human Rights Law Journal* 1, at 5. The better position notes the clearly open-ended nature of the reference to "discrimination of any kind as to . . . other status," and concludes that the list of prohibited grounds is illustrative: M. Craven, *The International Covenant on Economic, Social and Cultural Rights: A Perspective on its Development* (1995) (Craven, *ICESCR Commentary*), at 168. See also A. Chapman, "A 'Violations Approach' for Monitoring the International Covenant on Economic, Social and Cultural Rights," (1996) 18 *Human Rights Quarterly* 23, at 54–55: "It is notable that in a world which offers few protections of 'illegal immigrants,' the [Economic, Social and Cultural Rights] Committee has disagreed with the interpretation of at least one government (the government of Hong Kong) that asylum-seekers are not entitled to enjoy . . . rights in view of their status as 'illegal immigrants.'"

[977] Craven, *ICESCR Commentary*, at 169–170.

the Covenant is based upon an idea of the "equal and inalienable rights of all members of the human family."[978]

In relation to the right to food, for example, the Committee on Economic, Social and Cultural Rights has stressed that "any discrimination in access to food, as well as to means and entitlements for its procurement, on the grounds of race, color, sex, language, age, religion, political or other opinion, national or social origin, property, birth or other status with the purpose or effect of nullifying or impairing the equal enjoyment or exercise of economic, social and cultural rights constitutes a violation of the Covenant."[979] Because of their discriminatory character, Italy's arbitrary forty-five-day limit to the provision of assistance to refugees, as well as the decisions of Finland and the United Kingdom to provide refugees with less than the domestic standard of what is needed to meet basic needs, are presumptively in breach of their duties under the Economic Covenant. Bhutan's refusal to provide women refugees with food and other rations other than through a male family member is a particularly egregious breach, since it has in practice forced women to remain in abusive relationships in order to avoid starvation. In contrast, the French decision to give priority in admission to reception centers to women and families might well be reasonable (and hence non-discriminatory) in light of the evidence of their greater vulnerability to risk if denied shelter; this decision would not, however, excuse any lack of effort to meet the needs of single male refugees who are unable in practice to meet their needs by independent effort.

It remains, though, that duties under the Economic Covenant are not framed as obligations of result. State parties agree instead "to take steps,

---

[978] Ibid. at 153. To the extent that a host state government regulates the necessities of life, it is subject also to a more general duty of non-discrimination based on Art. 26 of the Civil and Political Covenant. See chapter 2.5.5 above, at pp. 125–127.

[979] UN Committee on Economic, Social and Cultural Rights, "General Comment No. 12: The right to adequate food" (1999), UN Doc. HRI/GEN/1/Rev.7, May 12, 2004, at 63, para. 18. See also UN Committee on Economic, Social and Cultural Rights, "General Comment No. 14: The right to the highest attainable standard of health" (2000), UN Doc. HRI/GEN/1/Rev.7, May 12, 2004, at 86, para. 18: "By virtue of article 2.2 and article 3, the Covenant proscribes any discrimination in access to health care and underlying determinants of health, as well as to means and entitlements for their procurement, on the grounds of race, color, sex, language, religion, political or other opinion, national or social origin, property, birth, physical or mental disability, health status (including HIV/AIDS), sexual orientation and civil, political, social or other status, which has the intention or effect of nullifying or impairing the equal enjoyment or exercise of the right to health." In its most recent elaboration of the scope of Art. 11, the Committee has specifically noted the duty to meet the needs of refugees on terms of equality with those of citizens: UN Committee on Economic, Social and Cultural Rights, "General Comment No. 15: The right to water" (2002), UN Doc. HRI/GEN/1/Rev.7, May 12, 2004, at 106, para. 16.

individually and through international assistance and co-operation ... to the maximum of [their] available resources, with a view to achieving progressively the full realization of the rights recognized in the present Covenant."[980] Thus, assuming the real logistical impossibility of, for example, delivering food and other essentials to refugees in remote parts of Guinea and Honduras during the rainy season, there would be no breach of any duty under the Economic Covenant. This duty of non-discriminatory, progressive implementation seeks to strike a delicate balance:

> It is on the one hand a necessary flexibility device, reflecting the realities of the real world and the difficulties involved for any country in ensuring full realization of economic, social and cultural rights. On the other hand, the phrase must be read in the light of the overall objective, indeed the *raison d'être*, of the Covenant which is to establish clear obligations for States parties in respect of the full realization of the rights in question. It thus imposes an obligation to move as expeditiously and effectively as possible towards that goal. Moreover, any deliberately retrogressive measures in that regard would require the most careful consideration and would need to be fully justified by reference to the totality of the rights provided for in the Covenant and in the context of the full use of the maximum available resources.[981]

There is therefore a duty to give priority to the realization of economic, social, and cultural rights,[982] and to ensure that their realization is subject to meaningful legal accountability and respectful of other requirements of human rights law:

---

[980] Economic, Social and Cultural Covenant, at Art. 2(1). "The term 'progressive realization' is often used to describe the intent of this phrase. The concept of progressive realization constitutes a recognition of the fact that full realization of all economic, social and cultural rights will generally not be able to be achieved in a short period of time": UN Committee on Economic, Social and Cultural Rights, "General Comment No. 3: The nature of states parties' obligations" (1990), UN Doc. HRI/GEN/1/Rev.7, May 12, 2004, at 15, para. 9.

[981] UN Committee on Economic, Social and Cultural Rights, "General Comment No. 3: The nature of states parties' obligations" (1990), UN Doc. HRI/GEN/1/Rev.7, May 12, 2004, at 15, para. 9.

[982] See D. Trubek, "Economic, Social, and Cultural Rights in the Third World," in T. Meron ed., *Human Rights in International Law: Legal and Policy Issues* 205 (1984), at 215: "I believe the available resources language should be read as establishing a priority for social welfare. Given the purpose of the Economic Covenant, it is hard to see how the alternative reading would make any sense. It is clear that the drafters of the Economic Covenant wished to impose obligations on states. Yet if the only obligation arising from the Economic Covenant was that a state could spend what it wanted on social welfare, then this would be no obligation at all and the drafters would have failed in their goal. This reasoning from purpose is supported by the legislative history."

[T]his flexibility coexists with the obligation upon each State party to use all the means at its disposal to give effect to the rights recognized in the Covenant. In this respect, the fundamental requirements of international human rights law must be borne in mind. Thus the Covenant norms must be recognized in appropriate ways within the domestic legal order, appropriate means of redress, or remedies, must be available to any aggrieved individual or group, and appropriate means of ensuring governmental accountability must be put in place.[983]

In line with this understanding, a state does not meet its obligations under Art. 11 when an adequate standard of living is available only to refugees who renounce other rights. The Belgian, German, and Swiss policies of agreeing to meet basic needs only in the case of refugees who submit to confinement in a reception center – despite their right to enjoy internal freedom of movement once identity is verified and a refugee claim duly lodged[984] – are examples of policies that set an unlawful barrier to realization of Art. 11 duties.

A second constraint on the value for refugees of the rights set by the Economic Covenant is Art. 2(3). This paragraph authorizes "[d]eveloping countries, with due regard to human rights and their national economy, [to] determine to what extent they [will] guarantee the economic rights recognized in the present Covenant to non-nationals." Sadly, neither the notion of a "developing country," nor that of "economic" rights – presumably as contrasted with social or cultural rights – is defined in the Covenant.[985] In the view of one commentator, economic rights should be narrowly confined to only those rights "that enable a person to earn a living or that relate to that process,"[986] a perspective that would require even less developed states to address access by refugees to the necessities of life under Arts. 11 and 12. But there is still no authoritative interpretation of the Covenant which embraces this view, leaving open the possibility that a poorer state might argue that Art. 2(3) effectively exempts it from extending most rights under the Covenant to refugees and other aliens.

The response of the Committee on Economic, Social and Cultural Rights to the dilemmas posed by the duty of progressive implementation and the

---

[983] UN Committee on Economic, Social and Cultural Rights, "General Comment No. 9: The domestic application of the Covenant" (1998), UN Doc. HRI/GEN/1/Rev.7, May 12, 2004, at 55, para. 2.

[984] See chapter 4.2.4 above.

[985] This leads Warren McKean to conclude that the language of Art. 2(3) "is unconscionably vague. It must therefore be regarded as an unfortunate inclusion in a covenant of this nature and likely to cause invidious and unreasonable distinctions to be made against aliens on the ground of their foreign nationality": W. McKean, *Equality and Discrimination under International Law* (1983), at 201.

[986] E. Dankwa, "Working Paper on Article 2(3) of the International Covenant on Economic, Social and Cultural Rights," (1987) 9 *Human Rights Quarterly* 230, at 240.

potential reach of Art. 2(3) has been indirect. First, the Committee has adopted the construct of "core content" of particularly essential rights. This core content is effectively treated as an obligation of result. Second, it has read the duty of progressive implementation in tandem with the clear duty of non-discrimination to impose a duty to take affirmative steps to ensure at least the core content of Covenant rights to those who are most socially marginalized or most vulnerable. As elaborated below, these interpretive developments provide a solid foundation from which to argue that all states have a duty to provide refugees under their jurisdiction with the necessities of life, including at least access to basic food, water, clothing, shelter, and physical and mental healthcare.

The notion of core content of key rights was first elaborated by the Committee in 1990, as a creative application of empirical evidence to the progressive implementation standard:

> On the basis of the extensive experience gained by the Committee, as well as by the body that preceded it, over a period of more than a decade of examining States parties' reports, the Committee is of the view that a minimum core obligation to ensure the satisfaction of, at the very least, minimum essential levels of each of the rights is incumbent upon every State party. Thus, for example, a State party in which any significant number of individuals is deprived of essential foodstuffs, of essential primary health care, of basic shelter and housing, or of the most basic forms of education is, *prima facie*, failing to discharge its obligations under the Covenant. If the Covenant were to be read in such a way as not to establish such a minimum core obligation, it would be largely deprived of its *raison d'être*.[987]

In other words, it is the Committee's view that virtually no state – if it *really* did what the Covenant requires, namely give clear priority in resource allocation to the realization of economic, social, and cultural rights, and never allocate those funds on a discriminatory basis – could fail to realize at least the most basic levels of these four, most vital rights.[988] While a state can still justify its failure fully to implement Covenant rights by reference to

---

[987] UN Committee on Economic, Social and Cultural Rights, "General Comment No. 3: The nature of states parties' obligations" (1990), UN Doc. HRI/GEN/1/Rev.7, May 12, 2004, at 15, para. 10.

[988] The Committee has reaffirmed its commitment to the notion of core rights. "Should a State party argue that resource constraints make it impossible to provide access to food for those who are unable by themselves to secure such access, the State has to demonstrate that every effort has been made to use all the resources at its disposal in an effort to satisfy, as a matter of priority, those minimum obligations. This follows from article 2.1 of the Covenant, which obliges a State party to take the necessary steps to the maximum of its available resources, as previously pointed out by the Committee in its General Comment No. 3, paragraph 10": UN Committee on Economic, Social and Cultural Rights, "General

Art. 2(1)'s duty of progressive implementation, the Committee has made clear that no state is immune from the duty to respect the core content of rights.[989] Specifically, every state "must demonstrate that every effort has been made to use all resources that are at its disposition in an effort to satisfy, as a matter of priority, those minimum obligations."[990] It follows, therefore, that Uganda and Tanzania may be held to account under this standard for the starvation-induced repatriation of refugees from their territory, as may countries such as Ethiopia, Iran, and Zambia where refugees were given grossly inadequate access to food or water.

Of critical importance in the refugee context, this duty will not be met unless a state claiming resource insufficiency proves that it has sought out, and been denied, international aid sufficient to meet its core obligations under the Covenant.[991] The Committee has specifically insisted on this duty in relation to the right to shelter[992] and, most emphatically, the right to food:

> Comment No. 12: The right to adequate food" (1999), UN Doc. HRI/GEN/1/Rev.7, May 12, 2004, at 63, para. 17. See also UN Committee on Economic, Social and Cultural Rights, "General Comment No. 14: The right to the highest attainable standard of health" (2000), UN Doc. HRI/GEN/1/Rev.7, May 12, 2004, at 86, para. 43: "In General Comment No. 3, the Committee confirms that States parties have a core obligation to ensure the satisfaction of, at the very least, minimum essential levels of each of the rights enunciated in the Covenant, including essential primary health care. Read in conjunction with more contemporary instruments, such as the Programme of Action of the International Conference on Population and Development, the Alma-Ata Declaration provides compelling guidance on the core obligations arising from article 12."

[989] In relation to the right to water, for example, the Committee has determined that "[t]o demonstrate compliance with their general and specific obligations, States parties must establish that they have taken the necessary and feasible steps towards the realization of the right to water. In accordance with international law, a failure to act in good faith to take such steps amounts to a violation of the right. It should be stressed that a State party cannot justify its non-compliance with the core obligations ... which are non-derogable": UN Committee on Economic, Social and Cultural Rights, "General Comment No. 15: The right to water" (2002), UN Doc. HRI/GEN/1/Rev.7, May 12, 2004, at 106, para. 40.

[990] UN Committee on Economic, Social and Cultural Rights, "General Comment No. 3: The nature of states parties' obligations" (1990), UN Doc. HRI/GEN/1/Rev.7, May 12, 2004, at 15, para. 10.

[991] "A final element of article 2(1), to which attention must be drawn, is that the undertaking given by all States parties is 'to take steps, individually and through international assistance and cooperation, especially economic and technical'": ibid. at para. 13. The Committee notes that the phrase "to the maximum of its available resources" was intended by the drafters of the Covenant to refer to both the resources existing within a state and those available from the international community through international cooperation and assistance: ibid.

[992] "As recognized in the Global Strategy for Shelter and in other international analyses, many of the measures required to promote the right to housing would only require the abstention by the Government from certain practices and a commitment to facilitating

In determining which actions or omissions amount to a violation of the right to food, it is important to distinguish the inability from the unwillingness of a State party to comply. Should a State party argue that resource constraints make it impossible to provide access to food for those who are unable by themselves to secure such access, the State has to demonstrate that every effort has been made to use all the resources at its disposal in an effort to satisfy, as a matter of priority, those minimum obligations. This follows from article 2.1 of the Covenant, which obliges a State party to take the necessary steps to the maximum of its available resources, as previously pointed out by the Committee in its General Comment No. 3, paragraph 10. *A State claiming that it is unable to carry out its obligation for reasons beyond its control therefore has the burden of proving that this is the case and that it has unsuccessfully sought to obtain international support to ensure the availability and accessibility of the necessary food* [emphasis added].[993]

But if poorer states are required to seek out international aid in order to ensure the necessities of life to refugees and other vulnerable persons, is there a corresponding obligation on the part of wealthier countries to provide the needed resources? For example, were wealthier countries required to assist in meeting the basic needs of desperate refugees in Zambia, or to enable Namibia to provide for the Angolan refugees it hosted?

The regrettable answer, bound up with the failure of the effort to promote a binding human right to development,[994] is that there is no more than a principled obligation to assist poorer states.[995] While all parties to the Economic Covenant with adequate resources agree to provide international aid to promote the implementation of Covenant rights – and while the aid given by Sweden and the United States to provide for Angolan refugees in Namibia was a commendable example of principled implementation of the Covenant – there is no clear or enforceable legal obligation to provide

---

'self-help' by affected groups. To the extent that any such steps are considered to be beyond the maximum resources available to a State party, it is appropriate that a request be made as soon as possible for international cooperation in accordance with articles 11(1), 22 and 23 of the Covenant, and that the Committee be informed thereof": UN Committee on Economic, Social and Cultural Rights, "General Comment No. 4: The right to adequate housing" (1991), UN Doc. HRI/GEN/1/Rev.7, May 12, 2004, at 19, para. 10.

[993] UN Committee on Economic, Social and Cultural Rights, "General Comment No. 12: The right to adequate food" (1999), UN Doc. HRI/GEN/1/Rev.7, May 12, 2004, at 63, para. 17. The Commission on Human Rights voted 52–1 to endorse the understanding of the right to food set out in General Comment No. 12 as authoritative: UN Commission on Human Rights Res. 2001/25, Apr. 20, 2001.

[994] To date, only a non-binding declaration on this subject has been adopted. See "Declaration on the Right to Development," UNGA Res. 41/128 (1986).

[995] "Although there seems to be agreement that the rights in the Covenant are contingent, to a degree, on the provision of international assistance, the nature, scope, and obligatory nature of such assistance is unclear": Craven, *ICESCR Commentary*, at 145.

aid.[996] In particular, there is no consensus on which states are subject to the duty to assist set by Art. 2(1), or the sorts of action which are encompassed by the obligation to engage in "international assistance and cooperation, especially economic and technical."[997] Most important, Art. 2(1) does not define how much assistance is required to meet a state's obligation, or to whom that assistance should be directed.[998] The tentative nature of the duty is evident also from the rather soft language used in relevant general comments issued by the Committee on Economic, Social and Cultural Rights. States "should" provide aid to realize the right to food;[999] they "should" facilitate realization

---

[996] The Committee on Economic, Social and Cultural Rights has framed the duty in typically vague terms. "The Committee wishes to emphasize that in accordance with Articles 55 and 56 of the Charter of the United Nations, with well-established principles of international law, and with the provisions of the Covenant itself, international cooperation for development and thus for the realization of economic, social and cultural rights is an obligation of all States. It is particularly incumbent upon those States which are in a position to assist others in this regard. The Committee notes in particular the importance of the Declaration on the Right to Development adopted by the General Assembly in its resolution 41/128 of 4 December 1986 and the need for States parties to take full account of all of the principles recognized therein. It emphasizes that, in the absence of an active programme of international assistance and cooperation on the part of all those States that are in a position to undertake one, the full realization of economic, social and cultural rights will remain an unfulfilled aspiration in many countries": UN Committee on Economic, Social and Cultural Rights, "General Comment No. 3: The nature of states parties' obligations" (1990), UN Doc. HRI/GEN/1/Rev.7, May 12, 2004, at 15, para. 14.

[997] The most direct conclusion of the Committee is that "given that some diseases are easily transmissible beyond the frontiers of a State, the international community has a collective responsibility to address this problem. The economically developed States parties have a special responsibility and interest to assist the poorer developing States in this regard": UN Committee on Economic, Social and Cultural Rights, "General Comment No. 14: The right to the highest attainable standard of health care" (2000), UN Doc. HRI/GEN/1/ Rev.7, May 12, 2004, at 86, para. 40. See generally Craven, *ICESCR Commentary*, at 146–147.

[998] At the 2001 session of the UN Commission on Human Rights, a Cuban proposal to establish an independent expert to monitor the fulfillment by developed countries of their political pledge to allocate 0.7 percent of their GNP to development assistance was abandoned for lack of support: M. Dennis, "The Fifty-Seventh Session of the UN Commission on Human Rights," (2002) 96(1) *American Journal of International Law* 181.

[999] "In the spirit of Article 56 of the Charter of the United Nations, the specific provisions contained in articles 11, 2.1, and 23 of the Covenant and the Rome Declaration of the World Food Summit, States parties should recognize the essential role of international cooperation and comply with their commitment to take joint and separate action to achieve the full realization of the right to adequate food. In implementing this commitment, States parties should take steps to respect the enjoyment of the right to food in other countries, to protect that right, to facilitate access to food and to provide the necessary aid when required. States parties should, in international agreements whenever relevant, ensure that the right to adequate food is given due attention and consider the development of further international legal instruments to that end": UN Committee on

of the right to water in other countries;[1000] they "should" provide the funds to facilitate access by all to basic healthcare;[1001] and of most direct relevance to this study, they "should" provide disaster assistance and humanitarian assistance to meet the needs of refugees.[1002] In no case, however, has the Committee found that the Economic Covenant imposes precise and directly enforceable obligations to provide a given quantum or kind of assistance to states in any specified predicament.[1003] Craven helpfully summarizes the historical basis for this caution in suggesting any duty to provide development assistance:

> During the drafting of the Covenant, Chile claimed that "international assistance to under-developed countries had in a sense become mandatory as a result of commitments assumed by States in the United Nations." This was almost universally challenged by other representatives of all the groupings involved. The general consensus was that developing States were entitled to ask for assistance but not claim it as a legal right. The text of article 11 bears out this conclusion. In recognizing the role of international

Economic, Social and Cultural Rights, "General Comment No. 12: The right to adequate food" (1999), UN Doc. HRI/GEN/1/Rev.7, May 12, 2004, at 63, para. 36.

[1000] UN Committee on Economic, Social and Cultural Rights, "General Comment No. 15: The right to water" (2002), UN Doc. HRI/GEN/1/Rev.7, May 12, 2004, at 106, para. 34.

[1001] "Depending on the availability of resources, States should facilitate access to essential health facilities, goods and services in other countries wherever possible and provide the necessary aid when required. States parties should ensure that the right to health is given due attention in international agreements and, to that end, should consider the development of further legal instruments. In relation to the conclusion of other international agreements, States parties should take steps to ensure that these instruments do not adversely impact upon the right to health. Similarly, States parties have an obligation to ensure that their actions as members of international organizations take due account of the right to health": UN Committee on Economic, Social and Cultural Rights, "General Comment No. 14: The right to the highest attainable standard of health" (2000), UN Doc. HRI/GEN/1/Rev.7, May 12, 2004, at 86, para. 39.

[1002] "States have a joint and individual responsibility, in accordance with the Charter of the United Nations, to cooperate in providing disaster relief and humanitarian assistance in times of emergency, including assistance to refugees and internally displaced persons. Each State should contribute to this task in accordance with its ability": UN Committee on Economic, Social and Cultural Rights, "General Comment No. 12: The right to adequate food" (1999), UN Doc. HRI/GEN/1/Rev.7, May 12, 2004, at 63, para. 38. "In disaster relief and emergency assistance, including assistance to refugees and displaced persons, priority should be given to Covenant rights, including the provision of adequate water": UN Committee on Economic, Social and Cultural Rights, "General Comment No. 15: The right to water" (2002), UN Doc. HRI/GEN/1/Rev.7, May 12, 2004, at 106, para. 34.

[1003] "While there would appear to be considerable scope for strengthening States' external obligations ... it is an area in which States are unlikely, in the foreseeable future, to agree to specific demands on the amount of distribution of aid to third countries": Craven, *ICESCR Commentary*, at 150.

co-operation in the realization of rights, it stipulates that it should be based upon "free consent."[1004]

The one legal constraint which does appear to exist, however, is that whatever international aid is provided must be granted and administered on a non-discriminatory basis. In line with the substantive content traditionally understood to comprise the duty of non-discrimination,[1005] the importance of allocating aid on the basis of relative need has been affirmed.[1006] In particular, Art. 26 of the Civil and Political Covenant requires that there be no discrimination, in law or in fact, in the allocation of any public goods on the basis of, for example, race, nationality, social origin, or other status.[1007] A dynamic interpretation of this overarching duty would suggest that since international aid provided under Art. 2(1) of the Economic Covenant is expressly intended to advance Covenant rights where states are least able to ensure those rights independently, political or other distortions of aid are violations of the duty of non-discrimination.[1008] Thus, the decision of donor states to cut critical aid to refugees in Tanzania in order to redirect funds to meet the needs of less desperate refugees from Kosovo arriving in European states seems plausibly discriminatory.

Yet even this minimal constraint may be undermined by the practice of the Human Rights Committee to afford states an exceedingly broad margin of appreciation before a given resource allocation is deemed to be unreasonable and hence potentially discriminatory.[1009] It is thus unlikely that the

---

[1004] Ibid. at 148–149.   [1005] See generally chapter 2.5.5 above.

[1006] While still employing irresolute language, the Committee has concluded that "[p]riority in the provision of international medical aid, distribution and management of resources, such as safe and potable water, food and medical supplies, and financial aid should be given to the most vulnerable or marginalized groups of the population": UN Committee on Economic, Social and Cultural Rights, "General Comment No. 14: The right to the highest attainable standard of health" (2000), UN Doc. HRI/GEN/1/Rev.7, May 12, 2004, at 86, para. 40. With respect to the aid provided by international organizations, see ibid. at para. 65.

[1007] See chapter 2.5.5 above, at pp. 125–127.

[1008] There is, of course, also the question of whether the duty of non-discrimination binds a state in its extraterritorial actions. It has been persuasively argued that there is no principled reason to release states which act extraterritorially from legal obligations that would otherwise circumscribe the scope of their authority. According to Meron, "[i]n view of the purposes and objects of human rights treaties, there is no a priori reason to limit a state's obligation to respect human rights to its national territory. Where agents of the state, whether military or civilian, exercise power and authority (jurisdiction, or de facto jurisdiction) over persons outside national territory, the presumption should be that the state's obligations to respect the pertinent human rights continues. That presumption could be rebutted only when the nature and content of a particular right or treaty language suggest otherwise": T. Meron, "Extraterritoriality of Human Rights Treaties," (1995) 89(1) American Journal of International Law 78, at 80–81.

[1009] See chapter 2.5.5 above, at pp. 128–145.

Committee would find a state in breach because of a politically inspired decision to shift aid resources from one group of refugees to another. And even if a wealthy government were to decide simply to end aid to refugees or other impoverished persons abroad in favor of spending resources on its own (less needy) citizenry, the current jurisprudence suggests that no violation of Art. 26 would be found. This is because most distinctions between citizens and aliens have been found to be reasonable and therefore not discriminatory.[1010]

In the end, then, under present interpretations of international human rights law, the failure of a government to provide foreign aid or to allocate its foreign aid resources to meet relative needs is probably not legally actionable. On the other hand, where a state such as India refuses foreign aid which could have enabled it more fully to meet the subsistence needs of refugees, it likely violates Art. 11 of the Economic Covenant for reasons previously described.[1011] There is therefore what amounts to an asymmetrical approach to foreign aid in international law. A government must accept available aid to enable it to provide the necessities of life to persons under its jurisdiction, but states with the means to satisfy even the most basic survival interests of destitute persons abroad are under no concomitant legal duty to share their wealth.

Normally a state is considered to be in breach of its obligations under the Economic Covenant only where there is evidence that it has prevented access to a right, failed to stop private actions from denying access to a right, or neglected to facilitate efforts by individuals to secure their rights.[1012] In all of these cases, there is an underlying expectation of individual initiative which allows the state's duty to be conceived as secondary. The assumption of states

---

[1010] See chapter 2.5.5 above, at pp. 130–133.   [1011] See text above, at pp. 490–491.

[1012] See e.g. UN Committee on Economic, Social and Cultural Rights, "General Comment No. 12: The right to adequate food" (1999), UN Doc. HRI/GEN/1/Rev.7, May 12, 2004, at 63, para. 15: "The right to adequate food, like any other human right, imposes three types or levels of obligations on States parties: the obligations to respect, to protect and to fulfil. In turn, the obligation to fulfil incorporates both an obligation to facilitate and an obligation to provide. The obligation to respect existing access to adequate food requires States parties not to take any measures that result in preventing such access. The obligation to protect requires measures by the State to ensure that enterprises or individuals do not deprive individuals of their access to adequate food. The obligation to fulfil (facilitate) means the State must pro-actively engage in activities intended to strengthen people's access to and utilization of resources and means to ensure their livelihood, including food security." As Eide points out, "this is the most important aspect of the right to food and other survival rights: not the State as provider, but as protector. This is a function similar to the role of the State as protector in regard to civil and political rights: protecting the right to life, to freedom from slavery and servitude, from violence and maltreatment by third parties": A. Eide, "Article 25," in A. Eide et al. eds., The Universal Declaration of Human Rights: A Commentary 385 (1992) (Eide, "Article 25"), at 388.

such as Canada and Norway that asylum-seekers will ordinarily meet their
own needs by earning money through engagement in employment – which
the government authorizes – is therefore precisely in line with the spirit of the
Economic Covenant. It follows also that Argentina would not be in violation
of the Covenant by virtue of its decision to issue asylum-seekers with a
provisional form of work permit viewed with some measure of suspicion by
employers – unless, of course, the practical result were to bar refugees from
virtually all work, making it impossible for them to meet their most basic
needs.

Conversely, the Dutch system, under which asylum-seekers may work for
no more than twelve weeks each year, is not oriented to meeting the needs of
refugees. As such, it – like the complete prohibitions on work by refugee
claimants imposed by such countries as Denmark, France, Germany, and
Italy, and the delayed access to work imposed by Finland and Sweden – would
give rise to a breach of Art. 11 of the Covenant if refugee claimants are not
provided with alternative means of support.[1013] Indeed, the South African
Supreme Court of Appeal has determined that the denial of the right to work
in such circumstances may amount to degrading treatment:

> [W]here employment is the only reasonable means for the person's support
> other considerations arise. What is then in issue is not merely a restriction
> upon the person's capacity for self-fulfilment, but a restriction upon his or
> her ability to live without positive humiliation and degradation. For it is
> not disputed that this country, unlike some other countries that receive
> refugees, offers no State support to applicants for asylum . . .
>
>   Thus a person who exercises his or her right to apply for asylum, but who
> is destitute, will have no alternative but to turn to crime, or to begging, or to
> foraging. I do not suggest that in such circumstances the State has an

---

[1013] This conclusion is in line with the view of the English Court of Appeal that regulations
which denied some refugee claimants both access to work and to social support
"necessarily contemplate for some a life so destitute that . . . no civilised nation can
tolerate it . . . [S]ome basic provision should be made, sufficient for genuine claimants
to survive and pursue their claims . . . Parliament cannot have intended a significant
number of genuine asylum-seekers to be impaled on the horns of so intolerable a
dilemma: the need either to abandon their claims to refugee status or alternatively to
maintain them as best they can but in a state of utter destitution": *R v. Secretary of State
for Social Security, ex parte Joint Council for the Welfare of Immigrants*, [1996] 4 All ER
385 (Eng. CA, June 21, 1996), per Simon Brown LJ, at 401–402. As subsequently
affirmed, "[t]he *ratio* of the *Joint Council* case was . . . that asylum-seekers were
being *deprived* of their right to appeal . . . and to remain in the country meanwhile
since the impugned regulations made those rights *nugatory*; they inevitably not merely
prejudiced but on occasion *defeated* those rights, and made the exercise of those rights
not merely difficult but *totally impossible* [emphasis in original]": *Secretary of State for
the Home Department v. Jammeh*, [1999] Imm AR 1 (Eng. CA, July 30, 1998), per
Hobhouse LJ, at 7.

obligation to provide employment ... but only that the deprivation of the freedom to work assumes a different dimension when it threatens positively to degrade rather than merely to inhibit the realisation of the potential for self-fulfilment.[1014]

For similar reasons, the refusal of Namibia and Zambia to waive their food import restrictions in order to allow international agencies to feed desperate refugees was a violation of the core content of the right to food.

But the obligations of states go beyond simply to respect and to protect access to the necessities of life. The Committee on Economic, Social and Cultural Rights has also recognized an explicit duty on states to take steps to fulfill this right, particularly where marginalized individuals and social groups are concerned.[1015] The Committee has recognized that vulnerable individuals and groups cannot always meet their basic needs by independent action, in consequence of which state parties are under a legal duty to take affirmative steps to realize their rights:

> States parties are also obliged to fulfil (provide) a specific right contained in the Covenant when individuals or a group are unable, for reasons beyond their control, to realize that right themselves by the means at their disposal.[1016]

In relation to the right to healthcare, for example, the Committee has noted that

---

[1014] *Minister of Home Affairs v. Watchenuka*, (2004) 1 All SA 21 (SA SCA, Nov. 28, 2003), at para. 32, per Nugent JA.

[1015] "The approach of the Committee towards the realization of the rights in the Covenant is marked by its insistence upon a process of equalization. As an initial step towards the realization of the rights in the Covenant, States are required to identify the disadvantaged sectors of the population. Those groups should be the focus of positive State action aimed at securing the full realization of their rights": Craven, *ICESCR Commentary*, at 159.

[1016] UN Committee on Economic, Social and Cultural Rights, "General Comment No. 14: The right to the highest attainable standard of health care" (2000), UN Doc. HRI/GEN/1/Rev.7, May 12, 2004, at 86, para. 37. See also Committee on Economic, Social and Cultural Rights, "General Comment No. 12: The right to adequate food" (1999), UN Doc. HRI/GEN/1/Rev.7, May 12, 2004, at 63, para. 15: "Finally, whenever an individual or group is unable, for reasons beyond their control, to enjoy the right to adequate food by the means at their disposal, States have the obligation to fulfil (provide) that right directly. This obligation also applies for persons who are victims of natural or other disasters"; and UN Committee on Economic, Social and Cultural Rights, "General Comment No. 15: The right to water" (2002), UN Doc. HRI/GEN/1/Rev.7, May 12, 2004, at 106, para. 37(b), which defines the core content of the right to water to include the obligation "[t]o ensure the right of access to water and water facilities and services on a non-discriminatory basis, especially for disadvantaged or marginalized groups."

[v]iolations of the obligation to fulfil occur through the failure of States parties to take all necessary steps to ensure the realization of the right to health. Examples include ... insufficient expenditure or misallocation of public resources which results in the non-enjoyment of the right to health by individuals or groups, particularly the vulnerable or marginalized.[1017]

Similarly, the duty to ensure access to housing requires "States parties [to] give due priority to those social groups living in unfavourable conditions by giving them particular consideration."[1018] Refugees are frequently a clear example of such a group:

> Asylum-seekers, refugees, and displaced persons do not have the same opportunity as others to achieve an adequate standard of living on the basis of their own efforts. They therefore require, to a larger extent than the ordinary public, direct provisions, until conditions are established in which they can obtain their own entitlements.[1019]

This direct obligation of states to provide the substance of basic survival rights to the most vulnerable – what Eide refers to as an obligation of "last recourse"[1020] – inheres even when a state is faced with extraordinary resource constraints.[1021] It should moreover be interpreted to apply once a state becomes aware of an imminent risk to vulnerable persons, not simply once

---

[1017] UN Committee on Economic, Social and Cultural Rights, "General Comment No. 14: The right to the highest attainable standard of health" (2000), UN Doc. HRI/GEN/1/Rev.7, May 12, 2004, at 86, para. 52.

[1018] UN Committee on Economic, Social and Cultural Rights, "General Comment No. 4: The right to adequate housing" (1991), UN Doc. HRI/GEN/1/Rev.7, May 12, 2004, at 19, para. 11.

[1019] Eide, "Standard of Living," at 105. Thus, for example, the Committee on Economic, Social and Cultural Rights has observed that "[w]hereas the right to water applies to everyone, States parties should give special attention to those individuals and groups who have traditionally faced difficulties in exercising this right, including ... refugees [and] asylum-seekers": UN Committee on Economic, Social and Cultural Rights, "General Comment No. 15: The right to water" (2002), UN Doc. HRI/GEN/1/Rev.7, May 12, 2004, at 106, at para. 16.

[1020] Eide, "Article 25," at 388.

[1021] "[T]he Committee underlines the fact that even in times of severe resources constraints, whether caused by a process of adjustment, of economic recession, or by other factors, the vulnerable members of society can and indeed must be protected by the adoption of relatively low-cost targeted programmes": UN Committee on Economic, Social and Cultural Rights, "General Comment No. 3: The nature of states parties' obligations" (1990), UN Doc. HRI/GEN/1/Rev.7, May 12, 2004, at 15, para. 12. See also UN Committee on Economic, Social and Cultural Rights, "General Comment No. 12: The right to adequate food" (1999), UN Doc. HRI/GEN/1/Rev.7, May 12, 2004, at 63, para. 28: "Even where a State faces severe resource constraints, whether caused by a process of economic adjustment, economic recession, climatic conditions or other factors, measures should be undertaken to ensure that the right to adequate food is especially fulfilled for vulnerable population groups and individuals."

the necessities of life have already been denied. In interpreting a comparable affirmative duty under European human rights law in a successful challenge to the United Kingdom's policy of denying income support to persons who failed to claim refugee status immediately upon arrival, the English Court of Appeal observed that

> The obligation "to take measures" [under the European Convention on Human Rights] seems to me to imply more than simply acting as a long-stop in individual cases as they arise. That may be sufficient if the alternative system of charitable support is able to cope with the generality of cases, so that ... suffering ... is truly the exception. However, if on the available information, the scale of the problem is such that the system is unable to cope, then it is the responsibility of the State to take reasonable measures to ensure that it can cope. How that is done, for example whether by direct support or by financial assistance to charities working in the field, is a policy matter for the State.[1022]

In sum, the rights set out in the Covenant on Economic, Social and Cultural Rights – including to the necessities of life, and to physical and mental healthcare – inhere in everyone under a state's jurisdiction, including refugees. Any discrimination in the allocation of the enumerated rights is automatically a violation of the Covenant. The essential duty of states is to implement the rights in the Covenant progressively and as matters of priority, though it is understood that genuine resource constraints may preclude full realization of all rights immediately in some countries. Retrogression is, however, presumptively in breach of the Covenant, as is the failure to implement rights in accordance with human rights standards and with real accountability. Less developed countries may determine the extent to which they will extend "economic" rights to non-citizens, including refugees. But that flexibility does not apply to the core content of the most basic rights set by the Covenant.[1023] Non-fulfillment of the core content of these rights on

---

[1022] *R (Limbuela) v. Secretary of State for the Home Department*, [2004] EWCA Civ 540 (Eng. CA, May 21, 2004), per Carnwath LJ, at para. 121. See also Jacob LJ, ibid. at para. 149: "It follows that although one may not be able to say of any particular individual that there is more than a very real risk that denial of food and shelter will take that individual across the threshold, one can say that collectively the current policy of the Secretary of State will have that effect in the case of a substantial number of people. It seems to me that it must follow that the current policy (which includes having no policy save in the case of heavily pregnant women) is unlawful as violating Art. 3. And it follows that the treatment of the particular individuals the subject of these appeals in pursuit of that policy is also unlawful."

[1023] Thus, "in so far as the Covenant establishes the rights of 'everyone,' non-nationals would have a right to the enjoyment of the minimum core content of those rights ... [I]n practice, the Committee will censure situations where aliens enjoy few rights and are the objects of exploitation": Craven, *ICESCR Commentary*, at 174.

economic grounds by even the poorest states is in breach of the Covenant unless the government is able to demonstrate that it has unsuccessfully made best efforts to secure international aid to implement these rights, and has distributed whatever resources are available without discrimination. This obligation to respect the core content of basic rights in virtually all circumstances includes a duty of affirmative implementation, at least where it is foreseeable that individuals and groups are unlikely to be able to secure their rights by autonomous effort.

Turning first to the specific content of the right to food, paragraph 2 of Art. 11 establishes the right of everyone to be free from hunger as a "fundamental right," the only right so defined in either Covenant.[1024] The most basic goal of ensuring "that individuals have a right not to die from hunger and not to suffer (either physically or mentally) from malnutrition . . . "[1025] is undisputed,[1026] as is clear from the view of the Committee on Economic, Social and Cultural Rights that "a State party in which any significant number of individuals is deprived of essential foodstuffs . . . is, *prima facie*, failing to discharge its obligations under the Covenant."[1027] In accordance with the general approach to economic and social rights set out above, the core right to food may be breached "through the direct action of States or other entities insufficiently regulated by States," including by "the prevention of access to humanitarian food aid in internal conflicts or other emergency situations."[1028] There is therefore little doubt that Ethiopian diversion of refugee

---

[1024] P. Alston, "International Law and the Human Right to Food," in P. Alston and K. Tomasevski eds., *International Law and the Human Right to Food* 10 (1984) (Alston, "Right to Food"), at 32.

[1025] Ibid. at 13–14.

[1026] "[A]ny proposed limitations on the right to food which could result in death by starvation are clearly unacceptable. Apart from violating the right to food provisions, such limitations would also violate the right to life which, according to the Human Rights Committee, is 'the supreme right from which no derogation is permitted even in times of public emergency which threatens the life of the nation'": ibid. at 21.

[1027] UN Committee on Economic, Social and Cultural Rights, "General Comment No. 3: The nature of states parties' obligations" (1990), UN Doc. HRI/GEN/1/Rev.7, May 12, 2004, at 15, para. 10. See also UN Committee on Economic, Social and Cultural Rights, "General Comment No. 12: The right to adequate food" (1999), UN Doc. HRI/GEN/1/Rev.7, May 12, 2004, at 63, para. 17: "Violations of the Covenant occur when a State fails to ensure the satisfaction of, at the very least, the minimum essential level required to be free from hunger."

[1028] UN Committee on Economic, Social and Cultural Rights, "General Comment No. 12: The right to adequate food" (1999), UN Doc. HRI/GEN/1/Rev.7, May 12, 2004, at 63, para. 19. The African Commission on Human and Peoples' Rights observed that the core content of the right to food could be violated by, for example, government actions which destroy or contaminate food sources (or which allow private parties to do so), as well as by the promotion of terror which poses a significant obstacle to the efforts of individuals to feed themselves: *Social and Economic Rights Action Center and Center for* food aid to rebel soldiers was in breach of the core right to food. On the other hand, Malawi was not in violation of the Covenant when food deliveries to refugees were halted by rebel Mozambican forces operating in its territory, since these armies could not be subdued by the government. Moreover, "whenever an individual or group is unable, for reasons beyond their control, to enjoy the right to adequate food by the means at their disposal, States have the obligation to fulfil (provide) that right directly. This obligation also applies for persons who are victims of natural or other disasters."[1029]

The Committee has defined the core content of the right to food to include "[t]he availability of food in a quantity and quality sufficient to satisfy the dietary needs of individuals, free from adverse substances, and acceptable within a given culture [as well as] [t]he accessibility of such food in ways that are sustainable and that do not interfere with the enjoyment of other human rights."[1030] The accessibility branch of this core duty means that failure to supervise food distribution adequately in camps where cultural norms dictate that men should eat their fill before women and children are fed is in breach of the Covenant. Equally clearly, the requirement of dietary sufficiency suggests a failure to meet Covenant requirements when refugees are provided with no milk, fruit, or vegetables, or when niacin shortages in food cause refugees to develop pellagra. And because cultural acceptability is also an aspect of the core duty, Botswana's refusal to provide refugees from the Democratic Republic of Congo with either fish or meat, and the insistence that Burundian refugees in Tanzania survive by consuming culturally unpalatable food, are also of doubtful legality.

Second and more generally, states are under a duty to promote a more complete right to "adequate food" under Art. 11(1). This branch of the right to food goes beyond concerns of immediate access to quantities of food required for survival,[1031] focusing instead on the sufficiency of diet over time to maintain health and to enable individuals to lead a normal, active life,[1032] including the establishment of food security for the medium to long

---

Economic and Social Rights v. Nigeria, Case ACPHR/COMM/A044/1 (May 27, 2002), at para. 65, reported at (2002) 96(4) *American Journal of International Law* 937.

[1029] UN Committee on Economic, Social and Cultural Rights, "General Comment No. 12: The right to adequate food" (1999), UN Doc. HRI/GEN/1/Rev.7, May 12, 2004, at 63, para. 15. In addition, however, all states "have a joint and individual responsibility ... to cooperate in providing disaster relief and humanitarian assistance in times of emergency, including assistance to refugees and internally displaced persons": ibid. at para. 38.

[1030] Ibid. at para. 8.

[1031] "The right to adequate food ... shall ... not be interpreted in a narrow or restrictive sense which equates it with a minimum package of calories, proteins and other specific nutrients": ibid at para. 6.

[1032] Alston, "Right to Food," at 22–23.

term.[1033] This broader right to adequate food is not, however, part of the core content of the right to food. A state therefore breaches its obligations under Art. 11(1) only when it fails to give priority in the allocation of available resources to the progressive and non-discriminatory realization of the right.[1034]

The Committee on Economic, Social and Cultural Rights has more recently set out detailed standards relating specifically to the right to water,[1035] determined to be a component of the duties set by both Arts. 11 and 12 of the Covenant.[1036] In line with its approach to the right to food, the right to water is defined as the entitlement of "everyone to sufficient, safe, acceptable, physically accessible and affordable water for personal and domestic uses."[1037] More specifically, it has been determined that "[r]efugees and asylum-seekers should be granted the right to water on the same conditions as granted to nationals."[1038]

The core content of the right to water, specifically said to be opposable even in relation to the poorest states,[1039] includes a number of components of frequent relevance to refugees. Most basically, it includes the duty "[t]o ensure access to the minimum essential amount of water, that is sufficient and safe for personal and domestic uses to prevent disease [and] [t]o ensure the right of access to water and water facilities and services on a non-discriminatory basis, especially for disadvantaged or marginalized groups."[1040] The provision to refugees in western Ethiopia of less than

---

[1033] "The notion of sustainability is intrinsically linked to the notion of adequate food or food security, implying food being accessible for both present and future generations. The precise meaning of 'adequacy' is to a large extent determined by prevailing social, economic, cultural, climatic, ecological and other conditions, while 'sustainability' incorporates the notion of long-term availability and accessibility": UN Committee on Economic, Social and Cultural Rights, "General Comment No. 12: The right to adequate food" (1999), UN Doc. HRI/GEN/1/Rev.7, May 12, 2004, at 63, para. 7.

[1034] In practice, however, the Committee is reported not to have directed much of its attention to non-core concerns. "That Committee members have only rarely requested information about the nutritional status of the population, or about food quality and safety, may be criticized as being unduly cautious. However, the Committee does face considerable problems in assessing the level of enjoyment of the right to food even in so far as it relates even to malnutrition": Craven, *ICESCR Commentary*, at 309.

[1035] UN Committee on Economic, Social and Cultural Rights, "General Comment No. 15: The right to water" (2002), UN Doc. HRI/GEN/1/Rev.7, May 12, 2004, at 106.

[1036] Ibid. at para. 3.   [1037] Ibid. at para. 2.   [1038] Ibid. at para. 16(f).

[1039] "A State which is unwilling to use the maximum of its available resources for the realization of the right to water is in violation of its obligations under the Covenant. If resource constraints render it impossible for a State party to comply fully with its Covenant obligations, it has the burden of justifying that every effort has nevertheless been made to use all available resources at its disposal in order to satisfy, as a matter of priority, the obligations outlined above": ibid. at para. 41.

[1040] Ibid. at para. 37(a), (b).

1 liter of water per day therefore amounted to a presumptive breach of the Covenant. More explicitly, at least in the case of vulnerable populations, states are required to ensure that there are "a sufficient number of water outlets to avoid prohibitive waiting times; and that are at a reasonable distance from the household"[1041] – a standard not met when there was only one borehole for all the Angolan refugees at the Maheba camp in Zambia. The core content of the right to water comprises as well the obligation "[t]o ensure [that] personal security is not threatened when having to physically access water."[1042] This standard is clearly not met when state parties require refugee women to collect water in circumstances that risk both their physical security and their health by exposure to such diseases as malaria or yellow fever.

The right to adequate clothing has not been authoritatively elaborated. In drafting the predecessor Universal Declaration of Human Rights,[1043] the specific reference to adequate food and clothing was the result of a well-received amendment by China to give substance to the notion of an "adequate standard of living."[1044] The language appears simply to have been carried forward into the Economic Covenant.[1045] The right to adequate clothing was, however, briefly considered by the Committee on Economic, Social and Cultural Rights in preparing its general comment on the rights of persons with disabilities. The Committee interpreted Art. 11 to require access to clothing that allows disabled persons "to function fully and effectively in society,"[1046] suggesting a purposive and contextualized understanding of adequacy.[1047] In line with this approach, Art. 11 should be understood to require that refugees have access to clothing which is, for example, suited to the climate and to the work and other roles which they undertake in the host country. They should also not be compelled to wear clothing which stigmatizes them as foreign to the host society, since this may amount to an

---

[1041] Ibid. at para. 37(c).   [1042] Ibid. at para. 37(d).

[1043] "Everyone has the right to a standard of living adequate for the health and well-being of himself and of his family, including food, clothing, housing and medical care and necessary social services": Universal Declaration, at Art. 25(1).

[1044] Eide, "Article 25," at 394.   [1045] Eide, "Standard of Living," at 89.

[1046] "The right to adequate clothing also assumes a special significance in the context of persons with disabilities who have particular clothing needs, so as to enable them to function fully and effectively in society. Wherever possible, appropriate personal assistance should also be provided in this connection. Such assistance should be undertaken in a manner and spirit which fully respect the human rights of the person(s) concerned": UN Committee on Economic, Social and Cultural Rights, "General Comment No. 5: Persons with disabilities" (1994), UN Doc. HRI/GEN/1/Rev.7, May 12, 2004, at 25, para. 33.

[1047] The Committee has thus far declined to issue a general definition of "adequacy," preferring to provide context-specific interpretive guidance (but the right to adequate clothing has not yet been the subject of a general comment).

invitation to discrimination[1048] or, at the very least, impede their ability to function in the asylum state. On the other hand, the right of refugees to choose to wear the clothing of their society or country of origin is logically protected by the right to cultural expression under Art. 27 of the Civil and Political Covenant,[1049] unless there are reasonable countervailing concerns, such as for the safety and well-being of the refugee.[1050]

Like the right to food, the Committee has identified the duty to provide "basic shelter and housing" as a core obligation of all state parties, whatever their circumstances.[1051] It has not, however, gone on specifically to elaborate the substance of that minimum obligation, except in a negative sense. The Committee determined in 1990 "that instances of forced eviction are *prima facie* incompatible with the requirements of the Covenant and can only be justified in the most exceptional circumstances, and in accordance with the

---

[1048] In another context, the Committee has seen a commitment to non-discrimination as relevant to the notion of "adequacy." In considering the right to education under Art. 13, the Committee held that "[t]he requirement that 'an adequate fellowship system shall be established' should be read with the Covenant's non-discrimination and equality provisions; the fellowship system should enhance equality of educational access for individuals from disadvantaged groups": UN Committee on Economic, Social and Cultural Rights, "General Comment No. 13: The right to education" (1999), UN Doc. HRI/GEN/1/Rev.7, May 12, 2004, at 71, para. 26.

[1049] "In those cases where aliens constitute a minority within the meaning of article 27, they shall not be denied the right, in community with other members of their group, to enjoy their own culture, to profess and practise their own religion and to use their own language. Aliens are entitled to equal protection by the law. There shall be no discrimination between aliens and citizens in the application of these rights. These rights of aliens may be qualified only by such limitations as may be lawfully imposed under the Covenant": UN Human Rights Committee, "General Comment No. 15: The position of aliens under the Covenant" (1986), UN Doc. HRI/GEN/1/Rev.7, May 12, 2004, at 140, para. 7.

[1050] In its decision in *Bhinder v. Canada*, UNHRC Comm. No. 208/1986, UN Doc. CCPR/C/37/D/208/1986, decided Nov. 9, 1989, the Human Rights Committee considered the case of a Sikh who, by reason of his religion, refused to wear safety headgear at work. Arguing that any safety risk was confined to himself, the Sikh claimed his freedom of religion was violated. The government countered that it was obliged by Art. 7(b) of the Economic Covenant to ensure a safe working environment for all. In dismissing the claim as inadmissible, the Human Rights Committee held that "[i]f the requirement that a hard hat be worn is seen as a discrimination de facto against persons of the Sikh religion ... then, applying criteria now well established in the jurisprudence of the Committee, the legislation requiring that workers in federal employment be protected from injury and electric shock by the wearing of hard hats is to be regarded as reasonable and directed towards objective purposes that are compatible with the Covenant": ibid. at para. 62.

[1051] UN Committee on Economic, Social and Cultural Rights, "General Comment No. 3: The nature of states parties' obligations" (1990), UN Doc. HRI/GEN/1/Rev.7, May 12, 2004, at 15, para. 10. See generally text above, at pp. 488–490.

relevant principles of international law."[1052] It has since developed this
position in a free-standing general comment.[1053] Perhaps most obviously,
"[f]orced eviction and house demolition as a punitive measure are ...
inconsistent with the norms of the Covenant."[1054] More generally, forced
eviction is to be an option of last resort,[1055] carefully regulated by law,[1056] and
"should not result in individuals being rendered homeless or vulnerable to
the violation of other human rights."[1057] The right to be protected against
forced eviction is specifically said to inhere in refugees and other involuntary
migrants:

> [T]he practice of forced evictions ... also takes place in connection with
> forced population transfers, internal displacement, forced relocations in
> the context of armed conflict, mass exoduses and refugee movements. In all
> of these contexts, the right to adequate housing and not to be subjected to
> forced eviction may be violated through a wide range of acts or omissions
> attributable to States parties. Even in situations where it may be necessary
> to impose limitations on such a right, full compliance with article 4 of the

[1052] UN Committee on Economic, Social and Cultural Rights, "General Comment No. 3:
The nature of states parties' obligations" (1990), UN Doc. HRI/GEN/1/Rev.7, May 12,
2004, at 15, para. 18.

[1053] UN Committee on Economic, Social and Cultural Rights, "General Comment No. 7:
The right to adequate housing (forced evictions)" (1997), UN Doc. HRI/GEN/1/Rev.7,
May 12, 2004, at 46. Interestingly, the African Commission on Human and Peoples'
Rights relied on General Comment No. 7 in a complaint brought on behalf of the people
of Ogoniland against Nigeria: *Social and Economic Rights Action Center and Center for
Economic and Social Rights v. Nigeria*, Case ACPHR/COMM/A044/1 (May 27, 2002), at
para. 63, reported at (2002) 96(4) *American Journal of International Law* 937.

[1054] UN Committee on Economic, Social and Cultural Rights, "General Comment No. 7:
The right to adequate housing (forced evictions)" (1997), UN Doc. HRI/GEN/1/Rev.7,
May 12, 2004, at 46, para. 12. The Committee observes that this right is grounded not
only in Art. 11 of the Economic Covenant, but also in "the Geneva Conventions of 1949
and Protocols thereto of 1977 concerning prohibitions on the displacement of the
civilian population and the destruction of private property": ibid.

[1055] "States parties shall ensure, prior to carrying out any evictions, and particularly those
involving large groups, that all feasible alternatives are explored in consultation with the
affected persons, with a view to avoiding, or at least minimizing, the need to use force":
ibid. at para. 13.

[1056] "Although the Committee has indicated in its General Comment No. 3 (1990) that such
measures may not be indispensable in relation to all rights, it is clear that legislation
against forced evictions is an essential basis upon which to build a system of effective
protection ... The legislation must also apply to all agents acting under the authority of
the State or who are accountable to it. Moreover, in view of the increasing trend in some
States towards the Government greatly reducing its responsibilities in the housing
sector, States parties must ensure that legislative and other measures are adequate to
prevent and, if appropriate, punish forced evictions carried out, without appropriate
safeguards, by private persons or bodies": ibid. at para. 9.

[1057] Ibid. at para. 16.

Covenant is required so that any limitations imposed must be "determined by law" only insofar as this may be compatible with the nature of these [i.e. economic, social, and cultural] rights and solely for the purpose of promoting the general welfare in a democratic society.[1058]

Beyond the duty stringently to curb resort to forced eviction, the affirmative content of the right to adequate housing "should not be interpreted in a narrow or restrictive sense which equates it with, for example, the shelter provided by merely having a roof over one's head or views shelter exclusively as a commodity. Rather it should be seen as the right to live somewhere in security, peace and dignity."[1059] This fundamental standard was clearly not met when Turkey forced Iraqi Kurds to live in open-air camps or uninsulated tents for prolonged periods, when Ethiopian refugees in Sudan failed to receive promised tents from UNHCR, or when Kosovar refugees were left without shelter in Albania. But the "security, peace and dignity" dimension of the right means that the right to housing was also infringed when Pakistan effectively forced Afghan refugees to choose between living in a place where their right to physical security could be respected (but where they would be given no rations) or moving to a place where they were at risk (but would be given food and other key supplies).

The "adequacy" of housing is moreover determined not only "by social, economic, cultural, climatic, ecological and other factors,"[1060] but also by reference to legal security of tenure, the availability of facilities and infrastructure, affordability, habitability, accessibility, location, and cultural adequacy.[1061] This standard was not met when Sahrawi refugees in Algeria received tents which could not withstand climatic conditions, in the case of refugees forced by the Bahamas to live in squalor in congested trailers, when Sudanese refugees in Ethiopia were granted no access to facilities for bathing or dishwashing, or when Roma refugees from Kosovo were provided with no sanitary facilities in Macedonia. The de facto relegation of Roma refugees to the periphery of Italian towns also raises concerns about access to basic services, as does the arbitrary assignment of refugee claimants in the United Kingdom to public housing in areas far from counseling and legal services critical to them.

[1058] Ibid. at para. 5.

[1059] UN Committee on Economic, Social and Cultural Rights, "General Comment No. 4: The right to adequate housing" (1991), UN Doc. HRI/GEN/1/Rev.7, May 12, 2004, at 19, para. 7.

[1060] Ibid. at para. 8.

[1061] Ibid. at para. 8(a)–(g). The Committee's general comment specifically endorses the conclusion of the Commission on Human Settlements and the Global Strategy for Shelter that "[a]dequate shelter means ... adequate privacy, adequate space, adequate security, adequate lighting and ventilation, adequate basic infrastructure and adequate location with regard to work and basic facilities – all at a reasonable cost": ibid. at para. 7.

In line with the general understanding of economic, social, and cultural rights set out above,[1062] the obligation of states to take affirmative action to ensure access to adequate housing applies with particular stringency in relation to marginalized or disadvantaged individuals and groups.[1063] Among the matters most vital to refugees, adequate shelter

> must contain certain facilities essential for health, security, comfort and nutrition. All beneficiaries of the right to adequate housing should have sustainable access to natural and common resources, safe drinking water, energy for cooking, heating and lighting, sanitation and washing facilities, means of food storage, refuse disposal, site drainage and emergency services.[1064]

It must also be habitable, in the sense that it provides the inhabitants "with adequate space and protect[s] them from cold, damp, heat, rain, wind or other threats to health, structural hazards, and disease vectors. The physical safety of occupants must be guaranteed as well."[1065] It is doubtful that this duty was met when refugee claimants in the United Kingdom were forced to live in areas where there were known risks of violent physical assaults. Nor was the habitability standard met when Honduras forced ten Nicaraguan refugees to share a single room, or when Spain and the Netherlands required refugees to live in grossly overcrowded refugee reception centers.

4.4.3 Access to healthcare

It is not surprising that inadequacies of food, water, and shelter take a major toll on refugee health.[1066] As previously described, the death rate among Angolan refugees in Zambia tripled when they lost access to clean water, while Iraqi refugees in Turkey forced to draw water from a polluted stream developed cholera and typhoid. In one particularly tragic example, the leading cause of death among children under the age of five in Tanzania's Lukole refugee camp was found to be acute respiratory tract infection. UNHCR's medical coordinator determined that the children's respiratory infections were the result of exposure to the cold, which usually took place

---

[1062] See text above, at pp. 497–499.

[1063] "States parties must give due priority to those social groups living in unfavourable conditions by giving them particular consideration. Policies and legislation should correspondingly not be designed to benefit already advantaged social groups at the expense of others": UN Committee on Economic, Social and Cultural Rights, "General Comment No. 4: The right to adequate housing" (1991), UN Doc. HRI/GEN/1/Rev.7, May 12, 2004, at 19, para. 11.

[1064] Ibid. at para. 8(b).   [1065] Ibid. at para. 8(d).

[1066] N. Van Hear and B. Harrell-Bond, "Refugees and Displaced People: Health Issues," in UN Institute for Training and Research ed., *The Challenge of African Disasters* (1991) (Van Hear and Harrell-Bond, "Health Issues"), at 61.

because mothers needed to go farming early in the morning, taking their children with them because no alternative care was available.[1067] In thinking about how best to secure the necessities of life for refugees, it is therefore critical to focus on the interrelationship between food, shelter, and health. As David Keen cogently observed,

> Filling the refugees' bowls may not keep them alive. Typically, it is not simply hunger that kills refugees, but a complicated interaction between hunger and disease. Disease prevention and treatment has a critical role to play. This need not cost the earth. In fact, simple health initiatives can save more lives than high-tech medical treatments – in part because they focus on prevention and in part because they can reach much larger numbers.[1068]

Particularly successful refugee primary healthcare initiatives, such as that undertaken in Somalia during the late 1980s, therefore focus on providing food, water, and shelter, as well as on immunizing refugees against common diseases, and treating at least the most prevalent post-flight health concerns.[1069] More generally, some asylum countries have been quick to respond to the need of refugees for access to medical care. Malawi, for example, integrated refugee healthcare with the national health service, ensuring equal access to refugees in camps and those who had moved into the population at large.[1070] And when confronted with millions of Afghan refugees, Iranian authorities wisely minimized the risk of epidemic by mobilizing doctors and medicine to treat the refugees for malaria, tuberculosis, and other diseases upon arrival, and by granting them completely free access to their own hospitals.[1071]

In stark contrast, virtually no healthcare was provided to Chakma refugees in India.[1072] The 1,200 Liberian refugees in a Nigerian camp had access to a doctor only one day per week, with no emergency access to hospitals.[1073] Thai authorities provided no medical care to even severely ill patients in Khmer Rouge refugee camps.[1074] Shortages of drugs and other medical supplies were

---

[1067] (2001) 86 *JRS Dispatches* (Feb. 3, 2001).   [1068] Keen, *Right to Life*, at 20.

[1069] Van Hear and Harrell-Bond, "Health Issues," at 69. See also World Health Organization and UNICEF, *Primary Health Care* (1978) and UNHCR, *Handbook for Emergencies* (1982).

[1070] D. Kuntz and Refugee Policy Group, "Serving the Health Needs of Refugees in Malawi: An Integrated Approach" (1990).

[1071] A. Billard, "Afghan Refugees: Health the Number One Concern," (1986) 26 *Refugees* 12.

[1072] B. S. Chimni, *International Academy of Comparative Law National Report for India* (1994), at 27.

[1073] A nursing superintendent and assistant were available at the camp five days per week, during working hours: P. Tiao and Nigerian Civil Liberties Organization, "The Status of Refugee Rights in Nigeria" (1992) (Tiao, "Refugee Rights in Nigeria"), at 10.

[1074] Banbury, "Kampuchean Displaced Persons in Thailand," at 27.

also pervasive in refugee camps inside Ethiopia and the Sudan.[1075] In particular, the failure to immunize refugees in Sudan in 1985 resulted in "a major epidemic, with the death rate from measles in one camp as high as one in every three cases diagnosed."[1076] In South Africa, refugees in principle enjoy the right to access healthcare, but "many refugees are finding a vast chasm between theory and practice, with medical personnel at many facilities acting as self-appointed 'gatekeepers' who restrict and even deny their access to health care."[1077] One South African nurse reportedly chased an Angolan refugee seeking immunization of her child away from a Mpumalanga clinic, shouting that "she, a foreigner, was eating South African medicines."[1078]

Even when healthcare is provided, it may fail to take account of linguistic, cultural, and social barriers. For example, none of the four doctors assigned to the Kiziltepe camps for Iraqi Kurds in Turkey spoke Kurdish.[1079] The health needs of women refugees are perhaps most frequently neglected. In order to secure permission to leave camps in Zambia, many refugee women have agreed to marriages of convenience to Zambian men. Yet until UNHCR organized funding for an education initiative in 2001, these women received none of the HIV/AIDS education provided by Zambia to its own citizens, roughly 20 percent of whom are HIV-positive.[1080] Female Afghan refugees in Pakistan felt unable personally to visit doctors in public health units because of the need to respect *purdah* rules (requiring the seclusion of females). Instead, a male relative was sent to explain the female's ailment to a doctor.[1081] A camp for Liberian refugees in Nigeria was reported to lack "virtually

---

[1075] US, "Living Conditions," at 14, 22. In the case of Sudan, problems attributable to resource insufficiency were exacerbated by logistical barriers imposed by the government. "[T]he denial of flight clearance to the area resulted in a shortage of medicine for the treatment of ongoing epidemic diseases and immunization programmes for children": UN Operation Lifeline Sudan, "Sudan Monthly Information Report," Apr. 1, 1997.

[1076] Keen, *Right to Life*, at 20.

[1077] *Mail & Guardian*, Sept. 25, 2000. "Even though refugees are entitled to the same constitutional rights as South Africans, they often end up competing with locals for access to essential social services provided by the government, and losing. 'Often they run into anti-foreign sentiments at clinics or other places where they should receive services. Also, they often do not have the papers they need to access services to which they are entitled,' explained Vincent Williams of the Southern African Migration Project": "Xenophobia, red tape hurts refugees," *IOL (Independent Online)*, June 20, 2003.

[1078] *Mail & Guardian*, Sept. 25, 2000. The same report notes that "[i]n some hospitals, particularly those not in the urban centers of the country, refugees are treated as so-called private patients and forced to pay exorbitant fees for medical treatment": ibid.

[1079] IHRK, "Kurdish Refugees," at 15.

[1080] *UN Integrated Regional Information Networks*, Sept. 6, 2001.

[1081] US, "Living Conditions," at 51. In response to this problem, a system of home visits by "lady health visitors" was successfully established: D. Wulf, *Refugee Women and Reproductive Health Care: Reassessing Priorities* (1994) (Wulf, *Refugee Women*), at 41.

all child-birth equipment and facilities, and [was] also deficient in important pre-natal and post-natal drugs and supplements."[1082] Even seemingly gender-neutral issues such as poor sanitation in overcrowded refugee camps affect women the most "because it is they who have to cope with frequent pregnancies and with children's illnesses."[1083] In the end, "[t]he issue of women's health care is of particular importance because, when a woman becomes ill or incapacitated, or dies, the whole family structure is likely to collapse."[1084]

Access to healthcare also varies considerably for refugee claimants across developed states. Some countries, including France, the Netherlands, and Norway provide refugees full access to their national healthcare systems.[1085] Yet even in such countries, refugee health needs may not really be met. In Britain, the mandatory dispersal policies mean that some asylum-seekers are required to live in parts of the country where, for example, there are no facilities for the treatment of victims of torture.[1086] There have also been reports that refugee claimants have been refused psychological treatment by National Health Service doctors "on the grounds that they are too trauma-tised, too time consuming and have little grasp of the English language."[1087]

In Germany and Sweden, access to public health services is granted only for emergencies.[1088] In the United States, where there is no national healthcare system even for citizens, refugees must usually turn to whatever emergency healthcare facilities have been established by particular municipalities or organizations to assist the domestic poor. Nor are refugees in the United States exempted from the effect of the 1996 welfare law reform, under which lawful immigrants have only limited access to health, nutrition, and other public benefits.[1089]

[1082] Tiao, "Refugee Rights in Nigeria," at 13. See generally Wulf, *Refugee Women.*
[1083] Camus-Jacques, "Forgotten Majority," at 148.   [1084] Ibid.
[1085] Liebaut, *Conditions 2000*, at 97, 216, and 234.
[1086] A. Travis, "'Patchy' refugee checks a health risk, warns BMA," *Guardian*, April 24, 2001, at 9; H. Carter, "Christmas charity appeal: Hard life in exile for women's rights pioneers," *Guardian*, Dec. 8, 2001, at 15. A 2001 study of service provision to refugee claimants housed in West Yorkshire found that "[m]ental health needs are often unmet": R. Wilson, "Dispersed: A Study of Services for Asylum Seekers in West Yorkshire" (2001), at 2–3.
[1087] J. Carvel, "Mental health care denied to refugees," *Guardian*, June 4, 2002, at 6. The same report noted that doctors "working with refugees in north London were shocked by a confidential letter from Barnet, Enfield and Haringey mental health NHS trust saying it would accept no more refugees for psychological therapy": ibid.
[1088] Liebaut, *Conditions 2000*, at 117, 282.
[1089] William Branigin, "'Chilling effects' seen from welfare reform: Caseload drops sharper among immigrants," *Washington Post*, Mar. 9, 1999, at A-06. See J. Frederiksson, "Bridging the Gap Between Rights and Responsibilities: Policy Changes Affecting Refugees and Immigrants in the United States Since 1996," (2000) 14(3) *Georgetown Journal of Immigration Law* 757, at 760–761.

Economic, Social and Cultural Covenant, Art. 12(1)
The States Parties to the present Covenant recognize the right of everyone to the enjoyment of the highest attainable standard of physical and mental health.

Art. 12 of the Economic Covenant is not, of course, a right to "be healthy," in the sense of imposing a duty to eradicate all disease or infirmity.[1090] Art. 12 defines a more limited right, consisting of certain immediately applicable freedoms from interference – for example, to non-interference with sexual and reproductive choices, as well as not to be subjected to medical experimentation[1091] – and an affirmative entitlement to access on a timely basis to a system of health protection which is both of good quality and respectful of cultural and individual concerns.[1092] Art. 12(2) sets out a non-exhaustive list of steps to be taken by states in implementing the right to health, including the improvement of infant and child healthcare, environmental and industrial hygiene, prevention and control of epidemics and disease, and medical service in the event of sickness.[1093]

The affirmative element of the right to health is by and large subject to the usual duty of progressive implementation. The supervisory committee has accordingly held that "[t]he notion of 'the highest attainable standard of health' in article 12.1 takes into account both the individual's biological and

---

[1090] A broader understanding of "health" is endorsed by the World Health Organization: see K. Tomasevski, "Health Rights," in A. Eide et al. eds., *Economic, Social and Cultural Rights: A Textbook* 125 (1995), at 128. But as the Committee on Economic, Social and Cultural Rights has confirmed, "[i]n drafting article 12 of the Covenant, the Third Committee of the United Nations General Assembly did not adopt the definition of health contained in the preamble to the Constitution of WHO, which conceptualizes health as 'a state of complete physical, mental and social well-being and not merely the absence of disease or infirmity'": UN Committee on Economic, Social and Cultural Rights, "General Comment No. 14: The right to the highest attainable standard of health" (2000), UN Doc. HRI/GEN/1/Rev.7, May 12, 2004, at 86, para. 4.

[1091] UN Committee on Economic, Social and Cultural Rights, "General Comment No. 14: The right to the highest attainable standard of health" (2000), UN Doc. HRI/GEN/1/Rev.7, May 12, 2004, at 86, para. 8. At its 2001 session, the UN Commission on Human Rights "note[d] with interest" General Comment No. 14 of the Committee on Economic, Social and Cultural Rights: UNCHR Res. 2001/30, UN Doc. E/CN.4/RES/2001/30, Apr. 20, 2001, at para. 2(b).

[1092] The elements of availability, accessibility, acceptability, and quality are defined in some detail in UN Committee on Economic, Social and Cultural Rights, "General Comment No. 14: The right to the highest attainable standard of health" (2000), UN Doc. HRI/GEN/1/Rev.7, May 12, 2004, at 86, paras. 12(a)–(d).

[1093] "The non-exhaustive catalogue of examples in article 12.2 provides guidance in defining the action to be taken by States. It gives specific generic examples of measures arising from the broad definition of the right to health contained in article 12.1, thereby illustrating the content of that right": ibid. at para. 13.

socio-economic preconditions and a State's available resources."[1094] As such, state parties with the resources to implement the right to health may not lawfully decide to refrain from taking the necessary steps fully to implement Art. 12. Because of its comparative wealth, Nigeria would therefore have a difficult time justifying its failure to provide emergency medical facilities or reasonable access to doctors to Liberian refugees.[1095] It would similarly not be open to countries such as Germany or Sweden to deny refugees access to other than purely emergency healthcare, nor to the United States to avoid its responsibility to treat healthcare for refugees and others as an essential public service.

Even states with insufficient resources must nonetheless give priority to the realization of the right to health without discrimination of any kind.[1096] Indeed, the Committee has expressly held that governments are under an "obligation to respect the right to health by, *inter alia*, refraining from denying or limiting equal access [to healthcare] for all persons, including . . . asylum-seekers and illegal immigrants."[1097] This critical duty of

---

[1094] Ibid. at para. 9. This flexibility has led two commentators to the perhaps overstated conclusion that "the amount a nation can afford to spend on the pursuit of health is what it chooses to spend": P. Townsend and N. Davidson, "The Black Report: Inequalities in Health" (1982), at 27. In fact, the Committee on Economic, Social and Cultural Rights has made clear that "[t]he central obligation in relation to the Covenant is for States parties to give effect to the rights recognized therein. By requiring Governments to do so 'by all appropriate means,' the Covenant adopts a broad and flexible approach which enables the particularities of the legal and administrative systems of each State, as well as other relevant considerations, to be taken into account . . . But this flexibility coexists with the obligation upon each State party to use all the means at its disposal to give effect to the rights recognized in the Covenant": UN Committee on Economic, Social and Cultural Rights, "General Comment No. 9: The domestic application of the Covenant" (1998), UN Doc. HRI/GEN/1/Rev.7, May 12, 2004, at 55, paras. 1–2.

[1095] "A State which is unwilling to use the maximum of its available resources for the realization of the right to health is in violation of its obligations under article 12": UN Committee on Economic, Social and Cultural Rights, "General Comment No. 14: The right to the highest attainable standard of health" (2000), UN Doc. HRI/GEN/1/Rev.7, May 12, 2004, at 86, para. 47.

[1096] "While the Covenant provides for progressive realization and acknowledges the constraints due to the limits of available resources, it also imposes on States parties various obligations which are of immediate effect. States parties have immediate obligations in relation to the right to health, such as the guarantee that the right will be exercised without discrimination of any kind (art. 2.2) and the obligation to take steps (art. 2.1) towards the full realization of article 12. Such steps must be deliberate, concrete and targeted towards the full realization of the right to health": ibid. at para. 30. See chapter 4.4.2 above, at pp. 485–486.

[1097] UN Committee on Economic, Social and Cultural Rights, "General Comment No. 14: The right to the highest attainable standard of health" (2000), UN Doc. HRI/GEN/1/Rev.7, May 12, 2004, at 86, para. 34.

non-discrimination means that India's decision to deny healthcare to Chakma refugees and Thailand's refusal to allow Khmer refugees to receive medical treatment were not lawful.

Of particular importance to refugees in the less developed world, the right to "essential primary health care" is one of the four core entitlements of all persons, whatever the circumstances of the host state.[1098] Indeed, the Committee on Economic, Social and Cultural Rights has taken the unprecedented step of declaring that "a State party cannot, under any circumstances whatsoever, justify its non-compliance with the core obligations [to provide healthcare], which are non-derogable."[1099] The substance of this non-derogable responsibility to provide essential primary healthcare comprises the duty of non-discrimination in access to healthcare, as well as freedom from hunger and access to basic shelter, sanitation, and water.[1100] South Africa was therefore under a duty to ensure that healthcare professionals ceased acting as vigilante gatekeepers seeking to limit scarce medical resources for citizens only. More specifically, the right to essential primary healthcare binds all state parties to "provide essential drugs, as from time to time defined under the WHO Action Program on Essential Drugs."[1101]

To ensure accountability for its duty to implement the right to health, no government may be excused from enacting and implementing a transparent and socially inclusive public health strategy, which must give priority to the needs of vulnerable or marginalized groups.[1102] It is highly doubtful that Turkey's unwillingness to provide Iraqi Kurds with access to doctors able to speak their language would meet this standard. Nor would the British decision to implement a dispersal policy which effectively prevented refugees

---

[1098] See chapter 4.4.2 above, at pp. 489–490.

[1099] UN Committee on Economic, Social and Cultural Rights, "General Comment No. 14: The right to the highest attainable standard of health" (2000), UN Doc. HRI/GEN/1/Rev.7, May 12, 2004, at 86, para. 47.

[1100] "[T]hese core obligations include at least the following obligations: (a) To ensure the right of access to health facilities, goods and services on a non-discriminatory basis, especially for vulnerable or marginalized groups; (b) To ensure access to the minimum essential food which is nutritionally adequate and safe, to ensure freedom from hunger to everyone; (c) To ensure access to basic shelter, housing and sanitation, and an adequate supply of safe and potable water; ... (e) To ensure equitable distribution of all health facilities, goods and services": ibid. at para. 43.

[1101] Ibid. at para. 43(d).

[1102] "[T]hese core obligations include at least the following obligations ... (f) To adopt and implement a national public health strategy and plan of action, on the basis of epidemiological evidence, addressing the health concerns of the whole population; the strategy and plan of action shall be devised, and periodically reviewed, on the basis of a participatory and transparent process; they shall include methods, such as right to health indicators and benchmarks, by which progress can be closely monitored; the process by which the strategy and plan of action are devised, as well as their content, shall give particular attention to all vulnerable or marginalized groups": ibid. at para. 43(f).

from accessing torture victim and other specialized health treatment facilities be in line with Art. 12. And perhaps most important, this requirement leaves no room to argue that the right to healthcare is respected when little or no attention is given to the specific reproductive and other health needs of women. For example, there was a clear duty on Pakistan to make female doctors available to female Afghan refugees who otherwise were culturally barred from any direct access to healthcare.

Finally, the Committee has established what amounts to a policy of strict scrutiny of another set of steps, defined as being of "comparable priority" to the non-derogable duties within the core of the duty to provide all with essential primary healthcare. These presumptive duties of immediate implementation include the provision of reproductive, pre-natal, and maternal healthcare; immunization against prevalent diseases; the control of epidemic and endemic diseases; and education and training on the prevention and control of disease and on health and human rights more generally.[1103] While a state is not held to an absolute standard of achievement in relation to these rights, non-implementation can be justified only on the basis of a true resource insufficiency.[1104] Thus, Sudan's failure to immunize refugees against a major measles outbreak was presumptively in breach of the Economic Covenant. Nigeria would be hard pressed to explain its failure to provide even basic maternal and post-natal care facilities to Liberian refugees. And Zambia, fully aware of the vital health risks for refugee women posed by widespread HIV infection in that country, would be held to a very high standard to justify its refusal to extend its general program of HIV education for women to refugee women as well.

4.5 Property rights

On occasion, refugees may be the victims of confiscation of their property. For example, refugee-specific legislation in both Uganda and Kenya provides for the confinement and slaughter of any animal brought into the country by

---

[1103] "The Committee also confirms that the following are obligations of comparable priority: (a) To ensure reproductive, maternal (pre-natal as well as post-natal) and child health care; (b) To provide immunization against the major infectious diseases occurring in the community; (c) To take measures to prevent, treat and control epidemic and endemic diseases; (d) To provide education and access to information concerning the main health problems in the community, including methods of preventing and controlling them; (e) To provide appropriate training for health personnel, including education on health and human rights": ibid. at para. 44.

[1104] "If resource constraints render it impossible for a State to comply fully with its Covenant obligations, it has the burden of justifying that every effort has nevertheless been made to use all available resources at its disposal in order to satisfy, as a matter of priority, the obligations outlined above": ibid. at para. 47.

a refugee.[1105] The net proceeds, if any, from the sale of the slaughtered animal are to be paid to the refugee if possible, and otherwise used for the support of refugees in general.[1106] This procedure is distinct from the right of authorities to slaughter diseased animals, in which case no compensation is payable to the refugee.[1107] The laws of these same countries also provide that any vehicle in which a refugee arrives may be commandeered by authorities to move refugees or stores or equipment for their use. No compensation is payable either for use of the vehicle, or for any consequential damage to it.[1108]

While confiscations of this kind are comparatively rare, refugees more frequently face restrictions on their ability to acquire and deal with personal property in asylum states. Restrictions may be refugee-specific, as in the case of the refusal by Botswana to allow refugees to own cattle.[1109] Refugees in Malawi enjoyed only restricted access to "natural resources – trees, land, natural building materials and wild woods ... [E]ven some types of wild edible insects and rodents were 'owned' by local landowners."[1110] More commonly, however, refugees are subject to general limitations on the acquisition of personal property applied to all foreigners. In the United States, for example, non-citizens may not own commercial radio stations[1111] or atomic energy facilities,[1112] and may not acquire federal mineral rights.[1113]

[1105] E. Khiddu-Makubuya, *International Academy of Comparative Law National Report for Uganda* (1994), at 7–8.

[1106] C. Maina Peter, "Rights and Duties of Refugees under Domestic Law: The Case of Tanzania," (1995) (Maina Peter, "Tanzania"), at 7–8; A. Kiapi, "The Legal Status of Refugees in Uganda: A Critical Study of Legislative Instruments" (1993) (Kiapi, "Uganda"), at 14.

[1107] Kiapi, "Uganda," at 14.   [1108] Maina Peter, "Tanzania," at 8; Kiapi, "Uganda," at 14.

[1109] J. Zetterqvist, *Refugees in Botswana in the Light of International Law* (1990), at 40.

[1110] Keen, *Right to Life*, at 56. In 2001, Malawi proposed a policy under which only citizens would be allowed to own freehold land, with non-citizens expected to become citizens in order to retain long-term title to their land: "Proposals to prohibit foreign land ownership," *UN Integrated Regional Information Networks*, Dec. 5, 2001.

[1111] "No broadcast ... radio station license shall be granted to or held by ... any alien or the representative of any alien": 47 USC §310(b)(1). In *Campos v. Federal Communications Commission*, (1981) 650 F 2d 890 (US CA7, June 3, 1981), it was determined that the section prohibiting the granting of radio operator licenses to non-citizens did not violate due process guarantees.

[1112] "No license may be issued to an alien or any corporation or other entity if the [Atomic Energy] Commission knows or has reason to believe it is owned, controlled, or dominated by an alien": 42 USC §2133(d). This prohibition applies even in the case of non-citizens seeking an atomic energy license for medical therapy purposes: 42 USC §2134(d).

[1113] "Except as otherwise provided, all valuable mineral deposits in lands belonging to the United States ... shall be free and open to exploration and purchase, and the lands in which they are found to occupation and purchase, by citizens of the United States and those who have declared their intention to become such": 30 USC §22.

Land ownership and tenure is undoubtedly the most sensitive area of all. In some countries, including Kenya,[1114] Sudan,[1115] Bulgaria,[1116] and Hungary,[1117] non-citizens are simply prohibited from owning land. Luxembourg and Venezuela limit the right of property ownership to citizens and persons authorized to reside in the state.[1118] Mexico[1119] and San Marino[1120] are among the nations which insist on the right to impose restrictions on the scope of the right of non-nationals to own land. In Namibia, it is a crime to sell agricultural land to a non-Namibian without

[1114] In Kenya, "land is not granted to foreigners irrespective of status because of the sensitivity of the land issue": "Implementation of the OAU/UN Conventions and Domestic Legislation Concerning the Rights and Obligations of Refugees in Africa," Final Report of a Conference sponsored by the Refugee Studies Programme, Oxford University, Sept. 14–28, 1986, at 33. "[T]he Kenya Government has in the past opposed any attempts to allow refugees access to land on the pretext that it is a very scarce and sensitive commodity. The new regime has, however, made a statement of intent to give land for resettling refugees so as to make them a little more self-reliant. Nothing has yet taken shape": J. Okamu (Center for Refugee Studies, Moi University), personal communication, Oct. 2, 2003.

[1115] G. Kibreab, *Refugees and Development in Africa: The Case of Eritrea* (1987) (Kibreab, *Development*), at 73.

[1116] "No foreign physical person or foreign legal entity shall acquire ownership over land, except through legal inheritance. Ownership thus acquired shall be duly transferred": Constitution of the Republic of Bulgaria, Art. 22, cited in Reservation of Bulgaria to the First Protocol to the European Convention on Human Rights and Fundamental Freedoms, Sept. 7, 1992, available at www.coe.fr (accessed Nov. 19, 2004).

[1117] D. Weissbrodt, "Final report of the Special Rapporteur on the rights of non-citizens," UN Doc. E/CN.4/Sub.2/2003/23/Add.3, May 26, 2003, at para. 20.

[1118] "The right of everyone to own property alone as well as in association with others, completed final report submitted by Mr. Luis Valencia Rodríquez, Independent Expert, to the United Nations Commission on Human Rights," UN Doc. E/CN.4/1994/19, Nov. 25, 1993, at paras. 86 and 103.

[1119] "The Mexican constitution regulates the ownership of its territory and establishes that '... in a zone of 100 km along the border or 50 km along the coast, a foreigner cannot acquire direct domain of the land and waters'": B. Walsten and D. Christi, "Foreigners Can Own Property in Mexico," available at www.flash.net/~mexis (accessed Nov. 18, 1997). See also I. Head, *International Law, National Tribunals, and the Rights of Aliens* (1971), at 237, citing Honduras and Peru as insisting upon restrictions comparable to those imposed by Mexico.

[1120] "The Government of the Republic of San Marino declares that having regard to the provisions of law in force which govern the use of goods in conformity with the general interest, the principle set forth in Article 1 of the Additional Protocol to the Convention for the Protection of Human Rights and Fundamental Freedoms, opened for signature, in Paris, on 20 March 1952, has no bearing on the regulations in force concerning the real estate of foreign citizens": Reservation of San Marino to the First Protocol to the European Convention on Human Rights and Fundamental Freedoms, Mar. 22, 1989, available at www.coe.fr (accessed Nov. 19, 2004).

the permission of the Minister of Lands.[1121] Similarly, New Zealand law allows foreign investment in farmland only if it can be proved to result in "substantial and identifiable benefits" to New Zealand.[1122]

In other countries, refugees face difficulties in even leasing land. Officials in both Honduras and Mexico, for example, often prevented refugees from renting land during the late 1980s.[1123] Refugees in much of Africa have been granted the use of land, but subject to limited rights of occupancy determined by customary law. In Sudan, for example, the security of land tenure for refugees is limited to between twelve and twenty-five years,[1124] and arbitrary eviction by fellow refugees has not been effectively constrained.[1125] Elsewhere in Africa the maximum plot size allocated to refugees has often been insufficient to be economically viable,[1126] or has been conditional on the growing of compulsory types of crops.[1127]

4.5.1 Movable and immovable property rights

Refugee Convention, Art. 13   Movable and immovable property
The Contracting States shall accord to a refugee treatment as favourable as possible and, in any event, not less favourable than that accorded to aliens generally in the same circumstances, as regards the acquisition of movable and immovable property and other rights pertaining thereto, and to leases and other contracts relating to movable and immovable property.

[1121] "The person who sold or otherwise disposed of that agricultural land to the foreign national or nominee owner shall ... be guilty of an offence and be liable on conviction to a fine not exceeding N$100,000 or to imprisonment for a term not exceeding five years or to both": "Foreigners face farmland squeeze," *Namibian*, Sept. 18, 2002.

[1122] D. Weissbrodt, "Final report of the Special Rapporteur on the rights of non-citizens," UN Doc. E/CN.4/Sub.2/2003/23/Add.3, May 26, 2003, at para. 21.

[1123] Keen, *Right to Life*, at 56.

[1124] "Implementation of the OAU/UN Conventions and Domestic Legislation Concerning the Rights and Obligations of Refugees in Africa," Final Report of a Conference sponsored by the Refugee Studies Programme, Oxford University, Sept. 14–28, 1986, at 33.

[1125] G. Kibreab, "Rural Refugee Land Settlements in Eastern Sudan: On the Road to Self-Sufficiency?," in P. Nobel ed., *Refugees and Development in Africa* 63 (1987), at 65.

[1126] Keen, *Right to Life*, at 56.

[1127] "[I]n the Sudan's New Halfa scheme ... tenancies were distributed to the newcomers to grow compulsory crops of cotton, wheat and ground-nuts. Lack of control over their allocated farms discourages settlers from fully committing themselves to agricultural production": V. Lassailly-Jacob, "Government-Sponsored Agricultural Schemes for Involuntary Migrants in Africa: Some Key Obstacles to Their Economic Viability," in H. Adelman and J. Sorenson eds., *African Refugees: Development Aid and Repatriation* 209 (1994), at 217.

The human right to own and to possess property enjoys a tenuous place in international law. It is usually said that controversy about the status of the right to property derives from a capitalist–socialist philosophical divide,[1128] with the right to property championed predominantly by Western countries.[1129] And it is certainly true that the status of property rights is more highly contested in the less developed world. As Gudmundur Alfredsson has observed,

> Property rights have been criticized as standing in the way of progress: from the owning of slaves to the exploitation of others through *apartheid* and transnational corporations. The importance of property rights is often deemed to pale against the background of other problems, such as hunger, poverty and misery ... The overall concentration of most of the world's property in the hands of a comparative few, especially in times of population growth and scarcity of resources, makes property rights seem more part of the problem than an interest entitled to protection.[1130]

Indeed, when the assets of the three richest individuals in the world exceed the combined GNP of all the least developed countries and their 600 million inhabitants,[1131] it is difficult to question this deep-seated skepticism about the value of private property rights.

Even in avowedly market-oriented countries, however, the content and legal standing of the right to own private property is significantly less robust than, for example, Locke's classic notion that the advancement of property rights is at the core of a state's responsibility.[1132] It is particularly noteworthy

---

[1128] See e.g. C. Krause, "The Right to Property," in A. Eide et al. eds., *Economic, Social and Cultural Rights: A Textbook* 143 (1995) (Krause, "Property"), at 144–145: "Western countries, with the United States in the forefront, have tended to proclaim a strong protection of the right to property, whereas the socialist countries and the Third World have emphasized the social function of property, allowing for interference with property rights in the name of public interest ... In spite of decreasing ideological and political tensions concerning property rights, the protection of property rights will remain a matter of controversy ... Property rights are closely connected with the social and economic policies of States and thus there will always be a certain amount of reluctance towards international supervision of these rights."

[1129] See A. Rosas, "Property Rights," in A. Rosas and J. Helgesen, *The Strength of Diversity: Human Rights and Pluralist Democracy* 133 (1992), at 146. "The Constitution and basic laws of most if not all Western countries have long guaranteed the right to property. This right is part and parcel of their very form of government": G. Alfredsson, "Article 17," in A. Eide et al. eds., *The Universal Declaration of Human Rights: A Commentary* 255 (1992) (Alfredsson, "Article 17"), at 255.

[1130] Alfredsson, "Article 17," at 260.

[1131] United Nations Development Program, *Human Development Report 1999* (1999), at 3.

[1132] "The great and chief end ... of men's uniting into commonwealths, and putting themselves under government, is the preservation of their property; to which in the state of nature there are many things wanting ... The reason why men enter into that property rights were not originally included even in the European Convention on Human Rights and Fundamental Freedoms.[1133] When ultimately enacted in Europe as part of Protocol No. 1 to the Convention, the right to property was meekly framed as a right of "[e]very natural or legal person ... to the peaceful enjoyment of his possessions. No one shall be deprived of his possessions except in the public interest and subject to the conditions of international law."[1134] Not only is the right to acquire property not explicitly enacted, but the right of peaceful enjoyment can be trumped by "the right of a State to enforce such laws as it deems necessary to control the use of property in accordance with the general interest."[1135]

The only general and universal formulation of the right to property is found in Art. 17 of the non-binding Universal Declaration of Human Rights, which proclaims a right both to own property individually and collectively, and to be protected against the arbitrary deprivation of property.[1136] This is clearly a fairly rudimentary version of a right to private property. In particular, unlike even the European norm, it does not specifically require undisturbed enjoyment of property. Nor does it take a position on the historically contentious issue of the standard of compensation that must be paid in the event of confiscation.[1137] And it certainly does not posit the right of every

society, is the preservation of their property; and the end why they choose and authorize a legislative, is, that there may be laws made, and rules set, as guards and fences to the properties of all the members of the society, to limit the power, and to moderate the dominion, of every part and member of the society: for since it can never be supposed to be the will of the society, that the legislative should have the power to destroy that which every one desires to secure, by entering into society, and for which the people submitted themselves to the legislators of their own making": J. Locke, *The Second Treatise on Civil Government and a Letter Concerning Toleration* (1690), at ss. 124, 222.

[1133] Krause notes that "[t]he right to property was included in the draft text passed by the Consultative Assembly. However, the Committee of Ministers felt ... that inclusion of the right to property would delay the entering into force of the Convention": Krause, "Property," at 146, n. 13.

[1134] Protocol No. 1 to the Convention for the Protection of Human Rights and Fundamental Freedoms, done Mar. 20, 1952, at Art. 1, incorporated in the European Convention for the Protection of Human Rights and Fundamental Freedoms, 213 UNTS 221, done Nov. 4, 1950, entered into force Sept. 3, 1953 (ECHR Protocol No. 1). As elaborated in the caselaw of the European Court of Human Rights, however, the notion of "possessions" includes the full range of property interests, and the right of peaceful enjoyment has been held to constrain even de facto expropriation: Krause, "Property," at 150–151.

[1135] ECHR Protocol No. 1.

[1136] "Everyone has the right to own property alone as well as in association with others. No one shall be arbitrarily deprived of his property": Universal Declaration, at Art. 17.

[1137] The essential difference of view has been between those (mostly capitalist) states which assert the right to "prompt, adequate and effective compensation," contrasted with the preference of other (mostly developing) countries for a less rigorous standard of compensation. See generally R. Higgins, "The Taking of Property by the State," (1982) *Recueil des Cours* 259.

person actually to own property.[1138] In part because agreement could not be reached on these more specific concerns that would have to be addressed before the right to property could be made legally enforceable, the right to property was one of only two standards[1139] in the Universal Declaration which failed to attract support for codification as a binding legal standard in either of the two Covenants on Human Rights.[1140]

Nor has the end of the Cold War resolved these tensions. The centrality of property to each state's understanding of its basic political and social values[1141] continues to make it exceedingly difficult to arrive at a universally binding standard acceptable to all. Property rights can be understood as a classic civil right mandating no more than non-interference – freedom from deprivation, or at least from arbitrary or inadequately compensated confiscation. But they can also be understood as affirmative socioeconomic rights – access to the means by which human needs are satisfied. While virtually every state is to some extent committed to the property rights project, many states are not yet prepared to bind themselves to respect both the negative and positive meanings of a right to property.[1142] Thus, the jurisprudence of the Human Rights Committee has confirmed that property rights are not a specifically protected interest under the Civil and Political Covenant,[1143] and a more recent initiative in the Commission on Human Rights to promote

---

[1138] Interestingly, however, the French language text suggests a stronger basis for an affirmative right to property ("droit à la propriété," rather than "right to own property").

[1139] The other right that was not made binding is the right to be protected against unemployment, found in Art. 23 of the Universal Declaration of Human Rights.

[1140] "Notwithstanding several proposals, no such article was adopted. In lengthy debates there was disagreement on practically every aspect of the topic . . . including such issues as the scope of property, conformity with State laws, expropriation and other allowable limitations, due process of law, compensation and indeed the very inclusion of the right": Alfredsson, "Article 17," at 259.

[1141] "The importance of the concept of property goes far beyond the legal sphere, as it constitutes the basic factor in the prevailing economic system within a specific society and the most fundamental variable of its social order. Its links with the political programme accepted within that society are therefore manifest. Furthermore, its philosophical and ethical implications are obvious": "The right of everyone to own property alone as well as in association with others, completed final report submitted by Mr. Luis Valencia Rodríquez, Independent Expert, to the United Nations Commission on Human Rights," UN Doc. E/CN.4/1994/19, Nov. 25, 1993, at para. 63.

[1142] "The varying opinions on and approaches to the right to property stand as textbook examples of the different cultures and economic systems of our modern world. Rich and poor, free marketeers and socialists, all see it with their own eyes. Needless to say, the conflict remains unresolved": Alfredsson, "Article 17," at 261.

[1143] "The right to property . . . is not protected by the International Covenant on Civil and Political Rights": *OJ v. Finland*, UNHRC Comm. No. 419/1990, UN Doc. CCPR/C/40/D/419/1990, decided Nov. 6, 1990, at para. 3.2. Property rights may, however, be indirectly protected by virtue of the duty of non-discrimination: see chapter 2.5.5 above, at pp. 126–128.

property rights within a socioeconomic context[1144] did not result in any new normative consensus.[1145] We are therefore left with little more than a patchwork of regional guarantees of property rights.[1146]

While universal treaties do not set a right to property as such, they do require respect for the principle of non-discrimination in relation to whatever property rights may be enacted in a given state.[1147] The guarantee of non-discrimination can, in practice, be an important means to contest the legal validity of restrictions on property rights imposed on aliens generally, or

---

[1144] The Universal Declaration, the International Convention on the Elimination of All Forms of Racial Discrimination, UNGA Res. 2106A(XX), adopted Dec. 21, 1965, entered into force Jan. 4, 1969 (Racial Discrimination Convention), and the regional instruments attribute this right to civil and political rights. However, the Commission on Human Rights has treated property rights as an issue of the realization in all countries of economic, social, and cultural rights, in line with General Assembly resolution 45/98 of December 1991. "The right of everyone to own property alone as well as in association with others, completed final report submitted by Mr. Luis Valencia Rodríguez, Independent Expert, to the United Nations Commission on Human Rights," UN Doc. E/CN.4/1994/19, Nov. 25, 1993, at para. 98.

[1145] In response to the final report submitted by the independent expert (see note 1142 above), the Commission on Human Rights "[r]ecommend[ed] that all relevant United Nations bodies take into consideration the recommendations of the independent expert ... and [c]onclude[d] its consideration of this matter": UN Doc. E/CN.4/1994/19, Nov. 25, 1993, at paras. 4–5.

[1146] In addition to ECHR Protocol No. 1 (discussed above, at pp. 518–519), see also African Charter on Human and Peoples' Rights, OAU Doc. CAB/LEG/67/3 rev. 5, 21 ILM 58 (1982), entered into force Oct. 21, 1986 (African Charter), at Art. 14; and the American Convention on Human Rights, 1144 UNTS 123, entered into force July 18, 1978 (American Convention), at Art. 21.

[1147] See Convention on the Elimination of All Forms of Discrimination Against Women, UNGA Res. 34/180, adopted Dec. 18, 1979, entered into force Sept. 3, 1981 (Discrimination Against Women Convention), at Art. 16; International Convention on the Protection of the Rights of All Migrant Workers and Members of their Families, UNGA Res. 45/158, UN Doc. A/45/49 (1990), adopted Dec. 18, 1990, entered into force July 1, 2003, at Art. 15. Of the several non-discrimination standards, the guarantee in the Racial Discrimination Convention, in which "the right to own property alone as well in association with others" and "the right to inherit" are both subject to a guarantee of non-discrimination on the basis of "national or ethnic origin," is potentially of greatest relevance to the whole refugee class, so long as the state of asylum is a party to that agreement: Racial Discrimination Convention, at Arts. 1(1) and 5(d)(v). In the context of refugee repatriation, the Committee on the Elimination of Racial Discrimination has relied on Art. 5 in order to reach the conclusion that "refugees ... have, after their return to their homes of origin, the right to be restored to them property of which they were deprived in the course of the conflict and to be compensated for any such property that cannot be restored to them. Any commitments or statements relating to such property made under duress are null and void": UN Committee on the Elimination of Racial Discrimination, "General Recommendation No. XXII: Refugees and displaced persons" (1996), UN Doc. HRI/GEN/1/Rev.7, May 12, 2004, at 214, para. 2(c).

on refugees specifically. As analyzed above,[1148] Art. 26 of the Civil and Political Covenant governs the allocation of all rights, and prohibits discrimination on the basis of both "national origin" and "other status." Legal distinctions between citizens and non-citizens must be justifiable on the basis of real differences of capability or potentiality to pass muster under the Covenant's guarantee of equal protection of the law. As interpreted by the Human Rights Committee, Art. 26 presumes the illegitimacy of any rights allocation made on the basis of any form of status, specifically understood to include alien status.[1149]

Thus, while some exclusions on property ownership by aliens may be deemed "reasonable" under international law,[1150] others may not. For example, while a case might be made that Mexican restrictions on alien property ownership along its borders are reasonable security measures,[1151] and perhaps even that the efforts of Namibia and New Zealand to ensure continued domestic control over agricultural land, and of the United States to limit access to atomic energy, are reasonable limitations to ensure important domestic security concerns, it is difficult to imagine how the absolute denial of non-citizen property ownership in Bulgaria, Hungary, Kenya, or Sudan would be similarly justified. Even less far-reaching prohibitions, such as the American denial of radio licenses and federal mineral rights to non-citizens, and the decisions of Luxembourg and Venezuela to limit land ownership to resident non-citizens, would also have to pass the test of a reasonable limitation on grounds of "other status." The denial of some key property rights to refugees may therefore be most effectively challenged on the grounds of unreasonable differentiation against the generic class of non-citizens.

Because of the absence of a clear right to private property in human rights law, however, the property rights specifically guaranteed in the Refugee Convention are of continuing importance. First, a right to protection against confiscation of property without compensation can be derived from Art. 7(1) of the Convention. Because the overarching duty to accord refugees "the same treatment as is accorded to aliens generally" is not limited to the rights specifically set out in the Refugee Convention,[1152] Art. 7(1) incorporates by reference the duty to adhere to customary norms of international aliens law.[1153] In essence, Art. 7(1) ensures that refugees are not denied the benefit of these

---

[1148] See chapter 2.5.5 above, at pp. 125–128.   [1149] See chapter 2.5.5 above, at p. 127.
[1150] See chapter 2.5.5 above, at pp. 128–145.
[1151] The IRO was prepared to recognize that "special regulations excluding aliens, based on security considerations, e.g. [from] property in frontier or strategic areas" were reasonable: Comments of the International Refugee Organization, UN Doc. E/AC.32/L.40, Aug. 10, 1940, at 40. The drafters did not, however, choose to restrict the scope of property rights on the basis of such considerations, opting instead to guarantee refugees whatever property rights are granted to "aliens generally in the same circumstances."
[1152] See chapter 3.2.1 above, at p. 197.   [1153] Ibid.

foundational rights simply because their own state of nationality cannot be counted on to exercise its notional responsibility to undertake enforcement action.[1154] In the case of property rights, Art. 7(1)'s indirect incorporation of the duty to comply with international aliens law helpfully clarifies the rights of refugees. This is because it is well established that even though there is no duty under general principles of aliens law to allow refugees or other non-citizens to acquire property, there is a clear obligation to provide adequate compensation for any denial of property rights.[1155] As this duty falls upon state parties by virtue of Art. 7(1), alien-specific confiscatory regimes, including those applied simply against refugees, are violations of the Refugee Convention.

But because international aliens law does not establish a right to be free from property deprivation as such (but only to be fairly compensated for any such loss), it does not prohibit even a refugee-specific rule such as that requiring the slaughter of all animals brought into Kenya and Uganda by refugees, so long as adequate compensation is paid to the refugees.[1156] On the other hand, Kenya and Uganda presumptively breach international law by authorizing officials to commandeer refugee vehicles without compensation. While there is an argument that general principles of law now authorize the subordination of property rights to important social or public needs,[1157] confiscation imposed only on refugees is discriminatory, thus vitiating any such justification.

Complementing Art. 7's incorporation of a prohibition of property confiscation, Art. 13 of the Refugee Convention requires non-discrimination in relation to an inclusive notion of the right to acquire and deal with property.[1158] The article explicitly protects the right to acquire both movable

---

[1154] See chapter 2.1 above, at p. 79.   [1155] See chapter 2.1 above, at p. 77.

[1156] Even the strongest advocates of the protection of refugee property rights conceded the logic of exceptions "based on security considerations": Comments of the International Refugee Organization, UN Doc. E/AC.32/L.40, Aug. 10, 1940, at 40.

[1157] An exception to the duty to respect private property rights in such circumstances is included in each of the three regional human rights treaties. ECHR Protocol No. 1 provides that "[t]he preceding provisions shall not, however, in any way impair the right of a State to enforce such laws as it deems necessary to control the use of property in accordance with the general interest": ibid. at Art. 1. The African Charter stipulates that "[i]t may only be encroached in the interest of public need or in the general interest of the community and in accordance with the provisions of appropriate laws": ibid. at Art. 14. Under the American Convention, "[t]he law may subordinate such use and enjoyment to the interest of society": ibid. at Art. 21. See Krause, "Property," at 153: "All three Conventions require that the interference must be taken in the public interest and it must be provided for by law. The formulations vary slightly, but in terms of substance there appear to be no major differences. The question of public interest is indeed a question where the State is given a wide margin of appreciation."

[1158] A broad reading of the scope of "property" is consistent with the general approach in international human rights law. "The absence of a definition of the concept of property in international conventions is not surprising. None of the Conventions limit the (personal) and immovable (real) property, including acquisition by lease.[1159] Specific reference was made during the drafting debates to the importance of enabling refugees to purchase securities (stocks)[1160] and land,[1161] to acquire a home,[1162] and to lease premises for accommodation or in which to carry on a business.[1163] Robinson and Weis logically add that Art. 13 encompasses the right to hold money, and to establish bank accounts.[1164] Under this broad-ranging construction, both Botswana's prohibition of cattle ownership by refugees and the refusal of Honduran and Mexican officials to allow refugees to rent land were presumptively in violation of Art. 13. Similarly, the type of refugee-specific prohibition on the leasing of plots of an economically viable size found in various parts of Africa is also contrary to the Refugee Convention.

Art. 13 not only protects the right to acquire all forms of property, but also guarantees non-discrimination in regard to "other rights pertaining thereto," specifically including related contractual interests. Robinson elaborates this

protection of property to any particular kind of property. In practice, the Strasbourg organs have given 'possessions' under Protocol No. 1 to the [European Convention on Human Rights and Fundamental Freedoms] a wide interpretation and held that it covers both immovable and movable property, including immaterial rights, such as contractual rights with economic value, various economic interests, and goodwill": Krause, "Property," at 150.

[1159] In view of the fact that Art. 17 of the Universal Declaration of Human Rights had been approved by the General Assembly just over one year before the preparation of the Secretary-General's draft of the Refugee Convention, it is surprising that no express reference is made in the Refugee Convention to the right of property "ownership." While the focus on the right to "acquire" property in the Refugee Convention might be argued to exclude protection of rights of ownership in property brought into the asylum country, the express language of Art. 30 (which permits refugees to transfer "assets which they have brought into [the asylum country's] territory") must negate that interpretation. In the result, the right to acquire property "and other rights pertaining thereto" should be understood in context to include protection of the rights of ownership in all property brought into, and acquired within, the asylum state.

[1160] Secretary-General, "Memorandum," at 26.

[1161] Statement of Sir Leslie Brass of the United Kingdom, UN Doc. E/AC.32/SR.36, Aug. 15, 1950, at 13.

[1162] In response to an American proposal to insert a new right of refugees to "housing accommodation," the Chairman of the Ad Hoc Committee advised that in the view of the Secretariat "the provisionally adopted article [13] might be considered to cover the question in a certain sense": Statement of the Chairman, Mr. Chance of Canada, UN Doc. E/AC.32/SR.15, Jan. 27, 1950, at 11. The representative of the United States "replied that article [13] dealt with the rights of refugees regarding immovable property and leases," leading him to constrain the scope of what became Art. 21 to "social welfare matters taken by States with a view to providing housing accommodation for certain categories of persons": Statement of Mr. Henkin of the United States, ibid. See generally chapter 6.4 below with respect to the latter issue.

[1163] Secretary-General, "Memorandum," at 26.

[1164] Robinson, *History*, at 106; Weis, *Travaux*, at 116.

notion by suggesting that such related activities as "sale, exchange, mortgaging, pawning, administration, [and] income"[1165] are protected interests. Another example of "rights pertaining" to property mentioned during the drafting debates is the ability of refugees to benefit from rent controls.[1166] Logically, then, the practice of some host states of imposing a refugee-specific requirement that only certain crops may be grown on rented land is in breach of Art. 13.

Critically, however, not even Art. 13 establishes an absolute guarantee of property rights for refugees. The original drafts suggested that property rights might be guaranteed either at the level of "the most favorable treatments accorded under treaty to foreigners"[1167] or even to require "treatment similar to that accorded to their nationals."[1168] But the drafters rejected pleas fully to enfranchise refugees in order to promote their speedy assimilation.[1169] Some states took the view that there was no good reason to privilege refugees relative to other non-citizens.[1170] Others simply wanted to be able to reserve some property rights for either their own citizens,[1171] or for the

---

[1165] Robinson, *History*, at 105–106.

[1166] "It may be noted that in certain countries foreigners are not covered by rent laws for the protection of tenants, save by virtue of treaties. If, therefore, refugees, who are usually destitute, are not to enjoy the treatment accorded under treaty to foreigners, they will be debarred from the benefits of such laws, which will spell disaster for them": Secretary-General, "Memorandum," at 27. The representative of the IRO suggested that rent controls might be a form of property to be excluded from the protection of Art. 13, a view expressed in the hope of persuading delegates to adopt a national treatment standard for property rights: Statement of Mr. Weis of the International Refugee Organization, UN Doc. E/AC.32/SR.36, Aug. 15, 1950, at 11. States opted instead for a broad definition of relevant property interests (presumably rejecting the IRO's bid to exclude some interests), but the standard of treatment was set as "aliens generally in the same circumstances."

[1167] Secretary-General, "Memorandum," at 26. A bracketed alternative form of words would allow states to commit themselves only to "the treatment accorded to foreigners generally": ibid.

[1168] France, "Draft Convention," at 4.

[1169] "In view of the desirability that refugees should be assimilated as quickly as possible into the economic life of their country of residence, refugees should be granted the same property rights as nationals subject to any special regulations excluding aliens, e.g. property in frontier or strategic areas, government or central bank bonds, shares of shipping companies, mines, etc.": Comments of the International Refugee Organization, UN Doc. E/AC.32/L.40, Aug. 10, 1950, at 40. See also Statement of Mr. Henkin of the United States, UN Doc. E/AC.32/SR.36, Aug. 15, 1950, at 10.

[1170] Statement of Mr. Kural of Turkey, UN Doc. E/AC.32/SR.10, Jan. 24, 1950, at 4. See also Statement of Sir Leslie Brass of the United Kingdom, ibid. at 7: "[W]hile the Committee was trying as it should to protect refugees against discrimination, it should not go to the other extreme of establishing discrimination in favour of refugees. He shared the uneasiness of other members regarding the most-favoured-nation clause."

[1171] Statement of Mr. Rain of France, ibid. at 6–7.

citizens of states with which they were allied in an economic or political association.[1172] In keeping with the traditional deference afforded states to define their own notions of property, Art. 13 requires only that refugees enjoy protected interests at a low contingent standard of treatment,[1173] namely treatment "as favourable as possible and, in any event, not less favourable than that accorded to aliens generally in the same circumstances."[1174] There is therefore clearly no basis to contest restrictions on property ownership which apply generally, such as Sudan's insistence that refugees are bound by customary limitations on land tenure, or Malawi's refusal to allow refugees to gather wild rodents and insects, said to be owned by the landowners on whose property they are found. Assuming these definitions of the nature of property ownership to be of general application (or at least applied to all other non-citizens), they may in most cases govern the rights of refugees as well.

In two ways, however, the Refugee Convention does allow refugees to contest such generally applicable restrictions. First, the actual duty under Art. 13 is to accord to a refugee "treatment as favourable as possible," though in no case less favorable than that afforded aliens generally. As noted above, this standard of treatment imposes a duty on states to consider in good faith the exemption of refugees from even rules applied generally to non-citizens.[1175] Second, limitations imposed on non-citizens may in any event only be validly applied to refugees who are "in the same circumstances" as other aliens. This proviso requires states to exempt refugees from requirements which may simply not be realistic in view of impediments that follow from the refugee's uprooting and dislocation.[1176]

One clear strength of Art. 13 is that it inheres immediately in all refugees. Perhaps because the primary goal of withholding certain rights for citizens and most-favored foreigners was met by the use of the low contingent standard for property rights, the initial limitations on the scope of the beneficiary class by reference to level of attachment[1177] fell by the wayside. Thus, even as it embraced the low contingent standard, the Ad Hoc Committee's Working Group recommended the extension of property rights

---

[1172] "Belgium . . . placed nationals of the Benelux countries for certain purposes on a quasi-equal footing with Belgian citizens. It was not the intention of the article under consideration, he hoped, to ask the same treatment for refugees": Statement of Mr. Cuvelier of Belgium, ibid. at 5. See also Statement of Mr. Larsen of Denmark, ibid. at 5: "[T]he Scandinavian countries . . . did accord special treatment to Scandinavian nationals which they would not be prepared to give to other foreigners, including refugees."

[1173] "Decisions of the Working Group Taken on 9 February 1950," UN Doc. E/AC.32/L.32, Feb. 9, 1950, at 5. This standard was adopted without further debate by the Ad Hoc Committee on a 5–1 (5 abstentions) vote: UN Doc. E/AC.32/SR.25, Feb. 10, 1950, at 5.

[1174] See chapter 3.2.1 above.   [1175] See chapter 3.2.1 above, at pp. 198–200.

[1176] See generally chapter 3.2.3 above.   [1177] See text above, at pp. 525–526.

to "a refugee" without qualification.[1178] In the result, the benefits of Art. 13 can now be invoked by any refugee under a state's authority, including those not yet formally recognized as refugees.[1179] Indeed, no objection was voiced to the conclusion of the Chairman of the Ad Hoc Committee that Art. 13 "make[s] no distinction between refugees in countries adhering to the Convention and refugees resident elsewhere ... [S]ome countries whose laws imposed restrictions on the property rights of aliens might feel some apprehension that article [13] would give the same rights to refugees living in other countries as to aliens living in the country where the property was."[1180] The only recorded response was the affirmation of the British representative that "[a] refugee abroad would presumably receive the same treatment as an alien abroad"[1181] by virtue of the fact that the contingent standard "not less favourable than that accorded to aliens generally in the same circumstances" allows state parties to apply to refugees whatever distinctions are ordinarily used to define the scope of non-citizen beneficiaries. Thus, non-resident refugees are entitled to the same protection of property rights as is afforded comparably situated non-resident aliens.[1182]

4.5.2 Tax equity

Countries of refuge rarely apply special rules for the taxation of refugees; when they do, the goal may actually be to assist refugees. For example, UNHCR reports that refugees are occasionally exempted from customs duties on the importation of their personal effects.[1183] Less formal

---

[1178] "Decisions of the Working Group Taken on 9 February 1950," UN Doc. E/AC.32/L.32, Feb. 9, 1950, at 5, adopted by the Ad Hoc Committee at UN Doc. E/AC.32/SR.25, Feb. 10, 1950, at 5.

[1179] See chapter 3.1.1 above, at pp. 169–170.

[1180] Statement of the Chairman, Mr. Larsen of Denmark, UN Doc. E/AC.32/SR.36, Aug. 15, 1950, at 19–20.

[1181] Statement of Sir Leslie Brass of the United Kingdom, ibid. at 20.

[1182] See Robinson, *History*, at 105: "Article 13 does not contain a requirement of domicile or residence for the enjoyment of the rights conferred by it on refugees. In other words, it applies to refugees regardless of whether they have their domicile or residence in the country in which they wish to acquire property or elsewhere"; and Weis, *Travaux*, at 116: "The provision applies to all refugees, whether resident in the territory of the Contracting State or not." The notion of "'in the same circumstances' implies that any requirements (including requirements as to length and conditions of sojourn or residence) which the particular individual would have to fulfil for the enjoyment of the right in question, if he were not a refugee, must be fulfilled by him, with the exception of requirements which by their nature a refugee is incapable of fulfilling": Refugee Convention, at Art. 6. See generally chapter 3.2.3 above.

[1183] UNHCR, "Information Note on Implementation of the 1951 Convention and the 1967 Protocol relating to the Status of Refugees," prepared for the Sub-Committee of the Whole on International Protection, Forty-second Session, July 22, 1991, at para. 94.

dispensation from taxation may also occur. For example, refugees arriving in the Qala en Nahal settlement in Sudan "were exempted from all taxes, and tractor service charges were also waived."[1184] Similarly, Somali and Sudanese refugees living in Kukuma camp in Kenya were allowed to conduct business free of taxation until the local business community put pressure on the government to end what was perceived as an unfair advantage.[1185] More commonly, however, refugees are simply taxed in the same way as nationals. As Brian Arnold observes, "[t]ax is rarely levied on the basis of nationality, and tax discrimination between citizens and aliens is rare."[1186]

Differences based on residence, rather than citizenship, are more common, though even this practice has been attenuated by the pervasive influence of Art. 24 of the OECD model tax treaty. This clause, which served as the model for the 1980 UN model tax treaty,[1187] requires the equal treatment of resident aliens with resident citizens, and of non-resident aliens with non-resident citizens.[1188] But not all interstate tax treaties incorporate this principle. For example, Australia has refused to include an article prohibiting non-discrimination on the basis of residence in most of its tax treaties.[1189]

In practice, however, refugees are frequently situated differently from citizens in ways that may expose them to increased tax liability on the basis of facially non-discriminatory tax laws. For example, most treaties modeled on the OECD draft do not provide any protection against tax discrimination on the basis of the geographical location of property, expenditures, or activities.[1190] A refugee who has spent most of his or her life in a state other than the asylum country will often have their primary asset base abroad. To the extent that refugees are more likely than citizens to derive a substantial share of their income from overseas property, they will be more adversely impacted than citizens by the failure of most tax treaties to proscribe discrimination on the basis of the geographical source of income.

[1184] Kibreab, *Development*, at 83.   [1185] Verdirame, "Kenya," at 68–69.

[1186] B. Arnold, *Tax Discrimination Against Aliens, Non-Residents, and Foreign Activities: Canada, Australia, New Zealand, the United Kingdom, and the United States* (1991) (Arnold, *Tax Discrimination*), at 27.

[1187] United Nations, *United Nations Model Double Taxation Convention Between Developed and Developing Countries* (1980) (UN Tax Treaty).

[1188] "The nationals of a Contracting State shall not be subjected in the other Contracting State to any taxation or any requirement connected therewith which is other or more burdensome than the taxation and connected requirements to which nationals of that other State in the same circumstances may be subjected": Organization for Economic Cooperation and Development, *Draft Double Taxation Convention on Income and Capital: Report of the OECD Fiscal Committee* (1963) (OECD Tax Treaty), at Art. 24(1).

[1189] Arnold, *Tax Discrimination*, at 258.   [1190] Ibid. at 46.

Refugee Convention, Art 29   Fiscal charges

1. The Contracting States shall not impose upon refugees duties, charges or taxes, of any description whatsoever, other or higher than those which are or may be levied on their nationals in similar situations.

2. Nothing in the above paragraph shall prevent the application to refugees of the laws and regulations concerning charges in respect of the issue to aliens of administrative documents including identity papers.

Art. 29 continues the pattern set by earlier treaties[1191] of protecting refugees against the possibility of "special taxes, duties and charges."[1192] Most non-citizens avoid the prospect of differential tax[1193] by reliance on the near-universal provision in bilateral tax treaties assimilating citizens and non-citizens for purposes of fiscal liability.[1194] In the case of refugees, a protection void might arise from either of two circumstances. First, there might simply be no tax treaty with the refugee's country of citizenship, or that treaty might not include the usual guarantee of non-discrimination based on citizenship.[1195] Second, as tax treaties are typically enforced on the basis of reciprocity, refugees might be denied tax equality because of the actions of the very government from which they had fled.[1196] The goal of the Refugee Convention is to put refugees in the same position as the nationals of a

---

[1191] Arrangement concerning the Extension to Other Categories of Refugees of Certain Measures taken in favour of Russian and Armenian Refugees, 2006 LNTS 65, done June 30, 1928, at Art. 8; Convention relating to the International Status of Refugees, 159 LNTS 3663, done Oct. 28, 1933, at Art. 13; Convention concerning the Status of Refugees Coming from Germany, 4461 LNTS 61, done Feb. 10, 1938, at Art. 16.

[1192] "In principle foreigners residing in a country are subject to the duties, taxes and charges to which nationals are liable. They may also be subject to special taxes, duties and charges. A large number of bilateral treaties concluded on the basis of reciprocity stipulate that nationals of the co-contracting country shall enjoy the same treatment in fiscal matters as nationals. Stateless persons cannot invoke these treaties": United Nations, "Statelessness," at 31.

[1193] Brian Arnold, for example, argues that "domestic and customary international law do not constrain a country's power to discriminate for tax purposes. In this respect, aliens ... are fair game for a legislature with protectionist tendencies": Arnold, *Tax Discrimination*, at 23.

[1194] This rule is contained in the two most influential model tax treaties: OECD Tax Treaty, at Art. 24; and UN Tax Treaty, at Art. 24. The text of the two rules is identical: see text above, at p. 528, n. 1188.

[1195] It is noteworthy that Australia, Canada, and New Zealand entered a reservation to the non-discrimination clause of the OECD Model Convention: OECD Tax Treaty.

[1196] This risk is, however, attenuated by Art. 7(2) of the Refugee Convention, which exempts refugees who have lived in an asylum country for three years from requirements of legislative reciprocity. See generally chapter 3.2.2 above.

contracting state which is in compliance with its duties under a tax treaty prohibiting discrimination based on nationality.[1197]

Art. 29 is very broadly framed. Refugees must receive national treatment with respect to "duties, charges or taxes, of any description whatsoever." The more cautiously framed duty under model tax treaties, which only applies to "any taxation or any requirement connected therewith," is authoritatively defined to require equality in regard to "taxes on income, on total capital, or on elements of income or of capital, including taxes on gains from the alienation of movable or immovable property, taxes on the total amounts of wages or salaries paid by enterprises, as well as taxes on capital appreciation."[1198] The more expansive language of Art. 29 of the Refugee Convention logically includes at least all of these forms of tax.[1199]

Robinson argues that the duty under Art. 29 extends also to "every kind of public assessment, be it of a general nature (taxes and duties) or for specific services rendered by the authorities to a given person (charges)."[1200] There is support for this broad reading not only in the unusually sweeping language of the article itself, but also in the rejection by the Conference of Plenipotentiaries of a proposed exception which would have allowed governments to continue to impose a refugee-specific stamp duty to issue identity cards, residence permits, and travel documents. Even though such levies were to be "wholly applied for the relief of refugees,"[1201] the drafters viewed them as an unacceptable infringement of the duty to tax refugees and nationals on the same basis.[1202] The duty to assimilate refugees to nationals does not, of

---

[1197] Refugees are therefore "not obliged to pay taxes or other charges levied on aliens only": Weis, *Travaux*, at 272.

[1198] OECD Tax Treaty, at Art. 2; UN Tax Treaty, at Art. 2.

[1199] The one area in which there is a sound argument not to incorporate general understanding of non-discrimination based on citizenship into the duty under Art. 29 of the Refugee Convention is with regard to taxes assessed by political sub-units of an asylum state. The general rule is that the duty to tax citizens and non-citizens equally applies not only to relevant charges made by the national government, but also to "taxes imposed by their political subdivisions or local authorities": UN Tax Treaty, at 47. On the other hand, Art. 41 of the Refugee Convention expressly provides that "[i]n the case of a Federal or non-unitary State ... [w]ith respect to those articles of this Convention that come within the legislative jurisdiction of [sub-units] ... the Federal Government shall bring such articles with a favourable recommendation to the notice of the appropriate authorities of States, provinces or cantons at the earliest possible moment": Refugee Convention, at Art. 41(b).

[1200] Robinson, *History*, at 148.

[1201] Secretary-General, "Memorandum," at 31.

[1202] "[R]efugees had already been assimilated to nationals in respect of public assistance and labour legislation and social security. Was it therefore absolutely necessary also to contemplate imposing *a tax* to provide relief for refugees? He thought not [emphasis added]": Statement of Mr. Miras of Turkey, UN Doc. A/CONF.2/SR.12, July 9, 1951, at 14. In earlier discussion in the Ad Hoc Committee, the Chinese representative had observed that "[r]efugees are not especially wealthy persons, and if the only course, prevent governments from assessing fees for services not required by nationals. Specifically, para. 2 of Art. 29 confirms that refugees may be required to pay a modest amount to cover the actual costs of delivering documentation required by non-citizens, such as identity papers.[1203]

Not only may refugees not be subjected to different assessments than nationals, but they must not be treated less well than nationals in relation to any given charge. This is clear from the textual prohibition of both "other *or higher*" charges or taxes. The parallel phrase in model tax treaties, which prohibits "other or more burdensome" taxation, requires "that when a tax is imposed on nationals and foreigners in the same circumstances, it must be in the same form as regards both the basis of charge and the method of assessment, its rate must be the same and, finally, the formalities connected with the taxation (returns, payment, prescribed times, etc.) must not be more onerous for foreigners than for nationals."[1204]

The duty to treat refugees on terms of equality with nationals applies, however, only to the extent that refugees and nationals can be said to be "in similar situations." In Robinson's view, differences in tax liability between citizens and refugees that are attributable to "deriving a certain amount of income, having income abroad, [or] having special income sources . . ."[1205] therefore do not infringe Art. 29. The equality guaranteed by this article of the Refugee Convention is, in other words, formal equality. There is no violation of Art. 29 if refugees in practice pay more tax than citizens not because they are refugees or non-citizens, but instead because their primary source of income is universally taxed in the asylum country at a higher rate than other sources of income. Thus, even though refugees are more likely than others to derive income from overseas property, Art. 29 would not prohibit a

---

intention . . . was to help them, it would be better to approach the rich": Statement of Mr. Cha of China, UN Doc. E/AC.32/SR.39, Aug. 21, 1950, at 23.

[1203] "[P]aragraph 2 . . . state[d] expressly that identity papers were included. He would therefore interpret it as applying to all the documents, including identity papers, referred to in the draft Convention. There might be other articles necessitating the issue of other administrative documents, and Contracting States should reserve the right to charge *a small fee for delivering them* [emphasis added]": Statement of the President, Mr. Larsen of Denmark, UN Doc. A/CONF.2/SR.12, July 9, 1951, at 15. As Weis observes, "[p]aragraph 2 must be read in conjunction with Article 25, paragraph 4 and paragraphs 3 and 10 of the Schedule. The documents referred to are those mentioned in Articles 25 and 27, but also other documents required under the Convention": Weis, *Travaux*, at 272. Specifically, para. 3 of the Schedule requires that "[t]he fees charged for issue of the [travel] document shall not exceed the lowest scale of charges for national passports"; and para. 10 stipulates that "[t]he fees for the issue of exit, entry or transit visas shall not exceed the lowest scale of charges for visas on foreign passports": Refugee Convention, at Schedule.

[1204] OECD Tax Treaty, at Art. 24(1) commentary; UN Tax Treaty, at Art. 24(1) commentary.

[1205] Robinson, *History*, at 148.

regime that taxes income from overseas property (for all) more severely than it does income from domestic property.

Similarly, if nationals who are not residents are taxed differently from nationals who are residents, there can be no complaint if non-resident refugees are taxed differently from resident refugees.[1206] But any attempt to treat non-resident citizens and non-resident aliens differently for income tax purposes would run afoul of the Refugee Convention. The 1951 Refugee Convention, unlike its predecessors, does not limit the duty of tax equality only to resident refugees.[1207] Every person who is in fact a refugee, even if his or her presence in a state party is only transient, must be equated to citizens for purposes of the imposition of taxes and related charges. While most forms of tax do not apply to non-residents, duties on imports or exports are examples of charges which are assessed against non-residents, in relation to which non-resident refugees must be treated on terms of equality with non-resident citizens.[1208]

[1206] This is clear from an exchange at the Conference of Plenipotentiaries. In response to the Swedish representative's comment that his country taxed non-citizen commercial travelers and performing artists differently from nationals, the President of the Conference affirmed that only differences grounded in substance, not in nationality, would be allowed under Art. 29. "[T]he problem referred to by the Swedish representative, which was a question of domicile or habitual residence rather than nationality, could be solved within the framework of paragraph 1. For example, if a Swedish artiste resident in Denmark went back to Sweden to perform for a short period, he would be subject to the same taxes as, for instance, a Danish artiste in the same position": Statement of the President, Mr. Larsen of Denmark, UN Doc. A/CONF.2/SR.12, July 9, 1951, at 16. The principle is also endorsed in the Commentary to the UN model tax treaty. "Consequently if a Contracting State, in giving relief from taxation on account of family responsibilities, distinguishes between its own nationals according to whether they reside in its territory or not, that State cannot be obliged to give nationals of the other State who do not reside in its territory the same treatment as it gives its resident nationals [so long as it] undertakes to extend to them the same treatment as is available to its non-resident nationals": UN Tax Treaty, at 208.

[1207] As initially proposed, the Convention continued the traditional practice of reserving the benefit of the tax equality rule for resident refugees. "The High Contracting Parties undertake not to impose upon refugees (or stateless persons) residing in their territory duties, charges or taxes, under any denomination whatsoever, other or higher than those which are or may be levied on their nationals in similar situations": Secretary-General, "Memorandum," at 31. As reframed by the Ad Hoc Committee, however, the residency requirement was deleted. "The Contracting States shall not impose upon refugees in their territory duties, charges or taxes": Ad Hoc Committee, "First Session Report," at 7. With no explicit discussion of the matter, the Conference of Plenipotentiaries deleted the reference to "refugees in their territory" in favor of "refugees." Theoretically, then, even refugees not in a state party's territory, but who are nonetheless under its authority for tax purposes, must be granted the benefit of Art. 29. See generally chapter 3.1.1 above.

[1208] "Art. 29 deals with refugees in general; in other words, to enjoy equal status with nationals 'in similar circumstances' of the country where the fiscal charges are payable,

4.6 Family unity

A critical imperative for most refugees is to avoid separation from their families. As UNHCR has observed, "family members together have more strength to face adversity than those apart."[1209] While family relations are important means of satisfying physical and psychological needs during normal times, these attachments take on even greater significance when involuntary migration deprives refugees of their traditional range of support networks.[1210] The more threatening the environment, the more family members will look to each other for intimacy and security.[1211]

Yet the very crises that force refugees to flee often shatter the unity of their families. Family members may not be able to leave together,[1212] or may be separated in the chaos of flight.[1213] Refugees separated from their families are not only less equipped to cope with life in an asylum state, but are often prone to loneliness, despair, and anxiety over the fate of their loved ones left behind in dangerous situations.[1214] As Dixon-Fyle has observed, "[t]heir relief at having reached safety may be so overshadowed by distress, guilt and worry about those who remain behind that the chances of their settling down and becoming fully integrated in their host country may be seriously reduced."[1215]

There are few legal impediments to family reunification in most less developed asylum states. Because these countries normally rely on group status determination of refugees, the acceptance of members of refugee families able to reach their territory tends to occur as a matter of course, with no differentiation made between the arrival of some family members as part of an initial influx and the subsequent arrival of others.[1216] In the South, the more serious obstacle to refugee family unity results from practical

---

the refugees need not reside in either the state concerned or in another Contracting State": Robinson, *History*, at 148.

[1209] UNHCR, "Families in Exile: Reflections from the Experience of UNHCR" (1995) (UNHCR, "Families"), at 3.

[1210] H. Williams, "Families in Refugee Camps," [Summer 1990] *Human Organization* 103.

[1211] J. Barudy, "The Therapeutic Value of Solidarity and Hope," in D. Miserz ed., *Refugees – The Trauma of Exile* 142 (1988). In particular, children have an increased need for physical contact with their parents, and often fear separation from their family above all else: E. Ressler et al., *Unaccompanied Children: Care and Protection in Wars, Natural Disasters and Refugee Movements* (1988) (Ressler et al., *Unaccompanied Children*), at 133, 147, and 150.

[1212] "Facing persecution and often death, refugee families are frequently forced to separate while fleeing amid mass destruction, spraying bullets, bombs, and guerilla warfare": UNHCR, "Families," at 1.

[1213] "Refugees often flee under chaotic, violent and traumatic circumstances, leaving all or part of their families behind": K. Dixon-Fyle, "Reunification: Putting the Family First," (1994) 95 *Refugees* 6 (Dixon-Fyle, "Reunification"), at 10.

[1214] "Year of the Family," (1994) 95 *Refugees* 3, at 5.

[1215] Dixon-Fyle, "Reunification," at 9.   [1216] Ibid. at 7.

difficulties in tracing family members who may be in another camp, or even in another country.

Most critically, there are often large numbers of unaccompanied children in massive refugee flows.[1217] Part or all of a child's family may be killed or accidentally separated from the child. Children may be sent out of the country, sometimes with siblings and sometimes alone, while the parents remain. Alternatively, children may remain behind temporarily while part of the family leaves to get established in a new land, or they may have been abducted into the army.[1218] In some truly extreme situations, parents are compelled voluntarily to become separated from their children as part of a survival strategy,[1219] or to enable their children to take advantage of superior opportunities often available to unaccompanied minors.[1220] In addition to such emergency-related circumstances, refugee families may become separated because of the same sorts of social, psychological, and cultural problems that arise generally in families. In other situations, "the separations are the unplanned result of the way relief assistance is provided. For example, relief workers have sometimes removed children from a dangerous area or to a medical facility without notifying the family or others in the vicinity."[1221] When resource constraints or logistical concerns conspire to keep family members apart – and particularly when children are missing – there is always a fear that "[s]ome family members [will] spontaneously repatriate to their homeland in precarious political circumstances to find their loved ones – and never return."[1222]

In the developed world, as in the South, family unity concerns more commonly arise in relation to reunification efforts, rather than as refusals of entry at the border.[1223] In contrast to the situation in poorer states,

---

[1217] For example, more than 20 percent of the Burundian refugees who sought asylum in Tanzania were unaccompanied children: C. Berthiaume, "Alone in the World," (1994) 95 *Refugees* 14, at 17.

[1218] F. Ahearn and J. Athey, *Refugee Children: Theory, Research, and Services* (1991), at 11.

[1219] For example, older boys may be encouraged to fend for themselves, and older girls "to attach themselves to more prosperous and safe families as helpers": L. Bonnerjea, "Disasters, Family Tracing and Children's Rights: Some Questions About the Best Interests of Separated Children," (1994) 18 *Disasters* 277 (Bonnerjea, "Disasters"), at 278.

[1220] Ressler et al., *Unaccompanied Children*, at 119.   [1221] Ibid. at 118–119.

[1222] UNHCR, "Families," at 3.

[1223] See also G. Fourlanos, *Sovereignty and the Ingress of Aliens* (1986) (Fourlanos, *Sovereignty*), at 111: "When it comes to immigration rights deriving from the principle of family unity, the situation is rather obscure. A specific right to enter and/or to reside is not very often mentioned in international agreements, but it seems that, in practice, States understand the individual right to family unity as including the right to enter their territory and to reside there (i.e. not to be expelled)." Hong Kong officials, however,

however, much of the difficulty faced by refugees seeking to reunite their families tends to result from the application of administrative requirements governing such issues as the point at which refugees should be allowed to sponsor the admission of their family members, which family members may be admitted, and what criteria must be met.

Virtually all Northern states decline family reunification to refugees awaiting the results of status determination.[1224] On the other hand, once formally recognized as a Convention refugee, most developed countries grant refugees a formal legal right to be reunited with family members.[1225] There is more ambiguity where a refugee is granted some alternative status, rather than full Convention refugee status. In Australia, for example, refugees who arrive in that country unlawfully, or who are intercepted offshore or in part of the territory deemed "excised" by Australia, are granted only temporary protected status which does not entitle them to be reunited with family members.[1226] Similar practices were once common in relation to persons granted alternative forms of protected status in much of Europe. In Germany, for example, those recognized as de facto refugees (*Duldung* status) were allowed to sponsor the admission of family members only on a discretionary basis.[1227] Refugees admitted under so-called "temporary protection" schemes were traditionally allowed access to family reunification in Italy, Norway, and

forcibly deported a pregnant asylum-seeker who was born in Vietnam, but who was considered Chinese by virtue of her resettlement in that country, even as they admitted her Vietnamese husband to a detention facility to await the outcome of his application to be recognized as a refugee: M. Eager, "Expectant mother split from spouse," *South China Morning Post*, Aug. 27, 1992. In contrast, a British High Court judge compelled the Home Office not to enforce a crime-based deportation order against the ex-spouse of an asylum applicant on the grounds that to do so would create the risk of violating the ex-spouse's right to respect for family life (as he would be separated from his children, who were in the custody of the asylum applicant, his ex-wife): C. Dyer, "HIV father wins human rights asylum case," *Guardian*, Oct. 25, 2000, at 12.

[1224] See generally Intergovernmental Consultations on Asylum, Refugee and Migration Policies in Europe, North America and Australia, *Report on Family Reunification: Overview of Policies and Practices in Participating States* (1997) (IGC, *Family Reunification*). The new European Union standards on family reunification are explicitly stated not to apply to "a third-country national applying for recognition of refugee status whose application has not yet given rise to a final decision": Council Directive on the Right to Family Reunification, Doc. 6912/03 (Feb. 28, 2003) (EU Family Reunification Directive), at Art. 3(2)(a).

[1225] For example, the Swiss *Asylum Act* authorizes a grant of asylum to the spouse and children of recognized refugees, even if these persons do not themselves have a well-founded fear of being persecuted: W. Kälin, *International Academy of Comparative Law National Report for Switzerland* (1994), at 7.

[1226] Mathew, "*Tampa*," at 673.

[1227] F. Liebaut and J. Hughes, *Legal and Social Conditions for Asylum Seekers and Refugees in Western European Countries* (1997), at 101.

Sweden,[1228] but not in Finland, the Netherlands, or Spain.[1229] Under the European Union's 2001 Directive on Temporary Protection, however, a clear right to family reunification is now established for the beneficiaries of temporary protection in member states.[1230]

Even if entitled to sponsor the entry of family members, a second question is the definition of the specific relationships which qualify as family members for purposes of reunification. Some states resist any understanding of "family" that goes beyond an opposite-sex spouse and minor, dependent children.[1231] For example, under the new European Union standards, a refugee's right to family reunification extends only to his or her "spouse" and minor, unmarried children.[1232] If the refugee is not formally married to his or her spouse, it is up to each state to decide for itself whether or not to permit reunification.[1233] A second or subsequent spouse in a polygamous marriage cannot be sponsored at all.[1234] Beyond this narrow category of family members, even the discretionary authority of European Union states is now limited. They may only elect to admit other first-degree relatives who are dependent on the refugee, and adult unmarried children who are incapacitated.[1235] Such a narrow construct may bear little resemblance to the de facto familial structures of emotional and economic interdependence of the refugees themselves.[1236] It is ironically also a less generous standard than that which governs reunification within the European Union for persons granted

---

[1228] IGC, *Family Reunification*, at 170, 207, 244.   [1229] Ibid. at 122, 186, 233, 326.

[1230] EU Temporary Protection Directive, at Art. 15.

[1231] For example, in the context of resettlement under the Comprehensive Plan of Action for Indochinese Refugees, reception states took different views on the validity of in-camp marriages and common law relationships: S. Bari, "Refugee Status Determination Under the Comprehensive Plan of Action: A Personal Assessment," (1992) 4(4) *International Journal of Refugee Law* 487, at 503–504.

[1232] EU Family Reunification Directive, at Art. 4(1).   [1233] Ibid. at Art. 4(3).

[1234] Ibid. at Art. 4(4).

[1235] Ibid. at Art. 4(2). This policy will result in a diminution of refugee rights in, for example, Greece, where refugees were entitled to sponsor their parents (provided they lived with the refugee in the country of origin): A. Skordas, "The New Refugee Legislation in Greece," (1999) 11(4) *International Journal of Refugee Law* 678, at 693.

[1236] Indeed, the strict definition of a "nuclear family" is not consistent with the historical understanding of "family" even in the developed countries which now embrace it. As Bonnie Fox has observed, "[b]efore the eighteenth century in Europe, there was no term of reference for persons related by blood, marriage, or common residence: the term 'family' was not used . . . Even in cultures and historical times when the nuclear unit was present, it was not necessarily distinguished from the larger groupings of which it was a part. Yet, through history, children have been raised and adults' need for food, shelter, and basic care have been met – although the way these were defined has varied tremendously": B. Fox, *Family Patterns, Gender Relations* (1993), at 23. See generally J. Hathaway, *Toward a Contextualized System of Family Class Immigration: A Study for the Government of Canada* (1994).

temporary protection in the event of a mass influx (including refugees). Such persons have the additional right to sponsor the admission of an unmarried partner, and may apply to be reunited with any other close relatives who were part of the family unit and dependent upon the refugee in the country of origin.[1237]

Even where a refugee is in principle entitled to reunification with particular family members, there may be additional criteria to be met. Australia and Canada, for example, require the refugee to prove his or her financial ability and willingness to meet the needs of some or all categories of sponsored family members.[1238] The European Union, in contrast, does not condition family reunification on such considerations so long as the application is filed within three months of the formal recognition of refugee status. After that time, however, family reunification may be subject to investigation of the sponsoring refugee's ability to provide his or her family with accommodation and health insurance, and to meet their other financial needs.[1239] More generally, the European Union authorizes the rejection of any application for family reunification on the sweeping basis of "public policy, public security or public health."[1240]

Finally, there are often prolonged delays in authorizing family reunification in developed states. Complex procedures absorb tremendous amounts of time and energy, and "keep refugees' minds riveted to the past and to trauma, instead of allowing them and their families to start thinking of the future and rebuilding their lives."[1241] In Australia, a Pakistani man recognized as a refugee in 1996 had still not received permission as of 2001 to be reunited with his wife and three daughters, one of whom suffered from cerebral palsy. His level of desperation was such that he set himself alight outside Parliament to protest the government's delays.[1242] Many Guatemalan and Salvadoran refugees in the United States were kept waiting for as many as twenty years after their arrival before being granted the formal status that entitled them to

[1237] EU Temporary Protection Directive, at Art. 15.

[1238] Under Australian law, refugees must agree to meet the needs of sponsored family members for two years, and provide a bond of A$3,500 for the principal applicant and A$1,500 for each other member of the family unit. In Canada, the sponsor of extended family members must undertake "to provide housing, care and maintenance and normal settlement needs of the applicant and accompanying dependants for up to ten years": IGC, *Family Reunification*, at 37, 91.

[1239] EU Family Reunification Directive, at Arts. 7(1), 12(1).

[1240] Ibid. at Art. 6(1). Somewhat ominously, a footnote to this provision makes clear that "[t]he notion of public policy and public security covers also cases in which a third-country national belongs to an association which supports international terrorism, supports such an association or has [extremist] aspirations": ibid.

[1241] Dixon-Fyle, "Reunification," at 9.

[1242] E. MacDonald, "Daughter to reunite with father 'to give him strength,'" *Canberra Times*, Apr. 11, 2001, at A-3.

sponsor the arrival of close family members.[1243] In some cases, delays may defeat the very possibility or logic of reunification as children reach the age of majority and are no longer eligible for admission, parents die, or marital relationships break down under the strain of separation.[1244]

Even once admitted to a state of refuge, family unity may on occasion be forcibly disrupted by the application of formal state policy. For example, hundreds of male refugees from Bosnia and Croatia were taken from their families in informal conscription "raids" conducted by the Serbian government during the mid-1990s.[1245] Another extreme example was the *en masse* detention and expulsion of Chadian refugees accused by Nigerian authorities of engaging in subversive activities against the Chadian regime. Male refugees in Maiduguri, the majority of whom were the primary breadwinners for their families, were arrested, tried, and expelled without being afforded any opportunity to defend themselves.[1246] In the United States, refugee husbands and wives have traditionally been sent to separate detention facilities while their claims are being assessed, with their children often sent to juvenile jails.[1247]

[1243] "Until recently, [Immigration and Naturalization Service] officials were estimating that it could take as many as 20 more years to process thousands of Salvadorans and Guatemalans ... who fled their homelands in the 1980s and have lived for years in legal limbo ... The hardest moment [for Salvadoran refugee Juana Fuentes] occurred in 1996, when her daughter, who lived with her grandmother, needed a stomach operation. Intensely worried, Fuentes considered going back to El Salvador. 'I could go to the operation,' Fuentes said. 'But then I couldn't come back ...' ... The daughter tried to obtain a visa to visit her in Washington but was turned down": M. Sheridan, "For many seeking asylum, a long wait; Immigration and Naturalization Service pledges faster processing of cases," *Washington Post*, Jan. 17, 2002, at T-09.

[1244] Dixon-Fyle, "Reunification," at 10.

[1245] "The Serbian Ministry of the Interior ran the conscription-by-force operation, with assistance from the Yugoslav army and ... [sometimes] with that of the military police from Krajina. Serb refugees from Bosnia and Croatia have been the main targets of the mass conscription ... Men have been taken off the streets, from farmers' markets, restaurants and university dormitories; they have been taken off buses, from work, even from high school proms": Humanitarian Law Center, "Spotlight Report No. 18: The Conscription of Refugees in Serbia" (1995), at 1. Forcible conscription has also been a risk for Liberian refugees in Guinea: Médecins sans frontières USA, "A voice from the field: Liberian refugees pay a high price for crossing into Guinea" (Dec. 2002); and for refugees in Pakistan living near the border with Afghanistan: Human Rights Watch, "Letter to General Pervez Musharraf," Oct. 26, 2001.

[1246] Nigerian Civil Liberties Organization, *The Status of Refugee Rights in Nigeria* (1992), at 30. "Most of those arrested are adult males who are now separated from the rest of their families who remain in Nigeria. The Nigerian police and army are believed to be responsible for the arrests, and they have reportedly extracted bribes from relatives for unfulfilled promises of the release of the detainees": (1992) 4(5) *News from Africa Watch* 11.

[1247] "Every year, hundreds of families arrive in the United States seeking asylum or refuge from persecution back home. Since immigration laws were made stricter in 1996, many

Less egregiously, family unity may also be adversely affected by host country policies which are simply not carefully designed or administered. For example, children and parents may become permanently separated by well-meaning but inadequately conceived efforts to "assist" children quickly to become reestablished,[1248] including putting unaccompanied child refugees up for adoption before adequate efforts to locate family members can be pursued.[1249] Even adoption systems in principle predicated on tracing and ensuring the consent of the birth family may be open to fraud or manipulation, particularly in times of crisis.[1250] Bureaucratic interference with family unity may also follow from the mechanistic administration of superficially reasonable policies. At the Ukwimi refugee settlement in Zambia, even close family members were prevented from living nearby one another by the rigid application of a policy that land parcels should be allocated strictly according to time of arrival.[1251] Similarly, only the immediate family members of

of them wind up in Immigration and Naturalization Service custody instead of out on bail while their cases are being considered. For the past five years, their arrival has meant domestic heartbreak. Husbands and wives are split up into separate detention facilities. Children are shipped to juvenile jails. In the best case scenario, a whole family would be escorted into a motel room by a round-the-clock guard, unable to use the phone or even walk down the hallway": H. Rossin, "Asylum seekers decry detention by Immigration and Naturalization Service; Agency's model shelter opened to meet family needs, but grievances remain," *Washington Post*, June 17, 2001, at A-06.

[1248] "[I]t has been quite common ... for programmes to separate children from their families as a way of 'targeting' them for help. However well meaning this is, it ignores the large body of evidence which shows that in most cases children are best off in their own families, that the needs of children through infancy and childhood are best met through constancy, continuity and stability of family membership": Bonnerjea, "Disasters," at 279.

[1249] "Adoption laws of the country of refuge may technically apply to them, but that country may not take the same interest in adoptions of refugee children as it does in adoptions of children of its nationality. In addition, in the turmoil that pervades many refugee situations, it may be difficult or impossible to get definitive proof that a child's parents are dead or have irrevocably relinquished him/her for adoption. Nonetheless, at least theoretically, some countries permit adoptions to occur without evidence of parental consent on the grounds that parents cannot be found and are not capable of giving their consent": M. McLeod, "Legal Protection of Refugee Children Separated From Their Parents: Selected Issues," (1989) 28(2) *Quarterly Review of the Intergovernmental Committee for Migration* 295, at 300.

[1250] "Unfortunately in the case of El Salvador, very little information was available and sometimes the information given to the adoptive family was false ... When informal adoptions took place, a war was going on ... However, such informal adoptions could also take place today, without raising many questions. The Salvadoran civil registration system is by no means fraud-proof. People often consider registering a child with a false identity as a more viable arrangement than trying to make an adoption or care arrangement through legal means": R. Sprenkels, *Lives Apart: Family Separation and Alternative Care Arrangements During El Salvador's Civil War* (2002), at 102–103.

[1251] "[O]ne refugee woman commented that when she came to Ukwimi, the lorry was full, so that her mother, father, four uncles and two brothers ended up in different villages":

Bosnian refugees admitted to Germany were exempted from the policy of distributing refugees throughout the country, creating real difficulties for newly arrived adult children and older relatives who, having been separated from their families for often extended periods, were prevented from reuniting even once safe from the risk of persecution.[1252] And because these refugees enjoyed no freedom of internal movement, they could not even travel within Germany to visit their relatives.[1253]

Recommendation "B", Final Act of the Conference of Plenipotentiaries

The Conference, [c]onsidering that the unity of the family, the natural and fundamental group of society, is an essential right of the refugee, and that such unity is constantly threatened, and [n]oting with satisfaction that, according to the official commentary of the *Ad Hoc* Committee on Statelessness and Related Problems the rights granted to a refugee are extended to members of his family, [r]ecommends Governments to take the necessary measures for the protection of the refugee's family, especially with a view to: (1) [e]nsuring that the unity of the refugee's family is maintained particularly in cases where the head of the family has fulfilled the necessary conditions for admission to a particular country, [and] (2) [t]he protection of refugees who are minors, in particular unaccompanied children and girls, with special reference to guardianship and adoption.

Civil and Political Covenant, Art. 17

No one shall be subjected to arbitrary or unlawful interference with his privacy, family, home or correspondence, nor to unlawful attacks on his honour and reputation. Everyone has the right to the protection of the law against such interference or attacks.

Civil and Political Covenant, Art. 23(1)–(2)

The family is the natural and fundamental group unit of society and is entitled to protection by society and the State. The right of men

R. Black and T. Mabwe, "Planning for Refugees in Zambia: The Settlement Approach to Food Self-Sufficiency," (1992) 14(1) *Third World Planning Review* 14.

[1252] A. Büllesbach, "War and Civil War Refugees in Germany: The Example of Refugees from Bosnia-Hercegovina" (1995), at 22. "It may be extremely difficult for family members who have come to Germany at different times to be reunited in the same district, if one part of the family has already been distributed to a local asylum center. In general there is also no consideration given in allocation of accommodation to where any asylum-seeker may have a family connection, although the possibility exists in exceptional cases": ECRE, "Limits," at 14.

[1253] ECRE, "Limits," at 18.

and women of marriageable age to marry and to found a family shall be recognized.

Civil and Political Covenant, Art. 24(1)
Every child shall have, without any discrimination as to race, colour, sex, language, religion, national or social origin, property or birth, the right to such measures of protection as are required by his status as a minor, on the part of his family, society and the State.

Economic, Social and Cultural Covenant Art. 10(1)
The States Parties to the present Covenant recognize that ... [t]he widest possible protection and assistance should be accorded to the family, which is the natural and fundamental group unit of society, particularly for its establishment and while it is responsible for the care and education of dependent children ...

The drafters of the Refugee Convention assumed that the family members of a refugee would benefit from the protection of the Refugee Convention, even if not able themselves to show a "well-founded fear of being persecuted." Under earlier refugee accords, there had been a consistent pattern of assimilating family members to the "head of the family" for purposes of defining entitlement to the benefits of refugee status.[1254] That practice was affirmed and broadened by the Conference of Plenipotentiaries, but only as a commitment in principle, not as a matter of clearly binding law.

Specifically, the Report of the Ad Hoc Committee observed that "[m]embers of the immediate family of a refugee should, in general, be considered as refugees if the head of the family is a refugee as here defined. Also, such members are to be regarded as refugees if the conditions set forth ... apply to them, even if the head of the family is not a refugee."[1255] This view not only affirmed traditional practice, but moreover eliminated the possibility of applying the notion of "family unity with a vengeance." That is, the novation of the Ad Hoc Committee's formulation was the ability of a dependent family member to claim refugee status in his or her own right,

---

[1254] Even as the approach of refugee law became more individualized with the advent of the IRO Constitution, respect for family unity continued. "[F]or reasons of equity as well as administrative convenience, families – not individuals – were considered the basic units with respect to determining who [was] within the Organization's mandate. Thus, if the head of a family was found to be within (or without) the mandate, the members of his family were also so considered, unless they fell under some constitutional provisions not applicable to the head of the family": Grahl-Madsen, *Status of Refugees I*, at 413.

[1255] "Comments of the Committee on the Draft Convention relating to the Status of Refugees," Annex II to Ad Hoc Committee, "First Session Report," at 2.

whether or not the "head of the family" was entitled to refugee status. Yet it was subject to no formal debate or discussion in the Ad Hoc Committee, with the result that no relevant article was proposed for the Convention itself.

At the Conference of Plenipotentiaries, however, a declaration was inserted into the Final Act of the Conference. On the initiative of the Holy See, the Conference agreed without dissent to recommend that governments take "the necessary measures for the protection of the refugee's family especially with a view to ... [e]nsuring that the unity of the refugee's family is maintained."[1256] They expressly affirmed the "essential right of the refugee" to family unity, and endorsed the understanding of that principle stated by the Ad Hoc Committee.[1257]

This declaration is in some ways a powerful, if non-binding, affirmation of the responsibility of states to avoid actions which might disturb the unity of a refugee's family. The language originally proposed[1258] was twice strengthened in order to avoid any impression of diluting the "categorical view of the Ad Hoc Committee that governments were under an obligation to take such action in respect of the refugee's family ... [I]t would be regrettable if governments were to take the action therein proposed only when they considered that circumstances enabled them to do so."[1259] Indeed, at least the German representative was of the view that the responsibility of states was not simply to avoid disrupting family unity, but also to facilitate the reunion of divided families.[1260] Yet it is also undeniable that – for reasons not explained by the drafters – they viewed the issue of the responsibility to respect family unity as "naturally not of a contractual nature."[1261] The High Court of Australia has thus determined that a domestic system which considers, but does not guarantee, the admission of a refugee's spouse and children amounts to "implementation in Australian law of Recommendation B ... [that goes] beyond observance of the international obligations imposed by the Refugees Convention."[1262]

[1256] Ibid.   [1257] See text of Recommendation "B", above at p. 540.

[1258] UN Doc. A/CONF.2/103.

[1259] Statement of Mr. Hoare of the United Kingdom, UN Doc. A/CONF.2/SR.34, July 25, 1951, at 7. The language had earlier been strengthened at the suggestion of Mr. Robinson of Israel, ibid. at 6.

[1260] "He felt it was appropriate that the Conference should emphasize the principle of the unity of the refugee's family, a principle of particular importance in a country like Germany where, by force of political circumstance, many German families had been split asunder. The German Government was making every effort to facilitate the reunion of such families": Statement of Mr. von Trutzschler of the Federal Republic of Germany, ibid. at 5–6.

[1261] Statement of Msgr. Comte of the Holy See, ibid. at 4.

[1262] *Re Minister for Immigration and Multicultural and Indigenous Affairs, ex parte Applicant S134/2002*, (2003) 195 ALR 1 (Aus. HC, Feb. 4, 2003). When this case was reviewed by

While it is possible to dismiss the Conference's recommendation as essentially hortatory,[1263] a plausible case can be made that at least the core elements of Recommendation B of the Final Act have ripened into customary international law. The Recommendation, reproduced and elaborated in the UNHCR *Handbook*,[1264] has inspired many resolutions of the UNHCR's Executive Committee. States have regularly affirmed the view that "the family is the natural and fundamental group unit of society and is entitled to protection by society and the state,"[1265] as well as the specific importance of the family "as the fundamental group of society concerned with the protection and well-being of children and adolescents."[1266] This centrality of the family requires that "family unity should be respected,"[1267] "maintained,"[1268] and "protected."[1269] There should be a "prioritization of family unity issues at an early stage in all refugee operations,"[1270] and "all action taken on behalf of refugee children must be guided by the principle of the best interests of the child as well as by the principle of family unity."[1271] And of most direct relevance to the question of the admission of family members, the Executive Committee has

> [u]nderline[d] the need for the unity of the refugee's family to be protected, *inter alia* by ... provisions and/or practice allowing that when the principal applicant is recognized as a refugee, other members of the family unit should normally also be recognized as refugees, and by providing each

the United Nations Human Rights Committee, however, it was determined that "to separate a spouse and children arriving in a State from a spouse validly resident in a State may give rise to issues under articles 17 and 23 of the Covenant": *Bakhtiyari v. Australia*, UNHRC Comm. No. 1069/2002, UN Doc. CCPR/C/79/D/1069/2002, decided Oct. 29, 2003, at para. 9.6. See discussion of relevant Covenant obligations below, at pp. 547–560.

[1263] "The 1951 Convention does little more than recommend measures to ensure family unity and protection": Goodwin-Gill, *Refugee in International Law*, at 257.

[1264] UNHCR, *Handbook*, at Annex I and paras. 181–188.

[1265] UNHCR Executive Committee Conclusions No. 85, "Conclusion on International Protection" (1998), at para. (u), and 88, "Protection of the Refugee's Family" (1999), at para. (b), both available at www.unhcr.ch (accessed Nov. 20, 2004).

[1266] UNHCR Executive Committee Conclusion No. 84, "Refugee Children and Adolescents" (1997), at para. (a)(i), available at www.unhcr.ch (accessed Nov. 20, 2004).

[1267] UNHCR Executive Committee Conclusion No. 22, "Protection of Asylum-Seekers in Situations of Large-Scale Influx" (1981), at para. (II)(B)(2)(h), available at www.unhcr.ch (accessed Nov. 20, 2004).

[1268] UNHCR Executive Committee Conclusion No. 85, "Conclusion on International Protection" (1998), at para. (v), available at www.unhcr.ch (accessed Nov. 20, 2004).

[1269] UNHCR Executive Committee Conclusion No. 88, "Protection of the Refugee's Family" (1999), at para. (b), available at www.unhcr.ch (accessed Nov. 20, 2004).

[1270] Ibid. at para. (b)(iv).

[1271] UNHCR Executive Committee Conclusion No. 47, "Refugee Children" (1987), at para. (d), available at www.unhcr.ch (accessed Nov. 20, 2004).

family member with the possibility of separately submitting any refugee claims that he or she may have.[1272]

Beyond the expectation that family members will be assimilated to the refugee for purposes of protection, "every effort should be made to ensure the reunification of separated refugee families."[1273] More recently, states have been "exhort[ed]" to pursue family reunification "in a positive and humanitarian spirit, and without delay,"[1274] and even to "consider[ ] ... liberal criteria in identifying those family members who can be admitted, with a view to promoting a comprehensive reunification of the family."[1275] Most generally, the Executive Committee has called upon states to consolidate their procedures for family unity and reunification in a "legal framework to give effect at the national level to a right to family unity for all refugees, taking into account the human rights of the refugees and their families."[1276] Indeed, in most state parties there is a long-standing jurisprudence affirming the principle of family unity,[1277] sometimes buttressed by policies that are explicitly based upon Recommendation B.[1278]

[1272] UNHCR Executive Committee Conclusion No. 88, "Protection of the Refugee's Family" (1999), at para. (b)(iii), available at www.unhcr.ch (accessed Nov. 20, 2004). To similar effect, see UNHCR Executive Committee Conclusion No. 85, "Conclusion on International Protection" (1998), at para. (v), available at www.unhcr.ch (accessed Nov. 20, 2004).

[1273] UNHCR Executive Committee Conclusion No. 24, "Family Reunification" (1981), at para. 1, available at www.unhcr.ch (accessed Nov. 20, 2004).

[1274] UNHCR Executive Committee Conclusion No. 85, "Conclusion on International Protection" (1998), at para. (w), available at www.unhcr.ch (accessed Nov. 20, 2004).

[1275] UNHCR Executive Committee Conclusion No. 88, "Protection of the Refugee's Family" (1999), at para. (b)(ii), available at www.unhcr.ch (accessed Nov. 20, 2004).

[1276] UNHCR Executive Committee Conclusion No. 85, "Conclusion on International Protection" (1998), at para. (x), available at www.unhcr.ch (accessed Nov. 20, 2004).

[1277] See generally Grahl-Madsen, *Status of Refugees I*, at 414–417. For example, the Belgian Conseil d'Etat refused to expel the spouse of a Zaïrian asylum-seeker on grounds of family unity: *Tshisuaka and Tshilele v. Belgium*, 3rd Chamber, Ref. No. 39227 (Apr. 2, 1992), reported at (1992) 68 *Revue du droit des étrangers* 66.

[1278] In the United Kingdom, for example, the position on family reunion "is entirely different where an asylum-seeker has been recognised as a refugee. The principle of family unity for refugees is contained in the Final Act of the instrument that established the 1951 Convention. Although family reunion does not form part of the Convention itself, the United Kingdom will normally permit the reunion of the immediate family, as a concession outside the immigration rules. Under that policy, people recognised as refugees immediately become eligible to be joined by their spouse and minor children, provided that they lived together as a family before the sponsor travelled to seek asylum. Families of refugees are not required to satisfy the maintenance and accommodation requirements that normally apply when families seek admission to join a sponsor here. Other dependent relatives may be admitted if there are compelling compassionate circumstances": *Munim v. Secretary of State for the Home Department*, Lexis Unreported Decisions (Eng. CA, May 3, 2000), quoting from the statement of Mr. Nicholas Baker MP to the House of Commons, Mar. 17, 1995.

There is therefore little doubt that there is ample raw material from which to derive the necessary *opinio juris* for recognition of a customary legal norm to protect the family unity of refugees. But on close examination, it is clear that while there is a continuing insistence that the family members of a primary applicant refugee should be admitted to protection,[1279] most refugee-specific formulations fail to define with any precision the content of an affirmative dimension of the principle of family unity. Standards in general human rights law similarly tend to limit the ambit of the principle to the avoidance of "arbitrary interference,"[1280] "arbitrary or unlawful interference,"[1281] or to the separation of children from their parents "except when competent authorities subject to judicial review determine, in accordance with the applicable law and procedures, that such separation is necessary for the best interests of the child."[1282] In other words, the *opinio juris* which achieves the specificity and precision needed to generate binding legal duties does not include norms mandating affirmative reunification,[1283] or even prohibiting all forms of interference with family unity. The sense of clear legal obligation instead extends only to a duty not to engage in *unlawful or arbitrary* interference with family unity.

Interestingly, this understanding of the scope of relevant *opinio juris* coincides with the core of state practice – this being, of course, the second critical element for establishment of a customary international legal

---

[1279] See Recommendation B of the Final Act of the Conference of Plenipotentiaries, above at p. 540; as well as Executive Committee Conclusions Nos. 85, "Conclusion on International Protection" (1998), at para. (v), and 88, "Protection of the Refugee's Family" (1999), at para. (b)(iii), both available at www.unhcr.ch (accessed Nov. 20, 2004).

[1280] Universal Declaration, at Art. 12.

[1281] Civil and Political Covenant, at Art. 17(1). "The term 'unlawful' means that no interference can take place except in cases envisaged by the law. Interference authorized by States can only take place on the basis of law, which itself must comply with the provisions, aims and objectives of the Covenant ... The expression 'arbitrary interference' is also relevant to the protection of the right provided for in article 17. In the Committee's view the expression 'arbitrary interference' can also extend to interference provided for under the law. The introduction of the concept of arbitrariness is intended to guarantee that even interference provided for by law should be in accordance with the provisions, aims and objectives of the Covenant and should be, in any event, reasonable in the particular circumstances": UN Human Rights Committee, "General Comment No. 16: Right to privacy" (1988), UN Doc. HRI/GEN/1/Rev.7, May 12, 2004, at 142, paras. 3–4.

[1282] Rights of the Child Convention, at Art. 9(1).

[1283] For example, UNGA Res. 51/89 (1996), which "reaffirms ... the vital importance of family reunification," was adopted on a vote of 89–4 (76 abstentions). The massive number of abstentions is cause for some caution on the question of consistent *opinio juris* favoring an affirmative duty to reunify families. For a discussion of the standards applicable to recognition of a norm of customary international law, see generally chapter 1.1.1 above.

obligation. While state practice nearly universally affirms the duty of states to act lawfully, and not to take steps which arbitrarily interfere with a refugee's family unity, the duty to take affirmative steps to facilitate family reunification is more controversial.[1284] At least in historical perspective, Goodwin-Gill is right to point to "[r]estrictions on family reunion ... [which] result from the conditions attached to certain types of status, such as temporary protection which, although they facilitate the grant of refuge, may be so circumscribed as to frustrate fundamental rights relating to the family."[1285]

The need to locate a core of relatively consistent state practice in support of the putative customary norm also results in a limitation on the scope of the beneficiary class of the duty to avoid unlawful or arbitrary interference with family unity. Practice suggests that the scope of "family" members who may

---

[1284] "The right of [family] unity is often distinguished from the right to reunification, which extends protection more specifically to families which have been separated and wish to reunite. Few international human rights instruments specifically designate a right of family reunification or otherwise elaborate on how the right to be treated as a unit should be implemented in cases of separated families": C. Anderfuhren-Wayne, "Family Unity in Immigration and Refugee Matters: United States and European Approaches," (1996) 8(3) *International Journal of Refugee Law* 347 (Anderfuhren-Wayne, "Family Unity"), at 349. In Canadian practice, for example, "[f]amilies are separated by reunion procedures which are protracted and unpredictable. Almost no refugee claimant or asylum-seeker has found any simple effective court remedy against these procedures": Inter-Church Committee for Refugees, "Rights to Protection of the Family and Refugees in Canada," May 1993, at 2.

[1285] Goodwin-Gill, *Refugee in International Law*, at 260. Under modern understandings of temporary protection within the European Union, however, the breadth of reunification rights may actually exceed that for Convention refugees: EU Temporary Protection Directive, at Art. 15. Goodwin-Gill also asserts the relevance of the fact that "[s]everal States have made reservations to the [Convention on the Rights of the Child] provisions on family reunion, despite the importance otherwise given to the family as the basic unit of society": ibid. at 259–260. In actuality, the relevant reservations to Arts. 10 and 22 are few, and are certainly insufficient to suggest a concern by governments to protect state practice significantly out of line with the duty of family reunification posited in the treaty. The only strong exception is Japan, which does not accept a duty to admit the families of refugees. Germany makes clear that the provisions do not authorize unlawful entry or stay (which they do not in any event); the Netherlands insists on the right to make admission subject to "certain conditions." Four countries – Indonesia, Liechtenstein, Switzerland, and Thailand – make the treaty-specific duty subject to their national laws. But more than 180 state parties have accepted the family reunification provisions of the Convention on the Rights of the Child without any qualification. See Anderfuhren-Wayne, "Family Unity," at 354: "[U]nder both US and European laws the right to family unity is a limited one. It is not only the doctrines of plenary power and State sovereignty which, in effect, circumscribe the right, but also the contradictions underlying these notions: That is, on the one hand, there is an emphasis placed upon the value and importance of families and family rights, including the right of reunification; on the other hand, there is a practice of limiting these rights in an effort to preserve State autonomy."

claim a right to be protected against even arbitrary or unlawful interference with family unity is limited to the refugee's opposite-sex spouse and any minor, dependent children.[1286] There is simply too much variation in state practice regarding members of the more extended family – including even parents, grandparents, and adult children – for a clear rule of customary international law to have emerged requiring respect for the unity of the broader family class.[1287] Yet even with all of these limitations, the ability of refugees to invoke a customary international legal duty prohibiting states from acting unlawfully or arbitrarily to disrupt the unity of at least their nuclear family is no small victory.

In state parties to the Human Rights Covenants, it makes more sense to rely upon those treaties to assert comparable entitlements. Both Covenants affirm the central place of the family in international law,[1288] and require

---

[1286] See Grahl-Madsen, *Status of Refugees I*, at 416, 418. This was also the understanding embraced by the drafters of the unsuccessful Convention on Territorial Asylum, which would have guaranteed reunification only for "the spouse and the minor or dependent children of any person to whom [the state] has granted the benefits of the Convention": UN Doc. A/CONF.78/DC.4, Jan. 31, 1977. Most recently, UNHCR observed that "[t]here is virtually universal consensus in the international community concerning the need to reunite members of [the] family nucleus": UNHCR, *Resettlement Handbook* (1996), at IV(12).

[1287] "The difficulty lies in the fact that a universally accepted concept of family can hardly be said to exist. The differences existing between the various regional-cultural family notions can be very large; sometimes the family is regarded as an institution, sometimes as a creation of contractual will, or it may be a part of religious life": Fourlanos, *Sovereignty*, at 88. For example, Swiss practice grants asylum-seekers no access to family reunification, and grants recognized refugees the right to be reunited only with a spouse and dependent children. More distant family members will be allowed to join the refugee only in exceptional cases, e.g. if they are disabled or otherwise dependent upon the support of the recognized refugee: W. Kälin, *International Academy of Comparative Law National Report for Switzerland* (1994), at 17. The UNHCR Executive Committee has, however, called on states to consider "liberal criteria in identifying those family members who can be admitted, with a view to promoting a comprehensive reunification of the family": UNHCR Executive Committee Conclusion No. 88, "Protection of the Refugee's Family" (1999), at para. (b)(iii), available at www.unhcr.ch (accessed Nov. 20, 2004). See also UNHCR, "Summary Conclusions on Family Unity," Global Consultations Expert Roundtable, Nov. 8–9, 2001, at para. 8: "International human rights law has not explicitly defined 'family' although there is an emerging body of international jurisprudence on this issue which serves as a useful guide to interpretation. The question of the existence or non-existence of family is essentially a question of fact, which must be determined on a case-by-case basis, requiring a flexible approach which takes account of cultural variations, and economic and emotional dependency factors. For the purposes of family reunification, 'family' includes, at the very minimum, members of the nuclear family (spouses and minor children)."

[1288] Civil and Political Covenant, Art. 23(1); Economic, Social and Cultural Covenant, Art. 10(1).

governments to take affirmative legislative steps to "protect" the family.[1289] It is also clear that refugees may not be denied protection of their familial rights on grounds of their status as non-citizens:

> The Covenant [on Civil and Political Rights] does not recognize the right of aliens to enter or reside in the territory of a State party. However, in certain circumstances an alien may enjoy the protection of the Covenant *in relation to entry or residence*, for example, when considerations of non-discrimination, prohibition of inhuman treatment and *respect for family life* arise ... [Non-citizens] may not be subjected to arbitrary or unlawful interference with their privacy, *family*, home, or correspondence [emphasis added].[1290]

The central concern, however, is just what type of concrete action by states is required in order to discharge this treaty-based duty of protection.

The most unambiguously framed protection is Art. 17 of the Civil and Political Covenant, the core of which mirrors the customary legal norm just described. It proscribes "arbitrary or unlawful interference with ... family" and grants "[e]veryone ... the right to the protection of the law against such interference or attacks." Thus, any interference with an individual's family unity not carried out on the basis of legal authority is a violation of the Covenant. As the Human Rights Committee has explained, "[i]nterference by States can only take place on the basis of law, which itself must comply with the provisions, aims and objectives of the Covenant."[1291] Because interference with the family unity is only "lawful" if conducted in a manner that respects "the provisions ... of the Covenant," both the Serbian break-up of refugee families from Bosnia and Croatia by informal conscription "raids," in which male family members were dragged away without any semblance of due process, and Nigeria's separation of Chadian refugee families by the *en masse* detention of male refugees without implementation of any process to

---

[1289] Civil and Political Covenant, Arts. 17(2), 23(1), 23(4), and 24(1); Economic, Social and Cultural Covenant, Art. 10(1).

[1290] UN Human Rights Committee, "General Comment No. 15: The position of aliens under the Covenant" (1986), UN Doc. HRI/GEN/1/Rev.7, May 12, 2004, at 140, paras. 5 and 7. See also UN Human Rights Committee, "General Comment No. 17: Rights of the child" (1989), UN Doc. HRI/GEN/1/Rev.7, May 12, 2004, at 144, para. 5: "The Covenant requires that children should be protected against discrimination on any grounds ... Reports by States parties should indicate how legislation and practice ensure that measures of protection are aimed at removing all discrimination in every field ... particularly as between children who are nationals and children who are aliens."

[1291] "The term 'unlawful' means that no interference can take place except in cases envisaged by the law": UN Human Rights Committee, "General Comment No. 16: Right to privacy" (1988), UN Doc. HRI/GEN/1/Rev.7, May 12, 2004, at 142, para. 3.

assess the legitimacy of subversion charges against them,[1292] amounted to indirect violations of this aspect of the duty under Art. 17.

But even if authorized by law, actions which interfere with family unity are still prohibited if they are "arbitrary." The drafting history of the predecessor provision in the Universal Declaration of Human Rights suggests that an interference is arbitrary if it is "not in accordance with well-established legal principles,"[1293] or if action is "taken at the will and pleasure of some person who could not be called upon to show just cause for it."[1294] In the context of the drafting of the Civil and Political Covenant, "it was stressed above all that 'arbitrary' clearly went beyond 'unlawful' and contained an element of 'capriciousness.'"[1295] Nowak elaborates:

> [R]egardless of its lawfulness, arbitrary interference contains elements of injustice, unpredictability, and unreasonableness. Moreover, the expression "arbitrary" suggests a violation by State organs. In evaluating whether interference ... by a State enforcement organ represents a violation of Art. 17, it must especially be reviewed whether, in addition to conformity with national law, the specific act of enforcement had a purpose that seems legitimate on the basis of the Covenant in its entirety, whether it was predictable in the sense of the rule of law and, in particular, whether it was reasonable (proportional) in relation to the purpose to be achieved.[1296]

This approach to Art. 17 is embraced by the Human Rights Committee, which insists that lawful interference is only non-arbitrary if it is "in accordance with the provisions, aims and objectives of the Covenant and ... in any event, reasonable in the particular circumstances."[1297]

The reference by the Human Rights Committee to "reasonableness" follows logically from the need for non-arbitrary acts to be consistent with other provisions of the Covenant, including the duty of equality before the law and equal protection of the law under Art. 26. While the Committee has generally afforded states a broad margin of appreciation in its assessment of reasonableness, particularly where non-citizens are concerned,[1298] it has nonetheless relied on Art. 17 to prevent the deportation of the family members of a

---

[1292] "No one shall be deprived of his liberty except on such grounds and in accordance with such procedures as are established by law": Civil and Political Covenant, at Art. 9(1).

[1293] L. Rehof, "Article 12," in A. Eide et al. eds., *The Universal Declaration of Human Rights: A Commentary* 187 (1992) (Rehof, "Article 12"), at 189–190, quoting from the New Zealand representative, Mrs. Newlands.

[1294] Ibid. at 190, quoting from the British representative, Mrs. Corbet.

[1295] Nowak, *ICCPR Commentary*, at 291.   [1296] Ibid. at 292–293.

[1297] UN Human Rights Committee, "General Comment No. 16: Right to privacy" (1988), UN Doc. HRI/GEN/1/Rev.7, May 12, 2004, at 142, para. 4.

[1298] See chapter 2.5.5 above, at pp. 130–132.

refugee whose claim had not yet been finally determined.[1299] The Committee recently considered a case in which a refugee's wife and children had arrived separately from him, and had been detained for nearly three years. The husband had initially been recognized as a Convention refugee, though the basis for that decision was under review. The Human Rights Committee determined that removal of the wife and children would amount to an arbitrary interference with family:

> Taking into account the specific circumstances of the case, namely the number and age of the children, including a newborn, the traumatic experiences Mrs. Bakhtiyari and her children would face if returned to Pakistan and the absence of arguments by the State party to justify removal in these circumstances, the Committee takes the view that removing Mrs. Bakhtiyari and her children without awaiting the final determination of Mr. Bakhtiyari's proceedings would constitute arbitrary interference in the family of the authors, in violation of articles 17, paragraph 1, and 23, paragraph 1, of the Covenant.[1300]

The fact-specific nature of the inquiry into arbitrariness suggests that Art. 17 will be most readily breached when there is capricious or unpredictable interference with family unity. For example, the refusal of Zambian authorities to take any account of family relationships in the assignment of refugees at Ukwimi to particular land parcels – insisting instead on an uncompromising application of a system of allocating plots based on the date of arrival – can readily be seen as an action in violation of Art. 17.[1301] The rigidity of the Zambian approach is demonstrative of the sort of capriciousness or unreasonableness that taints even a system authorized by law as "arbitrary," and therefore inconsistent with the protective responsibilities of Art. 17. A similar rigidity, and hence unreasonableness, also characterizes the traditional American approach of segregating the members of refugee families for indefinite detention while awaiting verification of their status. Art. 17 is also breached where a state engages in or promotes the adoption of

---

[1299] More generally, the Committee has been willing in the context of immigration-based removals to insist that a resultant interference with family life be not only lawful, but also not arbitrary. In considering a challenge to the deportation of a stateless married couple from Indonesia and their thirteen-year-old son who was a citizen of Australia, the Committee observed that "[i]t is certainly unobjectionable under the Covenant that a State party may require, under its laws, the departure of persons who remain in its territory beyond limited duration periods": *Winata v. Australia*, UNHRC Comm. No. 930/2000, UN Doc. CCPR/C/72/D/930/2000, decided July 26, 2001, at para. 7.3.

[1300] *Bakhtiyari v. Australia*, UNHRC Comm. No. 1069/2002, UN Doc. CCPR/C/79/D/1069/2002, decided Oct. 29, 2003, at para. 9.6.

[1301] It is noteworthy that "Art. 17 does not contain a legal proviso allowing for restrictions in the interest of public order or similar purposes": Nowak, *ICCPR Commentary*, at 290–291.

unaccompanied child refugees on the basis of inadequate efforts to trace the child's parents, or where – as in the case of El Salvador – it fails to take reasonable safeguards to avoid fraud and manipulation of the adoption process.[1302] Indeed, Germany's decision to exempt from its general aliens dispersal policy only "immediate" family members of Bosnian refugees likely also failed to comply with Art. 17 in view of the evolving domestic consensus against such a narrow construction of the "family."[1303]

As important as Art. 17 is as a means of contesting actions which disrupt family unity, the superficially less robust protection of Art. 23 of the Civil and Political Covenant may actually be of greater value to refugees seeking to compel states to take *affirmative* steps to unify their families.[1304] The key clause requires states to recognize "[t]he right of men and women of marriageable age to marry and *to found a family* [emphasis added]." In its General Comment on Art. 23, the Human Rights Committee determined that

> [t]he right to found a family implies, in principle, the possibility to procreate and live together ... [T]he possibility to live together implies the adoption of appropriate measures, both at the internal level and as the case may be, in cooperation with other States, to *ensure the unity or reunification of families*, particularly when their members are separated for *political, economic or similar reasons* [emphasis added]."[1305]

[1302] See also UNHCR Executive Committee Conclusion No. 85, "Conclusion on International Protection" (1999), available at www.unhcr.ch (accessed Nov. 20, 2004), at para. (c): "The Executive Committee ... [c]alls upon States, UNHCR and other relevant actors to give particular attention to the needs of unaccompanied refugee children pending their reunification with their families; and affirms, in this regard, that adoption of refugee children should only be considered when all feasible steps for family tracing have been exhausted, and then only in the best interests of the child and in conformity with international standards."

[1303] See e.g. *Kroon v. Netherlands*, (1994) 19 EHRR 263 (ECHR, Oct. 27, 1994), affirming the importance of biological and social realities in the definition of family relationships. More generally, see discussion of the duty under the Civil and Political Covenant universally to apply a state's own definition of family to all, below, at pp. 553–557. Moreover, Germany's refusal to allow refugee families the freedom to travel within Germany was likely in breach of the Convention: see chapter 4.2.4 above.

[1304] See Nowak, *ICCPR Commentary*, at 402, 406: "As an institutional guarantee, Art. 23 differs from negative protection against interference with private and family life guaranteed by Art. 17. The claim possessed by the institution 'family' under Art. 23 to protection by society and the State is stronger than that in Art. 12 of the [European Convention on Human Rights], which merely sets forth the right to marry and found a family ... [I]nstitutional guarantees always imply certain *privileges* on the part of the individuals affected by them. Since life together is an essential criterion for the existence of a family, members of a family are entitled to a stronger right to live together than other persons [emphasis in original]."

[1305] UN Human Rights Committee, "General Comment No. 19: The family" (1990), UN Doc. HRI/GEN/1/Rev.7, May 12, 2004, at 149, para. 5.

Clearly, the sorts of forces which cause refugee families to become separated are paradigmatic examples of "political . . . or similar reasons." Because refugee status manifestly precludes the family exercising its right to live together in the country of origin,[1306] the Human Rights Committee's conclusions should be read to compel measures to ensure the unity or reunification of refugee families in the state of asylum.

In practical terms, the most significant difficulty of relying on this official interpretation of Art. 23 to require states affirmatively to promote family unity parallels one of the constraints discussed above regarding the scope of a possible customary legal duty: some forms of "family" may be thought to be excluded from Art. 23's protection. One argument of this kind may, however, be dismissed. It is sometimes suggested that when Art. 23(2) is read as a whole – "[t]he right of men and women of marriageable age to marry and to found a family" – it follows that only persons who benefit from the first part of the right ("to marry") may claim the benefit of the second part of the right ("to found a family"). Thus, only persons who are "married" may assert the right to "found a family," entailing the right to "live together." This argument is, however, fallacious. As the drafting history of the clause makes clear, actual marriage is not required to invoke the right to found a family.[1307] The Human Rights Committee has recently made precisely this point in the context of its rejection of an argument by France that a refugee from Cameroon forfeited the right to be reunited with his wife by virtue of the absence of evidence of conjugal relations with her, and proof of his sexual infidelity with another woman:

> Article 23 of the Covenant guarantees the protection of family life including the interest in family reunification. The Committee recalls that the term "family," for purposes of the Covenant, must be understood broadly [so] as to include all those comprising a family in the society concerned. The protection of such family is not necessarily obviated, in any particular case, by the absence of formal marriage bonds, especially where there is a local practice of customary or common law marriage. Nor is the right to protection of family life necessarily displaced by geographical separation, infidelity, or the absence of conjugal relations.[1308]

[1306] This understanding parallels what has come to be known as the "elsewhere approach" under the jurisprudence interpreting the European Convention on Human Rights. While the legal duty is simply to allow families to live together, this may require the admission of family members where there is no possibility of safe reunification abroad. See generally H. Storey, "The Right to Family Life and Immigration Case Law at Strasbourg," (1990) 39 *International and Comparative Law Quarterly* 328.

[1307] Nowak makes reference to the failed motion submitted by the French government, which would have restricted the definition of the relevant family to a marital family: Nowak, *ICCPR Commentary*, at 413, n. 70.

[1308] *Ngambi and Nébol v. France*, UNHRC Comm. No. 1179/2003, UN Doc. CCPR/C/81/D/1179/2003, decided July 16, 2004, at para. 6.4. On the facts of the case, however, it was

While the Committee's reference to the duty to reunite families as understood in "the society concerned" is somewhat ambiguous,[1309] it is most likely that the duty is simply to facilitate the reunification of families as conceived in the country in which the refugee is now present. As Nowak frames the duty, "the protection of this provision covers cohabitation with or without children, the founding of a *polygamous marriage* with or without children in States that recognize polygamy, as well as the founding of all other familial forms consistent with the legal and cultural peculiarities of the respective State."[1310] Yet as this formulation suggests, the problem for refugees may well be that "the legal and cultural peculiarities" of the asylum country do not recognize *their* families – for example, the family of a refugee in a polygamous marriage or same-sex union, or an extended refugee family seeking protection from a society in which the nuclear family is the norm.[1311]

International law constrains the scope of a state's right to define family for itself in only a minimalist way. Most fundamentally, there is a presumptive duty of states arising from Art. 24 of the Covenant,[1312] significantly amplified

---

determined that the author of the communication had not effectively refuted evidence that the documents presented to substantiate the marriage were false: ibid.

[1309] That is, it is not textually clear whether the reference is to social constructions in the refugee's country of origin, or those which prevail in the state in which a duty of family reunification is being asserted. Nor does the subsequent reference to "local practice" clarify this issue.

[1310] Nowak, *ICCPR Commentary*, at 413. Since Nowak's analysis was prepared, however, it has been determined by the Human Rights Committee that "equality of treatment with regard to the right to marry implies that polygamy is incompatible with this principle. Polygamy violates the dignity of women. It is an inadmissible discrimination against women. Consequently, it should be definitely abolished wherever it continues to exist": UN Human Rights Committee, "General Comment No. 28: The equality of rights between men and women" (2000), UN Doc. HRI/GEN/1/Rev.7, May 12, 2004, at 178, para. 24. It might therefore logically be determined that Art. 23 of the Civil and Political Covenant compels reception states *not* to facilitate the reunification of families organized on the basis of unlawful discrimination.

[1311] "A *stricto senso* universality in international law hardly exists. There is always room for variations, and this is even more the case when it comes to culturally conditioned institutions, such as family. The differences from one region to another can be so big that what is normal and, thus, allowed in one society (e.g. a polygamous marriage), may be strongly disapproved of and legally forbidden somewhere else": Fourlanos, *Sovereignty*, at 92.

[1312] "Article 24 ... entails the adoption of special measures to protect children ... The Covenant requires that children should be protected against discrimination on any grounds such as ... national or social origin, property or birth ... Reports by States parties should indicate how legislation and practice ensure that measures of protection are aimed at removing all discrimination in every field ... particularly as between children who are nationals and children who are aliens": UN Human Rights Committee, "General Comment No. 17: Rights of the child" (1989), UN Doc. HRI/GEN/1/Rev.7, May 12, 2004, at 144, paras. 1, 5. Of particular importance, Nowak asserts that "Art. 24(3) ... grants at least a *subsidiary jus soli* for all children born or found on by the Convention on the Rights of the Child,[1313] to recognize children under the age of eighteen as part of the parental family unit.[1314] Second, it may also be argued that the agreement in principle of state parties to the International Covenant on Economic, Social and Cultural Rights that there is a special responsibility to meet the needs of aged family members[1315] should be read to compel the inclusion of such persons in the definition of the family unit. Third, the Human Rights Committee has suggested that the notion of "family" should be interpreted not in the abstract, but on the basis of social norms in the society concerned.[1316] But beyond these parameters, the asylum

the territory of a State Party and who would be stateless without recognition of this right": Nowak, *ICCPR Commentary*, at 434. A judge of the High Court of Australia arrived at a similar result on the basis of common law reasoning. In considering the deportation of the parent of an Australian-born child, Justice Gaudron commented that "it is arguable that citizenship carries with it a common law right on the part of children and their parents to have a child's best interest taken into account, at least as a primary consideration, in all discretionary decisions by governments, and government agencies which directly affect that child's individual welfare, particularly decisions which affect children as dramatically and as fundamentally as those involved in this case": *Minister for Immigration and Ethnic Affairs v. Teoh*, (1995) 183 CLR 273 (Aus. HC, Apr. 7, 1995), per Gaudron J. at 304.

[1313] "States Parties shall respect the right of the child who is separated from one or both parents to maintain personal relations and direct contact with both parents on a regular basis, except if it is contrary to the child's best interests ... [A]pplications by a child or his or her parents to enter or leave a State Party for the purpose of family reunification shall be dealt with by States Parties in a positive, humane and expeditious manner. States Parties shall further ensure that the submission of such a request shall entail no adverse consequences for the applicants and for the members of their family": Rights of the Child Convention, at Arts. 9(3) and 10(1).

[1314] "[T]he Covenant does not indicate the age at which [a child] attains his majority. This is to be determined by each State party in the light of the relevant social and cultural conditions. In this respect, States should indicate in their reports the age at which the child attains his majority in civil matters and assumes criminal responsibility. States should also indicate the age at which a child is legally entitled to work and the age at which he is treated as an adult under labour law ... However, the Committee notes that the age for the above purposes should not be set unreasonably low and that in any case a State party cannot absolve itself from its obligations under the Covenant regarding persons under the age of 18, notwithstanding that they have reached the age of majority under domestic law": UN Human Rights Committee, "General Comment No. 17: Rights of the child" (1989), UN Doc. HRI/GEN/1/Rev.7, May 12, 2004, at 144, para. 4.

[1315] "State parties should make all the necessary efforts to support, protect and strengthen the family and help it, in accordance with each society's system of cultural values, to respond to the needs of its dependent ageing members": UN Committee on Economic, Social and Cultural Rights, "General Comment No. 6: The economic, social and cultural rights of older persons" (1995), UN Doc. HRI/GEN/1/Rev.7, May 12, 2004, at 35, para. 31.

[1316] "Regarding the term 'family,' the objectives of the Covenant require that for purposes of article 17 this term be given a broad interpretation to include all those comprising the family as understood in the society of the State party concerned": UN Human Rights state has broad autonomy to interpret who qualifies as "family," and hence is entitled to "live together." The duty under international human rights law is simply to apply that definition to all, including when making decisions regarding the reunification of refugee families.[1317] It follows, therefore, that this provision cannot be relied upon, for example, to compel states to reverse their stand against reunification of multiple spouses in a polygamous marriage where such marriages are not recognized domestically.

Despite recognizing that family membership for reunification purposes should ordinarily be defined in line with the host state's own norms, Nowak nonetheless suggests that families organized around a same-sex union may face an additional hurdle. He argues that same-sex relationships do not qualify to benefit from the right to "found a family" (including the right to unity and to reunification of family), even in asylum states which authorize same-sex marriages:

> Given that the right to marry and *found* a family is, in contrast to all other rights of the Covenant, expressly provided to "men and women," the protection afforded the founding of a family presupposes at least that two persons of different sex and of marriageable age are living together. Persons of the same gender who live together with or without children, are, therefore, not protected by the right to found a family.[1318]

This seems an unduly restrictive interpretation. While there may be no practical choice but to defer to particular states' understandings of "family," there is no good reason to deny protection of the right to found a family to persons in a same-sex relationship in a state where such unions are lawful. Art. 23(2) extends its benefits to "men and women" – not to "a man and a woman" – and can therefore logically be read to require gender equality rather than to exclude homosexual relationships. Such an interpretation is moreover consistent with the position of the Human Rights Committee that

---

Committee, "General Comment No. 16: Right to privacy" (1988), UN Doc. HRI/GEN/1/Rev.7, May 12, 2004, at 142, para. 5.

[1317] "[T]he concept of the family may differ in some respects from State to State, and even from region to region within a State, and it is therefore not possible to give the concept a standard definition. However ... when a group of persons is regarded as a family under the legislation and practice of a State, it must be given the protection": UN Human Rights Committee, "General Comment No. 19: The family" (1990), UN Doc. HRI/GEN/1/Rev.7, May 12, 2004, at 149, para. 2. Comparable deference to national understandings is evident in, for example, UN Committee on the Elimination of Discrimination Against Women, "General Recommendation No. 21: Equality in marriage and family relations" (1994), UN Doc. HRI/GEN/1/Rev.7, May 12, 2004, at 253, para. 13: "The form and concept of the family can vary from State to State, and even between regions within a State. Whatever form it takes, and whatever the legal system, religion, or custom within the country, the treatment of women ... must accord with the principles of equality and justice for all people."

[1318] Nowak, *ICCPR Commentary*, at 413.

discrimination based on sexual orientation is discrimination based on sex, and is therefore prohibited.[1319] As such, Art. 23(2) may be a sound basis upon which to contest the failure of European Union member states to guarantee a right of reunification to unmarried (including same-sex) partners of refugees. Precisely because of its deference to domestic legal understandings, Art. 23(2) effectively requires the right of family reunification to extend to such relationships as are legally recognized as entitled to protection in a given state party. As the UN Human Rights Committee has determined,

> [T]he concept of the family may differ in some respects from State to State, and even from region to region within a State ... [I]t is therefore not possible to give the concept a standard definition. However, the Committee emphasizes that, when a group of persons is regarded as a family under the legislation and practice of a State, it must be given the protection referred to in article 23 [of the Civil and Political Covenant] ... In view of the existence of various forms of family, such as unmarried couples and their children or single parents and their children, States parties should also indicate whether and to what extent such types of family and their members are recognized and protected by domestic law and practice.[1320]

With both national and regional jurisprudence in Europe that recognizes non-married partners and other beyond the nuclear definition as family members,[1321] it is difficult to understand how their exclusion from the scope of family reunification could be justified on the basis of deference to local values.[1322] Nor is it a sufficient answer that particular European Union

---

[1319] "The State party has sought the Committee's guidance as to whether sexual orientation may be considered an 'other status' for the purposes of article 26. The same issue could arise under article 2, paragraph 1, of the Covenant. The Committee confines itself to noting, however, that in its view, the reference to 'sex' in articles 2, paragraph 1, and 26 is to be taken as including sexual orientation": *Toonen v. Australia*, UNHRC Comm. No. 488/1992, UN Doc CCPR/C/50/D/488/1992, decided Mar. 31, 1994, at para. 8.7. This decision was rendered by the Human Rights Committee after the publication of Nowak's treatise, which may account for his unduly cautious approach to the recognition of same-sex families.

[1320] UN Human Rights Committee, "General Comment No. 19: The family" (1990), UN Doc. HRI/GEN/1/Rev.7, May 12, 2004, at 149, para. 2.

[1321] Decisions of the European Court of Human Rights cast doubt on whether a narrow "nuclear" understanding of family can be sustained even in Europe, noting in particular the recognition of relationships between grandchildren and grandparents and between non-married partners to be within the realm of protected family interests: Nowak, *ICCPR Commentary*, at 300; and Jayawickrama, *Judicial Application*, at 765–767.

[1322] As much was impliedly recognized in the European Union's own position on the family reunification of temporarily protected persons, which grants a clear right to sponsor the admission of the applicant's "unmarried partner in a stable relationship, where the legislation or practice of the State concerned treats unmarried couples in a way states *may* choose to reunify such family members, in at least some circumstances: read in tandem with the guarantee of equal protection of the law found in Art. 26 of the Covenant,[1323] there is an obligation on state parties to define the *right* to family reunification in an even-handed way, without relegating any particular type of legally valid family relationship purely to the realm of discretion.

Drawing on the right under Art. 23(2) of families to "live together," the Human Rights Committee has determined that states are under a duty to take measures to "ensure the unity or reunification of [refugee] families."[1324] The question of when such affirmative efforts are sufficient will likely be measured in relation to the usual (and fungible) "reasonableness" standard.[1325] On this basis, it is doubtful that conditioning family reunification on the sponsor's ability to support his or her family members would be found to breach Art. 23(2), at least insofar as the requirements are fairly set in relation to a very basic cost of living, and the refugee has not been prevented from enjoying such rights as to work, to deal in property, etc.,[1326] which are key to giving him or her a fair chance of meeting that standard. Similarly, the European Union's policy of denying family reunification where public security or public health concerns are raised is likely justifiable, so long as those notions are interpreted in line with international standards.[1327] While also presumptively legitimate, greater scrutiny is nonetheless warranted of the ways in which the European Union's decision also to sanction denial of family reunification on "public policy" grounds is implemented: in practice, the breadth of this notion can raise the specter of measures that border on infringement of the prohibition of arbitrary conduct, and which therefore could not be considered reasonable limitations.[1328]

comparable to married couples under its law relating to aliens": EU Temporary Protection Directive, at Art. 15. For purposes of Art. 23 analysis, however, the relevant standard should be the treatment afforded such relationships under the state's general laws (not under its laws regarding non-citizens).

[1323] See chapter 2.5.5 above, at pp. 126–128.

[1324] UN Human Rights Committee, "General Comment No. 19: The family" (1990), UN Doc. HRI/GEN/1/Rev.7, May 12, 2004, at 149, para. 5.

[1325] "Problems with the positive obligation approach arise in establishing its scope. The point at which a State is obligated to act affirmatively to protect the right to family unity is unclear. Moreover, the interpretations of this notion also have a potential for ambiguity ... Such standards leave much in the hands of individual judicial opinion": Anderfuhren-Wayne, "Family Unity," at 380.

[1326] See chapters 5.3, 6.1, and 6.2 regarding the right of refugees to work; and chapters 4.5 and 6.5 regarding their property rights.

[1327] Compare Civil and Political Covenant, at Arts. 12(3), 19(3), 22(2). See chapter 6.7 below, at pp. 899, 901, for a discussion of the interpretation of these widely accepted limitations on the exercise of basic rights.

[1328] With respect to the potential breadth of the traditional notion of *ordre public*, this being the French-language equivalent of "Public Policy," see chapter 2.4.4 above, at pp. 102–103;

Most susceptible to successful challenge are limitations imposed on the right to family reunification based strictly on forms of status. In particular, many persons who are in fact Convention refugees have nonetheless been assigned "temporary protected" or other status by asylum countries, and denied full family reunification rights on the basis of that status. Despite its obvious connotation of limited duration, the "temporary protected" label has in practice not been routinely indicative of the actual duration of the refugees' stay in the asylum state. To the contrary, many "temporarily protected" refugees have in fact been compelled to remain in protection abroad for very long periods of time, even as some persons recognized as full Convention refugees have been able to repatriate in a short space of time.[1329] A particularly clear example of this concern was the American delay of more than twenty years to process the claims of many Guatemalan and Salvadoran refugees admitted under special regulatory regimes, during which time they were denied the right of family reunification. Indeed, the label "asylum-seeker" employed by some countries is similarly problematic. Because of the time which status verification may take in some systems – often stretching to several years – not even this label can be relied upon as a clearly reliable indicator of a short-term, transient position in the host state.

It follows that to the extent that a government relies strictly upon the label assigned a given individual – "asylum-seeker," "temporarily protected" person, or Convention refugee – to grant or to withhold rights to family reunification, it does not implement the right to family reunification in a reasonable way. This analysis calls into question the automatic denial of reunification rights in most developed countries to all persons awaiting the results of status verification, however long these inquiries take. It also raises doubts about the traditional practice of such countries as Finland, the Netherlands, and Spain to deny family reunification to all persons assigned to "temporary protected" status. Germany's traditional practice of allowing the holders of temporary (*Duldung*) status access to reunification on only a discretionary basis may similarly be adjudged an unacceptably formalist distinction.

A particularly egregious case is the decision of Australia to assign "temporary protected" status to all refugees arriving without pre-authorization or who are intercepted offshore or in so-called "excised" territories, and to rely on that status to prohibit such refugees from being reunited with their family members. In view of the legal right of refugees to seek protection without advance permission[1330] and the duty of states to protect all refugees under their de jure or de facto jurisdiction,[1331] it is difficult to imagine any plausible

---

chapter 5.1 below, at pp. 679–690; chapter 5.2 below, at p. 715; and in particular, chapter 6.7 below, at pp. 900–901.

[1329] See Hathaway, "Label."   [1330] See chapter 4.2 above, at pp. 386–388.
[1331] See chapter 3.1.1 above.

basis for stigmatizing all refugees arriving in these circumstances as entitled only to limited protection rights, and particularly to be denied any right of reunion with their families. In contrast to the European temporary protection policies, moreover, the temporary status assigned these refugees does not even purport to have any relationship to the anticipated duration of the need for protection in Australia – it is rather a punitively assigned label, earned on the basis of the refugee's internationally lawful, but domestically disapproved, actions. In such circumstances, the denial of all facilities for family reunification cannot be said to be reasonable under international law, with the result that Australia should be found in breach of its duties under Art. 23(2) of the Civil and Political Covenant.

To be clear, the argument here is not that the duty to act reasonably compels an immediate right of all refugees to family reunification; rather, it is simply that any delay in allowing refugees to access family reunification facilities must be based on rational, substantive considerations rather than simply on the basis of the formal status assigned to them. For example, assuming the existence of discretion to take account of the special psychological or other circumstances of the persons concerned, the Human Rights Committee's understandings would likely sanction an incremental approach under which a refugee (whatever his or her formal status) would be entitled to be reunited with a spouse and children after one year in the asylum state, and with other dependent family members after two years there. Under such a model, states would have ample time to avoid the reunification of families where the primary claim to protection is clearly unfounded, or where the need for protection is really short-lived. Yet refugees would not be indefinitely denied their right to family unity simply on the basis of a formal label assigned to them.

In sum, Art. 23(2) of the Civil and Political Covenant – in contrast to either the customary international legal duty to avoid unlawful or arbitrary interference with a refugee's family, or even the more elaborated Art. 17 with its concomitant duty to afford protection against such interference – is a standard against which the sufficiency of an asylum state's *affirmative* efforts to preserve refugee family unity, including by way of reunification efforts, can legitimately be measured.[1332] At the very least, authoritative interpretations of Art. 23(2) make it clear that an asylum state which either refuses to admit or to facilitate the reunification of a refugee's "family" – albeit as defined by

---

[1332] Fourlanos reaches a comparable conclusion on the basis of Art. 10(1) of the Covenant on Economic, Social and Cultural Rights. "If a State grants many kinds of protection to a family (e.g. financial, practical, education), but fails to ensure family unity, then that State has not complied with Article 10(1) of [the ESC] Covenant. This is especially so when minor children are living with the family": Fourlanos, *Sovereignty*, at 99.

the asylum country's own understanding of relevant relationships – is in breach of its international legal obligations.[1333]

4.7 Freedom of thought, conscience, and religion

Refugees who introduce a foreign religion into an asylum state are sometimes subjected to targeted restrictions on their freedom of religion. For example, Falasha Jews from Ethiopia were the objects of proselytization by Sudanese Christian camp administrators.[1334] In Chad, Nigerian and Senegalese members of the Faydal Djaria Muslim community were arrested at the behest of the Chadian Higher Council of Islamic Affairs, which took umbrage at this community's alleged failure to conform to the principles of Islam.[1335] Refugees of a minority religion may also experience pressure from other refugees to conform to dominant beliefs. The camps in which many Afghan refugees lived in Pakistan were controlled by conservative religious groups committed to strict enforcement of Islamic codes. Some refugees compelled to live in those camps were thus required to abide by religious standards in which they did not believe, and to which they had not subscribed in their home country.[1336] Bosnian Muslim refugees in Austria were accused of religious laxity by a Saudi-run relief agency when they refused to accept scarves for the women refugees to cover their heads.[1337]

More commonly, however, the religious freedom of refugees is constrained by limits which apply, at least in principle, to all persons in the asylum country. This dilemma clearly arises for refugees arriving in a theocratic state, in which all are expected to abide by a particular set of beliefs. For example, Taliban authorities in Afghanistan required all Muslims to adhere to an interpretation of Islam under which virtually all human rights of

---

[1333] Ibid. at 110: "Obviously, by imposing such duties on States, the principle of family unity limits the State exclusionary power with regard to admission of aliens. A State refusing admission to a family member will probably find itself in contravention of international law, unless there is a reason to justify such a deviation."

[1334] D. Kessler and T. Parfitt, *The Falashas: The Jews of Ethiopia* (1985), at 11.

[1335] "Report of the Special Rapporteur on the Elimination of All Forms of Intolerance and of Discrimination Based on Religion or Belief," UN Doc. E/CN.4/2001/63, Feb. 13, 2001, at para. 130.

[1336] N. Ahmad, *International Academy of Comparative Law National Report for Pakistan* (1994), at 9, citing as an example the required use of *purdah* (veil covering a woman's face). "Daily life in the camps strongly reflects the greater Islamification of society. There is peer pressure to conform and also pressure from the Mujahadeen": K. Clark, "Islamic Fundamentalism in the Afghan Camps in Peshawar," (1992) 3(1) *Women Against Fundamentalism Journal* 15, at 15.

[1337] K. Durán and J. Devon, "Saudi relief hypocrisy: How the Kingdom uses and abuses 'charity,'" *National Review Online*, May 13, 2003, available at www.nationalreview.com (accessed June 13, 2003).

women were denied.[1338] The opposite dilemma faces the nearly 300,000 Vietnamese refugees who settled in Southern China. These refugees face the same broad-ranging denials of any free religious practice as do Chinese citizens,[1339] defended by the Chinese government on the grounds that religious adherents in that country are "duty-bound to undergo patriotic re-education ... [R]eligion must adapt to the local society and to its development and operate within the confines of the Constitution and laws."[1340]

More commonly, however, states impose restrictions which target the adherents of minority religions.[1341] There are broad-ranging limits on

---

[1338] "[T]he Taliban's policy of intolerance and discrimination in the name of religion ... affects Afghan society as a whole and women and Shiite Muslims in particular. Two communications reveal that the Taliban has introduced what is in point of fact a system of apartheid in respect of women, based on its interpretation of Islam: exclusion of women from society, employment and schools, obligation for women to wear the burqa in public and restrictions on travel with men other than members of the family ... The Special Rapporteur believes that the maintenance, openly and publicly, of an apartheid policy of this nature is abnormal, from the standpoint of human rights": "Report of the Special Rapporteur on the Elimination of All Forms of Intolerance and of Discrimination Based on Religion or Belief," UN Doc. E/CN.4/1999/58, Jan. 11, 1999, at para. 26.

[1339] US Committee for Refugees, *World Refugee Survey 1996* (1996), at 81.

[1340] "Report of the Special Rapporteur on the Elimination of All Forms of Intolerance and of Discrimination Based on Religion or Belief," UN Doc. E/CN.4/1999/58, Jan. 11, 1999, at para. 48. "The Government continued its crackdown on unregistered churches, temples, and mosques ... Members of some unregistered religious groups, including Protestant and Catholic groups, were subjected to increased restrictions, including, in some cases, intimidations, harassment, and detention": US Department of State, *Annual Report on International Religious Freedom for 2002* (2002), at 197–198.

[1341] A helpful general overview of the religions subject to repression around the world was provided by the United Nations Special Rapporteur on the Elimination of All Forms of Intolerance and of Discrimination Based on Religion or Belief. "Religious minorities are affected primarily by the threat of their very existence as special communities, as exemplified by the deportation of Adventists and Protestants in Azerbaijan; the campaigns of repression against members of the Falun Gong, the arrest, imprisonment and expulsion of Tibetan monks and nuns from monasteries and the sentencing of Christians to death in China; the harassment of Christians in Myanmar; the sentencing to death of members of the Ismaili community in Saudi Arabia; and the arrest of Protestants and Adventists in Turkmenistan. Religious minorities are also subject to direct and indirect limitations on the manifestation of their religious identity or belief, as shown by the destruction of Tibetan Buddhist places of worship and the expulsion of nuns and monks from monasteries in China; the occupation and partial destruction of a property belonging to the Armenian Patriarchate in Israel; the closure of places of worship of religious minorities in Eritrea; threats to close Baptist places of worship in the Republic of Moldova and those of the Protestant communities in Turkey; and the prevention of non-recognition of conscientious objection, leading to the imprisonment of Jehovah's Witnesses, in the Republic of Korea": "Report of the Special Rapporteur on the Elimination of All Forms of Intolerance and of Discrimination Based on Religion or Belief," UN Doc. E/CN.4/2003/66, Jan. 15, 2003, at paras. 131 ff.

freedom of religion in Russia for persons who are not members of an officially recognized religion.[1342] Egypt[1343] and Iran[1344] are among the states which have criminalized practice of the Baha'i faith, while Pakistan has combated the appeal of Sufism by executing leaders of the faith on blasphemy

[1342] "The 1997 law on religion, which replaced a more liberal 1990 law, continues to be the focus of serious concern about the state of religious freedom in the country. One of the law's most controversial provisions is a requirement that a church must prove that it has existed for at least 15 years in the country before it is allowed to be registered as a full-fledged religious organization. (Registration as a religious organization is necessary in order for a religious community to rent or buy a facility, proselytize, publish literature, provide religious training, or conduct other activities.) In a November 1999 ruling, the Constitutional Court upheld the 15-year requirement but also permitted the registration of organizations that already were registered when the 1997 law was passed or that were willing to become a local branch of a larger registered denomination. The provision still severely restricts the activities of small, new, independent congregations": United States Department of State, *Annual Report on International Religious Freedom for 2000* (2000), at 357–358. "Despite court decisions that have liberalized its interpretation, [the 1997 law] seriously disadvantages religious groups that are new to the country by making it difficult for them to register as religious organizations. Unregistered groups lack the juridical status necessary to establish bank accounts, own property, invite foreign guests, publish literature, or conduct worship services in prisons, state-owned hospitals, and among the armed forces": US Department of State, *Annual Report on International Religious Freedom for 2002* (2002), at 449.

[1343] "According to another communication from the Special Rapporteur, the Supreme Religious Court in Cairo declared the Baha'i faith a dangerous heresy in 1925. In 1960, all Baha'i assemblies were dissolved, their property and other assets confiscated and their religious activities banned. Nevertheless, Baha'is supposedly remained free as individuals to practise their religion in accordance with the freedom of religion guaranteed to all under the Constitution. To this day, however, the Baha'i community is said to be subjected to constant close surveillance: Baha'is are not allowed to meet in groups, especially for religious observances, and their literature is destroyed. It is alleged that they cannot legally celebrate their marriages, which are deemed to constitute concubinage, while the children born of such unions are regarded as illegitimate": "Report of the Special Rapporteur on the Elimination of All Forms of Intolerance and of Discrimination Based on Religion or Belief," UN Doc. E/CN.4/2001/63, Feb. 13, 2001, at para. 33. "Baha'is also continued to face persecution, including being denied permission to worship or to carry out other communal affairs publicly. At least four Baha'is were serving prison terms for their religious beliefs": Human Rights Watch, *World Report 2003* (2003), at 446.

[1344] "An initial urgent appeal concerned the case of three Baha'is, namely, Mr. Ata'ullah Hamid Nasirizadih, Mr. Sirus Dhabihi-Muqaddam and Mr. Hidayat-Kashifi Najafabadi, who were reportedly condemned to death in secret because of their religious beliefs and ran the risk of execution. A second urgent appeal connected with the first alleged that Mr. Sirus Dhabihi-Muqaddam and Mr. Hidayat-Kashifi Najafabadi had been informed by the Mashad prison authorities that their sentence had been upheld. In these two communications, the Special Rapporteur 'urgently appealed to the Government of the Islamic Republic of Iran to ensure that the sentences were not carried out and that all judicial remedies and guarantees required by international human rights standards be provided to the above-mentioned persons.' A third urgent charges.[1345] Other states have employed only slightly less drastic tactics to discourage minority religions. In Turkmenistan, officials of the National Security Committee beat a Jehovah's Witness leader for failing to renounce his faith;[1346] Saudi Arabia arrested a member of the Ismaili religion on "sorcery" charges[1347] and expelled an Indian Christian for distributing a Christian videotape.[1348] Restrictions of this kind may mean that asylum is in no sense indicative of access to rights-regarding protection. For example, the Jehovah's Witness refugees who fled from Mozambique to Malawi

appeal concerned allegations of the hanging of a Baha'i, Mr. R. Rawahani, accused of converting a Muslim woman, even though the woman apparently claimed to be a Baha'i. This appeal also referred to a senior member of the Islamic Revolutionary Court, who allegedly described the report of the execution as a lie and stressed that no such sentence had been passed by the Iranian courts": "Report of the Special Rapporteur on the Elimination of All Forms of Intolerance and of Discrimination Based on Religion or Belief," UN Doc. E/CN.4/1999/58, Jan. 11, 1999, at para. 66.

[1345] "On 5 August 2000, Mohammed Yusuf Ali, a Sufi mystic accused of blasphemy, was reportedly condemned to death in Lahore. It appears that this decision was reached despite the fact that the persons who had accused Mohammed Yusuf Ali of proclaiming himself a prophet failed to back up their allegations with any hard evidence": "Report of the Special Rapporteur on the Elimination of All Forms of Intolerance and of Discrimination Based on Religion or Belief," UN Doc. E/CN.4/2001/63, Feb. 13, 2001, at para. 116. See generally D. Forte, "Apostasy and Blasphemy in Pakistan," (1994) 10 Connecticut Journal of International Law 27. "Government officials state that although religious minorities account for approximately 5 percent of the country's population, 25 percent of the cases filed under the blasphemy laws are aimed at religious minorities": US Department of State, Annual Report on International Religious Freedom for 2002 (2002), at 639.

[1346] "On 21 June 1999, in Gyzylarbat, members of the National Security Committee are reported to have arrested Annamammedov Yazmammed, a Jehovah's Witness ... Allegedly threatened with physical violence with the intention of forcing him to renounce his faith and to reveal the names of the Jehovah's Witnesses in Gyzylarbat, he was eventually beaten because of his refusal to comply. On 22 June 1999, he was reportedly sentenced by the Gyzylarbat court to 12 days' administrative detention for insulting the members of the National Security Committee": "Report of the Special Rapporteur on the Elimination of All Forms of Intolerance and of Discrimination Based on Religion or Belief," UN Doc. E/CN.4/2001/63, Feb. 13, 2001, at para. 132.

[1347] According to Saudi authorities, "[t]he facts were the following: information had reached the security forces about the illegal practice of sorcery on a large scale by an inhabitant of the kingdom, provoking reactions from a large number of citizens and residents ... The person who was at the origin of the incident was arrested for sorcery, which is forbidden by law in Saudi Arabia. According to Saudi Arabia, this had nothing to do with the person's affiliation with the Ismaili sect, whose members enjoy the same rights as others and are subject to the same obligations": ibid. at paras. 8–9.

[1348] "Saudi Arabia replied that George Joseph had been arrested for having engaged in activities that created a disturbance and in response to complaints from persons living in his neighbourhood. Mr. Joseph was allegedly distributing a video that was illegal, being contrary to the values and rules in force in Saudi Arabia": ibid. at paras. 10–11.

found that the Witnesses were one of five religious groups whose religious practice was banned by that country during the reign of President Hastings Banda.[1349]

The precise focus of efforts to repress religious practice varies considerably. In some states, the goal is to prohibit the actual holding of particular religious views, whether or not these views are put into practice. Nepal prohibits conversion to Seventh Day Adventism,[1350] while Laos has forced converted Christians to renounce their new faith.[1351] In one case, the Yemeni government agreed not to carry out a death sentence imposed for apostasy on a Somali refugee who had converted from Islam to Christianity; the "solution" arrived at in cooperation with UNHCR was to expel the refugee from the country to Djibouti.[1352]

[1349] Due to their precarious situation in Malawi, the Jehovah's Witnesses "have taken advantage of any chance to leave Malawi": D. Cammack, "Protection in a 'Model Program': Mozambican Refugees in Malawi" (1993), at 16–17. The one-party regime of President Hastings Banda ended in 1994, and religious freedom for minorities has now been restored, including provision for the payment of damages to persons dismissed from official employment on grounds of religion: US Department of State, *Annual Report on International Religious Freedom for 2002* (2002), at 60–61.

[1350] "The Seventh-Day Adventist church, which maintains several churches, a school and a hospital in Nepal, may conduct most religious activities with the exception of conversions, which are banned; the Church's right to own property is not officially recognized": "Report of the Special Rapporteur on the Elimination of All Forms of Intolerance and of Discrimination Based on Religion or Belief," UN Doc. E/CN.4/2001/63, Feb. 13, 2001, at para. 105.

[1351] "In October 2000 the Government reportedly launched a campaign to eradicate Christian churches and thereby curtail their role and influence in society. This campaign, styled a 'programme', seeks to monitor Christian organizations and accuses them of representing an alien religion controlled by enemy forces. The programme has already been partially implemented with security forces apparently forcing newly converted Christians to sign declarations renouncing the Christian faith": ibid. at para. 123.

[1352] "On 16 January 2000, Mohammed Omer Hadji, a Somali refugee resident in Yemen, was reportedly arrested and held at Tawahi police station on account of his conversion to Christianity. Following his release on 13 March 2000, he was allegedly beaten by the police and told that he would be killed unless he returned to the Muslim faith. He was reportedly rearrested two months later and condemned to death by a court for apostasy, although the court stated that the death sentence would not be carried out if he reconverted to Islam ... [T]he Government replied to the UN Special Rapporteur that '... such conduct constitutes an offence under Yemeni laws and legislation.' Accordingly, the said person was arrested and referred for trial on the charge of apostasy from Islam to another religion. However, in view of his status as a refugee in Yemen, the Yemeni Government decided that it would be more appropriate to expel him from the territory of Yemen in collaboration and coordination with the UNHCR office in Sana'a. This decision was put into effect and the said person was expelled to Djibouti on Friday, 25 August, as an alternative to the continuation of the trial proceedings": ibid. at paras. 147–148.

Even in asylum countries where there are no limits on religious belief, true freedom of religion may not exist. Simple adherence to (or refusal to adopt) a religion may not be prohibited, but religious worship or communal prayer may be barred. Christian church services are prohibited in Bhutan,[1353] and sometimes disrupted in Turkey.[1354] Police have broken up Baptist church services in Georgia[1355] and Turkmenistan;[1356] in Azerbaijan, Jehovah's Witnesses have been forced to conduct prayer meetings in private homes to avoid punishment

---

[1353] "Christian churches are not authorized to conduct religious activities. The Seventh-Day Adventist Church has reportedly complained that the authorities have refused to allow it to build a church even though Bhutanese citizens belong to that denomination": ibid. at para. 19. "The law provides for freedom of religion; however the Government limits this right in practice": US Department of State, *Annual Report on International Religious Freedom for 2002* (2002), at 618.

[1354] "As far as non-Muslims are concerned, with the exception of the Jewish minority, whose situation is entirely satisfactory, the situation of the Christian communities – Greek Orthodox, Armenian (Orthodox, Catholic and Protestant), Assyro-Chaldean and Turkish Catholic and Protestant – raises problems with regard to the principles of tolerance and non-discrimination. These communities have to endure many hardships and violations, including the confiscation of religious property, the banning of religious seminaries, interference at various times in procedures for electing religious dignitaries, restrictions on freedom of worship in public and, at times, even a climate of insecurity that affects Christians": "Report of the Special Rapporteur on the Elimination of All Forms of Intolerance and of Discrimination Based on Religion or Belief," UN Doc. E/CN.4/2001/63, Feb. 13, 2001, at para. 160.

[1355] "On 20 August 2000, in Tianeti, the chief of district police, assisted by three police officers, reportedly broke up a Baptist religious service. The police are reported to have destroyed objects of worship and taken Pastor Kalatozishvili to the police station in order to put pressure on him to give up his work in the Baptist Church in favour of the Orthodox Church": ibid. at para. 47. "Local police and security officials continued to harass at times non-traditional religious minority groups, especially members of the Jehovah's Witnesses. The police only sporadically intervened to protect such minorities from attacks by Orthodox extremists. In some cases, police actually participated in or facilitated the attacks": US Department of State, *Annual Report on International Religious Freedom for 2002* (2002), at 372.

[1356] "It is alleged that on 14 November 1999 the National Security Committee ordered a raid on the Baptist congregation of the Council of Evangelical Baptist Churches during the Sunday sermon. On 13 February 2000, the Committee reportedly interrupted a private religious meeting organized by the Baptist pastor Vitaly Tereshnev, on the grounds that the meeting was illegal ... On 2 February 2000, the Baptist pastor Anatoly Belyayev is said to have been arrested by members of the National Security Committee while he was peacefully performing his religious activities": "Report of the Special Rapporteur on the Elimination of All Forms of Intolerance and of Discrimination Based on Religion or Belief," UN Doc. E/CN.4/2001/63, Feb. 13, 2001, at para. 134. "As in previous years, the Russian Orthodox Church and Sunni Islam were the only religions permitted in Turkmenistan ... From November 2001 through February 2002, police dispersed Adventist, Baptist, and Jehovah's Witness prayer gatherings ... Dozens of worshippers were interrogated and faced verbal abuse and threats by police while in custody; several were beaten": Human Rights Watch, *World Report 2003* (2003), at 373.

by authorities.[1357] To counter "extremists," Egypt now controls all mosques in that country, and decides who is allowed to deliver sermons there.[1358]

Perhaps most frequently, authorities constrain religious practice by limiting the ability of minority religious organizations to establish a physical presence. For example, Chinese officials have invoked land use laws to justify the demolition of churches built by local inhabitants.[1359] Only Moslem mosques may be built in the Maldives,[1360] while Moslem mosques were effectively prohibited in Athens until 2000.[1361] Pentecostal churches have

---

[1357] In its response to the Special Rapporteur, the government observed that "[d]uring the inquiry, it also appeared that the activities of the Jehovah's Witnesses in the district were not limited to the refinery. Among other things, it was established that the members of the sect met regularly in an apartment located in an apartment building in Lokbatan. Those meetings, which were also attended by minors, were organized by the occupants of the apartment, Remi and Galina Remiev": "Report of the Special Rapporteur on the Elimination of All Forms of Intolerance and of Discrimination Based on Religion or Belief," UN Doc. E/CN.4/2001/63, Feb. 13, 2001, at para. 15. "Local law enforcement authorities regularly monitor religious services, and some observant Christians and Muslims are penalized for their religious affiliations": US Department of State, *Annual Report on International Religious Freedom for 2002* (2002), at 320.

[1358] "Management of all mosques and shrines has been centralized in the hands of the Ministry of Awqaf [Islamic endowments] ... Every person not expressly authorized to do so is prohibited from mounting a mosque pulpit and delivering a sermon, inasmuch as the law requires a statement from the Ministry of Awqaf": "Report of the Special Rapporteur on the Elimination of All Forms of Intolerance and of Discrimination Based on Religion or Belief," UN Doc. E/CN.4/2001/63, Feb. 13, 2001, at para. 35.

[1359] In defense of its actions, the Chinese government noted that "[a] thorough investigation has revealed that in 1998 the inhabitants of Cangnan County, Wenzhou, Zhejiang Province, acting without authorization from the public authorities, built a church on a plot of land in the village of Linguan, Pingdeng commune, Cangnan County, in serious violation of the Land Use Law of the People's Republic of China. On 31 December 1999, pursuant to the relevant provisions of that Law, the Cangnan County Office of Land Use had the church destroyed. Other inhabitants of the county, acting without authorization from the competent authorities, converted a factory into a church in Yanggong village, Lingqi commune, in violation of legislation of the People's Republic of China governing urban land use. On 15 December 1999 the Cangnan county authorities had the church destroyed, pursuant to the law": ibid. at para. 25.

[1360] "The law apparently restricts non-Muslim religious ceremonies. The public celebration of non-Muslim religious rites is forbidden and must be strictly limited to the private sphere. Consequently, only mosques may be built. School curricula include mandatory teaching of Islam": ibid. at para. 99.

[1361] M. Petronoti, "Greece as a Place for Refugees: An Anthropological Approach to Constraints Pertaining to Religious Practices," paper presented to the Conference on War, Exile and Everyday Life, Institute of Ethnology and Folklore Research, Zagreb, 1995. "In 2000, the Parliament approved a bill allowing construction for the first Islamic cultural center and mosque in the Athens area ... Members of the Orthodox Church oppose the cultural center, claiming it may 'spread the ideology of Islam and the Arab world'": US Department of State, *Annual Report on International Religious Freedom for 2002* (2002), at 385.

been destroyed by the government of Myanmar.[1362] Police in Sudan ransacked a Catholic college.[1363] Other tactics are more subtle, if equally effective. Nauru refuses to recognize the Seventh Day Adventist Church, by virtue of which it may not acquire property or hold public meetings.[1364] Hungary recently withdrew tax-exempt status from all but six favored churches.[1365]

Even if worship and the presence of organized religious institutions are not constrained, practices closely connected to religious belief may be restricted or prohibited. Proselytization is proscribed or heavily regulated in Bulgaria,[1366] Georgia,[1367] and France.[1368] And Uzbekistan defended its

---

[1362] "On 12 June 2000, the State Peace and Development Council allegedly ordered the demolition of a Pentecostal church in Cherry Street, Haka, capital of Chin State, even though the building had been erected in 1999 with the approval of the Ministry of Religious Affairs": "Report of the Special Rapporteur on the Elimination of All Forms of Intolerance and of Discrimination Based on Religion or Belief," UN Doc. E/CN.4/2001/63, Feb. 13, 2001, at para. 101.

[1363] "On 21 June 2000, at Khartoum, the police allegedly attacked the Comboni Catholic College and proceeded to destroy and commandeer property": ibid. at para. 125.

[1364] "It is reported that the authorities are refusing to allow the registration of the Seventh-Day Adventist Church. Owing to this lack of recognition, the said community is unable to purchase land and cannot hold public meetings or conduct baptisms, weddings or funerals. The Seventh-Day Adventist Church is therefore obliged to conduct its religious activities in private homes": ibid. at para. 104.

[1365] "In May 2000 tax and customs legislation was reportedly amended to limit the tax exemptions available to churches having contracts with the State. This modification allegedly stripped most religious communities (such as Seventh-Day Adventists, Evangelicals, Methodists and Pentecostalists) of their tax-exempt status, leaving only six churches exempt": ibid. at para. 52. "[C]riteria limit the tax benefit to only 14 of some 136 registered churches in the country. Several of the smaller churches whose members cannot participate in this tax deduction took the case to the Constitutional Court, which chose not to review it": US Department of State, *Annual Report on International Religious Freedom for 2002* (2002), at 390.

[1366] "According to a second communication, notwithstanding constitutional provisions guaranteeing freedom of religion and belief, such non-traditional minorities as the Jehovah's Witnesses and the Church of Jesus Christ of Latter-Day Saints face hurdles in conducting their activities. On 20 March 2000, two Jehovah's Witnesses in Turgovishte were reportedly arrested for disturbing the peace owing to their proselytizing in public. In April 2000, police in Plovdiv allegedly halted the distribution of religious tracts by missionaries from the Church of Jesus Christ of Latter-Day Saints, who were also charged with distributing documents without a permit": "Report of the Special Rapporteur on the Elimination of All Forms of Intolerance and of Discrimination Based on Religion or Belief," UN Doc. E/CN.4/2001/63, Feb. 13, 2001, at para. 22.

[1367] The Georgian government has reported "that there have been a number of citizens' complaints concerning the activity of Jehovah's Witnesses aimed at attracting new members by using bribes (money, food, etc.). In this connection, we are going to make amendments to the Criminal Code of Georgia in order to forbid unlawful proselytism, as has been done in some European countries. The elaboration of these amendments is under way": ibid. at para. 45.

[1368] Legislation passed in 2001 "provides up to three years' imprisonment for acts of 'serious and repeated pressure, or the use of techniques to alter the mind of a person, leading him refusal to allow Baptists to operate summer youth camps on the grounds that "members of the congregation were undesirables and should join the Russian Orthodox Church."[1369]

A particular concern is freedom of religious education. Norway insists on the teaching of Christianity and Christian ethics in its schools,[1370] Greece provides instruction in only the Greek Orthodox religion in its public schools,[1371] and Bhutan requires daily recitation in schools of a prayer

---

or her to commit a harmful act ... [or] ... to act in any way prejudicial to his interests.' Catholic, Protestant, Jewish and Muslim representatives objected that it could result in 'overzealousness and judicial excess' and might threaten established religions as well": J. Bosco, "China's French Connection," *Washington Post*, July 10, 2001, at A21. "Leaders of the four major religions, such as the president of the French Protestant Association and the president of the Conference of Bishops of France, raised concerns about the legislation. By the end of the period covered by this report, no cases had been brought under the new law": US Department of State, *Annual Report on International Religious Freedom for 2002* (2002), at 367.

[1369] "Report of the Special Rapporteur on the Elimination of All Forms of Intolerance and of Discrimination Based on Religion or Belief," UN Doc. E/CN.4/2001/63, Feb. 13, 2001, at para. 111.

[1370] "Pursuant to the Religious Knowledge and Education in Ethics Act of October 1995, the teaching of Christianity and Christian ethics is reported to be mandatory in primary and secondary schools. On special grounds, exemptions from specific religious activities such as prayer may be granted, but students may not forgo instruction in the subject as a whole": ibid. at para. 109. "The course [on 'Religious Knowledge and Education in Ethics'] covers world religions and philosophy and promotes tolerance and respect for all religious beliefs; however, based on the country's history and the importance of Christianity to society, the course devotes more time to Christianity. All children must attend this mandatory class, and there are no exceptions for children of other faiths ... The Norwegian Humanist Association contested the teaching of the subject in the courts, claiming that it is a breach of freedom of religion and parents' rights to provide religious instruction to their children. In August 2001, the Supreme Court unanimously rejected the claims from the Humanist Association": US Department of State, *Annual Report on International Religious Freedom for 2002* (2002), at 431.

[1371] "Primary and secondary school curricula include compulsory instruction in the Orthodox religion for pupils of that faith. This then raises the question as to whether pupils who were baptized Orthodox but are not observant or have become atheist should be exempted. Representatives of the Muslim community in Athens have reportedly complained of the absence of religious instruction in Islam in school curricula": "Report of the Special Rapporteur on the Elimination of All Forms of Intolerance and of Discrimination Based on Religion or Belief," UN Doc. E/CN.4/2001/63, Feb. 13, 2001, at para. 49. "Non-Orthodox students are exempted from [the duty to take the course, but] ... [t]he neighborhood schools offer no alternative supervision for the children during the period of religious instruction. The [Muslim] community has complained that this forces the parents to have their children attend Orthodox religious instruction by default": US Department of State, *Annual Report on International Religious Freedom for 2002* (2002), at 386.

common to Muslims and Hindus.[1372] The United Nations Special Rapporteur on Religious Intolerance criticized the former Afghan government for denying parents the right to ensure the religious and moral education of their children,[1373] and Sudan for forcing children of all faiths to study Islam in school on pain of corporal punishment or expulsion from school.[1374] In Malaysia, restrictions on freedom of religious education apply even to some adults. All Muslim civil servants are expected to attend continuing Islamic education courses, defended by that country's government on the grounds that "[w]hile civil servants are required to be politically neutral, all Malaysians are expected to play their role in the promotion of religious and cultural harmony ... [A]s Islam exhorts its believers to be fair and just to all regardless of religious and political belief, rather than impairing the neutrality of civil servants, these classes may in the end emphasize the principle of neutrality."[1375]

With rare exceptions, restrictions on the right to freedom of religion are not targeted at refugees as such. However, restrictions on belief or action directed at those who profess minority religions are more likely to have a disproportionate impact on refugees and other aliens, since most citizens will by definition be a part of the religious majority in their own country. Moreover, the vulnerability of refugees to loss of religious freedom may be heightened by the denial in some states of even formal guarantees of religious freedom to non-citizens. For example, A report of the United Nations Special Rapporteur on Religious Intolerance identified Bulgaria, Byelorussia, Cape Verde, Finland, Jordan, Pakistan, Rwanda, Sudan, Syria, Ukraine, and the United States as countries in which the religious freedom of non-citizens is less fully guaranteed than is that of citizens.[1376]

[1372] According to the Bhutanese government, "[s]chool curricula, with the exception of those of monastic schools, make no provision for religious instruction or practice; however, a prayer common to Buddhism and Hinduism is recited daily in all schools, and prayers are said in boarding schools at the secondary level": "Report of the Special Rapporteur on the Elimination of All Forms of Intolerance and of Discrimination Based on Religion or Belief," UN Doc. E/CN.4/1999/58, Jan. 11, 1999, at para. 45.

[1373] E. Benito, "Elimination of All Forms of Intolerance and Discrimination Based on Religion or Belief," UN Doc. E.89.XIV.3 (1989), at 12.

[1374] A. Amor, "Implementation of the Declaration on the Elimination of All Forms of Intolerance and of Discrimination Based on Religion or Belief," UN Doc. E/CN.4/1994/79, Jan. 20, 1994, at 110. See also Sudan Human Rights Voice, "The Right to Education: Limitations and Violations" (1995), at 3.

[1375] "Report of the Special Rapporteur on the Elimination of All Forms of Intolerance and of Discrimination Based on Religion or Belief," UN Doc. E/CN.4/2001/63, Feb. 13, 2001, at para. 97.

[1376] E. Benito, "Elimination of All Forms of Intolerance and Discrimination Based on Religion or Belief," UN Doc. E.89.XIV.3 (1989), at 35–46.

Refugee Convention, Art. 4   Religion
The Contracting States shall accord to refugees within their territories treatment at least as favourable as that accorded to their nationals with respect to freedom to practise their religion and freedom as regards the religious education of their children.

Civil and Political Covenant, Art. 18

1. Everyone shall have the right to freedom of thought, conscience and religion. This right shall include freedom to have or to adopt a religion or belief of his choice, and freedom, either individually or in community with others and in public or private, to manifest his religion or belief in worship, observance, practice and teaching.

2. No one shall be subject to coercion which would impair his freedom to have or to adopt a religion or belief of his choice.

3. Freedom to manifest one's religion or beliefs may be subject only to such limitations as are prescribed by law and are necessary to protect public safety, order, health, or morals or the fundamental rights and freedoms of others.

4. The States Parties to the present Covenant undertake to have respect for the liberty of parents and, when applicable, legal guardians to ensure the religious and moral education of their children in conformity with their own convictions.

Economic, Social and Cultural Covenant, Art. 13(3)
The States Parties to the present Covenant undertake to have respect for the liberty of parents and, when applicable, legal guardians, to ... ensure the religious and moral education of their children in conformity with their own convictions.

No predecessor refugee treaty included a specific reference to the right of refugees to enjoy religious freedom, and no such provision was contained in the working drafts of the Refugee Convention.[1377] The oversight seems to have been based on a belief in the Ad Hoc Committee that "no useful purpose"[1378] could be served by codifying a right so clearly understood to

---

[1377] Robinson, *History*, at 77.

[1378] Statement of Mr. Guerreiro of Brazil, UN Doc. E/AC.32/SR.11, Jan. 25, 1950, at 8. See also Statement of Sir Leslie Brass of the United Kingdom, ibid.: "[A] convention relating to refugees could not include an outline of all the articles of the Universal Declaration of Human Rights ... [B]y its universal character, the Declaration applied to all human groups without exception and it was pointless to specify that its provisions applied also to refugees."

be inalienable.[1379] Not only was the right affirmed in the Universal Declaration of Human Rights, but even under traditional aliens law there was a well-established duty to respect the non-citizen's "personal and spiritual liberty within socially bearable limits."[1380]

There was nonetheless overwhelming support at the Conference of Plenipotentiaries for the contrary view that "the text should impose a contractual obligation on states"[1381] to respect the religious liberties of refugees.[1382] In part, a formal obligation of this kind was felt to be warranted as a basic matter of principle, since lack of religious freedom was frequently a cause of refugee flight.[1383] But the delegates were also persuaded that "the spiritual and religious factor was of special significance, having regard to the material and moral distress prevailing among the majority of refugees."[1384] It

---

[1379] "The call for freedom of religion was undoubtedly one of the most important elements that led to the overcoming of medieval views of the world and the development of modern perceptions of basic and human rights. Therefore, it is not surprising that freedom of religion was set down in early, modern-day national and international documents ... [F]reedom of thought and religion is not infrequently termed, along with freedom of opinion, the core of the Covenant ... based on the philosophical assumption that the individual as a rational being is master of his (her) own destiny": Nowak, *ICCPR Commentary*, at 309–310.

[1380] See chapter 2.1 above, at p. 76.

[1381] Statement of Msgr. Comte of the Holy See, UN Doc. A/CONF.2/SR.30, July 20, 1951, at 11. See also Grahl-Madsen, *Commentary*, at 15: "The words 'shall accord' indicate a legal obligation. The right is due to all refugees within the territory, i.e. [it] is not conditioned on the presence of the refugee being lawful."

[1382] The Ad Hoc Committee deferred consideration of the issue, and ultimately failed to recommend an article on freedom of religion: UN Doc. E/AC.32/SR.11, Jan. 25, 1950, at 9. The idea was, however, resuscitated by a non-governmental observer, Pax Romana, at the Conference of Plenipotentiaries: Statement of Mr. Buensod of Pax Romana, UN Doc. A/CONF.2/SR.11, July 9, 1951, at 9–10.

[1383] "He believed that some of the pertinent provisions of the [Universal] Declaration had been overlooked and that it would be advisable to include ... two articles reproducing as closely as possible articles 18 and 19 ... which related to freedom of thought, conscience and religion, and freedom of opinion respectively. In his opinion, provisions relating to freedom of opinion would be most appropriate in a convention on refugees, as the latter, as a rule, had abandoned their country of origin because they no longer enjoyed that freedom there": Statement of Mr. Cuvelier of Belgium, UN Doc. E/AC.32/SR.11, Jan. 25, 1950, at 8.

[1384] Statement of Mr. Buensod of Pax Romana, UN Doc. A/CONF.2/SR.11, July 9, 1951, at 10. The representatives of Austria, Belgium, Canada, Colombia, Egypt, France, Germany, the Holy See, Luxembourg, the Netherlands, Sweden, the United Kingdom, and Venezuela spoke in favor of the adoption in principle of an article on the right of refugees to religious freedom: UN Doc. A/CONF.2/SR.11, July 20, 1951, at 10–18. The view of the Ad Hoc Committee that reference was not warranted because religious freedom was so obviously a core interest did not prevail, since there was evidence that in practice even core rights were not always respected: Statement of Mr. Rain of France, UN Doc. E/AC.32/SR.11, Jan. 25, 1950, at 9.

would clearly be unacceptable if refugees forced to flee religious persecution were to be required to accept as "protection" conditions of life which denied them the very freedom which forced them abroad, as was the case for the Jehovah's Witness refugees who fled to Malawi only to find their religion banned in that country. Indeed, such was the importance attached to religious freedom that the relevant article was given pride of place by locating it immediately after the duty of non-discrimination, prior to any other substantive rights.[1385]

Indeed, the right to religious freedom is the only article in the Convention which comprises a principled obligation on states to take steps for the benefit of refugees beyond even what is done for their own citizens. For reasons earlier elaborated,[1386] the standard of treatment for the right of refugees to religious freedom is defined as "treatment at least as favourable as that accorded to their nationals." Thus, while refugees may under no circumstance be afforded fewer religious rights than citizens, the drafters adopted what amounts to a principled commitment to go beyond simple formal equality in order to recognize "that, precisely on account of their position as refugees, they were frequently handicapped in the practice of their religion."[1387]

The proponent of this unique standard of treatment did not clearly define the substance of this duty of states to go beyond a "national treatment" standard. The representative of the Holy See initially argued that assimilation to the nationals of the asylum state was an inadequate standard of treatment, since "[t]here was ... a danger that in countries where religious liberty was circumscribed, refugees would suffer."[1388] Yet he later insisted that he was not "pressing for preferential treatment of refugees."[1389] All in all, there appears to have been agreement in principle that states should seek to provide what amounts to substantive equality of religious freedom for refugees. Recognizing that "religious freedom as an abstract principle might be of little value if divorced from the practical means of ensuring it,"[1390] governments accepted that they would in some circumstances need to make special efforts to enable refugees to practice their religion. As Weis observes, simple formal equality of treatment with nationals would be insufficient "particularly [in] countries in which there is a State religion to which the refugees do not belong

---

[1385] As initially proposed by Luxembourg, the provision on religious freedom would have been Art. 17(a): UN Doc. A/CONF.2/SR.30, July 20, 1951, at 10. The representatives of the Holy See, Venezuela, and Belgium advocated its placement at the start of the substantive rights in the Refugee Convention: ibid. at 11–12.

[1386] See chapter 3.3.2 above, at pp. 235–237.

[1387] Statement of Msgr. Comte of the Holy See, UN Doc. A/CONF.2/SR.33, July 24, 1951, at 8.

[1388] Ibid. at 7.   [1389] Ibid. at 8.

[1390] Statement of Mr. Petren of Sweden, ibid. at 9.

or where the refugees' religion is not represented in the local population."[1391] Thus, even *if* it were lawful to impose restrictions on minority religions of the kind now in place in Russia, to limit land use in ways that constrain the establishment of minority religions as is done in China and Nauru, or to use tax laws to benefit only established religions as is the case in Hungary, the Refugee Convention establishes an obligation on asylum states to take account of the specificity of the religious needs of refugees in pursuing such policies, rather than simply subsuming them within the more general application of policy.

The duty to go beyond the standard of treatment afforded citizens was, however, conceived as "a moral principle ... somewhat in the nature of an abstract recommendation, but one which was nevertheless entirely consonant with the Universal Declaration of Human Rights."[1392] There was no question of requiring asylum states to dismantle state churches,[1393] amend their constitutions,[1394] or even to commit financial resources to assist refugees to practice their religion.[1395] Thus, the responsibility to make accommodation for the special disadvantages faced by refugees in practicing their religion is recognized, but not defined with a degree of precision that admits of formal legal application. As a matter of binding law, there is only the understanding that the right of refugees to religious freedom "must be in no way inferior to

---

[1391] Weis, *Travaux*, at 43.

[1392] Statement of Mr. Rochefort of France, UN Doc. A/CONF.2/SR.33, July 24, 1951, at 7–8.

[1393] In calling for modifications to the original draft of Art. 4 tabled by Luxembourg, the French representative noted that "[t]he difficulty, however, lay in the precise form to be given to such a declaration of principle ... The problem also had a bearing on the question of the national church": Statement of Mr. Rochefort of France, UN Doc. A/CONF.2/SR.30, July 20, 1951, at 13. This matter was of particular concern to the Swedish representative, who referred "to the position in his own country, where there was an Established Church – the Lutheran Church – supported by the state ... Quite clearly, if there was a large influx of, for example, Roman Catholic refugees, Sweden could not be expected to give them the same treatment as members of the Lutheran Church. He presumed that under the provisions of article 4 such refugees would receive the same treatment as Swedish Roman Catholics": Statement of Mr. Petren of Sweden, UN Doc. A/CONF.2/SR.33, July 24, 1951, at 8.

[1394] "The text would have to be couched in such terms as would make allowance for the constitutional procedures providing for religious liberty in each country": Statement of Mr. Hoare of the United Kingdom, UN Doc. A/CONF.2/SR.30, July 20, 1951, at 15. See also concern in this regard expressed by Mr. Rochefort of France, ibid. at 13.

[1395] "Material facilities and economic assistance fell entirely outside the scope of the article": Statement of Mr. Hoare of the United Kingdom, UN Doc. A/CONF/2/SR.33, July 24, 1951, at 9. See also Statement of Mr. Petren of Sweden and Msgr. Comte of the Holy See, ibid. Earlier in the debate, the Canadian representative had proposed "that the provision might be drafted negatively in such terms that Contracting States would undertake not to restrict in any respect the freedom of refugees within their territories to practise their religion": Statement of Mr. Chance of Canada, UN Doc. A/CONF.2/SR.30, July 20, 1951, at 17.

that accorded to nationals."[1396] Yet even measured against this standard, the inferior protection of religious freedom for non-citizens found by the United Nations to exist in Bulgaria, Byelorussia, Cape Verde, Finland, Jordan, Pakistan, Rwanda, Sudan, Syria, Ukraine, and the United States is, to the extent it impacts refugees, an infringement of the Convention.

The content of the right of refugees "to practise their religion" is not spelled out in the Convention. The original formulation tabled by France on the initiative of the non-governmental organization Pax Romana stipulated that refugees should enjoy "full freedom to continue to practice and manifest their religion ... individually or jointly, in public and in private, through education, instruction, religious observance, worship and the carrying out of rites."[1397] The Working Party's reformulation deleted this catalog of protected religious interests in favor of a succinct reference to "complete" freedom of religious practice,[1398] which was in turn amended by the Style Committee to refer simply to "freedom to practice their religion." Importantly, however, nothing in the Conference discussion suggests an interpretation of the scope of religious freedom less robust than the original list proposed by Pax Romana.[1399] To the contrary, the representatives confirmed their intention to secure for refugees "a substantial measure of protection and the exercise of inalienable rights,"[1400] and "full freedom in the practice of religion."[1401]

A broad reading of the scope of protected religious practice is moreover compelled by Art. 18 of the Civil and Political Covenant. This protection, like nearly all rights set by general international human rights law, accrues to the benefit of non-citizens, including refugees,[1402] and is not subject to

---

[1396] Grahl-Madsen, *Commentary*, at 16.

[1397] Statement of Mr. Buensod of Pax Romana, UN Doc. A/CONF.2/SR.11, July 9, 1951, at 10. Mr. Rochefort of France agreed that this commitment should "be examined in principle": ibid. at 11, in consequence of which the proposal was referred to a working party.

[1398] UN Doc. A/CONF.2/94, introduced by the representative of Luxembourg, UN Doc. A/CONF.2/SR.30, July 20, 1951, at 10.

[1399] Grahl-Madsen suggests that the absence of a list of protected religious interests in Art. 4 "does not necessarily call for a more restrictive interpretation": Grahl-Madsen, *Commentary*, at 16.

[1400] Statement of Msgr. Comte of the Holy See, UN Doc. A/CONF.2/SR.30, July 20, 1951, at 11.

[1401] Statement of Mr. Montoya of Venezuela, ibid. at 12.

[1402] See chapter 2.5.4 above, at pp. 120–121. Even refugees subject to provisional or other detention enjoy the right to freedom of religion. "Persons already subject to certain legitimate constraints, such as prisoners, continue to enjoy their rights to manifest their religion or belief to the fullest extent compatible with the specific nature of the constraint": UN Human Rights Committee, "General Comment No. 22: Freedom of thought, conscience or religion" (1993), UN Doc. HRI/GEN/1/Rev.7, May 12, 2004, at 155, para. 8.

derogation, even in time of extreme national emergency.[1403] The Covenant textually protects "practice," which the Human Rights Committee has defined (in conjunction with the protected interests in religious "observance" and "teaching") to include

> not only ceremonial acts but also such customs as the observance of dietary regulations, the wearing of distinctive clothing or head coverings, participation in rituals associated with certain stages of life, ... the use of a particular language customarily spoken by a group ... [and] acts integral to the conduct by religious groups of their basic affairs, such as, *inter alia*, the freedom to choose their religious leaders, priests and teachers, the freedom to establish seminaries or religious schools and the freedom to prepare and distribute religious texts or publications.[1404]

Thus, the refusal of the Maldives to allow the construction of religious buildings other than mosques, the past refusal of Greece to allow the construction of mosques in Athens, as well as the destruction of Pentecostal churches in Myanmar and of Catholic schools in Sudan, are all actions in violation of the right of freedom to practice the religion of one's choice. On the other hand, Uzbekistan's refusal to allow Baptist summer camps may not involve activities sufficiently close to the core of religious observance to qualify as a violation of freedom of religion.

Religious freedom as defined under the Civil and Political Covenant moreover protects not just freedom to practice "religion," but more generally freedom of "thought, conscience and religion ... [including] freedom to have or to adopt a religion or belief of his choice."[1405] This formulation

---

[1403] Civil and Political Covenant, at Art. 4(2). Note, however, that the freedom to "manifest one's religion or beliefs" (as opposed to the right to have or to adopt a religion or belief) may be subject to certain limitations, pursuant to Art. 18(3). See text below, at pp. 579–581.

[1404] UN Human Rights Committee, "General Comment No. 22: Freedom of thought, conscience or religion" (1993), UN Doc. HRI/GEN/1/Rev.7, May 12, 2004, at 155, para. 4. In a recent decision, for example, the Human Rights Committee found a violation of Art. 18 in the case of a Muslim prisoner being held in Trinidad and Tobago on the grounds *inter alia* that "he has been forbidden from wearing a beard and from worshiping at religious services, and that his prayer books were taken from him ... [T]he Committee reaffirms that the freedom to manifest religion or belief in worship, observance, practice and teaching encompasses a broad range of acts and that the concept of worship extends to ritual and ceremonial acts giving expression to belief, as well as various practices integral to such acts": *Boodoo v. Trinidad and Tobago*, UNHRC Comm. No. 721/1996, UN Doc. CCPR/C/74/D/721/1996, decided Apr. 2, 2002, at para. 6.6.

[1405] "The Committee draws the attention of States parties to the fact that the freedom of thought and the freedom of conscience are protected equally with the freedom of religion and belief": UN Human Rights Committee, "General Comment No. 22:

makes it absolutely clear that the actual decision about whether to hold or not to hold a religion or belief is itself a protected interest:

> The right ... is far-reaching and profound; it encompasses freedom of thought on all matters, personal conviction and the commitment to religion or belief, whether manifested individually or in community with others ... Article 18 protects theistic, non-theistic and atheistic beliefs, as well as the right not to profess any religion or belief. The terms belief and religion are to be broadly construed.[1406]

There is thus no question that the Nepalese prohibition of conversion to Seventh Day Adventism, Laotian insistence on renunciation of Christianity by converts, the criminalization of the Baha'i faith in Egypt and Iran, prosecutions for apostasy in Pakistan and for "sorcery" in Saudi Arabia, as well as the attempt to force the conversion of Jehovah's Witness members by beatings in Turkmenistan are all violations of the Civil and Political Covenant.

More generally, the nature and scope of protected interests under the Covenant is quite wide-ranging:

> Although no definition of "thought" or "conscience" is provided, taken together with "religion" they include all possible attitudes of the individual toward the world, toward society, and toward that which determines his fate and the destiny of the world, be it a divinity, some superior being or just reason and rationalism, or chance.[1407]

Thus, the nature of relevant spiritual or intellectual commitments, and hence of the actions which follow from them, is arguably broader than under the Refugee Convention. By virtue of this conceptual expansion, for example, relevant educational freedoms under the Covenant on Economic, Social and Cultural Rights are now understood to include the right of parents and guardians "to ensure the religious *and moral* education of their children in conformity with their own convictions [emphasis added]."[1408] Nor can there be any question of excluding from protection actions taken within what is

---

Freedom of thought, conscience or religion" (1993), UN Doc. HRI/GEN/1/Rev.7, May 12, 2004, at 155, para. 1.

[1406] Ibid. at 155, paras. 1–2.

[1407] K. Partsch, "Freedom of Conscience and Expression, and Political Freedoms," in L. Henkin ed., *The International Bill of Rights* 208 (1981) (Partsch, "Freedom of Conscience"), at 213.

[1408] Economic, Social and Cultural Covenant, at Art. 13(3). In its General Comment on the right to education, the Committee on Economic, Social and Cultural Rights noted that "[t]he second element of article 13(3) is the liberty of parents and guardians to choose other than public schools for their children, provided the schools conform to 'such minimum educational standards as may be laid down or approved by the State.' This has to be read with the complementary provision, article 13(4), which affirms 'the liberty of individuals and bodies to establish and direct educational institutions,' provided the institutions conform to the educational objectives set out in article 13(1) and certain arguably a single "religious" tradition – for example, the arrest by Chad of Nigerian and Senegalese members of a minority Islamic sect on grounds of non-conformism with dominant understandings of Islam – since any variations in the scope of belief are clearly within the realm of the broadly framed freedom of thought, conscience, and religion.

Of particular relevance to refugees, the Civil and Political Covenant also makes clear that "[n]o one shall be subject to coercion which would impair his freedom to have or to adopt a religion or belief of his choice." There can be little question that desperate refugees confined to camps or settlements may feel compelled to repress their own religious views in the face of demands for compliance with divergent beliefs advocated by those with the power to control their access to food and other resources essential to their survival. Illicit forms of coercion include "the use of physical force or penal sanctions to compel believers or non-believers to adhere to their religious beliefs and congregations, to recant their religion or belief or to convert. Policies or practices having the same intention or effect, such as for example those restricting access to education, medical care, [and] employment ... are similarly inconsistent with article 18(2)."[1409] Thus, both the attempts of Sudanese officials to convert the Falasha Jewish refugees and the acquiescence of Pakistani officials in strict enforcement of Islamic precepts in Afghan refugee camps on its territory (albeit organized by refugee leaders themselves) violated the Covenant. Similarly, Bosnian refugee women who refused to wear the headscarves given to them by the Saudi Islamic organization charged with assisting them were entitled to turn to the state for relief against any recriminations grounded in that refusal.

minimum standards": UN Committee on Economic, Social and Cultural Rights, "General Comment No. 13: The right to education" (1999), UN Doc. HRI/GEN/1/Rev.7, May 12, 2004, at 71, para. 29. In respect to Art. 18(4) of the Civil and Political Covenant, the Human Rights Committee has observed simply that "[t]he liberty of parents or legal guardians to ensure that their children receive a religious and moral education in conformity with their own convictions ... is related to the guarantees of the freedom to teach a religion or belief stated in article 18(1)": UN Human Rights Committee, "General Comment No. 22: Freedom of thought, conscience or religion" (1993), UN Doc. HRI/GEN/1/Rev.7, May 12, 2004, at 155, para. 6. Indeed, the Convention on the Rights of the Child may actually have narrowed the scope of the parental prerogative, as the parental role is now conceived as auxiliary to the primary right of children to decide on the nature of their own religious or moral upbringing. "States Parties shall respect the right of the child to freedom of thought, conscience and religion. States Parties shall respect the rights and duties of the parents and, when applicable, legal guardians, to provide direction to the child in the exercise of his or her right in a manner consistent with the evolving capacities of the child": Rights of the Child Convention, at Art. 14(1)–(2).

[1409] UN Human Rights Committee, "General Comment No. 22: Freedom of thought, conscience or religion" (1993), UN Doc. HRI/GEN/1/Rev.7, May 12, 2004, at 155, para. 5.

Only two limitations on the scope of religious practice protected under the
Refugee Convention are clear. First, while the drafters rejected the prerogative of states to limit religious freedom in the interest of "public morality,"[1410]
they affirmed, in line with Art. 2 of the Convention,[1411] that states could
validly curtail activities which refugees might argue to be of a religious nature
under general limitations required to ensure "public order."[1412] With the
advent of the Civil and Political Covenant, however, even the right of states to
limit religious freedom in the interest of promoting public order is constrained. By relying on the cognate right to religious practice in the Covenant,
refugees can insist that any limitations be grounded not in the "concept of
ordre public under French civil law, but rather only to avoid disturbances to
the order in the narrow sense."[1413] Because the drafters of the Covenant chose
to deviate from precedent by avoiding reference to the broader civil law
construct of public order, the scope for limitation is significantly reduced,
as Partsch explains:

[1410] The Colombian representative urged that the religious freedom of refugees should be
subject to the requirements of "public morality": Statement of Mr. Giraldo-Jaramillo of
Colombia, UN Doc. A/CONF.2/SR.30, July 20, 1951, at 15. This proposal was not
pursued after the intervention of the French representative, Mr. Rochefort, ibid. at 16:
"[I]t would be undesirable to introduce into the text the words ... 'and of public
morality,' proposed by the Colombian representative, for clearly the practice of religion
went hand in hand with morality."

[1411] See chapter 2.4.4 above.

[1412] The Egyptian delegate proposed that the religious freedom of refugees should be
"limited by the requirements of national law": Statement of Mr. Mostafa of Egypt, UN
Doc. A/CONF.2/SR.30, July 20, 1951, at 14. The representative of the Netherlands was
initially disposed to this limitation, though he preferred the language "subject to the laws
and regulations and measures adopted to maintain public order": Statement of Baron
van Boetzelaer of the Netherlands, ibid. The Belgian representative was, however,
worried "that the phrase suggested by the Netherlands representative might prove
restrictive. Laws might be promulgated or regulations applied which would nullify the
provisions of the proposed new article. He would prefer the formula 'subject to the
requirements of public order' [emphasis added]": Statement of Mr. Herment of Belgium,
ibid. With the support of the representative of the Holy See, the delegate of the
Netherlands was persuaded that the Belgian formulation – predicated not just on the
invocation of public order reasons, but on the necessity for their invocation – was indeed
to be preferred: Statement of Baron van Boetzelaer of the Netherlands, ibid. In the end,
however, not even this more cautious language was inserted into Art. 4 based on the
recommendation of Msgr. Comte of the Holy See that "it was unnecessary to include the
words 'subject to the requirements of public order.' Article 2 of the draft Convention
already laid down that a refugee had the particular duty of conforming with measures
taken for the maintenance of public order in the country of refuge; that provision was of
a general nature, applicable to all the succeeding articles": ibid. at 17. Thus, only public
order measures which conform to the general requirements of Art. 2 (see chapter 2.4.4
above) are lawful limitations on the religious freedoms of refugees.

[1413] Nowak, *ICCPR Commentary*, at 327.

Article 18(3) permits limitations to protect "public safety, order, health or morals." Presumably "public" modifies "order" as well as "safety," but here it is used without the interpretative addition of the French term *ordre public*. Indeed, here even the French text does not speak of "*ordre public*" but of *la protection de l'ordre*. This clearly suggests that limitations on freedom to manifest one's religion cannot be imposed to protect *ordre public* with its general connotations of national public policy, but only where necessary to protect public order narrowly construed, i.e. to prevent public disorder. A state whose public policy is atheism, for example, cannot invoke Article 18(3) to suppress manifestations of religion or beliefs.[1414]

As such, China's invocation of "public order"[1415] to justify its efforts to minimize the influence of religion in its society is not within the realm of acceptable limitation. On the other hand, the decision by Egypt to manage and regulate the delivery of sermons in mosques in order to "prevent extremists from taking over mosques"[1416] may meet the standard for a public order limitation on religious freedom. As the UN Special Rapporteur on Religious Intolerance has impliedly recognized, so long as the risk of public violence is real and the steps taken are focused and proportional, some constraints on freedom of religious speech are permissible.[1417]

Interestingly, even as the duty simultaneously to respect obligations under the Covenant has effectively narrowed the scope for invocation of a public order limitation on religious practice under the Refugee Convention, the advent of the Covenant has sanctioned other forms of limitation – including those based on public safety, health, and respect for the fundamental rights and freedom of others.[1418] Of arguably greatest concern, the Covenant seems

---

[1414] Partsch, "Freedom of Conscience," at 212–213. See also Nowak, *ICCPR Commentary*, at 325: "The ground of national security is lacking altogether, [and] that of public order (*ordre public*) was substituted with the less far-reaching 'protection of order.'"

[1415] See e.g. the recent defense offered by the Chinese government to the Special Rapporteur on Religious Intolerance. "On 23 August 1999, Zhang Rongliang, Feng Jianguo, Wang Xincai and some other key members of cult organizations, flaunting the banner of 'unification of churches,' called together some people to set up a new cult organization in Tanghe county, Henan Province, and disturbed the public order there. The local public security department, acting on the local people's reports, banned their illegal activities according to law": "Report of the Special Rapporteur on the Elimination of All Forms of Intolerance and of Discrimination Based on Religion or Belief," UN Doc. E/CN.4/2001/63, Feb. 13, 2001, at para. 150.

[1416] Ibid. at para. 35.

[1417] "The Special Rapporteur thanks Egypt for the information concerning measures to combat the political exploitation of religion (particularly the posting of security personnel in places of worship) as part of a genuine medium- and long-term strategy for the prevention of religious extremism": ibid. at para. 36.

[1418] The Human Rights Committee has insisted however, that "[i]n interpreting the scope of permissible limitation clauses, States parties should proceed from the need to protect the rights guaranteed under the Covenant, including the right to equality and also to have validated one form of limitation specifically rejected by the drafters of the Refugee Convention – namely, restrictions based on "public morals."[1419] At first glance, then, the expulsion by Saudi Arabia of the Indian who distributed a Christian videotape contrary to host country "values," and even the rigid enforcement of an extreme version of Islam by the Taliban in Afghanistan, may appear to be consistent with the understanding of religious freedom codified in the Covenant. There are, however, two answers to this dilemma.

First, the potential risk stemming from the prerogative of states to limit religious freedom on grounds of public morals under the Covenant is in fact less serious than the treaty's broad language might suggest.[1420] As the Human Rights Committee has explained, "the concept of morals derives from many social, philosophical and religious traditions: consequently, limitations on the freedom to manifest a religion or belief for the purpose of protecting morals must be based on principles not deriving from a single tradition."[1421] This criterion makes Saudi actions, grounded in the promotion of only an Islamic understanding of morals, not justified. Moreover, a limitation for reasons of morals also has to be "directly related and proportionate to the specific need on which [it is] predicated."[1422] Thus, the decision of the Taliban in Afghanistan massively to violate the human rights of women in pursuit of its vision of a morally defined society – even if had not been based in a single vision of morality – could not in any event have been justified. Second, at least to the extent that the form of religious freedom at issue is within the arguably narrower

non-discrimination on all grounds specified in articles 2, 3 and 26. Limitations imposed must be established by law and must not be applied in a manner that would vitiate the rights guaranteed in article 18. The Committee observes that paragraph 3 of article 18 is to be strictly interpreted": UN Human Rights Committee, "General Comment No. 22: Freedom of thought, conscience or religion" (1993), UN Doc. HRI/GEN/1/Rev.7, May 12, 2004, at 155, para. 8. Moreover, "[t]he fact that a religion is recognized as a state religion or that it is established as official or traditional or that its followers comprise the majority of the population, shall not result in any impairment of the enjoyment of any of the rights under the Covenant, including articles 18 and 27, nor in any discrimination against adherents to other religions or non-believers": ibid. at para. 9.

[1419] Note, however, that "restrictions are not to be allowed on grounds not specified [in paragraph 3], even if they would be allowed as restrictions to other rights protected by the Covenant, such as national security": ibid. at para. 8.

[1420] "A Soviet proposal to make freedom of thought and religion subject to a mere formal legal proviso in accordance with 'the dictates of public morality' was deleted by the Human Rights Commission by a vote of 9:4, with 3 abstentions. Instead, agreement was reached on a proviso in Art. 18(3) listing all reasons for limitation, which relates only to public freedom of religion and belief and is narrower than comparable limitations clauses in the Covenant": Nowak, *ICCPR Commentary*, at 312.

[1421] UN Human Rights Committee, "General Comment No. 22: Freedom of thought, conscience or religion" (1993), UN Doc. HRI/GEN/1/Rev.7, May 12, 2004, at 155, para. 8.

[1422] Ibid.

ambit of Art. 4 of the Refugee Convention, a refugee can avoid the impact of public morality limitations on religious freedom by invoking the Refugee Convention's right to practice one's religion which, as explained above, does not admit of limitation for reasons of morals.[1423]

Beyond limitations grounded in securing public order, the second form of limitation on religious liberty accepted by the drafters of the Refugee Convention followed from the view of the representative of the Holy See that the right to "public worship" implied in Art. 4 need not be understood to require governments to authorize the performance by refugees of "external [religious] acts."[1424] There is no doubt that the Refugee Convention protects the rights of refugees to engage in public worship, for example in a church or mosque. As such, the Convention is violated when refugees are subject to the formal or de facto prohibition of minority worship in states such as Bhutan, Turkey, Georgia, Turkmenistan, and Azerbaijan. On the other hand, because the scope of religious freedom guaranteed under the Refugee Convention may not extend also to "external religious acts," the constraints on proselytization imposed by such countries as Bulgaria, Georgia, and France may not run afoul of Art. 4. But a refugee might choose instead to rely on the cognate right in the Civil and Political Covenant which, as noted above, has been interpreted to safeguard a variety of external practices, including the distribution of religious literature.[1425]

[1423] See text above, at p. 578. A refugee relying on the Covenant's protection of the right to manifest religion or beliefs could also face restrictions based on "public health," "public safety," or "the fundamental rights and freedoms of others." Nowak suggests that the public health limitation might include, for example, the right to require persons to be vaccinated against contagious diseases, religious convictions notwithstanding. The public safety limitation could justify a constraint on religious ceremonies which, if conducted, could engender a hostile confrontation. The exception for protection of the rights and freedoms of others would, in Nowak's view, validate the prohibition of acts such as female circumcision, even if based on a religious rite: Nowak, *ICCPR Commentary*, at 326–329. Except to the extent that comparable concerns amount to *ordre public* exceptions, however, a refugee could arguably avoid even these constraints on the right to practice religion by invoking Art. 4 of the Refugee Convention rather than Art. 18 of the Civil and Political Covenant.

[1424] "There was, in fact, a difference between external acts of worship and public worship. Public worship was not necessarily performed by external acts; while it did not exclude external acts of worship, it did not necessarily imply them, but it was possible to bring the two together": Statement of Msgr. Comte of the Holy See, UN Doc. A/CONF.2/SR.30, July 20, 1951, at 13.

[1425] See text above, at p. 575. In relying on the Covenant, however, the refugee would face the possibility of the various forms of limitation deemed permissible under Art. 18(3), even if these would not apply to constrain rights under Art. 4 of the Refugee Convention. This potential for restrictions would not, however, apply to communal religious observance in private. As Nowak has commented, "[w]hen an individual prays alone in his (her) home or performs together with those like-minded a religious observance, this

The most specific form of religious liberty protected by the Refugee Convention is the right of refugee parents "as regards the religious education of their children." This right, presented to the Conference of Plenipotentiaries as the right of refugees "to ensure that their children are taught the religion they profess,"[1426] was the subject of substantial debate. The main concern of states, in line with their view that their principled responsibility to facilitate the religious freedom of refugees should not entail a duty to fund such activities,[1427] was that the phrasing proposed "implied that the State would be committed to providing at its own expense facilities for teaching the religion of the refugee."[1428] To avoid this interpretation, it was agreed that the only obligation of states was "to grant refugees . . . freedom to ensure that their children were taught in the religion they professed."[1429] The duty was "permissive on [refugee] parents and not mandatory on governments."[1430] The implications of this understanding of the right to freedom of religious education are perhaps best understood in relation to a description of the Swedish approach to education, as given by that country's representative to the Conference of Plenipotentiaries:

> Primary education was compulsory in Sweden, and parents who could not afford to send their children to a private school were obliged to send them to a State school, where religious instruction was given according to the Lutheran faith. If a refugee belonged to a church other than the Lutheran church, he had full freedom to withdraw his children from the classes in religious instruction.[1431]

undoubtedly constitutes 'practice' . . . [P]rivate freedom to practice actively a religion or belief may not be subject to any restrictions pursuant to Art. 18(3). However, such practice may be termed private only so long as it does not leave that sphere of individual existence and autonomy that does not touch upon the freedom and sphere of privacy of others": Nowak, *ICCPR Commentary*, at 319.

[1426] UN Doc. A/CONF.2/94.   [1427] See text above, at p. 573.

[1428] Statement of Mr. Fritzer of Austria, UN Doc. A/CONF.2/SR.30, July 20, 1951, at 14–15.

[1429] Statement of Mr. van Heuven Goedhart of UNHCR, ibid. at 15.

[1430] Statement of Mr. Rees of the Commission of the Churches on International Affairs, ibid. at 17. See also Statements of Mr. Herment of Belgium and Mr. Fritzer of Austria, ibid. at 15.

[1431] Statement of Mr. Petren of Sweden, ibid. at 12. Mr. Petren went on to say that atheist parents did not enjoy the same right to withdraw their children from mandatory Lutheran education classes, a position now clearly inconsistent with the accepted position that freedom of religion includes the right to hold *or not to hold* particular convictions. See UN Human Rights Committee, "General Comment No. 22: Freedom of thought, conscience or religion" (1993), UN Doc. HRI/GEN/1/Rev.7, May 12, 2004, at 155, paras. 2, 6: "Article 18 protects theistic, non-theistic and atheistic beliefs, as well as the right not to profess any religion or belief . . . [A]rticle 18(4) permits public school instruction in subjects such as general history of religions and ethics if it is given in a neutral and objective way."

In essence, therefore, Art. 4 ensures that refugee parents are free (if they have the resources) to enrol their children in schools which provide their preferred form of religious instruction; and if they are not able to fund education of that kind, they enjoy the liberty to withdraw their children from any non-preferred form of religious instruction provided within the public school system. Thus, the Greek practice of requiring study of Greek Orthodoxy in all of its schools, Bhutanese insistence on recitation of a Muslim–Hindu prayer in its public classrooms, Sudanese infliction of corporal punishment on students who will not study Islam, and the absolute denial of freedom of religious education during the Taliban era in Afghanistan may all, albeit to varying degrees, result in violations of the Refugee Convention's right to freedom of religious education. Even the more nuanced Norwegian requirement for education in Christianity and Christian ethics, under which "exemptions from specific religious activities such as prayer may be granted, but students may not forgo instruction in the subject as a whole,"[1432] is not in compliance with the Refugee Convention because of the partial nature of the right of parents to withdraw their children from specifically Christian instruction. Much the same analysis follows from understandings of the right to religious education derived from the Civil and Political Covenant,[1433] though the Human Rights Committee has determined also that states may not discriminate in the funding of religious education.[1434]

[1432] "Report of the Special Rapporteur on the Elimination of All Forms of Intolerance and of Discrimination Based on Religion or Belief," UN Doc. E/CN.4/2001/63, Feb. 13, 2001, at para. 109.

[1433] "[T]he parental right in the Covenant on Civil and Political Rights is of a rather modest nature ... [In particular] it may be assumed that the parental right covers private school freedom. The States Parties are, of course, not obligated to subsidize private schools": Nowak, *ICCPR Commentary*, at 331–332. Similarly, under Art. 13(3) of the Covenant on Economic, Social and Cultural Rights, "[t]he State here is obliged merely to refrain from placing obstacles in the way of parents wishing to exercise this right": Craven, *ICESCR Commentary*, at 110. As neither Art. 4 of the Refugee Convention nor cognate rights under the Covenants specifically regulate the religious education of other than "children," a refugee seeking to contest subjection to the Malaysian policy of mandatory Islamic education for civil servants who self-define as Muslim would have to justify his or her complaint on the grounds of the more general right to practice one's religion in the manner of one's choosing. See text above, at p. 575.

[1434] "[T]he Committee observes that the Covenant does not oblige States parties to fund schools which are established on a religious basis. However, if a State party chooses to provide public funding to religious schools, it should make this funding available without discrimination. This means that providing funding for the schools of one religious group and not for another must be based on reasonable and objective criteria. In the instant case, the Committee concludes that the material before it does not show that the differential treatment between the Roman Catholic faith and the author's religious denomination is based on such criteria. Consequently, there has been a violation of the author's rights under article 26 of the Covenant to equal and effective

4.8 Education

The importance with which refugees view education is usually evident during their very earliest days in an asylum country.[1435] Anxious for their children's studies to resume before knowledge is lost, or simply to restore a sense of purpose in a situation otherwise without hope, refugees frequently establish classes for their children immediately upon reaching safety, using whatever resources are available to them.[1436] As most refugees anticipate eventual repatriation, resumption of the education of their children is also critical to providing them with a sense of continuity, enabling the children to retain their cultural identity which may be challenged by life in the host country. Of particular importance is preservation by children of facility in the language of the country of origin.[1437] As the mother tongue is often the first cultural characteristic to be lost, the viability of repatriation is undermined when children are unable to use their own language in school, particularly in the early grades.[1438]

Education takes on a different role if and when the prospect of return home becomes less real. When assimilation or resettlement is envisaged, education is instrumental in equipping both refugee children and adults to survive and succeed in their new environment. Learning the local language has been identified as one of the most important skills for newcomers,[1439] one that is essential to overcoming the "de-socialization" caused by communications problems.[1440] Training in productive skills can enable refugees to be

---

protection against discrimination": *Waldman v. Canada*, UNHRC Comm. No. 694/ 1996, UN Doc. CCPR/C/67/D/694/1996, decided Nov. 3, 1999, at para. 10.6.

[1435] International Extension College and World University Service (UK), "Refugee Education: The Case for International Action" (1986) (IEC and WUS, "Refugee Education"), at 8.

[1436] "Gathering primary school age children together and organizing some kind of educational activity for them immediately improves the morale of the community. It also gives parents, often single parents, the relief and time they need to carry out their other urgent responsibilities. Such 'schools' may be in tents or under trees or in any form of shelter, at least to start with": IEC and WUS, "Refugee Education," at 13. For example, the first classes for Mozambican refugees in Malawi were "held under trees in the absence of appropriate buildings, and teachers had to make do with whatever teaching materials had been brought with the refugees": D. Tolfree, "Refugee Children in Malawi: A Study of the Implementation of the UNHCR Guidelines on Refugee Children" (1991) (Tolfree, "Refugee Children in Malawi"), at 20.

[1437] UNHCR, "Refugee Children: Guidelines on Protection and Care" (1994), at 31.

[1438] UNHCR observes that it is also the case that refugee children tend to learn most quickly in their own language: ibid. at 113.

[1439] "Language is crucial to successful settlement. For young people it is the key to access to education; for adults it opens up a wide range of possibilities, not the least of which is managing everyday life": Joly, *Asylum*, at 59.

[1440] See generally M. Domanski, "Insights from the Refugee Experience: A Background Paper on Temporary Protection," in J. Hathaway ed., *Reconceiving International Refugee Law* 22 (1997).

employable and hence self-supporting in their new societies.[1441] Particularly where the transition is to a more developed economy, it will be important to assist refugees whose post-secondary academic training has been interrupted by flight.[1442] Refugee women not involved in the external workplace have unique needs for compensatory education to avoid social isolation, and to provide them with a measure of autonomy in their new community.[1443]

While the importance of refugee education is nearly universally recognized, UNHCR has estimated that fewer than half of refugee children receive even elementary education.[1444] The situation for refugee girls is worse still, as additional barriers such as family responsibilities and traditional values may lead to lower attendance for girls, leading to lower attendance and higher drop-out rates.[1445] Despite some extraordinary successes – notably among Afghan refugees in Pakistan[1446] – girls still make up only about 39 percent of refugee children attending UNHCR-assisted primary schools, and only about 29 percent of the secondary school population.[1447]

The inability of many refugee children to access education is perhaps not surprising in a world where the vast majority of refugees are the responsibility

---

[1441] IEC and WUS, "Refugee Education," at 17–18.   [1442] Ibid.

[1443] Forbes Martin, *Refugee Women*, at 49.

[1444] "While more refugee children are attending primary school – an estimated 44 percent in 2000, compared to 36 percent in 1993 – more can be done to increase primary education opportunities and ensure equal access for all refugee children, including adolescents": UNHCR, "Refugee Children," UN Doc. EC/GC/02/9, Apr. 25, 2002, at para. 19. "Only 50 percent of refugee children are enrolled in the four lowest grades and a mere 12 percent in the four highest grades": UNHCR, "Report of the United Nations High Commissioner for Refugees," UN Doc. E/2003/68, June 6, 2003, at para. 19.

[1445] "Refugee girls' enrolment decreases progressively; absenteeism among girls, who are obliged to assist with family chores, is higher than among boys; there is a high drop-out rate due in part to the lack of teachers properly trained and sensitive to girls' needs; families hold traditional values in which education is not seen as a goal for self-sufficiency or as being of assistance in the improvement of their daily life": Expert Group Meeting on Refugee and Displaced Women and Children, "Refugee and Displaced Women and Children," UN Doc. EGM/RDWC/1990/WP.2 (1990).

[1446] "The most dramatic success on behalf of girls' education was achieved in Pakistan, where resistance to it from Afghan men had to be overcome, but all UNHCR offices demonstrated a commitment to educating both boys and girls. Although girls still remain in school fewer years than do boys, hostility seems to be diminishing": Women's Commission for Refugee Women and Children, "UNHCR Policy on Refugee Women and Guidelines on their Protection: An Assessment of Ten Years of Implementation," May 2002, at 29. Just a decade earlier, less than 0.1 percent of school-age Afghan refugee girls in Pakistan were reported to be enrolled in school: Forbes Martin, *Refugee Women*, at 45.

[1447] UNHCR, "More refugee girls must go to school, says UNHCR on International Women's Day," Mar. 7, 2003.

586   4 RIGHTS OF REFUGEES PHYSICALLY PRESENT

of its poorest states.[1448] Unable in many cases to meet the educational needs of their own citizens, these countries simply lack the resources to provide adequate educational opportunities for refugees, whether within the national school system or through separate institutions.[1449] Cambodia, for example, has taken the view that because of its lack of resources it is entitled to prioritize the education of its own children over that of urban refugee children living in and around Phnom Penh.[1450] But financial constraints do not account for all failures to provide refugees with education. Education is sometimes denied as a means of discouraging refugee flows, or encouraging their premature repatriation. During the 1990s, for example, the Turkish government provided no educational facilities to the Iraqi Kurds in camps in southeastern Turkey, and prohibited refugee-organized educational programs for some 13,000 refugee children.[1451] Similarly, the Thai government was initially reluctant to approve any educational programs for Cambodian refugees in order "to prevent the institutionalization and perpetuation of the camps and the attendant likelihood of attracting more refugees from Cambodia."[1452] And before the South African Human Rights Commission intervened, the government of that country denied refugee children access to

---

[1448] "[I]n developing countries, 130 million children of school age are currently estimated to be without access to primary education, of whom about two-thirds are girls": UN Committee on Economic, Social and Cultural Rights, "General Comment No. 11: Plans of action for primary education" (1999), UN Doc. HRI/GEN/1/Rev.7, May 12, 2004, at 60, para. 3.

[1449] For example, the situation in Africa has been described as "mass movements of virtually illiterate peasantry fleeing to countries where educational resources are already over-burdened to meet even the basic needs of their own citizens, let alone those of outsiders": H. Pilkington, "The Higher Education of Refugees in Africa: Suggestions," [Nov. 1996] Refugee Issues 1 (Pilkington, "Higher Education"). See also S. Nkiwane, International Academy of Comparative Law National Report for Zimbabwe (1994), at 15, who writes that Zimbabwe has enough difficulty educating its own nationals, without taking on unlimited responsibilities for refugees.

[1450] "Public education is also inaccessible to refugee children. The UNHCR has been pushing for more rights for refugees though Cambodia, being a very poor country, prioritizes its own citizens' economic betterment over the enforcement of international treaty obligations relating to immigrants and asylum-seekers": "Cambodia: precarious position of refugees," (2002) 114 JRS Dispatches (June 28, 2002).

[1451] "The children are not receiving school instruction, nor are they being offered pedagogical supervision. The school instruction that was organized by the refugees themselves and took place in dark, stinking cellars has been prohibited. The makeshift school materials were confiscated": IHRK, "Kurdish Refugees," at 30.

[1452] P. Gyallay-Pap, "Reclaiming a Shattered Past: Education for the Displaced Khmer in Thailand," (1989) 2(2) Journal of Refugee Studies 257 (Gyallay-Pap, "Shattered Past"), at 265.

educational facilities until and unless their claims to refugee status (or those of their parents) were positively assessed.[1453]

When support for refugee education is provided, it often comes only after considerable delay,[1454] and is frequently inadequate.[1455] While refugee communities have proven capable of organizing their own education programs almost immediately upon reaching refuge,[1456] they often require support from national and international agencies in order to reach as many eligible children as possible, and to fund educational materials and teacher training.[1457] Continual financial shortfalls mean that, with notable exceptions,[1458] most refugee children in the less developed world who are fortunate enough to attend school still face daunting obstacles, such as overcrowded classrooms, shortages of teaching materials, and a dearth of qualified teachers.[1459] Teachers were particularly scarce among the Cambodian refugees in Thailand following the anti-intellectual massacres by the Khmer Rouge.[1460] Shortages of qualified teachers for Mozambican refugees in Malawi prevented

[1453] "Originally ... a prohibition on work and study was indicated in all asylum application papers ... The [South Africa Human Rights] Commission called this limitation into question as being unconstitutional, and the prohibition was eventually lifted in cases of children so that they would be entitled to start school immediately": L. Stone and S. Winterstein, *A Right or a Privilege? Access to Basic Education for Refugee and Asylum-Seeker Children in South Africa* (2003), at 28. The unconstitutionality of the prohibition was later confirmed in *Minister of Home Affairs v. Watchenuka*, (2004) 1 All SA 21 (SA SCA, Nov. 28, 2003), at para. 36.

[1454] It is reported that education is often a low priority among organizations assisting refugees, considered a luxury by agencies that "optimistically ignore the fact that most short-term refugee situations become long term": IEC and WUS, "Refugee Education," at 8. As a result, "[t]here are no examples where education has been provided to refugees in the early stage of their exile, along with emergency relief services, except where refugees themselves have mobilized what limited resources they have to set up schools and literacy classes": ibid. at 36.

[1455] "We are now reaching the stage where some budget restrictions may simply prove too severe to sustain ... In the educational sector, substantial cutbacks in the construction of new facilities and provision of materials will mean that many refugee children are denied access to schooling": Forbes Martin, *Refugee Women*, at 46, quoting from the UNHCR Head of Program Management Services.

[1456] Refugee-initiated schools were established, for example, in Djibouti, Thailand, Pakistan, and Sudan. "The spontaneity of such refugee self-help projects makes for speed ... They may have very few or no resources, but they are unhampered by bureaucratic delays and they thus provide the very first community development activities and the first injections of hope in the future which are so vital in the emergency stages of a refugee crisis": IEC and WUS, "Refugee Education," at 13.

[1457] Ibid. at 22.

[1458] Among the refugee education systems positively appraised by experts are those for Tibetans in India and for Palestinian refugees under the auspices of UNRWA: B. S. Chimni, *International Academy of Comparative Law National Report for India* (1994), at 28; Forbes Martin, *Refugee Women*, at 47.

[1459] Forbes Martin, *Refugee Women*, at 46.   [1460] Gyallay-Pap, "Shattered Past," at 270.

teacher–student ratios from improving beyond 1:100.[1461] Liberian refugees in Nigeria, restricted to their camp's makeshift school, suffered particularly from a shortage of teaching supplies and basic equipment such as desks and chairs.[1462] Some Sahrawi refugee children had only one textbook per class, and library resources were "practically nonexistent."[1463]

The nature of refugee education provided in the South is also sometimes contentious. UNHCR advocates "education for repatriation," with the curriculum to be based on that in the refugees' country of origin.[1464] This approach was adopted, for example, for Afghan refugees in Pakistan, Mozambican refugees in Malawi and Zimbabwe, and Rwandan refugees in Tanzania, Burundi, and Zaïre.[1465] But conflict may arise between the refugee community and host government when there is a divergence of views about whether repatriation, integration, or resettlement is the most appropriate goal. For instance, the Tanzanian government of the mid-1980s believed that it made most sense to attempt to integrate Burundian refugees into the Tanzanian national culture. The priority of the refugees themselves, however, was to be prepared for repatriation to Burundi.[1466] Similarly, the Sudanese government's policy of assimilating Eritrean refugees into its own schools conflicted with the refugees' aspiration for education that was relevant to the socioeconomic reality in their homeland, and which would prepare them to serve their people and country upon return.[1467] Differences in approach to education can also arise between refugees and international agencies. The curriculum developed by UNBRO for Cambodian refugees in the Thai border camps, for example, was based on Western methodology and Western

---

[1461] This ratio was considered a great success, and was only achieved after the hiring of hundreds of additional teachers: Tolfree, "Refugee Children in Malawi," at 20–21.

[1462] "In spite of the resourcefulness of the refugees, the school has many deficiencies caused by lack of adequate financial support. Interviews with the teaching staff revealed that there are insufficient chairs, desks and blackboards; and the school has virtually no books. From its inception, neither the teachers nor the students in grades 7–9 have had textbooks. The students in grades 1–6 have textbooks but very little else": Tiao, "Refugee Rights in Nigeria," at 14.

[1463] A. Velloso, "Palaces for Children: Education in the Refugee Camps of the Sahrawi Arab Democratic Republic," [Apr. 1996] Refugee Participation Network.

[1464] A. Avery, "Education: The Least of UNHCR's Priorities? UNHCR Responds," [Apr. 1996] Refugee Participation Network (Avery, "UNHCR Responds").

[1465] Ibid.

[1466] A. Ayok Chol, "Reflections on the Policies and Practices of Refugee Education in Tanzania," paper presented at the University of Dar es Salaam, Tanzania, July 29, 1987.

[1467] J. El Bushra, "Case Studies of Educational Needs Among Refugees II: Eritrean and Ethiopian Refugees in the Sudan" (1985), at 24. Because of the perceived inappropriateness of the Sudanese educational system, many refugees sent their children to schools set up by liberation groups or voluntary organizations: ibid.

industrialized standards, without reference to Khmer Buddhist culture and their traditional agrarian lifestyle. As Gyallay-Pap observed,

> The question [is] ... whether an education system based largely on western industrial development norms, with its emphasis on productivity and consumption (or "raising the standard of living"), is appropriate for a people who have steadfastly remained agriculturalists attached to the land and traditional culture. The disparity between the modern Khmer school curriculum and the realities of Khmer culture and society is seen in the near absence of artistic, religious, and other traditional cultural subjects through which the Khmer have traditionally self-understood themselves.[1468]

In developed countries, in contrast, recognized refugee children are nearly universally integrated into the national school systems of the asylum state.[1469] But until refugee status is formally recognized, refugee children may face barriers to accessing education. For example, the United Nations Committee on the Rights of the Child observed that in Greece there have been "[d]iffi-culties in gaining access to education for some groups of children, including asylum-seeking and refugee children."[1470] Under the British government's policy of dispersing asylum-seekers throughout the country, local school boards have sometimes refused to enroll refugee children for fear of reducing their schools' ranking based on student performance on standardized tests, or of having to fund language support for them.[1471] Even more seriously, British legislation passed in 2002 provides that the children of refugee claimants

---

[1468] Gyallay-Pap, "Shattered Past," at 273.

[1469] In the European Union it is now agreed that "[m]ember states shall grant full access to the education system to all minors granted refugee or subsidiary protection status, under the same conditions as nationals": Council Directive on minimum standards for the qualification and status of third country nationals or stateless persons as refugees or as persons who otherwise need international protection and the content of the protection granted, Doc. 2004/83/EC (Apr. 29, 2004) (EU Qualification Directive), at Art. 27(1).

[1470] UN Committee on the Rights of the Child, "Concluding Observations of the Committee on the Rights of the Child: Greece," UN Doc. CRC/C/15/Add.170, Feb. 1, 2002, at para. 66(e). The Committee therefore recommended that Greece "[e]nsure that asylum-seeking, refugee and illegal immigrant children have access to education": ibid. at para. 69(f).

[1471] A. Travis, "Asylum seekers suffer as dispersal system fails," *Guardian*, June 1, 2000, at 1. It is estimated "that 2,000 children of asylum-seekers are without school places ... [F]ewer than 12% of local authorities with a social services department had a refugee strategy": ibid. Writing in 1998, the chief executive of the British Refugee Council warned that "if in the future, asylum-seekers' families are dumped in areas where there is no experience of their needs, the number of children out of school will grow. Local community relations would suffer, particularly if the advance billing casts all asylum-seekers as bogus scroungers": N. Hardwick, "Asylum: Stairway to Hell," *Guardian*, Aug. 5, 1998, at 2. Interestingly, refugee children may actually contribute to an improvement of academic quality in schools, according to the head of education at will no longer be entitled to attend local schools, but may be limited to taking classes within refugee accommodation centers.[1472] From February 2005, however, the European Union's Reception Directive requires that the minor children of refugee applicants receive education "under similar conditions as nationals" beginning not later than three months after the filing of an application for protection by either the child or his or her parents.[1473]

Another contentious issue in developed countries is the language of instruction for refugee children. Whereas most jurisdictions in Canada[1474] and some European states, including Norway and Sweden,[1475] do provide mother tongue instruction to refugee children, other states, such as Belgium and France,[1476] offer little or no such instruction. In Ireland, for example, the decision was made that Vietnamese refugee children should be "left to either sink or swim"[1477] in English-language education.

Secondary and post-secondary education is usually less easily accessed by refugees than is elementary education. Most refugees in the South have no access whatever to advanced formal education;[1478] indeed, the Refugee

the British National Union of Teachers, who reported that "[a]ll the evidence we have is that in some of the toughest schools, it is the asylum-seekers' children who provide stability, because they are most dedicated to getting the best out of the system": L. Brooks, "Asylum: a special investigation," *Guardian*, May 1, 2003, at 2.

[1472] "For the purposes of section 13 of the Education Act 1996 (c. 56) (general responsibility of local education authority) a resident of an accommodation centre shall not be treated as part of the population of a local education authority's area": Nationality, Immigration and Asylum Act 2002, c. 41, at s. 36(1). An earlier report of a government-dominated committee on human rights had opined that educating refugee children outside mainstream schools would give rise "to troubling echos of educational regimes where children were educated separately on the basis of race or colour": G. Younge, "Villagers and the damned," *Guardian*, June 24, 2002, at 17.

[1473] EU Reception Directive, at Art. 10(2).

[1474] Half of the provinces of Canada (Quebec, Ontario, Manitoba, Saskatchewan, and Alberta) support heritage language programs, to which refugee children have access. In Ontario, for example, a heritage language program is provided when twenty-five or more students request it: Canadian Education Association, "Heritage Language Programs in Canadian School Boards" (1991).

[1475] ECRE, *Conditions 2003*. Italy also is in principle committed to providing mother-tongue instruction, but is reported not to do so in practice due to a lack of qualified teachers: ibid.

[1476] Ibid.

[1477] F. McGovern, "The Education of a Linguistic and Cultural Minority: Vietnamese Children in Irish Schools, 1979–1989," (1993) 12 *Irish Education Studies* 92, at 95. "No special language provision was made for the Vietnamese children of school-going age in the mainstream system ... The belief was that if children were submerged in the mainstream schooling system, they would pick up English language and somehow survive": ibid.

[1478] Pilkington, "Higher Education," at 1.

Education Trust has reported that of the 1.5 million teenage refugees living in less developed countries, only 50,000 – about 3 percent – are able to attend school beyond the primary level.[1479] There are notable exceptions, such as Sudan and Swaziland, which built secondary schools specifically for refugees.[1480] But the primary means for refugees in the less developed world to access secondary and university education has been through the award of scholarships provided by UNHCR and other agencies, the number of which is extremely limited.[1481] In the Osire refugee camp in Namibia, for example, rioting broke out when only three out of fifty-six applications for study grants were accepted.[1482] Even in states where refugees in principle have access to higher education, authorities who fear that the admission of a refugee effectively deprives a citizen of access to higher education therefore sometimes take action to restrict the educational opportunities of refugees.[1483] For example, Tanzania has set a limit of 2 percent non-citizens in post-elementary educational institutions.[1484] Other difficulties include recognition of academic credentials,[1485] accessing information about educational opportunities, and satisfaction of the requirements set by scholarship-granting agencies.[1486]

Non-formal education in the less developed world has also received insufficient attention and financial support.[1487] As a result, educational programs

---

[1479] Refugee Education Trust, "First International Symposium on Post-Primary Education for Refugees and Internally Displaced Persons, 18–19 September 2002, Geneva" (2003).

[1480] IEC and WUS, "Refugee Education," at 16.

[1481] For example, the number of scholarships provided to Afghan refugees in Pakistan has been described as "a drop in the bucket." As one UNHCR official explained, "[w]e have got to think about providing the new generation with a future. Afghans need doctors, teachers, engineers . . . We realize that a few scholarships are not going to do the trick": E. Girardet, "Urban Refugees in Peshawar," (1986) 27 *Refugees* 15 (Girardet, "Peshawar"), at 16–17.

[1482] "There are reportedly more than 3,000 students in pre-primary and primary schools as well as in adult education at the Osire camp. The exact number of students who would like to study from grades 10 and higher could not be established. There is no secondary school at Osire, which now houses over 17,000 refugees, more than five times the figure that the camp can officially accommodate": *Namibian*, Mar. 12, 2001.

[1483] "In Sudan, we encountered young Eritreans, many of high school age, who are desperate to continue their education but cannot. For most it is a question of funds or the refusal by local authorities to take more than a handful of students": T. Skari and E. Girardet, "Urban Refugees: Out of the Public Eye," (1985) 23 *Refugees* 14, at 14.

[1484] Forbes Martin, *Refugee Women*, at 47.

[1485] IEC and WUS, "Refugee Education," at 17. See also Tiao, "Refugee Rights in Nigeria," at 15, for a description of the problems faced by Liberian refugees seeking higher education in Nigeria.

[1486] Pilkington, "Higher Education," at 2–4.

[1487] IEC and WUS, "Refugee Education," at 31.

designed to impart basic skills to adult refugees, including literacy and numeracy training, have been in short supply.[1488] Where such programs have been established, they have at times been hampered by limited access,[1489] and by the failure to encourage refugee involvement in their development.[1490] In addition, the frequent absence of special compensatory programs for women refugees has at times been glaring.[1491] In contrast, a non-formal educational program for Bhutanese refugees in Nepal encouraged women's participation through the provision of separate male and female classes, held in "semi-public" space, and timed so as not to conflict with women's responsibilities such as ration collection, childminding, and other household activities.[1492]

Vocational programs tend to be more adequately funded by international agencies than are basic educational initiatives.[1493] The most common focus is the training of health workers and teachers,[1494] but some initiatives are more ambitious. For example, the self-help projects in Kenya's coastal refugee camps assisted many women, as well as men, to learn manual and management skills through such activities as craftwork, sewing, and agriculture.[1495] The ANC work unit program at their settlement in Tanzania provided opportunities for South African refugees to be trained in construction and agriculture, and in running small industries such as clothing, leather goods, carpentry, welding, and the repair of motor vehicles and electrical appliances.[1496] However, as refugees become settled, they frequently seek more expensive, institutionalized vocational training courses. Centers such as the Vocational Training Center in Angola for Namibians, the mechanical training center for Afghans in Pakistan, and the UNRWA/UNESCO Institute of

---

[1488] Ibid. An innovative success story is the Education Program for Sudanese Refugees (EPSR) established by Makerere University which provided refugees with library, reading, and training facilities, all at a location easily reached by foot from the area where more than half of the refugees lived: B. Sesnan, "Push and Pull: Education for Southern Sudanese in Exile, 1986–1996," in G. Retamal and R. Aedo-Richmond eds., *Education as a Humanitarian Response* 59 (1998), at 69–70.

[1489] For example, while several programs were run for refugees in Thailand, "only a small proportion of the eligible population has the possibility of participating in these activities": R. Preston, "Is There a Refugee-Specific Education?," (1990) 23(3) *Convergences* 3 (Preston, "Refugee-Specific"), at 7.

[1490] Educational programs for Mozambican refugees in Swaziland were criticized because refugees did "not generally participate in educational decision-making and program implementation, and many of the programs [were] generated within the offices of the UNHCR and other agencies": H. Woodbridge et al., "Education for Adult Refugees in Swaziland," (1990) 23(3) *Convergences* 23, at 33.

[1491] IEC and WUS, "Refugee Education," at 31–32.

[1492] T. Rahman, "Literacy for Refugee Women: A Case Study from Nepal," [Apr. 1996] *Refugee Participation Network.*

[1493] IEC and WUS, "Refugee Education," at 32.   [1494] Preston, "Refugee-Specific," at 6.

[1495] Avery, "UNHCR Responds."   [1496] IEC and WUS, "Refugee Education," at 18.

Education for Palestinian refugees have provided practical on-the-job train-ing, linked to needs in the host community.[1497] But the relatively high cost of such centers has limited their number.[1498]

In the developed world, access to secondary and post-secondary educa-tion, as well as to language courses, continuing education courses, and informal orientation courses is generally provided to recognized refugees on at least the same terms as that afforded other long-term lawful resi-dents.[1499] The form in which these latter adult-oriented programs is delivered varies considerably, including courses designed specifically for refugees, courses offered through national adult education systems, and courses orga-nized by NGOs. As in the South, one concern is that many refugee women have difficulty accessing educational opportunities truly suited to their needs. Due to conventional assumptions about which spouse is the "breadwinner," training courses have sometimes been unduly male-focused.[1500] For example, the British vocational education system has been found inadequate in addres-sing refugee women's family responsibilities,[1501] in particular the need for access to childcare facilities.[1502]

The most serious challenge for refugees seeking to avail themselves of educational opportunities in the developed world is the distinction some-times drawn between recognized refugees and those whose asylum claims have yet to be formally determined, or who are granted an alternative form of status. The European Union treats access to vocational training for refugees awaiting status verification as a matter of pure discretion for state parties.[1503] In the result, basic orientation programs, continuing education classes, and even language programs are denied to refugee claimants in some countries. For example, in Italy and Portugal, asylum-seekers must often depend on NGOs and community organizations to provide them with language

---

[1497] Ibid. at 18, 33; Girardet, "Peshawar," at 17.

[1498] IEC and WUS, "Refugee Education," at 18.

[1499] In the European Union, for example, "[m]ember states shall allow adults granted refugee or subsidiary protection status access to the general education system, further training or retraining, under the same conditions as third country nationals legally resident": EU Qualification Directive, at Art. 27(2).

[1500] "Because of the traditional assumption that heads of families are men, skill-training programmes and income-generating activities have been directed at them": Camus-Jacques, "Forgotten Majority," at 149.

[1501] V. Shawcross et al., *Women in Mind: The Educational Needs of Women Refugees in the UK* (1987), at 22.

[1502] Africa Educational Trust, "Education, Training, and Employment Needs of Refugees in London," available at www.africaed.org (accessed Sept. 16, 2003). See also A. Bloch, "Refugees' Opportunities and Barriers in Employment and Training," Research Paper No. 179, UK Department for Work and Pensions (2002).

[1503] "Member States may allow asylum-seekers access to vocational training irrespective of whether they have access to the labour market": EU Reception Directive, at Art. 12.

training.[1504] In Australia, the Chief Minister of the Australian Capital Territory defied the federal government's policy of denying language training to refugees holding temporary protection visas by arranging for their instruction at a Canberra technical institute.[1505]

Much the same pattern of differentiation holds for more formal sorts of advanced education. While recognized refugees in the North are for the most part assimilated to long-term residents for purposes of eligibility for grants and bursaries to attend university,[1506] refugees whose claims have not yet been formally assessed may be denied such access.[1507] Immigration officials frequently have discretion to authorize enrollment on an individual basis, and their decisions are typically non-reviewable.[1508]

> **Refugee Convention, Art. 22   Public education**
> 1. The Contracting States shall accord to refugees the same treatment as is accorded to nationals with respect to elementary education.
> 2. The Contracting States shall accord to refugees treatment as favourable as possible, and, in any event, not less favourable than that accorded to aliens generally in the same circumstances, with respect to education other than elementary education and, in particular, as regards access to studies, the recognition of foreign school certificates, diplomas and degrees, the remission of fees and charges and the award of scholarships.

[1504] In Italy, for example, "[l]anguage courses are organised on a large scale by NGOs and church organisations, including the Federation of Evangelical Churches, Caritas, the Communità di Sant' Egidio, the Salvation Army, and some reception centers": Liebaut, *Conditions 2000*, at 172. In Portugal, "[t]here are no state-funded language classes for asylum-seekers. For two years, the Portuguese Refugee Council has run a Program for asylum-seekers and refugees consisting in Portuguese language and computer classes. Due to a lack of funding, this has been stopped": ibid. at 249.

[1505] R. Macklin, "Stanhope defies Howard with English classes for asylum-seekers," *Canberra Times*, May 3, 2002, at A-5.

[1506] See, for example, EU Qualification Directive, at Art. 27(1).

[1507] F. Liebaut and J. Hughes, *Legal and Social Conditions for Asylum Seekers and Refugees in Selected European Countries* (1997). With the exception of minor children of refugees, access to advanced forms of education by persons seeking refugee status is simply not addressed by the European Union, leaving the matter to the discretion of state parties: EU Reception Directive, at Art. 10(1).

[1508] In Canada, for example, "[n]ot only has the Immigration Act failed to provide a clear way out of this ambiguity, but it has also left it to the whims and caprices of immigration officials. By what criteria are these officials supposed to grant permission when necessary? How do we ascertain whether such decisions are justifiable or not? How do we ensure that such a ruling, which has consequences for a refugee's future, will be made in the interest of a refugee?": E. Opoku-Dapaah, "Financial and Other Adjustment Assistance for Newcomers: Literature Review for the Center for Refugee Studies" (1994).

Economic, Social and Cultural Covenant, Art. 13

1. The States Parties to the present Covenant recognize the right of everyone to education. They agree that education shall be directed to the full development of the human personality and the sense of its dignity, and shall strengthen the respect for human rights and fundamental freedoms. They further agree that education shall enable all persons to participate effectively in a free society, promote understanding, tolerance and friendship among all nations and all racial, ethnic or religious groups, and further the activities of the United Nations for the maintenance of peace.

2. The States Parties to the present Covenant recognize that, with a view to achieving the full realization of this right:

(a) Primary education shall be compulsory and available free to all;

(b) Secondary education in its different forms, including technical and vocational secondary education, shall be made generally available and accessible to all by every appropriate means, and in particular by the progressive introduction of free education;

(c) Higher education shall be made equally accessible to all, on the basis of capacity, by every appropriate means, and in particular by the progressive introduction of free education;

(d) Fundamental education shall be encouraged or intensified as far as possible for those persons who have not received or completed the whole period of their primary education;

(e) The development of a system of schools at all levels shall be actively pursued, an adequate fellowship system shall be established, and the material conditions of teaching staff shall be continuously improved.

The Refugee Convention broke with precedent by making a clear commitment to provide at least the most basic forms of education to refugees (and their children[1509]) on terms of equality with nationals. While the predecessor

---

[1509] As Grahl-Madsen observes, "the present paragraph will on the whole only be meaningful if it is interpreted to give children of refugees the rights for which it provides, unless they have greater rights in their own right, i.e. as nationals of the country of residence": Grahl-Madsen, *Commentary*, at 86. Grahl-Madsen refers in this regard to Recommendation B of the Final Act of the Conference of Plenipotentiaries, in which the state representatives "[n]ot[ed] with satisfaction that, according to the official commentary of the Ad Hoc Committee on Statelessness and Related Problems, the rights granted to a refugee are extended to members of his family": ibid. See also, for example, the comment of the French representative in relation to Art. 22(2) that "[t]he fundamental purpose of article [22] was to prevent the *son* of a refugee from being forbidden to enter a given faculty [emphasis added]": Statement of Mr. Juvigny of France, UN Doc. E/AC.32/SR.37, Aug. 16, 1950, at 26.

treaties of 1933 and 1938 required only that educational rights be granted to refugees to the extent enjoyed by aliens in general,[1510] the drafters of the current Refugee Convention were firmly committed to the belief that public elementary education – meaning "elementary education over which the Contracting State concerned had direct control, whether financial or other"[1511] – should be made available to all refugees without qualification, and on terms of equality with citizens of the host state.

The Convention does not offer a clear definition of "elementary" education.[1512] One analysis of the Universal Declaration's right to "elementary" education suggests that "[t]here is no fixed border between elementary and fundamental education. Elementary education includes fundamental education such as literacy, arithmetic and basic orientation into society."[1513] On the other hand, the French representative to the Ad Hoc Committee seems to have equated the term with "primary education," as distinguished from "secondary and higher" education.[1514] Under this more formal and

---

[1510] The relevant provision in these earlier treaties stipulated that "[r]efugees shall enjoy in the schools, courses, faculties and universities of each of the Contracting Parties, treatment as favorable as other foreigners in general. They shall benefit in particular ... by the total or partial remission of fees and charges and the award of scholarships": United Nations, "Statelessness," at 58.

[1511] Statement of Mr. Hoare of the United Kingdom, UN Doc. A/CONF.2/SR.35, July 25, 1951, at 8. Mr. Hoare's position followed from the clarification of the American representative to the Ad Hoc Committee that "the words 'public education' ... were intended to apply not only to State-owned schools but also to private schools receiving Government subsidies": Statement of Mr. Henkin of the United States, UN Doc. E/AC.32/SR.23, Feb. 10, 1950, at 7. Indeed, while the general rule agreed to was that the headings for articles in the Convention should not have independent legal force, the President of the Conference of Plenipotentiaries noted that an exception should be made "in the case of article 22, 'Public education'": Statement of the President, Mr. Larsen of Denmark, UN Doc. A/CONF.2/SR.35, July 25, 1951, at 37.

[1512] See S. Blay and M. Tsamenyi, "Reservations and Declarations under the 1951 Convention and the 1967 Protocol relating to the Status of Refugees," (1990) 2(4) *International Journal of Refugee Law* 527 (Blay and Tsamenyi, "Reservations"), at 547: "The difficulty with Article 22(1) is that the Convention does not define what is 'elementary education.' Thus in the case of States where primary education stretches from primary school through to high school and therefore covers education before tertiary studies, Article 22(1) imposes a significant burden." While this critique may overstate the consequences of the definitional ambiguity, it is unclear whether, for example, "middle school," "junior high school" and other stages providing a transition between elementary and secondary education are encompassed by Art. 22(1). Perhaps most important for many refugees, it is not clear whether elementary education includes basic (adult) education in literacy and related matters. See text below, at pp. 596–597.

[1513] P. Arajäravi, "Article 26," in A. Eide et al. eds., *The Universal Declaration of Human Rights: A Commentary* 405 (1992) (Arajäravi, "Article 26"), at 408–409.

[1514] France, "Draft Convention," at 7. The French government appears to have seen no substantive divergence between its language and that proposed by the United Nations draft, and therefore withdrew its proposal: UN Doc. E/AC.32/SR.15, Jan. 27, 1950, at 9.

conservative interpretation, it is less clear that Art. 22(1) guarantees access to fundamental or basic education in all its forms (including, for example, adult education),[1515] but may be limited instead to participation in pre-secondary, grade school education.[1516]

There is, however, no mistaking the breadth of the beneficiary class.[1517] Rights under Art. 22(1) are granted to "refugees" – not, for example, only to refugees "lawfully in" or "lawfully staying in" a state party. Robinson thus logically concludes that "[i]t must be assumed that paragraph 1 is equally applicable to both resident and non-resident refugees, in view of the generally accepted nature of public elementary education."[1518] Indeed, the representative of the United Kingdom affirmed at the Conference of Plenipotentiaries that "[p]aragraph 1 was couched in very general terms, and the only limitation upon it was the title ('Public Education')."[1519]

Thus, the Greek failure to ensure access to elementary education by the children of asylum-seekers, as well as the failure of British authorities to ensure that local schools receiving refugees under dispersal policies in fact admit the children of asylum-seekers to primary education, were violations of Art. 22(1). More generally, the decision of the European Union to condition access to education by the children of refugee applicants on the lodging of a protection application, and even then to authorize a delay of as much as three months, are policies out of line with the requirements of Art. 22(1).[1520] Indeed, the European Union's decision to guarantee access to primary

---

[1515] The UN Committee on Economic, Social and Cultural Rights, for example, has taken the view that "[w]hile primary education is not synonymous with basic education, there is a close correspondence between the two. In this regard, the Committee endorses the position taken by UNICEF: 'Primary education is the most important component of basic education'": UN Committee on Economic, Social and Cultural Rights, "General Comment No. 13: The right to education" (1999), UN Doc. HRI/GEN/1/Rev.7, May 12, 2004, at 71, para. 9. The Committee on Economic, Social and Cultural Rights uses the terms "basic" and "fundamental" education interchangeably: ibid. at para. 22.

[1516] Grahl-Madsen suggests that "'[e]ducation other than elementary education' is normally understood as education beyond the grade school": Grahl-Madsen, *Commentary*, at 87.

[1517] This interpretation is borne out in state practice. In formulating their reservations to Art. 22(1) of the Convention, Egypt, Mozambique, Zambia, and Zimbabwe each noted their inability to assimilate refugees to their own citizens for purposes of access to public elementary education.

[1518] Robinson, *History*, at 123. See also Weis, *Travaux*, at 170: "The Article refers to 'refugees' without qualification such as 'lawfully stay[ing]'"; and Grahl-Madsen, *Commentary*, at 86: "Article 22 applies to 'refugees' – there is no condition as to residence, lawfulness of presence in territory, etc."

[1519] Statement of Mr. Hoare of the United Kingdom, UN Doc. A/CONF.2/SR.35, July 25, 1951, at 7.

[1520] Even under arguably difficult circumstances, there has been little tolerance of delay in ensuring that refugee children are granted access to education. For example, in its scrutiny of the report of Poland, the Committee on the Rights of the Child expressed education only under "similar conditions as nationals" – rather than, as the Refugee Convention requires, to guarantee "the same treatment as is accorded to nationals" – is also of doubtful validity. For the same reason, it is unlikely that the new British policy of denying the children of asylum applicants access to local schools, where the curriculum is almost surely more diverse,[1521] will pass muster under Art. 22(1). These policies stand in marked contrast to South Africa's recent reversal of its bar on the admission of the children of asylum-seekers to public primary schools, a decision taken in the face of social and economic circumstances significantly more challenging than those faced in any developed country. As that country's Supreme Court of Appeal pointedly observed, "[t]he freedom to study is . . . inherent in human dignity, for without it a person is deprived of the potential for human fulfilment."[1522]

In part, the decision of the drafters that all refugees should have immediate and unconditional access to the same forms of public elementary education as nationals was the product of an awareness that "schools are the most rapid and most effective instruments of assimilation."[1523] Equally important, however, it was recognized that access to elementary education "satisfies an urgent need (it is for this reason that most States have made it compulsory)."[1524] The Secretary-General's background study for the Convention thus explicitly referenced the conceptual breakthrough on this point that had been recently been achieved by Art. 26 of the Universal Declaration of Human Rights, which provides that "[e]veryone has the right to education.

its "concern[] that children waiting for their refugee claims to be processed do not have opportunities for education if they are housed in emergency blocks": UN Committee on the Rights of the Child, "Concluding Observations on the Report of Poland," UN Doc. CRC/C/121 (2002), 120, at para. 539.

[1521] For example, one fourteen-year-old Kurdish refugee girl in a British reception center reported, "I should be studying for my GCSEs now, but we are only taught English, history and art here for a few hours a day. We don't have the opportunity to learn every subject and if the teacher is away or on holiday we don't have any lessons. We are learning things we already know and because all . . . of us learn together, the standard is set at that of a seven-year-old. My ambition is to be a lawyer, but if I don't get my GCSEs I won't be able to do that": D. Taylor, "Education: Worlds apart: Is it right for asylum-seeking children to be taken out of school and taught in detention centers?," *Guardian*, Jan. 7, 2003, at 6, quoting Beriwan Ay.

[1522] *Minister of Home Affairs v. Watchenuka*, (2004) 1 All SA 21 (SA SCA, Nov. 28, 2003), per Nugent JA at para. 36. The same court was clear that while the right to education could not be universally guaranteed by any state to all who might wish to live in it, "where, for example, the person concerned is a child who is lawfully in this country to seek asylum (there might be other circumstances as well), I can see no justification for limiting that right so as to deprive him or her of the opportunity for human fulfilment at a critical period . . . A general prohibition that does not allow for study to be permitted in appropriate circumstances is in my view unlawful": ibid.

[1523] Secretary-General, "Memorandum," at 40.   [1524] Ibid.

Education shall be free, at least in the elementary and fundamental stages. Elementary education shall be compulsory."[1525] Importantly, the Universal Declaration's duty to provide elementary education to "everyone" is restricted neither to nationals, nor even to children:[1526]

> As "elementary education shall be compulsory," also adults who have not received elementary education must be educated ... The compulsion obliges society to attend to the existence of access to schools to see to it that either through the education offered by the society or otherwise the knowledge and skills provided by the elementary education are received.[1527]

It follows that under Art. 22(1), refugees and refugee children who have not completed their elementary education are entitled to receive it on terms of equality with the citizens of an asylum state, and without waiting for formal status determination procedures to be commenced or concluded.[1528] It is therefore likely that at least some of the adult asylum-seekers denied access to basic education programs pending verification of their status are not being granted their full rights under Art. 22(1). While limitations may be validly placed on access to the full range of adult education programs,[1529] any initiative which provides adult citizens with elementary school equivalency education (e.g. in basic literacy or numeracy) must be available to refugees, whether formally recognized as such or not, on terms of equality with nationals.

Importantly, the Refugee Convention's guarantee of access to elementary education is more comprehensive than the cognate right under Art. 13(2)(a) of the Covenant on Economic, Social and Cultural Rights. Under the Covenant, some flexibility in achieving free primary education for all is

---

[1525] Universal Declaration, at Art. 26(1).

[1526] This approach is consistent with the recent affirmation by the Committee on Economic, Social and Cultural Rights that the duty to provide education "to everyone" includes, for example, a duty towards the elderly. "Article 13, paragraph 1, of the Covenant recognizes the right of everyone to education. In the case of the elderly, this right must be approached from two different and complementary points of view: (a) the right of elderly persons to benefit from educational programmes; and (b) making the know-how and experience of elderly persons available to younger generations": UN Committee on Economic, Social and Cultural Rights, "General Comment No. 6: The economic, social and cultural rights of older persons" (1995), UN Doc. HRI/GEN/1/Rev.7, May 12, 2004, at 35, para. 36.

[1527] Arajärvi, "Article 26," at 408–409.

[1528] "Paragraph 1 was inspired by Art. 26(1) of the Universal Declaration of Human Rights which proclaimed that elementary education should be compulsory and free. It is obvious that in compulsory and free education refugees cannot be treated differently from nationals": Robinson, *History*, at 122.

[1529] See text below, at pp. 607–611.

available, at least to poorer states, as rights under that treaty need only be implemented progressively,[1530] albeit without discrimination.[1531] Even though primary education has been recognized as a "core" entitlement,[1532] meaning that any generalized failure to meet the standard is *prima facie*

[1530] "The term 'progressive realization' is often used to describe the intent of this phrase. The concept of progressive realization constitutes a recognition of the fact that full realization of all economic, social and cultural rights will generally not be able to be achieved in a short period of time. In this sense the obligation differs significantly from that contained in article 2 of the International Covenant on Civil and Political Rights which embodies an immediate obligation to respect and ensure all of the relevant rights. Nevertheless, the fact that realization over time, or in other words progressively, is foreseen under the Covenant should not be misinterpreted as depriving the obligation of all meaningful content. It is on the one hand a necessary flexibility device, reflecting the realities of the real world and the difficulties involved for any country in ensuring full realization of economic, social and cultural rights. On the other hand, the phrase must be read in the light of the overall objective, indeed the raison d'être, of the Covenant which is to establish clear obligations for States parties in respect of the full realization of the rights in question. It thus imposes an obligation to move as expeditiously and effectively as possible towards that goal. Moreover, any deliberately retrogressive measures in that regard would require the most careful consideration and would need to be fully justified by reference to the totality of the rights provided for in the Covenant and in the context of the full use of the maximum available resources": UN Committee on Economic, Social and Cultural Rights, "General Comment No. 3: The nature of states parties' obligations" (1990), UN Doc. HRI/GEN/1/Rev.7, May 12, 2004, at 15, para. 9.

[1531] The flexibility to implement the right to primary education is, however, significantly constrained by Art. 14 of the Covenant. This provision requires state parties which do not offer free and compulsory primary education upon accession to the Covenant to prepare and file – within two years – a "detailed plan of action for the progressive implementation, *within a reasonable number of years, to be fixed in the plan*, of the principle of compulsory education free of charge for all [emphasis added]": Economic, Social and Cultural Covenant, at Art. 14. The supervisory committee has therefore held that "the plan must specifically set out a series of targeted implementation dates for each stage of the progressive implementation of the plan. This underscores both the importance and the relative inflexibility of the obligation in question. Moreover, it needs to be stressed in this regard that the State party's other obligations, such as non-discrimination, are required to be implemented fully and immediately": UN Committee on Economic, Social and Cultural Rights, "General Comment No. 11: Plans of action for primary education" (1999), UN Doc. HRI/GEN/1/Rev.7, May 12, 2004, at 60, para. 10.

[1532] "In its General Comment 3, the Committee confirmed that States parties have 'a minimum core obligation to ensure the satisfaction of, at the very least, minimum essential levels' of each of the rights enunciated in the Covenant, including 'the most basic forms of education.' In the context of article 13, this core includes an obligation: to ensure the right of access to public educational institutions and programmes on a non-discriminatory basis; to ensure that education conforms to the objectives set out in article 13(1); [and] to provide primary education for all in accordance with article 13(2)(a)": UN Committee on Economic, Social and Cultural Rights, "General Comment No. 13: The right to education" (1999), UN Doc. HRI/GEN/1/Rev.7, May 12, 2004, at 71, para. 57.

evidence of a breach of the Covenant,[1533] states may nonetheless seek to justify their failure to provide universal primary education by reference to a true lack of resources.[1534] There is moreover a basis for argument that the Covenant's duty to provide primary education is an "economic right," thus allowing less developed countries legitimately to withhold it from non-citizens pursuant to Art. 2(3) of the Covenant.[1535] Even this flexibility would not, however, be a basis to justify the Thai government's reluctance to educate Khmer refugees, much less the refusal of the Turkish government

---

[1533] "Thus, for example, a State party in which any significant number of individuals is deprived of essential foodstuffs, of essential primary health care, of basic shelter and housing, or of the most basic forms of education is, prima facie, failing to discharge its obligations under the Covenant. If the Covenant were to be read in such a way as not to establish such a minimum core obligation, it would be largely deprived of its raison d'être": UN Committee on Economic, Social and Cultural Rights, "General Comment No. 3: The nature of states parties' obligations" (1990), UN Doc. HRI/GEN/1/Rev.7, May 12, 2004, at 15, para. 10. Thus, a recent report noted that "[w]hen discussing, for example, the report of Zaïre, the Committee made it clear that charging fees for primary education is contrary to article 13, paragraph 2(a). A State party cannot justify such a measure by referring to severe economic circumstances": "The right to education as a human right: an analysis of key aspects: Background paper submitted by Fons Coomans," UN Doc. E/C.12/1998/16, Sept. 29, 1998, at para. 5.

[1534] "In order for a State party to be able to attribute its failure to meet at least its minimum core obligations to a lack of available resources it must demonstrate that every effort has been made to use all resources that are at its disposition in an effort to satisfy, as a matter of priority, those minimum obligations. The Committee wishes to emphasize, however, that even where the available resources are demonstrably inadequate, the obligation remains for a State party to strive to ensure the widest possible enjoyment of the relevant rights under the prevailing circumstances. Moreover, the obligations to monitor the extent of the realization, or more especially of the non-realization, of economic, social and cultural rights, and to devise strategies and programmes for their promotion, are not in any way eliminated as a result of resource constraints": UN Committee on Economic, Social and Cultural Rights, "General Comment No. 3: The nature of states parties' obligations" (1990), UN Doc. HRI/GEN/1/Rev.7, May 12, 2004, at 15, paras. 10–11.

[1535] "Developing countries, with due regard to human rights and their national economy, may determine to what extent they would guarantee the economic rights recognized in the present Covenant to non-nationals": Economic, Social and Cultural Covenant, at Art. 2(3). On one reading, the right to education is *not* an "economic" right, and therefore not subject to derogation by less developed countries under Art. 2(3). "The right to education . . . is the most outstanding example of the 'cultural rights' category, although some scholars maintain that it is a social right": M. Nowak, "The Right to Education," in A. Eide et al. eds., *The Universal Declaration of Human Rights: A Commentary* 189 (1992), at 196. Yet the Committee on Economic, Social and Cultural Rights has recently muddied the waters by asserting that the right to education "has been variously classified as an economic right, a social right and a cultural right. It is all of these": UN Committee on Economic, Social and Cultural Rights, "General Comment No. 11: Plans of action for primary education" (1999), UN Doc. HRI/GEN/1/Rev.7, May 12, 2004, at 60, para. 2.

to allow non-governmental organizations to provide schooling to the children of Iraqi Kurdish refugees. Because these policies were intended to discourage refugee arrivals – and perhaps even indirectly to *refouler* refugees already present to their country of origin – they fail absolutely to meet the stringent criteria for justifiable non-compliance based purely on a genuine resource insufficiency.[1536]

But even if the fungibility of relevant obligations under the Economic Covenant were to be found to justify the withholding of primary education from non-citizens, the duty to provide elementary education under Art. 22 of the Refugee Convention admits of no such discretion. The right of refugees to access elementary education is rather a simple duty of result. While refugees are entitled to no greater access to elementary education than are nationals of the host country,[1537] they may not be denied access to education on the grounds that all nationals are entitled to be admitted before any refugees are provided for. Unless an express reservation of the kind entered by eight states – Egypt, Ethiopia, Malawi, Monaco, Mozambique, Papua New Guinea, Zambia, and Zimbabwe – is in place, the duty to assimilate refugees to nationals under Art. 22(1) means that the receiving country must share out whatever facilities and resources for elementary education it has on terms of equality between refugees and citizens. Thus, Malawi's reservation saved it from being in breach of Art. 22(1) when the number of primary school teachers made available for Mozambican refugees resulted in a 1:100 teacher–student ratio. But when Nigeria provided only meager educational facilities and supplies to Liberian refugees, or when Cambodia refused to provide any education facilities to urban refugee children, these states acted

---

[1536] The truly exceptional nature of a legitimate failure to provide primary education can be seen in the Committee on Economic, Social and Cultural Rights' approach to Art. 14 of the Covenant, under which states which do not already have universal and free primary education are "required to adopt a plan of action within two years ... This obligation is a continuing one and States parties to which the provision is relevant by virtue of the prevailing situation are not absolved from the obligation as a result of their past failure to act within the two-year limit. The plan must cover all of the actions which are necessary in order to secure each of the requisite component parts of the right and must be sufficiently detailed so as to ensure the comprehensive realization of the right ... A State party cannot escape the unequivocal obligation to adopt a plan of action on the grounds that the necessary resources are not available. If the obligation could be avoided in this way, there would be no justification for the unique requirement contained in article 14 which applies, almost by definition, to situations characterized by inadequate financial resources": UN Committee on Economic, Social and Cultural Rights, "General Comment No. 11: Plans of action for primary education" (1999), UN Doc. HRI/GEN/1/Rev.7, May 12, 2004, at 60, paras. 8–9.

[1537] Thus, for example, there would be no breach of Art. 22 in a state such as Mauritania, which is unable to provide even its own citizens with free elementary education. See C. Lindstrom, "Urban Refugees in Mauritania," (2003) 17 *Forced Migration Review* 46.

contrary to the Convention – even if their actions might have been saved by Art. 2(1) or 2(3) of the Economic Covenant. Under the theory of the Refugee Convention, refugee children are not to be made to pay the price for resource insufficiency in the host state. Whatever financial insufficiencies are present are instead to be addressed by burden-sharing among states.[1538]

For developed countries, the duties to provide elementary education under the Refugee Convention and the Economic Covenant are essentially indistinguishable,[1539] as wealthier states cannot easily meet the test for valid failure to satisfy such a core right.[1540] In interpreting Art. 13 of the Covenant, the Committee on Economic, Social and Cultural Rights has made clear that

[1538] See chapter 3.3.2 above. See also UNHCR Executive Committee Conclusion No. 47, "Refugee Children" (1987), at para. (o), available at www.unhcr.ch (accessed Nov. 20, 2004), in which the Executive Committee "[r]eaffirmed the fundamental right of refugee children to education and called upon all States, individually and collectively, to intensify their efforts, in cooperation with the High Commissioner, to ensure that all refugee children benefit from primary education of a satisfactory quality, that respects their cultural identity and is oriented towards an understanding of the country of asylum"; UNHCR Executive Committee Conclusion No. 59, "Refugee Children" (1989), at para. (f), available at www.unhcr.ch (accessed Nov. 20, 2004), in which the Executive Committee "encouraged UNHCR to strengthen its efforts in assisting host country governments to ensure the access of refugee children to education, *inter alia* through the involvement of new organizations and governmental and non-governmental donors, and where necessary through the incorporation of appropriate arrangements in its programmes of assistance"; and UNHCR Executive Committee Conclusion No. 74, "General Conclusion on International Protection" (1994), at para. (gg), available at www.unhcr.ch (accessed Nov. 20, 2004), in which the Executive Committee "[u]rges UNHCR, in cooperation with Governments, other United Nations and international and non-governmental organizations, especially UNICEF and ICRC, to continue its efforts to give special attention to the needs of refugee children, ensuring, in particular, that arrangements are made for their immediate and long-term care, including ... education." The problem, of course, is that developed countries have not always met this ethical responsibility in a complete or timely way. UNHCR has assembled advice on how best to meet this challenge in J. Crisp et al. eds., *Learning for a Future: Refugee Education in Developing Countries* (2001).

[1539] "[T]here are a number of other provisions in the International Covenant on Economic, Social and Cultural Rights, including article ... 13(2)(a) ... which would seem to be capable of immediate application by judicial and other organs in many national legal systems. Any suggestion that the provisions indicated are inherently non-self-executing would seem to be difficult to sustain": UN Committee on Economic, Social and Cultural Rights, "General Comment No. 3: The nature of states parties' obligations" (1990), UN Doc. HRI/GEN/1/Rev.7, May 12, 2004, at 15, para. 5.

[1540] See text above, at pp. 599–602. As Craven has written, "[a]lthough economic considerations will always play a part in any calculation relating to the implementation of the rights, the presumption is that developed States are under an obligation to implement the provisions of the Covenant immediately, the progressive nature of the obligations applying only to those States that lack sufficient resources to do so themselves": Craven, *ICESCR Commentary*, at 132–133.

compliance requires, *inter alia*, that primary education be completely free,[1541] and that there be no discrimination in accessing primary education, specifically on grounds of sex.[1542] The impermissibility of discrimination based on refugee (or "asylum-seeker") status is clear from Concluding Observations of the Committee on Economic, Social and Cultural Rights on the report of the United Kingdom:

> The Committee is deeply concerned by the information it has received concerning the treatment of Vietnamese asylum-seekers in Hong Kong. It is particularly concerned about the situation of the children and is alarmed by the statements made by the Government that these children have no entitlement to the enjoyment of the right to education or to other rights in

[1541] "The nature of this requirement is unequivocal. The right is expressly formulated so as to ensure the availability of primary education without charge to the child, parents or guardians. Fees imposed by the Government, the local authorities or the school, and other direct costs, constitute disincentives to the enjoyment of the right and may jeopardize its realization. They are also often highly regressive in effect. Their elimination is a matter which must be addressed by the required plan of action. Indirect costs, such as compulsory levies on parents (sometimes portrayed as being voluntary, when in fact they are not), or the obligation to wear a relatively expensive school uniform, can also fall into the same category": UN Committee on Economic, Social and Cultural Rights, "General Comment No. 11: Plans of action for primary education" (1999), UN Doc. HRI/GEN/1/Rev.7, May 12, 2004, at 60, para. 7.

[1542] "The element of compulsion serves to highlight the fact that neither parents, nor guardians, nor the State are entitled to treat as optional the decision as to whether the child should have access to primary education. Similarly, the prohibition of gender discrimination in access to education, required also by articles 2 and 3 of the Covenant, is further underlined by this requirement": ibid. at 60, para. 6. See also UN Committee on Economic, Social and Cultural Rights, "General Comment No. 13: The right to education" (1999), UN Doc. HRI/GEN/1/Rev.7, May 12, 2004, at 71, para. 5: "The Committee notes that since the General Assembly adopted the Covenant in 1966, other international instruments have further elaborated the objectives to which education should be directed. Accordingly, the Committee takes the view that States parties are required to ensure that education conforms to the aims and objectives identified in article 13(1), as interpreted in the light of the World Declaration on Education for All (Jomtien, Thailand, 1990) (art. 1), the Convention on the Rights of the Child (art. 29(1)), the Vienna Declaration and Program of Action (Part I, para. 33 and Part II, para. 80), and the Plan of Action for the United Nations Decade for Human Rights Education (para. 2). While all these texts closely correspond to article 13(1) of the Covenant, they also include elements which are not expressly provided for in article 13(1), such as specific references to gender equality and respect for the environment. These new elements are implicit in, and reflect a contemporary interpretation of, article 13(1)." The UNHCR Executive Committee has similarly expressed its concern that "all refugee women and girls [should be granted] effective and equitable access to basic services, including . . . education and skills training": UNHCR Executive Committee Conclusion No. 64, "Refugee Women and International Protection" (1990), at para. (a)(ix), available at www.unhcr.ch (accessed Nov. 20, 2004).

view of their status as "illegal immigrants." The Committee considers the situation inconsistent with obligations set forth in the Covenant.[1543]

Finally, and perhaps most interesting, the Committee has determined that ... the form and substance of education, including curricula and teaching methods, have to be acceptable (e.g. relevant, culturally appropriate and of good quality) to students ... [E]ducation has to be flexible so it can adapt to the needs of changing societies and communities and respond to the needs of students within their diverse social and cultural settings.[1544]

This interpretation raises interesting questions about whether the curriculum should, as UNHCR normally advocates, be presumptively oriented to preparation for repatriation, rather than designed to immerse refugees in the culture and society of the host country. Inflexibility in the opposite direction – for example, the UN's decision to implement a Western curriculum for Cambodian refugees in Thailand in order to prepare them for resettlement – may also be legally problematic.

[1543] "Concluding Observations of the Committee on Economic, Social and Cultural Rights: United Kingdom of Great Britain and Northern Ireland," UN Doc. E/C.12/1994/19, Dec. 21, 1994. This is in line with the general position of the Committee that non-citizen status is not usually to be understood as a legitimate ground for discrimination. "[T]he State party's other obligations, such as non-discrimination, are required to be implemented fully and immediately": UN Committee on Economic, Social and Cultural Rights, "General Comment No. 11: Plans of action for primary education" (1999), UN Doc. HRI/GEN/1/Rev.7, May 12, 2004, at 60, para. 10. The content of this duty of non-discrimination was subsequently elaborated to include access "to all, especially the most vulnerable groups, in law and fact, without discrimination on any of the prohibited grounds ... The prohibition against discrimination enshrined in article 2(2) of the Covenant ... encompasses all internationally prohibited grounds of discrimination. The Committee interprets articles 2(2) and 3 in the light of the UNESCO Convention against Discrimination in Education, the relevant provisions of the Convention on the Elimination of All Forms of Discrimination against Women, the International Convention on the Elimination of All Forms of Racial Discrimination, the Convention on the Rights of the Child and the ILO Indigenous and Tribal Peoples Convention, 1989 (Convention No. 169)": UN Committee on Economic, Social and Cultural Rights, "General Comment No. 13: The right to education" (1999), UN Doc. HRI/GEN/1/Rev.7, May 12, 2004, at 71, paras. 6(b)(i) and 31. The Committee on Economic, Social and Cultural Rights has moreover traditionally treated nationality as a prohibited ground of discrimination. "Certainly, in so far as the Covenant establishes the rights of 'everyone,' non-nationals would have a right to the enjoyment of the minimum content of those rights. Thus, in practice, the Committee will censure situations where aliens enjoy few rights and are the object of exploitation": Craven, *ICESCR Commentary*, at 174.

[1544] UN Committee on Economic, Social and Cultural Rights, "General Comment No. 13: The right to education" (1999), UN Doc. HRI/GEN/1/Rev.7, May 12, 2004, at 71, paras. 6(c)–(d).

Similar concerns arise where, as in the case of Burundians in Tanzania or Eritreans in Sudan, refugee parents wish education to focus on preparation for repatriation, but the host state prefers to orient teaching towards integration of the refugees. On balance, though, so long as the delivery of integration-oriented education proceeds from a genuine and reasonable belief that durable asylum is both needed and likely to be available in the host country, it is difficult to conceive of a basis upon which to criticize states such as Tanzania or Sudan for pursuing the integrative approach. If repatriation is unlikely, a focus on integration is very much adapted "to the changing societies and communities and respon[sive] to the needs of students within their diverse social and cultural settings."[1545] In line with Art. 13(3)–(4) of the Covenant,[1546] however, refugee parents should be allowed to establish alternative (repatriation-oriented) primary schools for their children if they wish, so long as minimum qualitative standards are met and the host state is not expected to fund those schools.

Much the same logic applies to the question arising in many Northern states of whether there is a duty to provide education in the native language of refugee children. While often a sensible policy, there is no consensus that governments have a duty to fund minority language education.[1547] While there would arguably be such a duty if repatriation were probable,[1548] the very nature of refugee status (in which there can be no such certainty, given the duty to protect refugees for as long as there is a real chance of persecution

---

[1545] Ibid. at paras. 6(c)–(d).

[1546] "The States Parties to the present Covenant undertake to have respect for the liberty of parents and, when applicable, legal guardians to choose for their children schools, other than those established by the public authorities, which conform to such minimum educational standards as may be laid down or approved by the State ... No part of this article shall be construed so as to interfere with the liberty of individuals and bodies to establish and direct educational institutions, subject always to the observance of the principles set forth in paragraph 1 of this article and to the requirement that the education given in such institutions shall conform to such minimum standards as may be laid down by the State": Economic, Social and Cultural Covenant, at Art. 13(3)–(4).

[1547] "[A] State must respect the freedom of individuals to teach, for instance, a minority language in schools established and directed by members of that minority. This does not imply, however, that a State must allow the use of this language as the only medium of instruction; this would be dependent on the educational policy of the State. As a minimum, however, States must not frustrate the right of members of national, ethnic or linguistic minorities to be taught in their mother tongue at institutions outside the official system of public education. However, there is no State obligation to fund these institutions": "The right to education as a human right: an analysis of key aspects: Background paper submitted by Fons Coomans," UN Doc. E/C.12/1998/16, Sept. 29, 1998, at para. 15.

[1548] See text above, at p. 605, n. 1544.

in the home state) argues against this being a universal position. Thus, the failure of states such as Belgium and France to provide instruction in the refugees' mother tongue is not clearly in violation of the Covenant so long as refugee parents are not prevented, if they wish, from establishing institutions to provide education in that language.

While there was ready agreement that refugees should have unconditional access to elementary education, the drafters of the Refugee Convention debated at some length the extent to which refugees should be entitled to rights in regard to secondary and other non-elementary forms of education. The initial proposal on this issue assumed that refugees were already entitled to enter higher institutions of learning, but needed to be assimilated to the citizens of most-favored states in order to have access to scholarship and other funds to pay their tuition and fees.[1549] The drafters were made aware of "the difficulties which might arise in connection with the award of scholarships to refugees. It seemed that most scholarships were administered by a foundation and granted according to special provisions."[1550] Thus, the UN's strategy coming into the drafting process was predicated on the de jure accessibility of non-elementary education to refugees, and sought simply to overcome the practical impediments to higher education by enfranchising refugees within the ranks of privileged non-citizens.

Sadly, most governments took a distinctly less liberal view on advanced forms of education than they had on elementary education. While the German and Yugoslav delegations proposed sweeping amendments that would have granted refugees full national treatment in regard to advanced education,[1551] the majority of representatives were determined to limit the

---

[1549] "The [non-elementary] grades of education are generally speaking open to foreigners; refugees will therefore receive the benefit of this circumstance if they are placed on the same footing as other foreigners. [But] [s]ince refugees are in a precarious economic position and the Government of their country of origin takes no interest in them, it would be desirable to do more than merely accord them the ordinary rights enjoyed by foreigners; otherwise in practice although secondary and higher education is open to them, they will be unable, for want of money, to take advantage of it. For this reason it is proposed to grant refugees the most favourable treatment accorded to nationals of a foreign country": Secretary-General, "Memorandum," at 40.

[1550] Statement of the Chairman, Mr. Chance of Canada, UN Doc. E/AC.32/SR.15, Jan. 27, 1950, at 9.

[1551] Comparable proposals were tabled by Yugoslavia (UN Doc. A/CONF.2/31) and Germany (UN Doc. A/CONF.2/45). "[T]he purpose of his amendment ... was to grant refugees facilities in higher as well as in elementary education. Such generosity would not only benefit refugees, but also the countries in which they resided. Indeed, there was a kind of moral obligation on public authority to help young people who, through no fault of their own, had been placed in unfavourable conditions. Moreover, although assimilation was difficult for the elderly, everything should be done to make it scope of entitlement. First, as in regard to elementary education, it was made clear that only *public* forms of post-elementary education are regulated by Art. 22(2).[1552] Second, while it was agreed that the Refugee Convention should specifically regulate "access to studies,"[1553] it was acknowledged that post-elementary educational institutions would retain significant autonomy to make merit-based evaluations of a refugee applicant's qualifications for admission,[1554] including the assessment of foreign credentials on the usual basis.[1555] And third, the governments were emphatic that the right of access to post-elementary education cannot be invoked as an indirect means to

possible and easy for young people to share fully in the life of the country of their adoption. They should consequently be allowed access to all educational opportunities in their new homeland": Statement of Mr. von Trutzschler of the Federal Republic of Germany, UN Doc. A/CONF.2/SR.10, July 6, 1951, at 11.

[1552] "In the United Kingdom, higher education was in the hands of schools and universities, which were for the most part private institutions with their own regulations which could not be overruled by a Convention, particularly where fees were concerned. If it was understood that the provisions of paragraph 2 applied to public education only, his delegation would see no objection to accepting that text": Statement of Sir Leslie Brass of the United Kingdom, UN Doc. E/AC.32/SR.15, Jan. 27, 1950, at 9. See also the remarks of the representatives of Canada, France, Israel, and Belgium, ibid. at 9–10. The French delegate thus concluded "that there could not be any doubt concerning the interpretation of paragraph 2: it referred solely to public education and State scholarships. Private institutions could obviously not be compelled against their will to admit refugees or to grant them reduced rates": Statement of Mr. Rain of France, ibid. at 10. At the Conference of Plenipotentiaries, the British representative insisted that "[w]hat the Conference must do was to bind states to give equality of treatment to refugees in the institutions over which the State had control": Statement of Mr. Hoare of the United Kingdom, UN Doc. A/CONF.2/SR.10, July 6, 1951, at 14.

[1553] The Belgian representative to the Ad Hoc Committee "suggested that the words 'access to education' be inserted ... since access to education was a matter of considerable importance": Statement of Mr. Herment of Belgium, UN Doc. E/AC.32/SR.38, Aug. 17, 1950, at 9.

[1554] This was a matter of particular concern to the Belgian representative, who was anxious to safeguard "the distinction [in Belgium] that study abroad qualified the candidate for admission to schools of a certain grade only if such study was recognized by an examining board as being equivalent to Belgian elementary or secondary education": Statement of Mr. Herment of Belgium, UN Doc. E/AC.32/SR.37, Aug. 16, 1950, at 25. In response, the French representative opined that "the instances cited by the Belgian representative were of minor importance and an explicit reservation could not in any way reflect badly upon the country making it": Statement of Mr. Juvigny of France, ibid. at 26. But in the end, it was agreed that so long as the assessment "was one not of nationality but rather of qualifications," it did not infringe the Convention: Statement of the Chairman, Mr. Larsen of Denmark, ibid. at 25.

[1555] Statement of Mr. van Heuven Goedhart of UNHCR, UN Doc. A/CONF.2/SR.35, July 25, 1951, at 6. The General Comment on the cognate right in the Economic, Social and Cultural Covenant allows for screening "by reference to all their relevant expertise and experience": UN Committee on Economic, Social and Cultural Rights, "General Comment No. 13: The right to education" (1999), UN Doc. HRI/GEN/1/Rev.7, May 12, 2004, at 71, para. 19.

insist on admission to a trade or profession for which the education acquired is the usual prerequisite. As the French representative explained,

> [T]he two questions should not be linked together, since the practice of a profession was dealt with in other articles. A scientific standpoint had to be adopted in the present case, whereas the question of exercising a profession should be decided on a non-scientific basis. The fundamental purpose of article [22(2)] was to prevent the son of a refugee from being forbidden to enter a given faculty. For example, a student who became a refugee after completing two years of medical studies should be allowed to continue those studies.[1556]

Concluding the discussion on this point, the Chairman of the Ad Hoc Committee observed that

> it would seem to him an unhappy solution if the State of residence were to refuse a refugee the right to obtain an education only on the ground that he would be unable as an alien to practice his profession. He might wish to get an education merely for his private scientific enjoyment, or he might wish to emigrate to another country and there to practice his profession. It was also possible that a person studying some science was not eligible for citizenship at the time when he was a student, for instance because he was not able to support himself; but he might nevertheless be interested in getting an education and a degree, hoping to be naturalized afterwards, whereupon he would be able to use the degree. So, in any event, the question of education and degrees covered by article [22(2)] should not be combined with the exercise of liberal professions dealt with in article [19].[1557]

But by far the most significant decision taken was to reject the duty to assimilate refugees to most-favored foreigners, and instead to grant them post-elementary education rights only to the extent these are enjoyed by "aliens generally." Because Art. 22(2) regulates "the remission of fees and charges and the award of scholarships," governments attending the Conference of Plenipotentiaries resurrected concerns which had been over-come in the Ad Hoc Committee[1558] that the provision would require the

---

[1556] Statement of Mr. Juvigny of France, UN Doc. E/AC.32/SR.37, Aug. 16, 1950, at 26. Thus, Grahl-Madsen concludes that "[o]nce a child of a refugee has been given the benefit of Article 22(2), he should continue to [enjoy that right] until he has finished the school to which he has been admitted, and until his diploma etc. has been superseded by another one of higher standing": Grahl-Madsen, *Commentary*, at 86.

[1557] Statement of the Chairman, Mr. Larsen of Denmark, UN Doc. E/AC.32/SR.37, Aug. 16, 1950, at 27–28. See also Statement of Mr. Henkin of the United States, ibid. at 28: "[I]t was better to allow an opportunity for study to a refugee, even if afterwards he could not practise a liberal profession, rather than prevent him from obtaining an education at all."

[1558] In response to arguments for redrafting to accommodate states anxious to preserve the right to award special bilateral and other scholarships, the United States insisted that "he did not think that preferential treatment had been excluded from the most favourable assimilation of refugees to students for whom special arrangements had been made under bilateral funding agreements.[1559] For example, the United Kingdom had made special provision to grant scholarships to Polish citizens,[1560] while Venezuela had particular scholarship arrangements with the "Bolivar countries, with which it was linked by ties of history and consanguinity."[1561] The general sense was that states should be free to make such special arrangements without fear that they were thereby indirectly assuming significant obligations to fund the education of refugees. On the initiative of the British government,[1562] the required standard of treatment was therefore reduced to "treatment as favorable as possible, and, in any event, not less favorable than that accorded to aliens generally in the same circumstances."[1563] Moreover, while there is nothing in the drafting history to suggest an intention by states to apply this lower standard of treatment to

treatment clause and would not like that interpretation adopted. If the Benelux countries, for example, were not prepared to accord their special treatment to refugees, he would prefer it to be stated in the form of a reservation": Statement of Mr. Henkin of the United States, ibid. at 24. See also Statement of Mr. Weis of the IRO, ibid.; and the Chairman, Mr. Larsen of Denmark, ibid. This led to the adoption of the more generous standard, under which states agreed to "accord to refugees the most favorable treatment accorded to nationals of a foreign country with respect to education other than elementary education and, in particular, as regards access to studies, the remission of fees and charges and the award of scholarships": "Report of the Ad Hoc Committee on Refugees and Stateless Persons, Second Session," UN Doc. E/1850, Aug. 25, 1950 (Ad Hoc Committee, "Second Session Report"), at 21.

[1559] "[I]n France there was a distinction between scholarships awarded under bilateral treaties, and those by which refugees could benefit ... [A]lthough the French Government was prepared to give refugees all possible assistance in that direction, it would not go beyond the measures already taken": Statement of Mr. Rochefort of France, UN Doc. A/CONF/2/SR.10, July 6, 1951, at 14.

[1560] Statement of Sir Leslie Brass of the United Kingdom, UN Doc. E/AC.32/SR.37, Aug. 16, 1950, at 23; repeated in the Statement of Mr. Hoare of the United Kingdom, UN Doc. A/CONF.2/SR.10, July 6, 1951, at 14.

[1561] Statement of Mr. Perez Perozo of Venezuela, UN Doc. E/AC.32/SR.37, Aug. 16, 1950, at 23.

[1562] "In the United Kingdom Government's view the legal effect of paragraph 2 would be to impose upon it the obligation of treating all refugees as favourably as it had done one particular group. The countries linked by the Brussels Treaty were also endeavouring to extend reciprocal arrangements between them to a large number of fields. It might be that schemes for the exchange of students and for scholarships would be developed. There again, such special arrangements would be inapplicable to refugees ... [H]e could not help but feel that it would be preferable to redraft the text so as to make it generally acceptable rather than to adopt it as it stood and oblige a number of governments to enter reservations": Statement of Mr. Hoare of the United Kingdom, UN Doc. A/CONF.2/SR.10, July 6, 1951, at 14–15.

[1563] Indeed, it was only when reminded by the UNHCR of the way in which this level of attachment had ordinarily been framed elsewhere in the Convention that the reference to "treatment as favourable as possible" was included in Art. 22(2): Statement of Mr. van Heuven Goedhart of UNHCR, UN Doc. A/CONF.2/SR.35, July 25, 1951, at 5.

the other matters regulated by Art. 22(2) – specifically, access to post-elementary education and the recognition of academic credentials[1564] – the text as adopted nonetheless makes clear that on these questions also, the duty of states is simply to treat refugees at least as well as they do aliens in general.

Under the Refugee Convention, then, there is no basis for contesting Tanzania's requirement that refugees be admitted to post-elementary education only as part of the overall 2 percent of places assigned to non-citizens; or Zambia's policy that refugees apply for the same costly student permit required of other aliens; or Canada's insistence that persons seeking recognition of refugee status seek the same exercise of particularized discretion to attend college or university that is required of all other non-citizens. On the other hand, Australia's policy of denying access to English-language education to refugees granted a "temporary protection" visa, but not to other refugees (or to resident non-citizens in general), puts it in breach of the duty to grant *all* persons who are in fact Convention refugees at least the same access to education (other than elementary education) as is enjoyed by aliens generally.

Because of the various limitations inherent in Art. 22 of the Refugee Convention,[1565] refugees seeking to benefit from other than elementary education will in many cases do well to invoke Art. 13(2) of the Economic Covenant. Under clauses (b) and (c), "secondary" and "higher" education must be made "generally available and accessible *to all* [emphasis added]." While poorer states may rely upon the Economic Covenant's general duty of progressive implementation to justify an overall insufficiency of secondary education opportunities or the failure progressively to make such education free of charge,[1566] there must be no discrimination against non-citizens in

---

[1564] The French representative, for example, had made clear that "[t]he reservations made by his delegation concerned the award of scholarships to aliens, and in that connection it should be noted that in France all aliens had access to all educational establishments, except for certain large schools which prepared candidates for posts from which aliens were excluded ... although they might, in certain conditions, be admitted with alien status": Statement of Mr. Rochefort of France, UN Doc. A/CONF.2/SR.10, July 6, 1951, at 17.

[1565] The weakness of the Refugee Convention on this point is clear from the framing of UNHCR Executive Committee Conclusion No. 37, "Central American Refugees and the Cartagena Declaration" (1985), at para. (p), available at www.unhcr.ch (accessed Nov. 20, 2004), in which the Executive Committee "*[r]ecognized the need* of refugee children to pursue further levels of education and *recommended* that the High Commissioner *consider* the provision of post-primary education within the general Program of assistance [emphasis added]."

[1566] Note, however, that "[t]he realization of the right to education over time, that is 'progressively,' should not be interpreted as depriving States parties' obligations of all meaningful content. Progressive realization means that States parties have a specific and granting access to secondary or higher forms of education.[1567] Because education at these levels, in contrast to primary education, need not be immediately free of charge,[1568] it is plausible that under the UN's "reasonableness" approach to the assessment of discrimination[1569] an equitable system of cost-recovery from non-citizens who have yet to contribute to the public funding base for advanced education might be found to be justifiable.[1570] It is, however, less clear that the European Union's decision to grant refugees post-secondary education opportunities only to the same extent provided to "third country nationals legally resident" would also be found to be reasonable, since in contrast to other non-citizens refugees cannot freely and safely avail themselves of such opportunities in their country of nationality.

The formulation of post-elementary education rights in the Economic Covenant is also valuable to refugees in several additional ways. First, it is clear that technical and vocational education is within the scope of guaranteed "secondary education."[1571] Second, whereas the Refugee Convention authorizes merit-based assessments to govern access to all post-elementary

---

continuing obligation 'to move as expeditiously and effectively as possible' towards the full realization of article 13": UN Committee on Economic, Social and Cultural Rights, "General Comment No. 13: The right to education" (1999), UN Doc. HRI/GEN/1/Rev.7, May 12, 2004, at 71, para. 44.

[1567] "[E]ducational institutions and programmes have to be accessible to everyone, without discrimination, within the jurisdiction of the State party": UN Committee on Economic, Social and Cultural Rights, "General Comment No. 13: The right to education" (1999), UN Doc. HRI/GEN/1/Rev.7, May 12, 2004, at 71, para. 6(b). See text above, at p. 600. If, however, the interpretation of the right to education as an "economic" right is accepted, less developed countries are entitled under Art. 2(3) of the Covenant to withhold any such protection from non-citizens. See text above, at. p. 601.

[1568] In regard to secondary and higher education, the relevant obligation is simply to increase accessibility "by the *progressive* introduction of free education [emphasis added]." While this duty does not allow for inaction (see text above, at pp. 600–601), neither does it set an immediate obligation of result.

[1569] See chapter 2.5.5 above, at pp. 128–145.

[1570] If, however, tuition or similar educational fees are deductible expenses or otherwise wholly or partially rebated to citizens of the asylum state, refugees must receive the same benefit by virtue of Art. 29 of the Refugee Convention: see chapter 4.5.2 above.

[1571] "Technical and vocational education (TVE) forms part of both the right to education and the right to work (art. 6(2)). Article 13(2)(b) presents TVE as part of secondary education, reflecting the particular importance of TVE at this level of education": UN Committee on Economic, Social and Cultural Rights, "General Comment No. 13: The right to education" (1999), UN Doc. HRI/GEN/1/Rev.7, May 12, 2004, at 71, para. 15. This is not to say that such education is clearly excluded from the requirements of the Refugee Convention, simply that it is not explicit there. In Grahl-Madsen's view, "[t]he phrase ["education other than elementary education" in the Refugee Convention] comprises general higher education as well as vocational training": Grahl-Madsen, *Commentary*, at 87.

education, Art. 13(2)(b) of the Covenant requires that access to secondary education – as distinguished from higher (e.g. college and university) education[1572] – be subject to no such evaluations. The Committee on Economic, Social and Cultural Rights has made clear that "[t]he phrase 'generally available' signifies ... that secondary education is not dependent on a student's apparent capacity or ability."[1573] Third, the reference in Art. 13(2)(d) of the Covenant to the importance of "[f]undamental education ... for ... persons who have not received or completed the whole period of their primary education" is, while not formally binding,[1574] a clear signal that adult education in literacy, numeracy, and social orientation education is a matter of international concern.

Finally, it is particularly interesting that Art. 13(2)(e) goes some distance to meeting the original concern of the drafters of the Refugee Convention, namely that legal access to education would be meaningless to most refugees if not provided with the financial wherewithal to pay their tuition and fees. Under this clause, governments commit themselves ("shall") to establish "an adequate fellowship system" applicable at all levels of education – primary, secondary, higher, and fundamental. Of critical importance to refugees, "[t]he requirement that 'an adequate fellowship system shall be established' should be read with the Covenant's non-discrimination and equality provisions; the fellowship system should enhance equality of educational access for individuals from disadvantaged groups."[1575] To the extent that refugees are forced to rely on an inferior scholarship system in order to access any level of education, they may therefore invoke Art. 13(2)(e) to contest their exclusion.[1576] At least in developed countries not entitled to withhold economic rights from aliens in reliance upon Art. 2(3) of the Covenant, any attempt to limit refugees to educational funding sources established by UNHCR or other agencies would require justification in relation to norms of non-discrimination law.

[1572] Access to higher education is governed by Art. 13(2)(c), which does allow restrictions to access "on the basis of capacity."

[1573] UN Committee on Economic, Social and Cultural Rights, "General Comment No. 13: The right to education" (1999), UN Doc. HRI/GEN/1/Rev.7, May 12, 2004, at 71, para. 13.

[1574] In contrast to access to secondary and higher education – which "shall be made equally accessible to all" – fundamental education "shall be encouraged or intensified as far as possible."

[1575] UN Committee on Economic, Social and Cultural Rights, "General Comment No. 13: The right to education" (1999), UN Doc. HRI/GEN/1/Rev.7, May 12, 2004, at 71, para. 26.

[1576] Thus, for example, the Committee on Economic, Social and Cultural Rights critiqued the Canadian practice of excluding refugees not yet in receipt of permanent resident status from eligibility for post-secondary education loan programs: "Concluding Observations: Canada," UN Doc. E/C.12/1/Add.31 (1998), at paras. 37, 39, 49.

4.9 Documentation of identity and status

Whatever rights are held by refugees may be of little value if their refugee status cannot be proved. The critical importance of documentary proof of identity was described in an information note submitted to UNHCR's Executive Committee in 1984:

> For a refugee, the lack of identity documents may be far more than a source of inconvenience. In almost all countries an alien must be able to prove not only his identity, but also that his presence in the country is lawful. In some countries aliens without appropriate documentation are subject to detention and sometimes even to summary expulsion. Such measures are particularly serious for a refugee, for whom they could involve the risk of being returned to his country of origin. Even where the consequences of being without documentation are less drastic, the refugee, in order to benefit from treatment in accordance with internationally accepted standards, needs to be able to establish vis-à-vis government officials not only his identity, but also his refugee character. Due to circumstances in which they are sometimes forced to leave their home country, refugees are perhaps more likely than other aliens to find themselves without identity documents. Moreover, while other aliens can turn to the authorities of their country of origin for help in obtaining documents, refugees do not have this option.[1577]

While most refugees do have access to state-issued documentation that confirms both their personal identity and legal status,[1578] there are three major exceptions.

First, a few host states refuse to distinguish between the legal status of refugees and that of other non-citizens. Burmese refugees in Thailand, for example, have not been considered "refugees" at all, but rather "displaced persons."[1579] Because their presence is unauthorized, they have been given no

---

[1577] UNHCR, "Identity Documents for Refugees," UN Doc. EC/SCP/33, July 20, 1984 (UNHCR, "Identity Documents"), at paras. 2–3.

[1578] Ibid. at para. 12. Progress has moreover been achieved on this front in many states. "In Kenya, for instance, the government initiated a major exercise to issue 100,000 adult refugees with laminated photographic identity cards. In Ecuador, a shared government–UNHCR database paved the way for personal documents for all Colombian asylum-seekers and refugees. In other operations, such as those in Côte d'Ivoire, Georgia, Guinea, and Yemen, UNHCR reached agreements with the government that photographic identity cards should be issued not only to all adult men, but also to women, thereby enhancing protection of refugee women in particular ... In another positive development, UNHCR began in late 2002 issuing asylum-seekers documentation with the cooperation of Egyptian authorities, helping prevent detention for illegal stay": UNHCR, "Note on International Protection," UN Doc. A/AC.96/975, July 2, 2003, at para. 5.

[1579] Thailand "has never recognized as refugees the Burmese ethnic minority refugees living near the Burmese border": US Committee for Refugees, *World Refugee Survey 1997* (1997), at 119.

identity documentation of any kind. Only a small minority of the Burmese refugees – primarily former students active in Burma's democracy movement – were recognized as "persons of concern" by UNHCR, and issued UNHCR identity documents. The government's insistence in 1989 that UNHCR cease providing documentation of status even to this group resulted in arrests, detention, and instances of forced repatriation by Thai authorities.[1580]

A second and more general concern is the unwillingness of authorities in many states to provide identity documentation until and unless an asylum-seeker's refugee status has been formally verified. Indeed, a majority of states which responded to a UNHCR survey on implementation of the Refugee Convention indicated that the provision of documentation to refugees is dependent on a positive determination of refugee status.[1581] In Russia, for example, refugees from non-CIS states are routinely denied identity documents. The Russian government refuses to accept their applications for asylum,[1582] and local authorities deny them the residence permits needed to legalize their presence.[1583] While the UNHCR does register such asylum-seekers, Russian authorities do not always respect this form of

---

[1580] "With no written document, Burmese have no way of identifying themselves as 'persons of concern to UNHCR' to Thai police. 'Persons of concern' facing arrest, trial, detention and deportation often have difficulty contacting UNHCR, leaving the refugee in an even more vulnerable position vis-à-vis the police": Asia Watch, "Abuses Against Burmese Refugees in Thailand" (1992), at 6. "Thailand has allowed UNHCR to assess the refugee claims of some Burmese, but it regards UNHCR-recognized refugees as illegal immigrants": US Committee for Refugees, *World Refugee Survey 2003* (2003), at 134. In the result, "[d]ue to the absence of official government recognition of their situation, the Shan refugees in the Shan State–Thailand border continue to languish in desperate conditions . . . Their protection needs are largely unmet": (2002) 122 *JRS Dispatches* (Nov. 22, 2002).

[1581] UNHCR, "Information Note on Implementation of the 1951 Convention and the 1967 Protocol relating to the Status of Refugees," UN Doc. EC/SCP/66, July 22, 1991, at para. 38.

[1582] "Many asylum-seekers . . . are left in legal limbo for years, unable to even register their asylum claim and obtain documents identifying them as asylum-seekers": Amnesty International, "Russian Federation: Failure to Protect Asylum Seekers" (1997). "By law, registration of applicants should take no more than five days. The [government], however, continued to place asylum-seekers on a pre-registration waiting list without issuing them documents confirming their applicant status. The waiting period, on average, lasted 18 months to two years, leaving asylum-seekers vulnerable to police harassment": US Committee for Refugees, *World Refugee Survey 2003* (2003), at 214.

[1583] "In some cities, official refugee status is required for a residence permit, while at the same time refugee status cannot be obtained without a resident permit": US Committee for Refugees, *World Refugee Survey 1997* (1997), at 206. Other obstacles to obtaining a residence permit include exorbitant fees, which in Moscow equate to 500 times the legal minimum wage. Residence registration systems have remained in use despite the Constitutional Court ruling of April 1996 which struck down the notorious *propiska* system: ibid.

identification.[1584] In the result, refugees are often treated as illegal immigrants, and subjected to extortion, harassment, arbitrary detention, physical abuse, and the threat of *refoulement*.[1585] They are "denied most rights, including the right to work, to receive public assistance and non-emergency health care, or even to register marriages and births. Many schools do not accept the children of far-abroad asylum-seekers because of their illegal status."[1586] South Africa, in contrast, issues a formal "asylum-seeker permit" to all refugees arriving in its territory. There have, however, been complaints that these permits are not in fact issued within the two weeks required by law, during which time refugees are "at risk of being apprehended, detained or even deported."[1587]

Even where some form of documentation is provided to asylum-seekers, it may not be generally recognized within the community at large. In Argentina, for example, the certificate of "precarious presence" issued to asylum-seekers pending assessment of the refugee claim is not considered to be valid by most employers, often resulting in exploitative employment relationships.[1588] Similarly, Canada's practice during the late 1990s of not processing Somali and Afghan refugees for permanent residency until five years after arrival in

---

[1584] Amnesty International quotes Lt.-Gen. Ivan Rakmanin of the border guards of Kaliningrad district as saying that "[UNHCR] identity cards given out to these people are not considered as documents by our law enforcement officials": Amnesty International, "Russian Federation: Failure to Protect Asylum Seekers" (1997). "Because most far-abroad asylum-seekers, including those registered with UNHCR, never receive refugee status, Russian authorities consider them to be illegal migrants": US Committee for Refugees, *World Refugee Survey 2003* (2003), at 216. See also R. Redmond, "Old Problem in a New World," (1993) 94 *Refugees* 28, at 30.

[1585] "[R]andom identity checks on the streets of cities in Russia are common and asylum-seekers without the proper residence registration papers often report being threatened with detention or even *refoulement* to their country of origin": Amnesty International, "Russian Federation: Failure to Protect Asylum Seekers" (1997).

[1586] US Committee for Refugees, *World Refugee Survey 2003* (2003), at 216.

[1587] *The Sowetan* (Johannesburg), May 11, 2000. This is confirmed by Jesuit Refugee Service advocacy and information officer in Johannesburg, Paulin Mbecke, who reported a "protest . . . against the blatant hostility shown by Home Affairs officials towards asylum-seekers and their failure to provide documentation for new arrivals. Among their grievances, asylum-seekers underlined the arbitrary use of power by officials and the failure to treat immigrants in a humane and dignified manner. The response from the Home Affairs Braamfontein officer in charge, Mr. Nkululeko, was that due to a shortage of staff and equipment, the office is unable to be more helpful": (2000) 83 *JRS Dispatches* (Dec. 2, 2000). Importantly, however, the Durban High Court intervened to order the Minister of Immigration and his Director-General to issue identity documents to two Rwandan refugees, failing which they would be held in contempt of court: "Court gives Buthelezi ultimatum over Rwandan students' documents," *Business Day*, May 28, 2003; "Buthelezi narrowly escapes jail sentences," *The Mercury*, June 5, 2003.

[1588] S. Fraidenraij, *International Academy of Comparative Law National Report for Argentina* (1994), at 9.

Canada – in contrast to its usual practice of moving immediately to assimilate recognized refugees – meant that these refugees, who lacked the permanent resident documentation normally possessed by refugees, were less likely to receive good job offers from employers.[1589] In Egypt, not even government officials have always respected refugee identification cards. During a police campaign of mass arrests of foreigners in early 2003, "[i]ndividuals carrying blue identification cards issued by the UNHCR were arrested alongside undocumented foreigners. Refugees explained to Human Rights Watch that the police repeatedly told them the UNHCR cards were 'useless.'"[1590]

A third set of problems arises in those states which do not ordinarily engage in the formal assessment of refugee status, but which simply acquiesce in the presence of refugees on their territory. The system which prevailed in Pakistan until 1992 required Afghan refugees who wished to procure an identity document ("Shanakti pass") to provide a recommendation from one of seven registered Afghan political parties. This process resulted in the denial of documentation to many non-partisan Afghan refugees in Pakistan.[1591] The failure of authorities in Côte d'Ivoire to provide identity documents to its Liberian refugee population prevented them from traveling outside of designated reception areas, and "[e]ven within the reception area, refugees [could] face harassment or arrest by the police for not carrying

---

[1589] "In 1996, Immigration Minister Lucienne Robillard decreed that Somali and Afghani refugees must wait for five years after coming to Canada before they can be considered for permanent status. They need time, she said, 'to demonstrate respect for the laws of Canada and for us to detect those who may be guilty of crimes against humanity or acts of terrorism.' Most Somali refugees don't have any kind of identification or travel documents. 'Many Somalis have never had such documents,' says one man angrily. 'And there is no government in Somalia, not for years. So who would issue documents?' Without permanent status, says Abdirahman Aden Sabriye, a community development worker ... 'you can't get a decent job. No employer is willing to give you training. You are stuck. You become helpless. There is depression, stress, mental problems'": B. Taylor, "The school where pupils look forward to Mondays," *Toronto Star*, Mar. 7, 1999. The "Undocumented Convention Refugees in Canada Class," by virtue of which this practice was implemented, was abolished with the entry into force of the *Immigration and Refugee Protection Act 2002*. "UCRCC, by the Department's own figures and evaluation, has been a colossal failure, and at the practical level it created new problems. Since the introduction of the UCRCC there was a reported escalation in the rate at which Somali and Afghan documents, including passports, were being summarily rejected without proper consideration": H. Mohamed and H. Kits, "Protecting the Unprotected: Submission to the House of Commons Standing Committee on Citizenship and Immigration," Feb. 14, 2002, at 7.

[1590] Human Rights Watch, "Egypt: Mass Arrests of Foreigners, African Refugees Targeted in Cairo," Feb. 10, 2003.

[1591] Letter from Mr. Ray Fell of UNHCR Islamabad to Ms. Nausheen Ahmad of Shirkat Gah, Aug. 18, 1994, cited in N. Ahmad, *International Academy of Comparative Law National Report for Pakistan* (1994).

proper identification."[1592] Rwandan refugee leaders voiced their concern that Tanzania would not issue them with generic refugee status identification cards, fearing that the purpose of the alternative "refugee labor card" issued only to refugees employed by UNHCR and other agencies was "to identify [an] elite group in Tanzania for the Government of Kigali ... This kind of action could constitute [an indirect] way to fulfill a plan of forced repatriation of the Rwandan refugees."[1593] Nepal has failed to register a whole generation of Tibetan refugees born in Nepal (but not granted Nepali citizenship),[1594] and declined to register refugees from Bhutan for more than a decade. It agreed to issue identity certificates only when the prospect of repatriation was in sight, and when it had secured the agreement of Bhutan to assist in the verification process.[1595] And in late 2000, Zambia implemented a computerized system to issue refugee identity cards in cooperation with UNHCR, but its purpose is strictly to identify the minority of refugees authorized to reside in urban areas.[1596]

> **Refugee Convention, Art. 27   Identity papers**
> The Contracting States shall issue identity papers to any refugee in their territory who does not possess a valid travel document.

Under the early generations of refugee treaties, refugees were issued a single identity document – originally known as a "Nansen passport" in honor of the first High Commissioner for Refugees, later simply as a "travel

---

[1592] Lawyers' Committee for Human Rights, *African Exodus: Refugee Crisis, Human Rights and the 1969 OAU Convention* (1995), at 50. "[M]ost refugees in Côte d'Ivoire lacked identity documents, leaving the refugee population vulnerable to harassment and arbitrary detention by police. A joint program by the government and UNHCR to issue identity cards began in 1999, but little progress was made during 2000 and 2001 because many police regarded the document as invalid. Refugees living in the capital, Abidjan, continued to receive new identity cards, however": US Committee for Refugees, *World Refugee Survey 2002* (2002), at 68.

[1593] Letter from Faustin Nkomati and two colleagues to the UNHCR Ngara Office, Jan. 30, 1996. In a letter of Jan. 6, 1996 written to the NGO Forum in Ngara, UNHCR had defended the labor card system, noting the importance of its secondary purpose – namely, to identify persons excluded from refugee status because they were reasonably believed to have contributed to the genocide.

[1594] "In 1963, Tibetan refugees who were 18 years of age or older were registered and issued identification cards ... Since then, however, there have not been any further registrations, and a whole generation of Tibetans born in Nepal – but not Nepali citizens – remains unregistered": US Committee for Refugees, "Tibetan Refugees: Still at Risk" (1990), at 12.

[1595] (2001) 89 *JRS Dispatches* (Mar. 22, 2001).

[1596] *Pana* (Lusaka), Nov. 10, 2000. Ironically, this system which facilitates denial of the right of refugees to internal freedom of movement (see chapter 4.2.4) was celebrated by the UNHCR Representative in Lusaka, who noted that "Zambia is among the first countries in the world where the system of registering refugees will be fully operational": ibid.

document" – which served both to facilitate international travel by refugees, and also to identify its holder as a refugee authorized to reside in the asylum country.[1597] For reasons elaborated below,[1598] the drafters of the 1951 Refugee Convention elected to provide themselves with some discretion to refuse to issue refugees with international travel documents on national security or public order grounds, as well as to standardize the format of those documents. A separate draft article was therefore proposed to stipulate the duty to provide refugees with a more general form of identification, essentially for use within the asylum country.[1599]

The working drafts of what became Art. 27 assumed that the general identity document would, as under the earlier treaties, only be issued to "refugees authorized to reside" in the state party, in consequence of which the duty under Art. 27 would ordinarily be met by issuance of a residence card to the refugee.[1600] This proposal did not survive the scrutiny of the Ad Hoc Committee, however, which insisted that not all refugees would necessarily be granted a right of residence in the state party[1601] (and indeed, no binding duty to grant residence was made part of the Convention[1602]). Yet, as the French representative observed, there was nonetheless a need to document the status of persons

> whose presence was merely tolerated on a temporary basis following an illegal crossing of the frontier. The latter only enjoyed the right of asylum

---

[1597] UNHCR, "Identity Documents," at para. 4.   [1598] See chapter 6.6 below.

[1599] "The 'identity papers' with which Art. 27 deals are for internal use, as contrasted with 'travel documents' to be used for journeys abroad. It is a paper certifying the identity of a refugee": Robinson, *History*, at 133.

[1600] "The High Contracting Parties undertake to issue identity papers (residence card, identity card, etc.) to refugees (and stateless persons) authorized to reside in their territory": Secretary-General, "Memorandum," at 41. The commentary noted that "[i]t is the practice to issue identity papers, under various designations, which serve both as identity cards and residence permits. This practice, which meets an essential requirement, should be generalized": ibid. The relevant provision in the French working draft for the Convention (draft Art. 16) was identical: France, "Draft Convention," at 7.

[1601] "Mr. Rain [of France] urged that the Committee could not decide on a text for the question of residence permits until a satisfactory formula on the right of residence had been adopted": Statement of Mr. Rain of France, UN Doc. E/AC.32/SR.15, Jan. 27, 1950, at 13. See also Statement of Mr. Henkin of the United States, ibid. at 14, who went so far as to propose "that in order to avoid any misinterpretation the first part of the article should be drafted to read: 'Without prejudice to the right of the High Contracting Parties to regulate the right of entry for permanent residence in the country.'" The same view prevailed at the Conference of Plenipotentiaries, where the Dutch representative insisted that the official record confirm that "[t]he High Commissioner had made it clear that the duty imposed on States by article [27] in no way impaired their right to control the admission and sojourn of refugees": Statement of Baron van Boetzelaer of the Netherlands, UN Doc. A/CONF.2/SR.11, July 9, 1951, at 17.

[1602] See chapter 7.4 below.

until such time as their position had been regularized by the issuance of a temporary and later of a permanent residence permit. While ... such permits would in practice serve them primarily as identity cards, there was a secondary aspect of the problem, since a variety of documents could serve as proof of identity. The residence permit was thus only secondarily an identity card; *it primarily constituted permission to reside in the reception country* [emphasis added].[1603]

As this makes clear, the purpose of what became Art. 27 was not to document identity in some abstract sense, but rather to document – albeit on a provisional basis – the refugee status of the person concerned.[1604] Indeed, the revised formula which emerged from a Working Group of the Committee seems explicitly to have been based on the French delegate's approach:

> The Contracting States shall issue identity papers to any refugee in their territory who does not possess a valid passport issued pursuant to Article [28, i.e. a Convention Travel Document].[1605]

This formula, which was adopted by the Ad Hoc Committee without comment,[1606] is noteworthy in two respects.

First, in contrast both to the working drafts and to all prior refugee treaties, the identity document in question is not to be withheld until a refugee is "lawfully staying" in the asylum country.[1607] The drafting history leaves no room for doubt that this formulation was intended to enfranchise asylum-seekers immediately upon their arrival.[1608] Indeed, at the Second Session of

---

[1603] Statement of Mr. Rain of France, UN Doc. E/AC.32/SR.15, Jan. 27, 1950, at 13.

[1604] The Canadian representative, for example, initially expressed some discomfort at Art. 27's duty to issue a certificate "guaranteeing re-admission to its territory": Statement of Mr. Winter of Canada, UN Doc. E/AC.32/SR.38, Aug. 17, 1950, at 23. Canada agreed at the Conference of Plenipotentiaries that it would meet its Art. 27 obligations by issuance of an "immigrant's record of landing," reflecting the then-prevailing practice of assimilating refugees immediately upon arrival: Statement of Mr. Chance of Canada, UN Doc. A/CONF.2/SR.11, July 9, 1951, at 17.

[1605] "Decisions of the Working Group Taken on 9 February 1950," UN Doc. E/AC.32/L.32, Feb. 9, 1950, at 10.

[1606] UN Doc. E/AC.32/SR.23, Feb. 10, 1950, at 8.

[1607] This view is confirmed by state practice in Malta, the only country which has entered a reservation to Art. 27. While identity cards are not issued to refugees immediately upon arrival, "[a]ll refugees and asylum-seekers who are in Malta for a period over six months have the possibility of obtaining an official Maltese I.D. card": C. Buttigieg, *International Academy of Comparative Law National Report for Malta* (1994), at 8.

[1608] See Robinson, *History*, at 134: "Contrary to other articles, Art. 27 deals with 'any refugee in their territory,' thus indicating verbally that neither residence nor even lawful presence is required. All that is necessary is that the refugee be physically in the territory of the given state"; Weis, *Travaux*, at 213: "The provision applies to all refugees physically present in the territory, whether legally or illegally there"; and Grahl-Madsen, *Commentary*, at 115: "The identity papers envisaged in Article 27 shall not only be the Ad Hoc Committee, the Belgian representative questioned the intent behind the amendment of Art. 27 to require the issuance of an identity certificate to "any refugee in their territory." He inquired

> whether the authors of the draft Convention would have any objection to the insertion of the word "lawfully" before the words "in their territory." He failed to see how any contracting party could agree to issue identity papers to refugees who were unlawfully in its territory or who were there on an essentially temporary basis. He assumed that the text referred to refugees who had been granted permission to reside in a country.[1609]

The response was swift and unequivocal. The American representative observed that "the Committee had agreed to extend the provisions of article [27] to all refugees, so that a refugee illegally present in any country, though still subject to expulsion, would be free from the extra hardships of a person in possession of no papers at all."[1610] Mr. Weis of the IRO insisted that "the intention of the Committee had been that every refugee should be provided with some sort of document certifying his identity, without prejudice to the right of the Government of any country in which he might be illegally present to expel him."[1611] And most forcefully of all, the French representative

> thought that was undoubtedly what the members of the Committee had in mind. When an alien whose position was irregular entered a country and the authorities of that country decided not to expel him immediately, he would be given a provisional document which he could produce if, say, he were stopped in the street; such a document would be purely provisional and its owner's stated identity might even prove to be false, but he would not be entirely an outcast and he would hold a provisional document enabling him to be identified.[1612]

The Belgian delegate accepted these explanations.[1613] The scope of the beneficiary class for Art. 27 was only once more alluded to during the drafting debates, resulting in a confirmation that the duty to issue identity papers "could not be refused to anyone, whatever his status or the legality of his presence in a given territory ... [T]he identity papers ... were not a legal document, but merely a temporary certificate of identity, in no way prejudging the future position of a refugee, or even his actual status as a refugee."[1614]

---

available to refugees lawfully in the territory, but also to those whose entry was illegal or whose position has not been regularized, however temporary their stay."
[1609] Statement of Mr. Herment of Belgium, UN Doc. E/AC.32.SR.38, Aug. 17, 1950, at 23.
[1610] Statement of Mr. Henkin of the United States, ibid. at 24.
[1611] Statement of Mr. Weis of the IRO, ibid. at 24.
[1612] Statement of Mr. Juvigny of France, ibid. at 24.
[1613] Statement of Mr. Herment of Belgium, ibid. at 24.
[1614] Statement of Mr. Juvigny of France, UN Doc. E/AC.32/SR.42, Aug. 24, 1950, at 23.

Thus, Russia's refusal to provide documents to non-CIS asylum-seekers is clearly in breach of Art. 27. On the other hand, the South African system, which mandates the delivery of provisional documentation to asylum-seekers within two weeks of arrival, seems a reasonable accommodation of the Art. 27 duty to administrative realities. It is critical, however, that even during such a brief delay, there be a means in place to meet refugees' most basic needs, and in particular to protect them from *refoulement*.

Art. 27's goal of ensuring that all refugees arriving in a state party receive provisional proof of their refugee status is affirmed by the second important change adopted by the Ad Hoc Committee. Rather than positing a general duty to issue identity documents, the text as adopted required states to provide such papers only to refugees not in possession of a Convention Travel Document (CTD) ("to any refugee in their territory who does not possess a valid passport issued pursuant to Article [28]").[1615] A CTD, issued under Art. 28, need only be issued to refugees "lawfully staying in their territory,"[1616] meaning in most cases refugees whose status has been verified and who have been granted the right to remain in the asylum country.[1617] Once in possession of the more authoritative CTD, the need for provisional documentation of refugee status would logically disappear – the holder of the CTD could use the document for travel, but it is also more than sufficient to substantiate the individual's status as a refugee for all domestic purposes, in line with pre-Second World War practice.[1618]

At the Conference of Plenipotentiaries, however, a drafting change was made that, if construed literally, has the potential to obscure the true purpose of Art. 27. On the motion of the delegate from France, the phrase "issued pursuant to article 28" was deleted as "superfluous in view of paragraph 2 of article 28."[1619] The latter paragraph requires that travel documents issued to refugees under earlier refugee treaties "be recognized and treated by the Contracting States in the same way as if they had been issued pursuant to this article."[1620] The evident concern of the French representative was to avoid the need to provide identity documents to the large number of refugees

---

[1615] See Art. 27 as adopted by the Ad Hoc Committee, text above, at p. 620, n. 1605.
[1616] See generally chapter 6.6 below.   [1617] See chapter 3.1.4 above, at pp. 189–190.
[1618] See text above, at pp. 618–619. There is, however, one circumstance in which this analysis may not hold. Because a state has the discretion (but not the duty) to provide even persons whose refugee status has not been formally verified with a CTD (see chapter 6.6 below, at pp. 847–851.), some persons in possession of a CTD may not, in fact, be recognized by the granting state as Convention refugees. In practical terms, however, it is unlikely that a state would both grant an individual a refugee travel document and simultaneously treat him or her as a non-refugee.
[1619] Statement of Mr. Rochefort of France, UN Doc. A/CONF.2/SR.35, July 25, 1951, at 9.
[1620] Refugee Convention, at Art. 28(2).

who already held a travel document certifying their refugee status, albeit not one issued under the 1951 Refugee Convention.

But the text as adopted has been considered by many commentators to have much more drastic consequences. Specifically, because Art. 27 now requires identity documents to be issued only to refugees "who do not possess a valid travel document," it is sometimes argued that the only duty is to provide documentation of *identity*, not of *identity as a refugee*.[1621] Thus, it is said that a refugee who still possesses the passport of his or her country of origin, or who holds a visa from third state, need not be provided with identity documentation under Art. 27.[1622] Yet it is manifestly clear that documents of this kind – in contrast to either the CTD or equivalent refugee travel documents issued under earlier treaties intended by the drafters to limit the Art. 27 duty – in no way serve the purpose of Art. 27, namely to establish the refugee's provisional entitlement to be treated as a refugee.

The linguistic confusion is such that it is suggested even by UNHCR that "[i]dentity papers which show only the name, the date and place of birth, and the current address of the refugee would satisfy the literal requirements of Article 27."[1623] The agency clearly understands that documents of this kind have little value as a tool of international protection,[1624] and appreciates the vital importance of the real purpose of Art. 27 – namely, documenting on an

---

[1621] See Grahl-Madsen, *Commentary*, at 113: "The identity papers to which Article 27 refers ... are simply papers which show the identity of the refugee[ ], without conferring on him any rights at all."

[1622] "The provision applies only if the refugee does not possess a valid travel document, whether issued by the State in which he or she finds themself or by another State; it may even be their national passport": Weis, *Travaux*, at 213. "The expression ['travel documents'] – as used in Article 27 – probably also applies to aliens' passports, if duly visaed. It is important to note that Article 27 does not require that the travel document must be issued by the State in whose territory the refugee is present, and upon whom the duty to issue an identity paper would devolve if the refugee possessed no valid travel document. In other words, the State in whose territory a refugee finds himself is not obliged to issue identity papers if the refugee possesses a valid travel document, issued by the authorities of that State or of a foreign State": Grahl-Madsen, *Commentary*, at 116.

[1623] UNHCR, "Identity Documents," at para. 9.

[1624] "For purposes of international protection, however, it is often essential that such identity papers also indicate the holder's refugee status. Proof of refugees status may be of vital importance, for example, in situations where refugees are caught up in police operations directed against aliens whose presence in the country is considered unlawful": ibid. More generally, the Executive Committee has "[a]cknowledge[d] the importance of registration as a tool of protection, including protection against *refoulement*, protection against forcible recruitment, protection of access to basic rights, family reunification of refugees and identification of those in need of special assistance, and as a means to enable the quantification and assessment of needs and to implement the appropriate durable solutions": UNHCR Executive Committee Conclusion No. 91, "Conclusion on Registration of Refugees and Asylum-Seekers" (2001), at para. (a), available at www.unhcr.ch (accessed Nov. 20, 2004).

interim basis the holder's status as an asylum-seeker.[1625] Yet because of its failure to interpret the text in its context, UNHCR feels compelled to state its case as a recommendation,[1626] rather than an assertion of legal entitlement under Art. 27. In its Conclusion No. 35, the Executive Committee

> *Recommended* that asylum applications whose applications cannot be decided without delay be provided with provisional documentation sufficient to ensure that they are protected against expulsion or *refoulement* until a decision has been taken by the competent authorities with regard to their application.[1627]

Similarly, in Conclusion No. 91, the Executive Committee merely

> *[r]equests* States, which have not yet done so, to take all necessary measures to register and document refugees and asylum-seekers on their territory as quickly as possible upon their arrival, bearing in mind the resources available, and where appropriate to seek the support and co-operation of UNHCR.[1628]

In truth, however, these statements largely reflect the essence of the legal *duty* of states pursuant to Art. 27. There was absolutely no discussion at the Conference of Plenipotentiaries to suggest any desire to depart from the purposive interpretation adopted by the Ad Hoc Committee; to the contrary, the French representative's suggestion to amend the language to its present form was explicitly predicated solely on concern to take account of "travel documents issued by countries which, though non-Contracting States,

---

[1625] "During the period preceding the determination of refugee status, asylum applicants clearly have the same need for appropriate identity documents as recognized refugees": UNHCR, "Identity Documents," at para. 18.

[1626] "The risk of expulsion or *refoulement* may indeed be greater for the asylum applicant – whose status has not yet been regularized and whose entitlement to refugee status has yet to be determined – than for the recognized refugee. It follows therefore that the asylum-seeker *should* be provided with documentation adequate to ensure that his provisional right to protection against *refoulement* will be respected and that he will be treated in accordance with his status as a person who may in fact be a refugee [emphasis added]": ibid.

[1627] UNHCR Executive Committee Conclusion No. 35, "Identity Documents for Refugees" (1984), at para. (d), available at www.unhcr.ch (accessed Nov. 20, 2004).

[1628] UNHCR Executive Committee Conclusion No. 91, "Conclusion on Registration of Refugees and Asylum-Seekers" (2001), at para. (g), available at www.unhcr.ch (accessed Nov. 20, 2004). See also Executive Committee of the High Commissioner's Programme, "Agenda for Protection," UN Doc. EC/52/SC/CRP.9/Rev.1 (June 26, 2002), at Part III, Goal 1, Point 11: "In keeping with the Conclusion on Registration of Refugees and Asylum-Seekers (No. 91, 2001), and bearing in mind confidentiality requirements regarding the use of data, States are to register and document female and male refugees and asylum-seekers on their territory on an individual basis as quickly as possible upon their arrival, in a manner which contributes to improving their security, their access to essential services, and their freedom of movement."

nevertheless wished to accept refugees outside the framework of the Convention."[1629] In other words, provisional refugee identification would not be required by persons in possession of a travel document issued to refugees (under the Convention or otherwise), since a person in possession of a refugee travel document already had sufficient proof of his status as a refugee. But asylum-seekers – whether present legally or illegally, whether their claims were verified or not – are entitled to certification of their provisional right to be treated as refugees. This duty is equally applicable to states which do not routinely assess refugee status, with the result that the failures of Côte d'Ivoire to document Liberian refugees and of Nepal to provide identity certificates to the Tibetans and Bhutanese are inconsistent with the requirements of Art. 27.

There is no particular form which the identity document must take.[1630] Thus, Rwanda could validly choose to issue a "refugee labor card" rather than an identity certificate as such. Whatever its title, the document must simply enable refugees to avail themselves of the rights to which they are entitled. As such, there is no reason to see the Canadian decision to delay issuance of permanent resident documentation to Somali and Afghan refugees as a violation of Art. 27 (so long as some alternative proof of their refugee status was provided), since there is no obligation under the Refugee Convention to grant permanent entry to refugees.[1631] Nor is it impermissible for Argentina to issue asylum-seekers with a "certificate of precarious presence" if the only objection taken is that employers are reluctant to accept that document for employment purposes; refugees only acquire the right to engage in employment once they are "lawfully staying" in the host country.[1632]

Zambia's system, in contrast, is not in compliance with Art. 27, since it illegitimately purports to document only a minority of refugees as entitled to internal freedom of movement contrary to Art. 26 of the Convention.[1633] Egypt's delegation of authority to UNHCR to issue refugee identification seems similarly problematic, in that not even its own police officers appear to have understood the legal authority of the documentation issued. Even more fundamentally, both the Thai refusal to recognize the Burmese as refugees, and the former Pakistani practice of allowing expatriate Afghan political parties to decide who should be granted refugee status identification,

---

[1629] Statement of Mr. Rochefort of France, UN Doc. A/CONF.2/SR.35, July 25, 1951, at 9.

[1630] "Identity cards did not necessarily mean identity cards like those issued in European countries; they might simply consist of a document showing the identity of the refugee": Statement of Mr. Herment of Belgium, UN Doc. A/CONF.2/SR.11, July 9, 1951, at 17. The Canadian government, for example, indicated that it planned simply to use its ordinary immigrant landing documents for this purpose: Statement of Mr. Chance of Canada, ibid.

[1631] See chapter 7.4 below.   [1632] See chapter 6.1.1 below.

[1633] See chapter 5.2 below.

were in violation of the Convention. States may not avoid their obligation to document refugees by willful blindness, or by purporting to delegate that role to agencies not under the effective control of a state with accountability under international law.

In sum, any refugee in the territory of a state party and not in possession of a refugee travel document is, pursuant to Art. 27, entitled to receive a provisional refugee identity certificate to use until his or her claim to refugee status is finally refused, or until it is accepted and eligibility for a refugee travel document established. This is consistent with the basic approach of the Convention under which a state party has essentially two choices when an asylum-seeker arrives on its territory. It may exercise its right under Art. 32 to expel an asylum-seeker not yet "lawfully in" its territory,[1634] if this can be done consistent with its immediate duty to avoid the prospect of *refoulement*, direct or indirect, to the refugee's country of origin;[1635] or it may provide the asylum-seeker with provisional documentation of refugee status, which entitles that person to be treated as a refugee pending the completion of any procedures established to verify claims to refugee status. Precisely because some refugee rights inhere by virtue of either simple physical presence,[1636] or lawful presence (e.g. while undergoing status determination or in receipt of temporary protection) yet before refugee status is formally acknowledged,[1637] Art. 27 is the vital link between theory and reality. If a person legally entitled to the benefit of refugee rights could not document his or her entitlement to same, the Refugee Convention would be of little practical value. The right to receive provisional refugee identification set out in Art. 27 is therefore the essential key to enabling refugees to in fact benefit from the protections which states have determined should be their due.

4.10 Judicial and administrative assistance

As important as it is to insist that persons claiming to be refugees are both identified and provisionally treated as entitled to the protection of the Convention, the practical reality is that refugees will often be unable to enforce their rights without assistance from state or international authorities.

[1634] See chapters 3.1.3 above and 5.1 below.

[1635] See chapter 4.1 above.

[1636] These include the rights elaborated in this chapter: protection from *refoulement*; freedom from arbitrary detention or penalization for illegal entry; physical security rights; access to the necessities of life; basic property rights; the right to family unity; freedom of thought, conscience, and religion; access to basic primary education; and the right to administrative assistance from host state authorities.

[1637] These rights are elaborated in chapter 5 below, and include protection from expulsion; internal freedom of movement; and the right to engage in self-employment.

As described above,[1638] the early generations of refugee accords were predicated on a recognition that "the characteristic and essential feature of the problem was that persons classed as 'refugees' have no regular nationality and are therefore deprived of the normal protection accorded to the regular citizens of a State."[1639] Like all non-citizens, refugees were essentially at the mercy of the institutions of a foreign state. In contrast to other foreigners, however, refugees clearly could not seek the traditional remedy of diplomatic protection from their country of nationality.

The various High Commissioners appointed by the League of Nations were therefore authorized to name the equivalent of consular representatives to state parties.[1640] These representatives not only issued a variety of forms of documentation required by refugees to effectuate their rights, but also "[s]upport[ed] the various requests submitted by refugees to the authorities of their place of residence."[1641] While the formal system of internationally rendered diplomatic protection for refugees came to an end with the onset of the Second World War, "in a number of countries certain quasi-consular functions ... continued to be rendered to refugees and displaced persons, first by representatives of the PCIRO, and subsequently by the IRO. If such persons came within the mandate of IRO, the representatives of IRO, where necessary, lent them assistance in a variety of forms, ranging from material aid to intervention with the authorities of the country of residence or with the Consuls of the countries of immigration."[1642]

In contrast, the Statute of the United Nations High Commissioner for Refugees, drafted contemporaneously with the Refugee Convention,[1643] does not expressly mandate the organization to provide refugees with consular

---

[1638] See chapter 2.3 above.

[1639] "Report by the Secretary-General on the Future Organisation of Refugee Work," LN Doc.1930.XIII.2 (1930), at 3.

[1640] Weis writes that "the question of administrative assistance to refugees arose with the establishment of the Soviet Union. As long as the Soviet Union was not recognized, the Czarist consuls continued to render administrative assistance to Russian nationals and refugees. With the recognition of the Soviet Union, these consuls lost their official character. They continued, however, to render assistance to refugees and it was then required that the documents and certifications issued by them should be countersigned by the local representative of the League of Nations High Commissioner for Refugees. The Arrangement concerning the Legal Status of Russian and Armenian Refugees of 30 June 1928 recommended that the League of Nations High Commissioner for Refugees [should], by appointing representatives in the greatest possible number of countries, render the services enumerated in the Arrangement, in so far as such services [did] not come within the exclusive competence of the national authorities": Weis, *Travaux*, at 203–204.

[1641] United Nations, "Statelessness," at 44.   [1642] Ibid. at 46.

[1643] The UNHCR Statute was adopted by the General Assembly as Res. 428(V), Dec. 14, 1950 (UNHCR Statute).

assistance of this kind. More generally, the Statute does not grant UNHCR any clear power to champion the enforcement of refugee rights. The agency is authorized to engage in the "promotion" of "the admission of refugees";[1644] it may moreover seek authority from specific states to engage in consular-type work under its mandate to "promot[e] through special agreements with Governments the execution of any measures calculated to improve the situation of refugees ... [and to] assist[ ] governmental and private efforts to promote ... assimilation within new national communities."[1645] At most, the agency may assert its general responsibility to "supervise the application" of the Refugee Convention.[1646] But unlike its institutional predecessors, UNHCR is not specifically tasked to act as agent for the enforcement of refugee rights.[1647] It was rather the expectation of the drafters of the Refugee Convention that primary responsibility to assist refugees to enforce their rights should fall to the state parties themselves:

> [E]ven if the Government of the country of asylum grants the refugee a status which ensures him treatment equivalent to or better than that enjoyed by foreigners, it does not follow that on that account alone he will be allowed to enjoy the rights granted to him. If the refugee is actually to enjoy these rights, he must obtain the assistance of an authority which will perform for him the services performed by national authorities in the case of persons with a nationality. In the absence of an international authority, the High Contracting Parties must appoint a national authority which will furnish its assistance to refugees and deliver the documents they require.[1648]

In practice, refugees have often looked to their host country's courts to secure respect for their rights. Even in states where the courts have no clear role in refugee-status determination, judges have at times intervened to ensure the protection of refugees. In one recent Japanese decision, for example, the court initially ordered the government to pay ¥9,500,000 in damages to a Burmese refugee in respect of what it determined to have been his unlawful

---

[1644] UNHCR Statute, at Art. 8(d).   [1645] Ibid. at Art. 8(b)–(c).

[1646] Ibid. at Art. 8(a), and Refugee Convention, Art. 35. This authority was not, however, intended to displace the primary role of states in oversight of the Refugee Convention. See J. Hathaway, "Who Should Watch Over Refugee Law?," (2002) 14 *Forced Migration Review* 23, and more generally, chapter 2.5.2 above and Epilogue below, at pp. 992–998.

[1647] Thus, for example, when Swaziland threatened the (unlawful) deportation of refugees because they had exercised their international legal entitlement to internal freedom of movement, UNHCR could do little more than request "an extended grace period" within which to arrange alternative protection for the refugees: "Unhappy refugees to stay a little longer," *Times of Swaziland*, Aug. 2, 2002.

[1648] Secretary-General, "Memorandum," at 43–44.

detention subsequent to a legally erroneous rejection of his protection claim.[1649] While the decision was successfully appealed on the basis that the required standard of wrongfulness for the award of damages against the state had not been proved,[1650] the underlying finding that the detention was in breach of the refugee's rights was not disturbed. Even in India, which has not acceded to either the Refugee Convention or Protocol, judges have shown remarkable creativity in crafting remedies for refugees which effectively vindicate Convention rights.[1651]

But in other contexts, the host government may effectively deny refugees access to its legal system. Verdirame reports an extreme case, in which the Kenyan government, acting through UNHCR and its implementing partner, simply left a refugee community to administer justice for itself, effectively ignoring its responsibility to ensure that the rights of refugees on its territory were respected:

> In theory, Kenyan law applies to Kakuma Camp. In practice, this seldom happens. In Kakuma, refugees have been allowed to establish their own "court" system which is funded by [UNHCR's implementing partner], Lutheran World Federation . . .
>
> Punishment meted out by these courts in camps . . . includes flogging. During a visit in July 1997, the obvious human rights implications of such decisions were brought to the attention of agency staff. This concern was dismissed with the observation that "this is their culture" . . .
>
> The population of Kakuma Camp, although living on the territory of Kenya, is administered by humanitarian organizations, independently of the government, outside its judicial system, with no checks on powers and, in effect, without legal remedies against abuses.[1652]

The same result can accrue by virtue of a legislative deficit. In Uganda, Art. 22 of the Constitution formally guarantees full access by all to that country's courts. But the Control of Alien Refugees Act allows authorities to order refugees to be relocated in their absolute discretion, with no provision for refugees to contest such a decision before the courts. Nor may refugees

---

[1649] The award included ¥8,000,000 in respect of emotional distress suffered during the period of unlawful detention, and a further ¥1,500,000 to cover his legal fees: *Z v. Japan*, 1819 HANREI JIHO 24 (Tokyo DC, Apr. 9, 2003).

[1650] Specifically, it was determined that while the detention was itself unlawful, a stricter standard of illegality is required before damages may be awarded in accordance with the terms of the State Redress Act: *Japan v. Z*, No. Heisei 16 Gho Ko 131 (Tokyo HC, Jan. 14, 2004), appeal denied No. Heisei 16 Gyo Tsu 106, Heisei 16 Gyo Hi 115 (Jap. SC, May 16, 2004).

[1651] See e.g. *National Human Rights Commission v. State of Arunachal Pradesh*, (1996) 83 AIR 1234 (India SC, Jan. 9, 1996).

[1652] Verdirame, "Kenya," at 62–64.

detained on public order grounds challenge an executive detention order before a judge.[1653]

Clearly, judicial assistance may be of greatest value to a refugee seeking recognition of his or her status as a refugee: unless refugee status is not contested by the host state, a fair assessment of refugee status is the indispensable means by which to vindicate Convention rights.[1654] Yet even on this vitally important question, refugees do not always enjoy clear access to the courts. In the United States, for example, national security concerns have been invoked to order the denial of asylum in secret hearings in which the persons seeking recognition of refugee status were not allowed to see the evidence, hear the testimony, or even know what charges were being brought against them.[1655] An administrative decision to detain a refugee claimant for the duration of the status assessment process is moreover not subject to appeal or review by American courts.[1656] Australia has gone farther still, actually "excising" some more remote parts of its territory from what it calls its "migration zone," with refugees arriving in such excised areas "treated as if they were in an overseas refugee camp – with their visas processed under (discretionary) rules, no rights to appeal to court, and no right to come to Australia if accepted as refugees."[1657]

[1653] E. Khiddu-Makubuya, *International Academy of Comparative Law National Report for Uganda* (1994), at 9–10.

[1654] See Kälin, "Temporary Protection," at 218: "Although the 1951 Convention does not contain any provisions relating to national status determination procedures, the principle of good faith in fulfilling treaty obligations requires, as has been stressed by the German Constitutional Court [citing the case of *EZAR 208*, 2 BvR 1938/93; 2 BvR 2315/93 (Ger. FCC, May 14, 1996), abstracted in (1997) 9 *International Journal of Refugee Law* 292], that States Parties to the Convention institute a procedure which allows for a determination of who is entitled to the guarantees of that treaty."

[1655] J. Risen, "Evidence to deny 6 Iraqis asylum may be weak, files show," *New York Times*, Oct. 13, 1998, at A-9.

[1656] "While the expedited removal provisions of the 1996 immigration law require the detention of asylum-seekers during the expedited removal process, they do not prohibit parole once asylum-seekers have established a credible fear of persecution and are therefore no longer subject to expedited removal proceedings. The authority to parole arriving asylum-seekers, however, is entrusted to the detaining authority, the Immigration and Naturalization Service. If the Immigration and Naturalization Service denies parole, that decision cannot be appealed to an independent judicial authority. While immigration judges can review Immigration and Naturalization Service custody decisions with respect to various other categories of non-citizens, immigration judges are precluded from reviewing issues relating to detention of 'arriving' aliens, a category which includes all arriving asylum-seekers": E. Acer, "Living up to America's Values: Reforming the US Detention System for Asylum Seekers," (2002) 20(3) *Refuge* 44, at 45–46.

[1657] K. Lawson, "Christmas Island plan to divide Labor MPs," *Canberra Times*, Dec. 3, 2002, at A-6. Extraordinarily, the United Nations High Commissioner for Refugees has endorsed a variant of this plan under which determination for some applicants would

The ability of refugees to seek an appeal or review of a negative decision on status determination is even more frequently stymied. An extraordinary British plan, which came to light in February 2003, proposed to remove asylum-seekers from the United Kingdom to so-called "regional protection zones" in places such as Iran, Iraq, and Somalia, where their claims to refugee status would be processed by UNHCR or another agency. One of the asserted strengths of this approach was said to be that "[t]here would not need to be a right to a legal challenge to the [refugee status] decision."[1658] Less ambitiously, the British government has already put in place a system under which all rejected asylum claims from listed countries are required to be certified as "clearly unfounded," meaning that no appeal can be pursued prior to deportation.[1659] As a former solicitor-general observed, "[i]t is difficult enough to appeal within the UK, where advisers can be based miles from dispersed applicants, but from overseas, appeals would be impossible. And this presumes the countries to which they are sent are safe."[1660]

The review of rejected refugee claims may also be foreclosed in practice by the setting of rigid deadlines within which an individual is required to seek judicial intervention. A clear example is provided by the Full Federal Court of Australia's decision in *Sahak*,[1661] in which the Court affirmed the application of a twenty-eight-day, non-reviewable filing deadline in the case of a rejected asylum-seeker from Afghanistan. It did so despite having found that his failure to comply "was not due to any personal default." Indeed, the applicant

---

occur at a common site within the European Union without any clear commitment to judicial review. "Under the 'EU Prong,' the UNHCR proposes separating out asylum-seekers from countries that produce hardly any genuine refugees. These asylum-seekers would be sent to one or more reception centers somewhere within the EU, where their claims would be *rapidly examined* by joint EU teams. Those judged not to have any sort of refugee claim *would be sent straight home* [emphasis added]": R. Lubbers, "Put an end to their wandering: Europe should do more to support refugees in their regions of origin," *Guardian*, June 20, 2003, at 22.

[1658] A. Travis, "Asylum report: Shifting a problem back to its source," *Guardian*, Feb. 5, 2003, at 6, quoting from the report, "A New Vision for Refugees."

[1659] "If the Secretary of State is satisfied that a person who makes ... an asylum claim is entitled to reside in a State listed in subsection (7), he shall issue a certificate under subsection (1) to the effect that that person might not bring an appeal under sections 65 or 69 of the Immigration and Asylum Act 1999 while in the United Kingdom unless satisfied that the claim is not clearly unfounded": Nationality, Immigration and Asylum Act 2002, at s. 115(6).

[1660] "A new iron curtain: The Lords must reform the asylum bill," *Guardian*, Oct. 9, 2002, at 19, quoting Lord Archer. So long as the initial consideration of their claims was fair, the English Court of Appeal has nonetheless held that the procedures envisaged by s. 115 are not unfair: *R (ZL) v. Secretary of State for the Home Department*, [2003] 1 WLR 1230 (Eng. CA, Jan. 24, 2003), at paras. 38, 49.

[1661] *Sahak v. Minister for Immigration and Multicultural Affairs*, [2002] FCAFC 215 (Aus FFC, July 18, 2002).

was detained during the relevant time by the government in a remote location. He was not provided with the forms on which to appeal even though he had written to the Minister in his native language requesting same; he had no access to counsel to assist him in applying to the Court; he did not speak English; and when the appeal forms were finally completed due to the intervention of an interpreter, the business manager of the detention facility failed to file them until after the deadline for appeal had expired.[1662] The Court, however, found no basis for relief from the literal application of the filing deadline.[1663] There are, however, signs that at least some courts have begun decisively to challenge legislative efforts to curtail their right to review rejected asylum claims. The High Court of Australia recently considered sweeping privative legislation in relation to the review of refugee claims, and determined that "if read literally, ... [the new law] would purport to oust the jurisdiction of this court."[1664] In rejecting such an interpretation, the High Court noted that "[i]f tribunals were to be at liberty to exceed their jurisdiction without any check by the courts, the rule of law would be at an end."[1665] And more generally, the European Union has codified the right of refugee claimants to "an effective remedy," including in particular the right to apply to a court or tribunal to review a refusal or withdrawal of refugee status.[1666]

[1662] Motta reports that under s. 193 of the Australian Migration Reform Act 1992, "there is no requirement for the Minister or any officer to provide a detained person with an application form for a visa; or to advise a person that they may apply for a visa; or to allow a person access to advice (whether legal or otherwise) in connection with applications for visas, unless the detainee should specifically request it. The ramifications of this 'cone of silence' built around asylum-seekers in detention was almost instantly obvious. In 1993–1994, 100% of unauthorized arrivals by boat made refugee claims. In 1994–1995 only 10.4% did. In 1996–1997, 80% of unauthorized boat entrants were removed without requesting legal assistance": Motta, "Rock," at 16.

[1663] Despite a creative effort to argue that the literal application of the rules for filing would amount to racial discrimination, the majority of the court declined to intervene, noting that "such discrimination or disadvantage as arose from the practical operation of ... the Act was not racial discrimination ... Any differential effect which the application of ... the Act produces is not based on race, color, descent or national or ethnic origin, but rather on the individual personal circumstances of each applicant": *Sahak v. Minister for Immigration and Multicultural Affairs*, [2002] FCAFC 215 (Aus FFC, July 18, 2002). While a concurring member of the court did find that the differential impact of the law was clearly on grounds of national origin, he nonetheless dismissed the application on the questionable grounds that the right to judicial review could still be pursued before the High Court. While true, restriction to one opportunity for prerogative review in a country's top court still amounts to a substantial disadvantage relative to the review rights enjoyed by persons not disadvantaged on the grounds of their national origin.

[1664] *S157/2002 v. Commonwealth of Australia*, [2003] HCA 2 (Aus. HC, Feb. 4, 2003), per Gleeson CJ.

[1665] Ibid.   [1666] EU Procedures Directive, at Art. 38.

Refugee Convention, Art. 16(1)   Access to courts
A refugee shall have free access to the courts of law on the territory
of all Contracting States.

Civil and Political Covenant, Art. 14(1)
All persons shall be equal before the courts and tribunals. In the
determination ... of his rights and obligations in a suit at law,
everyone shall be entitled to a fair and public hearing by a competent, independent and impartial tribunal established by law ...

Refugee Convention, Art. 25   Administrative assistance
1. When the exercise of a right by a refugee would normally
require the assistance of authorities of a foreign country to whom
he cannot have recourse, the Contracting States in whose territory
he is residing shall arrange that such assistance be afforded to him
by their own authorities or by an international authority.

2. The authority or authorities mentioned in paragraph 1 shall
deliver or cause to be delivered under their supervision to refugees
such documents or certifications as would normally be delivered
to aliens by or through their national authorities.

3. Documents or certifications so delivered shall stand in the
stead of the official instruments delivered to aliens by or through
their national authorities, and shall be given credence in the
absence of proof to the contrary.

4. Subject to such exceptional treatment as may be granted to
indigent persons, fees may be charged for the services mentioned
herein, but such fees shall be moderate and commensurate with
those charged to nationals for similar services.

5. The provisions of this article shall be without prejudice to
articles 27 and 28.

One possible means of assisting refugees to vindicate their rights would have
been to return to the pre-Second World War precedent of empowering the
international supervisory agency, presently the UNHCR, to undertake quasi-
consular representation on behalf of refugees. Yet in line with the more
general determination of states to decentralize authority for the implementation of refugee protection,[1667] no such proposal was tabled. Indeed, the
strongest endorsement of an international mechanism for effectuating the
exercise of refugee rights was contained in the French draft of Art. 25, under
which UNHCR would have had automatic residual authority to provide

---

[1667] See J. Hathaway, "A Reconsideration of the Underlying Premise of Refugee Law," (1990)
31(1) *Harvard International Law Journal* 129, at 166–168.

administrative assistance to refugees – but only if a state failed to devise its own system for facilitating the implementation of refugee rights.[1668]

The failure to grant UNHCR a general responsibility to assist refugees to vindicate their rights largely reflects a deference to the decision of the General Assembly not specifically to include this responsibility in the agency's mandate.[1669] There was also a clear disinclination to tie the hands of the future Office of the High Commissioner, which might not wish to undertake protection work in precisely the same way as had its predecessors.[1670] Because of these operational uncertainties, the drafters insisted that states assume the basic responsibility to facilitate the exercise of rights by refugees.

[1668] "In all cases in which the exercise of a right by the foreigner normally requires the administrative assistance of the authorities of his country or of its representatives abroad, the High Contracting Parties undertake either to appoint a national authority or, failing that, to empower the High Commissioner for Refugees to furnish assistance to refugees": France, "Draft Convention," at 8.

[1669] The relevant discussions occurred in the Ad Hoc Committee several months before UNHCR was established, and the representatives were understandably reluctant to usurp the jurisdiction of the General Assembly to define the agency's role. "The High Commissioner had not yet been appointed, the nature of his functions was not known, and it was still not clear whether he would administer them through offices in various countries or through a central agency": Statement of Mr. Henkin of the United States, UN Doc. E/AC.32/SR.19, Feb. 1, 1950, at 2. See also Statement of Sir Leslie Brass of the United Kingdom, ibid. at 3: "[I]t was beyond the competence of this Committee to attribute functions to the High Commissioner or to imply that his office would exercise functions in various countries." At the meeting of the Conference of Plenipotentiaries – which occurred after the enactment of the UNHCR Statute – one delegate expressed resignation that nothing could be done to reverse the decision of the General Assembly not to entrust UNHCR with the duty to render administrative assistance to refugees. "The Belgian Government regretted that a task of this nature had not been entrusted exclusively to an international authority. Under his mandate, the High Commissioner could protect only groups of refugees, and that was where the tragedy lay in certain cases, where the refugee needed not only the protection which the relations established between the High Commissioner and national authorities afforded him, but individual protection as well": Statement of Mr. Herment of Belgium, UN Doc. A/CONF.2/SR.11, July 9, 1951, at 12.

[1670] "[T]he language still appeared to retain a certain weakness inasmuch as it might be interpreted as granting a country the right, if it so desired, to designate an international authority to furnish assistance to refugees, regardless of the wishes of the international authority concerned": Statement of Mr. Henkin of the United States, UN Doc. E/AC.32/SR.19, Feb. 1, 1950, at 6. The immediate reply of the Israeli delegate – which the drafters agreed "should be incorporated into the Committee's report in order to meet the point of the United States representative" – was that "[o]bviously [states] could not arbitrarily designate an international body as the authority in question against its wishes. The reference to international authorities could be invoked only if an appropriate international organ existed and was willing to assume the obligation envisaged in the paragraph. Where no such organization existed, the Contracting Party would have to designate an authority to furnish requisite assistance to refugees": Statement of Mr. Robinson of Israel, ibid. at 7.

While a government might validly delegate its duty to provide administrative assistance to a willing international agency, the government ultimately remains responsible to ensure that refugees actually receive the assistance they require.[1671] As framed by the American representative,

> There was a danger that some countries might seek to relieve their own agencies of administrative responsibility by referring refugees to an international authority ... In order to eliminate the risk of leaving refugees unprotected, it seemed advisable to make it mandatory upon Governments to assume responsibility except when an international authority functioning in their territory was in a position to do so. In the latter event, States should retain the option of accepting the authority of an international organ.[1672]

In line with this perspective, the Refugee Convention requires each state party to conceive an administrative mechanism by which to facilitate the exercise of Convention rights by all refugees living in its territory. The nature of the duty of administrative "assistance" to be provided by a refugee's country of residence under Art. 25(1) is not, however, set out in the Convention. While the Committee deleted a parenthetical reference to consular assistance as an unnecessary refinement,[1673] it indicated no intention to vary the sorts of administrative assistance traditionally provided to refugees. As Grahl-Madsen suggests, the duty to provide administrative assistance to refugees under paragraph 1 of Art. 25 therefore goes beyond the responsibility to issue documents set out in paragraph 2, and logically includes "correspondence, investigations, recommendations, counseling, [and] personal

---

[1671] At the commencement of debate on this issue, the French delegate quickly assured his colleagues that even the French proposal "would leave each state free to decide whether administrative assistance should be furnished by its own national authorities or by an international authority, if such authority existed. It was not intended to impose duties upon the High Commissioner nor to give him exclusive competence in the matter": Statement of Mr. Ordonneau of France, ibid. at 2.

[1672] Statement of Mr. Henkin of the United States, ibid. at 2–3. Sir Leslie Brass of the United Kingdom, ibid. at 3, also emphasized that a consular role for an international agency on behalf of refugees "was not contemplated by the United Kingdom government." See also Statements of the Chairman, Mr. Chance of Canada, and Mr. Perez Perozo of Venezuela, ibid.

[1673] The original draft provided that "[i]n all cases in which the exercise of a right by a foreigner requires the assistance of the authorities of his country (in particular of the consular authorities) the High Contracting Parties shall designate an authority which shall furnish assistance to refugees": Secretary-General, "Memorandum," at 43. The reference to consular assistance was said by the Belgian representative to lack "clarity," leading the Brazilian delegate to suggest its deletion on the grounds that "the introductory clause of paragraph 1 was sufficiently clear in that respect": Statements of Mr. Cuvelier of Belgium and Mr. Guerreiro of Brazil, UN Doc. E/AC.32/SR.19, Feb. 1, 1950, at 4.

assistance"[1674] needed to enable refugees to benefit from their Convention rights.[1675] Thus, a state party may not validly limit respect for refugee rights to only such refugees as are somehow able to advance those rights independently; governments have an affirmative responsibility under Art. 25(1) to establish a mechanism by which refugees may benefit in practice from their legal entitlements.[1676]

One means of fulfilling this duty is for the host state to make arrangements with UNHCR or another international agency[1677] to act as intermediary in assisting refugees to secure their rights.[1678] A state might alternatively choose to establish or empower an independent national authority to assist refugees,[1679] or to include refugee protection within the mandate of one or

---

[1674] Grahl-Madsen, *Commentary*, at 103. Weis asserts at least as broad an understanding, noting that "[t]he term 'administrative assistance' is wider than the functions enumerated in the Arrangement of 1928. It may include investigations, counseling and personal assistance. It includes the functions normally exercised by consuls": Weis, *Travaux*, at 204.

[1675] The Belgian representative to the Conference of Plenipotentiaries stressed the importance of Art. 25 as mandating a mechanism to provide "individual protection" to refugees beyond the group-based protection role granted to UNHCR under its Statute: Statement of Mr. Herment of Belgium, UN Doc. A/CONF.2/SR.11, July 9, 1951, at 12.

[1676] "[T]he language of article [25] [is] mandatory, rather than permissive. It placed upon Governments the obligation to provide administrative assistance to refugees who could not obtain it through normal consular channels since they no longer enjoyed the protection of their country of origin": Statement of Mr. Robinson of Israel, UN Doc. E/AC.32/SR.19, Feb. 1, 1950, at 4. At the first session of the Ad Hoc Committee, the text of Art. 25(1) was amended to make this affirmative duty clear by adding the words "shall arrange" (so that it read, "The Contracting State . . . shall arrange that such assistance be afforded"): Ad Hoc Committee, "First Session Report," at Annex I.

[1677] "Article 25 does not specify any particular international authority. A Contracting State is therefore free to choose any international authority it likes, which is able and willing to carry out the task. It is, however, clear that the drafters of the Convention had in particular the Office of the High Commissioner for Refugees in mind. It was decided, however, not to mention this Office by name, because it was felt that the Contracting States should not impose any tasks on it, this being a matter for the United Nations to decide, and because there was a possibility that the Convention would survive the Office": Grahl-Madsen, *Commentary*, at 105.

[1678] See text above, at pp. 627–628. "A Government may itself provide such assistance by creating an authority to do so or by assigning the task to an existing national authority, or a country may prefer to make arrangements for an international authority to render such assistance. If, for example, the United Nations High Commissioner for Refugees should deal with administrative assistance, a country may arrange with the High Commissioner to have such assistance rendered in its territory. In any event, however, there is an obligation on the Contracting State to see that such assistance is provided": Ad Hoc Committee, "First Session Report," at Annex I.

[1679] "In some countries, such as the United Kingdom, no special machinery had been set up. In others, however, special offices had been established for that purpose. In fact, the more[1680] existing governmental agencies.[1681] In view of the explicit language of Art. 25(1),[1682] however, it would not be sufficient to entrust the provision of administrative assistance to a non-governmental organization unless that organization receives delegated power from the state, or from an international organization acting at the state's behest. The critical concern is to ensure that the entity charged with assisting refugees be genuinely in a position to act authoritatively.[1683]

All refugees, whether or not their status has been formally verified, are entitled to benefit from administrative assistance.[1684] Some confusion on this point could arise from the fact that this duty falls on a refugee's state of "residence," which might suggest that only refugees who meet one of the higher degrees of attachment (e.g. lawful presence, or lawful stay) may assert a right to assistance.[1685] On balance, however, this conclusion is not justified.

Not only does the text not qualify the beneficiary class by reference to a level of attachment, but the drafters at times used the phrase "residence" (as

---

provision was based on the practice of Belgium and France": Statement of Mr. Robinson of Israel, UN Doc. E/AC.32/SR.19, Feb. 1, 1950, at 4.

[1680] "[I]nasmuch as refugees might have to apply to several authorities in order to secure administrative documents, the words 'an authority' in the final clause of the paragraph should be in the plural": Statement of Mr. Cha of China, ibid. at 4. See also Statements of Mr. Kural of Turkey, ibid., and Mr. Perez Perozo of Venezuela, ibid. at 5.

[1681] "[T]he word 'designate' did not imply that an authority to furnish assistance to refugees was necessarily to be established; such authority or authorities might already exist in certain countries, in which case they need merely be designated": Statement of Mr. Cuvelier of Belgium, ibid. at 5. See also Statement of Mr. Robinson of Israel, ibid.: "[T]he reference [in the Secretary-General's draft] to the Arrangement of 30 January 1928 [under which the responsibility to provide administrative assistance was entrusted to a High Commissioner for Refugees] would in itself appear to make the creation rather than the mere designation of a special authority mandatory; as that was not the intention of the Committee, the reference to the Arrangement of 1928 should be deleted."

[1682] It is the duty of states to "arrange that such assistance be afforded ... by their own authorities or by an international authority": Refugee Convention, at Art. 25(1).

[1683] "If the refugee is actually to enjoy these rights, he must obtain the assistance of an authority which will perform for him the services performed by national authorities in the case of persons with a nationality. In the absence of an international authority, the High Contracting Parties must appoint a national authority which will furnish its assistance to refugees": Secretary-General, "Memorandum," at 43–44. See also Statement of Mr. Herment of Belgium, UN Doc. A/CONF.2/SR.11, July 9, 1951, at 12, who "stressed the importance of article [25], which was designed to meet one of the most constant and essential needs of refugees ... In many European countries refugees ... would like to be able to get into direct touch with someone *who was responsible for protecting them* [emphasis added]."

[1684] The text of Art. 25 grants "refugees" without qualification the right to a state's administrative assistance. See generally chapter 3.1.1 above.

[1685] See generally chapter 3.1 above.

opposed to habitual residence, or domicile[1686]) in a way that implied no more than transient presence in a state party.[1687] Significantly, the original draft text imposed the duty of administrative assistance simply on "the High Contracting Parties."[1688] This was amended by the Ad Hoc Committee to assign the duty to "[t]he Contracting State in whose territory the exercise of a right by aliens would normally require the assistance of the authorities of the country of nationality."[1689] The goal of this change was to make clear that there was a duty to assist refugees not just in their asylum country, but also in any country to which the refugee might travel or have dealings.[1690] At the Conference of Plenipotentiaries, however, the Belgian representative observed that it would make more sense to assign the duty of administrative assistance to a single state.[1691] Because a refugee might need to exercise a right in a non-contracting state, "the country of residence should lend its good offices. The concept of territory should, for those

---

[1686] "The word 'habitual' (Arts. 14, 16(2)) is not used, indicating that a permanent residence is not required": Robinson, *History*, at 131. See also Grahl-Madsen, *Commentary*, at 104: "The State 'in whose territory he is residing,' or the country of residence, is not the same as the country where a refugee has domicile or where he is 'lawfully staying' or allowed to settle."

[1687] For example, in debate on Art. 12 of the Convention, the Belgian representative expressed his concern about how to deal with the case of "a refugee domiciled in China, where he had his family and his business, [but] who might visit Belgium on a business trip. If he should happen to die in Belgium, it would be ludicrous to determine his status on the basis of the law of the *country of residence*. He would normally be subject to the law of China, his country of domicile [emphasis added]": Statement of Mr. Cuvelier of Belgium, UN Doc. E/AC.32/SR.8, Jan. 23, 1950, at 7. Significantly, it was also a representative of Belgium who introduced the notion of "residence" into Art. 25 at the Conference of Plenipotentiaries: see text below, at pp. 638–639.

[1688] Secretary-General, "Memorandum," at 43.

[1689] Ad Hoc Committee, "First Session Report," at Annex I.

[1690] "Refugees do not enjoy the protection and assistance of the authorities of their country of origin. Consequently, even if the government of the country of asylum grants the refugee a status which ensures him treatment equivalent to or better than that enjoyed by aliens, *he may not in some countries be in a position to enjoy the rights granted him*. Often he will require the assistance of an authority which will perform for him the services performed by national authorities in the case of persons with a nationality. In this article, *governments* undertake to assure that refugees obtain required assistance ... [T]here is an obligation *on the Contracting States* to see that such assistance is provided [emphasis added]": Ad Hoc Committee, "First Session Report," at Annex II.

[1691] "He did not consider that the obligation on Contracting States to afford refugees the necessary administrative assistance was brought out with sufficient clarity in that paragraph ... In the opinion of the Belgian delegation ... the responsibility should be placed squarely on the authorities of the country of residence, who were better able to come to the assistance of refugees": Statement of Mr. Herment of Belgium, UN Doc. A/CONF.2/SR.11, July 9, 1951, at 12–13.

reasons, be omitted from the provisions governing the exercise of a right by refugees."[1692]

Thus, the amendment of the text of Art. 25 to assign responsibility for the provision of administrative assistance to a refugee's country of residence was in no sense an effort to restrict the beneficiary class of Art. 25, but was rather intended simply to make clear that the country in which the refugee is staying should assist him or her, even when necessary for the exercise of a right outside that state's jurisdiction.[1693] This interpretation most readily advances the purposes of the Refugee Convention: since there is no doubt that some rights inhere in refugees prior to their being granted a right of ongoing residence in an asylum country,[1694] it would be nonsensical to allow states effectively to avoid their reciprocal duties towards refugees by refusing refugees the assistance required to invoke their rights.

One of the most basic concerns of refugees is to acquire the sorts of official documentation often required to function in the asylum country. Art. 25(2) is expressly addressed to this matter. It requires the refugee's state of residence to provide the refugee with "such documents or certifications as would normally be delivered to aliens by or through their national authorities."[1695] The explanatory note to the Secretary-General's original proposal for Art. 25(2) provides a helpful sense of both the scope of the duty, and the rationale for such a provision:

> In order to perform the acts of civil life (marriage, divorce, adoption, settlement of succession, naturalization, acquisition of immovable property, constitution of associations, opening of bank accounts, etc.), a person must produce documents to certify his identity, position, civil status, nationality, etc., and if he is a foreigner, to testify to the provisions of his former or present national law and the conformity of instruments executed in his country of origin with the legislation of that country . . .

[1692] Statement of Mr. Herment of Belgium, ibid. at 13. Both the Colombian delegate and the High Commissioner for Refugees voiced their approval of this change (see Statements of Mr. Giraldo-Jaramillo of Colombia and of Mr. van Heuven Goedhart of UNHCR, ibid. at 14), which was adopted by the Conference without further debate: ibid. at 15.

[1693] Weis notes that "[a]dministrative assistance is not limited to the territorial authorities of the country of residence. Diplomatic or consular authorities may be designated to render this assistance to refugees while abroad or they may furnish such assistance provided it is furnished 'under the supervision' of the designated authority": Weis, *Travaux*, at 204.

[1694] See chapter 3.1 above.

[1695] "The words 'by or through' (their national authorities) . . . indicate that it is either the local authority which ordinarily renders the service or the consula[r] authorities through which the documents or certifications are procured or delivered": Robinson, *History*, at 130. See also Grahl-Madsen, *Commentary*, at 105: "Paragraph 2 allows a flexible system to be established, on the [sole] condition that there is some supervision by a competent authority."

It is easy for a foreigner to obtain such documents. He merely has to apply to the national services which operate in his country of origin or which are accredited abroad and they will deliver the documents which he requires. A refugee whose links with his country of origin are broken cannot obtain such papers from the authorities of that country. In the absence of any international authority, a national authority designated for the purpose will be required to issue to refugees all the documents of which they stand in need.[1696]

This responsibility does not, however, include the issuance of either refugee identity or travel documents, matters regulated by Arts. 27 and 28 of the Convention respectively.[1697] Nor does it amount to a duty to issue documents which the refugee could readily acquire by independent effort,[1698]

[1696] Secretary-General, "Memorandum," at 44. Note, however, that the substance of a refugee's personal status is governed by the rules which pertain in his or her country of domicile, in accordance with Art. 12 of the Refugee Convention. See generally chapter 3.2.4 above.

[1697] These matters are expressly excluded by Art. 25(5). The duty to issue identity documents is discussed at chapter 4.9 above; the issuance of travel documents is considered in chapter 6.6 below. Art. 25(5) was added to the text to respond to concerns of some representatives that its scope might otherwise appear to be overly broad. The American delegate, for example, credited the Swiss observer "for pointing out that article [25] might appear to cover travel documents, which were properly the subject of article [29]. The Drafting Committee might wish to make some change to remove the possibility of confusion": Statement of Mr. Henkin of the United States, UN Doc. E/AC.32/SR.38, Aug. 17, 1950, at 21. Similarly, the Chairman of the Ad Hoc Committee confirmed that "the 'certifications' referred to in article [25] were not identity papers but evidence of such matters as marital status or medical proficiency": Statement of the Chairman, Mr. Larsen of Denmark, ibid.

[1698] For example, the British delegate asked whether "if a Spanish refugee currently in England required a birth certificate, would the United Kingdom Government be obliged to attempt to procure the certificate for him, although in such a case the refugee might presumably obtain the document simply by requesting it from the Spanish Government's Registrar of Births?": Statement of Sir Leslie Brass of the United Kingdom, UN Doc. E/AC.32/SR.19, Feb. 1, 1950, at 6. The response was "that the hypothesis just mentioned by the United Kingdom representative automatically fell outside the scope of paragraph 1 which would operate only in the case of a refugee unable to secure the necessary documents from the authorities of his country": Statement of Mr. Cuvelier of Belgium, ibid. As this exchange makes clear, the duty to provide refugees with documents under Art. 25(2) is appropriately considered a subset of the more general duty of administrative assistance set out in Art. 25(1). See Grahl-Madsen, *Commentary*, at 106: "Whereas Paragraph 1 deals with administrative assistance of any description, Paragraph 2 is restricted to 'documents or certifications.'" But as Grahl-Madsen insists, "[a] refugee cannot be expected to ask the authorities of his country of origin for assistance, and the authorities of the country of residence consequently cannot refuse to afford assistance on the ground that the refugee has not first tried [to see] if the former can help him. The same must apply if the refugee needs documentation relating to acts which have taken place in countries with a regime similar to that prevailing in [the refugee's] country of origin, e.g. if a refugee from Hungary or which are not genuinely necessary to the conduct of daily life or for the vindication of a refugee's rights. For example, it was noted by the drafters that in most common law states, non-citizens were normally allowed to rely on an affidavit attesting to relevant facts, rather than securing official documentation from governmental authorities. Refugees could, of course, do the same.[1699] But where official documentation is required, a commitment from the authorities of the refugee's host state to provide the refugee with substitute documentation is often critical.[1700] As observed by the Belgian delegate to the Conference of Plenipotentiaries, "[t]he object of paragraph 2 of article [25] was to enable refugees to procure documents which they would not be able to obtain from the countries which would normally provide them ... That was a most important provision, and it was therefore right that it should be safeguarded to the greatest possible extent."[1701] The drafters therefore agreed that states should enjoy no latitude to refrain from issuing such documents or certifications as are truly required by a

needs a certificate from Czechoslovakia or Romania. If, on the other hand, administrative assistance is required from some other country where a refugee cannot fear any persecution, e.g. a country where he formerly enjoyed asylum, the refugee must try [to] get what he needs from that country": ibid. at 103.

[1699] "No difficulties arose in countries of common law, where the affidavit system was applied": Statement of Mr. van Heuven Goedhart of UNHCR, A/CONF.2/SR.11, July 9, 1951, at 14. As confirmed by the representative of the United Kingdom, Art. 25(2) would "in point of fact have no practical effect in the United Kingdom": Statement of Mr. Hoare of the United Kingdom, ibid. at 15. He later amplified this position, noting that he "wished to make it clear that the Government of the United Kingdom, where the system envisaged in paragraph 2 of article 25 did not exist, would not interpret the paragraph as mandatory in the sense that it would require the United Kingdom Government to invent and introduce a system for supplying documents of the type which would be supplied by other countries. The United Kingdom Government would, however, render every assistance to refugees by continuing to apply its own system – which was based on the personal affidavit – and to other countries by seeing that documents of that type were duly legalized if required by refugees for transmission to other countries": Statement of Mr. Hoare of the United Kingdom, UN Doc. A/CONF.2/ SR.35, July 25, 1951, at 9.

[1700] The concern is, of course, documentation related to matters which occurred outside the asylum country. "If an act has taken place in the country of residence, the refugee will be able to get a certificate from the appropriate authority just like anybody else": Grahl-Madsen, *Commentary*, at 103.

[1701] Statement of Mr. Herment of Belgium, UN Doc. A/CONF.2/SR.11, July 9, 1951, at 13. Thus, in response to an Austrian amendment which would have made the duty to provide refugees with substitute documentation purely an optional matter, the High Commissioner for Refugees replied that he "would very much regret it if the Conference were to adopt the Austrian amendment, which would so weaken article [25] as to deprive it of all significance": Statement of Mr. van Heuven Goedhart of UNHCR, ibid. at 14. The Austrian government thereupon withdrew its proposal: ibid.

refugee.[1702] As the earlier discussion of the beneficiary class of Art. 25 makes clear, it is the responsibility of the refugee's state of residence to issue these documents, even if they are required by the refugee for purposes outside its borders.[1703]

What sorts of documentation does Art. 25(2) envisage? A decision was taken not to enumerate specific categories of documents, but rather to leave it to each state to provide refugees with whatever documents are "required in the performance of the acts of civil life."[1704] The list of documents in the Secretary-General's original draft, itself based on the sorts of documents provided to refugees by international authorities under earlier treaties,[1705] was recommended by the drafters as illustrative of the scope of the duty under Art. 25(2).[1706] It includes documents certifying "the position" of the refugees or their "family position and civil status," attestations of "the regularity" of documents issued in the refugee's home country, certifications to "the good character and conduct of the individual refugee, to his previous record, to his professional qualifications[1707] and to his university degrees or academic diplomas," and even recommendations "with a view to obtaining visas, permits to reside in the country, admission to schools, libraries, etc."[1708] The duty under Art. 25(2) extends to all documents and certifications

[1702] The Chairman of the Ad Hoc Committee, in his capacity as representative of Canada, proposed that the duty under Art. 25(2) should inhere only "as far as possible" or "when possible": Statement of the Chairman, Mr. Chance of Canada, UN Doc. E/AC.32/SR.19, Feb. 1, 1950, at 7, 8. He subsequently withdrew his suggestions: UN Doc. E/AC.32/SR.25, Feb. 10, 1950, at 8.

[1703] "If a refugee resident in the territory of country A happened to marry, and so exercised a right in the territory of country B, the question would arise as to which authorities were responsible for giving him the administrative assistance which he required. In the opinion of the Belgian delegation, as expressed in its amendment . . . the responsibility should be placed squarely on the authorities of the country of residence": Statement of Mr. Herment of Belgium, UN Doc. A/CONF.2/SR.11, July 9, 1951, at 13. See text above, at pp. 638–639. Robinson adds that "[a]lthough par. 3 does not say so, it must be assumed that such documents or certifications are valid in all Contracting States even if delivered by the authorities of one Contracting State (not an international authority). This conclusion is based on the equal force of documents or certifications issued by either the international authority or the local authorities": Robinson, *History*, at 132.

[1704] Statement of Mr. Cuvelier of Belgium, UN Doc. E/AC.32/SR.19, Feb. 1, 1950, at 8.

[1705] Statement of Mr. Weis of the International Refugee Organization, ibid. at 8.

[1706] "As an indication of the types of document which refugees may require according to the varying practices of countries, a list is given below. This list is not intended to be exhaustive, nor does it imply that these documents are necessary to refugees in all countries": Ad Hoc Committee, "First Session Report," at Annex II.

[1707] The Chairman of the Ad Hoc Committee also specifically mentioned documentation of "medical proficiency" as an example of the type of documentation within the scope of Art. 25(2): Statement of the Chairman, Mr. Larsen of Denmark, UN Doc. E/AC.32/SR.38, Aug. 17, 1950, at 21.

[1708] Secretary-General, "Memorandum," at 43.

typically issued "either by the judicial or administrative authorities of [the refugee's] country of nationality or by its consular authorities,"[1709] including those "relating to material and legal rights."[1710]

Documents issued pursuant to Art. 25(2) "shall be given credence in the absence of proof to the contrary."[1711] The initial drafts of Art. 25 had been framed in more emphatic terms. Under the Secretary-General's proposal, "certificates so delivered shall take the place of the original acts and documents and shall be accorded the same validity."[1712] The French proposal went even further, proposing that Art. 25 documents "shall rank as authentic documents and shall take the place of the acts and documents issued in the refugee's country of origin."[1713] However, as a consensus emerged in the Ad Hoc Committee that even the English affidavit system would meet the requirements of Art. 25(2),[1714] the French representative expressed his unwillingness to accept at face value the authenticity of all such documents.[1715] The Committee's conclusions note as well that documents issued under Art. 25 could not really be said to have the same validity as original documents; the point was rather that they were as authentic as the secondary certifications or attestations that would ordinarily be issued to a non-citizen by his or her consular authorities.[1716] Thus, "[s]uch documents would be accepted as evidence of the facts or acts certified, in accordance with the laws of the country in which the document is presented."[1717] In positing this clarification, the report notes that "the Committee in no way intended

[1709] Ad Hoc Committee, "First Session Report," at Annex II. Robinson goes farther, arguing that under Art. 25(2) "Contracting States would be called upon to deliver also documents and certifications which are to be supplied by authorities other than those of the country of nationality of the refugee (for instance, if the refugee was born outside the country of his nationality or married there) because in such instances the documents and certifications are usually provided through the authorities of a person's home country which act[s] as intermediar[y]": Robinson, *History*, at 130.

[1710] Statement of Mr. Fritzer of Austria, UN Doc. A/CONF.2/SR.11, July 9, 1951, at 11.

[1711] Refugee Convention, at Art. 25(3).   [1712] Secretary-General, "Memorandum," at 43.

[1713] France, "Draft Convention," at 8.   [1714] See text above, at p. 641.

[1715] "[I]n inserting the provision that the certificates delivered should rank as authentic documents, his delegation had intended to give them the highest possible value. On considering the type of certificates envisaged, however, he had come to the conclusion that they could not all rank as authentic documents in the accepted meaning of that term under French law ... He therefore withdrew the French version of paragraph 3 in favor of the Secretariat draft": Statement of Mr. Ordonneau of France, UN Doc. E/AC.32/ SR.19, Feb. 1, 1950, at 8–9.

[1716] "The purpose of this clause is to have the Contracting States give documents issued to refugees the same validity as if the documents had been issued by the competent authority of the country of nationality (within the country or by a consular agent abroad) of an alien, or as if the act had been certified by such authority": Ad Hoc Committee, "First Session Report," at Annex II.

[1717] Ibid.

to reduce the value which such documents have under existing arrangements."[1718]

This equivocation was nonetheless clearly of concern to the Belgian delegate to the Conference of Plenipotentiaries who introduced the final wording of Art. 25(3). He insisted that the Ad Hoc Committee's draft should be replaced "by some text easily capable of dispelling any doubts arising out of such documents; that was why [Belgium] had suggested that they should be regarded as authentic in the absence of proof to the contrary."[1719] His proposal was adopted without opposition,[1720] in consequence of which the onus must be understood to fall squarely on a government to whom an Art. 25 document is presented to show why it ought not to be relied upon. As Robinson concludes, "such documents or certifications possess a lesser degree of validity than ordinary documents (which is inherent in the circumstance that their delivery is often based on insufficient proofs) and may be annulled or modified by contrary evidence. However, as long as such contrary evidence is not available, the documents and certifications are to serve the same purpose as official instruments of the national authorities."[1721]

Despite the importance of each state party's commitment to provide administrative assistance to refugees, the downside of this approach, cogently observed by Mr. Herment of Belgium, is that "when the authorities of the receiving country were called upon to consider a complaint or a protest from a refugee, they would always be both judge and party to the dispute."[1722] In view of this potential conflict of interest, it was to be expected that refugees would in at least some instances turn to the courts of a state party to enforce their rights, whether based specifically on Convention entitlements or on Art. 7(1)'s attribution to refugees of the rights inhering in aliens generally.[1723] To this end, there was general agreement to adopt Art. 16(1), derived almost literally from the guarantee in both the 1933 and 1938 treaties of "free and ready access to the courts of law" in the territory of any state party.[1724]

[1718] Ibid.

[1719] Statement of Mr. Herment of Belgium, UN Doc. A/CONF.2/SR.11, July 9, 1951, at 14.

[1720] Both the representative of Colombia and the High Commissioner for Refugees expressed their support for the Belgian amendment: Statements of Mr. Giraldo-Jaramillo of Colombia and Mr. van Heuven Goedhart of UNHCR, ibid. at 14. The Belgian amendment was adopted without dissent on a 17–0 (5 abstentions) vote: ibid. at 15.

[1721] Robinson, *History*, at 132. See also Grahl-Madsen, who notes that "[t]aking into consideration the basis on which the documents . . . often shall have to be issued (corroborated or uncorroborated statements by the persons concerned) it seems that the Conference has made a sound ruling": Grahl-Madsen, *Commentary*, at 108.

[1722] Statement of Mr. Herment of Belgium, UN Doc. A/CONF.2/SR.11, July 9, 1951, at 12.

[1723] See chapter 3.2 above.

[1724] Ad Hoc Committee, "First Session Report," at Annex I. This right is, in any event, part of customary international law on the protection of aliens: see chapter 2.1 above, at p. 77.

Importantly, Art. 16(1) is not limited to a right to access the courts of the country in which the refugee is located. In the words of the President of the Conference of Plenipotentiaries, Art. 16(1) "stipulated that a refugee should not only have free access to the courts in the country where he resided, but to the courts in the territory of all contracting States."[1725] Nor do rights inhere only in refugees once they are granted a right to enter or remain in a given state. To the contrary, the drafting history makes quite clear that Art. 16(1) rights inhere in all refugees, whether or not they have been admitted to a state.[1726] As the American representative observed, "persons who had only recently become refugees and therefore had no habitual residence were ... covered by the provisions of ... paragraph 1."[1727] Indeed, as the English High Court (Queen's Bench Division) has observed, any other interpretation might well frustrate the essential purposes of the Convention:

> The use of the word "refugee" [in Art. 16(1)] is apt to include the aspirant, for were that not so, if in fact it had to be established that he did fall within the definition of "refugee" in article 1, he might find that he could have no right of audience before the court because the means of establishing his status would not be available to him.[1728]

Thus, subject only to the issue of subject-matter jurisdiction noted below,[1729] the efforts of an increasing number of countries to deny access to their courts to refugees seeking the review or appeal of a negative assessment of refugee status are *prima facie* incompatible with Art. 16(1) of the Convention.

[1725] Statement of the President, Mr. Larsen of Denmark, UN Doc. A/CONF.2/SR.8, July 5, 1951, at 13. The mechanics of this duty were explained in comments by the Israeli representative, Mr. Robinson, ibid. at 12: "Assuming, for instance, that the Governments of the United Kingdom and Yugoslavia were both parties to the Convention, and that a refugee resident in the United Kingdom wished to sue a debtor in Yugoslavia, the legal authorities in the latter country would ask the United Kingdom authorities whether the claimant was a refugee. If the answer was in the affirmative, the problem would be solved for the Yugoslav Court. It seemed to him that the issue was perfectly straightforward."

[1726] As framed in the Secretary General's original proposal, "[r]efugees are to have free access to justice, not only in their own country of residence, but in any other country party to the Convention": Secretary-General, "Memorandum," at 30.

[1727] Statement of Mr. Henkin of the United States, UN Doc. E/AC.32/SR.25, Feb. 10, 1950, at 6.

[1728] *R v. Secretary of State for the Home Department, ex parte Jahangeer et al.*, [1993] Imm AR 564 (Eng. QBD, June 11, 1993), per Jowitt J at 566.

[1729] See text below, at p. 647. The subject-matter jurisdiction concern may, however, be remedied by reliance on the Civil and Political Covenant: see text below, at pp. 647–650.

Only two, fairly modest, amendments were made to the original proposal for what became Art. 16(1).[1730] First, the English language text was altered to refer only to "free access" to the courts (rather than "free and ready access") on the grounds that "in English, the words 'free' and 'ready' were synonymous in the context if used alone, but in conjunction 'free' might mean without payment of court fees."[1731] The clear intention, affirmed by the decision not to amend the French language text (which continues to refer to "libre et facile accès devant les tribunaux"),[1732] is that while refugees may be expected to pay the usual fees to access the courts,[1733] state parties must not seek in any way to impede their resort to the courts. The effective denial of any access to domestic courts by Kenya to refugees in Kakuma camp was therefore clearly an infringement of Art. 16(1).

The second amendment made by the drafters was to vary the title of Art. 16 to the more general "access to the courts," rather than the arguably more constrained "right to appear before the courts as plaintiff or defendant."[1734] While this change of title does not resolve the interpretive question (particularly since the shift does not appear to have been formally debated by the Ad Hoc Committee),[1735] the new title nonetheless neatly affirms the ordinary meaning of the language used in Art. 16(1). While clearly the provision entitles refugees to engage in private litigation as a means of enforcing their rights – specific reference was made, for example, to the right of refugees to sue for divorce[1736] or to recover a debt[1737] – the right of access to the courts is framed as a general right, in no sense limited to access for purposes of launching or defending a civil suit.[1738] In principle, Art. 16(1) therefore

---

[1730] France, "Draft Convention," at 4. The members of the Ad Hoc Committee preferred this draft to that presented by the Secretary-General: UN Doc. E/AC.32/SR.11, Jan. 25, 1950, at 7–8.

[1731] Statement of Sir Leslie Brass of the United Kingdom, ibid. at 7.

[1732] On the motion of the Israeli representative, the English version of Art. 16(1) was amended to meet the British delegate's concerns, though the French language text was explicitly left unamended: Statement of Mr. Robinson of Israel, ibid. at 7.

[1733] Only refugees who have established "habitual residence" in a state party may claim the right to dispensation from some of the usual financial barriers to accessing the courts, in particular the duty to post security for costs and to receive legal aid. These matters are addressed by Art. 16(2)–(3) of the Convention: see chapter 6.8 below.

[1734] France, "Draft Convention," at 4. The title proposed in the Secretary-General's draft was even more narrow ("the right to sue and be sued"): Secretary-General, "Memorandum," at 29.

[1735] The change first appears in Ad Hoc Committee, "First Session Report," at Annex I.

[1736] Statement of Mr. Larsen of Denmark, UN Doc. E/AC.32/SR.11, Jan. 25, 1950, at 7.

[1737] Statement of Mr. Robinson of Israel, UN Doc. A/CONF.2/SR.8, July 5, 1951, at 12.

[1738] The First Court of Appeal of Paris rendered a judgment which appears to dispute this proposition. In sensibly rejecting the view that Art. 16(2)'s obligation to grant refugees "the same treatment as a national in matters pertaining to access to the courts" should be read to grant a refugee immunity from extradition proceedings, the Court observed that governs when refugees seek to litigate their Convention or any other rights before domestic courts.

The challenge, however, is that Art. 16(1) is only a guarantee that refugees may access whatever judicial remedies exist in the state party. The Refugee Convention does not stipulate the subject-matter jurisdiction of a state's courts, but requires simply that whenever the courts have competence over a given matter, refugees must have unimpeded access to the courts to enforce relevant claims. As such, where the courts lack subject-matter jurisdiction to entertain claims of the kind being advanced by refugees, Art. 16(1) does not afford refugees a remedy.[1739] The dilemma of the Ugandan courts – in theory open to all, but not legislatively empowered to adjudicate refugee rights – is thus quite real. Similarly, the failure of United States law to authorize the judicial review of an administrative decision to detain a refugee claimant deprives refugees of the ability to invoke Art. 16 in aid of any effort to contest their indefinite detention before that country's courts.

A domestic jurisdictional stalemate of this kind may, however, be at odds with the requirements of the Civil and Political Covenant. Art. 14(1) of the Covenant, which expressly inheres in "[a]ll persons," affords a sound basis for arguing the entitlement of refugees to a formal legal determination of their rights, at least by way of review or appeal if these are denied by more informal decision-making structures. Specifically, the Covenant requires *inter alia* that "in the determination . . . of his rights and obligations in a suit at law, every-one shall be entitled to a fair and public hearing by a competent, independent and impartial tribunal established by law." The understanding of a "suit at

"the mere reading of this text is sufficient to indicate that it refers solely to civil courts . . . [T]he Geneva Convention merely intended that the refugee should have the opportunity of bringing or defending civil proceedings": *Drago*, Decision of the Cour d'appel de Paris, 1ère Chambre d'accusation, Nov. 29, 1961, reported at (1963) 90(1) *Journal du Droit International* 719. Not only is this finding expressly based on a "mere reading" of Art. 16(2), rather than taking account of its context, object, and purpose, but the case could readily have been determined on the basis that Art. 16(2) relates to the right to bring or to defend proceedings, not to immunity from prosecution.

[1739] UNHCR nonetheless significantly overstates the challenge posed by the need to establish subject-matter jurisdiction when it opines that the "[p]rovisions [of the Convention] that define the legal status of refugees and their rights . . . have *no influence* on the process of determination of refugee status [emphasis added]": UNHCR, *Handbook*, at para. 12(ii). UNHCR provides no argument in support of this overly broad position which is, for reasons set out here, at odds with the general ambit of Art. 16(1) of the Convention. At least one court, however, has taken note of UNHCR's views on this subject: *Krishnapillai v. Minister of Citizenship and Immigration*, [2002] 3(1) FC 74 (Can. FCA, Dec. 6, 2001), at para. 26 – though it nonetheless proceeded to analyze whether Canadian refugee procedures met the Art. 16(1) standard: ibid. at paras. 30–32. See also *R v. Secretary of State for the Home Department, ex parte Jahangeer et al.*, [1993] Imm AR 564 (Eng. QBD, June 11, 1993).

law" adopted by the Human Rights Committee is quite broad,[1740] including matters such as a claim for a disability pension,[1741] an application to dissolve a labor contract,[1742] and professional conduct regulation.[1743] In line with this inclusive approach, an expert study approved by the Commission on Human Rights observed that

> Immigration hearings and deportation proceedings may be suits at law. The [UN Human Rights] Committee considered a Salvadoran's claim that Canada violated his right to a fair hearing in deportation proceedings. Canada argued that deportation proceedings were not suits at law and thus not subject to Article 14(1). The Committee did not accept Canada's argument and stated explicitly that such proceedings were suits at law.[1744]

[1740] "The *travaux préparatoires* do not resolve the apparent discrepancy in the various [official] language texts [of Art. 14(1)]. In the view of the Committee, the concept of a 'suit at law' . . . is based on the nature of the right in question rather than on the status of one of the parties (governmental, parastatal or autonomous statutory entities), or else on the particular forum in which individual legal systems may provide that the right in question is to be adjudicated upon": *YL v. Canada*, UNHRC Comm. No. 112/1981, decided Apr. 8, 1986, at para. 9.2; *Deisl v. Austria*, UNHRC Comm. No. 1060/2002, UN Doc. CCPR/C/81/D/1060/2002, decided Aug. 23, 2004, at para. 11.1. See also UN Human Rights Committee, "General Comment No. 13: Administration of justice" (1984), UN Doc. HRI/GEN/1/Rev.7, May 12, 2004, at 135, paras. 2, 4: "In general, the reports of States parties fail to recognize that article 14 applies not only to procedures for the determination of criminal charges against individuals but also to procedures to determine their rights and obligations in a suit at law . . . The provisions of article 14 apply to all courts and tribunals within the scope of that article, whether ordinary or specialized."

[1741] *YL v. Canada*, UNHRC Comm. No. 112/1981, decided Apr. 8, 1986.

[1742] *Van Meurs v. Netherlands*, UNHRC Comm. No. 215/1986, decided July 13, 1990.

[1743] *JL v. Australia*, UNHRC Comm. No. 491/1992, UN Doc. CCPR/C/45/D/491/1992, decided July 29, 1992. "[W]henever . . . a judicial body is entrusted with the task of deciding on the imposition of disciplinary measures, it must respect the guarantee of equality of all persons before the courts and tribunals as enshrined in article 14, paragraph 1, and the principles of impartiality, fairness and equality of arms implicit in this guarantee": *Perterer v. Austria*, UNHRC Comm. No. 1015/2001, UN Doc. CCPR/C/81/D/1015/2001, decided July 20, 2004, at para. 9.2.

[1744] UN Sub-Commission on Prevention of Discrimination and Protection of Minorities, "The Right to a Fair Trial: Current Recognition and Measures Necessary for its Strengthening," UN Doc. E/CN.4/Sub.2/1991/29, July 5, 1991, at para. 80, citing the decision of the Committee on Human Rights in *VMRB v. Canada*, decided July 18, 1988, Annex VIII.F. A follow-up report containing a draft Body of Principles to promote the right to a fair trial similarly indicated that because the relevant consideration is "the character of the rights at issue," the right to a fair trial inheres not just in the context of formal judicial action, but also in "proceedings before administrative tribunals": UN Sub-Commission on Prevention of Discrimination and Protection of Minorities, UN Doc. E/CN.4/Sub.2/1994/24, June 3, 1994, at Annex II, para. 74(b). More generally, the same follow-up report concluded that "[i]f a person's rights and obligations may be adversely affected in a suit at law or by particularized actions or inactions taken or

On the basis of this understanding, it would be difficult to conceive a reason to exclude a determination of entitlement to claim refugee rights from the ambit of Art. 14(1) scrutiny.[1745] This principled concern to ensure an effective means to vindicate Convention rights is similarly clear from an important decision of the English Court of Appeal which rejected the view that there is no duty to allow an appeal or review of the denial of refugee status simply because the person concerned would not in fact be at risk of *refoulement*:

> The Convention requires [state parties] to grant certain rights to refugees, who have fled from their home countries ... Refugees who arrive in this country are anxious to have their status as refugees established. This is not merely because recognition of their refugee status will carry with it the entitlement to remain here, but because it will ensure they are accorded Convention rights while they are here ... There is no doubt that this country is under an obligation under international law to enable those who are in truth refugees to exercise their Convention rights ...
>
> An interpretation of the Rules which permitted the Secretary of State to refuse asylum to a refugee on the ground that he had been granted [permission to remain] would ... be in conflict with the UK's obligations

proposed by a public authority, the court or the public authority shall give the person ... a fair and public hearing by a competent, independent and impartial tribunal established by law": ibid. at Annex II, para. 4. The expert reports by Special Rapporteurs Chernichenko and Treat were endorsed by the Sub-Commission in Res. 1994/35, Aug. 26, 1994; and subsequently by the Commission on Human Rights, UN Doc. E/CN.4/1997/2, Nov. 25, 1996, at para. 5.

[1745] While dismissing the claim on the merits, the Human Rights Committee's view that the Covenant requires that refugee claimants be afforded a fair hearing before an impartial tribunal is clear from its holding in *Adu v. Canada*, UNHRC Comm. No. 654/1995, UN Doc. CCPR/C/60/D/654/1995, decided July 18, 1997, at para. 6.3: "The author claims that the hearing was not fair, as one of the two Commissioners who participated was of Ghanaian origin and a member of the Ewe tribe whose hostile attitude towards Ghanaian refugees was said to be well known among members of the Ghanaian community in Montreal. However, neither the author nor his counsel raised objections to the participation of the Commissioner in the hearing until after the author's application for refugee status had been dismissed despite the fact that the grounds for bias were known to the author and/or his counsel at the beginning of the hearing. The Committee is therefore of the opinion that the author has failed to substantiate, for purposes of admissibility, his claim that his right to a fair hearing by an impartial tribunal was violated." Similarly, the Committee Against Torture determined in its review of Venezuela's compliance with that treaty that "[t]he State party should regulate procedures for dealing with and deciding on applications for asylum and refugee status which envisage the opportunity for the applicant to attend a formal hearing and to make such submissions as may be relevant to the right which he invokes, including pertinent evidence, with protection of the characteristics of due process of law": UN Committee Against Torture, "Concluding Observations on the Report of Venezuela," UN Doc. A/54/44 (1999), 16, at para. 147.

under the Convention in relation to the treatment of refugees living within this country.[1746]

While access itself is not specifically mentioned in Art. 14(1) of the Covenant, it is generally acknowledged to be inherent in the duty to ensure equality before courts and tribunals:

> If the right extends only to the conduct of an action which has already been initiated before a court, a state can do away with its courts, or transfer their jurisdiction to other bodies which do not possess the minimum attributes of a judicial tribunal. It is inconceivable that international human rights instruments should prescribe in detail the procedural guarantees afforded to parties in a pending proceeding without guaranteeing that which alone makes it possible for them to benefit from such guarantees. The fair, public and expeditious characteristics of a judicial proceeding are of no value at all if there is no judicial proceeding. Accordingly, the right to a fair trial embodies the "right to a court"; of which the right to institute proceedings, i.e. the right of access, constitutes one aspect.[1747]

Because Art. 14(1) rights inhere in "all persons" under a state's jurisdiction, apply to suits at law broadly conceived, and must be read to require access to a tribunal, the Australian attempt to avoid due process rights by the fictitious "excision" of parts of its territory is in breach of its duties under the Covenant. This conclusion is moreover consistent with the approach of the European Court of Human Rights in *Amuur v. France*,[1748] in which the Court ruled against the validity of a French law that purported to deny refugees access to protection by domestic courts in a so-called "international zone":

> Although by the force of circumstances the decision to order holding [of refugees seeking protection] must necessarily be taken by the administrative or police authorities, its prolongation requires speedy review by the courts, the traditional guardians of personal liberties.[1749]

[1746] *Saad v. Secretary of State for the Home Department*, [2001] EWCA Civ 2008 (Eng. CA, Dec. 19, 2001), per Lord Phillips MR at paras. 1, 2, 11, and 65. The approach of the European Union to this question comes close to meeting the requirements of international law. It is proposed that an appeal or review of the denial or withdrawal of refugee status need not be provided "[w]here an applicant has been granted a status, which offers the same rights and benefits under national and Community law as . . . refugee status": EU Procedures Directive, at Art. 38(5). Reliance on this provision would be lawful only if the rights and benefits "under national and Community law" are in fact no less generous than those which must be provided under the Refugee Convention.

[1747] Jayawickrama, *Judicial Application*, at 481–482.

[1748] [1996] ECHR 25 (ECHR, June 25, 1996).

[1749] *Amuur v. France*, [1996] ECHR 25 (ECHR, June 25, 1996), at para. 43. In the same case, the French Constitutional Council had opined on Feb. 25, 1992 that "the legislature must make appropriate provision for the courts to intervene, so that they may carry out

Despite the general importance of access to justice, reasonable limitations on access, particularly where these serve the broader purpose of ensuring access to courts and tribunals for all, are not inconsistent with Art. 14(1). But these limitations must not undermine the general right to have justiciable claims settled by a competent tribunal that meets the standards of Art. 14. As Jayawickrama observes,

> [w]hat counts is the sufficiency or insufficiency, the adequacy or inadequacy, of the room which the limitation leaves open in the beginning for the exercise of the right. The consistency of [a] limitation with the right depends upon the availability of an initial opportunity to exercise the right that amounts, *in all the circumstances characterizing the class of case in question, to a real and fair one* [emphasis added].[1750]

The flaw in the new British system of denying an appeal in the United Kingdom to refugee claimants from listed states is thus clear: the ability to appeal a negative status determination from within the very country where there is alleged to be a real risk of persecution is cold comfort to a genuine refugee, as it will expose him or her to the very threats which induced flight in the first instance.[1751] Nor can a rigid cut-off time for making an application or seeking review or appeal be reconciled to Art. 14(1). The facts in the Australian case of *Sahak* – where the failure to meet a filing deadline was the direct result of the circumstances of the applicant's detention and "was not due to any personal default"[1752] – illustrate vividly that an ironclad filing deadline is inherently incapable of taking account of the sort of individuated circumstances which must be considered in evaluating the existence of a real and fair ability to access a court or tribunal. On the other hand, there is no reason to contest the international legality of a fairly administered requirement to seek leave or permission to present one's case to a court. As the

---

their responsibilities and exercise the supervisory power conferred on them": ibid. at para. 21.

[1750] Jayawickrama, *Judicial Application*, at 483.

[1751] The UN Human Rights Committee has determined that "[t]he right to a fair trial in a suit at law, guaranteed under article 14, paragraph 1, may require that an individual be able to participate in person in court proceedings. In such circumstances the State party is under an obligation to allow that individual to be present at the hearing, even if the person is a non-resident alien": *Ben Said v. Norway*, UNHRC Comm. No. 767/1997, UN Doc. CCPR/C/68/D/767/1997, decided Mar. 20, 2000, at para. 11.3. In an earlier decision reached on admissibility grounds, however, the Committee denied that expulsion of a refugee claimant prior to the completion of an appeal procedure constituted a breach of the duty of non-discrimination under Art. 2 of the Covenant, noting simply that "it emerges from the author's own submission that he was given ample opportunity in formal proceedings, including oral hearings, to present his case for sojourn in the Netherlands": *MF v. Netherlands*, UNHRC Comm. No. 173/1984, decided Nov. 2, 1984, at para. 4.

[1752] See text above, at pp. 631–632.

Canadian Federal Court of Appeal helpfully observed in an analysis of Art. 16 of the Refugee Convention,

> Article 16 does not define a special procedure nor does it provide for special procedures for refugees. Quite to the contrary: in granting refugees the right to equal treatment before the courts, it implicitly recognizes that refugees are subject to the procedures available in the country in which [they reside]. Article 16 does not impose on the state the obligation to make available to refugees because they are refugees the most favorable procedures that can be put in place.
>
> There is no doubt that the right to apply for leave is a right of access to courts. Leave requirement is a usual procedure in Canadian law and it is, in Canadian terms, an accepted form of access to the courts of the country.[1753]

As the foregoing analysis suggests, the right of all persons seeking adjudication of a suit at law to go before a court or tribunal that meets the requirements of Art. 14 may be secured by way of appeal or review.[1754] There is therefore no objection to entrusting initial oversight of refugee rights to officials or an administrative body, so long as their actions are ultimately subject to scrutiny on the merits by a tribunal that meets the standards of Art. 14(1).[1755] But unless the initial decision is taken by a body which itself meets the requirements of Art. 14(1),[1756] the review or appellate tribunal must have "full jurisdiction. This includes the power to quash in all respects, on questions of fact and law, the decision of the administrative authority."[1757] The strong position taken on this question by the High Court of Australia, while framed as a matter of domestic constitutional law, is thus equally required by international human rights law.[1758] Because of this

---

[1753] *Krishnapillai v. Minister of Citizenship and Immigration*, [2002] 3(1) FC 74 (Can. FCA, Dec. 6, 2001), at paras. 31–32, per Décary JA.

[1754] "A rule that requires an [individual] to apply for and obtain leave before pursuing an appeal does not infringe his right of access to a court, particularly where if leave is refused, a petition procedure allows the [individual] to approach a higher court for a reassessment of the issues": Jayawickrama, *Judicial Application*, at 483.

[1755] For example, the Human Rights Committee found that Art. 14(1) had been complied with where entitlement to a disability pension was determined by the Canadian Pension Commission – said not to be impartial (as an executive branch of government, comprised entirely of civil servants) – so long as the decision reached was subject to "judicial supervision and control" by the Federal Court of Canada: *YL v. Canada*, UNHRC Comm. No. 112/1981, decided Apr. 8, 1986.

[1756] "[A]dministrative authorities that are largely independent and free of directives may, under certain circumstances, satisfy the requirements of a tribunal pursuant to Art. 14": Nowak, *ICCPR Commentary*, at 245.

[1757] Jayawickrama, *Judicial Application*, at 490, citing to decisions of the European Court of Human Rights on the cognate provision of the European Convention on Human Rights.

[1758] Interestingly, the only member of the High Court to comment on the relevance of international law, Justice Callinan, noted simply that "[d]espite the Universal requirement, the British proposal to avoid judicial review or appeal by mandatory removal to an extraterritorial processing site is unworkable as a matter of international law. The courts of the country ordering the removal would by virtue of Art. 14(1) be required to entertain applications for appeal or review of the administrative decision to expel them to the processing site, and the courts of any country in which processing occurs would be similarly bound with respect to reviewing a decision not to recognize refugee status.[1759]

The essential qualitative requirements of Art. 14(1) are, first, that the tribunal adjudicating entitlement to refugee rights be "established by law."[1760] The notion of "law" in this context is "to be understood in the strict sense of a general-abstract parliamentary law or an equivalent, unwritten norm of common law, which must be accessible to all persons subject to it [and which must] define the subject matter and territorial scope of [the tribunal's] jurisdiction."[1761] Second, and closely related, the tribunal must be "competent," meaning that its "jurisdiction has been previously established by law, and arbitrary action so avoided."[1762] Third, the tribunal must be independent. Particularly relevant in this regard are "the manner in which judges are appointed, the qualifications for appointment, and the duration of their terms of office; [as well as] the conditions governing promotion,

---

Declaration of Human Rights, itself still in many respects an aspirational rather than an effective and enforceable instrument, there is no unanimity throughout the world ... as to what claims, practices, benefits and values are deserving of protection": *S157/2002 v. Commonwealth of Australia*, [2003] HCA 2 (Aus. HC, Feb. 4, 2003). While these observations with respect to the legal authority of the Universal Declaration are certainly true (see chapter 1.2.3 above, at pp. 44–46), it is to be regretted that no reference was made in this judgment to the clearly binding standard set by Art. 14(1) of the Civil and Political Covenant.

[1759] Art. 16(1) of the Refugee Convention is also relevant, since it requires access by a refugee to the courts of any state party, not simply those of a state in which the refugee is resident: see text above, at p. 645.

[1760] Nowak's analysis implies that whatever court or tribunal is ultimately entrusted with the responsibility to determine or to oversee the enforcement of refugee rights must not be established solely for the benefit of refugees (or any other protected sub-population). Specifically, "[e]stablishing separate courts for the groups of persons listed in Art. 2(1) ... violates Art. 14": Nowak, *ICCPR Commentary*, at 239. While conceding the risk that a separate court or tribunal may be less subject to scrutiny and thus more inclined to fall below the requirements of Art. 14, it nonetheless seems to overstate the case to deem any separate tribunal to be *per se* discriminatory. There may very well be good reasons, e.g. relevant legal expertise, special access of applicants to interpreters, cross-cultural sensitivity on the part of decision-makers, etc., that argue in favor of a specialized adjudicative structure. The relevant issue should therefore not be separateness *per se*, but rather that the relevant tribunal delivers substantive equality of treatment. See generally chapter 2.5.5 above, at pp. 126–128.

[1761] Nowak, *ICCPR Commentary*, at 245.   [1762] Jayawickrama, *Judicial Application*, at 514.

transfer and cessation of [the decision-makers'] functions."[1763] Fourth, the tribunal must be impartial, meaning not only that its members are not personally prejudiced, but also that the tribunal itself is, and appears to be, disinterested in the outcome of the cases that come before it.[1764] In this regard, the Human Rights Committee has insisted on its need to be informed about "the actual independence of the judiciary from the executive branch and the legislative."[1765] As Nowak concludes, rights and obligations "are not to be heard and decided by political institutions or by administrative authorities subject to directives."[1766]

Beyond these structural qualities, the tribunal must be positioned to deliver a "fair and public hearing." First, access to a tribunal must be without undue delay.[1767] Second, there must be respect for principles of natural justice, including the rights to submit and to contest evidence, and to a hearing before the decision-maker.[1768] Third, the tribunal must ensure the principle of procedural equality between the parties, often referred to as "equality of arms."[1769] Fourth, there should be "a reasonable opportunity to present [one's] case – under conditions that do not place [the individual concerned] at a substantial disadvantage vis à vis his opponent, and to be represented by counsel for that purpose."[1770] Respect for this principle may, for example, require the provision of an interpreter.[1771] Fifth, the hearing

---

[1763] UN Human Rights Committee, "General Comment No. 13: Administration of justice" (1984), UN Doc. HRI/GEN/1/Rev.7, May 12, 2004, at 135, para. 3. The Supreme Court of Canada has defined three essential conditions for judicial independence. These are security of tenure, financial security, and institutional independence: *Valente v. R*, [1985] 2 SCR 673 (Can. SC, Dec. 19, 1985).

[1764] See by way of analogy the decision of the European Court of Human Rights in *Gregory v. United Kingdom*, (1997) 25 EHRR 577 (ECHR, Feb. 25, 1997).

[1765] UN Human Rights Committee, "General Comment No. 13: Administration of justice" (1984), UN Doc. HRI/GEN/1/Rev.7, May 12, 2004, at 135, para. 3.

[1766] Nowak, *ICCPR Commentary*, at 244.

[1767] *Muñoz v. Peru*, UNHRC Comm. No. 203/1986, decided Nov. 4, 1988, at para. 11.3. Jayawickrama notes that the European Court of Human Rights has held that not even "chronic overload" justifies a violation of the duty for expeditious access to a tribunal: Jayawickrama, *Judicial Application*, at 508.

[1768] See the individual opinion of members Cooray, Dimitrijevic, and Lallah in *Muñoz v. Peru*, UNHRC Comm. No. 203/1986, decided Nov. 4, 1988, at para. 3.

[1769] In *Robinson v. Jamaica*, UNHRC Comm. No. 223/1987, decided Mar. 30, 1989, a violation of Art. 14 was found when adjournments were granted to the government, but not to the accused person: ibid. at para. 104.

[1770] Jayawickrama, *Judicial Application*, at 507.

[1771] *Guesdon v. France*, UNHRC Comm. No. 219/1986, decided July 25, 1990, at para. 10.2; *Cadoret and Bihan v. France*, UNHRC Comm. Nos. 221/1987 and 323/1988, decided Apr. 11, 1991, at para. 5.6. The Canadian Federal Court of Appeal presumed that the right to an interpreter may also be grounded in Art. 16(1) of the Refugee Convention. "Items such as free assistance of an interpreter are contemplated by the use of the word must be public "in the interest of the individual and of society at large."[1772] While some circumstances may justify all or part of a hearing not being open to the public, "even in cases in which the public is excluded from the trial, the judgement must, with certain strictly defined exceptions, be made public."[1773]

Because national security and other exceptional concerns are only listed as the basis for the exclusion of the press and the public, they cannot be invoked to justify a wholesale violation of multiple aspects of the due process rights guaranteed by Art. 14(1). The breadth of the American departures from accepted norms in refusing the asylum requests of Iraqis on the basis of completely secret evidence, described above, is thus presumptively invalid. Indeed, as the European Court of Human Rights made clear in its decision of *Chahal v. United Kingdom*, national security concerns cannot be allowed to run roughshod over the right to a fair hearing before a court:

> The Court recognises that the use of confidential material may be unavoidable where national security is at stake. This does not mean, however, that the national authorities can be free from effective control by the domestic courts whenever they choose to assert that national security and terrorism are involved ... The Court attaches significance to the fact that, as the interveners pointed out ... in Canada a more effective form of judicial control has been developed in cases of this type. This example illustrates that there are techniques which can be employed which both accommodate legitimate security concerns about the nature and sources of intelligence information and yet accord the individual a substantial measure of procedural justice.[1774]

It remains, however, that reliance upon access to the general courts is not an entirely satisfactory means of enabling refugees to bring their internationally derived rights to bear. Most fundamentally, not all courts have subject-matter jurisdiction over international treaties: it may be the case that neither the Refugee Convention nor the Civil and Political Covenant is directly enforceable at the suit of the refugee himself or herself. Particularly in common law countries, courts may therefore be able to take account of international law only indirectly by reliance on principles of statutory

'including' in that paragraph": *Krishnapillai v. Minister of Citizenship and Immigration*, [2002] 3(1) FC 74 (Can. FCA, Dec. 6, 2001), at para. 30.

[1772] UN Human Rights Committee, "General Comment No. 13: Administration of justice" (1984), UN Doc. HRI/GEN/1/Rev.7, May 12, 2004, at 135, para. 6.

[1773] Ibid. at para. 6. The reasons for excluding the public from a hearing are set out in Art. 14(1) of the Civil and Political Covenant, namely "reasons of morals, public order (*ordre public*) or national security in a democratic society, or when the interest of the private lives of the parties so requires, or to the extent strictly necessary in the opinion of the court in special circumstances where publicity would prejudice the interests of justice": ibid.

[1774] *Chahal v. United Kingdom*, (1996) 23 EHRR 413 (ECHR, Nov. 15, 1996), at para. 131.

interpretation, unless the treaty has in some sense been domesticated by the state party.[1775] In addition, litigation is often a very expensive process. While the drafters of the Refugee Convention did ultimately agree to help refugees overcome some of the practical impediments to accessing the courts (including by assimilating them to nationals for purposes of the duty to post security for costs, and under legal aid schemes), these more sophisticated rights are reserved for refugees who have established habitual residence in a state party.[1776]

[1775] See e.g. D. Bederman, *International Law Frameworks* (2001), at 151 ff.
[1776] See chapter 6.8 below.

Rights of refugees lawfully present

As the degree of attachment between a refugee and a state party increases, so too do the rights which the refugee may claim. All of the rights acquired by simple physical presence – to enter and remain in the asylum state; freedom from arbitrary detention or penalization for illegal entry; protection of physical security; access to the necessities of life; protection of property; respect for family unity; free exercise of thought, conscience, and religion; access to basic education; documentation of identity and status; and to benefit from administrative assistance and access to the courts – continue for the duration of refugee status. But once a refugee is not only in fact under the jurisdiction of a state party to the Convention, but also *lawfully present* in that country, he or she acquires three additional rights.

First, a refugee who is lawfully present enjoys both substantive and procedural protections against expulsion. These guarantees govern any effort to remove the refugee to any country, and are in addition to the right not to be sent to a country in which there is a risk of being persecuted.[1]

Second, lawfully present refugees enjoy a presumptive right to freedom of internal movement. As previously observed, the Refugee Convention grants states only a limited prerogative to detain a person seeking refugee status until his or her identity is established, basic security concerns are investigated, and the asylum-seeker's cooperation is secured for purposes of conducting all necessary investigations into his or her claim to protection. Once these concerns have been addressed, the refugee's presence has been regularized in the receiving state, and refugee-specific restrictions on freedom of movement must come to an end.[2]

Third and finally, refugees who are lawfully present are explicitly entitled to engage in self-employment. While permission to engage in employment or professional practice may be withheld until the refugee is authorized to remain in the asylum state (for example, consequent to the formal recognition of refugee status), mere lawful presence entitles the refugee to engage in independent income-generating activities. This right is a pragmatic means by

---

[1] See chapter 4.1 above.   [2] See chapter 4.2.4 above, at pp. 415–419.

which to allow refugees to fund their own necessities of life,[3] but without thereby sanctioning integration into the more organized structures of the asylum state's economic life.

As addressed earlier,[4] a refugee is lawfully present in any of three circumstances. First, a refugee is lawfully present for the duration of any period of time for which his or her admission is authorized, even if only for a few hours.[5] Second, and of greater contemporary relevance, a refugee is lawfully present while his or her claim to refugee status is being verified, including the time required for exhaustion of any appeals or reviews.[6] Third, a refugee is lawfully present if the reception state opts not to verify his or her refugee status, including when formal status determination procedures are suspended in favor of so-called temporary protection regimes.[7]

It is important briefly to repeat the logic behind this critical third point. Simply put, a government cannot avoid its duty to grant refugees the benefit of rights which accrue upon "lawful presence" by refusing to admit them to a lawful procedure to verify their claims to be refugees.[8] While a state may decide that it does not wish, either generally or as an exceptional measure, to engage in formal status assessment, that decision not to authenticate refugee status exists against the backdrop of the government's legal duty to grant Convention rights to all persons in its territory who are in fact refugees, whether or not their status has been assessed. The nature of those rights increases as the refugee's attachment to the receiving state increases over time.[9]

The fundamental expectation that a refugee will either be resettled or have his or her status somehow normalized in the receiving state is particularly clear from the text of Art. 31(2) of the Refugee Convention. This article authorizes host states to impose constraints on a refugee's freedom of movement only "until their status in the country is regularized or they obtain admission into another country."[10] But if no inquiry is ever undertaken into refugee status, a refugee will never be able to escape what are expressly stated to be purely provisional constraints.[11] As such, the state's legal obligation to implement its treaty duties in good faith can be reconciled to its decision not to assess refugee status only if the latter decision does not prejudice

---

[3] See chapter 4.4 above.   [4] See chapter 3.1.3 above.

[5] See chapter 3.1.3 above, at p. 174.   [6] See chapter 3.1.3 above, at pp. 175–183.

[7] See chapter 3.1.3 above, at pp. 183–185.   [8] See chapter 3.1.3 above, at pp. 184–185.

[9] See generally chapter 3.1 above.   [10] See chapter 4.2.4 above.

[11] The logic of this system led the European Court of Human Rights to hold that a person claiming to be a refugee has "the right to gain effective access to the procedure for determining refugee status": *Amuur v. France*, [1996] ECHR 25 (ECHR, June 25, 1996), at para. 43. While not precisely true, this conclusion would nonetheless be accurate in those states which condition access to refugee rights on a formal process of refugee status determination.

enjoyment by the refugee claimant, at least on a provisional basis, of those rights that require no more than lawful presence. As Grahl-Madsen has explained,

> It has never been envisaged that there should be any group of under-privileged refugees, subject to the whims of the authorities. Quite to the contrary, so many of the provisions of the Refugee Convention ... are based on the appreciation of the very special situation of refugees ... as aliens incapable of gaining admission to any other country than the one in which they find themselves ... After a time, the humanitarian considerations underlying the Refugee Convention and similar instruments must be held to override other considerations of a more traditional legal nature.[12]

5.1 Protection from expulsion

During the early part of the twentieth century, refugees allowed to enter an asylum state nonetheless often found themselves vulnerable to expulsion on grounds that they had committed even minor criminal offenses, or were deemed "public charges" because they were unable to meet their own needs due to indigence or ill health. As Grahl-Madsen describes the problem,

> [I]t became the habit of certain States to expel refugees ... and to push those so expelled across the frontier to a neighbouring country. This practice caused considerable hardship to the refugees, who were often pushed back and forth between two or more countries and punished each time for illegal entry, but it also caused considerable inconvenience for the countries into whose territory the expelled refugees were sent in the first place. It [was] therefore quite natural that expulsion of refugees became a matter of concern to the international community. The question has been dealt with in all international instruments relating to the status of refugees [since 1928].[13]

In essence, the concern is that unlike other aliens, refugees subject to expulsion generally have no safe place to go. Yet this principled concern has continued to run up against the determination of some states to rid themselves of refugees whose continued presence is adjudged incompatible with their own interests.

For example, the United Kingdom authorizes the Secretary of State for the Home Department to expel an alien whose continued presence is not conducive to the public good. In reliance on this authority, the British government attempted to expel an Indian Sikh refugee believed to have supported terrorist activities,[14] and to force a Saudi asylum-seeker whose activities

---

[12] A. Grahl-Madsen, *The Status of Refugees in International Law* (vol. II, 1972) (Grahl-Madsen, *Status of Refugees II*), at 442–443.

[13] A. Grahl-Madsen, *Commentary on the Refugee Convention 1951* (1963, pub'd. 1997) (Grahl-Madsen, *Commentary*), at 185–186.

[14] *Chahal v. United Kingdom*, (1996) 23 EHRR 413 (ECHR, Nov. 15, 1996).

threatened British commercial interests to accept residence on the Caribbean island of Dominica.[15] Canadian courts have sanctioned the expulsion of, for example, a Chilean refugee convicted in Canada of sexually assaulting two young teenagers.[16] On the basis of secret testimony provided to its security police, Sweden authorized the Egyptian government to send a plane to its territory to take away two Egyptian refugees believed to be involved with international terrorism. Ahmed Hussein Agaiza had been sentenced by Egypt in absentia for having taken part in an attack on the Egyptian embassy in Pakistan, while Muhammad Zari faced a long term of imprisonment in that country for membership of an Islamic terrorist group. Both men denied the charges, but were granted no hearing before removal.[17]

Among the states of the developed world, however, Australia has traditionally pursued the expulsion of refugees on the most systematic basis. The Federal Court has endorsed a general right of the government to expel asylum-seekers to any non-persecutory country willing to admit and to protect them. On the basis of domestic legislation mandating the protection not of refugees, but instead only of persons to whom Australia owes a duty of protection, it has until the recent intervention of the High Court been accepted that even claimants who clearly meet the Convention refugee definition may legitimately be removed to any state so long as there is no real chance of *refoulement* from that country back to the asylum-seeker's own state.[18]

---

[15] "The British government ... bowed to pressure from the Saudi regime, the United States government and British arms companies when it ordered the deportation of Saudi Arabia's most prominent dissident to a tiny Caribbean island. Mohammed al-Mas'ari, leader of the influential London-based Islamic opposition group, the Committee for the Defence of Legitimate Rights – who last year applied for political asylum in Britain – was given 10 days to appeal against his removal to Dominica ... Mr. Mas'ari's removal would be an enormous relief to the Foreign Office, which has found his presence in Britain an embarrassment in relations with Saudi Arabia, a key export market and political ally in the region": S. Milne and I. Black, "UK bows to pressure over dissident," *Guardian Weekly*, Jan. 14, 1996, at 1. But the Chief Immigration Adjudicator overturned the deportation order, citing concerns about his safety in Dominica and the inappropriateness of the government's decision to refuse to consider his refugee claim: S. Milne, "Mas'ari's victory humiliates Howard," *Guardian Weekly*, Mar. 17, 1996, at 9.

[16] *Barrera v. Canada*, (1992) 99 DLR 4th 264 (Can. FCA, Dec. 14, 1992).

[17] P. Finn, "Europe tossing terror suspects out the door," *Washington Post*, Jan. 29, 2002, at A-01.

[18] This understanding of Convention duties derives from a series of decisions applying the judgment of the Full Federal Court in *Minister for Immigration and Multicultural Affairs v. Thiyagarajah*, (1997) 80 FCR 543 (Aus. FFC, Dec. 19, 1997), now incorporated in s. 36 of the Australian Migration Act. That body of law has been summarized as being "to the effect that, where a country other than the country of the claimant for refugee status, and other than Australia, would provide for that applicant effective protection, the person is not a person to whom Australia owes protection obligations": *Al Toubi v. Minister for Immigration and Multicultural Affairs*, [2001] FCA 1381 (Aus. FFC, Sept. 28, 2001). The High Court of Australia has recently determined, however, that Australia owes

More recently, the Australian government has implemented its so-called "Pacific Solution," under which many persons wishing to seek refugee status in Australia may be expelled from its territorial waters or contiguous zone to neighboring countries which, in exchange for often substantial development assistance and other payments, agree to receive them. This program began with the expulsion of several hundred Afghan and other refugee claimants who sought to enter Australian waters aboard the *KM Palapa I* in late August 2001. Some particularly vulnerable individuals were admitted to New Zealand's refugee status determination procedure, but the majority were taken aboard an Australian naval vessel to the tiny and impoverished island nation of Nauru. That country agreed to admit them for status verification by UNHCR and eventual resettlement in exchange for a payment of A$10 million worth of fuel, A$3 million for new generators, the cancellation of A$1 million worth of hospital bills run up by Nauruans in Australia, refurbishment of the island's sports oval, and the provision of sporting and educational scholarships for Nauruans to come to Australia.[19]

The expulsion of refugees in the less developed world is regrettably both more common and even less likely to be carried out under formal legal procedures. For example, many refugees were among the thousands of Rwandans "chased" from Uganda in an outbreak of anti-Rwandan hostility in 1982–1983. Arguing that "Uganda was for Ugandans," local government officials instigated public antipathy through accusations that Rwandans had displaced locals economically, engaged in cattle thefts, participated in paramilitary groups, and supported anti-government guerrillas.[20] Relying on

"protection obligations" to any person in Australia who meets the definition of a refugee, not simply to those refugees who cannot safely be sent elsewhere: *NAGV and NAGW of 2002 v. Minister for Immigration and Multicultural and Indigenous Affairs*, [2005] HCA 6 (Aus. HC, Mar. 2, 2005), at paras. 29, 33, 42, 47. The joint reasons of six members of the High Court expressly invited the Federal Court to reconsider the approach previously adopted in *Thiyagarajah*: ibid. at paras. 52–53. In his separate opinion, Justice Kirby moreover emphasized that the traditional Australian approach renders the entitlement of refugees "hostage to arrangements purportedly made affecting their nationality by countries with which they may have no real connection. It ... shift[s] obligations clearly imposed by international law to contingencies that, in some cases, may be imponderable": ibid. at para. 93.

19 P. Barkham, "Paradise lost awaits asylum-seekers," *The Guardian*, Sept. 11, 2001, at 3. Australia subsequently entered into negotiations with Papua New Guinea and Kiribati to receive interdicted refugees for processing: K. Lawson, "PNG next in line to process Australia-bound refugees," *Canberra Times*, Oct. 11, 2001, at A-1. See generally J. Hathaway, "Refugee Law is Not Immigration Law," (2002) *Proceedings of the Canadian Council on International Law* 134, edited version reprinted in US Committee for Refugees, *World Refugee Survey 2002* (2002), at 38; and P. Mathew, "Australian Refugee Protection in the Wake of the *Tampa*," (2002) 96(3) *American Journal of International Law* 661.

20 E. Khiddu-Makubuya, *International Academy of Comparative Law National Report for Uganda* (1994), at 14.

security agreements signed with countries such as Tunisia and Iran, Turkey rounded up and expelled hundreds of non-European refugees, including many recognized by UNHCR and awaiting resettlement.[21] In the aftermath of the first Gulf War, Kuwait ordered the expulsion of foreigners from countries deemed sympathetic to Iraq, including Palestinian and Iraqi refugees; it was reported that "even those who were cleared of charges without trial or were acquitted by martial law courts [were] deported."[22] In 1990, Kenyan President Moi ordered Rwandan, Ugandan, and "all refugees engaged in illegal activities" to leave the country. Police and "youth wingers" swept through major towns, indiscriminately arresting refugees and confiscating their property. Without being granted access to lawyers, trainloads of refugees were shipped to the Ugandan border and handed over to that country's security officials.[23] In 1997, soldiers of the Democratic Republic of Congo summarily expelled hundreds of Rwandan and Burundian refugees who had been awaiting processing of their claims at UNHCR's Kisangani transit camp.[24] And in 2002, Kenyan authorities threatened summarily to repatriate hundreds of Ethiopian and Somali refugees rounded up in a police sweep of Nairobi.[25]

Particularly in Africa, the expulsion of refugees is often linked to fear that their presence will embroil the host state in armed conflict, or retaliatory attack. For example, the threat of military attacks from *apartheid*-era South Africa led some neighboring countries, including Botswana, Mozambique, and Swaziland, to expel South African refugees. As Mtango observed, "because of their inability to defend themselves [from armed attack by South Africa], they [were] inclined instead to return refugees to South Africa or force them to seek resettlement in other countries."[26] Beginning in 1992, Nigerian officials began arresting and expelling Chadian refugees on the grounds that they were using northeastern Nigeria as a base for launching attacks on Chad. The Nigerian government adduced no evidence of rebel

---

[21] "In April 1996, [Turkey and Iran] reportedly signed an agreement stipulating the reciprocal exchange of opposition activists. The information available to Amnesty International indicates that after signing of this agreement, the numbers of Iranian asylum-seekers sent back to Iran increased sharply": Amnesty International, "Turkey: *Refoulement* of Non-European Refugees: A Protection Crisis" (1997). Turkey has also relied on new readmission treaties to return persons seeking refugee status to such states as Iraq and Syria: US Committee for Refugees, *World Refugee Survey 2002* (2002), at 251.

[22] Middle East Watch, "A Victory Turned Sour: Human Rights in Kuwait Since Liberation" (1991), at 43.

[23] Africa Watch, "Kenya: Illegal Expulsion of More than 1000 Refugees," Dec. 11, 1990, at 1–5.

[24] UNHCR, "UNHCR condemns refugee expulsion from ex-Zaïre," Press Release, Sept. 4, 1997.

[25] Human Rights Watch, "Kenyan Government Sweep of Foreigners Puts Refugees at Risk," June 8, 2002.

[26] E. Mtango, "Military and Armed Attacks on Refugee Camps," in G. Loescher and L. Monahan eds., *Refugees and International Relations* 92 (1990), at 95. See also J. Molefi, "Few Safe Havens for Apartheid's Exiles," 29(1) *Africa Report* 14, at 15.

activity by the refugees, however, and denied the refugees a public trial and access to legal representation.[27] And in the early months of 2001, Zimbabwean police ordered the expulsion of some thirty Central African refugees suspected of being rebels from the Democratic Republic of Congo sent to assassinate senior Zimbabwean officials, including President Mugabe.[28]

Refugee Convention, Art. 32   Expulsion

1. The Contracting States shall not expel a refugee lawfully in their territory save on grounds of national security or public order.

2. The expulsion of such a refugee shall be only in pursuance of a decision reached in accordance with due process of law. Except where compelling reasons of national security otherwise require, the refugee shall be allowed to submit evidence to clear himself, and to appeal to and be represented for the purpose before competent authority or a person or persons specially designated by the competent authority.

3. The Contracting States shall allow such a refugee a reasonable period within which to seek legal admission into another country. The Contracting States reserve the right to apply during that period such internal measures as they may deem necessary.

Civil and Political Covenant, Art. 13

An alien lawfully in the territory of a State Party to the present Covenant may be expelled therefrom only in pursuance of a decision reached in accordance with law and shall, except where compelling reasons of national security otherwise require, be allowed to submit the reasons against his expulsion and to have his case reviewed by, and be represented for the purpose before, the competent authority or a person or persons especially designated by the competent authority.

When a refugee first arrives in search of protection, he or she enjoys a very limited right of non-return. At this stage, the only safeguards which an unauthorized asylum-seeker may claim derive from the duty of *non-refoulement* set by Art. 33,[29] and the right to be exempted from arbitrary detention and from penalties for unlawful entry pursuant to Art. 31.[30] These duties do not necessarily preclude a state party from expelling a refugee claimant from its territory during the earliest phases of refugee reception.[31] Governments are then only barred from

---

[27] P. Tiao and Nigerian Civil Liberties Organization, "The Status of Refugee Rights in Nigeria" (1992) (Tiao, "Refugee Rights in Nigeria"), at 23–25.

[28] *Independent Online* (Harare), Feb. 1, 2001.   [29] See chapter 4.1 above.

[30] See chapter 4.2 above.

[31] See chapter 4.2.3 above.

effecting expulsion which is at odds with the duty of *non-refoulement*, inter-preted in the light of the Convention's context, object, and purpose. As previously described, this means that there must be no real chance that the expulsion will lead, directly or indirectly, to the refugee being persecuted, or of being denied such international rights as he or she may already have acquired.[32] Where these requirements are met, a refugee whose presence is not yet lawful – for example, because he or she has yet to apply for recognition of refugee status, or to comply with the formalities necessary to that end – may be expelled to another country. It would thus be possible in principle to design a system that pursues goals akin to those of Australia's "Pacific Solution" without breaching the Refugee Convention.[33]

As this discussion makes clear, an appreciation of the continuing relevance of the duty of *non-refoulement* is essential to understanding Art. 32's constraints on the expulsion of lawfully present refugees. The duties of *non-refoulement* and non-expulsion were never conceived as mutually exclu-sive; indeed, they were originally proposed as two aspects of a common obligation.[34] Thus, in describing the protection that refugees lawfully present would receive by virtue of Art. 32's protection against expulsion, the American representative referred to it as a "supplement" to the duty of *non-refoulement*.[35] Israel similarly insisted that the foundation for discussion

---

[32] See chapter 4.1.2 above, at pp. 322–335.

[33] A more detailed discussion of the requirements for lawful implementation of such a regime is found at chapter 4.1.2 above, at pp. 327–333.

[34] See United Nations, "Memorandum by the Secretary-General to the Ad Hoc Committee on Statelessness and Related Problems," UN Doc. E/AC.32/2, Jan. 3, 1950 (Secretary-General, "Memorandum"), at 45. This approach was modeled on Art. 3 of the 1933 Convention, under which each state party agreed to protect refugees against efforts "to remove or keep [them] from its territory by application of police measures, such as expulsion or non-admittance at the frontier (*refoulement*)": Convention relating to the International Status of Refugees, 159 LNTS 3663, done Oct. 28, 1933, entered into force June 13, 1935 (1933 Refugee Convention). The decision to separate the duties of *non-refoulement* and non-expulsion into separate articles was reached by the Ad Hoc Committee without clear explanation. It may, however, have followed from the decision to broaden the class of persons entitled to protection against *refoulement* to encompass all refugees, including those not yet admitted to an asylum country (in contrast to the more limited beneficiary class for protection against expulsion): see "Report of the Ad Hoc Committee on Statelessness and Related Problems," UN Doc. E/1618, Feb. 17, 1950 (Ad Hoc Committee, "First Session Report"), at Annex II. The British representative, for example, had made clear that "the notion of *refoulement* could apply to (a) refugees seeking admission, (b) refugees illegally present in a country, and (c) refugees admitted temporarily or conditionally": Statement of Sir Leslie Brass of the United Kingdom, Doc. E/AC.32/SR.21, Feb. 2, 1950, at 5.

[35] Statement of Mr. Henkin of the United States, UN Doc. E/AC.32/SR.20, Feb. 1, 1950, at 12. "Whatever the case might be, whether or not the refugee was in a regular position, he must not be turned back to a country where his life or freedom could be threatened. No consideration of public order should be allowed to overrule that guarantee, for if the State

of the duty of non-expulsion was that "[t]he Committee had already settled the humanitarian question of sending any refugee whatever back to a territory where his life or liberty might be in danger."[36] The official comments of states on the Ad Hoc Committee's draft are equally clear. Both the Chilean and British governments argued for a generous interpretation of the scope of permissible expulsion precisely because the duty of *non-refoulement* had already limited their removal options.[37] And perhaps most emphatically, the Canadian representative to the Conference of Plenipotentiaries (and former chairman of the Ad Hoc Committee) affirmed that "the exercise of [expulsion] powers would be tempered with compassion, and never be at variance with the spirit of the Convention or with the terms of article [33], which related to the prohibition of expulsion to territories where the life or freedom of a refugee was threatened."[38] Because the duty of *non-refoulement* is not displaced once a refugee is lawfully present in a state party, even a state which has entered a reservation to Art. 32 cannot expel a refugee without consideration of the consequences of that act. Thus, while Uganda's purported reservation of its "unfettered right to expel any refugee in [its] territory" means that it did not violate Art. 32 when it "chased" Rwandans back to their country of origin, its actions were nonetheless in breach of Art. 33.[39]

concerned wished to get rid of the refugee at all costs, it could send him to another country or place him in an internment camp": ibid.

[36] Statement of Mr. Robinson of Israel, ibid. at 13. See also Statement of Mr. Guerreiro of Brazil, UN Doc. E/AC.32/SR.21, Feb. 2, 1950, at 7, who felt that amendment of Art. 32 to establish protections against expulsion to persecution was not necessary because the duty of *non-refoulement* "covered the fundamental aspect of the problem and its provisions were applicable to all refugees."

[37] "It should also be taken into consideration that Article [33] limits the countries to which the expelled person may be sent, since it provides, and rightly so, that he may not be expelled to countries where he might be persecuted for political, social, or religious reasons": United Nations, "Compilation of the Comments of Governments and Specialized Agencies on the Report of the Ad Hoc Committee on Statelessness and Related Problems," UN Doc. E/AC.32/L.40, Aug. 10, 1950 (United Nations, "Compilation of Comments"), at 55 (Chile). See also comments of the British government, which made clear that it sought greater operational flexibility in relation to expulsion only "[i]n any case where a refugee is returnable to a country where he has no reason to fear persecution": ibid. at 57.

[38] Statement of Mr. Chance of Canada, UN Doc. A/CONF.2/SR.15, July 11, 1951, at 8.

[39] This is in fact acknowledged in the text of Uganda's reservation, which provides that "[w]ithout recourse to legal process the Government of the Republic of Uganda shall, in the public interest, have the unfettered right to expel any refugee in her territory and may at any time apply such internal measures as the Government may deem necessary in the circumstances; so however that, any action taken by the Government of the Republic of Uganda in this regard shall not operate to the prejudice of the provisions of article 33 of this Convention": available at www.unhcr.ch (accessed Nov. 19, 2004). Blay and Tsamenyi argue further that summary expulsion by Uganda violates Art. 16(1) of the Convention requiring that refugees have access to the courts of law of all state parties: S. Blay and M. Tsamenyi, "Reservations and Declarations under the 1951 Convention and the 1967 Protocol relating to the Status of Refugees," (1990) 2(4) *International Journal of Refugee Law* 527 (Blay and Tsamenyi, "Reservations"), at 544–545.

As originally conceived, this supplementary protection against expulsion was to be granted only to refugees who were "authorized to reside regularly in the territory" of a state party.[40] If subject to this level of attachment, protection against expulsion would inhere only in refugees who benefit from some form of officially sanctioned, ongoing presence in a state party; refugees undergoing status verification and those present only for a limited period of time would, for example, be excluded from the beneficiary class.[41] The drafters of Art. 32, however, opted to delete the requirement for refugees to be residing in a state party in order to benefit from protection against expulsion. Instead, Art. 32 rights now inhere in all refugees "lawfully in [a state party's] territory," which includes those undergoing status verification, admitted for a set period of time, or whose claim to refugee status the asylum state has opted not to assess.[42]

The change seems to have been motivated by an effort to bring Art. 32 into line with the draft version of Art. 13 of the Civil and Political Covenant, which proposed granting a less robust form of protection against expulsion to all non-citizens who are "lawfully in the territory of a State Party."[43] The Report of the Ad Hoc Committee's first session made the change to grant Art. 32 protection to refugees "lawfully in their territory,"[44] with only a footnoted explanation citing the language proposed by the Commission on Human Rights for the draft Covenant.[45] At the Conference of Plenipotentiaries, the Swedish representative made reference to the "difficulty" of extending protection against expulsion to all refugees lawfully in a state's territory:

> What criterion would in fact be applied to decide whether a refugee was indeed lawfully in a territory? Sweden distinguished between aliens to whom a right of establishment had been granted, and aliens possessing only a right of temporary residence. The question did not arise in respect of the former, but, in respect of the latter, the Swedish Government wished to be able to expel them if it so decided when the authorization granted to them expired.[46]

Yet because a temporarily admitted refugee whose authorization to remain has expired is clearly no longer lawfully present in the state party,[47] the fact that no amendment was made to Art. 32 to accommodate the Swedish concern is not necessarily probative of the scope of the beneficiary class. This intervention does make clear, however, that the drafters were on notice that the language of Art. 32 could be construed to include refugees who had not been granted permission to stay in the asylum state.

---

[40] Secretary-General, "Memorandum," at 45.   [41] See chapter 3.1.4 above.
[42] See chapter 3.1.3 above.   [43] Civil and Political Covenant, at Art. 13.
[44] Ad Hoc Committee, "First Session Report," at Annex I.   [45] Ibid. at Annex II.
[46] Statement of Mr. Petren of Sweden, UN Doc. A/CONF.2/SR.14, July 10, 1951, at 21.
[47] See chapter 3.1.3 above, at pp. 185–186.

The most significant indication that Art. 32's beneficiary class should be broadly interpreted occurred on second reading of the Convention at the Conference of Plenipotentiaries. The Swedish delegate this time pointed out the inconsistency between the English language title of Art. 32 ("Expulsion of refugees lawfully admitted") and the French language equivalent, which used the phrase "résidant régulièrement au pays d'accueil." Referring to an earlier decision of the Style Committee which had defined the equivalent English and French language terms for the various levels of attachment,[48] Mr. Petren observed that the English title did not correspond to the French title (indeed, "lawfully admitted" had not been accepted by the Style Committee at all as a relevant term of art).[49] Acknowledging the discrepancy, the Conference deleted the reference to the level of attachment in Art. 32's title without making any change to the corresponding language of the text.[50] Art. 32 was therefore approved on the basis that protection against expulsion inheres in refugees "lawfully in their territory" (in French, "se trouvant régulièrement sur leur territoire"). Because this vote was taken immediately after attention had been drawn by the Swedish delegate to the fact that the personal scope of Art. 32 required clarification, with explicit reference to the fact that being "lawfully in the territory" implies a lesser attachment to the asylum state than does "lawfully staying in the territory,"[51] it is difficult to imagine that there was any doubt among the drafters about the significance of the Conference's decision.[52]

There is, moreover, a particular logic to interpreting Art. 32 so as to grant protection against expulsion to refugees who are awaiting the results of their status verification inquiry. Because such persons have by definition complied with the host state's legal requirements and have not been finally determined to fall outside the Convention refugee definition, allowing them to remain in the country pending the results of the inquiry seems very much a matter of basic fairness. This can be seen, for example, against the backdrop of the

---

[48] "Draft Convention relating to the Status of Refugees, Report of the Style Committee," UN Doc. A/CONF.2/102, July 24, 1951, at para. 5.

[49] Statement of Mr. Petren of Sweden, UN Doc. A/CONF.2/SR.35, July 25, 1951, at 20.

[50] The vote in favor was 21–0 (1 abstention): ibid.

[51] "Draft Convention relating to the Status of Refugees, Report of the Style Committee," UN Doc. A/CONF.2/102, July 24, 1951, at para. 5. The attention of delegates was expressly drawn to this report immediately prior to the vote on Art. 32: Statement of Mr. Petren of Sweden, UN Doc. A/CONF.2/SR.35, July 25, 1951, at 20.

[52] See G. Stenberg, *Non-Expulsion and Non-Refoulement* (1989) (Stenberg, *Non-Expulsion*), at 92: "Based on the fact that the drafters intended that a refugee should be regarded as lawfully in the territory regardless of the period of time for which his sojourn has been authorized it may nevertheless tentatively be submitted that neither did the drafters intend that protection in accordance with Article 32 should be extended only to those whose refugee status had already been recognized by the expelling State and not to those refugees whose status had not yet been recognized."

Democratic Republic of Congo's refusal to respect the duty of non-expulsion in the case of the Rwandan and Burundian refugees awaiting processing of their claims by UNHCR at the Kisangani refugee camp: it surely offended basic norms of fairness to deny interim protection against removal to these persons simply because the formalities of status verification had yet to be completed.

In insisting upon this interpretation, it is important to remember that asylum states genuinely unable to cope with refugee arrivals always retain the option under Art. 33 initially to redirect those refugees to other states where their acquired rights will be respected, and in which there is no direct or indirect risk of being persecuted. But once the refugee has been allowed to enter a refugee status determination procedure and has acquitted himself or herself of all responsibilities to contribute to the inquiry into his or her claim (thereby regularizing his or her presence, and becoming "lawfully present" in the state), it would be unnecessarily harsh to force him or her away before a final answer is given. Indeed, such an act may well run the very risk of concern to the drafters of Art. 32, namely that of the refugee being "[c]aught between two sovereign orders, one ordering him to leave the country and the other forbidding his entry into the neighbouring country, [causing him or her to] lead[ ] the life of an outlaw and . . . in the end becom[ing] a public danger."[53] This duty to desist from expulsion is, of course, purely provisional, since the refugee's "lawful presence" comes to an end if and when refugee status is denied. In the interim, the legitimate concerns of the host state are surely adequately safeguarded by the right to expel a refugee on national security or public order grounds as described above.[54]

The basic rationale for going beyond the duty of *non-refoulement* to impose limits on the right of states to expel refugees[55] to even non-persecutory countries was elegantly stated in the Secretary-General's background study for the Convention:

> There is little likelihood that a foreign country will consent to receive a refugee whose expulsion has been ordered and who is thereby stamped as undesirable. As every frontier is barred to a refugee whose expulsion has

---

[53] Secretary-General, "Memorandum," at 46.

[54] State practice is largely in accordance with this position: Stenberg, *Non-Expulsion*, at 119.

[55] "Expulsion means any measure which obliges the refugee to leave the territory of a Contracting State, for instance, a residence ban": P. Weis, *The Refugee Convention, 1951: The Travaux Préparatoires Analysed with a Commentary by Dr. Paul Weis* (posthumously pub'd., 1995) (Weis, *Travaux*), at 322. This broad reading is in line with the authoritative interpretation of the cognate duty under the Civil and Political Covenant which defines expulsion to include "all procedures aimed at the obligatory departure of an alien, whether described in national law as expulsion or otherwise": UN Human Rights Committee, "General Comment No. 15: The position of aliens under the Covenant" (1986), UN Doc. HRI/GEN/1/Rev.7, May 12, 2004, at 140, para. 9.

been ordered, only two possibilities are open to him, either not to obey the order and go into hiding to avoid being caught or to cross a frontier illegally and clandestinely enter the territory of a neighbouring country. In that country, too, he must go into hiding to avoid being caught. In either case, after a certain time he is discovered, arrested, prosecuted, sentenced and escorted to the frontier after serving his sentence. Caught between two sovereign orders, one ordering him to leave the country and the other forbidding his entry into the neighbouring country, he leads the life of an outlaw and may in the end become a public danger. In this way measures of expulsion, ... intended to protect law and order, achieve opposite results when an attempt is made to apply them to refugees without taking account of their particular position.[56]

In line with this profound concern about the risks of expelling a refugee,[57] the Secretary-General's draft of the combined duty of *non-refoulement* and non-expulsion disallowed either act unless "dictated by reasons of national security or public order."[58] The expulsion of refugees was further constrained at a procedural level: only "a judicial authority"[59] could expel a refugee.[60] The competing French draft for Art. 32, on the other hand, sought to give governments much more leeway to expel refugees to non-persecutory states. Under its proposal, there would be no substantive limits on the right to expel refugees (though *refoulement* would be limited to "national security" cases), and there would be no guarantee of an opportunity to appear in court. It would be enough if the refugee were allowed "to submit evidence to clear himself, and to be represented before the competent judicial or administrative authority."[61]

In the end, a third approach suggested by a non-governmental organization, the Agudas Israel World Organization, was selected as the working draft of Art. 32.[62] This draft presented states with two options: the right to expel

---

[56] Secretary-General, "Memorandum," at 46.

[57] As Grahl-Madsen notes, the practice of expelling refugees not only caused real hardship to refugees, "but it [also] caused ... considerable inconvenience for the countries into whose territory the expelled refugees were sent in the first place": Grahl-Madsen, *Commentary*, at 185.

[58] Secretary-General, "Memorandum," at 45. [59] Ibid.

[60] This right to contest expulsion before a court was based on a generous interpretation of the draft of what became Art. 13 of the International Covenant on Civil and Political Rights, UNGA Res. 2200A(XXI), adopted Dec. 16, 1966, entered into force Mar. 23, 1976 (Civil and Political Covenant), then framed to require the expulsion of any alien to be ordered "according to such procedure and safeguards as are provided by law": Secretary-General, "Memorandum," at 47.

[61] France, "Proposal for a Draft Convention," UN Doc. E/AC.32/L.3, Jan. 17, 1950 (France, "Draft Convention"), at 9.

[62] The decision to work from the non-governmental draft was reached on the basis of a proposal from the British representative, who found that it "presented the question of expulsion and non-admittance in a more logical form than did the others": Statement of Sir Leslie Brass of the United Kingdom, UN Doc. E/AC.32/SR.20, Feb. 1, 1950, at 2–3.

refugees could be constrained on substantive grounds (limited to "national security") or procedurally (by requiring that any expulsion decision be reached "in pursuance of a decision of a judicial authority," presumably for a broader range of reasons).[63] The gist of the proposal was that refugees could be adequately protected in either of two ways. Their basic interests would be safeguarded so long as refugees could only be expelled for very grave ("national security") reasons; but sufficient protection would also exist if even a broadranging expulsion power were always subject to judicial oversight. In either event, the non-governmental draft proposed that the refugee would be entitled to the minimal due process guarantees stated in the French draft.

Over the course of the ensuing debates, it was decided to revert to a more flexible version of the approach initially proposed by the Secretary-General, that being that the expulsion of refugees would be subject to both substantive and procedural limits. But a broader range of substantive concerns would suffice – either national security or public order grounds could be invoked – and not only courts, but also administrative decision-makers, could be entrusted to afford the refugee basic due process guarantees.

The procedure by which refugees could be expelled was the first concern of the drafters. While acknowledging the general right of states to remove noncitizens from their territory,[64] safeguards were felt necessary because

> [e]xperience had shown that a large number of expulsion orders are due to false accusations and the malice of ousted competitors. Sometimes the orders are due to an error *de persona*. So long as expulsion proceedings are secret and so long as the expelled person is deprived of any means of presenting his case, mistaken decisions are inevitable.[65]

As noted above, the Secretary-General's view was that entrusting all expulsion cases to the courts would best ensure refugees due process. The American representative championed this approach; he was adamant that allowing lesser tribunals or authorities to expel a refugee "would deprive the refugee of the safeguards which every individual was entitled to expect from judicial authority. He would be left to the discretion of police measures."[66] It was soon clear, however, that most governments were unwilling to guarantee judicial oversight of refugee expulsion.[67] The American representative thus

---

[63] "Communication from the Agudas Israel World Organization," UN Doc. E/C.2/242, Feb. 1, 1950, at para. 2.

[64] "The sovereign right of a State to remove ... from its territory foreigners regarded as undesirable cannot be challenged": Secretary-General, "Memorandum," at 45.

[65] Ibid. at 47. See also Ad Hoc Committee, "First Session Report," at Annex II.

[66] Statement of Mr. Henkin of the United States, UN Doc. E/AC.32/SR.20, Feb. 1, 1950, at 6.

[67] See comments of the representatives of Canada, Turkey, France, and Belgium, ibid. at 6–7; and comments of the government of Austria in United Nations, "Compilation of Comments," at 55.

acquiesced in a Canadian compromise,[68] under which governments could leave expulsion decisions to administrative authorities but would formally commit themselves to ensure that expulsion would be ordered "only in pursuance of a decision reached by due process of law."[69]

Importantly, Art. 32 establishes a stronger guarantee of due process than does the general standard set by the Civil and Political Covenant,[70] in that it explicitly entitles refugees "to *appeal to* ... competent authority or ... persons specially designated by the competent authority."[71] This standard was chosen "to avoid the possibility of a [refugee] being expelled on the decision of a mere policeman, for example"[72] – precisely the approach Kenya sought to impose on Ethiopian and Somali refugees rounded up in a sweep of Nairobi. While the language was not intended to require access to a formal appellate court[73] or even directly to the

---

[68] "The essential thing was that it should not be possible to expel refugees other than in accordance with a regular procedure provided by the law, whether administrative or judicial": Statement of Mr. Henkin of the United States, UN Doc. E/AC.32/SR.20, Feb. 1, 1950, at 12.

[69] Statement of the Chairman, Mr. Chance of Canada, ibid. at 7.

[70] Under Art. 13 of the Civil and Political Covenant, in contrast, aliens enjoy only a right to have their case "reviewed by" the competent authority or its designate. Nowak, however, interprets Art. 13 of the Covenant to provide for "an express right to *an appeal* to a higher authority [emphasis added]": M. Nowak, *UN Covenant on Civil and Political Rights* (1993) (Nowak, *ICCPR Commentary*), at 229. This conclusion may be overstated. For example, in *Hammel v. Madagascar*, UNHRC Comm. No. 155/1983, decided Apr. 3, 1987, the Committee found a violation of Art. 13 because "in the circumstances of the present case, the author was not given an effective remedy to challenge his expulsion and ... the State party has not shown that there were compelling reasons of national security to deprive him of that remedy": ibid. at para. 19.2. While a review is clearly required, no reference is made to the specific necessity of an "appeal."

[71] Despite the generality of the language used in Art. 13 of the Civil and Political Covenant, the Human Rights Committee has found that standard to be infringed when a French national was expelled by Madagascar with only two hours' notice, and with no opportunity to challenge his removal: *Hammel v. Madagascar*, UNHRC Comm. No. 155/1983, decided Apr. 3, 1987.

[72] Statement of the Chairman, Mr. Chance of Canada, UN Doc. E/AC.32/SR.20, Feb. 1, 1950, at 18. The Chairman had originally referred to the need for a "final decision rendered by due process of law": ibid. at 17.

[73] "The position of the United Kingdom was similar to that of Italy, since there was no specially constituted appeals tribunal. But the reference to the procedure of appeal, at least in the English version ... was not so specific as to make the text unacceptable to the United Kingdom Government": Statement of Mr. Hoare of the United Kingdom, UN Doc. A/CONF.2/SR.15, July 11, 1951, at 13. In some circumstances, however, it was recognized that appeal to a court might be required. At the Conference of Plenipotentiaries, the Danish Chairman asked, "How, for example, would an appeal be possible if the decision had been taken by the King in Council? He assumed that the meaning of the text was that, in the event of expulsion pronounced by the highest authority, the refugee would be given the chance of having his case re-examined. In countries where such a sentence would have been passed by local authority, the appeal

ultimate decision-maker,[74] there was agreement that a refugee should be entitled to appeal his or her case to an authority of some seniority. A simple administrative review by, for example, the supervisor of a border guard will not suffice.[75] The appeal provided should instead be a more formal reevaluation of the kind implied by the notion of the right to "présenter un recours."[76] As succinctly summarized by the British representative to the Conference of Plenipotentiaries, "[w]hat mattered was that a refugee should have full opportunity of presenting his case to the proper authority."[77]

Thus, the body or person entrusted with the ultimate decision on expulsion should, at the very least, be explicitly empowered to take account of all the circumstances of the case, including the special vulnerabilities and rights of refugees. The appellate authority must, of course, have real authority over the expulsion process. This requirement is met where, as in Canada, judicial

would be addressed to a court of higher instance": Statement of the Chairman, Mr. Larsen of Denmark, ibid. at 14–15.

[74] The British delegate was insistent that there could be no question of requiring the personal involvement of the ultimate decision-maker on expulsion cases, that being the Home Secretary in the United Kingdom: Statement of Sir Leslie Brass of the United Kingdom, UN Doc. E/AC.32/SR.20, Feb. 1, 1950, at 20. His government introduced an amendment adopted at the Conference of Plenipotentiaries, which resulted in the clarification in Art. 32(2) that the appeal could be to "competent authority or a person or persons specially designated by the competent authority": UN Doc. A/CONF.2/60.

[75] In the Ad Hoc Committee, the French representative reacted to the original wording of the Canadian amendment by observing that "he had not grasped the exact meaning of the words 'final decision.' In France an expulsion order was issued by the Prefect, and no administrative authority could usurp his right. His order was therefore final": Statement of Mr. Ordonneau of France, UN Doc. E/AC.32/SR.20, Feb. 1, 1950, at 18. The Chairman responded that the amendment had, in fact, been intended to ensure that the ultimate decision could *not* be made by a police officer: Statement of the Chairman, Mr. Chance of Canada, ibid. At its second session, the Ad Hoc Committee dropped the (arguably ambiguous) reference to a "final decision" in favor of an explicit requirement to allow a refugee to "appeal," noting that "[t]he procedural safeguards accorded to refugees were clarified and are now contained wholly in paragraph 2": "Report of the Ad Hoc Committee on Refugees and Stateless Persons, Second Session," UN Doc. E/1850, Aug. 25, 1950 (Ad Hoc Committee, "Second Session Report"), at 13.

[76] The authoritative nature of the French text is clear from the remarks of the British representative, who had been the most ardent opponent of access to an appellate court in cases of expulsion. The French representative suggested that the French notion of "présenter un recours" could most readily be translated into English as "to lodge an appeal": Statement of Mr. Rochefort of France, UN Doc. A/CONF.2/SR.15, July 11, 1951, at 14. The British representative replied that the notion of "présenter un recours" "was in fact equivalent to the English word 'appeal'": Statement of Mr. Hoare of the United Kingdom, ibid. The decision to employ the term "appeal" in Art. 32(2) should therefore be understood in context to require access to a procedure of reevaluation of the kind implied by the French concept of "présenter un recours."

[77] Statement of Mr. Hoare of the United Kingdom, ibid. at 13.

authority over expulsion is exercised on a discretionary basis.[78] But Kuwait's decision to expel refugees suspected of collaboration with Iraq even though the charges against them had either been withdrawn or dismissed makes clear that its courts did not, in fact, possess the degree of authority required by Art. 32.

The importance of granting refugees enhanced protection against erroneous or otherwise unjustified expulsion is emphasized as well by the specificity of the Refugee Convention's procedural requirements. Like all aliens, refugees are presumptively entitled to claim the benefit of the Civil and Political Covenant's right to submit reasons against their expulsion,[79] and to be represented on the review of any decision to expel them.[80] But Art. 32's more explicit language unambiguously affirms the right of refugees to "submit evidence" in support of their case, not merely to state their reasons for resisting expulsion. The breadth of relevant evidence moreover includes any evidence which may assist the refugee to "clear himself," not just evidence "against expulsion."[81] There can therefore be no question that the person or body considering a refugee's appeal against expulsion must consider evidence relevant to, for example, the soundness of a criminal conviction which underpins the expulsion order, rather than limiting itself simply to the consideration of evidence about the propriety of the expulsion order itself.

Another striking difference between the Civil and Political Covenant and the Refugee Convention is that the latter expressly requires that the decision to expel a refugee "shall be only in pursuance of a decision reached in accordance with due process of law." The more general formulation in the Civil and Political Covenant requires only that the expulsion decision be "reached in accordance with law."[82] In Nowak's view, the Civil and Political Covenant's formulation means that "such a decision must be made by a court or an administrative authority on the basis of a law affording protection against arbitrary expulsion through the establishment of corresponding procedural guarantees."[83] In contrast, the drafters of the Refugee Convention were emphatic that a stronger guarantee of safeguards was

---

[78] *Krishnapillai v. Minister of Citizenship and Immigration*, [2002] 3(1) FC 74 (Can. FCA, Dec. 6, 2001), at para. 33.

[79] Nowak observes that "[e]ven though the reasons against a pending expulsion should, as a rule, be asserted in an oral hearing, Art. 13 does not … give rise to a right to personal appearance": Nowak, *ICCPR Commentary*, at 228.

[80] "[A] person threatened with expulsion is not entitled to *legal* counsel or to the appointment of an attorney [emphasis in original]": ibid. at 231.

[81] While Nowak may be right that the more constrained language of the Civil and Political Covenant "did not change the substance of the right" as conceived in the Refugee Convention (ibid. at 228) the greater precision of Art. 32 of the Refugee Convention more readily forecloses debate on these points.

[82] Civil and Political Covenant, at Art. 13.   [83] Nowak, *ICCPR Commentary*, at 226.

required[84] in order to ensure a meaningful "legal check on the powers of the administration."[85] The Israeli delegate, in particular, insisted that the specific protection needs of refugees justified stronger protections against expulsion than afforded aliens generally:

> [T]here should be a great distinction between the treatment of aliens in general and the treatment of refugees. The stage had now been reached in social legislation when social cases could be spoken of, and the great problem was, who was responsible for the social cases represented by the refugee. In the case of aliens, the answer was their own country; in the case of refugees, the answer was no country. If refugees were not nationals in the political sense of the country where they were resident, however, they were in a moral sense. It seemed to him that countries should accept refugees as human beings, with all the infirmities and weaknesses inherent in the human condition, and treat them accordingly when they offended against national laws.[86]

To this end, the Chinese representative endorsed the Canadian proposal to require respect for due process,[87] remarking that "[t]he concept of due process, familiar to those who understood Anglo-American common law, would be easily acceptable."[88] At its most basic level, due process embraces a duty to respect a range of technical, procedural requirements associated with basic fairness. For example, the High Commissioner for Refugees noted during the Conference of Plenipotentiaries that he "assumed that it was understood that a refugee would not be expelled while his case was *sub judice*."[89] But as Weis has correctly observed, due process also has a fundamental substantive dimension which "means that the [expulsion] decision must be based on law, that it may not be unreasonable, arbitrary or capricious and must have a real and substantive relation to its object."[90]

The drafters did not simply agree that adherence to due process norms was desirable, but formally bound themselves to respect these standards. There was little support for an effort by Italy to delete the reference to respect for due process,[91] nor even for a French proposal that decisions be reached "with

---

[84] Statement of Mr. Weis of the International Refugee Organization, UN Doc. E/AC.32/SR.40, Aug. 22, 1950, at 15.

[85] Statement of Mr. Juvigny of France, ibid. at 12.

[86] Statement of Mr. Robinson of Israel, ibid. at 16.

[87] Statement of the Chairman, Mr. Chance of Canada, UN Doc. E/AC.32/SR.20, Feb. 1, 1950, at 7.

[88] Statement of Mr. Cha of China, UN Doc. E/AC.32/SR.40, Aug. 22, 1950, at 24.

[89] Statement of Mr. van Heuven Goedhart of UNHCR, UN Doc. A/CONF.2/SR.15, July 11, 1951, at 16.

[90] Weis, *Travaux*, at 322.

[91] UN Doc. A/CONF.2/57. Italy withdrew its proposal: Statement of Mr. Theodoli of Italy, UN Doc. A/CONF.2/SR.15, July 11, 1951, at 13.

regard for" (rather than "in accordance with") due process of law.[92] Noting that he thought the Italian and French proposals "went rather further than their authors had intended,"[93] the Belgian delegate proffered an amendment that would have required respect for the three specific aspects of due process mentioned in Art. 32(2) – the right to submit evidence, to appeal, and to be represented – only "[i]nsofar as national security permits."[94] But even this approach was generally felt to be too risky for refugees. Baron van Boetzelaer of the Netherlands successfully persuaded the Conference that limitations on the three due process rights should not be possible simply because national security was involved, but rather only when "imperative" national security concerns so required.[95] The text of Art. 32 was thus amended to allow state parties exceptionally to justify limits on a refugee's right to submit evidence, to appeal, and to be represented, but only "where compelling reasons of national security [so] require."

Three key notions therefore circumscribe the possibility of procedural constraints on the applicability of Art. 32(2). First, as the drafting history makes clear, there is no general right to avoid respect for due process norms even when compelling national security concerns require derogation: only the three rights set out in the second sentence of Art. 32(2) may be constrained. Thus, for example, not even compelling national security concerns would justify the expulsion of a refugee under a procedure which is unreasonable, arbitrary, or capricious. Whatever concerns Kenya had about the "illegal activities" of Ugandan and Rwandan refugees, or which Nigeria had about the support of Chadian refugees for rebels launching attacks on their home country from its territory, could not justify elimination of the right to a hearing altogether. Similarly, Turkey's decision summarily to expel refugees under secret "security agreements" with their states of origin clearly goes significantly beyond what Art. 32(2) allows.

---

[92] Statement of Mr. Juvigny of France, UN Doc. E/AC.32/SR.40, Aug. 22, 1950, at 29. France had formally tabled comments to similar effect, observing that "[t]his modification would make the text more flexible and cover urgent cases which might require a simpler procedure": Comments of France in United Nations, "Compilation of Comments," at 56. It had also tabled a formal amendment to this end (see UN Doc. A/CONF.2/63), which it subsequently withdrew: Statement of Mr. Rochefort of France, UN Doc. A/CONF.2/SR.15, July 11, 1951, at 13.

[93] Statement of Mr. Herment of Belgium, UN Doc. A/CONF.2/SR.15, July 11, 1951, at 12.

[94] UN Doc. A/CONF.2/68. The Belgian representative "understood the motives that had prompted the French and Italian delegations to submit their amendments ... He wondered whether a reservation concerning national security would not meet the points that the French and Italian delegations had in mind": Statement of Mr. Herment of Belgium, UN Doc. A/CONF.2/SR.15, July 11, 1951, at 12.

[95] Statement of Baron van Boetzelaer of the Netherlands, UN Doc. A/CONF.2/SR.15, July 11, 1951, at 15.

Second, and equally fundamentally, because this is a highly constrained, necessity-based exception to a fundamental norm, the state party seeking to avail itself of the right to avoid its usual responsibilities must establish that respect for one or more of the three due process rights cannot be reconciled to "compelling reasons of national security." The corollary to this principle is that the asylum state must logically limit its restrictions on these rights to only what is objectively necessary to safeguard its compelling security interests. This understanding is consistent with the finding of the European Court of Human Rights in the case of *Chahal v. United Kingdom*, in which the Court found that limitations on due process even when considering the expulsion of an alleged terrorist asylum-seeker must be conceived in the least intrusive fashion possible.[96] There is therefore little doubt that Sweden's peremptory expulsion of refugees suspected of terrorist affiliations or acts without any hearing, and strictly on the basis of secret evidence, was unlawful.[97]

Third, the exception to Art. 32(2) is logically difficult to invoke outside the more formal judicial arena. As Grahl-Madsen has observed,

> It is difficult to see that this exception is of much relevance in a system where the power to expel lies exclusively with administrative authorities. Even if they have reached their decision on the basis of confidential material, the nature of which may not be disclosed without endangering national security, there is hardly any reason why the refugee should not be allowed to submit evidence, appeal or be represented. This will, after all, not force the authorities to disclose their sources of information.
>
> If, on the other hand, the law provides for hearings before or appeals to a judicial or semi-judicial authority, it may be necessary for the administration to plead that certain evidence, an appeal or presentations by counsel are non-receivable by the tribunal, because if the latter received such pleas,

---

[96] "The Court recognises that the use of confidential material may be unavoidable where national security is at stake. This does not mean, however, that the national authorities can be free from effective control by the domestic courts whenever they choose to assert that national security and terrorism are involved ... The Court attaches significance to the fact that ... in Canada a more effective form of judicial control has been developed in cases of this type. This example illustrates that there are techniques which can be employed which both accommodate legitimate security concerns about the nature and sources of intelligence information and yet accord the individual a substantial measure of procedural justice": *Chahal v. United Kingdom*, (1996) 23 EHRR 413 (ECHR, Nov. 15, 1996), at para. 131.

[97] More generally, the UN Human Rights Committee expressed its concern "at cases of expulsion [by Sweden] of asylum-seekers suspected of terrorism to their countries of origin. Despite guarantees that their human rights would be respected, those countries could pose risks to the personal safety and lives of the persons expelled, especially in the absence of sufficiently serious efforts to monitor the implementation of those guarantees (two visits by the embassy in three months, the first only some five weeks after the return and under the supervision of the detaining authorities)": UN Human Rights Committee, "Concluding Observations: Sweden," UN Doc. A/57/40, vol. I (2002) 57, at para. 79(12).

the administration would be forced to counter them by submitting classified material. Being an exception, this provision is subject to restrictive
interpretation.[98]

While respect for due process before deciding to expel a refugee is clearly
important, the Refugee Convention does not limit itself (as does Article 13 of
the Civil and Political Covenant) to purely procedural constraints on expulsion. Under some of the early proposals for Art. 32, there were either no
substantive limits on the power to expel refugees,[99] or only tribunal-dependent
substantive strictures.[100] But as finally adopted, the Refugee Convention
establishes a presumptive immunity from expulsion of refugees lawfully in an
asylum state. The expulsion of a refugee may be lawfully pursued in only two
cases, namely when either "national security" or "public order" grounds justify
such action. As successfully argued by the representative of the International
Refugee Organization, substantive limits on refugee expulsion make ethical
and practical good sense:

> Several representatives had said that there was no reason for granting
> special privileges to refugees [in relation to expulsion]. He submitted that
> there were strong grounds for doing so, above all the ground that aliens
> possessing an effective nationality could return to their country of nation-
> ality in case of expulsion, whereas for a refugee it was a matter of life and
> death, as he had no other country to go to.[101]

The drafters therefore agreed that refugees would be entitled to assert both
procedural and substantive limitations on the usual right of states to expel
non-citizens:

> [T]he measure of expulsion should be decreed only after regular procedure.
> Such a safeguard did not, however, appear to be sufficient, for a refugee
> could then be expelled in due and proper form for even a slight offence.
> States would have to undertake not to resort to the *ultima ratio* of expulsion
> except for very grave reasons, namely, actions endangering national secur-
> ity or public order. Thus the refugee would be protected both in the matter
> of procedure and in that of grounds, which was not the least important
> consideration.[102]

Because an expulsion is lawful only where based on national security or
public order grounds, the British effort to expel the Saudi dissident asylum-
seeker Mohammed al-Mas'ari in order to safeguard its trade links or to
promote international comity was in contravention of Art. 32. Similarly,
the Australian legal regime authorization of the expulsion of asylum-seekers

---

[98] Grahl-Madsen, *Commentary*, at 222.   [99] See the French proposal above, at p. 669, n. 61.
[100] See the Agudas Israel World Organization proposal above, at pp. 669–670.
[101] Statement of Mr. Weis of the IRO, UN Doc. E/AC.32/SR.40, Aug. 22, 1950, at 15.
[102] Statement of Mr. Robinson of Israel, UN Doc. E/AC.32/SR.20, Feb. 1, 1950, at 10.

simply on the grounds of their admissibility to a state in which no risk of *refoulement* exists cannot be reconciled to Art. 32: because persons undergoing verification of their refugee status are lawfully in the state party, the presumption against expulsion inheres until and unless they are found not so to qualify. Only a removal affirmatively grounded in national security or public order concerns, as described below, is compatible with the requirements of the Refugee Convention.

The clearest situation in which a refugee may lawfully be expelled is when his or her presence in the asylum state poses a risk to that country's national security. Because a threat to national security is also grounds for *refoulement* under Art. 33(2),[103] a refugee expelled on national security grounds may be removed even to his or her country of origin, if no alternative destination can be identified.[104] The core meaning of "national security" has already been discussed at some length in the context of the right of asylum states to take provisional measures under Art. 9 of the Refugee Convention,[105] and noted in relation to the right of states to engage in individuated *refoulement*.[106] The cases most readily identified as justifying expulsion on grounds of national security are those involving a refugee who seeks directly to attack the political integrity of the host state. For example, in the discussions leading to the adoption of Art. 32, the Venezuelan representative was emphatic that "young countries . . . subject to internal upheavals and revolutions" would be unlikely to sign the Convention unless guaranteed the right to expel refugees who attacked their basic democratic institutions:

> Venezuela had experienced disturbances, accompanied by violence, in which refugees from various countries had taken part; the people of Venezuela had suffered a great deal during and following those upheavals and they would not accept a convention for refugees which contained any provisions that would prevent them from defending their own institutions.[107]

Thus, if Zimbabwe had followed the required procedures before expelling the Central African refugees who were intending to murder key political

---

[103] See chapter 4.1.4 above, at pp. 345–348.

[104] There may be, however, legal obligations beyond those set by the Refugee Convention which limit the right of a state to return an individual to the risk of persecution: see, in particular, Convention against Torture and Other Cruel, Inhuman or Degrading Treatment or Punishment, UNGA Res. 39/46, adopted Dec. 10, 1984, entered into force June 26, 1987 (Torture Convention), at Art. 3; the Civil and Political Covenant, at Art. 7; and the European Convention for the Protection of Human Rights and Fundamental Freedoms, 213 UNTS 221, done Nov. 4, 1950, entered into force Sept. 3, 1953, at Art. 3.

[105] See chapter 3.5.1 above, at pp. 263–267.   [106] See chapter 4.1.4 above, at pp. 345–348.

[107] Statement of Mr. Perez Perozo of Venezuela, UN Doc. E/AC.32/SR.20, Feb. 1, 1950, at 8.

leaders, expulsion on national security grounds would have been reconcilable to Art. 32.

But under modern conceptions endorsed by senior courts, the threat to national security need be neither direct nor immediate. Instead, a refugee is understood to pose a risk to the host state's national security if his or her presence or actions give rise to an objectively reasonable, real possibility of directly or indirectly inflicted substantial harm to the host state's most basic interests, including the risk of an armed attack on its territory or its citizens, or the destruction of its democratic institutions.[108] While this test clearly leaves states a substantial margin of appreciation, a threat to national security must be capable of objective justification.[109] As the Supreme Court of Canada has put it, the threat to a state's most basic interests must be "grounded on objectively reasonable suspicion."[110] There is no requirement, though, that the refugee already have been convicted or even charged with a criminal offense. Indeed, as Grahl-Madsen notes, "an alien may offend against national security even if he cannot be considered guilty of any crime."[111] Under this approach, and assuming the credibility of the *apartheid*-era South African government's threats to invade neighboring states which provided asylum to ANC and other refugees, their expulsion in line with due process guarantees would not have violated Art. 32.[112] Of greater contemporary relevance, objection could also not be taken to the expulsion of a refugee whose terrorist acts against other states indirectly pose a credible threat to the security of the host state.

While the French representative to the Ad Hoc Committee made a valiant attempt to limit refugee expulsions to cases required by national security concerns,[113] the majority of states favored the inclusion of a second, more

---

[108] See chapter 3.5.1 above, at pp. 264–266.

[109] The American representative to the Ad Hoc Committee was of the view, for example, that there was a difference between the simple declaration of a national emergency by a head of state and the existence of national security grounds for the expulsion of a refugee: Statement of Mr. Henkin of the United States, UN Doc. E/AC.32/SR.40, Aug. 22, 1950, at 14.

[110] *Suresh v. Canada*, [2002] 1 SCR 3 (Can. SC, Jan. 11, 2002), at para. 90.

[111] Grahl-Madsen, *Commentary*, at 203.

[112] As Maluwa writes in relation to one such neighboring state, "Botswana's commitment and *bona fides* with regard to the protection of refugees from other States in the region, and in particular those from South Africa, cannot be doubted. Nor, judging from its official pronouncements, can one charge Botswana with a failure to appreciate the duties and obligations incumbent upon it under international law with regard to the granting of asylum and protection to South African and other refugees. Responsibility for the breach of international law in this regard, therefore, must be placed squarely upon South Africa alone": T. Maluwa, "The Concept of Asylum and the Protection of Refugees in Botswana: Some Legal and Political Aspects," (1990) 2(4) *International Journal of Refugee Law* 587, at 607.

[113] Statement of Mr. Ordonneau of France, UN Doc. E/AC.32/SR.20, Feb. 1, 1950, at 16, 20.

fluid ground for expulsion: "public order." The essential concern of the drafters was to allow an asylum state to expel refugees who pose a fundamental risk to the safety and security of their citizens. Whereas national security primarily addresses threats emanating from outside the host state's borders, public order was understood as a general category of concerns focusing on the importance of maintaining basic internal security.[114]

Refugees who committed serious crimes,[115] or who "obstinately refused to abide by the laws,"[116] were the main objects of public order exclusion under Art. 32. Reference was made, for example, to the right of states to expel a refugee who had committed larceny[117] or trafficked in narcotics.[118] Canada's expulsion of refugees convicted of serious sexual assaults is therefore readily

---

[114] "[I]n [Venezuela], 'public order' was synonymous with internal order, while 'national security' implied 'international order' . . . [T]he two ideas complemented each other and were closely linked": Statement of Mr. Perez Perozo of Venezuela, ibid. at 18. This led the Israeli delegate to propose "the adoption of the words 'internal and external national security' as the words 'public order' could in fact give rise to different interpretations": Statement of Mr. Robinson of Israel, ibid. at 19. This suggestion was not taken up, however, as there was a strong preference among delegates not to abandon the traditional term of art, "public policy." Even the British representative supported retention of this civil law construct. He "objected to the introduction of new, and hitherto unknown, terms": Statement of Sir Leslie Brass of the United Kingdom, ibid.

[115] Some references to the right of states to expel refugees on public order grounds were not clearly limited to serious offenses. Belgium "pointed out that a refugee who broke the laws also undermined public order": Statement of Mr. Cuvelier of Belgium, ibid. at 16. Sir Leslie Brass advised that "[i]n the United Kingdom, deportations were ordered on grounds of national security or public order only, which included offences against the law": Statement of Sir Leslie Brass of the United Kingdom, ibid. at 17. Yet the importance of not authorizing expulsion for "even a slight offence" was insisted upon by the Israeli representative: Statement of Mr. Robinson of Israel, ibid. at 10. See also text below, at p. 681, in which concern was expressed about the potential over-breadth of substitute language that would have authorized the expulsion of refugees for "commission of illegal acts" rather than on public policy grounds.

[116] Statement of Sir Leslie Brass of the United Kingdom, UN Doc. E/AC.32/SR.20, Feb. 1, 1950, at 14.

[117] In explaining why he preferred reference to persons who had committed criminal acts to a proposal from the Chairman to replace "public order" by "public safety" expulsion, the American representative noted that "in the United States of America, the term 'public safety' was closely related to the term 'national security,' and could therefore not be made to cover even such serious offences as larceny": Statement of Mr. Henkin of the United States, UN Doc. E/AC.32/SR.40, Aug. 22, 1950, at 20.

[118] Replying to a Canadian concern, the Chairman of the Ad Hoc Committee insisted that "the term 'public order' would certainly cover the deportation of aliens convicted under the [Canadian] Opium and Narcotic Drugs Act. In view of the public injury which resulted from traffic in drugs, there could be no possible objection to that interpretation": Statement of the Chairman, Mr. Larsen of Denmark, ibid. at 22. The Canadian preoccupation was repeated at the Conference of Plenipotentiaries: Statement of Mr. Chance of Canada, UN Doc. A/CONF.2/SR.14, July 10, 1951, at 18.

justifiable under the public order exception to Art. 32. But there was resistance to inserting a reference to criminality concerns instead of to the traditional civil law notion of public order.[119] In the view of most representatives, a simple entitlement to expel refugees for the "commission of illegal acts"[120] was both too broad, and too narrow.

It was too broad in that some criminal acts really do not pose a serious risk to the peace and stability of the state:[121] the Chairman of the Ad Hoc Committee mentioned the case of a refugee convicted for "riding a bicycle on a footpath" as an example of a "smaller illegal act"[122] that could not justify expulsion on public order grounds.[123] On the other hand, states ought to be allowed to expel a refugee who had not engaged in criminal activity, but who refused to conform his or her conduct to the basic manners and customs of

[119] The British representative, for example, responded to a proposal for deletion of the reference to "public order" in favor of "internal and external national security" by stating that "neither the Chairman nor he himself could accept [that language], as they both had criminal offences in mind": Statement of Sir Leslie Brass of the United Kingdom, UN Doc. E/AC.32/SR.20, Feb. 1, 1950, at 19. The IRO's representative then "advised the Committee that if it had in mind criminal offences, it should say so clearly": Statement of Mr. Weis of the International Refugee Organization, ibid. at 19. This led various delegations, including those of Venezuela, Turkey, and Belgium, to insist that there was no need for additional clarity, as the meaning of "public order" was not in doubt: Statements of Mr. Perez Perozo of Venezuela, Mr. Kural of Turkey, and Mr. Cuvelier of Belgium: ibid.

[120] Statement of Mr. Henkin of the United States, UN Doc. E/AC.32/SR.40, Aug. 22, 1950, at 19. In the view of the American representative, refugees "should be expelled only on the grounds that they had committed crimes, which should be as explicitly defined as possible": Statement of Mr. Henkin of the United States, ibid. at 14.

[121] "So far as his own government was concerned, 'public order' was directly related to the maintenance of the peace and stability of the State": Statement of Mr. Perez Perozo of Venezuela, ibid. at 13. Grahl-Madsen suggests that the focus of public order exclusion on grounds of criminality should be persons who have committed crimes which "are particularly dangerous, because they demonstrate contempt for normal human and social values or at least a clear antisocial or reckless attitude on the part of its perpetrators, e.g. poisoning, arson. One may also have to draw a distinction between wilful and negligent acts": Grahl-Madsen, *Commentary*, at 214.

[122] "It would be better to change the term 'public order' to 'public safety,' which was also a vague term, and would fail to cover extreme cases on both sides, but would not, like the wording proposed by the representative of the United States of America, cover both extremes and permit the deportation of any refugee who had committed the smallest illegal act": Statement of the Chairman, Mr. Larsen of Denmark, UN Doc. E/AC.32/SR.40, Aug. 22, 1950, at 19. This suggestion was rejected by the American delegate on the grounds that some forms of criminal conduct which did not endanger public safety (e.g. larceny) should nonetheless be grounds for expulsion: Statement of Mr. Henkin of the United States, ibid. at 20.

[123] "But just as a conviction does not ... in itself justify expulsion, a criminal conviction cannot be considered a condition *sine qua non* for expulsion": Grahl-Madsen, *Commentary*, at 217.

the host state. Mention was made, for example, of refugees who engaged in political activism against the asylum country,[124] though the American delegation thought such concerns would have to amount to a threat to national security before they justified expulsion.[125] The Chinese representative, however, offered a particularly striking example of what he viewed as a circumstance in which it would be permissible to expel a refugee on public order grounds:

> [T]he concept of public order was important to China where manners and customs differed greatly from those of other countries, and also differed from one region to another. He himself came from a mountainous area where husbands were obliged to travel great distances to work, and were able to visit their wives only once in three years. Wives generally remained extremely faithful to their absent husbands, and if any one were to receive a visit from a stranger it would cause a considerable sensation. The concept of public order was important in relation to such peculiarities of circumstance and custom.[126]

This example was apparently welcomed by the French representative, who "remarked that the observation of the representative of China showed what different interpretations might be given to the notion of public order."[127] The Chairman also stated that "there would be general agreement that, owing to differences of custom, what would be a question of public order in one country would not in another."[128] He offered the additional example of

---

[124] "[T]he political activity of a refugee might also be regarded as undesirable for reasons of 'public order'": Statement of Mr. Herment of Belgium, UN Doc. E/AC.32/SR.40, Aug. 22, 1950, at 11. More bluntly, the Venezuelan representative felt that the possibility of expulsion on public order grounds "could be considered as a warning to refugees not to indulge in political activities against the State. It was essential that the term should be retained": Statement of Mr. Perez Perozo of Venezuela, ibid. at 13.

[125] "The representative of Venezuela, who had implied that 'public order' in his country meant something related to national emergency, could feel assured that in the opinion of the United States delegation, the requirements of national emergency were taken into account in the term 'national security'": Statement of Mr. Henkin of the United States, ibid. at 18. At the Conference of Plenipotentiaries, the delegate of the Netherlands also opposed an understanding of public order expulsion based on "activities of a subversive nature": Statement of Baron van Boetzelaer of the Netherlands, UN Doc. A/CONF.2/SR.14, July 10, 1951, at 23. By way of parallel, it is interesting that the New Zealand Court of Appeal recently determined that "[i]t is also important that the interpretation of the term 'danger to the security of the country' takes account of a person's right to freedom of association and expression": *Attorney General v. Zaoui*, Dec. No. CA20/04 (NZ CA, Sept. 30, 2004), at para. 151.

[126] Statement of Mr. Cha of China, UN Doc. E/AC.32/SR.40, Aug. 22, 1950, at 24.

[127] Statement of Mr. Juvigny of France, ibid.

[128] Statement of the Chairman, Mr. Larsen of Denmark, ibid.

"illegal distillation of spirits, [which] was in some countries merely a fiscal problem, but in others a problem of public order."[129]

The various efforts to justify reliance on the traditional, civil law understanding of public order expulsion met with strong opposition from the American representative. Mr. Henkin was quite distraught, observing that "[h]is main fear was that the term 'public order' might mean much more than what it appeared to mean on the surface."[130] He worried that the right to expel a refugee based on public order concerns was so vague that some states would undoubtedly abuse this authority,[131] a fear clearly held by the non-governmental community as well.[132] Henkin was blunt in asserting that the explanations provided of the content of public order expulsion in civil law states "had not dispelled his doubts, but had in fact increased them, because of the examples ... given. It seemed that the term 'public order' could be used as a pretext for getting rid of any refugee on the ground that he was, for one reason or another, an undesirable person."[133] While representatives had asserted that there was a clear meaning attached to "public order" in the civil law world,[134] the American representative was skeptical that there really was much agreement on the substance of the concept outside a small number of European states.[135] It most certainly was a notion that had no resonance in common law states.[136]

[129] Statement of the Chairman, Mr. Larsen of Denmark, ibid.

[130] Statement of Mr. Henkin of the United States, ibid. at 14.

[131] "He was glad to hear that, vague though the concept of public order was, it was not liable to abuse, at least in France, Belgium, and Venezuela. He would make no invidious remarks about the possibility of a less liberal application of the term in other countries, but would merely point to the importance of defining legal notions exactly in a legal instrument": Statement of Mr. Henkin of the United States, ibid. at 18.

[132] "[T]he proviso contained in article [32] relating to 'national security' and especially that relating to 'public order' seemed to his organization to be far too vague, and consequently harmful to the interests of refugees ... Moreover, the Commission on Human Rights had on several occasions noted that the term 'public order' was vague and general and – as indeed history testified – capable of serving as a justification for glaring abuse": Statement of Mr. Braun of Caritas International, UN Doc. A/CONF.2/SR.15, July 11, 1951, at 5.

[133] Statement of Mr. Henkin of the United States, ibid. at 12.

[134] Typical of the bald assurances was the statement of the representative of the Netherlands to the Conference of Plenipotentiaries, who "said that the term *ordre publique* was acceptable to the Netherlands government as its meaning was perfectly clear": Statement of Baron van Boetzelaer of the Netherlands, UN Doc. A/CONF.2/SR.14, July 10, 1951, at 23.

[135] "[C]ontrary to the impression he had formed in earlier discussions in the Committee, the term 'public order,' which in British and American law was more or less equivalent to 'public policy,' was not so understood in certain other countries": Statement of Mr. Henkin of the United States, ibid. at 18.

[136] The American representative "confessed that his delegation still felt concern at the use of the term 'public order,' partly because of its ambiguity, partly because it feared that it

Interestingly, the French delegation conceded the accuracy of much of the concern about the definition of "public order." France "admitted the contention of the United States representative that the notion of public order might stir up unpleasant memories, since it was on that notion that certain totalitarian States had based their claim to absolute discretionary powers."[137] Moreover, while the civil law states of Europe could look to detailed jurisprudential understandings of the term,[138] "the expression 'public order' was not interpreted in all countries in the same way ... Consequently the inclusion of that expression would not ... restrict the right of expulsion to any considerable extent."[139] Yet it was generally felt that the notion of public order provided states with a necessary source of reassurance, and gave them the flexibility required to accommodate their unique social concerns, as well as to meet future contingencies.[140] And in any event, the inclusion of a power to expel on public order grounds was effectively a deal-breaker:

> [Mr. Herment of Belgium] wondered whether the discussion was not animated by a spirit of mistrust of Governments. After all, the States which would sign and ratify the Convention would undoubtedly have the intention of according reasonably favourable treatment to refugees.
>
> He would like to urge that the long accepted notion of public order should not be set aside ... Powers of expulsion should be left to Governments, even in cases the circumstances of which could not be foreseen, since such might in fact arise. If that were not done, the article would only be accepted with a number of reservations which would deprive it of all value.[141]

embraced too much": Statement of Mr. Henkin of the United States, ibid. at 11. At the Conference of Plenipotentiaries, the Canadian delegate stated that his government "found some difficulty with regard to the expression 'public order,' which was a term which had a more precise legal connotation in continental countries than in common law countries": Statement of Mr. Chance of Canada, UN Doc. A/CONF.2/SR.14, July 10, 1951, at 18. Even the British government, which had supported use of the 'public order' language at the Ad Hoc Committee, took the position at the Conference that "the expression 'public order' presented definite difficulties to common law countries, where it did not possess the legal connotation it bore in continental jurisprudence": Statement of Mr. Hoare of the United Kingdom, ibid. at 24.

[137] Statement of Mr. Juvigny of France, UN Doc. E/AC.32/SR.40, Aug. 22, 1950, at 17.

[138] "[A]n administrative and judicial case law had been developed such as enabled jurists and even public opinion to know what was meant by 'public order'": Statement of Mr. Juvigny of France, ibid. at 17–18.

[139] Statement of Mr. Ordonneau of France, UN Doc. E/AC.32/SR.20, Feb. 1, 1950, at 18.

[140] "There might possibly – though he hoped not – be countries where it was considered to be a man's private affair if he chose to poison himself with drugs. It would be impossible therefore to define precisely questions of public order for all countries": Statement of the Chairman, Mr. Larsen of Denmark, UN Doc. E/AC.32/SR.40, Aug. 22, 1950, at 25.

[141] Statement of Mr. Herment of Belgium, ibid. at 20.

The French representative was, if anything, even more candid. The civil law states with a long tradition of expelling non-citizens on public order grounds simply would not agree to be bound by a treaty that did not allow them to continue these practices:

> There were laws in existence in which threats or actions prejudicial to public order were explicitly cited as grounds for expulsion. It was naturally not the intention of the Committee that States should be required to alter their legislation on so important a subject, especially at the present time. Accordingly, whatever formula was adopted, the notion of public order would inevitably raise its head in those code law countries where it was traditionally accepted. Any other formula the Committee might endeavour to evolve would therefore run the risk of proving illusory.[142]

In the end, those who opposed the "public order" clause appear simply to have given in to the impossibility of persuading civil law states to abandon their traditional attachment to public order expulsion.[143] But in a spirit of compromise, there was general agreement that public order should be given a narrow interpretation,[144] with the *travaux préparatoires* serving as a definitive point of reference for state parties in interpreting their authority to expel refugees on public order grounds.[145] Thus, only the commission of a serious crime (not any crime) is grounds for public order expulsion,[146] and other

---

[142] Statement of Mr. Juvigny of France, ibid. at 21.

[143] "[S]ince it appeared that in certain countries there was a provision of law that an alien could be expelled on grounds of public order, the only solution to the present difficulties of the Committee would be to retain the present text ... and perhaps add thereto a number of specific exclusions, stating, for example, that a refugee might not be expelled on grounds of indigency or ill health": Statement of Mr. Henkin of the United States, ibid. at 21.

[144] Mr. Robinson of Israel made the point that "it had to be remembered that considerations of national security and public order were interpreted differently in different countries. In the sense of a narrow interpretation, however, there could be no argument in favour of treating refugees differently from other aliens": Statement of Mr. Robinson of Israel, ibid. at 16. His speech was hailed by the French representative as a "brilliant statement": Statement of Mr. Juvigny of France, ibid. at 17.

[145] At the first session of the Ad Hoc Committee, the Belgian representative "asked that the discussion should be recorded in the summary record of the meeting so as to make clear what the Committee understood by the concept of public order": Statement of Mr. Cuvelier of Belgium, UN Doc. E/AC.32/SR.20, Feb. 1, 1950, at 19. Similarly, at the Conference of Plenipotentiaries, the British representative noted that "if any difficulty occurred as to the meaning of ['public order'], it would presumably arise in connexion with some specific case and the court concerned would have the records of the proceedings leading up to the adoption of the Convention. It would therefore be in a position to ascertain the interpretation placed on those words": Statement of Mr. Hoare of the United Kingdom, UN Doc. A/CONF.2/SR.14, July 10, 1951, at 24.

[146] Belgium, for example, insisted that only refugees "convicted of a fairly serious offence" should be subject to public order expulsion: Statement of Mr. Herment of Belgium, UN

concerns – such as basic affronts to public morality or social norms of the asylum country[147] – are to be deemed grounds for expulsion only in truly grave cases.[148] In Grahl-Madsen's words, "it was obviously the intention of the drafters that expulsion should only be resorted to where the continued presence of the refugee would to some extent upset the very equilibrium of society."[149]

The clear goal of the drafters not to authorize the expulsion of refugees for every reason potentially within traditional civil law understandings of public order is especially clear from the drafters' decision not to amend the English language version of Art. 32 to refer to "public policy," which the Secretariat made clear was the real equivalent of the broad-ranging civil law notion of "*ordre public*."[150] The English notion of "public order," while not a formal

Doc. E/AC.32/SR.40, Aug. 22, 1950, at 11. Most important, the report of the second session of the Ad Hoc Committee records the view that Art. 32 "would permit the deportation of aliens who had been convicted of certain serious crimes where in that country such crimes are considered violations of 'public order'": Ad Hoc Committee, "Second Session Report," at 13. See also details of the objections voiced to the American proposal which would have allowed for the expulsion of refugees who had committed any criminal act: text above, at pp. 681–683. Grahl-Madsen helpfully concludes that "only where normal punishment could not save the maintenance of public order or help to restore it would one resort to the measure of expulsion": Grahl-Madsen, *Commentary*, at 208.

[147] While an Egyptian draft which made specific reference to expulsion on grounds of "public morals" was not pursued (UN Doc. A/CONF.2/44), and the representative of the Netherlands voiced his concern with any refugee expulsion predicated on moral concerns (Statement of Baron van Boetzelaer of the Netherlands, UN Doc. A/CONF.2/SR.14, July 10, 1951, at 23), the British representative to the Conference of Plenipotentiaries affirmed that "the United Kingdom had accepted the words 'public order' in international instruments, while making a reservation that they were deemed to include matters relating to crime and public morals. That interpretation had not so far been challenged": Statement of Mr. Hoare of the United Kingdom, ibid. at 24.

[148] "States would have to undertake not to resort to the *ultima ratio* of expulsion except for very grave reasons, namely, actions endangering national security or public order. Thus the refugee would be protected both in the matter of procedure and in that of grounds, which was not the least important consideration": Statement of Mr. Robinson of Israel, UN Doc. E/AC.32/SR.20, Feb. 1, 1950, at 10.

[149] Grahl-Madsen, *Commentary*, at 209.

[150] "In civil law countries, the concept of '*l'ordre public*' is a fundamental legal notion used principally as a basis for negating or restricting private agreements, the exercise of police power, or the application of foreign law. The common law counterpart of '*l'ordre public*' is not 'public order,' but rather 'public policy.' It is this concept which is employed in common law countries to invalidate or limit private agreements of the application of law. In contrast to this concept of public policy, the English expression 'public order' is not a recognized legal concept. In its ordinary English sense, it would presumably mean merely the absence of public disorder. This notion is obviously far removed from the concept of '*l'ordre public*' or 'public policy'": UN Doc. E/L.68, tabled at the Conference of Plenipotentiaries by its Executive Secretary, UN Doc. A/CONF.2/SR.14, July 10, 1951, at 19–20.

legal construct, authorizes expulsion only for the narrower range of concerns necessary to avoid public disorder.[151] The significance of the failure to opt for the English language equivalent of the broader civil law notion was not lost on states. Australia, for example, unsuccessfully sought to amend the English language version of Art. 32 in order to refer to the broader notion of "public policy."[152] As such, when Ireland acceded to the Convention in 1956, it quite rightly felt the need to enter a formal understanding that it "understands the words 'public order' in article 32(1) . . . to mean . . . 'public policy'"[153] in order to avoid the strictures on its expulsion authority otherwise implied by the narrower notion of "public order."

Most specifically, there is no doubt that an effort to expel a refugee on grounds of poverty or ill health – matters felt by some to fall within the traditional civil law *ordre public* expulsion authority – cannot be reconciled to the requirements of the Convention.[154] At the first session of the Ad Hoc Committee, the Danish representative insisted that it must be clear that "social considerations, such as destitution, should not come under the heading of public order."[155] Mr. Cuvelier of Belgium agreed, explaining that "it was naturally impossible to expel a refugee for economic reasons, as in the case of destitution he could not be returned to his country of origin as could an ordinary emigrant."[156] The rationale for a distinctive approach to the expulsion of refugees was eloquently explained by the Israeli representative:

> If refugees were not nationals in the political sense of the country where they were resident, however, they were in a moral sense . . . [C]ountries should accept refugees as human beings, with all the infirmities and weaknesses inherent in the human condition.[157]

All the members of the Ad Hoc Committee who spoke to the question agreed with the view that no refugee should ever be expelled "on grounds of

---

[151] See text above, at p. 686, n. 150.

[152] Statement of Mr. Shaw of Australia, UN Doc. A/CONF.2/SR.14, July 10, 1951, at 22.

[153] The text of declarations and reservations of state parties is available at www.unhcr.ch (accessed Nov. 19, 2004).

[154] As Grahl-Madsen notes, "[t]he drafters . . . were on the whole keenly aware of the vagueness of the term 'public order' in general. However, they expressed clearly their desire to delimit[ ] the meaning of the term as used in Article 32. Mr. Rochefort's emphatic statement in the Conference of Plenipotentiaries, to the effect that it would not be worthwhile to take part in the work of the Conference if it were not clear that 'public order' could not justify expulsion of indigent refugees [see text below, at p. 689] is clear proof that [it was] desired to give the term a technical meaning, without regard to the interpretation given the term in the municipal law of various countries": Grahl-Madsen, *Commentary*, at 205.

[155] Statement of Mr. Larsen of Denmark, UN Doc. E/AC.32/SR.20, Feb. 1, 1950, at 16.

[156] Statement of Mr. Cuvelier of Belgium, ibid.

[157] Statement of Mr. Robinson of Israel, UN Doc. E/AC.32/SR.40, Aug. 22, 1950, at 16.

indigency or ill health."[158] But because of concern that a formal limitation to this effect in Art. 32 could encourage states to take an aggressive attitude toward forms of public order expulsion not expressly disallowed,[159] it was decided simply to note this implied limitation in the Committee's report.[160]

The importance of protecting refugees from public order expulsion on social grounds was emphasized again at the Conference of Plenipotentiaries. Every attempt to assert the propriety of public order expulsion by reason of ill health or poverty was soundly denounced by, in particular, the French representative. An Egyptian amendment that would have authorized the expulsion of a refugee "because he is indigent and is a charge on the State"[161] led Mr. Rochefort to assert that "[p]overty was not a vice, and indigence could not be considered a crime."[162] The Egyptian proposal was swiftly withdrawn.[163] The Canadian government's rather apologetic effort to

---

[158] Statement of Mr. Henkin of the United States, ibid. at 21. See also Statement of Mr. Juvigny of France, ibid.; Statement of Sir Leslie Brass of the United Kingdom, ibid. at 23; and Statement of Mr. Giraud of the Secretariat, ibid. at 26.

[159] "If . . . a country really had the intention of expelling refugees because, by reason of their state of health, for instance, they were a burden on the public purse, such a country would of necessity be obliged, when ratifying the Convention, to make reservations with regard to article [32] . . . [H]e considered that however vague the notion of public order might be, it . . . offer[ed] greater safeguards for refugees than would be given by a hastily drafted formula which would not cover all possible cases and which, moreover, would lend itself to interpretation *a contrario*": Statement of Mr. Juvigny of France, ibid. at 22. See also Statement of the Chairman, Mr. Larsen of Denmark, ibid. at 26, who expressed his concern "that the Committee might be considering the inclusion in an international convention of a provision which appeared to suggest that 'social reasons' were a question of public order."

[160] "[S]ince there was obvious agreement that 'social reasons' should not be grounds [for] expulsion, the only question which remained was whether to provide specifically for such exclusion, or to let the records of the Committee indicate that interpretation of 'public order.' He felt that the Drafting Committee should take that decision": Statement of Mr. Henkin of the United States, ibid. at 26. With the proposal for an explicit reservation defeated on a 5–2 (4 abstentions) vote (ibid. at 27), the Committee's report stipulated that "[t]he phrase 'public order' would not . . . permit the deportation of aliens on 'social grounds' such as indigence or illness": Ad Hoc Committee, "Second Session Report," at 13.

[161] UN Doc. A/CONF.2/44.

[162] Statement of Mr. Rochefort of France, UN Doc. A/CONF.2/SR.14, July 10, 1951, at 21. See also the remarks of Baron van Boetzelaer of the Netherlands, ibid. at 23: "He hoped the Conference would not adopt the Egyptian amendment which introduced somewhat indefinite concepts . . . He feared the adoption of such an amendment would excessively restrict the freedom of refugees." (In addition to its provisions on expulsion for reasons of indigence, the Egyptian amendment would have authorized expulsion on grounds of, for example, subversion, public morality, and health.)

[163] The Egyptian representative "noted with regret that his amendment did not seem to command general support . . . He therefore withdrew it": Statement of Mr. Mostafa of Egypt, ibid. at 25.

safeguard its domestic laws authorizing the discretionary expulsion of refugees who became public charges or who were committed to psychiatric institutions[164] prompted a similarly emphatic rebuke:

> The French delegation could not admit that the indigence of a refugee could constitute one of those reasons [for expulsion], and, if the idea of indigence was to be interpreted as a factor detrimental to public order, would no longer consider it worthwhile to take part in the work of the Conference. In France, indeed, refugees and persons who were a charge on the State were frequently synonymous terms. Tens of thousands of people were in receipt of assistance of that kind ... If there was neither the desire nor the courage on the part of governments to embark upon the legislative changes required by the application of the Convention, it seemed pointless to draft it.[165]

Canada, like Egypt, readily conceded the force of the French government's argument.[166] Undeterred, the Australian delegate insisted that states should be allowed to expel refugees "for instance, when the alien became an inmate of a charitable institution or a mental asylum."[167] Once more, the French representative replied caustically that "the fact that a refugee was penniless should most certainly not constitute one of the reasons which ... would justify the expulsion of a refugee; on the contrary, the French Government felt it was a fundamental reason for showing greater leniency."[168] Australia did not press its point.

In the end, there was a general recognition that sanctioning a right to expel refugees on grounds of poverty would create a vicious circle which would deter any state party from meeting its duty to provide refugees with basic social assistance.[169] Taking account of the prevailing view that not even aliens

---

[164] "In all frankness, however, he must state that Canadian law – and probably the laws of other countries too – provided in ... discretionary clauses for deportation on the grounds that the person concerned had become a public charge or was an inmate of a mental asylum or a public charitable institution": Statement of Mr. Chance of Canada, UN Doc. A/CONF.2/SR.15, July 11, 1951, at 8.

[165] Statement of Mr. Rochefort of France, ibid. at 8–9.

[166] The Canadian representative "heartily endorsed the French view that expulsion on the grounds of indigency alone would be entirely out of keeping with the ideals and hopes entertained by the Conference. He had merely pointed out how difficult it would be to amend the relevant Canadian legislation, and could only repeat that he could conceive of no circumstances in which the Canadian authorities would expel a refugee on grounds of indigency alone": Statement of Mr. Chance of Canada, ibid. at 9.

[167] Statement of Mr. Shaw of Australia, ibid. at 11.

[168] Statement of Mr. Rochefort of France, ibid. at 11.

[169] The French representative "apologized if he had expressed himself too forcefully; but he nevertheless wished to emphasize that the French delegation had no intention of concluding a one-sided bargain which, for the French Government, would mean the assumption of multilateral obligations with respect to countries the legislation of which would not grant refugees rights equivalent to those which the French

in general should be expelled on grounds of indigence[170] and of the legal obligation to meet at least the basic needs of refugees,[171] the British representative aptly concluded that "[t]he discussion had been useful in making it clear that the words 'public order' could not be construed as including mere indigency."[172]

Just how salient must the reasons of national security or public order be in order to justify the expulsion of a refugee? The Secretary-General's draft of Art. 32 recommended the standard from the 1933 Refugee Convention, namely that expulsion be "dictated by" reasons of national security or public order.[173] The alternative formulation proposed by the Agudas Israel World Organization, which was selected as the Ad Hoc Committee's working draft,[174] used what may on first impression appear to be less demanding language: "save on" grounds of national security.[175] It is the latter formulation ("save on") that was adopted. Yet both Grahl-Madsen[176] and

Government would undertake to guarantee them upon signing the Convention. It was by no means a theoretical consideration, since France very frequently had to take in refugees who had been expelled from other countries simply because they were penniless, or possibly, stateless": Statement of Mr. Rochefort of France, ibid. at 12. This led the Canadian delegate to reply that he "regretted that he had caused so much trouble": Statement of Mr. Chance of Canada, ibid.

[170] The President referred to resolutions of the Economic and Social Council which recommended against expulsion based on indigency: Statement of the President, Mr. Larsen of Denmark, ibid. at 9–10.

[171] See chapters 4.4 above and 6.3 below.

[172] Statement of Mr. Hoare of the United Kingdom, UN Doc. A/CONF.2/SR.15, July 11, 1951, at 10. One possible exception, noted by Grahl-Madsen, is the situation where a refugee sets out explicitly to make himself or herself a public charge. "The refugee who is able to work and still continually refuses to do so with the clear intent of living off public funds may, under certain circumstances, set such a bad example that it might seem necessary to apply sanctions of some kind or another. But it goes without saying that the situation must be nothing short of extraordinary in order to justify the invoking of public order – as understood in the Refugee Convention – in such a case": Grahl-Madsen, *Commentary*, at 211.

[173] Secretary-General, "Memorandum," at 45.

[174] See text above, at pp. 669–670.

[175] As described above (see text above, at pp. 669–670), the recommendation of the Agudas Israel World Organization was that the expulsion of refugees be subject to either procedural or substantive limitations. The latter option provided that a refugee could not be expelled "save on grounds of national security": "Communication from the Agudas Israel World Organization," UN Doc. E/C.2/242, Feb. 1, 1950, at para. 2.

[176] "[T]here was hardly any intention behind the change of wording. And in view of the meaning of the terms 'national security' and 'public order,' it seems possible to submit that the change of wording has not caused any change of meaning. If the concepts of national security and public order are to be understood in the sense that they imply a public necessity to rid oneself of the objectionable person, it is clear that it does not make any difference whether one uses the words 'dictated by' or simply says 'on grounds of'": Grahl-Madsen, *Commentary*, at 199.

Stenberg[177] take the view that there is no reason to suggest that the use of this form of words was intended to deviate from the traditional understanding that the host state must show some imperative or genuine necessity for expulsion, rather than simply that there is a plausible case for removal on grounds of national security or public order. Indeed, given the history of the drafting of Art. 32, it is probable that when the Chairman of the Ad Hoc Committee recommended what became the final language of Art. 32 ("save on grounds of national security or public order")[178] he was simply following the phrasing of the Agudas draft from which the Committee had been working, and which had not been said to posit any shift from traditional evidentiary standards.

But even if significance is attributed to the decision to use the words "save on" rather than "dictated by," the former wording also implies an evidentiary imperative, albeit one that is somewhat less demanding. As Grahl-Madsen observes, under Art. 32(1) "expulsion is not justified unless it will have a salutary effect with regard to [national security or public order]. It is not something to which one [should] resort lightly, but rather ... one must consider whether the measure will serve its end – in other words, that it is necessary."[179] This interpretation is in line with the view of UNHCR's Executive Committee that "expulsion measures against a refugee should only be taken in very exceptional circumstances and after due consideration of all the circumstances."[180]

If a determination is made that reasons of national security or public order require a refugee's expulsion, it does not follow that the host state may immediately effect the refugee's removal. First and most critically, the safeguards against *refoulement* described above continue to apply unless the more exacting standards of Art. 33(2) for removal to a country where there is a risk of being persecuted have been met.[181] While this is unlikely to pose a

---

[177] "The words 'are dictated by' in the 1933 Convention serve, much more than the corresponding wording of Article 32(1) of the 1951 Convention, to stress the *ultima ratio* character of the exceptions. Nevertheless, it is quite clear, on the basis of the preparatory work of the 1951 Convention, that the change of wording in Article 32(1) was not intentional": Stenberg, *Non-Expulsion*, at 132.

[178] Statement of the Chairman, Mr. Chance of Canada, UN Doc. E/AC.32/SR.20, Feb. 1, 1950, at 17.

[179] Grahl-Madsen, *Commentary*, at 200.

[180] UNHCR Executive Committee Conclusion No. 7, "Expulsion" (1977), at para. (c), available at www.unhcr.ch (accessed Nov. 20, 2004).

[181] See text above, at pp. 663–665. Indeed, the French representative to the Ad Hoc Committee remarked that the provisions of what became Art. 32(3), allowing refugees subject to expulsion a reasonable period within which to identify a state willing to accept them, were a useful practical means of meeting the duty of *non-refoulement* in such circumstances. "It had, in fact, been agreed that a refugee could not be sent back to a country where his life would be threatened. But a refugee who had been expelled from one

difficulty in national security cases,[182] the combined effect of Arts. 33(2) and 32 is that all but the most egregious forms of public order expulsion are effectively proscribed unless removal can be effected to a non-persecutory state.[183] Because it is ordinarily only the refugee's country of origin (in which the risk of being persecuted has been established) to which return may be effected as of right, the right to expel a refugee found to pose a lesser public order risk may therefore be foreclosed as a practical matter.[184]

Second, in line with the position that the expulsion of a refugee must clearly be a matter of final recourse, Art. 32(3) expressly requires the state contemplating expulsion to grant the refugee a reprieve for purposes of organizing his or her own admission to some other (presumably safe) country. This paragraph is innovative in two ways. In contrast to earlier conventions, it imposes a duty on state parties to delay expulsion while the refugee pursues his or her own options, rather than simply acknowledging the logic of delay.[185] In addition, while the Secretary-General's draft had predicated the right to secure a delay of expulsion solely on non-receipt of the authorizations

country had little chance of being admitted elsewhere": Statement of Mr. Ordonneau of France, UN Doc. E/AC.32/SR.20, Feb. 1, 1950, at 21.

[182] This is because Art. 33(2) authorizes particularized *refoulement* in the case of a refugee "whom there are reasonable grounds for regarding as a danger to the security of the country in which he is", a test which is essentially indistinguishable from Art. 32's authorization for the expulsion of a refugee "on grounds of national security" so long as due process norms are respected (including the substantive due process norm prohibiting unreasonable or arbitrary action). See chapter 4.1.4 above, at pp. 345–348.

[183] This is because Art. 33(2), unlike Art. 32(1), does not allow particularized *refoulement* on grounds of public order *per se*. Only a subset of public order concerns – namely, those relating to a person who "having been convicted by a final judgment of a particularly serious crime, constitutes a danger to the community of [the host] country" – is a basis for *refoulement*. See chapter 4.1.4 above, at pp. 349–352.

[184] See Weis, *Travaux*, at 323: "No expulsion order may be carried out unless another country is willing to admit [the] refugee."

[185] The Belgian representative had observed that the wording proposed by the Secretary-General "afforded no guarantee to refugees, and left governments free to act as they pleased, in so far as the refugees were concerned": Statement of Mr. Cuvelier of Belgium, UN Doc. E/AC.32/SR.20, Feb. 1, 1950, at 22. The final wording of the paragraph as ultimately adopted was proposed by the American representative to the Ad Hoc Committee who "asked whether the Committee thought it advisable to include in article [32] certain words which, without placing any obligation on the High Contracting Parties, would express the hope that any refugee . . . would have the opportunity of trying to obtain legal admission into another country before the expulsion order was put into effect": Statement of Mr. Henkin of the United States, ibid. at 23. The proposal which Mr. Henkin then drafted (UN Doc. E/AC.32/L.23) actually went farther, using the mandatory form "shall" to define the duty to allow a refugee to seek admission to another state. The approach advocated by the Secretary-General's draft had provided simply for the right of states to impose constraints on refugees allowed to remain in the country while exploring options to expulsion. See Secretary-General, "Memorandum," at 45.

or visas needed to enter another country,[186] Art. 32(3) as adopted is not narrowly constrained in this way.[187] Its broader scope is intended to recognize that even when permission to enter another state has been received, an additional delay in departure may be required to take account of compelling personal reasons, such as "a pregnant wife or a sick child."[188] Thus, even if the Swedish decision to expel the Egyptian refugees suspected of having terrorist affiliations had been both substantively justifiable and pursued in accordance with due process, the peremptory nature of their removal was in clear violation of Art. 32(3).

Art. 32(3) should, however, be interpreted in light of its primary purpose to enable refugees to pursue non-coercive departure options. Thus, the American drafter of the paragraph readily conceded the logic of the British representative's point that states were under no obligation to grant refugees a stay of expulsion if the refugee had already sought and secured valid documentation for entry into a safe country to which expulsion could be effected.[189] Nor is there a duty to grant refugees such a prolonged delay that their travel documents expire, making their expulsion a practical impossibility.[190]

During a delay in effecting expulsion, state parties may "apply . . . such internal measures as they deem necessary."[191] It is clear that such measures

---

[186] The relevant part of the draft defined the beneficiary class as refugees "who are unable to leave its territory because they have not received, at their request or through the intervention of Governments or through the High Commissioner for Refugees or non-governmental agencies, the necessary authorizations and visas permitting them legally to proceed to another country": Secretary-General, "Memorandum," at 45.

[187] The Danish and French representatives took the view that this limitation was superfluous: Statements of Mr. Larsen of Denmark and Mr. Ordonneau of France, UN Doc. E/AC.32/SR.20, Feb. 1, 1950, at 21.

[188] Statement of Mr. Larsen of Denmark, ibid.

[189] The British representative had expressed his concern that "the wording of the proposed new paragraph was slightly too sweeping. For example, in some cases when a refugee left a country it had been agreed that he could return if he wished within a certain time limit. If the country where he went decided to expel him and had to allow a 'reasonable period' to elapse before enforcing that decision, the time limit within which he was allowed to return to the first country might have expired in the interval": Statement of Sir Leslie Brass of the United Kingdom, UN Doc. E/AC.32/SR.21, Feb. 2, 1950, at 3. The American representative replied succinctly that "when there was a country prepared to admit the refugee, it would be unnecessary to grant him a reasonable period within which to seek legal admission": Statement of Mr. Henkin of the United States, ibid.

[190] "It was obvious that if the travel document of a refugee returnable to another country had almost expired, he could not be given the same opportunity to find another country willing to receive him as a refugee whose travel document was still valid for a considerable period": Statement of Sir Leslie Brass of the United Kingdom, UN Doc. E/AC.32/SR.40, Aug. 22, 1950, at 30.

[191] States are granted a substantial margin of appreciation in deciding what internal measures should be taken. "The second sentence of para. 3 is less liberal than Art. 31, para. 2,

may include detention.[192] This is contextually logical, since once a refugee has been finally determined to be amenable to expulsion, his or her presence in the host state ceases to be lawful. In consequence, the presumptive right to freedom of internal movement under Art. 26 can no longer be invoked.[193] The refugee's presence is now simply tolerated on the state's territory, meaning that constraints on freedom of movement in line with Art. 31(2) are once again permitted.[194] Art. 32(3) would, however, be contravened were the constraints to be such as to negate the refugee's ability to pursue his or her applications for onward travel as an alternative to expulsion.[195]

To summarize, Art. 32 is a supplement to the protection against *refoulement* set by Art. 33. It is intended to limit the right of states to expel refugees to even non-persecutory states on both procedural and substantive grounds. At a procedural level, the expulsion of a refugee may be ordered by an administrative agency, but the refugee must be guaranteed the right to appeal that decision to an authority of some seniority which has the power to consider all the circumstances of the case, including the refugee's special vulnerabilities and rights, and to issue an authoritative decision governing expulsion. The appeal must moreover be conducted in line with norms of due process, including both the requirements of procedural fairness and substantive protections against a result not based on law or which is not related to the true objects of Art. 32 or is otherwise unreasonable, arbitrary, or capricious. The right of the refugee to submit evidence, to appeal, or to be represented, may, however, be constrained to the extent required by compelling reasons of national security.

---

first sentence: the former speaks of measures as 'they *may deem* necessary' ... while the latter mentions measures 'which *are* necessary' ... The difference is in the subjective appraisal of the measures: in the case of Art. 31, they must appear to be necessary to an objective observer ... [Under] Art. 32, it suffices if the competent authorities consider them to be required": N. Robinson, *Convention relating to the Status of Refugees: Its History, Contents and Interpretation* (1953) (Robinson, *History*), at 159–160.

[192] The Chairman of the Ad Hoc Committee expressed his worry that "temporary detention might constitute a punitive measure for deported refugees who could not proceed elsewhere": Statement of the Chairman, Mr. Chance of Canada, UN Doc. E/AC.32/SR.20, Feb. 1, 1950, at 22. The representative of the IRO pointedly responded "that a refugee would not regard a period in prison or in an internment camp as a punitive measure, as he might otherwise run the risk of being sent back to a country where his life would be threatened": Statement of Mr. Weis of the International Refugee Organization, ibid. While Mr. Weis' assertion is not legally correct in view of the continuing force of Art. 33, his essential point – that detention while arranging a preferred departure option is likely to be seen by a refugee as preferable to expulsion – is nonetheless sound.

[193] See chapter 5.2 below.   [194] See chapter 4.2.4 above. See also Robinson, *History*, at 159.

[195] Robinson notes that the restrictions "cannot be of such nature as to make it impossible for the refugee to secure admission elsewhere because the Convention considers expulsion a measure to be taken only if the refugee is unable to leave the country on his own motion": Robinson, *History*, at 160.

Substantively, the expulsion of a refugee is lawful only if shown to be based on grounds of national security or public order. Expulsion on the basis of national security requires the host state to show an objective, reasonable possibility that the refugee's actions or presence expose the host state to the risk of direct or indirect substantial harm to its most basic interests. This test would be met, for example, where there is a real risk of an armed attack on that state's territory or its citizens, or of the destruction of its essential democratic institutions. Expulsion may also be based on public order concerns – a term of art not coterminous with traditional civil law notions of *ordre public*, a notion understood to include a wide range of public policy concerns. Under the Refugee Convention, relevant public order concerns are those which bespeak a threat to the internal security of the host country. Public order concerns may be based, for example, on the fact that a refugee has committed a serious crime or is a recidivist, or that he or she has engaged in activity which amounts to a grave affront to public morality or social norms. But social concerns such as poverty or ill health are not to be invoked as public order grounds to expel a refugee.

5.2 Freedom of residence and internal movement

The range of constraints on freedom of movement to which refugees may be subjected immediately upon arrival has been addressed in chapter 4.[196] Detention is particularly common in the case of refugees who come as part of a mass influx. In addition, governments sometimes provisionally detain persons they believe may pose a risk to their own safety or security, whose identity is unclear, or who have yet to provide authorities with the basic information needed in order to begin the process of verifying their claim to refugee status.

The focus here is instead on limitations on freedom of residence and internal movement that are imposed after the initial reception stage. A refugee may be granted some form of time-limited right to stay in the host state, or be admitted to a formal procedure to verify his or her refugee status. In many less developed states which do not formally assess refugee status, persons claiming to be refugees are simply allowed to remain. Despite the explicit or tacit authorization granted to stay in the reception country in each of these circumstances, limits on the right to decide where to live or on internal travel may still be imposed. So pervasive is the belief that refugees may lawfully be confined away from local populations that outrage has at times been expressed when refugees seek even a modicum of mobility. For example, a senior Malawian official is quoted as having expressed his anger

---

[196] See chapter 4.2.4 above.

that "refugees were violating local regulations that they remain in holding camps and were instead 'roaming free through Malawi's city streets ... These refugees are insulting their hosts by breaking the rules. They are not allowed to wander about freely ... They should appreciate Malawi's hospitality and not spoil our attitude towards all refugees.'"[197]

Most seriously, some countries – including Australia and the United States – routinely continue the imprisonment of many refugees even after they have complied with all formalities required to investigate their claims to protection.[198] While prolonged detention of this kind is not common in the industrialized world, it is widespread in many less developed countries. Kenya and Uganda are among the states which generally restrict refugees to camps and criminalize any attempt to escape from them.[199] Indeed, Kenya has gone so far as to detain refugees found in urban areas on the grounds of their failure to register there, even when no registration service was in fact available.[200] It has even forcibly relocated some of the small minority of refugees granted formal permission to live in urban areas.[201] In the late 1980s, Zimbabwe designated certain areas where refugees were required to reside, then forced its growing population of Mozambican refugees to relocate to five large

---

[197] *African Eye News Service*, Nov. 8, 2000, quoting Deputy Commissioner for Relief and Rehabilitation Willy Gidala.

[198] The Australian and American practices are described in chapter 4.2 above, at pp. 375–377. The practice of general or mandatory detention begins upon arrival, and normally continues until and unless refugee status is formally recognized. The Australian immigration minister, Philip Ruddock, has remained unmoved by massive protests and strong international legal criticism directed against his country's regime. "'Detention policy is public policy in Australia which will not be unwound,' Mr. Ruddock said": P. Barkham, "Refugees dig their own graves in Australian detention protest," *Guardian*, Mar. 8, 2002, at 17.

[199] Refugees in these countries who violate the rules requiring them to live in camps and who move to urban areas – Nairobi and Kampala in particular – have been essentially abandoned by the host governments, and have been subjected "to beatings, sexual violence, harassment, extortion, arbitrary arrest and detention": Human Rights Watch, "Hidden in Plain View," Nov. 2002.

[200] "The 145 refugees have been charged with failing to register with the government of Kenya, a statutory violation that is being enforced for the first time. But no refugee is able to comply with the statute because there has been no governmental registration service for the refugees since 1991": Human Rights Watch, "Kenyan Government Sweep of Foreigners Puts Refugees at Risk," June 8, 2002.

[201] "In the largest group arrest on November 29 [2002] ... 20 Kenyan police officers began house-to-house arrests in Kawangware, a so-called slum neighborhood to the southwest of Nairobi. More than 50 refugees were arrested, and some described being beaten during the arrests ... Among those arrested were two Congolese women with UNHCR-issued documents granting them permission to remain in Nairobi for security reasons": Human Rights Watch, "Kenya: Crackdown on Nairobi's Refugees after Mombassa Attacks," Dec. 6, 2002.

camps on its eastern border.[202] It took much the same approach in response to a rise in refugee arrivals during 2002, deciding to "round up all refugees not employed or attending school and confine them to Tongogara camp in Chipinge," apparently with UNHCR's approval.[203] Similarly, during the late 1990s and early part of this century, Pakistan forcibly relocated millions of settled Afghan refugees into camps in the northwest frontier province near the border with their country of origin, notwithstanding evidence that their security was at risk there.[204]

Forcible residence in refugee camps is not always the result of direct coercion, but may sometimes be achieved indirectly. For example, Malawian officials used their control over relief supplies, especially food, as a means of inducing reluctant Mozambican refugees to "accept" relocation to camps.[205] India refused to allow separated refugee families in Tamil Nadu to live together, threatening to cut off the minimal ($3 per month) refugee subsistence allowance to anyone who moved away from his or her assigned camp.[206]

While refugees sent to so-called "open" refugee camps may still enjoy at least some measure of freedom of movement,[207] it is otherwise in "closed"

---

[202] Lawyers' Committee for Human Rights, *African Exodus* (1995) (LCHR, *African Exodus*), at 100–101; S. Nkiwane, *International Academy of Comparative Law National Report for Zimbabwe* (1994), at 15–20. "The justification for this policy [was] that it is easier to cater to the refugees' needs when they are grouped together. A further reason for these security measures is that the recent RENAMO incursions ... have claimed many victims among the local population and left a trail of devastation in their wake. These attacks have terrorized the inhabitants and engendered hostility towards the Mozambican refugees, who are held responsible for them": M. El-Chichini, "Four Crowded Camps," (1988) 55 *Refugees* 38, at 38.

[203] "Government rounds up refugees," *Daily News* (Harare), May 20, 2002. "The United Nations High Commissioner for Refugees (UNHCR) in Zimbabwe is expanding Tongogara camp to accommodate the refugees ... 'In the urban areas the cost of living is high,' [UNHCR assistant programme officer Tapiwa] Huye said. 'Some of the refugees could end up being destitute or getting involved in illegal activities and prostitution for survival. Besides, it is government policy that only those refugees who are attending school or in employment will remain in the urban centres'": ibid.

[204] Human Rights Watch, "Letter to General Pervez Musharraf," Oct. 26, 2001; and "Pakistan: Refugees Not Moving Voluntarily," Dec. 5, 2001.

[205] "Refugees in Zobwe, Thyolo, and Machinga, and on the east side of Lake Malawi were told that they must go to Lisungwe if they wanted to receive food aid": LCHR, *African Exodus*, at 102.

[206] "64 year old Rafael ... has his daughter in another camp 100 km away ... 'I cannot move to the other camp, the authorities ban refugee movements, and if I move I will lose my registration and won't receive any assistance from the government'": (1999) 41 *JRS Dispatches* (Jan. 15, 1999). Concerns regarding interference with family unity are addressed in detail at chapter 4.6 above.

[207] For example, Liberian refugees housed in Nigerian refugee camps enjoyed the right to leave the camps, though not to abandon them as their residence: Tiao, "Refugee Rights in

camp settings. Kurdish refugees from Iraq were confined in southeast Turkey in guarded camps, surrounded by barbed wire, with strict limitations on external movement.[208] Burundians in Tanzania were not only forced into camps, but "said their requests to leave the camp in order to locate their spouses and children or to return to their home areas to sell their possessions were repeatedly ... denied by camp commanders."[209] Even Vietnamese refugees formally "screened in" as genuine refugees under the Comprehensive Plan of Action were not always released from mandatory confinement in Hong Kong and other processing states.[210] Cambodian and Burmese refugees in Thailand have been subjected to a similarly restrictive regime, unable to leave the military-controlled camps except to resettle in third states.[211] Indeed, in July 2003 it was announced that the UNHCR had agreed to fund

Nigeria," at 5. Mozambican refugees in Zimbabwean camps had some flexibility to leave the camps, as did Guatemalan refugees assigned to refugee settlements: K. Jacobsen, "Factors Influencing the Policy Responses of Host Governments to Mass Refugee Influxes," (1996) 30 *International Migration Review* 655 (Jacobsen, "Host Governments"), at 661; F. Stepputat, "Self-Sufficiency and Exile in Mexico: Report on a Field Study among Relocated Guatemalan Refugees in South-East Mexico, August–November 1988," UN Research Institute for Social Development Discussion Paper No. 9, Aug. 1989 (Stepputat, "Exile in Mexico"), at 13, 14, 17.

[208] US Committee for Refugees, *World Refugee Survey 1992* (1992), at 81. "In late 2002, the Turkish government feared a new influx, and established a series of camps within the 9-mile (15 km) Turkish-occupied strip in northern Iraq. When it introduced this plan in November, the Turkish government stated that its main goal would be to send foreigners in the camps either back to their region of origin or to third countries": US Committee for Refugees, *World Refugee Survey 2003* (2003), at 229.

[209] Human Rights Watch, "In the Name of Security: Forced Round-Ups of Refugees in Tanzania," July 1999, at 28.

[210] "Even for those screened in as refugees under the 1951 Convention, there was not complete recognition of the rights enumerated in that Convention. They had limited freedom of movement and selective access to employment, and there was a tendency to keep them in semi-closed camps, pending resettlement. Often they needed passes to leave the camps on a daily basis for activities outside the camps": V. Muntarbhorn, *The Status of Refugees in Asia* (1992), at 155. Hong Kong's practices were particularly harsh. "Vietnamese who succeeded in proving their status as a refugee were to be sent to closed camps": Lawyers' Committee for Human Rights, "Inhumane Detention: The Treatment of Vietnamese Boat People in Hong Kong" (1989), at 10–11. As of 1995, 1,500 persons determined to qualify for Convention refugee status remained incarcerated in Hong Kong: Lawyers' Committee for Human Rights, "Hong Kong Critique 1995" (1995).

[211] "The Thai Defense Force associated the refugees with a variety of security threats, and then sought to control strictly the refugees' movements and location. Refugees were obliged to remain in camps close to the Thai–Cambodian border; they were not permitted to work and could only leave the camps when they were to be resettled in third countries": Jacobsen, "Host Governments," at 661. "In the mid-1990s, Thailand improved its relations with Burma's government, and began restricting refugees' movements in and out of the camps in Thailand and curtailing their ability to work on nearby farms or to rent land and grow crops": US Committee for Refugees, *World Refugee Survey 2003* (2003), at 135.

the building of a camp for the mandatory detention of some 1,500 Burmese refugees in Thailand. The Thai government announced that "[i]f [the refugees] resist the relocation . . . their registration with UNHCR will be revoked and they will be prosecuted."[212]

Despite the prevalence of such policies, it is increasingly recognized that laws forcing refugees to live in camps are often difficult to enforce in practice. For example, the Zambian Deputy Minister of Home Affairs was reduced to "appeal[ing] to [escaped refugees] to return to the camp because it was an offence under the law to leave it."[213] More generally, and despite the determination of most African states to detain refugees, Sommers reports that most refugees simply become self-settled in violation of the law:

> In legal terms . . . the local government usually gives them no alternative because virtually all refugees are ordered to live in camps or settlements. Yet almost from the outset, the reality of refugee lives confounds common perceptions of them as passive, compliant victims of violence. Given a chance, refugees turn entrepreneurial, violating camp regulations along the way. They are risk-takers who prefer to conceal illegal activities rather than constrict their lives inside camp or settlement enclosures . . .
>
> Despite institutional attempts to keep refugees and host populations separate . . . most refugees in Africa are spontaneously settled . . . Local governments and UNHCR have long been aware of this . . . UNHCR, whose mandate is to protect and assist all refugees, tends to focus on camp refugees both because their funding is usually constrained and because they prefer not to challenge African government policies that commonly restrict urban residence for refugees. This presents refugees with a clear choice: choosing between the protection and provisions that settlements promise to provide and UNHCR is mandated to assure on the one hand, and accepting considerable risks for the chance to pursue a life outside the camps on the other. Many, if not most, refugees willingly accept the risk of living outside the camps.[214]

Beyond their impracticality, laws confining refugees to camps may have unintended negative consequences not only for refugees, but also for surrounding communities. In Zambia, for example, women refugees began to marry local men in order to gain automatic access to citizenship, entitling them to leave the refugee camps. This practice, in turn, "excited a backlash from concerned locals . . . Zambian women . . . lodged a formal complaint with the Ministry of Home Affairs about refugee women 'stealing' their

[212] "Thais to intern 1,500 Burmese," *International Herald Tribune*, July 3, 2003, at 1.

[213] "Ex-combatants from Angola, DRC desert refugee camp in Zambia," *SAPA-AP*, Apr. 22, 2002. "'Most of them have deserted the camp and joined the Zambian communities in villages,' [a Zambian official] said": ibid.

[214] M. Sommers, "Young, Male and Pentecostal: Urban Refugees in Dar es Salaam, Tanzania," (2001) 14(4) *Journal of Refugee Studies* 347, at 348–350.

husbands."[215] And when Tanzania commenced its policy of requiring refugees to live in camps, both the self-reliance of refugees and the economic prosperity of surrounding communities were compromised:

> During the height of the refugee presence in Ngara and Karagwe districts in 1994 and 1995, there were few restrictions on the mobility of refugees and hosts. Tanzanian- and refugee-owned businesses thrived. Refugees provided labor on Tanzanian farms throughout the area, and Tanzanians moved in and out of the camps to conduct business, socialize, and make use of camp-based resources such as water taps and hospitals ...
>
> After 1996, however, the government controlled more carefully the movement of refugees within its borders ... In Kibondo, Kasulu and Kigoma rural districts, where the refugee populations did not peak until later, the tighter controls on refugee–host interactions affected the extent to which hosts could benefit ... Villagers complained that they were prevented from exchanging goods in refugees' markets and that refugees were restricted from leaving camps to work as laborers on their farms.[216]

Even if not detained in prisons or refugee camps, refugees may still be compelled to reside in a location not of their choosing. In the early 1970s, the government of Sudan worked with UNHCR to relocate Eritrean refugees from border camps to new, permanent settlements in the Qala en Nahal area. The relocation was justified as requisite to enabling the refugees to become self-sufficient by taking advantage of under-utilized agricultural land. But it was opposed by the refugees themselves as incompatible with their desire to repatriate.[217] Much the same rationale was given for Mozambique's decision to force refugees to abandon their homes near Maputo and to relocate them thousands of kilometers away in the northern provinces, where there was access to arable land for agricultural purposes.[218] In an effort to promote a regional peace plan and to avoid the risk of cross-border raids, Mexico forced

---

[215] "UNHCR tackles HIV/AIDS in refugee camps," *UN Integrated Regional Information Networks*, Sept. 6, 2001.

[216] B. Whitaker, "Refugees in Western Tanzania: The Distribution of Burdens and Benefits among Local Hosts," (2002) 15(4) *Journal of Refugee Studies* 339, at 351–352.

[217] G. Kibreab, *Refugees and Development in Africa: The Case of Eritrea* (1987), at 80–83. See also A. Karadawi, *Refugee Policy in Sudan, 1967–1984* (1999), at 138: "This was thought to be an appropriate political option that minimised the security risk created by the presence of the refugees inside Sudan and the political tensions between Sudan and Ethiopia." The duty of refugees to live in camps is codified in Sudanese law, with "[n]on-compliance ... punishable with imprisonment not exceeding one year ... Camps and settlements in the Sudan are thus established to perpetuate, rather than to bring to an end, refugee status and to block the incorporation of refugees into Sudanese society": G. Kibreab, "Resistance, Displacement, and Identity: The Case of Eritrean Refugees in Sudan," (2000) 34(2) *Canadian Journal of African Studies* 249, at 268–270.

[218] The Mozambican Foreign Minister responded to protests by indicating "that he thought some of [the refugees] had an exaggerated idea of their rights. 'There have been frequent

Guatemalan refugees away from their border camps, and towards interior locations. To ensure the success of the relocation drive, "[s]ettlements were burned, food supplies were severed, and forced evictions were carried out by the Mexican Navy."[219] Also arguing operational necessity, during the late spring of 2000 India forced some 3,000 settled Tamil refugees away from their homes and into distant areas so as to make room for expected new arrivals from Sri Lanka. The refugees were given no choice about where they were to be sent, and were moved without clear regard for their physical safety.[220]

One of the most notorious systems for restricting the residence of refugees in the developed world has been implemented by Germany. While not confining refugees to prisons or camps, Germany's 1982 Asylum Procedure Act authorizes the dispersal around the country of persons awaiting verification of their refugee status, argued to be the best means by which fairly to share the responsibility for their protection and support among the various *Länder*. The designated area of residence can be as small as 15 square kilometers, and the duration of the enforced residence as long as two to seven years. With limited exceptions, not even travel outside the assigned area is allowed without a special permit. Failure to obtain the required authorization may result in a fine of up to €2,500, with repeat offenders unable to pay the fine liable to imprisonment for up to one year.[221]

There is moreover reason to believe that other European states may soon begin to impose tough limits on freedom of residence and movement along the lines of the German system. Under the European Union's recently agreed Reception Directive, EU states enjoy the right to "decide on the residence of the applicant for asylum for reasons of public interest, public order or, when necessary, for the swift processing and effective monitoring of his or her application."[222] Moreover, if a refugee abandons the assigned place of

---

cases of demands that go beyond the obligations that states have towards them,' he said. [Minister] Simao explained that the decision to transfer the refugees to northern provinces was taken to allow them space to carry out self-support activities": Agencia de Informaçao de Mozambique, "Mozambique committed to assisting refugees," Mar. 27, 2003.

[219] J. Simon and B. Manz, "Representation, Organization, and Human Rights Among Guatemalan Refugees in Mexico – 1980–1992," (1992) 5 *Harvard Human Rights Journal* 95, at 109–110.

[220] "On 24 May, during the transfer of some refugees to another camp, a six-month-old child suffocated to death in a scuffle in a bus. When the mother of the dead child wanted the bus to be stopped, the reply of the police escort was, 'Let us keep moving. Even if we stop the bus, the dead child will not be alive'": (2000) 73 *JRS Dispatches* (June 19, 2000).

[221] European Council on Refugees and Exiles, "Setting Limits" (2002) (ECRE, "Limits"), at 11–15. See also F. Liebaut, *Legal and Social Conditions for Asylum Seekers in Western European Countries* (2000) (Liebaut, *Conditions 2000*), at 115–116.

[222] The relevant portions of Art. 7 provide that "[a]sylum seekers may move freely within the territory of the host Member State *or within an area assigned to them by that Member State* ... Member States may decide on the residence of the asylum-seeker for reasons of public interest, public order or, when necessary, for the swift processing and effective

residence without permission, the Directive purports to authorize the host state to "reduce or withdraw the reception conditions"[223] – a euphemism for the various rights otherwise guaranteed to persons awaiting a decision on their refugee claim,[224] including, for example, the rights to family unity, education, and healthcare.[225]

To date, however, most developed countries have imposed few formal restrictions on the residence or mobility of refugees. Belgian law assimilates refugees to non-citizens generally, all of whom may be subject to restrictions on mobility or residence on public order or national security grounds.[226] Spain and Sweden are among the countries which allow refugees to settle and travel wherever they choose, subject only to a duty to inform police of any change of residence.[227] Refugees who have complied with the requirements for verification of their status are otherwise free to choose their home and to travel inside the country as they wish.[228]

The only significant trend away from this respect for mobility rights in the developed world has been the imposition in some states of de facto constraints on the mobility of refugees by tying access to public housing or income support to residence in designated areas or facilities. In Austria, for example, refugee claimants who leave their place of accommodation for more than three days without permission lose their entitlement to federal assistance.[229] In the United Kingdom, refugees must agree to dispersal to an assigned residence if they do not have the financial resources to meet their own needs. Only one offer of accommodation is made; if not accepted by the

---

monitoring of his or her application … When it proves necessary, for example for legal reasons or reasons of public order, Member States may confine an applicant to a particular place in accordance with their national law [emphasis added]": Council Directive laying down minimum standards for the reception of asylum-seekers, Doc. 2003/9/EC (Jan. 27, 2003) (EU Reception Directive), at Art. 7.

[223] Ibid. at Art. 16(1)(a). Beyond concerns of freedom of movement and residence, the withdrawal of rights as punishment is inconsistent with decisions taken in drafting Art. 2 of the Refugee Convention. See chapter 2.4.4 above, at pp. 104–107.

[224] "'[R]eception conditions' shall mean the full set of measures that Member States grant to asylum-seekers in accordance with this Directive": EU Reception Directive, at Art. 2(i).

[225] These rights are set out in Chapter II of the Directive, "General Provisions on Reception Conditions": EU Reception Directive, at Arts. 8, 10, and 13. The right to benefit from emergency healthcare is, however, under no circumstances to be withdrawn: ibid. at Art. 16(4).

[226] "Like any other alien, a refugee may be placed under forced residence restrictions, whereby the Minister of Justice can require an individual alien who has breached public order or national security to leave a specific location, to remain away from that location, or to reside in a specified place": F. Liebaut and J. Hughes, "Legal and Social Conditions for Asylum Seekers and Refugees in Western European Countries" 39 (2000).

[227] ECRE, "Limits," at 29.   [228] France and Italy are typical in this regard: ibid. at 35, 37.

[229] European Council on Refugees and Exiles, *Legal and Social Conditions for Asylum Seekers in Western European Countries, 2003* (2003) (ECRE, *Conditions 2003*), at 23.

refugee claimant, no alternative housing is offered.[230] Changes introduced in 2001 required refugees to arrive at their designated residence within forty-eight hours, or risk being permanently barred from the public welfare system.[231] The way in which the dispersal system has been administered has moreover been criticized as grossly insensitive:

> The dispersal system itself is pure harassment. Recently, a refugee was sent from the Tees Valley to Leicester, away from his best friend and only known contact in the UK, on the pretext that there was no single male accommodation available. The same day, a man in Leicester was dispersed to the Tees Valley.[232]

A softer approach is implemented in the Netherlands. Those refugees who agree to live in a reception center, or *Asielzoekerscentrum*, receive comparatively generous income support, as well as language classes and assistance to find work outside the center. But some income support – albeit insufficient to pay a market rent – is still provided to those refugees who prefer to live on their own, or with friends or family members.[233]

Even where refugees are not subject to efforts to confine them in camps or particular regions, they may still not enjoy real freedom of movement within the whole of the territory of the host country. Refugees in the Sudan, for instance, have generally been allowed to reside in Khartoum only if they already had employment, were referred by a qualified doctor for medical reasons, secured admission to a university, or were the spouse or dependant of a lawful resident of Khartoum.[234] Zambia has traditionally taken much the same approach, allowing only students, professionals, and traders to live in urban areas. Yet not even these persons have been able readily to move internally, since the permit required to live in a city is typically granted only upon payment of an exorbitant fee.[235]

The relevance of financial concerns to freedom of movement is borne out also in the experience of some refugees in developed states. Because in France

---

[230] ECRE, "Limits," at 21.

[231] "Until now, those who have failed to travel – 'without good cause' – have had a second chance to move before their support was stopped ... According to Home Office rules, the only valid reasons for failure to travel are illness or the need to maintain contact with the charity, the Medical Foundation for the Care of Victims of Torture": R. Prasad, "'One strike' rule: Asylum seekers face tough new code," *Guardian*, July 25, 2001, at 4.

[232] J. Hardy, "Tough on toys, tough on the causes of toys: How we ensure that asylum-seekers stick to life's bare essentials," *Guardian*, Dec. 20, 2000, at 18.

[233] ECRE, "Limits," at 38.

[234] G. Kibreab, "Refugees in the Sudan: Unresolved Issues," in H. Adelman and J. Sorenson eds., *African Refugees: Development Aid and Repatriation* 58 (1994).

[235] "Several refugees interviewed for this article at the Commissioner for Refugees' offices revealed that the fees for employment (K250,000) and study permits (K100,000) issued by the government cost 'too much money.' 'Imagine asking a person working as a store

no social assistance is paid to refugees until after registration with a *préfecture*, a process that may take several months, movement outside their place of arrival for virtually any reason is essentially beyond reach for most refugees.[236] In the United Kingdom, welfare payments made to refugees awaiting a decision on their claim expressly exclude any allocation for travel.[237] The protection consequences can sometimes be quite direct:

> [T]here have been problems with travel to attend immigration interviews. Asylum seekers are issued with travel vouchers to cover the cost of the train journey, but there have been problems with travel vouchers not arriving in time for the interviews. This has had a direct effect on the outcome of asylum applications since the number of refusals for "non-compliance" – i.e. not attending interviews, has risen dramatically since the dispersal system was introduced.[238]

Refugee Convention, Art. 26   Freedom of movement
Each Contracting State shall accord to refugees lawfully in its territory the right to choose their place of residence and to move freely within its territory, subject to any regulations applicable to aliens generally in the same circumstances.

Civil and Political Covenant, Art. 12
   1. Everyone lawfully within the territory of a State shall, within that territory, have the right to liberty of movement and freedom to choose his residence.

   . . .

   3. The above-mentioned rights shall not be subject to any restrictions except those which are provided by law, are necessary to protect national security, public order (*ordre public*), public health or morals or the rights and freedoms of others, and are consistent with the other rights recognized in the present Covenant.

   . . .

The drafters of the Refugee Convention were firmly committed to the view that once lawfully in the territory of a state party, refugees should be subject

---

attendant or vegetable vendor . . . to pay K250,000,' lamented a DRC refugee . . . Before 1999, refugees were allowed to reside in urban areas provided they had a valid refugee identity card, and could prove to authorities that they had means of support": *Daily Mail of Zambia*, June 16, 2000.
[236] ECRE, "Limits," at 36.
[237] "[W]hile travel is not prohibited, the welfare payment is set at a level that is not expected to make travel possible. In reality, asylum-seekers have experienced acute difficulties in meeting basic needs . . . and the ability to travel is one of the first casualties": ibid. at 22.
[238] Ibid. at 22.

only to whatever restrictions govern the freedom of internal movement and residence of other non-citizens. The presumptive right of refugees to be assimilated to other aliens for purposes of freedom of movement can lawfully be suspended or limited in only two circumstances: during a mass influx, or while investigating the identity of and possible security threat posed by an individual seeking recognition of refugee status. The more general rule prohibits refugee-specific policies or practices which curtail the ability of refugees to choose the place where they wish to live, or to move about the territory of a state party.

This compromise position was awkwardly arrived at. Despite the precedent of the 1938 Convention, which expressly provided for the right of refugees to enjoy freedom of internal movement,[239] the working draft for the 1951 Convention did not even mention the issue. This omission was noted during discussion of the right of refugees to receive identity papers, when the Belgian and French representatives suggested that the failure to codify freedom of internal movement would amount to "a gap in the draft."[240] It emerged that the reason for the omission had been to avoid a situation in which states would not enjoy the right to impose restrictions on freedom of movement during a mass influx:

> The Secretariat had had in mind the case of the Spanish refugees who presented themselves in large numbers at the French frontier towards the end of the Spanish Civil War and for whom it had been necessary to set up reception camps to meet their immediate needs before regularizing their position and arranging for their dispersal throughout the country. The obligation to remain in these camps was clearly a considerable limitation on the right of movement ... Such a practice might, however, prove essential in certain circumstances.[241]

Elaborating this concern later in the debate, the representative of the International Refugee Organization implored representatives who favored

---

[239] "Without prejudice to the power of any High Contracting State to regulate the right of sojourn and residence, a refugee shall be entitled to move about freely, to sojourn or reside in the territory the present Convention applies to, in accordance with the laws and internal regulations applying therein": Convention governing the Status of Refugees coming from Germany, 4461 LNTS 61, done Feb. 10, 1938 (1938 Refugee Convention), at Art. 2.

[240] Statement of Mr. Rain of France, UN Doc. E/AC.32/SR.15, Jan. 27, 1950, at 12. See also Statement of Mr. Cuvelier of Belgium, ibid. at 11: "Such a provision was included in article 2 of the 1938 Convention, which gave refugees the right to move about freely, to sojourn and to reside in the territory to which they had been admitted. He would like to know why the Secretariat had omitted to include those provisions in its draft, and also whether the Committee would be prepared to have them in the Convention."

[241] Statement of Mr. Rain of France, ibid. at 14.

an article that would codify the right of refugees to enjoy freedom of movement to be realistic:

> Realities must be faced and it must be remembered that the problem which had arisen in France when vast numbers of Spanish refugees had arrived was reappearing, or was liable to reappear in other countries, such as Switzerland, Italy, and so forth.[242]

In addition to the need to be able lawfully to restrict freedom of movement while organizing the reception of a mass influx of refugees, the Danish representative to the Ad Hoc Committee argued that governments should also be entitled to detain dangerous refugees. Mr. Larsen was concerned about "the case of refugees who, having been admitted to a country, had to be expelled from it but could not leave immediately. It was clear that the two situations had certain points in common."[243] He therefore proposed an amendment that

> Internment and restricted residence may be enforced only in individual cases and for imperative reasons of national security and order. The conditions of internment and the treatment of interned refugees shall, both morally and materially, be consistent with human dignity.[244]

In the end, it was agreed that the right of states to detain refugees who pose a threat to host state security, as well as to resort to provisional detention during a mass influx, should be addressed in the context of the proposed rule governing expulsion and non-admittance.[245] The result was Art. 31(2), which grants states some flexibility to limit the freedom of movement of refugees in both situations of concern.[246] As previously described, Art. 31(2) authorizes the provisional detention of refugees arriving in the context of a mass influx for a period of days to enable the receiving state to organize the logistics of emergency reception and dispersal in a way that minimizes disruptions to

---

[242] Statement of Mr. Weis of the IRO, ibid. at 18.

[243] Statement of Mr. Larsen of Denmark, ibid. at 22. The original concern of the Danish representative really does not raise an issue of concern to refugee law. If it is determined that the person seeking recognition of refugee status is subject to exclusion on the grounds of, for example, having committed an extraditable crime or posing a threat to national security, he or she is not a refugee and is therefore subject to the state's general immigration detention rules. But because of the declaratory nature of refugee status, an exception to the general right to freedom of movement was required to authorize detention while the circumstances which might justify exclusion from refugee status are being investigated. This is the function of Art. 31(2). See chapter 4.2.4 above, at pp. 420–424.

[244] Statement of Mr. Larsen of Denmark, ibid. at 23.

[245] Statements of Mr. Henkin of the United States and Mr. Rain of France, ibid. at 23–24.

[246] The scope of these exceptions is addressed at chapter 4.2.4 above, at pp. 419–429.

public order.[247] More generally, it also allows host states to limit freedom of movement during the time needed to ensure that an individual seeking entry as a refugee does not pose a threat to national security, for example while investigating his or her identity and circumstances of arrival.[248]

Importantly, however, the right of a state to limit freedom of movement on either ground comes to an end when a refugee's status is "regularized." As previously analyzed, regularization is not synonymous with recognition of

---

[247] See chapter 4.2.4 above, at pp. 419–420. The French representative insisted that any right to detain refugees arriving in a mass influx *not* be included as a limitation on the Convention's right of freedom of movement, but instead be carefully placed within the article addressing the question of expulsion and admittance (now Art. 31). He observed that "[t]he admission that refugees could be placed in camps was only due to the fact that such measures were sometimes inevitable if the refugees were in such vast numbers that a State felt that to allow them to scatter throughout its territory might be detrimental to public order": Statement of Mr. Rain of France, UN Doc. E/AC.32/SR.15, Jan. 27, 1950, at 24. In introducing the right of states to restrict freedom of movement under Art. 31(2), the representative of the International Refugee Organization confirmed that it "concerned primarily the position of refugees admitted provisionally as an emergency measure. He recognized that it was sometimes impossible for Governments to allow such refugees full freedom of movement and the paragraphs proposed were intended to define the restrictions which might be necessary and to reduce them to the minimum": Statement of Mr. Weis of the IRO, UN Doc. E/AC.32/SR.21, Feb. 2, 1950, at 3. Robinson observes in a footnote that "Art. 26 would also not conflict with *special situations* where refugees have to be accommodated in special camps or in special areas even if this does not apply to aliens generally [emphasis added]": Robinson, *History*, at 133, n. 207. Goodwin-Gill cites Robinson's position without analysis, noting simply that "[s]uch measures are now the usual response, *especially on the occasion of large-scale influx* [emphasis added]": G. Goodwin-Gill, "International Law and the Detention of Refugees," (1986) 20(2) *International Migration Review* 193, at 207. But in light of the drafting history and context of Arts. 31(2) and 26 described here, the exceptional right to detain should be understood to be fully codified in Art. 31(2). Otherwise refugees may be confined to camps only in accordance with rules applicable to aliens generally, and which meet the requirements of Art. 12 of the Civil and Political Covenant: see text below, at pp. 711–718.

[248] See UNHCR Executive Committee Conclusion No. 44, "Detention of Refugees and Asylum-Seekers" (1986), at para. (a), available at www.unhcr.ch (accessed Nov. 20, 2004), which "[n]oted with deep concern that large numbers of refugees and asylum-seekers in different areas of the world are currently the subject of detention or similar measures by reason of their illegal entry or presence in search of asylum, pending resolution of their situation." The Executive Committee then agreed that "detention should normally be avoided. If necessary, detention may be resorted to only on grounds prescribed by law to verify identity; to determine the elements on which the claim to refugee status or asylum is based; to deal with cases where refugees or asylum-seekers have destroyed their travel and/or identity documents in order to mislead the authorities of the State in which they intend to claim asylum; or to protect the national security or public order": ibid. at para. (b). While the reference to public order is not justified under Art. 31(2), the balance of this formulation is a helpful summary of the scope of permissible provisional denial of freedom of movement.

refugee status.[249] To the contrary, "[a]ny person in possession of a residence permit was in a regular position. In fact, the same was true of a person who was not yet in possession of a residence permit but who had applied for it and had the receipt for the application. *Only those persons who had not applied, or whose application had been refused, were in an irregular position* [emphasis added]."[250] Once status is regularized, including by the lodging of an application for recognition of refugee status and completion by the individual concerned of the necessary steps to enable a state to assess his or her claim,[251] all refugee-specific restrictions on the right to move freely and to choose one's residence must end in accordance with Art. 26.[252]

In the result, general policies of post-regularization refugee detention of the kind pursued by Australia and the United States, as well as the long-term confinement of refugees by such countries as Kenya, Pakistan, Uganda, and Zimbabwe, are in breach of the Refugee Convention. While significant latitude is available prior to regularization of status under the terms of Art. 31, there is no legal basis for refugee-specific detention once the individual concerned has complied with his or her obligations to provide authorities with the information needed to assess the claim to be a refugee.

This prohibition on refugee-specific constraints on choice of residence is no less offended when the approach of authorities is indirect, such as the issuance of threats by Malawi and India to deny food and subsistence allowances to coerce refugees to remain in assigned camps, or the Austrian and British rules which withdraw income support from refugees who choose to exercise internal freedom of movement.[253] Because no state may lawfully withhold the essentials of life from refugees,[254]

---

[249] See chapter 3.1.3, above, at pp. 178–183.

[250] This statement of the representative of France was made during the course of the discussion on the right of refugees to enjoy freedom of internal movement and choice of residence: Statement of Mr. Rain of France, UN Doc. E/AC.32/SR.15, Jan. 27, 1950, at 20. See generally chapter 3.1.3 in which the logical and legal reasons for endorsing this understanding are set out in detail.

[251] See chapter 3.1.3 above, at pp. 175–178.

[252] "The freedom of movement as [defined] by Article 26 is not dependent on any particular purpose. The refugee may move around for business or for pleasure": Grahl-Madsen, *Commentary*, at 111.

[253] Indeed, in the cases where the United Kingdom forced a refugee to live in a remote location but failed to provide the individual in a timely way with the funds required to travel to the refugee status interview, resulting in the dismissal of the claim to protection, there is a basis to argue that the duty of *non-refoulement* has been indirectly violated: see chapter 4.1.2 above, at pp. 319–321. More generally, however, Art. 26 is simply a prohibition of constraints as opposed to a duty to facilitate the right of a refugee to choose his or her residence, or to enjoy internal freedom of movement. Thus, to the extent that these rights are compromised in practice by the French decision to delay access to the social welfare system until registration with the local *préfecture*, Art. 26 is not violated.

[254] See chapter 4.4 above.

there is no legal difference between the use of such threats to compel a refugee to reside in a place not of his or her choosing and a direct order of confinement.[255]

In a similar vein, governments may not lawfully rely on the terms of refugee resettlement or temporary admission in order indirectly to limit the freedom of movement and choice of residence of refugees. This possibility was raised directly by the representative of Venezuela to the Ad Hoc Committee, who noted that granting refugees complete freedom to choose their residence might allow them to ignore the terms of resettlement agreements under which refugees were admitted to residence in return for agreeing to work on a particular farm for a period of years.[256] Similarly, the Danish delegate sought to safeguard systems under which refugees are required to live in a particular location while acquiring the skills that would enable them to be resettled.[257] The example given was Denmark's decision during the Nazi era to admit to its territory "certain young German Jews on the condition that after they had completed their agricultural training there, they would leave for other countries, Israel for example, in order to follow their occupation."[258] In a bid to accommodate concerns of this kind, the Chairman of the Ad Hoc Committee proposed that the right of refugees to enjoy freedom of internal movement and residence be "subject to the conditions under which they were admitted."[259]

The Chairman's proposal was, however, rejected on the grounds that it could be invoked to sanction refugee-specific constraints. Because "such an addition would provide few safeguards for refugees,"[260] the Committee voted to prohibit all refugee-specific limitations on freedom of movement or

---

[255] In contrast, the Dutch system – under which basic income support is provided to all refugees awaiting the results of status verification, but superior benefits are offered to those willing to live in a refugee reception center – is not legally problematic. By offering an enhanced level of support to those who agree to reside in a designated place, the Netherlands promotes the reception center option without any unlawful coercion.

[256] The Venezuelan representative "drew attention to the problem with which the authorities of a signatory State might be faced in the event of the article's adoption, if, for example, refugees admitted as agricultural workers were to leave the farms to which they had been assigned and engage in trade in the towns, refusing to return to agricultural work. Although the refugees would thereby have infringed the conditions of their admission to the territory, the reception State might find itself powerless to take any action against them by virtue of the provisions of the article which the Committee was proposing to adopt": Statement of Mr. Perez Perozo of Venezuela, UN Doc. E/AC.32/SR.15, Jan. 27, 1950, at 15.

[257] Statement of Mr. Larsen of Denmark, ibid. at 16.

[258] Statement of Mr. Larsen of Denmark, ibid. at 16.

[259] Statement of the Chairman, Mr. Chance of Canada, ibid. at 21.

[260] Statement of Sir Leslie Brass of the United Kingdom, ibid. at 21.

residence, including those implemented indirectly by terms and conditions of admission,[261] unless generally applied to all non-citizens:[262]

> If new restrictions were introduced into a provision which was intended to grant refugees simple equality of treatment with aliens – an equality which, it seemed to him, should be taken for granted – it would look as though States were being invited to treat the refugees with less consideration than was accorded to aliens.[263]

[261] The use of indirect limitations was identified as problematic by the American representative early in the discussions. In response to a Belgian proposal to incorporate the rule on freedom of movement from the 1938 Convention, Mr. Henkin "pointed out that the first phrase of that article, 'Without prejudice to the power of any High Contracting Party to regulate the right of sojourn and residence' appeared to nullify in advance the rights granted to refugees in the latter part of the text": Statement of Mr. Henkin of the United States, ibid. at 13. Interestingly, even though the discussions noted above had clearly resulted in a decision that terms and conditions of admission could not be relied upon to restrict freedom of movement, the draft adopted by the First Session of the Ad Hoc Committee still contained the reference to "the conditions under which such refugees were admitted": Ad Hoc Committee, "First Session Report," at Annex I, Art. 21. Without any recorded debate, however, the report of the Second Session of the Ad Hoc Committee deleted the reference, allowing only "regulations applicable to aliens generally in the same circumstances" to delimit a refugee's freedom of movement and residence: Ad Hoc Committee, "Second Session Report," at Annex I, Art. 21. But see Weis, *Travaux*, at 210: "Article 26 ... does not affect the conditions imposed on refugees for their admission."

[262] At the Conference of Plenipotentiaries, it was suggested by Canada and Australia that requiring refugees admitted under general immigration schemes to remain in a given job for a period of time should not be understood to violate Art. 26: Statements of Mr. Shaw of Australia and Mr. Chance of Canada, UN Doc. A/CONF.2/SR.11, July 9, 1951, at 16. This is a plausible interpretation, since refugees resettled as immigrants would only face the same (indirect) constraints on freedom of movement as any other non-citizen admitted under the general program. As Grahl-Madsen observed, Art. 26 "does not relate to employment. The rules regulating employment are found in Articles 17 through 19 [see text below at chapters 5.3, 6.1, and 6.2]. It will be appreciated that in so far as there are restrictions on the freedom to seek whatever employment one might desire, the right to choose one's place of residence may be restricted in fact though not in law": Grahl-Madsen, *Commentary*, at 111. It would be otherwise, however, if a resettlement program were directed only to refugees, or if a variant of a general program addressed to refugees imposed more significant limitations on freedom of movement or residence than the general scheme for non-citizens wishing to immigrate. Indeed, Australia recognized as much by entering a reservation, providing that Art. 26 would not be understood to preclude "the imposition of conditions upon which a refugee may enter the Commonwealth ... [or] the making of arrangements with a refugee under which he is required to undertake employment under the direction of the Government": 189 UNTS 200–202, since withdrawn.

[263] Statement of Mr. Rain of France, UN Doc. E/AC.32/SR.15, Jan. 27, 1950, at 21. See also Statements of Mr. Guerreiro of Brazil and Mr. Cuvelier of Belgium, ibid. Providing an example of a limit which appears to have been found acceptable by the Committee, the Brazilian delegate pointed out that "it was true that refugees authorized to enter Brazil as farm workers were required to remain so for a certain number of years, [but] the same provisions applied equally to aliens": Statement of Mr. Guerreiro of Brazil, ibid.

In line with this firm commitment to assimilate refugees to other non-citizens,[264] not even a proposal introduced at the Conference of Plenipotentiaries to authorize refugee-specific constraints on place of residence where necessary to avoid friction between states was pursued.[265] Thus, Mexico's forcible relocation of Guatemalan refugees away from its southern border in order to promote regional peace was not justified under the Convention.[266] There is, of course, no legal impediment to the promotion of residence in areas safe from border incursion or incitement to hostility, so long as refugees are not forcibly moved or confined to their new homes. As much is clear from the softer language of Art. II(6) of the OAU Refugee Convention, which provides that "[for] reasons of security, countries of asylum shall, *as far as possible*, settle refugees at a reasonable distance from the frontier of their country of origin [emphasis added]."[267] But if mandatory constraints on freedom of residence are deemed essential, they must be directed to all non-citizens (or to all persons). Even Art. 9 of the Convention, which does allow strictly provisional and genuinely essential restrictions on freedom of movement and residence in response to "war or other grave and exceptional circumstances," does not authorize a general policy of refugee-specific constraints after the verification of refugee status.[268]

This does not mean, however, that there can be no limits on the freedom of movement of lawfully present refugees (including those awaiting a decision on their application for recognition of refugee status). To the contrary, Art. 26

---

[264] "Article 26 makes it clear beyond doubt that a Contracting State may not impose such restrictions applicable only to refugees": Grahl-Madsen, *Commentary*, at 110.

[265] "[T]he Yugoslav delegation had submitted an amendment ... to cover cases where the fact that refugees resided near the frontier of their country of origin might cause friction between the States. Contracting States should be empowered to prescribe zones in which residence would be forbidden to refugees": Statement of Mr. Makeido of Yugoslavia, UN Doc. A/CONF.2/SR.11, July 9, 1951, at 16. The proposal was, however, withdrawn: ibid.

[266] The harshness with which the relocation was enforced also raises issues of the violation by Mexico of its duty to ensure the physical security of refugees: see chapter 4.3.3 above.

[267] Convention governing the Specific Aspects of Refugee Problems in Africa, UNTS 14691, done Sept. 10, 1969, entered into force June 20, 1974, at Art. II(6). The concern expressed by Blay and Tsamenyi that "[t]he Convention overlooks these issues [of the need for security-based limitations on movement], which may be very significant in the case of some States" is therefore not entirely accurate: Blay and Tsamenyi, "Reservations," at 551.

[268] More specifically, any decision to invoke Art. 9 must be predicated on a good faith assessment that restrictive measures are essential to protection of the receiving state's most vital national interests. The steps taken must be logically connected to eradication of the security concern, may not be of indefinite duration, and may be continued after an individual's refugee status is affirmatively verified only on the basis of unresolved case-specific security concerns. In order to avail itself of even this discretion, a state much proceed in good faith to investigate the security concerns and to verify refugee status. See generally chapter 3.5.1 above.

allows state parties to subject refugees to "any regulations applicable to aliens generally in the same circumstances." For example, where all non-citizens in a state for more than a brief period are required to register their place of residence – as in Spain and Sweden – there is no legal concern where refugees are required to meet the same requirement. Because the internal movement of refugees is limited only by a measure that is generally applied to other non-citizens,[269] the requirements of Art. 26 are met.[270] The same is true where restrictions on freedom of movement are less broadly conceived. Belgium, for example, complies with Art. 26 by limiting the freedom of residence and movement of refugees who present national security or public order threats only on the basis of its general laws addressed to all non-citizens.

In particular, it was noted by the drafters that refugees would be required to respect "the existence in most countries of frontier or strategic zones, access to which [is] forbidden to aliens."[271] As Grahl-Madsen suggests, refugees may also be subject to general rules which impose limits on freedom of movement "because of a natural catastrophe, or because of a rebellion, civil war or large scale police operation, that is to say areas where strangers may be in the way, or where their safety cannot be guaranteed."[272] But the constraints must not be targeted solely at refugees. Thus, the lawfulness of any effort to exclude refugees from border areas prone to armed conflict depends on the scope of the prohibition. So long as all persons, or at least all non-citizens, are excluded from that area, refugees may similarly be barred from entry. But if the prohibition is targeted solely at refugees, it is in breach of the Refugee Convention.

[269] See chapter 3.2.1 above.

[270] The Turkish representative to the Ad Hoc Committee posed a question of direct contemporary relevance to many states. He "wondered what the position would be in the case of a State which, having adopted a very liberal attitude with regard to aliens, who were subject to no restrictions of time or place, received refugees and wished in some way to restrict the conditions of residence of those refugees. Such a State might be prompted to modify its legislation concerning aliens, which would be a highly regrettable measure": Statement of Mr. Kural of Turkey, UN Doc. E/AC.32/SR.15, Jan. 27, 1950, at 19. No reply was offered. While the risk posed was real at the time of the Convention's drafting, the subsequently enacted Art. 12 of the Civil and Political Covenant constrains the risk of downgrading the mobility rights of non-citizens generally in order to be able lawfully to restrict the movements of refugees: see text below, at pp. 713–718. Mr. Kural's intervention is helpful as a clear indication that it was understood by the drafters that the approach taken to Art. 26 would allow no room for refugee-specific limitations.

[271] Statement of Mr. Kural of Turkey, ibid. at 14. A limitation of this kind can also be applied to refugees, assuming that it is not itself found to infringe the general duty not to discriminate against non-citizens, including refugees: see chapter 2.5.5 above.

[272] Grahl-Madsen, *Commentary*, at 111. In such circumstances, however, any distinction in the freedom of movement enjoyed by citizens and that allowed aliens would have to be consistent with the duty of non-discrimination: see text below, at pp. 717–718.

As a matter of logic and fairness, this duty not to stigmatize refugees makes good sense. While there are often good reasons for a government to deny a right of entry into, or residence in, a given place, it is difficult to see how the fact of being a refugee – as contrasted with simply being a person, or at least a non-citizen – can be relevant to the imposition of a categorical exclusion of this very fundamental freedom.[273]

There are two exceptions to the principle that refugees may be subject to the same constraints on freedom of movement which apply to aliens generally. First, because freedom of movement and residence may be limited under Art. 26 only in accordance with "any regulations applicable to aliens generally *in the same circumstances* [emphasis added]," the Refugee Convention requires the non-mechanistic application to refugees of even limits routinely applied to other non-citizens. This form of words requires states to temper the application to refugees of generally applicable rules in order to compensate for any disadvantages faced by refugees in consequence of their refugeehood – for example, because of the urgency of flight, the severing of ties with the home state, or the inability to plan for relocation.[274] Thus, if a reception country normally limits the freedom of internal movement to aliens able to produce a satisfactory security attestation from their country of origin, or grants non-citizens the right to choose their place of residence only after a certain period of residence or sojourn in the host state, it must make some dispensation in administering those rules for refugees whose situation makes perfect compliance an untenable proposition. The Zambian rule requiring possession of a (very expensive) permit to live as a student, professional, or trader in an urban area is a clear example of a general norm which, if strictly applied, would fail to take account of the general inability of refugees (relative to other non-citizens) to plan and save funds in anticipation of their new circumstances.

Second and more generally, Art. 12 of the Civil and Political Covenant delimits the general right of states to control the freedom of internal movement and residence of non-citizens lawfully inside a state's territory.[275] Because most aliens cannot insist on a right of entry into a foreign state,[276]

---

[273] "Without the freedom to move and to take up residence without official permission, personal freedom would indeed be curtailed": A. Grahl-Madsen, "Article 13," in A. Eide et al. eds., *The Universal Declaration of Human Rights: A Commentary* 203 (1992), at 205. See generally the discussion of the duty not to discriminate in imposing limits on freedom of movement and residence set by Art. 12 of the Civil and Political Covenant, below, at pp. 717–718.

[274] See chapter 3.2.3 above, at pp. 207–208.

[275] See generally UN Human Rights Committee, "General Comment No. 27: Freedom of movement" (1999), UN Doc. HRI/GEN/1/Rev.7, May 12, 2004, at 173.

[276] It has recently been determined, however, that persons who "because of [their] special ties to or claims in relation to a given country cannot be considered to be a mere alien,"

it is sometimes suggested that non-citizens may "bargain away" their rights under Art. 12 by assenting to conditions of entry which deny them freedom of internal movement or residence.[277] This is a difficult position to justify in law, based as it is on the notion that individuals may somehow elect to decline rights which are explicitly defined to be inalienable.[278] But in any event, it has no application to refugees, as the drafting discussions recounted above make abundantly clear.[279] By virtue of the non-negotiability of access[280] and the presumptive lawfulness of a refugee who has met a state party's procedural requirements for verification of refugee status,[281] limits on a refugee's freedom of movement or residence derived from rules generally applicable to all aliens must meet the requirements of Art. 12 of the Civil and Political Covenant.

At first glance, the need to comply with the rules on permissible limitation set by Art. 12 of the Covenant appears not to be much of a constraint, as the

including in particular "long-term residents, including but not limited to stateless persons arbitrarily deprived of the right to acquire the nationality of the country of such residence," may invoke the right to enter their "own country" under Art. 12(4) of the Civil and Political Covenant: ibid. at para. 20.

[277] Nowak asserts, without any analysis, that "the lawful residency of aliens may be limited to a part of a State's territory, such that the freedom of movement and residency is locally restricted": Nowak, *ICCPR Commentary*, at 201–202. The view of the UN Human Rights Committee on this issue is awkwardly framed. "Consent for entry may be given subject to conditions relating, for example, to movement, residence and employment. A State may also impose general conditions upon an alien who is in transit. However, once aliens are allowed to enter the territory of a State party they are entitled to the rights set out in the Covenant": UN Human Rights Committee, "The position of aliens under the Covenant" (1986), UN Doc. HRI/GEN/1/Rev.7, May 12, 2004, at 140, para. 6. This formulation could be read to suggest that the non-citizen (once allowed to enter the state's territory) is able to refuse to comply with terms or conditions of admission which conflict with Art. 12.

[278] "The States Parties to the present Covenant, considering that, in accordance with the principles proclaimed in the Charter of the United Nations, recognition of the inherent dignity and of the equal *and inalienable rights* of all members of the human family is the foundation of freedom, justice and peace in the world ... [a]gree upon the following articles [emphasis added]": Civil and Political Covenant, at Preamble. It is difficult to imagine anyone making the argument that a non-citizen could agree to become a slave, or to be subjected to cruel or inhuman treatment, in exchange for permission to enter a foreign state's territory. Yet under the Covenant, the only legal difference between these rights and Art. 12 is that the latter is derogable during time of national emergency, not a distinction which is relevant to the question of renouncing inalienable rights.

[279] See text above, at pp. 709–710. Any effort to condition access to protection on the refugee's preparedness to accept constraints on freedom of movement or residence is unlawful because refugees, unlike most non-citizens, have a legal right to claim protection in a state party under the terms of the Refugee Convention.

[280] See chapter 4.1 above.

[281] Refugees, including those awaiting the results of verification of their status, are by definition "lawfully in" the reception state (see chapter 3.1.3 above, at pp. 175–183).

list of approved purposes for restricting the mobility rights of non-citizens is quite broad. For example, a limitation may be imposed where necessary "to protect national security," now understood to include measures necessary to avoid an objectively reasonable, real possibility of directly or indirectly inflicted substantial harm to the host state's most basic interests, including the risk of an armed attack on its territory or its citizens, or the destruction of its democratic institutions.[282] In addition, restrictions on freedom of movement may be imposed where necessary to protect public order (*ordre public*), a wide-ranging notion that includes the prevention of crime and the promotion of general democratic standards of conduct.[283] Germany might, for example, argue that the assignment of refugees to live in a specific region is compelled by the basic tenets of its federal system. And even if the host government's goal cannot be brought within the scope of a general public order concern, states may also limit freedom of movement where required by considerations of "public health or morals or the rights and freedoms of others." Thus, India might take the view that forcing Tamil refugees to move in order to open up reception places for new (and more vulnerable) refugees expected to arrive on its territory was also justifiable under Art. 12 of the Covenant. Indeed, even Sudan and Mozambique might suggest that the forcible relocation of refugees to areas where they could meet their own subsistence needs was dictated by the need to avoid a huge drain on their resources, thus enabling them to meet the basic needs of their own citizens.

As these examples make clear, the Civil and Political Covenant authorizes limitations on non-citizens' freedom of movement for quite a broad-ranging set of reasons. But Art. 12(3) is not without limits. For example, it is unlikely that Sudan's decision to ban most refugees from residing in Khartoum could be justified on the basis of any of the purposes authorized by the Covenant. It is moreover difficult to see how European Union restrictions on the residence and movement of refugee claimants in order simply to advance the "public interest," much less to enhance "swift processing and effective monitoring" of

---

[282] See chapter 3.5.1 above, at pp. 264–266. For example, the Danish delegate to the Ad Hoc Committee which drafted the Refugee Convention noted that "Denmark and Czechoslovakia, for example, would undoubtedly have hesitated to admit German refugees in 1938 if they had been obliged to allow them to settle in areas already inhabited by minorities, whose ranks would, in the first place, have been swelled by the refugees and in whose political activity against the unity of the country the refugees might subsequently have participated": Statement of Mr. Larsen of Denmark, UN Doc. E/AC.32/SR.15, Jan, 27, 1950, at 16.

[283] But "the purpose for interference does not relate to the specific *ordre public* of the state concerned but rather to an international standard of the democratic society. For instance, the far-reaching restrictions on freedom of internal movement and residency for reasons of *apartheid* that were proposed by South Africa ... not only contravene the prohibition of discrimination under Arts. 2(1) and 26 in conjunction with Art. 12, but also the international *ordre public* under Art. 12(3)": Nowak, *ICCPR Commentary*, at 213.

refugees, can be brought within the terms of Art. 12(3). Such overly broad formulations may well infringe the duty to ensure

> that the restrictions ... not impair the essence of the right; the relation between right and restriction, between norm and exception must not be reversed. The laws authorizing the application of restrictions should use precise criteria and may not confer unfettered discretion on those charged with their execution.[284]

And in any event, there is little doubt that the European Union's purported authorization to withdraw even basic human rights from refugees who disobey limits on their freedom of internal movement contravenes the obligation to ensure that any limits on freedom of movement be administered in a way that is "consistent with all other rights recognized in the Covenant."[285]

Even where the goals of a given restriction on movement or residence can be linked to one of the approved purposes defined by the Covenant, the restriction must still meet Art. 12(3)'s quite demanding legal provisos. First and most basic, a restriction is valid only if it is "provided in law." As the Human Rights Committee has held, "[t]he law itself has to establish the conditions under which the rights may be limited."[286] This is in line with Nowak's appraisal that "[m]ere administrative provisions are insufficient ... [unless they] follow[ ] from the enforcement of a law that provides for such interference with adequate certainty."[287] The informality of the forced relocation of Eritreans by Sudan, even if otherwise lawful, would therefore not meet the standard of the Civil and Political Covenant.

Second, the legal restriction must be substantively justifiable as "necessary" to meet one of the listed goals. This language, intended by the drafters of the Covenant to be intentionally strict, requires that a restriction on freedom of movement or residence be objectively justifiable as essential to one of the approved purposes:[288]

> Article 12, paragraph 3, clearly indicates that it is not sufficient that the restrictions serve the permissible purposes; they must also be necessary to protect them. Restrictive measures must conform to the principle of proportionality; they must be appropriate to achieve their protective

---

[284] UN Human Rights Committee, "General Comment No. 27: Freedom of movement" (1999), UN Doc. HRI/GEN/1/Rev.7, May 12, 2004, at 173, para. 13.

[285] Ibid. at para. 11.   [286] Ibid. at para. 12.

[287] Nowak, *ICCPR Commentary*, at 209. He concludes that "[a] broad interpretation that ... seeks to sweep so-called 'executive legislation' or administrative provisions under the term ['prescribed by law'] would ... correspond with neither the purpose of a legal proviso nor the intentions of its drafters": ibid.

[288] "A restriction on this right is ... consistent with the legal provision in Art. 12(3) not when the State concerned believes it serves one of the listed purposes for interference but rather when it is necessary for achieving this purpose": ibid. at 211.

function; they must be the least intrusive instrument amongst those which might achieve the desired result; and they must be proportionate to the interest to be protected.

The principle of proportionality has to be respected not only in the law that frames the restrictions, but also by the administrative and judicial authorities in applying the law.[289]

In light of this understanding, Germany would likely find it impossible to show that its federal system could not withstand the strain of, for example, the shift to a system of fiscal burden-sharing among the *Länder* to replace the current policy of enforced dispersal of refugees.[290] The necessity requirement makes it particularly difficult ever to establish the legality of closed refugee camps, such as those operated by Hong Kong, Thailand, and Turkey. Unless it can be shown that only the absolute denial of freedom of movement would suffice to meet an approved objective – that is, that an open camp, or a camp from which absences of even limited time and purpose were allowed, could not meet the state's legitimate goals – then the necessity requirement is not satisfied.

Third, the restriction must be one that is consistent with the general rights regime established by the Covenant ("and are consistent with the other rights recognized in the present Covenant").[291] As such, even if Tanzania's closed camp policy for Burundians were otherwise lawful, its administration of the camps in a way that contravened the duty of states to protect family unity (under Art. 23 of the Covenant[292]) would render the detention unlawful. The drafters were particularly concerned that any limitation on freedom of movement – even if legally sanctioned and objectively justifiable as necessary to meet one of the approved goals – must nonetheless not violate the duty of non-discrimination.[293] This preoccupation has recently been affirmed by the Human Rights Committee:

---

[289] UN Human Rights Committee, "General Comment No. 27: Freedom of movement" (1999), UN Doc. HRI/GEN/1/Rev.7, May 12, 2004, at 173, paras. 14–15.

[290] By way of comparison, the Human Rights Committee has "note[d] that asylum-seekers in Denmark are often restricted or discouraged from choosing a residence in specific municipalities or from moving from one municipality to another. Denmark should ensure that any such measures are applied in strict compliance with article 12 of the Covenant": UN Human Rights Committee, "Concluding Observations: Denmark," UN Doc. CCPR/C/70/DNK (2000), at para. 16.

[291] "The permissible limitations which may be imposed on the rights protected under article 12 ... are governed ... by the need for consistency with the other rights recognized in the Covenant ... [T]o be permissible, restrictions must ... be consistent with all other rights recognized in the Covenant": UN Human Rights Committee, "General Comment No. 27: Freedom of movement" (1999), UN Doc. HRI/GEN/1/Rev.7, May 12, 2004, at 173, paras. 2, 11.

[292] See generally chapter 4.6 above.

[293] Nowak, *ICCPR Commentary*, at 210. The meaning of the duty of non-discrimination is canvassed in depth in chapter 2.5.5 above.

> [I]t would be a clear violation of the Covenant if the rights enshrined in article 12, paragraphs 1 and 2, were restricted by making distinctions of any kind, such as race, colour, sex, language, religion, political or other opinion, national or social origin, property, birth or other status.[294]

In the case of its decision to evict Tamil refugees in order to make room for newly arriving refugees, India would thus be required to show that the eviction of non-citizens of a single ethnic group was objectively justifiable on the basis of an assessment of their relative needs and ability to reestablish themselves elsewhere.

Despite its principled constraints, there is however no reason to believe that the scope of permissible limitations on freedom of internal movement presents a serious challenge to the ability of host countries to ensure their most basic interests. The flexibility of Art. 12 is nicely illustrated by a decision of the Human Rights Committee rendered in response to the complaint of a Tunisian refugee against France. The complainant was co-founder of the political movement Ennahdha, and fled Tunisia where he was sentenced to death by trial in absentia. After being recognized by France as a refugee, it came to light that the refugee was an active supporter of groups which engaged in violence against civilian populations. Rather than effecting his expulsion on public security grounds, the decision was made to confine him to the Digne-les-Bains region, and to require him to report daily to police there. This limitation on his internal freedom of movement was upheld by the Committee, though clearly only on the basis of a determination that it was a restriction that was not unduly broad, and which was open to careful scrutiny by national courts:

> [T]he State party produced evidence to the domestic courts that Mr. Karker was an active supporter of a movement which advocates violent action. It should also be noted that the restrictions of movement on Mr. Karker allowed him to reside in a comparatively wide area. Moreover, the restrictions on Mr. Karker's freedom of movement were examined by the domestic courts which, after reviewing all the evidence, held them to be necessary for reasons of national security.[295]

In sum, host governments enjoy reasonable latitude lawfully to limit the freedom of movement and residence of refugees arriving in their territory. Under Art. 31(2), both persons arriving as part of a mass influx and individuals seeking recognition of refugee status whose identity and circumstances

---

[294] UN Human Rights Committee, "General Comment No. 27: Freedom of movement" (1999), UN Doc. HRI/GEN/1/Rev.7, May 12, 2004, at 173, para. 18.

[295] *Karker v. France*, UNHRC Comm. No. 833/1998, UN Doc. CCPR/C/70/D/833/1998, decided Oct. 26, 2000, at para. 9.2. See also *Celepli v. Sweden*, UNHRC Comm. No. 456/1991, UN Doc. CCPR/C/51/D/456/1991, decided Mar. 19, 1993, in which it was determined that it was reasonable to confine a non-citizen terrorist suspect to his home town of 10,000 persons, and to require him to report to the police three times weekly.

of arrival are under investigation may lawfully be detained on a strictly provisional basis. But once the refugee is lawfully present – which includes admission to a procedure for verification of refugee status, as well as so-called temporary admission – Art. 26 requires the termination of all refugee-specific limits on choice of residence and freedom of movement. From that point, only constraints applied to aliens generally may be enforced against refugees, and even then only in a way that takes account of the specificity of the refugee's predicament. Any such limits are moreover only validly enforced to the extent they are based on unambiguous legislative authority, are objectively necessary to attain one of the purposes defined by the Civil and Political Covenant, and are administered in a non-discriminatory way that is consistent with respect for civil and political rights.

5.3 Self-employment

There is little doubt that the inherent trauma of the refugee experience can be exacerbated by enforced idleness and dependence.[296] Ohaegbulom has written of the refugee's need "to become a whole person again, one who earns his own living and the respect of those around him."[297] Simply put, "[s]elf-reliance can improve the refugee's self-image and therefore his or her ability to cope with being a refugee."[298] More fundamentally, the refugee's ability to engage in productive economic activity in the asylum country may also be critical to survival. While international human rights law has evolved to recognize the duty of states affirmatively to assist all persons under their authority – including refugees – to access the necessities of life,[299] refugees too often find that in practice they must fend for themselves.

The focus of this section is the right of refugees to engage in independent economic activity. Under the Refugee Convention's structure of incremental entitlement, this right accrues at an earlier stage than the right of refugees either to be employed, or to engage in professional practice.[300] Because these

---

[296] Gorman makes the case against what he calls the 'Palestinization' of refugees who are forced to remain in dependent situations and are denied the opportunity to pursue self-reliance through economic activity, resulting in their alienation, resentment, and exasperation: R. Gorman ed., *Refugee Aid and Development* (1993), at 8. See also D. Miserz ed., *Refugees – The Trauma of Exile: The Humanitarian Role of the Red Cross and the Red Crescent* (1987), at 92.

[297] F. Ohaegbulom, "Human Rights and the Refugee Situation in Africa," in G. Shepherd and V. Nanda eds., *Human Rights and Third World Development* (1985), at 197.

[298] S. Forbes Martin and E. Copeland, *Making Ends Meet? Refugee Women and Income Generation* (1988), at 3.

[299] See chapter 4.4 above.

[300] Each of these rights accrues only once a refugee is "lawfully staying" in the country of reception, while the right to engage in self-employment is owed to refugees who are simply "lawfully in" a state party. See generally chapters 3.1.3 and 3.1.4 above for an

two means of earning a livelihood may lawfully be withheld from refugees for a period of time, the ability of refugees to survive through their own efforts – for example, by raising food for consumption or sale, trading, or launching their own business – takes on a particular importance for refugees awaiting a decision on refugee status recognition, or on access to some alternative mechanism of durable protection.

In the less developed world, the right to engage in agricultural activities is usually the most pressing concern. There are sometimes blunt refusals to allow refugees to farm. Pakistan, for example, not only denied Afghan refugees the right to own land or other property, but was unwilling to allocate vacant land on which they might engage in food production.[301] Exclusion from agriculture may also be the more subtle result of the refugees' assignment to an area in which there is no available land, or where cultural norms prevent them from farming. A study of Sudanese and Somali refugees living in camps in northwest Kenya observed that "there is little possibility of [the refugees] engaging in agricultural activities, and refugees cannot normally keep cattle. This would be unacceptable to the local population, given the existing fierce competition among different groups for ownership of cattle. These factors conspire to render the refugee population almost completely dependent on aid for survival."[302]

In contrast, Guinea allowed traditional land allocation systems – under which land is made available by appeal to a village "friend," with no government or other involvement – to function as Liberian refugees arrived in that country. Because it was largely in the economic interests of those controlling access to land to promote its cultivation by refugees, the net result was an increase in overall food production.[303] More affirmative efforts were undertaken by Tanzania to respond to the needs of Hutu refugees from Burundi during the 1990s. Upon arrival, refugee families were granted plots of land to clear for cultivation. Refugees began farming basic subsistence crops, later incorporating cash crops. They were also encouraged to undertake poultry farming, brick-making, and carpentry.[304] Refugees at Namibia's Osire camp

---

elaboration of the meaning of these terms. The substance of the rights to engage in employment and professional practice is detailed in chapters 6.1 and 6.2 below.

[301] H. Christensen and W. Scott, "Survey of the Social and Economic Conditions of Afghan Refugees in Pakistan," UN Research Institute for Social Development Report No. 88.1 (1988), at 2–3.

[302] G. Verdirame, "Human Rights and Refugees: The Case of Kenya," (1999) 12(1) *Journal of Refugee Studies* 54, at 62.

[303] R. Black and M. Sessay, "Forced Migration, Land-Use Change and Political Economy in the Forest Region of Guinea," (1997) 96 *African Affairs* 587, at 602–604.

[304] J. Sterkenburg et al., "Refugees and Rural Development: A Comparative Analysis of Project Aid in Sudan and Tanzania," in H. Adelman and J. Sorenson eds., *African Refugees: Development Aid and Repatriation* (1994), at 199–200.

were allowed to take up agricultural activities and to form small businesses to alleviate their poverty and hunger.[305] Botswana has similarly promoted efforts by refugees to engage in income-generating and agricultural activities in settlements such as that at Dukwe,[306] and allowed those refugees who wished to start their own business outside the settlement to apply for a permit (normally reserved for citizens) to do so – though a journey of some 460 km to Gabarone is required to make the necessary application.[307] Mexico is another state which has established planned agricultural settlements for refugees. Guatemalan refugees were settled in Campeche, where they were allowed to grow fruits and vegetables for their own consumption and sale. Refugees also had the opportunity to engage in small-scale projects such as handicraft production, carpentry, and tailoring.[308]

Some countries have taken a similarly open view of the right of refugees to engage in handicrafts and various forms of trading or commerce. Refugees assigned to camps in Ghana have been allowed to supplement their rations by independent commercial activity, including by operating restaurants and other independent business ventures.[309] Switzerland allows only non-citizens with durable status in that country to undertake self-employment, but nonetheless extends that right to all refugees.[310] In Belgium, both recognized refugees and those awaiting verification of their status are eligible to secure an authorization to engage in self-employment.[311] Indeed, Joly describes a range of affirmative efforts by European states to promote independent economic activity by refugees, including rural projects in France, a Spanish initiative to provide funds for refugees seeking to start businesses, and refugee craft cooperatives in the United Kingdom launched with government loans and local council grants.[312] To the extent that limitations are imposed, they tend to be fairly specific. France, for example, subjects refugees to its general rules prohibiting non-citizens from engaging in such businesses as arms

---

[305] "Self-help initiative at Osire refugee camp," *Namibia Economist*, June 7, 2002.

[306] "Examples of income-generating projects in the settlement are a brick-moulding unit, knitting groups, a carpentry unit, a bakery, a restaurant, an art and craft group, and several small shops throughout the settlement ... Examples of successful agricultural activities are poultry projects with broilers and laying hens": J. Zetterqvist, *Refugees in Botswana in the Light of International Law* (1990), at 39–40.

[307] Ibid. at 63.   [308] Stepputat, "Exile in Mexico," at 13–17.

[309] A. Essuman-Johnson, *International Academy of Comparative Law National Report for Ghana* (1994), at 13–14. Thus, for example, UNHCR determined that refugees in the Buduburam refugee camp were economically self-sufficient, and ended assistance to them in 2000: US Committee for Refugees, *World Refugee Survey 2003* (2003), at 72.

[310] W. Kälin, *International Academy of Comparative Law National Report for Switzerland* (1994), at 15.

[311] K. Leus and G. Vermeylen, *International Academy of Comparative Law National Report for Belgium* (1994), at 11.

[312] D. Joly, *Refugees: Asylum in Europe?* (1992), at 59.

manufacturing, mining and oil production, banking, the serving of alcohol, and truck driving.[313]

There are, however, countries that take a harder line on self-employment. In many countries, there are "very limited provisions ... for refugee craftsmen and artisans to re-establish their trades and exploit new markets."[314] While the law authorizes the issuance of permits to refugees who wish to start their own enterprises in Greece, authorities there are reported to delay the issuance of the required permits in the hope of avoiding early integration.[315] Refugees in Botswana have complained that there are no funds available to start up independent enterprises.[316] Indeed, Botswana issued by-laws in 2002 which deny all non-citizens the right to operate hair salons and barber shops in the Central District – thereby depriving refugees and others of access to one of the few successful options for self-support.[317] Costa Rica will allow refugees to undertake self-employment, but only if the applicant has relevant prior experience and can show that Costa Rican citizens will not be displaced by the refugee's business.[318] Zambia has made it practically impossible for refugees lawfully to start a business:

> Until now, refugees had to show a viable registered business in order to get a self-employment permit. Now, new regulations for issuing or renewing a self-employment permit will require that the refugee show at least US$25,000 in assets.[319]

Even more bluntly, Denmark simply refuses to allow refugees awaiting the results of status verification to engage in any form of self-employment or commercial activity,[320] and Malawi insists that refugees have no right to

---

[313] N. Guimezanes, *International Academy of Comparative Law National Report for France* (1994), at 18.

[314] R. Zetter, "Shelter Provision and Settlement Policies for Refugees: A State of the Art Review," Nordic Africa Institute Studies on Emergencies and Disaster Relief Working Paper No. 2 (1995), at 39.

[315] Z. Papassiopi-Passia, *International Academy of Comparative Law National Report for Greece* (1994), at 50.

[316] *Botswana Daily News*, Sept. 13, 2000.   [317] *Gazette* (Gabarone), July 3, 2002.

[318] "To assess this displacement factor, a refugee official must make a geographical reconnaissance of the *barrio* in which the refugee lives, and generally works, to see if there are Costa Ricans engaged in the same trade. Where there are Costa Rican businesses (usually small workshops attached to living quarters) of the type requested by the refugee, the government may deny the work permit. This procedure ensures that the refugee business does not compete with Costa Rican business": E. Larson, "Costa Rican Government Policy on Refugee Employment and Integration, 1980–1990," (1992) 4(3) *International Journal of Refugee Law* 326, at 338.

[319] (2001) 90 *JRS Dispatches* (Apr. 7, 2001).

[320] J. Vedsted-Hansen, *International Academy of Comparative Law National Report for Denmark* (1994), at 2.

establish or to operate businesses.[321] Under the new rules applicable throughout the European Union, states are required to allow refugees to undertake "self-employed activities subject to rules generally applicable to the profession and to the public service," but only once "refugee status has been granted."[322]

> **Refugee Convention, Art. 18   Self-employment**
> The Contracting States shall accord to a refugee lawfully in their territory treatment as favourable as possible and, in any event, not less favourable than that accorded to aliens generally in the same circumstances, as regards the right to engage on his own account in agriculture, industry, handicrafts and commerce and to establish commercial and industrial companies.

This rarely invoked article of the Refugee Convention is in several respects quite extraordinary. First, it is not derived from either of the usual sources, those being prior refugee conventions and the Universal Declaration of Human Rights. The 1951 Refugee Convention was the first international instrument to speak to the right of refugees to undertake independent economic activity, a notion not even alluded to in the subsequently drafted Human Rights Covenants.[323] Second, particularly in view of its legal novelty, it is astonishing that the drafters of the Refugee Convention viewed it as essentially uncontroversial, confining most of their discussions on Art. 18 to the question of the appropriate contingent standard for measuring compliance with the right. Yet as an explicit acknowledgment of the right to participate in entrepreneurial activities at the heart of the market economy, this provision is of potentially enormous importance to refugees. It is, in this

---

[321] Malawi's Deputy Commissioner for Relief and Rehabilitation, Willy Gidala, is reported to have stated emphatically that "refugees are insulting their hosts by breaking the rules. They are not allowed to wander about freely or engage in business": *African Eye News Service*, Nov. 8, 2000.

[322] Council Directive on minimum standards for the qualification and status of third country nationals or stateless persons as refugees or as persons who otherwise need international protection and the content of the protection granted, Doc. 2004/83/EC (Apr. 29, 2004) (EU Qualification Directive), at Art. 26(1). There is no rule specifically addressed to the ability to undertake any form of independent economic activity prior to recognition of refugee status; the general principle relevant to employment is that "Member States shall determine a period of time, starting from the date on which an application for asylum was lodged, during which an applicant shall not have access *to the labour market* [emphasis added]": EU Reception Directive, at Art. 11.

[323] The closest provision is Art. 6 of the Economic, Social and Cultural Covenant, which affirms "the right of everyone to the opportunity to gain his living by work which he freely chooses or accepts": International Covenant on Economic, Social and Cultural Rights, UNGA Res. 2200A(XXI), adopted Dec. 16, 1966, entered into force Jan. 3, 1976 (Economic, Social and Cultural Covenant), at Art. 6(1).

sense, a critical complement to the right of refugees to acquire, and to deal with, both movable and immovable forms of private property, and to be treated fairly under host state taxation schemes.[324]

The rationale for the novel provision was blandly said to be that "a certain number of refugees are handicraft workers with special knowledge and occupational skills, or manufacturers familiar with manufacturing processes peculiar to their country of origin."[325] The case for allowing refugees to make use of their entrepreneurial talents appears to have been considered self-evident. Nor was there any real consideration given to the substantive scope of Art. 18 – including the right of refugees to participate in "agriculture, industry, handicrafts and commerce and to establish commercial and industrial companies." This list is precisely the same as that proposed in the Secretary-General's initial draft,[326] and was not even debated by the drafters.[327]

The textual reference to the right to establish "companies" clearly grants refugees the right to incorporate their enterprises, thereby securing the usual benefits of limited liability. We know also that the competing French version of Art. 18, which would have omitted the right of refugees to engage in agricultural self-employment,[328] was withdrawn even before debate was commenced.[329] There can therefore be no question of excluding agriculture from the range of permissible activities for refugees. But because Art. 18 does not mandate affirmative agricultural resettlement efforts of the kind laudably undertaken by such states as Tanzania, Botswana, Namibia, and Mexico, neither the failure of Pakistan to grant Afghan refugees access to vacant farmland, nor even the assignment by Kenya of Somali and Sudanese refugees to camps where agriculture was unviable and raising livestock was culturally contentious, amounts to a breach of Art. 18.[330] It is enough if the usual

---

[324] The rights of refugees to own property and to be dealt with equitably under taxation schemes are canvassed at chapters 4.5.1 and 4.5.2 above.

[325] Secretary-General, "Memorandum," at 35.   [326] Ibid.

[327] Grahl-Madsen suggests only that "[i]t is apparent that the expression used ['self-employment'] must be given the widest possible interpretation": Grahl-Madsen, *Commentary*, at 76.

[328] France, "Draft Convention," at 6.

[329] Statement of the Chairman, Mr. Chance of Canada, UN Doc. E/AC.32/SR.13, Jan. 26, 1950, at 13.

[330] This does not mean, however, that such actions are insulated from legal challenge. To the contrary, to the extent that the Pakistani actions were targeted at Afghan refugees, they likely breach the duty of non-discrimination: see chapters 2.5.5 and 3.4 above. Similarly, the fact that Kenya required the refugees to live in a place where they could not pursue agricultural production is presumptively in violation of the right of refugees freely to choose their place of residence: see chapter 5.2 above. And in each case, the host government was under an affirmative obligation to provide refugees with the essentials of life, particularly in view of the clear link between official policies and the inability of the refugees to provide for their own needs: see chapter 4.4 above.

market or other rules are allowed to govern access to land, as was the case for Liberian refugees arriving in Guinea.

The drafting history of Art. 18 does assist us to understand the level of attachment at which the right to engage in self-employment inheres. The proposal was initially that only refugees "regularly resident" (*résidant régulièrement*) in a state would be entitled to undertake independent economic activity.[331] While that level of attachment, subsequently translated into English as "lawfully staying,"[332] still governs the rights to undertake employment and to engage in professional practice,[333] the text of Art. 18 was amended by the Ad Hoc Committee to grant the right to self-employment at an earlier stage, namely when a refugee is simply "lawfully in" the territory of a state party (*se trouvant régulièrement*).[334] In view of this clear, if unremarked, change, there can be little doubt that all refugees who have regularized their presence in the host state – including those whose short-term presence is authorized, who have been admitted into a process for refugee status verification, or who are present in a state party which elects not to verify status[335] – may rely on Art. 18.[336] As Robinson writes,

> The expression "lawfully in their [territory]" cannot be only verbally different from "lawfully staying in the country." It must mean in substance something else, viz. the mere fact of lawfully being in the territory, even without any intention of permanence, must suffice.[337]

This duty is clearly recognized in the Belgian policy of making self-employment permits available to persons awaiting the results of refugee status verification. Danish practice, as well as the comparable new European Union rules (in the EU Qualification Directive) – each of which purports to withhold the right to engage in independent economic activity until status has been recognized – are, in contrast, out of step with the requirements of the Convention.

---

[331] Secretary-General, "Memorandum," at 35.

[332] See chapter 3.1.4 above. [333] See chapters 6.1 and 6.2 below.

[334] There is no record of debate on this point, the revised text having appeared for the first time in Ad Hoc Committee, "First Session Report," at Annex I. The point was not dealt with in the subsequent session of the Ad Hoc Committee, nor at the Conference of Plenipotentiaries.

[335] See chapter 3.1.3 above.

[336] Robinson accurately observes, however, that "Art. 18 is not applicable to refugees residing outside the country where the self-employed activity is to be exercised; applicable in such cases is Art. 7(1), i.e. refugees not residing in the country in which they want to engage in self-employment or establish commercial or industrial companies will be permitted to do so only if, under the laws of the country, aliens in general, residing abroad, are authorized to do so and under the same conditions": Robinson, *History*, at 116–117.

[337] Ibid. at 117. See also Weis, *Travaux*, at 152: "[P]hysical presence, even a temporary stay or visit, [is] sufficient, in distinction to 'lawfully staying,' the terminology used in other Articles."

There is, in fact, a real logic to this decision to grant refugees early access to independent economic activity. The Refugee Convention was drafted prior to the advent of modern social welfare systems, and even before the elaboration of the Economic Covenant's duty to provide the essentials of life to all persons unable to meet their own basic needs.[338] Absent some means of enabling refugees to survive economically in the asylum state while awaiting a formal decision on refugee status or other durable protection, it is clear that extraordinary hardship would have been inflicted on the many destitute refugees. Yet the drafters were profoundly concerned not to provide for the economic needs of refugees at the expense of the citizenry of reception states. The British delegate, for example, insisted that refugee rights could not compromise the "planned economy" of his country.[339]

The drafters achieved a workable compromise of interests by authorizing governments to delay refugees' access to both employment and professional practice – areas in which the potential for conflict with the domestic labor market is probably both most acute and most visible – while at the same time agreeing to allow refugees to survive economically through their own entrepreneurship. In essence, refugees are allowed to meet their needs by the generation of new economic activity, though they may initially be barred from competing with citizens for a share of extant employment opportunities. This determination to ensure that refugees have early access only to self-generated economic activity is clear from the only amendment to Art. 18 made at the Conference of Plenipotentiaries. At the suggestion of the Dutch and British representatives, it was agreed that a refugee would have the right to engage in self-employment only "on his own account,"[340] thereby clearly distinguishing this right from a right to undertake activities approximating either employment or investment in a concern established or operated by others.

A true balance between respecting the need of refugees to survive economically and not subjecting the host community to undue competition from refugees was, however, never really established. While it was agreed that the right to engage in self-employment would inhere at an early stage, the value to refugees of the right was significantly compromised by the decision to define the standard for compliance as simply "treatment as favourable as possible and, in any event, not less favourable than that accorded to aliens generally in the same circumstances." This contingent standard builds on the residual minimum standard in Art. 7 ("the same treatment as is accorded to aliens generally").[341] It clearly disallows any restrictions on self-employment aimed

---

[338] See generally chapter 4.4.1 above.
[339] Statement of Sir Leslie Brass of the United Kingdom, UN Doc. E/AC.32/SR.13, Jan. 26, 1950, at 13.
[340] UN Doc. A/CONF.2/SR.9, July 6, 1951, at 19.   [341] See chapter 3.2.1 above.

strictly at refugees, rather than at non-citizens generally. Thus, the Costa Rican regime under which *refugees* alone were denied the right to self-employment if their activities were deemed likely to compete with indigenous enterprises was in breach of Art. 18. More generally, where there is truly generality of access by non-citizens to self-employment or other independent economic activity – as evinced by, for example, relevant domestic laws or practices, a pervasive pattern of bilateral or multilateral agreements, or de facto enjoyment of the right by most aliens – the right to engage in self-employment automatically accrues to refugees as well.[342]

On the other hand, if non-citizens are only rarely allowed to engage in self-employment, or if self-employment is strictly a special right genuinely associated with unique bilateral or similar arrangements, it is not a right that necessarily inheres in refugees. Thus, Botswana's refusal to allow any non-citizen to operate a hair salon or barber shop may not infringe Art. 18, since refugees are caught by what appears to be a rule generally applicable to all non-citizens. Under this standard, it is also clear that refugees should normally be expected to comply with routine requirements to undertake self-employment, such as the acquisition of a license, and be subject to the normal constraints on the scope of such activity.[343] As such, the French rules barring non-citizens generally from self-employment in certain sensitive fields may reasonably be applied to refugees as well (though some forms of activity on the prohibited list – such as truck driving or the serving of alcohol – would likely be difficult to sustain as reasonable constraints in keeping with the duty of non-discrimination[344]). On the other hand, Art. 18 is not respected by the practice of Greek authorities intentionally to prolong the bureaucratic process for issuing self-employment permits to refugees in the hope of slowing down their assimilation. Refugees may only be subject to the *usual* rules governing the treatment of non-citizens, applied in the *usual* way.

The exclusion of refugees from independent economic activity where it is not a right generally enjoyed by other non-citizens may not, however, be implemented in a mechanistic way. This is because the drafters of Art. 18 devised what they intended to be an intermediate contingent standard between the baseline of Art. 7 and the assimilation of refugees to either nationals or the citizens of most-favored states. Specifically, the American representative had criticized reliance simply on the residual contingent standard, noting that granting refugees the same right to engage in self-employment as foreigners generally "would confer no real benefit on refugees."[345] He therefore "wondered whether it might not be possible to find a third solution,

---

[342] See chapter 3.2.1 above, at pp. 199–200.   [343] See Robinson, *History*, at 117.
[344] See chapter 2.5.5 above, at pp. 129–145.
[345] Statement of Mr. Henkin of the United States, UN Doc. E/AC.32/SR.13, Jan. 26, 1950, at 14.

whereby refugees would be granted not the most favourable treatment, but a treatment more favourable than that given to foreigners generally."[346] This proposal met with general agreement,[347] resulting in amendment of the draft article to include the current standard of treatment.

Art. 18's duty to afford refugees "treatment as favourable as possible and, in any event, not less favourable than that accorded to aliens generally in the same circumstances" as regards self-employment thus requires a state party to give consideration in good faith to the non-application to refugees of limits generally applied to other aliens.[348] While exigent circumstances clearly suffice to withhold the right from refugees,[349] refugees should not be barred from independent economic activity on purely formalistic grounds. As such, Malawi's blanket refusal even to consider allowing refugees to undertake self-employment breaches Art. 18 because of its rigid, mechanistic nature. In contrast, Switzerland's decision not to apply its usual rules restricting self-employment by non-citizens to refugees is an example of the thoughtful and humanitarian approach intended by the drafters.

Second, as previously analyzed, the duty to grant refugees access to self-employment on terms not less favorable than those enjoyed by aliens generally "in the same circumstances" means that there is a duty to exempt refugees from general requirements which the refugee cannot meet by virtue of his or her refugeehood – for example, because of the urgency of flight, the severing of ties with the home state, or the inability to plan for relocation.[350] Ideally, states would be inspired to go beyond the strict scope of this duty and, for example, provide start-up funds and other forms of compensatory assistance to refugees wishing to establish businesses in line with the practices of such countries as France, Spain, and the United Kingdom. But because Art. 18 read in the light of Art. 6 requires only the exemption of refugees from insurmountable restrictions (rather than the provision of positive aid to launch a business), Botswana's failure to provide comparable start-up assistance is not in breach of the Convention.

---

[346] Ibid.
[347] Mr. Kural of Turkey "appreciated the humanitarian motives of the United States representative and felt that a formula should be found urging States to accord to refugees treatment more favourable than that given to foreigners generally": Statement of Mr. Kural of Turkey, ibid. at 15. See also Statement of Sir Leslie Brass of the United Kingdom, ibid. Indeed, the Brazilian representative would have preferred an even stronger standard: ibid.
[348] See chapter 3.2.1 above, at p. 200.
[349] During the drafting of Art. 18, the Belgian representative noted his concern regarding an overly liberal contingent standard on the grounds that his country "had an acute middle class problem": Statement of Mr. Cuvelier of Belgium, UN Doc. E/AC.32/SR.13, Jan. 26, 1950, at 14.
[350] See chapter 3.2.3 above.

The legal duty to exempt refugees from insurmountable requirements does, however, provide reason to question the legality of Botswana's failure to make it possible for refugees to secure the required business permit without traveling 460 km to Gabarone. Even if this is the usual practice applied to other non-citizens, Botswana is under a legal duty to tailor generally applicable requirements which fail to take account of the hardships already endured by refugees, logically including a responsibility to minimize the usual bureaucratic hurdles to undertaking independent economic activity.

Even more serious are the distinctly punitive regulations enacted by Zambia, under which only refugees with a net worth of US$25,000 – more than sixty times the average per capita income in that country – may secure a self-employment permit. As the Jesuit Refugee Service has explained, "[t]his condition is insurmountable for most refugees, who have lost their previously accumulated capital in the process of fleeing their country."[351] As such, it would be difficult to conceive a much clearer example of a situation in which a constraint on access to self-employment – even if applied generally to non-citizens – may not lawfully be enforced against refugees. Because even general limitations on the self-employment of non-citizens may be applied only to refugees who are, in fact, "in the same circumstances" as other aliens, governments are under a legal duty to vary or eliminate constraints which fail to take real account of the disadvantages that accrue from involuntary alienage.[352]

---

[351] (2001) 90 *JRS Dispatches* (Apr. 7, 2001).

[352] Indeed, restrictions such as the Zambian regulations, which are aimed solely at refugees, are even more flagrant violations of the Refugee Convention. Whatever the flexibility granted states by virtue of Art. 18's comparatively low contingent standard of treatment, it simply cannot be read to authorize refugee-specific constraints of any kind: see text above, at pp. 726–727.

6

Rights of refugees lawfully staying

A significant number of important rights accrue to refugees only once they are "lawfully staying" in a state party. These include the right to engage in wage-earning employment and to practice a profession, freedom of association, access to housing and welfare, to benefit from labor and social security legislation, intellectual property rights, and the entitlement to receive travel documentation.

As previously described, a refugee is lawfully staying (*résidant régulièrement*) when his or her presence in a given state is ongoing in practical terms.[1] This may be because he or she has been granted asylum consequent to formal recognition of refugee status. But refugees admitted to a so-called "temporary protection" system or other durable protection regime are also lawfully staying. So long as the refugee enjoys officially sanctioned, ongoing presence in a state party, he or she is lawfully staying in the host country; there is no requirement of a formal declaration of refugee status, grant of the right of permanent residence, or establishment of domicile.[2] On the other hand, rights which require lawful stay do not accrue to refugees awaiting the results of a formal process of status verification, as the purely provisional nature of such persons' presence in the host state is at odds with the Convention's reservation of these more integration-oriented rights for those who are expected to remain in the state party for a significant period of time.

6.1 Right to work

In most of the less developed world, access to the national labor market is either denied altogether or extremely limited for refugees. Host states are often concerned that allowing refugees to work will drive down wages for

---

[1] See chapter 3.1.4 above, at pp. 186–187.

[2] This understanding is consistent with the basic structure of the Refugee Convention, which does not require states formally to adjudicate status or assign any particular immigration status to refugees, which does not establish a right to permanent "asylum," and which is content to encourage, rather than to require, access to naturalization. See Convention relating to the Status of Refugees, 189 UNTS 2545, done July 28, 1951, entered into force Apr. 22, 1954 (Refugee Convention), at Art. 34.

their own citizens, thereby creating tensions between the refugees and their hosts. As UNHCR has observed,

> The arrival of large numbers of asylum-seekers and the absorption of some or even all of them as refugees, even on a temporary basis, can create serious strains for host countries. This is particularly the case for poorer communities where the ability of the people and the inclination of the government to shoulder the resultant burden may be severely diminished by economic difficulties, high unemployment, declining living standard, and shortages in housing and land ... Inevitably there are tensions between international obligations and national responsibilities in such circumstances, with the result, in a number of States, that priority is accorded to nationals over all aliens, including refugees, in fields such as employment.[3]

Thus, for example, refugees in Cambodia are granted no work authorizations, "reducing them to little more than illegal immigrants."[4] Tanzania, anxious to avoid the prospect of the de facto integration of Hutu refugees from Burundi, imposed an effective ban on their employment.[5] An only slightly more subtle approach was adopted by Zambia, which set an exorbitant fee for issuance of a work permit to refugees, well beyond the means of nearly all.[6] This tack was defended by immigration officials on the grounds of "the Zambian government's decision to 'push back' some refugees to control crime in towns, attributed largely to the presence of 'aliens.'"[7]

In some circumstances, however, formal bans on the employment of refugees may be of little practical significance. While Mauritania disallows work by refugees, the country's lack of administrative infrastructure means that in practice work can usually be found in informal sectors of the

---

[3] UNHCR, "Implementation of the 1951 Convention and the 1967 Protocol relating to the Status of Refugees," UN Doc. EC/SCP/54, July 7, 1989, at para. 11.

[4] "Cambodia: precarious position of refugees," (2002) 114 *JRS Dispatches* (June 28, 2002).

[5] J. Astill, "UN refugee work in crisis as world ignores Burundi," *Guardian*, Feb. 14, 2001, at 18. Despite the recommendations of a study conducted in 2001 by the Centre for the Study of Forced Migration at the Faculty of Law, University of Dar es Salaam, the Tanzanian government decided not to expand the employment rights of refugees. Instead, the 2003 National Refugee Policy provided only that the government would "continue to look for solutions to its unemployment problem and this calls for all stakeholders to join hands in developing a conducive environment for more employment opportunities. As far as refugees are concerned, the government will allow small income generating activities to be undertaken within the camps": personal communication with Cheggy Mziray of the Centre for the Study of Forced Migration, Faculty of Law, University of Dar es Salaam, Dec. 3, 2003.

[6] "'Imagine asking a person working as a store attendant or vegetable vendor ... to pay K250,000,' lamented a DRC refugee ... The absence of permits often resulted in detention by police, a fact that worried ... [the] regional representative for UNHCR. More than 30 refugees are presently languishing in detention centres, while two Congolese refugees died recently while in detention": *Daily Mail of Zambia*, June 16, 2000.

[7] Ibid. quoting Zambian immigration department spokesperson Danny Lungu.

economy.[8] And some poorer states do allow refugees to work, though usually under the same conditions as other non-citizens. In Zimbabwe, for example, domestic law provides that refugees "shall, in respect of wage-earning employment, be entitled to the same rights and subject to the same restrictions, if any, as are conferred or imposed generally on persons who are not citizens of Zimbabwe."[9]

There are, however, important exceptions to the exclusion of refugees from authorized employment in less developed states. In South Africa, judicial intervention has ensured that even persons awaiting refugee status verification are entitled to work.[10] In Pakistan, Afghan refugees have been allowed to work, with the result that more than 87 percent of Afghan refugee households could claim at least one income earner.[11] And in Western Africa, the governments of ECOWAS states have agreed to allow refugees from within that region to work while in receipt of protection.[12] But even here, reality does not always match commitments. In Senegal, for example, Mauritanian refugees remained unrecognized and hence forced to survive on food aid,[13] while Liberian refugees in Côte

---

[8] "[N]ot one refugee interviewed had been granted a work permit nor heard of any others who had obtained such a permit. Most refugees do not believe, however, that a work permit is necessary for them to carry out labor in the informal sectors of the economy where they have found work; due to weak administrative infrastructure and a lack of enforcement resources, the government has adopted a laissez-faire approach": C. Lindstrom, "Urban Refugees in Mauritania," (2003) 17 *Forced Migration Review* 46.

[9] *Zimbabwe Refugees Act* (Law No. 13, 1983), at s. 12(3), cited in Lawyers' Committee for Human Rights, *African Exodus* (1995) (LCHR, *African Exodus*), at 104.

[10] *Watchenuka Case*, Dec. No. 1486/02 (SA Cape Prov. Div., Nov. 18, 2002); affirmed in *Minister of Home Affairs v. Watchenuka*, (2004) 1 All SA 21 (SA SCA, Nov. 28, 2003).

[11] But Pakistan has deemed refugees from other countries, including Iraq, Iran, Somalia, and Bosnia, simply to be illegal immigrants, and denied them the right to work: N. Ahmad, *International Academy of Comparative Law National Report for Pakistan* (1994), at 6–7; US Committee for Refugees, *World Refugee Survey 2003* (2003), at 153.

[12] LCHR, *African Exodus*, at 108. Pursuant to the Protocol relating to Free Movement of Persons, Residence and Establishment, UNTS 32496 (1996), done at Dakar, May 29, 1979, member governments of the Economic Community of West African States agreed to ensure that by the end of a fifteen-year transitional period "Community citizens have the right to enter, reside and establish in the territory of Member States": ibid. at Art. 2(1). Pursuant to the Supplementary Protocol on the Second Phase (Right of Residence) of the Protocol on Free Movement of Persons, the Right of Residence and Establishment, UNTS 32496 (1996), done at Abuja, July 1, 1986, "each of the Member States shall grant to citizens of the Community who are nationals of other Member States, the right of residence in its territory for the purpose of seeking and carrying out income earning employment": ibid. at Art. 2.

[13] LCHR, *African Exodus*, at 108. "In 2000, the Senegalese government abruptly halted efforts to register Mauritanian refugees and provide them with identity cards. The government initially cited planned changes in its refugee administrative system as the reason for the delay. The registration process remained stalled in 2002": US Committee for Refugees, *World Refugee Survey 2003* (2003), at 88.

d'Ivoire lost their right to food aid if they left their assigned place of residence in search of employment.[14]

Some countries, while insisting on stringent limitations on the right of refugees to work, have nonetheless taken affirmative steps to enable refugees to become economically productive. In Costa Rica, refugees enjoyed no right to work until 1984, at which time the rules were changed to allow refugees to work solely as wage-laborers, and under strict conditions.[15] Because of the limited nature of the right granted, refugees were able to survive only by virtue of an internationally financed effort to establish opportunities for refugee self-employment, particularly in workshops producing leather goods and clothes.[16] Elsewhere refugees have been settled in areas near to large-scale agricultural plantations so that they would be able to earn their living as wage-laborers, simultaneously providing a much-needed source of labor for local farming enterprises.[17]

But when access to work or other economic activity is conditioned on relocation to camps or planned settlements, many refugees will resist such constraints and choose instead to self-settle, typically in rural villages near the border with their country of origin.[18] Often sharing the ethnic origin of their neighbors, and settling in a geographic and economic environment similar to that which they left behind, self-settled refugees enjoy certain advantages in their efforts to integrate into the local economy.[19] Yet because they exist outside the national legal framework, generally remaining unregistered with national or international agencies for fear of discovery, they do not receive

---

[14] LCHR, *African Exodus*, at 108. "Refugees living outside the official refugee zone were ineligible for material assistance, UNHCR reported": US Committee for Refugees, *World Refugee Survey 1998* (1998), at 66.

[15] Specifically, 90 percent of the workers in every business were required to be Costa Rican nationals, and no Costa Rican citizen could be displaced in order to facilitate the employment of a refugee: T. Basok, *Keeping Heads Above Water: Salvadorean Refugees in Costa Rica* (1993) (Basok, *Heads Above Water*), at 35–36, 61.

[16] The widespread failure of the initiative led the government to focus on smaller urban enterprises, such as shoe-making and tailoring, but that program too suffered from a very high failure rate: Basok, *Heads Above Water*, at xvii, 66–67, 74–84. A more recent survey determined that "while legal aspects have improved – every refugee in Costa Rica is legally entitled to work with the refugee ID card – some employers are still unclear about the significance of such documentation and about refugees' right to work in general": G. Monge, "Survey indicates refugee profile, integration in Costa Rica," *UNHCR Behind the Headlines*, Oct. 31, 2002.

[17] T. Kuhlman, "Organized Versus Spontaneous Settlement of Refugees in Africa," in H. Adelman and J. Sorenson eds., *African Refugees: Development Aid and Repatriation* 117 (1994) (Kuhlman, "Organized Versus Spontaneous"), at 128–129.

[18] Ibid. at 124.

[19] E. Brooks, "The Social Consequences of the Legal Dilemma of Refugees in Zambia," paper presented to the Silver Jubilee Conference of the African Studies Association of the United Kingdom, Sept. 1988 (Brooks, "Refugees in Zambia"), at 4. See also Kuhlman, "Organized Versus Spontaneous," at 135.

food or other forms of refugee assistance.[20] In particular, the uncertainty of their legal status often inhibits their efforts to achieve self-reliance, and particularly to undertake longer-term economic planning. Angolan refugees in Zambia, for example, initially survived by a combination of selling their possessions, working as casual agricultural labor, and charity. Three years after their arrival, more than 80 percent were still dependent on others for assistance.[21] Moreover, as Brooks has observed, "[r]elations with local residents will be stressful as long as the uncertainty lasts. After all, it is pretty hard to put much effort into crop production if one is expecting to be shifted at any moment."[22]

Self-settled refugees in the South who defy restrictions on their freedom of movement in order to secure work in urban settings often find that the illegality of their presence means that they are at the mercy of their employers, and must accept much lower wages than locals receive.[23] Even when their work is legally authorized, refugees often have difficulty actually securing employment because of language barriers and cultural differences.[24] As a result, work for urban refugees is generally concentrated in the informal sector despite the often highly employable skills which refugees have to offer.[25]

Most developed states place few restrictions on the right to work of persons formally recognized as refugees. Indeed, the European Union has determined that "Member States shall authorise beneficiaries of refugee status to engage in employed ... activities subject to rules generally applicable to the profession and to the public service, immediately after ... refugee status has been granted."[26] Despite their generally good record on allowing recognized refugees full access to employment opportunities, many countries, including France,[27]

---

[20] Brooks, "Refugees in Zambia," at 2.

[21] H. Williams, "Self-Settled Refugees in North-Western Zambia: Shifting Norms of Assistance from Social Networks," in M. Hopkins and N. Donnely eds., *Selected Papers on Refugee Issues II* (1993), at 145.

[22] Brooks, "Refugees in Zambia," at 6.

[23] G. Kibreab, "Refugees in the Sudan: Unresolved Issues," in H. Adelman and J. Sorenson eds., *African Refugees: Development Aid and Repatriation* 58 (1994) (Kibreab, "Sudan"); Kuhlman, "Organized Versus Spontaneous," at 133.

[24] A. Karadawi, "The Problem of Urban Refugees in Sudan," in J. Rogge ed., *Refugees: A Third World Dilemma* 124 (1987) (Karadawi, "Urban Refugees in Sudan").

[25] J. El Bushra, "Case Studies of Educational Needs Among Refugees II: Eritrean and Ethiopian Refugees in the Sudan," unpublished manuscript, Mar. 1985 (El Bushra, "Educational Needs"), at 22. See also Karadawi, "Urban Refugees in Sudan," at 126.

[26] Council Directive on minimum standards for the qualification and status of third country nationals or stateless persons as refugees or as persons who otherwise need international protection and the content of the protection granted, Doc. 2004/83/EC (Apr. 29, 2004) (EU Qualification Directive), at Art. 26(1).

[27] "Asylum seekers are not allowed to work, although significant numbers work illegally, particularly once their allowance has expired": European Council on Refugees and Exiles, "Setting Limits" (2002) (ECRE, "Limits"), at 36.

Germany,[28] Italy,[29] and the United Kingdom,[30] have nonetheless traditionally denied persons undergoing refugee status assessment the right to undertake employment. In the case of Ireland, the policy seems to have pleased virtually nobody:

> Despite pleas from business and labour leaders and the Association for the Unemployed, the [Irish] Government refuses to allow asylum-seekers to work in the booming economy. They draw the dole while waiting for a hearing, which can take more than a year, prompting accusations of sponging.[31]

Despite such concerns, the member states of the European Union have agreed that they will each set a period of time during which applicants for asylum are barred from entering the labor market.[32] Those limits will, however, normally be lifted if a decision on the refugee claim is not reached within one year. Even at that point, however, states are still allowed to grant priority in employment to EU and European Economic Area nationals, as well as to legally resident

---

[28] "While they await a final verdict on their application, asylum-seekers are sent to hostels or camps, often in extremely isolated locations. They are not allowed to work. They are not allowed to study. And for as long as their case takes to decide – normally several years – they are obliged to remain within the boundaries of the local police authority": J. Hooper, "Welcome to Britain: Fortress Germany," *Guardian*, May 23, 2001, at 8.

[29] "The country's clogged bureaucracy takes more than six months to provide a modest sustenance allowance and more than a year to hear asylum claims. In the meantime, refugees are barred from working officially, and their children are barred from attending public school": J. Smith, "Europe bids immigrants unwelcome," *Washington Post*, July 23, 2000, at A-01.

[30] "Home Secretary David Blunkett talked recently about broadening the work permit system to help deal with skill shortages, but there was nothing in his proposals to help asylum-seekers already in the UK. A Home Office spokesman confirmed asylum-seekers' worst fears. 'I think the answer is no – work permits would not be aimed at those already in the country'": C. Cottell, "Asylum seekers: Would you flee the land of your birth for this?," *Guardian*, Oct. 27, 2001, at 22.

[31] R. Carroll, "Dublin curbs Romanian immigration," *Guardian*, Aug. 5, 1998, at 4. Under ss. 9(4)(b) and 9(7) of the Refugee Act 1996 as amended, "[a]n applicant shall not seek or enter employment ... during the period before the final determination of his or her application for a declaration [to be a Convention refugee] ... A person who contravenes [this limitation] ... shall be guilty of an offence and shall be liable on summary conviction to a fine not exceeding €635 or to an imprisonment for a term not exceeding one month, or both."

[32] This approach mirrors the practice of such countries as the Netherlands, where employment is denied for the first six months, and Sweden, where there is a bar on work for the first four months after filing of the request for protection: ECRE, "Limits," at 27, 38. The United Kingdom previously allowed refugees to work if their claims remained undecided six months after submission; that policy was, however, revoked in July 2002: "UK asylum-seekers' right to work withdrawn," (2002) 117 *JRS Dispatches* (Aug. 29, 2002).

third country nationals[33] – an approach that has been followed for several years in Greece.[34]

Similarly, refugees channeled into "temporary protection" systems have not always enjoyed the right to work. While many states – including Australia, Belgium, Finland, Italy, Norway, Sweden, the United Kingdom, and the United States – have normally granted the beneficiaries of temporary protected status the right to work,[35] other developed countries have been less generous. A delay of up to six months has generally been imposed in Switzerland and the Netherlands before work is authorized;[36] and France applied a similar rule to Kosovar Albanian refugees provisionally admitted to its territory in the late 1990s.[37] Refugees diverted into temporary protection systems in states such as Denmark and Germany have faced even more severe restrictions. In Denmark, refugees granted temporary protected status have not been issued work permits, and are forbidden from accepting employment other than in a job that has been advertised through the employment office and relevant publications for three months without having been filled by a Danish resident or holder of a work permit.[38] Similarly, Bosnian refugees in receipt of temporary protection in Germany were allowed to work after a three-month waiting period, but then only if a labor market assessment confirmed that there was no "privileged employee" – that is, a German or

[33] Council Directive laying down minimum standards for the reception of asylum-seekers, Doc. 2003/9/EC (Jan. 27, 2003) (EU Reception Directive), at Art. 11.

[34] "The right to work of [persons seeking recognition of refugee status] ... is granted under the condition that no interest has been shown in this specific occupation by a Greek citizen, a citizen of another member state of the European Union, by a recognized refugee, or by an emigrant Greek with foreign citizenship [citing to Article 4 of Presidential Decree 189/1998]": A. Skordas, "The Regularization of Illegal Immigrants in Greece," in P. deBruycker ed., *Regularization of Illegal Immigrants in the European Union* 343 (2000), at 381.

[35] Intergovernmental Consultations on Asylum, Refugee and Migration Policies in Europe, North America and Australia, *Report on Temporary Protection in States in Europe, North America and Australia* (1995) (IGC, *Temporary Protection*), at 8.

[36] Ibid. at 153, 210. In Switzerland, the delay may be as little as three months: T. Armyros, "Migration und Xenephobie in der Schweiz," available at www.raben-net.ch (accessed Feb. 28, 2005). In the Netherlands, "[a]sylum seekers are allowed to work, but not during the first six months of their stay and only for periods of limited duration (like the summer season)": US Committee for Refugees, *World Refugee Survey 2003* (2003), at 210.

[37] B. Philippe, "L'embarras des authorités," *Le Monde*, Apr. 9, 1999.

[38] Prior to revisions to the Yugoslav Act in June 1994, not even these exceptional opportunities were open to persons in receipt of temporary protection. Between the time of the 1994 amendments and April 1995, only 366 refugees found employment under the new arrangements: G. Brochmann, "Bosnian Refugees in the Nordic Countries: Three Routes to Protection," paper prepared for the Norwegian Institute for Social Research, Mar. 1995, at 18–19. See also IGC, *Temporary Protection*, at 74, 82; and F. Liebaut ed., *Legal and Social Conditions for Asylum Seekers in Western European Countries* (2000) (Liebaut, *Conditions 2000*), at 63.

other EU national, or non-citizen with a permanent residence or work permit – available to fill the job.[39] Work permits were normally restricted to a specific activity at a particular company, and limited to a duration of one year before reassessment. This approach resulted in very high unemployment rates for Bosnians in Germany, as well as widespread "under-employment" in unskilled jobs not subject to the "privileged employee" priority system.[40]

In response to the real problems faced by refugees diverted into temporary protection regimes as an alternative to seeking Convention refugee status, the Parliamentary Assembly of the Council of Europe recommended that employment rights should be granted to such refugees "where . . . stay is prolonged."[41] This position has now been formally adopted in European Union law, which since 2001 has required that "persons enjoying temporary protection [shall be authorized] to engage in employed or self-employed activities."[42] Priority may, however, be given "to EU citizens and citizens of States bound by the Agreement on the European Economic Area, and also to legally resident third-country nationals who receive unemployment benefits."[43]

Even where refugees in developed countries do not face legal barriers to seeking work, they nonetheless often encounter practical barriers to securing employment. Some barriers may be specific to the situation of refugees, as a study by the Dutch Refugee Council suggests:

> An estimated 40% of [refugees are] looking for a job. By comparison, the Dutch population unemployment figure for 2000 was around 3%, and among immigrants around 12%. The level of education among refugees is virtually the same as that for Dutch people, and many refugees have had work experience in their countries of origin. Why is the unemployment rate so high?
>
> There are a few reasons for this. Refugees are relatively old when they enter the labour market, and their work experience does not match what is required on the Dutch labour market. The long asylum procedure forces asylum-seekers into long years of idleness. When they finally are allowed to work, the gap between them and the labour market is already very large. Refugees have no network of family, friends, neighbours and acquaintances

---

[39] IGC, *Temporary Protection*, at 116.

[40] A. Büllesbach, "War and Civil War Refugees in Germany: The Example of Refugees from Bosnia-Hercegovina," May 1995 (Büllesbach, "Civil War Refugees"), at 54–60.

[41] Parliamentary Assembly of the Council of Europe, "Temporary Protection of Persons Forced to Flee Their Country," Rec. 1348 (1997), at para. 9.

[42] Council Directive on minimum standards for giving protection in the event of a mass influx of displaced persons and on the measures promoting a balance of efforts between Member States in receiving such persons and bearing the consequences thereof, Doc. 2001/55/EC (July 20, 2001) (EU Temporary Protection Directive), at Art. 12.

[43] Ibid. Equally important, persons who prefer to be assessed for formal Convention refugee status may no longer be forced by a state to accept temporary protected status instead: ibid. at Art. 17(1).

who can help them to find a job informally. Employers are not familiar with refugees and have difficulties acknowledging their qualities.[44]

More generally, differences of culture and language, local unemployment, and discrimination may all work against a refugee's success in the job market.[45] In Spain, it has been suggested that "as in other Western societies, situations and circumstances of racial discrimination against immigrants occur at each and every step of their efforts to enter the labour market."[46] Labor market statistics from Sweden, showing higher unemployment among Iranian, Iraqi, and African refugees than for refugees from Eastern Europe and Latin America, have similarly been interpreted as revealing "concealed discrimination." While measures were introduced in Sweden to combat discrimination in the workforce, concerns have been raised that "currently legal rules in Sweden do not provide job applicants and employees with adequate protection against ethnic discrimination, and there is a risk that discrimination will increase in the future."[47]

In response, many developed host states have established programs designed to assist refugees to adapt to local labor markets. Employment schemes involving local employers have been established in the Netherlands and the United Kingdom, self-employment projects are available to refugees in France and Spain, and training programs are commonly available in many other countries.[48] The United States places tremendous emphasis on early employment for refugees; indeed, some arrangements between government and voluntary agency partners require refugees to accept any reasonable job offer to remain eligible for assistance.[49]

[44] Dutch Refugee Council, "Living in Freedom: Work," available at www.vluchtelingen werk.nl (accessed Feb. 28, 2005).

[45] Joly decries "the discrimination experienced by refugees, especially if they come from the third world. They frequently have to accept the most menial and worst paid jobs": D. Joly, *Refugees: Asylum in Europe?* (1992) (Joly, *Asylum*), at 58. See generally H. Lambert, *Seeking Asylum: Comparative Law and Practice in Selected European Countries* (1995) (Lambert, *Seeking Asylum*), at 171.

[46] C. Solé and S. Parella, "The Labour Market and Racial Discrimination in Spain," (2003) 29(1) *Journal of Ethnic and Migration Studies* 121, at 122.

[47] M. Eriksson, *International Academy of Comparative Law National Report for Sweden* (1994), at 39.

[48] Joly, *Asylum*, at 58–59. Issues of access to vocational training are discussed in more detail in chapter 4.8 above, at pp. 607–613.

[49] Tang Thanh Trai Le, *International Academy of Comparative Law National Report for the United States* (1994), at 33 and Annex, at 2–3. "[A]ll refugees are eligible for [Temporary Assistance for Needy Families] assistance for their first five years in the country ... States must ensure that recipients are involved in some form of work-related activity. However, the work requirement might not take effect immediately, and some recipients may be exempted from the work requirement": Institute for Social and Economic Development, Refugee Welfare and Immigration Reform Project, "Fact Sheet: Refugees and Temporary Assistance for Needy Families (TANF)," Sept. 1, 1999, at 2–3.

6.1.1 Wage-earning employment

Refugee Convention, Art. 17   Wage-earning employment

1. The Contracting States shall accord to refugees lawfully staying in their territory the most favourable treatment accorded to nationals of a foreign country in the same circumstances, as regards the right to engage in wage-earning employment.

2. In any case, restrictive measures imposed on aliens or the employment of aliens for the protection of the national labour market shall not be applied to a refugee who was already exempt from them at the date of entry into force of the Convention for the Contracting State concerned, or who fulfils one of the following conditions:

(a)   He has completed three years' residence in the country;
(b)   He has a spouse possessing the nationality of the country of residence. A refugee may not invoke the benefit of this provision if he has abandoned his spouse;
(c)   He has one or more children possessing the nationality of the country of residence.

3. The Contracting States shall give sympathetic consideration to assimilating the rights of all refugees with regard to wage-earning employment to those of nationals, and in particular of those refugees who have entered their territory pursuant to programmes of labour recruitment or under immigration schemes.

Economic, Social and Cultural Covenant, Art. 6

1. The States Parties to the present Covenant recognize the right to work, which includes the right of everyone to the opportunity to gain his living by work which he freely chooses or accepts, and will take appropriate steps to safeguard this right.

2. The steps to be taken by a State Party to the present Covenant to achieve the full realization of this right shall include technical and vocational guidance and training programmes, policies and techniques to achieve steady economic, social and cultural development and full and productive employment under conditions safeguarding fundamental political and economic freedoms to the individual.

Under even contemporary general standards of international human rights law, non-citizens cannot be said to enjoy any meaningful right to engage in wage-earning employment.[50] It is true that Art. 6 of the Economic Covenant

---

[50] There is no international guarantee of a right actually to secure work, only freely to seek work: M. Craven, *The International Covenant on Economic, Social and Cultural Rights: A Perspective on its Development* (1995) (Craven, *ICESCR Commentary*), at 203.

speaks in general terms, and that it expressly confirms that the specific right not to be forced to undertake particular work against one's will inheres in "everyone." But except in fairly extreme cases bordering on exploitation, treaty supervisory bodies, including the Committee on Economic, Social and Cultural Rights, have generally been slow to critique exclusions from employment based on citizenship.[51] Craven attributes this reluctance to the overwhelming weight of state practice, noting that "it is somewhat unlikely that States would consider themselves bound by a provision forcing them to eliminate any restrictions on the employment of aliens."[52]

More fundamentally, apart from the core content of Art. 6[53] – normally understood to include protection against unjust denial of work, and the right not to be subjected to forced labor[54] – this provision of the Economic Covenant imposes only a duty of progressive, non-discriminatory implementation, not of immediate result.[55] More seriously still, there can be little doubt that all but the core content of the right to work is an "economic right," meaning that states of the less developed world – home to the overwhelming majority of the world's refugees – "may determine to what extent they [will] guarantee [the right to work] to non-nationals."[56] Nor is there much force to the rather creative argument that the flip-side of Art. 2(3) is logically a

---

[51] For example, a member of the Economic, Social and Cultural Rights Committee did pursue the issue of whether Jordanian restrictions on the employment of non-citizens were in breach of the duty of non-discrimination, particularly because there appeared to be no economic basis for the restrictions: UN Doc. E/C.12/1988/SR.4, at para. 45. But more generally, the Committee has been described as exhibiting a "[r]eluctance . . . to be unequivocal in its defence of the equal treatment of aliens": Craven, *ICESCR Commentary*, at 173. The Human Rights Committee has shown a comparable preparedness to assume the legitimacy of distinctions in the allocation of rights based on citizenship: see chapter 2.5.5 above, at pp. 131–133. More generally, "job requirements may not in themselves be deemed to be discrimination . . . [I]t is not an easy task to establish a clear line making it legitimate to resort to 'inherent requirements' or 'security of the State'": K. Drzewicki, "The Right to Work and Rights in Work," in A. Eide et al. eds., *Economic, Social and Cultural Rights: A Textbook* 169 (1995), at 178.

[52] Craven, *ICESCR Commentary*, at 174. It is possible, however, that the argument against discrimination would be better received if predicated on the overarching obligation set by Art. 26 of the Civil and Political Covenant: see generally chapter 2.5.5 above, particularly at pp. 125–128.

[53] "[E]ven if non-nationals are not entitled to equal treatment in all respects, it is important to stress that this does not deprive them of all rights under the Covenant. Certainly, in so far as the Covenant establishes the rights of 'everyone,' non-nationals would have a right to the enjoyment of the minimum core content of those rights": Craven, *ICESCR Commentary*, at 174. The notion of "core content" of economic rights is discussed in detail at chapter 4.4.2 above, at pp. 488–490.

[54] Craven, *ICESCR Commentary*, at 205.

[55] See generally chapter 2.5.4 above, at p. 123 and, in particular, chapter 4.4.2 above, at pp. 486–488.

[56] See chapter 2.5.4 above, at p. 122 and chapter 4.4.2 above, at p. 488.

presumption that states of the developed world *do* have a duty to allow non-citizens to work: even though some countries have entered reservations to guard against such an interpretation, neither state practice nor the pattern of inquiry before supervisory bodies is in line with such a construction.[57]

In practical terms, then, refugees might look to the Economic Covenant as a source of protection against arbitrary dismissal (though recognizing that preferring unemployed citizens to aliens is unlikely to be deemed arbitrary), and in particular against forced labor (which may include situations of perceived serious exploitation).[58] Tanzanian employment restrictions, apparently aimed in practice only at Hutu non-citizens, might well breach the UN Charter's prohibition of discrimination on grounds of race,[59] thereby qualifying them as being in breach of the "unjust denial of work" component of the non-derogable core of Art. 6. It might also be determined that the US policy of requiring a refugee to accept "any available job" in order to remain eligible for assistance payments amounts to unlawful forced labor, assuming the assistance scheme is critical to enabling the refugee to secure access to the necessities of life.[60] Because in such a case the refugee would effectively face a Hobson's choice – either take the available job at the pay offered, or forfeit the necessities of life – he or she would not be able in any meaningful sense "freely [to] choose[ ]or accept[ ]" the job offered. But apart from such extreme situations, the provisions of the Economic Covenant are unlikely to be of great value to refugees.

In light of the minimalist import of the Economic Covenant, the scope of the right to work guaranteed by the Refugee Convention is truly impressive. Of particular note, Art. 17 of the Refugee Convention is *not* conceived as a duty of progressive implementation: once its requirements are met, the obligation to allow refugees to work accrues immediately. More important still, Art. 17 binds all states, whatever their level of economic development. Thus, even assuming that less developed countries may rely on Art. 2(3) of the Economic Covenant to insulate themselves from breach of that treaty where

---

[57] "The effects of the UK and French reservations, which may be said to be tacitly approved, are to modify the obligations of those States under the Covenant in relation to other States parties. They do not imply, however, that the provisions of the Covenant in general allow for such an interpretation": Craven, *ICESCR Commentary*, at 213–214.

[58] There is agreed to be a special obligation to facilitate access to the core content of rights by the members of vulnerable groups, which may include refugees: see chapter 4.4.2 above, at pp. 497–499. Craven also suggests that reliance might be placed upon Art. 4 of the Economic Covenant, which requires that any restriction on rights be "solely for the purpose of promoting the general welfare in a democratic society": Craven, *ICESCR Commentary*, at 213–214.

[59] See chapter 1.2.3 above, at p. 44.

[60] This is because there is a binding duty under international law to provide particularly vulnerable populations with at least the most basic necessities of life: see chapter 4.4.1 above, at pp. 497–499.

non-citizens are not allowed to work,[61] the application of such policies to refugees will likely be in breach of the Refugee Convention. Only six countries of the less developed world – Botswana, Burundi, Ethiopia, Iran, Papua New Guinea, and Sierra Leone – maintain reservations to Art. 17 of the Refugee Convention which are broad enough to allow them to enforce a general policy of excluding refugees from wage-earning employment altogether.[62] For the overwhelming majority of less developed state parties, including several known to exclude refugees from the legal right to work – for example, Cambodia, Côte d'Ivoire, Mauritania, and Senegal – the possible right to exclude refugees from work under Art. 2(3) of the Economic Covenant is effectively trumped by Art. 17 of the Refugee Convention.

This result is in keeping with the intentions of the drafters of the Refugee Convention, who were determined to provide refugees with better than the lowest common denominator of state practice, under which non-citizens are often excluded from the labor market.[63] The drafters clearly recognized, and intended, that Art. 17 would require states to grant refugees preferential access to work opportunities, even though this had not been the case under earlier refugee treaties. As the American delegate observed, "the mere fact that the provisions of a convention required a change in the existing laws of any country was not a valid argument against them. If all national laws were to remain unchanged, why should there be a convention?"[64]

This is not to say that Art. 17 was conceived in naïveté. Then as now, governments were keenly aware of the domestic political and other risks of allowing refugees to compete with their own citizens for employment opportunities. The Austrian representative, for example, insisted that "[e]very state had the duty of giving its own nationals priority consideration."[65] While it

---

[61] See chapter 2.5.4 above, at p. 122.

[62] See reservations and declarations of state parties, available at www.unhcr.ch (accessed Nov. 20, 2004). Three other less developed countries – Malawi, Zambia, and Zimbabwe – have entered reservations requiring only treatment at the same level as is afforded aliens generally which, in the light of Art. 2(3) of the Economic Covenant, may be no access to work at all. In each of these countries, however, the more specific duties under Art. 17(2) still apply, subject to the reservation to that paragraph entered by all three countries requiring that refugees entitled to the benefit of Art. 17(2) secure a work permit. Austria and Latvia maintain a blanket reservation to Art. 17 of the Refugee Convention, but as developed countries are bound by the duty progressively to implement the right to work under Art. 6 of the Economic Covenant. The nature of that duty is described at chapter 2.5.4 above, at p. 123 and, in particular, chapter 4.4.2 above, at pp. 486–488.

[63] "[I]f the Committee merely granted to refugees the treatment granted to foreigners generally, it would actually bring about no improvement in their lot": Statement of Mr. Henkin of the United States, UN Doc. E/AC.32/SR.13, Jan. 26, 1950, at 3.

[64] Statement of Mr. Henkin of the United States, UN Doc. E/AC.32/SR.37, Aug. 16, 1950, at 15. See also Statement of Mr. Weis of the IRO, ibid. at 16.

[65] Statement of Mr. Fritzer of Austria, UN Doc. A/CONF.2/SR.9, July 6, 1951, at 8.

might be reasonable to enfranchise refugees in the domestic labor market during times of economic expansion,[66] the same was not true when host countries were confronted with high domestic unemployment.[67] As the Italian government explained,

> A country such as Italy, which was over-populated and therefore had a great deal of unemployment, and whose frontiers and Adriatic coast lay adjacent to areas which formed an inexhaustible source of refugees, could definitely not consider assuming commitments regarding the employment ... of foreign refugees, which could only add to the difficulties already confronting the Italian economy.[68]

The French and Belgian representatives worried that a generous approach to the right of refugees to work "would be unfavourably received by the trade unions concerned in the country of reception and that, in fact, might work against the refugees."[69] Indeed, the observer from the American Federation of Labor explicitly invoked the importance for workers of a "defence of their rights against foreign competition."[70] His organization therefore pressed for language that made refugee rights subject to "the laws and regulations for the protection of the national labour market."[71]

More generally, governments just recovering from the Second World War were anxious not to jeopardize their plans for economic recovery by allowing the free entry of refugees into the workforce. The situation of the United Kingdom was typical of that faced by many European countries. While

---

[66] "Refugees must be guaranteed normal living conditions, which implied freedom to engage in work. The existing state of the labour market allowed the country to observe that principle. Nevertheless his country could not undertake to apply the provisions [of Art. 17(2)] for an indefinite period": Statement of Mr. Schurch of Switzerland, ibid. at 6.

[67] "It should not be forgotten that a large number of Swiss nationals were obliged to leave their own country to find work": Statement of Mr. Schurch of Switzerland, ibid. at 6. See also Statement of Mr. Juvigny of France, UN Doc. E/AC.32/SR.37, Aug, 16, 1950, at 14: "France ... desired to be able to control the movement of labour, and the refusal to permit a refugee to take employment in an overcrowded branch of activity in which there were already thousands of French subjects unemployed did not amount to a denial of the right to work."

[68] Statement of Mr. Del Drago of Italy, UN Doc. A/CONF.2/SR.9, July 6, 1961, at 9. Earlier in the drafting process, Italy had expressed its willingness to allow refugees to work "as soon as unemployment has fallen back to the average figure recorded for a certain number of pre-war years to be determined": United Nations, "Compilation of the Comments of Governments and Specialized Agencies on the Report of the Ad Hoc Committee on Statelessness and Related Problems," UN Doc. E/AC.32/L.40, Aug. 10, 1950 (United Nations, "Compilation of Comments"), at 14.

[69] Statement of Mr. Rain of France, UN Doc. E/AC.32/SR.13, Jan. 26, 1950, at 4. Mr. Cuvelier of Belgium "shared the view of the representative of France": ibid.

[70] Statement of Mr. Stolz of the American Federation of Labor, ibid. at 12.   [71] Ibid.

emphasizing that Britain had previously authorized refugees to work and "that the favourable treatment provided for them had caused no serious hardship for British workers,"[72] Sir Leslie Brass nonetheless explained the salience of changed circumstances:

> [T]he war had altered the economic situation of the United Kingdom which was currently facing serious difficulties resulting both from the material damages it had sustained and from the fact that its economy had been geared to war production over a period of several years. To remedy the situation, the United Kingdom, in agreement with the employers and trade union representatives concerned, and for the common good of the people, had had to adopt a system of planned economy. The United Kingdom had had, for example, to subject wage-earners who were its own nationals to certain restrictions.[73]

In other countries, recovery efforts had been pursued by strategies more directly targeted at the regulation of non-citizen labor. French law, for example, "authorized the fixing of a maximum percentage of aliens employable in each branch of activity,"[74] while Sweden "had been obliged for domestic reasons to introduce a system of labour permits for all aliens which, at the present juncture, it was unable to abandon."[75]

Concerns such as these could very easily have resulted in either the failure to guarantee refugees the right to work, or no more than a minimalist commitment at the lowest common denominator. But the opposite occurred. To begin, the drafters decided not to work from the draft article proposed by the Secretary-General, under which a full right to work would ordinarily be denied during the refugee's first three years in the host state, and even then would be only a right to claim exemption from the full "severity" of general limits on the employment of non-citizens.[76] Instead, they selected as their model the competing French proposal,[77] which began with a much stronger, affirmative statement of entitlement. Once a refugee was "regularly resident" in a state party, he or she would be entitled to benefit from "the most favourable treatment given in the country in question to nationals of a foreign country as regards the right to engage in wage-earning

---

[72] Statement of Sir Leslie Brass of the United Kingdom, ibid. at 5.

[73] Ibid. See also Statement of Mr. Larsen of Denmark, ibid. at 6–7.

[74] Statement of Mr. Juvigny of France, UN Doc. E/AC.32/SR.37, Aug. 16, 1950, at 13.

[75] Statement of Mr. Petren of Sweden, UN Doc. A/CONF.2/SR.9, July 6, 1951, at 6.

[76] United Nations, "Memorandum by the Secretary-General to the Ad Hoc Committee on Statelessness and Related Problems," UN Doc. E/AC.32/2, Jan. 3, 1950 (Secretary-General, "Memorandum"), at 34. This approach was based on that previously adopted in earlier refugee conventions.

[77] Reliance on the French draft was proposed by the Chairman of the Ad Hoc Committee, Mr. Chance of Canada, UN Doc. E/AC.32/SR.13, Jan. 26, 1950, at 2.

employment."[78] The difference of approach is key: not only did the French model provide that the right to work would accrue on the basis of a more flexible (and usually earlier attained) level of attachment,[79] but the right was conceived as having affirmative content at a fairly high contingent level, namely the same right to work as enjoyed by "most-favored foreigners."[80] Despite all of their concerns about domestic unemployment and the requirements of their planned economies, the drafters did not depart from these two baseline principles in fleshing out the content of Art. 17.

What accounts for this apparently courageous stand? Fundamentally, there seems to have been a clear awareness among the drafters that there are few rights more central to refugee self-sufficiency than the right to work.[81] As the American representative observed, "without the right to work all other rights were meaningless. Without that right no refugee could ever become assimilated in his country of residence."[82] It was therefore decided that it made more sense to set the right to work at a meaningfully high level, recognizing that states not yet in a position to enfranchise refugees within their domestic labor market would feel compelled to enter a reservation to the treaty.[83] As the Chairman of the Ad Hoc Committee explained,

[78] France, "Proposal for a Draft Convention," UN Doc. E/AC.32/L.3, Jan. 17, 1950 (France, "Draft Convention"), at 6.

[79] Under neither proposal, however, was there a suggestion that most refugees should be allowed to work from the beginning of their time in a host country.

[80] Under the Secretary-General's standard, in contrast, refugees would only have been entitled to relief from restrictions on the employment of non-citizens. This would not have entitled them to the special privileges often enjoyed by the citizens of most-favored countries. The general meaning of this contingent standard is set out in detail at chapter 3.3.1 above, and analyzed in relation to the right to work below, at pp. 749–752.

[81] The South African Supreme Court of Appeal has recently determined that, as a matter of domestic constitutional law, even persons seeking recognition of refugee status may in some circumstances be entitled to undertake employment. In reaching this conclusion, the Court observed that "[t]he freedom to engage in productive work – even where that is not required in order to survive – is indeed an important part of human dignity ... for mankind is pre-eminently a social species with an instinct for meaningful association. Self-esteem and the sense of self-worth – the fulfilment of what it is to be human – is most often bound up with being accepted as socially useful": *Minister of Home Affairs v. Watchenuka*, (2004) 1 All SA 21 (SA SCA, Nov. 28, 2003), per Nugent JA at para. 27.

N. B.

[82] Statement of Mr. Henkin of the United States, UN Doc. E/AC.32/SR.37, Aug. 16, 1950, at 12. This thinking is shared by Craven, who writes that "[n]ot only is [work] crucial to the enjoyment of 'survival rights' such as food, clothing, or housing, [but] it affects the level of satisfaction of many other human rights such as the rights to education, culture, and health ... [W]ork is an element integral to the maintenance of the dignity and self-respect of the individual": Craven, *ICESCR Commentary*, at 194.

[83] In response to a suggestion by the Chairman of the Ad Hoc Committee that "the question was whether article [17] should remain unchanged, thereby risking numerous reservations, or, with a view to obviating reservations, ... an attempt should be made to restrict

It had, of course, been realised that the inclusion of provisions which, without representing ideals to strive for, were too generous for some Governments to accept, would lead to their making reservations, but it had been thought that such a course might in the long run have a good effect even on Governments which felt themselves unable to accord the treatment prescribed in the Convention upon signing it. Other such cases had arisen in the past where refugees and those who had the interests of refugees at heart had addressed appeals to Governments applying low standards, pointing to the higher standards applied by other Governments, and so had gradually produced an improvement in their policies.[84]

This strategy of setting a relatively high standard with awareness that some reservations would initially be likely, was affirmed by the President of the Conference of Plenipotentiaries:

[T]he Conference ... could aim either at perfection or at reaching the lowest common denominator of agreement. If the latter course were adopted, the government which insisted on the most restrictive conditions would be in a position to dictate the final form that the provisions of the draft Convention should take. If, on the other hand, the former course was followed, many governments would probably be obliged to enter reservations ... Neither of these solutions seemed very desirable, and he therefore appealed to representatives to seek the golden mean, and, if possible, by precept and example, to encourage others to withdraw their reservations at a later stage. If the Conference worked along those lines, he believed it might be possible to arrive at a just and effective instrument.[85]

With the benefit of hindsight, this strategy was extraordinarily insightful.[86] While there is no doubt that Art. 17 has attracted many reservations, more

the provisions concerning wage-earning employment to a minimum," the Belgian representative answered that he "was in favour of the first alternative": Statements of the Chairman, Mr. Larsen of Denmark, and of Mr. Herment of Belgium, UN Doc. E/AC.32/SR.37, Aug. 16, 1950, at 17. See also Statement of Mr. Robinson of Israel, ibid. at 18.

84 Statement of the Chairman, Mr. Larsen of Denmark, ibid. at 11–12.

85 Statement of the President, Mr. Larsen of Denmark, UN Doc. A/CONF.2/SR.9, July 6, 1951, at 14. In response, the British representative to the Conference of Plenipotentiaries withdrew an amendment that would have constrained the scope of Art. 17, noting that "the aim of the Conference should be to frame as liberal a text as could be achieved in the light of practical possibilities": Statement of Mr. Hoare of the United Kingdom, ibid. at 14–15.

86 "[I]t would be better to incorporate in the convention a clause providing for a real improvement in refugees' situation ... even if that clause were to result in reservations, which, it might be hoped, would be neither very numerous or extensive": Statement of Mr. Henkin of the United States, UN Doc. E/AC.32/SR.13, Jan. 26, 1950, at 8. Weis has noted that "[a] number of States made reservations to Article 17. They either withdrew them later, however, or put its provisions into force in spite of the reservation. Thus, the provisions of Article 17 can today be regarded as the general standard as regards the

than 80 percent of state parties have accepted the provision without qualification of any kind.[87] Most reservations are moreover fairly tightly conceived:[88] only eight states (Austria, Botswana, Burundi, Ethiopia, Iran, Latvia, Papua New Guinea, and Sierra Leone) maintain what amounts to a blanket reservation denying the applicability of the article as a whole. Equally important, seven countries which originally constrained their acceptance of Art. 17 – Australia, Brazil, Denmark, Greece, Italy, Malta, and Switzerland – have either withdrawn or significantly narrowed the scope of their reservations,[89] just as the drafters hoped would occur. Because no new reservations can be made after a country has ratified the Convention,[90] the decision to adopt a realistically high standard has resulted in what amounts to the strongest guarantee at the universal level of the right of any group of noncitizens to undertake employment.

In substantive terms, the essence of the obligation to allow refugees to work, contained in the first paragraph of Art. 17, is "of a more categorical nature"[91] than that found in any of the predecessor refugee conventions. While the drafters did not elaborate the scope of "wage-earning employment," Grahl-Madsen concludes that taking account of both the plain meaning of the term and the fact that self-employment and professional practice are the only types of work addressed elsewhere in the Convention,[92]

---

right of refugees to engage in wage-earning employment": P. Weis, *The Refugee Convention, 1951: The Travaux Préparatoires Analysed with a Commentary by Dr. Paul Weis* (posthumously pub'd., 1995) (Weis, *Travaux*), at 149.

[87] Specifically, only 27 of the 145 state parties maintain any reservation or qualification with respect to Art. 17: see text of reservations and declarations of state parties available at www.unhcr.ch (accessed Nov. 20, 2004). This fact bears out the intuition of the drafters that a simple cost–benefit analysis would prove the value of setting a relatively high standard. As the French delegate to the Ad Hoc Committee put it, "[i]f it was thought that 'x' States would accede and that 'x-2' States would express reservations . . . it would be preferable to modify [the article]. If, on the other hand, the majority of states would accept article [17] . . . without any reservations, it would make sense to retain the article": Statement of Mr. Juvigny of France, UN Doc. E/AC.32/SR.37, Aug. 16, 1950, at 14.

[88] This tendency to enter fairly specific reservations was predicted by the American representative to the Ad Hoc Committee, who observed that "an article to which all or most countries made reservations would be pointless. However, if only some countries, even four or five, made reservations, those reservations would not all be equal in their nature and scope": Statement of Mr. Henkin of the United States, ibid. at 15.

[89] See reservations and declarations of state parties, available at www.unhcr.ch (accessed Nov. 20, 2004).

[90] Refugee Convention, at Art. 42(1). This understanding was affirmed at the Conference of Plenipotentiaries: Statement of the President, Mr. Larsen of Denmark, UN Doc. A/CONF.2/SR.9, July 6, 1951, at 13.

[91] N. Robinson, *Convention relating to the Status of Refugees: Its History, Contents and Interpretation* (1953) (Robinson, *History*), at 114.

[92] See chapter 5.3 above regarding the right to engage in self-employment, and chapter 6.2 below regarding the right to engage in professional practice.

> there can be no doubt that [the term "wage-earning employment"] must be understood in its broadest sense, so as to include all kinds of employment which cannot properly be described as self-employment, or [professional practice] ... It ... comprises employment as factory workers, farmhands, office workers, salesmen, domestics and any other kind of work the remuneration for which is in the form of a salary as opposed to fees or profits. It seems reasonable to include waiters, salesmen and others who are remunerated to a greater or smaller extent in the form of tips, commissions or percentages; the crucial point is apparently whether they may be said to have an employer and are not free agents.[93]

In view of the breadth of this definition, the decision of some less developed countries to permit refugees to work only as wage laborers on agricultural plantations is clearly in breach of Art. 17. Nor may a country indirectly limit the right of refugees to look for work, as for example Zambia did to Angolan refugees when it set a prohibitive fee to secure the registration needed lawfully to approach employers.[94]

Refugees not only have the right to work, but also to look for and to accept any offer of "wage-earning employment" which is extended to them. This is not to say that refugees have the right to secure the form of employment which they prefer. As Craven explains in the context of Art. 6 of the Economic Covenant,

> In theory, the concept of freely chosen employment extends to ensuring the fullest opportunity for each worker to use his or her skills in a suitable job. There is a possible tension here between absolute individual choice and the limited options that might be open to him or her in the employment market. It is not realistic to suggest, for example, that the State has to create work opportunities that correspond entirely to the wishes of individuals seeking work.[95]

Thus, the mere fact that refugees face linguistic, cultural, or other barriers to effective competition in the domestic labor market does not bespeak a violation of the Refugee Convention.[96] It remains, however, that refugees may in

---

[93] A. Grahl-Madsen, *Commentary on the Refugee Convention 1951* (1963, pub'd. 1997) (Grahl-Madsen, *Commentary*), at 70. See also Robinson, *History*, at 114; and Weis, *Travaux*, at 147.

[94] With regard to the duty of states to provide refugees with documentation of their identity and status, see chapter 4.9 above. Nor may the failure to provide refugees with documentation be based on the refusal of refugees to comply with restrictions on internal freedom of movement, since the latter are presumptively invalid. See chapter 5.2 above.

[95] Craven, *ICESCR Commentary*, at 217–218.

[96] At best, it might be argued that developed countries have a duty under the International Covenant on Economic, Social and Cultural Rights, UNGA Res. 2200A(XXI), adopted Dec. 16, 1966, entered into force Jan. 3, 1976 (Economic, Social and Cultural Covenant), at Art. 6(2), progressively to take affirmative steps within the bounds of their available resources to promote "full and productive employment" of all persons under their jurisdiction.

some cases be entitled to invoke the duty of non-discrimination, including in particular the responsibility of states to "guarantee to all persons equal and effective protection against discrimination on any ground," in order to contest such exclusions.[97]

The contingent standard by which enjoyment of the right to work is to be measured – namely "the most favourable treatment accorded to nationals of a foreign country in the same circumstances" – amounts to a particularly important advance over earlier treaties. To be sure, not all states felt it was appropriate to enfranchise refugees in the ranks of most-favored foreigners. Austria argued that "[t]he number of persons to whom the most favoured nation clause applies is as a rule relatively small. Since Austria has hundreds of thousands of refugees, their automatic inclusion in a most favoured nation clause . . . would make it impossible for Austria to conclude such agreements in the future."[98] On the other hand, Yugoslavia would have gone much farther in the opposite direction, advocating a national treatment standard because "in most countries the number of refugees was smaller than the number of unemployed . . . [U]nless the former were accorded the freedom to seek employment on equal terms with the nationals of the country concerned, they would be unable to find work."[99]

Each of these extreme positions was rejected. While France congratulated the Yugoslav delegation for its "generous display of liberalism,"[100] there was nearly universal consensus that it would be unrealistic to ask reception states to assimilate refugees to their own citizens for purposes of access to employment opportunities.[101] Canada therefore "urged the Yugoslav representative not to press his amendment; otherwise the Conference would probably find itself involved in an endless discussion."[102] Even UNHCR argued against the more generous Yugoslav approach, insisting that "certain delegations would then be obliged to enter reservations to the entire article."[103]

---

[97] See chapter 2.5.5 above, at pp. 126–128.

[98] United Nations, "Compilation of Comments," at 43.

[99] Statement of Mr. Makiedo of Yugoslavia, UN Doc. A/CONF.2/SR.9, July 6, 1951, at 15.

[100] Statement of Mr. Rochefort of France, ibid. at 10.

[101] For example, Norway "could not agree to put refugees on the same footing as its own nationals in respect of wage-earning employment": Statement of Mr. Anker of Norway, ibid. at 13. The French reaction was more blunt, asserting that "[t]he Yugoslav amendment jeopardized the very existence of [the right to asylum], and did not therefore reflect a very realistic attitude": Statement of Mr. Rochefort of France, ibid. at 10. Interestingly, Germany – which today maintains perhaps the least generous policy in Europe on the right of refugees to work – voiced the strongest support for the Yugoslav initiative, noting that a clause "similar in purport to the Yugoslav amendment had been incorporated in the legislation of the Federal Republic of Germany": Statement of Mr. von Trutzschler of the Federal Republic of Germany, ibid. at 4.

[102] Statement of Mr. Chance of Canada, ibid. at 8.

[103] Statement of Mr. van Heuven Goedhart of UNHCR, ibid. at 12. The Yugoslav amendment was soundly defeated on a 16–1 (4 abstentions) vote: ibid. at 16.

At the same time, however, there was surprisingly strong support for the view that unless refugees benefited from at least most-favored-national treatment, Art. 17 would be of little practical value.[104] In responding to a Belgian query whether the most-favored-national standard might not be too generous, the French representative was emphatic that no less could be granted to refugees:

> [I]t was legitimate and desirable to accord the most favourable treatment to refugees as regards the right to engage in wage-earning employment, and not only the treatment accorded to foreigners generally because refugees by their very nature were denied the support of their Governments and could not hope for governmental intervention in their favour in obtaining exceptions to the general rule by means of conventions. France was therefore merely being faithful to the spirit which had heretofore guided United Nations action in favour of refugees: the purpose of that action was to obtain for refugees the advantages which Governments sought to have granted to their own subjects.[105]

In the end, even those countries which were uncomfortable with the higher contingent standard were persuaded to accept it, and to make whatever reservation was deemed necessary to accommodate their particular national circumstances. Belgium, for example, "considered the right to work as one of the fundamental rights to be accorded to refugees and, despite the amount of unemployment in Belgium, it accepted article [17]."[106]

The drafting history therefore leaves no room for doubt that the most-favored-national standard is intended to secure for refugees the same right to seek employment as is enjoyed by the nationals of states with which the host country has a regional economic or customs union, or other special form of association. As Grahl-Madsen concluded,

> If a country concludes an international agreement, passes a law or institutes a practice, whereby nationals of a certain foreign State are entitled to an especially favourable treatment with regard to wage-earning employment, refugees shall be entitled to the same treatment. It does not matter if there

---

[104] "[I]f the Committee merely granted to refugees the treatment granted to foreigners generally, it would actually bring about no improvement in their lot because it was impossible to give them less than that general treatment": Statement of Mr. Henkin of the United States, UN Doc. E/AC.32/SR.13, Jan. 26, 1950, at 3.

[105] Statement of Mr. Rain of France, ibid. at 2–3.

[106] Statement of Mr. Herment of Belgium, UN Doc. E/AC.32/SR.37, Aug. 16, 1950, at 16. See also Statement of Mr. Anker of Norway, UN Doc. A/CONF.2/SR.9, July 6, 1951, at 13, in which he indicated "that Norway accepted the principle [of most-favored-national treatment] laid down in article [17] of the draft Convention. It could do so all the more readily in that its labour legislation granted refugees more favourable treatment than aliens in general."

are special ties between the two States, as long as they both are States in the eyes of international law.[107]

Consensus on this point is particularly clear from the fact that during the drafting process, Belgium, Norway, and Sweden all expressed their intention to enter reservations to protect their special regional arrangements from the language of Art. 17.[108] And indeed, a significant number of countries have entered reservations intended to avoid the duty to grant refugees the same right to work as the citizens of partner states: in addition to the six countries which grant refugees only the same employment rights as aliens generally,[109] a further eighteen have accepted the general standard but denied refugees work benefits associated with particular customs, economic, or political unions.[110]

It follows, therefore, that the decisions of Denmark and Germany to grant work rights to Bosnian and other refugees in receipt of so-called "temporary protection" only when nationals or other EU citizens were not available to

[107] Grahl-Madsen, *Commentary*, at 70. See also Robinson, *History*, at 109–110: "Most favorable treatment includes also rights granted under bilateral or multilateral conventions whether on the basis of specific conventional provisions or on that of the 'most favored nation' clause. This was made clear by the Belgian representative, who proclaimed that his country would have to enter a reservation to [Art. 17] in view of the economic and customs agreements existing between Belgium and certain neighboring countries"; and Weis, *Travaux*, at 129–130: "Most favourable treatment means the best treatment which is accorded to nationals of another country by treaty or usage. It also includes rights granted under bilateral or multilateral treaties on the basis of special provisions or the 'most favoured nation' clause."

[108] Statements of Mr. Herment of Belgium, UN Doc. E/AC.32/SR.37, Aug. 16, 1950, at 16 ("[H]e would, however, like to express a reservation relating to countries members of a regional union"), and UN Doc. A/CONF.2/SR.9, July 6, 1951, at 8 ("However, the Belgian delegation would have to enter reservations in respect of paragraph 1 of that article in view of the economic and customs agreements between Belgium and certain neighbouring countries"); Statement of Mr. Petren of Sweden, ibid. at 6 (Sweden "could not undertake to extend to refugees the preferential treatment granted to nationals of other Scandinavian countries under existing special treaties"); and Statement of Mr. Anker of Norway, ibid. at 14 ("He desired to associate himself with the statements made by the Swedish and Danish representatives on the regional policy of the Scandinavian countries in respect of the labour market. Accordingly, he would be compelled to enter reservations on article [17] when the Convention was signed").

[109] The six countries are Ireland, Liechtenstein, Malawi, Mexico, Zambia, and Zimbabwe: see reservations and declarations of state parties, available at www.unhcr.ch (accessed Nov. 20, 2004). Because of this reservation, the legislation of Zimbabwe described earlier, which grants refugees only the same right to work as enjoyed by aliens generally, is not in violation of the Convention.

[110] These countries are Angola, Belgium, Brazil, Burundi, Cape Verde, Denmark, Finland, Iran, Latvia, Luxembourg, Moldova, Netherlands, Norway, Portugal, Spain, Sweden, Uganda, and Venezuela: see reservations and declarations of state parties, available at www.unhcr.ch (accessed Nov. 20, 2004).

take relevant jobs did not comply with the requirements of Art. 17(1). More generally, all state parties which are members of the European Union – excepting only Austria and Latvia (which have entered a blanket reservation to Art. 17), and Belgium, Luxembourg, and the Netherlands (which have entered a relevant reservation[111]) – must grant refugees lawfully staying in their territory the same access to employment as is provided to citizens of other European Union countries. While this requirement does not impact the position of refugees awaiting status verification (who are in most cases merely lawfully present, not yet lawfully staying), it does govern the entitlement of refugees present on an ongoing basis, including both those recognized as refugees and those admitted to a temporary protection regime. While this is the approach now taken under the European Union's Qualification Directive with respect to recognized refugees,[112] the provision allowing the right to work of refugees admitted to a temporary protection regime to be subordinated to the claims of European Union and European Economic Area citizens, as well as to those of legally resident third-country nationals, is in breach of the Refugee Convention. Once a refugee is lawfully staying, he or she must be treated on par with the citizens of most-favored states, not ranked hierarchically after them.

Importantly, though, because the contingent standard for the right to work is framed not simply as most-favored-national treatment, but rather as "the most favourable treatment accorded to nationals of a foreign country *in the same circumstances* [emphasis added]," refugees must generally qualify for the right to work in the same way as do most-favored non-citizens, unless the general requirements are effectively insurmountable for refugees because of the uniqueness of their circumstances.[113] It was logically suggested, for example, that this language means that a refugee may not legitimately refuse to comply with the terms of a resettlement program[114] under which the beneficiary (whether a refugee, or simply an immigrant) agrees to undertake particular employment for a period of years in the host country in return for preferential admission, transportation assistance, or comparable

---

[111] None of the reservations entered by other EU states to preserve privileges granted to citizens of special partner states (Denmark, Finland, Portugal, Spain, and Sweden) purports to deny to refugees the special privileges afforded the citizens of EU states; all are rather of a more limited character: see reservations and declarations of state parties available at www.unhcr.ch (accessed Nov. 20, 2004).

[112] EU Qualification Directive, at Art. 26(1).   [113] See generally chapter 3.2.3 above.

[114] "IRO had concluded agreements with certain countries of reception providing for a mass influx of refugees into those countries under a special scheme for manpower recruitment. Those agreements stipulated that after completion of their original contracts, refugees would be entitled to the same conditions as nationals as regards the right to engage in wage-earning employment": Statement of Mr. Weis of the IRO, UN Doc. E/AC.32/SR.13, Jan. 26, 1950, at 3–4.

immigration benefits.[115] (The drafters did, however, incorporate language in Art. 17(3) which affirms their hope that at least upon conclusion of the period of assigned work, refugees admitted under immigration-based schemes would be assimilated to citizens for purposes of access to the full range of employment opportunities.[116]) More generally, the "in the same circumstances" language of Art. 17(1) easily accommodates the concerns of some states that refugees should obtain work permits, or otherwise satisfy routine administrative requirements for the employment of non-citizens.[117] But it is otherwise where, as in the case of Zambia, the exorbitant fee imposed to

[115] At the Conference of Plenipotentiaries, the Australian representative expressed grave concerns regarding his country's ability to enforce the terms of labor restrictions under resettlement agreements if Art. 17 were adopted. "He also had his doubts about the words 'in the same circumstances' in the third line of paragraph 1, and in that connexion, recalled his earlier statement regarding Australia's position as a country of immigration ... Australia's aim was to assimilate the refugees within its territory, but its immigration scheme provided for labour contracts for certain types of migrants ... It had been asserted by some representatives that the Australian delegation's reservations would be covered by the words 'in the same circumstances,' those words being taken to mean that refugees should have the same treatment as other aliens in the same circumstances, in the sense that the refugees would have to satisfy the requirements prescribed for nationals of foreign States resident in Australia": Statement of Mr. Shaw of Australia, UN Doc. A/CONF.2/SR.9, July 6, 1951, at 11. Indeed, because a refugee who is admitted under an immigration-style relocation scheme (often providing affirmative assistance to travel and becoming reestablished) is in essentially the same position as an immigrant in receipt of the same benefits, it is not unreasonable to treat the immigrant and the refugee comparably.

[116] The representative of the International Refugee Organization expressed his desire to see "a clause in the convention safeguarding [the] position in the future" of "refugees in special categories which fell within the framework of plans for the recruiting of foreign manpower and of immigration plans": Statement of Mr. Weis of the IRO, UN Doc. E/AC.32/SR.13, Jan. 26, 1950, at 9–10. Specifically, he had sought to ensure that once the terms of the labor contract were completed, refugees would automatically receive the same right to compete for jobs as citizens: ibid. at 4. The French representative was among those who felt such a rigid prescription "would go beyond the intentions of his Government": Statement of Mr. Rain of France, ibid. at 4. Thus, the American delegate proposed a middle ground position under which states would agree simply to give "favourable consideration" to the assimilation of refugees who had honored the terms of their immigration contracts to nationals for purposes of work: Statement of Mr. Henkin of the United States, ibid. at 5. Paragraph 3 of Art. 17 was drafted by the US representative, and requires that "sympathetic consideration" be given to granting national treatment to refugees, "in particular ... those refugees who have entered their territory pursuant to programmes of labour recruitment or under immigration schemes."

[117] In general international human rights law as well, "[i]t is readily accepted that foreign workers may be required to obtain special authorizations (or permits) in order to be able to work": Craven, *ICESCR Commentary*, at 213. Interestingly, several states – Malawi, Mexico, Mozambique, Sweden, Zambia, and Zimbabwe – nonetheless felt it necessary to enter a reservation to Art. 17 of the Refugee Convention to safeguard their right to require refugees to secure a work permit: see reservations and declarations of state parties, available at www.unhcr.ch (accessed Nov. 20, 2004). Because these reservations do not

secure a work permit amounts to a de facto bar on access to work by virtually all refugees. The duty under Art. 6 to exempt refugees from insurmountable requirements applies in such a case,[118] meaning that refugees must receive administrative dispensation sufficient to offset the disadvantages they face in meeting the requirement to secure a work permit.[119]

The right to be assimilated to most-favored non-citizens as regards a broad-ranging right to seek wage-earning employment is, of course, reserved for refugees who are "lawfully staying" in the host country. At one point, it had been agreed that a lower level of attachment – simply being "lawfully in" a state party – would suffice to have access to employment.[120] But in keeping with the general decision to translate rights defined in the French text to inhere in refugees "résidant régulièrement"[121] as requiring "lawful stay,"[122] the text as finally adopted requires a refugee to show de facto ongoing residence in a state (whether or not domicile or a right of permanent residence has been acquired) before claiming Art. 17(1) rights. Thus, the President of the Conference of Plenipotentiaries accurately concluded that a refugee temporarily visiting a country "should not be accorded the right to engage in wage-earning employment to any greater extent than other aliens."[123]

The more important contemporary concern addressed by this level of attachment is the perceived need to deter the filing of unfounded refugee claims in order simply to gain access, albeit only provisionally, to employment opportunities in the host country. As the English Court of Appeal has noted,

> Part of the purpose of immigration policy is to exclude economic migrants: the removal of the restriction upon the right to work merely because someone has claimed asylum would jeopardize that policy.[124]

indicate an intention to deviate from the substantive requirements of Art. 17, they should be interpreted simply to require refugees to comply with the state's administrative requirements. That is, the reservations cannot be relied upon as a means of indirectly avoiding the substantive obligations set by Art. 17, absent specific words to that effect.

[118] See generally chapter 3.2.3 above.

[119] Zambia's justification for its policy – namely, as a means of "pushing back" refugees – may also be a basis for challenging the policy as an indirect tool of *refoulement*. See chapter 4.1.2 above, at p. 318.

[120] "Report of the Ad Hoc Committee on Statelessness and Related Problems," UN Doc. E/1618, Feb. 17, 1950 (Ad Hoc Committee, "First Session Report"), at Annex I.

[121] "[I]n the first paragraph of the French text, the expression 'refugiés résidant habituellement' should be replaced by the phrase already accepted: 'refugiés résidant régulièrement'": Statement of Mr. Cuvelier of Belgium, UN Doc. E/AC.32/SR.13, Jan. 26, 1950, at 10.

[122] See chapter 3.1.4 above, at p. 189.

[123] Statement of the President, Mr. Larsen of Denmark, UN Doc. A/CONF.2/SR.9, July 6, 1951, at 14.

[124] *Secretary of State for the Home Department v. Jammeh*, [1999] Imm AR 1 (Eng. CA, July 30, 1998). The same decision less accurately suggests the lawfulness of withholding the right to work until "status has been established." Art. 17 of the Refugee Convention requires simply that a refugee be "lawfully staying" in the state party in order to acquire

Because the right to undertake wage-earning employment does not ordinarily inhere in persons who have simply claimed refugee status, the failure by such states as France, Germany, Ireland, Italy, and the United Kingdom to authorize refugees to work while undergoing refugee status verification (assuming those procedures are not unduly prolonged[125]) is not in breach of the Convention.[126] Nor can objection be taken on the basis of Art. 17 to the traditional practice of some European countries, including France, the Netherlands, and Switzerland, of delaying the right to work of refugees in receipt of temporary protection for a period of several months (now superseded in EU states by a duty of immediate access to the labor market[127]). While persons admitted to so-called temporary protection systems are appropriately treated as "lawfully staying" in the host country,[128] it has always been understood that the notion of lawful "stay" (as opposed to mere lawful presence) can be said to begin on the last date that an individual is allowed to remain in a country without securing a residence permit (usually three to six months).[129] So long as the right to work is granted once the refugee's presence becomes ongoing in practical terms (whatever the label assigned by the host country), the requirements of Art. 17 are met.[130]

There are, however, some circumstances in which even refugees not yet lawfully staying in a state party may claim a right of exemption from a critical subset of the limits imposed by many states on the employment of non-citizens. Indeed, these specific exemptions may be of value to refugees lawfully staying in a country where even most-favored nationals face real constraints on access to wage-earning employment.[131] Under Art. 17(2),

the right to work. While a person recognized as a refugee clearly meets this standard, a refugee may also be lawfully staying in some circumstances prior to formal recognition of refugee status. See chapter 3.1.4, at pp. 186–188.

[125] But where, as is reported to be the case in Senegal, the formal status recognition procedure cannot be relied upon to function in a reasonably timely way, a state may not rely upon the absence of formal status to contradict the de facto reality of ongoing presence in the state party. See chapter 3.1.4 above, at pp. 189–190.

[126] If, however, these procedures do not result in a decision within three years, there is nonetheless a duty under Art. 17(2)(a) to provide at least exemption from labor-market-based restrictions on access to employment. See text below, at pp. 756–757.

[127] EU Temporary Protection Directive, at Art. 12. This new European Union policy complies with the Refugee Convention's duty to grant the right to work once a refugee is lawfully staying in the host country, but breaches the duty to assimilate refugees to the citizens of most-favored states (in that it grants EU and EEA citizens priority in employment over refugees).

[128] See chapter 3.1.4 above, at p. 188.   [129] Ibid. at pp. 186–187.   [130] Ibid. at pp. 189–190.

[131] Arts. 17(1) and 17(2) are not, in other words, alternative provisions. A refugee who is lawfully staying in a state party and therefore entitled to the benefit of Art. 17(1) may also claim rights under Art. 17(2). Conversely, a refugee who has met one of the conditions for relief from labor-market-based employment restrictions under Art. 17(2) also acquires rights under Art. 17(1) at such time as he or she is lawfully staying in the country.

refugees in any of four situations described below – whether or not they are also "lawfully staying" in the host state – must not be subjected to "restrictive measures . . . for the protection of the national labour market."

In general terms, the grounds for entitlement to invoke Art. 17(2) identify "refugees who ha[ve] already established some ties with a country."[132] First and most straightforward, the opening clause of Art. 17(2) makes clear that refugees who already enjoyed exemption from labor restrictions in the host state before the Convention entered into force continued to benefit from such exemption.[133] Second and of greater contemporary relevance, any refugee who has been "resident" in a host state for three years,[134] even if it cannot yet be said that he or she is lawfully staying there, is entitled to exemption from labor-market-based restrictions. Because the term "residence" is used in the Convention to refer to de facto ongoing presence rather than to legal notions such as the establishment of domicile,[135] time spent in the reception state since the lodging of an application for refugee status verification should be understood to count toward satisfaction of the three-year threshold. So conceived, Art. 17(2) provides an important safeguard for refugees: while it may offer less protection than the most-favored-national treatment which refugees lawfully staying receive under Art. 17(1), Art. 17(2) rights at least accrue both automatically and at an earlier stage (even if provisionally),[136] thereby mitigating to some extent the hardship which can follow when status assessment procedures are prolonged. The recent European Union directive allowing persons awaiting the results of a refugee status determination

[132] Statement of Mr. Henkin of the United States, UN Doc. E/AC.32/SR.37, Aug. 16, 1950, at 12.

[133] As Robinson explains, "the purpose of this provision is to bind the Contracting States to continue applying . . . favourable treatment": Robinson, *History*, at 115.

[134] As originally framed, Art. 17(2)(a) required "at least" three years' residence: France, "Draft Convention," at 6. The text was amended by France at the suggestion of the representative of the IRO, who feared that "the expression 'at least' might lead to misunderstanding. It might be understood to mean that what was involved was a period of undetermined duration that was, however, in excess of three years": Statement of Mr. Weis of the IRO, UN Doc. E/AC.32/SR.13, Jan. 26, 1950, at 3. The French representative "saw no objection to the deletion of the expression 'at least,' if its retention might lead to debate": Statement of Mr. Rain of France, ibid. On the basis of this exchange, it is clear that states have no discretion to prolong the three-year delay set by Art. 17(2)(a).

[135] "It seems that the term 'residence' must be interpreted as liberally as possible, so as to include anyone who has been physically present in the country for a period of three years, irrespective of whether his presence has been lawful or not. The period of residence will not be interrupted by short periods spent in travelling or visiting other countries": Grahl-Madsen, *Commentary*, at 72. Weis takes a similarly broad approach, arguing that "[t]he term 'residence' . . . is not qualified and might, therefore, include residence which may have been illegal for a certain time but which was subsequently legalized; short absences should not be taken into account": Weis, *Travaux*, at 148. See generally chapter 3.1.3 above, at pp. 182–183.

[136] See chapter 3.1 above, at pp. 158–160.

procedure the right to work after one year reflects a commitment to the purpose advanced by Art. 17(2)(a), and implements it at an earlier time than the Refugee Convention requires.[137]

Significantly greater debate was elicited in regard to paragraphs (b) and (c) of Art. 17(2). Under the first of these provisions, a refugee who is married to a citizen of the host country is immediately entitled to relief from employment restrictions based on labor market considerations. There was little support for the view that an immediate exemption should be withheld unless the refugee automatically acquires the host state's nationality by marriage.[138] To the contrary, the dominant view was that the fact of marriage was itself a sufficient pragmatic basis for exemption, since it clearly showed that the refugee had "some roots in the country, whatever might be the basis of these roots under the nationality laws of that country."[139] The only limitation, reflected in the explicit caveat to Art. 17(2)(b), is that abandonment of the citizen spouse deprives a refugee of the benefit of this provision. An effort was made to authorize the withdrawal of Art. 17(2)(b) benefits also for violation of family obligations falling short of abandonment,[140] but the complexity of defining the relevant circumstances with precision appears to have led the drafters to forsake that effort.[141] Thus, the best view is that a

---

[137] EU Reception Directive, at Art. 11. There are, however, two concerns with the approach adopted by the European Union. First, as described below, no provision is made for earlier access to the right to work required by paras. (b) and (c) of Art. 17(2): see text below, at pp. 757–760. Second, to the extent that a given refugee is entitled to the benefit of any part of Art. 17(2), the European Union standard unlawfully makes access by refugees subordinate to that afforded European citizens and long-term residents. The freedom from "restrictive measures imposed on aliens" set by Art. 17(2) is framed in general terms, not simply as freedom from restrictive measures imposed on "all but most favored" non-citizens. See text below, at p. 761.

[138] This concern was raised by the Chinese representative, who objected to Art. 17(2)(b) on the grounds that "China applied the *jus sanguinis* [principle] ... under which the nationality of the spouse was not changed by marriage. There was, therefore, no reason in law to favour a refugee who married a person of Chinese nationality": Statement of Mr. Cha of China, UN Doc. E/AC.32/SR.13, Jan. 26, 1950, at 8.

[139] Statement of Mr. Henkin of the United States, UN Doc. E/AC.32/SR.37, Aug. 16, 1950, at 13.

[140] The Belgian representative to the Conference of Plenipotentiaries "said that it was known that marriages were at times contracted solely with a view to securing certain advantages. It would be paradoxical if a refugee was able to benefit from his marital status without observing his marital obligations": Statement of Mr. Herment of Belgium, UN Doc. A/CONF.2/SR.9, July 6, 1951, at 17–18. The precise form of the Belgian amendment was rephrased by the French representative to focus on either abandonment or failure "to honour their family obligations": Statement of Mr. Rochefort of France, ibid. at 18, and adopted by the Conference on a 6–5 (9 abstentions) vote "subject to appropriate drafting changes by the Style Committee": ibid. As finally presented and adopted, however, the text of Art. 17(2)(b) refers only to abandonment.

[141] The remarks of the British representative make clear the difficulty of a complete definition of the circumstances in which Art. 17(2)(b) benefits should be withdrawn. "The French

refugee may rely on Art. 17(2)(b) even if he or she does not in fact cohabit with his or her spouse.[142] Indeed, taking account of the recognition that the clause should not be interpreted so as to deprive the citizen spouse of practical access to support payments ordered by a court upon marital break-down,[143] it makes sense to embrace Grahl-Madsen's view that a refugee who is separated (but not yet divorced) may also rely upon Art. 17(2)(b).[144] As he suggests, a purposive understanding of the notion of abandonment should focus on "whether there is still a community of interests between [the refugee and his or her spouse] e.g. that the refugee supports the spouse."[145] If not, and only then, should Art. 17(2)(b) exemption be denied.

Finally, Art. 17(2)(c) allows the parent of a child who is a citizen of the host country also to claim exemption from labor-market-based employment restrictions. Opposition to this clause came primarily[146] from the United

---

representative's attempt to improve on the Belgian amendment raised difficulties of its own. For example, a refugee might not abandon his wife, but he might treat her with such cruelty that she was forced to leave him . . . It would be extremely difficult to allow for all possible contingencies": Statement of Mr. Hoare of the United Kingdom, ibid. at 17.

[142] Belgium took the view that "a stipulation obviously had to be made that, in order to be exempt from the application of the restrictions imposed on aliens, the refugee must reside with the spouse . . . on whose account he or she enjoyed that exemption": Statement of Mr. Herment of Belgium, ibid. at 8. But he later withdrew this suggestion on the basis of the French delegate's comment that "[i]t might be physically impossible for the refugee to reside with his wife, in which case the wording of the Belgian amendment, if adopted, would be unfair to him": Statement of Mr. Rochefort of France, ibid. at 16. Most obviously, for example, the refugee might be able to secure employment only by living apart from his or her spouse for some or much of the time; it would defeat the purpose of Art. 17(2)(b) were the refugee to be prevented from supporting his or her family in such circumstances.

[143] "Moreover, if the wife were able to obtain from the courts a maintenance order against her husband, it would clearly be desirable that the husband should continue to enjoy rights in relation to employment so as to be able to support her": Statement of Mr. Hoare of the United Kingdom, ibid. at 17.

[144] "[A] refugee may invoke Article 17(2)(b) if he is married to a national of the country concerned, also if they live apart, and even if they are factually or legally separated; but not after a divorce, for in that case he (she) has no spouse any longer": Grahl-Madsen, *Commentary*, at 73.

[145] Ibid.

[146] China also opposed the clause, though probably not for sound reasons. "With regard to children, only those who were born of a Chinese mother or father became Chinese. It was therefore unlikely that sub-paragraph (c) would be applied frequently in [China] and the Chinese Government could not be expected to alter its legislation on nationality merely to improve the situation of refugees. The Chinese delegation would therefore find it hard to accept [clause (c)]": Statement of Mr. Cha of China, UN Doc. E/AC.32/SR.13, Jan. 26, 1950, at 8. This intervention suggests that the Chinese representative really did not understand the purport of Art. 17(2)(c) since, if the children of a refugee did not in fact acquire Chinese citizenship under its laws, the refugee parent would receive no exemption from employment restrictions.

Kingdom, which initially opposed the rule on the grounds that it would result in "capricious discrimination"[147] in countries where nationality is acquired in accordance with the principle of *jus soli*. Because a refugee's child born on the territory of such a state would automatically be a citizen, whereas a child born to the same parents before arrival in the host state would not, clause (c) would "favour[ ] those who had children born after their arrival."[148] Yet as the delegate from the United States (also a *jus soli* state) countered, the preferred treatment was logical because the bond of citizenship gave rise to a greater attachment between at least part of the refugee family and the host country.[149] This led the British representative to adopt a somewhat different (and arguably more candid) tack. He expressed his worry that refugees might exploit Art. 17(2)(c) by timing their arrival in the United Kingdom to coincide with the birth of a child, thereby indirectly securing immediate access to the labor market.[150] The Danish chairman provocatively "wondered whether that was the fault of the draft Convention or of *jus soli*,"[151] and suggested that such concerns should logically be addressed by reservation[152] (a position ultimately accepted by the United Kingdom). But the American representative was adamant in defense of the principled logic of allowing the refugee parent of a child citizen to avoid labor market restrictions: "The capriciousness of the provision in question . . . was not as real as it might appear . . . [I]t was clearly in the national interest that the mother of a citizen of the country should have some means of sustenance."[153] The British effort to delete clause (c) was thereupon defeated in the Ad Hoc Committee.[154]

---

[147] Statement of Sir Leslie Brass of the United Kingdom, ibid. at 6.   [148] Ibid.

[149] Statement of Mr. Henkin of the United States, UN Doc. E/AC.32/SR.37, Aug. 16, 1950, at 13.

[150] "A case which had arisen recently would answer the question of the United States representative. A woman who had come to the United Kingdom with a permit to engage in one particular sort of employment had given birth to a child two days after arrival. If the United Kingdom accepted article [17] with no reservations, such a woman would be free of all the restrictions imposed by her work permit since her child would be a citizen of the United Kingdom. That was why it was fair to say that in countries whose nationality laws were based on *jus soli* the principle in paragraph 2(c) would operate very oddly": Statement of Sir Leslie Brass of the United Kingdom, ibid. at 15. He later continued that "[i]t was hardly necessary to point out that to relieve a woman, who entered the country and later gave birth to a child, of all restrictions with regard to employment might be an inducement to such conduct": ibid. at 17. Yet as the Belgian representative immediately noted, it was doubtful that "the example quoted by the United Kingdom was well chosen. The lady in question had a labour contract and, after the birth of her child, the authorities might have insisted on the contract being respected": Statement of Mr. Herment of Belgium, ibid. at 16. This is clearly right: see text above, at pp. 752–753.

[151] Statement of the Chairman, Mr. Larsen of Denmark, ibid. at 15.   [152] Ibid. at 16.

[153] Statement of Mr. Henkin of the United States, ibid. at 17.   [154] Ibid. at 19.

Despite efforts by the United Kingdom again to press its concerns at the Conference of Plenipotentiaries,[155] clause (c) was maintained. The scope of the provision was moreover clarified in response to a suggestion from the President of the Conference that he assumed that Art. 17(2)(c) "covered illegitimate as well as legitimate children, in view of the provisions contained in Article 25(2) of the Universal Declaration of Human Rights."[156] While the Israeli representative believed that absent an amendment only the parents of children born in wedlock would be covered by Art. 17(2)(c),[157] the majority of representatives appear to have been persuaded by the French delegate's assurance "that the existing text of the sub-paragraph was satisfactory. It would be difficult to make it clearer."[158] This seems clearly to be correct, since the ordinary meaning of "children" is not limited to the offspring of a married couple.

Where a refugee falls into one of these categories – he or she has been present in the asylum state for at least three years, or has a spouse or children with the host state's nationality – "restrictive measures imposed on aliens or the employment of aliens for the protection of the national labour market" are prohibited, whether or not the refugee in question is also lawfully staying in the state party.[159] This duty to exempt refugees applies whether the restriction is formally directed at non-citizens themselves, or at

---

[155] "Although he recognized that the purpose of sub-paragraph 2(c) was to ensure that a refugee with a family, who was firmly established in his country of refuge, should be accorded his due rights, he could not accept the arbitrary conditions stipulated in that sub-paragraph": Statement of Mr. Hoare of the United Kingdom, UN Doc. A/CONF.2/ SR.9, July 6, 1951, at 5. The United Kingdom has, however, entered and maintained a reservation to Art. 17(2)(c): see reservations and declarations of state parties, available at www.unhcr.ch (accessed Nov. 20, 2004).

[156] Statement of the President, Mr. Larsen of Denmark, UN Doc. A/CONF.2/SR.9, July 6, 1951, at 15. The relevant part of the Universal Declaration provides that "[a]ll children, whether born in or out of wedlock, shall enjoy the same social protection": Universal Declaration of Human Rights, UNGA Res. 217A(III), Dec. 10, 1948 (Universal Declaration), at Art. 25(2).

[157] "[A]s sub-paragraph 2(c) opened with the word 'He' it could only apply to legitimate children. He would suggest that if the intention was that the provision should be applicable to illegitimate children as well, the words 'or she' should be inserted after the word 'He' in this particular case": Statement of Mr. Robinson of Israel, UN Doc. A/ CONF.2/SR.9, July 6, 1951, at 15. The implication seems to be that a man cannot have an "illegitimate" child. As a factual matter, this is clearly not true. If, on the other hand, this position is taken because the father of a child born out of wedlock has no parental rights, then the argument is anachronistic.

[158] Statement of Mr. Rochefort of France, ibid.

[159] Grahl-Madsen argues for an implied restriction on access to Art. 17(2)(c) exemption in the case of "a father, who has never made any attempt to support his illegitimate child, and [who may] never [have] shown any interest in it": Grahl-Madsen, *Commentary*, at 73. But Grahl-Madsen's conclusion fails to take account of the fact that para. (c), unlike para. (b), does not provide for the withdrawal of entitlement consequent to abandonment. While it would clearly be undesirable in policy terms for a father who provides no

employers.[160] By way of example, France noted that by virtue of Art. 17(2), it could not subject all refugees to its system of issuing restricted work authorizations based on labor market conditions in particular fields.[161] Perhaps most obviously, refugees entitled to the benefit of Art. 17(2) must not be subject to "provisions that aliens may only be employed if no nationals are available for the job in question."[162] The European Union's new Reception Directive, in contrast, <u>fails both to take account of the duty to allow more</u> <u>immediate access to work by the spouses and parents of host country minor</u> <u>citizens, and specifically to ensure that such refugees are not subject to its</u> <u>usual policy of subordinating the right to work of refugee claimants to those</u> <u>of European citizens and resident third-country nationals.</u>[163]

N. B.

On the other hand, as was the case for Art. 17(1), Art. 17(2) provides no relief against the duty to respect the terms of resettlement agreements;[164] much less does it excuse refugees from compliance with restrictive measures

> support to his citizen child to rely upon his status as father to secure exemption from employment restrictions, it is nonetheless difficult to find a textual basis for the approach suggested by Grahl-Madsen. Moreover, in view of the legal duty in most countries for the father of a child born out of wedlock to provide support for his child, application of Grahl-Madsen's interpretation might also defeat the ability of the child's mother to secure access to the funds she requires in order to support the child.

[160] "The first category may relate to measures taken by the authorities directly against the foreigner ... The second group apparently deals with restrictions imposed on the employer: he may be prohibited from hiring foreigners, who are generally permitted to do the work in question, unless he can prove that no national is available for the position or he may be permitted to accept only a certain number or percentage of alien employees or only such who are not engaged elsewhere. In order to cover all the possibilities, the authors of the Convention combined both cases of restrictions": Robinson, *History*, at 115.

[161] "If article [17] remained as it stood, France would be obliged to enter a reservation to ... part of paragraph 2 ... [Its domestic law], enacted in 1932 in view of the economic situation, and in 1946 in order to regulate the labour market, did not have the effect of denying refugees the right to work ... All [France] desired was to be able to control the movement of labour, and the refusal to permit a refugee to take employment in any overcrowded branch of activity in which there were already thousands of French subjects unemployed ...": Statement of Mr. Juvigny of France, UN Doc. E/AC.32/SR.37, Aug. 16, 1950, at 13–14. France did enter such a reservation, which it maintains at the time of writing: see reservations and declarations of state parties, available at www.unhcr.ch (accessed Nov. 20, 2004). Interestingly, though Venezuela suggested that it had a comparable system in place (Statement of Mr. Perez Perozo of Venezuela, UN Doc. E/AC.32/SR.37, Aug. 16, 1950, at 19), it did not enter a reservation to protect its domestic regime.

[162] Weis, *Travaux*, at 148.   [163] EU Reception Directive, at Art. 11.

[164] "[T]he restrictions referred to in the second paragraph were certainly not those stipulated in agreements between certain countries and IRO. They were restrictions deriving from the domestic law of various countries": Statement of Mr. Rain of France, UN Doc. E/AC.32/SR.13, Jan. 26, 1950, at 9. See also Statement of Mr. Henkin of the United States, UN Doc. E/AC.32/SR.37, Aug. 16, 1950, at 13; Statement of Mr. Herment of Belgium, ibid. at 16; and Weis, *Travaux*, at 148: "The preoccupation of Australia about refugees

which bind even nationals of the host country.[165] More generally, there is no exemption from measures which have a purpose other than the protection of national workers.[166] As the French representative insisted, "the measures in question were the result of laws and regulations for the protection of the labour market. It was therefore only a question of restrictive measures to protect national labour against foreign competition. There could be no possible doubts on that point."[167] Grahl-Madsen concurs, observing that Art. 17(2) "only deals with measures for the protection of the national labour market. Measures which have another purpose, e.g. prohibition of employment of aliens in industries working for the national defence, based on considerations of national security, are not affected."[168]

The last paragraph of Art. 17 requires the governments of state parties to "give sympathetic consideration to assimilating the rights of *all refugees* with regard to wage-earning employment to those of *nationals* [emphasis added]." As this text makes clear, Art. 17(3) does not impose a duty of result.[169] It nonetheless mandates a process of "sympathetic consideration" which

who had been admitted with a work contract obliging them to perform specific work for two years was not well-founded."

[165] In response to concerns expressed by the United Kingdom regarding its right to apply measures imposed on its own citizens "in agreement with the employers and trade union organizations concerned . . . for the common good of the people" (Statement of Sir Leslie Brass of the United Kingdom, UN Doc. E/AC.32/SR.13, Jan. 26, 1950, at 5), the representative of the IRO was unambiguous. "[T]he French text was, in fact, identical with that of the Convention of 1933 which was designed to ensure equal treatment for refugees and nationals. At that time, no restrictive measures had been applied against refugees in the matter of employment. The situation had since changed and it was obvious that the text to be adopted should indicate that restrictive measures which were applicable in the case of nationals, applied equally to refugees": Statement of Mr. Weis of the IRO, ibid. at 11.

[166] This is not to say that restrictions on the right to work for *any* other reason are valid. The policy of Côte d'Ivoire of taking away a refugee's right to work if he or she moves without authorization is, for example, not valid because it is predicated on enforcement of an illegal constraint on internal freedom of movement: see chapter 5.2 above.

[167] Statement of Mr. Rain of France, UN Doc. E/AC.32/SR.13, Jan. 26, 1950, at 11. See also Statements of Mr. Cuvelier of Belgium, Mr. Stolz of the American Federation of Labor, and Mr. Metall of the International Labor Organization: ibid. at 11–12. Indeed, the British representative proposed a more direct fromulation of the purpose of Art. 17(2), namely to ensure the "protection of national workers": Statement of Sir Leslie Brass of the United Kingdom, ibid. at 12.

[168] Grahl-Madsen, *Commentary*, at 71.

[169] Indeed, it was opposed by the Netherlands for precisely this reason. The Dutch representative to the Conference of Plenipotentiaries "considered that the provisions of paragraph 3 of article [17] constituted a recommendation to, rather than an obligation on, Contracting States. It was undesirable to make recommendations in a convention. It would therefore be desirable to relegate *voeux* [aspirations] and recommendations appearing in the draft Convention as it then stood to a separate draft resolution, which the Conference could adopt later when the instrument itself was signed": Statement of Baron van Boetzelaer of the Netherlands, UN Doc. A/CONF.2/SR.9, July 6, 1951, at 15.

may, or may not, ultimately provide refugees with a full-fledged right to work.[170] While the primary goal of Art. 17(3) as initially conceived was to provide some relief to refugees admitted under immigration schemes or labor contracts once the terms of their initial agreements are satisfied,[171] its scope is not narrowly conceived. In light of the debates on Art. 17 taken as a whole, the third paragraph seems very much to be a principled recognition of the centrality of employment to the ability of refugees to reestablish their lives,[172] which states regrettably felt unable fully to permit in the context of their own difficult domestic circumstances. Importantly, the constrained approach taken by the drafters to definition of the right of refugees to work was never promoted on grounds of lack of need or merit, but simply on the grounds that state parties could not do better by refugees without sacrificing their own critical national interests. When and if conditions allow, Art. 17(3) signals the commitment of governments to allowing refugees both earlier and more complete access to the full range of wage-earning opportunities.[173]

6.1.2 Fair working conditions

Refugee Convention, Art. 24 Labour legislation and social security

   1. The Contracting States shall accord to refugees lawfully staying in their territory the same treatment as is accorded to nationals in respect of the following matters:

(a) In so far as such matters are governed by laws or regulations or are subject to the control of administrative authorities:

---

[170] Significantly, para. 3 does not take the approach initially advocated in the Secretary-General's draft, under which state parties simply "reserve[d] the right to accord the treatment given to national wage-earners to specified categories of refugees": Secretary-General, "Memorandum," at 34. Rather, as proposed by the American representative, it requires states to give favorable consideration to the assimilation of refugees to citizens for purposes of work, instead of just allowing them to do so: Statement of Mr. Henkin of the United States, UN Doc. E/AC.32/SR.13, Jan. 26, 1950, at 5.

[171] See text above, at pp. 752–753.

[172] See UNHCR Executive Committee Conclusion No. 50, "General Conclusion on International Protection" (1988), available at www.unhcr.ch (accessed Nov. 20, 2004), at para. (j): "[T]he enhancement of basic economic and social rights, including gainful employment, is essential to the achievement of self-sufficiency and family security for refugees and is vital to the process of re-establishing the dignity of the human person and of realizing durable solutions to refugee problems."

[173] The Executive Committee has affirmed this obligation in principle by "[e]ncourag[ing] all States hosting refugees to consider ways in which refugee employment in their countries might be facilitated and to examine their laws and practices, with a view to identifying and to removing, to the extent possible, existing obstacles to refugee employment": ibid. at para. (k).

remuneration, including family allowances where these form part of remuneration, hours of work, overtime arrangements, holidays with pay, restrictions on home work, minimum age of employment, apprenticeship and training, women's work and the work of young persons, and the enjoyment of the benefits of collective bargaining.

. . .

Economic, Social and Cultural Covenant, Art. 7
The States Parties to the present Covenant recognize the right of everyone to the enjoyment of just and favourable conditions of work, which ensure, in particular:

(a) remuneration which provides all workers, as a minimum, with:
  (i) fair wages and equal remuneration for work of equal value without distinction of any kind, in particular women being guaranteed conditions of work not inferior to those enjoyed by men, with equal pay for equal work;
  (ii) a decent living for themselves and their families in accordance with the provisions of the present Covenant;
(b) safe and healthy working conditions;
(c) equal opportunity for everyone to be promoted in his employment to an appropriate higher level, subject to no considerations other than those of seniority and competence;
(d) rest, leisure and reasonable limitation of working hours and periodic holidays with pay, as well as remuneration for public holidays.

The right of refugees to enjoy fair working conditions is a novel feature of the 1951 Refugee Convention. It was not guaranteed in any of the predecessor refugee treaties, nor was it proposed in the French government's draft of the 1951 Convention. The decision of the Secretary-General to promote such a right was likely inspired by the contemporaneously drafted Arts. 23 and 24 of the Universal Declaration of Human Rights[174] which, in turn, were based upon the detailed work of the International Labor Organization.[175] In

---

[174] Art. 23 of the Universal Declaration refers *inter alia* to "just and favourable conditions of work," to "equal pay for equal work" without discrimination, to "just and favourable remuneration ensuring for [the worker] and his family an existence worthy of human dignity," and to the right "to form and to join trade unions." This is complemented by Art. 24 which posits "the right to rest and leisure, including reasonable limitation of working hours and periodic holidays with pay."

[175] See generally K. Källström, "Article 23," in A. Eide et. al. eds., *The Universal Declaration of Human Rights: A Commentary* 373 (1992); and G. Melander, "Article 24," in ibid. at 379 (Melander, "Article 24"). For example, "[t]he rights mentioned in article 24 are among

presenting his proposal for what became Art. 24 of the Refugee Convention, the Secretary-General insisted that it had both a principled[176] and a pragmatic rationale:

> The placing of foreigners and national workers on the same footing not only met the demands of equity but was in the interests of national wage-earners who might have been afraid that foreign labour, being cheaper than their own, would have been preferred.[177]

In line with this thinking, it was proposed that refugees – at least once they are "lawfully staying" in the host country[178] – should be able to insist upon guarantees of fair working conditions not simply on par with those extended to aliens generally or even to most-favored foreigners, but rather at a level of equivalency with the protections enjoyed by citizens of the asylum state itself.

While the commitment to assimilating refugees to nationals was maintained, the substantive breadth of Art. 24(1)(a) as originally proposed by the Secretary-General was reduced to bring it into line with the approach taken in the Migration for Employment Convention, drafted by the International

---

the original concerns of the labour movement and among the early standards established by international labour law": Melander, ibid. at 379.

[176] Craven neatly captures the ethical dimension, arguing that "[i]f, on the one hand, work is seen as a necessary evil, then humanity requires that the conditions under which it is undertaken are as tolerable as possible": Craven, *ICESCR Commentary*, at 226.

[177] Secretary-General, "Memorandum," at 37. The Ad Hoc Committee specifically referenced these considerations as underpinning para. 1(a): Ad Hoc Committee, "First Session Report," at Annex II.

[178] This level of attachment was implied in the original draft prepared by the Secretary-General, which made Art. 24 "subject to the provisions of Article [17, on wage-earning employment]": Secretary-General, "Memorandum," at 37. The Ad Hoc Committee, however, proposed a more relaxed standard based on the approach of the cognate provision of the ILO's Migration for Employment Convention of 1949, which granted labor protections to migrants "lawfully within [the state party's] territory." It therefore agreed that Art. 24 rights be granted to refugees "lawfully in their territory": Ad Hoc Committee, "First Session Report," at Annex I. Without engaging in any plenary debate on the issue, the Conference of Plenipotentiaries reverted to the present, more restrictive formulation. The timing of entitlement to access wage-earning employment and to the protection and labor standards is in principle the same, namely when the refugee is lawfully staying in the state party. But it is arguable that in the event access to employment is granted at an earlier time than required by the Convention, the state party may still refuse to grant refugees the benefit of Art. 24(1)(a) until lawful stay is established. If it were to do so, it would of course create precisely the competitive advantage for refugee workers over nationals which the drafters sought to avoid. In addition, refugees working in such circumstances would still be entitled to assert the right to basic labor protections under Art. 7 of the Economic Covenant, discussed below, at pp. 770–771. An argument could also be made that the refusal to refugees authorized to work of the protection of labor laws would breach the general duty of non-discrimination set by Art. 26 of the Civil and Political Covenant, since it would be difficult to justify as a reasonable exclusion: see chapter 2.5.5 above.

Labor Organization in 1949.[179] As explained by the Belgian representative, who had also chaired the conference that produced the ILO's convention, that treaty "had been prepared by experts after long and careful study. They had been guided by a desire to apply to migrant workers or refugees the same regulations which governed nationals."[180] Because not all states that would sign the Refugee Convention were also members of the ILO, "the draft convention on refugees would lose nothing by duplicating the provisions of the ILO convention, with the drafting changes required to adapt the latter to refugees."[181]

As the Danish representative feared,[182] however, the decision to follow the ILO's approach meant that some protections proposed by the Secretary-General fell by the wayside. First, the Secretary-General had proposed that governments grant refugees the benefit of "all the labour regulations applicable to nationals,"[183] whereas Art. 24(1)(a) follows the ILO's lead of requiring respect for only a finite – if nonetheless quite extensive – list of protections.[184] Second and more specifically, two types of standard mentioned in the original draft as examples of laws from which refugees would benefit were not found in the ILO's list, and were therefore not included in the Refugee Convention.[185] These are "guarantees of employment" and standards directed to "health and safety in employment."[186] While the latter protection now accrues to refugees in many countries by virtue of the subsequently adopted Art. 7 of the Economic Covenant,[187] the loss of a specific right to be treated as a citizen in enforcing guarantees of employment may be of particular concern to refugees who are resettled under a labor migration program. This omission of an explicit reference to this right to enforce a private arrangement is, however, consistent with a third shift occasioned by the decision to follow the ILO's approach: it explicitly grants access to the listed forms of labor protection only "in so far as such matters are governed by laws or regulations

---

[179] Convention concerning Migration for Employment (Revised) (ILO Conv. 97), 120 UNTS 70, done July 1, 1949, entered into force Jan. 22, 1952, at Art. 6.

[180] Statement of Mr. Cuvelier of Belgium, UN Doc. A/AC.32/SR.14, Jan. 26, 1950, at 5.

[181] Statement of Mr. Metall of the International Labor Organization, ibid. at 6.

[182] "[T]he draft convention on refugees was intended to deal specifically with that particular category of persons and the special circumstances in which they found themselves. It seemed pointless to copy the provisions of a convention applicable to foreigners in general": Statement of Mr. Larsen of Denmark, ibid. at 5.

[183] Secretary-General, "Memorandum," at 37.

[184] These are described below, at pp. 768–770.

[185] One right included in the Convention, but not mentioned in the original draft by the Secretary-General, is the right to benefit from "overtime arrangements." It might, however, be argued that this entitlement is implied in the duty to grant refuges protections related to wages and working hours.

[186] Secretary-General, "Memorandum," at 37.   [187] See text below, at pp. 770–771.

or are subject to the control of administrative authorities." This clause, now included in Art. 24(1)(a), makes it clear that only public domain labor protection must be extended to refugees.[188] Where particular forms of labor protection are granted and governed solely by private agreement between employer and employee, there is no duty to provide refugees the same rights as nationals.[189]

Moreover, in "adapting" the ILO Convention to meet the particular circumstances of refugees, the drafters retreated from full incorporation of that treaty in at least two respects. First, the ILO treaty requires that migrant workers be granted national treatment with regard to worker "accommodation."[190] The Belgian representative to the Ad Hoc Committee proposed the deletion of this protection for purposes of the Refugee Convention,[191] a move supported in particular by the British representative who worried that "it would be difficult to guarantee exactly equal treatment for refugees in the matter of housing, since the housing shortage was acute and the matter had to be dealt with on the basis of need. It was also felt that a certain degree of preference as regards housing should be given to some categories of nationals, such as ex-servicemen."[192] The drafters therefore declined to grant refugee workers any special housing rights, meaning that they benefit only from the general entitlement of refugees to access housing on the same terms as aliens generally set by Arts. 13 and 21 of the Refugee Convention.[193]

The second area in which refugee entitlements are framed to require less than the ILO Convention was the commitment to migrant workers of equality with nationals as regards "membership of trade unions and enjoyment of

---

[188] Under parallel provisions of the Economic Covenant, "[i]n the case of those States that operated a system of collective bargaining, it would be impossible for the State to assume responsibility for matters that were negotiated by the trade unions": Craven, *ICESCR Commentary*, at 227, quoting from the statement of a British drafter of the Covenant at UN Doc. E/CN.4/SR.206 (1951), at 10.

[189] "The State could not intervene, for example, where agreements existed between employees and employers": Statement of Mr. Cuvelier of Belgium, UN Doc. E/AC.32/SR.14, Jan. 26, 1950, at 5.

[190] One of the concerns was whether, in fact, the ILO Convention required equal treatment only with respect to *worker* accommodation, or with regard to accommodation in general: Statements of Mr. Henkin of the United States and Mr. Rain of France, ibid. at 9.

[191] Statement of Mr. Cuvelier of Belgium, ibid. at 8.

[192] Statement of Sir Leslie Brass of the United Kingdom, ibid. at 8. See also Statement of Mr. Cha of China, ibid. at 9–10: "His own country, devastated by war and suffering from a grave shortage of housing, had taken urgent measures, following the end of the Second World War, to relieve the suffering of the refugees; those measures had often placed the refugees in a more advantageous position, from the point of view of housing, than many Chinese nationals. He felt that the matter of housing should be left to the initiative and control of the individual Governments."

[193] See chapter 4.5.1 above and chapter 6.4 below. This conflict was noted by the Chairman, Mr. Larsen of Denmark, UN Doc. E/AC.32/SR.38, Aug. 17, 1950, at 9.

the benefits of collective bargaining." The focus of concern was the first part of the clause, which conflicted with the lower standard of treatment (assimilation to most-favored nationals) granted to refugees by Art. 15's guarantee of the right of association (including trade unions).[194] If the ILO's precedent of assimilating refugees to nationals were followed, France feared that refugees might be entitled to establish and run trade unions:

> [The French] Government ... would be unable to accept a provision which would make it possible for refugees to participate in the administration or management of unions comprising French nationals and aliens, or which would, by implication, make it possible to organize unions of workers or employees consisting entirely of aliens ... His Government was prepared to accord refugees most-favoured-nation treatment, but was not prepared to accord them treatment equal to that accorded to its own nationals.[195]

The ILO's observer accurately insisted, however, that his organization's treaty actually spoke only to "membership of trade unions; it was not a question of providing in the Convention for equal treatment with regard to the organization of trade unions and participation in their administration."[196] Nonetheless, some states clearly objected to even allowing refugees the same access as citizens to join trade unions. China, for instance, asserted that "because of the presence of surplus labour in [that] country, there was no question of any alien joining a trade union there."[197] It was therefore agreed that while Art. 24(1)(a) would assimilate refugees to nationals for purposes of enjoying the benefits of collective bargaining,[198] the right to join and participate in the work of trade unions would be governed by the more general rules of Art. 15.

Reliance on the ILO treaty as a precedent nonetheless had some important advantages for refugee workers, even as compared with the subsequently enacted cognate provision of the Economic Covenant. Neither the Secretary-General's original draft for the Refugee Convention nor Art. 7 of the Economic Covenant requires that refugees be assimilated to nationals for purposes of the right to benefit from overtime arrangements, restrictions on

---

[194] See chapter 6.7 below.
[195] Statement of Mr. Juvigny of France, UN Doc. E/AC.32/SR.38, Aug. 17, 1950, at 10.
[196] Statement of Mr. Oblath of the International Labor Organization, ibid. at 11.
[197] Statement of Mr. Cha of China, ibid. at 10. China was, however, prepared to accept the most-favored-national level of attachment provided for in Art. 15's guarantee of freedom of association, presumably because it did not intend to grant the nationals of any country the right to join trade unions: ibid.
[198] The American representative had earlier proposed "that the words 'enjoyment of the benefits of collective bargaining' ... should be added at the end of sub-paragraph 1(a)(i)": Statement of Mr. Henkin of the United States, UN Doc. E/AC.32/SR.14, Jan. 26, 1950, at 8.

home work, minimum age of employment rules, opportunities for apprenticeship and training, or rules governing the work of young persons – all matters now governed by Art. 24(1)(a).

The core protections of Art. 24(1)(a), in contrast, are today mirrored by similar duties in Art. 7 of the Covenant on Economic, Social and Cultural Rights. Where there is overlap, it is clear that a fused obligation may be advanced by refugee workers in at least the majority of developed states which have acceded to both treaties. In the less developed world, where duties under the Economic Covenant are often avoided by reliance either on the Covenant's duty of progressive implementation or on its authorization for poor states to exclude non-citizens from the scope of economic rights,[199] the obligations under Art. 24(1)(a) of the Refugee Convention – which are immediately binding, and applicable to all state parties – provide an important source of entitlement for refugees who might otherwise not have been able to insist on access to any form of labor protection.

First, Art. 24(1)(a) of the Refugee Convention requires that refugees be treated as citizens for purposes of the regulation of "remuneration, including family allowances where these form part of remuneration." The parallel right in the Economic Covenant is more explicit, requiring governments to commit themselves to a minimum qualitative standard of remuneration – sufficient to provide for a "decent living for themselves and their families," at least to the level guaranteed by Art. 11 of the Covenant;[200] and, in any event, "fair wages and equal remuneration for work of equal value *without distinction of any kind* [emphasis added]." This guarantee of *equal* pay for *equal* work logically imports a theory of comparable worth,[201] and leaves no room for the application of a margin of appreciation which might defeat the claims of refugees brought under general duties of non-discrimination.[202]

Second, the Refugee Convention requires that refugee workers be treated as nationals where there are protections addressed to "hours of work . . . [and] holidays with pay." The Economic Covenant requires further that

---

[199] See chapter 2.5.4 above, at pp. 122–123.

[200] "The text indicates that the term 'decent living' is to be read in the light of the other provisions of the Covenant. Particular reference could be made to article 11 which refers to 'an adequate standard of living.' More specifically, however, the phrase 'a decent living' appears to refer to those rights that depend for their enjoyment upon personal income such as rights to housing, food, clothing, and perhaps health, education, and culture": Craven, *ICESCR Commentary*, at 235. The ambit of Art. 11 of the Economic Covenant is discussed in some detail in chapter 4.4.2 above.

[201] See Craven, *ICESCR Commentary*, at 237.

[202] See chapter 2.5.5 above, at pp. 139–145. "The requirement of equal remuneration in the Covenant is broader than that found in other instruments . . . First, whereas the ILO Convention No. 100 and article 119 of the Treaty of Rome provide for equal pay only in relation to men and women, article 7(1) applies to 'all workers . . . without distinction of any kind'": Craven, *ICESCR Commentary*, at 238.

hours of work be subject to "reasonable limitations," a standard which at least one member of the supervisory committee found would not ordinarily be met in the case of a fifty-four-hour working week.[203] The Covenant also requires that work be constrained to allow for "rest [and] leisure," said by one expert to impose a bifurcated duty:

> The word "rest" . . . is intended to guarantee a real cessation of activities, giving the individual [the] possibility to regain his strength. "Leisure" on the other hand should make it possible for the individual to cultivate his mind and interests.[204]

More specifically, the Covenant stipulates also that all workers receive "periodic holidays with pay" and "remuneration for public holidays."[205]

A third area of overlap between the Refugee Convention and the Economic Covenant is the regulation of "women's work." While the drafters of the Refugee Convention likely had in mind regulations which traditionally limited the hours or conditions of work of women to enable them to meet family and other responsibilities, in contemporary context refugees must benefit from rules intended to implement the Economic Covenant's commitment to "women being guaranteed conditions of work not inferior to those enjoyed by men, with equal pay for equal work." Importantly, the supervisory committee has taken a particular interest in the plight of migrant women, insisting that they must benefit from this duty to promote sex equality in the workplace in the same way as citizens.[206]

There are also three aspects of Art. 7 of the Economic Covenant that provide protections not granted under the Refugee Convention. First, the Covenant guarantees equal opportunity "for everyone to be promoted in his employment," with no criteria other than seniority and competence deemed relevant. The Committee on Economic, Social and Cultural Rights has held that Art. 7(c) imposes a duty on state parties to establish objective norms for promotion in the public sector, as well as legislation to counter private sector discrimination in promotion.[207] By virtue of this clause, a refugee worker may not ordinarily be passed over for advancement in favor of a citizen of the host state on grounds of his refugee (or non-citizen) status.[208]

---

[203] See Craven, *ICESCR Commentary*, at 245, referring to the comments of expert Mratchov, UN Doc. E/C.12/1989/SR.8, at 7.

[204] Melander, "Article 24," at 380.

[205] Economic, Social and Cultural Covenant, at Art. 7(d).

[206] See Craven, *ICESCR Commentary*, at 240.   [207] Ibid. at 243–244.

[208] That is, there would be a duty to show the reasonableness of the differential treatment on objective grounds. While it might be possible to make this argument in relation to security-sensitive fields of work, it would otherwise be difficult to justify why lack of citizenship makes an otherwise employable refugee ineligible for promotion on the basis of competence and seniority. See chapter 2.5.5 above, at pp. 130–133.

A second provision of the Economic Covenant ironically requires states to grant refugees a form of protection that was deleted from the Secretary-General's draft of Art. 24 when the decision was made to work from the ILO precedent,[209] namely to benefit from "safe and healthy working conditions." The drafting history of Art. 7(b) makes clear only that there was a commitment that workers be protected from conditions "injurious to health,"[210] though the Committee on Economic, Social and Cultural Rights has in practice required states to demonstrate both non-exclusion of various categories of workers from protection and progressive achievement in advancing the standards of worker health and safety.[211]

Finally, the Economic Covenant effectively reestablishes the formula originally proposed by the Secretary-General for the Refugee Convention, namely that the listed entitlements are merely examples of what should be done to promote the more general obligation to provide workers with "just and favourable conditions of work." Because Art. 7 of the Economic Covenant applies to "everyone," state parties are duty-bound to recognize its standards for all workers under their jurisdiction, including refugees.

In sum, at least in developed countries bound by both the Refugee Convention and the Economic Covenant, the scope of the guarantee of fair working conditions may be said to derive from a fusion of norms – the best of both worlds, since each treaty provides for some rights not set by the other. Most important, the generality of the duty under the Economic Covenant implied in its recognition of the "right of everyone to the enjoyment of just and favourable conditions of work" means that refugees may claim the benefit of any public domain protection of workplace fairness, whether or not it is of a type specifically mentioned in Art. 24(1)(a) of the Refugee Convention. But while it is true that there is now significant overlap between Art. 24(1)(a) of the Refugee Convention and the subsequently enacted Art. 7 of the Economic Covenant, the Refugee Convention's guarantees remain of real importance for at least two reasons.

First, the substantive ambit of the Refugee Convention's guarantees of workplace fairness is in some ways broader than that of the Economic Covenant, explicitly including the right to benefit from rules and procedures related to overtime arrangements, restrictions on home work, minimum age of employment, apprenticeship and training, the work of young persons, and enjoyment of the benefits of collective bargaining. Thus, even in developed states, Art. 24(1)(a) is a source of entitlement beyond what is granted by general norms of international human rights law.

---

[209] See text above, at p. 766.
[210] Craven, *ICESCR Commentary*, at 230, citing the Statement of the Yugoslav representative, UN Doc. E/CN.4/AC.14/Add.2, at 2.
[211] Craven, *ICESCR Commentary*, at 142.

Second and most important, less developed states may normally elect not to extend an economic right set by the Covenant to non-citizens by reliance on Art. 2(3) of that treaty, but enjoy no such discretion where the same right appears in the Refugee Convention. Thus, the fact that Art. 24(1)(a) guarantees refugees the same public domain safeguards of fair treatment in the workplace as accrue to citizens of the host country – whatever that country's economic circumstances – is enormously important to the majority of the world's refugees who live outside the developed world. Indeed, because the Refugee Convention repeats three of the most critical forms of protection required by the Economic Covenant (namely those related to remuneration, hours of work and holidays, and the employment of women), the Refugee Convention effectively trumps Art. 2(3) of the Covenant to the extent of that overlap.

6.1.3 Social security

Refugee Convention, Art. 24   Labour legislation and social security

1. The Contracting States shall accord to refugees lawfully staying in their territory the same treatment as is accorded to nationals in respect of the following matters: . . .

(b) Social security (legal provisions in respect of employment injury, occupational diseases, maternity, sickness, disability, old age, death, unemployment, family responsibilities and any other contingency which, according to national laws or regulations, is covered by a social security scheme), subject to the following limitations.
  (i) There may be appropriate arrangements for the mainte-nance of acquired rights and rights in course of acquisition;
  (ii) National laws or regulations of the country of residence may prescribe special arrangements concerning benefits or portions of benefits which are payable wholly out of public funds, and concerning allowances paid to persons who do not fulfil the contribution conditions prescribed for the award of a normal pension.

2. The right to compensation for the death of a refugee result-ing from employment injury or from occupational disease shall not be affected by the fact that the residence of the beneficiary is outside the territory of the Contracting State.

3. The Contracting States shall extend to refugees the benefits of agreements concluded between them, or which may be con-cluded between them in the future, concerning the maintenance of acquired rights and rights in the process of acquisition in regard to

social security, subject only to the conditions which apply to nationals of the States signatory to the agreements in question.

4. The Contracting States will give sympathetic consideration to extending to refugees so far as possible the benefits of similar agreements which may at any time be in force between such Contracting States and non-contracting States.

Economic, Social and Cultural Covenant, Art. 9
The States Parties to the present Covenant recognize the right of everyone to social security, including social insurance.

While the structure of the Refugee Convention anticipates that refugees lawfully staying in an asylum country will support themselves by undertaking work, the drafters logically took account of the possibility that refugees, like citizens, might sometimes be prevented by circumstances beyond their control from earning their own living. Most of the states which prepared the Refugee Convention had established social security systems funded largely by contributions from workers and employers to compensate persons unable to work for more than strictly temporary reasons.[212] But refugees were not always in a position meaningfully to benefit from these social security systems. In Switzerland, for example,

> With regard to old-age and widows' and orphans' insurance, refugees were treated as favourably as aliens generally. They had to be insured if they carried on any gainful activity, but were entitled to a grant only if they had paid contributions for at least 10 years, and the grant they received was only two-thirds of that received by Swiss nationals. In addition, they were not entitled to temporary grants.[213]

In many other countries, the situation was worse still, as non-citizens frequently had no right to access social security at all unless a treaty was in place between the host state and the non-citizen's country of origin.[214] An

---

[212] "A distinction is often made between *social security* and *social welfare*. Through such a classification one wishes to separate between the 'earned' social security benefits of workers and their families, and any individual or group receiving need-based assistance from public funds, raised through tax revenues": M. Scheinin, "The Right to Social Security," in A. Eide et al. eds., *Economic, Social and Cultural Rights: A Textbook* 159 (1995) (Scheinin, "Social Security"), at 159. The issue of access to need-based (publicly funded) social assistance is addressed below, at chapter 6.3.

[213] Statement of Mr. Schurch of Switzerland, UN Doc. E/AC.32/SR.38, Aug. 17, 1950, at 11.

[214] "A number of bilateral treaties and certain international treaties, notably those concluded under the auspices of the International Labour Office, place foreigners who are nationals of State Parties to the Agreements on the same footing as nationals in respect of social security ... In these circumstances, the same equality should be ensured to refugees": Secretary-General, "Memorandum," at 38.

injured or incapacitated refugee worker might therefore be left with no means of support, based simply on the failure of his or her country of origin to sign an agreement with the new country of residence. In line with their general commitment to compensate refugees for the disadvantages of involuntary alienage, and their particular concern that the welfare of refugees should not be held hostage to the whims of the states they had been compelled to flee, the drafts presented by both the Secretary-General[215] and the French government[216] proposed the assimilation of refugees lawfully staying in a state party to citizens of the host country for purposes of entitlement to social security. Subject only to the understanding that the actual mechanisms by which social security benefits are delivered to refugees might be distinct,[217] this basic principle was never called into question during the drafting process.[218]

As in the case of guarantees of workplace fairness,[219] the members of the Ad Hoc Committee were persuaded to model the social security rules of the Refugee Convention on the precedent of the ILO's Migration for

---

[215] The Secretary-General's draft contained two separate articles. The first, Art. 16(2), provided that States would "accord to the victims of industrial accidents or their beneficiaries the same treatment that is granted to their nationals." The second and more general provision, Art. 17, required further that refugees would receive national treatment "in respect of social security ... (sickness, maternity, invalidity, old-age insurance, insurance against the death of the breadwinner, and unemployment insurance)": Secretary-General, "Memorandum," at 37–38.

[216] "While regularly resident in the territory of one of the High Contracting Parties, refugees shall receive the same treatment as nationals in respect of insurance and social security (including industrial accident compensation)": France, "Draft Convention," at 7.

[217] "[I]n Denmark an insured person only made a formal contribution to the social security scheme ... [so] that it was in reality the State that contributed to the various funds. The Danish Government was prepared to extend social security to refugees, but under the Danish system it would be necessary for the benefits to be paid to refugees on that count to come from funds other than the old age pension fund and the like": Statement of Mr. Larsen of Denmark, UN Doc. A/CONF.2/SR.10, July 6, 1951, at 19. See also Statement of Mr. Hoare of the United Kingdom, ibid.: "[A] similar situation arose in the United Kingdom. There were certain old age pensions for which foreigners were not eligible, but their grant depended on the applicants' means, and a foreigner whose means were the same would get the equivalent under the general social security legislation. He had assumed that article [24] could be interpreted broadly enough to meet the requirements of Denmark and the United Kingdom in that respect."

[218] Some countries, including Switzerland, maintained the view that certain social security payments would be made to refugees only on the same terms as granted to aliens generally: see Statement of Mr. Zutter of Switzerland, ibid. at 20. The Swiss reservation to this effect has since been withdrawn, though several other countries maintain comparable reservations: see reservations and declarations of state parties, available at www.unhcr.ch (accessed Nov. 20, 2004).

[219] See chapter 6.1.2 above.

Employment Convention.[220] The substantive reach of Art. 24(1)(b) is there-fore quite broad, extending to legal schemes to provide for assistance in the event of "employment injury, occupational diseases, maternity, sickness, disability, old age, death, unemployment, family responsibilities and any other contingency which, according to national laws or regulations, is cov-ered by a social security scheme." The notion of "social security," in other words, includes the full range of contribution-based initiatives designed to compensate workers unable to continue working. As the intervention of the International Labor Organization made clear, nothing turns on the label assigned to the program since "[p]resent-day legislation and treaties made no distinction between industrial accidents and social security and it would be difficult to discuss the two matters separately."[221] Subsequent exchanges, for example, establish that any scheme to provide compensation for employ-ment injury – whether called "social security" or something else – is covered by the terms of Art. 24(1)(b).[222]

The only form of social security protection which elicited any significant discussion by the drafters was assistance to be paid in the event of "disability." The ILO precedent used the term "invalidity," said by that organization to mean "permanent disability, while 'disability' also covers temporary disabil-ity."[223] Despite the ILO's plea to incorporate the narrower term ("invalidity")

---

[220] See chapter 6.1.2 above, at pp. 765–767. Not all countries supported this approach. The British representative, for example, "did not feel satisfied that the ILO text under consideration entirely covered, or could be made to cover, the situation of refugees": Statement of Sir Leslie Brass of the United Kingdom, UN Doc. E/AC.32/SR.14, Jan. 26, 1950, at 7. Even the Belgian representative who had chaired the conference that produced the ILO Convention was cautious in his endorsement of using that treaty as the model for the Refugee Convention. He "wished to make it clear that he did not advocate the adoption of article 6 of the Migration for Employment Convention as it stood; he merely felt that it would be a more useful basis for discussion than the Secretariat's text": Statement of Mr. Cuvelier of Belgium, ibid.

[221] Statement of Mr. Metall of the International Labor Organization, UN Doc. E/AC.32/SR.14, Jan. 26, 1950, at 4.

[222] The Belgian delegate insisted that the Refugee Convention should be understood to give "refugees general security against social and other risks": Statement of Mr. Cuvelier of Belgium, UN Doc. E/AC.32/SR.24, Feb. 3, 1950, at 3. The American representative suggested that an amendment to clarify this point was not required "as Mr. Cuvelier's explanation would appear in the summary record": Statement of Mr. Henkin of the United States, ibid. That report notes explicitly that "[t]his article includes provision for payment in cases of employment injury even if in a particular country such payments do not constitute a part of a social security system": Ad Hoc Committee, "First Session Report," at Annex II.

[223] "Comments submitted by the Director-General of the International Labour Office on the Draft Convention relating to the Status of Refugees," UN Doc. E/AC.32/7, Aug. 15, 1950, at 3.

in the Refugee Convention, the drafters were content to allow refugees to benefit from a more comprehensive duty:

> [T]he reason for the change to the word "disability" was that "invalidity" apparently had no connection in English with the state of being an invalid. As "disability" was in any event wider in its meaning than what was meant by "invalidity," [the representative of the United States] saw no reason why the International Labour Office should object to it.[224]

It was thereupon agreed that the broader meaning of social security in the event of disability – including programs to provide compensation in the event of either permanent or temporary incapacity – should be recorded as authoritative.[225]

Not only does Art. 24(1)(b) require that refugees be assimilated to citizens for purposes of benefiting from all forms of social security protection,[226] but it also sets one duty to assist refugees in a way that may not be open to nationals. As several delegates confirmed, their general laws or regulatory practices normally prohibited the payment of a social security survivor

---

[224] Statement of Mr. Henkin of the United States, UN Doc. E/AC.32/SR.38, Aug, 17, 1950, at 9. As Mr. Henkin suggested, the word "invalidity" simply does not have a relevant meaning in English. See also Statement of Sir Leslie Brass of the United Kingdom, ibid. at 16: "[T]he word 'invalidity' had no connection with health. If it was desired to indicate that the disability was permanent, then the words 'permanent disability' should be used. 'Invalidity' was obviously a mistranslation of a French term, which had crept into previous instruments." The Chairman then proposed the use of the term "permanent disability" in Art. 24(1)(b), but abandoned that notion when no support was expressed for the idea: ibid.

[225] The Canadian representative "supported the proposal previously made by the United States representative that the Committee's interpretation ... quoted by the International Labour Office in paragraph 5 of its comments should be included in that article": Statement of Mr. Winter of Canada, ibid. at 15. This proposal was supported by the representatives of the United Kingdom, Denmark, and France: ibid.

[226] In consequence of this duty, for example, the United States is in *prima facie* breach by opting to deny social security benefits to refugees who failed to acquire US citizenship within seven years of arrival in that country: "Thousands of refugees face loss of US benefits," *Seattle Post-Intelligencer*, Nov. 12, 2003. While refugees are to be assimilated to citizens for purposes of determining their entitlement to social security, states enjoy no right to *require* refugees to become citizens in order to participate in social security schemes. In the case of the United States, however, a finding of non-compliance is probably avoided by the terms of a US reservation to Art. 24(1)(b) which provide that the obligation is accepted "except insofar as that paragraph may conflict in certain instances with any provisions of title II (old age, survivors' and disability insurance) or title XVIII (hospital and medical insurance for the aged) of the Social Security Act. As to any such provision, the United States will accord to refugees lawfully staying in its territory treatment no less favorable than is accorded aliens generally in the same circumstances": see reservations and declarations of state parties, available at www.unhcr.ch (accessed Nov. 20, 2004).

benefit to a non-resident. The President of the Conference of Plenipotentiaries, for example, noted that "Danes were not allowed to draw pensions when resident abroad, so that it would not be possible, for instance, to allow the compensation payable on the death of a refugee to be transferred to his widow resident outside the country."[227] Similar rules existed in the United Kingdom, Germany, and Norway.[228] Even though a rule of general application, the refusal to pay social security to a non-resident surviving spouse or child was said by the International Refugee Organization to have a disproportionate impact on the survivors of refugee workers:

> Difficulties had arisen in cases of fatal accidents to refugees whose beneficiaries resided abroad. Since those beneficiaries were not regular residents of the country where the accident had occurred, they had not received the benefits.[229]

As such, "[t]he dispensation of a residential qualification is of particular importance to refugees whose families are often split in their search for re-establishment in a country other than their country of origin."[230]

Art. 24(2) provides precisely that dispensation. It sets an absolute duty, whatever the host state's general rules, that compensation in the event of the death of a refugee worker occasioned by employment injury or occupational disease be made to the refugee's survivors whether they live in the host country or elsewhere.[231] Importantly, none of the governments which voiced concern about their non-conforming social security laws actually opposed this provision, agreeing instead simply to enter a reservation on point.[232] In the result,

> Paragraph 2 of Article 24 ... goes beyond national treatment. Even if the [surviving] dependants of nationals are not entitled to benefit if they stay outside the country concerned, surviving dependants of refugees shall be allowed to enjoy such benefits and have them transferred out of the country.[233]

---

[227] Statement of Mr. Larsen of Denmark, UN Doc. A/CONF.2/SR.10, July 6, 1951, at 21.

[228] Statements of Mr. Hoare of the United Kingdom, Mr. von Trutzschler of the Federal Republic of Germany, and Mr. Anker of Norway, ibid. at 21–22.

[229] Statement of Mr. Weis of the International Refugee Organization, UN Doc. E/AC.32/SR.14, Jan. 26, 1950, at 6.

[230] United Nations, "Compilation of Comments," at 49.

[231] Weis notes, however, that "[a]s to the actual transfer of the compensation, currency regulations are preserved but they should, as far as possible, be interpreted in such a way as to make transfer possible": Weis, *Travaux*, at 192.

[232] Germany did not, in fact, enter a relevant reservation; Denmark and Norway initially reserved on this point, but have since withdrawn their reservations to Art. 24(2). In addition to the United Kingdom (which maintains its reservation), New Zealand and Poland have also entered a reservation specifically to Art. 24(2): see reservations and declarations of state parties, available at www.unhcr.ch (accessed Nov. 20, 2004).

[233] Grahl-Madsen, *Commentary*, at 96–97.

In at least this one way, the Convention's rules on social security clearly accommodate the specificity of the refugee predicament.

Apart from this one enhancement, the refugee is generally entitled to receive only the same access to social security as is enjoyed by citizens of the host country. And even this general principle is attenuated by the rules set out in clauses (i) and (ii) of Art. 24(1)(b), read in conjunction with Arts. 24(3) and (4). These rules are in response to the general expectation of states that where an individual has contributed to the social security system of more than one country, certain benefits (such as an old age or retirement benefit) are routinely cost-shared by the various governments in which some measure of entitlement has accrued. As the representative of the International Labor Organization explained, "agreements were often concluded in order to enable workers who moved from one country to another to accumulate the insurance benefits earned in both countries. The two countries concerned would each agree to pay their share according to the time worked in their territory."[234] This is the case for nearly all refugees, who have generally spent part of their working life in their country of origin, and the rest in one or more asylum states. But because of their status as refugees, there is the possibility that partner states will not in fact be willing to cost-share the social security to be paid by the asylum country.

Most obviously, the ruptured relationship between the refugee and his or her country of origin means that there is no guarantee that the country of origin will be willing to make its contribution to the refugee's social security benefit.[235] But it is also frequently the case that refugees work in a country of transit or first asylum which may be similarly disinclined to contribute to the social security benefit.[236] In either of these situations, and unless express provision were made in the text of Art. 24, the drafters were concerned that the asylum state might be in the unhappy position of being asked to pay a full

---

[234] Statement of Mr. Metall of the ILO, UN Doc. E/AC.32/SR.14, Jan. 26, 1950, at 11.

[235] "Such agreements could benefit the nationals of the countries concerned but it was difficult to see how they could benefit a refugee who had lost the protection of his Government and had cut himself off from the social security system of his country of origin": Statement of Mr. Metall of the ILO, ibid. See also Statement of Mr. Cuvelier of Belgium, ibid. at 12: "[S]uch arrangements were always the result of special arrangements . . . [R]efugees could not expect to receive any insurance benefits from their countries of origin."

[236] This situation was raised by the observer from the American Federation of Labor. "[A]lthough refugees could not expect to benefit from any rights acquired in their countries of origin, some of them had acquired rights in Germany before moving to some other country for resettlement. Arrangements were being made to obtain recognition for those rights. He fully agreed with the representative of Belgium that it was essential to mention the limitation [in para. 14(1)(b)(i)] since all the arrangements were the result of special agreements": Statement of Mr. Stolz of the American Federation of Labor, ibid. at 12.

social security benefit to the refugee, but being unable to recover any contribution from the governments of other states where the refugee had accrued social security entitlements.[237] As Grahl-Madsen explains, this predicament could arise because

> [i]t follows from sub-paragraph [(1)(b)] that a refugee shall as a rule receive national treatment with regard to social security in the country where he is lawfully staying. That is to say, if nationals, by virtue of being nationals, are entitled to the full benefit of a social security scheme even if they have spent most of their life abroad and only resided in the country for a marginal period, whereas aliens must have resided in the country and contributed to the scheme for a considerable period of time in order to become eligible, refugees shall be assimilated to the former.[238]

The essential goal of clauses (i) and (ii) of Art. 24(1)(b), read together with paragraphs (3) and (4) of the same article, is therefore to delimit the general right of refugees to be treated as citizens for purposes of entitlement to social security by authorizing state parties to reduce the refugee's social security benefit to the extent of any unfunded contribution which should in principle have been made by one or more other countries in which the refugee has worked. The Belgian delegate to the Ad Hoc Committee provided a simple example of the approach ultimately adopted:

> He took as an example the case of a Polish miner in France. If the miner had worked ten years in Poland and twenty years in France, under the existing bilateral agreement Poland would pay one-third and France two-thirds of his pension. If the miner became a refugee, however, Poland could hardly be asked to pay the share which normally ought to have been paid by Poland. The miner would therefore receive in France only the two-thirds which that country had originally undertaken to pay.[239]

The text which implements this principle is somewhat awkwardly drafted, but is actually quite sensible if its various parts are viewed as a whole.

First, and in line with the Belgian representative's example just cited, it was agreed that there could be no question of denying refugees such social security benefits as are owed them under the general rules of the host state, taking into account relevant requirements based on such factors as the time spent working and/or contributions made while working in the asylum state. On the basis of a firm assurance that "even in the absence of bilateral

---

[237] This can be seen in the blunt response of the American representative to an amendment proposed by the American Federation of Labor: "Mr. Stolz's amendment would ensure a refugee the rights he had acquired by virtue of bilateral agreements before becoming a refugee. He did not consider it possible to adopt such a proposal."

[238] Grahl-Madsen, *Commentary*, at 94.

[239] Statement of Mr. Cuvelier of Belgium, UN Doc. E/AC.32/SR.24, Feb. 3, 1950, at 4.

agreements, [a refugee's] acquired rights would be safeguarded,"[240] a non-governmental amendment to Art. 24(1)(b) designed explicitly to safeguard the portion of a social security benefit payable under the host state's own laws was withdrawn.[241]

Second, clause (i) is predicated on the understanding that refugees should in principle receive the benefit of any bilateral or other arrangements in place to preserve their "acquired rights and rights in course of acquisition."[242] As the Belgian representative explained, "A Polish miner residing in France would normally receive the insurance benefits he had accumulated in both countries, assuming there was close cooperation between the two countries in respect of insurance."[243] But the fact that clause (i) is a limitation clause makes clear that where there are no such arrangements in place, the country in which the refugee is staying cannot be expected to pay a benefit to the extent it is owed as the result of work not carried out on its territory, or for which worker or other contributions have not been made to its coffers. As Robinson writes, these rights acquired abroad "may either be disregarded or recognized in part only."[244]

It was also agreed that governments could lawfully exclude refugees from certain special arrangements funded by the state and designed to "top up" social security payments to their own citizens.[245] But the right of

[240] Statement of Mr. Henkin of the United States, UN Doc. E/AC.32/SR.14, Jan. 26, 1950, at 12.

[241] In response to Mr. Henkin's assurance (see text above, at p. 780, n. 240), the representative of the American Federation of Labor withdrew his amendment, noting that he had proposed it "only because he had feared that becoming a refugee might deprive a person of the share to be paid by the country of reception": Statement of Mr. Stolz of the American Federation of Labor, UN Doc. E/AC.32/SR.24, Feb. 3, 1950, at 4.

[242] "Maintenance of 'acquired rights' relates to rights to social security benefits acquired in one country and to be recognized, within the existing accumulation, by another country; maintenance of 'rights in [course] of acquisition' refers to a partial accumulation of rights which in itself is not sufficient to grant benefits and which represents part of the necessary amount of accumulation required for the enjoyment of benefits": Robinson, *History*, at 126.

[243] Statement of Mr. Cuvelier of Belgium, UN Doc. E/AC.32/SR.23, Feb. 3, 1950, at 12.

[244] Robinson, *History*, at 126. Grahl-Madsen takes a more extreme position, arguing that a refugee who is subject to a treaty pertaining to a social security scheme is excluded from the general right to be assimilated to nationals for purposes of entitlement to social security: Grahl-Madsen, *Commentary*, at 94. There was, however, no discussion among the drafters that supports this view. Moreover, if the goal of clause (i) had been to exclude refugees covered by interstate social security treaties from the scope of the basic duty to assimilate refugees to nationals, it is surprising that it was framed merely in descriptive terms ("There may be appropriate agreements . . . ") rather than as a definitive exclusion from the basic duty set by Art. 24(1)(b).

[245] Grahl-Madsen clarifies that this clause normally refers to "allowances paid over and above the partial pension to which a person may be entitled by virtue of contributions paid, so that his total benefit shall be equal to a normal (or only slightly less than a normal) pension": Grahl-Madsen, *Commentary*, at 96.

governments to deny refugees access to such additional benefits is limited to circumstances in which the supplementary benefit is paid *entirely* from state funds, that is, from a fund not based even in part on contributions from workers or employers. This restriction is clear from the text of Art. 24(1)(b)(ii), which resulted from the defeat of an Austrian proposal that refugees not receive the benefit of special arrangements funded "wholly or partially out of public funds."[246] While sympathetic to the right of a state to provide special support to its citizens, the drafters feared that if any leeway were granted states to exclude refugees from special payments funded even in part from employer and worker contributions, "refugees would lose certain rights deriving from their contributions."[247] As the French government insisted,

> It was ... possible that under certain social security systems the contributions paid by employers and workers were not sufficient to ensure financial stability; in such cases there was often a system of State assistance to redress the balance. If the Austrian proposal were accepted, in countries where the system was financed partly by the State but mainly by contributions from the persons insured, wage-earning refugees who paid contributions might find themselves deprived of all right to benefits, that was to say, of the counterpart of the contributions they had paid.[248]

Because it could be seen that the Austrian approach was open to an interpretation that might deprive a refugee worker "of the benefits of his own or his employer's contributions,"[249] sub-paragraph (ii) of Art. 24(1)(b) disallows any exclusion of refugees from special arrangements funded in whole or in part from such contributions.

One of the most important protections of Art. 24 is the guarantee in paragraph (3) that refugees benefit automatically from any social security arrangements made between or among state parties to the Refugee Convention. As conceived by the Ad Hoc Committee, Art. 24(3) would have gone farther still, entitling refugees to claim the benefit of any interstate agreement binding their host country, including one with a state not bound by the Refugee Convention.[250] There was, however, concern that such a

---

[246] United Nations, "Compilation of Comments," at 48.

[247] Statement of Mr. Oblath of the International Labor Organization, UN Doc. E/AC.32/SR.38, Aug. 17, 1950, at 17.

[248] Statement of Mr. Juvigny of France, ibid. at 17–18.

[249] Statement of Sir Leslie Brass of the United Kingdom, ibid. at 18.

[250] "The Contracting States whose nationals enjoy the benefits of agreements for the maintenance of acquired rights and rights in the process of acquisition in regard to social security, shall extend the benefits of such agreements to refugees subject only to the conditions which apply to their nationals": "Report of the Ad Hoc Committee on Refugees and Stateless Persons, Second Session," UN Doc. E/1850, Aug. 25, 1950 (Ad Hoc Committee, "Second Session Report"), at 22.

broadly framed duty could effectively compel state parties to pay out a combined social security benefit even when the partner country refused to cost-share the benefit. Governments were willing to commit themselves fully to enfranchise refugees only where there was a sufficiently solid guarantee that cost-sharing rules would apply also to benefits paid to refugees – and only state parties to the Refugee Convention would clearly be bound in this regard. As explained by the British representative to the Conference of Plenipotentiaries:

> He had no objection to the principle that those agreements [on transfer of social security rights] ... should apply equally to refugees and to nationals, but the text ... [should not] permit of the possibility that, under a bilateral agreement concluded between a State Party and a State non-Party to the Convention, the former would be required to apply to refugees from the latter the same conditions as it would apply to its own nationals. Such a unilateral obligation would be an unjustifiable burden on the State Party to the Convention, and he doubted whether it would be practicable without the co-operation of the non-Contracting State. He believed the original intention had been that where such agreements existed between Contracting States, they should automatically be applied to refugees from both countries.[251]

The text of Art. 24(3) was therefore amended to limit the legal duty of states to enfranchise refugees under interstate arrangements for the protection of social security benefits to such agreements as are made between or among state parties to the Refugee Convention.[252] This provision clearly responds to one of the two circumstances of initial concern to the drafters, namely the cases of refugees who had worked in one or more countries of asylum before ultimately settling in a different state party:[253]

---

[251] Statement of Mr. Hoare of the United Kingdom, UN Doc. A/CONF.2/SR.10, July 6, 1951, at 22.

[252] Grahl-Madsen takes the view that para. 3 applies also where two or more contracting states are parties to a multilateral treaty to which non-contracting states are also parties, but only as regards "rights acquired or in the process of acquisition in countries parties to the [Refugee] Convention": Grahl-Madsen, *Commentary*, at 97. This is a sensible interpretation, as the mutuality of obligation to enfranchise refugees upon which para. 3 is based would exist in such circumstances.

[253] Robinson argues that para. 3 "refers *only* to rights which a refugee accumulated in a Contracting State where he first found asylum and which he would like to make use of in another such country [emphasis added]": Robinson, *History*, at 127. While this was clearly the focus of concern to the drafters, there is no basis in the language adopted or purposes pursued to exclude a similar approach to, for example, social security entitlement acquired by a refugee in respect of work undertaken in a state party different from that in which he or she has established residence.

Taking the case of the social security agreement between France and Belgium, and assuming that there was no additional protocol extending the benefits of that agreement to refugees, and further assuming that both France and Belgium ratified the draft Convention at present before the Conference, refugees moving from France to Belgium and *vice versa* would enjoy the benefits accruing to nationals even though there was no special agreement to that effect.

Consequently, benefits enjoyed by nationals would be extended to refugees whose countries of domicile or of habitual residence were parties to the Convention and to a bilateral agreement relating to the maintenance of acquired rights and rights in the process of acquisition for their nationals, provided such refugees were able to fulfil the requirements to which such benefits were subject so far as nationals were concerned.[254]

Moreover, refugees are entitled to benefit not only from contributory arrangements which are in place between state parties when the refugee arrives in the asylum country, but also from any future arrangements which may come into force.[255] No special measures are required to enfranchise refugees, since "[t]he intention of paragraph 3 of article [24] was, of course, to extend such benefits to refugees *ipso facto*, without any special provisions to that end."[256]

---

[254] Statement of Mr. Robinson of Israel, UN Doc. A/CONF.2/SR.11, July 9, 1951, at 5. This statement was made in response to a request from the Conference that Mr. Robinson review the drafting records of the Ad Hoc Committee on this point, and "enlighten the Conference at its next meeting": Statement of the President, Mr. Larsen of Denmark, UN Doc. A/CONF.2/SR.10, July 6, 1951, at 24.

[255] Speaking to his amendment, which was adopted by the Conference (UN Doc. A/CONF.2/SR.11, July 9, 1951, at 7), the Belgian representative affirmed that his goal in proposing an amendment to para. 3 to include agreements "which may be concluded between them in the future" was "to enable refugees to benefit not only from existing social security measures, but also from any subsequent arrangements": Statement of Mr. Herment of Belgium, ibid. at 6.

[256] Statement of Mr. Robinson of Israel, ibid. at 7. This clarification was offered in response to a question from the Belgian delegate who wished to know "whether [the Israeli] representative thought that the agreements referred to should become automatically applicable to refugees as soon as the Convention had been ratified": Statement of Mr. Herment of Belgium, ibid. at 6. Upon receiving the quoted response from Mr. Robinson, the Belgian delegate "accepted the Israeli representative's interpretation": ibid. at 7. The fact that no specific mention of refugees in a relevant interstate agreement is required to enfranchise refugees does not, however, mean that the international agreement is automatically enforceable in domestic law. As Weis observes, "[w]hether the provision of [para.] 3 is self-executing depends on the national law of the Contracting State concerned. Where the provision is not self-executing, the Contracting State is obliged to take the necessary measures to extend the benefits of the agreement to refugees, be it by arrangement with the other Party to the agreement or by measures on the national level": Weis, *Travaux*, at 192–193.

States were, however, unwilling to undertake a comparable legal commitment where combined social security benefits should in principle be cost-shared with a state that is not a party to the Refugee Convention, including the refugee's country of origin. In these circumstances, governments were prepared to agree only that, as a matter of principle,[257] they would endeavor to provide refugees with the benefits stipulated under relevant social security agreements. Thus, paragraph 4 speaks to the situation of an individual:

> who, having accumulated certain social security rights in his home country and having moved to another country which had a social security benefits agreement with the former, then renounced the protection of his country of origin and became a refugee. Under what circumstances the contractual right to the benefits accruing under the bilateral agreement would be forfeited was a matter that could only be determined by the parties to the agreement in the light of its letter and of its spirit. A State, granting asylum to a refugee of the nature just described, would, however, not be prevented from granting benefits of its own free will to a person towards whom it might have no contractual obligations. The purpose of paragraph 4 was to provide for such a contingency, but, unlike paragraph 3, it took the form, not of a binding provision but of a recommendation.[258]

In contrast to the form in which it was proposed by the Ad Hoc Committee, paragraph 4 as adopted is not restricted only to agreements which may exist with a refugee's country of origin,[259] but extends also to agreements between the host country and any "non-contracting State." Thus, for example, a refugee's country of residence should make best efforts to secure additional social security benefits for the refugee based on work and social security contributions in a country of first asylum that is not a party to the Convention.[260] Also in contrast to the Ad Hoc Committee's approach,

---

[257] The American representative referred to para. 4 as "merely a recommendation, [and therefore] . . . not [a matter] in respect of which a reservation was justified": Statement of Mr. Henkin of the United States, UN Doc. E/AC.32/SR.38, Aug. 17, 1950, at 9.

[258] Statement of Mr. Robinson of Israel, UN Doc. A/CONF.2/SR.11, July 9, 1951, at 6.

[259] "The Contracting States will give sympathetic consideration to extending to individual refugees so far as possible the benefits of similar agreements which may have been concluded by such Contracting States with the country of the individual's nationality or former nationality": Ad Hoc Committee, "Second Session Report," at 22.

[260] Indeed, Robinson sees this as the primary purpose of para. 4. "Para. 4 deals with rights accumulated in the refugee's first country of asylum, a non-Contracting State, to be exercised in his second country of asylum, a Contracting State. In such instances the Convention does not impose on the Contracting State an obligation to treat the refugee as if he were a national of the non-Contracting State, but only recommends such a treatment to the parties to the Convention": Robinson, *History*, at 127.

such efforts are expected to be made on behalf of all refugees similarly situated, not simply in individual cases.[261]

In sum, the general rule is that refugees lawfully staying in a state party are to be assimilated to that country's citizens for purposes of entitlement to all forms of social security. Indeed, refugees are entitled to better than national treatment where necessary to ensure that a social security death benefit is paid out to non-resident dependants. The major limitation on the right of refugees to national treatment in regard to social security involves the situation where a portion of the benefit due a refugee would ordinarily be paid at least in part by another country in which the refugee has accrued some measure of social security entitlement. Where there is no arrangement in place between the relevant governments to combine the entitlements to social security of persons who have worked and contributed in each jurisdiction, the refugee is entitled only to receive whatever benefits are owed under the domestic rules of the host country.

On the other hand, where there is a cost-sharing arrangement in place between the refugee's host state and the other country in which entitlement has accrued, the refugee should in principle receive the combined benefit. But if in fact the other country refuses to pay its share, the host state is liable to pay out only the part of the social security benefit to which the refugee is entitled under its domestic laws. This is so even if the citizens of the host country would, in similar circumstances, receive a supplementary payment from the government to "top up" the domestic portion – thus amounting to a departure from the basic principle of Art. 24 that refugees should be afforded national treatment.

The only circumstance in which a refugee is effectively insulated against the prospect of a reduced social security benefit based on the default of a country under an agreement for shared social security responsibility is where that other country is also a party to the Refugee Convention. If so, the host government must pay the refugee the whole of any combined benefit due to the refugee pursuant to its arrangement with the defaulting state, then rely on its right to seek redress from the defaulting government based on the latter's duty to extend the benefit of the arrangement to refugees under Art. 24 of the Refugee Convention. Where, however, the defaulting government is not a party to the Refugee Convention (and therefore may not be legally required to extend the benefit of social security cooperation agreements to refugees), the

---

[261] The amendment approved by the Ad Hoc Committee (see note 243 above) occurred in response to the proposal of Mr. Robinson of Israel, UN Doc. A/CONF.2/SR.11, July 9, 1951, at 8–9: "[T]he Style Committee might consider the desirability of deleting the word 'individual' before the word 'refugees' in the second line of paragraph 4, particularly if there was any risk of the retention of that word leading to discrimination between one refugee and another."

host state is under no legal duty to make up the shortfall. Art. 24(4) encourages, but does not require, state parties to do what they can to assist refugees in such a predicament.

6.2 Professional practice

While it is increasingly rare, the governments of some asylum states still do not allow refugee professionals to work in their territory. UNHCR observed in 1991 that

> [t]he majority of States require that aliens generally (including refugees) possess the necessary professional qualifications and that these be validated or recognized by the competent authorities before they are allowed to practise ... [However] [s]ome states have reserved the practice of certain professions such as law, medicine, engineering, architecture and teaching to their own nationals while, in some cases, allowing aliens to be employed in these fields on a contractual basis.[262]

The refusal to allow refugees to contribute their professional skills may have truly grave consequences. Despite both the shortage of medical care for most refugee groups, and the importance of understanding the language, culture, and health context of a specific refugee population,[263] some asylum countries have even prohibited refugee doctors from assisting their own people. For example, Ugandan refugee doctors were refused the opportunity to work among the Ugandan refugee population,[264] and Turkey denied Iraqi Kurdish doctors permission to work in the Kurdish refugee camps.[265]

More generally, refugees with professional qualifications in the less developed world face general barriers on access to work, including bars on noncitizens engaging in many or most forms of work,[266] or confinement to camps or settlements where the opportunities for professional practice may simply not exist.[267] In Nairobi, for example, "[t]rained teachers or civil administrators are forced to do sweeping jobs, if they are lucky."[268] In Sudan, Eritrean

---

[262] UNHCR, "Information Note on Implementation of the 1951 Convention and the 1967 Protocol relating to the Status of Refugees," UN Doc. EC/SCP/66, July 22, 1991 (UNHCR, "Implementation"), at para. 84.

[263] See chapter 4.4.3 above, at pp. 507–511.

[264] N. Van Hear and B. Harrell-Bond, "Refugees and Displaced People: Health Issues," in UN Institute for Training and Research ed., *The Challenge of African Disasters* 61 (1991), at 65.

[265] Initiative for Human Rights in Kurdistan, "Silence is Killing Them: A Report on the Situation of the Kurdish Refugees in Turkey" (1990), at 12.

[266] See chapter 6.1 above, at pp. 730–738.   [267] See chapter 5.2 above, at pp. 696–704.

[268] T. Skari and E. Girardet, "Urban Refugees: Out of the Public Eye," (1985) 14 *Refugees* 14.

and Ethiopian medical doctors were able to work only under the auspices of healthcare programs sponsored by international aid agencies.[269]

Some states of the developed world also bar non-citizens from engaging in certain professions, most commonly including the civil service and military, but sometimes including also the legal profession, judiciary, law enforcement, medicine, engineering, architecture, and teaching.[270] France goes farther still, prohibiting non-citizens from working even as pharmacists or chartered accountants.[271] The Supreme Court of the United States has upheld bars on the employment of non-citizens as public school teachers,[272] but struck down citizenship requirements for lawyers, engineers, and notaries.[273] Switzerland denies most non-citizens the right to work as doctors, dentists, veterinarians, or pharmacists, but has enacted a specific legislative exception in favor of refugees who wish to engage in such work.[274] Similarly, Italy bars non-citizen journalists from working in its territory absent a reciprocity agreement favoring its own journalists, but it exempts refugee journalists from this restriction.[275] Belgium has traditionaly pursued a still more liberal policy, allowing refugees, including those awaiting verification of their claims, to secure a permit authorizing them to engage in professional practice for up to five years.[276]

Even where formal bars do not exist, the nearly universal practice of professional accreditation poses a significant barrier in practical terms for refugees who wish to resume their professional life in the asylum state. Professions may refuse to recognize certifications obtained outside the reception country, or require substantial apprenticeship in the host state; they may require that candidates be licensed in the particular discipline in their country of origin, effectively excluding applications for refugees whose home states did not regulate their profession; or they may subject foreign-trained individuals to certification examinations not required of citizens.[277] The result of

---

[269] El Bushra, "Educational Needs," at 23.

[270] UNHCR, "Implementation," at paras. 82, 84.   [271] Lambert, *Seeking Asylum*, at 172.

[272] *Ambach v. Norwick*, 441 US 68 (US SC, Apr. 17, 1979).

[273] *In re Griffiths*, 413 US 717 (US SC, June 25, 1973), re lawyers; *Examining Board of Engineers v. Flores de Otero*, 426 US 572 (US SC, June 17, 1976), re engineers; *Bernal v. Fainter*, 467 US 216 (US SC, May 30, 1984), re notaries public.

[274] W. Kälin, *International Academy of Comparative Law National Report for Switzerland* (1994), at 15.

[275] G. D'Orazio, *International Academy of Comparative Law National Report for Italy* (1994), at 36.

[276] K. Leus and G. Vermeylen, *International Academy of Comparative Law National Report for Belgium* (1994), at 11.

[277] P. Cumming, *Access: Task Force on Access to Professions and Trades in Ontario* (1989). The report cites by way of example the fact that the Canadian province of Ontario requires foreign-trained dentists successfully to complete a four-part dental licensing examination from which the graduates of Canadian or American dental schools are exempt. The failure rate for the examination is said to be substantial: ibid. at 161.

these many requirements is that professional refugees "often cannot practice because there is no equivalence of degrees and qualifications, and they experience severe downward social mobility."[278]

By way of example, while Germany has lifted most citizenship requirements for professional practice, "asylees usually will have to pass special exams in order to be able to practise a liberal profession notwithstanding the fact that they might have longstanding professional experience."[279] A refugee from Afghanistan who was medical director and a consultant gynaecologist at the university hospital in Kabul explained the difference of treatment she experienced in France and in the United Kingdom:

> In France, working as a doctor was easy. After a language course and a voluntary hospital attachment, I was offered a part-time position running an obstetrics, gynaecology and family planning outpatients clinic ... In 1995, my husband was offered a position in the UK and we moved ...
>
> First I applied for Senior House Officer positions but apparently I'm overqualified. But for more senior positions I must pass the Membership of the Royal College of Obstetricians and Gynaecology exams. I've passed Part I, but now I'm told I can't sit Part II unless I have two to four years of work experience, so it's Catch 22. Without an interview, or even any feedback, I can't display my experience. In Kabul, I worked as a GP and a gynaecologist. I saw patients daily; I performed hundreds of operations; I lectured students; I published research papers. Here that counts for nothing.[280]

Even with significant support, the manager of the Skills Match program in the United Kingdom reported that only about 5 percent of refugee professionals found work truly commensurate with their qualifications. He observed that "demotion is the biggest problem for qualified asylum-seekers ... In my experience, the odd-job man can get cash jobs with little problem, but professional barriers prevent people such as lawyers and teachers getting work."[281]

Refugee Convention, Art. 19   Liberal professions

1. Each Contracting State shall accord to refugees lawfully staying in their territory who hold diplomas recognized by the competent authorities of that State, and who are desirous of practising

---

[278] Joly, *Asylum*, at 58.

[279] R. Hofmann, *International Academy of Comparative Law National Report for Germany* (1994), at 19. See also R. Haines, *International Academy of Comparative Law National Report for New Zealand* (1994), at 37; and J. Vedsted-Hansen, *International Academy of Comparative Law National Report for Denmark* (1994), at 2.

[280] "Bordering on the ridiculous: The doctor who's not wanted," *Guardian*, Sept. 30, 2000, at 29, quoting Dr. Zhargona Tanin.

[281] R. Prasad, "Raekha Prasad on a scheme to harness the much-needed skills of refugees," *Guardian*, Jan. 24, 2001, at 6, quoting David Forbes of the Manchester-based organization, Skills Match.

a liberal profession, treatment as favourable as possible and, in any event, not less favourable than that accorded to aliens generally in the same circumstances.

2. The Contracting States shall use their best endeavours consistently with their laws and constitutions to secure the settlement of such refugees in the territories, other than the metropolitan territory, for whose international relations they are responsible.

It seems clear that the Secretary-General's draft of what became Art. 19 was motivated by a genuine concern for the predicament of refugees who found themselves in reception states where they could not exercise the only livelihood familiar to them:

> Access to the liberal professions, which are the most highly regulated of all and generally speaking, overcrowded in European countries, is, in principle, barred to foreigners. Where, however, treaty provisions exist, these professions are open to foreigners to some extent. It should be noted that there is a high proportion of members of the liberal professions among the refugees, including qualified and experienced scientists, engineers, architects and doctors holding diplomas equivalent to those required in the reception country. Such professional men, moreover, are not suited to any other occupation than their own.[282]

It was therefore recommended that professionally qualified refugees be assimilated to most-favored foreigners, allowing them access to at least those professional opportunities open to the citizens of partner and other closely affiliated countries.[283]

The drafters, however, showed little enthusiasm to guarantee even this fairly narrow opportunity for refugees to have privileged access to professional practice. To begin with, they decided not to work from the Secretary-General's proposal for Art. 19, but instead to base their drafting on the French government's proposal. The latter did not require most-favored-national treatment, but stipulated simply that governments would provide refugees with "as favourable treatment as possible" in accessing the professions.[284] The only concession made by France was that whatever treatment was granted would "be in no case inferior to the treatment afforded to foreigners generally."[285] This approach was contrary to the advice of the Secretary-General, who had noted that granting refugees only the same access to professions as

---

[282] Secretary-General, "Memorandum," at 35–36.
[283] The Secretary-General recognized that the alternative would be simply to grant refugees the same treatment as afforded aliens generally, but warned against that approach: Secretary-General, "Memorandum," at 36.
[284] France, "Draft Convention," at 6–7.
[285] Statement of Mr. Rain of France, UN Doc. E/AC.32/SR.13, Jan. 26, 1950, at 16.

aliens generally "would in practice be of little help to refugees, since in point of fact access to the professions is normally only accorded to foreigners – and even then with reservations – by virtue of treaty provisions."[286] The International Refugee Organization also opposed the "aliens generally" standard, arguing that "[i]n countries where the rights of aliens ... depend on reciprocity arising out of treaty arrangements it is doubtful that the formula as it now stands would ensure any rights for refugees."[287]

In what can only be described as an extraordinary contrast with discussion of the appropriate contingent standard for access to wage-earning employment,[288] no state representative at any stage of the drafting process advocated moving beyond the baseline ("aliens generally") standard of treatment. As the Chairman of the Ad Hoc Committee observed, "there was no question of according refugees the most favourable treatment given to foreigners by virtue of treaties, but merely the most favourable treatment possible."[289] Much less was there any interest in giving refugees the same rights as citizens to practice a profession: the Conference of Plenipotentiaries even rejected an Egyptian amendment that would have made explicit that refugees were *not* entitled to access professions reserved for citizens on the grounds that "it might be dangerous to refer to rights which could be covered by special regulations ... inasmuch as it might suggest to States the possibility of taking such action in respect of refugees."[290] As the Belgian representative to the Conference of Plenipotentiaries concluded, "the draft Convention gave refugees [only] the status of aliens"[291] with regard to the right to engage in professional practice.

The duty to assimilate refugees only to aliens generally requires, however, that where there is in practice true generality of access to a given right, the right in question automatically accrues to refugees as well. This means that if access to professional practice is only formally reserved for citizens (or subject to reciprocity arrangements) but in fact is generally granted to non-citizens, such access must be extended also to refugees.[292] The decision of Italy to allow refugee journalists to work in its territory, though that right is formally predicated on reciprocity, is thus in accord with this principle: given the generality of reciprocal arrangements, the right to journalistic practice is in fact open to most non-citizens, and thus owed to refugees as well.

---

[286] Secretary-General, "Memorandum," at 36.
[287] United Nations, "Compilation of Comments," at 39, 45.
[288] See chapter 6.1.1 above, at pp. 744–747.
[289] Statement of the Chairman, Mr. Chance of Canada, UN Doc. E/AC.32/SR.13, Jan. 26, 1950, at 17.
[290] Statement of Mr. Hoare of the United Kingdom, UN Doc. A/CONF.2/SR.9, July 6, 1951, at 21.
[291] Statement of Mr. Herment of Belgium, ibid. at 21.
[292] See chapter 3.2.1 above, at pp. 199–200.

As well, the "treatment as favourable as possible" clause requires state parties to give consideration in good faith to the non-application to refugees of limits generally applied to aliens.[293] The Belgian decision to grant refugees free access to professional life, as well as the Swiss decision to exempt refugees from more particular exclusions applied to other non-citizens, are examples of action that is very much in accord with this expectation. But since the duty to consider preferential treatment of refugees is an obligation of process, not a duty of result,[294] Art. 19 provides little solid assistance to refugees in asylum states where only nationals (or privileged non-citizens) are entitled to engage in some or all forms of professional practice. As a matter of law, the Refugee Convention requires only that a refugee be granted access to professional practice to the same extent that, in law or in practice, such access is normally granted to most non-citizens.[295] Where states give due consideration to the issue, but decide ultimately to limit particular kinds of professional practice to their own citizens, there is no violation of the Refugee Convention. As such, it is possible that the refusals of Uganda and Turkey to allow refugee doctors to attend to the needs of refugee populations in their territories were not contrary to Art. 19, assuming that medical practice in those countries is effectively not open to non-citizens. But given the urgency of the situations faced by the refugees there and the failure to provide them with access to local medical assistance, those states would have a very difficult time demonstrating that they truly gave good faith consideration to the exemption of refugee doctors from the general prohibition of practice by non-citizen physicians.[296]

The Refugee Convention provides no significant relief from the most common impediment faced by non-citizens wishing to engage in a profession, that being the need to meet often quite exacting standards for licensing or accreditation. These rules are frequently administered by professional associations authorized by the government to regulate access to professional life. A non-citizen wishing to continue his or her professional life in a new country may be required to meet a variety of standards, including possession of particular academic qualifications, a positive assessment of experience or standing in the applicant's home country, and satisfactory completion of a period of local training or testing.

---

[293] See chapter 3.2.1 above, at p. 200.

[294] As the Chinese representative insisted, "the provisions of article [19] as proposed by France had been applied in China already. It had done so of its own free will, but would hesitate to accept such provisions if they were imposed on it by a convention": Statement of Mr. Cha of China, UN Doc. E/AC.32/SR.13, Jan. 26, 1950, at 17.

[295] See chapter 3.2.1 above, at pp. 198–200.

[296] Given the failure of the host states to provide medical attention in truly extreme cases, it is also likely that Uganda and Turkey breached Art. 12 of the Economic Covenant. See chapter 4.4.3 above, at p. 513.

The drafters of the Refugee Convention recognized that not all accreditation requirements were really designed to protect the public interest. Indeed, the Chairman of the Ad Hoc Committee candidly conceded that "in the United Kingdom and Canada liberal profession bodies admitted holders of local diplomas only ... [T]hat was because they wished to maintain a certain level of tradition ... [I]t was true, of course, that such a requirement reflected too rigid a spirit of exclusiveness."[297] But in contrast to the approach taken to wage-earning employment,[298] the drafters showed no interest in exempting refugees from even accreditation requirements designed simply to avoid competition with domestic professionals.[299] To the contrary, they made access to Art. 19 rights contingent on the refugee possessing a "diploma[ ] recognized by the competent authorities of [the host] state,"[300] thereby explicitly sanctioning the practice in many states of leaving such decisions to the professional bodies themselves. More generally, they adopted language under which Art. 19 rights inhere in "refugees ... desirous of practising a liberal profession" in order to signal that the mere possession of formal qualifications could under no circumstance give rise to an international legal entitlement to engage in professional life:

> [T]he form of words was vague, but ... it should remain so. The Committee was faced with two separate considerations: on the one hand, the recognition of diplomas and, on the other, the exercise of the professions. In Belgium a foreigner could practise medicine if he held a Belgian diploma or a diploma recognized as equivalent; on the other hand, no foreigner, no matter what his diploma, was allowed to practise as a lawyer.

[297] Statement of the Chairman, Mr. Chance of Canada, UN Doc. E/AC.32/SR.13, Jan. 26, 1950, at 16.

[298] See chapter 6.1 above, at pp. 741–747.

[299] "The Italian Government could not agree to a clause which might aggravate the existing internal situation caused by over-population and unemployment": Statement of Mr. Theodoli of Italy, UN Doc. E/AC.32/SR.37, Aug. 16, 1950, at 20. Earlier, the French representative had similarly remarked "that the question gave rise to grave difficulties in France where there was a considerable number of refugees belonging to the liberal professions ... It should be understood that there were two types of interests: on the one hand, national interests which tended to reserve for some nationals exclusively, or to a very large extent, the exercise of liberal professions; on the other hand, the material interests of persons exercising those professions who were stubbornly defending their positions. It was the Committee's duty to see that States accorded refugees the most favourable treatment possible provided it did not conflict with national interests": Statement of Mr. Rain of France, UN Doc. E/AC.32/SR.13, Jan. 26, 1950, at 17–18.

[300] It was clarified, however, that the refugee need not arrive in the asylum state with a relevant diploma in order to benefit from Art. 19, but could invoke his or her rights once in possession of a diploma acquired in the host country or elsewhere: Statement of Mr. Cuvelier of Belgium, UN Doc. E/AC.32/SR.13, Jan. 26, 1950, at 16.

> It would be impossible therefore to adopt a definite form of words, as it could not be applied to all cases.[301]

At best, some value is secured by the obligation to assimilate refugees to aliens generally "in the same circumstances," which requires those undertaking an examination of professional qualifications to exempt refugees from general requirements which the refugee's particular circumstances render effectively insurmountable.[302] For example, a state which ordinarily requires proof that a non-citizen has been licensed in his or her discipline in the country of origin for accreditation would be required to waive this requirement in the case of a refugee who came from a state in which no system of professional regulation exists, or where professional registration was not open to the refugee for reasons related to his or her need for protection.

As if these several constraints were not enough, it was ultimately determined that Art. 19 could not be invoked by a refugee until he or she is "lawfully staying" in the territory of a state party. Interestingly, neither of the original drafts proposed any delay in the right to access professional practice based on attachment.[303] The report of the first session of the Ad Hoc Committee, however, limited professional practice to refugees "lawfully resident in their territory."[304] The only substantive debate on this question occurred at the Committee's second session, where it was agreed to revise the level of attachment downward simply to "lawfully in their territory"[305] in order to ensure that the right could be invoked by "persons entering a territory even for a few hours, provided that they had been duly authorized to enter."[306] As the American representative insisted, "his delegation wished to cover all refugees for however short a time they were lawfully in a territory."[307] Under this approach, Art. 19 could have been invoked, for example,

---

[301] Statement of Mr. Cuvelier of Belgium, ibid. at 18. The Chairman of the Ad Hoc Committee immediately concurred, noting that he "also thought that it was impossible to adopt a more definite formula; the High Contracting Parties should simply be invited to do their best to make the most liberal provisions possible": Statement of the Chairman, Mr. Chance of Canada, ibid.

[302] See chapter 3.2.3 above, at p. 208.

[303] The drafts prepared by the Secretary-General and by France simply granted Art. 19 rights to "refugees" without qualification: Secretary-General, "Memorandum," at 35; France, "Draft Convention," at 6.

[304] Ad Hoc Committee, "First Session Report," at Annex I.   [305] Ibid.

[306] Statement of Mr. Henkin of the United States, UN Doc. E/AC.32/SR.41, Aug. 23, 1950, at 14. The Chairman gave the example of "a person travelling through a country on his way back to his own country" who would be lawfully in the country of transit, and therefore entitled to exercise his or her profession there: Statement of the Chairman, Mr. Larsen of Denmark, ibid. at 15.

[307] Statement of Mr. Henkin of the United States, ibid. at 15.

by "a German refugee lawyer who periodically travelled from Sweden to Denmark to give consultations in a hotel for a period of three hours."[308]

In the end, however, the more restrictive view prevailed. While not formally debated there, the Conference of Plenipotentiaries reversed the Ad Hoc Committee's approach, deciding that Art. 19 rights would accrue only once a refugee is "lawfully staying" in a state party. In adopting this level of attachment, the Conference was probably influenced by the French view that the purpose of Art. 19 should be "to protect refugees residing in foreign territory, not merely staying there for a few hours."[309] But this more exacting level of attachment allows the right of professional practice to be denied not only to refugees present on a short-term basis, but also to most refugees awaiting the results of their refugee status claim and to refugees present in a state which opts not to assess refugee status,[310] at least until an ongoing presence is established in practical terms by the passage of time.[311]

It is therefore difficult to see Art. 19 as having any significant positive value for refugees. If no specific rule on access to the liberal professions had been included in the Refugee Convention, the ability of refugees to work in a professional capacity would presumably have been regulated by either the rule on self-employment, or by that dealing with wage-earning employment. Either of these approaches would have been more beneficial to refugees. Under Art. 18's provisions on self-employment, the refugee professional would have received no better standard of treatment than that now granted by Art. 19 ("treatment as favourable as possible and, in any event, not less favourable than that accorded to aliens generally in the same circumstances"), but that right would have accrued at an earlier point in time, namely when the refugee was simply "lawfully in" (rather than "lawfully staying") there.[312] If, on the other hand, the refugee professional's right to work had been governed by Art. 17's general rules on wage-earning employment, he or she would have been faced with the same contingent standard as that which governs Art. 19 ("lawfully staying"), but once qualified he or she would at least have been entitled to a higher standard of treatment, namely assimilation to the nationals of most-favored countries.[313] Under Art. 19, in contrast, the refugee professional is faced with the worst of both worlds: the point at which entitlement accrues is significantly delayed, and the right which is ultimately received is of little value. In pith and substance, then, Art. 19 is therefore most appropriately understood not so much as a source of refugee entitlement, but as a clawback provision directed to a subset of refugees who would otherwise have been able to invoke the more generous

---

[308] Statement of the Chairman, Mr. Larsen of Denmark, ibid. at 18.
[309] Statement of Mr. Juvigny of France, ibid. at 15.
[310] See chapter 3.1.3 above, at pp. 183–185.   [311] See chapter 3.1.4 above, at pp. 186–187.
[312] See chapter 5.3 above.   [313] See chapter 6.1 above.

provisions of either Art. 17 on wage-earning employment or Art. 18 on self-employment.[314]

The disinterest of the drafters in committing themselves to the meaningful enfranchisement of refugee professionals is perhaps most clear from the second paragraph of Art. 19, requiring government to "use their best endeavours" to secure the resettlement of professionally qualified refugees in affiliated territories. This approach seems to have been considered something of a "win–win" approach for both refugees and their host countries:

> Many countries were under pressure not to admit to their metropolitan territories refugees who might compete with professional workers resident there. In some colonial areas, however, there was an urgent need for qualified persons, and nationals of the metropolitan country were often reluctant to respond to that need. Colonial Governments which would not be willing to give refugees the opportunity of gainful employment in their profession in the metropolitan country might be quite prepared to send them into overseas territories.[315]

While the drafters rejected both a British effort to delete the paragraph altogether[316] and a French effort to frame Art. 19 as no more than vaguely hortatory,[317] not even this part of Art. 19 provides professional refugees with any significant benefit.

---

[314] Robinson reaches a comparable conclusion, at least in part. "It will make little difference (except for the diploma) whether a person is labelled a 'professional' or 'self-employed' because the treatment is the same. But it would make a considerable difference if he were classified as wage-earner instead of professional or *vice versa*": Robinson, *History*, at 118. The first part of Robinson's conclusion is, for reasons set out above, not accurate: the fact that self-employment rights accrue at a lower level of attachment than does the right to practice a liberal profession is a significant difference in many cases, e.g. refugees awaiting the results of status verification or present in a country that does not formally verify refugee status.

[315] Statement of Mr. Robinson of Israel, UN Doc. E/AC.32/SR.14, Jan. 26, 1950, at 3. See also Statement of Mr. Guerreiro of Brazil, ibid., who "agreed that the need for such qualified workers justified the settlement in colonial areas of refugees practising liberal professions."

[316] The British concern was that the duty amounted to an intrusion on the autonomy of subordinate territories: Statements of Sir Leslie Brass of the United Kingdom, UN Doc. E/AC.32/SR.13, Jan. 26, 1950, at 19; and at UN Doc. E/AC.32/SR.14, Jan. 26, 1950, at 2.

[317] The original language of the Secretary-General's proposal (Secretary-General, "Memorandum," at 35) required governments to "promote" resettlement, while a much softer approach was taken in the French draft (France, "Draft Convention," at 7), namely "as far as possible [to] facilitate" resettlement. The United States then advanced an intermediate view, under which the duty would have been to "encourage" resettlement: Statement of Mr. Henkin of the United States, UN Doc. E/AC.32/SR.13, Jan. 26, 1950, at 20. While this proposal was adopted by the Ad Hoc Committee, ibid., the language used by the Ad Hoc Committee is based on the subsequent suggestion of the

First, the duty under Art. 19(2) is really only to do whatever can already be done under the asylum country's own laws and policies.[318] While even the Secretary-General's draft did not attempt to require resettlement other than in accordance with national laws,[319] the British government persuaded governments to narrow the duty to require only such efforts as are "consistent[ ] with their laws and constitutional practices."[320] This language was further modified to refer simply to consistency with national laws and "constitutions" in order to make clear that no effort at odds with "constitutional usage"[321] would be expected. These changes were based on concern that "care should be taken not to offend the local authorities"[322] who in most cases were said to enjoy substantial autonomy in making immigration decisions. In the end, the duty of state parties under Art. 19(2) is really only to "do their best to convince the administrations of overseas territories that it [is] in their interest to attract refugees belonging to the liberal professions."[323]

Second, this duty to attempt to persuade does not apply to all subordinate territories of a state party. The broad approach taken by the Ad Hoc Committee,[324] based on the Secretary-General's rather expansive list of the entities which state parties should seek to influence,[325] was significantly constrained by the Conference of Plenipotentiaries. In keeping with the logical concern not to infringe the autonomy of administrators in subordinate territories, Art. 19(2) was reframed to refer only to a duty to exercise influence in relation to "territories for whose international relations [the state party is] responsible."[326] Even this formula was narrowed, based on British unwillingness to promote the establishment of professional refugees in

representative of the United Kingdom that governments commit themselves to "use their best endeavours . . . to secure the settlement of such refugees": Statement of Sir Leslie Brass of the United Kingdom, UN Doc. E/AC.32/SR.14, Jan. 26, 1950, at 2, adopted by the Committee, ibid. at 4.

[318] "It imposes upon [states] the moral obligation to try to secure such employment but only within the limits of existing legislation and the special rules governing the rights of the Contracting State in the dependent territory": Robinson, *History*, at 118.

[319] Secretary-General, "Memorandum," at 35.

[320] Statement of Sir Leslie Brass of the United Kingdom, UN Doc. E/AC.32/SR.14, Jan. 26, 1950, at 2.

[321] Statement of Mr. Cuvelier of Belgium, ibid. at 3. This understanding was agreed to by the proponent of the amendment, Sir Leslie Brass of the United Kingdom, ibid. at 4.

[322] Statement of Mr. Rain of France, UN Doc. E/AC.32/SR.13, Jan. 26, 1950, at 20. See also Statement of Sir Leslie Brass of the United Kingdom, ibid. at 19.

[323] Statement of Mr. Rain of France, ibid. at 20.

[324] The obligation of states was to encourage the resettlement of professional refugees to "colonies, protectorates or in Trust Territories under their administration": Ad Hoc Committee, "Second Session Report," at 20.

[325] The original proposal extended to "colonies, protectorates and overseas territories, and . . . mandated or trust territories": Secretary-General, "Memorandum," at 35.

[326] Statement of Mr. Rochefort of France, UN Doc. A/CONF.2/SR.34, July 25, 1951, at 24–25.

subordinate territories located near to the state party, and from which they might pose a competitive threat to nationals. Specifically, the British representative objected to any duty which might see more refugee professionals in "adjacent territories, like the Channel Islands, where the settlement of [professional] refugees must of necessity be governed by the same conditions as those obtaining in the United Kingdom itself."[327] The text as agreed therefore sets no duty to promote the settlement of refugee professionals in even dependent territories which might broadly be considered part of the state party's "metropolitan territory."

In sum, Art. 19(2) is no more than a minimalist form of compensation for the exclusion of refugee professionals from the benefit of the usual rules on either self-employment or wage-earning employment. It imposes only a duty to exercise suasion in line with existing national laws and constitutional usage, taking account in particular of the largely autonomous authority which many dependent territories enjoy over immigration. Even that duty of process applies only to those dependent territories whose international relations are under the authority of the state party, and which are not sufficiently proximate to the main territory of the state party to be considered part of its metropolitan territory.

There are potentially two means by which the rather bleak picture conceived by Art. 19 may be challenged. First, the limits of Art. 19 do not speak to all refugee professionals, but only to refugees who wish to practice a "liberal profession." While the notion of a "profession" as a branch of work is itself rather vague,[328] there is even less consensus on which professions may be said to be "liberal." Under the Secretary-General's proposal, for example, the term included, at a minimum, "qualified and experienced scientists, engineers, architects and doctors."[329] The drafters referred to lawyers and medical doctors as examples of persons who exercise a liberal profession,[330] but otherwise did not elucidate the term. Robinson, Weis, and Grahl-Madsen agree on a list of six liberal professions – physicians, dentists, veterinarians, lawyers, engineers, and architects – but otherwise disagree on the ambit of the term.[331]

---

[327] Statement of Mr. Hoare of the United Kingdom, ibid. at 25.

[328] For example, a profession may be defined simply as "a vocation or calling, especially one that involves some branch of advanced learning or science": *Concise Oxford Dictionary* 1092 (9th edn, 1995).

[329] Secretary-General, "Memorandum," at 36.

[330] See e.g. Statements of Mr. Cha of China, UN Doc. E/AC.32/SR.13, Jan. 26, 1950, at 17; Mr. Cuvelier of Belgium, ibid. at 18; and the Chairman, Mr. Larsen of Denmark, UN Doc. E/AC.32/SR.41, Aug, 23, 1950, at 18.

[331] Specifically, Robinson and Weis would add pharmacists and artists to the list of liberal professions, in at least some circumstances; Weis and Grahl-Madsen would include accountants; Robinson alone would include teachers; and Grahl-Madsen alone would

As a general principle, Grahl-Madsen suggests a fairly generous understanding of a liberal profession, focusing on two basic criteria. First, a
"profession" is a type of work which requires formal qualification "normally
confirmed by a diploma from a university, or a similar institution, or a licence
from a State agency, a chartered society or some other legally competent body
allowing him to practise."[332] Second, a "liberal" profession is one in which
the individual "acts on his own, not as an agent of the State or as a salaried
employee."[333] As he clearly insists, it would not make sense to classify an
individual as a member of a liberal profession if, despite the possession of
relevant formal qualifications, the work he or she proposes to undertake is
not characterized by the independence of action which marks a liberal
profession. Thus, "certain holders of academic diplomas are excluded from
the application of the term, e.g. the clergy, judges, teachers, [and]
scientists."[334]

Grahl-Madsen's relatively broad definition of a liberal profession was
likely inspired by his desire to read Art. 19 in a way that would allow
professional refugees "to receive the benefit of Article 19."[335] However,
since Art. 19 is more accurately understood not as conferring a substantive
benefit, but rather as limiting access to more generous rights which would
otherwise accrue under Arts. 17 or 18, the human rights context of the
Refugee Convention actually argues against giving this exception a broad
reading. Helpful guidance on a somewhat more constrained approach to the
definition of a "liberal profession" has recently been provided in a tax law
decision of the European Court of Justice. In the Court's view, a liberal
profession is an activity (1) of a marked intellectual character, (2) requiring
a high-level qualification, (3) normally subject to clear and strict professional
regulation, and (4) incorporating a personal element and a significant level of
independence.[336] While clearly the Court did not have the particular objects
and purposes of refugee law in mind when arriving at this formula, its
guidance should nonetheless be instructive in that Art. 19 of the Refugee
Convention appears to incorporate by reference a general term of art from
outside the field of refugee law. Indeed, as Robinson observed, the intent was
that "local authorities will decide in each case whether a person falls under the
rubric 'liberal profession' or any other heading."[337]

---

treat interpreters and translators as members of a liberal profession: Robinson, *History*, at
118; Weis, *Travaux*, at 158; and Grahl-Madsen, *Commentary*, at 78. Weis would also
include the salaried assistants to members of a liberal profession as liberal professionals
themselves, while Grahl-Madsen would do so only if there are certain qualifications set by
the state for undertaking such work: Weis, *Travaux*, at 158; Grahl-Madsen, *Commentary*,
at 78–79.

[332] Grahl-Madsen, *Commentary*, at 78.   [333] Ibid.   [334] Ibid.   [335] Ibid. at 79.

[336] *Urbing-Adam v. Administration de l'Enregistrement et des Domaines*, Dec. No. C-267/99
(ECJ, 2nd Ch., Oct. 11, 2001).

[337] Robinson, *History*, at 118.

To the extent that the European Court's logic is found persuasive, it helpfully limits the risk that any form of work requiring advanced education and involving largely independent activity is, for those reasons alone, deemed a liberal profession, thereby depriving the refugee of the more favorable treatment set out in Arts. 17 and 18. For example, neither France's restrictive approach to the employment of non-citizens, including refugees, as accountants and pharmacists, nor the refusal in parts of the United States to hire non-citizens as teachers could be justified on the basis of Art. 19. As wage-earners, refugees engaged in these forms of work would be entitled to benefit from the same treatment afforded most-favored foreigners in those countries, including the citizens of partner states.[338]

Even if the work which the refugee wishes to pursue cannot be classified as other than a liberal profession, a second and more general concern is that domestic laws or practices based on Art. 19 may breach the general duty of non-discrimination set by Art. 26 of the Civil and Political Covenant.[339] Art. 26 speaks to distinctions based on any form of status, and governs in any field regulated (directly or indirectly) by public authorities.[340] Its guarantee of equal protection of the law essentially requires that any distinction in the allocation of rights based on status be grounded in reasonable criteria. Thus, unless it can be shown that it is reasonable to disfranchise refugees who are liberal professionals relative to all other refugees,[341] the guarantee of equal protection of the law should operate to invalidate their exclusion from the more liberal rules on access to work set by Arts. 17 and 18.[342]

Showing the reasonableness of this sort of exclusion would likely be a difficult task. As Robinson warned, "[t]here is no clear-cut distinction between certain liberal professions (for instance, pharmacists, engineers) and either self-employment (owner of an engineering firm or a pharmacy)

---

[338] See chapter 6.1 above.

[339] See generally chapter 2.5.5 above. The duty of non-discrimination set by Art. 3 of the Refugee Convention itself is not relevant to this question, as it is textually limited to the prohibition of discrimination "as to race, religion, or country of origin": see chapter 3.4 above.

[340] See chapter 2.5.5 above, at pp. 123–125.

[341] While the UN Human Rights Committee has established an extraordinarily broad margin of appreciation for distinctions based on citizenship, there is no reason to believe that comparable deference would be forthcoming when the distinctions made govern the allocation of rights within the class of refugees, none of whom can claim the arguably special bond which citizenship entails: see chapter 2.5.5 above, at pp. 127–133. On the other hand, because of this margin of appreciation, it is less clear that the duty of non-discrimination would prove of assistance to refugee professionals faced with accreditation processes applied generally to non-citizens, but which set standards for qualification that appear significantly greater than required to ensure professional competence.

[342] See chapter 2.5.5 above, at pp. 126–128.

or wage-earner (non-self-employed engineer, pharmacist, chemist)."[343] Because the "bright line" is so unclear, it is difficult to imagine the principled basis for the much more rigorous approach adopted in Art. 19. If there is no sound basis for denying refugees who are liberal professionals the right to earn a livelihood on terms as favorable as those granted to all other refugee workers (who are either self-employed, wage-earners, or indeed members of professions not defined as liberal), then the duty of non-discrimination is a presumptive barrier to the establishment or continuation of policies based on the approach stipulated in Art. 19 of the Refugee Convention. If reliance on Art. 19 were to be invalidated, the right to work of refugees who are liberal professionals would be determined not by their status as liberal professionals, but on the basis of an objective assessment of the work to be undertaken as either self-employment or wage-earning employment.[344]

6.3 Public relief and assistance

Consideration was previously given to the various predicaments faced by refugees seeking to meet their basic needs upon arrival in an asylum country, or while waiting for a decision to be taken on the verification of their claim to refugee status.[345] For the most part, persons recognized as refugees, or who are otherwise allowed to stay in the host country on an ongoing basis, are less vulnerable than those in the early stages of seeking a state's protection, primarily because refugees lawfully staying are entitled to earn their living through work.[346] But for refugees unable to work, or for whom work is either unavailable or too poorly paid, it may still be impossible to meet even basic needs. Nor does the right of refugees to access social security programs necessarily provide an answer to their dilemma, as most such programs base entitlement on employment-based contributions. The refugee may not yet have been in a position to have worked and contributed in the host country, and his or her contributions made abroad may not be relevant to the qualification calculus.[347] As such, the question of access by refugees to a country's general system of social support is often key.

---

[343] Robinson, *History*, at 118.

[344] The invalidation of Art. 19 would, perhaps ironically, further the goal set by the Final Act of the Conference of Plenipotentiaries, which "[e]xpress[ed] the hope that the Convention ... will have value as an example exceeding its contractual scope": "Final Act of the United Nations Conference of Plenipotentiaries on the Status of Refugees and Stateless Persons," 189 UNTS 37, adopted July 28, 1951, at Art. E.

[345] See generally chapter 4.4 above, and in particular discussion of the right of all refugees to be free from deprivation, to access food and shelter, and to receive basic healthcare in chapters 4.4.1, 4.4.2, and 4.4.3 respectively above.

[346] See chapter 6.1 above.   [347] See chapter 6.1.3 above.

As earlier described, refugees in much of the less developed world are expected to meet their own needs by independent economic activity undertaken in organized settlements.[348] Yet because self-sufficiency is rarely immediately achieved, refugees are typically provided for some period of time with food rations, as well as educational, health, and other basic community services.[349] For example, the Eastern Sudan Refugee Program focused on enabling refugees to meet their needs through the cultivation of sorghum and provision of seasonal labor to others, but nonetheless provided the members of vulnerable groups (that is, refugees with low incomes, pregnant women, nursing mothers, and young children) with access to preventative healthcare programs, medical services, and food supplements.[350] But it is not always possible for refugees ever to achieve real self-sufficiency. For example, the land assigned for farming may be too small, environmentally degraded, or too far from markets. In such circumstances, there is often a long-term need for a more general economic supplement program.

Too often there are no local funds to meet such needs and international donors cannot be found to fill the void. In the Ikafe refugee settlement in Uganda, for example, most refugees were able to grow some food, but drought and rocky conditions limited the success of harvests. Other refugees, including the old, sick, and injured, were unable to farm at all. Yet the World Food Program was unable to secure pledges sufficient to meet even basic nutritional requirements, forcing it to impose significant reductions in supplementary maize distributions to the refugees.[351]

There are also frequently real difficulties when a decision is taken by local or international authorities that refugees in a given settlement have reached an adequate level of self-sufficiency, such that assistance can be terminated. UNHCR and the Mexican government decided in 1986 that Guatemalan refugees should be able to meet their own needs from their increasing harvest

---

[348] See chapter 6.1 above, at p. 733.

[349] V. Lasailly-Jacob, "Government-Sponsored Agricultural Schemes for Involuntary Migrants in Africa: Some Key Obstacles to Their Economic Viability," in H. Adelman and J. Sorenson eds., *African Refugees: Development Aid and Repatriation* 213 (1994).

[350] As a result of these services, "the population's health and nutrition standards have improved, and immunization programmes have been very successful": J. Sterkenburg et al., "Refugees and Rural Development: A Comparative Analysis of Project Aid in Sudan and Tanzania," in H. Adelman and J. Sorenson eds., *African Refugees: Development Aid and Repatriation* 197 (1994).

[351] N. van der Gaag, "Food and Fair Shares," [Sept. 1996] *New Internationalist* 14. Comparable problems persist. "Despite the dangers [of armed attack], the overwhelming majority of Sudanese refugees continued to live in nearly two dozen designated settlements in northern Uganda, where they had access to farmland. Farming plots were small and only semi-fertile, however, and the unsafe conditions forced some refugees to curtail their agricultural activities": US Committee for Refugees, *World Refugee Survey 2003* (2003), at 102.

yields, though the refugees protested that they were in fact only barely making ends meet.[352] Similarly, the World Food Program strictly enforced a two-year limit on the provision of food rations to Ethiopian refugees in Sudan on the grounds that self-sufficiency should be achieved within that timeframe. In fact, the refugees were not yet able to meet their own needs, forcing other agencies to step in to continue a food program for the members of vulnerable groups with no possibility of earning a living.[353] The problems may be particularly acute where transitional support has been provided to refugee settlements through a parallel support system (often internationally funded), rather than as part of the general system for meeting the needs of nationals. The separateness and consequent relative invisibility of such parallel programs frequently means that local officials fail to see themselves as in any sense responsible for refugee welfare when international aid ends, particularly when faced with their own endemic problems of limited resources and other pressing priorities.[354]

Refugees in less developed countries not living in organized settlements may receive even less public assistance than those who agree to live in organized settlements. A notable exception is South Africa, where the Constitutional Court struck down as unconstitutional laws which denied destitute Mozambican refugees the full benefit of national assistance programs, including child support and old-age dependency grants.[355] Elsewhere there are sometimes successful assistance projects directed towards self-settled refugees, including initiatives undertaken in the Kigoma region of Tanzania, in the Western Province of Zambia, and in Bas Zaïre.[356] But much more commonly, whatever assistance is available tends to be directed to refugees residing in government-approved settlements. In the result, "[a]n estimated 60 percent of the total number of refugees [in Africa] receive no aid of any sort."[357]

---

[352] "'We don't starve,' the refugees say, but often they have to be content with 'tortilla with salt,' which is rock bottom and the symbol of poverty": F. Stepputat, "Self-Sufficiency and Exile in Mexico: Report on a Field Study Among Relocated Guatemalan Refugees in South-East Mexico, August–November 1988," UN Research Institute for Social Development Discussion Paper No. 9, Aug. 1989, at 20.

[353] El Bushra, "Educational Needs," at 22.

[354] L. Clark, "Key Issues in Post-Emergency Refugee Assistance in Eastern and Southern Africa," paper presented at the UNHCR/DMC Emergency Managers Training Workshop (1987) (Clark, "Post-Emergency"), at 16.

[355] The Court determined that the constitutional right of "everyone" to enjoy equality, social security, and the protection of children meant that laws that withheld relevant social benefits from non-citizens should be struck down: *Khosa et al. v. Minister of Social Development*, (2004) 6 BCRR 569 (SA CC, Mar. 4, 2004).

[356] Clark, "Post-Emergency," at 22.

[357] S. Ricca, *International Migration in Africa: Legal and Administrative Aspects* (1989), at 139. See also A. Hansen, "African Refugees: Defining and Defending Their Human Rights," in R. Cohen et al. eds., *Human Rights and Governance in Africa* (1993), at 153.

To some extent, UNHCR has sought to fill the assistance gap for self-settled refugees, particularly those living in urban areas. Despite the agency's efforts, the aid made available to urban and other self-settled refugees normally does not meet the refugees' real needs.[358] In Costa Rica, UNHCR cash allowances to Salvadoran refugees amounted at times to less than half the cost of basic food, and were then eliminated entirely.[359] Urban refugees in Cairo received 72 percent less assistance from UNHCR in 2002 than in 1998, leaving many refugee families well below Egypt's poverty line. As one Sudanese refugee living there explained,

> We now receive less than 100 Egyptian pounds a month. I could not find an apartment with an address. The only place I found is a tiny room in the shantytown with 20 people, where there is no running water and most definitely no electricity.[360]

Circumstances were so dire for refugees in Zimbabwe in 1998 that some 100 refugees besieged the UNHCR office in Harare to protest the lack of "meaningful allowances," taking two UNHCR officials hostage until funds were disbursed.[361]

For the most part, comparable problems do not exist in the developed world. Once their refugee status is recognized, most refugees in the North benefit from the same public assistance programs as are available to citizens. A notable exception is Denmark, which amended its laws in 2002 to withhold

---

[358] UNHCR "faces significant funding shortfalls. Based on the agency's original budget appeal, UNHCR last year suffered a deficit of about $160 million. However, the agency continues to reduce its budget in response to donor demands ... Budget problems consistently delay food deliveries, impede repairs to refugee schools and water systems, deprive refugee women of sanitary supplies, and impede efforts to move refugees to safer locations": Immigration and Migration Services of America, "Advocates Push for Increased Funding for MRA and ERMA in FY 2003," (2002) 23(4) *Refugee Reports*.

[359] Such was the case in 1983; assistance was increased in 1984, then cut off completely in 1985: Basok, *Heads Above Water*, at 57–58.

[360] "Hard times for Cairo's refugees," *UNHCR News Stories*, Nov. 25, 2002, quoting Marta Bole. More specifically, "[s]ix years ago, UNHCR assisted more than 4,400 refugees in Cairo with a $2.9 million budget, doling out on average $660 to each person over the year. [In 2002], with more than 9,000 refugees assessed to be in need of aid, UNHCR Cairo has only $1.5 million for its urban assistance program, or about $171 for each refugee": ibid.

[361] "Two senior local UNHCR officials, who were kept hostage for one night by the demonstrating refugees, were only set free yesterday afternoon after the Zimbabwean government intervened, and the refugees' delayed stipends were disbursed": L. Machipisa and J. Deng, "Refugees in Zimbabwe face hard times," *InterPress Service*, June 3, 1998. "While the refugees in Zimbabwe say they understand the problems facing UNHCR, they argue that their allowances in Zimbabwe should reflect the movement of the Zimbabwean dollar and the rising prices in the Southern African nation. The refugees say that their monthly stipends are paid late, and several have been evicted from their places of residence as a result": *SAPA*, June 4, 1998.

full welfare benefits from refugees until they are eligible for permanent resident permits – thus effectively excluding refugees from full social support for seven years.[362] But under the European Union's new rules, "Member States shall ensure that beneficiaries of refugee status ... receive, in the Member State that has granted such status[ ], the necessary social assistance, as provided to nationals of that Member State."[363] Similarly, Canada assimilates refugees to citizens for purposes of its public assistance programs,[364] and Australia amended its rules governing disability support pensions in 1995 to ensure that refugees are exempted from the ten-year residence requirement imposed before benefits are paid to most immigrants.[365] In practice, however, even states which recognize the entitlement of refugees to be treated as citizens for purposes of public assistance may not always take the procedural steps needed to provide that access on terms of genuine equality. For example, in the United Kingdom the transition from the less generous regime governing assistance to persons awaiting the results of their claim to full entitlement is reported to be problematic for many refugees:

> Destitute families are having to wait six months or more for national insurance numbers, which should arrive in a fortnight. Without these numbers, the refugees cannot receive benefits, so they have no income and are unable to apply for any government help ... The benefits agency needs immigration identification forms to allocate financial support. But ... many of these forms are being misplaced or badly written, resulting in benefits being withheld.[366]

The situation in the North is much less positive for refugees channeled by states into so-called "temporary protection" or other auxiliary categories. The extent to which public relief and assistance are granted has traditionally varied significantly from one state to another.[367] Refugees in receipt of

---

[362] A. Osborn, "Danes justify harshest asylum laws in Europe," *Guardian*, June 29, 2002, at 15.

[363] EU Qualification Directive, at Art. 28. The practice of most European countries has traditionally been in line with this standard. For example, Denmark, France, Germany, Sweden, and the United Kingdom routinely granted formally recognized refugees the same treatment as citizens under their welfare laws: Lambert, *Seeking Asylum*, at 174–177.

[364] F. Crépeau and M. Barutciski, "The Legal Condition of Refugees in Canada," (1994) 7(2/3) *Journal of Refugee Studies* 239.

[365] "By an internal Departmental circular dated May 1994, it was noted that the Government was to introduce amending legislation, effective from 1 January 1995, providing that persons with refugee status could have access to DSP notwithstanding less than ten years' residence": *Scott v. Secretary, Department of Social Security*, [2000] FCA 1241 (Aus. FFC, Sept. 7, 2000).

[366] A. Chrisafis, "Christmas charity appeal: Beaten in Kabul, then left derelict in Leicester," *Guardian*, Dec. 12, 2001, at 11.

[367] IGC, *Temporary Protection*, at 96, 109, 153, 220, 245.

temporary protection in the United States have been granted access to some forms of food aid, but not to the major income support programs.[368] Refugees in receipt of temporary protection visas in Australia now receive special benefits, medical care, and trauma counseling, but cannot access the mainstream social welfare system.[369] This general approach to temporary protection replaced a variable system of entitlements, under which, for example, Australia allowed temporarily protected Chinese refugees access to its medical care system, but gave temporarily protected refugees from Sri Lanka and the former Yugoslavia access only to emergency healthcare.[370]

In Europe, the beneficiaries of temporary protection have also traditionally received inferior access to public assistance compared with persons formally recognized as refugees. Denmark, Germany, the Netherlands, and Sweden have provided the beneficiaries of temporary protection with only a minimal maintenance allowance, similar to that granted persons seeking recognition of their refugee status.[371] In Italy, temporarily protected refugees have been eligible only for employment-related social security.[372] This general pattern of differential treatment of persons in receipt of temporary protection was codified by the European Union in 2001. The new Council directive does not set a national treatment standard, but instead requires only that "Member States shall ensure that persons enjoying temporary protection have access to suitable accommodation or, if necessary, receive the means to obtain housing. The Member States shall make provision for persons enjoying temporary protection to receive necessary assistance in terms of social welfare and means of subsistence, if they do not have sufficient resources, as well as for medical care."[373]

---

[368] Ibid. at 234–235. "Under the new welfare law, these restrictions continue and others are added (no job training or federal share of unemployment insurance, for example) because TPS beneficiaries are considered to be 'non-qualified aliens' for purposes of public benefits": S. Martin and A. Schoenholtz, "Fixing Temporary Protection in the United States," in US Committee for Refugees, *World Refugee Survey 1998* (1998), at 40.

[369] J. Centenera, "ACT to help refugees with adjustment," *Canberra Times*, July 12, 2000, at A-1. Whereas refugees holding permanent visas have "[i]mmediate access to the full range of social security benefits," temporary protection visa holders have "[a]ccess only to Special Benefits for which a range of eligibility criteria apply": Refugee Council of Australia, "Position on Temporary Protection Visas," Nov. 1999. "Any Special Benefit entitlement [for TPV holders] is stringently means-tested and is reviewed every 13 weeks": Australian Department of Immigration and Multicultural and Indigenous Affairs, "Factsheet No. 64: Temporary Protection Visas," Aug. 28, 2003.

[370] IGC, *Temporary Protection*, at 49, 235.

[371] Liebaut, *Conditions 2000*, at 62–63, 122, 221, 286. See also IGC, *Temporary Protection*, at 83, 122, 153, 195. German courts were reported sometimes to have denied even this modest allowance to Bosnian refugees on grounds that their presence in Germany was motivated by a search for social assistance: Büllesbach, "Civil War Refugees," at 51.

[372] IGC, *Temporary Protection*, at 49, 132.

[373] EU Temporary Protection Directive, at Art. 13.

Refugee Convention, Art. 23   Public relief
The Contracting States shall accord to refugees lawfully staying in their territory the same treatment with respect to public relief and assistance as is accorded to their nationals.

In view of the controversy which frequently exists regarding the right of refugees to benefit from public assistance programs, both the simplicity of Art. 23 and the ease with which its adoption was secured are quite astounding. Not only did Art. 23 effect a significant enhancement in entitlement beyond the standard of earlier refugee conventions, but it remains a provision without parallel in general international human rights law.

Under both the 1933 and 1938 treaties, certain refugees residing in state parties were entitled to "such relief and assistance as they may require, including medical attendance and hospital treatment."[374] But the right to receive relief and assistance was limited to several categories of refugees deemed inherently unable to earn their own living,[375] and was payable only to the same extent that relief and assistance were provided to most-favored foreigners. The drafters of the 1951 Convention abolished both limitations, opting to guarantee public relief and assistance to all refugees lawfully staying in a state's territory, and setting the standard for compliance as "the same treatment . . . as is accorded to their nationals."[376] Because there is nothing in the drafting history to suggest any implied limitation on Art. 23's broadly framed and inclusive text, Grahl-Madsen logically concludes that the provision requires that "refugees get the same material benefits [as citizens], with the same minimum of delay."[377] The provisions in the European Union's Qualification Directive which guarantee access to welfare by recognized refugees,[378] traditional Canadian practice, the inclusive approach to social welfare eligibility mandated by the South African Constitutional Court, and Australia's decision to exempt refugees from the waiting period for disability support imposed on other immigrants are all policies in line with this standard.

---

[374] Convention relating to the International Status of Refugees, 159 LNTS 3663, done Oct. 28, 1933, entered into force June 13, 1935 (1933 Refugee Convention), at Art. 9; Convention concerning the Status of Refugees coming from Germany, 4461 LNTS 61, done Feb. 10, 1938 (1938 Refugee Convention), at Art. 11.

[375] Specifically, the two treaties enfranchised "unemployed persons, persons suffering from physical or mental disease, aged persons or infirm persons incapable of earning a livelihood, children for whose upkeep no adequate provision is made either by their families or by third parties, pregnant women, women in childbed or nursing mothers": 1933 Refugee Convention, at Art. 9; 1938 Refugee Convention, at Art. 11.

[376] This approach was recommended in the French draft of Art. 23, which would have required national treatment for refugees regularly resident in a state party with regard to "insurance and social security (including industrial accident compensation) and all forms of public relief": France, "Draft Convention," at 7.

[377] Grahl-Madsen, *Commentary*, at 89.   [378] EU Qualification Directive, at Art. 28.

On the other hand, Art. 23 was clearly contravened by the Danish decision to withhold access to the full national welfare system for the seven years required for a refugee to become eligible for a permanent resident permit. Similarly, Costa Rica acted contrary to Art. 23 when it failed to grant refugees access to its domestic family allowance system as UNHCR assistance to the refugees was reduced, and then ended altogether.[379] Indeed, the requirements of Art. 23 also call into question the administrative practices of the United Kingdom to the extent that they delay implementation of that country's formal commitment to the assimilation of recognized refugees to citizens for purposes of social welfare entitlement.

There are, however, two critical constraints on the right of a refugee to claim full access to national systems of public relief and assistance. First, this is a right only of a refugee who is "lawfully staying" in the state party concerned. Prior to that time, including both when a refugee is simply under a state's authority and even while status verification is not yet completed, the refugee may claim only the more modest guarantee of access to the necessities of life, previously considered in some depth.[380] In brief, the Convention requires that all refugees, whatever their attachment to the host country, be treated as nationals under whatever rationing systems may exist,[381] while the Economic Covenant sets a duty of progressive, non-discriminatory implementation of a more broadly framed right to an adequate standard of living, as well as an immediate duty to provide everyone with the essential core of the rights to food, shelter, healthcare, and education.[382] But none of these rights require the full assimilation of refugees to citizens for purposes of comprehensive access to social welfare systems.

This issue of attachment sometimes arises in the developed world when refugees are diverted into so-called "temporary protection." For reasons previously discussed, such refugees are "lawfully staying" and thus entitled to the benefit of Art. 23.[383] As such, Australia's new system under which many refugees are granted temporary protection visas which exclude them from access to the mainstream social support system is presumptively in breach of Art. 23. Unless the government can show that the various benefits offered under its special income support regime for such refugees are substantively equal to those available to its own citizens under general programs,[384] the program does not respect the duty to assimilate refugees to nationals for

---

[379] Since 1974, Costa Rica has relied on a combination of sales tax revenue and payroll taxes to fund a system of relief for indigent persons not entitled to a contributory pension: US Social Security Administration, "Social Security Programs throughout the World" (1999), available at www.ssa.gov (accessed Feb. 28, 2005).

[380] See chapter 4.4 above.   [381] See chapter 4.4.1 above.

[382] See chapters 4.4.2, 4.4.3, and 4.8 above.   [383] See chapter 3.1.4 above, at p. 188.

[384] See text below, at p. 812.

purposes of public relief and assistance.[385] Similarly, the terms of a settlement granting protection to Salvadoran and Guatemalans in the United States denied them access to the US asylum system, and diverted them into a temporary protection regime.[386] In such circumstances, application of the American rules that deny certain benefits to temporarily protected refugees, including access to its major income support programs, cannot be reconciled to Art. 23. The same was true of many traditional temporary protection initiatives in Europe which effectively gave some refugees, such as those from Bosnia, no choice but to accept protection under a temporary protection regime with less-than-full-Convention welfare rights.[387] While the new European Union rules on temporary protection also fail to ensure access to public welfare on terms of equality with citizens, they do not breach the Convention by virtue of the critical right of any person entitled to temporary protection to opt instead to claim Convention refugee status, including of course access to the Convention's right to benefit from public relief and assistance programs on the same terms as citizens.[388]

The other key limitation is that Art. 23 does not require a state to grant refugees any public relief or assistance unless it provides relief or assistance to its own citizens. It is a matter of some contention whether states are under any duty to establish a public welfare system,[389] and in practice many poorer

---

[385] The earlier Australian approach, under which temporarily protected refugees of different nationalities received different social welfare benefits, was likely in breach of both Art. 3 of the Refugee Convention and Art. 26 of the Civil and Political Covenant. See chapters 2.5.5 and 3.4 above.

[386] *American Baptist Churches v. Thornburgh*, 760 F Supp 796 (US DCNDCa, Jan. 31, 1991).

[387] See e.g. D. Sopf, "Temporary Protection in Europe After 1990: The 'Right to Remain' of Genuine Convention Refugees," (2001) 6 *Washington University Journal of Law and Policy* 109.

[388] EU Temporary Protection Directive, at para. 17(1). This provision ensures that a genuine refugee may not be compelled to accept protection under a lesser regime.

[389] Art. 9 of the Economic, Social and Cultural Covenant requires state parties to "recognize the right of everyone to social security, including social insurance." Both "social security" and "social insurance," however, are terms of art that are generally understood to refer to "the 'earned' ... benefits of workers and their families [as contrasted with] ... need-based assistance from public funds, raised through tax revenues": Scheinin, "Social Security," at 159. The best argument that there is at least a principled duty to "recognize" the right of everyone to a broader notion of (non-contributory) social assistance is that the Committee on Economic, Social and Cultural Rights has required states to report on compliance with Art. 9 by providing information on a broad range of "social security" initiatives, including "medical care, cash sickness benefits, old age benefits, invalidity benefits, survivors' benefits, employment injury benefits, unemployment benefits, [and] family benefits": "Revised Guidelines Regarding the Form and Content of Reports to be Submitted by States Parties under Articles 16 and 17 of the International Covenant on Economic, Social and Cultural Rights," UN Doc. E/1991/23 (1992). Clearly some of these matters are more likely to be social assistance programs than true social security

states have failed to do so. Because Art. 23 requires only equivalency of treatment with that afforded citizens, there is no case to be made under Art. 23 in respect of the failure by asylum states such as Kenya,[390] Sudan,[391] and Uganda[392] to provide welfare assistance to refugees, since these states lack a meaningful social assistance program for their own nationals. In such situations, refugees can invoke only the more general guarantee of the right to an adequate standard of living, in particular to benefit from the four core rights – to basic food, shelter, education, and healthcare – which, as described earlier, must be provided to all persons whatever the circumstances of the host country.[393] The situation is not improved for refugees where the shortfall occurs because of the insufficiency of internationally funded aid, as there is presently no more than a principled obligation on the part of wealthier states to provide aid to poorer countries.[394]

But where social welfare systems do exist, even at a rudimentary level, the Refugee Convention is breached to the extent that refugees are not fully enfranchised under national initiatives. Thus, refugees lawfully staying in Mexico are entitled to benefit from that country's recently established education-based welfare program, which provides healthcare and cash payments to the mothers of poor children who remain in school.[395] It would no longer be lawful for the government and UNHCR to say, as they did in the 1980s, that

programs. To the extent that governments accede to this understanding of Art. 9, state practice may provide the basis for asserting a more general duty to establish a public welfare system, albeit in the context of the general duty to abide by the treaty only through progressive, non-discriminatory implementation.

[390] Kenya lacks any major social support programs. While officially the country supports a National Social Security Fund and a National Hospital Insurance Fund, both programs appear to be near collapse and provide no real support to the poor: A. Obondoh, "Economic Inequalities and Social Exclusion – The Core Objects of the Structural Reform Agenda," *Eco News Africa*, Nov. 2001.

[391] Sudan operates pension funds for public and private sector workers (the National Pensions Fund and the National Social Insurance Fund) but appears not otherwise to operate any form of social welfare program: United States Social Security Administration, "Social Security Programs throughout the World" (1999), available at www.ssa.gov (accessed Feb. 28, 2005).

[392] Most social welfare programs within Uganda appear to be funded by international organizations and missionaries, which operate hospitals and rural clinics. Social welfare as such is not provided by the government: Microsoft Encarta, "People and Society – Uganda 2000," available at www.magic-safaris.com (accessed Aug. 12, 2002).

[393] See chapter 4.4.2 above, at pp. 488–490.   [394] Ibid. at pp. 491–494.

[395] A. Krueger, "Economic sense," *New York Times*, May 2, 2002, at C2; J. Egan, "Mexico's welfare revolution," *BBC News Online*, Oct. 15, 1999, available at www.bbc.co.uk (accessed Feb. 28, 2005). "[B]y the start of 2000, the program had enlisted two million families in Mexico, or about one-tenth of the entire Mexican population": T. Schultz, "School Subsidies for the Poor: Evaluating a Mexican Strategy for Reducing Poverty," International Food Policy Research Institute FCND Discussion Paper No. 102, Mar. 2001, at 3.

refugees should sustain themselves without access to state support. This is so despite any shortfall of funds, or lack of international assistance. In this sense, Art. 23 of the Refugee Convention effectively enables refugees to avoid the general right under the Economic Covenant of poorer countries to limit the extent to which they will grant economic rights to non-citizens.[396] But this does not mean that the needs of refugees will necessarily be satisfied. For example, in Zimbabwe the only relief system not funded by private sector contributions is a basic healthcare program for low-paid workers.[397] So long as the benefits of this program are extended to refugees, the fact that cash allowances granted to refugees are viewed as inadequate does not infringe Art. 23.

As these examples make clear, the scope of the entitlement to benefit from public welfare programs under Art. 23 is quite broad.[398] The decision was made by the drafters not to define the intended beneficiaries of "public relief and assistance" in the text of the Convention since "such an enumeration was of necessity incomplete."[399] Instead, the drafters opted to defer to each state's own decision, "since it was, in point of fact, national legislation which determined the categories of persons eligible for public relief."[400] During the debates, however, no objection was taken to the Secretary-General's proposal that public relief would ordinarily be understood to include benefits paid to persons "suffering from physical or mental disease and incapable because of their condition or age of earning a livelihood for themselves and their families, and also to children without support."[401] Specific reference was also made to assistance to the blind,[402] hospital care,[403] and emergency relief[404] as forms of public relief or assistance.[405] Indeed, the only subject

---

[396] See chapter 2.5.4 above, at p. 122.

[397] The healthcare program "[c]overs about 75% of the population. [It provides] [f]ree primary health care for those earning below Z$400 per month; proof must be provided. Government and mission hospitals serve rural areas; government and private hospitals and doctors are available in urban areas": US Social Security Administration, "Social Security Programs throughout the World" (1999), available at www.ssa.gov (visited Feb. 28, 2005).

[398] See Weis, *Travaux*, at 174: "What is meant by public relief and assistance depends on national law, but the concept should be interpreted widely."

[399] Statement of Mr. Metall of the International Labor Organization, UN Doc. E/AC.32/SR.15, Jan. 27, 1950, at 7.

[400] Statement of Mr. Weis of the International Refugee Organization, ibid.

[401] Secretary-General, "Memorandum," at 39.

[402] Statement of Mr. Metall of the International Labor Organization, UN Doc. E/AC.32/2, Jan. 3, 1950, at 7; and Statement of Mr. Rain of France, ibid. at 8.

[403] Statement of Mr. Malfatti of Italy, UN Doc. E/AC.32/SR.38, Aug. 17, 1950, at 4.

[404] Ibid.

[405] Grahl-Madsen concludes that "[d]uring the discussion in the Ad Hoc Committee it was firmly stressed that public relief encompasses hospital treatment, measures of relief for

which generated any controversy was whether Art. 23 covered compensation in the event of unemployment. But the difference of view really reflected only the variant ways in which unemployment benefits are delivered in different states – in some via a contributory scheme, therefore more logically understood as a form of social security, in others via a state-funded program, thus properly deemed public relief or assistance.[406] In the end, the distinction will usually be of no practical significance to refugees, since refugees lawfully staying are entitled to national treatment under *both* social security and public relief and assistance initiatives.[407]

Not only are refugees entitled to access all of the same public relief and assistance benefits provided to citizens, but they may not be denied that relief or assistance on the grounds that under a particular country's system such benefits are provided only to citizens with a close affiliation to a particular region or community. Indeed, the drafters formally recorded the view that "refugees should not be required to meet any conditions of local residence or affiliation which may be required of nationals."[408] To the extent that a common system for implementation of the duty to treat refugees on terms of equality with citizens is felt inappropriate – for example, where the usual local residence requirement reflects the fact that it is the community itself that funds the public relief and assistance – it is open to the government to organize the logistics of equal treatment in whatever way it deems appropriate.[409]

---

the blind, as well as emergency relief. It may be taken for granted that the Article also covers the cases specified in Article [9] of the 1933 Convention": Grahl-Madsen, *Commentary*, at 88–89. The scope of Art. 9 of the 1933 Refugee Convention is set out above, at p. 806.

[406] "[I]t would be difficult to mention the unemployed in article [23], because legislation concerning the unemployed varied according to the country; in Belgium, for example, unemployment was covered by insurance rather than by assistance": Statement of Mr. Cuvelier of Belgium, UN Doc. E/AC.32/SR.15, Jan. 27, 1950, at 5. On the other hand, the British representative felt that unemployment benefits should be mentioned in Art. 23 because under his country's system the insurance component of unemployment benefits "did not take effect until a certain number of contributions had been paid and it was granted for a specific period only, after which the unemployed person would, if necessary, receive assistance from public relief. That example would suffice to show that it was not superfluous to mention the unemployed in article [23]": Statement of Sir Leslie Brass of the United Kingdom, ibid. at 6–7.

[407] See Robinson, *History*, at 124: "No difficulties will, as a rule, arise in practice concerning the delimitation between public relief and assistance on the one hand, and social security on the other, because the Convention provides for the same treatment, in both instances, except for the cases enumerated in Art. 24(1)(b)(i) and (ii)." With regard to the meaning of the latter limitations, see chapter 6.1.3 above, at pp. 778–781.

[408] Ad Hoc Committee, "Second Session Report," at 13.

[409] "The article, however, permitted the grant of relief and assistance in whatever way States desired; it did not specify the way": Statement of Mr. Henkin of the United States, UN

This matter was of particular concern to the Swiss delegate, who observed that in his country "indigent Swiss nationals were helped by the cantons and communes, whereas refugees were helped by charitable organizations to which the Confederation refunded all or 60% of the cost of the relief given. In that way, refugees did not have to apply to officials in small communes for whom it was perhaps more difficult to understand their special position."[410] To this, the Chairman of the Ad Hoc Committee replied that

> the Committee had not intended to interfere with the administrative systems of any country. It had merely endeavoured to secure the same public relief and assistance for refugees as for nationals. It did not matter whether relief and assistance were provided out of federal, cantonal, or municipal funds; the only thing that mattered was that the State should guarantee that in some way relief would be given to refugees.[411]

In short, it is the end result that counts:

> [T]he principle of article [23] was clear: the refugees should be accorded the same treatment with respect to public relief and assistance as was accorded to nationals, and it did not matter how the treatment was accorded, provided the results were the same.[412]

Perhaps the most interesting question is just what accounted for the decision of the drafters so comprehensively to embrace refugees in the public relief and assistance systems of state parties, even though they were well aware of the potential magnitude of the commitment being made.[413] Their decision was in part driven by pragmatic considerations, rooted in the view that the

---

Doc. E/AC.32/SR.38, Aug. 17, 1950, at 6. A state's right to design the mechanism for implementation must, of course, not breach any other duty under the Convention. For example, the Venezuelan representative noted that in his country refugees with infectious diseases were sometimes not treated in public hospitals and institutions, but were instead sent to medical facilities outside the country (something "[t]hat could not of course be done to a national"): Statement of Mr. Perez Perozo of Venezuela, ibid. at 7. The American and Canadian representatives seemed generally to view this practice as not contrary to Art. 23, though suggesting that its legality would be subject to Art. 32's rules on expulsion: Statements of Mr. Henkin of the United States and Mr. Winter of Canada, ibid.

[410] Statement of Mr. Schurch of Switzerland, ibid. at 5.

[411] Statement of the Chairman, Mr. Larsen of Denmark, ibid. at 5.

[412] Statement of Mr. Henkin of the United States, ibid. at 6. As Grahl-Madsen put it, "what interested the drafters was the material situation, not procedure": Grahl-Madsen, *Commentary*, at 89.

[413] At the Conference of Plenipotentiaries, the Italian delegate explicitly raised the issue of the real cost to state parties of complying with Art. 23. He noted that Italy had signed a specific agreement with the IRO under which it had admitted "a large number of refugees, 1,000 of whom had been hard-core cases requiring hospital treatment. In respect of those cases, the Italian Government had agreed to pay the same benefits as to Italians in respect of public assistance, for as long as the refugees concerned lived. That

provision of public relief and assistance to refugees lawfully staying in a state party is, at least over time, an economically efficient response.[414] But more fundamentally, there was clearly a strong sense that assimilating refugees to citizens for purposes of public relief and assistance was simply the right thing to do. As the Secretary-General's background study cogently observed, destitute refugees could not expect their country of origin to assume liability for their support in the host country, as most bilateral treaties on point required. Yet, unlike most non-citizens, they could not safely return home to benefit from their own country's support systems.[415] Since the needs of refugees are no less than those of citizens and their options for external support are essentially non-existent, it was recognized that there really was no ethical option but to assimilate them to citizens for purposes of access to public relief and assistance. In the simple but poignant words of the French representative to the Ad Hoc Committee, "it would be inhuman to deny such assistance to refugees."[416]

6.4 Housing

The majority of refugees who seek protection in the less developed world are expected to live in organized camps or settlements, even after the emergency reception phase has passed.[417] Indeed, some refugees must make do for substantial periods of time with makeshift dwellings. Refugees in Ethiopia,

represented a very considerable burden, particularly as there was small probability of their being able to work. Thus it would be very difficult for the Italian Government to give an undertaking in the terms of article [23] in respect of an indefinite number of refugees": Statement of Mr. Theodoli of Italy, UN Doc. A/CONF.2/SR.10, July 6, 1951, at 18. (In the result, Italy opted to enter a reservation to Art. 23, which it withdrew on Oct. 20, 1964.) Immediately after this comment by Italy, Art. 23 was unanimously adopted by the Conference without change: ibid. at 19.

[414] "Apart from the humanitarian aspect of the matter, it was in the national interest to grant public relief to refugees, for the slight assistance provided at home involved much less expense than hospital treatment": Statement of Mr. Rain of France, UN Doc. E/AC.32/SR.15, Jan. 27, 1950, at 6.

[415] "Most of the conventions dealing with public assistance contain certain stipulations which cannot be satisfied in the case of refugees, such as the requirement that the State of which the recipient of relief is a national should either repatriate him or assume liability for the cost of assistance": Secretary-General, "Memorandum," at 39.

[416] Statement of Mr. Rain of France, UN Doc. E/AC.32/SR.15, Jan. 27, 1950, at 6.

[417] "It is often host governments, who in their desire to have control over refugees and to discourage their permanent settlement, insist on the camp or organised settlement solution . . . It is apparent that camp-confined refugees make better pawns in the international power play for donor assistance, both for host governments and for aid providers": T. Hoerz, "Refugees and Host Environments: A Review of Current and Related Literature," [Aug. 1995] *Deutsche Gesellschaft für Technische Zusammenarbeit* 18. The housing rights of refugees immediately upon arrival are discussed in chapter 4.4.2 above, at pp. 504–507.

for example, were left sheltering under the remaining shreds of eight-year-old plastic sheeting when funds ran out for UNHCR's Horn of Africa operation in the early 1990s.[418] Others are more fortunate: Afghan refugees in Pakistan were initially given only tents for shelter, but were later able to replace them with traditional mud-brick buildings.[419]

Settlements located in remote or marginal areas may be confronted with absolute shortages of essential building materials, or rising demand may drive the price of materials beyond what refugees or the agencies assisting them can afford to buy.[420] When aid is available, some donors are reluctant in practice to involve refugees in the design or building of housing, or to use local materials,[421] insisting instead on the use of foreign technologies and designs.[422] These have at times proved culturally inappropriate,[423] too expensive to maintain,[424] and even dangerous.[425] Many camps and settlements in which refugees live also suffer from shortcomings in design and layout. As Clark has written,

---

[418] "Violent winds blasting Hartisheik [refugee camp] have since torn the tarpaulin to shreds, although its tattered remains can still be seen woven into a patchwork quilt of old rags and wheat sacks that cover the *takul* from the ground up": "Shelter: No Place Like Home," (1996) 105 *Refugees* 12, at 12.

[419] H. Christensen, "Afghan Refugees in Pakistan," in H. Adelman and M. Lanphier eds., *Refuge or Asylum?* 178 (1990).

[420] "Access to building materials is the crucial element in the process of shelter consolidation; but these materials quickly become commodified and locally scarce. Even where materials like poles, mats, thatch and mud can be locally garnered, supply constraints and environmental degradation caused by excess demand in countries like Malawi ... and Rwanda ... can be exceptionally severe": R. Zetter, "Shelter Provision and Settlement Policies for Refugees: A State of the Art Review," Nordic Africa Institute Studies on Emergencies and Disaster Relief Working Paper No. 2 (1995) (Zetter, "Shelter Provision"), at 39–40.

[421] "[T]he global experience is that [housing] is best provided by the settlers themselves – first as temporary housing and then, as their incomes rise, as permanent housing": T. Scudder, "From Relief to Development: Some Comments on Refugee and Other Settlements in Somalia," Institute for Development Anthropology Working Paper, June 1981, at 35. Among the advantages of using local materials are lessened need for imports, reduced transportation costs, and lower capital investment: O. Sherrer, "Afghan Refugee Housing," (1990) 34 *Mimar* 43, at 47.

[422] "[T]oo often international agencies and donors, in their concern for the rapid deployment of emergency assistance, import foreign technologies and professional capacity because these are most readily at hand": Zetter, "Shelter Provision," at 37.

[423] Imported "A-frame" technology for refugees in Bangladesh, for example, was "culturally inappropriate without adaptation of the physical and social space around the dwelling": ibid. at 38.

[424] The maintenance of timber-framed buildings designed by European architects for refugees in Costa Rica was "unaffordable [for] many refugees": ibid.

[425] "[A] ... recent evaluation of shelter construction in Somali refugee camps in Kenya illustrates how, with insufficient technical advice and limited NGO capability, prefabricated shelter was being erected which was structurally dangerous": ibid.

The spacial layout and design of a settlement can obviously have a profound effect on its viability and on the quality of life of the settlers. Too
often these decisions reflect little input as to how they would prefer to live.
It is ironic to listen to aid officials complain about the lack of community
spirit in a settlement where the residents have been forced to live spread out
along the roadways, with no village structure to draw them together in the
first place.[426]

Once settlements are established, they have a tendency to grow to an
unwieldy size and to suffer from overcrowding. This can be the result of
government policies which fail to acknowledge the need for additional refugee accommodation:

> Once a settlement has opened there is a great temptation to continue to
> send newly arrived refugees (or spontaneously settled refugees who have
> been rounded up by the host government) to the site. The plan may be to
> expand the settlement, or to use it as a transit center or holding camp, while
> planning an additional settlement or hoping for repatriation. The govern-
> ment is often reluctant to accept the need for additional settlements, feels
> constrained by the lack of staff resources, or is disinclined to go through the
> search and negotiations to provide another settlement site.[427]

Such policies led Zetter to conclude that typical camps, comprising between
20,000 and 30,000 refugees, are far too large "to function effectively either as
social communities or for the logistical and managerial requirements for
which they are established."[428] With services stretched beyond capacity,
problems of water supply, sanitation, and waste disposal frequently lead to
a serious deterioration of health.[429] The lack of privacy and the inability
effectively to patrol sprawling refugee settlements is moreover a major con-
tributor to the exposure of refugees to violent attacks.[430]

The location of refugee camps and settlements is also a key determinant of
their success. But political considerations and the assumed temporariness of
the refugees' presence means "almost invariably, that refugees are settled in
the most marginal areas."[431] In the cases of Croatia and Bosnia, for example,
short-term administrative convenience led to the assignment of refugees to
inexpensive government-owned land which lacked the topography, natural

---

[426] Clark, "Post-Emergency," at 16. A positive example is, however, provided by the settlements for Angolan refugees in Zaïre, where "the decision was made to design the
settlement to reflect the culture of the refugees as closely as possible": ibid.

[427] B. Stein and L. Clark, "Older Refugee Settlements in Africa," Refugee Policy Group Paper
(1986), at 21.

[428] Zetter, "Shelter Provision," at 49.

[429] This was the case, for example, for refugees from Togo in Benin and for Bhutanese
refugees in Nepal: ibid.

[430] See chapter 4.3 above, at pp. 443–444.   [431] Zetter, "Shelter Provision," at 78.

ecology or climatic conditions to enable the refugees to become self-sustaining.[432] Clearly, the viability of settlements is undermined in locations "where the carrying capacity of the land is most fragile, building materials are scarcest, access to productive resources and alternative sources of employment [are] most limited, and the environment is vulnerable to degradation."[433] This was true of the refugee settlements in Eastern Sudan, which were located on marginal land with inadequate water supply.[434] Most seriously, refugee camps located near border areas may be prone to attack of the kind that occurred when Thai authorities denied Burmese refugees the right to move away from the frontier.[435]

Refugees in the South who avoid living in organized camps or settlements tend to replicate the settlement patterns of their host villages,[436] and to adapt more successfully to their new life circumstances.[437] There are notable exceptions, however. Chakma refugees from Bangladesh, settled in the Indian state of Arunachal Pradesh for more than two decades, were threatened in the 1990s with eviction from their homes by a union of student activists which the regional government was unwilling to counter.[438] Even when not confronted with such

---

[432] Ibid. at 56. See also S. Ellis and S. Barakat, "From Relief to Development: The Long-Term Effects of the 'Temporary' Accommodation of Refugees and Displaced Persons in the Republic of Croatia," (1996) 20(2) *Disasters* 111, at 113–114, observing that accommodation for refugees included "re-used postal trains that have been shunted on to a sideline and refitted to accommodate refugees ... This emergency, temporary accommodation has, due to the political and financial pressures on the Croatian government, become permanent."

[433] Zetter, "Shelter Provision," at 78.

[434] The lack of rainfall in eastern Sudan "makes life in the settlements highly precarious ... The fact that most land settlements are located in marginal areas means that the risk of crop failure is very high": Kibreab, "Sudan," at 49. "[M]ost settlements were located in marginalised barren lands where rainfall was inadequate, unevenly distributed, and absolutely undependable": T. Yousif, "Encampment at Abu Rakham in Sudan: A Personal Account," (1998) 2 *Forced Migration Review* 15, at 15.

[435] "Attacks in January on three refugee camps resulted in at least three deaths and left 7,000 homeless. Despite the obvious danger, Thai authorities refused to allow the refugees to move. Again in April, Burmese troops attacked the Ta Per Poo refugee camp, razing eighteen houses. The international outcry ... prompted Thai authorities to move some of the camps away from the border, but most of the approximately twenty-five camps remained where they were": Human Rights Watch, *World Report 1998* (1998), at 211–212. See chapter 4.3 above, at pp. 445–446.

[436] In Malawi, for example, self-settled refugee housing is "in the form of dense clusters grouped around small open spaces, usually indistinguishable from and often integrated with host villages": Zetter, "Shelter Provision," at 55.

[437] "[T]he empirical evidence demonstrates that spontaneous settled refugees exercise far greater flexibility than their encamped counterparts in selecting more environmentally sustainable locations in which to locate, or in adopting more sustainable settlement practices": ibid. at 74.

[438] *National Human Rights Commission v. State of Arunachal Pradesh*, (1996) 83 AIR 1234 (India SC, Jan. 9, 1996).

direct aggression, self-settled refugees may still have difficulty meeting their housing needs because of shortages of building materials and of property.[439] These challenges are often compounded by the decision of many governments to deny self-settled refugees access to the relief programs made available to refugees who agree to live in organized camps or settlements.[440]

Refugees attempting self-settlement in urban areas may face even greater difficulty in securing adequate housing. They tend to concentrate in neighborhoods with dilapidated housing and which lack basic services such as water, electricity, and sanitation.[441] An influx of refugees onto the housing market also tends to drive rents upward and to result in the imposition of unfair rental conditions. In the Pakistani city of Peshawar, for example, the property shortages that followed from the arrival of many Afghan refugees led "not surprisingly, to escalating rents and inequitable leasing conditions. Refugees adopted strategies to minimize costs, such as leasing property in groups."[442] In Sudan, the plight of urban refugees was increased by the decision to prohibit non-citizens from purchasing housing, which left them entirely dependent on the rental sector.[443]

In the developed world, there are few formal barriers to accessing accommodation for settled refugees.[444] An important exception is those refugees granted "temporary protected" or another form of auxiliary status, who are sometimes treated only on par with persons seeking recognition of refugee status and required to live in reception centers.[445] In the German federal state of Saxony-Anhalt, "temporarily protected" Bosnians were granted access to subsidized housing and rent subsidies, but only if this arrangement was determined to be less expensive than accommodation in a collective center.[446] Local authorities in parts of Bavaria refused to provide welfare assistance to meet the private housing costs of the Bosnians, forcing many to turn to homeless shelters. Indeed, Bavarian authorities refused to provide even

---

[439] Zetter, "Shelter Provision," at 73.

[440] See chapter 6.1 above, at pp. 733–734. A notable exception is Malawi, which included self-settled refugees in its relief and assistance programs: Zetter, "Shelter Provision," at 75.

[441] Kuhlman, "Organized Versus Spontaneous," at 130. Kuhlman adds that the reverse "could have been achieved if the aid spent on [settlements] had been used to assist self-settled refugees": ibid.

[442] Zetter, "Shelter Provision," at 73.

[443] "Because they do not possess Sudanese citizenship they cannot buy houses and are dependent on the rental sector. However, the lack of rented houses has led to a sharp rise in rents": J. Post, "Considerations on the Settlement of Urban Refugees in Eastern Sudan" (1983), at 6.

[444] The accommodation challenges and rights of refugees seeking recognition of their status are addressed in chapter 4.4.2 above, at pp. 480–484.

[445] This has been the traditional practice in Belgium, the Netherlands, Norway, and Sweden: IGC, Temporary Protection, at 7–8.

[446] Büllesbach, "Civil War Refugees," at 45–46.

such emergency housing to Bosnian refugees until forced by the courts to do so.[447] Under the recent European Union directive, however, there is a general, if vaguely framed, obligation to "ensure that persons enjoying temporary protection have access to suitable accommodation or, if necessary, receive the means to obtain housing."[448]

The housing options in the North for persons recognized as Convention refugees are less constrained. For example, European Union law now requires that states "ensure that beneficiaries of refugee ... status have access to accommodation under equivalent conditions as other third country nationals legally resident in their territories."[449] Yet those who choose to live in large urban centers are frequently confronted by generalized shortages of affordable housing.[450] Coupled with the refugees' usually limited financial resources, lack of contacts, unfamiliarity with neighborhoods, and lack of awareness of services,[451] the challenge of locating affordable and decent housing in large cities is often quite real. Refugees' efforts to locate housing may also be frustrated by practices such as those reported in Canada, where real estate agents tend to direct refugees of particular ethnic backgrounds into specific neighborhoods,[452] or by racist refusals to rent to people of color. In Italy, for example, many apartment advertisements specifically state that no "stranieri" – foreigners – need apply, and non-citizens are not given standing in the courts to contest their exclusion.[453]

In the Netherlands and Scandinavia, responsibility to meet the housing needs of refugees is often assigned to a particular municipality.[454] Chronic shortages of accommodation in many states often result in long delays before

---

[447] Ibid. at 45.

[448] EU Temporary Protection Directive, at Art. 13(1). An earlier proposal for this rule was framed simply in aspirational terms, providing that states "shall, where necessary, endeavour to offer suitable housing facilities, or adequate means to obtain such housing": "Note from the Presidency of the European Union to the Working Party on Asylum," EU Doc. 12617/98, Nov. 9, 1998.

[449] EU Qualification Directive, at Art. 31.

[450] Lambert, *Seeking Asylum*, at 184. Lambert notes that Belgium is an exception, being "one of the rare countries where modest accommodation can be found for reasonable prices": ibid.

[451] See generally R. Murdie et al., "Housing Issues Facing Immigrants and Refugees in Greater Toronto: Initial Findings from the Jamaican, Polish and Somali Communities," in E. Komut ed., *Housing Question of the "Others"* (1996) (Murdie, "Housing Issues"), at 179–183.

[452] Ibid. at 185–188.

[453] "[T]hey of course have no standing to sue in courts. So some immigrants turn to crime. Foreigners now constitute roughly a quarter of all those in jail or out on bail in Italy": J. Smith, "Europe bids immigrants unwelcome; Natives resent changes in 'their way of life,'" *Washington Post*, July 23, 2000, at A-01.

[454] While refugees who are able to find their own accommodation may settle where they wish, severe housing shortages make this option unrealistic in practice for most refugees: Liebaut, *Conditions 2000*, at 219, 58, 77, 235, and 283.

accommodation is located. In Sweden, for example, refugees have been required to wait as long as two to three years to acquire a permanent residence.[455] Refugees may also face real discrimination in accessing public housing. In Denmark, some local councils declared refugees non-admissible to housing facilities,[456] while the Swedish municipality of Sjöbo gained international notoriety for its refusal to allow fifteen refugees to access its subsidized accommodation.[457]

In other countries, including Austria, Canada, France, New Zealand, and Spain, refugees have access to subsidized public housing on the same terms as citizens. Refugees are often also eligible for supplemental assistance, such as the loans generally available in Germany for a rental deposit, and in-kind donations of furniture, kitchen equipment, and other essentials.[458] In Canada, public housing is often located far from basic amenities, and may not be designed to accommodate the extended families of many refugee groups.[459] In the United Kingdom, the challenge of finding subsidized housing is reported to have reached crisis proportions, especially for many single people and members of minority groups.[460]

Some Northern states make little effort to provide housing assistance to refugees. In Italy, refugees may be able to find shelter in one of the limited number of accommodation centers open to foreigners generally, which are free for the first sixty days. Most refugees, however, must seek accommodation on the private market, as only some regions allow refugees and other non-citizens to access the general stock of public housing.[461] Malta similarly provides refugees with little assistance to acquire adequate housing, in consequence of which "[m]any have to rent at exorbitant prices and others live in terrible conditions":[462]

---

[455] Lambert, *Seeking Asylum*, at 186.

[456] The Ministry of the Interior halted the practice: J. Vedsted-Hansen, *International Academy of Comparative Law National Report for Denmark* (1994), at 3.

[457] T. Hammar, "The Integration or Non-Integration of Refugee Immigrants," in G. Rystad ed., *Uprooted: Forced Migration as an International Problem in the Post-War Era* 179 (1990), at 181.

[458] See European Council on Refugees and Exiles, *Legal and Social Conditions for Asylum Seekers in Western European Countries, 2003* (2003) (ECRE, *Conditions 2003*); Liebaut, *Conditions 2000*; and Lambert, *Seeking Asylum*, at 184–188.

[459] Murdie, "Housing Issues," at 188.

[460] Lambert observes that refugees with families are given preferred housing benefits, and that blacks are often housed in inferior accommodation by local authorities: Lambert, *Seeking Asylum*, at 187.

[461] Liebaut, *Conditions 2000*, at 174.

[462] (1999) 57 *JRS Dispatches* (Oct. 1, 1999). Indeed, the United Nations Committee on the Rights of the Child "expressed [concern] . . . at the limited access of refugee children to . . . housing": Committee on the Rights of the Child, "Concluding Observations of the Committee on the Rights of the Child: Malta," UN Doc. CRC/C/15, Add.129, June 2, 2000, at para. 43.

I recently visited one refugee who is sharing a two roomed "flat" with two other refugees. The flat has tiles which are black with damp, the walls dark with filth, with mice and cockroaches crawling through a grating which leads to a neighbour's basement. The drain pipes in the yard leak so the floor is always wet, and the walls of the yard are green with slime. The toilet is in a room built of wood and corrugated iron in the yard, the roof is missing in places and so are some bits of the wall ... [The] toilet is out of order. To top it all, this yard is actually a passage to upper flats which house more refugees. So even if it was in use, it would still be embarrassing to use it.[463]

While the housing programs of Portuguese municipalities are in principle open to all persons in need, in practice applicants have often been denied assistance unless they have at least one Portuguese family member.[464] In Russia, refugees have no right to rent housing; in the result, many are destitute and homeless.[465]

> **Refugee Convention, Art. 21   Housing**
> As regards housing, the Contracting States, in so far as the matter is regulated by laws or regulations or is subject to the control of public authorities, shall accord to refugees lawfully staying in their territory treatment as favourable as possible and, in any event, not less favourable than that accorded to aliens generally in the same circumstances.

> **Economic, Social and Cultural Covenant, Art. 11(1)**
> The States Parties to the present Covenant recognize the right of everyone to an adequate standard of living for himself and his family, including adequate ... housing ...

It was not initially intended that the Refugee Convention would expressly address the right of refugees to housing. None of the predecessor treaties had done so,[466] and the Secretary-General did not propose any change from past

---

[463] (1999) 57 *JRS Dispatches* (Oct. 1, 1999).

[464] "[T]his requirement makes housing almost impossible for refugees [to obtain]": F. Liebaut and J. Hughes eds., *Legal and Social Conditions for Asylum Seekers and Refugees in Western European Countries* (1997), at 194.

[465] R. Redmond, "Old Problems in a New World," (1993) 94 *Refugees* 28, at 29–30. "The asylum problems for the 'foreigner refugees' are exacerbated by a series of technical and substantive problems on the ground: for instance, there is no settlement or provision for staying before, during, or after the asylum claim is made ... In one situation, when Somalis were evicted from ... [a] home in a district of Moscow, the act was legitimised on the grounds of their unworthiness": E. Voutira, "Vestiges of Empire: Migrants, Refugees and Returnees in Post-Soviet Russia," (1996) 7(3) *Oxford International Review* 52, at 56.

[466] Weis, *Travaux*, at 163.

practice. Indeed, because the right of refugees to acquire housing was considered to be an aspect of Art. 13's guarantee of movable and immovable property rights,[467] the Secretariat was initially skeptical that any further reference to housing would be helpful.[468]

This is an important starting point, since many housing concerns are in fact most appropriately addressed by invocation of other Convention-based or general international human rights. In line with the Secretariat's observation, both Sudan's denial to refugees of the right to buy a home and Russia's refusal to allow refugees freely to rent apartments or other accommodation raise property rights concerns. Art. 13 of the Convention expressly includes not only the right of refugees to own property, but also to benefit from "leases and other contracts relating to movable and immovable property."[469]

Nor is the right to property the only basis for insistence upon what may broadly be thought of as housing rights. The duty of states to ensure the physical security of refugees is breached by those African states that require refugees to live in overcrowded camps which cannot be effectively patrolled, and by the Thai assignment of Burmese refugees to live in a border zone prone to armed conflict.[470] In at least the latter case, the right to life is also jeopardized.[471] The forcible expulsion of refugees from their homes is another clear example of activity that may breach the duty to protect life and basic physical security, as was observed by the Supreme Court of India in response to efforts by private groups to drive Chakma refugees from their homes:

> The State is bound to protect the life and liberty of every human being, be he a citizen or otherwise, and it cannot permit anybody or any group of persons ... to threaten the Chakmas ... No State Government worth the name can tolerate such threats ... The State Government must act impartially and carry out its legal obligation to safeguard the life, health and well-being of Chakmas residing in the State without being inhibited by local politics ...
>
> Except in accordance with law, the Chakmas shall not be evicted from their homes and shall not be denied domestic lives and comfort therein. The quit notices and ultimatums issued ... [are] tantamount to threats to the life and liberty of each [and] every Chakma, [and] should be dealt with ... in accordance with law.[472]

---

[467] See chapter 4.5.1 above, at pp. 523–525.

[468] "[I]n Mr. Humphrey's opinion, the provisionally adopted article [13] might be considered to cover the question in a certain sense": Statement of the Chairman, Mr. Chance of Canada, UN Doc. E/AC.32/SR.15, Jan. 27, 1950, at 11.

[469] Refugee Convention, at Art. 13. See chapter 4.5.1 above, at pp. 523–524.

[470] See chapter 4.3.3 above.   [471] See chapter 4.3.1 above, at p. 452.

[472] *National Human Rights Commission v. State of Arunachal Pradesh*, (1996) 83 AIR 1234 (India SC, Jan. 9, 1996).

When Togolese refugees in Benin and Bhutanese refugees in Nepal became ill because they were forced to live in overcrowded camps lacking water, sanitation, and waste disposal services, their right to health was violated.[473] And the right of refugees to enjoy freedom of residence and internal movement is infringed by the practice of many Southern countries to confine refugees in camps or settlements, and by the traditional insistence of some European countries, including Belgium, the Netherlands, Norway, and Sweden, that refugees granted "temporary protection" live in state-sanctioned centers.[474] More generally, the Committee on the Elimination of Racial Discrimination has invoked the duty of non-discrimination to insist upon fair access to housing, specifically in the context of Italian treatment of the Roma.[475] When any of these more general rights is infringed, there is no need to rely upon a right to housing in order to secure protection.

The incorporation in the Refugee Convention of a specific provision addressed to housing rights resulted from the decision described earlier to adopt the text of the ILO's Migration for Employment Convention as the basis for the Refugee Convention's Art. 24(1)(a) guaranteeing fair conditions of employment to refugee workers.[476] One of the ILO guarantees not imported into the Refugee Convention was the right of migrant workers to benefit from national treatment with regard to employee accommodation.[477] In agreeing to the omission of this provision from the Refugee Convention, the American representative to the Ad Hoc Committee gave notice that "although he did not think the reference to housing should be inserted at that point in the convention, he felt it should be included at a later stage. It might form the subject of a separate article which would apply to the whole draft convention and not only to the provisions regarding labour."[478]

---

[473] See chapter 4.4.3 above, particularly at p. 513 (regarding the duty to ensure basic healthcare in even very poor states).

[474] See chapter 5.2 above, at pp. 707–708.

[475] UN Committee on the Elimination of Racial Discrimination, "Concluding Observations on the Report of Italy," UN Doc. CERD/C/5/Misc.32/Rev.3, Mar. 18, 1999.

[476] See chapter 6.1.2 above, at pp. 765–769.   [477] Ibid. at note 183.

[478] Statement of Mr. Henkin of the United States, UN Doc. E/AC.32/SR.14, Jan. 26, 1950, at 10. Several governments were opposed to this initiative. Denmark, for example, argued that "the *Migration for Employment Convention* had been prepared in the interests of a group who desired to become productive members of a national community. Refugees constituted a different group; many of them were unfitted to make any constructive contribution to the life of the community. For that reason he was uncertain whether the provisions of the ILO document could be made to apply to the case of refugees": Statement of Mr. Larsen of Denmark, ibid. at 9. The Chinese representative did not wish to accept any obligation on this matter, noting that "[h]is own country, devastated by war and suffering from a grave shortage of housing, had taken urgent measures, following the end of the Second World War, to relieve the suffering of the refugees; these measures had often placed the refugees in a more advantageous position, from the point

The goal of the American project was not to reiterate the property rights protections of Art. 13. Mr. Henkin wished instead to ensure that "refugees might benefit under any social welfare measures taken by States with a view to providing housing accommodation for certain categories of persons."[479] Thus, as Robinson opines, Art. 21 "deals with rent control and assignment of apartments and premises."[480] Similarly, Grahl-Madsen logically contends that the right of refugees to housing under Art. 21 includes "not only the obtaining of [a] dwelling-place, but also participation in schemes for financing of the construction of dwelling-places (cf. the expression 'housing schemes')."[481]

These examples help to establish a workable boundary between rights grounded in Art. 21's provisions on housing, and those more appropriately conceived as aspects of a public relief program governed by Art. 23. The distinction will often be important, since refugees lawfully staying in an asylum country must be assimilated to nationals for purposes of public relief,[482] whereas Art. 21's provisions on housing require only that they receive "treatment as favourable as possible and, in any event, not less favourable than that accorded to aliens generally in the same circumstances." For reasons described below,[483] this standard of treatment clearly falls short of a duty to treat refugees on par with citizens of the kind set by the public relief provisions of Art. 23.

In practice, the boundary between a housing program and a public relief initiative will often be blurred, requiring the delineation between Arts. 21 and 23 to be made on the basis of the essential goal of the official initiative in question. Despite the American delegate's reference to Art. 21 as focused on the "social welfare" aspect of housing, it is difficult to see why a state that assists the destitute or disabled by direct cash payments should be bound to the higher standard of Art. 23, whereas a government that provides such persons with in-kind access to free or subsidized accommodation would have to meet only the lower test of Art. 21. For this reason, and taking particular

---

of view of housing, than many Chinese nationals. He felt that the matter of housing should be left to the initiative and control of the individual Governments": Statement of Mr. Cha of China, ibid. at 10. The decision to include an article on housing was only narrowly approved on a 5–2 (4 abstentions) vote: ibid.

[479] Statement of Mr. Henkin of the United States, UN Doc. E/AC.32/SR.15, Jan. 27, 1950, at 11.

[480] Robinson, *History*, at 120. Weis goes still farther, arguing that Art. 13 includes "housing schemes and allocation of premises for the exercise of one's occupation": Weis, *Travaux*, at 163. Weis provides no justification, however, for his view that the right of refugees to "housing" includes the right to premises from which to engage in business; as a matter of ordinary construction, this conclusion is suspect.

[481] Grahl-Madsen, *Commentary*, at 84.   [482] See chapter 6.3 above, at p. 806.

[483] See text below, at pp. 826–827.

account of the broad scope of Art. 23,[484] initiatives which provide housing benefits to sub-populations on the basis of need should be deemed in pith and substance to be forms of relief or assistance subject to the requirements of Art. 23. Thus, the denial of public housing to refugees by some Danish and Swedish municipalities, as well as the refusal of Saxony and Bavaria to extend generally available housing assistance benefits to temporarily protected refugees, are examples of policies in breach of the duty to assimilate lawfully staying refugees to citizens for welfare purposes. Art. 23 similarly requires Italy and Malta to enfranchise refugees within any scheme to assist homeless or poorly housed nationals – not simply to provide them with whatever aid is normally afforded to other non-citizens.

In contrast, policies or programs which regulate or control housing in general terms – for example, rent controls, landlord–tenant laws, or schemes to assist in the construction or purchase of a home – are more appropriately understood to be governed by the provisions of Art. 21. As originally proposed, Art. 21 would have regulated only housing matters "regulated by laws *and* regulations or . . . subject to the control of *Governmental* authorities [emphasis added]."[485] But the Ad Hoc Committee decided that the provisions of Art. 21 should apply also "in so far as [housing] lies within the discretion of local governmental authorities."[486] This view is reflected in the decision to amend the text initially to refer to matters subject to the control "of *governmental* authorities [emphasis added],"[487] then finally to speak simply to matters under the control "of public authorities."[488] In the result, the Refugee Convention's guarantee of housing rights applies whenever a refugee claims the benefit of a housing policy or program over which some level of government[489] exercises authority, whether that official control is formal (by law or regulation) or simply practical (administration, oversight, or review).[490] Thus, the fact that public housing is administered by regional

---

[484] See chapter 6.3 above, at pp. 810–811.

[485] This was the language submitted to the Ad Hoc Committee by Mr. Henkin of the United States, UN Doc. E/AC.32/SR.24, Feb. 3, 1950, at 12.

[486] Statement of the Chairman, Mr. Chance of Canada, ibid. at 13. Speaking as the representative of Canada, Mr. Chance had earlier voiced his approval for Art. 21 "on the condition that it was compatible with the federal laws in force in his country": ibid. at 12.

[487] "Decisions of the Committee on Statelessness and Related Problems taken at the meetings of 3 February 1950," UN Doc. E/AC.32/L.28, Feb. 3, 1950, at 2.

[488] Ad Hoc Committee, "First Session Report," at Annex I. This language is consistent with the text of the predecessor ILO Convention on migrant worker rights: see chapter 6.1.2 above, at p. 767.

[489] "It is an obligation incumbent not only on the state but also on all other public authorities (municipalities, regional self-governments)": Robinson, *History*, at 120.

[490] The agreement that regulatory (as opposed to statutory) involvement is sufficient to bring Art. 21 into play is clear from the change to a disjunctive formulation ("regulated

authorities in the Netherlands, the United Kingdom, and most of Scandinavia is sufficient to engage Art. 21.

Indeed, while there is little doubt about the principle that purely private housing programs are exempt from the requirements of the Convention's provision on housing,[491] the breadth of modern-day regulation of private activity in the field of housing, particularly to guard against discrimination, may mean that in practice there are few aspects of housing policy that will escape scrutiny under Art. 21. For example, the real estate profession is officially regulated in Canada, and there is landlord–tenant law in Italy. The fact that Art. 21's scope extends to any aspect of housing "regulated by laws or regulations or . . . subject to the control of public authorities" may well mean that refugees should be able to invoke the article to require Canada to take action in response to the propensity of some real estate agents to direct refugees into ethnic neighborhoods with substandard accommodation, or to insist that Italy counter the refusal of many Italian landlords to rent to refugees.[492]

The real value of Art. 21 is nonetheless limited in two fundamental ways. First, an amendment late in the drafting process raised the required level of attachment for access to housing rights from simply refugees "lawfully in" a state's territory[493] to refugees "lawfully staying in" the territory. The benefit of Art. 21 may therefore be claimed only by refugees present on an ongoing basis, including, for example, recognized refugees and refugees granted so-called "temporary" or other durable forms of status.[494] No explanation was given for this shift.[495] While likely prompted by concern not to exacerbate acute postwar housing shortages for their own citizens,[496] the result is that Art. 21 – in essence, an auxiliary property rights provision – is accessible to only a subset of refugees able to invoke the more general guarantee of property rights set by Art. 13 of the Convention.[497]

---

by laws or regulations"): "Decisions of the Committee on Statelessness and Related Problems taken at the meetings of 3 February 1950," UN Doc. E/AC.32/L.28, Feb. 3, 1950, at 2. This amended text was in line with the original ILO precedent: see chapter 6.1.2 above, at pp. 766–767.

[491] See Grahl-Madsen, *Commentary*, at 84: "If housing is left entirely to private enterprise, the State is not obliged to interfere and pass laws simply in order to ensure that refugees will find suitable accommodation."

[492] The challenge in each of these situations is that a state party need only provide refugees with the same protection as is afforded aliens generally in the same circumstances. Where this is little or nothing, Art. 21 provides little practical value to refugees. See text below, at pp. 826–827.

[493] This formulation was endorsed at all stages of the work of the Ad Hoc Committee, including in its final report: Ad Hoc Committee, "Second Session Report," at 20.

[494] See chapter 3.1.4 above.

[495] The altered language seems to have been agreed to in the Style Committee: "Report of the Style Committee," UN Doc. A/CONF.2/102.

[496] See the comments of the British and Chinese delegates at note 410 above.

[497] See chapter 4.5.1 above, at pp. 526–527.

Second, Art. 21 sets no firm qualitative guarantee of any rights beyond those which inhere in "aliens generally in the same circumstances." This duty is "not merely [an obligation] not to discriminate against refugees."[498] It rather has affirmative content in the sense of incorporating by reference all general sources of relevant rights,[499] and requiring that governments consider in good faith the more complete enfranchisement of refugees.[500] But in practice, it may nonetheless amount to a guarantee of very little, if any, protection.[501] Despite the early plea of the French government,[502] and a Yugoslav initiative advanced at the Conference of Plenipotentiaries,[503] most governments were not prepared to grant refugees all of the housing rights provided to their own citizens, preferring to reserve the right to limit special housing programs to at least some parts of their own populations. For example, the representative of the United Kingdom argued that

> In his own country it would be difficult to guarantee exactly equal treatment for refugees in the matter of housing, since the housing shortage was acute and the matter had to be dealt with on the basis of need. It was also felt that a certain degree of preference as regards housing should be given to some categories of nationals, such as ex-servicemen.[504]

---

[498] Statement of Mr. Cuvelier of Belgium, UN Doc. E/AC.32/SR.24, Feb. 3, 1950, at 13.

[499] See chapter 3.2.1 above, at p. 197.

[500] See chapter 3.2.1 above, at p. 200. It may also be relevant that there is a duty to exempt refugees from the application of general requirements for access to housing which cannot in practice be met in view of the refugee's particular circumstances: see chapter 3.2.3 above.

[501] This point was made by the International Refugee Organization, which argued that "in many countries it is not possible to speak of general treatment in relation to . . . housing. These matters are frequently subject to administrative regulations which are often framed with other objects in view than the distinction between nationals and aliens, e.g. service in national armies, local residential qualifications, etc., or leave much discretion to the competent authorities": United Nations, "Compilation of Comments," at 40.

[502] The French delegate "had altered his opinion and was now convinced that the reference [in the ILO migrant workers treaty used as a precedent] was to general housing . . . and that in cases where such legislation existed, equal treatment should be accorded to refugees and nationals. That was the more liberal interpretation, which . . . he believed his Government would endorse": Statement of Mr. Rain of France, UN Doc. E/AC.32/SR.14, Jan. 26, 1950, at 9.

[503] "[I]t would be unfair to refugees in countries where housing was controlled by the public authorities if they were treated differently from nationals in respect of housing. Unless refugees were given identical treatment, it would be impossible for them to secure accommodation": Statement of Mr. Makiedo of Yugoslavia, UN Doc. A/CONF.2/SR.10, July 6, 1951, at 10–11. His amendment to this effect (UN Doc. A/CONF.2/31, at 2) was defeated on a 9–1 (7 abstentions) vote: ibid. at 11.

[504] Statement of Sir Leslie Brass of the United Kingdom, UN Doc. E/AC.32/SR.14, Jan. 26, 1950, at 8.

The vagueness of the new European Union directive applicable to temporarily protected refugees – requiring only that they receive "access to suitable accommodation" – cannot therefore be criticized by reference to Art. 21 for failing to codify any particular qualitative standard.[505] Indeed, the European Union's decision to enfranchise recognized refugees on par with legally resident third-country nationals, as well as the traditional practice of states such as Austria, Canada, France, and Spain to assimilate refugees to citizens for purposes of access to public housing are, while commendable, clearly standards in excess of the requirements of the Refugee Convention. As described above,[506] while the concomitant duty to treat refugees "as favourably as possible" is not purely hortatory, neither does it compel governments to grant refugees special benefits, even relative to other non-citizens. Thus, there is no violation of Art. 21 when refugees must endure the same hardships in accessing housing as other non-citizens. This is the case, for example, under the Portuguese practice of giving preference in accessing public housing to families – including refugee families – with at least one citizen member.[507]

On the other hand, the "aliens generally" standard of treatment does incorporate by reference all general sources of legal entitlement,[508] including notably Art. 11 of the Covenant on Economic, Social and Cultural Rights. While of most critical importance to those refugees unable to satisfy Art. 21's level of attachment (and therefore analyzed previously in some depth in defining the right of all refugees – even those who have no legal status in an asylum state – to be assisted in acquiring the necessities of life[509]), Art. 11 of the Economic Covenant is of value even to those refugees able to satisfy the higher attachment criterion of Art. 21 of the Refugee Convention. This is because the guarantees set by the Economic Covenant establish an authoritative qualitative baseline for the attribution of housing rights to refugees, thereby compensating somewhat for the substantive fungibility of Art. 21.

Invoking Art. 11 of the Economic Covenant to establish the minimum acceptable content of the housing rights of aliens generally (and all other persons), refugees may lawfully insist that an asylum country grant them not less than the housing rights set by general international law. Importantly, the Committee on Economic, Social and Cultural Rights has emphasized that

---

[505] The regional notion of "suitability" must not, however, fall below the international legal standard of "adequacy": see text below, at pp. 827–829.

[506] See chapter 3.2.1 above, at pp. 198–200.

[507] The better argument in this situation would be that the duty of non-discrimination has not been met. But even here, the margin of appreciation afforded states to privilege their own nationals may foreclose any remedy: see chapter 2.5.5 above, at pp. 130–133.

[508] See chapter 3.2.1 above, at p. 197.   [509] See chapter 4.4.2 above.

Art. 11 of the Economic Covenant does not simply establish a right to housing, but rather to "an *adequate* standard of living ... including *adequate* ... housing [emphasis added]."[510] Governments are moreover required to provide all persons under their jurisdiction with an effective domestic remedy against violation of their core housing rights.[511] Because international law defines the right to housing as requiring governments to meet at least this basic qualitative standard ("adequacy"), the Committee has observed that the essential requirement of Art. 11(1) is that "everyone"[512] must enjoy the right "to live somewhere in security, peace and dignity."[513] It has moreover elaborated a set of standards against which to assess compliance.

Thus, the Committee has determined that housing is only adequate if it is affordable; accessible to all, including in particular the disadvantaged; and located in a place that is not impractically remote and which affords reasonable access to services, materials, facilities, and infrastructure.[514] This standard is not met when governments, such as those of Bosnia, Croatia, and Sudan, force refugees to live in marginal areas where they have little chance of becoming self-sustaining. The refusal of some asylum countries to allow refugee settlements to expand in a way that ensures the continuing viability of infrastructure to meet the needs of their inhabitants is also a failure to ensure adequate housing.

More specifically, the accommodation itself must be habitable, meaning that it provides protection from the elements and other hazards, and it must be culturally appropriate.[515] This standard was clearly not met when refugees in Ethiopia were left for prolonged periods attempting to shelter under old plastic sheeting. The Canadian practice of providing little or no public housing sufficient to meet the needs of the traditional extended families of many refugee groups, while clearly less egregious, is nonetheless a failure to provide culturally adequate housing. Housing is also adequate only if it can be enjoyed with reasonable security of tenure.[516] In particular, the Committee has concluded that "instances of forced eviction are *prima facie* incompatible with the requirements of the Covenant and can only be justified in the most exceptional circumstances, and in accordance with the relevant

---

[510] "The human right to adequate housing, which is thus derived from the right to an adequate standard of living, is of central importance for the enjoyment of all economic, social and cultural rights": UN Committee on Economic, Social and Cultural Rights, "General Comment No. 4: The right to adequate housing" (1991), UN Doc. HRI/GEN/1/Rev.7, May 12, 2004, at 19, para. 1.

[511] Ibid. at para. 18.

[512] "The right to adequate housing applies to everyone ... In particular, enjoyment of this right must, in accordance with Article 2(2) of the Covenant, not be subject to any form of discrimination": ibid. at para. 6.

[513] Ibid. at para. 7.   [514] Ibid. at para. 8.   [515] Ibid. at para. 8.   [516] Ibid. at para. 8.

principles of international law."[517] The efforts to expel Chakma refugees from their homes in India were therefore in breach not only of basic security rights as described above, but also of the right to adequate housing.

In implementing housing rights, governments are under a duty to give special attention to the housing needs of "social groups living in unfavorable conditions";[518] they are expected to seek out international aid where necessary to comply with the duty to ensure adequate housing;[519] and they are bound to engage in "extensive genuine consultation with, and participation by, all of those affected, including the homeless."[520] There is therefore no basis for receiving states to cut off housing aid to refugees who prefer to self-settle, rather than to live in organized camps or refugee communities. This is particularly so since, as previously noted, refugees lawfully present enjoy the right to choose their own place of residence.[521] There is also a failure to respect the right to adequate housing when local authorities and the aid agencies working with them fail meaningfully to involve refugees in the planning of their homes and communities.

6.5 Intellectual property rights

As in the case of housing rights, no prior refugee treaty expressly dealt with the issue of intellectual property rights. This is likely because such protection was thought to have been unnecessary. Refugees would not typically have encountered any difficulty claiming intellectual property rights, since non-citizens have routinely been understood to be entitled to assert such interests. And while some states condition the enforcement of intellectual property rights in their courts on the existence of reciprocity – meaning that the citizens of the state in which enforcement is sought can claim comparable protections in the refugee's country of citizenship – these barriers to enforcement abroad of intellectual property claims did not apply to refugees. This is because earlier refugee treaties included a general duty to exempt refugees from any requirements of reciprocity.[522]

---

[517] Ibid. at para. 18. The duty to avoid forced eviction has been elaborated in a specific general comment: UN Committee on Economic, Social and Cultural Rights, "General Comment No. 7: The right to adequate housing: forced evictions" (1997), UN Doc. HRI/GEN/1/Rev.7, May 12, 2004, at 46. The applicability of this protection to refugees is described in detail in chapter 4.4.2 above, at pp. 504–506.

[518] UN Committee on Economic, Social and Cultural Rights, "General Comment No. 4: The right to adequate housing" (1991), UN Doc. HRI/GEN/1/Rev.7, May 12, 2004, at 19, para. 11.

[519] Ibid. at para. 10.   [520] Ibid. at para. 12.   [521] See chapter 5.2 above.

[522] See chapter 3.2 above, at p. 195.

But the 1951 Convention ended this blanket exemption of refugees from reciprocity requirements (diplomatic reciprocity requirements now being preserved, and even legislative and de facto reciprocity requirements being waived only after three years' residence in a state party).[523] Without the benefit of an exemption from reciprocity rules, many refugees would, in practice, have been unable to protect their intellectual property rights outside their country of origin.[524]

> **Refugee Convention, Art. 14   Artistic rights and industrial property**
> In respect of the protection of industrial property, such as inventions, designs or models, trade marks, trade names, and of rights in literary, artistic and scientific works, a refugee shall be accorded in the country in which he has his habitual residence the same protection as is accorded to nationals of that country. In the territory of any other Contracting State, he shall be accorded the same protection as is accorded in that territory to nationals of the country in which he has his habitual residence.

> **Economic, Social and Cultural Covenant, Art. 15(1)(c)**
> The States Parties to the present Covenant recognize the right of everyone . . . to benefit from the protection of the moral and material interests resulting from any scientific, literary or artistic production of which he is the author.

Both the Secretary-General and French government drafts of the Refugee Convention proposed avoiding the effect of reciprocity requirements by mandating the assimilation of refugees to most-favored foreigners for purposes of enforcing intellectual property rights.[525] That is, refugees present in any state party would have been automatically entitled to invoke whatever mechanisms to protect intellectual property that country was willing to make available to the citizens of any foreign country "by treaty or usage,"[526]

---

[523] See chapters 3.2.1 and 3.2.2 above.

[524] There was agreement that this would be inequitable, since intellectual property "is the creation of the human mind and recognition is not a favour": Secretary-General, "Memorandum," at 27.

[525] "In respect of industrial and intellectual property (copyright, industrial property, patents, licences, trademarks, designs and models, trade names, etc.), refugees (and stateless persons) shall enjoy the most favourable treatment accorded to nationals of foreign countries": ibid. The French draft of the convention took essentially the same approach, though with a slightly different list of the interests to be protected. Specifically, the French proposal omitted the protection of "licences" found in the Secretary-General's draft and added a reference to "scientific property": France, "Draft Convention," at 4.

[526] Ad Hoc Committee, "First Session Report," at Annex II.

including procedures open only to the nationals of countries united in special economic or other associations. This approach would not have imposed any particular model on a given state party, but would have required that every refugee be granted the best protection afforded any non-citizen.

Even at the first session of the Ad Hoc Committee, however, the British delegate expressed concern about this approach. Despite his acceptance of the clear need to exempt refugees from reciprocity requirements in the enforcement of intellectual property rights, he questioned whether the assimilation of refugees to most-favored foreigners was the right mechanism to adopt.[527] Additional force was given to this argument when the Chairman of the Ad Hoc Committee drew the attention of representatives to an expert report addressing the Berne Convention on the Protection of Literary and Artistic Works.[528] The gist of this analysis was that the Berne Convention, the main treaty regulating the transnational enforcement of rights in literary and artistic property, did not provide for the enfranchisement of non-citizens on the same terms as the nationals of most-favored countries.[529] Instead, it established a uniform standard for the enforcement of intellectual property claims abroad, based on whether the individual seeking enforcement was a citizen of a state party to the relevant treaty:

> Taking Denmark as an example, any Dane who wrote a book had the Danish copyright wherever the book might be published. The same was true if the author was a national of a country adhering to the Berne Convention. If the author was a national of a country not adhering to the Convention, his rights were safeguarded in Denmark only if the book was first published there. Finally, the rights of a stateless author had no protection anywhere. With regard to the last of those situations, some change was certainly needed; but supposing that a national of a country not adhering to the Berne Convention became a refugee and fled to another country not adhering to that Convention, it would be unfair if merely by becoming a refugee he were to receive better treatment than a citizen of his country of refuge.[530]

[527] "[W]hile the Committee was trying, as it should, to protect refugees against discrimination, it should not go to the other extreme of establishing discrimination in favour of refugees. He shared the uneasiness of other members regarding the most-favoured-nation clause": Statement of Sir Leslie Brass of the United Kingdom, UN Doc. E/AC.32/SR.10, Jan. 24, 1950, at 7.

[528] 828 UNTS 221, done Sept. 9, 1886, revised in Stockholm, July 14, 1967 (Berne Convention). Statement of the Chairman, Mr. Larsen of Denmark, UN Doc. E/AC.32/SR.36, Aug. 15, 1950, at 20.

[529] "[E]xisting conventions on the subject ... applied to nationals rather than to refugees, hence such a clause was needed for the protection of the latter": Statement of Mr. Weis of the International Refugee Organization, UN Doc. E/AC.32/SR.10, Jan. 24, 1950, at 8.

[530] Statement of the Chairman, Mr. Larsen of Denmark, UN Doc. E/AC.32/SR.36, Aug. 15, 1950, at 20–21.

Concern about fairness arose because if a refugee's asylum country were not itself a party to the Berne Convention, its nationals would have no guarantee of most-favored-national treatment when seeking to enforce intellectual property rights in a third country. But a refugee residing in that asylum state, if entitled to most-favored-national treatment in any state party to the Refugee Convention, would be able to claim preferred rights in the third country and, to that extent, would enjoy a benefit not open to the citizens of his or her host state. It was generally felt that the Refugee Convention should compensate for the disadvantages of refugeehood, but not operate in a way that was significantly different from the general approach under the Berne Convention.[531]

Thus, the Ad Hoc Committee affirmed that it was entirely reasonable to avoid the penalization of a refugee because of the failure of his or her country of origin to assist other countries to enforce the intellectual property rights of their citizens – after all, since a refugee is by definition a person who no longer enjoys the protection of the home state, there is little logic to holding him or her hostage to the whims of that country. On this basic point, the drafters went beyond what the Secretary-General had proposed, deciding that in the asylum state refugees should be assimilated to citizens (not just most-favored foreigners) for purposes of enforcing their intellectual property rights. But since the enforcement *abroad* of intellectual property rights was generally contingent on the individual coming from a state party to the intellectual property treaty regime, refugees should not be able to avoid that essential premise set by the Berne Convention.[532] It was felt that justice could be done to refugees simply by substituting their country of residence for their country of citizenship in determining where, and to what extent, they could enforce

---

[531] The United Kingdom, for example, "cannot agree to accord refugees in respect of these matters the most favourable treatment accorded to nationals of foreign countries. They would, however, be prepared to consider sympathetically the possibility of according refugees the same protection as the nationals of the country in which they are resident, subject to the same conditions and formalities as apply to such nationals": United Nations, "Compilation of Comments," at 41.

[532] "If a book was first published in the United Kingdom, any author could secure the United Kingdom copyright; if it was published in a country adhering to the Berne Convention, the author could also secure that copyright . . . The United Kingdom proposal was therefore that refugees in their country of residence should receive the rights normally accorded to nationals of that country . . . The rights they would receive for books first published in other countries would not depend on whether those countries were signatories to the Convention or not": Statement of Sir Leslie Brass of the United Kingdom, UN Doc. E/AC.32/SR.36, Aug. 15, 1950, at 21–22. See also Statement of Mr. Herment of Belgium, ibid. at 22: "[T]he difficulties referred to could perhaps be avoided by according a refugee the same treatment as was accorded to nationals of the country in which he found himself ('national treatment')."

their intellectual property claims in foreign countries.[533] The Drafting Committee therefore recommended a text based on these points of consensus,[534] and which provided the essential model approved for the Convention:[535]

> In respect of the protection of industrial property, such as inventions, designs of models, trade marks, trade names, etc., and of rights in literary, scientific and artistic works, a refugee shall be accorded in the country in which he is resident, the same protection as is accorded to nationals of that country. In the territory of another Contracting State, he shall be accorded the same protection as is accorded in that territory to nationals of the country in which he is resident.[536]

As such, Art. 14 entitles a refugee to enforce intellectual property rights, whether in the asylum country or in another state party to the Refugee Convention, to exactly the same extent as a citizen of his or her asylum country.[537] In essence, it effected an indirect amendment of the Berne Convention for state parties to the Refugee Convention, requiring those states to assimilate refugees living in their country to their own citizens for purposes of the reciprocal enforcement of intellectual property rights.

---

[533] "'[N]ational treatment' should not ... apply to refugees resident in a country not a signatory to the Convention": Statement of Mr. Herment of Belgium, ibid. at 22. While the Chairman based his remarks on the assumption that the Berne Convention was designed to protect the rights of publishers as well as those of authors, his analysis is comparable. "The fairest solution would be to provide for 'national treatment' in the country where the publisher was resident, and in other countries for the same treatment as was normally accorded to citizens of that country, and also to provide for protection of the copyright in any country where the book might first be published": Statement of the Chairman, Mr. Larsen of Denmark, ibid.

[534] "Article [14] was revised by the Committee to bring this provision into conformity with existing Conventions on the subject": Ad Hoc Committee, "Second Session Report," at 12.

[535] The President of the Conference of Plenipotentiaries observed that "[t]he question of nationality entered into the matter, inasmuch as the recognition, for example, of a person's rights in his literary, scientific or artistic works depended on whether the country of which he was a national or in which he resided had signed the relevant international convention. To quote an example, it might reasonably be asked why a refugee from a country which had not acceded to such a convention and who resided in a country of asylum which had also not signed the convention should, when residing in Switzerland for a few days, be given the same protection in that respect as a Swiss national": Statement of the President, Mr. Larsen of Denmark, UN Doc. A/CONF.2/SR.7, July 5, 1951, at 21.

[536] "Report of the Drafting Committee," UN Doc. E/AC.32/L.40, Aug. 10, 1950 at Art. 9.

[537] As Weis concludes, "[t]he scope of the rights depends on the municipal law of the country concerned and the international conventions to which it is a party": Weis, *Travaux*, at 122.

The substantive scope of the interests protected by Art. 14 is not, however, restricted to the issue of literary and artistic rights on which debate focused.[538] To the contrary, the Refugee Convention expressly protects "industrial property," and was amended to add a reference to "inventions."[539] More generally, the nature of the interests protected includes the refugee's "literary, artistic *and scientific* rights [emphasis added]."[540] The only substantive reduction from the scope of protection originally proposed by the Secretary-General was to eliminate the references to "licences,"[541] "copyright,"[542] and "patents,"[543] decisions prompted by a desire to refer only to "the thing protected" and not to "a method of protection."[544] Instead of guaranteeing refugees access simply to these particular modes of protecting intellectual property rights, the drafters opted to insert a more comprehensive duty to grant refugees "the same protection" as enjoyed by citizens of the host country. Thus, refugees are entitled to protect and assert their intellectual property rights via licenses, patents, or copyright, in addition to any other means of protecting their interests which may be made available to nationals.[545]

[538] "The scope of Art. 14 does not produce any doubts: it is the totality of creations of the human mind": Robinson, *History*, at 108.

[539] The addition of this reference was not formally debated, but was included in the draft adopted at the second session of the Ad Hoc Committee: Ad Hoc Committee, "Second Session Report," at 18.

[540] Ad Hoc Committee, "First Session Report," at Annex I. The initial drafts were concerned predominantly with industrial property: see text above, at p. 830, n. 525.

[541] No reference to "licenses" was made in the French government's initial proposal for what became Art. 14: see text above, at p. 830, n. 525. While there was no debate specifically on this point, the reference was omitted from the text as adopted at the second session of the Ad Hoc Committee: Ad Hoc Committee, "Second Session Report," at 18.

[542] The British representative "reserved the position of his government regarding copyright provisions in the article" at the first session of the Ad Hoc Committee: Statement of Sir Leslie Brass, UN Doc. E/AC.32/SR.10, Jan. 24, 1950, at 8. While not the subject of a recorded discussion, the reference to copyright was omitted in the text adopted at that first session: Ad Hoc Committee, "First Session Report," at Annex I.

[543] The French representative expressed some concern at the decision of the Drafting Committee to delete the express reference to patents: Statement of Mr. Juvigny of France, UN Doc. E/AC.32/SR.41, Aug. 23, 1950, at 8. The American representative agreed with this concern: Statement of Mr. Henkin, ibid.

[544] Statement of Sir Leslie Brass of the United Kingdom, ibid. at 9. In response to the French and American proposal to reinsert a reference to patents, "[t]he Chairman felt that such an insertion would be illogical, since article [14] made no reference to the means of affording protection. In English, a 'patent' was a means of protecting an invention": Statement of the Chairman, Mr. Larsen of Denmark, ibid. at 8.

[545] For example, the British representative noted that "[i]n the case of a trademark, it was the registration which afforded protection and in the case of an invention it was the patent": Statement of Sir Leslie Brass of the United Kingdom, ibid. at 9.

The net utility of Art. 14 in assisting refugees to enforce their *industrial property* rights was nonetheless, at least initially, quite limited.[546] This is because the provisions of Berne's parallel treaty, the Paris Convention for the Protection of Industrial Property,[547] already provided protection superior to that granted by Art. 14 at the time of the Refugee Convention's adoption:

> Persons *within the jurisdiction* of each of the countries of the Union shall, as regards the protection of industrial property, enjoy in all other countries of the Union the advantages that their respective laws now grant, or may hereafter grant, to their nationals [emphasis added].[548]

In contrast, Art. 14 of the Refugee Convention only provides an exemption from reciprocity for refugees who are "habitually resident" in a state party, and entitles such refugees to enforce their rights abroad only to the same extent as citizens of their host country are able to do. At least in 1951, the only net benefit of Art. 14 for refugees residing in a state party to the Paris Convention would have been the Refugee Convention's insistence that the asylum country protect resident refugees' industrial property rights domestically on the same terms as it did those of its own citizens (but this was not generally a problem in any event).

Ironically, the benefits secured by refugees under Art. 14 of the Refugee Convention have today been effectively reversed. The Berne Convention was amended in 1967 to provide that "[a]uthors who are not nationals of one of the countries of the Union but who have their habitual residence in one of them shall, for the purposes of this Convention, be assimilated to nationals of that country."[549] Art. 14 of the Refugee Convention therefore does not improve upon this general language for purposes of enabling refugees to enforce their literary and artistic claims abroad.[550] On the other hand, amendments to the Paris Convention may have given rise to at least some need for the protections of Art. 14. The earlier language of that treaty, under which it was sufficient simply to be "within the jurisdiction" of a state party to claim exemption from reciprocity in other countries, was deleted.

---

[546] The debates of the Ad Hoc Committee were suspended on the motion of the Israeli delegate to obtain expert advice on the best way to protect intellectual property interests beyond those covered by the Berne Convention, but there is no indication of any effort substantively to tailor Art. 14 to address the broader range of issues: UN Doc. E/AC.32/SR.36, Aug. 15, 1950, at 23.

[547] 828 UNTS 11851, done Mar. 20, 1883, revised in Stockholm July 14, 1967 (Paris Convention).

[548] This is the language of the treaty as it existed at the time of the Refugee Convention's drafting, subsequent to the London Amendment of June 2, 1934: (1938) 4459 LNTS 19, at Art. 2(1).

[549] Berne Convention, at Art. 3(2).

[550] The Berne Convention is today subscribed to by 157 states: status of ratifications available at www.wipo.int (accessed Nov. 20, 2004).

Non-citizens must today be "domiciled . . . in the territory of one of the countries of the Union" to be treated as a citizen for purposes of enforcing their industrial property rights abroad. This is a marginally more exacting requirement than the Refugee Convention's rule that Art. 14 rights inhere in refugees who are "habitually resident" in a state party.[551]

The "habitual residence" language of Art. 14 was adopted just after the decision was made to grant refugees the same protection of intellectual property rights as enjoyed by citizens of their host country. Against the backdrop of that expansion of the scope of Art. 14, the drafters felt compelled to ensure that the beneficiary class was not "too wide in scope."[552] The Conference of Plenipotentiaries therefore dropped the reference to granting refugees the same rights as the nationals of their country of "residence" – understood in some European countries to include even a country of short-term de facto presence[553] – in favor of the present rule, which requires that intellectual property rights be protected by state parties on the same terms as those of the citizens of the refugee's country of "habitual residence."[554] Importantly, however, "habitual residence" was agreed not to be the equivalent of the more formal notion of "domicile."[555] While the drafters clearly intended that refugees who had stayed for no more than a short time in any

---

[551] On the other hand, the Paris Convention has been subscribed to by 168 states, more than are parties to the Refugee Convention: status of ratifications available at www.wipo.int (accessed Nov. 20, 2004).

[552] Statement of Mr. Fritzer of Austria, UN Doc. A/CONF.2/SR.7, July 5, 1951, at 19.

[553] For example, the Austrian representative noted that "[u]nder the existing text [which granted rights to refugees based on 'residence'], a refugee would be entitled to enjoy the protection referred to even if he only stayed in the country for a few days. In the opinion of the Austrian delegation, it was necessary to specify in the text that a refugee must be more than a temporary visitor. He was therefore proposing that the words 'in which he is resident' should be replaced by the phrase 'in which he has his habitual residence or, if he has no habitual residence, in which he resides'": Statement of Mr. Fritzer of Austria, ibid. See also Statement of Mr. Herment of Belgium, UN Doc. A/CONF.2/SR.8, July 5, 1951, at 5: "Two types of residence were indeed recognized: habitual residence and temporary residence."

[554] "The term 'habitual residence' was introduced to distinguish it from purely temporary residence": Weis, *Travaux*, at 123. See also Robinson, *History*, at 107: "The change [to refer to 'habitual residence'] was made to denote that a stay of short duration was not sufficient."

[555] Sweden pressed for the incorporation of the notion of domicile (see Statement of Mr. Petren of Sweden, UN Doc. A/CONF.2/SR.7, July 5, 1951, at 19), but the French government objected that "the concept of 'domicile,' entailing as it did certain disadvantages from the legal point of view, involved difficulties": Statement of Mr. Rochefort of France, ibid. at 20. The Belgian representative similarly argued that "it would not be possible to require of a refugee that he possess a domicile": Statement of Mr. Herment of Belgium, UN Doc. A/CONF.2/SR.8, July 5, 1951, at 5. More fundamentally, the representative of Colombia provided a principled rationale for referring to habitual residence rather than to domicile in the context of Art. 14. "There was a difference between rights

asylum country could not yet benefit from Art. 14,[556] they were equally emphatic that intellectual property rights should be protected as soon as the refugee had established some form of de facto ongoing presence in a state party.[557] As such, the Refugee Convention has present-day value as a means

dependent on personal status and other civil rights, for example, property rights such as those under discussion. In the former case, the concept of 'domicile' might be suitable, but the concept of 'residence' was preferable so far as artistic rights and industrial property were concerned": Statement of Mr. Giraldo-Jaramillo of Colombia, UN Doc. A/CONF.2/SR.7, July 5, 1951, at 20. This reasoning was endorsed by the representative of the United Kingdom, who observed that "[t]he use of the well-known and clearly defined term 'domicile' was appropriate in article [12], as it constituted a criterion for determining the laws that should apply in respect of the personal status of a refugee. As, however, the restriction aimed at in article [14] was merely in respect of the period of residence in a receiving country, he considered it would be wrong to introduce the term 'domicile' into the text of that article": Statement of Mr. Hoare of the United Kingdom, UN Doc. A/CONF.2/SR.8, July 5, 1951, at 6. Thus, Robinson concludes that "the exercise of the right was not made dependent on 'permanent residence' or 'domicile' because it was felt that it was too far-reaching [a] concept for the enjoyment of civil rights": Robinson, *History*, at 107.

[556] The approach initially proposed to the Conference of Plenipotentiaries by the Austrian representative would have granted intellectual property rights equivalent to those enjoyed by the nationals of the country "in which [the refugee] has his habitual residence or, if he has no habitual residence, in which he resides": Statement of Mr. Fritzer of Austria, UN Doc. A/CONF.2/SR.7, July 5, 1951, at 19, citing UN Doc. A/CONF.2/38. In eventually agreeing to drop his opposition to this form of words, the Swedish representative insisted that "the words 'or, if he has no habitual residence, in which he resided' [be] deleted": Statement of Mr. Petren of Sweden, UN Doc. A/CONF.2/SR.8, July 5, 1951, at 7. The Austrian representative "accepted the Swedish amendment to his proposal": Statement of Mr. Fritzer of Austria, ibid.

[557] "[I]f 'domicile' seemed too narrow, and 'residence' too wide a concept, 'habitual residence' constituted a happy medium ... While it was true that [the phrase] might lack legal precision, it should be remembered that refugees found themselves in a *de facto* position before they enjoyed a *de jure* position": Statement of Mr. Rochefort of France, UN Doc. A/CONF.2/SR.8, July 5, 1951, at 7–8. See also Statement of Mr. Hoare of the United Kingdom, ibid. at 6: "[T]he restriction aimed at in Article [14] was merely in respect of the period of residence in a receiving country." Even the Swedish representative, who had argued for the alternative language of "domicile," acknowledged that "the Swedish delegation was mainly concerned with eliminating the idea of residence pure and simply," in consequence of which it could accept the Austrian reference to "habitual residence": Statement of Mr. Petren of Sweden, ibid. at 5. In line with these understandings, Grahl-Madsen concludes that "refugees do not have to have a permanent residence or domicile. With the exception of new refugees who have not yet habitual residence anywhere, it is difficult to envisage a refugee having no habitual residence": Grahl-Madsen, *Commentary*, at 60. Robinson notes simply that "'[h]abitual residence' means residence of a certain duration, but it implies much less than permanent residence": Robinson, *History*, at 107. This leads him logically to conclude that "it is difficult to envisage a refugee having no habitual residence except new refugees who did not yet succeed in establishing 'habitual residence' anywhere": ibid.

of protecting the literary and artistic property rights of refugees who are habitually resident, but not domiciled, in a state party.

More critically, Art. 14 also grants refugees rights in relation to systems for the protection of intellectual property which have emerged since the drafting of the Refugee Convention, such as the specialized treaty regime for the protection of the performers and producers of "phonograms" (audio recordings). Under the Rome Convention of 1961, the ability of producers and performers to enforce abroad their intellectual property interests in phonograms – that is, in the performance itself, rather than in the musical score on which the performance was based – is reserved for persons who are "nationals" of a contracting state party.[558] The same is true of the more specialized treaties which build upon the Rome Convention, including the 1971 accord prohibiting the unauthorized duplication of phonograms[559] and the more recent 1996 World International Property Organization treaty on the same subject.[560] Yet in any state party to the Refugee Convention, Art. 14 requires that refugees be treated as citizens of their state of habitual residence. In the result, refugees are entitled to enforce their phonogram rights in a country that is also a party to the Rome Convention on the same terms as a national of their host country.

This ability of Art. 14 to provide a safeguard against any enforcement regime that might not enfranchise refugees is of continuing importance. Arguably the most important contemporary treaty on the subject, the World Trade Organization's recent Agreement on Trade-Related Aspects of Intellectual Property Rights, Including Trade in Counterfeit Goods ("TRIPS Agreement"),[561] requires only that the "nationals" of state parties be

---

[558] International Convention for the Protection of Performers [and] Producers of Phonograms and Broadcasting Organisations, done Oct. 26, 1961, entered into force May 18, 1964 (Rome Convention), at Art. 2(1).

[559] "Each Contracting State shall protect producers of phonograms who are nationals of other Contracting States against the making of duplicates without the consent of the producer and against the importation of such duplicates, provided that any such making or importation is for the purpose of distribution to the public, and against the distribution of such duplicates to the public": Convention for the Protection of Producers of Phonograms Against Unauthorized Duplication of their Phonograms, done Oct. 29, 1971, at Art. 2.

[560] "Contracting Parties shall accord the protection provided under this Treaty to the performers and producers of phonograms who are nationals of other Contracting Parties": WIPO Performances and Phonograms Treaty, done Dec. 20, 1996, at Art. 3(1).

[561] 33 ILM 81, Dec. 15, 1993 (TRIPS Agreement). "TRIPS expands the scope of GATT's most-favored nation and national-treatment principles to intellectual property rights as they affect the trade in products protected by such rights. Most-favored nation treatment requires that any protection and rights granted to *nationals* of any Member must be accorded to *nationals* of all Members [emphasis added]": N. Telecki, "The Role of Special 301 in the Development of International Protection of Intellectual Property Rights After the Uruguay Round," (1996) 14 *Boston University International Law Journal* 187, at 193.

guaranteed the right to enforce their intellectual property rights,[562] except to the extent that one of the core predecessor intellectual property treaties contains rules to assimilate non-citizen residents.[563] In the case of phonograms, the TRIPS Agreement simply defers to the narrow definition of the Rome Convention. Yet by virtue of Art. 14 of the Refugee Convention, this definition cannot be relied upon to exclude habitually resident refugees from access to enforcement procedures.

It remains, however, as both Weis and Grahl-Madsen conclude, that a refugee who has yet to establish habitual residence in any state party would be entitled only to whatever protection of intellectual property rights is enjoyed by aliens generally, in line with the residual standard of Art. 7(1) of the Refugee Convention.[564] Those who view the Universal Declaration of Human Rights as a source of law[565] have suggested that this residual protection might be based on its Art. 27(2),[566] said to establish that "copyright ... has been given the rank of a human right."[567] This position is, however, difficult to reconcile to the more cautious approach taken in the formally binding Covenant on Economic, Social and Cultural Rights. Art. 15(1)(c) of the Covenant, which comes closest to a duty to protect intellectual property rights, actually establishes only a "recognition" of the right of everyone "*[t]o benefit from the protection of* the moral and material interests resulting from any scientific, literary or artistic production of which he is the author [emphasis added]."[568]

Effectively, this amounts to a duty of non-discrimination,[569] requiring only that any exclusion of non-citizens from systems for enforcing

---

[562] "Each Member shall accord to the nationals of other Members treatment no less favourable than that it accords to its own nationals with regard to the protection of intellectual property": TRIPS Agreement, at Art. 3.

[563] Ibid. at Art. 1(3).

[564] Grahl-Madsen, *Commentary*, at 61; Weis, *Travaux*, at 123.

[565] A more cautious position on this question is taken here: see chapter 1.2.3 above, particularly at pp. 44–46.

[566] "Everyone has the right to the protection of the moral and material interests resulting from any scientific, literary or artistic production of which he is the author": Universal Declaration of Human Rights, UNGA Res. 217A(III), Dec. 10, 1948 (Universal Declaration), at Art. 27(2).

[567] I. Szabo, *Cultural Rights* (1974), at 45.

[568] Economic, Social and Cultural Covenant, at Art. 15(1)(c).

[569] As Melander writes, "[i]n spite of the impression given by reading the UN Charter, stressing cultural rights as an essential part of UN activities, it must be admitted that little attention has been paid to cultural rights, at least in comparison with other human rights": G. Melander, "Article 27," in A. Eide et al. eds., *The Universal Declaration of Human Rights: A Commentary* 429 (1992), at 429. Nor have private property rights been codified as a matter of binding international law: see chapter 4.5.1 above, at pp. 518–521. But it may be difficult for a state to justify withholding the protection of the law from non-citizens under general norms of non-discrimination law: see chapter 2.5.5 above.

intellectual property rights be justifiable. In view of the breadth of the "reasonableness" doctrine as conceived in international law and, in particular, taking account of the broad margin of appreciation granted states,[570] it is not self-evident that an asylum country's decision to withhold enforcement rights until habitual residence is established would be deemed discriminatory. Much less is there any guarantee that the refusal of a third state to allow refugees to enforce intellectual property rights in their courts would be adjudged discriminatory, given the accepted pattern of dispensing with reciprocity requirements only on the basis of express treaty obligations to that effect. As Eide concludes, the substantive bedrock for claims of this kind will normally need to be found in the more specialized intellectual property treaties,[571] assuming these have been adhered to by the country in which the refugee seeks to advance his or her claim.

In sum, the primary purpose of Art. 14 as conceived by the drafters – to allow refugees to enforce their literary and artistic rights outside their country of citizenship despite the prevalence of reciprocity requirements – is today largely superseded by the amended Berne Convention and the TRIPS Agreement (which incorporates by reference the expanded Berne definition, assimilating habitually resident non-citizens to nationals). But Art. 14 remains of value in ensuring that the industrial property rights of refugees who are habitually resident, even if not domiciled, in a state party can be enforced outside the asylum country. It also ensures that refugees benefit from new forms of intellectual property protection, such as that established to protect performance rights (phonograms), even when, as in the case of the pertinent Rome Convention, non-citizens are not otherwise enfranchised. Finally, the Refugee Convention's Art. 14 expressly precludes any effort by an asylum state to deny habitually resident refugees access to any system it offers its own citizens for enforcing their intellectual property rights, thereby avoiding the need for refugees to seek access on the basis of more fungible non-discrimination rules.

6.6 International travel

With few exceptions, international travel has long required the possession of a passport issued by a national government. Yet refugees often arrive without a passport from their country of origin, either because they were incapable of (safely) securing that document before departure, or because its destruction was effectively compelled to avoid visa controls, carrier sanctions, or other

---

[570] See chapter 2.5.5 above, at pp. 129–145.
[571] A. Eide, "Cultural Rights as Individual Human Rights," in A. Eide et al. eds., *Economic, Social and Cultural Rights: A Textbook* 236 (1995).

impediments to their escape and entry into an asylum state.[572] Even once inside the asylum country, refugees are not free to apply for a passport from the consular authorities of their country of origin, since to do so risks the cessation of their refugee status in accordance with Art. 1(C)(1) of the Convention.[573] In such circumstances, a refugee "would therefore be unable to leave the initial reception country if a document replacing the passport had not been established for their benefit."[574]

The Refugee Convention therefore provides for the issue to refugees of a Convention Travel Document (CTD) intended to serve the purpose of a national passport. UNHCR reports that while most state parties to the Refugee Convention make these documents available,[575] some states have failed to implement the legislative or administrative changes required to ensure the provision of travel documents to refugees.[576] Zambia, for example, has issued only internal identification documents to refugees for fear of incurring responsibility for their welfare while abroad.[577] Nigeria has refused to issue travel documents to refugees wishing to study abroad, purportedly on

---

[572] The drafters recognized that the use of false documents to seek asylum was sometimes unavoidable, and was not a basis for the penalization of refugees so long as the requirements of Art. 31(1) are met: see chapter 4.2.2 above, at pp. 405–406.

[573] "This Convention shall cease to apply to any person falling under the terms of section A if . . . [h]e has voluntarily re-availed himself of the protection of the country of his nationality": Refugee Convention, at Art. 1(C)(1). Indeed, the same clause may even be interpreted to authorize the termination of refugee status in the event a refugee who arrived with a national passport presents his or her national passport in order to secure entry into a third country. UNHCR seeks to limit the scope of Art. 1(C)(1) by, for example, arguing that there is "re-availment" only when a passport is both applied for and received, not simply when it is used for travel abroad: see UNHCR, *Handbook on Procedures and Criteria for Determining Refugee Status* (1979, re-edited 1992) (UNHCR, *Handbook*), at paras. 118–125. But this construction may be contested on the grounds that the presentation of a government's passport in order to secure entry into a third state amounts, in law, to an invocation of the issuing state's protective authority. Lambert observes that "[t]he Convention Travel Document (CTD) should be used in place of a national passport or identity card by the refugee; otherwise there is a serious risk that he or she will lose refugee status": Lambert, *Seeking Asylum*, at 163.

[574] Secretary-General, "Memorandum," at 41.

[575] UNHCR, "Note on follow-up to the earlier Conclusion of the Executive Committee on Travel Documents for Refugees," UN Doc. EC/SCP/48, July 3, 1987 (UNHCR, "Travel Documents Follow-Up"), at para. 2.

[576] Ibid. at para. 4. More recently, UNHCR pointed to administrative difficulties experienced by refugees in Slovenia (but "this problem has now been resolved"), and delays in the issuance of CTDs in states such as Poland: UNHCR, *Integration Rights and Practices with Regard to Recognized Refugees in the Central European Countries*, Eur. Series, vol. 5(1), July 2000, at 327.

[577] F. Ohaegbulom, "Human Rights and the Refugee Situation in Africa," in G. Shepherd and V. Nanda eds., *Human Rights and Third World Development* 197 (Ohaegbulom, "Refugee Situation in Africa") (1994), at 197.

the grounds that such documents are only to be granted to permanent residents.[578] A more common problem, however, is the provision to refugees of only non-standardized travel documents which do not include a clause guaranteeing the right of the refugee to reenter the issuing country. Kenya, Tanzania, and Uganda are among the states "that issue one-way travel documents that do not include an automatic right of return."[579] As UNHCR reports, "restrictions on the validity of the return clause or refusal of readmission can seriously reduce the value of the travel documents by discouraging other States from granting visas, and could even have wider consequences, e.g. jeopardizing educational schemes for refugees."[580]

In some states, including Switzerland and the United Kingdom, a travel document is not issued until refugee status has been formally recognized.[581] UNHCR reports that most governments will not issue a refugee travel document to a refugee who lives in another country, though they may do so in exceptional circumstances where it cannot be obtained from the country of residence.[582] There may also be geographical restrictions on the validity of refugee travel documents. Those issued by the United States, for example, are not valid for travel to a list of countries from which that country is politically estranged.[583] More frequently, travel is simply prohibited to the country of origin.[584]

There are often significant delays in the granting[585] or renewal[586] of travel documents. The ability of a refugee to secure a travel document may also be

---

[578] P. Tiao and Nigerian Civil Liberties Organization, "The Status of Refugee Rights in Nigeria" (1992), at 16.

[579] Ohaegbulom, "Refugee Situation in Africa." See also P. van Krieken, "African Refugee Law," (1981) 45/46 *Yearbook of the Association of Attenders and Alumni of the Hague Academy of International Law* 133, at n. 37, who writes that in Africa, "the regulations concerning the return clauses are quite often not applied correctly." The same point has been made by UNHCR, "Travel Documents for Refugees," paper presented at the Conference on the Legal and Social Aspects of African Refugee Problems, Oct. 1967, UN Doc. AFR/REF/CONF.1967/No.5, at 1.

[580] UNHCR, "Travel Documents Follow-Up," at para. 11.

[581] Lambert, *Seeking Asylum*, at 167.   [582] UNHCR, "Implementation," at 10.

[583] G. Goodwin-Gill, *The Refugee in International Law* (1994) (Goodwin-Gill, *Refugee in International Law*), at 302, n. 44.

[584] This is the case for Austria, Belgium, Denmark, France, Germany, Greece, Ireland, Italy, Luxembourg, the Netherlands, Spain, Sweden, and the United Kingdom: European Council on Refugee and Exiles, "Survey Provisions on Travel Documents and Visas for Refugees in the European Union" (2000), at 5, 9, 15, 26, 31, 35, 39, 42, 46, 51, 61, 64, and 68.

[585] "In certain countries . . . applications can take from six to twelve months to process. Such protracted periods lead to obvious hardship for refugees, and may delay resettlement and lead to loss of educational or employment opportunities": UNHCR, "Travel Documents Follow-Up," at para. 7.

[586] A number of states have not empowered their diplomatic or consular authorities to renew or extend travel documents: ibid. at para. 12.

compromised by disagreements between governments about which has the responsibility to issue documents when a particular refugee is thought to have ties to more than one state party.[587] Only in Europe has a comprehensive set of arrangements been put in place to resolve the details of transfer of responsibility to issue refugee travel documents.[588]

Valid refugee travel documents are reported to be routinely recognized by governments as the equivalent of a passport.[589] With the exception of state parties to the 1959 European Agreement on the Abolition of Visas for Refugees,[590] however, most countries require refugees granted a CTD also to hold valid transit or entry visas.[591] In general, issuing governments guarantee the right of the CTD holder to reenter their territory for the duration of the document's validity, though one state is reported to require all refugees to secure a reentry visa, while another requires a reentry visa only of refugees returning from a country whose nationals also need a visa.[592]

> **Refugee Convention, Art. 28   Travel documents**
>
> 1. The Contracting States shall issue to refugees lawfully staying in their territory travel documents for the purpose of travel outside their territory, unless compelling reasons of national security or public order otherwise require, and the provisions of the Schedule to this Convention shall apply with respect to such documents. The Contracting States may issue such a travel document to any other refugee in their territory; they shall in particular give sympathetic consideration to the issue of such a travel document to refugees in their territory who are unable to obtain a travel document from the country of their lawful residence.
>
> 2. Travel documents issued to refugees under previous international agreements by parties thereto shall be recognized and treated by the Contracting States in the same way as if they had been issued pursuant to this article.

---

[587] Ibid. at paras. 13, 14.

[588] Under the European Agreement on Transfer of Responsibility for Refugees, 107 ETS, done Oct. 16, 1980 (European Agreement on Transfer of Responsibility for Refugees), responsibility is considered to be transferred after two years of legal and continuous stay in a second state, or sooner if the refugee has been granted a permanent stay, or allowed to stay for a period that exceeds the validity of the travel document upon which he or she entered the country.

[589] UNHCR, "Implementation," at 10.

[590] 31 ETS, done Apr. 20, 1959, entered into force Apr. 9, 1960. This agreement exempts refugees from visa requirements for visits of under three months. There are also various bilateral arrangements among European states to similar effect: UNHCR, "Travel Documents Follow-Up," at para. 20.

[591] UNHCR, "Implementation," at 11.   [592] Ibid. at 10–11.

Refugee Convention, Schedule

1. (1) The travel document referred to in article 28 of this Convention shall be similar to the specimen annexed hereto.

    (2) The document shall be made out in at least two languages, one of which shall be English or French.

2. Subject to the regulations obtaining in the country of issue, children may be included in the travel document of a parent or, in exceptional circumstances, of another adult refugee.

3. The fees charged for issue of the document shall not exceed the lowest scale of charges for national passports.

4. Save in special or exceptional cases, the document shall be made valid for the largest possible number of countries.

5. The document shall have a validity of either one or two years, at the discretion of the issuing authority.

6. (1) The renewal or extension of the validity of the document is a matter for the authority which issued it, so long as the holder has not established lawful residence in another territory and resides lawfully in the territory of the said authority. The issue of a new document is, under the same conditions, a matter for the authority which issued the former document.

    (2) Diplomatic or consular authorities, specially authorized for the purpose, shall be empowered to extend, for a period not exceeding six months, the validity of travel documents issued by their Governments.

    (3) The Contracting States shall give sympathetic consideration to renewing or extending the validity of travel documents or issuing new documents to refugees no longer lawfully resident in their territory who are unable to obtain a travel document from the country of their lawful residence.

7. The Contracting States shall recognize the validity of the documents issued in accordance with the provisions of article 28 of this Convention.

8. The competent authorities of the country to which the refugee desires to proceed shall, if they are prepared to admit him and if a visa is required, affix a visa on the document of which he is the holder.

9. (1) The Contracting States undertake to issue transit visas to refugees who have obtained visas for a territory of final destination.

    (2) The issue of such visas may be refused on grounds which would justify refusal of a visa to any alien.

10. The fees for the issue of exit, entry or transit visas shall not exceed the lowest scale of charges for visas on foreign passports.

11. When a refugee has lawfully taken up residence in the territory of another Contracting State, the responsibility for the issue of a new document, under the terms and conditions of article 28, shall be that of the competent authority of that territory, to which the refugee shall be entitled to apply.

12. The authority issuing a new document shall withdraw the old document and shall return it to the country of issue if it is stated in the document that it should be so returned; otherwise it shall withdraw and cancel the document.

13. (1) Each Contracting State undertakes that the holder of a travel document issued by it in accordance with article 28 of this Convention shall be readmitted to its territory at any time during the period of its validity.

(2) Subject to the provisions of the preceding sub-paragraph, a Contracting State may require the holder of the document to comply with such formalities as may be prescribed in regard to exit from or return to its territory.

(3) The Contracting States reserve the right, in exceptional cases, or in cases where the refugee's stay is authorized for a specific period, when issuing the document, to limit the period during which the refugee may return to a period of not less than three months.

14. Subject only to the terms of paragraph 13, the provisions of this Schedule in no way affect the laws and regulations governing the conditions of admission to, transit through, residence and establishment in, and departure from, the territories of the Contracting States.

15. Neither the issue of the document nor the entries made thereon determine or affect the status of the holder, particularly as regards nationality.

16. The issue of the document does not in any way entitle the holder to the protection of the diplomatic or consular authorities of the country of issue, and does not confer on these authorities a right of protection.

Refugee Convention, Art. 11   Refugee seamen

In the case of refugees regularly serving as crew members on board a ship flying the flag of a Contracting State, that State shall give sympathetic consideration to their establishment on its territory and the issue of travel documents to them or their temporary admission to its territory particularly with a view to facilitating their establishment in another country.

Recommendation A of the Conference of Plenipotentiaries
The Conference, [c]onsidering that the issue and recognition of travel documents is necessary to facilitate the movement of refugees, and in particular their resettlement; [u]rges Governments which are parties to the Inter-Governmental Agreement on Refugee Travel Documents signed in London [on] 15 October 1946, or which recognize travel documents issued in accordance with the Agreement, to continue to issue or to recognize such travel documents, and to extend the issue of such documents to refugees as defined in article 1 of the Convention relating to the Status of Refugees or to recognize the travel documents so issued to such persons, until they shall have undertaken obligations under article 28 of the said Convention.

Civil and Political Covenant, Art. 12
    . . .
    2. Everyone shall be free to leave any country, including his own.
    3. The above-mentioned right[ ] shall not be subject to any restrictions except those which are provided by law, are necessary to protect national security, public order (*ordre public*), public health or morals or the rights and freedoms of others, and are consistent with the other rights recognized in the present Covenant.
    4. No one shall be arbitrarily deprived of the right to enter his own country.

Despite its rather simple title, Art. 28 of the Convention is about much more than just the issuance to refugees of a Convention Travel Document (CTD). In line with earlier refugee treaties, this article commits governments to administer an interstate system which dispenses with the need for passports for travel by refugees between and through state parties. By virtue of Art. 28 and its Schedule, governments oblige themselves not only to issue CTDs, but more importantly to honor the refugee travel documents issued by other state parties, to make transit visas available to refugees as required, and to re-admit the holders of refugee travel documents issued by them. The net result is to establish a unified regime for international freedom of movement that exists in parallel to the more general passport-based system.

The CTD system is intended both to enable refugees "to travel on business or on a holiday"[593] and, perhaps more importantly, to make it possible for refugees to move beyond their state of first asylum in search of a durable home. As the British representative to the Ad Hoc Committee succinctly

---

[593] Statement of Mr. Hoeg of Denmark, UN Doc. A/CONF.2/SR.17, July 12, 1951, at 9.

observed, "[o]ne object of a travel document [is] to allow a refugee to go out and find his feet in another country."[594] The facilitation of onward movement was, indeed, the primary goal of earlier refugee treaties, some of which provided refugees with few benefits beyond a travel document.[595]

In line with most earlier treaties, states are only obliged to issue a travel document to a refugee who is lawfully staying in their territory. The practice of states such as Britain and Switzerland, which issue the CTD only after formal status verification, is therefore in compliance with the Convention. So too may be the Nigerian decision to deny CTDs to refugees with no more than a temporary right to stay in that country. But the importance attached to enabling refugees to seek a home beyond the first asylum country is particularly clear from the decision taken to grant states the right – though not to impose a duty upon them – to issue CTDs even to refugees not "lawfully staying" in their territory, and therefore not able formally to claim the benefit of Art. 28. The authorization of states to issue travel documents to "any other refugee in their territory" was a departure from predecessor agreements, which allowed no more than transitional exceptions to the rule that only refugees who were "lawfully staying" in a state party were entitled to receive a travel document.[596]

The origin of the expanded authority was an intervention by the Danish representative to the Ad Hoc Committee, who raised the question of travel documents for refugees "who had just arrived in the initial reception country":[597]

---

[594] Statement of Sir Leslie Brass of the United Kingdom, UN Doc. E/AC.32/SR.39, Aug. 21, 1950, at 10.

[595] "The problem of travel documents was the one with which the concern of the comity of nations for refugees actually began. The July 5, 1922 Arrangement ... , that of May 31, 1924 ... , [and] the Arrangements of May 12, 1926, June 30, 1928, and July 30, 1935, dealt exclusively with travel documents. The 1933 and 1938 Conventions also imposed on the Contracting Parties the obligations to issue travel documents, and the first post-World War II agreement, that of October 15, 1946, again treated of travel documents only": Robinson, *History*, at 135.

[596] Under the Agreement relating to the issue of a travel document to refugees who are the concern of the Inter-Governmental Committee on Refugees, 11 UNTS 150, at 73 (London Agreement), at Art. 2, there was only a transitional exception for refugees already present in a state party (though not "lawfully staying" there) as of the date the agreement entered into force. The same approach was taken in the 1938 Refugee Convention, at Art. 3(1)(b). The 1933 Refugee Convention, however, took a more general liberal stance, requiring the issuance of a refugee travel document to any refugee "residing regularly" in a state's territory: 1933 Refugee Convention, at Art. 2.

[597] Statement of Mr. Larsen of Denmark, UN Doc. E/AC.32/SR.16, Jan. 30, 1950, at 11. Interestingly, though, the Secretary-General had proposed a lower general standard of attachment for issuance of a CTD, namely that a refugee be only "regularly resident" in the territory of a state party: Secretary-General, "Memorandum," at 41. See also France,

He took as an example the hypothetical case of a German refugee arriving clandestinely in Denmark, without identity papers, and anxious to travel to the United States for family or other reasons. In accordance with paragraph 1 of article [28] as adopted, Denmark would not issue him travel documents, because he did not reside regularly in that country. If, therefore, the real objective was to protect the interests of refugees effectively, it seemed expedient to make some provision whereby Denmark would be able to grant such a refugee a travel document ...

He therefore proposed that article [28] should be so amended that the High Contracting Parties would be able to grant travel documents to all refugees in their territory, whatever their status in the eyes of the law, with the sole stipulation that they should not be regularly resident in another country.[598]

Mr. Larsen concluded his plea by noting the critical importance of travel documents to enabling refugees to "test the waters" in their intended country of asylum:

A refugee who arrived in Denmark, for example, and was immediately granted a travel document, could go for a certain period of time to the country where he intended to settle; while there, he could obtain authorization to reside there regularly. On the other hand, if such a refugee had no freedom of movement but was confined to Denmark owing to the lack of a travel document, it would be very difficult for him to study the possibility of settling elsewhere.[599]

It was therefore agreed that in the interest of promoting freedom of onward movement, the authority to issue travel documents should extend to all refugees in a state's territory,[600] even if there only for a brief period of

---

"Draft Convention," at 7. Thus, the decision to adopt a higher mandatory standard (lawful stay) together with a lower optional standard (any refugee) was in some sense reflective of a more general desire among some delegates to liberalize access to the CTD system overall.

[598] Statement of Mr. Larsen of Denmark, UN Doc. E/AC.32/SR.16, Jan. 30, 1950, at 11–12.

[599] Ibid. at 14.

[600] States are not, however, entitled to issue a CTD to a refugee not physically present on their territory. At the Conference of Plenipotentiaries, the President opined that "the phrase 'in their territory' ... was unnecessarily restrictive. He failed to see why a Contracting State should be prevented from issuing a travel document to a refugee outside its borders": Statement of the President, Mr. Larsen of Denmark, UN Doc. A/CONF.2/SR.12, July 9, 1951, at 5. No other state expressed support for this view, and no relevant amendment to the text of Art. 28 was proposed. The insistence on a territorial connection may reflect the view, articulated in the Ad Hoc Committee, that "the article would be weakened if it were framed [by deleting the words 'in their territory'] so as to permit Contracting States to issue travel documents to refugees who were in no way connected with them ... [There were] obvious difficulties of obtaining reliable certificates of identity": Statement of Sir Leslie Brass of the United Kingdom, UN Doc. E/AC.32/SR.42, Aug. 24, 1950, at 6.

time,[601] and whether their refugee status has been formally verified or not.[602] Indeed, it was subsequently decided that any state party might rely on this discretionary authority to issue travel documents to a refugee faced with practical impediments to obtaining them from his or her country of usual residence,[603] as well as to refugee seamen who in many cases lack a sufficient territorial connection to any country to entitle them to a travel document.[604] But each state is entitled to decide for itself[605] whether it wishes to issue a CTD to a refugee not

[601] The representative of the International Refugee Organization "warmly supported the opinion of the representative of Denmark. If the High Contracting Parties could grant travel documents to refugees not regularly resident in their territory, that would give many refugees an opportunity to settle permanently, in full knowledge of the circumstances, and therefore in the best possible conditions": Statement of Mr. Weis of the IRO, UN Doc. E/AC.32/SR.16, Jan. 30, 1950, at 14–15.

[602] Robinson opines that a state may issue travel documents to, for example, refugees who "are there on a temporary basis only or even illegally": Robinson, *History*, at 136. See also Weis, *Travaux*, at 266; and Grahl-Madsen, *Commentary*, at 128–129. UNHCR also clearly views it as permissible to issue a CTD before recognition of refugee status, as it has observed that "*[s]ome states restrict the issue of CTDs to persons who have been formally determined by them to be Convention refugees* . . . Thus persons who have been allowed to remain in the country under 'humanitarian' programmes or who have been admitted under non-refugee quotas are not eligible for CTDs, even though they may, in fact, fulfil the criteria for refugee status. These persons are normally granted certificates of identity or other aliens travel documents, which may have . . . disadvantages[emphasis added]": UNHCR, "Travel Documents Follow-Up," at para. 5.

[603] "Under the recommendation, if a person were in the United Kingdom, for example, he could, though lawfully resident elsewhere, apply to the United Kingdom for travel documents": Statement of Mr. Henkin of the United States, UN Doc. E/AC.32/SR.41, Aug. 23, 1950, at 20.

[604] "It was . . . suggested that the time spent by seamen serving in a ship belonging to a given country should count towards the period of residence necessary to secure the right to travel documents. He realized that it might be difficult for many governments represented at the Conference to enter into a specific commitment of that kind; if so, perhaps the suggestion might be incorporated in a separate recommendation": Statement of Mr. Mowat of the International Labor Organization, UN Doc. A/CONF.2/SR.12, July 9, 1951, at 5. When the ILO again raised this issue, it was determined that "the issue it raised was wider than that dealt with in article [28], and should perhaps form the subject of a special general article": Statement of the President, Mr. Larsen of Denmark, UN Doc. A/CONF.2/SR.17, July 12, 1951, at 16. In response to a French proposal, it was agreed that time spent aboard a state party's vessel "would count" towards establishing lawful stay, but not if the seaman "had never set foot on [the state party's] soil": Statement of Mr. Hoare of the United Kingdom, UN Doc. A/CONF.2/SR.30, July 20, 1951, at 9–10. To enable refugee seamen to establish at least this minimum physical connection to the primary territory of the vessel's flag state, Art. 11 as ultimately approved recommends "their temporary admission to [the flag state's] territory particularly with a view to facilitating their establishment in another country": Refugee Convention, at Art. 11.

[605] "It would, however, be going too far to make such a thing obligatory, since to do so would involve States in the further obligation of re-admitting refugees, who might have spent only a few weeks in their territory, if they were unable to remain in the country to which they went": Statement of Sir Leslie Brass of the United Kingdom, UN Doc. E/AC.32/SR.16, Jan. 30, 1950,

able to meet the lawful stay requirement[606] because of the duty, described below, to readmit any refugee to whom a travel document has been issued.[607]

This broader discretionary authority under Art. 28(1) may today be of value to states in a way not initially considered. Since the drafting of the Refugee Convention, states have adopted Art. 12(2) of the Civil and Political Covenant, which provides that "[e]veryone shall be free to leave any country, including his own." Recognizing that the right to leave one's country is essentially meaningless without access to the documentation required for travel abroad, the Human Rights Committee has determined that Art. 12(2) entails a positive duty on the part of a state to issue its citizens with travel documents, unless there is valid justification to withhold same.[608] While the Committee's relevant holdings to date have been addressed only to the rights of citizens, Nowak correctly observes that "[f]reedom to leave and emigrate is available to *everyone*, i.e. to nationals and aliens alike, and is not conditioned on lawful residency within the territory of a State Party."[609] It thus follows

---

at 12–13. He subsequently successfully proposed the use of the word "may" in the second sentence of Art. 28(1), making it clear that the authority is strictly permissive: ibid. at 15.

[606] A difficult issue is whether a state may exercise its discretion to issue a CTD to a refugee denied a CTD in his or her country of lawful stay on grounds of a threat to public order or national security (as is expressly authorized by Art. 28). In Grahl-Madsen's view, the discretionary authority to issue a CTD to a refugee who is physically present, though not lawfully staying, in a country's territory "applies if the country of lawful residence is not a party to the Refugee Convention or any of the other arrangements relating to travel documents for refugees ... or if the country of lawful residence has made reservations to the effect that it will not issue travel documents to refugees ... But what if the country of lawful residence has refused to issue travel documents by invoking 'compelling reasons of national security or public order'? The question was, possibly by an oversight, not discussed by the Conference ... [But] if a person is considered a 'security risk' or worse in one country, another State may consider him otherwise, and two different States do not necessarily have to see eye to eye on matters listed under the admittedly vague term 'public order.' Very often one State will not be able to know why a travel document has not been issued by another State ... [Therefore] if a country chooses to issue a travel document under any of these provisions, it seems that it has every right to do so, and that the validity of the travel document will not be the least affected by the fact that the issue of a travel document has been refused for cogent reasons by the country of lawful residence": Grahl-Madsen, *Commentary*, at 129–130. There is, however, no duty on the second state to issue a travel document in such circumstances. "It could hardly be the intention of the Conference to request one state to issue a travel document to a resident of another state if the latter refuses to issue the document for compelling reasons of national security or public order": Robinson, *History*, at 137.

[607] See text below, at pp. 865–870.

[608] M. Mubanga-Chipoya, "Analysis of the current trends and developments regarding the right to leave any country including one's own, and to return to one's own country, and to some other rights or considerations arising therefrom," UN Doc. E/CN.4/Sub.2/1987/10, at 21 ff.

[609] M. Nowak, *UN Covenant on Civil and Political Rights* (1993) (Nowak, *ICCPR Commentary*), at 204.

logically that a state in which a refugee is present (even if not lawfully staying there) must find some means by which to enable him or her to travel beyond its borders. To this end, the discretionary authority under Art. 28(1) of the Refugee Convention to issue CTDs to any refugee physically present on a state party's territory[610] affords a useful means by which to implement duties under Art. 12(2) of the Civil and Political Covenant in relation to any refugee.[611]

As this flexibility demonstrates, the issuance of a CTD is conceived in purely functional terms – specifically, to enable refugees to travel for business or pleasure, and most particularly to seek out opportunities for resettlement in a preferred country of asylum.[612] It does not entitle the holder to the diplomatic protection of the issuing state, nor does it even authorize that state to assert protective authority.[613] More controversially, the travel document does not amount to documentation of refugee status as such.[614] State practice, however, has often been to "recognize the Convention Travel Document not only as a document on which a visa may be given but also as evidence of the holder's refugee status."[615] At one level, this practice bespeaks a liberal preparedness to defer to the judgement of a fellow state party's interpretation of entitlement to protection. Moreover, some support for

---

[610] See text above, at pp. 847–851.

[611] This more general duty to facilitate international movement may, however, be restricted for a broader range of concerns than can be invoked in relation to refugees lawfully staying in a state party to the Refugee Convention. National security and public order concerns need not rise to the level of "compelling" reasons for restriction, and other considerations – "public health or morals or the rights and freedoms of others" – may also be invoked to deny the right to leave a country. See text below, at pp. 860–865, regarding the scope of permissible limits on the duty to issue refugees with a CTD under Art. 28(1) of the Refugee Convention.

[612] The UN High Commissioner for Refugees "emphasized the great importance of travel documents both to refugees and to States. Even countries of resettlement were in favour of travel documents": Statement of Mr. van Heuven Goedhart of UNHCR, UN Doc. A/CONF.2/SR.18, July 12, 1951, at 14.

[613] "The issue of the document does not in any way entitle the holder to the protection of the diplomatic or consular authorities of the country of issue, and does not confer on these authorities a right of protection": Refugee Convention, at Schedule, para. 16. The primary rationale for this rule, imported from the London Agreement, was "that the Contracting Parties wished to avoid disputes over protection": Statement of Mr. Robinson of Israel, UN Doc. E/AC.32/SR.24, Feb. 3, 1950, at 5. This goal leads Weis to conclude that para. 16 "does not preclude the State which has issued the travel document [from granting] such protection to a refugee, provided the State vis à vis which this protection is to be exercised admits such protection": Weis, *Travaux*, at 267.

[614] "Neither the issue of the document nor the entries made thereon determine or affect the status of the holder, particularly as regards nationality": Refugee Convention, at Schedule, para. 15.

[615] UNHCR, "Note on Travel Documents for Refugees," UN Doc. EC/SCP/10, Aug. 30, 1978 (UNHCR, "Travel Documents"), at para. 23.

this view can be garnered from Art. 27 of the Convention, which requires states to issue identity papers – which *are* intended to be treated as at least provisional evidence of refugee status[616] – to "any refugee in their territory *who does not possess a valid travel document* [emphasis added]." If the CTD were not understood to be evidence of refugee status, why would a person holding a travel document not also be entitled to receive identity papers?

A plausible answer is that because identity papers are intended only to enable an individual to claim the benefits of refugee status *inside the asylum state*,[617] they are of little net value to the holder of a CTD. This is because there is little practical likelihood that a given government would issue an individual with a CTD (or grant entry on that basis), yet treat him or her in other respects as a non-refugee. In truth, however, the drafters' decision not to require the issuance of identity documents to refugees already holding a travel document seems really to have been predicated on expediency. At the time of the Convention's drafting there were already many refugees resident in state parties who held one of the earlier refugee travel documents – which *were* specifically designed to serve both as a form of domestic identification and to facilitate international travel[618] – to whom states did not wish to be obliged to issue new documentation.[619] Art. 27's exclusion of refugees holding a travel document from the beneficiary class for identity paper purposes was intended essentially to promote administrative simplicity in circumstances understood not to pose a risk to refugees.

This explanation has the advantage of avoiding a genuine hardship to a segment of the refugee population clearly intended to benefit from access to the CTD, namely those recent arrivals who wish to seek protection in a state other than that in which they first arrived.[620] By seeing the travel document only as a means of facilitating international movement (rather than as a means of certifying Convention refugee status), the intended flexibility of the travel document system is safeguarded. This purely pragmatic position is in line with the views advocated by Grahl-Madsen:

---

[616] See chapter 4.9 above, at p. 620.   [617] Ibid. at p. 619.   [618] Ibid. at pp. 618–619.

[619] Indeed, the drafters were at one point inclined to decide that the CTD should be issued only in French and the issuing state's language "in order to use up the stocks of travel documents already printed in French": Statement of Mr. Herment of Belgium, UN Doc. E/AC.32/SR.39, Aug. 21, 1950, at 5. Even the representative of the IRO argued against including a second mandatory language on the CTD, since "it would be necessary to print new [CTDs], which would involve waste of time and expenditure": Statement of Mr. Weis of the IRO, ibid. at 6. The solution – insisting that use of *either* French or English, in addition to the language of the issuing state, would be adequate – was in part fashioned in order to allow "all stocks [to be] used": Statement of Mr. Juvigny of France, ibid. at 7. As this exchange makes clear, what should arguably have been a principled decision was, in fact, driven by a determination to avoid a short-term administrative concern.

[620] See text above, at pp. 847–850.

The travel document is issued for the purpose of travelling outside the issuing country. It is not designed to be a proof of refugee status or any other status, and it is not at all certain that the holder of a travel document at any given time is a refugee according to the definition in Article 1 of the Refugee Convention. It is noteworthy that in contrast with the *London* travel document [of 1946], which sets out that the holder "is the concern of the Intergovernmental Committee of Refugees," the Convention travel document contains no confirmation of the holder's eligibility under the Convention or the Statute of the High Commissioner's Office. If some authority . . . wants to ascertain whether a person is a refugee according to some relevant definition, that authority would be well advised not to make its decision solely on the basis of the travel document presented to it.[621]

A CTD may not be denied on the grounds that the refugee seeking it already possesses, or could secure, an alternative form of travel documentation from the host or another country. Much less can it be denied on the grounds, as is the case in Zambia, that the host government is prepared to issue an internal certificate of identity. While some governments would have preferred each country to issue refugees special travel documents of purely national authority,[622] most of the drafters shared the view of the Chairman of the Ad Hoc Committee that "even if all Governments had adopted some such practice, it would be an advantage to adopt [a] unified system."[623] The establishment of a single, uniform system of refugee travel documents was thought important to avoid the risk of non-recognition of purely national documents by destination and transit states.[624] The fundamental goal of the CTD system was to provide

---

[621] Grahl-Madsen, *Commentary*, at 160. It is noteworthy that the text of Art. 28 as proposed by the Secretary-General did not expressly define the purpose to be served by a CTD: Secretary-General, "Memorandum," at 41. The present language of Art. 28, which makes clear that travel documents are issued "for the purpose of travel outside [the issuing state's] territory," was inserted on the motion of the United Kingdom: "United Kingdom: Draft Proposal for Article [28]," UN Doc. E/AC.32/L.17, Jan. 30, 1950, at 1.

[622] "Chile . . . already has a special passport which is issued not only to refugees, but to any other foreigner not in possession of the usual documents. This passport is issued for the specific purpose of facilitating travel . . . There would in consequence be no advantage in replacing our present legislation by the provisions of the proposed Convention": United Nations, "Compilation of Comments," at 51–52.

[623] Statement of the Chairman, Mr. Larsen of Denmark, UN Doc. E/AC.32/SR.39, Aug. 21, 1950, at 4. See also Statement of Mr. Henkin of the United States, ibid., who "hoped that countries like Chile would accept the provisions of article [28], both for the reasons given by the Chairman and because he doubted whether the kind of document provided by such countries contained any provisions permitting the holder to re-enter the country." Weis succinctly concludes that "if the applicant is a refugee . . . the Contracting State must issue him or her with a Convention travel document and not with any other document such as an aliens passport": Weis, *Travaux*, at 265.

[624] "The Nansen certificate and the travel document established pursuant to the London Agreement are completely satisfactory, while the other documents ['the various travel

refugees with a more broadly based alternative to a patchwork of nationally issued travel documents which "would prevent the bearer being asked to produce special credentials during the journey."[625] Moreover,

> There was no need to stress the practical advantages which would result from the standardization of travel documents for refugees. The work of passport control and immigration officers would be considerably simplified if all such documents were based on a single model.[626]

In the interests of "achieving uniformity,"[627] the drafters adopted a very detailed Schedule setting out binding formal and operational details of the CTD system, which all agreed to respect.[628] Most critically, they established a system of reciprocal recognition of travel documents, under which all state parties commit themselves to honor a CTD issued by any other state party[629]

---

documents issued by the administrative authorities of certain countries'] are not accepted by many countries": Secretary-General, "Memorandum," at 42.

[625] Statement of Mr. Rain of France, UN Doc. E/AC.32/SR.16, Jan. 30, 1950, at 10. UNHCR reports that this goal has been effectively attained, since the CTD "is accepted for visa purposes, not only by States parties to the 1951 Convention and/or the 1967 Protocol, but in practice by all countries to which refugees wish to travel": UNHCR, "Travel Documents," at para. 11.

[626] Statement of Sir Leslie Brass of the United Kingdom, UN Doc. E/AC.32/SR.16, Jan. 30, 1950, at 7.

[627] Ibid. at 3.

[628] The Schedule is incorporated by reference in Art. 28. It was essentially drawn from the London Agreement: "United Kingdom: Draft Proposal for Article [28]," UN Doc. E/AC.32/L.17, Jan. 30, 1950. "The 1946 Agreement had been signed and put into effect by a large number of countries. It therefore seemed that its provisions might be acceptable to the future contracting parties of the new convention": Statement of Sir Leslie Brass of the United Kingdom, UN Doc. E/AC.32/SR.16, Jan. 30, 1950, at 4. On the suggestion of the French representative, these details were moved to a Schedule, as "[t]o include [them] in the convention itself would be to destroy its harmony, for then it would contain, side by side with articles setting forth the principles of administrative solutions, one single article containing very detailed rules to cover one specific point": Statement of Mr. Rain of France, ibid. at 5.

[629] Once issued, all state parties are bound to "recognize the validity" of any CTD issued "in accordance with the provisions of article 28 of this Convention": Refugee Convention, at Schedule, para. 7. The French draft of Art. 28 had proposed a more explicit reference in the body of the primary article itself, specifically that "[e]ach of the High Contracting Parties shall recognize the documents issued by the other High Contracting Parties": France, "Draft Convention," at 8. Similarly, Israel pressed for formal incorporation of the duty of mutual recognition in the text of Art. 28: Statement of Mr. Robinson of Israel, UN Doc. E/AC.32/SR.39, Aug. 21, 1950, at 13. But while ultimately included in the Schedule, there seems to have been a general view that the obligation of mutual recognition was inherent in the system established. The representative of the International Refugee Organization, for example, "thought that, though from a purely legal point of view, paragraph 7 was perhaps unnecessary, it might have some psychological value in stimulating recognition of travel documents issued under the present and previous agreements": Statement of Mr. Weis of the IRO, ibid. at 13.

(including pursuant to its expanded discretionary authority[630]). Indeed, the drafters even agreed that state parties to the Refugee Convention would treat all refugee travel documents issued under any of the predecessor treaties as though they had been issued under the terms of the Refugee Convention[631] – including documents issued by a state that might choose not to accede to the Refugee Convention.[632] There can therefore be little doubt about the depth of the commitment to "replac[ing] all previous instruments, the

[630] "[O]ther parties cannot question the right of a Contracting State to issue a document if this is done under the powers granted to it by Art. 28, even if, in their estimation, the person is not a 'refugee' in the sense of the Convention, so long as the document was issued legally": Robinson, *History*, at 143. See also Goodwin-Gill, *Refugee in International Law*, at 156. This deference to the decision of the issuing state to issue a CTD to refugees who did not meet the "lawful stay" requirement was possible by virtue of the correlative duty of the issuing state to receive back the holder of *any* CTD issued by it during the validity of that document: see text below, at pp. 865–870. See also Statement of Mr. Larsen of Denmark, UN Doc. E/AC.32/SR.16, Jan. 30, 1950, at 13: "All travel documents ... would be subject to the provisions of paragraph 13 of the schedule ... That provided the country in which the refugee wished to travel with a safeguard that would apply in all cases: the country issuing a travel document to a refugee would be responsible for him and would be obliged to readmit him, whatever his legal status in that country, if he was not accepted elsewhere." Grahl-Madsen takes a somewhat more cautious approach to this issue, basing his opinion that all states should respect CTDs issued to refugees broadly conceived on Recommendation E of the Final Conference that adopted the Refugee Convention, in which the signatories express their hope that the Convention "will have value as an example exceeding its contractual scope." He observes that "[t]he recommendation, which was unanimously adopted by the Conference, is not legally binding on any government; nevertheless it may be said to express the spirit of the Convention, and if governments do issue Convention travel documents to certain extra-Convention refugees, they may claim to be acting in keeping with that spirit ... On the other hand, whereas Paragraph 7 of the Schedule must be interpreted so broadly as to include all travel documents issued in accordance with the Convention or the Schedule, and not only those issued pursuant to the express provisions in Article 28, it can hardly be stretched so far as to compel governments to recognize the validity of Convention travel documents issued to refugees who are clearly outside the scope of Article 1 of the Convention. However, if the issue of Convention travel documents to extra-Convention refugees is not against international law, it is not either based on international law, but is outside the scope of international law. The recognition of such travel documents therefore comes within the sphere of comity": Grahl-Madsen, *Commentary*, at 124–125. In his more detailed analysis of para. 7 of the Schedule, however, Grahl-Madsen agrees with the dominant view set out above that "[t]he conclusion seems inevitably to be that the Contracting States are obliged to recognize on an equal footing travel documents issued under any of the cited provisions [Art. 28, Art. 11, or para. 6(3)]": ibid. at 145.

[631] Refugee Convention, at Art. 28(2).

[632] "[P]aragraph 2 ... provided for recognition of the validity of travel documents which would continue to be issued by countries signatories of previous conventions which were not parties to the new convention: that was a provision of a lasting nature": Statement of Mr. Cuvelier of Belgium, UN Doc. E/AC.32/SR.16, Jan. 30, 1950, at 9. There was,

diversity and vaguely defined field of application of which merely served to confuse the issue."[633]

While, as previously described, any state party *may* choose to issue a CTD to a refugee simply physically present in its territory,[634] the Convention sets a presumptive duty[635] on the state with which a given refugee has the strongest territorial connection – namely, the country of his or her lawful stay – to issue

however, some confusion on this point at the Conference of Plenipotentiaries, where comments made by the French representative suggested a duty to recognize travel documents issued under prior treaties *only* to the extent that the state party to the 1951 Convention was also a party to the relevant earlier treaty, or where the issuing state was also a party to the 1951 Convention: Statement of Mr. Rochefort of France, UN Doc. A/ CONF.2/SR.17, July 12, 1951, at 14. On the other hand, the British representative was emphatic that "[t]he meaning of paragraph 2 was surely perfectly clear. It stated that parties to the Convention undertook to recognize all travel documents issued under previous agreements by the parties to those agreements": Statement of Mr. Hoare of the United Kingdom, ibid. at 13. The President agreed, observing that "at least for some time to come, certain States parties to the previous agreements would not be parties to the present Convention ... He was ready to admit that from a strictly juridical point of view it might be somewhat unorthodox to allow a refugee to enter with a travel document in which reference was made to an international instrument to which the State of entry was not a party. But he believed that on the whole the advantages of paragraph 2 outweighed its slight legal disadvantages": Statement of the President, Mr. Larsen of Denmark, ibid. at 15. On the basis of this interpretation, paragraph 2 was immediately adopted on a 23–1 vote: ibid. See also Robinson, *History*, at 137–138: "[P]ara. 2 is a 'one-way' provision, imposing an obligation on the parties to this Convention to recognize travel documents issued by non-parties thereto, while the latter are not bound to do the same in regard to signatories of this Convention, not parties to the earlier agreements." In point of fact, seven state parties to the 1946 London Agreement did not ratify the Refugee Convention until at least the 1960s: Brazil (1960), Chile (1972), Dominican Republic (1978), Greece (1960), Liberia (1964), South Africa (1996), and Venezuela (1986: Protocol only). Moreover, one party to the London Agreement, India, is still not a party to either the Refugee Convention or Protocol, raising the interesting question of whether India could today still issue a travel document under the London Agreement which state parties to the Refugee Convention would be obliged to recognize. (As among state parties to the Refugee Convention, that treaty replaces the London Agreement: Refugee Convention, at Art. 37.) See also Recommendation A of the Final Act of the Conference of Plenipotentiaries on the Status of Refugees and Stateless Persons, 189 UNTS 37, in which governments participating in earlier refugee travel document systems were urged "to continue to issue or to recognize such travel documents, and to extend the issue of such documents to refugees as defined in article 1 of the Convention ... or to recognize the travel documents so issued to such persons."

[633] Statement of Mr. Rain of France, UN Doc. E/AC.32/SR.16, Jan. 30, 1950, at 5.

[634] See text above, at pp. 847–851.

[635] "[A] Contracting State may not refuse to issue a travel document to a refugee if, for example, it regards the proposed travel as inappropriate ... [A] refugee is not required to 'justify' the proposed travel in order to receive a travel document to which he is entitled 'for travel purposes'": UNHCR, "Travel Documents," at para. 14.

a travel document.[636] The language of Art. 28(1), providing that a state party "*shall* issue [a CTD] to refugees lawfully staying in their territory [emphasis added]," was adopted in preference to a proposal from Yugoslavia to leave open the question of which state, if any, was expected to issue a CTD to a particular refugee.[637] As the British representative to the Conference of Plenipotentiaries pointed out, this territorially based principle is critical to ensure that, at some point, every refugee can hold at least one state party accountable to issue him or her with a travel document.[638] The locus of responsibility automatically changes if and when a refugee may be said to be lawfully staying in a new country.[639]

[636] At the Conference of Plenipotentiaries, the French representative voiced his concern that para. 11 of the Schedule – which then granted "the power" to issue a CTD to the country of lawful residence – might be read to preclude other countries from issuing a CTD to a refugee simply physically present in their territory. He therefore proposed that para. 11 be amended in a way that left the broader discretionary authority of other state parties intact, but which assigned "the obligation" to issue a CTD to the state of lawful residence: Statement of Mr. Rochefort of France, UN Doc. A/CONF.2/SR.32, July 24, 1951, at 9. Because Venezuela felt that the term "obligation" might unduly tie the hands of the state of lawful stay, para. 11 was amended both to reference the scope of the duty under the text of Art. 28 itself, and to refer to the state of lawful stay's "responsibility," rather than to its obligation: Statements of Mr. Montoya of Venezuela, Mr. Rochefort of France, and Mr. Hoare of the United Kingdom, ibid. at 9–12.

[637] The Belgian representative "was unable to accept the Yugoslav amendment; the substitution of the words 'may issue' for the words 'shall issue' would deprive paragraph 1 of all force": Statement of Mr. Herment of Belgium, UN Doc. A/CONF.2/SR.12, July 9, 1951, at 7.

[638] In response to a proposal that would have amended Art. 28 to provide simply for a general right of state parties to issue a CTD to any refugee, including those outside its borders, but which would not have required any particular state to take responsibility for the issuance of a CTD to any given refugee, the British representative appropriately insisted "that adoption of that suggestion would weaken article [28] by making it no longer the primary obligation of the Contracting State in whose territory the refugee was resident to issue travel documents": Statement of Mr. Hoare of the United Kingdom, ibid. at 8.

[639] Refugee Convention, at Schedule, para. 11. Detailed rules for ascertaining the time at which this transfer of responsibility occurs may be agreed between states, e.g. pursuant to the European Agreement on Transfer of Responsibility for Refugees, at Art. 2. In proposing the amendment of para. 11, the American representative suggested that "[s]ome such phrase as 'becomes transferred' should be employed [in contrast to the language of the draft then under discussion, 'will be transferred'] to show that the transfer was automatic and required no action on the part of anyone": Statement of Mr. Henkin of the United States, UN Doc. E/AC.32/SR.39, Aug. 21, 1950, at 13. The automatic nature of the transfer contemplated in the revised text of para. 11 was confirmed by the Belgian representative to the Conference of Plenipotentiaries who, in response to a Venezuelan proposal to delete the word "désormais" from the French language version of para. 11 of the Schedule, noted that "[t]he retention of the word 'désormais' was necessary so that there would be a transfer of responsibility under the terms of paragraph 11": Statement of

The state which issues a CTD is allowed substantial administrative autonomy.[640] While the CTD issued must conform to the specimen travel document included in the Convention,[641] it is for the issuing country to decide whether it is valid for a period of one or two years,[642] and which refugee children are to be included on the passport of a parental refugee or other adult refugee.[643] The issuing government also determines the scope of its geographical validity, though the Schedule encourages state parties to make the travel document "valid for the largest possible number of countries."[644] As such, the Convention is not breached by the many states, including Belgium, which issue a CTD which is not valid for travel to the refugee's

Mr. Herment of Belgium, UN Doc. A/CONF.2/SR.33, July 24, 1951, at 6. It was hoped that having a single state designated as the holder of the responsibility to issue a CTD to any given refugee would "prevent the issue of several travel documents to one and the same refugee by different authorities of different countries": Robinson, *History*, at 144. Yet this reasoning was not entirely sound since any state remains *entitled* (though not required) to issue a CTD to a refugee in its territory, thereby providing a means by which a single refugee could obtain more than one travel document. It is moreover ironic that the Conference of Plenipotentiaries elected to omit one requirement for issuance of a CTD approved by the Ad Hoc Committee, namely that the applicant "not possess a valid travel document issued pursuant to article [28]": Ad Hoc Committee, "Second Session Report," at 23. This omission was the result of a Belgian amendment (UN Doc. A/CONF.2/61). The only delegate to speak to the matter supported the omission on the rather simplistic basis that "there would obviously be no need to issue a document if the refugee already had one": Statement of Mr. Arff of Norway, UN Doc. A/CONF/2/SR.17, July 12, 1951, at 5.

[640] For an extremely detailed analysis of the provisions of the various paragraphs of the Schedule, see Grahl-Madsen, *Commentary*, at 132–161.

[641] Refugee Convention, at Schedule, para. 1.

[642] Refugee Convention, at Schedule, para. 5. An effort was made to authorize CTDs with a validity of less than one year: Statements of Mr. Herment of Belgium and Mr. Makiedo of Yugoslavia, UN Doc. A/CONF.2/SR.18, July 12, 1951, at 4. This proposal was rejected on a 15–4 (6 abstentions) vote, ibid. at 5, though it was conceded that an issuing state might achieve much the same end by invoking its authority under para. 13(3) "in exceptional cases, or in cases where the refugee's stay is authorized for a specific period . . . to limit the period during which the refugee may return [to the issuing country] to a period of not less than three months": Statement of Mr. Zutter of Switzerland, ibid. at 4.

[643] Refugee Convention, at Schedule, para. 2. "[I]t would be wise for the Conference to take a liberal attitude in the matter. The families of refugees were often scattered, and it might be that a child would have to travel in the company of a grandparent or a relative": Statement of Mr. Hoeg of Denmark, UN Doc. A/CONF.2/SR.17, July 12, 1951, at 17. Thus, "[p]ara. 2 leaves it to individual countries to define the word 'children,' i.e. to prescribe the age at which a person may obtain his own document and below which he may be included in the travel document of another, adult refugee": Robinson, *History*, at 141.

[644] Refugee Convention, at Schedule, para. 4. "[T]he vast majority of States . . . endorse the CTD as valid for all countries with the exception of the country of origin. A few States, however, restrict the geographical validity of CTDs to certain named countries, usually for political or security reasons": UNHCR, "Travel Documents Follow-Up," at para. 8.

country of origin, nor even by the American prohibition of travel on a refugee travel document to countries it deems enemy states. And while an effort was made to require the issuing government to renew a CTD, at least if the refugee had no state of lawful stay at the date of its expiration,[645] para. 6(3) of the Schedule as finally adopted merely directs state parties to "give sympathetic consideration" to renewing, extending, or replacing travel documents in the case of persons unable to secure them from the country in which they are lawfully residing.[646]

A particularly important form of authority reposed in the territorial state is the right to withhold travel documents from a refugee. The Conference of Plenipotentiaries was clear that not every refugee lawfully staying in a state party has an absolute right to be issued a travel document. To the contrary, it was felt that a balance should be struck between the usual duty of the state of lawful stay to issue a travel document and the fact that there were some "cases in which Contracting States could legitimately refuse to do so."[647] As the High Commissioner for Refugees advised,

> The issue of travel documents was one of the most essential aspects of the treatment accorded to refugees ... The adoption of the Yugoslav

[645] The American representative to the Ad Hoc Committee "was also afraid that situations might arise in which one country was not willing to extend any longer the validity of a travel document issued to a refugee, while the country of his new residence was not yet prepared to issue him one for the first time. To prevent the refugee from thus falling between the stools, he proposed the addition to paragraph 6(1) of the following words: 'No travel document shall be cancelled or its prolongation refused so long as a refugee should not have received a new one from the country of his new residence'": Statement of Mr. Henkin of the United States, UN Doc. E/AC.32/SR.39, Aug. 21, 1950, at 10.

[646] Refugee Convention, at Schedule, para. 6(3). The British representative argued "that the United States proposal went too far ... If the country of his first residence was forced to wait until a document had been issued by the country of new residence before cancelling its own document, it would probably never be released from its obligations": Statement of Sir Leslie Brass of the United Kingdom, UN Doc. E/AC.32/SR.39, Aug. 21, 1950, at 10–11. As Grahl-Madsen writes, the duty to "give sympathetic consideration" "means that the authorities of the country concerned are obliged not to reject out of hand, without considering the merits, or to make it their policy to reject such applications. On the other hand, a State is not obliged to issue travel documents to persons covered by the provisions here considered. The obligation entered into is only to consider applications fairly and with understanding for the difficult situation of the persons involved": Grahl-Madsen, *Commentary*, at 129. Regrettably, UNHCR is therefore in error to suggest that "[t]he State which first issued the CTD retains responsibility for the refugee and for the renewal of the travel documents until such time as this responsibility is effectively transferred to another State": UNHCR, "Travel Documents Follow-Up," at para. 13. The notion of "residing" used in para. 6(3) should be understood to identify refugees who are lawfully present in another state, many of whom will not also be lawfully staying there and hence entitled to claim the benefit of Art. 28: see chapter 3.1.4 above, at p. 188.

[647] Statement of the President, Mr. Larsen of Denmark, UN Doc. A/CONF.2/SR.12, July 9, 1951, at 8.

amendment, for example, would virtually vitiate its intention, for the article would then mean that refugees would have no guarantee that they would be able to secure travel documents. However, he realized the cogency of the objections raised by certain representatives concerning the mandatory obligation by the first sentence of article [28]. They might be disposed of by substituting the words "undertakes to issue to refugees" for the words "shall issue, on request, to a refugee." The principle would then be more clearly stated, and the acquisition of travel documents would not be defined as a right belonging to the individual ... [But] [h]e earnestly appealed to representatives to refrain from weakening the article as a whole.[648]

The approach adopted by the Conference closely parallels this recommendation. The mandatory language contained in the Ad Hoc Committee's draft, "shall issue," was retained, though without the additional phrase approved by the Ad Hoc Committee, "on request."[649] More fundamentally, the Conference added an express caveat to Art. 28(1), the effect of which is to set a legal duty on the country of lawful stay to issue a CTD "unless compelling reasons of national security or public order otherwise require."

There was a great deal of discussion about this qualifying phrase. While Austria argued that there was no need for the Convention to address the circumstances in which a CTD might be withheld,[650] the general preference was to be clear about the grounds for non-issuance to avoid "a risk of lowering the status of refugees vis à vis national authorities."[651] The British representative successfully persuaded the Conference that "[i]f modifications were to be introduced ... their proper place was in article [28], where the circumstances in which refugees had a right to acquire travel documents were broadly defined."[652] This approach was adopted.

One view was that states should be entitled to withhold issuance of a refugee travel document only on the same grounds that would justify denial

---

[648] Statement of Mr. van Heuven Goedhart of UNHCR, ibid. at 9.

[649] In the version of Art. 28 originally presented to the Conference of Plenipotentiaries, Art. 28 read, "The Contracting States shall issue, on request ... a travel document": "Texts of the Draft Convention and the Draft Protocol to be Considered by the Conference," UN Doc. A/CONF.2/1, Mar. 12, 1951, at 15.

[650] "[E]ach country had specific legislation or regulations governing the issue of passports, which stipulated, no doubt, the cases in which issue could be refused. Such regulations presumably extended to the issue of passports to refugees. No provision in the Convention could impair that sovereign right of States. He therefore believed that article [28] should prove acceptable as it stood": Statement of Mr. Fritzer of Austria, UN Doc. A/CONF.2/SR.12, July 9, 1951, at 11.

[651] Statement of Mr. Hoare of the United Kingdom, UN Doc. A/CONF.2/SR.17, July 12, 1951, at 8.

[652] Statement of Mr. Hoare of the United Kingdom, UN Doc. A/CONF.2/SR.12, July 9, 1951, at 13.

of a passport to a citizen.[653] Under an amendment presented jointly by Australia and Canada, states might "as an exceptional measure" elect to withhold issue of a travel document from a refugee "if the circumstances are such that the issue of a passport would be withheld from a national of that state."[654] As the Australian delegate observed,

> The issue of travel documents was a matter for the discretion of each government. There might be cases where a Contracting State, for good reason, refused a passport to one of its own nationals to travel for a certain purpose. It would be anomalous in the extreme if a refugee wishing to travel for a similar purpose was entitled to be issued with a travel document.[655]

Canada similarly insisted that the assimilation of refugees to nationals for purposes of travel document eligibility was a clear matter of basic fairness:

> Passports were issued in pursuance of the royal prerogative, and no citizen had an inalienable right to receive a passport ... It was obvious that refugees could not be given preferential treatment over nationals in that respect.[656]

This approach was not adopted, based on opposition rooted in both liberal and restrictionist thinking. On the one hand, it was argued that reliance on the same criteria applied to the issuance of a passport to citizens would pose a risk to refugees. The Belgian representative made the case that refugees "could not be expected to conform to the same conditions as nationals,"[657] and should therefore be denied travel documents only for reasons of "national security or public order."[658] He insisted that this approach

> was more in the interests of refugees than was the joint amendment [proposed by Australia and Canada]. The Norwegian representative had mentioned the case of a government refusing to issue passports to persons who had not paid their taxes. Such a case was one of the "circumstances" in

---

[653] "The general obligation laid on States would be interpreted as being to respect a right to which the individual refugee was entitled, and refugees might thus be in a position to claim something which was denied to nationals": Statement of Mr. Shaw of Australia, ibid. at 10. See also Statement of Mr. Zutter of Switzerland, ibid.

[654] UN Doc. A/CONF.2/66. This approach received the grudging support of the representative of the United Kingdom who conceded that "there would be circumstances in which it would be desirable to allow states a certain amount of latitude. The joint Australian/Canadian amendment was preferable ... inasmuch as it provided for the application to the issue of travel documents to refugees of the same criteria as were applied in the issue of passports": Statement of Mr. Hoare of the United Kingdom, UN Doc. A/CONF.2/SR.17, July 12, 1951, at 5. See also Statement of Mr. Hoeg of Denmark, ibid.

[655] Statement of Mr. Shaw of Australia, UN Doc. A/CONF.2/SR.12, July 9, 1951, at 7.

[656] Statement of Mr. Chance of Canada, UN Doc. A/CONF.2/SR.12, July 9, 1951, at 7.

[657] Statement of Mr. Herment of Belgium, ibid.   [658] UN Doc. A/CONF.2/61.

which a State withheld the issue of passports to its own nationals and, if the joint amendment was adopted, it would be possible to invoke a similar reason for denying the issue of travel documents to a refugee. In the same way, if the national of a State had not done his military service, his application for a passport was usually refused. Logically, therefore, such an application should also be refused if made by a refugee in the same position. Hence it was clear that the text of the joint amendment submitted by the delegations of Australia and Canada allowed of a very wide interpretation. The Belgian delegation therefore preferred its own text.[659]

On the other hand, and perhaps more candidly, the case for the "national security or public order" test was made on the basis of a need to grant states more flexibility to deny travel documents to refugees on grounds not applicable to their own citizens.[660] France insisted that "circumstances might make it necessary for her to keep a check on the movements of refugees and aliens."[661] To adopt the approach envisaged by the joint amendment proposed by Australia and Canada "would simply be tying the hands of the French government so far as the issue of travel documents was concerned."[662] Indeed, France went so far as to claim that while "the fact that a French citizen [who] expressed extremist views did not preclude him from holding a passport . . . [i]t might, however, be necessary in certain cases to treat refugees differently."[663] Even when this position was soundly denounced by the British representative as "tantamount to discrimination on the grounds of political opinion,"[664] the French government was not moved, insisting that if it were to grant a travel document to a refugee with extremist views, the refugee's state of destination would likely deport him or her back to France.[665]

The compromise which emerged reflects substantial deference to the French position. The text as adopted allows a CTD to be denied on public order or national security grounds, even if such concerns do not govern the issuance of a passport to citizens. But because Art. 28 allows a CTD to be denied to refugees *only* on these grounds, it follows that a travel document

---

[659] Statement of Mr. Herment of Belgium, UN Doc. A/CONF.2/SR.17, July 12, 1951, at 6–7.

[660] The first state to propose this approach was Italy, which suggested that states retain the right, also expressed as "a purely exceptional measure," to withhold travel documents from a refugee "suspected on reasonable grounds of engaging in illicit traffic": UN Doc. A/CONF.2/56.

[661] Statement of Mr. Colemar of France, UN Doc. A/CONF.2/SR.12, July 9, 1951, at 6.

[662] Statement of Mr. Rochefort of France, UN Doc. A/CONF.2/SR.17, July 12, 1951, at 6. He concluded that "[t]he Belgian amendment was, therefore, the only one which the French delegation could support": ibid.

[663] Statement of Mr. Rochefort of France, ibid. at 9.

[664] Statement of Mr. Hoare of the United Kingdom, ibid. at 9.

[665] Statement of Mr. Rochefort of France, ibid. at 9–10.

may not be refused to refugees for the sorts of reasons, e.g. insolvency, or failure to perform military service or to pay taxes, argued by the proponents of the "public order and national security" approach to be uniquely applicable to citizens.[666] As Weis concludes,

> There is ... a difference between nationals and refugees in favour of the latter. While the issuance of a passport to a national is often a matter of discretion, the issue of a travel document is an obligation, unless compelling reasons of public security or public order justify a refusal. There is good reason for this distinction between nationals and refugees, since refugees may have to travel, for example, from the country of first asylum to a country of resettlement.[667]

Moreover, not any public order or national security reason is sufficient to deny a CTD. Responding to British concerns that these concepts could justify excessive restrictions,[668] states agreed to emphasize the exceptional nature of any refusal to grant refugees a travel document,[669] and to authorize such refusal only in situations in which there are *compelling* reasons of national

---

[666] See text above, at pp. 861–862.

[667] Weis, *Travaux*, at 265. See also Grahl-Madsen, *Commentary*, at 127: "[I]t seems clear, on the basis of the firm statement of the Belgian representative, that the Belgian proposal would not justify the refusal of issuing a travel document in the cases enumerated by the Norwegian delegate, viz. 'for reasons of insolvency, failure to pay taxes and so on.'" Yet "'public order' (*ordre public*) still remains a relatively fluid concept, and certain states have not excluded the possibility of applying to the issue of Convention travel documents the same restrictions as they would apply with regard to national passports": Goodwin-Gill, *Refugee in International Law*, at 155.

[668] "If the holding of extremist views was accepted as a valid ground for not issuing travel documents, certain States might take advantage of that facility in order to put obstacles in the way of legitimate travel on the part of a refugee, and that would be a marked deterioration in the status of refugee from the position obtaining under the London Agreement of 1946": Statement of Mr. Hoare of the United Kingdom, UN Doc. A/CONF.2/SR.17, July 12, 1951, at 10.

[669] Under the Belgian draft, consideration of public order and national security concerns would have been a routine and intrinsic part of the decision about whether to issue a refugee travel document. "*Subject to the requirements of national security or public order*, the Contracting States shall issue to refugees [emphasis added]": UN Doc. A/CONF.2/61. In contrast, the text as adopted makes clear that the starting point is the duty to issue the travel document, subject only to clear exceptions. "The Contracting States shall issue to refugees lawfully staying in their territory travel documents ... unless compelling reasons of national security or public order otherwise require": Refugee Convention, at Art. 28(1). The exceptional nature of this authority includes a temporal dimension. As the Belgian representative insisted, "the limiting clause ... did not mean that the issue of travel documents to refugees would be categorically refused. It was merely intended to allow for the temporary discontinuance of the issue of such documents. That action would no longer be necessary once the consideration of national security or public order which had led States to suspend the issue of travel documents had ceased to hold": Statement of Mr. Herment of Belgium, UN Doc. A/CONF.2/SR.17, July 12, 1951, at 5.

security or public order which *require* non-issuance of the travel document.[670] As Grahl-Madsen concludes, this means "that it is only in grave and exceptional circumstances that a Contracting State may refuse to issue a travel document to a refugee lawfully staying in its territory."[671]

The specific reason for including reference in Art. 28 to the "public order" ground was to authorize denial of a travel document to a refugee "who was being prosecuted for an offence under civil law."[672] As explained by the Danish representative,

> [T]ravel documents were used not only for immigration purposes, but also to allow a person to travel on business or on holiday. It might well be that, if in possession of a travel document, a refugee suspected of having committed a crime in a particular country would be able to obtain a visa from the Consul of another country without the Consul being aware of the facts of the case. It would consequently be undesirable to issue a travel document to such a person before the alleged offence had been fully investigated.[673]

This justification is very much in line with thinking on the notion of public order employed in Art. 32 of the Convention, said in that context to justify restrictions in the interests of internal security, particularly to the safety and security of the host country's citizens.[674] The logic of refusing a travel document to a refugee on national security grounds is perhaps less clear, since that expression was traditionally understood to relate to a threat to the host country emanating from outside the host state's borders.[675] But under

---

[670] "[T]he United Kingdom fully appreciated the French representative's difficulties, and the need for doing something to meet his point. In order, however, to avoid any abuse of the formula finally adopted, he would suggest that the phrase, 'Subject to the requirements of national security and public order' in the Belgian amendment ... should be replaced by the words 'Except where imperative reasons of national security or public order otherwise require'": Statement of Mr. Hoare of the United Kingdom, UN Doc. A/CONF.2/SR.17, July 12, 1951, at 11. "The word 'imperative' was changed [to] 'compelling' by the style committee without any reason being given, and it was clearly nobody's intent that this change of words should imply a change of substance": Grahl-Madsen, *Commentary*, at 128. As Robinson observes, "[t]he words 'compelling reasons' are to be understood as a restriction upon 'reason of national security and public order,' i.e. not every case which would ordinarily fall under the latter concept could be used to refuse a document, but only very serious cases": Robinson, *History*, at 136.

[671] Grahl-Madsen, *Commentary*, at 128.

[672] Statement of Mr. Herment of Belgium, UN Doc. A/CONF.2/SR.17, July 12, 1951, at 7.

[673] Statement of Mr. Hoeg of Denmark, ibid. at 9.

[674] See chapter 5.1 above, at pp. 679–690.

[675] It might be that denying a refugee the right to leave the host country would, for example, prevent him or her from consorting with persons abroad who might intend to do damage to the basic institutions of the host country. But such circumstances would, one presumes, be rare. To the contrary, denial of departure to a refugee in some sense posing a

more recent understandings of national security – in which it is recognized that national security may be implicated even in distant events which may have an indirect impact on the host state[676] – there may be greater scope to deny refugees a travel document on this basis. For example, if a refugee is traveling to raise funds for, or otherwise to contribute to the endeavors of, a terrorist organization, the state in which he or she lawfully resides would be justified in refusing a travel document.

Underlying the determination of states to enjoy some right to refuse travel documents to "risky" refugees seems to be a recognition that a unified travel document system can only survive if care is taken by the issuing state not to facilitate the international movement of refugees who could jeopardize the interests of a transit or destination state – even though the logical alternative, effectively requiring the refugee to remain in the country,[677] at least pending lawful removal under Arts. 32 and 33, is hardly in the immediate self-interest of the issuing state.[678] Governments were prepared to shoulder additional burdens at the time of considering the issuance of a CTD out of a recognition that some vetting was essential to safeguard the safety and security of partner states whose cooperation was required to make the travel document system workable. Because the country in which the refugee was resident was usually in a better position to know whether he or she posed a risk, the credibility of the travel document system depended in part on that state's knowledge being brought to bear.

It is important, however, not to overstate the level of confidence reposed in the issuing country. Fundamentally, the practical viability of a common travel document system which left so much discretion to the issuing state rested on two decisions which left significant authority to both destination and transit states. First, it was agreed that the issuing government would be under a clear duty to readmit the holder of a CTD issued by it, subject only to temporal limitations set out in the document itself. Second, both countries of destination and of passage – while

---

threat to the host country would normally be thought counterproductive to that country's security.

[676] See chapter 3.5.1 above, at pp. 263–266.

[677] "Since ordinarily a refugee cannot leave the country without a travel document ... [the right to withhold issuance of a travel document] means in essence that every Contracting State may forbid the egress of a refugee if this prohibition appears to be in the interest of national security or public order": Robinson, *History*, at 135.

[678] It is noteworthy that the original draft of para. 13(1) of the Schedule, drawn from the 1946 London Agreement, specifically "entitle[d] the holder to leave the country where it had been issued": "United Kingdom: Draft Proposal for Article [28]," UN Doc. E/AC.32/L.17, Jan. 30, 1950, at 3. With the omission of this language from the final text of para. 13, the issuing state is entitled, in accordance with para. 14 of the Schedule, to apply its general "laws and regulations" to govern "departure from" its territory: Refugee Convention, at Schedule, para. 14.

required to honor every CTD as the equivalent of a valid passport[679] – were nonetheless entitled to apply their usual rules with respect to the issuance of visas. With these safeguards in hand, governments felt that their interests were adequately protected.

At the very start of debate on the travel document system, the British representative opined that the goal of the regime had to be "to enable a refugee who had no passport to return within a given period to the country that issued his travel document. Without that provision, the refugee would probably not be allowed to enter other countries, for they would hesitate to admit him for fear that they might be obliged to keep him permanently on their territory."[680] More bluntly, the Chairman of the Ad Hoc Committee warned that

> When a refugee ... travelled out of his country of residence, the first question which rose in the minds of the authorities of any country which admitted him was whether it would be possible to get rid of him. They knew that if they kept him after his travel document had expired, the country which had issued that document could disclaim any further responsibility for him, but as long as that travel document remained valid he would be admitted on the understanding that at least one country would accept him again. If that last protection for countries admitting refugees in possession of travel documents issued by their country of residence was removed, entry visas would be supplied only after careful study of the probability of the refugee being permitted to return to his country of residence. The purpose of article [28] was to make it possible for a refugee to travel away from his country of residence with the same relative facility as nationals of most countries, and, if the countries in which he travelled were deprived of their only safeguard, his travel document would become worthless.[681]

The approach adopted therefore enshrined the principle of presumptive duty to readmit[682] during the period of the travel document's validity (either one or two years[683]):

---

[679] Statement of Mr. Henkin of the United States, UN Doc. E/AC.32/SR.42, Aug. 23, 1950, at 20.

[680] Statement of Sir Leslie Brass of the United Kingdom, UN Doc. E/AC.32/SR.16, Jan. 30, 1950, at 4. The practical importance of codifying this principle is clear from the view expressed by the Chairman of the Ad Hoc Committee that, as a matter of general law, he had "doubt concerning the principle that the country issuing the travel document was under an obligation to readmit the refugee if the country of destination would not permit him to remain there": Statement of the Chairman, Mr. Chance of Canada, ibid. at 12.

[681] Statement of the Chairman, Mr. Larsen of Denmark, UN Doc. E/AC.32/SR.39, Aug. 21, 1950, at 14.

[682] "Each Contracting State undertakes that the holder of a travel document issued by it in accordance with article 28 of this Convention shall be readmitted to its territory at any

[T]he country issuing a travel document to a refugee would be responsible for him and would be obliged to readmit him, whatever his legal status in that country, if he was not accepted elsewhere.[684]

As such, state parties may not lawfully issue only a "one-way" travel document with no return clause, as has been the case in Kenya, Tanzania, and Uganda. Governments concerned that they may be subject to readmission obligations of an unacceptably long duration[685] can exercise the option "in exceptional cases, or in cases where the refugee's stay is authorized for a specific period" to limit the right of reentry to a period not less than three months from the date of issue.[686] But any such limitation must be noted explicitly in clause 1(2) of the CTD, thus ensuring that there is no question of

time during the period of its validity": Refugee Convention, at Schedule, para. 13(1). This was in line with prevailing state practice. "[A]ny holder of a Danish travel document was entitled to re-enter Denmark, provided the document was still valid": Statement of the President, Mr. Larsen of Denmark, UN Doc. A/CONF.2/SR.18, July 12, 1951, at 11. See also Statement of Mr. Rochefort of France, ibid. at 14: "In point of fact, the travel document conferred the right both of exit and of re-entry"; and Statement of Mr. Herment of Belgium, ibid. at 11: "[T]he terms on which the document was conceived implicitly covered authorization to return."

[683] "The document shall have a validity of either one or two years, at the discretion of the issuing authority": Refugee Convention, at Schedule, para. 5.

[684] Statement of Mr. Larsen of Denmark, UN Doc. E/AC.32/SR.16, Jan. 30, 1950, at 13. When a refugee reenters the issuing state, "the refugee need be accorded no better status than he had before he left. For example, a refugee authorized to remain in a country for a limited period who leaves that country with a travel document could, on his return, claim to remain only for the unexpired period granted in the original permission, unless the government concerned decided to extend the period": Ad Hoc Committee, "First Session Report," at Annex II.

[685] Canada, for example, was worried about "the question of [refugees'] return ... The re-admission clause, as proposed, might raise certain difficulties. Nevertheless Canada would be ready to accept provisionally a solution whereby the proposed travel document would, during the period of validity, give the bearer considerable possibility of returning to the country of residence": Statement of the Chairman, Mr. Chance of Canada, UN Doc. E/AC.32/SR.16, Jan. 30, 1950, at 7–8.

[686] "The Contracting States reserve the right, in exceptional cases, or in cases where the refugee's stay is authorized for a specific period, when issuing the document, to limit the period during which the refugee may return to a period of not less than three months": Refugee Convention, at Schedule, para. 13(3). "These 'exceptional cases' are not defined. In view, however, of the basic purpose of issuing travel documents to refugees (i.e. to facilitate their movement), it is evident that such exceptions should be limited to cases where there are very special reasons for restricting the validity of the return clause to a period less than that of the validity of the travel document": UNHCR, "Travel Documents," at para. 22. See also Grahl-Madsen, *Commentary*, at 156: "[T]he word 'exceptional' makes it quite clear that the provision of subparagraph 3 is not one which should be easily invoked, and a Contracting State cannot make it its practice or policy to issue travel documents with a limited return clause."

the admitting state being taken unawares by any special temporal limitation on reentry to the issuing country.[687]

Apart from such an express limitation, the right of a refugee holding a CTD to reenter the issuing country may only be subjected to compliance with return "formalities."[688] The language proposed by the Ad Hoc Committee, under which the issuing state might have conditioned reentry on compliance with "those regulations which apply to returning resident aliens bearing duly visaed passports or re-entry permits,"[689] as well as a more far-ranging French effort that would have subjected reentering refugees to the possibility of substantive visa controls,[690] were rejected by the Conference of Plenipotentiaries on grounds that these approaches "would raise doubts as to whether holders of travel documents could, in fact, return."[691] As the British delegate cautioned,

---

[687] This approach resulted from an amendment proposed by Canada: Statement of Mr. Chance of Canada, UN Doc. A/CONF.2/SR.18, July 12, 1951, at 11. As the President of the Conference of Plenipotentiaries observed, adoption of this approach ensured that "[i]t would then be perfectly clear what the possession of a travel document entailed": Statement of the President, Mr. Larsen of Denmark, ibid. at 12.

[688] "[A] Contracting State may require the holder of the document to comply with such formalities as may be prescribed in regard to exit from or return to its territory": Refugee Convention, at Schedule, para. 13(2). Nor may the issuing state rely on the general authority under para. 14 to apply its laws and regulations governing admission to its territory to impose substantive visa controls on returning CTD holders, as para. 14 is expressly made "[s]ubject ... to the terms of paragraph 13": Refugee Convention, at Schedule, para. 14.

[689] Ad Hoc Committee, "Second Session Report," at Schedule, para. 13(1). This language, in turn, had replaced a provision that would have subjected refugees to "those laws and regulations which apply to the bearers of duly visaed passports": Ad Hoc Committee, "First Session Report," at Schedule, para. 13(1). The amendment at the second session of the Ad Hoc Committee was prompted by concern that it might otherwise have allowed the denial of entry to a refugee "if they were penniless or suffering from infectious disease": Statement of the Chairman, Mr. Larsen of Denmark, UN Doc. E/AC.32/SR.39, Aug. 21, 1950, at 16.

[690] France proposed the deletion of the language in the Ad Hoc Committee's draft that expressly granted a right of return "without a visa from the authorities of that country": Statement of Mr. Rochefort of France, UN Doc. A/CONF.2/SR.18, July 12, 1951, at 9.

[691] Statement of Mr. Warren of the United States, ibid. at 12. A similar preoccupation was expressed in the Ad Hoc Committee by its Chairman, Mr. Larsen of Denmark, UN Doc. E/AC.32/SR.39, Aug, 21, 1950, at 14, who "feared that paragraph 13 in its present form might lead to something in the nature of mental reservations on the part of the authorities issuing travel documents." Even the French representative to the Conference of Plenipotentiaries conceded that it was important to signal that "exit implied subsequent return. As things were at present, a travel document which had no return clause would be completely meaningless": Statement of Mr. Rochefort of France, UN Doc. A/CONF.2/SR.18, July 12, 1951, at 12.

[T]he Conference should consider further the implications of the French amendment. The basic principle underlying the provisions of paragraph 13 [of the Schedule] was that States issuing travel documents to refugees resident within their territory would bind themselves to allow such refugees re-entry during the period of validity of the document. He was anxious that that principle not be tampered with.[692]

Indeed, even a less wide-ranging provision that would have allowed the readmission of refugees to be subject to the same requirements as those imposed on returning citizens[693] was deleted on the motion of its Turkish proponent.[694]

In the end, it was decided that an issuing state should be entitled to "exercise supervision over the comings and goings of the refugees in its territory,"[695] including by requiring them to obtain a reentry visa. But the right to exercise such supervisory authority must not rebound to the detriment of the states that relied on a CTD to admit a refugee to their territory:

[T]wo considerations were involved: the respective obligations of the issuing country and those of the country admitting the refugees for temporary sojourn; and the relations between the issuing country and the holder of the travel document. Issuing countries could impose any regulations they wished covering the exit and entry of refugees, but what he was concerned to ensure was that they should assume an unconditional commitment to re-admit holders of their own travel documents. He did not think that such a principle was incompatible with a certain amount of supervision, such as was envisaged by the French representative, but care

---

[692] Statement of Mr. Hoare of the United Kingdom, UN Doc. A/CONF.2/SR.18, July 12, 1951, at 13. In the Ad Hoc Committee, the Chairman had expressed a comparable concern. "A refugee would not take out a travel document unless he intended to travel abroad and there was no reason why the return visa should not be supplied when the document was issued. If the refugee was obliged to apply for the visa after leaving the country, his passport might perhaps have expired when the visa was issued, and again the responsibility would pass to another country": Statement of the Chairman, Mr. Larsen of Denmark, UN Doc. E/AC.32/SR.39, Aug. 21, 1950, at 16.

[693] "Where a visa is required of a returning national, a visa may be required of a returning refugee, but shall be issued to him on request and without delay": Ad Hoc Committee, "Second Session Report," at Schedule, para. 13(1).

[694] Statement of Mr. Miras of Turkey, UN Doc. A/CONF.2/SR.18, July 12, 1951, at 15. The clause had originally been inserted to avoid conflict with Turkish law, amended prior to the conclusion of the Refugee Convention, which imposed a visa requirement on returning Turkish citizens: Statement of Mr. Weis of the IRO, UN Doc. E/AC.32/SR.39, Aug. 21, 1950, at 16. While there was substantial support even in the Ad Hoc Committee for the deletion of this clause, it was left in the draft out of consideration for the views of the Venezuelan representative, whose country also imposed a visa requirement on returning citizens: see Statements of Mr. Perez Perozo of Venezuela, ibid. at 17, and Sir Leslie Brass of the United Kingdom, ibid. at 18.

[695] Statement of Mr. Rochefort of France, UN Doc. A/CONF.2/SR.18, July 12, 1951, at 10.

should be taken to ensure that countries admitting refugees for short periods were not penalized or placed in difficulties by the regulations of the States issuing the travel documents.[696]

The Conference therefore adopted the proposal of a working group for the present language of para. 13 of the Schedule.[697] It stipulates the duty of the issuing state to readmit the holder of a CTD issued by it during the period of its validity, subject only to compliance with any "formalities" for return. This authority allows the issuing state to impose requirements that enable it to monitor the international travel of refugees, but disallows any substantive requirement which could result in a denial of reentry.[698]

In addition to the duty of readmission, the CTD system was made palatable to potential destination and transit states by its explicit recognition of their right to apply general visa policies to the holders of refugee travel documents. Importantly, this authority does not include a right to scrutinize the underlying refugee status of the holder of a CTD:

> Because there is no international eligibility procedure and it is left to each State to decide whether it considers a particular person as a refugee within the meaning of Article 1 . . . there may be differences of opinion between governments with regard to factual circumstances, as well as on points of law. A person who is considered a bona fide refugee in one country may on factual or legal grounds be considered ineligible in another country. Paragraph 7 of the Schedule [which requires states to recognize the validity of documents issued under Art. 28] must be considered in view of the fact that the drafters were fully aware that such differences of opinion might occur; nevertheless they made it an unconditional obligation on the part of Contracting States to recognize travel documents issued by one of them.[699]

On the other hand, para. 14 of the Schedule grants states a broad-ranging right to apply their usual "laws and regulations" to holders of a CTD seeking "admission, transit through, residence and establishment in, and departure

---

[696] Statement of the President, Mr. Larsen of Denmark, ibid. at 15. This understanding was expressly endorsed by the French delegate, who had previously promoted greater restrictions: Statement of Mr. Rochefort of France, ibid. at 15.

[697] "Report of the Working Group appointed to study paragraph 13 of the Schedule," UN Doc. A/CONF.2/95, July 19, 1951, adopted by the Conference on an 18–0 vote: UN Doc. A/CONF.2/SR.31, July 20, 1951, at 4.

[698] This is clear from the text of para. 13. The authorization of the state of issue to require compliance with exit or return formalities, set out in sub-paragraph (2), is expressly "subject to the provision of the preceding sub-paragraph," in which state parties undertake to readmit the holder of a CTD issued by them "at any time during the period of its validity."

[699] Grahl-Madsen, *Commentary*, at 122–123.

from" its territory.[700] As the British delegate to the Ad Hoc Committee observed, "the issue of a travel document imposed an obligation on the State of issue only. No other State assumed any obligation whatsoever until it affixed a visa to that document."[701] As set out in detail in paras. 8 and 9 of the Schedule, states are, in particular, fully entitled to apply their usual criteria for the issue of either an entry or a transit visa.[702]

There was little discussion of the right of destination countries to require an entry visa, the only amendment to the draft of para. 8 of the Schedule being to make clear that whether an entry visa is required or not is strictly a matter for the destination state to decide. That is, it may choose to admit the holder of a CTD without a visa if it wishes to do so.[703] The issue of transit visas, however, elicited more discussion. The primary concern was "the serious difficulties which would arise if a refugee applied for a transit visa to a certain country, and then, instead of proceeding to the country of final destination, remained in the territory for which he had been granted a transit visa

---

[700] Refugee Convention, at Schedule, para. 14. In explaining the net value of this general authority, the British representative to the Conference of Plenipotentiaries suggested that para. 14's right of a state to apply its "'laws and regulations' [was] of far broader application than formalities": Statement of Mr. Hoare of the United Kingdom, UN Doc. A/CONF.2/SR.33, July 24, 1951, at 4. The only reference to the ability to apply "formalities," however, is contained in para. 13(2)'s grant to the issuing state of the right to supervise conditions of reentry. Because para. 14 is expressly stated to be "[s]ubject only to the terms of paragraph 13," the British representative's remarks are inaccurate if meant to suggest that the issuing state can apply its laws and regulations to condition reentry in other than the purely formal and supervisory sense authorized by para. 13. Thus, para. 14 adds nothing to that authority. The issuing state may, however, apply its usual laws and regulations to govern other matters covered by para. 14, e.g. residence and establishment in its territory.

[701] Statement of Sir Leslie Brass of the United Kingdom, UN Doc. E/AC.32/SR.16, Jan. 30, 1950, at 14.

[702] Refugee Convention, at Schedule, paras. 8, 9. In discussion of the right of states to insist on visa requirements in the Ad Hoc Committee, the Belgian representative "drew attention to paragraph 7 of the schedule ... under the terms of which the High Contracting Parties would recognize the validity of travel documents issued in accordance with the provisions of article [28]": Statement of Mr. Cuvelier of Belgium, UN Doc. E/AC.32/SR.16, Jan. 30, 1950, at 14. The British proponent of the Schedule "admitted that the text of the paragraph could be made more explicit: it should be understood that the High Contracting Parties would not be required to recognize travel documents which did not bear their visa": Statement of Sir Leslie Brass of the United Kingdom, ibid. It is nonetheless regrettable that no effort was made to revise the text of para. 7 clearly to indicate its qualification by paras. 8 and 9.

[703] Refugee Convention, at Schedule, para. 8. As originally proposed, the phrase "and if a visa is required" was not contained in para. 8, which could therefore have been read to suggest a duty to issue a visa to the holder of a CTD allowed to enter a state party: "United Kingdom: Draft Proposal for Article [28]," UN Doc. E/AC.32/L.17, Jan. 30, 1950, at para. 8. The language was amended to its present form without debate at the first session of the Ad Hoc Committee: Ad Hoc Committee, "First Session Report," at para. 8.

only."[704] In the result, state parties "could not assume an unconditional obligation" to issue transit visas to all CTD holders.[705]

To safeguard the interests of transit states, Venezuela wanted to be able to require "firm evidence that they possessed the means of reaching their countries of destination,"[706] for example, "an air or sea ticket to his country of final destination as evidence of his good faith."[707] Denmark sought the right to apply its usual rule that a transit visa would only be issued upon presentation of a valid travel document with a duration of at least two months beyond the expiry of the entry visa to the state of destination.[708] Most generally, Egypt argued for some latitude in the issuance of transit visas in the event that public security in the transit state were threatened by a mass influx of refugees.[709]

The agreement reached sets a presumptive right of the refugee to pass through the territory of any state party as required. In keeping with the mandatory system of mutual recognition,[710] a state party through which a refugee has to pass en route to a "territory of final destination"[711] is generally obliged by para. 9 of the Schedule to honor a validly issued CTD.[712] But the transit country may refuse a transit visa to the holder of a CTD on the same grounds that might be invoked to justify refusal of a transit visa to non-citizens in general.[713] A state party will thus need to rely on generic rules or

---

[704] Statement of Mr. Montoya of Venezuela, UN Doc. A/CONF.2/SR.32, July 24, 1951, at 7.

[705] Statement of Mr. Makiedo of Yugoslavia, UN Doc. A/CONF.2/SR.18, July 12, 1951, at 5.

[706] Statement of Mr. Montoya of Venezuela, ibid. at 7.   [707] Ibid. at 6.

[708] Statement of Mr. Hoeg of Denmark, ibid. at 6–7.

[709] "Where such immigration occurred, transit countries might experience difficulties in applying the provisions of the paragraph, which should therefore include certain limitations based upon considerations of public security": Statement of Mr. Mostafa of Egypt, ibid. at 6.

[710] See text above, at pp. 854–856.

[711] Grahl-Madsen reads the "final destination" language to suggest that a transit visa need only be issued in the case of a refugee seeking resettlement "or some serious travel purpose, not for holiday trips or other pleasure travels": Grahl-Madsen, *Commentary*, at 147–148. There is, however, nothing in the *travaux* that requires this meaning. Moreover, in view of the general goals of the CTD system, which include the facilitation of business and holiday travel (see text above, at p. 846), there is no good reason to conceive the notion of "final destination" as meaning other than the final destination for the particular travel intended (which may or may not be a permanent destination).

[712] "The Contracting States undertake to issue transit visas to refugees who have obtained visas for a territory of final destination": Refugee Convention, at Schedule, para. 9(1). Since destination states are entitled to authorize entry without a visa (see text above, at pp. 870–871), the presumptive duty to issue a transit visa logically arises as well once it is established that no visa is required to enter the country of final destination.

[713] An amendment proposed by Yugoslavia (UN Doc. A/CONF.2/31) was adopted in part by the Ad Hoc Committee, which resulted in the addition of the second sentence of para. 9 of the Schedule ("The issue of such visas may be refused on grounds which would justify refusal of a visa to any alien"): UN Doc. A/CONF.2/SR.18, July 12, 1951, at 7.

standards to limit or restrict the issuance of transit visas to the holders of a CTD, and may not impose refugee-specific constraints.[714]

The Egyptian delegate seems clearly to have believed that this approach precludes a decision to suspend the issuance of transit visas in the case of a mass influx of refugees. After passage of the amended text of para. 9, he indicated that the rule adopted "did not fully meet his point."[715] At one level, this seems right: the existence of a mass influx may have little bearing on whether the transit state is likely to face the risk of non-departure from its territory of refugees who gain entry on the basis of an intention to travel onward. But despite the primary motivation for its adoption, the text of the second sentence of para. 9 of the Schedule is not limited to the authorization of measures necessary to ensure the departure of refugees in transit. If a state were comprehensively to curtail the issuance of transit visas in the event of a public security threat (of any kind), there would be no impediment to relying upon that generic authority to suspend the issuance of transit visas to the holders of CTDs (including where public security was threatened by a mass influx of refugees). This may explain the view of the Colombian representative that he "appreciated the difficulties of the Egyptian and Venezuelan representatives, but felt they were met by the Yugoslav amendment."[716] This understanding moreover allows para. 9(2) to be read in consonance with the general rule in para. 14, pursuant to which state parties are entitled to apply their usual migration control rules governing, *inter alia*, "transit through" their territory.[717]

In sum, the CTD system codified in Art. 28 and its Schedule is not only a critical means of facilitating ordinary, short-term travel by refugees, but is of fundamental value in providing refugees with the documentation often required to seek out opportunities for onward movement in search of their preferred durable solution. In this sense, it is the practical complement to

---

[714] "[A] State cannot refuse to grant a transit visa simply because it considers such a visa as a privilege which it may grant or refuse at will without having to give reasons for a refusal. The State in question must show grounds which can justify its refusal in the individual case or in the special circumstances. That is to say that the refusal must refer to a specific exclusion ground in its Aliens Law or pertinent regulations, or at least be rooted in a general policy": Grahl-Madsen, *Commentary*, at 148.

[715] Statement of Mr. Mostafa of Egypt, UN Doc. A/CONF.2/SR.18, July 12, 1951, at 7.

[716] Statement of Mr. Giraldo-Jaramillo of Colombia, ibid. at 7.

[717] Indeed, the view was expressed that para. 9(2) was superfluous in view of para. 14: Statement of Mr. van Heuven Goedhart of UNHCR, UN Doc. A/CONF.2/SR.32, July 24, 1951, at 7. It seems to have been retained essentially to avoid any ambiguity on this point. "[T]he second sentence in paragraph 9 was a natural corollary to the first. It was impossible to envisage the unconditional granting of transit visas, but that was what paragraph 9 could mean, in the present context, if the second sentence were deleted": Statement of Mr. Rochefort of France, ibid.

Art. 31(2)'s express contemplation of resettlement beyond the state of first reception.[718]

The workability of the CTD system is attributable to a careful balance between the rights of individual states, and a shared commitment to making the sorts of compromise needed for a collective regime to work in practice. On the one hand, there is extraordinary flexibility and autonomy in the system. Subject only to the presumptive responsibility to issue travel documents to refugees lawfully staying in their territory, states may issue travel documents to a broader class of refugees if they wish; they decide independently whether the test for withholding of issuance on public order or national security grounds is met; and they are largely responsible for determining the terms of validity and renewal of the travel documents issued. Yet because this independence of action is neatly balanced by a commitment to readmit the holders of any CTD issued by them, it has been possible to secure the commitment of all state parties to recognize the validity of any refugee travel document issued by a partner state, and to regulate the transit and entry of CTD holders on the basis of only their usual migration control policies. In the result, most refugees are entitled to enjoy international freedom of movement on terms that are not appreciably different from those that govern the more general, passport-based system of travel.

6.7 Freedom of expression and association

In the liberal tradition, freedom of expression is thought to be "an indispensable prerequisite for life in society based on the principles of rationality and mutual respect for human dignity."[719] Individuals are allowed to participate in a two-way flow of information and ideas, and then to stimulate both attention to, and discussion of, their views. As a practical matter, meaningful

---

[718] See chapter 4.2.4 above, at p. 414. More generally, Executive Committee Conclusion No. 15 requires that even efforts among states to avoid gaps in the assignment of protective responsibility should observe the principle that "[t]he intentions of the asylum-seeker as regards the country in which he wishes to request asylum should as far as possible be taken into account": UNHCR Executive Committee Conclusion No. 15, "Refugees Without an Asylum Country" (1979), at para. (h)(iii), available at www.unhcr.ch (accessed Nov. 20, 2004). These principles are not reflected in regimes such as the European Convention Determining the State Responsible for Examining Applications for Asylum Lodged in One of the Member States of the European Communities, June 15, 1990, 30 ILM 425 (1991) (Dublin Convention) and the Agreement between the Government of Canada and the Government of the United States Regarding Asylum Claims Made at Land Borders, Aug. 30, 2002, (2002) 79(37) *Interpreter Releases* 1446 (Canada–US Agreement), an express goal of which is to prohibit asylum-seekers from seeking protection in other than the country of first arrival.

[719] Nowak, *ICCPR Commentary*, at 337.

engagement in this process of exchange is often possible only where there is scope for individuals to act collectively. As Jayawickrama explains,

> [T]he attainment of individual goals, through the exercise of individual rights, is generally impossible without the aid and co-operation of others. Uniting protects individuals from the vulnerability of isolation. It enables those who would otherwise be ineffective to meet on more equal terms the power and strength of those with whom their interests interact and, perhaps, conflict.[720]

The motivation to organize is found no less among refugees. In fact, the circumstances of their flight and exile often lead refugees to value their expressive rights particularly highly:

> Exiles are under enormous pressure to organize politically, and their status alone is proof of their political disenfranchisement at home. Within the asylum country as well, exiles are likely to be politically, economically, and socially vulnerable. They rarely have representation within the asylum State's political system, and the national and international agencies chartered to assist them typically give inadequate consideration to their views. Members of an exile community will also likely share a racial, national, religious, or social characteristic which marked them as a target for persecution in the country of origin. Such circumstances make some level of political organization inevitable.[721]

In practice, refugees organize for many reasons. Participation in associations may help them counteract feelings of isolation, increase their self-esteem, and lessen their sense of alienation.[722] Refugee associations may also play a role in preserving values and elements of identity of the refugee community within the context of a dominant host culture – for example, language, family structure, and religious beliefs. Such associations, while obviously incapable of rendering refugees impervious to acculturation, may nonetheless play a critical role in allowing refugees better to position themselves for successful readjustment in the event repatriation proves ultimately to be possible.[723]

One of the most fundamental reasons leading refugees to form associations is the need to work collectively to provide for their necessities of

---

[720] N. Jayawickrama, *The Judicial Application of Human Rights Law* (2002) (Jayawickrama, *Judicial Application*), at 738–739.

[721] S. Corliss, "Asylum State Responsibility for the Hostile Acts of Foreign Exiles," (1990) 2(2) *International Journal of Refugee Law* 181 (Corliss, "Hostile Acts"), at 192.

[722] J. Sorenson, "Opposition, Exile and Identity: The Eritrean Case," (1990) 3 *Journal of Refugee Studies* 298, at 313.

[723] M. Castillo and J. Hathaway, "Temporary Protection," in J. Hathaway ed., *Reconceiving International Refugee Law* 1 (1997), at 11. See also R. Hofmann, *International Academy of Comparative Law National Report for Germany* (1994), at 30–31.

life.[724] Refugee groups which have successfully organized to achieve significant self-reliance include Tibetan refugees in India, Angolan refugees in Zambia, and Mozambican refugees in Swaziland, to name only a few examples.[725] Refugees have also organized so as to be represented before host country and international authorities, and to facilitate the establishment and delivery of education, healthcare, and other social services. Bhutanese refugees in Nepal, for example, formed groups to advocate for refugee education and healthcare, to establish professional and technical organizations, to aid victims of violence, and to provide opportunities for sub-populations such as women, young people, and students to share concerns and devise coping strategies.[726] Salvadoran refugees in Honduras created a structure of elected representatives to self-govern their camps, including the running of health campaigns, workshops, and schools, the distribution of food and clothing, and delivery of pastoral services.[727] Eritrean nationalist groups represented the refugee population before the Sudanese government and international relief organizations, operated health clinics and schools, and orchestrated community development initiatives.[728]

Most states do not restrict such activities by refugee associations.[729] To the contrary, they often find such organizations helpful in facilitating the provision of assistance and services to the refugee community.[730] The United States, for example, determined in the mid-1970s that there was value in funding Southeast Asian refugee organizations to provide employment, language, vocational, and other services to refugees from Vietnam.[731] Not all host governments welcome refugee participation, however. For example, the Meheba Management Committee was excluded from the planning of projects

---

[724] See generally P. Van Arsdale, "The Role of Mutual Assistance Associations in Refugee Acculturation and Service Delivery," in M. Hopkins and N. Donnelly eds., *Selected Papers on Refugee Issues II* 156 (1993).

[725] D. Keen, *Refugees: Rationing the Right to Life* (1992), at 60–61.

[726] These organizations included the Bhutanese Refugees Educational Coordinating Committee, Bhutan Health Organization, Association of Bhutanese Professionals and Technicians, Bhutanese Refugees Aiding Victims of Violence, Bhutan Women's Association, Refugee Women Committee, Youth Organization of Bhutan, Students Union of Bhutan, as well as several Bhutanese human rights organizations: G. Siwakoti, *International Academy of Comparative Law National Report for Nepal* (2002), at 10.

[727] J. Hammond, "War-Uprooting and the Political Mobilization of Central American Refugees," (1993) 6(2) *Journal of Refugee Studies* 105, at 110.

[728] Corliss, "Hostile Acts," at 192.

[729] UNHCR, "Implementation," at para. 76.

[730] Corliss, "Hostile Acts," at 192.

[731] C. Mortland, "Patron–Client Relations and the Evolution of Mutual Assistance Associations," in P. Van Arsdale ed., *Refugee Empowerment and Organizational Change: A Systems Perspective* 15 (1993), at 16.

with UNHCR implementing partners in Zambia.[732] The participation of refugees in economic associations, particularly trade unions, may also be strictly regulated by way of special registration requirements, limitations on the number of non-citizens in a union, or the expulsion of refugees who participate in an unlawful strike.[733] In the more explicitly political realm, the main concern of host states is generally that refugee associations not raise the risk of destabilization. For example, while Switzerland has scrapped its formal ban on refugees engaging in political activities, it nonetheless adopted a policy of requiring refugees to secure special authorization to make a political speech in order to ensure that refugees not interfere in Swiss internal affairs.[734] Namibian authorities ordered the arrest of several refugee members of a musical group on the grounds that they had illicitly participated in domestic politics by performing at a Congress of Democrats function.[735] And in Zimbabwe, refugees accused of funding political parties opposed to the government have been expelled.[736]

Refugee organizations have at times engaged in efforts to overthrow the government of their country of origin. As Corliss notes, "[f]ew exiles want to remain exiles, and a change in the political *status quo* is usually the only truly secure way to return home."[737] Such activities may be non-violent, including the establishment of opposition groups, or the conduct of public awareness campaigns such as those organized by Kurdish refugees in the United Kingdom.[738] But refugees may also establish armed bands, terrorist attacks, assassinations, and outright invasions – for example, the mobilization of

[732] E. Brooks, "The Social Consequences of the Legal Dilemma of Refugees in Zambia" (1988), at 8. Ten years later, however, progress had been made on this front. Refugees were allowed to select Road Chairmen to present their views to a tripartite administration comprised of government, UNHCR, and the lead non-governmental partner, Lutheran World Foundation: M. Barrett, "Tuvosena: 'Let's Go Everybody': Identity and Ambition Among Refugees in Zambia," Uppsala University Department of Cultural Anthropology Working Paper (1998), at 14.

[733] UNHCR, "Implementation," at para. 76.

[734] W. Kälin, *International Academy of Comparative Law National Report for Switzerland* (1994), at 16.

[735] *Namibian*, June 16, 2000. While the Namibian courts subsequently intervened to prohibit the government from punishing the refugees by detaining or deporting them, the Minister of Home Affairs "responded to the order . . . by issuing statements attacking the judiciary, and to the effect that despite the order he would seek to arrest [the refugees] . . . Following a few tense weeks, an agreement was reached [providing that the refugees] would apply for work permits while returning to Osire [refugee camp] voluntarily": Legal Assistance Centre, "Constitutional and Human Rights Unit Annual Report" (2000), at 5–6.

[736] LCHR, *African Exodus*, at 95.   [737] Corliss, "Hostile Acts," at 195.

[738] O. Wahlbeck, "Community Work and Exile Politics: Kurdish Refugee Associations in London," (1998) 11(3) *Journal of Refugee Studies* 215, at 226.

Rwandese refugees in Uganda prior to the invasion of 1990,[739] and the repeated violation of Cuban airspace by refugees from that country based in the United States.[740]

State responses to political activity directed at the refugees' country of origin range from toleration or even support of the refugees, to harsh "crack-downs." It has been noted that "[w]hether or not a host government restricts the political activities of refugees depends almost entirely on its own alignments and preferences."[741] For example, Kenya has alternated between restricting and allowing the political activities of successive generations of Ugandan refugees, depending upon whether the party benefiting from their support was in domestic political favor.[742] The same has been true for Liberian refugees in Côte d'Ivoire.[743] In some situations, refugees have even played key roles in advancing the international political goals of their host state. Pakistan actively supported the use of its territory by Afghan rebels engaged in anti-Soviet assaults, even to the point of delivering military aid from the United States to the refugee fighters.[744] Similarly,

---

[739] C. Watson and US Committee for Refugees, "Exile from Rwanda: Background to an Invasion," Feb. 1991. See also Corliss, "Hostile Acts," at 199: "The use of external bases to mount an actual insurgency has ... become more pervasive in recent decades. Foreign sanctuaries permit an otherwise unviable insurgent movement to mature and gain strength. Without the burden of having to maintain territorial control, the insurgents can train, expand their numbers, and develop international political and material support links without hindrance."

[740] "The Cuban attack on the unarmed civilian planes used by 'Brothers to the Rescue,' a refugee organization, is one more sad chapter in Castro's 35-year antagonistic relationship with the United States. In the past, Brothers pilots have blatantly violated US and international law by crossing into Cuban airspace. But even if they did so again last weekend, as the Cuban government claims, shooting them down was inexcusable. However, blame must be shared by rabid expatriates determined to overthrow Castro's communist government. [The US government] must rein in these forces – or at least make sure they don't use the United States as the launching pad for their incursions": "Retaliation by force is not answer in Cuba," *Chicago Sun–Times*, Feb. 28, 1996, at 25.

[741] LCHR, *African Exodus*, at 94.

[742] Ibid. Of perhaps greater concern, the local UNHCR representative, Reinier Thiadens, is reported to have declared that "our position is that political activities should not take place within the refugee camps": R. Oduol, "Ethiopian refugees need not fear harassment in camps," *East African*, July 2, 2001.

[743] LCHR, *African Exodus*, at 94.

[744] N. Ahmad, *International Academy of Comparative Law National Report for Pakistan* (1994), at 10. "Pakistan offered not only generous humanitarian assistance to the Afghan refugees, but also military aid and training to the mujahiddin – allowing its territory to be used as an arms pipeline – and diplomatic support for the resistance ... The multinational aid effort led by the US and Pakistan gave the Afghan resistance the support it needed to continue to fight, thus creating a refugee-based insurgency along the Pakistan–Afghanistan border": L. Goodson, *Afghanistan's Endless War: State Failure, Regional Politics, and the Rise of the Taliban* (2001), at 147.

Honduras allowed its territory to be used as a staging ground for attacks on Nicaragua by exiles from the Sandinista government supported by the United States.[745]

Conversely, while the Indian government initially tolerated the subversive activities of the Tamil refugees who arrived from Sri Lanka in the mid-1980s,[746] militant groups were disarmed and the LTTE banned after the assassination of Rajiv Gandhi.[747] Thai police arrested Burmese refugees for planning a peaceful protest in front of the Burmese Embassy against the unlawful detention by that country's military junta of opposition leader Aung San Suu Kyi. In doing so, they explicitly cited "the Prime Minister's policy to keep order in the country by restricting the political activities of Burmese refugees in Thailand."[748] Tanzania detained Burundian refugees engaged in a campaign for Hutu majority rule in their country because they had "assembled and drilled unlawfully with political intent which could create disharmony between Tanzania and its neighbouring countries."[749] Indeed, such is the intensity of concern about the risk to interstate relations in Africa that the 1969 OAU Refugee Convention requires refugees to "abstain from any subversive activities against any Member State of the OAU"; signatory governments moreover "undertake to prohibit refugees residing in their respective territories from attacking any State Member of the OAU, by any activity likely to cause tension between Member States, and in particular by use of arms, through the press, or by radio."[750]

---

[745] E. Ferris, *The Central American Refugees* (1987), at 106. "[W]hen the United States in 1979 lost Nicaragua, its closest ally in Central America, to a regime that favored ties to Havana and Moscow over Washington ... Honduras was transformed into a 'Pentagon Republic,' a military sanctuary from which to launch a covert war against Nicaragua": F. Terry, *Condemned to Repeat? The Paradox of Humanitarian Action* (2002), at 86.

[746] Indira Gandhi's administration was accused of actively assisting Sri Lankan guerrillas with aid and training, as well as turning a blind eye to smuggling and other illegal activities: B. Bastiampillai, "Sri Lankan Tamil Refugees in Tamilnadu: Trouble to the Host," paper presented at the International Seminar on Refugees and Internal Security in South Asia, Colombo, July 1994 (Bastiampillai, "Tamil Refugees"), at 10.

[747] Ibid. at 12; US Committee for Refugees, *World Refugee Survey 1993* (1993), at 93. Even today, "[t]he LTTE is banned in India ... and its leader is among those wanted by Indian courts to stand trial in the case [of the assassination of Rajiv Gandhi]": V. Sambandan, "India, US urged to 'rethink' on LTTE," *Hindu*, Apr. 10, 2003.

[748] S. Phasuk, "Old habits die hard," *Irrawaddy*, July 4, 2003. The Prime Minister had earlier "threatened to repatriate pro-democracy activists after openly acknowledging that most would be persecuted on arrival in military-ruled Burma": ibid.

[749] Amnesty International, "Tanzania: Burundi Nationals Detained in Tanzania," Sept. 1990.

[750] Convention governing the Specific Aspects of Refugee Problems in Africa, UNTS 14691, done Sept. 10, 1969, entered into force June 20, 1974 (OAU Refugee Convention), at Art. III.

Refugee Convention, Art. 15   Right of association

As regards non-political and non-profit-making associations and trade unions, the Contracting States shall accord to refugees lawfully staying in their territory the most favourable treatment accorded to nationals of a foreign country, in the same circumstances.

Civil and Political Covenant, Art. 19

1. Everyone shall have the right to hold opinions without interference.

2. Everyone shall have the right to freedom of expression; this right shall include freedom to seek, receive and impart information and ideas of all kinds, regardless of frontiers, either orally, in writing or in print, in the form of art, or through any other media of his choice.

3. The exercise of the rights provided for in paragraph 2 of this article carries with it special duties and responsibilities. It may therefore be subject to certain restrictions, but these shall only be such as are provided by law and are necessary:

(a) For respect of the rights or reputations of others;

(b) For the protection of national security or of public order (*ordre public*), or of public health or morals.

Civil and Political Covenant, Art. 20

1. Any propaganda for war shall be prohibited by law.

2. Any advocacy of national, racial or religious hatred that constitutes incitement to discrimination, hostility or violence shall be prohibited by law.

Civil and Political Covenant, Art. 21

The right of peaceful assembly shall be recognized. No restrictions may be placed on the exercise of this right other than those imposed in conformity with the law and which are necessary in a democratic society in the interests of national security or public safety, public order (*ordre public*), the protection of public health or morals or the protection of the rights and freedoms of others.

Civil and Political Covenant, Art. 22

1. Everyone shall have the right to freedom of association with others, including the right to form and join trade unions for the protection of his interests.

2. No restrictions may be placed on the exercise of this right other than those which are prescribed by law and which are

necessary in a democratic society in the interests of national security or public safety, public order (*ordre public*), the protection of public health or morals or the protection of the rights and freedoms of others . . .

Economic, Social and Cultural Covenant, Art. 8

1. The States Parties to the present Covenant undertake to ensure:

    (a) the right of everyone to form trade unions and join the trade union of his choice, subject only to the rules of the organization concerned, for the promotion and protection of his economic and social interests. No restrictions may be placed on the exercise of this right other than those prescribed by law and which are necessary in a democratic society in the interests of national security or public order or for the protection of the rights and freedoms of others;

        . . .

    (d) the right to strike, provided that it is exercised in conformity with the laws of the particular country.

        . . .

The wording initially proposed by the Secretary-General for Art. 15 of the Refugee Convention provided that "[r]efugees . . . shall have the right to join non-profit-making associations, including trade unions."[751] This was a clear advance on the rather narrow approach taken in predecessor treaties, which had authorized refugees to establish only "associations for mutual relief and assistance."[752] So framed, the provision would have been subject to no contingency, and would have inhered in all refugees without qualification. The more inclusive formulation proposed was said to have been based upon a desire to bring the Refugee Convention into line with Art. 20(1) of the Universal Declaration of Human Rights, a broadly framed provision acknowledging that "[e]veryone has the right to freedom of peaceful assembly and association."[753]

Yet it must be conceded that even the initial formulation of Art. 15 fell significantly short of the standard which the drafters cited as their inspiration. Not only did the first draft of Art. 15 fail to make any mention of the

---

[751] Secretary-General, "Memorandum," at 27.

[752] 1933 Refugee Convention, at Art. 11; 1938 Refugee Convention, at Art. 13.

[753] Universal Declaration, at Art. 20(1). "The ordinary law of the democratic countries includes freedom of association which, in principle, is enjoyed by foreigners as well as by nationals . . . [as set out in] Article 20 of the Universal Declaration of Human Rights . . . In these circumstances, there can be no objection to [refugees] joining non-profit-making associations": Secretary-General, "Memorandum," at 27–28.

branch of Art. 20 of the Universal Declaration requiring freedom of peaceful assembly, but it made no attempt to codify the Declaration's Art. 19, stipulating the arguably more basic right to freedom of opinion and expression.[754] Even the content of the right to freedom of association proposed for the Refugee Convention was narrowly conceived: refugees would have been granted the right to join only "non-profit-making associations, including trade unions," said to include "associations pursuing cultural, sports, social or philanthropic aims, as distinct from associations 'for pecuniary gain,' whose aim is the making of profits."[755] Yet the cognate provisions in general human rights law are generally understood to include the right to belong to all forms of association.[756]

The lack of consonance between Art. 15 and the principles of the Universal Declaration intensified over the course of the drafting process. Most critically, the decision was taken not to guarantee the right of refugees to belong to political associations. And even though the Universal Declaration's guarantee inheres in "everyone," the Refugee Convention's right to freedom of association extends only to refugees who are lawfully staying in a state party, and even then must be honored only to the same extent that such rights are granted to most-favored foreigners.

The reluctance of the drafters to establish a comprehensive right of refugees to freedom of association appears to have been driven by genuine concern about the risk of political destabilization, both in receiving states and internationally. As the Belgian delegate remarked, refugees were seen to present a political risk which distinguished them from other non-citizens:

> [T]he position of some Governments *vis à vis* foreigners generally was essentially different from their attitude towards refugees. It was not too difficult to ask a foreign national to leave the country, but it was often virtually impossible to expel a refugee. Different measures had to be taken

---

[754] "Everyone has the right to freedom of opinion and expression; this right includes freedom to hold opinions without interference and to seek, receive and impart information and ideas through any media and regardless of frontiers": Universal Declaration, at Art. 19. As Jayawickrama observes, the freedoms of opinion, assembly, and association combine in practice to "require[ ] the acceptance of the public airing of disagreements and the refusal to silence unpopular views": Jayawickrama, *Judicial Application*, at 666.

[755] Secretary-General, "Memorandum," at 28. Oddly, the Secretary-General's draft assumed that "[p]rofit-making associations are covered by the provisions dealing with the exercise of the professions": ibid. Yet this approach seems to leave out the right to join a non-professional profit-making association, e.g. a business council or non-unionized workers' collective.

[756] Specifically, Art. 22 of the Civil and Political Covenant, which is the legally binding codification of Art. 20 of the Universal Declaration, has a "protective scope [which] is broad. Religious societies, political parties, commercial undertakings and trade unions are as protected by Art. 22 as cultural or human rights organizations, soccer clubs or associations of stamp collectors": Nowak, *ICCPR Commentary*, at 386.

for the two groups. Moreover, it had been the experience of some States that foreign nationals rarely engaged in political activity, while refugees frequently did so.[757]

Indeed, the constrained approach taken to the associational rights of refugees was explicitly defended by the French government on the grounds that "[w]hile it was embarrassing to favour the withdrawal of rights from a group of people, it would be better to do that than to expose that group of people – refugees – to the more drastic alternative of deportation (on grounds of national security or public order)."[758] The denial of a complete right to freedom of association was therefore said to be "a warning to refugees in their own interest."[759]

The international political concerns of states derived in part from a fear that refugees might prove to be infiltrators determined "to serve the interests of some other country."[760] Thus, Denmark, Egypt, and France expressly invoked national security concerns to justify the denial of freedom of political association to refugees.[761] More generally, Austria expressed its worry that "recognition of the right of refugees to form associations could readily cause strained or aggravated relations between the countries of residence and those of origin."[762] While amendments based on such concerns did not garner majority support in the Ad Hoc Committee,[763] the Conference of

---

[757] Statement of Mr. Cuvelier of Belgium, UN Doc. E/AC.32/SR.23, Feb. 3, 1950, at 10–11.

[758] Statement of Mr. Devinat of France, ibid. at 9.

[759] Statement of Mr. Cuvelier of Belgium, ibid. at 11.

[760] Statement of Mr. Rain of France, UN Doc. E/AC.32/SR.10, Jan. 24, 1950, at 10.

[761] "[T]he French amendment should not be regarded as a discriminatory measure against refugees, but rather as a security measure": Statement of Mr. Devinat of France, UN Doc. E/AC.32/SR.23, Feb. 3, 1950, at 9. See also Statement of Mr. Larsen of Denmark, UN Doc. E/AC.32/SR.10, Jan. 24, 1950, at 10: "[R]efugees who had found freedom and security in another country should not be permitted to engage in political activity which might endanger that country"; and Statement of Mr. Mostafa of Egypt, UN Doc. A/CONF.2/SR.8, July 5, 1951, at 10: "Refugees admitted to a country should not be in a position to engage in political activities prejudicial to the security of that country."

[762] United Nations, "Compilation of Comments," at 41. The Austrian government concluded that "[i]t would be preferable, therefore, to leave as a matter of principle to the administrative authorities in the country of refuge the decision as to the right of refugees to form associations": ibid.

[763] "The Chairman feared that the Committee was reopening questions discussed at the first session, when a proposal of the French delegation to allow, in providing for freedom of association, for the possibility of forbidding political activities had found small favour as it had been felt that article 2 covered the point sufficiently. Many delegates, moreover, remembering that the Universal Declaration of Human Rights imposed no conditions on the right of association, had thought that in some countries, especially those proud of their democratic institutions, the Committee might be suspected of a desire to limit actions which were certainly legal": Statement of the Chairman, Mr. Larsen of Denmark, UN Doc. E/AC.32/SR.37, Aug. 16, 1950, at 9.

Plenipotentiaries formally amended Art. 15 to exclude political associations from its ambit.[764] The rationale for doing so was the determination of Switzerland to ensure that refugees did not jeopardize its position of international political neutrality:

> In principle, aliens in Switzerland enjoyed freedom of association as one of the basic rights guaranteed by the Swiss Federal Constitution. [But] past experience had shown that the policy of neutrality pursued by Switzerland in implementation of her international obligations made it necessary to impose certain limits on the political activity of aliens resident in the country ... They also applied to political groups of aliens. It had proved necessary to establish a slightly stricter regulation in respect of refugees. In principle, the regulations ... debarred refugees from engaging in any political activity of any kind while in Switzerland: hence refugees had no right to participate in the activity of political groups or to form such groups themselves. That was just one of the conditions attached to the granting of asylum, and its justification could not be disputed.[765]

Similar concerns to avoid interstate tension are evident today in, for example, Tanzania's detention of activist Hutu refugees from Burundi, and Thailand's arrest of pro-democracy Burmese refugees. More generally, the duty of state parties to the OAU Convention to ensure that refugees are prohibited from engaging in "any activity likely to cause tension between Member States" shows the continuing salience of this preoccupation.

Even though interstate concerns were the express reason for the successful effort to exclude political associations from the scope of Art. 15, the broadly framed amendment appealed also to governments anxious to deny refugees the right to participate in domestic political associations of absolutely no international significance. From the beginning, concern was expressed that the Secretary-General's draft of Art. 15 "might even imply that refugees were to enjoy the unqualified right to [engage in] political activities,"[766] in which case "it might be conveniently invoked by [refugees] in order to sanction undesirable political activity."[767] In much the same way that Switzerland viewed abstention from internationally significant political activity as "just one of the conditions attached to the granting of asylum,"[768] so too other countries felt justified in withholding purely domestic political rights from

---

[764] The amendment to insert the words "non-political" into the definition of protected associational activities was adopted on a 10–0 (9 abstentions) vote: UN Doc. A/CONF.2/SR.8, July 5, 1951, at 11.

[765] Statement of Mr. Schurch of Switzerland, ibid. at 8–9.

[766] Statement of Mr. Kural of Turkey, UN Doc. E/AC.32/SR.10, Jan. 24, 1950, at 9.

[767] Statement of Mr. Kural of Turkey, UN Doc. A/AC.32/SR.23, Feb. 3, 1950, at 11.

[768] Statement of Mr. Schurch of Switzerland, UN Doc. A/CONF.2/SR.8, July 5, 1951, at 9.

refugees as the *quid pro quo* for the granting of protection. France, in particular, argued that

> [a]lthough France had always taken a very liberal attitude towards the many refugees who had found shelter and protection within its borders, it felt that in return they were under an obligation to refrain from taking part in its internal politics until they had become naturalized citizens. In the meantime, they had neither the full duties nor the full rights of nationals.[769]

The Refugee Convention does not, therefore, prevent Zimbabwe from denying refugees the right to fund domestic political parties. While that country may not implement such a ban on a discriminatory basis (that is, applied only against those who fund opposition parties),[770] or violate the duty either of non-expulsion[771] or of *non-refoulement*[772] in enforcing it, the Convention affords refugees no presumptive right to join or otherwise support their host state's political associations. On the other hand, the Namibian arrest of members of a musical group simply because they had performed at a political gathering is surely at odds with even a broad understanding of the prohibition of political association.

This concern to exclude refugees from the internal politics of asylum states is evident also in the debates regarding the scope of permissible trade union activities. While there was no dissent from the view that refugees should be entitled to join existing national trade unions,[773] there was disagreement about whether refugees should also be allowed to engage in the more

---

[769] Statement of Mr. Rain of France, UN Doc. E/AC.32/SR.10, Jan. 24, 1950, at 10.

[770] Art. 26 of the Civil and Political Covenant prohibits discrimination on the grounds of *inter alia* political opinion: see chapter 2.5.5 above, at p. 125.

[771] See chapter 5.1 above. While states have the right to expel refugees on "public order" grounds, this notion does *not* include all concerns within the civil law understanding of *ordre public*: ibid. at pp. 685–690. Moreover, lawful expulsion under Art. 32 requires scrupulous attention to due process norms: ibid. at pp. 670–677.

[772] See chapters 4.1.2 and 4.1.4 above.

[773] "It will be noted that the text expressly refers to trade unions, in order that there should be no doubt with respect to them": Secretary-General, "Memorandum," at 28. For example, even as it proposed restrictive amendments to Art. 15, the Belgian representative "wished to emphasize that his Government's reservation referred precisely to non-profit-making associations other than trade unions. If only trade unions were in question, it was quite clear that the Belgian delegation would approve of the provision, but there were other associations involved whose activities might give rise to legitimate concern": Statement of Mr. Herment of Belgium, UN Doc. E/AC.32/SR.37, Aug. 16, 1950, at 9. The French representative similarly observed that "he was glad to see that [Art. 15] contained the words 'trade unions'": Statement of Mr. Juvigny of France, UN Doc. E/AC.32/SR.36, Aug. 15, 1950, at 26. Reflecting this view, the Second Session of the Ad Hoc Committee adopted the portion of Art. 15 referring to trade union rights on a 7–0 (4 abstentions) vote, even as the article as a whole passed by a less powerful 7–4 (0 abstentions) margin: UN Doc. E/AC.32/SR.37, Aug. 16, 1950, at 10.

politicized acts of assuming leadership roles within unions,[774] or establishing unions of their own.[775] In the end, the rather vague language of Art. 15 – in which refugees are granted rights "[a]s regards … trade unions" – was adopted as a means of encouraging (but not requiring) states to grant broad associational rights to refugees.[776] But if and when a refugee's role in

[774] For example, "[i]n France, refugees could join trade unions, but they could not assume leadership or hold executive positions. He thought the problem could be solved by suitable drafting": Statement of Mr. Rain of France, UN Doc. E/AC.32/SR.10, Jan. 24, 1950, at 9.

[775] The original language proposed by the Secretary-General referred only to the right "to join" trade unions: Secretary-General, "Memorandum," at 27. Denmark proposed the amendment of Art. 15 to provide that refugees would have the right "to form and to join" trade unions: Statement of Mr. Larsen of Denmark, UN Doc. E/AC.32/SR.10, Jan. 24, 1950, at 10. As explained by the supportive Belgian representative, the amendment "would then conform to the Universal Declaration of Human Rights, which accorded both rights to everyone": Statement of Mr. Cuvelier of Belgium, ibid. at 11. But the American Federation of Labor sought to justify a withholding of this right on the grounds that "in practice, it might well work to [refugees'] disadvantage, as the existing trade unions in various countries might grow suspicious and possibly hostile … Trade unions in Canada and the United States might hesitate to allow refugees to join if they were also permitted to form their own trade unions": Statement of Mr. Stolz of the American Federation of Labor, ibid. at 11. While the amendment expressly referring to a right "to form" as well as to join trade unions was thereupon defeated, the Chairman adopted an American interpretation "that the negative vote on the Danish amendment did not mean that refugees should be prohibited from forming either trade unions or other non-profit-making associations": Statement of Mr. Henkin of the United States, ibid. at 12, affirmed by the Chairman, Mr. Chance of Canada, ibid.

[776] As remarked by the French representative, "[t]he very general formula used left open the question whether membership or organization of a trade union was meant, and left room for whatever interpretation might be put upon it by the various national legislations": Statement of Mr. Juvigny of France, UN Doc. E/AC.32/SR.36, Aug. 15, 1950, at 26. The drafting history set out at note 775 above affirms the lack of a clear consensus on this question. The ambiguity inherent in the framing of Art. 15 was also remarked upon by the Israeli representative, who observed that he "saw a notable disparity between article [15] and the comment of the Committee [on its content]. If that comment [suggesting that 'although not expressly stated, this article recognizes the right of refugees to form as well as to join associations': Ad Hoc Committee, 'First Session Report,' at Annex II] correctly set forth the intention of the article, the words 'As regards non-profit-making associations' should be replaced by the words 'As regards their right to form or join non-profit-making associations'": Statement of Mr. Robinson of Israel, UN Doc. E/AC.32/SR.36, Aug. 15, 1950, at 24. The Chairman replied that "the suggestion of the representative of Israel recalled one he himself had made during the first session. His suggestion had not been favourably received by the Committee, which had seen in it the suggestion of encouraging refugees to establish special trade unions instead of joining the regular trade unions of their countries of residence": Statement of the Chairman, Mr. Larsen of Denmark, ibid. at 25. While the American representative maintained his position that "the article … covered both types of activity," even he conceded the diversity of views on the issue and opposed

a union (or other association) becomes more political than strictly associational, governments have the right under the Refugee Convention to circumscribe the scope of the refugee's activities.[777]

The same determination to constrain the involvement of refugees in the internal politics of receiving states can be seen in the decision taken to impose a high level of attachment – lawful stay – before even the fairly constrained right to freedom of association is granted to refugees. While less exigent than the French representative's view that refugees should be "under an obligation to refrain from taking part in its internal politics until they had become naturalized citizens,"[778] the increasingly strict standard set – which evolved from no attachment in the original draft, to a requirement that a refugee be "lawfully in" a state's territory as the result of the Ad Hoc Committee's work, to the eventual decision of the Conference of Plenipotentiaries to require "lawful stay" before the granting of associational

any effort to amend its wording expressly to refer to a right "to form" (as well as to join) trade unions: Statement of Mr. Henkin of the United States, ibid. at 25. Yet the issue arose again at the Conference of Plenipotentiaries, where the British representative observed that it was not "clear whether the article related to joining associations alone, or to forming them also": Statement of Mr. Hoare of the United Kingdom, UN Doc. A/CONF.2/SR.8, July 5, 1951, at 10. The President – arguably inaccurately, in light of the French representative's statements above – "recalled that the Ad Hoc Committee had changed the text of article [15] in order to make it consistent with Article 23(4) of the Universal Declaration of Human Rights [which protects both the rights to form and to join trade unions]. That was why the words 'As regards' had been used": Statement of the President, Mr. Larsen of Denmark, ibid. There is thus a conflict between the actual decision taken by the Ad Hoc Committee – which was neither to protect nor to prohibit refugees from forming trade unions – and the report of that decision to the Conference of Plenipotentiaries, upon which representatives may well have based their vote in favor of the adoption of Art. 15.

[777] "It was common knowledge that some countries did not allow refugees to engage in any sort of political activity ... The non-profit-making associations to which article [15] referred might often be political in character": Statement of Mr. Perez Perozo of Venezuela, UN Doc. E/AC.32/SR.37, Aug. 16, 1950, at 6. The reluctance of the drafters to sanction overt political activity by refugees is evident as well from the debate about whether the Refugee Convention should codify Art. 19 of the Universal Declaration, which guarantees freedom of opinion and expression. In (successfully) advocating that no such right be included, the French representative observed that "refugees, residing in a country which was not their own, might wish, under article 19, to engage in political activities which it would be difficult to allow. If article 19 were mentioned in the convention, many States would have to make reservations, which would greatly weaken the scope of the article not only in the convention, but also in the Declaration itself": Statement of Mr. Rain of France, UN Doc. E/AC.32/SR.11, Jan. 25, 1950, at 9.

[778] Statement of Mr. Rain of France, UN Doc. E/AC.32/SR.10, Jan. 24, 1950, at 10. The same approach had been proposed in the French government's draft of the Refugee Convention, which would have limited associational rights to refugees "permanently settled" in a state's territory: France, "Draft Convention," at 4.

rights[779] – is consistent with a determination to delay as much as possible the acquisition of the only essentially political right contained in the Refugee Convention.

This distancing of the approach to freedom of association in the Refugee Convention from the more liberal standard set by the Universal Declaration of Human Rights was clearly troubling to some delegates. As proposals were tabled to exclude political associations from the scope of Art. 15, the American representative protested that constraints on freedom of association "did not seem to be in keeping with the principles of the United Nations":[780]

> It might, in fact, be interpreted as forbidding refugees even to express political opinions, and would certainly deny them access to an area of human activity in which they should have at least as much right to engage as any other aliens ... Like all other residents of a country, they would be forbidden to engage in illegal political activity, and should not be singled out and denied the right to engage in legal activity.[781]

The American representative insisted that it was clearly "undesirable to include in a United Nations document a clause prohibiting political activities – a very broad and vague concept indeed."[782] He argued that the legitimate concerns of states could readily be met by reliance on the general duty of refugees to obey the laws of the host state,[783] coupled with judicious resort to the right to expel refugees for reasons of public order.[784] Yet only

---

[779] Interestingly, neither of the shifts to require a higher level of attachment appears to have been formally debated in plenary session. The shift to require lawful presence first appeared in Ad Hoc Committee, "First Session Report," at Annex I. While the comments of the Committee helpfully define the notion to "exclude a refugee who, while lawfully admitted, has over-stayed the period for which he was admitted or was authorized to stay or who has violated any other conditions attached to his admission or stay" (ibid. at Annex II), no indication of the precise reason for the shift is provided. Similarly, the Conference of Plenipotentiaries did not formally debate the increase in the level of attachment to require lawful stay.

[780] Statement of Mr. Henkin of the United States, UN Doc. E/AC.32/SR.10, Jan. 24, 1950, at 10.

[781] Ibid.

[782] Statement of Mr. Henkin of the United States, UN Doc. E/AC.32/SR.23, Feb. 3, 1950, at 8.

[783] "[N]othing in the draft convention prohibited a state from exercising its authority in respect of the political activity of its residents": Statement of Mr. Henkin of the United States, ibid. at 10. Clearly, the American delegate did not feel that Arts. 19 and 20 of the Universal Declaration were a significant constraint on this authority, suggesting as he did that "[i]n the absence of any specific clause on the subject, [host states] would still have the right to restrict political activities of refugees as of any other foreigners": ibid. at 8. The Chinese representative was even more adamant, insisting that "[n]othing in the draft convention could be construed as a derogation of the sovereign right of a State to restrict political activity": Statement of Mr. Cha of China, ibid. at 10.

[784] "Perhaps the points raised by the French and Turkish representatives were already met in the clause recognizing the right to expel refugees for violations of public order. While 'public order' was likewise a vague term, and one not to be invoked indiscriminately, it

the Canadian representative voiced any support for these highly principled views.[785]

Nor can the decision to grant only a minimalist freedom of association to refugees be ascribed simply to a reluctance on the part of the drafters to be the first to codify in law the liberal standard set by the Universal Declaration. To the contrary, the representative of the International Labor Organization drew their attention to the fact that state parties to the Migration for Employment Convention had already committed themselves to grant migrant workers the same trade union rights as enjoyed by national workers.[786] This led the American representative to suggest that "if an international organization affiliated with the United Nations had decided to give special treatment to migrant workers, the Committee should ... consider whether refugees might be in even greater need."[787] Only the Italian delegate responded, noting simply that his government "felt that refugees should not receive preferential treatment, but [only] the same treatment normally accorded to aliens in general."[788]

In fact, the sole liberalizing concession which the American representative was able to wrest from his colleagues was rejection of the "aliens generally" contingent standard[789] in favor of a duty to assimilate refugees' right to freedom of association to that granted to the nationals of most-favored states[790] – this having been the contingent standard which had governed associational rights under both the 1933 and 1938 refugee conventions.[791] While Belgium[792] and

would probably cover most of the cases envisaged by the French amendment": Statement of Mr. Henkin of the United States, ibid. at 8.

[785] "The Chairman, speaking as the Canadian representative, said that he fully shared Mr. Henkin's views": Statement of the Chairman, Mr. Chance of Canada, UN Doc. E/AC.32/SR.10, Jan. 24, 1950, at 10.

[786] Statement of Mr. Oblath of the International Labor Organization, UN Doc. E/AC.32/SR.36, Aug. 15, 1950, at 23–24.

[787] Statement of Mr. Henkin of the United States, ibid. at 27.

[788] Statement of Mr. Theodoli of Italy, ibid. at 27.

[789] This standard had been provisionally adopted at the first session of the Ad Hoc Committee, on the motion of the Chairman, in an effort to meet the concerns expressed, in particular, by France and Turkey: Statement of the Chairman, Mr. Chance of Canada, UN Doc. E/AC.32/SR.10, Jan. 24, 1950, at 9; unanimously adopted, ibid. at 12. A working group formed to revise the draft for approval by the Committee opted nonetheless to reinsert the "most-favored-national" standard: "Decisions of the Working Group Taken on 9 February 1950," UN Doc. E/AC.32/L.32, Feb. 9, 1950, at 5.

[790] The American representative "emphasized that when the Convention gave refugees the same privileges as aliens in general, it was not giving them very much": Statement of Mr. Henkin of the United States, UN Doc. E/AC.32/SR.37, Aug. 16, 1950, at 7.

[791] This precedent was noted in Ad Hoc Committee, "First Session Report," at Annex II, n. 9.

[792] "[H]is Government would like the words 'nationals of foreign countries' to be replaced by the words 'aliens in general'": Statement of Mr. Herment of Belgium, UN Doc. E/AC.32/SR.36, Aug. 15, 1950, at 23.

Venezuela[793] joined Italy[794] in pressing for a less generous contingent standard, the American representative prevailed upon those unwilling to extend to refugees the benefits afforded the citizens of special partner states simply to enter a reservation to the article on freedom of association.[795] As a general matter, he persuaded his colleagues that the "most-favored-national" standard was a fair compromise between the competing views of states:

> He questioned whether, with regard to the right of association, most governments were really not prepared to grant better treatment to refugees than to aliens in general ... The Committee would recall that at the previous meeting, the representative of the International Labor Organization had proposed that refugees be granted even better treatment in connection with trade union membership than was laid down in article 10, that they should receive in fact the same treatment as was guaranteed to nationals, as was provided under the *Migration for Employment Convention*. The representatives of Venezuela and Belgium were proposing to amend the article in the opposite direction. It might be possible to arrive at a compromise, but he hoped that more consideration would first be given to the proposal of the International Labor Organization.[796]

France rejected the American representative's suggestion to align the Refugee Convention with the ILO's national treatment standard, accurately asserting that the right to freedom of association in general was a significantly broader right than the ILO's guarantee of trade union rights.[797] The most-favored-national standard was retained by the slimmest of margins upon final consideration by the Ad Hoc Committee,[798] and not reconsidered at the Conference of Plenipotentiaries. The Refugee Convention is therefore infringed, for example, if refugees are not granted the same dispensation

---

[793] "There was no need in any case to provide for most-favoured-nation treatment under article [15] since the privileges granted under that article would only very rarely be made subject to reciprocity, even more rarely to treaty reciprocity": Statement of Mr. Perez Perozo, UN Doc. E/AC.32/SR.37, Aug. 16, 1950, at 6.

[794] Statement of Mr. Theodoli of Italy, UN Doc. E/AC.32/SR.36, Aug. 15, 1950, at 27.

[795] "[T]he reservation mentioned by the Belgian representative was exactly the kind that the Committee had recognized that some countries might find it necessary to make, especially with regard to other countries with which they had entered into specially close relationship. Benelux had in fact been cited as an example": Statement of Mr. Henkin of the United States, ibid.

[796] Statement of Mr. Henkin of the United States, UN Doc. E/AC.32/SR.37, Aug. 16, 1950, at 7.

[797] "The right to form a trade union and the right of association were two very different things. Trade union rights were derived from a more general right, that of association, but the purposes of a trade union and those of an association were different ... The orbit of associations and that of trade unions did not therefore exactly coincide and in national legislation they were often governed by different laws. He did not consider it superfluous to make special mention of the right of association. Article [15] had its place in the Convention": Statement of Mr. Juvigny of France, ibid. at 8.

[798] A Belgian proposal to revert to the "aliens generally" standard was rejected on a 6–5 (0 abstentions) vote: UN Doc. E/AC.32/SR.41, Aug. 23, 1950, at 11.

from citizenship quotas on trade union membership that is afforded the nationals of any partner or other favored state.

Overall, the best that can be said for Art. 15 is that it is an important affirmation of the right of refugees – at least once they are lawfully staying, and to the same extent as most-favored foreigners – to undertake quite a broad range of associational activities, including not only the right to join trade unions, but also to participate in the activities of a diverse array of associations, including those with cultural, sporting, social, or philanthropic aims. For example, in view of the drafters' clear aim to improve upon the associational rights granted in the conventions of 1933 and 1938 – which already allowed refugees to establish "associations for mutual relief and assistance" – there can be no doubt that the self-help associations established by Tibetan refugees in India, Angolan refugees in Zambia, and Mozambican refugees in Swaziland are protected by Art. 15. And while the disinclination of the drafters to sanction the participation of refugees in political associations means that the Refugee Convention falls short of the goals set by the Universal Declaration,[799] the drafters did not seek to limit purely individuated forms of political expression[800] (though neither did they opt expressly to protect such rights[801]).

Because of its critical deficiencies, however, the right of refugees to freedom of association – and to its closely related rights to freedom of opinion, expression, and assembly – is more effectively vindicated by reliance upon the subsequently

[799] Robinson correctly observes that the right to participate in the work of political associations is "not covered by Art. 15 but would come under Art. 7(1) [pursuant to which refugees must receive treatment not less favorable than that granted to aliens generally]": Robinson, *History*, at 108–109.

[800] The Venezuelan representative affirmed that Art. 15 "did not apply to political activity which might be carried on outside of associations": Statement of Mr. Perez Perozo of Venezuela, UN Doc. E/AC.32/SR.23, Feb. 3, 1950, at 11.

[801] In debates regarding codification in the Refugee Convention of Arts. 18 and 19 of the Universal Declaration of Human Rights [dealing with freedom of thought, opinion, and expression], the Belgian representative argued that "[i]n his opinion, provisions relating to freedom of opinion would be most appropriate in a convention on refugees, as the latter, as a rule, had abandoned their country of origin because they no longer enjoyed that freedom there": Statement of Mr. Cuvelier of Belgium, UN Doc. E/AC.32/SR.11, Jan. 25, 1950, at 8. But the French representative countered that "[f]reedom of opinion and expression was no doubt a right which should be granted to all, but the exercise of that right might sometimes lead to serious difficulties. For instance, refugees residing in a country which was not their own might wish, under article 19, to engage in political activities which it would be difficult to allow": Statement of Mr. Rain of France, ibid. at 9. Some comfort may nonetheless be taken from the view of the British representative, who opined that "a convention relating to refugees could not include an outline of all the articles of the Universal Declaration of Human Rights; furthermore, by its universal character, the Declaration applied to all human groups without exception and it was pointless to specify that its provisions applied also to refugees": Statement of Sir Leslie Brass of the United Kingdom, ibid. at 8. The Brazilian representative and the Canadian Chairman expressly concurred in the views of the British delegate: Statements of Mr. Guerreiro of Brazil and the Chairman, Mr. Chance of Canada, ibid. at 8–9.

codified Arts. 19–22 of the Civil and Political Covenant. Critically, and in contrast to the rather grudging approach taken by the Refugee Convention, the UN Human Rights Committee has expressly affirmed that non-citizens have

> the right to hold opinions and to express them. Aliens receive the benefit of the right of peaceful assembly and of freedom of association . . . There shall be no discrimination between aliens and citizens in the application of these rights.[802]

The foundational right is Art. 19(1) of the Covenant, which guarantees the "right to hold opinions without interference." Because freedom to hold opinions is a purely private matter, it is an absolute right "to which the Covenant permits no exception or restriction."[803] Importantly, the drafters of Art. 19(1) rejected a proposal to frame the right as simply one to hold opinions "without *governmental* interference,"[804] in favor of the more general right to freedom of opinion "without interference." As such, Art. 19(1) not only prohibits official efforts to force individuals to change their opinions, but also sets an affirmative duty of states to prevent private parties from coercing individuals to renounce their views.[805]

Not only may individuals freely hold opinions, but they are simultaneously entitled under Art. 19(2) to "seek, receive and impart information and ideas of all kinds." This article "requires the acceptance of the public airing of disagreements and the refusal to silence unpopular views,"[806] and extends to

---

[802] UN Human Rights Committee, "General Comment No. 15: The position of aliens under the Covenant" (1986), UN Doc. HRI/GEN/1/Rev.7, May 12, 2004, at para. 7.

[803] UN Human Rights Committee, "General Comment No. 10: Freedom of expression" (1983), UN Doc. HRI/GEN/1/Rev.7, May 12, 2004, at 133, para. 1. As Nowak observes, "[t]he private freedom to have and form opinions thus overlaps with freedom of thought guaranteed by Art. 18": Nowak, *ICCPR Commentary*, at 339. Partsch suggests that "'[t]hought' may be nearer to religion or other beliefs, 'opinion' nearer to political convictions. 'Thought' may be used in connection with faith and creed, 'opinion' for conviction in secular and civil matters": K. Partsch, "Freedom of Conscience and Expression, and Political Freedoms," in L. Henkin ed., *The International Bill of Rights* 208 (1981) (Partsch, "Freedom of Conscience"), at 217. With regard to freedom of thought and conscience, see generally chapter 4.7 above.

[804] This wording was proposed by the British government in UN Doc. E/CN.4/365.

[805] The narrower approach "floundered in the [Commission] due to the support voiced by the majority of the delegates for protection against every form of interference. This recognition of horizontal effects implies that State Parties are also obligated pursuant to Art. 2(1) to protect freedom of opinion against interference by third parties . . . Normally it is possible to speak of an interference with the right of freedom of opinion only when an individual is influenced against his (her) will or at least without his (her) implicit approval, and when this is effected by coercion, threat or similar, unallowed means": Nowak, *ICCPR Commentary*, at 340.

[806] Jayawickrama, *Judicial Application*, at 666, citing in this regard the decision of the Constitutional Court of South Africa in *South African National Defence Union v. Minister of Defence*, [2000] LRC 152 (SA CC, May 26, 1999).

"every form of subjective idea[ ] and opinion[ ] capable of transmission to others."[807] As Nowak observes, "[i]t is thus impossible to attempt to close out undesirable content, such as pornography or blasphemy, by restrictively defining the scope of protection."[808] Unless the information or idea in question either breaches the duty of states to prohibit war propaganda and hate speech, or can be brought under one of the explicit limitations allowed by Art. 19(3),[809] it must be protected. The duty of protection does not mean that there can be no regulation of freedom of expression, but a regulatory regime may not be unduly onerous.[810] Thus, a regime such as that implemented by Switzerland – requiring refugees to secure authorization to make a political speech – is not inherently unlawful so long as the grounds for denial of authorization are based upon the terms of Art. 19(3) or 21, and the nature of the approval procedure itself does not pose an unreasonable impediment to exercise of freedom of expression.[811]

The forms of protected expression include not only communications made orally, in writing, or in print, but also those transmitted by "any . . . media of [the individual's] choice." The Human Rights Committee has thus held, for example, that the raising of a banner condemning human rights abuse is a form of protected expression.[812] Of particular importance to refugees, the right to freedom of expression is guaranteed "regardless of frontiers," in consequence of which the transmission of information and opinions across national borders cannot lawfully be prohibited.[813] Thus, the broad-ranging prohibition set by Art. III of the OAU Refugee Convention – under which state parties "undertake to prohibit refugees residing in their respective territories from attacking any State Member of the OAU, by any activity

---

[807] *Ballantyne and Davidson v. Canada* and *McIntyre v. Canada*, UNHRC Comm. Nos. 359/ 1989 and 385/1989 (joined on Oct. 18, 1990), UN Docs. CCPR/C/40/D/359/1989 and CCPR/C/40/D/385/1989, decided Mar. 31, 1993.

[808] Nowak, *ICCPR Commentary*, at 341.

[809] The scope of permissible limitation is discussed below, at pp. 897–903.

[810] *Laptsevich v. Belarus*, UNHRC Comm. No. 780/1997, UN Doc. CCPR/C/68/D/780/1997, decided Mar. 20, 2000.

[811] The duty of non-discrimination could be invoked to argue the inappropriateness of requiring authorization in the case of non-citizens only. But in view of the substantial margin of appreciation traditionally afforded states in deciding whether distinctions between citizens and aliens are reasonable, it is not clear that such a challenge would succeed: see chapter 2.5.5 above, at pp. 129–133. If, on the other hand, the duty were imposed simply on refugees (but not all non-citizens), Art. 7(1) of the Refugee Convention could be relied upon to strike down the refugee-specific requirement: see chapter 3.2.1 above.

[812] *Kivenmaa v. Finland*, UNHRC Comm. No. 412/1990, UN Doc. CCPR/C/50/D/412/1990, decided Mar. 31, 1994.

[813] "The rights of freedom of opinion and expression may be exercised not only in one's own country but internationally. They are international rights": Partsch, "Freedom of Conscience," at 217.

likely to cause tension between Member States, and in particular by use of arms, through the press, or by radio" – is not in conformity with duties under the Civil and Political Covenant. Because the communication of ideas by press or the radio, even across borders, is protected by Art. 19(2), the onus is on a state party seeking to prohibit such transmission of ideas to meet the standard for valid limitation of the right, considered below.[814]

Beyond the rights to hold and to communicate opinions and information, the Civil and Political Covenant also guarantees more collective forms of expressive freedom. The right to peaceful assembly, established by Art. 21, "brings the public into direct contact with those expressing opinions, and thereby stimulates both attention and discussion."[815] The requirement that an assembly be "peaceful" "refers exclusively to the conditions under which the assembly is held, i.e. 'without uproar, disturbance, or the use of arms,'"[816] and is not limited, for example, to pro-democratic assemblies.[817] The protected interests include the right to prepare, conduct, and participate in an assembly,[818] understood to be an "intentional, temporary gathering[ ] of several persons for a specific purpose."[819] States are obliged not only to allow peaceful assemblies, but also "to ensure through adequate police protection, perhaps also by the prohibition of counter-demonstrations, that clashes or riots do not occur."[820] While Art. 21, unlike Art. 19, does not expressly grant the right to freedom of assembly to "everyone,"[821] the Human Rights Committee has nonetheless affirmed that freedom of assembly must be granted "without discrimination between citizens and aliens."[822] Refugees are therefore entitled to undertake campaigns and to hold rallies intended to

---

[814] See text below, at pp. 897–903.

[815] Jayawickrama, *Judicial Application*, at 723.

[816] Partsch, "Freedom of Conscience," at 231, citing the statement of the Uruguayan representative, Eduardo Jimenez de Arechaga, UN Doc. A/C.3/SR.61.

[817] "[A] clear majority in the [Commission] rejected ... the patronizing tendencies of socialist States, which proposed that freedom of assembly be exercised only 'in the interests of democracy' and be prohibited for 'anti-democratic' purposes ... [B]ecause experiences in all corners of the world demonstrate that democracy is such a vague concept, its interests are too easily equated with those of the political power holders, which would mean that assemblies might only have been permissible when they supported the respective system": Nowak, *ICCPR Commentary*, at 371.

[818] Ibid. at 372.   [819] Ibid. at 373.

[820] Ibid. at 376. Nowak reports that "[w]hereas a US draft sought to limit this right to the negative freedom from State interference, the vast majority of the delegates ... were of the view that the individual should be protected against all kinds of interference with the exercise of his freedom of assembly": ibid.

[821] It merely provides that "[t]he right of peaceful assembly shall be recognized": Civil and Political Covenant, at Art. 21.

[822] UN Human Rights Committee, "General Comment No. 15: The position of aliens under the Covenant" (1986), UN Doc. HRI/GEN/1/Rev.7, May 12, 2004, at paras. 2, 7.

raise awareness of conditions in their country of origin, even to the point of advocating the ouster of that country's government.[823]

Finally, Art. 22 of the Civil and Political Covenant addresses freedom of association. In contrast to the cognate right in Art. 15 of the Refugee Convention, this right explicitly inheres in "everyone" without qualification, and extends to all forms of association.[824] States must not only refrain from direct interference with associational freedom,[825] but are required both to implement a legal framework for the legal establishment of associations[826] and to take steps to prevent private parties from interfering with associational activities.[827] Freedom of association may also take a negative form, meaning that "no one may be forced, either directly or indirectly, by the State or by private parties, to join a political party, a religious society, a commercial undertaking or a sports club."[828]

Nor may freedom of association be constrained on the grounds that an association already exists to pursue a given interest or activity. Individuals have the right to choose between belonging to an existing association and forming one of their own design:

[823] "So long as exiles act within the scope of these broadly accepted rights [freedom of thought, expression, assembly, and association], they can injure no legally protected interest of the state of origin": Corliss, "Hostile Acts," at 193. The duty of states to prevent acts of aggression is discussed below, at pp. 903–905.

[824] "Religious societies, political parties, commercial undertakings and trade unions are as protected by Art. 22 as cultural or human rights organizations, soccer clubs or associations of stamp collectors. Moreover, the legal form of an association is basically unrestricted. In addition to such juridical persons as clubs, parties or societies under trade or civil law, mere *de facto* associations are likewise protected": Nowak, *ICCPR Commentary*, at 386–387.

[825] Art. 22 was, for example, found to have been violated by Uruguay in the context of official efforts to intimidate and persecute a trade union activist: *Burgos v. Uruguay*, UNHRC Comm. No. 52/1979, decided July 29, 1981.

[826] "That individuals should be able to form a legal entity in order to act collectively in a field of mutual interest is one of the most important aspects of the right to freedom of association": Jayawickrama, *Judicial Application*, at 738. See also Nowak, *ICCPR Commentary*, at 387: "Because groups of persons usually seek to pursue their longer-term interests in a legally recognized form (usually as juridical persons), States Parties are also under a positive duty to provide the legal framework for founding juridical persons."

[827] "As with freedom of expression and assembly, the US was unsuccessful with its motion in the [Commission] to protect freedom of association only against 'governmental interference' [citing UN Doc. E/CN.4/365]": Nowak, *ICCPR Commentary*, at 387, n. 15.

[828] Ibid. at 388. "Although motions by France and Uruguay in the [Commission] and by Somalia in the Third Committee of the General Assembly to set down an express prohibition on compulsory membership modelled on Art. 20(2) of the Universal Declaration of Human Rights were defeated in both organs, the discussions surrounding them make clear that negative freedom of association was protected as well. The reasons why this prohibition was not adopted have solely to do with considerations for the interests of trade unions": ibid.

When a country has only one organization for promoting human rights but I am not in agreement with its methods and objectives, my freedom of association is not exhausted simply because I am not forced to join this organization. On the contrary, Art. 22(1) also guarantees my right to found a second human rights organization with other, like-minded persons corresponding more to my liking. In other words, when a State Party creates an association (with or without compulsory membership) in a certain economic, political, cultural, etc. field, it has in no way fulfilled its duties under Art. 22(1). Subject to the limitations set down in para. 2, it must make it legally and factually possible for all persons to choose between existing (State and private) organizations and, should none of these appeal to them, to found a new one.[829]

As such, Bhutanese refugees in Nepal and Eritrean refugees in Sudan were entitled to form their own associations to advocate for their particular educational, health, and other interests. On the other hand, freedom of association is not tantamount to a right to self-govern. Because only citizens of a state have the right to take part in the conduct of public affairs, to vote, and to hold elected office,[830] Honduras was under no duty to allow Salvadoran refugees to govern their own camps, and Zambia was not required to include the refugees' Meheba Management Committee in refugee aid and development planning. While refugee self-governance often makes good practical and economic sense, it cannot be insisted upon as a matter of international law.

As under the Refugee Convention, the Civil and Political Covenant's provision on freedom of association specifically protects trade union rights. But in contrast to the Refugee Convention's vague formulation – intended to leave open the question of whether refugees are entitled not only to join unions, but also to lead and even to form them[831] – Art. 22 of the Covenant expressly guarantees "the right to form and join trade unions," and further stipulates that "[n]o restrictions" are presumptively to be placed on the exercise of this right.[832] Two possible qualifications may, however, be implied. First, the European Court of Human Rights has suggested that so-called "closed shop agreements" – under which there is legally sanctioned, compulsory membership in a trade union designated to represent workers at a given work site – may not infringe the right to freedom of association, at least where the sanction for refusal to join is reasonable.[833] Second, a

---

[829] Ibid. at 388.   [830] Civil and Political Covenant, at Art. 25.

[831] See text above, at pp. 885–887.

[832] The scope of permissible restrictions is discussed below, at pp. 897–903.

[833] See *Gustafsson v. Sweden*, (1996) 22 EHRR 409 (ECHR, Apr. 25, 1996); *Sibson v. United Kingdom*, (1994) 17 EHRR 193 (ECHR, Apr. 20, 1993); and *Young, James and Webster v. United Kingdom*, (1981) 4 EHRR 38 (ECHR, Aug. 13, 1981). The UN Human Rights Committee has not yet specifically addressed this question.

controversial decision of the UN Human Rights Committee has held that the right to strike is not guaranteed under Art. 22.[834] While the right to strike is nonetheless expressly guaranteed by Art. 8(1)(d) of the Economic Covenant, this provision – unlike Art. 22 of the Civil and Political Covenant – admits of the possibility that, as an economic right, less developed countries may decide not to recognize this right in the case of non-citizens.[835]

Despite the fact that the expressive freedom provisions of the Covenant on Civil and Political Rights are generally broadly framed and guaranteed to non-citizens, including refugees, each of the interests protected by Arts. 19, 21, and 22 may be subject to restrictions. Most fundamentally, none of these provisions is immune from emergency derogation by state parties.[836] But more generally, these articles[837] authorize governments to limit expressive rights so long as that limitation is established by law, and can be objectively assessed as necessary to protect an enumerated interest.

The first requirement for restriction of an expressive freedom – that the limitation be provided or prescribed by law (in the case of the rights to freedom of expression, and of association) – is "designed to assure the rule of law, the principle of legality, a knowledge of the existence of the law and accessibility to it by those affected, and sufficient definiteness as to its content and meaning."[838] In Nowak's view, this standard is not met in the case of "[i]nterference based solely on an administrative provision or a vague statutory authorization."[839] The standard of lawfulness for limits on the right to freedom of assembly is, however, less exacting than that for limits on freedom of expression and association.[840] Because a constraint on freedom of

---

[834] *JB et al. v. Canada*, UNHRC Comm. No. 118/1982, decided July 18, 1986. This decision is, however, highly controversial. "[F]ive members of the committee disagreed. In their view, Civil and Political Covenant [Art.] 22 guaranteed the broad right of freedom of association. There is no mention not only of the right to strike but also of the various other activities, such as holding meetings, or collective bargaining, that a trade unionist may engage in to protect his interests. However, the exercise of this right requires that some measure of concerted activities be allowed; otherwise it could not serve its purposes": Jayawickrama, *Judicial Application*, at 753–754.

[835] See chapter 2.5.4 above, at p. 122.

[836] Civil and Political Covenant, at Art. 4(2). See chapter 2.5.4 above, at p. 121.

[837] As previously noted, only the purely private right to hold opinions without interference is not subject to limitations of this kind. See text above, at p. 892.

[838] Partsch, "Freedom of Conscience," at 220. Drawing on caselaw of the European Court of Human Rights, Partsch opines that this requirement may be satisfied either by statute or by unwritten common law: ibid.

[839] Nowak, *ICCPR Commentary*, at 351.

[840] The more flexible definition of lawfulness applies, however, only if the gathering is appropriately defined as an "assembly." The more rigorous standard ("provided by law") which governs Art. 19(2) is applicable to public expressions of opinion which fall short of the organized nature of an "assembly." For example, the Human Rights Committee did not agree that the presence of some twenty-five members of the Social

assembly need only be "imposed in conformity with the law," it is sufficient if it is ordered by administrative officials acting on the basis of some general statutory or common law authority.[841]

The second requirement is that the constraint be imposed in order to advance one of several enumerated interests. A restriction is only valid if its purpose is to protect the rights and freedoms of others; to ensure respect for national security, public order, public health, or morals; or, in the case of the rights to assembly and association, to ensure public safety. In addition, by virtue of the duty of state parties under Art. 20 to prohibit propaganda of war[842] and the advocacy of hatred,[843] a constraint on an expressive freedom necessary to meet either of those obligations is presumptively lawful.[844]

Democratic Youth Organization amidst a larger crowd of persons permitted by the state to gather near the Presidential Palace constituted a "demonstration" which could be constrained under the less exacting standards of Art. 21: *Kivenmaa v. Finland*, UNHRC Comm. No. 412/1990, UN Doc. CCPR/C/50/D/412/1990, decided Mar. 31, 1994.

[841] "Elsewhere the restriction must be 'provided' or 'prescribed' by law; here it seems sufficient that restrictions are 'imposed in conformity with law,' doubtless in order to allow wider discretion to administrative authorities acting under general authorizations. Presumably, the police may act on the basis of a general clause authorizing them to act in the interests of public safety": Partsch, "Freedom of Conscience," at 232–233.

[842] This includes "propaganda threatening or resulting in an act of aggression or breach of peace contrary to the Charter of the United Nations": UN Human Rights Committee, "General Comment No. 11: Prohibition of propaganda for war and advocacy of hatred" (1983), UN Doc. HRI/GEN/1/Rev.7, May 12, 2004, at 133, para. 2. Nowak thus concludes that "Art. 20(1) does not affect the right of individual or collective self-defence guaranteed in Art. 51 of the UN Charter and other measures consistent with chapter VII or the right of all peoples to self-determination and independence. Consequently, Art. 20(1) prohibits only propaganda for so-called 'wars of aggression' but not for wars waged out of merely defence or for liberation. In addition, internal 'civil wars' do not fall under its scope of application, so long as they do not develop into an international conflict ... [W]hat is decisive is that the propaganda aims at creating or reinforcing the willingness to conduct a war of aggression": Nowak, *ICCPR Commentary*, at 364.

[843] The object of this part of the duty is to prohibit "any advocacy of national, racial or religious hatred that constitutes incitement to discrimination, hostility or violence": UN Human Rights Committee, "General Comment No. 11: Prohibition of propaganda for war and advocacy of hatred" (1983), UN Doc. HRI/GEN/1/Rev.7, May 12, 2004, at 133, para. 2. For example, it has been held that the failure to stop the dissemination of anti-Semitic tape-recorded messages by telephone was contrary to Art. 20's duty to prohibit hate speech: *Taylor and the Western Guard Party v. Canada*, UNHRC Comm. No. 104/1981, decided Apr. 6, 1983.

[844] "In the opinion of the Committee, these required prohibitions are fully compatible with the right of freedom of expression as contained in article 19, the exercise of which carries with it special duties and responsibilities": UN Human Rights Committee, "General Comment No. 11: Prohibition of propaganda for war and advocacy of hatred" (1983), UN Doc. HRI/GEN/1/Rev.7, May 12, 2004, at 133, para. 2. As Nowak observes, "Art. 20 differs from the permissible purposes for interference ... only in that States Parties are internationally obligated to interfere in certain cases, whereas in others they are merely entitled to do so": Nowak, *ICCPR Commentary*, at 368.

One basis for restrictions on expressive freedoms is the need to protect the "rights and freedoms of others." This authority should not, however, be interpreted in a way that breaches the duty of non-discrimination by privileging the views or concerns of the majority, or of those in power.[845] In keeping with the overall goal of the Covenant, the purpose of any limitation should instead be to promote a more rights-regarding society. Thus, for example, the Human Rights Committee upheld a French law which prohibited speech denying that crimes against humanity had occurred during the Holocaust as a restriction necessary to allow the Jewish community to live free from the fear of anti-Semitism.[846] The additional authority under Art. 19(3) to limit freedom of expression where necessary to protect the "reputation of others" authorizes also the imposition of constraints on free speech where necessary to avoid "intentional infringement on honour and reputation by untrue assertions,"[847] e.g. by the enforcement of laws on defamation.

Expressive rights may also be constrained if required by considerations of national security. The contemporary meaning of this notion has already been developed in some detail.[848] In essence, the limitation imposed on expressive freedom must be in response to an objectively reasonable, real possibility of directly or indirectly inflicted substantial harm to the host state's most basic interests, including the risk of an armed attack on its territory or its citizens, or the destruction of its democratic institutions.[849] Importantly, the Human Rights Committee has not been willing simply to accept the assurances of states that restrictions are required to prevent "subversive activities,"[850] but has insisted on the presentation of specific information enabling it to evaluate the soundness of a state's claim that a restriction on national security grounds is necessary.[851]

---

[845] A helpful analogy may be made to the right to restrict freedom of religion under Art. 18(3) of the Covenant. In this context, the Human Rights Committee has observed that "[i]n interpreting the scope of permissible limitation clauses, States parties should proceed from the need to protect the rights guaranteed under the Covenant, including the right to equality and non-discrimination on all grounds specified in articles 2, 3 and 26 ... Restrictions may not be imposed for discriminatory purposes or applied in a discriminatory manner": UN Human Rights Committee, "General Comment No. 22: Freedom of thought, conscience or religion" (1993), UN Doc. HRI/GEN/1/Rev.7, May 12, 2004, at 155, para. 8.

[846] *Faurisson v. France*, UNHRC Comm. No. 550/1993, UN Doc. CCPR/C/58/D/550/1993, decided Nov. 8, 1996.

[847] Nowak, *ICCPR Commentary*, at 353.

[848] See chapter 3.5.1 above, at pp. 264–266.

[849] See chapter 3.5.1 above, at p. 266.

[850] *Weinberger v. Uruguay*, UNHRC Comm. No. 28/1978, decided Oct. 29, 1980; *Burgos v. Uruguay*, UNHRC Comm. No. 52/1979, decided July 29, 1981.

[851] "Bare information from the State party that [the applicant] was charged with subversive association ... is not in itself sufficient, without details of the alleged charges and copies

Third, limits may be set where necessary to ensure "public order (*ordre public*)." This is quite a broad-ranging notion, allowing restrictions beyond those authorized by the narrower concept of "public order" which is used, for example, to define the scope of permissible limitations on freedom of thought, conscience, and religion under Art. 18 of the Covenant.[852] The bilingual formulation employed in Arts. 19, 21, and 22 instead incorporates by reference the traditional civil law notion of "*ordre public*" – roughly equivalent to the common law construct of public policy.[853] The drafters of the Covenant were not prepared even to replace the notion of "public order (*ordre public*)" with that of "prevention of disorder or crime,"[854] leading Nowak to conclude that "in addition to prevention of disorder and crime, it is possible to include under the term *ordre public* all of those 'universally accepted fundamental principles, consistent with respect for human rights, on which a democratic society is based.'"[855]

The Human Rights Committee has thus suggested that a fair and transparent restriction on the right of the media to seek and receive information could be justified on grounds of public order (*ordre public*) where necessary to ensure the effective operation of Parliament and the safety of its members.[856] On the other hand, not even *ordre public* was found to be a sufficiently fungible concept to justify Cameroon's efforts to stifle pro-democracy advocacy, allegedly in the interests of ensuring national unity under difficult circumstances.[857] Under this approach, the efforts of Kenya and Côte d'Ivoire to limit the activities of refugee populations based simply upon

---

of the court proceedings": *Pietraroia v. Uruguay*, UNHRC Comm. No. 44/1979, decided Mar. 27, 1981, at para. 15.

[852] See chapter 4.7 above, at pp. 578–579.

[853] In rejecting the civil law construct for purposes of the right of expulsion under the Refugee Convention (Art. 32), it was observed that "[i]n civil law countries, the concept of '*l'ordre public*' is a fundamental legal notion used principally as a basis for negating or restricting private agreements, the exercise of police power, or the application of foreign law. The common law counterpart of '*l'ordre public*' is not 'public order,' but rather 'public policy'": UN Doc. E/L.68, tabled at the Conference of Plenipotentiaries by its Executive Secretary, UN Doc. A/CONF.2/SR.14, July 10, 1951, at 19–20.

[854] This proposal was narrowly defeated on a 7–6 (2 abstentions) vote: UN Doc. E/CN.4/SR.167.

[855] Nowak, *ICCPR Commentary*, at 356, citing the definition in Art. 4(e) of the Strasbourg Declaration on the Right to Leave and Return (1986), 1987 HRLJ 481.

[856] *Gauthier v. Canada*, UNHRC Comm. No. 633/1995, UN Doc. CCPR/C/65/D/633/1995, decided Apr. 7, 1999. On the facts of the case, however, it was determined that the effective grant of a monopoly over access to parliamentary press facilities to a single organization, the Canadian Press Gallery Association, had not been shown to be a necessary and proportionate restriction.

[857] *Mukong v. Cameroon*, UNHRC Comm. No. 458/1991, UN Doc. CCPR/C/51/D/458/1991, decided July 2, 1994.

whether the refugees' views corresponded with their host government's prevailing foreign policy preferences would also contravene the Covenant.

In view of the breadth of the public order (*ordre public*) exception, it may seem unnecessary that the drafters also authorized a fourth category of limitation on the rights of assembly and association, namely constraints required to ensure "public safety." The language derives from a British proposal intended to allow assemblies to be prohibited or broken up where there is a specific risk to persons or property.[858] By way of example, Partsch suggests that "[i]n a country where different groups of political refugees exiled from their homeland are fighting with each other, it would seem legitimate to impose some restrictions on their right of assembly in the interest of public safety."[859] Similarly, the duty of refugees living in camps and settlements "to abstain from any activity likely to detract from the exclusively civilian and humanitarian character of the camps and settlements"[860] might logically entail some constraints on expressive freedom to ensure public safety.

Fifth, expressive freedom may be limited for reasons of public health. While primarily of import in restricting commercial free speech (e.g. in the marketing of hazardous products), there is regional caselaw in Europe suggesting its applicability also to constrain the advocacy of euthanasia in order to protect the right to life of vulnerable persons.[861] One could similarly imagine the logic of invoking this ground to prohibit the advocacy of traditional practices known to pose a serious risk to health, including many forms of female genital mutilation, or to deny a right of assembly based on the need to prevent the spread of a serious airborne disease, such as SARS.

The final reason authorized for limiting expressive freedom is the protection of "public morals." The understanding of this notion embraced by the Human Rights Committee in the context of defining the scope of permissible restrictions on freedom of thought, conscience, and religion is instructive:

> [T]he concept of morals derives from many social, philosophical and religious traditions: consequently, limitations . . . for the purpose of protecting morals must be based on principles not deriving from a single tradition . . . [They must also be] directly related and proportionate to the specific need on which they are predicated.[862]

---

[858] UN Doc. E/CN.4/L.145.   [859] Partsch, "Freedom of Conscience," at 234.

[860] UNHCR Executive Committee Conclusion No. 48, "Military or Armed Attacks on Refugee Camps and Settlements" (1987), at para. 4(a), available at www.unhcr.ch (accessed Nov. 20, 2004). States further commit themselves "to do all within their capacity to ensure that the civilian and humanitarian character of such camps and settlements is maintained": ibid. at para. 4(b).

[861] *Application No. 10083/82 v. United Kingdom*, (1983) 6 EHRR 140 (Eur. Comm. HR, July 4, 1983).

[862] UN Human Rights Committee, "General Comment No. 22: Freedom of thought, conscience or religion" (1993), UN Doc. HRI/GEN/1/Rev.7, May 12, 2004, at para. 8.

The universalism of this standard is appropriate to a treaty intended to establish global standards,[863] while the insistence on a constrained application of this potentially all-encompassing ground is critical to ensuring that no limitation on expressive freedom may "put in jeopardy the right itself."[864]

Despite the breadth of some of these grounds, the possibility of fundamental erosion of expressive freedom by the imposition of relevant limitations is significantly constrained by the third general requirement set by the Covenant. It is not enough for a given restriction to be set by law and related to one of the permitted grounds of limitation; it must rather be demonstrably "necessary" (freedom of expression) or "necessary in a democratic society" (rights of assembly and association) to secure the enumerated interest. As previously described, the drafters of the Covenant conceived the necessity standard as requiring that a restriction be objectively justifiable as essential to the attainment of one of the approved purposes.[865] In the result, a right should not be abridged if some other, non-rights-violative option is available. Even where there is no alternative but to infringe a right, the abridgement should be kept to the absolute minimum required by the circumstances. Thus, "the restriction must be proportional in severity and intensity to the purpose being sought, and may not become the rule."[866] For example, the complete ban imposed by India on all LTTE-related activities of refugees after the assassination of Rajiv Gandhi might reasonably be deemed overly broad.

Moreover, any restriction on two forms of expressive freedom – the rights to freedom of assembly and association – must not only be "necessary," but be also demonstrably "necessary in a democratic society." The drafters did not define this notion with precision, opting instead to endorse a flexible but nonetheless internationalist standard:

> It was objected [by some members of the Commission on Human Rights] that it was impossible to discern a uniform understanding of democracy common to all countries of the world. On the other hand, it was submitted that freedom of assembly [and association] cannot be effectively protected if the limitations proviso is not applied in conformity with certain minimum democratic principles, which stem, *inter alia*, from the respect for the

---

[863] The approach in General Comment No. 22 may be contrasted with the more relativist perspective adopted by the Committee in its 1982 decision of *Hertzberg et al. v. Finland*, UNHRC Comm. No. 61/1979, decided Apr. 2, 1982. In dismissing a claim based on state efforts to censor the broadcast of material dealing with homosexuality, the Committee opined that "public morals differ widely. There is no universally applicable common standard. Consequently, in this respect, a certain margin of discretion must be accorded national authorities": ibid. at para. 10.3.

[864] UN Human Rights Committee, "General Comment No. 10: Freedom of expression" (1983), UN Doc. HRI/GEN/1/Rev.7, May 12, 2004, at para. 4.

[865] See chapter 5.2 above, at pp. 716–717.   [866] Nowak, *ICCPR Commentary*, at 351.

principles of the UN Charter, the Universal Declaration of Human Rights, and the two Covenants.[867]

Thus, as Partsch concludes, "the government has a margin of appreciation, but the standards are international standards and a government's reliance on the limitation clause is subject to international scrutiny."[868] It would, for example, be difficult to imagine that this standard would be met in the case of Tanzania's detention of Burundian refugees simply because they were campaigning for majority rule in their home country, or when Burmese refugees were detained simply for calling attention to the internationally condemned detention of opposition leader Aung San Suu Kyi.

Beyond limitations imposed by international human rights law, the political activities of refugees, like those of all persons subject to the host state's authority, may also be constrained to meet that state's obligations to maintain international peace and security.[869] Regrettably, host states are unlikely to be inclined to take this obligation seriously when refugees are used as the instruments of the host state's own aggressive policies[870] – for example, Pakistan's arming of Afghan rebels in exile, or Honduras' support for Nicaraguan contras on its territory. Scenarios of this kind, however, represent the clearest example of a situation in which the host government is itself liable for the aggressive actions of refugees, and hence under a concomitant duty to restrain them.[871]

Where, in contrast, the host state is not itself the progenitor of the aggression – for example, when Rwandan refugees planned an invasion of their home country while enjoying refugee protection in Uganda, or when

---

[867] Ibid. at 378–379. More specifically, Nowak suggests that the litmus test for a valid limitation should be whether the constraint is "oriented along the basic democratic values of pluralism, tolerance, broad-mindedness, and peoples' sovereignty": ibid. at 394.

[868] Partsch, "Freedom of Conscience," at 233.

[869] All states are required by the Charter of the United Nations to "refrain in their international relations from the threat or use of force against the territorial integrity or political independence of any state": UN Charter, 1 UNTS 16, adopted June 26, 1945, at Art. 2(4).

[870] The UN General Assembly has affirmed that states are under a duty to prevent aggression, defined to include "[t]he sending by or on behalf of a State of armed bands, groups, irregulars or mercenaries, which carry out acts of armed force against another State of such gravity as to amount to [aggression], or its substantial involvement therein": UNGA Res. 3314(XXIX), Dec. 14, 1974.

[871] As recently suggested by the International Law Commission, "[t]he conduct of a person or group of persons shall be considered an act of a State under international law if the person or group of persons is in fact acting on the instructions of, or under the direction or control of, that State in carrying out the conduct": "Draft Articles on Responsibility of States for Internationally Wrongful Acts," UN Doc. A/56/10, Ch. IV.E.1, adopted Nov. 2001, at Art. 8. The duty to take corrective action follows from the principle that "[e]very internationally wrongful act of a State entails the international responsibility of that State": ibid. at Art. 1.

anti-communist Cuban refugees based in the United States sent harassing aircraft into Cuban airspace – the host state is liable for acts of aggression committed by private groups only "if and to the extent that the State acknowledges and adopts the conduct in question as its own."[872] There is moreover no responsibility of any kind where the actions undertaken by refugees do not amount to a form of international wrongdoing. For example, because it is generally accepted that there is no breach of international law in the case of an armed intervention necessary to ensure the right of a people to political self-determination, the host country of refugees undertaking attacks of this kind cannot be said to be under a duty to prevent such action.[873] All in all, the scope for limitation of expressive freedom based on the need to avoid international legal liability is thus fairly narrow.

Where the refugees' host state is not legally obligated to prevent the refugees' activities, any constraints on their freedom of expression, assembly, and association must be justified on the basis of the usual criteria described above.[874] So long as the limitations are set by law, and are truly necessary – including considerations of minimal intrusiveness and proportionality – considerations of national security may well be relevant, at least where the target state is able and disposed to retaliate against the host country. More generally, the host country may also in at least some circumstances assert public order (*ordre public*) considerations given the importance ascribed today to the principles of non-intervention in the affairs of other countries,[875] and more generally to the maintenance of friendly relations among

[872] Ibid. at Art. 11.
[873] Grahl-Madsen, "Political Rights and Freedoms of Refugees," in G. Melander and P. Nobel eds., *African Refugees and the Law* 47, (1978) at 54–55. See also O. Eze, *Human Rights in Africa* (1984), at 606: "[A]s a result of provisions of the UN Charter recognizing the right of self-determination of colonial peoples and subsequent United Nations General Assembly resolutions elaborating the content of this right, it is now well accepted that refugees from colonial territories who have decided to resort to armed struggle have a right to use force and that the country aiding them by, for example, granting them a base from which to operate, is in fact fulfilling its obligations under the UN Charter." Tacit support for this position can be located in *obiter dicta* of the decision of the International Court of Justice in *Military and Paramilitary Activities in and Against Nicaragua*, [1986] ICJ Rep 14, at para. 98, in which the Court was careful not to deem an attack necessary for self-determination to be unlawful: "The Court is not here concerned with the process of decolonization; this question is not an issue in the present case." But in view of the strong dissent of Judge Schwebel in that decision, Corliss concludes that "[t]he complex question of intervention in support of self-determination remains unsettled in international law. There is a fundamental conflict between the universalist and statist principles set forth in the United Nations Charter. The international legal order cannot simultaneously pay equal respect to self-determination and human rights on the one hand, and sovereignty and non-intervention on the other": Corliss, "Hostile Acts," at 205–206.
[874] See text above, at pp. 897–903.
[875] The Declaration on Territorial Asylum, UNGA. Res. 2312(XXII), adopted Dec. 14, 1967, provides at Art. 4 that "[s]tates granting asylum ... not permit persons who have

states.[876] While the absolutist nature of Art. III of the OAU Refugee Convention – under which there is a blanket duty on states "to *prohibit* refugees ... from attacking *any* State Member of the OAU, by *any* activity likely to cause tension between Member States [emphasis added]" – makes that standard unlawful, a more selective and context-sensitive invocation of the public order (*ordre public*) limitation authority will allow states legitimately to constrain refugee activities at odds with basic international legal and political commitments.

6.8 Assistance to access the courts

As earlier described,[877] refugees are entitled to assert their rights before the courts[878] of any state party,[879] even before admission to a status

received asylum to engage in activities contrary to the principles and purposes of the United Nations." More generally, states have agreed "to ensure that [their] territory is not used in any manner which would violate the sovereignty, political independence, territorial integrity and national unity or disrupt the political, economic, and social stability of another State": Declaration on the Inadmissibility of Intervention in the Internal Affairs of States, UNGA. Res. 103(XXVI), adopted Dec. 9, 1981, at Art. II(b). While not binding as a matter of international law (see chapter 1.1.2 above, at pp. 26–27), these resolutions of the General Assembly nonetheless have significant political authority.

[876] By virtue of the Declaration on Principles of International Law Concerning Friendly Relations and Cooperation Among States, UNGA Res. 2625(XXV), adopted Nov. 4, 1970, governments have committed themselves not to "organize, assist, foment, finance, incite, or tolerate subversive terrorist or armed activities directed toward the violent overthrow of another State." This formally non-binding standard exceeds the legal duty described above: see text above, at pp. 903–904.

[877] See chapter 4.10 above.

[878] Grahl-Madsen opines that "[t]he paragraph is limited to courts of law and does, therefore, not apply to administrative authorities. However, in certain other articles of the Convention a right to appear before administrative authorities has been established": Grahl-Madsen, *Commentary*, at 66. Weis agrees with this position, and gives Art. 32 (duty of non-expulsion) as an example of a provision in which access to administrative authorities *is* expressly guaranteed: Weis, *Travaux*, at 134. In line with Weis' position on the right to access to tribunals by virtue of Art. 32, see UNHCR Executive Committee Conclusion No. 22, "Protection of Asylum Seekers in Situations of Large-Scale Influx" (1981), at para. II(B)(2)(f), available at www.unhcr.ch (accessed Nov. 20, 2004), which affirms that "asylum-seekers who have been temporarily admitted pending arrangements for a durable solution ... are to be considered as persons before the law, enjoying free access to courts of law *and other competent administrative authorities* [emphasis added]." But the general understanding of Art. 14(1) of the Covenant on Civil and Political Rights – which also impliedly guarantees a right of access to the courts by everyone (see chapter 4.10 above, at pp. 647–650) – is that this right applies "to all courts and tribunals which determine criminal charges or rights and obligations in a suit at law, whether ordinary or specialized": Jayawickrama, *Judicial Application*, at 481.

[879] "[A]rticle [16] stipulated that a refugee should not only have free access to the courts in the country where he resided, but to the courts of all contracting states": Statement of the

determination procedure. The drafters agreed that even "persons who had only recently become refugees and therefore had no habitual residence were ... covered by the provisions of ... paragraph 1 [of Art. 16]."[880] The qualitative dimension of that access to the courts is now regulated by Art. 14(1) of the Civil and Political Covenant.[881] In brief, the body before which refugees are entitled to present their claims must be established by law, jurisdictionally competent, independent, and impartial. It must moreover be positioned to deliver a fair and public hearing, meaning that access is reasonably expeditious, the rules of natural justice are respected, there is procedural equality between the parties, it is possible reasonably to present one's case, and the hearing (or at least the judgment, where special circumstances exist) is accessible to all.

Yet the drafters were keenly aware that the basic guarantee of the right to bring a case to court could often prove illusive in practical terms:

> Although in principle the right of a refugee to sue and be sued is not challenged, in practice there are insurmountable difficulties to the exercise of this right by needy refugees: the obligation to furnish *cautio judicatum solvi* and the refusal to grant refugees the benefit of legal assistance makes the right illusory. In many countries, legal assistance is available solely to nationals and only foreigners who can invoke a treaty of reciprocity are granted the benefit of such assistance. Refugees should therefore be exempted, as was done in the Conventions of 1933 and 1938, from the obligation to furnish *cautio judicatum solvi* and should enjoy the benefit of legal assistance on the same conditions as nationals.[882]

President, Mr. Larsen of Denmark, UN Doc. A/CONF.2/SR.8, July 5, 1951, at 13. Furthermore, "[p]aragraph 1 applies to any refugee ... If he has his habitual residence in a non-Contracting State, he shall nevertheless have access to courts of law in any of the Contracting States, subject only to the rule that each Contracting State must determine for its own purposes whether a person is to be considered as a refugee or not": Grahl-Madsen, *Commentary*, at 64. As drafted, refugees are to have the right of access to courts, even if the citizens of the host state do not. Thus, Grahl-Madsen observes that "[t]he rule is interesting because it is of an absolute character and does not refer to any standard relating to nationals or most favoured aliens or any other group or category of aliens": Grahl-Madsen, *Commentary*, at 66.

[880] Statement of Mr. Henkin of the United States, UN Doc. E/AC.32/SR.25, Feb. 10, 1950, at 6. This position was thought largely uncontroversial, since "[u]nder present day practice foreigners are usually granted the right to appear before courts of law as plaintiffs or defendants ... [But] [t]o avoid difficulties in such countries where free access to courts is not granted to all foreigners, the Convention explicitly imposes such an obligation on the Contracting States": Robinson, *History*, at 112. See chapter 4.10 above, at pp. 646–647.

[881] See chapter 4.10 above, at pp. 647–650.

[882] Secretary-General, "Memorandum," at 30.

These concerns persist in some jurisdictions to the present day. In Uganda, for example, there is no general legal aid system to which refugees may apply. UNHCR has, however, often assisted refugees to pay their lawyers' bills.[883] In Italy, refugees without independent means may access the general legal aid plan to assist them in presenting their cases for refugee status, but are entitled to legal assistance for other kinds of cases only after formal recognition of their claim.[884] Britain's decision to reduce legal aid for refugee claimants from a maximum of 100 hours to no more than 5 hours' work provoked a protest by UNHCR directly to the Lord Chancellor.[885] Under the European Union's Procedures Directive, state parties are required to provide free "legal assistance and/or representation" for purposes of at least the first review or appeal of a negative status determination.[886] They may, however, limit access to such assistance on the basis of financial need; limit its applicability to designated counsel; set monetary and/or time limits; and, perhaps most ominously, deny such assistance altogether where authorities determine that the appeal or review is not "likely to succeed."[887] In Belgium, refugees

---

[883] E. Khiddu-Makubuya, *International Academy of Comparative Law National Report for Uganda* (1994), at 9. Yet according to the Refugee Law Project at Makarere University, which provides some support to persons claiming refugee status, "asylum-seekers are not allowed legal representation in presenting their case. It has been argued by UNHCR that legal representation would infringe upon the confidentiality of the asylum-seeker": Refugee Law Project, "Refugees in the City: Status Determination, Resettlement, and the Changing Nature of Forced Migration in Uganda," Refugee Law Project Working Paper No. 6, July 2002, at 15.

[884] G. D'Orazio, *International Academy of Comparative Law National Report for Italy* (1994), at 29. Despite legislative change in 2001, a substantively inclusive right of access to legal aid has not been established for refugee claimants in Italy. "Under the 2001 Immigration and Asylum Bill, asylum-seekers are entitled to free legal aid when appealing the Commission's decision and can request this aid from the Commission for Free Legal Aid ... Other than these measures, there is no right to legal aid for asylum-seekers": Lawyers' Committee for Human Rights, "Country Review 2002," available at www.lchr.org/refugees/reports (accessed Oct. 19, 2003) (LCHR, "Country Review 2002").

[885] "The UN's high commissioner for refugees has written to the lord chancellor, Lord Falconer, warning that the proposal to limit the hours of legal advice will harm deserving and vulnerable asylum-seekers who have to navigate an unfamiliar legal system without English language skills ... The asylum changes which will restrict publicly funded advice to four hours for the initial decision and four hours for any subsequent appeal are designed to save £30 million a year": A. Travis, "UN attacks plans to limit legal aid for asylum-seekers," *Guardian*, Sept. 1, 2003, at 6.

[886] Council Directive on minimum standards of procedures in Member States for granting and withdrawing refugee status, Doc. 8771/04, Asile 33 (Apr. 29, 2004) (EU Procedures Directive), at Art. 13. Time limits for access to review are, however, allowed: ibid. at Art. 38(4).

[887] Ibid. at Art. 13(3)–(5). It is stipulated, however, that access to legal assistance "shall not be arbitrarily restricted" on the basis of a determination that an appeal or review is not likely to succeed: ibid. at Art. 13(3).

face the requirement to post security for costs under the doctrine of *cautio judicatum solvi* until and unless their claims to refugee status are recognized;[888] in France, on the other hand, all non-citizens, including refugees, are now exempt from the requirement.[889]

Refugee Convention, Art. 16   Access to courts

. . .

2. A refugee shall enjoy in the Contracting State in which he has his habitual residence the same treatment as a national in matters pertaining to access to the courts, including legal assistance and exemption from *cautio judicatum solvi*.

3. A refugee shall be accorded in the matters referred to in paragraph 2 in countries other than that in which he has his habitual residence the treatment granted to a national of the country of his habitual residence.

Over the course of the drafting debates, it was decided that the more sophisticated rights relevant to accessing the courts – in particular, eligibility for legal assistance, and exemption from *cautio judicatum solvi* – would be reserved for refugees who had established a "habitual residence" in some state. Thus, refugees who have yet to establish a habitual residence need only receive the benefit of Art. 16(1) in addition to whatever access to the courts is afforded non-citizens generally.[890] They may, for example, bring an action to secure a divorce[891] or recover a debt,[892] but need not be granted the forms of practical assistance in accessing the courts envisaged by paras. 2 and 3 of Art. 16.[893] Much less is there any duty to exempt refugees from the usual court or other fees to pursue a court action.[894]

---

[888] K. Leus and G. Vermeylen, *International Academy of Comparative Law National Report for Belgium* (1994), at 7.

[889] N. Guimezanes, *International Academy of Comparative Law National Report for France* (1994), at 18.

[890] See generally chapter 4.10 above, at pp. 644–656. At this point, the operative provisions of the Refugee Convention are Arts. 16(1) and 7(1), the latter stipulating that "[e]xcept where this Convention contains more favourable provisions, a Contracting State shall accord to refugees the same treatment as is accorded to aliens generally." See chapter 3.2.1 above.

[891] Statement of Mr. Larsen of Denmark, UN Doc. E/AC.32/SR.11, Jan. 25, 1950, at 7.

[892] Statement of Mr. Robinson of Israel, UN Doc. A/CONF.2/SR.8, July 5, 1951, at 12.

[893] "[R]efugees who have not established habitual residence in any country will not benefit from the provisions of paragraphs 2 and 3": Grahl-Madsen, *Commentary*, at 67.

[894] "Free access" to the courts, as required by Art. 16(1), does not imply a right of refugees to access courts without the payment of the usual court fees. In the French government's proposal for the Convention, adopted as the working model for Art. 16, refugees were to have received "free and ready" access to the courts of law: France, "Draft Convention,"

The "habitual residence" requirement for access to the additional benefits set by paras. 2 and 3 of Art. 16 was not intended to limit those rights to refugees who are formally domiciled in a state party.[895] Instead, a refugee's presence need only be ongoing in practical terms.[896] But because mere lawful presence is insufficient to give rise to entitlement under Art. 16(2), that provision does not provide a basis to contest Italy's decision to delay general access to the legal aid system or Belgium's continued application of the *cautio judicatum solvi* regime until refugee status is formally recognized.[897] Indeed, even the British rules establishing reduced access to legal aid and the European Union requirements to provide free legal aid

at 4. This led the British representative to observe that "the first paragraph of the French draft spoke of 'free and ready access'; ... in English the words 'free' and 'ready' were synonymous in the context if used alone, but in conjunction 'free' might mean without payment of court fees": Statement of Sir Leslie Brass of the United Kingdom, UN Doc. E/AC.32/SR.11, Jan. 25, 1950, at 7. On the motion of the Israeli delegate, the English language text was amended to refer solely to "free" access in order to avoid this interpretation: Statement of Mr. Robinson of Israel, ibid. However, "Article 16 should ... be read in conjunction with Article 29, according to which refugees shall not be obliged to pay higher or other charges than nationals of the State concerned": Grahl-Madsen, *Commentary*, at 64. Thus, "'free access' to courts does not mean that a refugee is free from the payment of any fees which nationals have to pay in the same circumstances ... [S]uch fees and charges may not be higher than those levied on nationals": Weis, *Travaux*, at 134.

[895] The drafters rejected the early draft which granted rights under Art. 16(2) and (3) on the basis of "domicile or regular residence" in favor of the present language of "habitual residence" based upon the view of the British representative that "the aim was to give refugees the right to sue and be sued in the country of their residence whether it was the country of their domicile or not": Statement of Sir Leslie Brass of the United Kingdom, UN Doc. E/AC.32/SR.11, Jan. 25, 1950, at 7. The revised draft adopted at the first session of the Ad Hoc Committee refers only to "habitual residence": Ad Hoc Committee, "First Session Report," at Annex I. Robinson observes that the "habitual residence" language was chosen "to denote that a stay of short duration was not sufficient. On the other hand, the exercise of the right was not made dependent on 'permanent residence' or on 'domicile' because it was felt that it was a too far-reaching concept for the enjoyment of civil rights. 'Habitual residence' means residence of a certain duration, but it implies much less than permanent residence": Robinson, *History*, at 107.

[896] The language of "habitual residence" was debated in the context of Art. 14, which establishes artistic rights and rights to industrial property: see chapter 6.5 above, at pp. 836–838. As Robinson affirms, "[t]he scope of the rights accorded to refugees under para. 2 is the same as in Art. 14": Robinson, *History*, at 113. See also Weis, *Travaux*, at 134. Because "habitual residence" is not intended to focus on legal status, "[w]ith the exception of new refugees who have not yet habitual residence anywhere, it is difficult to envisage a refugee having no habitual residence": Grahl-Madsen, *Commentary*, at 60.

[897] In certain extreme circumstances, economic barriers to accessing the courts may nonetheless amount to an infringement of the duty to provide a "fair hearing" under Art. 14(1) of the Civil and Political Covenant: see chapter 4.10 above, at pp. 654–655.

only on a review or appeal set standards in excess of what Art. 16(2) requires.[898]

The enhanced aspects of the right to access the courts which accrue at this point have both an internal and an external dimension.[899] Within the country of habitual residence, refugees are to enjoy the same practical means of accessing the courts as do citizens of their host country.[900] In other countries, refugees are to be treated as citizens of their host country.[901] Thus, whatever dispensations are afforded citizens of the host country, including by virtue of treaties of reciprocity, must be extended to refugees from that country as well.[902] This duty inheres even if the refugee seeking access to the courts is habitually resident in a state which is not a party to the Refugee Convention.[903]

While the enhanced obligations under paras. 2 and 3 are general in scope,[904] the two practical impediments of greatest concern to the drafters – the need for exemption from *cautio judicatum solvi*, and access to legal assistance – are expressly referenced in the text of Art. 16. First, under the rules of *cautio judicatum solvi* some "countries admit foreigners to their courts of law, but request them, in the absence of reciprocity, to deposit an amount at the court's discretion [which] is sufficient to cover the costs he will be compelled to pay the other party if he loses the case."[905] Thus, if treated on par with other non-citizens, refugees could be required to post security for costs in a civil action under a procedure not applicable to citizens of the host

---

[898] Issues may still arise, however, with respect to the cognate requirements of the Civil and Political Covenant. See text below, at pp. 911–912.

[899] The external dimension, found in para. 3, is a net addition over the cognate protections established by the 1933 and 1938 refugee conventions: Robinson, *History*, at 112.

[900] Refugees are to be "subject to the same conditions as nationals": Statement of Sir Leslie Brass of the United Kingdom, UN Doc. E/AC.32/SR.11, Jan. 25, 1950, at 7. Thus, "they will be considered more favourably than aliens who are not enjoying such favourable treatment": Grahl-Madsen, *Commentary*, at 67.

[901] "Refugees are to have free access to justice, not only in their country of residence but in any other country party to the convention": Secretary-General, "Memorandum," at 30.

[902] "They would be entitled in this respect to benefit under the system applied to nationals of the country of asylum in pursuance of the treaties in force": ibid.

[903] "Just as in paragraph 1, this paragraph also applies to refugees residing in non-Contracting States": Grahl-Madsen, *Commentary*, at 64.

[904] The Belgian representative, for example, observed that "the exemption from *cautio judicatum solvi* was already provided for under the first sentence of paragraph 2, which provided that a refugee should enjoy in that respect the same rights and privileges as a national": Statement of Mr. Herment of Belgium, UN Doc. A/CONF.2/SR.8, July 5, 1951, at 13. Weis cites to Federal Court of Germany Decision No. ATF 83 (1951) I, at p. 16, as having relied on Art. 16(2) to reach the conclusion that it had competence to grant a refugee from Yugoslavia, resident in Germany, a divorce from her non-resident spouse on the same terms as it would for a German citizen: Weis, *Travaux*, at 135.

[905] Grahl-Madsen, *Commentary*, at 63.

state.[906] By virtue of Arts. 16(2) and (3), however, any such rules may no longer be invoked against refugees.[907] As a practical matter, however, the net benefit of this rule may be marginal. The Belgian representative to the Conference of Plenipotentiaries observed that even in 1951 "the practice of demanding *cautio judicatum solvi* was dying out,"[908] a view affirmed by more recent developments,[909] including the decision by France to end this requirement for all non-citizens.

Second, and of greater contemporary importance, refugees are to be assimilated to nationals of their country of residence with respect to "legal assistance."[910] This right to equal treatment is, of course, of no practical benefit to refugees where, as in Uganda, not even nationals benefit from a legal aid program. Yet for refugees living in countries where legal aid is generally available, Art. 16(2) may be of real value. Without the benefit of this provision (and this is still the case for refugees who have yet to establish an habitual residence), a refugee seeking to vindicate a right to legal aid would be required to rely upon the very general language of Art. 14 of the Civil and Political Covenant, in addition to the duty of non-discrimination. The difficulty is that Art. 14's guarantee to all persons of equality before courts

---

[906] The Court of Appeal of Paris has taken the position that while Art. 16(2) exempts refugees from the being the *object* of a request for *cautio judicatum solvi*, it is not a source of positive entitlement for refugees to seek *cautio judicatum solvi* in relation to a suit being brought against them by a non-citizen. Because the right to seek *cautio judicatum solvi* was determined to be "a privilege of nationality," a refugee resident in France was not allowed to seek *cautio judicatum solvi* against American plaintiffs: *Fliegelman*, reported at (1963) 90 *Journal du droit international* 723 (Fr. Cour d'Appel de Paris, 1ère Chambre, Nov. 29, 1961).

[907] The result under Art. 14(1) of the Civil and Political Covenant would be less clear. "The assessment of whether the deposit of security raises an unacceptable barrier to a person's access to court should be based on the total sum required as security": Jayawickrama, *Judicial Application*, at 484. The duty to post security for costs is not, therefore, impermissible *per se*. Whether an otherwise valid requirement applied only to non-citizens is allowable would be determined by reference to the duty of non-discrimination. See chapter 2.5.5 above, at pp. 129–133, for a discussion of the margin of appreciation enjoyed by states in providing enhanced benefits to their own citizens.

[908] Statement of Mr. Herment of Belgium, UN Doc. A/CONF.2/SR.8, July 5, 1951, at 13.

[909] In the draft of the ALI/UNIDROIT Principles and Rules of Transnational Civil Procedure (Discussion Draft No. 4, 2003), Principle 3.3 provides that "[a] person should not be required to provide security for costs, or security for liability for pursuing provisional measures, solely because that person is not a national or resident of the forum state." Draft Rule 32.9 similarly provides that "[s]ecurity should not be required solely because a party is not domiciled in the forum state."

[910] "With regard to legal aid or legal assistance, it is clear that the Article can only apply to such benefits which are granted by the State under a State-supported scheme. In countries where legal aid is solely granted by bar associations, the Article will certainly not apply": Grahl-Madsen, *Commentary*, at 67.

and tribunals is exceedingly general,[911] in consequence of which "[a] state has a free choice of the means to be used towards guaranteeing to litigants an effective right of access to the courts. The institution of a legal aid scheme constitutes one of those means, but there are others."[912] Still, a host country which has opted to establish a system of legal aid would be under a significant burden by virtue of Arts. 2(1) and 26 of the Civil and Political Covenant to explain why the failure to extend the benefit of the system to refugees is justifiable differentiation, rather than impermissible discrimination.[913] The risk is that it might be determined that the margin of appreciation regularly afforded states with regard to the treatment of non-citizens should prevail.[914]

The clear strength of the Refugee Convention is that, at least once habitual residence has been established, none of these questions needs to be addressed. If a system of legal aid is in place in the host country, refugees must have access to it on precisely the same terms as citizens. And in any other state party to the Convention, refugees must receive legal aid under the same conditions as do citizens of their country of habitual residence. Arguments concerning the scope of the duty to provide access to the courts and the difficult issue of establishing discrimination are avoided by virtue of the clear language of paras. 2 and 3 of Art. 16.

---

[911] See chapter 4.10 above, at pp. 647–655.

[912] Jayawickrama, *Judicial Application*, at 488, citing in support the decision of the European Court of Human Rights in *Andronicus and Constantinou v. Cyprus*, (1997) 25 EHRR 491 (ECHR, Oct. 9, 1997). But "[w]hile the right to free legal aid in civil cases is not expressly guaranteed, its denial may, in certain circumstances, infringe the principle of 'equality of arms' and [therefore] constitute a violation of the right to a fair hearing": ibid. at 507.

[913] See generally chapter 2.5.5 above, and in particular *Avellanal v. Peru*, UNHRC Comm. No. 202/1986, decided Oct. 28, 1988, at para. 10.2, in which the right to a fair trial was deemed to have been contravened by a procedure predicated on sex discrimination.

[914] See chapter 2.5.5 above, at pp. 129–133.

Rights of solution

There is increasing impatience with the duty simply to honor the rights of persons who are Convention refugees. The focus of much contemporary discourse is instead on the importance of defining and pursuing so-called "durable solutions" to refugee flight.[1] The main goal of a refugee protection regime oriented towards durable solutions is effectively to find a way to bring refugee status to an end – whether by means of return to the country of origin, resettlement elsewhere, or naturalization in the host country. Indeed, those who focus on achieving durable solutions increasingly regard respect for refugee rights as little more than a "second best" option, to be pursued only until a durable solution can be implemented. UNHCR's Executive Committee, for example, has recently endorsed a conclusion

> Recognizing the need for Governments, UNHCR and the international community to continue to respond to the asylum and assistance needs of refugees *until durable solutions are found* [emphasis added].[2]

---

[1] UNHCR records more than fifty resolutions of the General Assembly between 1959 and 2000 which call upon states to find "durable solutions" to refugee situations; it provides by way of a "sample text" GA Res. 38/121, para. 8, which "[u]rges all States to support the High Commissioner in his efforts to find durable solutions to refugee problems, primarily through voluntary repatriation, including assistance to returnees, as appropriate, or, wherever appropriate, through integration in countries of asylum or resettlement in third countries": UNHCR, "Durable Solutions," available at www.unhcr.ch (accessed Nov. 20, 2004). In response to these and similar calls, including the mandate set by the Declaration of States Parties to the 1951 Convention and/or its 1967 Protocol relating to the Status of Refugees, UN Doc. HCR/MMSP/2001/09, Dec. 13, 2001, incorporated in Executive Committee of the High Commissioner's Program, "Agenda for Protection," UN Doc. EC/52/SC/CRP.9/Rev.1, June 26, 2002, the agency released a "Framework for Durable Solutions for Refugees and Persons of Concern" in May 2003.

[2] UNHCR Executive Committee Conclusion No. 89, "Conclusion on International Protection" (2000), at Preamble, available at www.unhcr.ch (accessed Nov. 20, 2004). The special concern of UNHCR to promote durable solutions is arguably compelled by its Statute, which requires UNHCR to "seek[ ] permanent solutions for the problem of refugees by assisting Governments ... to facilitate the voluntary repatriation of such refugees, or their assimilation within new national communities": Statute of the Office of

In contrast to this emphasis on the pursuit of durable solutions, the Refugee Convention gives priority to allowing refugees to make their own decisions about how best to respond to their predicament. As a non-governmental advocate astutely observed, one of the strengths of the refugee rights regime is that it eschews "the false notion of 'durable solutions' to refugee problems, especially as refugees [may] have no idea as to how long they are likely to stay in a particular country."[3] Rather than propelling refugees towards some means of ending their stay abroad, the Refugee Convention emphasizes instead the right of refugees to take the time they need to decide when and if they wish to pursue a durable solution. In some cases, refugees will choose not to pursue any solution right away, but will prefer simply to establish a reasonably normal life in the state party where they sought protection. This is a fully respectable alternative, which may not lawfully be interfered with by either governments or international agencies. Because refugee rights inhere as the result of the individual's predicament and consequent status – rather than as a result of any formal process of adjudication by a state – they provide refugees with a critical, self-executing arsenal of entitlements which may be invoked in any of the state parties to the Refugee Convention. They afford refugees a real measure of autonomy and security to devise the solutions which they judge most suited to their own circumstances and ambitions, and to vary those decisions over time.[4]

the United Nations High Commissioner for Refugees, UNGA Res. 428(V), adopted Dec. 14, 1950 (UNHCR Statute), at Art. 1(1).

[3] Comments of M. Barber of the British Refugee Council, "Final Report: Implementation of the OAU/UN Conventions and Domestic Legislation Concerning the Rights and Obligations of Refugees in Africa, 14–28 September 1986," Refugee Studies Programme, Oxford University (1988), at 34.

[4] The alternative of simply respecting refugee rights is moreover practical because it is not one-sided. As shown in previous chapters, the structure of the refugee rights regime neatly reconciles the interest of refugees in having an array of protection options to the legitimate concerns of the states and communities called upon to receive them. For example, the qualitative measure of respect for refugee rights is absolute in relation to only a few, truly essential rights. Otherwise, it is measured by reference to the protection afforded others residing in the host country, resulting in a flexible, but nonetheless quantifiable, standard of compliance. See generally chapters 3.2 and 3.3 above. Equally important, the Refugee Convention embraces the sensible proposition that not all rights are immediately due upon arrival in the territory of a state party. Instead, enhanced rights accrue to refugees as a function of the passage of time, and the establishment of a deeper connection between them and their hosts: see generally chapter 3.1 above. On the other hand, these two sources of flexibility for receiving states are themselves constrained by basic principles required to ensure fairness to refugees: refugees may not be the objects of discrimination, they must be exempted from expectations which they are inherently unable to fulfill, they may not be penalized by exceptional measures applied against the citizens of their state of origin, and they must not lose their basic rights even in times of war or serious emergency. See generally chapters 2.5.5, 3.4, and 3.5 above. All in all, the careful balance struck by the Refugee Convention remains in many ways an ideal mechanism for reconciling the

This is not to suggest that there is any inherent contradiction between a commitment to honoring refugee rights and the pursuit of durable solutions to refugeehood. As analysed in detail below, each of the options described as a durable solution is, to a greater or lesser degree, reconcilable to the requirements of the Refugee Convention. The concern is rather that much current practice reverses the emphasis of refugee law on the primacy of respect for refugee rights in favor of the pursuit of durable solutions. For example, a senior official of the United Nations High Commissioner for Refugees (UNHCR) opined that

> protection should be seen as a temporary holding arrangement between the departure and return to the original community, or as a bridge between one community and another. Legal protection is the formal structure of that temporary holding arrangement or bridge.[5]

Despite the technical accuracy of the view that protection is a duty which inheres only for the duration of risk, that duty may be inadvertently degraded by referring to it as simply an "arrangement or bridge" rather than as a fully legitimate alternative to the pursuit of a durable solution to refugee status. This very simple notion – that the recognition and honoring of refugee rights is itself a fully respectable, indeed often quite a desirable response to involuntary migration – can too easily be eclipsed by the rush to locate and implement so-called durable solutions.[6]

Under the Refugee Convention, the refugee himself or herself normally determines whether a solution beyond respect for refugee rights is to be pursued. Indeed, the only circumstance under which a solution to refugee

refugee's individual autonomy to communal expectations and capacities in receiving states. The broader issue of modern challenges to the viability of the refugee rights regime is briefly taken up below in the Epilogue. In considering responses to refugeehood, the most basic answer of all is therefore simply to honor the requirements of refugee law itself. Particularly where the standard of protection is derived by a synthesis of refugee law and cognate norms of international human rights law (as the analysis in preceding chapters has proposed), many, perhaps most, refugees will require no more. If refugees are genuinely able freely to access a place where they are allowed to remain for the duration of risk and are granted a solid array of both civil and socioeconomic rights that enable them to live in dignity there, that may well be all that is required by way of an international response to their predicament.

[5] G. Arnaout, "International Protection of Refugees' Rights," remarks delivered at the Training Course on International Norms and Standards in the Field of Human Rights, Moscow, 1989 (Arnaout, "Refugees' Rights"), at 7. Arnaout was at the time the Director of the Division of Law and Doctrine of UNHCR.

[6] See, for example, Arnaout, "Refugees' Rights," at 7: "It is not adequate to consider as a solution to the [refugee] problem ... mere 'self-sufficiency.' The problem of the refugee has always been seen as *de iure* or *de facto* statelessness, and the solution to this problem, therefore, must be either the reacquiring of the normal 'community' benefits of the original nationality or the acquisition of a new nationality with all its normal benefits ... Without a community, the individual is isolated, deprived and vulnerable."

status may lawfully be undertaken without the consent of the refugee is where there has been a fundamental change of circumstances in the refugee's state of origin, which change has eliminated the refugee's need for surrogate protection. Refugee status comes to an end in such a case, and the former refugee may be mandatorily repatriated to the country of origin. So long as the requirements of international human rights law are met, there is no requirement that repatriation in such circumstances be voluntary. The label often attached to this option – "voluntary repatriation" – is thus not appropriate. For reasons set out below, the solution of requiring a refugee's departure once the need for protection comes to an end is better referred to simply as *repatriation*, thus avoiding confusion with the second solution, *voluntary reestablishment*.

While repatriation involves the return of a person who is no longer a refugee (and hence need not be voluntary), a person who remains a refugee may voluntarily decide to reestablish himself or herself in the country of origin despite the risk of being persecuted there. A refugee is, of course, always free in law to opt for return to his or her own country. Return under such circumstances must, however, be the result of the refugee's free choice if the state of asylum is to avoid breach of the duty of *non-refoulement*. Once there is evidence of both a genuinely voluntary return and of the refugee's de facto reestablishment in his or her own country, the Refugee Convention deems refugee status to have come to an end. This is so because the refugee's own clear actions signal that he or she no longer wishes to benefit from the surrogate protection of an asylum country that is the concern of refugee law.

Beyond repatriation and voluntary reestablishment, the third solution to refugee status is resettlement. This solution acknowledges the reality that time spent in an asylum state may afford a refugee the opportunity to explore and secure access to durable protection options better suited to his or her needs. The Refugee Convention explicitly envisages the possibility of onward movement by way of resettlement from the first country of arrival, and requires the government in the refugee's initial host state to facilitate that process. Once resettlement has occurred, the continuing need for refugee protection is, of course, at an end.

Fourth, and as a logical extension of the Convention's core commitment to affording refugees greater rights as their attachment to the asylum country increases over time, a point may be reached where the refugee and the authorities of that country agree to the refugee's formal naturalization by the host state. If a refugee opts to accept an offer of citizenship there, with entitlement fully to participate in all aspects of that state's public life, his or her need for the surrogate protection of refugee law comes to an end. There is no need for surrogate protection in such a case, as the refugee is able and entitled to benefit from the protection of his or her new country of nationality.

Having focused in chapters 4–6 on the primary duty of states to respect refugee rights for the duration of risk, this chapter now takes up the question of the rights of refugees when a decision is made to pursue their repatriation, or when the refugee opts for voluntary reestablishment, resettlement, or naturalization.

7.1 Repatriation

There is strong support for regarding repatriation as the best solution to refugeehood. UNHCR's Executive Committee, for example, has "not[ed] that [while] voluntary repatriation, local integration and resettlement are the traditional durable solutions for refugees, ... voluntary repatriation is *the preferred solution*, when feasible [emphasis added]."[7] As the language of the Executive Committee makes clear, support is not normally expressed for "repatriation" as a solution to refugeehood, but rather for "voluntary repatriation."[8] The routine use of this terminology is, however, problematic. While anchored in the language of the UNHCR Statute,[9] and hence logically taken into account in determining the focus of *institutional* practice,[10] the rights of state parties to the Refugee Convention are quite differently conceived. Whereas UNHCR is mandated to promote voluntary repatriation, the Convention posits two distinct options to bring refugee status to an end:

[7] UNHCR Executive Committee Conclusion No. 89, "Conclusion on International Protection" (2000), at Preamble, available at www.unhcr.ch (accessed Nov. 20, 2004).

[8] See e.g. UNHCR Executive Committee Conclusions Nos. 18, "Voluntary Repatriation" (1980); 41, "General Conclusion on International Protection" (1986); 46, "General Conclusion on International Protection" (1987); 55, "General Conclusion on International Protection" (1989); 62, "Note on International Protection" (1990); 68, "General Conclusion on International Protection" (1992); 74, "General Conclusion on International Protection" (1994); 79, "General Conclusion on International Protection" (1996); 81, "General Conclusion on International Protection" (1997); 85, "Conclusion on International Protection" (1998); 87, "General Conclusion on International Protection" (1999); and 89, "Conclusion on International Protection" (2000), all available at www.unhcr.ch (accessed Nov. 20, 2004). The Executive Committee has recently "[r]eaffirm[ed] the voluntary character of refugee repatriation, which involves the individual making a free and informed choice through, *inter alia*, the availability of complete, accurate and objective information on the situation in the country of origin": UNHCR Executive Committee Conclusion No. 101, "Conclusion on Legal Safety Issues in the Context of Voluntary Repatriation of Refugees" (2004), at Preamble, available at www.unhcr.ch (accessed Nov. 20, 2004).

[9] "The High Commissioner shall provide for the protection of refugees falling under the competence of his Office by ... [a]ssisting governmental and private efforts to promote *voluntary* repatriation [emphasis added]": UNHCR Statute, at Art. 8(d).

[10] See e.g. UNHCR, "Handbook: Voluntary Repatriation: International Protection" (1996) (UNHCR, "Voluntary Repatriation Handbook").

voluntary reestablishment, and repatriation consequent to a fundamental change of circumstances. Neither is the same as voluntary repatriation.[11]

On the one hand, it may be the case that a person who is a refugee – that is, who continues to be objectively at risk of being persecuted – nonetheless decides to go back to the country where that risk exists. In so doing, the refugee is simply exercising the right of every person to return to his or her own country.[12] But as a matter of refugee law, refugee status comes to an end by operation of Art. 1(C)(4) of the Convention if the voluntary return amounts to reestablishment in the country of origin.[13] As a matter of logic, this must be so: the refugee's actions signal that an essential requirement of refugee status, the presence of the putative refugee *outside* the territory of his or her own country, will no longer be satisfied.[14] But this voluntary act of return and reestablishment is not appropriately referred to as "repatriation," since there is no requirement at law that the result of the return home be the restoration of a normal relationship between the (former) refugee and the government of the home state. As Stein has rightly insisted, "In many situations, 'repatriation' is the wrong term, because there has been no restoration of the bond between citizen and fatherland. 'Return' is a better term because it relates to the fact of going home without judging its content."[15]

Critically, state parties are not entitled to rely upon the simple fact of return to the home country, even if clearly voluntary, to terminate Convention refugee

[11] See M. Barutciski, "Involuntary Repatriation when Refugee Protection is no Longer Necessary: Moving Forward after the 48th Session of the Executive Committee," (1998) 10(1/2) *International Journal of Refugee Law* 236 (Barutciski, "Involuntary Repatriation"), at 249: "[T]he concept of voluntary repatriation is incoherent if taken as a legally binding standard. Its value appears in terms of recommending that a State take into account the individual's desire to return home. Although this is undoubtedly a reasonable recommendation, it cannot be a coherent legally binding standard according to international principles of refugee protection."

[12] "No one shall be arbitrarily deprived of the right to enter his own country": International Covenant on Civil and Political Rights, UNGA Res. 2200A(XXI), adopted Dec. 16, 1966, entered into force Mar. 23, 1976 (Civil and Political Covenant), at Art. 12(4).

[13] "The Convention shall cease to apply to any person falling under the terms of section A if ... [h]e has voluntarily re-established himself in the country which he left or outside [of] which he remained owing to fear of persecution": Convention relating to the Status of Refugees, 189 UNTS 2545, done July 28, 1951, entered into force Apr. 22, 1954 (Refugee Convention), at Art. 1(C)(4).

[14] The refugee definition limits protection to a person "*outside* the country of his nationality ... [or in the case of a stateless person] *outside* the country of his former habitual residence" owing to a well-founded fear of being persecuted for a Convention reason: Refugee Convention, at Art. 1(A)(2).

[15] B. Stein, "Policy Challenges Regarding Repatriation in the 1990s: Is 1992 the Year for Voluntary Repatriation?," paper presented at the Conference on Global Refugee Policy: An Agenda for the 1990s, at the Aspen Institute, Feb. 1992, at 2.

status. Under Art. 1(C)(4), it is only if and when the refugee is *reestablished* in the country of origin that refugee status comes to an end. As analyzed below,[16] this more demanding test provides refugees with significant protection not available under the voluntary repatriation paradigm.[17]

> **Refugee Convention, Art. 1(C)(5)–(6)**
> This Convention shall cease to apply to any person falling under the terms of section A if:
>
> . . .
>
> (5) He can no longer, because the circumstances in connection with which he has been recognized as a refugee have ceased to exist, continue to refuse to avail himself of the protection of the country of his nationality;
>
> Provided that this paragraph shall not apply to a refugee falling under section A(1) of this article who is able to invoke compelling reasons arising out of previous persecution for refusing to avail himself of the protection of the country of nationality; [or]
> (6) Being a person who has no nationality he is, because the circumstances in connection with which he has been recognized as a refugee have ceased to exist, able to return to the country of his former habitual residence.

The other notion generally subsumed under the label of "voluntary repatriation," the subject of this section, is more sensibly referred to simply as repatriation. Because refugee protection is conceived as protection for the

---

[16] See chapter 7.2 below.
[17] In brief, under Art. 1(C)(4), the voluntariness of the return and subsequent reestablishment is an essential element of this solution, both because it is part of the test for cessation of refugee status under Art. 1(C)(4), and more fundamentally because any involuntary return may amount to a breach of the host state's duty of *non-refoulement*. In view of the right of all individuals to return to their country of citizenship, the truly voluntary decision of a refugee to become reestablished in his or her state of origin – including to risk his or her life in so doing – does not violate any duty of the state which has granted protection. But if return is not really based on the refugee's free consent, including in situations where it has been coerced by threat of sanction or the withdrawal of rights, the duty of *non-refoulement* is infringed. As such, the voluntariness of the decision to return must be considered in assessing the legality of any return in circumstances where refugee status has not come to an end. The question of voluntariness of return has accordingly been taken up in the earlier analysis of the duty of *non-refoulement*: see chapter 4.1.2 above. An effort is made to build on that understanding and to develop the further requirement of reestablishment in the country of origin in the next section: see chapter 7.2 below.

duration of risk in the country of origin,[18] state parties are not obliged to honor refugee rights when the underlying risk comes to an end. Under Art. 1(C)(5)–(6) of the Refugee Convention, refugee status is lost once the refugee can no longer claim surrogate international protection "because the circumstances in connection with which he has been recognized as a refugee have ceased to exist."[19] When this standard is met, the host government is ordinarily entitled to require the former refugee to depart its territory, even if the only option is return to his or her state of origin.[20] Without the protection

[18] As recently observed in the House of Lords, "[r]efugee status is a temporary status for as long as the risk of persecution remains": *R v. Secretary of State for the Home Department, ex parte Yogathas*, [2002] UKHL 36 (UK HL, Oct. 17, 2002), per Lord Scott. More explicitly, the English Court of Appeal has noted "that the Convention only requires this country to grant asylum for so long as the person granted asylum remains a refugee. It would be enough to satisfy the Convention if the Secretary of State were to grant refugees temporary leave to remain for so long as their refugee status persisted": *Saad v. Secretary of State for the Home Department*, [2001] EWCA Civ 2008 (Eng. CA, Dec. 19, 2001). See generally J. Hathaway, "The Meaning of Repatriation," (1997) 9(4) *International Journal of Refugee Law* 551; also published in European University Institute ed., *Legal and Policy Issues Concerning Refugees from the Former Yugoslavia* 4 (1997) (Hathaway, "Repatriation").

[19] "We should not lose sight of the fact that international law concerns the imposition of obligations on States. It may be in the individual's best interest actually to remain in the host country and continue his or her life in exile, but is the State obliged to provide refuge if conditions in the country of origin have become safe within a reasonable time period? Clearly, States never agreed to such legal obligations": Barutciski, "Involuntary Repatriation," at 245.

[20] While the range of issues to be considered in initially assessing the existence of a well-founded fear and at the cessation stages is similar, Art. 1(C)(5)–(6) nonetheless insists upon a higher standard of scrutiny in the context of adjudicating cessation. The Canadian Federal Court has sensibly taken the view that while the criteria for cessation due to changed circumstances are not technically binding at the time of initial status assessment, nonetheless "when a panel is weighing changed country conditions, together with all the evidence in an applicant's case, factors such as durability, effectiveness and substantiality are still relevant. The more durable the changes are demonstrated to be, the heavier they will weigh against granting the applicant's claim": *Penate v. Canada*, [1994] 2 FC 79 (Can. FCA, Nov. 26, 1993). See also *Villalta v. Canada*, [1993] FCJ 1025 (Can. FC, Oct. 8, 1993), holding that the cessation criteria "are a small subset of a larger circle of circumstances in which status will not be found to exist. This small subset is what must be proven by the government if it wishes to take status away from someone but it does not control the framework of the analysis ... in determining whether status exists ... I do not mean to suggest that in assessing the significance of changed country conditions, for the purposes of deciding whether to grant status, the [decision-maker] should not consider factors such as the significance, the likely effectiveness and likely durability of the changed conditions. But I do not think the [decision-maker] needs to apply the *more demanding criteria*, which it is necessary to meet when one is considering removal of status [emphasis added]." But see *Minister for Immigration and Multicultural Affairs v. Betkhoshabeh*, 55 ALD 609 (Aus. FFC, July 20, 1999), in which the court took the view that there is no difference between the initial test for determining the existence of a well-founded fear and that for the cessation of refugee status under Art. 1(C). Because cessation involves the withdrawal of

of refugee law, the former refugee is in the same position as any other non-citizen: he or she is subject to removal, so long as the removal can be accomplished without breach of any relevant norm of international human rights law.[21]

Because the rationale for cessation due to a fundamental change of circumstances is the existence of a government in the home state able and willing to protect the refugee,[22] it makes sense to refer to return in this context as "repatriation." That is, the legal basis for deeming refugee status to have ended is precisely the restoration of a bond or social contract between citizen and state. It follows that where the state of origin is shown to be able and willing to protect the individual concerned, there is no legal basis to insist that repatriation consequent to cessation of status under Art. 1(C)(5)–(6) also be *voluntary*.[23] Because the repatriation of the former refugee cannot by

an acquired status from a refugee – based upon an already proved or assumed risk of being persecuted – the refugee should be subjected to uprooting and enforced departure only where there is particularly clear evidence that protection is no longer required. To similar effect, see UNHCR, "Note on the Cessation Clauses," UN Doc. EC/47/SC/CRP.30 (1997) (UNHCR, "Cessation"), at paras. 8–9: "Given that the application of the cessation clauses would result in the withdrawal of refugee status, the clauses should be interpreted in a restrictive way ... UNHCR recommends that in deciding whether to invoke the cessation clauses, States should take into account the consequences of cessation of refugee status. Difficulties which may follow from the invocation of the cessation clauses should be considered in both the decision and the timing of cessation. In particular, States should avoid a situation where the former refugee remains in the country of asylum without a definite legal status or with an illegal status. Human rights factors should be taken into account as well as previously acquired rights of refugees, particularly in regard to those who, due to their long stay in the country of asylum, have developed strong family, social and economic links there."

[21] The limitations on lawful repatriation set by international human rights law are discussed below, at pp. 944–952.

[22] This is most clear in the case of (the overwhelming majority of) refugees who hold the citizenship of that country, who lose their refugee status only if the change of circumstances means that the refugee "can no longer ... continue to refuse to avail himself of the protection of the country of his nationality": Refugee Convention, at Art. 1(C)(5). In the case of stateless refugees, only the ability to return to the country of former habitual residence is required for cessation to ensue: ibid. at Art. 1(C)(6). Cessation under Art. 1(C)(1)–(2), while less common, is similarly predicated on the reestablishment of a protective bond between the refugee and his or her country of origin. See generally J. Hathaway, *The Law of Refugee Status* (1991) (Hathaway, *Refugee Status*), at 191–197.

[23] The situation is somewhat more ambiguous for state parties to the Convention governing the Specific Aspects of Refugee Problems in Africa, 10011 UNTS 14691, done Sept. 10, 1969, entered into force June 20, 1974 (OAU Refugee Convention). While Art. I(4)(e) of this treaty is largely comparable to the right of cessation due to a fundamental change of circumstances found in the Refugee Convention, Art. V(1) of the OAU Refugee Convention expressly provides that "[t]he essentially voluntary character of repatriation shall be respected *in all cases* and *no refugee* shall be repatriated against his will [emphasis added]." The OAU Refugee Convention does not make clear how this provision is to be related to the cessation clauses. On the one hand, the reference to the duty to respect the voluntary character of repatriation "in all cases" could be read to limit the right of states to

definition involve a risk of *refoulement* (it having been found that there is no longer an objective risk of being persecuted in the country of origin), repatriation does not require the former refugee's consent.[24]

There are three requirements for invocation of the change of circumstances cessation clause of Art. 1(C)(5)–(6).[25] As advocated by the UNHCR, the first requirement is that the change in the country of origin be genuinely *fundamental*.[26] Second, it must be *enduring*.[27] Third, it must result not just in the eradication of a well-founded fear of being persecuted, but also in the *restoration of protection*.[28] Taken together, these tests give substance to the UNHCR Executive Committee's view that the cessation of refugee status is warranted only "where a change of circumstances in a country is of such a profound and enduring nature that refugees from that country no longer require international protection and can no longer

repatriate even a person who is no longer a refugee by virtue of cessation of status. On the other hand, the final clause more clearly stipulates that the requirement of voluntarism may in fact be invoked only by a person who is a "refugee," thereby excluding a (former) refugee whose status has validly ceased. If read to apply only to (present) refugees, then the OAU provision can not only be reconciled to its own cessation clauses, but also applied in consonance with Art. 1(C)(4) of the Refugee Convention, which does require voluntary reestablishment by a person otherwise entitled to refugee status before the duty to protect him or her comes to an end: see chapter 7.2 below.

[24] Insistence on consent to repatriation could easily grant (former) refugees what amounts to a veto over their return to the home state, based on reasons which may have nothing to do with the criteria for cessation under Art. 1(C)(5)–(6). For example, spokespersons for Chakma refugees from Bangladesh articulated a thirteen-point charter of demands before they would agree to go back to Chittagong (in Bangladesh). While many of the demands related to cessation criteria, others – including compensation for the refugees, and the eviction of Muslim settlers from traditional tribal lands – did not: *Times of India*, Jan. 17, 1994, cited in B. S. Chimni, *International Academy of Comparative Law National Report for India* (1994), at 12. Moreover, even in the context of decisions regarding the UNHCR mandate itself, it has been noted that "the means do not yet exist to enable the wishes and choices of the refugees themselves to play a decisive part in determining their own future": "Refugees Returning Home: Report of the Symposium for the Horn of Africa on the Social and Economic Aspects of Mass Voluntary Return Movements of Refugees, Addis Ababa, 15–17 September 1992" (1993), at 14. See UNHCR, "Guidelines on International Protection No. 3: Cessation of Refugee Status under Articles 1(C)(5) and (6) of the 1951 Convention relating to the Status of Refugees (the 'Ceased Circumstances Clauses')," UN Doc. HCR/GIP/03/03, Feb. 10, 2003 (UNHCR, "Ceased Circumstances Guidelines"), at para. 7: "Cessation under Article 1C(5) and 1C(6) does not require the consent of or a voluntary act by the refugee. Cessation of refugee status terminates rights that accompany that status."

[25] UNHCR, "Ceased Circumstances Guidelines," at paras. 10–16. This language is an overall improvement on the test proposed in Hathaway, *Refugee Status*, at 200–202, requiring that the change be "of substantial political significance ... truly effective ... [and] shown to be durable." In particular, UNHCR's insistence on a restoration of protection affords valuable clarity on the meaning of effectiveness.

[26] UNHCR, "Ceased Circumstances Guidelines," at paras. 10–12.

[27] Ibid. at paras. 13–14.   [28] Ibid. at paras. 15–16.

continue to refuse to avail themselves of the protection of their country."[29] This restrictive approach to cessation is very much in line with the intentions of the drafters of the Refugee Convention, who showed no inclination to authorize the withdrawal of refugee status on the basis of changes that are insufficiently fundamental to justify the conclusion that "the circumstances in connection with which [a refugee] has been recognized . . . *have ceased to exist* [emphasis added]." Indeed, the type of circumstance which they had in mind in proposing Art. 1(C)(5)–(6) was the reversion of a totalitarian state to democratic governance:

> To take the case of the aged belonging to the "hard core" of refugees, it could hardly be agreed that the government of a country which had returned to democratic ways should fail to take over the burden of that category of refugees . . . [France] was quite prepared to continue to assist such refugees so long as such assistance was necessary. But if their country reverted to a democratic regime, the obligation to assist them should not fall perforce upon the French Government . . . France merely said that she did not wish to be under an obligation to continue to provide assistance to refugees who could seek the protection of their country of origin.[30]

To meet the first requirement of "fundamental change," UNHCR has opined that "[a] complete political change remains the most typical situation in which this cessation clause has been applied. Depending on the grounds for flight, significant reforms altering the basic legal or social structure of the State may also amount to fundamental change, as may democratic elections, declarations of amnesties, repeal of oppressive laws and dismantling of former security ser-vices."[31] Caution of this kind is appropriate in order to ensure that a refugee's life not be disturbed simply because there is evidence of movement in a peaceful or rights-regarding direction: the basic reforms must rather be in place before cessation is contemplated. Thus, for example, the German Administrative Court in 1992 refused to recognize a fundamental change of circumstances in Romania – where the Communist era secret police had been reestablished – in contrast to the more radical structural reforms undertaken in Poland, Czechoslovakia, and Hungary, which were appropriately considered of sufficient magnitude to justify a cessation inquiry.[32]

---

[29] UNHCR Executive Committee Conclusion No. 65, "General Conclusion on International Protection" (1991), at para. (q), affirmed in Executive Committee Conclusion No. 69, "Cessation of Status" (1992), both available at www.unhcr.ch (accessed Nov. 20, 2004).

[30] Statement of Mr. Rochefort of France, UN Doc. A/CONF.2/SR.28, July 19, 1951, at 12–14.

[31] UNHCR, "Cessation," at para. 20.

[32] *An 17 K 91 42844; An 17 K 91 42845* (Ger. AC, Ansbach), reported as Abstract No. IJRL/ 0193 in (1994) 6(2) *International Journal of Refugee Law* 282. See also *Nkosi v. Canada*, (1993) FCJ 629 (Can. FC, June 23, 1993), declining to refuse refugee status on the basis of a "hesitant and equivocal finding that certain limited changes in circumstances in Zaïre had occurred."

The fundamental nature of a reform is moreover not a function simply of its social and political significance. Rather, it must also be determined that whatever changes have occurred genuinely "address the causes of displacement which led to the recognition of refugee status."[33] Even major political reforms do not warrant cessation unless they are causally connected to the risk upon which refugee status was recognized, or could presently be justified. Clearly, whatever general view may be taken of the significance of a change of circumstances must be tested by reference to the particularized circumstances of the applicant:

> [W]hen one says that "change" in circumstances is an important consideration, one is not speaking of any change. The [decision-maker] must not be content in simply noting that changes have taken place, but must assess the impact of those changes on the person of the applicant.[34]

The importance of contemplating cessation only when there is evidence of fundamental change – in the sense that it is both truly significant and substantively relevant – is closely connected to the second requirement: the reform must be shown to be enduring. In the case of an Indian Sikh at risk under the regime of Indira Gandhi, for example, a reviewing court was satisfied that a relevant change of circumstances had occurred because "six years had passed since the assassination of Indira Gandhi and the incidents of alleged persecution, and . . . a new government was in place in India."[35] While twelve to eighteen months since a fundamental reform is argued by UNHCR to be the minimum time which should elapse before cessation is contemplated,[36] the more basic rule is "that all developments which would appear to evidence significant and profound changes be given time to consolidate before any decision on cessation is made."[37] Because the process of consolidation is context-specific, the time required to establish the durability of change will inevitably be longer where the reform was the result of

---

[33] UNHCR, "Ceased Circumstances Guidelines," at para. 10. "Fundamental changes are considered as effective only if they remove the basis of the fear of persecution; therefore, such changes must be assessed in light of the particular cause of fear, so as to ensure that the situation which warranted the grant of refugee status has ceased to exist": UNHCR, "Cessation," at para. 19.

[34] *Arugello Garcia v. Canada*, (1993) FCJ 635 (Can. FC, June 23, 1993).

[35] *Virk v. Canada*, (1992) FCJ 119 (Can. FC, Feb. 14, 1992).

[36] "In the *Discussion Note on the Application of the "ceased circumstances" cessation clause in the 1951 Convention* (EC/SCP/1992/CRP.1), it was advocated that a period of twelve to eighteen months elapse after the occurrence of profound changes before such a decision is made. It is UNHCR's recommendation that this period be regarded as a minimum for assessment purposes. Recent applications of the cessation clause by UNHCR show that the average period is around four to five years from the time fundamental changes commenced": UNHCR, "Cessation," at para. 21.

[37] Ibid.

conflict,[38] and hence less likely to be quickly and whole-heartedly embraced by all:

> Occasionally, an evaluation as to whether fundamental changes have taken place on a durable basis can be made after a relatively short time has elapsed. This is so in situations where, for example, the changes are peaceful and take place under a constitutional process, where there are free and fair elections with a real change of government committed to respecting fundamental human rights, and where there is relative political and economic stability in the country. A longer period of time will need to have elapsed before the durability of change can be tested where the changes have taken place violently, for instance, through the overthrow of a regime. Under the latter circumstances, the human rights situation needs to be especially carefully assessed. The process of national reconstruction must be given sufficient time to take hold and any peace arrangements with opposing militant groups must be carefully monitored.[39]

Third and most important, the fundamental and durable reform must be shown to have dependable, practical protection consequences. In many cases, courts have shown an unhealthy willingness to defer to formal evidence of fundamental change without carefully assessing the resultant ground reality.[40] For example, the fall of the Mengistu regime in Ethiopia,[41] the existence

---

[38] As such, cessation should clearly not be contemplated simply because there is presently peace in an area previously prone to conflict. This point was neatly made by the Federal Court of Canada. "The very article in *The Economist* cited by the [decision-maker] states merely, 'for now there is peace . . . ', leaving it an open question to the reader how long this *status quo* will last. Given this result, we do not find it necessary to consider the other matters raised": *Abarajithan v. Canada*, (1992) FCJ 54 (Can. FC, Jan. 28, 1992).

[39] UNHCR, "Ceased Circumstances Guidelines," at paras. 13–14. In contrast, for example, refugees from the Democratic Republic of Congo were told to prepare for return only two months after the signing of a peace accord: "DRC refugees reluctant to go home," *Daily News*, Oct. 1, 2002. The result of a premature termination of refugee status can simply be that refugees end up coming back to the former host state, as was the case for many Burundians removed from Tanzania who were forced once more to flee fighting between the government and rebel forces: "Hundreds more flee Burundi as conflict escalates," *UN Integrated Regional Information Networks*, Oct. 2, 2002. Alternatively, they may feel compelled to seek protection in another state party, as was the case for Rwandans deported from Tanzania, many of whom then sought asylum in Zimbabwe: "Zimbabwe hit by influx of refugees," *Daily News*, Feb. 15, 2003.

[40] Governments may also focus unduly on the formalities of change. Australian immigration minister Philip Ruddock was quoted in April 2003 as having said that "Australia has no obligation to take into account the safety of [Iraq] when it comes to returning the refugees," despite the fact that the military victory there was of recent date and the political transition barely commenced: G. Barns, "Sheik's advice for Howard and Bush," *Canberra Times*, Apr. 25, 2003, at A-15.

[41] "The Mengistu regime has fallen. The successor government stated that its aim was a 'broad-based transitional government, representative of Ethiopia's various tribes and factions, as a prelude to fair elections and multi-party democracy'": *U91–05190* (Can. IRB, Feb. 21, 1992), reported at (1992) *RefLex* 113–114.

of a formal cease-fire in Somalia,[42] as well as the signing of peace accords in El Salvador[43] and Guatemala[44] have all been treated as a sufficient basis to find the need for refugee status to have dissipated. Other courts, however, have properly insisted on the need for patience before finding a fundamental reform to be relevant to the cessation of refugee status.[45] The Federal Court of Canada thus reversed a decision to deny refugee status to an Iranian applicant on the basis of political reforms in that country, it having been determined that the reforms had not, in fact, put an end to the practice of politically inspired arrests and executions.[46]

---

[42] Despite its recognition of the need to avoid the premature determination of durability of change, the Full Federal Court of Australia nonetheless deferred to a determination by the tribunal that a Somali claim could be dismissed on the grounds that a cease-fire in the civil war in that country had been announced by warlords eleven days prior to the hearing: *Ahmed v. Minister for Immigration and Multicultural Affairs*, 55 ALD 618 (Aus. FFC, June 21, 1999). Justice Branson, however, took serious issue with this approach: "First, the cease-fire upon which the Tribunal placed reliance was of recent origin . . . A conclusion by a decision-maker as to the likely effectiveness of the cease-fire, having regard to the preceding seven years of civil war in Somalia, called for some caution. Secondly, the material before the Tribunal upon which it based its conclusion that peace had existed in Somalia since January 31, 1998 was, at best, tentative in character": ibid.

[43] "The documentary evidence describes the peace accord and provides details with respect to its implementation and progress. It is a fact that some documentary evidence also shows that the changes in El Salvador are conservative in nature and that human rights abuses continue. However, it is apparent to me that the Board concluded that as a result of the changed circumstances, the applicant as a union member no longer had cause for a well-founded fear of persecution, and I believe it was open to the Board on the evidence before it to conclude as it did": *Caballos v. Canada*, (1993) FCJ 623 (Can. FC, June 22, 1993).

[44] See e.g. *Gomez Garcia v. Immigration and Naturalization Service*, 1999 US App. Lexis 12096 (US CA8, June 11, 1999); *Mazariegos v. Immigration and Naturalization Service*, 241 F 3d 320 (US CA11, Feb. 12, 2001).

[45] In assessing the claim of a Ugandan Arab, the Canadian Immigration and Refugee Board had determined that the Ugandan government "intended to restore democracy, the rule of law and respect for human rights." In response, the Federal Court noted succinctly that "[t]hese may well have been Museveni's intentions, but these intentions have not materialized": *Ahmed v. Canada*, (1993) FCJ 1035 (Can. FC, Oct. 8, 1993). Similarly, in rejecting the sufficiency of the fall of the Siad Barré regime in Somalia as a basis for finding there to have been a fundamental and durable change of circumstances, the same court observed that "[t]hat finding . . . must be linked with the further finding that the country continues to be divided along tribal lines and to be torn by civil war": *Abdulle v. Canada*, (1992) FCJ 67 (Can. FC, Jan. 27, 1992). In a particularly succinct admonishment of the official propensity to seek premature revocation of status, the Federal Court of Canada observed that "[i]f the political climate in a country changes to the extent that it adversely affects the status of a refugee, the Minister may make an application to . . . determine whether the person has ceased to be a Convention refugee. Presumably, the Minister would only seek such a determination after monitoring the effects of any political change in the subject country": *Salinas v. Canada*, (1992) FCJ 231 (Can. FC, Mar. 20, 1992).

[46] *Oskoy v. Canada*, (1993) FCJ 644 (Can. FC, June 25, 1993).

This qualitative dimension of effective reform has recently been helpfully described by UNHCR as linked to the core concern of the refugee definition itself, namely whether it can truly be said that the refugee can presently "avail himself [or herself] of the protection" of his or her home state:

> In determining whether circumstances have changed so as to justify cessation under Article 1C(5) or (6), another crucial question is whether the refugee can effectively re-avail him- or herself of the protection of his or her own country. Such protection must therefore be effective and available. It requires more than mere physical security or safety. It needs to include the existence of a functioning government and basic administrative structures, as evidenced for instance through a functioning system of law and justice, as well as the existence of adequate infrastructure to enable residents to exercise their rights, including their right to a basic livelihood. An important indicator in this respect is the general human rights situation in the country.[47]

As such, it is not sufficient to find simply that the fundamental and durable reform has eliminated the particular well-founded fear of the refugee. Cessation is warranted only if and when an affirmative situation has been established,[48] namely the "restoration of protection"[49] to the refugee.[50] In line with this approach, the UN Committee on the Elimination of Racial Discrimination has adopted the view that "refugees ... have, after their return to their homes of origin, the right to participate fully and equally in public affairs at all levels and to have equal access to public services and to receive rehabilitation assistance."[51] Equally important, the principle that

---

[47] UNHCR, "Ceased Circumstances Guidelines," at paras. 15–16.

[48] In line with this understanding, four of the nineteen signatories to the Burundi peace agreement prevailed upon Tanzania to avoid the premature repatriation of refugees to Burundi, arguing that "tension was still high in Burundi, in spite of [the] recent installation of a transitional government as a formula for lasting peace conceived by the leaders of the Great Lakes region. They ... call[ed] for the formation of a special protection unit to protect all Burundians as [a] pre-condition[ ] for [repatriation]": "Dar es Salaam urged not to repatriate Bujumbura refugees," *TOMRIC*, Nov. 12, 2001.

[49] UNHCR, "Ceased Circumstances Guidelines," at paras. 15–16.

[50] The Executive Committee of UNHCR has endorsed the agency's Agenda for Protection, which calls upon "[c]ountries of origin ... to commit themselves to respecting the right to return and [to] receiving back their refugees within an acceptable framework of physical, legal and material safety, achievable, for example, through amnesties, human rights guarantees, and measures to enable the restitution of property, all of which should be appropriately communicated to refugees": Executive Committee of the High Commissioner's Program, "Agenda for Protection," UN Doc. EC/52/SC/CRP.9/Rev.1, June 26, 2002 (UNHCR Executive Committee, "Agenda for Protection"), at Part III, Goal 5, Point 2.

[51] UN Committee on the Elimination of Racial Discrimination, "General Recommendation No. XXII: Refugees and displaced persons" (1996), UN Doc. HRI/GEN/1/Rev.7, May 12,

protection must actually be "available" ensures that refugee status cannot be withdrawn in circumstances where the country of origin refuses to readmit the individual concerned.[52] For example, Bhutan has questioned the citizenship of many Bhutanese refugees awaiting repatriation from Nepal, in consequence of which they have been unable to return for more than a decade.[53] There clearly has been no restoration of protection in such circumstances, and hence refugee status should not be deemed to have come to an end.

Despite the clarity of its views on when cessation due to a fundamental change of circumstances is justified, UNHCR has not made the obvious – but critical – linkage between satisfaction of the test for cessation of status under Art. 1(C)(5)–(6) and the right of state parties mandatorily to repatriate former refugees to their country of origin.[54] While it is perhaps understandable that the agency is uncomfortable being seen to encourage governments to promote mandated repatriation, the failure to be explicit about the lawful consequence of valid cessation is intellectually disingenuous.[55] Because

2004, at 214, para. 2(d). Thus, for example, it is doubtful that protection was reestablished while reliance continued to be placed on Bosnian wartime property legislation which effectively precluded the return by refugees to their pre-1992 homes: "Two Years after Dayton: A View from Bosnia's Ombudsperson," (1988) 22 *Forced Migration Monitor* 1.

[52] "In some cases, persons who are not in need of international protection can, nonetheless, not be returned to their country. Return may be impossible even for those who did not leave for refugee-related reasons. Countries of origin may refuse to readmit nationals who do not volunteer to return, or who do not apply for travel documents; in some cases, the authorities may deny that the individual is their national, a dispute which may be difficult to resolve": UNHCR, "Return of Persons Not in Need of International Protection," UN Doc. EC/46/SC/CRP.36, May 28, 1996, at para. 7. In the context of Bosnia, the International High Representative reported that the rate of refugee return was dramatically slowed by both legal and bureaucratic impediments. "Closing loopholes in property legislation and firing foot-dragging officials (I removed 22 in one day alone) boosted the rate of minority returns": W. Petritsch, "In Bosnia, an 'entry strategy,'" *Washington Post*, July 2, 2002, at A-15.

[53] After many rounds of talks, only about 2.5 percent of the population seeking repatriation has been recognized by Bhutan as having its citizenship, and hence entitled to return: Human Rights Watch, "Nepal: Bhutanese refugees rendered stateless, leading global NGOs criticize screening process," June 18, 2003. As the Jesuit Refugee Service explained, "[m]ore than 70% [of the refugees] were classed as Category 2 or voluntary migrants, who would have to re-apply for citizenship if they wished to return; and this would involve a two-year probation period, following which their chances of being accepted as Bhutanese citizens are unclear": (2003) 135 *JRS Dispatches* (July 1, 2003).

[54] UNHCR indirectly recognizes the legality of enforced repatriation by observing that valid cessation of refugee status under Art. 1(C)(5)–(6) involves "loss of refugee status and the rights that accompany that status, and it may contemplate the return of persons to their countries of origin": UNHCR, "Ceased Circumstances Guidelines," at para. 25.

[55] "The promotion of involuntary repatriation if and when refugee protection ceases to be necessary is a pragmatic approach that represents an acceptable compromise between legitimate State concerns and the protection needs of refugees": Barutciski, "Involuntary Repatriation," at 254.

refugee status is a transitory status which survives only for the duration of risk, the right of states to require persons no longer in need of protection to return home needs explicitly to be acknowledged.[56] Not only is the failure to do so intellectually dishonest but, as elaborated below, it can have negative protection consequences for persons who remain refugees, as well as for former refugees subject to removal to their country of origin.

The rules which govern mandated repatriation are in fact fairly simple. Once the criteria for valid cessation of refugee status under Art. 1(C)(5)–(6) are satisfied, state parties are entitled to enforce the departure from their territory of any person who previously benefited from Convention refugee status. The only qualification on this right is the duty of the state to meet other requirements of international human rights law. In particular, account must be taken of the former refugee's rights to security of person; to be free from cruel, inhuman, or degrading treatment; and not to be subjected to arbitrary or unlawful interference with his or her family life.[57]

In contrast, however, UNHCR routinely insists that repatriation is lawful only if it is "voluntary,"[58] and if it can be accomplished "in safety, and with dignity."[59] This approach likely reflects a failure to distinguish between the right of states to undertake repatriation under the terms of the Convention (which is constrained principally by considerations of risk and the availability of protection, but not of voluntariness) and the institutional mandate of the UNHCR. In contrast to the Convention, UNHCR as an agency is expressly authorized to take part only in repatriation efforts which are "voluntary."[60] Because its mandate does not clearly distinguish between different kinds of

---

[56] This approach is readily reconcilable to respect for all rights set by the Refugee Convention: see J. Hathaway and A. Neve, "Making International Refugee Law Relevant Again: A Proposal for Collectivized and Solution-Oriented Protection," (1997) 10 *Harvard Human Rights Journal* 115.

[57] The implications of these duties are elaborated below, at pp. 944–952.

[58] See e.g. Lawyers' Committee for Human Rights, "General Principles Relating to the Promotion of Refugee Repatriation" (1992), at Principle 3, which erroneously insists that "[r]efugee repatriations must be voluntary." Rather than insisting on voluntariness as a legal requirement, the more defensible position is to refer to its logic as a barometer of protection. Amnesty International, for example, has sensibly suggested that a focus on voluntariness "helps ensure that refugees' rights and dignity are respected. It increases the likelihood that the returning population will be able to successfully reintegrate and rebuild. Voluntariness also recognizes that it is refugees themselves who are generally the best judges of whether conditions have become sufficiently safe in the country of origin. In that respect it plays an important protection role": Amnesty International, "Great Lakes Region: Still in Need of Protection: Repatriation, *Refoulement* and the Safety of Refugees and the Internally Displaced," Doc. No. AFR/02/07/97 (1997) (Amnesty, "Great Lakes Report"), at 4.

[59] UNHCR, "Voluntary Repatriation Handbook," at 11. See text below, at pp. 944–945.

[60] "The High Commissioner shall provide for the protection of refugees falling under the competence of his Office by ... [a]ssisting governmental and private efforts to promote

repatriation – namely, those of persons who remain refugees, and those who have ceased to be refugees – UNHCR has opted to err on the side of caution, adopting the view that it will only become involved with repatriation (of any population) if there is consent by the persons to be repatriated.[61]

Because the overwhelming majority of repatriations of former refugees have to date involved returns from one less developed country to another,[62] this institutional position – setting voluntariness as the core criterion for UNHCR involvement in the return of any population, including both refugees and persons whose refugee status has ceased – has eclipsed the development of a clear understanding of the rules of repatriation rooted in the principles of the Refugee Convention. Lacking the resources to effectuate repatriation on their own, poorer countries have generally turned to UNHCR to underwrite and/or conduct the repatriation effort.[63] When it chooses to participate, UNHCR understandably takes the view that it must operate in

voluntary repatriation": UNHCR Statute, at Art. 8(c). Beyond this authority, UNHCR may engage in other repatriation activities only with the authorization of the General Assembly of the United Nations: UNHCR Statute, at Art. 9. The Executive Committee of UNHCR has recently gone beyond this constraint in a modest way, calling upon the agency to "tak[e] clear public positions on the acceptability of return of persons found not to be in need of international protection": UNHCR Executive Committee Conclusion No. 96, "Conclusion on the Return of Persons Found Not to be in Need of International Protection" (2003), at para. (j)(ii), available at www.unhcr.ch (accessed Nov. 20, 2004). The reference to persons not in need of international protection refers, however, only to persons not initially entitled to recognition of Convention refugee status.

[61] See UNHCR, "Voluntary Repatriation Handbook," at 5–8. While this is undoubtedly a very cautious reading of its authority, UNHCR's disinclination to become involved in mandatory repatriation may well be critical to its ability to secure and maintain the trust of refugees, and more generally to avoid any possible conflict of interest with its overarching responsibility to champion the protection of refugees. Art. 8(c) of its Statute clearly does not prohibit participation by UNHCR in the mandated repatriation of persons who are no longer refugees, since these persons presumptively cease to be persons under the competence of UNHCR: UNHCR Statute, at Art. 6. But neither is the agency expressly authorized to lend its assistance to mandated repatriation efforts absent authorization from the General Assembly under Art. 9.

[62] For example, in 2002 more than 2,250,000 Afghans returned home from Pakistan and Iran. Other large-scale returns in that year included those of more than 80,000 Angolans from Zambia and the Democratic Republic of Congo; more than 50,000 Burundians returning from Tanzania; over 75,000 Sierra Leoneans from Guinea and Liberia; and more than 30,000 East Timorese from Indonesia. In the same year, the only developed country to achieve five-figure return statistics was Bosnia Herzegovina, which effected nearly 17,000 returns to Serbia and Montenegro: UNHCR, "2002 UNHCR Population Statistics," Aug. 4, 2003, at Table 10.

[63] In 2002, for example, the governments of Burundi and Tanzania announced that they would "send a delegation to UNHCR headquarters in Geneva to petition for allowing repatriation to all areas in Burundi ... [A UNHCR spokesperson] said that at a recent tripartite meeting, a request had been made to the UN for funding to allow both governments to conduct the repatriations themselves": UN Integrated Regional Information Networks, July 8, 2002.

line with what it reads as its statutory mandate to effect only *voluntary* repatriation. As such, fiscal reality in much of the South has meant that the dominant standard for repatriation is not truly Convention-based at all, but is rather structured to meet the requirements of UNHCR's institutional mandate to undertake only "voluntary repatriation."[64]

It might be thought that the resultant absence of a Convention-based understanding of the norms governing repatriation would be of little more than academic interest. If anything, reliance on the voluntary repatriation standard might be thought to compel the host country to recognize a continuing duty to protect a person whose refugee status had ceased, but who refused to be repatriated. While arguably unfair to state parties, insistence on compliance with UNHCR's institutional precondition to repatriation would at least have the virtue of erring on the side of protection. But in practice, this is not necessarily so.

Most fundamentally, state practice in the less developed world is not simply to inject a voluntarism requirement into the inquiry under Art. 1(C)(5)–(6) regarding whether refugee status can lawfully be withdrawn due to a fundamental change of circumstances in the country of origin. Instead, the pattern is for governments in most of the less developed world to take UNHCR involvement in a given repatriation effort as a sufficient *imprimatur* for the termination of their own duty to protect the refugees in question, without any real attention being paid to the criteria for cessation of status. This practice can result in the de facto premature termination of refugee status.[65] This confusion occurs because UNHCR as an agency

---

[64] As Zieck has observed, "[i]n comparison to the time when 'voluntary repatriation' functioned predominantly in the form of the possibility to refuse repatriation, as an eligibility criterion in order to protect those who were considered to have valid reasons against returning, 'voluntary repatriation' now functions as a mode of cessation of refugee status": M. Zieck, *UNHCR and Voluntary Repatriation of Refugees: A Legal Analysis* (1997) (Zieck, *Voluntary Repatriation*), at 430. The historical reasons for undue attention being paid to UNHCR's approach to repatriation, in contrast to the development of an authentic understanding of repatriation based upon the terms of the Refugee Convention itself, are set out in Hathaway, "Repatriation."

[65] "UNHCR has organized itself to facilitate repatriation ... As evidenced by its healthy and thoroughgoing debate over how far it could venture toward repatriation without violating refugee rights, UNHCR was no mere plaything in the hands of states, but rather had the capacity for reasoned reflection and exhibited some relative autonomy ... But soon there developed a repatriation culture that left refugees at greater risk ... [A] repatriation culture means that UNHCR is oriented around concepts, symbols, and discourse that elevates the desirability of repatriation, coats it in ethical luster, and makes it more likely that repatriation will occur under more permissive conditions": M. Barnett, "UNHCR and Involuntary Repatriation: Environmental Developments, the Repatriation Culture, and the Rohingya Refugees," paper presented at the 41st Annual Convention of the International Studies Association, Los Angeles, Mar. 14–18, 2000, available at www.ciaonet.org/isa (accessed Nov. 22, 2003).

frequently becomes involved with repatriation before the requirements of the Convention's change of circumstances cessation clause are met.[66] Indeed, its Executive Committee has instructed UNHCR that "[f]rom the outset of a refugee situation, the High Commissioner should at all times keep the possibility of voluntary repatriation for all or part of a group under active review and the High Commissioner, whenever he deems that the prevailing circumstances are appropriate, should actively pursue the promotion of this solution."[67] In reliance on this instruction, UNHCR has adopted a spectrum of institutional positions on repatriation, which explicitly includes the facilitation of return "even where UNHCR does not consider that, objectively, it is safe for most refugees to return":[68]

> While the condition of fundamental change of circumstances in the country of origin will usually not be met in such situations, UNHCR may consider facilitating return in order to have a positive impact on the safety of refugees/returnees as well as to render assistance which the refugees may require in order to return. Such assistance may have to be given in the absence of formal guarantees or assurances by the country of origin for the safety of repatriating refugees, and without any agreement or understanding having been concluded as to the basic terms and conditions of return.[69]

Critically, this *institutional* preparedness to facilitate repatriation before cessation due to change of circumstances is established is explicitly predicated on ascertainment that the refugees themselves understand the risks of going home, but are nonetheless determined to do so. Because no UNHCR

---

[66] For example, UNHCR justified its facilitation of repatriation to northern Burundi in 2002 on the grounds that the region (though not the country as a whole) was "deemed relatively secure": "Dwindling numbers of refugees opting for repatriation," *UN Integrated Regional Information Networks*, July 8, 2002. The agency launched a repatriation exercise for refugees in Zambia "because the peace process[es] in war-torn neighbouring countries are progressing well": "UNHCR to begin repatriation of refugees in Zambia," *Zambezi Times*, Sept. 17, 2002, quoting UNHCR Country Representative Ahmed Gubartala.

[67] UNHCR Executive Committee Conclusion No. 40, "Voluntary Repatriation" (1985), at para. (e), available at www.unhcr.ch (accessed Nov. 20, 2004). See also UNHCR Executive Committee Conclusion No. 101, "Conclusion on Legal Safety Issues in the Context of Voluntary Repatriation of Refugees" (2004), at para. (e), available at www.unhcr.ch (accessed Nov. 20, 2004), in which it is "[r]eaffirm[ed] that voluntary repatriation should not necessarily be conditioned on the accomplishment of political solutions in the country of origin in order not to impede the exercise of the refugees' right to return."

[68] UNHCR, "Voluntary Repatriation Handbook," at 15.

[69] Ibid. Indeed, the Executive Committee has "[e]mphasiz[ed] that some legal or administrative issues may only be addressed over time; and recogniz[ed] that voluntary repatriation can and does take place without all of the legal and administrative issues . . . having first been resolved": UNHCR Executive Committee Conclusion No. 101, "Conclusion on Legal Safety Issues in the Context of Voluntary Repatriation of Refugees" (2004), at Preamble, available at www.unhcr.ch (accessed Nov. 20, 2004).

repatriation can lawfully occur absent the refugee's free and informed consent, it cannot sensibly be suggested that UNHCR's facilitation of what is arguably premature repatriation is rights-violative. Indeed, particularly where it is clear that refugees will in any event go home, UNHCR assistance may well be key to avoiding unnecessary risks to their safety or security.[70] But governments accustomed to taking their cue on repatriation from UNHCR – or, less charitably, anxious to exploit an opportunity for rationalization provided by UNHCR – have invoked the agency's participation in the repatriation of a given refugee population to justify their own less-than-truly-voluntary repatriation initiatives.

In an extreme case, the Tanzanian government announced in early December 1996 that "all Rwandese refugees in Tanzania are expected to return home by 31 December 1996."[71] This announcement, "endorsed and co-signed by the UNHCR,"[72] resulted in the return of more than 500,000 refugees within the month.[73] Yet the criteria for cessation under Art. 1(C)(5)–(6) could not possibly have been met in the circumstances: fair trials were only beginning in Rwanda, disappearances and deliberate killings were continuing there, and there was no reason to believe that Rwanda could meet

[70] "For UNHCR, charged with protecting refugees and finding durable solutions for their problems, the standard criteria for return are 'voluntary repatriation in safety and dignity,' preferably in an organized fashion and with the co-operation of the governments of both the host country and the country of origin. But refugees often decide to return independently, according to their own pace and criteria. UNHCR is then left with the choice of refusing to assist in the process, which would undermine the refugees' autonomy and jeopardize their chances of successful return, or of facilitating it despite reservations. In practice, the only forms of repatriation that UNHCR refuses to assist are those that are enforced": UNHCR, *The State of the World's Refugees 1993* (1993), 104–106.

[71] Amnesty, "Great Lakes Report", at 2.

[72] "On December 5, 1996 . . . UNHCR distributed information sheets to refugees about the repatriation exercise, including the immediate suspension of economic and agricultural activities in the camps . . . During the repatriation exercise, UNHCR provided both financial and logistical assistance to the Tanzanian government": B. Whitaker, "Changing Priorities in Refugee Protection: The Rwandan Repatriation from Tanzania," UNHCR New Issues in Refugee Research Working Paper No. 53, Feb. 2002, at 1–2. UNHCR pronounced itself satisfied that the returns were in fact voluntary despite solid evidence to the contrary. See Amnesty, "Great Lakes Report," at 2; US Committee for Refugees, *World Refugee Survey 1997* (1997), at 99–100.

[73] "Initially tens of thousands of refugees fled the [Tanzanian] camps and attempted to move further into Tanzania, in the hope of reaching neighbouring countries. The Tanzanian security forces intercepted the fleeing refugees and 'redirected' them towards the Rwandese border . . . Reports now indicate that some refugees who refuse to go back are being arrested and held in a detention camp . . . Other refugees who wished to remain were undoubtedly forced back in the rush": Amnesty, "Great Lakes Report," at 2. Importantly, it was only *after* the returns occurred that UNHCR "expressed hope that Tanzania [would] institute a screening procedure to evaluate the claims of individuals too fearful to return": ibid.

the basic needs of the returning refugees.[74] Again, in 2002, UNHCR announced that it had received "assurances [from] the Tanzanian and Rwandan governments that security in Rwanda *had improved* [emphasis added],"[75] and sanctioned the *voluntary* repatriation of the remaining 20,000 Rwandan refugees living in Tanzania.[76] Yet even the spokesperson for a partner agency participating in the ensuing "voluntary" repatriation conceded that the repatriation actually conducted by Tanzania relied upon an "impetus" in the form of "verbal pressure"[77] – in particular, a firm year-end deadline for the refugees' departure.[78] In at least some instances, officials implementing the program used brute force to compel even long-term Rwandan residents to leave the country.[79]

---

[74] Ibid. at 5–6.

[75] It is noteworthy that at this time, the training of judges who would preside over the trial of persons accused of all but the highest category of genocide crimes had only been commenced. It was therefore not surprising that Rwandan refugees continued to express grave reservations about the practical efficacy of commitments to protect them from retaliation: "Focus on Rwanda refugees in Tanzania," *UN Integrated Regional Information Networks*, May 9, 2002.

[76] "Rwandan refugees to be out by December 31," *East African*, Oct. 14, 2002.

[77] "Thousands more refugees seek repatriation," *UN Integrated Regional Information Networks*, Jan. 9, 2002, quoting Mark Wigley, deputy director of Norwegian People's Aid. In the context of a subsequent effort by Tanzania to repatriate refugees to Burundi, a consortium of US-based non-governmental organizations called upon the Tanzanian government to "cease placing political and psychological pressure" on the refugees to return: "NGOs concerned over voluntary repatriation of refugees," *UN Integrated Regional Information Networks*, May 15, 2002.

[78] "In late September 2002, UNHCR and the governments of Tanzania and Rwanda convened a tripartite meeting in Geneva ... to discuss durable solutions for refugees living in Tanzania. The officials ... found that, *inter alia*, '[p]ressure exerted by the governments of Tanzania and Rwanda on Rwandan refugees living in Tanzania and on UNHCR officials in Tanzania and Rwanda played a significant role in unnecessarily hurrying the voluntary repatriation program'": J. Frushone, "Repatriation of Rwandan Refugees Living in Tanzania," US Committee for Refugees, Jan. 10, 2003. Indeed, "[n]ewspapers in Eastern Africa have reported that Tanzania will forcibly send 2,000 Rwandan refugees living in the camps in western Tanzania back to Rwanda. The 2,000 are those who refused to return home during the recent voluntary repatriation, citing insecurity in their home country as the reason for remaining ... The feeling in the Tanzanian government is that there is no need for the refugees to remain because the security situation in Rwanda is now stable. Earlier this month, Tanzania's Home Affairs Minister, Mr. Omar Ramadhan Mapuri, warned that Tanzania might be forced to repatriate all the refugees living in the country if the international community does not intervene in the serious food crisis facing the refugees": (2003) 127 *JRS Dispatches* (Feb. 28, 2003).

[79] "The President of the National Repatriation Commission ... [said] that the move by the Tanzanian government had caught more than the evictees by surprise. 'We had not anticipated this. We asked them to stop the process for some time so that we can talk with them and work out the modalities of how it should be done' ... [Tanzanian ambassador to Rwanda] Mwakalindile admits that the forced repatriation may not have

In short, because of the failure clearly to articulate the standards which govern mandated repatriation – indeed, because of what amounts to a conflation of the rules for what are substantively distinct frameworks for return under the singular rubric of "voluntary repatriation"[80] – it is too easy for governments simplistically to invoke UNHCR repatriation activities as authorization for repatriation in general, thereby avoiding the more exacting requirements for cessation of status which in fact bind them.[81]

Second, even host states not seeking to avoid their protection obligations may be misled by the failure clearly to distinguish between UNHCR's institutional policies on repatriation and the repatriation authority of state parties. In particular, the existence of a large-scale UNHCR-authorized repatriation effort can be taken to suggest the propriety of repatriation as a general policy, equally open to state parties.[82] Despite the formal requirements of the Refugee Convention for cessation of refugee status, there is in practice a

been handled appropriately": "Forced to go home: Rwandan immigrants in Tanzania," *Internews*, Apr. 15, 2003. "The last convoy [of Rwandan refugees] to depart Tanzania carried refugees who alleged that Tanzanian authorities threatened to burn down their homes if they refused to leave the country. UNHCR insisted, however, that 'those repatriated were refugees who had voluntarily signed up . . . to return home'": US Committee for Refugees, *World Refugee Survey 2003* (2003), at 100.

[80] The confusion on this point is reinforced by UNHCR itself. For example, in its discussion of repatriation consequent to the application of Art. 1(C)(5)–(6), the agency notes that the "Convention does not address the question of *voluntary* repatriation of refugees directly [emphasis added]": UNHCR, "Voluntary Repatriation Handbook," at 8–10. Not only is there no explicit recognition of the right of states to enforce involuntary repatriation when the criteria of Art. 1(C)(5)–(6) are met, but the Handbook obfuscates by making the (technically accurate) general assertion that "[t]he principle of voluntariness is the cornerstone of international protection with respect to the return of refugees" (ibid. at 10) without simultaneously acknowledging its non-applicability to persons who have ceased to be refugees. Despite a recent and more candid approach to the issue of cessation itself (see UNHCR, "Ceased Circumstances Guidelines," at para. 7), no comparable frankness on the consequential right of mandated repatriation has been forthcoming.

[81] Even as UNHCR has acknowledged the difference between its own standards for voluntary repatriation and the right of states to invoke the cessation clauses, its own language contributes to confusion on this point. See e.g. UNHCR, "Ceased Circumstances Guidelines," at para. 29: "Voluntary repatriation can take place at a lower threshold of change in the country of origin, occurring as it does at the express wish of the refugee, who may also have personal reasons for repatriating, regardless of the situation prevailing in the country of origin. Therefore, the facilitation or promotion of voluntary repatriation by UNHCR does not necessarily mean that the cessation clause should be applied. However, where large-scale voluntary repatriation is organized against a backdrop of fundamental changes and providing that such fundamental changes stabilize and can eventually be considered as durable, the cessation clause may be invoked at an appropriate later time."

[82] The point is not that UNHCR intends to provide comfort to states anxious to avoid the strictures of Art. 1(C)(5)–(6); to the contrary, as discussed above, at pp. 922–928, its formal positions clearly adumbrate strict requirements for cessation. But because these requirements are not linked to the right of states to effect mandated repatriation, the opportunity for confusion and obfuscation arises.

common assumption that state parties should look to UNHCR's positions to determine when refugee status may legitimately be ended. For example, the Zambian Home Affairs Permanent Secretary was quoted as having said that his country was "not in a hurry to repatriate the more than 5,000 Rwandan refugees currently in the country until the United Nations signs a cessation clause *to strip them of their status* ... He said the repatriation procedures and endorsement were done by the international community and the host nation *only gave a helping hand* to the UNHCR [emphasis added]."[83]

The difficulty with deference of this kind is that UNHCR as an agency will on occasion be under pressure to proceed quickly to repatriate refugees – albeit on a voluntary basis – particularly where there is a perceived need to be supportive of more broadly based political and social transitions. For example, Mafwe refugees from Namibia anxious for their security by reason of their pro-secessionist activities were assured by UNHCR that they should accept repatriation because the situation in Namibia was "calm," and the Namibian government deserved "a pat on the back."[84] Similarly, UNHCR launched a regional initiative in 2003 to promote the voluntary repatriation of some 500,000 Angolan refugees from Zambia, Namibia, and the Democratic Republic of Congo. The exercise – referred to as "organized voluntary repatriation"[85] – was predicated on the existence of "current peace"[86] in a country just emerging from more than a quarter of a century of civil war, and UNHCR's view that "acceptable conditions"[87] prevailed there. While promoted as integral to the success of a national reconstruction

---

[83] "Repatriation of Rwandan refugees voluntary," *Times of Zambia*, Mar. 3, 2003.

[84] "Scared refugees reluctant to return home," *African Church Information Service*, Mar. 24, 2003, quoting Cosmos Chanda, UNHCR representative to Botswana.

[85] "Authorities sign repatriation accords with Zambia and Namibia," *Angola Press Agency*, Nov. 28, 2002.

[86] "Angolan refugees leave for home in May," *Times of Zambia*, Mar. 5–13, 2003, quoting Zambian Home Affairs Permanent Secretary Peter Mumba. Not even UNHCR appears to have believed that a definitive peace had been established when the promotion of repatriation was agreed to. UNHCR spokesperson Lucia Teoli observed that "[p]revious attempts to bring people back home failed because of the ongoing war, but since the cease-fire in April, most people and leaders believe that peace is irreversible in the country. *The UNHCR is optimistic about this attempt* [emphasis added]": "First wave of Angolan refugees to go home next year," *UN Integrated Regional Information Networks*, Nov. 28, 2002.

[87] "UNHCR prepares to start repatriating Angolans," *Namibian*, Apr. 23, 2003, quoting an interview with UNHCR Senior Protection Officer Magda Medina and Public Information Officer David Nthengwe. "The regional coordinator for the Angolan Refugees Repatriation Operations, Kallu Kalumiya, who is based in Geneva ... said despite progress made so far, there was still insecurity in Angola and also millions of land mines were laid during Angola's long civil war": "Angolan refugees to head home," *Namibian Economist*, Dec. 6, 2002.

program for Angola,[88] some refugees were deeply opposed to the initiative, particularly in view of the disastrous attempt to promote their repatriation based upon another cease-fire in 1994.[89] Clearly, no sound case could be made that conditions in either Namibia or Angola were such as to allow state parties validly to deem their refugee status to have come to an end. Yet this point was not made to governments, which enthusiastically embraced repatriation as the right response in the circumstances.

Even less happily, UNHCR's determination to end its mandate in relation to particular refugee groups, and to promote their repatriation, may at times reflect no more than the need to reduce long-term-care expenditures in an era of shrinking budgets, financial insecurity, and increased political pressure from states.[90] Indeed, the Angolan repatriation was reported to have been driven in part by concerns "to ease logistical pressure on both the [host] government[s] and UNHCR, which have had to look after a rapidly expanding refugee population in a time of dwindling resources."[91] More clearly still, UNHCR's decision to end assistance to, and step up the "voluntary" repatriation of, Muslim Rohingya refugees to Burma – despite the continued reality of grave and systematic discrimination, including the denial to them of citizenship – really cannot be explained on protection grounds.[92] Particularly

[88] "UNHCR addresses returnee concerns," *UN Integrated Regional Information Networks*, Mar. 14, 2003, quoting UNHCR regional spokesperson Fidelis Swai.

[89] "Most refugees from the former Portuguese colony are reluctant to go back to the land of their forefathers unless they are assured of a durable cease-fire between Unita and the MPLA government. Even the news that former Unita leader Jonas Savimbi is dead and buried, and [that] the country is on a reconstruction course, is not good enough to convince them. But you would not blame them entirely for dragging their feet over their return to their homeland. Their fears may be well-founded ... [Some] are jittery [because] someone told them in 1994, shortly after the Lusaka Peace Protocol was signed between Unita and the MPLA government, that there was peace in Angola and they, therefore, could return to their country. They are fearful because most of those, if not all, who returned received a rude shock when they were greeted with barrels of guns": "Angolan refugees reluctant to return home," *Times of Zambia*, Mar. 18–26, 2003.

[90] As Amnesty International noted in a stinging critique of UNHCR's decision to assist Tanzania's December 1996 enforced repatriation of Rwandans, "[t]hat [protection] oversights were possible, were legitimized by UNHCR, and were so readily accepted by the international community speaks volumes. Does the world remain committed to protecting refugees, or do we now emphasize return, for political and financial reasons, over safety?": Amnesty, "Great Lakes Report," at 3.

[91] "40,000 refugees return home from Zambia," *Zambezi Times*, Apr. 16, 2003.

[92] "While conditions for Rohingya inside Burma have hardly changed in the last decade, what appears to have changed is UNHCR's policy towards Rohingya concerning rights to UNHCR protection and support. By stepping up repatriation efforts and reducing assistance to refugees ... UNHCR has created an environment in which protection for the Rohingya is virtually untenable": Refugees International, "Lack of Protection Plagues Burma's Rohingya Refugees in Bangladesh," May 30, 2003. "The aid group Doctors Without Borders (MSF) has accused Bangladesh's government of harassing thousands

when the language of enthusiasm for return is embraced by UNHCR – for example, its decision in early 2003 to "change its policy from merely facilitating to *actively promoting* repatriation to Rwanda ... [under a plan] *harmonised and implemented across Africa* [emphasis added]"[93] – a signal is sent to governments that repatriation is really the appropriate course of action for states themselves to pursue.

In sum, the importation of UNHCR's more fungible voluntary repatriation standard into what should be decisions about repatriation consequent to a change of circumstances in countries of origin has in many cases proved a less than sanguine development. While the reliance on voluntarism – whether or not there has been a fundamental change of circumstances in the country of origin – may well be appropriate as a standard for agency involvement in repatriation, a clear line needs to be drawn between the standard governing UNHCR institutional efforts and that which sets the contours for repatriation conducted by state parties. Whether expressly or by tacit implication, the institutional standard has in practice been relied upon to justify the premature repatriation of refugees by state parties without full benefit of the safeguards upon which UNHCR insists for the conduct of its own repatriation work.

In fairness to host governments, it must be said that UNHCR has recently taken positions which suggest that governments *should be* guided by its institutional decisions about when to pursue repatriation. Indeed, such deference is now said by UNHCR to be part of the "responsibilities of the host country."[94] Against the backdrop of such pronouncements, even host governments firmly committed to protection may on occasion feel under pressure to acquiesce in the agency's repatriation plans. For example, Zambia raised concerns about the risks of land mines for Angolan refugees slated for repatriation by UNHCR, but was reportedly lobbied by UNHCR to acquiesce

---

of Muslim refugees from Myanmar in an attempt to force them to return home. 'In recent months, staff from MSF received over 550 complaints of coercion from the refugees,' MSF said in a statement, adding that complaints ranged from 'incidents of intimidation to outright threats of physical abuse to push people to repatriate.' The aid agency also called into question the voluntary nature of the repatriation of the remaining 19,000 refugees from Myanmar's Rohingya minority, which is being supervised by the UN refugee agency": "Bangladesh forcing out Myanmar refugees: MSF," *Agence France Presse*, Sept. 18, 2003.

[93] "5,000 refugees to be repatriated from Zambia," *UN Integrated Regional Information Networks*, Jan. 20, 2003, quoting UNHCR's Regional Coordinator for the Great Lakes Region, Wairimu Karago. This policy shift was apparently justified on the basis of a belief that the Rwandan justice system was positioned to deal with genocide allegations more quickly and fairly: ibid.

[94] UNHCR, "Voluntary Repatriation Handbook," at 12. Specifically, UNHCR asserts that "[t]he country of asylum should respect the leading role of UNHCR in promoting, facilitating and coordinating voluntary repatriation": ibid.

in the return. The agency sought to reassure Zambia that even though many areas were "heavily mined ... '[w]ith the funding UNHCR has received, we will be expanding our presence in those areas of resettlement to ensure that people are *reminded of the threat* of land mines. So the problem *is addressed* [emphasis added].'"[95]

The blurring of the line between the circumstances under which UNHCR may legitimately promote the genuinely voluntary return of refugees and the conditions which justify the withdrawal of protection by a state party is most intense when UNHCR opts not simply to withdraw its assistance from a group of refugees, or even to encourage their repatriation, but instead to issue what it refers to as a "formal declaration of general cessation."[96] The legal relevance of such declarations is understandably ambiguous to states and others. Subject to the views of the Economic and Social Council, UNHCR may apply the changed circumstances cessation clause to refugees in receipt of its institutional protection or assistance.[97] On the other hand, states – and only states – are entrusted with the responsibility conscientiously to apply the cessation clause to refugees in receipt of their protection.[98] Despite this clear

---

[95] "UNHCR addresses returnee concerns," *UN Integrated Regional Information Networks*, Mar. 14, 2003, quoting UNHCR regional spokesperson Fidelis Swai; see also "Zambia: Plans for return of refugees finalised," *Africa News*, Mar. 17, 2003, confirming UNHCR's efforts to downplay Zambian concerns regarding the safety and security of conditions for return in Angola. In fact, even after UNHCR had announced that the road linking Maheba refugee settlement in Zambia with Cazombo in Angola was free of mines, "the return of more than 400 Angolan refugees ... was postponed due to the discovery of a mine on June 10, two days before the beginning of the planned repatriation": "Angola: Preparations for the Beginning of the Organised Repatriation of Refugees," (2003) 135 *JRS Dispatches* (July 1, 2003).

[96] UNHCR, "Ceased Circumstances Guidelines," at n. 3. Historical examples include "Applicability of the Cessation Clauses to Refugees from Poland, Czechoslovakia and Hungary," Nov. 15, 1991, "Applicability of Cessation Clauses to Refugees from Chile," Mar. 28, 1994, "Applicability of the Cessation Clauses to Refugees from the Republics of Malawi and Mozambique," Dec. 31, 1996, "Applicability of the Cessation Clauses to Refugees from Bulgaria and Romania," Oct. 1, 1997, "Applicability of the Ceased Circumstances Cessation Clauses to pre-1991 Refugees from Ethiopia," Sept. 23, 1999, and "Declaration of Cessation – Timor Leste," Dec. 20, 2002: ibid.

[97] But despite prevailing practice, the UNHCR's Statute does not actually foresee the possibility of an *en bloc* withdrawal of protection by the agency from an entire group of refugees, at least where the refugees concerned fall within its core competence. To the contrary, it is provided simply that "[t]he competence of the High Commissioner shall cease to apply to *any person* [emphasis added]" who falls within one of six cessation clauses, all expressly framed in individuated terms: UNHCR Statute, at Art. 6(A)(ii).

[98] In the same year during which they debated the issue of legal standards for repatriation, the states that make up UNHCR's Executive Committee affirmed that "refugee protection is primarily the responsibility of States, and ... UNHCR's mandated role in this regard cannot substitute for effective action, political will, and full cooperation on the part of States": UNHCR Executive Committee Conclusion No. 81, "General Conclusion on

delineation of responsibilities, the agency has recently sought to give more weight to its own institutional positions on cessation:

> The Executive Committee Conclusion 69 affirms that any declarations by UNHCR that its competence ceases to apply in relation to certain refugees may be useful to States in connection with the application of the cessation clauses. Where UNHCR has made a declaration of cessation of its competence in relation to any specified group of refugees, States may resort to the cessation clauses for a similar group of refugees if they deem it appropriate and useful for resolving the situation of these refugees in their territory.[99]

This ambition effectively to determine the issue of cessation for state parties is most clearly seen in the way in which UNHCR speaks about changes to the application of its institutional mandate. For example, the High Commissioner for Refugees is reported to have stated during a visit to Africa that "Rwanda is safe for refugees in Tanzania and Uganda ... 'In Tanzania, we informed the refugees that they could return to Rwanda. Some have returned, but many remain,' he said ... Such people, he said, were 'not refugees anymore* [emphasis added].'"[100] A similar elision of institutional and Convention-based determinations can be seen even in UNHCR's more formal statements. For example, a press release of May 8, 2002 was headed, "UNHCR Declares Cessation of Refugee Status for Eritreans," and stated:

> UNHCR announced ... that it is ending refugee status for all Eritreans who fled their country as a result of the war of independence or the recent border conflict between Ethiopia and Eritrea. The world-wide cessation will take effect on December 31 and will affect hundreds of thousands of Eritreans in neighbouring countries.[101]

Only near the end of the statement is the true scope of the declaration made clear, though still in language which suggests the logic of its more general applicability, and followed immediately by a reference to the process of cessation under the Refugee Convention:

International Protection" (1997), at para. (d), available at www.unhcr.ch (accessed Nov. 20, 2004).

[99] UNHCR, "Cessation," at para. 33. The same document candidly recognized, however, that "[t]he decision to apply the 'ceased circumstances' cessation clause lies with the State of asylum concerned": ibid. at para. 36. Its most recent statement on the issue, however, fails even to note that cessation decisions are, in fact, the duty of state parties to adjudicate: UNHCR, "Ceased Circumstances Guidelines."

[100] "Rwanda is safe for returning refugees, says UNHCR head," *UN Integrated Regional Information Networks*, Apr. 16, 2003.

[101] UNHCR, "UNHCR declares cessation of refugee status for Eritreans," Press Release, May 8, 2002, available at www.unhcr.ch (accessed July 14, 2003).

"I believe that these two groups of refugees from Eritrea should no longer have a fear of persecution or other reasons to continue to be regarded as refugees," said Ruud Lubbers, UN High Commissioner for Refugees. "They will, therefore, cease to be regarded as refugees by my Office with effect from the end of this year."[102]

The critical point, however, is that there is no legal basis for state parties simply to defer to UNHCR's views on cessation as an alternative to domestic adjudication of the issue.

Perhaps ironically, reliance on UNHCR views regarding cessation of refugee status may also result in continued protection for persons no longer entitled to refugee status under the Convention. This dissonance follows from the fact that the cessation criteria which govern the work of UNHCR as an agency are very similar to, but not identical with, those which apply to the actions of state parties to the Refugee Convention. UNHCR enjoys a broader authority to retain under its competence persons who no longer face the risk of being persecuted so long as their reasons for refusing to accept the renewed protection of their own country are not simply rooted in economic or other considerations of personal convenience.[103] Under the Refugee Convention, in contrast, cessation of status is to follow once the changed circumstances test is met.[104] By virtue of an explicit compromise between the majority of drafters who favored a purely objective test of risk for refugee status and the minority who wished to allow refugees to retain their status based upon purely emotional or psychological reasons,[105] pre-1951 refugees were granted the right to invoke a proviso regarding "compelling reasons arising out of previous persecution" to retain their refugee status even after a relevant change of circumstances.[106] But for the future, refugee status was

---

[102] Ibid. The immediate next paragraph reads, "Both the 1951 Refugee Convention and the 1969 OAU Convention, which is applied in Africa, stipulate that the convention shall cease to apply to any refugee '... if he can no longer, because the circumstances in connection with which he was recognised as a refugee have ceased to exist, continue to refuse to avail himself of the protection of the country of his nationality'": ibid.

[103] "The competence of the High Commissioner shall cease to apply to any person ... if ... [h]e can no longer, because the circumstances in connection with which he has been recognized as a refugee have ceased to exist, *claim grounds other than personal convenience* for continuing to refuse to avail himself of the protection of the country of his nationality. *Reasons of a purely economic nature may not be invoked* [emphasis added]": UNHCR Statute, at Art. 6(f).

[104] "This Convention shall cease to apply to any person ... if ... [h]e can no longer, because the circumstances in connection with which he has been recognized as a refugee have ceased to exist, continue to refuse to avail himself of the protection of the country of his nationality": Refugee Convention, at Art. 1(C)(5).

[105] Hathaway, *Refugee Status*, at 66–69.

[106] "Provided that this paragraph shall not apply to a refugee *falling under section A(1) of this article* and who is able to invoke *compelling reasons arising out of previous persecution* for

reserved for those able to show a continuing objective risk of being persecuted. Because refugee status requires the ability to show "a present fear of
persecution,"[107] refugees must be able to show that they "are or may in the
future be deprived of the protection of their country of origin."[108]

Despite the clarity of the text of the Refugee Convention on this point,
UNHCR has regrettably invoked an unwieldy claim of customary international law to assert not only the duty of states to apply the "compelling
reasons" proviso to modern refugees,[109] but also to suggest a responsibility
(in principle, if not in law) to read the Convention as the effective equivalent
of its own Statute.[110] While all states have the sovereign authority to allow any
person they wish to remain on their territory, and while it will often be
humane and right to extend such generosity,[111] this is not a matter fairly
understood to be required by either the text or purposes of refugee law.[112]

refusing to avail himself of the protection of the country of nationality [emphasis
added]": Refugee Convention, at Art. 1(C)(5).

[107] Statement of Sir Leslie Brass of the United Kingdom, UN Doc. E/AC.32/SR.18, Feb. 8,
1950, at 6.

[108] Statement of Mr. Rochefort of France, UN Doc. A/C.3/529, Nov. 2, 1949, at 4.

[109] "Application of the 'compelling reasons' exception is interpreted to extend beyond the
actual words of the provision to apply to Article 1A(2) refugees. This reflects a general
humanitarian principle that is now well-grounded in State practice": UNHCR, "Ceased
Circumstances Guidelines," at para. 21. Yet in the same document, UNHCR concedes
that there is, in fact, a paucity of relevant state practice upon which to draw. "Due to the
fact that large numbers of refugees voluntarily repatriate without an official declaration
that conditions in their countries of origin no longer justify international protection,
declarations [of cessation due to changed conditions] are infrequent": ibid. at para. 3. It is
therefore questionable whether there is truly a sound basis to assert a clear norm of
customary international law which effectively supersedes the text of the Refugee
Convention.

[110] "In addition [to exemption based upon the effects of past persecution], the Executive
Committee, in Conclusion No. 69, recommends that States consider 'appropriate
arrangements' for persons 'who cannot be expected to leave the country of asylum, due
to a long stay in that country resulting in strong family, social and economic links.' In
such situations, countries of asylum are encouraged to provide, and often do provide, the
individuals concerned with an alternative residence status, which retains previously
acquired rights, though in some instances with refugee status being withdrawn.
Adopting this approach for long-settled refugees is not required by the 1951
Convention per se, but it is consistent with the instrument's broad humanitarian purpose
and with respect for previously acquired rights": UNHCR, "Ceased Circumstances
Guidelines," at para. 22.

[111] For example, the rationale for the extension of the proviso in US law to all refugees has
been stated to be as "an expression of humanitarian considerations that sometimes past
persecution is so horrific that the march of time and the ebb and flow of political tides
cannot efface the fear in the mind of the persecuted": *Lal v. Immigration and
Naturalization Service*, 255 F 3d 998 (US CA9, July 3, 2001).

[112] UNHCR has at times recognized as much. "The underlying rationale for the cessation
clauses was expressed to the Conference of Plenipotentiaries in the drafting of the 1951
Convention by the first United Nations High Commissioner for Refugees, G. J. van

This point was recently affirmed in a detailed decision of the English Court of Appeal:

> Aspirations are to be distinguished from legal obligations. It is significant that a number of the [arguments] relied upon by the appellants are expressed in terms of what "could" or "should" be done . . . This is not the language which one would expect if there was a widespread and general practice establishing a legal obligation . . .
>
> Where one has clear and express language imposing a restriction upon the scope of a particular provision, as is the case with the proviso to Art. 1(C)(5), it must require very convincing evidence of a widespread and general practice of the international community to establish that that restriction is no longer to be applied as a matter of international law . . . A number of states do adopt a more generous approach towards Art. 1(C)(5) than is required by the terms of the Convention itself, but they represent . . . a minority of the signatories . . .
>
> Moreover, it must be seen as significant that the international community did not take the opportunity at the time of the 1967 Protocol to amend the proviso to Art. 1(C)(5) when it was considering the temporal scope of the 1951 Convention . . .
>
> One might think it desirable that states should . . . recognise the humanitarian purpose which would be served by ignoring the restriction on the proviso to Art. 1(C)(5). But that is not enough to establish a legal obligation binding upon all parties to the Convention.[113]

This analysis is clearly compelling as a matter of law. But because UNHCR has been unwilling to distinguish between its own institutional cessation and repatriation authority and that of state parties to the Convention, the

---

Heuven Goedhart, who stated that refugee status should 'not be granted for a day longer than was absolutely necessary, and should come to an end . . . if, in accordance with the terms of the Convention or the Statute, a person had the status of de facto citizenship, that is to say, if he really had the rights and obligations of a citizen of a given country.' Cessation of refugee status therefore applies when the refugee, having secured or being able to secure national protection, either of the country of origin or of another country, no longer needs international protection": UNHCR, "Cessation," at para. 4. Indeed, a footnote to the same document recognizes the hortatory nature of the advice to extend the proviso clause beyond its textual ambit. "The proviso expressly covers only those refugees falling under section A(1) of Article 1 of the 1951 Convention, that is, those persons who are considered as refugees under the Arrangements of 12 May 1926 and 30 June 1928 or under the Conventions of 28 October 1933 and 10 February 1938, the Protocol of 14 September 1939 or the Constitution of the International Refugee Organization. However, the UNHCR Handbook on Procedures and Criteria for Determining Refugee Status suggests that the exception reflects a more general humanitarian principle and could also be applied to refugees other than those in Article 1A(1) of the 1951 Convention (see paragraph 136 of the Handbook)": ibid. at n. 8.

[113] *R (Hoxha) v. Secretary of State for the Home Department*, [2002] EWCA Civ 1403 (Eng. CA, Oct. 14, 2002).

authentic scope of the Refugee Convention was unnecessarily and unhelpfully muddied.

The risks of conflating the principles which govern UNHCR's decisions regarding voluntary repatriation and the requirements of refugee law binding on states are clear also from an examination of the rules which circumscribe the authority mandatorily to repatriate persons whose refugee status has ceased. Of contemporary relevance not only to governments in the less developed world, but also to industrialized countries increasingly prone to order mandated repatriation, there is real ambiguity in UNHCR's positions regarding the standards which govern the actual process by which lawful repatriation may be effected.

Because this is not a subject expressly addressed by the Convention, the agency has devised a series of policies for the guidance of states. In an early formulation, UNHCR's Executive Committee opined that repatriation must "be carried out under conditions of absolute safety."[114] The requirement for "absolute" safety has not, however, featured in more recent agency standards, which have instead posited the bifurcated duty to carry out repatriation "in safety, and with dignity."[115]

The first part of this notion – safety – is said specifically to require that repatriation be conducted so as to avoid "harassment, arbitrary detention or physical threats during or after return."[116] UNHCR has more recently noted as well that safety requires analysis of "physical security [during the process of return] ... including protection from armed attacks, and mine-free routes."[117] The second branch of the UNHCR standard, requiring that return be "with dignity," is frankly acknowledged by the agency to be "less

[114] UNHCR Executive Committee Conclusion No. 40, "Voluntary Repatriation" (1985), at para. (b), available at www.unhcr.ch (accessed Nov. 20, 2004).

[115] UNHCR Executive Committee Conclusion No. 65, "General Conclusion on International Protection" (1991), at para. (j); and UNHCR Executive Committee Conclusion No. 101, "Conclusion on Legal Safety Issues in the Context of Voluntary Repatriation of Refugees" (2004), at para. (a), both available at www.unhcr.ch (accessed Nov. 20, 2004). This standard is firmly incorporated in agency practice: UNHCR, "Voluntary Repatriation Handbook," at 11.

[116] UNHCR Executive Committee Conclusion No. 65, "General Conclusion on International Protection" (1991), at para. (j), available at www.unhcr.ch (accessed Nov. 20, 2004).

[117] UNHCR, "Voluntary Repatriation Handbook," at 11. The same standard regrettably refers also to considerations actually relevant to the determination of cessation itself, not of the safety of repatriation ("legal safety (such as amnesties or public assurances of personal safety, integrity, non-discrimination and freedom from fear of persecution or punishment upon return ... [and of] if not mine-free then at least demarcated settlement sites"): ibid. It similarly places considerations of material security ("access to land or means of livelihood") under the safety rubric, matters which ought instead to be addressed in the context of the requirement of a dignified return: see text below, at pp. 948 and 951–952.

self-evident than that of safety."[118] UNHCR defines "return with dignity" to require that "refugees are not manhandled; that they can return unconditionally ... ; that they are not arbitrarily separated from family members; and that they are treated with respect and full acceptance by their national authorities, including the full restoration of their rights."

In practice, however, the fungibility of the "in safety, and with dignity" standard – particularly the fact that this language is not directly rooted in any clear legal obligations of states – is likely to engender confusion.[119] Because the language stands apart from binding norms of human rights law, the "in safety, and with dignity" standard can inadvertently send the signal that UNHCR is merely recommending best practice to governments. As much is clear from the Executive Committee's most recent attempt comprehensively to address the "legal safety issues" involved in refugee repatriation.[120] The relevance of international human rights law is relegated to a brief preambular reference,[121] followed by a series of specific recommendations which are merely "recognized," "stressed," "encouraged," or "noted."[122] To ensure that they are taken seriously, protection concerns would be better served by an explicit linkage to binding legal standards. While these may not encompass every constraint seen as desirable by UNHCR or others, all core concerns are encompassed in a way that clearly commands the respect of governments.

---

[118] UNHCR, "Voluntary Repatriation Handbook," at 11.

[119] Even those who advocate reference to the "safety" standard impliedly concede its fungibility. See e.g. G. Goodwin-Gill, *The Refugee in International Law* (1996) (Goodwin-Gill, *Refugee in International Law*), at 276: "So far as safe return may have a role to play in the construction of policy, its minimum conditions include a transparent process based on credible information ... These or equivalent means seem most likely to ensure that the element of risk is properly appreciated, so reducing the chance of States acting in breach of their protection obligations."

[120] UNHCR Executive Committee Conclusion No. 101, "Conclusion on Legal Safety Issues in the Context of Voluntary Repatriation of Refugees" (2004), available at www.unhcr.ch (accessed Nov. 20, 2004).

[121] The Executive Committee "[n]ot[ed] the relevance for voluntary repatriation of the Universal Declaration of Human Rights, the International Covenant on Civil and Political Rights, the International Covenant on Economic, Social and Cultural Rights, the International Convention on the Elimination of All Forms of Racial Discrimination, the Convention on the Rights of the Child and the Convention on the Elimination of All Forms of Discrimination against Women": UNHCR Executive Committee Conclusion No. 101, "Conclusion on Legal Safety Issues in the Context of Voluntary Repatriation of Refugees" (2004), at Preamble, available at www.unhcr.ch (accessed Nov. 20, 2004). None of the requirements of these key human rights treaties are, however, expressly referenced in any of twenty paragraphs of specific recommendations of the Conclusion.

[122] UNHCR Executive Committee Conclusion No. 101, "Conclusion on Legal Safety Issues in the Context of Voluntary Repatriation of Refugees" (2004), at paras. (a)–(t), available at www.unhcr.ch (accessed Nov. 20, 2004).

Specifically, the duty to effect repatriation in safety can be said to be a matter of legal obligation, particularly in view of the requirements of Arts. 7 and 9(1) of the Civil and Political Covenant.[123] These binding standards require respectively that states not engage in "torture, or . . . cruel, inhuman or degrading treatment or punishment"[124] and that they affirmatively ensure "security of person."[125] Under the jurisprudence of the Human Rights Committee, a state party is liable for the actions of its agents – logically including those involved in the process of repatriation – even if those actions occur outside the state's own borders.[126] The rights to be protected from

[123] See generally UN Human Rights Committee, "General Comment No. 20: Prohibition of torture, or other cruel, inhuman or degrading treatment or punishment" (1992), UN Doc. HRI/GEN/1/Rev.7, May 12, 2004, at 150. The European Union has affirmed the centrality of human rights norms to defining the right of repatriation. In its Council Directive on minimum standards for giving protection in the event of a mass influx of displaced persons and on the measures promoting a balance of efforts between Member States in receiving such persons and bearing the consequences thereof, Doc. 2001/55/EC (July 20, 2001) (EU Temporary Protection Directive), the European Union agreed that protection should be ended only when "the situation in the country of origin is such as to permit safe and durable return . . . with due respect for human rights and fundamental freedoms": ibid. at Art. 6(2). In the official commentary included with the Directive, the Commission refers specifically to the importance of there being conditions "guaranteeing respect for . . . the rule of law": ibid., Commentary accompanying Art. 6(2).

[124] Civil and Political Covenant, at Art. 7. See generally chapter 4.3.2 above.

[125] Civil and Political Covenant, at Art. 9. See generally chapter 4.3.3 above.

[126] Under the Civil and Political Covenant, obligations inhere in "all individuals within [a state's] territory and subject to its jurisdiction": Civil and Political Covenant, at Art. 2(1). Rather than adopting a literal construction of this standard, the Human Rights Committee has embraced an interpretation oriented to respect for the objects and purposes of the Covenant. "Article 2(1) of the Covenant . . . does not imply that the State party concerned cannot be held accountable for violations of rights under the Covenant which its agents commit upon the territory of another State, whether with the acquiescence of the Government of that State or in opposition to it . . . [I]t would be unconscionable to . . . interpret the responsibility under article 2 of the Covenant as to permit a State party to perpetrate violations of the Covenant on the territory of another State, which violations it could not perpetrate on its own territory": Casariego v. Uruguay, UNHRC Comm. No. 56/1979, decided July 29, 1981, at para. 12.3. In an Individual Opinion, Committee member Tomuschat offered a helpful explanation of why this result was compelled despite the possibility of a literal construction to the contrary. "To construe the words 'within its territory' pursuant to their strict literal meaning as excluding any responsibility for conduct occurring beyond the national boundaries would . . . lead to utterly absurd results. The formula was intended to take care of objective difficulties which might impede the implementation of the Covenant in specific situations. Thus, a State party is normally unable to ensure the effective enjoyment of the rights under the Covenant to its citizens abroad, having at its disposal only the tools of diplomatic protection with their limited potential. Instances of occupation of foreign territory offer another example of situations which the drafters of the Covenant had in mind when they confined the obligations of States parties to their own territory. All of these factual patterns have in common, however, that they provide plausible grounds for

torture, as well as from cruel, inhuman, or degrading treatment, and to benefit from security of person moreover inhere equally in citizens and aliens.[127]

As previously analyzed, an action may be defined as "cruel or inhuman" if it meets most, but not all, of the criteria for torture; for example, the specific intent requirement may not be met, or the level of pain may not rise to the same level of severity.[128] But actions which are not cruel or inhuman are also prohibited if they are "degrading," meaning that they are intended to humiliate the victim, or show an egregious disregard for his or her humanity.[129] More generally, the duty to ensure "security of person" means that states are required to take measures to protect persons being repatriated from foreseeable attacks against their personal integrity, and perhaps also their property.[130] By way of example, the treatment afforded a long-term Rwandan resident of Tanzania by authorities enforcing a bilateral repatriation agreement likely amounted to both degrading treatment, and to a failure to ensure his security of person:

> I was grazing livestock; they came and beat me up. In the confusion, I was taken one way and the livestock in another. They took the money I had in my pocket, and told me, "Rwandan go home."[131]

denying the protection of the Covenant. It may be concluded, therefore, that it was the intention of the drafters, whose sovereign decisions cannot be challenged, to restrict the territorial scope of the Covenant in view of such situations where enforcing the Covenant would be likely to encounter exceptional obstacles. Never was it envisaged, however, to grant States parties unfettered discretionary power to carry out wilful and deliberate attacks against the freedom and personal integrity of their citizens living abroad": *Burgos v. Uruguay*, UNHRC Comm. No. 52/1979, decided July 29, 1981, per Member Tomuschat (concurring). This jurisprudence has been expressly affirmed by the International Court of Justice in *Legal Consequences of the Construction of a Wall in the Occupied Palestinian Territory* (2004) ICJ Gen. List No. 131, decided July 9, 2004.

[127] "Aliens . . . must not be subjected to torture or to cruel, inhuman or degrading treatment or punishment . . . Aliens have the full right to . . . security of the person": UN Human Rights Committee, "General Comment No. 15: The position of aliens under the Covenant" (1986), UN Doc. HRI/GEN/1/Rev.7, May 12, 2004, at 140, para. 7.

[128] See chapter 4.3.2 above, at pp. 454–455.

[129] Ibid. at pp. 456–457. Thus, for example, the UN Human Rights Committee has expressed its concern that "in the course of [Swiss] deportation of aliens there have been instances of degrading treatment and use of excessive force" in contravention of Art. 7 of the Covenant: "Concluding Observations of the Human Rights Committee: Switzerland," UN Doc. CCPR/CO/73/CH, Nov. 5, 2001, at para. 13.

[130] See chapter 4.3.3 above, at p. 458.

[131] *Internews*, Apr. 15, 2003. The same report noted that "[t]he President of the National Repatriation Commission, Sheik Abdul Karim Harerimana, [said] . . . that the move by the Tanzanian government caught more than the evictees by surprise. 'We had not anticipated this'": ibid.

The "in dignity" prong of the UNHCR repatriation standard is particularly unwieldy. Two of the concerns said to define whether repatriation can be conducted in dignity – the existence of an unconditional right to return, and acceptance of the returnee by authorities with restoration of rights – are more appropriately canvassed in the context of the protection prong of the cessation inquiry itself.[132] Nor is there any need to rely on the "in dignity" concept to proscribe the risk of "manhandling," since such concerns are encompassed by the duty to ensure a safe return grounded in Arts. 7 and 9(1) of the Civil and Political Covenant.[133] And while UNHCR is clearly right to argue that repatriation would be undignified if it leads to the arbitrary separation of family members, the real constraints on state actions would be made more clear if grounded in specific human rights obligations.[134] The Human Rights Committee has expressly observed that the right to freedom from arbitrary or unlawful interference with family life inheres despite the (former) refugee's status as a non-citizen:

> The Covenant [on Civil and Political Rights] does not recognize the right of aliens to enter or reside in the territory of a State party. However, in certain circumstances an alien may enjoy the protection of the Covenant *in relation to entry or residence*, for example, when considerations of non-discrimination, prohibition of inhuman treatment and *respect for family life* arise ... [Non-citizens] may not be subjected to arbitrary or unlawful interference with their privacy, *family*, home, or correspondence [emphasis added].[135]

Indeed, there is a firm basis to assert a customary legal duty on states to avoid acts which arbitrarily interfere with family unity, at least where family is defined to include only an opposite-sex spouse and minor, dependent children.[136]

---

[132] See text above, at pp. 925–928.   [133] See text above, at pp. 946–947.

[134] Reference should be made in particular to Art. 17 of the International Covenant on Civil and Political Rights, and to Arts. 10(1), 23, and 24 of the International Covenant on Economic, Social and Cultural Rights, UNGA Res. 2200A(XXI), adopted Dec. 16, 1966, entered into force Jan. 3, 1976 (Economic, Social and Cultural Covenant). See generally chapter 4.6 above.

[135] UN Human Rights Committee, "General Comment No. 15: The position of aliens under the Covenant" (1986), UN Doc. HRI/GEN/1/Rev.7, May 12, 2004, at 140, paras. 5 and 7. See also UN Human Rights Committee, "General Comment No. 17: Rights of the child" (1989), UN Doc. HRI/GEN/1/Rev.7, May 12, 2004, at 144, para. 5: "The Covenant requires that children should be protected against discrimination on any grounds ... Reports by States parties should indicate how legislation and practice ensure that measures of protection are aimed at removing all discrimination in every field ... particularly as between children who are nationals and children who are aliens."

[136] See chapter 4.6 above, at pp. 543–547.

By focusing on the human right to be free from *unlawful or arbitrary* interference with family unity, the legally binding nature of state obligations is made more clear. Lawful repatriation consequent to cessation of refugee status is, of course, not sensibly deemed either arbitrary or unlawful *per se*. The relevant question is thus whether the *way* in which repatriation is effected renders an otherwise permissible act either arbitrary or unlawful. It will ordinarily be possible to respect family unity even while pursuing repatriation, for example by ensuring that the family as a whole is safely returned to the home country. On the other hand, at least where the laws of the host state grant citizenship to all children born on its territory, it may be necessary to delay repatriation of the family unit until any citizen children reach the age of majority, since earlier removal would deny them the right to live in their own country.[137] Indeed, a recent decision of the Supreme Court of Canada invoked international law to require that account be taken of the rights of Canadian-born children before ordering the deportation of their non-Canadian mother.[138] A similar caution has been insisted upon by the UN Human Rights Committee in upholding a challenge to the deportation from Australia of a stateless married couple from Indonesia and their thirteen-year-old son (who was a citizen of Australia):

> It is certainly unobjectionable under the Covenant that a State party may require, under its laws, the departure of persons who remain in its territory beyond limited duration periods. Nor is the fact that a child is born, or that by operation of law such a child receives citizenship either at birth or at a later time, sufficient of itself to make a proposed deportation of one or both parents arbitrary. Accordingly, there is significant scope for States parties to

[137] Under the Convention on the Rights of the Child, UNGA Res. 44/25, adopted Nov. 20, 1989, entered into force Sept. 2, 1990 (Rights of the Child Convention), states "undertake to respect the right of the child to preserve his or her identity, including nationality ... [and to ensure that no] child is illegally deprived of some or all of the elements of his or her identity": ibid. at Art. 8. Governments agree to "ensure that a child is not separated from his or her parents against their will, except when ... such separation is necessary for the best interests of the child": ibid. at Art. 9. Moreover, "applications by a child or his or her parents to enter ... a State Party for the purpose of family reunification shall be dealt with by States Parties in a positive, humane and expeditious manner": ibid. at Art. 10. And under no circumstance may any of the rights guaranteed in the Convention be withheld on a discriminatory basis, including on the basis of "the child's or his or her parent's or legal guardian's ... national ... origin ... or other status": ibid. at Art. 2.

[138] "The United Nations Declaration of the Rights of the Child (1959), in its preamble, states that the child 'needs special safeguards and care.' The principles of the Convention [on the Rights of the Child] and other international instruments place special importance on protections for children and childhood, and on particular consideration of their interests, needs, and rights. They help show the values that are central in determining whether this decision was ... reasonable": *Baker v. Canada*, [1999] 2 SCR 817 (Can. SC, July 9, 1999).

enforce their immigration policy and to require departure of unlawfully present persons. That discretion is, however, not unlimited and may come to be exercised arbitrarily in certain circumstances. In the present case, both authors have been in Australia for over 14 years. The authors' son has grown [up] in Australia from his birth 13 years ago, attending Australian schools as an ordinary child would and developing the social relationships inherent in that. In view of the duration of time, it is incumbent on the State party to demonstrate additional factors justifying the removal of both parents that go beyond a simple enforcement of its immigration law in order to avoid a characterization of arbitrariness.[139]

Applying this principle, the Committee has gone on to determine that a deportation decision which interrupts family unity will ordinarily be deemed arbitrary where the significance of a state's reasons for removal does not outweigh the degree of hardship that would be occasioned to the family as the result of the deportation.[140]

---

[139] *Winata v. Australia*, UNHRC Comm. No. 930/2000, UN Doc. CCPR/C/72/D/930/2000, decided July 26, 2001, at para. 7.3.

[140] "[I]n cases where one part of a family must leave the territory of the State party while the other part would be entitled to remain, the relevant criteria for assessing whether or not the specific interference with family life can be objectively justified must be considered, on the one hand, in light of the significance of the State party's reasons for the removal of the person concerned and, on the other, [in light of] the degree of hardship the family and its members would encounter as a consequence of such removal. In the present case, the Committee notes that the State party justifies the removal of Mr. Madafferi by his illegal presence in Australia, his alleged dishonesty in his relations with the Department of Immigration and Multicultural Affairs, and his 'bad character' stemming from criminal acts committed in Italy twenty years ago. The Committee also notes that Mr. Madafferi's outstanding sentences in Italy have been extinguished and that there is no outstanding warrant for his arrest. At the same time, it notes the considerable hardship that would be imposed on a family that has been in existence for 14 years. If Mrs. Madafferi and the children were to decide to emigrate to Italy in order to avoid separation of the family, they would not only have to live in a country they do not know and whose language the children (two of whom are already 13 and 11 years old) do not speak, but would also have to take care, in an environment alien to them, of a husband and father whose mental health has been seriously troubled, in part by acts that can be ascribed to the State party. In these very specific circumstances, the Committee considers that the reasons advanced by the State party for the decision of the Minister overruling the Administrative Appeals Tribunal [ ] to remove Mr. Madafferi from Australia are not pressing enough to justify, in the present case, interference to this extent with the family and infringement of the right of the children to such measures of protection as are required by their status as minors. Thus, the Committee considers that the removal by the State party of Mr. Madafferi would, if implemented, constitute arbitrary interference with the family, contrary to article 17, paragraph 1, in conjunction with article 23, of the Covenant in respect of all of the authors, and additionally, a violation of article 24, paragraph 1, in relation to the four minor children due to a failure to provide them with the necessary measures of protection as minors": *Madafferi v. Australia*, UNHRC Comm. No. 1011/2001, UN Doc. CCPR/C/81/D/1011/2001, decided July 26, 2004, at para. 9.8.

A final concern with the free-standing "in safety, and with dignity" standard is that it likely overstates the real obligations of governments undertaking mandated repatriation.[141] As the preceding discussion makes clear, international human rights law precludes the right to effect an otherwise lawful repatriation only in circumstances of fairly clear risk.[142] Thus, for example, there is reason to question the legal authority for UNHCR's view that repatriation cannot lawfully be undertaken unless the (former) refugees have access in the destination to "material security (access to land or means of livelihood)."[143] To the contrary, international human rights law guarantees only a basic right to access the necessities of life,[144] not a full-blown right to have either property[145] or

[141] The difficulty stems in part from the tendency, discussed above at pp. 929–935, to conflate the rules that govern UNHCR's work as an agency with those that circumscribe the repatriation authority of state parties to the Refugee Convention. The elaboration of the meaning of repatriation in safety and with dignity is textually said to define the ways in which UNHCR will conduct *its* repatriation work. But the language of safety and dignity is included in resolutions of the Executive Committee addressed to the authority of states, and UNHCR follows the recitation of its institutional positions with the assertion that it is part of the "responsibilities of the host country" to "respect the leading role of UNHCR in promoting, facilitating and coordinating voluntary repatriation": UNHCR, "Voluntary Repatriation Handbook," at 8–10.

[142] The most extensive rights to non-return apart from those which follow from Convention refugee status are those which are based on application of the European Convention for the Protection of Human Rights and Fundamental Freedoms, 213 UNTS 221, done Nov. 4, 1950, entered into force Sept. 3, 1953. The House of Lords has recently suggested that in principle the breadth of such rights may in fact be quite extensive: see *R (Ullah) v. Special Adjudicator; Do v. Secretary of State for the Home Department*, [2004] UKHL 26 (UK HL, June 17, 2004). Yet, to date, the primary additional basis for implying a duty of non-return has in fact been the duty under Art. 8 of the European Convention, ibid., to the protection of private life: see *Boultif v. Switzerland*, (2000) 22 EHRR 50 (ECHR, Aug. 2, 2001).

[143] UNHCR, "Voluntary Repatriation Handbook," at 11.

[144] This may be derived from Arts. 6, 7, 9, and 10 of the Civil and Political Covenant, as well as from Art. 11 of the Economic, Social and Cultural Covenant. See generally chapter 4.4 above.

[145] See chapter 4.5.1 above, at pp. 518–521. Perhaps the strongest affirmation of a right to property, and specifically of a right of returning refugees to receive restitution for property of which they were deprived, is based on the provisions of the International Convention on the Elimination of All Forms of Racial Discrimination, UNGA Res. 2106A(XX), adopted Dec. 21, 1965, entered into force Jan. 4, 1969 (Racial Discrimination Convention). Under Art. 5(d)(v), state parties agree to eliminate racial discrimination (i.e. discrimination based on "race, color, or national or ethnic origin") in regard to "[t]he right to own property alone as well as in association with others." On the basis of this provision, the Committee on the Elimination of Racial Discrimination has "emphasize[d]" that "refugees . . . have, after their return to their homes of origin, the right to be restored to them property of which they were deprived in the course of the conflict and to be compensated appropriately for any such property that cannot be restored to them. Any commitments

a job.[146] Even the expert charged by the United Nations with studying the issue of the property rights of returning refugees has focused his work on housing rights, noting that these rights "are enshrined in international human rights and humanitarian law to a far greater degree and encompass far more under international law, substantively speaking, than . . . property rights more generally."[147] Second and more critically, the position that repatriation can be ordered only if it results in return to conditions of material security unhelpfully confuses the standards which should govern the way in which repatriation is *conducted* with considerations of the qualitative standards which must prevail in the place of destination. The latter questions are part of the cessation inquiry itself, not of the definition of permissible means of repatriation.[148]

The European Union's Temporary Protection Directive moves more closely towards the codification of a legally oriented set of constraints on the effectuation of repatriation. The Directive acknowledges that the repatriation of those no longer entitled to protection must be "conducted with due respect for human dignity."[149] But it implements that principle by way of two, quite specific injunctions. First, the Directive denies member states the right to repatriate persons no longer in need of protection if they "cannot, in view of their state of health, reasonably be expected to travel . . . where for example they would suffer serious negative effects if their treatment were interrupted."[150] A delay in repatriation is also sanctioned (though, regrettably, not required) so as to "allow families whose children are minors and attend school in a Member State . . . to complete the current school period."[151] The specificity of each of these constraints can readily be linked to a duty to conduct repatriation with due regard for human rights obligations –

---

or statements relating to such property made under duress are null and void": UN Committee on the Elimination of Racial Discrimination, "General Recommendation No. XXII: Refugees and displaced persons" (1996), UN Doc. HRI/GEN/1/Rev.7, May 12, 2004, at 214, para. 2(c). Art. 5 (in contrast to, for example, the Covenant on Civil and Political Rights) expressly recognizes property rights as a form of civil right. But it must be recalled that the purpose of this part of the Convention is clearly to proscribe race-based discrimination. It is legally doubtful that the duty not to discriminate in regard to property rights on grounds of race can be said to give rise to an affirmative obligation to recognize property rights in the first place.

[146] See chapter 6.1.1 above, at pp. 739–740.

[147] S. Pinheiro, "Housing and property restitution in the context of the return of refugees and internally displaced persons, Preliminary report of the Special Rapporteur submitted in accordance with Sub-Commission resolution 2002/7," UN Doc. E/CN.4/Sub.2/2003/11, June 16, 2003, at para. 5.

[148] It is likely that at least some core aspects of material security are relevant to whether or not protection is available in the refugee's state of origin, the third prong of UNHCR's recommended approach to assessment of Art. 1(C)(5)–(6): see text above, at pp. 927–928.

[149] EU Temporary Protection Directive, at Art. 22(1).

[150] Ibid. at Art. 23(1).   [151] Ibid. at Art. 23(2).

in the one case, the right to basic healthcare,[152] in the other the right of children to access primary education.[153] These constraints moreover do not confuse the question of whether repatriation is warranted at all with the distinct set of issues regarding whether repatriation may be lawfully carried out at a particular moment, and if so, what precautions are required given the circumstances of the individual concerned.[154] They are instead appropriately directed simply to averting the adverse effects of repatriation on the human rights (to access basic healthcare, and to benefit from primary education) of those to be repatriated by setting relevant constraints on the timing or means by which otherwise lawful repatriation may be effected.[155]

7.2 Voluntary reestablishment

It might be argued that reestablishment in the country of origin while the risk of being persecuted there persists should not sensibly be considered to be a solution to refugeehood. At one level, it is clearly no solution at all: the likelihood of harm befalling the refugee is made all the more real by reentry into the state where the threat exists. But it is a solution, at least if viewed from the perspective of the host state. That country's protection obligations have been "solved" by the decision of the refugee to assume the risks of life in the home state, so long as the decision to return home has truly been voluntary (that is, there was no direct or indirect *refoulement*) and the decision is firm (as evinced by reestablishment in, not simply return to, the country of origin).

---

[152] This right is guaranteed by Art. 12 of the Covenant on Economic, Social and Cultural Rights. See generally chapter 4.4.3 above.

[153] This right is guaranteed by Art. 13(2)(a) of the Covenant on Economic, Social and Cultural Rights. See generally chapter 4.8 above.

[154] While not required by law, it is both more practical and respectful of refugee autonomy to encourage (former) refugees to return home of their own initiative wherever possible. To this end, the extension to them of a generous deadline for departure, together with a readjustment allowance for voluntary compliance, may be of value. See M. Castillo and J. Hathaway, "Temporary Protection," in J. Hathaway ed., *Reconceiving International Refugee Law* 1 (1997) (Castillo and Hathaway, "Temporary Protection"), at 21. It is unlikely, however, that such a program will be successful when refugees are not convinced of the safety of return. For example, a British initiative for failed asylum-seekers from Afghanistan in early 2003 – under which individuals were offered £600 and families £2,500 to go back to a "safe area" inside Afghanistan – is reported to have attracted only thirty-nine applicants, far short of the target of 1,000: N. Morris, "Protests at first enforced return of Afghans since war," *Independent*, Apr. 29, 2003, at 6; R. Ford, "Afghan refugees put on aircraft back to Kabul," *Times*, Apr. 29, 2003, at 7.

[155] See text above, at pp. 945–950.

Refugee Convention, Art. 1(C)(4)
This Convention shall cease to apply to any person falling under the terms of section A if:

. . .

(4) He has voluntarily re-established himself in the country which he left or outside which he remained owing to fear of persecution.

Civil and Political Covenant, Art. 12

. . .

2. Everyone shall be free to leave any country, including his own.

3. The above-mentioned right[] shall not be subject to any restrictions except those which are provided by law, are necessary to protect national security, public order (*ordre public*), public health or morals or the rights and freedoms of others, and are consistent with the other rights recognized in the present Covenant.

4. No one shall be arbitrarily deprived of the right to enter his own country.

From the perspective of general international law, the cessation of refugee status upon voluntary reestablishment in the country of origin makes good sense. Most obviously, the alienage requirement of the refugee definition[156] reflects the legal limits of a state's right to project its protective authority on the international plane:[157] individual governments generally have no right to assert authority over non-citizens, even for positive purposes, outside their own jurisdiction.[158] When an individual otherwise entitled to be recognized as a refugee opts freely to leave the jurisdiction of a protecting state, that country is simply no longer positioned to assist him or her, at least in the direct sense envisaged by the Refugee Convention.

Equally important, cessation of refugee status upon voluntary reestablishment reflects the autonomous right of every refugee to decide for himself or

---

[156] The refugee definition limits protection to a person "*outside* the country of his nationality . . . [or in the case of a stateless person] *outside* the country of his former habitual residence" owing to a well-founded fear of being persecuted for a Convention reason: Refugee Convention, at Art. 1(A)(2). See generally Hathaway, *Refugee Status*, at 29–63.

[157] See generally chapter 3.1.1 above.

[158] There is, of course, a live debate about where the so-called right of humanitarian intervention persists (or has even been reinvented) in the post-UN Charter era. This debate does not, however, have any direct relevance to issues of jurisdiction relevant to refugee law. See chapter 3.1.1 above.

herself when protection abroad is no longer desired.[159] Under international law, a refugee has the presumptive right to return home – whether for reasons adjudged objectively sound, or not.[160] Under Art. 12 of the Civil and Political Covenant, "[e]veryone shall be free to leave any country."[161] As such, the primary duty of the host state is "to avoid interfering with the freedom to leave."[162] While the right to leave may be subject to limited forms of restriction,[163] it is doubtful that any of these could justify even a well-meaning refusal of departure on grounds of the risks that persist in the home country.[164]

[159] See e.g. UNHCR, "Ceased Circumstances Guidelines," at para. 19: "Voluntary repatriation can take place at a lower threshold of change in the country of origin, occurring as it does at the express wish of the refugee, who may also have personal reasons for repatriating, regardless of the situation prevailing in the country of origin."

[160] See generally H. Hannum, *The Right to Leave and Return in International Law and Practice* (1987). The well-established nature of the legal right to return to one's country as codified in the Civil and Political Covenant seems not always to be recognized even by senior officials. Commenting on the return of refugees to Bosnia, the International High Representative there claimed, "'We've invented a new human right here, the right to return after a war . . . It's absolutely astonishing, a huge success by Bosnians and the international community that has gone unrecognised'": J. Glover, "Absolute power," *Guardian*, Oct. 11, 2002.

[161] Civil and Political Covenant, at Art. 12(2).

[162] M. Nowak, *UN Covenant on Civil and Political Rights* (1993) (Nowak, *ICCPR Commentary*), at 206. The host state is also jointly responsible with the individual's state of citizenship to make any relevant travel documents available. "In order to enable the individual to enjoy the rights guaranteed by article 12, paragraph 2, obligations are imposed both on the State of residence and on the State of nationality. Since international travel usually requires appropriate documents, in particular a passport, the right to leave a country must include the right to obtain the necessary travel documents": UN Human Rights Committee, "General Comment No. 27: Freedom of movement" (1999), UN Doc. HRI/GEN/1/Rev.7, May 12, 2004, at 173, para. 9. Importantly, however, so long as the refugee remains under the host state's authority, that country remains responsible for protection of basic rights, such as physical security. There is therefore a duty to respond meaningfully to efforts by private parties to prevent refugees from exercising their right to return home, as when twenty-four Burundian refugees were killed in Tanzania's Kibondo district by persons apparently opposed to their effort to go home: "24 Burundian refugees killed in Tanzania," *UN Integrated Regional Information Networks*, Jan. 31, 2002. See generally chapter 4.3 above.

[163] This right may be subject only to "restrictions . . . which are provided by law, are necessary to protect national security, public order (*ordre public*), public health or morals or the rights and freedoms of others, and are consistent with the other rights recognized in the present Covenant": Civil and Political Covenant, at Art. 12(3).

[164] Specifically, the fact that Art. 12(3) allows restrictions necessary to protect "the rights and freedoms *of others* [emphasis added]" suggests that a restriction would not be permissible in order to protect the rights and freedoms of the refugee himself or herself. See Nowak, *ICCPR Commentary*, at 216–217, and N. Jayawickrama, *The Judicial Application of Human Rights Law* (2002) (Jayawickrama, *Judicial Application*), at 468–469.

Perhaps the only legally valid form of constraint on a refugee's decision to return home would be where such return would threaten the stability in the state to which the refugee plans to return. Because Art. 12(3) of the Covenant does not constrain the scope of valid limitation to relevant considerations which exist in the state from which departure is contemplated, a restriction on voluntary departure might be found valid if its purpose were to ensure public order (*ordre public*) or safety *in the destination state*. For example, it is arguable that return might be constrained where the destination country is faced with a massive return of refugees that it cannot immediately accommodate in a secure way, or without critical risk to the human rights of those already there. But the requirement that any restriction on departure be both necessary[165] and proportionate,[166] as well as the overarching duty to ensure that restrictions imposed "are consistent with the other rights recognized in the Covenant" (including, for example, the duty of non-discrimination[167] based on status as refugees[168]), means that any limitations on freedom to depart the host country would have to be both strictly provisional, and carefully implemented.[169]

[165] "Article 12, paragraph 3, clearly indicates that it is not sufficient that the restrictions serve the permissible purposes; they must also be necessary to protect them. Restrictive measures must conform to the principle of proportionality; they must be appropriate to achieve their protective function; they must be the least intrusive instrument amongst those which might achieve the desired result": UN Human Rights Committee, "General Comment No. 27: Freedom of movement" (1999), UN Doc. HRI/GEN/1/Rev.7, May 12, 2004, at 173, para. 14.

[166] "The principle of proportionality has to be respected not only in the law that frames the restrictions, but also by the administrative and judicial authorities in applying the law. States should ensure that any proceedings relating to the exercise or restriction of these rights are expeditious and that reasons for the application of restrictive measures are provided": ibid. at para. 15.

[167] "The application of the restrictions permissible under article 12, paragraph 3, needs to be consistent with the other rights guaranteed in the Covenant and with the fundamental principles of equality and non-discrimination. Thus, it would be a clear violation of the Covenant if the rights enshrined in article 12, paragraphs 1 and 2, were restricted by making distinctions of any kind, such as on the basis of race, color, sex, language, religion, political or other opinion, national or social origin, property, birth or other status": ibid. at para. 18. See also UN Committee on the Elimination of Racial Discrimination, "General Recommendation No. XXII: Refugees and displaced persons" (1996), UN Doc. HRI/GEN/1/Rev.7, May 12, 2004, at 214, para. 2(a): "All . . . refugees and displaced persons have the right freely to return to their homes of origin under conditions of safety."

[168] See chapter 2.5.5 above, at p. 127.

[169] Nowak similarly takes a cautious view of this authority. "It is more difficult to evaluate which *restrictions on the freedom to leave the country* . . . are permissible in the interests of public order. It is only clear from the historical background and the [Human Rights] Committee's holding in *González del Rio v. Peru* [UNHRC Comm. No. 263/1987, UN Doc. CCPR/C/40/D/263/1987, decided Nov. 6, 1990] that States have a limited right to

The home state of a refugee has even less legal authority to constrain return. Art. 12(4) is emphatic that "[n]o one shall be arbitrarily deprived of the right to enter his own country."[170] Specifically, none of the limitations available to constrain departure may be invoked by the refugee's own state to limit the right of return.[171] The only form of restriction which is allowed is one adjudged not to be "arbitrary," a notion included in the Covenant to validate restrictions consequent to lawful exile.[172] The contemporary stance of the Human Rights Committee affords states only slightly more latitude to impose restrictions on return:

> The reference to the concept of arbitrariness in this context is intended to emphasize that it applies to all State action, legislative, administrative and judicial; it guarantees that even interference provided for by law should be in accordance with the provisions, aims and objectives of the Covenant and should be, in any event, reasonable in the particular circumstances. *The Committee considers that there are few, if any, circumstances in which deprivation of the right to enter one's own country could be reasonable* [emphasis added].[173]

This firm stance on the duty to readmit is justified, in the view of the Committee, by the "special relationship" of an individual to his or her own country.[174]

Significantly, the Human Rights Committee has affirmed that "[t]he right to return is of the utmost importance for refugees seeking voluntary repatriation [*sic*]."[175] And by virtue of the language used, the duty to readmit under Art. 12(4) is not restricted to those who are the formal citizens of the state. Rather,

> [t]he wording of article 12, paragraph 4, does not distinguish between nationals and aliens ("no one"). Thus, the persons entitled to exercise this right can be identified only by interpreting the meaning of the phrase "his own country." The scope of "his own country" is broader than the concept "country of his nationality." It is not limited to nationality in a

---

prevent persons who have been accused of a crime from leaving the territory of the State [emphasis in original]": Nowak, *ICCPR Commentary*, at 213. More generally, the Human Rights Committee has warned that "[i]n adopting laws providing for restrictions permitted by article 12, paragraph 3, States should always be guided by the principle that the restrictions must not impair the essence of the right (cf. art. 5, para. 1); the relation between right and restriction, between norm and exception, must not be reversed. The laws authorizing the application of restrictions should use precise criteria and may not confer unfettered discretion on those charged with their execution": UN Human Rights Committee, "General Comment No. 27: Freedom of movement" (1999), UN Doc. HRI/GEN/1/Rev.7, May 12, 2004, at 173, para. 13.

[170] Civil and Political Covenant, at Art. 12(4).
[171] Nowak, *ICCPR Commentary*, at 218.   [172] Ibid. at 219.
[173] UN Human Rights Committee, "General Comment No. 27: Freedom of movement" (1999), UN Doc. HRI/GEN/1/Rev.7, May 12, 2004, at 173, para. 21.
[174] Ibid. at para. 19.   [175] Ibid. at para. 19.

formal sense, that is, nationality acquired at birth or by conferral; it embraces, at the very least, an individual who, because of his or her special ties to or claims in relation to a given country, cannot be considered to be a mere alien. This would be the case, for example, of nationals of a country who have there been stripped of their nationality in violation of international law, and of individuals whose country of nationality has been incorporated in or transferred to another national entity, whose nationality is being denied them. The language of article 12, paragraph 4, moreover, permits a broader interpretation that might embrace other categories of long-term residents, including but not limited to stateless persons arbitrarily deprived of the right to acquire the nationality of the country of such residence . . . [O]ther factors may in certain circumstances result in the establishment of close and enduring connections between a person and a country.[176]

There is thus a clear legal foundation for what appears, in any event, to be an essentially unstoppable social phenomenon: the preparedness of refugees to risk even their safety in order to go home. For example, refugees returned to Sarajevo even while the fighting there was still ongoing:

> No one – not UNHCR, not the International Committee of the Red Cross, not the Bosnian government's Ministry of Refugees – admits to knowing how many refugees or displaced people from Sarajevo have returned to the city . . . Some of the people trying to get back into the city, particularly after the Croats and Muslims began fighting each other, had a difficult time. Often they were pinned down on the road from Herzegovina to Sarajevo by the fighting . . . People still continue to come to Sarajevo, crossing Mount Igman by bus and using the tunnel to enter the city, although the Serbs now shell its entrance in Butmir.[177]

In making their own decisions about return, these refugees were opting for what is clearly the predominant solution to refugeehood: voluntary reestablishment in the state of origin. Indeed, Stein notes that between 1975 and 1991, more than 90 percent of refugee returns were self-directed efforts by refugees themselves, accomplished without any significant international assistance.[178]

From a practical perspective, there are many steps that can be taken to ensure that refugees make the best choices possible.[179] Most clearly, efforts to

---

[176] Ibid. at para. 20.

[177] P. Reed, *Sarajevo: Spontaneous Repatriation to a City Under Siege* (1995), at 20–22.

[178] B. Stein, "Policy Challenges Regarding Repatriation in the 1990s: Is 1992 the Year for Voluntary Repatriation?," paper presented at the Tufts University Fletcher School of Law and Diplomacy, Apr. 15, 1992. "The majority of refugees who repatriated voluntarily in past years did so spontaneously and it is likely that spontaneous repatriation will continue to be a regular feature of refugee return": UNHCR, "Voluntary Repatriation Handbook," at para. 3.3.

[179] Castillo and Hathaway, "Temporary Protection," at 19–21.

provide them with current and specific information about conditions in the home country are key. The UNHCR Executive Committee has also recommended the facilitation of carefully managed visits by home country representatives to meet with refugees abroad.[180] Of perhaps greatest value, representatives of a refugee population may be assisted to undertake a "look-see" visit to the home state, and to report back on conditions there to the community in exile. For example, in 2002 UNHCR helped five representatives of the Namibian refugee population in Botswana to return to their homes in Caprivi province to assess the suitability of return. Based on their positive assessment, nearly half of the refugee population opted to go home.[181] Other countries provide comparable assurances on a more individuated basis, guaranteeing refugees the right to resume their refugee status should efforts to reestablish themselves in the home country ultimately prove unviable.

Somewhat more controversially, host governments may offer financial incentives to refugees who agree to go home. Such initiatives can be sensible investments in human capital. For example, a British initiative administered in cooperation with the International Organization for Migration provided an "installation grant" of £210 and a modest salary top-up to well-educated Afghans living in the United Kingdom who agreed to return home and to contribute to the rebuilding of their home country.[182] But Britain later promoted a more assertive repatriation plan, under which Afghan families agreeing to go home would receive a grant of up to £2,500. The British Refugee Council and Amnesty International expressed their concern that despite the optional nature of the initiative, it could in practice prove too

---

[180] The Executive Committee "[a]cknowledge[d] the usefulness, in appropriate circumstances, of visits by representatives of the countries of origin to refugee camps in countries of asylum within the framework of information campaigns to promote voluntary repatriation": UNHCR Executive Committee Conclusion No. 74, "General Conclusion on International Protection" (1994), at para. (z), available at www.unhcr.ch (accessed Nov. 20, 2004).

[181] "Many refugees have expressed a strong desire to return home, especially after a 'go and see' visit by representatives of the refugee community in June. 'One young man who went on the go and see visit was so enthusiastic [that] he wanted UNHCR to take him immediately,' recalled a staff member of the UN refugee agency in Namibia": "UNHCR starts repatriating Namibian refugees in Botswana," *UNHCR News Stories*, Aug. 13, 2002. "The principle of go-and-see is as old as UNHCR itself, and aims at refugees making an on-the-spot assessment of the security situation, interacting with their relatives, seeing the state of their properties. The visits also ensure that there are adequate facilities in the areas of return – such as education, health, water supply and any other facilities necessary": "Repatriation of refugees from Botswana to Namibia begins," *UN Integrated Regional Information Networks*, Aug. 14, 2002.

[182] J. Steele, "Afghan exile puts his mind at his country's service," *Guardian*, June 19, 2002, at 13.

strong a motivation for refugees to opt for return at a time when conditions in Afghanistan were still far from secure.[183] A comparable Australian plan was even more aggressive, offering Afghan refugee families their cost of travel and a grant of up to A$10,000 to go home – a sum amounting to five years' income for the average Afghan. In announcing the program, the Immigration Minister gave refugees only twenty-eight days to accept the offer, with the warning that any Afghans not ultimately recognized as refugees would be subject to mandatory return without compensation.[184]

While such plans have been encouraged by UNHCR,[185] they raise the specter of an infringement of the cardinal requirement of voluntariness in a refugee's decision to go home. There may in practice be very little real space for self-determination when a poor refugee is offered a sum of money significantly beyond his or her own financial dreams, leading to allegations of bribery or blackmail.[186] Particularly when such an offer must be accepted within a short timeframe, and is made when conditions in the home country are not objectively safe,[187] there is reason to be concerned that a superficially generous offer may unfairly skew what should be a genuinely voluntary decision by the refugee to give up his or her protected status.

Fundamentally, a voluntary decision to go home should be a decision reached without external inducement, and certainly without coercion of any kind. In contrast, Burundian refugees in Tanzania reported that they returned home despite uncertainty about the security situation there in part because "they

---

[183] A. Travis, "Afghans offered £2,500 to go home," *Guardian*, Aug. 21, 2002, at 1.

[184] K. Lawson, "Afghan detainees to be offered $2,000 each to go home," *Canberra Times*, May 24, 2002, at A-3.

[185] Human Rights Watch, "Afghanistan Unsafe for Refugee Returns – UN Refugee Agency Sending 'Misleading' Message," July 23, 2002.

[186] This allegation was reportedly made by Simon O'Neil, a spokesperson for the Australian Refugee Action Collective: P. Barkham, "Australia offers Afghan asylum-seekers £3,800 to go home," *Guardian*, May 24, 2002, at 6.

[187] Even as the British and Australian plans to encourage Afghan repatriation were being promoted, for example, "Human Rights Watch investigations in recent months have found that conditions inside Afghanistan are still extremely unstable and that risk of persecution exists for certain groups. Continuing factional rivalry between General Abdul Rashid Dostrum's Junbish forces and General Atta Mohammed's Jamiat troops has created a security vacuum in northern Afghanistan, leading to a rise in attacks on humanitarian aid agencies and Afghan civilians. Armed conflict between the two factions has increased over a wider area of the north in recent weeks, affecting at least four different districts during the week of July 8. At the same time, ethnic Pashtuns, a minority in the north, continue to flee targeted violence, rapes of women and children, seizure of farmland and demands of money by local commanders in Farah and Faryab province. Human Rights Watch has also documented ongoing lawlessness and abuses by warlord forces in the south and west of the country": Human Rights Watch, "Afghanistan Unsafe for Refugee Returns – UN Refugee Agency Sending 'Misleading' Message," July 23, 2002.

were being 'encouraged' by Tanzania to go home."[188] It later came to light that the "encouragement" included actions in violation of international law, such as limiting access by the refugees to food rations, and restricting their movements outside of refugee camps.[189] The decision of some Angolan refugees to return home from Zambia was similarly tainted by a policy of cutbacks in food rations in the camps.[190] Despite the movement having been characterized by officials as a "spontaneous return," one returning refugee saw matters quite differently:

> We left Mahewa [refugee camp] to come here because there was no food there ... When we first went there, we got enough food. But later we suffered as the food we received was not enough. We thought, let's go back to our country, which could be better.[191]

In such circumstances, return cannot truly be said to be voluntary, with the result that the standard for cessation under Art. 1(C)(4) is not met, and refugee status does not come to an end. Indeed, violations of refugee rights as a tool of coercion can readily amount to acts of indirect *refoulement*.[192]

Importantly, refugee status does not come to an end simply because a refugee chooses, even with complete freedom, to return to his or her country of origin. The second requirement for valid cessation of refugee status is that the refugee be not just physically inside the country of origin, but rather that he or she be *reestablished* there. The original draft of this provision, which would have revoked the refugee status of any person who "returns to his country of former nationality,"[193] was rejected by the Ad Hoc Committee on the grounds that it might bar persons who had been forcibly repatriated to their state of origin, as well as those who had chosen to return to their country of origin only temporarily.[194] The substitute language, which sets the

---

[188] "Another 800 refugees to return home to Burundi," *UN Integrated Regional Information Networks*, May 30, 2002.

[189] "Burundian refugees returning home from Tanzania," (2003) 135 *JRS Dispatches* (July 1, 2003).

[190] "'Of course some refugees told us they will be returning to Angola because the half-ration of the food was not good for them,' [UNHCR local representative] Gubartalla told a news conference in Lusaka. 'But I believe that if we did not have the cease-fire and the peace process starting in Angola, nobody would have ... come and said they want to go back to Angola'": "Thousands of Angolan refugees living in Zambia return home," *SAPA-AP*, June 13, 2002.

[191] "Refugees returning, but little aid available," *UN Integrated Regional Information Networks*, July 5, 2002. "Officials are talking about a 'spontaneous' return. But it was prompted not only by a longing to be on home soil, but also by recent cutbacks in rations to refugees in the camps in Zambia": ibid.

[192] See chapter 4.1.2 above, at pp. 318–321.

[193] UN Doc. E/AC.32/L.4, Jan. 18, 1950, at 3.

[194] See e.g. Statement of the Director of the International Refugee Organization, UN Doc. E/AC.32/L.16, Jan. 30, 1950, at 2. In the result, the decision of the Swiss Federal Court in the *Romanian Refugee Case*, 72 ILR 580 (Sw. FC, Mar. 3, 1969), at 581, holding that "[w]here

cessation threshold at voluntary reestablishment in the country of origin,[195] was thus intended to ensure that only persons who have willingly resettled in their state of origin are subject to cessation of refugee status. As Weis observed, "[i]f a person returns to his country of origin for a temporary stay without re-establishing himself, and then returns to the country where he was recognized as a refugee, this should not lead to *ipso facto* loss of refugee status."[196]

It is therefore incumbent on state parties to afford refugees the opportunity to explain the reasons for their trip home, which may or may not evince reestablishment there. For example, a tribunal sensibly determined that the return of a Salvadoran refugee for two-and-a-half months in order to attempt to save her marriage did not amount to reestablishment there. In particular, there was evidence that she had never stayed more than three nights in the same place, had avoided public transportation, had identified herself as a foreigner, and had prepared answers to questions which might have exposed her real identity.[197] A similarly exceptional and transient presence was found to exist in the case of a Sri Lankan refugee who had returned home briefly to care for his ill mother.[198] In general, the potential for reestablishment arises either where the refugee has been present in the home state for a prolonged period of time, or regularly returns there for shorter periods of time. In such circumstances, the refugee bears the onus to demonstrate that he or she is objectively unable to benefit from protection of basic human rights in the country of origin, and thus continues to be a refugee.

Most critically, it would work against the goal of promoting autonomous solutions to refugee status for Art. 1(C)(4) to be treated as the basis for penalizing refugees who return home to "test the waters" in their country of origin. If refugees are to be encouraged to attempt to return home, they must have some assurance that they can resume refugee status in the event

---

a refugee returns, even temporarily, to the State from which he fled and thereby submits himself to its power, he expresses his conviction that the essential ground for obtaining the status of refugee – a well-founded fear of being persecuted – has disappeared," should be viewed as bad law. While it is legally doubtful that there is truly a subjective element to refugee status at all (see Hathaway, *Refugee Status*, at 66–75), whatever implications might arguably be drawn from a "subjective element" should in any event not be allowed to contradict the clear language and history of Art. 1(C)(4) of the Refugee Convention.

[195] Statement of Mr. Henkin of the United States, UN Doc. E/AC.7/SR.165, Aug. 19, 1950, at 16. The amendment was adopted on a vote of 13–0 (2 abstentions): ibid. at 18, and was addressed to the situations of both persons with formal nationality, and those who are stateless.

[196] P. Weis, "The Concept of the Refugee in International Law," (1960) 87 *Journal du Droit International* 928, at 978.

[197] *C89–00332* (Can. IRB, Aug. 27, 1991), reported at (1991) 5 *RefLex* 41.

[198] *Shanmugarajah v. Canada*, (1992) FCJ 583 (Can. FC, June 22, 1992). See also *Mitroi v. Canada*, (1995) FCJ 216 (Can. FC, Feb. 8, 1995), where no adverse inference was drawn from the decision of a refugee from Romania briefly to travel to that country as a tourist.

that actual conditions at home prove unviable for a safe reintegration. The drafters' insistence on evidence of reestablishment, rather than simply of return, sensibly ensures that this critical objective is safeguarded.

7.3 Resettlement

If a refugee cannot lawfully be repatriated and does not choose freely to resume life in his or her own country, a third solution to refugee status is for the refugee to move to another state which is willing to grant him or her a durable form of immigrant status. Resettlement has traditionally been contemplated either because the state in which a refugee first arrives declines to provide ongoing protection, or because a refugee wishes to make his or her home in some other country.

> **Refugee Convention, Art. 30   Transfer of assets**
>
> 1. A Contracting State shall, in conformity with its laws and regulations, permit refugees to transfer assets which they have brought into its territory, to another country where they have been admitted for the purposes of resettlement.
>
> 2. A Contracting State shall give sympathetic consideration to the application of refugees for permission to transfer assets wherever they may be and which are necessary for their resettlement in another country to which they have been admitted.

> **Refugee Convention, Art. 31   Refugees unlawfully in the country of refuge**
>
> . . .
>
> 2. The Contracting States shall not apply to the movements of [refugees coming directly from a territory where their life or freedom was threatened] restrictions other than those which are necessary and such restrictions shall only be applied until their status in the country is regularized or they obtain admission into another country. The Contracting States shall allow such refugees a reasonable period and all the necessary facilities to obtain admission into another country.

The first form of resettlement, based on the absence of a durable solution in the first country of arrival,[199] was foreseen as early as the 1936 and 1938

---

[199] As the representative of Italy noted in the Ad Hoc Committee, "[a]s a matter of fact, the question of naturalizing refugees did not generally arise in his country which, by reason of its geographical position and of certain other special considerations, could only offer them temporary hospitality": Statement of Mr. Malfatti of Italy, UN Doc. E/AC.32/SR.39, Aug. 21, 1950, at 29.

Refugee Conventions. In each case, it was agreed that any refugee required to leave a state's territory "shall be granted a suitable period to make the necessary arrangements."[200] Indeed, the 1938 Convention,[201] and more particularly the refugee regimes administered by the Intergovernmental Committee for Refugees (IGCR) and the International Refugee Organization (IRO), assumed that there was little likelihood that refugees would be accommodated in the first asylum country.[202] Under these arrangements, most persons recognized as refugees were instead expected to resettle in overseas states.

There has been a recent renaissance of interest by some governments in mandatory resettlement schemes similar to those pioneered by the IGCR and IRO. A crucial difference, however, is that these new initiatives have been conceived and operated by particular states, rather than by an international refugee agency. Most (in)famously, the so-called "Pacific Solution" administered by the Australian government saw refugees arriving to seek its protection being diverted for status assessment outside its territory, and presented with no alternative to accepting offers of resettlement negotiated on their behalf.[203] A similar initiative was proposed in 2003 by the British government, which sought to have refugees arriving in the European Union sent for processing to a non-EU country from which resettlement into the Union would be arranged for persons recognized as genuine refugees.[204] Both the UNHCR and an informal grouping of core members of the European Union, in addition to Australia, Canada, New Zealand, Norway, Switzerland, and the United States – the Intergovernmental Consultations on Refugees, Asylum and Migration Policies – have since taken up the call to devise organized resettlement schemes as part of a broader agenda to reform the mechanisms of refugee protection.[205]

---

[200] Provisional Arrangement concerning the Status of Refugees coming from Germany, 3952 LNTS 77, done July 4, 1936 (1936 Refugee Convention), at Art. 4(1); Convention concerning the Status of Refugees coming from Germany, 4461 LNTS 61, done Feb. 10, 1938 (1938 Refugee Convention), at Art. 5(1).

[201] "With a view to facilitating the emigration of refugees to oversea countries, every facility shall be granted to the refugees and to the organizations which deal with them for the establishment of schools for professional re-adaptation and technical training": 1938 Refugee Convention, at Art. 15.

[202] See generally J. Hathaway, "The Evolution of Refugee Status in International Law: 1920–1950," (1984) 33 *International and Comparative Law Quarterly* 348.

[203] Australia, Department of Immigration and Multicultural Affairs, "Refugees and Humanitarian Issues: Australia's Response" (Oct. 2001), at 5.

[204] The plan was designed "to achieve better management of the asylum process globally through improved management and transit processing centres": Letter from Tony Blair, UK Prime Minister, to Costas Smitis, European Council President, Mar. 10, 2003.

[205] The evolution of these recent initiatives is summarized in J. Hathaway, "Review Essay: N. Nathwani, Rethinking Refugee Law," (2004) 98(3) *American Journal of International Law* 616.

Such programs can in theory be operated without infringing the Refugee Convention if the non-consensual diversion into a resettlement scheme occurs before the refugee concerned is "lawfully in" a state party[206] and hence entitled to the more elaborate protections against expulsion found in Art. 32. So long as the requirements of Art. 33 (*non-refoulement*) are scrupulously observed, a refugee not yet lawfully in a state may be required to accept resettlement to another country, even one not of his or her choosing.[207] Importantly, however, a state which detains or otherwise restricts the movement of refugees pending their removal for purposes of status assessment or resettlement abroad is bound to respect the requirements of Art. 31(2) of the Refugee Convention, previously analyzed in some detail.[208] In particular, mirroring the provisions of the 1936 and 1938 treaties, "[t]he Contracting States shall allow such refugees a reasonable period and all the necessary facilities to obtain admission into another country."[209]

By virtue of this obligation, a refugee is legally entitled to an opportunity to devise his or her own resettlement solution before being required to accept the government's option. In particular, the refugee may insist upon a delay in his or her removal to enable him or her to pursue alternative resettlement options. Faced with such a request, the host government must suspend pursuit of its own plan for a "reasonable period," meaning "the period necessary to obtain a visa by a refugee who makes all reasonable efforts to obtain such a visa, possibly with the help of UNHCR or voluntary organizations."[210] As Robinson and Grahl-Madsen affirm, the definition of a "reasonable period" must further take into account all "existing circumstances," including the time required to process a resettlement application "for a person without a nationality and possessing given qualifications (skills, age, etc.)."[211]

In addition, the host state must ensure that the refugee has access to "all the necessary facilities to obtain admission into another country."[212] Thus, the refugee must "not be [so] restricted in his movement as not to [be able] to see foreign consulates, the representatives of UNHCR, or voluntary agencies."[213] While not ruling out the possibility of keeping the refugee in provisional

---

[206] See chapter 3.1.3 above, at pp. 175–183.

[207] See chapter 5.1 above and J. Hathaway, "Refugee Law is Not Immigration Law," (2002) *Proceedings of the Canadian Council on International Law* 134, edited version reprinted in US Committee for Refugees, *World Refugee Survey 2002* (2002), at 38.

[208] See chapter 4.2.4 above.   [209] Refugee Convention, at Art. 31(2).

[210] P. Weis, *The Refugee Convention, 1951: The Travaux Préparatoires Analysed with a Commentary by Dr. Paul Weis* (posthumously pub'd., 1995) (Weis, *Travaux*), at 304.

[211] N. Robinson, *Convention relating to the Status of Refugees: Its History, Contents and Interpretation* (1953) (Robinson, *History*), at 155; A. Grahl-Madsen, *Commentary on the Refugee Convention 1951* (1963, pub'd. 1997) (Grahl-Madsen, *Commentary*), at 184.

[212] Refugee Convention, at Art. 31(2).   [213] Weis, *Travaux*, at 304.

detention,[214] this obligation "will as a rule exclude confinement in a camp or prison or in remote places, and require the state to permit the refugee to travel and to communicate with the outside world and such bodies as are likely to assist him in obtaining admission into a country."[215]

There are therefore two fundamental challenges in the operation of a lawful mandatory resettlement system. First, the requirements of Art. 31(2) may detract from the efficient operation of such a system: unless those to be removed are not detained or otherwise restricted in their movements while under the receiving state's authority, they must be afforded the means and opportunity to pursue their preferred resettlement options. Second, the window of opportunity for such efforts is in any event quite short. It ends once lawful presence (not lawful stay) is established,[216] at which point the strict limitations on expulsion set by Art. 32 apply so as to make enforced resettlement unviable in most cases.[217]

Perhaps because of the legal difficulties inherent in mandatory resettlement, most resettlement is in practice effected with the consent of the refugee concerned. So long as resettlement is freely agreed to, there is no breach of the Refugee Convention. To the contrary, in line with Art. 12 of the Civil and Political Covenant, analyzed above,[218] any person – including a refugee – has the right to decide to leave any country, including a state of asylum.

Apart from the special steps required by Art. 31(2) when a refugee's freedom of movement has been curtailed, the country from which resettlement is contemplated is not ordinarily obliged to take affirmative steps to assist him or her to secure a resettlement offer.[219] Moreover, in line with the commitment of the drafters to safeguarding the sovereign right of states to decide which refugees should be permanently admitted to their territories,[220]

---

[214] Grahl-Madsen, *Commentary*, at 184.   [215] Robinson, *History*, at 155.

[216] Lawful presence (as contrasted with lawful stay) is a status that is usually quickly acquired. Lawful presence includes authorized temporary presence; presence while undergoing refugee status assessment, including the exhaustion of appeals and reviews; and presence in a state party to the Convention which has opted either not to establish a procedure to verify refugee status, or to suspend the operation of such a procedure: see chapter 3.1.3 above.

[217] A refugee entitled to the benefit of Art. 32 may not be removed from a state party "save on grounds of national security or public order" and subject to a variety of due process guarantees: see chapter 5.1 above. Moreover, once Art. 32 is applicable, para. 3 of the article imposes the same sort of duty of delay on expulsion to allow the refugee to arrange his or her preferred alternative that is foreseen by Art. 31(2).

[218] See chapter 7.2 above, at pp. 954–958.

[219] In the case of refugee seamen, however, governments do agree to "give sympathetic consideration to . . . the issue of travel documents to them or their temporary admission to [their] territory particularly with a view to facilitating their establishment in another country": Refugee Convention, at Art. 11.

[220] See chapter 4.1 above, at pp. 300–301.

no state is obliged to make an offer of resettlement to any refugee. The actual mechanics of the resettlement process are largely unregulated by the Refugee Convention.

The Refugee Convention nonetheless requires the facilitation of resettlement to a very limited degree. Under Art. 30, a refugee taking up an offer of resettlement enjoys certain privileges with respect to the export of assets to the resettlement state. The approach first advocated by Belgium would have entitled refugees being resettled to "take with them any funds which belong to them and which they might require for the purpose of settlement."[221] As proposed, this right was subject only to compliance with any "formalities prescribed ... with regard to the export and import of currencies."[222] The Belgian initiative sought to counter two related concerns. In some cases refugees were unable to convert their assets into hard currencies that would be honored in their resettlement state.[223] Even more seriously, some countries where the refugees' funds were held simply refused or significantly limited their export.[224] If subject to restrictions of this kind, it was clear that refugees seeking to make a new home would be effectively deprived of the benefit of their own resources.[225]

None of the drafters took serious issue with the basic premise of the Belgian initiative. As the American representative to the Conference of Plenipotentiaries observed, "[i]t was surely only fair that a refugee should be able to take out of the country of asylum whatever assets he had brought into it, as well as any money that he might have earned."[226] Moreover, while some were opposed to granting refugees treatment more favorable than that

---

[221] "Belgium: Proposed New Article," UN Doc. E/AC.32/L.24, Feb. 2, 1950.

[222] Ibid.

[223] "Australia was often used by refugees as a place of temporary residence before they re-settled elsewhere. Such refugees brought in money in various currencies. The Australian Government could not interpret [the proposed article] as overruling national laws and regulations in respect of hard currencies": Statement of Mr. Shaw of Australia, UN Doc. A/CONF.2/SR.13, July 10, 1951, at 10.

[224] "Extremely rigid currency control had been introduced in the United Kingdom not only to consolidate the country's economy, but in the interests of all countries. A person leaving the United Kingdom to settle in another country could transfer funds belonging to him up to a specified amount": Statement of Sir Leslie Brass of the United Kingdom, UN Doc. E/AC.32/SR.24, Feb. 3, 1950, at 7.

[225] In a 1991 UNHCR survey of state practice, a number of governments indicated that they still impose general restrictions on the export of foreign currency and other items of value. No government, however, imposed restrictions specifically on asset transfer by refugees: UNHCR, "Information Note on Implementation of the 1951 Convention and the 1967 Protocol relating to the Status of Refugees," UN Doc. EC/SCP/66, July 22, 1991 (UNHCR, "Implementation"), at para. 95.

[226] Statement of Mr. Warren of the United States, UN Doc. A/CONF.2/SR.13, July 10, 1951, at 10.

accorded other would-be migrants,[227] most drafters felt that the special predicament of refugees justified a more generous approach to the issue of asset transfer.[228]

There was, though, real concern that if the Convention were fully to "lift in the case of a refugee the restrictions imposed ... on the transfer of assets,"[229] the impact on the still-fragile, postwar economies of state parties could be severe. As the French representative argued,

> [T]he Belgian proposal might permit a somewhat artificially stimulated export of capital. Exchange control regulations were based on very serious considerations, which could hardly be set aside for the humanitarian reasons advanced by the Belgian representative ... Furthermore, application of the provisions recommended by the Belgian delegation might set very powerful financial interests in motion and make Governments liable to thaw without previous notice holdings which they had reasonably regarded as frozen.[230]

To meet these concerns, the Belgian proposal was reframed to require refugees wishing to export capital from the state of first asylum to comply not simply with export "formalities," but more generally with the "laws and regulations" of the host country.[231] It was nonetheless noted immediately

---

[227] The Canadian representative to the Ad Hoc Committee complained of the restrictions on capital transfers from the United Kingdom, which impeded immigration from that country. He was worried that "[a]daption of the Belgian proposal might give the impression that the Committee had wished to obtain more favourable treatment for refugees than accorded to nationals of the States signatory to the Convention": Statement of Mr. Chance of Canada, UN Doc. E/AC.32/SR.24, Feb. 3, 1950, at 8. Turkey agreed, noting that "the humanitarian considerations which the Belgian representative would like to see applied in favour of the refugees might well be applied to the nationals of a State who wished to settle on the territory of another State. If that were so, it was difficult to grant refugees a privilege which was refused to nationals": Statement of Mr. Kural of Turkey, ibid. at 9.

[228] At the Conference of Plenipotentiaries, the Egyptian representative inquired "whether the purpose of the Convention was to ensure that refugees should be given more favourable treatment than that enjoyed by aliens": Statement of Mr. Mostafa of Egypt, UN Doc. A/CONF.2/SR.13, July 10, 1951, at 10. The President of the Conference then "emphasized that the Ad Hoc Committee had wished to ensure that the conditions imposed on refugees should be less stringent than those imposed on nationals and other aliens": Statement of the President, Mr. Larsen of Denmark, ibid. See also Statement of Mr. Zutter of Switzerland, ibid. at 6.

[229] This was precisely the goal advanced by the Belgian proponent: Statement of Mr. Herment of Belgium, ibid. at 5.

[230] Statement of Mr. Devinat of France, UN Doc. E/AC.32/SR.24, Feb. 3, 1950, at 9.

[231] The American representative explicitly acknowledged that the article "had been somewhat weakened ... [so as to] induce some members to withdraw their reservations": Statement of Mr. Henkin of the United States, UN Doc. E/AC.32/SR.25, Feb. 10, 1950, at 10.

prior to the adoption of this change that "[i]t was to be hoped, however, that Contracting States would make appropriate changes in their laws and regulations so as to accord protection to refugees in the matter of the transfer of assets."[232] The positions taken at the Conference of Plenipotentiaries were to similar effect. The President of the Conference affirmed that states had a "duty to help a refugee to resettle permanently."[233] It would not be enough to apply existing currency control and related rules fairly to refugees; the rationale for Art. 30, framed in "mandatory terms in the interest of refugees,"[234] was rather to make clear that general rules must be applied to refugees with generous use of discretion.[235]

Despite the real value to refugees of these points of consensus, Robinson likely overstates the force of Art. 30. In his view, the right of state parties to invoke their laws and regulations "do[es] not free a Contracting State from its obligation to permit the transfer of assets ... even if it generally prohibits transfers in favor of other aliens or nationals, since the obligation is of a categorical nature":

> These words were inserted to regulate the manner of the transfer. In other words, the words ["in conformity with its laws and regulations"] require a refugee to obtain a license if such a document is required; they may in certain cases militate against total transfer at once if amounts of such magnitude cannot generally be exported in one lump sum; the transfer in certain currency may be subject to restrictions or can be made only through the intermediary of a certain agency or a payment union, if this is a general rule, etc. *A state, however, cannot refuse to permit the transfer if all such formalities are complied with*, on the grounds of lack of exchange or that other aliens or their own nationals do not enjoy the right of transfer [emphasis added].[236]

But this interpretation seems insufficiently attentive to the reasons for amending Art. 30 to include the "laws and regulations" proviso. In particular, there was real concern expressed that it would be going too far to require refugees only to comply with export "formalities," since this could be taken to suggest that no substantive limits of any kind could be set on the export of assets by a refugee.[237] Grahl-Madsen impliedly acknowledges as much, suggesting that the

---

[232] Ibid.

[233] Statement of the President, Mr. Larsen of Denmark, UN Doc. A/CONF.2/SR.13, July 10, 1951, at 7.

[234] Statement of Mr. Hoare of the United Kingdom, ibid. at 6.

[235] Statement of Mr. Hoare of the United Kingdom, ibid. at 6.

[236] Robinson, *History*, at 149–150.

[237] "[T]he Belgian proposal seemed to imply that a refugee need only apply, in accordance with the formalities prescribed by law, for authorization to export funds belonging to him, for the Government concerned to be obliged to give him such authorization": Statement of Sir Leslie Brass of the United Kingdom, UN Doc. E/AC.32/SR.24, Feb. 3, 1950, at 7.

proviso allows state parties "to prescribe a reasonable transformation of the assets to be taken out of the country."[238] Weis is still more explicit:

> The words "in conformity with its laws and regulations" do[] not mean that the application of these laws and regulations, particularly currency regulations, may frustrate the mandatory obligation. They have to be applied in such a way as to make the transfer possible, but there may be limitations such as . . . that the transfer shall take place in instalments or not in hard currency.[239]

Thus, host governments are not legally prevented from applying substantive, rather than simply formal, requirements on the export of a refugee's assets. But because it would frustrate the essential rationale of Art. 30 simply to apply all general rules with their full intensity,[240] state parties are legally bound to interpret and apply their general rules in a way that facilitates the transfer of assets for resettling refugees.[241]

Despite the relatively weak nature of the basic obligation in Art. 30(1), the scope of state obligations was expanded over the course of deliberations in at least two respects. First, on the basis of an American proposal, the right of export was broadened from simply a right to export "funds" to include the right to export all forms of "assets."[242] Second, it was made clear that the duty of the host state to permit the transfer of assets applies not simply to whatever assets actually accompanied the refugee upon arrival there, but to any assets brought into that state by the refugee at any time.[243] As the President of the

---

[238] Grahl-Madsen, *Commentary*, at 165.   [239] Weis, *Travaux*, at 277.

[240] "He appealed to the Committee to retain at least the idea upon which the Belgian proposal had been based and to seek the formula which would be of the greatest possible humanitarian value to the refugees and most acceptable to Governments": Statement of Mr. Cuvelier of Belgium, UN Doc. E/AC.32/SR.24, Feb. 3, 1950, at 9.

[241] "The purpose of paragraph 1 [is] to ensure that a refugee who entered a country with the intention and possibility of ultimately settling elsewhere should not be deprived of the material assets he had been able to bring with him, since such assets might be of considerable help to him in settling overseas": Statement of Mr. Chance of Canada, UN Doc. A/CONF.2/SR.13, July 10, 1951, at 6. See Weis, *Travaux*, at 277: "[Art. 30(1)] contains a mandatory obligation . . . [Domestic rules] have to be applied in such a way as to make the transfer possible, but there may be limitations such as . . . that the transfer shall take place in instalments or not in hard currency'; and Grahl-Madsen, *Commentary*, at 165: "Even [though] it was agreed to soften the original phraseology, it was clearly not the intention of the drafters to weaken the provision so much that it would make transfer of the assets concerned wholly subject to the discretion of the authorities."

[242] "[T]he article proposed by the Belgian delegation covered only currency belonging to the refugee, whereas they might have other forms of property. The wording of the article should, therefore, be amended": Statement of Mr. Henkin of the United States, UN Doc. E/AC.32/SR.24, Feb. 3, 1950, at 10.

[243] UNHCR convinced delegates to the Conference of Plenipotentiaries that the French language text – which spoke of a right to "transférer les avoirs qu'ils ont fait entrer sur leur territoire" – was preferable to the English language version, which then spoke of "assets

Conference of Plenipotentiaries put it, "the intention of the Ad Hoc Committee had been to allow the refugee to take out of the country of asylum the money and assets that he owned. It would not be fair to interpret the position in terms only of such assets as a refugee might have in his pocket."[244]

The drafters also broadened the scope of the article in ways that resulted in the addition of paragraph 2. France persuaded the Ad Hoc Committee that the Convention should promote the right of refugees to transfer not only assets held in the country from which resettlement is being effected (the subject of para. 1), but also assets held in any state party:[245]

> [I]f the Committee wished to recommend that the High Contracting Parties should grant facilities for the export of capital belonging to refugees, the recommendation should cover not only cases in which the refugee passed through the country where his property was before travelling to the country in which he settled, but also those in which a High Contracting Party withheld property belonging to a foreigner who, whatever the country in which he was, had acquired refugee status and had made an application in accordance with a procedure to be determined.[246]

Similarly, the view was expressed that the article should address the right of refugees to export not only assets brought into the first asylum state, but also assets acquired there.[247]

There was, however, no serious interest in imposing a specific, binding obligation to require states to permit the transfer of either assets acquired in the present state of residence,[248] or those located in other

---

which he has brought with him": Statement of Mr. van Heuven Goedhart of UNHCR, UN Doc. A/CONF.2/SR.13, July 10, 1951, at 7. Grahl-Madsen thus concludes that "[p]aragraph 1 applies to any and all assets which the refugee concerned has brought into the territory of a Contracting State, regardless of whether he brought the assets with him when he came to apply for asylum, or if he brought the assets into the country concerned before or after that time": Grahl-Madsen, *Commentary*, at 166.

[244] Statement of the President, Mr. Larsen of Denmark, UN Doc. A/CONF.2/SR.13, July 10, 1951, at 7–8.

[245] "[T]here was no apparent reason why refugees who had been able to go to the country in which they possessed property before settling in the country of final residence should be accorded treatment differing from that of refugees who had gone to a country other than that in which their property was": Statement of Mr. Devinat of France, UN Doc. E/AC.32/SR.24, Feb. 3, 1950, at 9.

[246] Ibid. at 10.

[247] "[D]uring his period of residence in the country of asylum a refugee might earn money. Should he not be allowed to transfer his earnings?": Statement of the President, Mr. Larsen of Denmark, UN Doc. A/CONF.2/SR.13, July 10, 1951, at 8.

[248] "[G]overnments would be reluctant to permit a refugee to export a larger sum than he had brought in for fear of injuring the general economy of the country and of encouraging the illegal export of capital": Statement of Mr. Kural of Turkey, UN Doc. E/AC.32/SR.24, Feb. 3, 1950, at 8. In response, Belgium proposed that "the Committee might

countries.[249] Despite Colombian opposition to adoption of a mere duty of process on the grounds of "the futility of wishes, no doubt full of goodwill but not mandatory in character,"[250] the drafters took precisely this approach. They agreed that the binding duty of the state from which the refugee intends to resettle (stated in para. 1) would be supplemented by a second paragraph addressed to all states, requiring them to "give sympathetic consideration" to a resettling refugee's application to transfer all forms of assets "wherever they may be."[251]

request Governments to show the greatest possible latitude in certain exceptional cases, in order to prevent refusals based upon the strict letter of existing laws": Statement of Mr. Cuvelier of Belgium, ibid. at 10.

[249] In the Ad Hoc Committee it was agreed "that the article should be divided into two paragraphs, the first laying down the principle that the refugee could take with him any property he had brought with him, and the second incorporating *the recommendation* to the High Contracting Parties [emphasis added]": Statement of Mr. Cuvelier of Belgium, ibid. at 11. Grahl-Madsen disputes this view, suggesting that "[i]t is noteworthy that paragraph 1 does not specify that the refugee concerned must himself be staying in the country where the assets are. The Contracting States have *the same obligations* towards refugees who have never set foot on their territory, but merely brought funds into it, as [they have] towards refugees who have stayed for a shorter or longer period in the country [emphasis added]": Grahl-Madsen, *Commentary*, at 166. This interpretation is, however, inconsistent with the drafting history that resulted in the addition of para. 2 to Art. 30. It also renders the purpose of para. 2 unclear. As Weis observes, "[p]aragraph 2 applies to all other assets, that is, those the refugee has acquired in the country of residence *or those which he possesses in the territory of other Contracting States* [emphasis added]": Weis, *Travaux*, at 277. Indeed, Grahl-Madsen himself concedes that his interpretation renders "the words 'wherever they may be' in paragraph 2 . . . more or less redundant", as para. 2 would apply only to "assets [in the refugee's state of residence] . . . acquired by labour, inheritance, or in any other lawful way": Grahl-Madsen, *Commentary*, at 167.

[250] Statement of Mr. Giraldo-Jaramillo of Colombia, UN Doc. A/CONF.2/SR.13, July 10, 1951, at 5.

[251] Refugee Convention, at Art. 30(2). The President of the Conference of Plenipotentiaries provided a helpful example of how Art. 30(2) should be applied in practice. "[T]he attitude of countries towards the export of funds by resident nationals or aliens inevitably depended on their currency position; for instance, States which suffered from a dollar shortage could not allow the export of dollars. Thus, a refugee who owned property in Denmark would not be able, on emigrating, to change the Danish currency he got from the sale of that property into dollars, but in the Danish Government's view it would be unfair to deprive a refugee of dollars which he had brought into Denmark and wished to take with him on emigrating, even if he had in the meantime sold those dollars in accordance with the Danish currency regulations. That, indeed, had been the attitude taken by the Ad Hoc Committee, and it was for that reason, and in order to cover such cases, that paragraph 2 had been included in article [30]": Statement of the President, Mr. Larsen of Denmark, UN Doc. A/CONF.2/SR.13, July 10, 1951, at 8–9. Despite the provisions of Art. 30(2), only one government indicated that it renders assistance to refugees in order to facilitate the transfer of their property upon departure from the country: UNHCR, "Implementation," at para. 95.

Two important qualifications should be noted with regard to Art. 30 as a whole. First, the provision does not purport to establish any general right of refugees to export their assets.[252] The duty in paragraph 1 applies only to transfers "to another country where they have been admitted for the purposes of resettlement."[253] Similarly, the obligation of sympathetic consideration in the second paragraph governs only such assets as "are necessary for their resettlement in another country to which they have been admitted."

Second, Art. 30 can under no circumstance be relied upon to justify granting refugees rights inferior to those of other non-citizens.[254] At the Conference of Plenipotentiaries, the representative of Colombia proposed an alternative formulation under which refugees would simply have the same rights to export assets as enjoyed by aliens generally.[255] In doing so, he expressed his concern that any "privileged" treatment for refugees could in fact be used as a pretext to restrict their options.[256] His amendment was withdrawn, however, based on the understanding that "refugees could in no case be treated less favourably than aliens, since that was expressly forbidden by article [7(1)] of the Convention."[257]

In sum, and in line with the remarks of the President of the Conference of Plenipotentiaries, two different kinds of obligation under Art. 30 can be identified.[258] First, whatever assets a refugee has brought into the state where he or she presently lives – whether the refugee arrived with those assets, or had them transferred to that state before or after entering as a refugee – should in principle be completely available for export by the refugee to his or her resettlement country. While the host state may apply its currency control

---

[252] See Robinson, *History*, at 149: "It imposes an obligation upon the Contracting States to permit the transfer of assets of refugees, provided these assets have been brought in by the refugee and the transfer is made to another country where he has been admitted for resettlement. Thus no obligation exists in cases where the refugee leaves the country of his residence for a temporary stay abroad"; and Grahl-Madsen, *Commentary*, at 166: "The Contracting States are not obliged to permit transfers of assets to any country of the refugee's choice, but merely to a country where the refugee concerned has been admitted for the purpose of resettlement."

[253] "[T]he Committee seemed to be in agreement that refugees who were so to speak in transit through a country could export the possessions they had brought with them to the country of final resettlement": Statement of Mr. Henkin of the United States, UN Doc. E/AC.32/SR.24, Feb. 3, 1950, at 10.

[254] See Grahl-Madsen, *Commentary*, at 164: "Article 30 must be read in conjunction with Article 7(1). Should the regime established for refugees by virtue of Article 30 in any set of circumstances not correspond to the same treatment as is accorded to aliens generally, [the refugee] may invoke the provisions set forth in Article 7(1)."

[255] UN Doc. A/CONF.2/54.

[256] Statements of Mr. Giraldo-Jaramillo of Colombia, UN Doc. A/CONF.2/SR.13, July 10, 1951, at 5–6, 9.

[257] Statement of Mr. Herment of Belgium, ibid. at 11.

[258] See Statement of the President, Mr. Larsen of Denmark, ibid. at 7–8.

and comparable regulations, it is bound to interpret those rules generously in the spirit of advancing the presumed entitlement of a refugee to "take out of the country of asylum whatever assets he had brought into it."[259] As Grahl-Madsen succinctly concludes, "[t]he underlying idea is that a State shall be neither richer nor poorer as a result of the fact that a refugee has spent a transitory period in the country until he found a possibility for resettlement in another country."[260]

Second, whatever assets a refugee acquired in the original host state (e.g. by savings from employment, investment, etc.), as well as assets held in other state parties, should also, in principle, be made available for export to the resettlement state. But the obligation of state parties in regard to the export of such assets is simply one of process – namely, sympathetic consideration. In contrast to the duty of result with regard to assets brought into the country of current residence, the Convention does not require governments to operate from a presumption that their ordinary rules should be applied less rigorously in the case of refugees undertaking resettlement.[261] In no case, however, may a refugee be treated less well than aliens generally with regard to the ability to export his or her assets.

In both political and practical terms, the importance of resettlement as a solution for refugees declined dramatically during the 1980s and 1990s.[262] As recently as the late 1970s resettlement was still highly valued by the international community: it was endorsed by the UNHCR Executive Committee as the logical alternative solution when local integration of refugees was not possible,[263] and was in fact the solution for about 5 percent of the world's

---

[259] Statement of Mr. Warren of the United States, ibid. at 10.

[260] Grahl-Madsen, *Commentary*, at 166.

[261] In at least one resolution, the UNHCR Executive Committee seems to have failed to make this distinction. In the context of its leading statement of the duties which follow in the event of a mass influx of refugees, the Executive Committee opined that "asylum-seekers who have been temporarily admitted pending arrangements for a durable solution should be treated in accordance with the following minimum basic human standards . . . (o) they should be permitted to transfer assets which they have brought *into a territory* to the country where the durable solution is obtained [emphasis added]": UNHCR Executive Committee Conclusion No. 22, "Protection of Asylum-Seekers in Situations of Large-Scale Influx" (1981), at para. II(B)(2)(o), available at www.unhcr.ch (accessed Nov. 20, 2004).

[262] J. Fredriksson, "Reinvigorating Resettlement: Changing Realities Demand Changed Approach," (2002) 13 *Forced Migration Review* 28 (Fredriksson, "Reinvigorating Resettlement").

[263] The Executive Committee "appealed to States . . . [t]o offer resettlement opportunities to those who had been unable to obtain permanent residence in the State of first asylum": UNHCR Executive Committee Conclusion No. 2, "Functioning of the Sub-Committee and General Conclusion on International Protection" (1976), at para. (h)(ii), available at www.unhcr.ch (accessed Nov. 20, 2004).

5 million refugees in the peak year of 1979.[264] But with the conclusion of the Comprehensive Plan of Action for Indochinese Refugees,[265] UNHCR embraced a hierarchy of solutions during the late 1980s and 1990s. Resettlement was then relegated to a purely auxiliary role, to be pursued "only as a last resort, when neither voluntary repatriation nor local integration is possible."[266] Specifically, resettlement came to be understood as an appropriate solution mainly for "individual refugees with special protection needs, including women at risk, minors, adolescents, elderly refugees, and survivors of torture":[267]

> Resettlement under UNHCR auspices is geared primarily to the *special needs* of refugees under the Office's mandate whose life, liberty, safety, health or fundamental human rights are at risk in the country where they sought refuge. It is also considered a durable solution for refugees who, although not in need of immediate protection, have *compelling reasons* to be removed from their country of refuge. The decision to resettle a refugee is normally made *only in the absence of other options* such as voluntary

---

[264] Fredriksson, "Reinvigorating Resettlement," at 29.

[265] See generally J. Hathaway, "Labeling the 'Boat People': The Failure of the Human Rights Mandate of the Comprehensive Plan of Action for Indochinese Refugees," (1993) 15(4) *Human Rights Quarterly* 686.

[266] UNHCR Executive Committee Conclusion No. 67, "Resettlement as an Instrument of Protection" (1991), at para. (g), available at www.unhcr.ch (accessed Nov. 20, 2004). Some UNHCR materials and commentators have more recently sought to distance themselves from the language of resettlement as a solution of "last resort," though in substance that is in fact what it remains. See e.g. A. Edwards, "Resettlement: A Valuable Tool in Protecting Refugee, Internationally Displaced and Trafficked Women and Girls," (2001) 11 *Forced Migration Review* 31, at 32: "By offering resettlement as a solution, one has *ipso facto* ruled out voluntary repatriation or local integration as solutions in an individual case. This is not to say that resettlement should be used as a solution of 'last resort.' Resettlement should be considered when 'it is the best, or perhaps *only*, solution' in an individual case (emphasis in original)."

[267] UNHCR Executive Committee Conclusion No. 85, "Conclusion on International Protection" (1998), at para. (jj), available at www.unhcr.ch (accessed Nov. 20, 2004). See also UNHCR Executive Committee Conclusions Nos. 47, "Refugee Children" (1987); 54, "Refugee Women" (1988); 55, "General Conclusion on International Protection" (1989); 67, "Resettlement as an Instrument of International Protection" (1991); 68, "General Conclusion on International Protection" (1992); 71, "General Conclusion on International Protection" (1993); and 81, "General Conclusion on International Protection" (1997), all available at www.unhcr.ch (accessed Nov. 20, 2004), which recognize this more limited role for resettlement. Thus, for example, "[r]esettlement of Central American refugees has not constituted a durable solution on par with ... repatriation, but has been reserved for particular cases involving persons who, for protection or family reunification reasons, need to be resettled elsewhere": H. Gros Espiell et al., "Principles and Criteria for the Protection of and Assistance to Central American Refugees, Returnees, and Displaced Persons in Central America," (1990) 2(1) *International Journal of Refugee Law* 83, at 108.

repatriation and local integration. It *becomes a priority* when there is no other way to guarantee the legal or physical security of the person concerned.

Resettlement may be necessary to ensure the security of refugees who are threatened with *refoulement* to their country of origin or those whose physical safety is seriously threatened in the country where they have sought sanctuary [emphasis added].[268]

There is little doubt that the residual role now officially attributed to resettlement is at least in part a practical accommodation to the absence of a binding duty of states to resettle refugees, coupled with a disinclination by most states to in fact make resettlement opportunities available on any significant scale.[269] But, as John Fredriksson has observed, the growing determination of states to manage the movement of refugees, and in particular to harmonize refugee protection with more general migration goals, may present a golden opportunity to reinvent resettlement as a viable option for many of the world's refugees:

The time is ripe to discard the notion that there is a hierarchy of durable solutions, i.e. dubbing some as "preferred" and others as "undesirable." Developing a clear policy on the intrinsic link between resettlement and the need for durable solutions will result in operational guidelines and criteria for this type of resettlement activity, which are now virtually absent from the UNHCR *Resettlement Handbook*. A reinvigorated debate about the role of resettlement for durable solutions purposes is also timely in many states. The challenge laid out in early 2001 by then British Home [Secretary] Jack Straw to substantially increase resettlement capacity in Europe needs to be taken up by policy makers.[270]

As much has recently been recognized by state parties meeting on the fiftieth anniversary of the Refugee Convention. These governments committed themselves "to examine how more flexible resettlement criteria could be applied with regard to refugees recognized on a *prima facie* basis in mass influx situations"; "to enhance protection through an expansion of the number of countries engaged in resettlement, as well as through more strategic use of resettlement"; and "to streamline requirements for the processing of applications for resettlement, with a stronger focus on

---

[268] UNHCR, "Refugee Resettlement: An International Handbook to Guide Reception and Integration" (2002) (UNHCR, "Resettlement Handbook"), at 2.

[269] "No country is legally obliged to resettle refugees. Only a small number of States do so on a regular basis; allocating budgets, devising programmes and providing annual resettlement targets. Some countries regularly accept refugees for resettlement, sometimes in relatively large numbers, but do not set annual targets. Accepting refugees for resettlement is a mark of true generosity on the part of Governments": ibid.

[270] Fredriksson, "Reinvigorating Resettlement," at 29.

protection needs."[271] UNHCR has responded with a series of discussions and initiatives designed to "enhance[ ] . . . resettlement as a tool of protection for individual refugees, as well as a durable solution for larger numbers of refugees and as a global responsibility-sharing mechanism."[272] It is to be hoped that a renewed debate about the viability of a strong commitment to resettlement will afford the opportunity to return to the fundamental question of whether this solution – clearly envisaged by the Refugee Convention, and in no sense treated by it as inferior to other options – may prove a vital means of ensuring the human dignity of refugees themselves.[273] In Fredriksson's words,

> [As] the "solution" pendulum swung from resettlement to repatriation . . . policy documents began to refer to repatriation as the "happiest" of durable solutions while resettlement was the "least desirable." The question remains: in whose eyes was it the "happiest" solution – refugees, individual states, or the international community, including UNHCR?[274]

7.4 Naturalization

In the usual formulation of solutions to refugeehood, reference is made to the possibility of "local integration."[275] Local integration means in essence that a refugee is granted some form of durable legal status that allows him or her to remain in the country of first asylum on an indefinite basis, and fully to

---

[271] "Declaration of States Parties to the 1951 Convention and/or its 1967 Protocol relating to the Status of Refugees," UN Doc. HCR/MMSP/2001/09, Dec. 13, 2001, incorporated in UNHCR Executive Committee, "Agenda for Protection," at Part III, Goal 3, Point 6; and Goal 5, Points 5 and 6.

[272] UNHCR, "Progress Report on Resettlement," UN Doc. EC/54/SC/CRP.10, June 7, 2004, at para. 1.

[273] See generally G. Noll and J. van Selm, "Rediscovering Resettlement," (2003) 3 *Migration Policy Institute Insight* 1.

[274] Fredriksson, "Reinvigorating Resettlement," at 29.

[275] See generally UNHCR Executive Committee Conclusions Nos. 29, "General Conclusion on International Protection" (1983); 50, "General Conclusion on International Protection" (1988); 58, "Problem of Refugees and Asylum-Seekers Who Move in an Irregular Manner from a Country in Which They Had Already Found Protection" (1989); 79, "General Conclusion on International Protection" (1996); 81, "General Conclusion on International Protection" (1997); 85, "Conclusion on International Protection" (1998); and 87, "General Conclusion on International Protection" (1999), all available at www.unhcr.ch (accessed Nov. 20, 2004). In the Agenda for Protection, state parties called upon the Executive Committee "to set out framework considerations for implementing the *solution of local integration*, in the form of a Conclusion sensitive to the specificities of refugee needs, international and national legal standards, as well as the socioeconomic realities of hosting communities [emphasis added]": UNHCR Executive Committee, "Agenda for Protection," at Part III, Goal 5, Point 4.

participate in the social, economic, and cultural life of the host community.[276]

So conceived, local integration is not really distinguishable from the primary solution envisaged by the Refugee Convention, namely simple respect for refugee rights.[277] That is, the rights which are said to be the hallmarks of the solution of local integration are essentially the same rights which actually accrue by virtue of refugee status itself.[278] Even the economic and social aspects of local integration[279] add little substantive content to the rights already guaranteed by the Convention. As previously set out, the refugee rights regime prohibits the isolation of refugees from their host

[276] "Local integration in the refugee context is the end product of a multifaceted and on-going process, of which self-reliance is but one part. Integration requires a preparedness on the part of the refugees to adapt to the host society, without having to forego their own cultural identity": UNHCR, "Local Integration," UN Doc. EC/GC/02/6, Apr. 25, 2002 (UNHCR, "Local Integration"), at para. 5. Harrell-Bond helpfully emphasizes that integration is a process that happens not only to refugees, but also to their host communities. While acknowledging it to be an over-simplification, she therefore proposes a working definition of integration as "a situation in which host and refugee communities are able to co-exist, sharing the same resources – with no greater mutual conflict than that which exists within the host community": B. Harrell-Bond, *Imposing Aid: Emergency Assistance to Refugees* (1986), at 7.

[277] See chapter 7.0 above, at pp. 913–914. It has been observed that "official discourse on 'integration' ... lacks clarity": E. Michel, "Leadership and Social Organization: The Integration of Guatemalan Refugees in Campeche, Mexico," (2002) 15(4) *Journal of Refugee Studies* 359 (Michel, "Guatemalan Refugees").

[278] "First, [local integration] is a legal process, whereby refugees are granted a progressively wider range of rights and entitlements by the host State that are broadly commensurate with those enjoyed by its citizens. These include freedom of movement, access to education and the labour market, access to public relief and assistance, including health facilities, the possibility of acquiring and disposing of property, and the capacity to travel with valid travel and identity documents. Realization of family unity is another important aspect of local integration. Over time the process should lead to permanent residence rights and in some cases the acquisition, in due course, of citizenship in the country of asylum": UNHCR, "Local Integration," at para. 6. As the analysis in chapters 4–6 above has shown, all of these rights apart from access to permanent residence or citizenship and to family unity are entitlements which follow from refugee status itself, rather than being part of a solution to refugee status.

[279] "Second, local integration is clearly an economic process. Refugees become progressively less reliant on State aid or humanitarian assistance, attaining a growing degree of self-reliance and becoming able to pursue sustainable livelihoods, thus contributing to the economic life of the host country. Third, local integration is a social and cultural process of acclimatization by the refugees and accommodation by the local communities, that enables refugees to live amongst or alongside the host population, without discrimination or exploitation, and contribute actively to the social life of their country of asylum. It is ... an interactive process involving both refugees and nationals of the host State, as well as its institutions. The result should be a society that is both diverse and open, where people can form a community, regardless of differences": UNHCR, "Local Integration," at paras. 7–8.

communities[280] and requires that they be granted a broad array of social, economic, and civil rights[281] on par with those enjoyed by others in the host state community.[282] Moreover, the duties of *non-refoulement*[283] and non-expulsion[284] effectively require the first host country to continue to host and to honor the rights of refugees on an indefinite basis, absent a protection alternative.[285] Contemporary formulations of local integration may add some value to the Convention by emphasizing the dynamic process necessary to transform these rights into a social reality.[286] But as a matter of law, even this activist dimension of local integration may reasonably be thought to be implicit in the duty to implement treaty obligations in good faith.

> **Refugee Convention, Art. 1(C)(3)**
> This Convention shall cease to apply to any person falling under the terms of section A if:
> . . .
> (3) He has acquired a new nationality, and enjoys the protection of the country of his new nationality.

> **Refugee Convention, Art. 34 Naturalization**
> The Contracting States shall as far as possible facilitate the assimi-lation and naturalization of refugees. They shall in particular make every effort to expedite naturalization proceedings and to reduce as far as possible the charges and costs of such proceedings.

Because local integration is not really an *alternative* solution to simple respect for refugee rights,[287] the focus here is instead on the possibility of moving beyond refugee status towards the acquisition of citizenship in the

---

[280] See in particular chapters 4.2.4 and 5.2 above.   [281] See generally chapters 4–6 above.

[282] See chapter 3.1 above. One difference between "local integration" and respect for refugee rights may be that refugees are to enjoy all relevant rights on par with citizens of the host country, rather than on the basis of the Refugee Convention's contingent rights structure. The UNHCR, however, requires only that rights associated with local integration be "broadly commensurate" with those enjoyed by citizens: UNHCR, "Local Integration," at para. 6.

[283] See chapter 4.1 above.   [284] See chapter 5.1 above.

[285] That is, the duty of protection continues absent one of the three alternative solutions previously discussed in this chapter – repatriation consequent to a fundamental change of circumstances in the home country, voluntary reestablishment there, or resettlement to a third state.

[286] "From the host society, [local integration] requires communities that are welcoming and responsive to refugees, and public institutions that are able to meet the needs of a diverse population. As a process leading to a durable solution for refugees in the country of asylum, local integration has three inter-related and quite specific dimensions [legal, economic, and socio-cultural]": UNHCR, "Local Integration," at para. 5.

[287] At best, "local integration" may refer to the recognition of rights equivalency for refugees, that is, the granting to them not simply of respect for rights at the contingent standard set

asylum country. In contrast to simple local integration, enfranchisement through citizenship is legally sufficient to bring refugee status to an end.[288] Becoming a citizen bespeaks a qualitatively distinct level of acceptance of the refugee by the host state. Once a citizen, not only is the refugee guaranteed the right to remain and to enjoy basic rights as required by the Refugee Convention and general norms of international human rights law, but he or she is entitled also to take part as an equal in the political life of the country.[289] By granting the refugee the right to participate in the public life of the state, naturalization eliminates the most profound gap in the rights otherwise available to refugees, since full political rights are not guaranteed to refugees under the Refugee Convention, nor to non-citizens under general principles of international human rights law.

For example, while associational freedoms do accrue to refugees,[290] the drafters of the Refugee Convention upheld the right of states to prohibit refugees from assuming even politicized roles within trade unions.[291] And despite the comparative breadth of associational freedoms guaranteed to non-nationals under general norms of international human rights law,[292] core political rights remain very much the province of citizens:

> The fact that Art. 25 [of the Civil and Political Covenant] is the only provision in the Covenant that does not guarantee a universal human right but rather a *citizen's right* clearly shows that the States Parties may deny *aliens* the right to vote [and to "take part in the conduct of public affairs" and to have "access ... to public service"]. The restriction to the "citizen" ("citoyen," "ciudadano") stems from the concept of the modern nation-State, namely, that only those individuals who are

by the Refugee Convention: see chapter 3.2 above. While not understating the value of enhanced protection of this kind, the ability of refugees to assert most generally applicable international human rights already results in a comparable duty of rights equivalency in regard to many entitlements: see generally chapter 2.5.5, at pp. 127–128, and generally chapters 4–6 above.

[288] "This Convention shall cease to apply to any person ... if ... [h]e has acquired a new nationality, and enjoys the protection of the country of his new nationality": Refugee Convention, at Art. 1(C)(3).

[289] Enfranchisement can be achieved, in principle, other than by the granting of citizenship. "The right to participate in public life ... is not restricted to citizens; a state may choose to extend its application to others who live within its territory": Jayawickrama, *Judicial Application*, at 793–794. But as the French representative to the Ad Hoc Committee insisted, "[t]he purpose of the recommendation in article [34] was to bring about the naturalization of the largest possible number of refugees": Statement of Mr. Juvigny of France, UN Doc. E/AC.32/SR.39, Aug. 21, 1950, at 25.

[290] Freedom of association is guaranteed under Art. 15 of the Refugee Convention: see chapter 6.7 above.

[291] See chapter 6.7 above, at pp. 885–887.

[292] Freedoms of opinion, expression, association, and assembly are guaranteed to non-citizens under international human rights law: see chapter 6.7 above, at pp. 891–903.

attached to "their" State by the special bond of citizenship may exercise political rights.[293]

Access to citizenship through naturalization[294] is addressed by Art. 34 of the Refugee Convention, a provision without precedent in international refugee law.[295] It is predicated on a recognition that a refugee required to remain outside his or her home country should at some point benefit from "a series of privileges, including political rights."[296] Art. 34 is not, however, framed as a strong obligation:[297] it neither requires that state parties ultimately grant their citizenship to refugees, nor that refugees accept any such offer made to them.[298] To the contrary, the Secretary-General was emphatic that it would be inappropriate to circumscribe the prerogative of governments to decide to whom, and under what circumstances, an offer of citizenship would be made:

[293] Nowak, *ICCPR Commentary*, at 445. See UN Human Rights Committee, "General Comment No. 25: Participation in public affairs and the right to vote" (1996), UN Doc. HRI/GEN/1/Rev.7, May 12, 2004, at 167, para. 3: "In contrast with other rights and freedoms recognized by the Covenant (which are ensured to all individuals within the territory and subject to the jurisdiction of the State), article 25 protects the rights of 'every citizen.'"

[294] The drafters did not debate the meaning of naturalization, it having been asserted simply that "[t]he word 'naturalization' was well known and bore a distinct meaning": Statement of Mr. Robinson of Israel, UN Doc. E/AC.32/SR.39, Aug. 21, 1950, at 26.

[295] Grahl-Madsen, *Commentary*, at 244.

[296] United Nations, "Memorandum by the Secretary-General to the Ad Hoc Committee on Statelessness and Related Problems," UN Doc. E/AC.32/2, Jan. 3, 1950 (Secretary-General, "Memorandum"), at 50.

[297] In Weis' perspective, "Article 34 is in the form of a recommendation. It contains, nevertheless, the obligation to facilitate the assimilation and naturalization of refugees as far as possible": Weis, *Travaux*, at 352. See also Robinson, *History*, at 166–167: "Art. 34 consists of two parts. One is a recommendation to or a general moral obligation on States to facilitate as far as possible the naturalization and assimilation of the refugees residing in their countries. The other is a more specific obligation to expedite proceedings whenever an application for naturalization can be or has been made and to reduce the costs involved."

[298] This is not to say, however, that persons legally entitled to acquire citizenship in their country of long-term residence may complain if they are denied privileges extended to those who are citizens. In a decision regarding whether a legally resident non-citizen could avail himself of the right to enter "his own country" under Art. 12(4) of the Civil and Political Covenant, the UN Human Rights Committee observed that "[c]ountries like Canada, which enable immigrants to become nationals after a reasonable period of residence, have a right to expect that such immigrants will in due course acquire all the rights and assume all the obligations that nationality entails. Individuals who do not take advantage of this opportunity and thus escape the obligations nationality imposes can be deemed to have opted to remain aliens in Canada. They have every right to do so, but must also bear the consequences": *Stewart v. Canada*, UNHRC Comm. No. 538/1993, UN Doc. CCPR/C/58/D/538/1993, decided Nov. 1, 1996, at para. 12.8.

> The decision of the State granting naturalization is ... absolute. It cannot
> be compelled to grant its nationality, even after a long waiting period, to a
> refugee settled in its territory.[299]

Similarly, the proposal for what became Art. 34 canvassed the possibility that a long-staying refugee who declined an offer of citizenship made by the host country might thereby forfeit refugee status.[300] Despite the argument that such an approach was warranted to combat the aberrational nature of de facto statelessness,[301] no state party advocated mandatory enfranchisement during the drafting of the Convention. This suggests the persuasiveness of the contrary view, predicated on the recognition that even long-time refugees "may remain fundamentally attached to [their] country of origin and cherish the hope of returning ... Nationality should not be imposed on a refugee in violence to his inmost feelings."[302] Indeed, as the Israeli representative insisted, enfranchisement "if it were not voluntary, ... would be an attack on the spiritual independence of the refugee."[303]

In the result, the drafters committed themselves simply to promote naturalization as an option that should in principle be made available to refugees,[304] stipulating that states "shall as far as possible ... facilitate the assimilation and naturalization of refugees." As the language of Art. 34

---

[299] Secretary-General, "Memorandum," at 50.

[300] "[T]he idea has been suggested that after a fairly long lapse of time (e.g. fifteen years) the authorities of the country in which the refugee ... had settled might propose to him that he should apply for naturalization. If he failed to do so within a year, or did not give valid reasons for such failure, the Contracting Party would be entitled to consider itself as released from the obligations of the Convention": ibid.

[301] "If, indeed, it is recognized that an individual has the right to a nationality, as a counterpart it should be the duty of the stateless person to accept the nationality of the country in which he has long been established – the only nationality to which he can aspire – if it is offered him": ibid.

[302] Ibid. at 51.

[303] Statement of Mr. Robinson of Israel, UN Doc. E/AC.32/SR.39, Aug. 21, 1950, at 26. See also Secretary-General, "Memorandum," at 51: "Compulsory naturalization would be particularly inappropriate in the case of persons who had been prominent politically and represent a cause or a party." As Joly observes, contemporary refugees may not seek citizenship in the asylum state, even when it is available to them. "Despite the advantages to be gained, many, if not most, refugees are reluctant to become citizens of the host country, or do so only after a long time has elapsed in exile. Several factors shape this attitude, of which the most important is loyalty to the homeland which they were forced to leave": D. Joly, *Refugees: Asylum in Europe?* (1992), at 64.

[304] A stronger argument is made by Frelick, based upon the physical structure of the Refugee Convention. "By placing the call for naturalization directly after the *non-refoulement* guarantee (Articles 33 and 34), the Convention's drafters indicated what they saw as *non-refoulement*'s corollary principle – that while not returning a refugee is a mandatory minimum, it is not sufficient as a solution to the refugee's plight; that, indeed, a solution entails permanent protection, and that such protection is best achieved through naturalization (for refugees not able or willing to return)": B. Frelick, "Secure and Durable

makes clear, the duty is largely one of principle rather than formally binding.[305]

The bifurcated objective – assimilation and naturalization – was the subject of some discussion. Objection was initially taken to use of the term "assimilation" on the grounds of its "rather unpleasant connotation closely related to the notion of force."[306] The French representative, whose country had submitted the draft language from which the drafters chose to work,[307] explained the importance of retaining the reference to assimilation:

> The term "assimilation" had, of course, a special connotation in sociology and might perhaps carry with it certain unpleasant associations. Nevertheless, in the sense it was used in the context, it was an apt description of a certain stage in the development of the life of the refugee. The Convention was intended to provide refugees with a means of existence and at the same time to accord more favourable treatment than that granted generally to aliens to those refugees desirous of settling in a country for a certain length of time. Its final aim was to permit the assimilation of refugees into a national community by means of naturalization proceedings. He accordingly considered that the term "assimilation" clearly corresponded to the condition that the refugee should fulfil in order to qualify for

Asylum: Article 34 of the Refugee Convention," in US Committee for Refugees, *World Refugee Survey 2001* 42 (2001) (Frelick, "Article 34"), at 42. While Frelick's argument is plausible, the *travaux* record neither a preference for naturalization over other alternative solutions (repatriation, reestablishment, or resettlement), nor any discussion suggesting that the physical placement of Art. 34 after the *non-refoulement* obligation was meant to signal its corollary nature.

[305] A comparable duty of principled consideration is set by Art. 11 of the Refugee Convention, which requires the flag state of the vessel on which a refugee seaman is serving to "give sympathetic consideration" to the "establishment on its territory" of such refugee seamen. As Grahl-Madsen summarizes the Art. 11 obligation, "the State cannot refuse such measures out of hand or as a matter of principle; moreover ... the State has obliged itself to weigh carefully the interest of the refugee in the measure under consideration against other legitimate interests which the State has to consider, and that it shall regard the situation of the refugee with sympathy and understanding. In other words, the State has undertaken to let itself be guided by considerations of humanity, as far as other important interests do not stand in the way": Grahl-Madsen, *Commentary*, at 52.

[306] Statement of Mr. Robinson of Israel, UN Doc. E/AC.32/SR.39, Aug. 21, 1950, at 26. A similar concern is noted in Michel, "Guatemalan Refugees," at 367: "Article 34 of the 1951 Refugee Convention uses the concept of assimilation to explain integration ... Nevertheless, more recent discussions about local integration mentioned that the reference to assimilation is inadequate because 'the international community has always rejected the notion that refugees should be expected to abandon their own culture and way of life.'"

[307] The decision was taken to work from the French draft, "Proposal for a Draft Convention," UN Doc. E/AC.32/L.3, Jan. 17, 1950 (France, "Draft Convention"), rather than from that submitted by the Secretary-General: UN Doc. E/AC.32/SR.22, Feb. 2, 1950, at 3.

> naturalization ... [I]t was an apt description of the intermediate stage
> between the establishment of the refugee on a particular territory and his
> naturalization.[308]

That is, if the naturalization objective were to be effectively pursued, it was necessary first to convince states that refugees could be "absorbed within the national community."[309] As the Canadian representative remarked, "a country might not be prepared to grant naturalization if the refugee were not assimilated."[310]

So conceived, assimilation is not about compelling refugees to change their ways,[311] but rather a means of giving refugees a fair chance to persuade states of their suitability for citizenship.[312] This is very much in line with Grahl-Madsen's perspective:

> What is meant ... is in fact the laying of foundations, or stepping stones,
> so that the refugee may familiarize himself with the language, customs and
> way of life of the nation among whom he lives, so that he – without any
> feeling of coercion – may be more readily integrated in the economic, social
> and cultural life of his country of refuge.[313]

As regards the facilitation of naturalization itself, Art. 34 commits state parties to show flexibility in relation to "the administrative formalities taking place between the submission of the application and the decision."[314] Thus,

---

[308] Statement of Mr. Juvigny of France, UN Doc. E/AC.32/SR.39, Aug. 21, 1950, at 27–28.

[309] Statement of Mr. Perez Perozo of Venezuela, ibid. at 27.

[310] Statement of Mr. Winter of Canada, ibid. at 28. See also Statement of Mr. Cha of China, ibid. For example, "[i]n 1996, Immigration Minister Lucienne Robillard decreed that Somali and Afghani refugees must wait for five years after coming to Canada before they can be considered for permanent status. They need time, she said, 'to demonstrate respect for the laws of Canada and for us to detect those who may be guilty of crimes against humanity or acts of terrorism'": B. Taylor, "The school where pupils look forward to Mondays," *Toronto Star*, Mar. 7, 1999.

[311] UNHCR appears uncomfortable with this historical understanding, which clearly rejects efforts to force refugees to adopt the ways of their host community. "While both Article 34 of the 1951 Convention and UNHCR's Statute make reference to 'assimilation,' the international community has always rejected the notion that refugees should be expected to abandon their own culture and way of life, so as to become indistinguishable from nationals of the host community. In this respect, 'local integration' is the more appropriate term and should be used when referring to this durable solution": UNHCR, "Local Integration," at n. 3.

[312] While still of the view that the terms "adaptation" or "adjustment" better captured this notion, the Israeli representative ultimately "agreed with the concept": Statement of Mr. Robinson of Israel, UN Doc. E/AC.32/SR.39, Aug. 21, 1950, at 28.

[313] Grahl-Madsen, *Commentary*, at 247. See also Robinson, *History*, at 167, who writes that assimilation "is used not in the usual meaning of loss of the specific identity of the persons involved but in the sense of integration into the economic, social and cultural life of the country."

[314] Statement of Mr. Ordonneau of France, UN Doc. E/AC.32/SR.22, Feb. 2, 1950, at 3.

Art. 34 does not require state parties to engage in the "mass naturalization" of refugees.[315] Nor even are governments expected to waive or reduce substantive requirements for the acquisition of citizenship, such as minimum periods of residence in the state.[316] On the other hand, state parties are expected to make a good faith effort to help refugees meet the usual requirements for acquisition of the host state's citizenship.[317] This duty to facilitate assimilation and naturalization is of a general character,[318] meaning that state parties are encouraged to dispense with as many formalities in their naturalization process as possible so that refugees are positioned to acquire citizenship with

---

[315] Statement of Mr. Malfatti of Italy, UN Doc. E/AC.32/SR.39, Aug. 21, 1950, at 29.

[316] The Canadian representative, for example, defended his country's policy of requiring five years' residence of any person seeking Canadian citizenship: Statement of the Chairman, Mr. Chance of Canada, UN Doc. E/AC.32/SR.22, Feb. 2, 1950, at 3. Similarly, Switzerland noted that "Swiss Federal legislation did not provide for any different treatment for refugees in the matter of naturalization. They were treated in the same way as other aliens who were required to have resided lawfully in Switzerland for six years during the twelve years preceding their application before they could submit a valid application for naturalization": Statement of Mr. Schurch of Switzerland, UN Doc. E/AC.32/SR.39, Aug. 21, 1950, at 29. While Art. 10 of the Convention is today only of hortatory value, debates on its adoption suggest that in the view of the drafters, the calculation of a period of residence is not a matter simply of ascertaining how long a refugee has resided outside his or her own country, but rather how much time the refugee has spent in the particular state party. The calculation of a period of residence should, however, be carried out with due regard to the particular disabilities faced by refugees, including a period of enforced presence in the state party, or the time during which continuous residence was interrupted by forces beyond the refugee's control. See chapter 3.2.3 above, at p. 208.

[317] A similar duty was recognized outside the context of the Refugee Convention by the Supreme Court of India, which ordered a state government to desist from efforts to prevent Chakma refugees from securing Indian citizenship on the basis of the usual legal requirements. "[B]y refusing to forward their applications, the Chakmas are denied rights, constitutional and statutory, to be considered for being registered as citizens of India. If a person satisfies the requirements of Section 5 of the *Citizenship Act*, he/she can be registered as a citizen of India": *National Human Rights Commission v. State of Arunachal Pradesh*, (1996) 83 AIR 1234 (India SC, Jan. 9, 1996).

[318] "The second sentence of Article 34 mentions but two of several modes of facilitating naturalization. The words 'in particular' make it clear that the scope of the Article is by no means limited to the two kinds of measures mentioned in the second sentence, but also that the drafters considered those measures as being of very great importance": Grahl-Madsen, *Commentary*, at 250. Thus, Weis suggests that a state implementing Art. 34 might reasonably waive requirements to produce evidence that the refugee's former nationality would be lost upon naturalization: Weis, *Travaux*, at 352. Grahl-Madsen advocates a somewhat more aggressive reading, opining that state parties should consider the adoption of provisions providing for "refugee children born in the country [to] acquire its nationality at birth, and [authorizing] refugee youngsters [to] opt for the nationality of the country of refuge upon reaching a certain age": Grahl-Madsen, *Commentary*, at 248.

the absolute minimum of difficulty. Two specific forms of expected facilitation are codified in Art. 34.

First, states are to "expedite" the processing of applications for naturalization received from refugees. Art. 34 is "an appeal to [state parties] to accelerate their procedure."[319] The present Hungarian law, under which refugees need only be continuously resident for three (rather than the usual eight) years in order to be eligible for citizenship, is therefore an excellent example of committed implementation of this standard.[320] More generally, European nationality law does set a decidedly minimalist ten-year deadline to allow lawfully resident persons (including, but not limited to, refugees) to access naturalization procedures.[321]

Second, states are expected to "reduce as far as possible the charges and costs of such proceedings." This general language was adopted in contrast to that of the Secretary-General's draft, which advocated the reduction of costs and charges only in relation to "destitute refugees."[322] As the Turkish representative made clear, the broader language was desirable because "it extended the reduction of costs to all refugees, instead of limiting it to those who were destitute."[323] In line with this commitment, Canada determined in

---

[319] Statement of Mr. Cuvelier of Belgium, UN Doc. E/AC.32/SR.22, Feb. 2, 1950, at 3. While the British representative initially opposed this duty on the grounds that it would "entail giving priority to the applications of refugees over those of other foreigners," he was persuaded to drop his objections to this clause: Statement of Sir Leslie Brass of the United Kingdom, UN Doc. E/AC.32/SR.22, Feb. 2, 1950, at 3. Blay and Tsamenyi are therefore justified in their conclusion that Art. 34 "effectively requires the States to give the refugees more favorable treatment than the States would normally give to other aliens": S. Blay and M. Tsamenyi, "Reservations and Declarations under the 1951 Convention and the 1967 Protocol relating to the Status of Refugees," (1990) 2(4) *International Journal of Refugee Law* 527, at 542.

[320] See M.-E. Fullerton, "Hungary, Refugees, and the Law of Return," (1996) 8(4) *International Journal of Refugee Law* 499, at 516–517. Less dramatically, but similarly of benefit to refugees, are the policies of Germany and Sweden, which reduce their usual residence periods to acquire permanent residence by two years in the case of refugees: "Factsheet Denmark: Refugees and Other Foreigners in Denmark, Seen in International Perspective," at Fig. 6, available at www.um.dk (accessed Sept. 1, 2003). On the other hand, a provision in Dutch law which allowed refugees to apply for Netherlands citizenship one year earlier than other non-citizens – hence very much in line with this aspect of Art. 34 – was abolished as of Apr. 1, 2003: personal communication with Prof. Kees Groenendijk, University of Nijmegen, Dec. 5, 2003.

[321] Under the 1997 European Convention on Nationality, each state party "shall provide in its internal law for the possibility of naturalisation of persons lawfully and habitually resident on its territory. In establishing the conditions for naturalisation, it shall not provide for a period of residence exceeding ten years before the lodging of an application": European Convention on Nationality, 166 ETS, done Nov. 6, 1997, entered into force Jan. 3, 2000, at Art. 6(3).

[322] Secretary-General, "Memorandum," at 50.

[323] Statement of Mr. Kural of Turkey, UN Doc. E/AC.32/SR.22, Feb. 2, 1950, at 2.

February 2000 that it would exempt refugees seeking permanent resident status (a required step before eligibility for citizenship) from the need to pay a "right-of-landing fee." Coupled with the usual processing fees, a family of four had been required to pay more than C$3,000, leading to concern that recognized refugees would be deterred from pursuing a more durable status.[324] In eliminating the right-of-landing fee, the Minister of Citizenship and Immigration declared that "[r]efugees have already faced enormous difficulties and stresses ... By eliminating this fee we help them to get on with their lives and to integrate successfully into Canadian society."[325] But in general, UNHCR has observed that "[i]n certain countries it is governmental policy to charge heavily for ... naturalization applications."[326] In less developed countries, UNHCR has at times had to make its own funds available to meet naturalization costs, as was the case for the 30,000 Rwandan refugees naturalized by Tanzania in 1980.[327]

Despite these two clear expectations, it remains that Art. 34 sets a duty only to "facilitate" assimilation and naturalization, not an obligation of result.[328] The version of Art. 34 ultimately adopted is moreover framed at a very low level,[329] combining the weakest language of obligation found in the drafts proposed by each of the Secretary-General and France. The French proposal under which states would "undertake" to facilitate assimilation and

[324] L. Sarick, "Increase in fees for immigrants called new 'Chinese head tax,'" *Globe and Mail* (Toronto), Mar. 1, 1995, at A-34. A refugee outreach worker observed that "[r]efugees know that they won't be deported, but an important part of their becoming comfortable in Canada is the fact of being granted permanent residence": L. Sarick, "New tax on refugees a hardship, critics say," *Globe and Mail* (Toronto), Mar. 25, 1995, at A-12, quoting Anab Osman of the Association of Somali Service Agencies.

[325] Citizenship and Immigration Canada, "Landing Fee Eliminated for Refugees," Feb. 28, 2000, quoting Minister of Citizenship and Immigration Elinor Caplan.

[326] UNHCR, "Implementation," at para. 19.

[327] UNHCR paid Shs. 500,000 to the Tanzanian government on the condition that it "shall submit to the UNHCR not later than 31st December 1980 a nominal roll of Rwandese refugees having acquired Tanzanian citizenship": A. Chol, "The Legal Dimensions of the Refugee Problem in Africa," (1992) 14 *Migration* 5 (Chol, "Refugee Problem in Africa"), at 23.

[328] More generally, "neither the [Civil and Political] Covenant nor international law in general spells out specific criteria for the granting of citizenship through naturalization": *Borzov v. Estonia*, UNHRC Comm. No. 1136/2002, UN Doc. CCPR/C/81/D/1136/2002, decided Aug. 25, 2004, at para. 7.4.

[329] While conceding the minimalist legal duty imposed by Art. 34, Bill Frelick argues that an emphasis on legal requirements "is overly narrow, focusing on the little that [the Convention] requires of contracting states and dismissing the suasive power of its non-binding language. It is quite unremarkable that the Convention does not attempt to compel states to facilitate the assimilation and naturalization of refugees, clearly an act within the sovereign's discretion. But the Convention's promotion of assimilation and naturalization is clearly its preferred solution for refugees unable or unwilling to return": Frelick, "Article 34," at 45.

naturalization was rejected in favor of the Secretary-General's less legally charged (though still mandatory) verb, "shall." In addition, the drafters declined to adopt the Secretary-General's proposal for a duty to facilitate assimilation and naturalization "to the fullest possible extent," deciding instead to adopt the somewhat weaker French formulation, referring to facilitation "as far as possible."[330] Given this minimalist obligation, it really cannot be said that even steps which diminish opportunities for refugees to obtain citizenship are clearly unlawful. For example, recent amendments to the Danish Aliens Act which effectively increased the waiting period for refugees and other aliens to acquire citizenship from six to nine years,[331] while clearly not supportive of the underlying aspirations of Art. 34, were nonetheless not so retrogressive as to amount to a refusal to facilitate the assimilation and naturalization of refugees.[332] In view of its very soft sense of obligation, it is perhaps not surprising that Art. 34 has propelled so few governments to make naturalization more readily accessible to refugees.[333]

It would, however, be a mistake to view Art. 34 as completely without force. As Grahl-Madsen has observed,

> It goes without saying that a State must judge for itself whether it is "possible" for it to naturalize a particular individual or any number of refugees. On the other hand, the decision must be taken in good faith. If, for

---

[330] Compare Secretary-General, "Memorandum," at 50, and France, "Draft Convention," at 10. While the French draft was in most respects the model from which the Ad Hoc Committee worked, a Working Group specifically recommended the use of "shall" rather than "undertake" in Art. 34: "Decisions of the Working Group Taken on 9 February 1950," UN Doc. E/AC.32/L.32, Feb. 9, 1950, at 13.

[331] Specifically, under amendments that came into force on July 1, 2002, the waiting period to acquire permanent residence was increased from three to seven years. After acquiring permanent resident status, a further two-year period of good behavior is required before citizenship may be granted: Danish Refugee Council, "The New Danish Policy in the Field of Asylum and Immigration," Feb. 11, 2002. These requirements apply to all non-citizens, not just to refugees.

[332] The UN Committee on the Elimination of Discrimination against Women has, however, expressed its concern that the extended period before permanent residence may be obtained may effectively entrap non-citizen women in abusive relationships: "Report of the Committee on the Elimination of Discrimination against Women," UN Doc. A/57/38, Part II (Oct. 8, 2002), at para. 347.

[333] For example, "[a]lthough only a few African states have introduced reservations to Article 34, the naturalization of refugees has to date not been widely practiced on the African continent. In many instances, the period of residence is very long, and it is sometimes difficult for refugees to establish the date at which they first took up residence in a particular country": Chol, "Refugee Problem in Africa," at 22. In the European Union, the effective residence requirement to acquire citizenship ranges from a low of three years in Belgium, to a maximum of ten years in Austria, Italy, Luxembourg, Portugal, and Spain: "Factsheet Denmark: Refugees and Other Foreigners in Denmark, Seen in International Perspective," at Fig. 8, available at www.um.dk (accessed Sept. 1, 2003).

example, a Contracting State outright fails to allow any refugee to be assimilated or naturalized, and is not able to show any other reason than unwillingness, the other Contracting States may have a ground for complaint.[334]

This seems a very sensible formulation. Despite the minimalist nature of the duties it sets, Art. 34 is breached where a state party simply does not allow refugees to secure its citizenship, and refuses to provide a cogent explanation for that inaccessibility.[335] Because a state "*shall* facilitate *as far as possible* the assimilation and naturalization of refugees [emphasis added],"[336] it is incumbent upon state parties, at the very least, to provide a good faith justification for the formal or de facto[337] exclusion of refugees from naturalization.

Thus, a law such as that in force in Zambia, under which refugees are excluded from applying for citizenship even if able to satisfy the criteria applicable to other non-citizens, is presumptively in breach of the Refugee Convention.[338] A successful challenge might also be made to the decision of Australia to deny naturalization to any refugee who has passed through another state en route to Australia, since it is difficult to discern any logical basis for assuming that all such persons are inherently unsuitable for enfranchisement.[339] Art. 34 has real legal force in at least extreme cases such as these where refugees are effectively barred without sound reasons from accessing the usual process to acquire citizenship.[340]

---

[334] Grahl-Madsen, *Commentary*, at 246–247.

[335] The fact that several states – Botswana, Chile, Honduras, Latvia, Malawi, Malta, Mozambique, Papua New Guinea, and Swaziland – have entered reservations to Art. 34 affirms that it is not perceived by states as completely without legal force. Indeed, the reservations of Botswana, Latvia, Papua New Guinea, and Swaziland expressly provide that a reservation is being entered because those states are not in a position to "accept obligations" with regard to assimilation and naturalization: see text of reservations and declarations of state parties, available at www.unhcr.ch (accessed Nov. 20, 2004).

[336] See Grahl-Madsen, *Commentary*, at 246: "The word 'shall' makes it clear that Article 34 imposes a duty on the Contracting States, not only a recommendation."

[337] For example, Belize is reported to have "an unwritten official policy that refugee residence cannot lead to naturalization": J.-F. Durieux, "Capturing the Central American Refugee Phenomenon: Refugee Law-Making in Mexico and Belize," (1992) 4(3) *International Journal of Refugee Law* 301, at n. 11.

[338] Extraordinarily, the Zambian government was forced to withdraw even a bill that would have allowed refugees to apply for citizenship after *thirty years'* residence in that country (in contrast to the ten-year requirement applied to other non-citizens). One member of parliament was reported to have referred to the proposed legislation as "national suicide": "Zambia debating citizenship for refugees," *Independent Online*, Feb. 9, 2001; "State withdraws refugees bill," *Times of Zambia*, Dec. 19, 2002.

[339] P. Barkham, "Australians toughen up refugee laws," *Guardian*, Sept. 22, 2001, at 17.

[340] Indeed, the UN Human Rights Committee has implied that states may be under a duty to enable persons lawfully resident in their territory ultimately to become citizens. In a decision regarding whether a legally resident non-citizen could avail himself of the right

In other than such egregious situations, Art. 34 is intended to promote, rather than to compel, access to naturalization.[341] Refugee status does not give rise to an entitlement to access citizenship, even after the passage of a long period of time. But the Refugee Convention does commit governments to assisting refugees to access whatever opportunities for naturalization may exist under the host state's general laws. As Frelick concludes, Art. 34 "is not limited to directing contracting states not to do bad, but positively directs them to do good: its underlying premise is about providing asylum, sharing the burdens among states, and seeking just and durable solutions."[342] The facilitation of naturalization is moreover a policy that has been shown to promote harmony within the host state as well:

> The danger of [host] countries not taking positive steps to promote the full social inclusion of people whom they accept as refugees is that this can lead to a withdrawal of their emotional commitment to, and social engagement with, the [host] country. Refugees who perceive themselves to be excluded ... may continue to reside there, but turn inwards and identify themselves in terms of their ethnic minority status ... [T]his leads to the racialization and ethnicization of social relations, which in turn leads to further experience of social exclusion for the group concerned. The downward spiral of a vicious circle becomes established. Logical outcomes are that the ethnic group adopts an oppositional stance vis-à-vis the mainstream, and that ghettos develop.[343]

to enter "his own country" under Art. 12(4) of the Civil and Political Covenant, it was observed that "[t]he question in the present case is whether a person who enters a given State under that State's immigration laws, and subject to the conditions of those laws, can regard that State as his own country when he has not acquired its nationality and continues to retain the nationality of his country of origin. The answer could possibly be positive were the country of immigration to place unreasonable impediments on the acquiring of nationality by new immigrants": *Stewart v. Canada*, UNHRC Comm. No. 538/1993, UN Doc. CCPR/C/58/D/538/1993, decided Nov. 1, 1996, at para. 12.5. See also *Canepa v. Canada*, UNHRC Comm. No. 558/1993, UN Doc. CCPR/C/59/D/558/1993, decided Apr. 3, 1997, at para. 11.3; and *Madafferi v. Australia*, UNHRC Comm. No. 1011/2001, UN Doc. CCPR/C/81/D/1011/2001, decided July 26, 2004, at para. 9.6.

[341] At the Conference of Plenipotentiaries, the British representative observed immediately prior to the vote to adopt Art. 34 that it "should be considered as a recommendation rather than as a binding legal obligation, particularly in view of the use of the words 'as far as possible' and 'make every effort'": Statement of Mr. Hoare of the United Kingdom, UN Doc. A/CONF.2/SR.16, July 11, 1951, at 18.

[342] Frelick, "Article 34," at 54.

[343] D. Barnes, "Resettled Refugees' Attachment to Their Original and Subsequent Homelands: Long-Term Vietnamese Refugees in Australia," (2001) 14(4) *Journal of Refugee Studies* 394, at 409–410, drawing on the analysis of S. Castles and A. Davidson, *Citizenship and Migration: Globalization and the Politics of Belonging* (2000).

Epilogue

Challenges to the viability of refugee rights

Despite its length, this book is no more than a first step in the development of a clear appreciation of how best to ensure the human rights of refugees under international law. The effort here to elaborate and illustrate application of the basic normative structure of the refugee rights regime rests on a thus-far unacknowledged assumption: namely, that governments which choose to become parties to the Refugee Convention intend rights defined therein to be treated as enforceable in fact, and more generally that their consent to be bound by the Convention is a signal that they are committed to managing involuntary migration on the basis of a rights-oriented framework. Each of these assumptions is sometimes questioned.

As a matter of strict law, there can be little doubt that the terms of Arts. 16 and 25 of the Refugee Convention, particularly when read in tandem with Art. 14 of the Civil and Political Covenant,[1] require state parties to implement the rights guaranteed under the Convention in good faith.[2] It is equally clear that when governments fail in practice to live up to this responsibility, they are often compelled to come into compliance with international law as the result of domestic legal remedies pursued before national courts or tribunals.[3] But as judicial oversight is neither always available nor reliably effective, there is the real risk that refugee rights not voluntarily implemented by states

---

[1] See chapter 4.10 above, at pp. 644–656.

[2] See chapter 1.3.3 above, at p. 62.

[3] See generally chapter 4.10 above, at pp. 644–656. The legal systems of many countries, particularly those that are based on civil law, provide for the direct incorporation of international law into domestic law, including any treaty obligation assumed in accordance with the national constitution. See generally I. Brownlie, *Principles of Public International Law* (2003), at 47–48; M. Shaw, *International Law* (2003), at 151–160. While most legal systems derived from British common law insist on the domestic transformation of international law as a condition for domestic enforceability, any ambiguity in national law is normally to be construed so as to avoid a conflict with international law. This is so because there is an assumption that "Parliament does not intend to act in breach of international law, including therein specific treaty obligations": *Salomon v. Commissioner of Customs and Excise*, [1967] 2 QB 116 (Eng. CA, Oct. 26, 1966), per Lord Diplock at 143. See generally Shaw, ibid. at 135–143; and Brownlie, ibid. at 45–46.

will be denied in practice. Because the Refugee Convention incorporates no clear oversight mechanism of the kind routinely established to promote compliance by governments with other international human rights treaties,[4] the real value of its rights regime may be seen as seriously compromised.

The second and more general concern is that whatever the intentions of the drafters, the nature, scope, and geopolitical setting of refugee protection today simply differ too fundamentally from the reality of 1951 for the Convention's rights regime to be taken seriously as the baseline of the international response to involuntary migration. With developed states increasingly able and determined to deter would-be refugees from ever arriving at their territory,[5] and with roughly 80 percent of the refugee population today located in states of the less developed world,[6] doubts are expressed about the soundness of a Convention that both assumes access to protection, and fails to address how states should reconcile refugee protection responsibilities to their own, often difficult, domestic circumstances.

While it is beyond the scope of this book to analyze these broader concerns in the detail they deserve, this Epilogue seeks at least to acknowledge the most critical political and economic challenges which impede full respect for even freely assumed obligations towards refugees. There are answers to each of these concerns, though clearly not answers provided by law alone.

The challenge of enforceability

Enforcement of Refugee Convention rights has earlier been addressed in significant detail.[7] In brief, the drafters of the 1951 Refugee Convention declined to give the international supervisory agency, now UNHCR, a general right to facilitate the enforcement of refugee rights in state parties. UNHCR was instead entrusted with a general duty "of supervising the application of the provisions of this Convention."[8] To the extent that a state party is willing, UNHCR may, of course, provide direct assistance to refugees to enforce their rights in the asylum country.[9] But under the decentralized implementation

---

[4] See generally P. Alston and J. Crawford eds., *The Future of UN Human Rights Treaty Monitoring* (2000).
[5] See chapter 4.1.3 above.   [6] See Introduction above, at p. 3.
[7] See chapter 4.10 above.
[8] Convention relating to the Status of Refugees, 189 UNTS 2545, done July 28, 1951, entered into force Apr. 22, 1954 (Refugee Convention), at Art. 35. This authority links neatly to UNHCR's statutory duty to "provide for the protection of refugees by . . . [p]romoting the conclusion and ratification of international conventions for the protection of refugees, supervising their application and proposing amendments thereto": Statute of the Office of the United Nations High Commissioner for Refugees, UNGA Res. 428(V), adopted Dec. 14, 1950 (UNHCR Statute), at Art. 8(b).
[9] See chapter 4.10 above, at pp. 634–636.

structure envisaged by the Convention, it is governments themselves which ultimately remain responsible to ensure that refugees are treated as the Convention requires.

In practice, and despite the externally imposed limits on its authority, there is no doubt that UNHCR plays an absolutely vital role in promoting respect for refugee rights around the world. Most generally, the agency's many standard-setting exercises referenced throughout this book have been literally indispensable to the implementation of Convention duties. UNCHR is regularly involved in the promotion of refugee rights on the ground as well. Invoking the duty of states to cooperate with the agency in its duty to oversee application of the Convention, and specifically to report legislative and practical steps taken to ensure refugee rights to it,[10] UNHCR has persuaded most governments to allow it to have a physical presence in their jurisdiction, to meet with and to counsel refugees, and ordinarily to be assured of access to officials with the authority to respond to concerns regarding the treatment of refugees.[11] Particularly in countries with limited resources or infrastructure to oversee the welfare of refugees, UNHCR may even be authorized to exercise what amounts to a more direct surrogate protector role analogous to that played by the League of Nations during the Minorities Treaties era.[12]

But it remains that the vital role played by UNHCR does not amount to a transparent system to ensure accountability by states for duties undertaken pursuant to the Convention. While UNHCR protection officers in the field provide confidential compliance reports to headquarters staff, states are not required to submit to public, or even collegial, scrutiny of their records. In the result, there is no forum within which to require governments to engage in the kind of dialogue of justification that is standard practice under nearly every other human rights instrument.[13] Nor has there been any effort by UNHCR to devise a formal mechanism to facilitate the presentation by refugees themselves of allegations of failure to respect Convention rights,[14] despite the precedent of other United Nations bodies which have relied on

---

[10] Refugee Convention, at Art. 35(1).

[11] See generally W. Kälin, "Supervising the 1951 Convention relating to the Status of Refugees: Article 35 and Beyond," in E. Feller et al. eds., *Refugee Protection in International Law* 613 (2003), at 623–624.

[12] See chapter 2.2 above.

[13] See e.g. L. Sohn, "Human Rights: Their Implementation and Supervision by the United Nations," in T. Meron ed., *Human Rights in International Law: Legal and Policy Issues* 369 (1984), at 373–379.

[14] In contrast, even the League of Nations Minorities Treaties enabled the intended beneficiaries to petition the League Council. While no formal standing was granted to the minorities themselves, the enforcement of interstate obligations relied in large part on the information generated from individual petitions. See chapter 2.2 above, at pp. 82–83.

lesser legal authority to establish individual petition systems.[15] The generality of UNHCR's Art. 35 authority notwithstanding, supervision of refugee rights by the agency remains very much a matter of standard-setting and private representations to states.[16]

This may, in fact, be precisely the approach intended by those who drafted the Refugee Convention and UNHCR's own Statute. The more direct enforcement role was in principle attributed to the community of state parties. Any state party may legitimately take up concerns regarding non-compliance directly with any other state party, and may in most cases require the non-compliant state to answer to the International Court of Justice.[17] In practice, there have been some formal protests, including those in response to the notorious push-back policy of states faced with the arrival of Vietnamese boat people in the late 1970s. More commonly, though, indifference or fear of bilateral disadvantage means that few direct efforts are made to correct even egregious breaches of Convention rights. In particular, no application has ever been made to the International Court of Justice as contemplated by Art. 38 of the Refugee Convention.[18]

The question then logically arises: why is it that the Refugee Convention, virtually alone among major human rights treaties, still has no free-standing mechanism to promote interstate accountability under the auspices of an independent expert supervisory body charged with the review of periodic reports from states and the consideration of individuated communications from those aggrieved?[19]

---

[15] The major petition systems established by Resolutions 728F (1959), 1235 (1967) and 1503 (1970), which have enabled the Commission on Human Rights to take account of individuated petitions, are grounded in no more than the general pledge of states in the Charter to promote respect for and observance of human rights: see H. Steiner and P. Alston, *International Human Rights in Context* (2000) (Steiner and Alston, *Rights in Context*), at 374–420.

[16] National implementing legislation is to be routinely supplied to the UNHCR and United Nations Secretary-General: Refugee Convention, at Arts. 35 and 36. More detailed information regarding the law and practice of constituent units of non-unitary states must also be provided to the United Nations upon the request of any other contracting state: Refugee Convention, at Art. 41(c).

[17] Refugee Convention, at Art. 38.

[18] The lack of interest among states in taking judicial action against another country based on the latter state's failure to respect human rights is borne out as well in the reluctance of governments to make use of interstate complaint procedures under major human rights treaties. See e.g. S. Leckie, "The Inter-State Complaint Procedure in International Human Rights Law: Hopeful Prospects or Wishful Thinking?," (1988) 10 *Human Rights Quarterly* 249.

[19] See J. Crawford, "The UN Human Rights Treaty System: A System in Crisis?," in P. Alston and J. Crawford eds., *The Future of UN Human Rights Treaty Monitoring* 1 (2000), at 1–2, noting that the universal approach to human rights treaty implementation is predicated on the establishment of a specialist supervisory body not of a judicial or quasi-judicial character, with regular reporting obligations leading to a dialogue between states and the

The failure to establish an independent supervisory mechanism for the Refugee Convention may be no more than an historical anomaly. The Refugee Convention was the second major human rights treaty adopted by the United Nations, having been preceded only by the Genocide Convention. It is noteworthy that the Genocide Convention, like the Refugee Convention, is not externally supervised. In part, then, the absence of an independent supervisory mechanism for the Refugee Convention is simply a reflection of the historical reality of the late 1940s and early 1950s, when the entire idea of interstate supervision of human rights was new, potentially threatening, and not truly accepted by states. Yet with the adoption of the Human Rights Covenants and more specialized treaties beginning in the mid-1960s, the establishment of independent mechanisms for interstate oversight of the human rights treaties has become routine. Whatever its accuracy, the historical explanation is thus surely insufficient to immunize the Refugee Convention from the contemporary general practice of meaningful independent supervision.

An alternative explanation for the continuing failure to establish an interstate supervisory mechanism for the Refugee Convention is that the UNHCR's agency-based oversight function provides all that is required by way of supervision. Refugee law is the only branch of international human rights law that can claim an exclusive international organization assigned to oversee its implementation. At best, other UN human rights treaties can rely on the generic authority of a seriously under-resourced UN High Commissioner for Human Rights to support the efforts of treaty supervisory bodies.[20] Because refugee law has its own institutional guardian in the person of the High Commissioner for Refugees, it might be thought that any additional mechanism for oversight would be superfluous.

Yet despite all of UNHCR's critical contributions to oversight of the Refugee Convention, there are at least three fundamental reasons why vesting UNHCR with sole responsibility to oversee the treaty is unwise. First, UNHCR has been fundamentally transformed during the 1990s from an agency whose job was essentially to serve as trustee or guardian of refugee rights as implemented by states to an agency that is now primarily focused on direct service delivery.[21] Simply put, UNHCR is no longer at arm's length

---

supervisory body. In addition, individual complaints are receivable under the terms of four major UN human rights treaties: see Steiner and Alston, *Rights in Context*, at 738–739.

[20] See generally M. Schmidt, "Servicing and Financing Human Rights Supervisory Bodies," in P. Alston and J. Crawford eds., *The Future of UN Human Rights Treaty Monitoring* 481 (2000).

[21] This transition is described in J. Hathaway, "New Directions to Avoid Hard Problems: The Distortion of the Palliative Role of Refugee Protection," (1995) 8(3) *Journal of Refugee Studies* 288; G. Goodwin-Gill,"Refugee Identity and Protection's Fading Prospects," in F. Nicholson and P. Twomey eds., *Refugee Rights and Realities: Evolving International Concepts and Regimes* 220 (1999); and M. Barutciski, "A Critical View on UNHCR's Mandate Dilemmas," (2002) 14(2/3) *International Journal of Refugee Law* 365.

from the implementation of refugee protection. In most big refugee crises around the world today, UNHCR is – in law or in fact – the means by which refugee protection is delivered on the ground. In seeking to exercise its traditional supervisory authority, UNHCR therefore faces a serious ethical dilemma, since it is often in the position of being responsible effectively to supervise itself.

Second, the failure to establish the usual form of interstate supervisory mechanism for the Refugee Convention encourages states to avoid the meaningful accountability between and among themselves that is at the root of the entire international human rights project. Because states presently take little, if any, direct responsibility for ensuring that their fellow states live up to international refugee law obligations, the dynamic of persuading, cajoling, and indeed shaming partner states – so critical to the success of the international human rights project in general – is largely absent in refugee law. It is just too easy to leave the task to UNHCR. Yet UNHCR is not really in a position to apply meaningful forms of pressure on states.[22] It is, after all, an entity with a tiny core budget and which is effectively dependent on the annual voluntary contributions of a very small number of powerful governments, virtually none of which has been predisposed to empower UNHCR to act autonomously in advancing a strong regime of international refugee protection. While these states have been generous in providing funds for refugee relief and for humanitarian assistance, they have too often either avoided or, on occasion, evaded UNHCR's insistence on the importance of protection principles. Because UNHCR is, and will remain, politically and fiscally constrained by design, it cannot reasonably be expected to provide the sort of strong voice in favor of unflinching attention to refugee protection that is now required.

Finally, and perhaps ironically, a third reason to establish an arms-length expert supervisory mechanism for the Refugee Convention is to facilitate UNHCR's basic work of protecting refugees. As a matter of practical reality, the agency's on-the-ground efforts to protect refugees frequently require compromise and even expediency in the interest of saving lives. In some truly egregious situations, UNHCR's pursuit of "least bad options" for refugees may leave the agency with little realistic choice but to turn a blind eye to breaches of the very norms it is charged with overseeing – clearly a difficult and often debilitating dilemma. As such, the welfare of refugees might be better served by the combination of a more flexible and operationally oriented international agency combined with an expert, arms-length supervisory body responsible to critique practice based on rules set by international law. This is not to say that UNHCR's statutory authority to *supervise*

---

[22] See generally G. Loescher, *The UNHCR and World Politics: A Perilous Path* (2001).

the application of the Convention should be reconsidered; there is, in particular, real value in its standard-setting and related legal work. But experience under other human rights treaties makes clear that there is a profound logic to the establishment of a complementary mechanism capable of engaging governments and refugees in a direct and transparent process of bringing rights to bear in real cases.

Despite the failure to establish a supervisory mechanism for the Refugee Convention itself, the central role of domestic remedies in enforcing refugee rights is nonetheless even now reinforced in critical ways by indirect supervision at the international level. Of particular value is the growing awareness of the value of invoking Convention-based refugee rights in briefs to global and regional bodies established to receive periodic compliance reports under other human rights treaties, in the hope of generating authoritative holdings to guide state practice.[23] In view of the significant points of overlap in the normative structures of these general human rights treaties and the Refugee Convention, supervisory bodies may reasonably draw on refugee-specific rights to inform their approach to the interpretation of general norms in the specific circumstances encountered by refugees. For example, it would be entirely appropriate for the Committee on Economic, Social and Cultural Rights to inquire of a state party to both the Economic Covenant and the Refugee Convention why it has not taken account of the Refugee Convention's duty to grant refugees the same access to elementary education as afforded nationals in implementing the Economic Covenant's right to education. Similarly, the Human Rights Committee might be expected to refer to the Refugee Convention's requirement that detention ordinarily be limited to the time prior to regularization of status in supervising a state's obligation under the Civil and Political Covenant to ensure liberty and security of the person.

Even more immediate opportunities to enforce refugee rights exist by virtue of the individuated complaints procedures established under regional human rights regimes, and also increasingly available under the auspices of United Nations human rights treaties. The communications mechanisms under each of the International Covenant on Civil and Political Rights, the

---

[23] The preparedness of the Committee on the Elimination of Racial Discrimination to take up refugee-related concerns is particularly evident: see e.g. UN Committee on the Elimination of Racial Discrimination, "General Recommendation No. XXII: Refugees and displaced persons" (1996), UN Doc. HRI/GEN/1/Rev.7, May 12, 2004, at 214. See also UN Human Rights Committee, "General Comment No. 15: The position of aliens under the Covenant" (1986), UN Doc. HRI/GEN/1/Rev.7, May 12, 2004, at 140. With regard to the potential value of activism in the context of periodic reporting procedures, see A. Clapham, "UN Human Rights Reporting Procedures: An NGO Perspective," in P. Alston and J. Crawford eds., *The Future of UN Human Rights Treaty Monitoring* 175 (2000).

Convention on the Elimination of All Forms of Racial Discrimination, the Convention against Torture, and the Convention on the Elimination of All Forms of Discrimination Against Women are open to refugees and other persons under the jurisdiction of a state party on terms of equality with nationals,[24] therefore affording a meaningful forum for the vindication of particularized grievances. While the subject matter of complaints to these bodies must involve a right set by the relevant treaty, refugee-specific rights may nonetheless be invoked to assist the adjudicative body to interpret generic rights in a way that takes special account of the unique predicament of refugees. Thus, even before there is agreement to establish an independent supervisory body for the Refugee Convention, there are still real opportunities to bring refugee rights to bear in international settings.

The challenge of political will

Even assuming that states ultimately agree to bring the Refugee Convention into line with the general expectation of independent oversight, a more fundamental challenge remains. As the empirical evidence presented in this book tragically attests, the reality today is that a significant number of governments in all parts of the world are withdrawing in practice from meeting the legal duty to provide refugees with the protection they require.[25] While states continue to proclaim a willingness to assist refugees as a matter of political discretion or humanitarian goodwill, many appear committed to a pattern of defensive strategies designed to avoid international legal responsibility toward involuntary migrants. Some see this shift away from a legal paradigm of refugee protection as a source of enhanced operational flexibility in the face of changed political circumstances. For refugees themselves, however, the increasingly marginal relevance of international refugee law has in practice signaled a shift to inferior or illusory protection. It has also

---

[24] "A State Party to the Covenant that becomes a Party to the present Protocol recognizes the competence of the Committee to receive and consider communications from *individuals subject to its jurisdiction* who claim to be victims of a violation by that State Party of any of the rights set forth in the Covenant [emphasis added]": Optional Protocol to the International Covenant on Civil and Political Rights, UNGA Res. 2200A(XXI), Dec. 16, 1966, entered into force Mar. 23, 1976, at Art. 1. See also International Convention on the Elimination of All Forms of Racial Discrimination, UNGA Res. 2106A(XX), adopted Dec. 21, 1965, entered into force Jan. 4, 1969, at Art. 14; Convention against Torture and Other Cruel, Inhuman or Degrading Treatment or Punishment, UNGA Res. 39/46, adopted Dec. 10, 1984, entered into force June 26, 1987, at Art. 22; and Optional Protocol to the Convention on the Elimination of All Forms of Discrimination Against Women, UNGA Res. 54/4, adopted Oct. 6, 1999, entered into force Dec. 22, 2000.

[25] The analysis here is based on J. Hathaway and A. Neve, "Making International Refugee Law Relevant Again: A Proposal for Collectivized and Solution-Oriented Protection," (1997) 10 *Harvard Human Rights Journal* 115.

imposed intolerable costs on many of the poorest countries, and has involved states in practices antithetical to their basic political values.

In the face of resistance of this kind, it must be recognized that no international oversight body (or international agency) will ever be positioned actually to *require* governments to implement rights perceived by states as fundamentally at odds with their fundamental interests. The real challenge is therefore to design a structure for the implementation of Convention rights which states will embrace, or at least see as reconcilable to their own priorities. Only with the benefit of an implementation mechanism of this kind will governments be persuaded normally to abide by even clear Convention duties; and only when compliance is the norm will it be realistic to expect any supervisory mechanism to be capable of responding dependably and effectively to instances of non-compliance.

To be clear, it is suggested here that the goal should be to reconceive the *mechanisms* by which international refugee law, including the refugee rights regime, are implemented – *not* to undertake a renegotiation of the Refugee Convention itself. Those who favor the latter course seem largely to misunderstand the nature and function of the Convention-based protection regime. The goal of refugee law, like that of public international law in general, is not to deprive states of either authority or operational flexibility. It is instead to enable governments to work more effectively to resolve problems of a transnational character, thereby positioning them better to manage complexity, contain conflict, promote decency, and avoid catastrophe.[26] Indeed, international refugee law was established precisely because it was seen to afford states a politically and socially acceptable way to maximize border control in the face of socially inevitable involuntary migration[27] – an objective which is, if anything, even more pressing today than it was in earlier times. Refugee law has fallen out of favor with many states not because there is any real belief either that governments can best respond to involuntary migration independently, or that the human dignity of refugees should be infringed in the interests of operational efficiency. Rather, there seems to be an overriding sentiment that there is a lack of balance in the mechanisms of the refugee regime which results in little account being taken of the legitimate interests of the states to which refugees flee.

First, some governments increasingly believe that a clear commitment to refugee protection may be tantamount to the abdication of their migration control responsibilities. They see refugee protection as little more than an uncontrolled "back door" immigration route which contradicts official efforts to tailor admissions on the basis of economic or other criteria, and

[26] R. Falk, *Revitalizing International Law* (1993), at 91–93.
[27] These points are developed in J. Hathaway, "A Reconsideration of the Underlying Premise of Refugee Law," (1990) 31(1) *Harvard International Law Journal* 129.

which is increasingly at odds with critical national security and related priorities. Second, neither the actual duty to admit refugees nor the real costs associated with their arrival are fairly apportioned among states. There is a keen awareness that the countries in which refugees arrive – overwhelmingly poor, and often struggling with their own economic or political survival – presently bear sole legal responsibility for what often amounts to indefinite protection. In short, the legal duty to protect refugees is understood to be neither in the national interest of most states, nor a fairly apportioned collective responsibility. It is therefore resisted.

There are ways to address both of these concerns. As a starting point, there needs to be a clear recognition that refugee protection responsibilities can be implemented without denying states the right to set their own immigration priorities. The refugee regime is not an immigration system; it rather establishes a situation-specific human rights remedy. When the violence or other human rights abuse that induced refugee flight comes to an end, so too does refugee status.[28] Equally important, even this right to protection is explicitly denied to serious criminals who pose a danger to the host community, and to persons who threaten national security.[29]

Nor is the duty of protection logically assigned on the basis of accidents of geography or the relative ability of states to control their borders. To the contrary, governments have regularly endorsed the importance of international solidarity and burden-sharing to an effective regime of refugee protection. While collectivized efforts to date have been ad hoc and usually insufficient, they provide an experiential basis for constructing an alternative to the present system of unilateral and undifferentiated state obligations.[30] It is particularly important to recognize that different states have differing capabilities to contribute to a collectivized process of refugee protection. Some states will be best suited to provide physical protection for the duration of risk. Other states will be motivated to assist by providing dependable guarantees of financial resources and residual resettlement opportunities. Still other governments will collaborate by funding protection or receiving refugees in particular contexts, on a case-by-case basis. Under a thoughtful system of common but differentiated responsibility, the net resources available for refugee protection could be maximized by calling on states to contribute in ways that correspond to their relative capacities and strengths.

In short, none of the legitimate concerns voiced by governments amounts to a good reason to question the underlying soundness of responding to

[28] See chapter 7.1 above, at pp. 919–928.   [29] See chapter 4.1.4 above, at pp. 345–352.

[30] The body of social science research in support of a renewed approach to implementation of the Refugee Convention is presented in J. Hathaway ed., *Reconceiving International Refugee Law* (1997).

involuntary migration in line with the rights-based commitments set by the Refugee Convention and other core norms of international law.

Today, more than ever before, governments are engaged in a variety of serious discussions regarding reform of the refugee law system.[31] Perhaps spurred on by the formal commitment made on the fiftieth anniversary of the Refugee Convention, there is clear interest in exploring both the operational flexibility which refugee law affords,[32] and the value of systems to share both the responsibilities and burdens inherent in refugee protection.[33] It is not at all clear, however, that these initiatives are predicated on the central importance of finding practical ways by which to respond to involuntary migration from within a rights-based framework. Poorer states are glad that there is, at last, some realization by governments in the developed world that ad hoc charity must be replaced by firm guarantees to share responsibilities and burdens. Governments of wealthier and more powerful countries are pleased that UNHCR and other states are now prepared to acquiesce in demands that their refugee protection responsibilities not be construed to impose ongoing obligations towards all who arrive at their territory. But potentially lost in the discussions as they have evolved to date is the central importance of reforming the mechanisms of refugee law not simply to avert perceived hardships for states, but also in ways that really improve the lot of refugees themselves. It is not enough to find sources of operational flexibility, nor even to devise mechanisms by which to share responsibilities and burdens. If the net result of these reforms is only to lighten the load of governments, or to signal the renewed relevance of international agencies to meeting the priorities of states, then an extraordinary opportunity to advance the human dignity of refugees themselves will have been lost.

[31] The various fora in which refugee protection reforms are presently under discussion are summarized in J. Hathaway, "Review Essay: N. Nathwani, Rethinking Refugee Law," (2004) 98(3) *American Journal of International Law* 616.

[32] The governments of state parties to the Refugee Convention agreed "to consider ways that may be required to strengthen the 1951 Convention and/or 1967 Protocol": "Declaration of States Parties to the 1951 Convention and/or its 1967 Protocol relating to the Status of Refugees," UN Doc. HCR/MMSP/2001/09, Dec. 13, 2001, incorporated in Executive Committee of the High Commissioner's Program, "Agenda for Protection," UN Doc. EC/52/SC/CRP.9/Rev.1, June 26, 2002, at Part II, Operative Paragraphs, para. 9.

[33] State parties to the Convention notably "[c]ommit[ted] [them]selves to providing, within the framework of international solidarity and burden-sharing, better refugee protection through comprehensive strategies, notably regionally and internationally, in order to build capacity, in particular in developing countries and countries with economies in transition, especially those which are hosting large-scale influxes or protracted refugee situations, and to strengthening response mechanisms, so as to ensure that refugees have access to safer and better conditions of stay and timely solutions to their problems": ibid. at para. 12.

The real challenge is to ensure that the reform process is actually driven by a determination fully and dependably to implement the agreed human rights of refugees, even as it simultaneously advances the interests of governments. There is no necessary inconsistency between these goals; to the contrary, they are actually mutually reinforcing priorities. The Convention's refugee rights regime elaborated here establishes a framework that can easily lay the groundwork for solutions to the current crisis of confidence in the value of refugee law.

CONVENTION RELATING TO THE STATUS OF REFUGEES (1951)

Preamble

The High Contracting Parties,

Considering that the Charter of the United Nations and the Universal Declaration of Human Rights approved on 10 December 1948 by the General Assembly have affirmed the principle that human beings shall enjoy fundamental rights and freedoms without discrimination,

Considering that the United Nations has, on various occasions, manifested its profound concern for refugees and endeavoured to assure refugees the widest possible exercise of these fundamental rights and freedoms,

Considering that it is desirable to revise and consolidate previous international agreements relating to the status of refugees and to extend the scope of and the protection accorded by such instruments by means of a new agreement,

Considering that the grant of asylum may place unduly heavy burdens on certain countries, and that a satisfactory solution of a problem of which the United Nations has recognized the international scope and nature cannot therefore be achieved without international co-operation,

Expressing the wish that all States, recognizing the social and humanitarian nature of the problem of refugees, will do everything within their power to prevent this problem from becoming a cause of tension between States,

Noting that the United Nations High Commissioner for Refugees is charged with the task of supervising international conventions providing for the protection of refugees, and recognizing that the effective co-ordination of measures taken to deal with this problem will depend upon the co-operation of States with the High Commissioner,

Have agreed as follows:

Chapter I General provisions

Article 1 Definition of the term "refugee"

A. For the purposes of the present Convention, the term "refugee" shall apply to any person who:

(1) Has been considered a refugee under the Arrangements of 12 May 1926 and 30 June 1928 or under the Conventions of 28 October 1933 and 10 February 1938, the Protocol of 14 September 1939 or the Constitution of the International Refugee Organization;

Decisions of non-eligibility taken by the International Refugee Organization during the period of its activities shall not prevent the status of refugee being accorded to persons who fulfil the conditions of paragraph 2 of this section;

(2) As a result of events occurring before 1 January 1951 and owing to well-founded fear of being persecuted for reasons of race, religion, nationality, membership of a particular social group or political opinion, is outside the country of his nationality and is unable or, owing to such fear, is unwilling to avail himself of the protection of that country; or who, not having a nationality and being outside the country of his former habitual residence as a result of such events, is unable or, owing to such fear, is unwilling to return to it.

In the case of a person who has more than one nationality, the term "the country of his nationality" shall mean each of the countries of which he is a national, and a person shall not be deemed to be lacking the protection of the country of his nationality if, without any valid reason based on well-founded fear, he has not availed himself of the protection of one of the countries of which he is a national.

B. (1) For the purposes of this Convention, the words "events occurring before 1 January 1951" in article 1, section A, shall be understood to mean either

(a) "events occurring in Europe before 1 January 1951"; or
(b) "events occurring in Europe or elsewhere before 1 January 1951";
and each Contracting State shall make a declaration at the time of signature, ratification or accession, specifying which of these meanings it applies for the purpose of its obligations under this Convention.

(2) Any Contracting State which has adopted alternative (a) may at any time extend its obligations by adopting alternative (b) by means of a notification addressed to the Secretary-General of the United Nations.

C. This Convention shall cease to apply to any person falling under the terms of section A if:

(1) He has voluntarily re-availed himself of the protection of the country of his nationality; or
(2) Having lost his nationality, he has voluntarily reacquired it; or
(3) He has acquired a new nationality, and enjoys the protection of the country of his new nationality; or
(4) He has voluntarily re-established himself in the country which he left or outside which he remained owing to fear of persecution; or

(5) He can no longer, because the circumstances in connection with which he has been recognized as a refugee have ceased to exist, continue to refuse to avail himself of the protection of the country of his nationality;

Provided that this paragraph shall not apply to a refugee falling under section A (1) of this article who is able to invoke compelling reasons arising out of previous persecution for refusing to avail himself of the protection of the country of nationality;

(6) Being a person who has no nationality he is, because the circumstances in connection with which he has been recognized as a refugee have ceased to exist, able to return to the country of his former habitual residence;

Provided that this paragraph shall not apply to a refugee falling under section A (1) of this article who is able to invoke compelling reasons arising out of previous persecution for refusing to return to the country of his former habitual residence.

D. This Convention shall not apply to persons who are at present receiving from organs or agencies of the United Nations other than the United Nations High Commissioner for Refugees protection or assistance.

When such protection or assistance has ceased for any reason, without the position of such persons being definitively settled in accordance with the relevant resolutions adopted by the General Assembly of the United Nations, these persons shall *ipso facto* be entitled to the benefits of this Convention.

E. This Convention shall not apply to a person who is recognized by the competent authorities of the country in which he has taken residence as having the rights and obligations which are attached to the possession of the nationality of that country.

F. The provisions of this Convention shall not apply to any person with respect to whom there are serious reasons for considering that:

(a) he has committed a crime against peace, a war crime, or a crime against humanity, as defined in the international instruments drawn up to make provision in respect of such crimes;

(b) he has committed a serious non-political crime outside the country of refuge prior to his admission to that country as a refugee;

(c) he has been guilty of acts contrary to the purposes and principles of the United Nations.

Article 2   *General obligations*

Every refugee has duties to the country in which he finds himself, which require in particular that he conform to its laws and regulations as well as to measures taken for the maintenance of public order.

Article 3   Non-discrimination

The Contracting States shall apply the provisions of this Convention to refugees without discrimination as to race, religion or country of origin.

Article 4   Religion

The Contracting States shall accord to refugees within their territories treatment at least as favourable as that accorded to their nationals with respect to freedom to practise their religion and freedom as regards the religious education of their children.

Article 5   Rights granted apart from this Convention

Nothing in this Convention shall be deemed to impair any rights and benefits granted by a Contracting State to refugees apart from this Convention.

Article 6   The term "in the same circumstances"

For the purpose of this Convention, the term "in the same circumstances" implies that any requirements (including requirements as to length and conditions of sojourn or residence) which the particular individual would have to fulfil for the enjoyment of the right in question, if he were not a refugee, must be fulfilled by him, with the exception of requirements which by their nature a refugee is incapable of fulfilling.

Article 7   Exemption from reciprocity

1. Except where this Convention contains more favourable provisions, a Contracting State shall accord to refugees the same treatment as is accorded to aliens generally.

2. After a period of three years' residence, all refugees shall enjoy exemption from legislative reciprocity in the territory of the Contracting States.

3. Each Contracting State shall continue to accord to refugees the rights and benefits to which they were already entitled, in the absence of reciprocity, at the date of entry into force of this Convention for that State.

4. The Contracting States shall consider favourably the possibility of according to refugees, in the absence of reciprocity, rights and benefits beyond those to which they are entitled according to paragraphs 2 and 3, and to extending exemption from reciprocity to refugees who do not fulfil the conditions provided for in paragraphs 2 and 3.

5. The provisions of paragraphs 2 and 3 apply both to the rights and benefits referred to in articles 13, 18, 19, 21 and 22 of this Convention and to rights and benefits for which this Convention does not provide.

Article 8   Exemption from exceptional measures

With regard to exceptional measures which may be taken against the person, property or interests of nationals of a foreign State, the Contracting States shall not apply such measures to a refugee who is formally a national of the said State solely on account of such nationality. Contracting States which, under their legislation, are prevented from applying the general principle expressed in this article, shall, in appropriate cases, grant exemptions in favour of such refugees.

Article 9   Provisional measures

Nothing in this Convention shall prevent a Contracting State, in time of war or other grave and exceptional circumstances, from taking provisionally measures which it considers to be essential to the national security in the case of a particular person, pending a determination by the Contracting State that that person is in fact a refugee and that the continuance of such measures is necessary in his case in the interests of national security.

Article 10   Continuity of residence

1. Where a refugee has been forcibly displaced during the Second World War and removed to the territory of a Contracting State, and is resident there, the period of such enforced sojourn shall be considered to have been lawful residence within that territory.

2. Where a refugee has been forcibly displaced during the Second World War from the territory of a Contracting State and has, prior to the date of entry into force of this Convention, returned there for the purpose of taking up residence, the period of residence before and after such enforced displacement shall be regarded as one uninterrupted period for any purposes for which uninterrupted residence is required.

Article 11   Refugee seamen

In the case of refugees regularly serving as crew members on board a ship flying the flag of a Contracting State, that State shall give sympathetic consideration to their establishment on its territory and the issue of travel documents to them or their temporary admission to its territory particularly with a view to facilitating their establishment in another country.

Chapter II Juridical status

Article 12 Personal status

1. The personal status of a refugee shall be governed by the law of the country of his domicile or, if he has no domicile, by the law of the country of his residence.

2. Rights previously acquired by a refugee and dependent on personal status, more particularly rights attaching to marriage, shall be respected by a Contracting State, subject to compliance, if this be necessary, with the formalities required by the law of that State, provided that the right in question is one which would have been recognized by the law of that State had he not become a refugee.

Article 13 Movable and immovable property

The Contracting States shall accord to a refugee treatment as favourable as possible and, in any event, not less favourable than that accorded to aliens generally in the same circumstances, as regards the acquisition of movable and immovable property and other rights pertaining thereto, and to leases and other contracts relating to movable and immovable property.

Article 14 Artistic rights and industrial property

In respect of the protection of industrial property, such as inventions, designs or models, trade marks, trade names, and of rights in literary, artistic and scientific works, a refugee shall be accorded in the country in which he has his habitual residence the same protection as is accorded to nationals of that country. In the territory of any other Contracting State, he shall be accorded the same protection as is accorded in that territory to nationals of the country in which he has his habitual residence.

Article 15 Right of association

As regards non-political and non-profit-making associations and trade unions the Contracting States shall accord to refugees lawfully staying in their territory the most favourable treatment accorded to nationals of a foreign country, in the same circumstances.

Article 16 Access to courts

1. A refugee shall have free access to the courts of law on the territory of all Contracting States.

2. A refugee shall enjoy in the Contracting State in which he has his habitual residence the same treatment as a national in matters pertaining to access to the courts, including legal assistance and exemption from *cautio judicatum solvi*.

3. A refugee shall be accorded in the matters referred to in paragraph 2 in countries other than that in which he has his habitual residence the treatment granted to a national of the country of his habitual residence.

Chapter III   Gainful employment

Article 17   *Wage-earning employment*

1. The Contracting States shall accord to refugees lawfully staying in their territory the most favourable treatment accorded to nationals of a foreign country in the same circumstances, as regards the right to engage in wage-earning employment.

2. In any case, restrictive measures imposed on aliens or the employment of aliens for the protection of the national labour market shall not be applied to a refugee who was already exempt from them at the date of entry into force of this Convention for the Contracting State concerned, or who fulfils one of the following conditions:

(a) He has completed three years' residence in the country;
(b) He has a spouse possessing the nationality of the country of residence. A refugee may not invoke the benefit of this provision if he has abandoned his spouse;
(c) He has one or more children possessing the nationality of the country of residence.

3. The Contracting States shall give sympathetic consideration to assimilating the rights of all refugees with regard to wage-earning employment to those of nationals, and in particular of those refugees who have entered their territory pursuant to programmes of labour recruitment or under immigration schemes.

Article 18   *Self-employment*

The Contracting States shall accord to a refugee lawfully in their territory treatment as favourable as possible and, in any event, not less favourable than that accorded to aliens generally in the same circumstances, as regards the right to engage on his own account in agriculture, industry, handicrafts and commerce and to establish commercial and industrial companies.

Article 19   Liberal professions

1. Each Contracting State shall accord to refugees lawfully staying in their territory who hold diplomas recognized by the competent authorities of that State, and who are desirous of practising a liberal profession, treatment as favourable as possible and, in any event, not less favourable than that accorded to aliens generally in the same circumstances.

2. The Contracting States shall use their best endeavours consistently with their laws and constitutions to secure the settlement of such refugees in the territories, other than the metropolitan territory, for whose international relations they are responsible.

Chapter IV   Welfare

Article 20   Rationing

Where a rationing system exists, which applies to the population at large and regulates the general distribution of products in short supply, refugees shall be accorded the same treatment as nationals.

Article 21   Housing

As regards housing, the Contracting States, in so far as the matter is regulated by laws or regulations or is subject to the control of public authorities, shall accord to refugees lawfully staying in their territory treatment as favourable as possible and, in any event, not less favourable than that accorded to aliens generally in the same circumstances.

Article 22   Public education

1. The Contracting States shall accord to refugees the same treatment as is accorded to nationals with respect to elementary education.

2. The Contracting States shall accord to refugees treatment as favourable as possible, and, in any event, not less favourable than that accorded to aliens generally in the same circumstances, with respect to education other than elementary education and, in particular, as regards access to studies, the recognition of foreign school certificates, diplomas and degrees, the remission of fees and charges and the award of scholarships.

Article 23   Public relief

The Contracting States shall accord to refugees lawfully staying in their territory the same treatment with respect to public relief and assistance as is accorded to their nationals.

Article 24   Labour legislation and social security

1. The Contracting States shall accord to refugees lawfully staying in their territory the same treatment as is accorded to nationals in respect of the following matters:

(a) In so far as such matters are governed by laws or regulations or are subject to the control of administrative authorities: remuneration, including family allowances where these form part of remuneration, hours of work, overtime arrangements, holidays with pay, restrictions on home work, minimum age of employment, apprenticeship and training, women's work and the work of young persons, and the enjoyment of the benefits of collective bargaining;

(b) Social security (legal provisions in respect of employment injury, occupational diseases, maternity, sickness, disability, old age, death, unemployment, family responsibilities and any other contingency which, according to national laws or regulations, is covered by a social security scheme), subject to the following limitations:

   (i)   There may be appropriate arrangements for the maintenance of acquired rights and rights in course of acquisition;
   (ii) National laws or regulations of the country of residence may prescribe special arrangements concerning benefits or portions of benefits which are payable wholly out of public funds, and concerning allowances paid to persons who do not fulfil the contribution conditions prescribed for the award of a normal pension.

2. The right to compensation for the death of a refugee resulting from employment injury or from occupational disease shall not be affected by the fact that the residence of the beneficiary is outside the territory of the Contracting State.

3. The Contracting States shall extend to refugees the benefits of agreements concluded between them, or which may be concluded between them in the future, concerning the maintenance of acquired rights and rights in the process of acquisition in regard to social security, subject only to the conditions which apply to nationals of the States signatory to the agreements in question.

4. The Contracting States will give sympathetic consideration to extending to refugees so far as possible the benefits of similar agreements which may at any time be in force between such Contracting States and non-contracting States.

Chapter V   Administrative measures

Article 25   Administrative assistance

1. When the exercise of a right by a refugee would normally require the assistance of authorities of a foreign country to whom he cannot have recourse, the Contracting States in whose territory he is residing shall arrange

that such assistance be afforded to him by their own authorities or by an international authority.

2. The authority or authorities mentioned in paragraph 1 shall deliver or cause to be delivered under their supervision to refugees such documents or certifications as would normally be delivered to aliens by or through their national authorities.

3. Documents or certifications so delivered shall stand in the stead of the official instruments delivered to aliens by or through their national authorities, and shall be given credence in the absence of proof to the contrary.

4. Subject to such exceptional treatment as may be granted to indigent persons, fees may be charged for the services mentioned herein, but such fees shall be moderate and commensurate with those charged to nationals for similar services.

5. The provisions of this article shall be without prejudice to articles 27 and 28.

Article 26   Freedom of movement

Each Contracting State shall accord to refugees lawfully in its territory the right to choose their place of residence and to move freely within its territory, subject to any regulations applicable to aliens generally in the same circumstances.

Article 27   Identity papers

The Contracting States shall issue identity papers to any refugee in their territory who does not possess a valid travel document.

Article 28   Travel documents

1. The Contracting States shall issue to refugees lawfully staying in their territory travel documents for the purpose of travel outside their territory, unless compelling reasons of national security or public order otherwise require, and the provisions of the Schedule to this Convention shall apply with respect to such documents. The Contracting States may issue such a travel document to any other refugee in their territory; they shall in particular give sympathetic consideration to the issue of such a travel document to refugees in their territory who are unable to obtain a travel document from the country of their lawful residence.

2. Travel documents issued to refugees under previous international agreements by parties thereto shall be recognized and treated by the Contracting States in the same way as if they had been issued pursuant to this article.

Article 29   Fiscal charges

1. The Contracting States shall not impose upon refugees duties, charges or taxes, of any description whatsoever, other or higher than those which are or may be levied on their nationals in similar situations.

2. Nothing in the above paragraph shall prevent the application to refugees of the laws and regulations concerning charges in respect of the issue to aliens of administrative documents including identity papers.

Article 30   Transfer of assets

1. A Contracting State shall, in conformity with its laws and regulations, permit refugees to transfer assets which they have brought into its territory, to another country where they have been admitted for the purposes of resettlement.

2. A Contracting State shall give sympathetic consideration to the application of refugees for permission to transfer assets wherever they may be and which are necessary for their resettlement in another country to which they have been admitted.

Article 31   Refugees unlawfully in the country of refuge

1. The Contracting States shall not impose penalties, on account of their illegal entry or presence, on refugees who, coming directly from a territory where their life or freedom was threatened in the sense of article 1, enter or are present in their territory without authorization, provided they present themselves without delay to the authorities and show good cause for their illegal entry or presence.

2. The Contracting States shall not apply to the movements of such refugees restrictions other than those which are necessary and such restrictions shall only be applied until their status in the country is regularized or they obtain admission into another country. The Contracting States shall allow such refugees a reasonable period and all the necessary facilities to obtain admission into another country.

Article 32   Expulsion

1. The Contracting States shall not expel a refugee lawfully in their territory save on grounds of national security or public order.

2. The expulsion of such a refugee shall be only in pursuance of a decision reached in accordance with due process of law. Except where compelling reasons of national security otherwise require, the refugee shall be allowed to submit evidence to clear himself, and to appeal to and be represented for the purpose before competent authority or a person or persons specially designated by the competent authority.

3. The Contracting States shall allow such a refugee a reasonable period within which to seek legal admission into another country. The Contracting States reserve the right to apply during that period such internal measures as they may deem necessary.

Article 33   Prohibition of expulsion or return ("refoulement")

1. No Contracting State shall expel or return ("refouler") a refugee in any manner whatsoever to the frontiers of territories where his life or freedom would be threatened on account of his race, religion, nationality, membership of a particular social group or political opinion.

2. The benefit of the present provision may not, however, be claimed by a refugee whom there are reasonable grounds for regarding as a danger to the security of the country in which he is, or who, having been convicted by a final judgment of a particularly serious crime, constitutes a danger to the community of that country.

Article 34   Naturalization

The Contracting States shall as far as possible facilitate the assimilation and naturalization of refugees. They shall in particular make every effort to expedite naturalization proceedings and to reduce as far as possible the charges and costs of such proceedings.

Chapter VI   Executory and transitory provisions

Article 35   Co-operation of the national authorities with the United Nations

1. The Contracting States undertake to co-operate with the Office of the United Nations High Commissioner for Refugees, or any other agency of the United Nations which may succeed it, in the exercise of its functions, and shall in particular facilitate its duty of supervising the application of the provisions of this Convention.

2. In order to enable the Office of the High Commissioner or any other agency of the United Nations which may succeed it, to make reports to the competent organs of the United Nations, the Contracting States undertake to provide them in the appropriate form with information and statistical data requested concerning:

(a) the condition of refugees,
(b) the implementation of this Convention, and
(c) laws, regulations and decrees which are, or may hereafter be, in force relating to refugees.

Article 36   Information on national legislation

The Contracting States shall communicate to the Secretary-General of the United Nations the laws and regulations which they may adopt to ensure the application of this Convention.

Article 37   Relation to previous conventions

Without prejudice to article 28, paragraph 2, of this Convention, this Convention replaces, as between parties to it, the Arrangements of 5 July 1922, 31 May 1924, 12 May 1926, 30 June 1928 and 30 July 1935, the Conventions of 28 October 1933 and 10 February 1938, the Protocol of 14 September 1939 and the Agreement of 15 October 1946.

Chapter VII   Final clauses

Article 38   Settlement of disputes

Any dispute between parties to this Convention relating to its interpretation or application, which cannot be settled by other means, shall be referred to the International Court of Justice at the request of any one of the parties to the dispute.

Article 39   Signature, ratification and accession

1. This Convention shall be opened for signature at Geneva on 28 July 1951 and shall thereafter be deposited with the Secretary-General of the United Nations. It shall be open for signature at the European Office of the United Nations from 28 July to 31 August 1951 and shall be re-opened for signature at the Headquarters of the United Nations from 17 September 1951 to 31 December 1952.

2. This Convention shall be open for signature on behalf of all States Members of the United Nations, and also on behalf of any other State invited to attend the Conference of Plenipotentiaries on the Status of Refugees and Stateless Persons or to which an invitation to sign will have been addressed by the General Assembly. It shall be ratified and the instruments of ratification shall be deposited with the Secretary-General of the United Nations.

3. This Convention shall be open from 28 July 1951 for accession by the States referred to in paragraph 2 of this article. Accession shall be effected by the deposit of an instrument of accession with the Secretary-General of the United Nations.

Article 40   Territorial application clause

1. Any State may, at the time of signature, ratification or accession, declare that this Convention shall extend to all or any of the territories

for the international relations of which it is responsible. Such a declaration shall take effect when the Convention enters into force for the State concerned.

2. At any time thereafter any such extension shall be made by notification addressed to the Secretary-General of the United Nations and shall take effect as from the ninetieth day after the day of receipt by the Secretary-General of the United Nations of this notification, or as from the date of entry into force of the Convention for the State concerned, whichever is the later.

3. With respect to those territories to which this Convention is not extended at the time of signature, ratification or accession, each State concerned shall consider the possibility of taking the necessary steps in order to extend the application of this Convention to such territories, subject, where necessary for constitutional reasons, to the consent of the Governments of such territories.

Article 41   Federal clause

In the case of a Federal or non-unitary State, the following provisions shall apply:

(a) With respect to those articles of this Convention that come within the legislative jurisdiction of the federal legislative authority, the obligations of the Federal Government shall to this extent be the same as those of parties which are not Federal States;

(b) With respect to those articles of this Convention that come within the legislative jurisdiction of constituent States, provinces or cantons which are not, under the constitutional system of the Federation, bound to take legislative action, the Federal Government shall bring such articles with a favourable recommendation to the notice of the appropriate authorities of States, provinces or cantons at the earliest possible moment;

(c) A Federal State Party to this Convention shall, at the request of any other Contracting State transmitted through the Secretary-General of the United Nations, supply a statement of the law and practice of the Federation and its constituent units in regard to any particular provision of the Convention showing the extent to which effect has been given to that provision by legislative or other action.

Article 42   Reservations

1. At the time of signature, ratification or accession, any State may make reservations to articles of the Convention other than to articles 1, 3, 4, 16 (1), 33, 36–46 inclusive.

2. Any State making a reservation in accordance with paragraph 1 of this article may at any time withdraw the reservation by a communication to that effect addressed to the Secretary-General of the United Nations.

Article 43   Entry into force

1. This Convention shall come into force on the ninetieth day following the day of deposit of the sixth instrument of ratification or accession.

2. For each State ratifying or acceding to the Convention after the deposit of the sixth instrument of ratification or accession, the Convention shall enter into force on the ninetieth day following the date of deposit by such State of its instrument of ratification or accession.

Article 44   Denunciation

1. Any Contracting State may denounce this Convention at any time by a notification addressed to the Secretary-General of the United Nations.

2. Such denunciation shall take effect for the Contracting State concerned one year from the date upon which it is received by the Secretary-General of the United Nations.

3. Any State which has made a declaration or notification under article 40 may, at any time thereafter, by a notification to the Secretary-General of the United Nations, declare that the Convention shall cease to extend to such territory one year after the date of receipt of the notification by the Secretary-General.

Article 45   Revision

1. Any Contracting State may request revision of this Convention at any time by a notification addressed to the Secretary-General of the United Nations.

2. The General Assembly of the United Nations shall recommend the steps, if any, to be taken in respect of such request.

Article 46   Notifications by the Secretary-General of the United Nations

The Secretary-General of the United Nations shall inform all Members of the United Nations and non-member States referred to in article 39:

(a) Of declarations and notifications in accordance with section B of article 1;
(b) Of signatures, ratifications and accessions in accordance with article 39;
(c) Of declarations and notifications in accordance with article 40;

(d) Of reservations and withdrawals in accordance with article 42;

(e) Of the date on which this Convention will come into force in accordance with article 43;

(f) Of denunciations and notifications in accordance with article 44;

(g) Of requests for revision in accordance with article 45.

IN FAITH WHEREOF the undersigned, duly authorized, have signed this Convention on behalf of their respective Governments,

DONE at Geneva, this twenty-eighth day of July, one thousand nine hundred and fifty-one, in a single copy, of which the English and French texts are equally authentic and which shall remain deposited in the archives of the United Nations, and certified true copies of which shall be delivered to all Members of the United Nations and to the non-member States referred to in article 39.

APPENDIX 2
PROTOCOL RELATING TO THE STATUS
OF REFUGEES (1967)

The States Parties to the present Protocol,

Considering that the Convention relating to the Status of Refugees done at Geneva on 28 July 1951 (hereinafter referred to as the Convention) covers only those persons who have become refugees as a result of events occurring before 1 January 1951,

Considering that new refugee situations have arisen since the Convention was adopted and that the refugees concerned may therefore not fall within the scope of the Convention,

Considering that it is desirable that equal status should be enjoyed by all refugees covered by the definition in the Convention irrespective of the dateline 1 January 1951,

Have agreed as follows:

Article I   General provision

1. The States Parties to the present Protocol undertake to apply articles 2 to 34 inclusive of the Convention to refugees as hereinafter defined.

2. For the purpose of the present Protocol, the term "refugee" shall, except as regards the application of paragraph 3 of this article, mean any person within the definition of article 1 of the Convention as if the words "As a result of events occurring before 1 January 1951 and . . . " and the words "as a result of such events", in article 1 A (2) were omitted.

3. The present Protocol shall be applied by the States Parties hereto without any geographic limitation, save that existing declarations made by States already Parties to the Convention in accordance with article 1 B (1) (a) of the Convention, shall, unless extended under article 1 B (2) thereof, apply also under the present Protocol.

Article II   Co-operation of the national authorities
with the United Nations

1. The States Parties to the present Protocol undertake to co-operate with the Office of the United Nations High Commissioner for Refugees, or any

other agency of the United Nations which may succeed it, in the exercise of its functions, and shall in particular facilitate its duty of supervising the application of the provisions of the present Protocol.

2. In order to enable the Office of the High Commissioner or any other agency of the United Nations which may succeed it, to make reports to the competent organs of the United Nations, the States Parties to the present Protocol undertake to provide them with the information and statistical data requested, in the appropriate form, concerning:

(a) The condition of refugees;
(b) The implementation of the present Protocol;
(c) Laws, regulations and decrees which are, or may hereafter be, in force relating to refugees.

Article III   Information on national legislation

The States Parties to the present Protocol shall communicate to the Secretary-General of the United Nations the laws and regulations which they may adopt to ensure the application of the present Protocol.

Article IV   Settlement of disputes

Any dispute between States Parties to the present Protocol which relates to its interpretation or application and which cannot be settled by other means shall be referred to the International Court of Justice at the request of any one of the parties to the dispute.

Article V   Accession

The present Protocol shall be open for accession on behalf of all States Parties to the Convention and of any other State Member of the United Nations or member of any of the specialized agencies or to which an invitation to accede may have been addressed by the General Assembly of the United Nations. Accession shall be effected by the deposit of an instrument of accession with the Secretary-General of the United Nations.

Article VI   Federal clause

In the case of a Federal or non-unitary State, the following provisions shall apply:

(a) With respect to those articles of the Convention to be applied in accordance with article I, paragraph 1, of the present Protocol that come within the legislative jurisdiction of the federal legislative authority, the obligations of the Federal Government shall to this extent be the same as those of States Parties which are not Federal States;

(b) With respect to those articles of the Convention to be applied in accordance with article I, paragraph 1, of the present Protocol that come within the legislative jurisdiction of constituent States, provinces or cantons which are not, under the constitutional system of the Federation, bound to take legislative action, the Federal Government shall bring such articles with a favourable recommendation to the notice of the appropriate authorities of States, provinces or cantons at the earliest possible moment;

(c) A Federal State Party to the present Protocol shall, at the request of any other State Party hereto transmitted through the Secretary-General of the United Nations, supply a statement of the law and practice of the Federation and its constituent units in regard to any particular provision of the Convention to be applied in accordance with article I, paragraph 1, of the present Protocol, showing the extent to which effect has been given to that provision by legislative or other action.

Article VII   Reservations and declarations

1. At the time of accession, any State may make reservations in respect of article IV of the present Protocol and in respect of the application in accordance with article I of the present Protocol of any provisions of the Convention other than those contained in articles 1, 3, 4, 16(1) and 33 thereof, provided that in the case of a State Party to the Convention reservations made under this article shall not extend to refugees in respect of whom the Convention applies.

2. Reservations made by States Parties to the Convention in accordance with article 42 thereof shall, unless withdrawn, be applicable in relation to their obligations under the present Protocol.

3. Any State making a reservation in accordance with paragraph 1 of this article may at any time withdraw such reservation by a communication to that effect addressed to the Secretary-General of the United Nations.

4. Declarations made under article 40, paragraphs 1 and 2, of the Convention by a State Party thereto which accedes to the present Protocol shall be deemed to apply in respect of the present Protocol, unless upon accession a notification to the contrary is addressed by the State Party concerned to the Secretary-General of the United Nations. The provisions of article 40, paragraphs 2 and 3, and of article 44, paragraph 3, of the Convention shall be deemed to apply *mutatis mutandis* to the present Protocol.

Article VIII   Entry into force

1. The present Protocol shall come into force on the day of deposit of the sixth instrument of accession.

2. For each State acceding to the Protocol after the deposit of the sixth instrument of accession, the Protocol shall come into force on the date of deposit by such State of its instrument of accession.

Article IX   Denunciation

1. Any State Party hereto may denounce this Protocol at any time by a notification addressed to the Secretary-General of the United Nations.

2. Such denunciation shall take effect for the State Party concerned one year from the date on which it is received by the Secretary-General of the United Nations.

Article X   Notifications by the Secretary-General of the United Nations

The Secretary-General of the United Nations shall inform the States referred to in article V above of the date of entry into force, accessions, reservations and withdrawals of reservations to and denunciations of the present Protocol, and of declarations and notifications relating hereto.

Article XI   Deposit in the archives of the Secretariat of the United Nations

A copy of the present Protocol, of which the Chinese, English, French, Russian and Spanish texts are equally authentic, signed by the President of the General Assembly and by the Secretary-General of the United Nations, shall be deposited in the archives of the Secretariat of the United Nations. The Secretary-General will transmit certified copies thereof to all States Members of the United Nations and to the other States referred to in article V above.

APPENDIX 3
UNIVERSAL DECLARATION OF HUMAN RIGHTS (1948)

Preamble

Whereas recognition of the inherent dignity and of the equal and inalienable rights of all members of the human family is the foundation of freedom, justice and peace in the world,

Whereas disregard and contempt for human rights have resulted in barbarous acts which have outraged the conscience of mankind, and the advent of a world in which human beings shall enjoy freedom of speech and belief and freedom from fear and want has been proclaimed as the highest aspiration of the common people,

Whereas it is essential, if man is not to be compelled to have recourse, as a last resort, to rebellion against tyranny and oppression, that human rights should be protected by the rule of law,

Whereas it is essential to promote the development of friendly relations between nations,

Whereas the peoples of the United Nations have in the Charter reaffirmed their faith in fundamental human rights, in the dignity and worth of the human person and in the equal rights of men and women and have determined to promote social progress and better standards of life in larger freedom,

Whereas Member States have pledged themselves to achieve, in cooperation with the United Nations, the promotion of universal respect for and observance of human rights and fundamental freedoms,

Whereas a common understanding of these rights and freedoms is of the greatest importance for the full realization of this pledge,

Now, therefore, The General Assembly,

Proclaims this Universal Declaration of Human Rights as a common standard of achievement for all peoples and all nations, to the end that every individual and every organ of society, keeping this Declaration constantly in mind, shall strive by teaching and education to promote respect for these rights and freedoms and by progressive measures, national and international, to secure their universal and effective recognition and observance, both among the peoples of Member States themselves and among the peoples of territories under their jurisdiction.

Article 1

All human beings are born free and equal in dignity and rights. They are endowed with reason and conscience and should act towards one another in a spirit of brotherhood.

Article 2

Everyone is entitled to all the rights and freedoms set forth in this Declaration, without distinction of any kind, such as race, colour, sex, language, religion, political or other opinion, national or social origin, property, birth or other status.

Furthermore, no distinction shall be made on the basis of the political, jurisdictional or international status of the country or territory to which a person belongs, whether it be independent, trust, non-self-governing or under any other limitation of sovereignty.

Article 3

Everyone has the right to life, liberty and security of person.

Article 4

No one shall be held in slavery or servitude; slavery and the slave trade shall be prohibited in all their forms.

Article 5

No one shall be subjected to torture or to cruel, inhuman or degrading treatment or punishment.

Article 6

Everyone has the right to recognition everywhere as a person before the law.

Article 7

All are equal before the law and are entitled without any discrimination to equal protection of the law. All are entitled to equal protection against any discrimination in violation of this Declaration and against any incitement to such discrimination.

Article 8

Everyone has the right to an effective remedy by the competent national tribunals for acts violating the fundamental rights granted him by the constitution or by law.

Article 9

No one shall be subjected to arbitrary arrest, detention or exile.

Article 10

Everyone is entitled in full equality to a fair and public hearing by an independent and impartial tribunal, in the determination of his rights and obligations and of any criminal charge against him.

Article 11

1. Everyone charged with a penal offence has the right to be presumed innocent until proved guilty according to law in a public trial at which he has had all the guarantees necessary for his defence.

2. No one shall be held guilty of any penal offence on account of any act or omission which did not constitute a penal offence, under national or international law, at the time when it was committed. Nor shall a heavier penalty be imposed than the one that was applicable at the time the penal offence was committed.

Article 12

No one shall be subjected to arbitrary interference with his privacy, family, home or correspondence, nor to attacks upon his honour and reputation. Everyone has the right to the protection of the law against such interference or attacks.

Article 13

1. Everyone has the right to freedom of movement and residence within the borders of each State.

2. Everyone has the right to leave any country, including his own, and to return to his country.

Article 14

1. Everyone has the right to seek and to enjoy in other countries asylum from persecution.

2. This right may not be invoked in the case of prosecutions genuinely arising from non-political crimes or from acts contrary to the purposes and principles of the United Nations.

Article 15

1. Everyone has the right to a nationality.

2. No one shall be arbitrarily deprived of his nationality nor denied the right to change his nationality.

Article 16

1. Men and women of full age, without any limitation due to race, nationality or religion, have the right to marry and to found a family. They are entitled to equal rights as to marriage, during marriage and at its dissolution.

2. Marriage shall be entered into only with the free and full consent of the intending spouses.

3. The family is the natural and fundamental group unit of society and is entitled to protection by society and the State.

Article 17

1. Everyone has the right to own property alone as well as in association with others.

2. No one shall be arbitrarily deprived of his property.

Article 18

Everyone has the right to freedom of thought, conscience and religion; this right includes freedom to change his religion or belief, and freedom, either alone or in community with others and in public or private, to manifest his religion or belief in teaching, practice, worship and observance.

Article 19

Everyone has the right to freedom of opinion and expression; this right includes freedom to hold opinions without interference and to seek, receive and impart information and ideas through any media and regardless of frontiers.

Article 20

1. Everyone has the right to freedom of peaceful assembly and association.

2. No one may be compelled to belong to an association.

Article 21

1. Everyone has the right to take part in the government of his country, directly or through freely chosen representatives.

2. Everyone has the right to equal access to public service in his country.

3. The will of the people shall be the basis of the authority of government; this will shall be expressed in periodic and genuine elections which shall be by universal and equal suffrage and shall be held by secret vote or by equivalent free voting procedures.

Article 22

Everyone, as a member of society, has the right to social security and is entitled to realization, through national effort and international co-operation and in accordance with the organization and resources of each State, of the economic, social and cultural rights indispensable for his dignity and the free development of his personality.

Article 23

1. Everyone has the right to work, to free choice of employment, to just and favourable conditions of work and to protection against unemployment.

2. Everyone, without any discrimination, has the right to equal pay for equal work.

3. Everyone who works has the right to just and favourable remuneration ensuring for himself and his family an existence worthy of human dignity, and supplemented, if necessary, by other means of social protection.

4. Everyone has the right to form and to join trade unions for the protection of his interests.

Article 24

Everyone has the right to rest and leisure, including reasonable limitation of working hours and periodic holidays with pay.

Article 25

1. Everyone has the right to a standard of living adequate for the health and well-being of himself and of his family, including food, clothing, housing and medical care and necessary social services, and the right to security in the event of unemployment, sickness, disability, widowhood, old age or other lack of livelihood in circumstances beyond his control.

2. Motherhood and childhood are entitled to special care and assistance. All children, whether born in or out of wedlock, shall enjoy the same social protection.

Article 26

1. Everyone has the right to education. Education shall be free, at least in the elementary and fundamental stages. Elementary education shall be compulsory. Technical and professional education shall be made generally available and higher education shall be equally accessible to all on the basis of merit.

2. Education shall be directed to the full development of the human personality and to the strengthening of respect for human rights and fundamental freedoms. It shall promote understanding, tolerance and friendship among all nations, racial or religious groups, and shall further the activities of the United Nations for the maintenance of peace.

3. Parents have a prior right to choose the kind of education that shall be given to their children.

Article 27

1. Everyone has the right freely to participate in the cultural life of the community, to enjoy the arts and to share in scientific advancement and its benefits.

2. Everyone has the right to the protection of the moral and material interests resulting from any scientific, literary or artistic production of which he is the author.

Article 28

Everyone is entitled to a social and international order in which the rights and freedoms set forth in this Declaration can be fully realized.

Article 29

1. Everyone has duties to the community in which alone the free and full development of his personality is possible.

2. In the exercise of his rights and freedoms, everyone shall be subject only to such limitations as are determined by law solely for the purpose of securing due recognition and respect for the rights and freedoms of others and of meeting the just requirements of morality, public order and the general welfare in a democratic society.

3. These rights and freedoms may in no case be exercised contrary to the purposes and principles of the United Nations.

Article 30

Nothing in this Declaration may be interpreted as implying for any State, group or person any right to engage in any activity or to perform any act aimed at the destruction of any of the rights and freedoms set forth herein.

APPENDIX 4

INTERNATIONAL COVENANT ON CIVIL AND POLITICAL RIGHTS (1966)

Preamble

The States Parties to the present Covenant,

Considering that, in accordance with the principles proclaimed in the Charter of the United Nations, recognition of the inherent dignity and of the equal and inalienable rights of all members of the human family is the foundation of freedom, justice and peace in the world,

Recognizing that these rights derive from the inherent dignity of the human person,

Recognizing that, in accordance with the Universal Declaration of Human Rights, the ideal of free human beings enjoying civil and political freedom and freedom from fear and want can only be achieved if conditions are created whereby everyone may enjoy his civil and political rights, as well as his economic, social and cultural rights,

Considering the obligation of States under the Charter of the United Nations to promote universal respect for, and observance of, human rights and freedoms,

Realizing that the individual, having duties to other individuals and to the community to which he belongs, is under a responsibility to strive for the promotion and observance of the rights recognized in the present Covenant,

Agree upon the following articles:

Part I

Article 1

1. All peoples have the right of self-determination. By virtue of that right they freely determine their political status and freely pursue their economic, social and cultural development.

2. All peoples may, for their own ends, freely dispose of their natural wealth and resources without prejudice to any obligations arising out of international economic co-operation, based upon the principle of mutual benefit, and international law. In no case may a people be deprived of its own means of subsistence.

3. The States Parties to the present Covenant, including those having responsibility for the administration of Non-Self-Governing and Trust Territories, shall promote the realization of the right of self-determination, and shall respect that right, in conformity with the provisions of the Charter of the United Nations.

Part II

Article 2

1. Each State Party to the present Covenant undertakes to respect and to ensure to all individuals within its territory and subject to its jurisdiction the rights recognized in the present Covenant, without distinction of any kind, such as race, colour, sex, language, religion, political or other opinion, national or social origin, property, birth or other status.

2. Where not already provided for by existing legislative or other measures, each State Party to the present Covenant undertakes to take the necessary steps, in accordance with its constitutional processes and with the provisions of the present Covenant, to adopt such legislative or other measures as may be necessary to give effect to the rights recognized in the present Covenant.

3. Each State Party to the present Covenant undertakes:

(a) To ensure that any person whose rights or freedoms as herein recognized are violated shall have an effective remedy, notwithstanding that the violation has been committed by persons acting in an official capacity;

(b) To ensure that any person claiming such a remedy shall have his right thereto determined by competent judicial, administrative or legislative authorities, or by any other competent authority provided for by the legal system of the State, and to develop the possibilities of judicial remedy;

(c) To ensure that the competent authorities shall enforce such remedies when granted.

Article 3

The States Parties to the present Covenant undertake to ensure the equal right of men and women to the enjoyment of all civil and political rights set forth in the present Covenant.

Article 4

1. In time of public emergency which threatens the life of the nation and the existence of which is officially proclaimed, the States Parties to the present Covenant may take measures derogating from their obligations under the

present Covenant to the extent strictly required by the exigencies of the situation, provided that such measures are not inconsistent with their other obligations under international law and do not involve discrimination solely on the ground of race, colour, sex, language, religion or social origin.

2. No derogation from articles 6, 7, 8 (paragraphs 1 and 2), 11, 15, 16 and 18 may be made under this provision.

3. Any State Party to the present Covenant availing itself of the right of derogation shall immediately inform the other States Parties to the present Covenant, through the intermediary of the Secretary-General of the United Nations, of the provisions from which it has derogated and of the reasons by which it was actuated. A further communication shall be made, through the same intermediary, on the date on which it terminates such derogation.

Article 5

1. Nothing in the present Covenant may be interpreted as implying for any State, group or person any right to engage in any activity or perform any act aimed at the destruction of any of the rights and freedoms recognized herein or at their limitation to a greater extent than is provided for in the present Covenant.

2. There shall be no restriction upon or derogation from any of the fundamental human rights recognized or existing in any State Party to the present Covenant pursuant to law, conventions, regulations or custom on the pretext that the present Covenant does not recognize such rights or that it recognize them to a lesser extent.

Part III

Article 6

1. Every human being has the inherent right to life. This right shall be protected by law. No one shall be arbitrarily deprived of his life.

2. In countries which have not abolished the death penalty, sentence of death may be imposed only for the most serious crimes in accordance with the law in force at the time of the commission of the crime and not contrary to the provisions of the present Covenant and to the Convention on the Prevention and Punishment of the Crime of Genocide. This penalty can only be carried out pursuant to a final judgement rendered by a competent court.

3. When deprivation of life constitutes the crime of genocide, it is understood that nothing in this article shall authorize any State Party to the present Covenant to derogate in any way from any obligation assumed under the provisions of the Convention on the Prevention and Punishment of the Crime of Genocide.

4. Anyone sentenced to death shall have the right to seek pardon or commutation of the sentence. Amnesty, pardon or commutation of the sentence of death may be granted in all cases.

5. Sentence of death shall not be imposed for crimes committed by persons below eighteen years of age and shall not be carried out on pregnant women.

6. Nothing in this article shall be invoked to delay or to prevent the abolition of capital punishment by any State Party to the present Covenant.

Article 7

No one shall be subjected to torture or to cruel, inhuman or degrading treatment or punishment. In particular, no one shall be subjected without his free consent to medical or scientific experimentation.

Article 8

1. No one shall be held in slavery; slavery and the slave-trade in all their forms shall be prohibited.

2. No one shall be held in servitude.

3. (a) No one shall be required to perform forced or compulsory labour.

  (b) Paragraph 3 (a) shall not be held to preclude, in countries where imprisonment with hard labour may be imposed as a punishment for a crime, the performance of hard labour in pursuance of a sentence to such punishment by a competent court.

  (c) For the purpose of this paragraph the term "forced or compulsory labour" shall not include:

    (i) Any work or service, not referred to in subparagraph (b), normally required of a person who is under detention in consequence of a lawful order of a court, or of a person during conditional release from such detention;

    (ii) Any service of a military character and, in countries where conscientious objection is recognized, any national service required by law of conscientious objectors;

    (iii) Any service exacted in cases of emergency or calamity threatening the life or well-being of the community;

    (iv) Any work or service which forms part of normal civil obligations.

Article 9

1. Everyone has the right to liberty and security of person. No one shall be subjected to arbitrary arrest or detention. No one shall be deprived of his

liberty except on such grounds and in accordance with such procedure as are established by law.

2. Anyone who is arrested shall be informed, at the time of arrest, of the reasons for his arrest and shall be promptly informed of any charges against him.

3. Anyone arrested or detained on a criminal charge shall be brought promptly before a judge or other officer authorized by law to exercise judicial power and shall be entitled to trial within a reasonable time or to release. It shall not be the general rule that persons awaiting trial shall be detained in custody, but release may be subject to guarantees to appear for trial, at any other stage of the judicial proceedings, and, should occasion arise, for execution of the judgement.

4. Anyone who is deprived of his liberty by arrest or detention shall be entitled to take proceedings before a court, in order that that court may decide without delay on the lawfulness of his detention and order his release if the detention is not lawful.

5. Anyone who has been the victim of unlawful arrest or detention shall have an enforceable right to compensation.

Article 10

1. All persons deprived of their liberty shall be treated with humanity and with respect for the inherent dignity of the human person.

2. (a) Accused persons shall, save in exceptional circumstances, be segregated from convicted persons and shall be subject to separate treatment appropriate to their status as unconvicted persons;

   (b) Accused juvenile persons shall be separated from adults and brought as speedily as possible for adjudication.

3. The penitentiary system shall comprise treatment of prisoners the essential aim of which shall be their reformation and social rehabilitation. Juvenile offenders shall be segregated from adults and be accorded treatment appropriate to their age and legal status.

Article 11

No one shall be imprisoned merely on the ground of inability to fulfil a contractual obligation.

Article 12

1. Everyone lawfully within the territory of a State shall, within that territory, have the right to liberty of movement and freedom to choose his residence.

2. Everyone shall be free to leave any country, including his own.

3. The above-mentioned rights shall not be subject to any restrictions except those which are provided by law, are necessary to protect national security, public order (*ordre public*), public health or morals or the rights and freedoms of others, and are consistent with the other rights recognized in the present Covenant.

4. No one shall be arbitrarily deprived of the right to enter his own country.

Article 13

An alien lawfully in the territory of a State Party to the present Covenant may be expelled therefrom only in pursuance of a decision reached in accordance with law and shall, except where compelling reasons of national security otherwise require, be allowed to submit the reasons against his expulsion and to have his case reviewed by, and be represented for the purpose before, the competent authority or a person or persons especially designated by the competent authority.

Article 14

1. All persons shall be equal before the courts and tribunals. In the determination of any criminal charge against him, or of his rights and obligations in a suit at law, everyone shall be entitled to a fair and public hearing by a competent, independent and impartial tribunal established by law. The Press and the public may be excluded from all or part of a trial for reasons of morals, public order (*ordre public*) or national security in a democratic society, or when the interest of the private lives of the parties so requires, or to the extent strictly necessary in the opinion of the court in special circumstances where publicity would prejudice the interests of justice; but any judgement rendered in a criminal case or in a suit at law shall be made public except where the interest of juvenile persons otherwise requires or the proceedings concern matrimonial disputes or the guardianship of children.

2. Everyone charged with a criminal offence shall have the right to be presumed innocent until proved guilty according to law.

3. In the determination of any criminal charge against him, everyone shall be entitled to the following minimum guarantees, in full equality:

(a) To be informed promptly and in detail in a language which he understands of the nature and cause of the charge against him;

(b) To have adequate time and facilities for the preparation of his defence and to communicate with counsel of his own choosing;

(c) To be tried without undue delay;

(d) To be tried in his presence, and to defend himself in person or through legal assistance of his own choosing; to be informed, if he does not have legal assistance, of this right; and to have legal assistance assigned to him, in any case where the interests of justice so require, and without payment by him in any such case if he does not have sufficient means to pay for it;

(e) To examine, or have examined, the witnesses against him and to obtain the attendance and examination of witnesses on his behalf under the same conditions as witnesses against him;

(f) To have the free assistance of an interpreter if he cannot understand or speak the language used in court;

(g) Not to be compelled to testify against himself or to confess guilt.

4. In the case of juvenile persons, the procedure shall be such as will take account of their age and the desirability of promoting their rehabilitation.

5. Everyone convicted of a crime shall have the right to his conviction and sentence being reviewed by a higher tribunal according to law.

6. When a person has by a final decision been convicted of a criminal offence and when subsequently his conviction has been reversed or he has been pardoned on the ground that a new or newly discovered fact shows conclusively that there has been a miscarriage of justice, the person who has suffered punishment as a result of such conviction shall be compensated according to law, unless it is proved that the non-disclosure of the unknown fact in time is wholly or partly attributable to him.

7. No one shall be liable to be tried or punished again for an offence for which he has already been finally convicted or acquitted in accordance with the law and penal procedure of each country.

Article 15

1. No one shall be held guilty of any criminal offence on account of any act or omission which did not constitute a criminal offence, under national or international law, at the time when it was committed. Nor shall a heavier penalty be imposed than the one that was applicable at the time when the criminal offence was committed. If, subsequent to the commission of the offence, provision is made by law for the imposition of a lighter penalty, the offender shall benefit thereby.

2. Nothing in this article shall prejudice the trial and punishment of any person for any act or omission which, at the time when it was committed, was criminal according to the general principles of law recognized by the community of nations.

Article 16

Everyone shall have the right to recognition everywhere as a person before the law.

Article 17

1. No one shall be subjected to arbitrary or unlawful interference with his privacy, family, home or correspondence, nor to unlawful attacks on his honour and reputation.

2. Everyone has the right to the protection of the law against such interference or attacks.

Article 18

1. Everyone shall have the right to freedom of thought, conscience and religion. This right shall include freedom to have or to adopt a religion or belief of his choice, and freedom, either individually or in community with others and in public or private, to manifest his religion or belief in worship, observance, practice and teaching.

2. No one shall be subject to coercion which would impair his freedom to have or to adopt a religion or belief of his choice.

3. Freedom to manifest one's religion or beliefs may be subject only to such limitations as are prescribed by law and are necessary to protect public safety, order, health, or morals or the fundamental rights and freedoms of others.

4. The States Parties to the present Covenant undertake to have respect for the liberty of parents and, when applicable, legal guardians to ensure the religious and moral education of their children in conformity with their own convictions.

Article 19

1. Everyone shall have the right to hold opinions without interference.

2. Everyone shall have the right to freedom of expression; this right shall include freedom to seek, receive and impart information and ideas of all kinds, regardless of frontiers, either orally, in writing or in print, in the form of art, or through any other media of his choice.

3. The exercise of the rights provided for in paragraph 2 of this article carries with it special duties and responsibilities. It may therefore be subject to certain restrictions, but these shall only be such as are provided by law and are necessary:

(a) For respect of the rights or reputations of others;
(b) For the protection of national security or of public order (*ordre public*), or of public health or morals.

Article 20

1. Any propaganda for war shall be prohibited by law.

2. Any advocacy of national, racial or religious hatred that constitutes incitement to discrimination, hostility or violence shall be prohibited by law.

Article 21

The right of peaceful assembly shall be recognized. No restrictions may be placed on the exercise of this right other than those imposed in conformity with the law and which are necessary in a democratic society in the interests of national security or public safety, public order (*ordre public*), the protection of public health or morals or the protection of the rights and freedoms of others.

Article 22

1. Everyone shall have the right to freedom of association with others, including the right to form and join trade unions for the protection of his interests.

2. No restrictions may be placed on the exercise of this right other than those which are prescribed by law and which are necessary in a democratic society in the interests of national security or public safety, public order (*ordre public*), the protection of public health or morals or the protection of the rights and freedoms of others. This article shall not prevent the imposition of lawful restrictions on members of the armed forces and of the police in their exercise of this right.

3. Nothing in this article shall authorize States Parties to the International Labour Organisation Convention of 1948 concerning freedom of association and protection of the right to organize to take legislative measures which would prejudice, or to apply the law in such a manner as to prejudice, the guarantees provided for in that Convention.

Article 23

1. The family is the natural and fundamental group unit of society and is entitled to protection by society and the State.

2. The right of men and women of marriageable age to marry and to found a family shall be recognized.

3. No marriage shall be entered into without the free and full consent of the intending spouses.

4. States Parties to the present Covenant shall take appropriate steps to ensure equality of rights and responsibilities of spouses as to marriage, during marriage and at its dissolution. In the case of dissolution, provision shall be made for the necessary protection of any children.

Article 24

1. Every child shall have, without any discrimination as to race, colour, sex, language, religion, national or social origin, property or birth, the right to

such measures of protection as are required by his status as a minor, on the part of his family, society and the State.

2. Every child shall be registered immediately after birth and shall have a name.

3. Every child has the right to acquire a nationality.

Article 25

Every citizen shall have the right and the opportunity, without any of the distinctions mentioned in article 2 and without unreasonable restrictions:

(a) To take part in the conduct of public affairs, directly or through freely chosen representatives;

(b) To vote and to be elected at genuine periodic elections which shall be by universal and equal suffrage and shall be held by secret ballot, guaranteeing the free expression of the will of the electors;

(c) To have access, on general terms of equality, to public service in his country.

Article 26

All persons are equal before the law and are entitled without any discrimination to the equal protection of the law. In this respect, the law shall prohibit any discrimination and guarantee to all persons equal and effective protection against discrimination on any ground such as race, colour, sex, language, religion, political or other opinion, national or social origin, property, birth or other status.

Article 27

In those States in which ethnic, religious or linguistic minorities exist, persons belonging to such minorities shall not be denied the right, in community with the other members of their group, to enjoy their own culture, to profess and practise their own religion, or to use their own language.

Part IV

Article 28

1. There shall be established a Human Rights Committee (hereafter referred to in the present Covenant as the Committee). It shall consist of eighteen members and shall carry out the functions hereinafter provided.

2. The Committee shall be composed of nationals of the States Parties to the present Covenant who shall be persons of high moral character and recognized

competence in the field of human rights, consideration being given to the usefulness of the participation of some persons having legal experience.

3. The members of the Committee shall be elected and shall serve in their personal capacity.

Article 29

1. The members of the Committee shall be elected by secret ballot from a list of persons possessing the qualifications prescribed in article 28 and nominated for the purpose by the States Parties to the present Covenant.

2. Each State Party to the present Covenant may nominate not more than two persons. These persons shall be nationals of the nominating State.

3. A person shall be eligible for renomination.

Article 30

1. The initial election shall be held no later than six months after the date of the entry into force of the present Covenant.

2. At least four months before the date of each election to the Committee, other than an election to fill a vacancy declared in accordance with article 34, the Secretary-General of the United Nations shall address a written invitation to the States Parties to the present Covenant to submit their nominations for membership of the Committee within three months.

3. The Secretary-General of the United Nations shall prepare a list in alphabetical order or all the persons thus nominated, with an indication of the States Parties which have nominated them, and shall submit it to the States Parties to the present Covenant no later than one month before the date of each election.

4. Elections of the members of the Committee shall be held at a meeting of the States Parties to the present Covenant convened by the Secretary-General of the United Nations at the Headquarters of the United Nations. At that meeting, for which two thirds of the States Parties to the present Covenant shall constitute a quorum, the persons elected to the Committee shall be those nominees who obtain the largest number of votes and an absolute majority of the votes of the representatives of States Parties present and voting.

Article 31

1. The Committee may not include more than one national of the same State.

2. In the election of the Committee, consideration shall be given to equitable geographical distribution of membership and to the representation of the different forms of civilization and of the principle legal systems.

Article 32

1. The members of the Committee shall be elected for a term of four years. They shall be eligible for re-election if renominated. However, the terms of nine of the members elected at the first election shall expire at the end of two years; immediately after the first election, the names of these nine members shall be chosen by lot by the Chairman of the meeting referred to in article 30, paragraph 4.

2. Elections at the expiry of office shall be held in accordance with the preceding articles of this part of the present Covenant.

Article 33

1. If, in the unanimous opinion of the other members, a member of the Committee has ceased to carry out his functions for any cause other than absence of a temporary character, the Chairman of the Committee shall notify the Secretary-General of the United Nations, who shall then declare the seat of that member to be vacant.

2. In the event of the death or the resignation of a member of the Committee, the Chairman shall immediately notify the Secretary-General of the United Nations, who shall declare the seat vacant from the date of death or the date on which the resignation takes effect.

Article 34

1. When a vacancy is declared in accordance with article 33 and if the term of office of the member to be replaced does not expire within six months of the declaration of the vacancy, the Secretary-General of the United Nations shall notify each of the States Parties to the present Covenant, which may within two months submit nominations in accordance with article 29 for the purpose of filling the vacancy.

2. The Secretary-General of the United Nations shall prepare a list in alphabetical order of the persons thus nominated and shall submit it to the States Parties to the present Covenant. The election to fill the vacancy shall then take place in accordance with the relevant provisions of this part of the present Covenant.

3. A member of the Committee elected to fill a vacancy declared in accordance with article 33 shall hold office for the remainder of the term of the member who vacated the seat on the Committee under the provisions of that article.

Article 35

The members of the Committee shall, with the approval of the General Assembly of the United Nations, receive emoluments from United Nations resources on such terms and conditions as the General Assembly may decide, having regard to the importance of the Committee's responsibilities.

Article 36

The Secretary-General of the United Nations shall provide the necessary staff and facilities for the effective performance of the functions of the Committee under the present Covenant.

Article 37

1. The Secretary-General of the United Nations shall convene the initial meeting of the Committee at the Headquarters of the United Nations.

2. After its initial meeting, the Committee shall meet at such times as shall be provided in its rules of procedure.

3. The Committee shall normally meet at the Headquarters of the United Nations or at the United Nations Office at Geneva.

Article 38

Every member of the Committee shall, before taking up his duties, make a solemn declaration in open committee that he will perform his functions impartially and conscientiously.

Article 39

1. The Committee shall elect its officers for a term of two years. They may be re-elected.

2. The Committee shall establish its own rules of procedure, but these rules shall provide, *inter alia*, that:

(a) Twelve members shall constitute a quorum;
(b) Decisions of the Committee shall be made by a majority vote of the members present.

Article 40

1. The States Parties to the present Covenant undertake to submit reports on the measures they have adopted which give effect to the rights recognized herein and on the progress made in the enjoyment of those rights:

(a) Within one year of the entry into force of the present covenant for the States Parties concerned;

(b) Thereafter whenever the Committee so requests.

2. All reports shall be submitted to the Secretary-General of the United Nations, who shall transmit them to the Committee for consideration. Reports shall indicate the factors and difficulties, if any, affecting the implementation of the present Covenant.

3. The Secretary-General of the United Nations may, after consultation with the Committee, transmit to the specialized agencies concerned copies of such parts of the reports as may fall within their field of competence.

4. The Committee shall study the reports submitted by the States Parties to the present Covenant. It shall transmit its reports, and such general comments as it may consider appropriate, to the States Parties. The Committee may also transmit to the Economic and Social Council these comments along with the copies of the reports it has received from States Parties to the present Covenant.

5. The States Parties to the present Covenant may submit to the Committee observations on any comments that may be made in accordance with paragraph 4 of this article.

Article 41

1. A State Party to the present Covenant may at any time declare under this article that it recognizes the competence of the Committee to receive and consider communications to the effect that a State Party claims that another State Party is not fulfilling its obligations under the present Covenant. Communications under this article may be received and considered only if submitted by a State Party which has made a declaration recognizing in regard to itself the competence of the Committee. No communication shall be received by the Committee if it concerns a State Party which has not made such a declaration. Communications received under this article shall be dealt with in accordance with the following procedure:

(a) If a State party to the present Covenant considers that another State Party is not giving effect to the provisions of the present Covenant, it may, by written communication, bring the matter to the attention of that State Party. Within three months after the receipt of the communication, the receiving State shall afford the State which sent the communication an explanation, or any other statement in writing clarifying the matter, which should include, to the extent possible and pertinent, reference to domestic procedures and remedies taken, pending, or available in the matter.

(b) If the matter is not adjusted to the satisfaction of both States Parties concerned within six months after the receipt by the receiving State of the initial communication, either State shall have the right to refer the matter to the Committee, by notice given to the Committee and to the other State.

(c) The Committee shall deal with a matter referred to it only after it has ascertained that all available domestic remedies have been invoked and exhausted in the matter, in conformity with the generally recognized principles of international law. This shall not be the rule where the application of the remedies is unreasonably prolonged.

(d) The Committee shall hold closed meetings when examining communications under this article.

(e) Subject to the provisions of subparagraph (c), the Committee shall make available its good offices to the States Parties concerned with a view to a friendly solution of the matter on the basis of respect for human rights and fundamental freedoms as recognized in the present Covenant;

(f) In any matter referred to it, the Committee may call upon the States Parties concerned, referred to in subparagraph (b), to supply any relevant information.

(g) The States Parties concerned, referred to in subparagraph (b), shall have the right to be represented when the matter is being considered in the Committee and to make submissions orally and/or in writing.

(h) The Committee shall, within twelve months after the date of receipt of notice under subparagraph (b), submit a report:

  (i) If a solution within the terms of subparagraph (e) is reached, the Committee shall confine its report to a brief statement of the facts and of the solution reached;

  (ii) If a solution within the terms of subparagraph (e) is not reached, the Committee shall confine its report to a brief statement of the facts; the written submissions and record of the oral submissions made by the States Parties concerned shall be attached to the report.

In every matter, the report shall be communicated to the States Parties concerned.

2. The provisions of this article shall come into force when ten States Parties to the present Covenant have made declarations under paragraph 1 of this article. Such declarations shall be deposited by the States Parties with the Secretary-General of the United Nations, who shall transmit copies thereof to the other States Parties. A declaration may be withdrawn at any time by notification to the Secretary-General. Such a withdrawal shall not prejudice the consideration of any matter which is the subject of a communication already transmitted under this article; no further communication by any State Party shall be received after the notification of withdrawal of the declaration has been received by Secretary-General, unless the State Party concerned has made a new declaration.

Article 42

1. (a) If a matter referred to the Committee in accordance with article 41 is not resolved to the satisfaction of the States Parties concerned, the Committee may, with the prior consent of the States Parties concerned, appoint an *ad hoc* Conciliation Commission (hereinafter referred to as the Commission). The good offices of the Commission shall be made available to the States Parties concerned with a view to an amicable solution of the matter on the basis of respect for the present Covenant.

   (b) The Commission shall consist of five persons acceptable to the States Parties concerned. If the States Parties concerned fail to reach agreement within three months on all or part of the composition of the Commission the members of the Commission concerning whom no agreement has been reached shall be elected by secret ballot by a two-thirds majority vote of the Committee from among its members.

2. The members of the Commission shall serve in their personal capacity. They shall not be nationals of the States Parties concerned, or of a State not party to the present Covenant, or of a State Party which has not made a declaration under article 41.

3. The Commission shall elect its own Chairman and adopt its own rules of procedure.

4. The meetings of the Commission shall normally be held at the Headquarters of the United Nations or at the United Nations Office at Geneva. However, they may be held at such other convenient places as the Commission may determine in consultation with the Secretary-General of the United Nations and the States Parties concerned.

5. The secretariat provided in accordance with article 36 shall also service the commissions appointed under this article.

6. The information received and collated by the Committee shall be made available to the Commission and the Commission may call upon the States Parties concerned to supply any other relevant information.

7. When the Commission has fully considered the matter, but in any event not later than twelve months after having been seized of the matter, it shall submit to the Chairman of the Committee a report for communication to the States Parties concerned.

(a) If the Commission is unable to complete its consideration of the matter within twelve months, it shall confine its report to a brief statement of the status of its consideration of the matter;

(b) If an amicable solution to the matter on the basis of respect for human rights as recognized in the present Covenant is reached, the Commission shall confine its report to a brief statement of the facts and of the solution reached;

(c) If a solution within the terms of subparagraph (b) is not reached, the Commission's report shall embody its findings on all questions of fact relevant to the issues between the States Parties concerned, and its views on the possibilities of an amicable solution of the matter. This report shall also contain the written submissions and a record of the oral submissions made by the States Parties concerned;

(d) If the Commission's report is submitted under subparagraph (c), the States Parties concerned shall, within three months of the receipt of the report, notify the Chairman of the Committee whether or not they accept the contents of the report of the Commission.

8. The provisions of this article are without prejudice to the responsibilities of the Committee under article 41.

9. The States Parties concerned shall share equally all the expenses of the members of the Commission in accordance with estimates to be provided by the Secretary-General of the United Nations.

10. The Secretary-General of the United Nations shall be empowered to pay the expenses of the members of the Commission, if necessary, before reimbursement by the States Parties concerned, in accordance with paragraph 9 of this article.

Article 43

The members of the Committee, and of the *ad hoc* conciliation commissions which may be appointed under article 42, shall be entitled to the facilities, privileges and immunities of experts on mission for the United Nations as laid down in the relevant sections of the Convention on the Privileges and Immunities of the United Nations.

Article 44

The provisions for the implementation of the present Covenant shall apply without prejudice to the procedures prescribed in the field of human rights by or under the constituent instruments and the conventions of the United Nations and of the specialized agencies and shall not prevent the States Parties to the present Covenant from having recourse to other procedures for settling a dispute in accordance with general or special international agreements in force between them.

Article 45

The Committee shall submit to the General Assembly of the United Nations, through the Economic and Social Council, an annual report on its activities.

Part V

Article 46

Nothing in the present Covenant shall be interpreted as impairing the provisions of the Charter of the United Nations and of the constitutions of the specialized agencies which define the respective responsibilities of the various organs of the United Nations and of the specialized agencies in regard to the matters dealt with in the present Covenant.

Article 47

Nothing in the present Covenant shall be interpreted as impairing the inherent right of all peoples to enjoy and utilize fully and freely their natural wealth and resources.

Part VI

Article 48

1. The present Covenant is open for signature by any State Member of the United Nations or member of any of its specialized agencies, by any State Party to the Statute of the International Court of Justice, and by any other State which has been invited by the General Assembly of the United Nations to become a party to the present Covenant.

2. The present Covenant is subject to ratification. Instruments of ratification shall be deposited with the Secretary-General of the United Nations.

3. The present Covenant shall be open to accession by any State referred to in paragraph 1 of this article.

4. Accession shall be effected by the deposit of an instrument of accession with the Secretary-General of the United Nations.

5. The Secretary-General of the United Nations shall inform all States which have signed this Covenant or acceded to it of the deposit of each instrument of ratification or accession.

Article 49

1. The present Covenant shall enter into force three months after the date of the deposit with the Secretary-General of the United Nations of the thirty-fifth instrument of ratification or instrument of accession.

2. For each State ratifying the present Covenant or acceding to it after the deposit of the thirty-fifth instrument of ratification or instrument of accession, the present Covenant shall enter into force three months after the date of the deposit of its own instrument of ratification or instrument of accession.

Article 50

The provisions of the present Covenant shall extend to all parts of federal States without any limitations or exceptions.

Article 51

1. Any State Party to the present Covenant may propose an amendment and file it with the Secretary-General of the United Nations. The Secretary-General of the United Nations shall thereupon communicate any proposed amendments to the States Parties to the present Covenant with a request that they notify him whether they favour a conference of States Parties for the purpose of considering and voting upon the proposals. In the event that at least one third of the States Parties favours such a conference, the Secretary-General shall convene the conference under the auspices of the United Nations. Any amendment adopted by a majority of the States Parties present and voting at the conference shall be submitted to the General Assembly of the United Nations for approval.

2. Amendments shall come into force when they have been approved by the General Assembly of the United Nations and accepted by a two-thirds majority of the States Parties to the present Covenant in accordance with their respective constitutional processes.

3. When amendments come into force, they shall be binding on those States Parties which have accepted them, other States Parties still being bound by the provisions of the present Covenant and any earlier amendment which they have accepted.

Article 52

Irrespective of the notifications made under article 48, paragraph 5, the Secretary-General of the United Nations shall inform all States referred to in paragraph 1 of the same article of the following particulars:

(a) Signatures, ratifications and accessions under article 48;
(b) The date of the entry into force of the present Covenant under article 49 and the date of the entry into force of any amendments under article 51.

Article 53

1. The present Covenant, of which the Chinese, English, French, Russian and Spanish texts are equally authentic, shall be deposited in the archives of the United Nations.

2. The Secretary-General of the United Nations shall transmit certified copies of the present Covenant to all States referred to in article 48.

IN FAITH WHEREOF the undersigned, being duly authorized thereto by their respective Governments, have signed the present Covenant, opened for signature at New York, on the nineteenth day of December, one thousand nine hundred and sixty-six.

APPENDIX 5

INTERNATIONAL COVENANT ON ECONOMIC, SOCIAL AND CULTURAL RIGHTS (1966)

Preamble

The States Parties to the present Covenant,

Considering that, in accordance with the principles proclaimed in the Charter of the United Nations, recognition of the inherent dignity and of the equal and inalienable rights of all members of the human family is the foundation of freedom, justice and peace in the world,

Recognizing that these rights derive from the inherent dignity of the human person,

Recognizing that, in accordance with the Universal Declaration of Human Rights, the ideal of free human beings enjoying freedom from fear and want can only be achieved if conditions are created whereby everyone may enjoy his economic, social and cultural rights, as well as his civil and political rights,

Considering the obligation of States under the Charter of the United Nations to promote universal respect for, and observance of, human rights and freedoms,

Realizing that the individual, having duties to other individuals and to the community to which he belongs, is under a responsibility to strive for the promotion and observance of the rights recognized in the present Covenant,

Agree upon the following articles:

Part I

Article 1

1. All peoples have the right of self-determination. By virtue of that right they freely determine their political status and freely pursue their economic, social and cultural development.

2. All peoples may, for their own ends, freely dispose of their natural wealth and resources without prejudice to any obligations arising out of international economic co-operation, based upon the principle of mutual benefit, and international law. In no case may a people be deprived of its own means of subsistence.

3. The States Parties to the present Covenant, including those having responsibility for the administration of Non-Self-Governing and Trust

Territories, shall promote the realization of the right of self-determination, and shall respect that right, in conformity with the provisions of the Charter of the United Nations.

Part II

Article 2

1. Each State Party to the present Covenant undertakes to take steps, individually and through international assistance and co-operation, especially economic and technical, to the maximum of its available resources, with a view to achieving progressively the full realization of the rights recognized in the present Covenant by all appropriate means, including particularly the adoption of legislative measures.

2. The States Parties to the present Covenant undertake to guarantee that the rights enunciated in the present Covenant will be exercised without discrimination of any kind as to race, colour, sex, language, religion, political or other opinion, national or social origin, property, birth or other status.

3. Developing countries, with due regard to human rights and their national economy, may determine to what extent they would guarantee the economic rights recognized in the present Covenant to non-nationals.

Article 3

The States Parties to the present Covenant undertake to ensure the equal right of men and women to the enjoyment of all economic, social and cultural rights set forth in the present Covenant.

Article 4

The States Parties to the present Covenant recognize that, in the enjoyment of those rights provided by the State in conformity with the present Covenant, the State may subject such rights only to such limitations as are determined by law only in so far as this may be compatible with the nature of these rights and solely for the purpose of promoting the general welfare in a democratic society.

Article 5

1. Nothing in the present Covenant may be interpreted as implying for any State, group or person any right to engage in any activity or to perform any act aimed at the destruction of any of the rights or freedoms recognized herein, or at their limitation to a greater extent than is provided for in the present Covenant.

2. No restriction upon or derogation from any of the fundamental human rights recognized or existing in any country in virtue of law, conventions, regulations or custom shall be admitted on the pretext that the present Covenant does not recognize such rights or that it recognizes them to a lesser extent.

Part III

Article 6

1. The States Parties to the present Covenant recognize the right to work, which includes the right of everyone to the opportunity to gain his living by work which he freely chooses or accepts, and will take appropriate steps to safeguard this right.

2. The steps to be taken by a State Party to the present Covenant to achieve the full realization of this right shall include technical and vocational guidance and training programmes, policies and techniques to achieve steady economic, social and cultural development and full and productive employment under conditions safeguarding fundamental political and economic freedoms to the individual.

Article 7

The States Parties to the present Covenant recognize the right of everyone to the enjoyment of just and favourable conditions of work, which ensure, in particular:

(a) remuneration which provides all workers, as a minimum, with:

   (i) fair wages and equal remuneration for work of equal value without distinction of any kind, in particular women being guaranteed conditions of work not inferior to those enjoyed by men, with equal pay for equal work;

   (ii) a decent living for themselves and their families in accordance with the provisions of the present Covenant;

(b) safe and healthy working conditions;

(c) equal opportunity for everyone to be promoted in his employment to an appropriate higher level, subject to no considerations other than those of seniority and competence;

(d) rest, leisure and reasonable limitation of working hours and periodic holidays with pay, as well as remuneration for public holidays.

Article 8

1. The States Parties to the present Covenant undertake to ensure:

(a) the right of everyone to form trade unions and join the trade union of his choice, subject only to the rules of the organization concerned, for the promotion and protection of his economic and social interests. No restrictions may be placed on the exercise of this right other than those prescribed by law and which are necessary in a democratic society in the interests of national security or public order or for the protection of the rights and freedoms of others;

(b) the right of trade unions to establish national federations or confederations and the right of the latter to form or join international trade-union organizations;

(c) the right of trade unions to function freely subject to no limitations other than those prescribed by law and which are necessary in a democratic society in the interests of national security or public order or for the protection of the rights and freedoms of others;

(d) the right to strike, provided that it is exercised in conformity with the laws of the particular country.

2. This article shall not prevent the imposition of lawful restrictions on the exercise of these rights by members of the armed forces or of the police or of the administration of the State.

3. Nothing in this article shall authorize States Parties to the International Labour Organisation Convention of 1948 concerning Freedom of Association and Protection of the Right to Organize to take legislative measures which would prejudice, or apply the law in such a manner as would prejudice, the guarantees provided for in that Convention.

Article 9

The States Parties to the present Covenant recognize the right of everyone to social security, including social insurance.

Article 10

The States Parties to the present Covenant recognize that:

1. The widest possible protection and assistance should be accorded to the family, which is the natural and fundamental group unit of society, particularly for its establishment and while it is responsible for the care and education of dependent children. Marriage must be entered into with the free consent of the intending spouses.

2. Special protection should be accorded to mothers during a reasonable period before and after childbirth. During such period working mothers should be accorded paid leave or leave with adequate social security benefits.

3. Special measures of protection and assistance should be taken on behalf of all children and young persons without any discrimination for reasons of parentage or other conditions. Children and young persons should be

protected from economic and social exploitation. Their employment in work harmful to their morals or health or dangerous to life or likely to hamper their normal development should be punishable by law. States should also set age limits below which the paid employment of child labour should be prohibited and punishable by law.

Article 11

1. The States Parties to the present Covenant recognize the right of everyone to an adequate standard of living for himself and his family, including adequate food, clothing and housing, and to the continuous improvement of living conditions. The States Parties will take appropriate steps to ensure the realization of this right, recognizing to this effect the essential importance of international co-operation based on free consent.

2. The States Parties to the present Covenant, recognizing the fundamental right of everyone to be free from hunger, shall take, individually and through international co-operation, the measures, including specific programmes, which are needed:

(a) to improve methods of production, conservation and distribution of food by making full use of technical and scientific knowledge, by disseminating knowledge of the principles of nutrition and by developing or reforming agrarian systems in such a way as to achieve the most efficient development and utilization of natural resources;

(b) taking into account the problems of both food-importing and food-exporting countries, to ensure an equitable distribution of world food supplies in relation to need.

Article 12

1. The States Parties to the present Covenant recognize the right of everyone to the enjoyment of the highest attainable standard of physical and mental health.

2. The steps to be taken by the States Parties to the present Covenant to achieve the full realization of this right shall include those necessary for:

(a) the provision for the reduction of the stillbirth-rate and of infant mortality and for the healthy development of the child;

(b) the improvement of all aspects of environmental and industrial hygiene;

(c) the prevention, treatment and control of epidemic, endemic, occupational and other diseases;

(d) the creation of conditions which would assure to all medical service and medical attention in the event of sickness.

Article 13

1. The States Parties to the present Covenant recognize the right of everyone to education. They agree that education shall be directed to the full development of the human personality and the sense of its dignity, and shall strengthen the respect for human rights and fundamental freedoms. They further agree that education shall enable all persons to participate effectively in a free society, promote understanding, tolerance and friendship among all nations and all racial, ethnic or religious groups, and further the activities of the United Nations for the maintenance of peace.

2. The States Parties to the present Covenant recognize that, with a view to achieving the full realization of this right:

(a) primary education shall be compulsory and available free to all;
(b) secondary education in its different forms, including technical and vocational secondary education, shall be made generally available and accessible to all by every appropriate means, and in particular by the progressive introduction of free education;
(c) higher education shall be made equally accessible to all, on the basis of capacity, by every appropriate means, and in particular by the progressive introduction of free education;
(d) fundamental education shall be encouraged or intensified as far as possible for those persons who have not received or completed the whole period of their primary education;
(e) the development of a system of schools at all levels shall be actively pursued, an adequate fellowship system shall be established, and the material conditions of teaching staff shall be continuously improved.

3. The States Parties to the present Covenant undertake to have respect for the liberty of parents and, when applicable, legal guardians, to choose for their children schools, other than those established by the public authorities, which conform to such minimum educational standards as may be laid down or approved by the State and to ensure the religious and moral education of their children in conformity with their own convictions.

4. No part of this article shall be construed so as to interfere with the liberty of individuals and bodies to establish and direct educational institutions, subject always to the observance of the principles set forth in paragraph 1 of this article and to the requirement that the education given in such institutions shall conform to such minimum standards as may be laid down by the State.

Article 14

Each State Party to the present Covenant which, at the time of becoming a Party, has not been able to secure in its metropolitan territory or other territories under its jurisdiction compulsory primary education, free of charge, undertakes, within two years, to work out and adopt a detailed plan of action for the progressive implementation, within a reasonable number of years, to be fixed in the plan, of the principle of compulsory education free of charge for all.

Article 15

1. The States Parties to the present Covenant recognize the right of everyone:

(a) to take part in cultural life;
(b) to enjoy the benefits of scientific progress and its applications;
(c) to benefit from the protection of the moral and material interests resulting from any scientific, literary or artistic production of which he is the author.

2. The steps to be taken by the States Parties to the present Covenant to achieve the full realization of this right shall include those necessary for the conservation, the development and the diffusion of science and culture.

3. The States Parties to the present Covenant undertake to respect the freedom indispensable for scientific research and creative activity.

4. The States Parties to the present Covenant recognize the benefits to be derived from the encouragement and development of international contacts and co-operation in the scientific and cultural fields.

Part IV

Article 16

1. The States Parties to the present Covenant undertake to submit in conformity with this part of the Covenant reports on the measures which they have adopted and the progress made in achieving the observance of the rights recognized herein.

2. (a) All reports shall be submitted to the Secretary-General of the United Nations, who shall transmit copies to the Economic and Social Council for consideration in accordance with the provisions of the present Covenant.

   (b) The Secretary-General of the United Nations shall also transmit to the specialized agencies copies of the reports, or any relevant parts therefrom, from States Parties to the present Covenant which are also members of these specialized agencies in so far as these reports, or parts therefrom, relate to any matters which fall within the responsibilities of the said agencies in accordance with their constitutional instruments.

Article 17

1. The States Parties to the present Covenant shall furnish their reports in stages, in accordance with a programme to be established by the Economic and Social Council within one year of the entry into force of the present Covenant after consultation with the States Parties and the specialized agencies concerned.

2. Reports may indicate factors and difficulties affecting the degree of fulfilment of obligations under the present Covenant.

3. Where relevant information has previously been furnished to the United Nations or to any specialized agency by any State Party to the present Covenant, it will not be necessary to reproduce that information, but a precise reference to the information so furnished will suffice.

Article 18

Pursuant to its responsibilities under the Charter of the United Nations in the field of human rights and fundamental freedoms, the Economic and Social Council may make arrangements with the specialized agencies in respect of their reporting to it on the progress made in achieving the observance of the provisions of the present Covenant falling within the scope of their activities. These reports may include particulars of decisions and recommendations on such implementation adopted by their competent organs.

Article 19

The Economic and Social Council may transmit to the Commission on Human Rights for study and general recommendation or as appropriate for information the reports concerning human rights submitted by States in accordance with articles 16 and 17, and those concerning human rights submitted by the specialized agencies in accordance with article 18.

Article 20

The States Parties to the present Covenant and the specialized agencies concerned may submit comments to the Economic and Social Council on any general recommendation under article 19 or reference to such general recommendation in any report of the Commission on Human Rights or any documentation referred to therein.

Article 21

The Economic and Social Council may submit from time to time to the General Assembly reports with recommendations of a general nature and a summary of the information received from the States Parties to the present Covenant and the specialized agencies on the measures taken and the progress made in achieving general observance of the rights recognized in the present Covenant.

Article 22

The Economic and Social Council may bring to the attention of other organs of the United Nations, their subsidiary organs and specialized agencies concerned with furnishing technical assistance any matters arising out of the reports referred to in this part of the present Covenant which may assist such bodies in deciding, each within its field of competence, on the advisability of international measures likely to contribute to the effective progressive implementation of the present Covenant.

Article 23

The States Parties to the present Covenant agree that international action for the achievement of the rights recognized in the present Covenant includes such methods as the conclusion of conventions, the adoption of recommendations, the furnishing of technical assistance and the holding of regional meetings and technical meetings for the purpose of consultation and study organized in conjunction with the Governments concerned.

Article 24

Nothing in the present Covenant shall be interpreted as impairing the provisions of the Charter of the United Nations and of the constitutions of the specialized agencies which define the respective responsibilities of the various organs of the United Nations and of the specialized agencies in regard to the matters dealt with in the present Covenant.

Article 25

Nothing in the present Covenant shall be interpreted as impairing the inherent right of all peoples to enjoy and utilize fully and freely their natural wealth and resources.

PART V

Article 26

1. The present Covenant is open for signature by any State Member of the United Nations or member of any of its specialized agencies, by any State

Party to the Statute of the International Court of Justice, and by any other State which has been invited by the General Assembly of the United Nations to become a party to the present Covenant.

2. The present Covenant is subject to ratification. Instruments of ratification shall be deposited with the Secretary-General of the United Nations.

3. The present Covenant shall be open to accession by any State referred to in paragraph 1 of this article.

4. Accession shall be effected by the deposit of an instrument of accession with the Secretary-General of the United Nations.

5. The Secretary-General of the United Nations shall inform all States which have signed the present Covenant or acceded to it of the deposit of each instrument of ratification or accession.

Article 27

1. The present Covenant shall enter into force three months after the date of the deposit with the Secretary-General of the United Nations of the thirty-fifth instrument of ratification or instrument of accession.

2. For each State ratifying the present Covenant or acceding to it after the deposit of the thirty-fifth instrument of ratification or instrument of accession, the present Covenant shall enter into force three months after the date of the deposit of its own instrument of ratification or instrument of accession.

Article 28

The provisions of the present Covenant shall extend to all parts of federal States without any limitations or exceptions.

Article 29

1. Any State Party to the present Covenant may propose an amendment and file it with the Secretary-General of the United Nations. The Secretary-General shall thereupon communicate any proposed amendments to the States Parties to the present Covenant with a request that they notify him whether they favour a conference of States Parties for the purpose of considering and voting upon the proposals. In the event that at least one third of the States Parties favours such a conference, the Secretary-General shall convene the conference under the auspices of the United Nations. Any amendment adopted by a majority of the States Parties present and voting at the conference shall be submitted to the General Assembly of the United Nations for approval.

2. Amendments shall come into force when they have been approved by the General Assembly of the United Nations and accepted by a two-thirds

majority of the States Parties to the present Covenant in accordance with their respective constitutional processes.

3. When amendments come into force they shall be binding on those States Parties which have accepted them, other States Parties still being bound by the provisions of the present Covenant and any earlier amendment which they have accepted.

Article 30

Irrespective of the notifications made under article 26, paragraph 5, the Secretary-General of the United Nations shall inform all States referred to in paragraph 1 of the same article of the following particulars:

(a) signatures, ratifications and accessions under article 26;
(b) the date of the entry into force of the present Covenant under article 27 and the date of the entry into force of any amendments under article 29.

Article 31

1. The present Covenant, of which the Chinese, English, French, Russian and Spanish texts are equally authentic, shall be deposited in the archives of the United Nations.

2. The Secretary-General of the United Nations shall transmit certified copies of the present Covenant to all States referred to in article 26.

IN FAITH WHEREOF the undersigned, being duly authorized thereto by their respective Governments, have signed the present Covenant, opened for signature at New York, on the nineteenth day of December, one thousand nine hundred and sixty-six.

SELECT BIBLIOGRAPHY

Books

Alston, P., and J. Crawford eds., *The Future of UN Human Rights Treaty Monitoring* (2000, Cambridge University Press)

Amerasinghe, C., *State Responsibility for Injuries to Aliens* (1967, Clarendon Press)

Anker, D., *The Law of Asylum in the United States* (1999, Refugee Law Center, Inc.)

Aust, A., *Modern Treaty Law and Practice* (2000, Cambridge University Press)

Borchard, E., *The Diplomatic Protection of Citizens Abroad* (1915, Banks Law Publishing Co.)

Bossuyt, M., *Guide to the "Travaux Préparatoires" of the International Covenant on Civil and Political Rights* (1987, Bruylant)

Brownlie, I., *Principles of Public International Law* (2003, Clarendon Press)

Byers, M., *Custom, Power and the Power of Rules: International Relations and Customary International Law* (1999, Cambridge University Press)

Craven, M., *The International Covenant on Economic, Social and Cultural Rights: A Perspective on its Development* (1995, Clarendon Press)

Crock, M., ed., *Protection or Punishment: The Detention of Asylum Seekers in Australia* (1993, Federation Press)

Danilenko, G., *Law-Making in the International Community* (1993, Martinus Nijhoff)

Eggli, A., *Mass Refugee Influx and the Limits of Public International Law* (2001, Martinus Nijhoff)

Eide, A., et al. eds., *Economic, Social and Cultural Rights: A Textbook* (1995, Martinus Nijhoff)

The Universal Declaration of Human Rights: A Commentary (1992, Scandinavian University Press)

Falk, R., *Revitalizing International Law* (1993, Iowa State University Press)

The Status of Law in International Society (1970, Princeton University Press)

Feller, E., et al. eds., *Refugee Protection in International Law* (2003, Cambridge University Press)

Forbes Martin, S., *Refugee Women* (1991, Zed Books)

Fourlanos, G., *Sovereignty and the Ingress of Aliens* (1986, Almqvist & Wiksell)

Fredman, S., *Discrimination Law* (2001, Oxford University Press)

Garcia Amador, F. V., et al., *Recent Codification of the Law of State Responsibility for Injuries to Aliens* (1974, Oceana Publications)

Goodwin-Gill, G., *The Refugee in International Law* (1996, Clarendon Press)

Grahl-Madsen, A., *Commentary on the Refugee Convention 1951* (1963, pub'd. 1997, UNHCR)

    The Status of Refugees in International Law (vol. I, 1966; vol. II, 1972, A. W. Sijthoff)

    Territorial Asylum (1980, Swedish Institute of International Affairs)

Guild, E., and C. Harlow eds., *Implementing Amsterdam: Immigration and Asylum Rights in EC Law* (2001, Hart Publishing)

Hathaway, J., *The Law of Refugee Status* (1991, Butterworths)

Hathaway, J., ed., *Reconceiving International Refugee Law* (1997, Kluwer)

Hathaway, J., and J. Dent, *Refugee Rights: Report on a Comparative Survey* (1995, York Lanes Press)

Helton, A., *The Price of Indifference: Refugees and Humanitarian Action in the New Century* (2002, Oxford University Press)

Henkin, L., ed., *The International Bill of Rights* (1981, Columbia University Press)

Jayawickrama, N., *The Judicial Application of Human Rights Law* (2002, Cambridge University Press)

Jennings, R., and A. Watts eds., *Oppenheim's International Law* (1992, Longman Publishers)

Joly, D., *Refugees: Asylum in Europe?* (1992, Minority Rights)

Julien-Laferrière, F., ed., *Frontières du droit, Frontières des droits* (1993, L'Harmattan)

Kälin, W., *Grundriss des Asylverfahrens* (1990, Helbing & Lichtenhahn)

    Das Prinzip des Non-Refoulement (1982, Peter Lang)

Keen, D., *Refugees: Rationing the Right to Life* (1992, Zed Books)

Kibreab, G., *Refugees and Development in Africa: The Case of Eritrea* (1987, Red Sea Press)

Lambert, H., *Seeking Asylum: Comparative Law and Practice in Selected European Countries* (1995, Martinus Nijhoff)

Lauterpacht, E., ed., *International Law: The Collected Papers of Hersch Lauterpacht* (1970, Cambridge University Press)

Lillich, R., *The Human Rights of Aliens in Contemporary International Law* (1984, Manchester University Press)

Loescher, G., *The UNHCR and World Politics: A Perilous Path* (2001, Oxford University Press)

Loescher, G., and L. Monahan eds., *Refugees and International Relations* (1990, Oxford University Press)

McKean, W., *Equality and Discrimination under International Law* (1983, Clarendon Press)

Martin, D., ed., *The New Asylum Seekers: Refugee Law in the 1980s* (1986, Martinus Nijhoff)

Melander, G., and P. Nobel eds., *African Refugees and the Law* (1978, Scandinavian Institute of African Studies)

Meron, T., *Human Rights and Humanitarian Norms as Customary Law* (1989, Clarendon Press)

Meron, T., ed., *Human Rights in International Law: Legal and Policy Issues* (1984, Clarendon Press)

Merrills, J., *The Development of International Law by the European Court of Human Rights* (1993, Manchester University Press)

Muntarbhorn, V., *The Status of Refugees in Asia* (1992, Clarendon Press)

Nicholson, F., and P. Twomey eds., *Refugees Rights and Realities: Evolving International Concepts and Regimes* (1999, Cambridge University Press)

Noll, G., *Negotiating Asylum: The EU Acquis, Extraterritorial Protection, and the Common Market of Deflection* (2000, Martinus Nijhoff)

Nowak, M., *UN Covenant on Civil and Political Rights* (1993, N. P. Engel)

Pellonpää, M., *Expulsion in International Law: A Study in International Aliens Law and Human Rights with Special Reference to Finland* (1984, Suomalainen Tiedeakatemia)

Ragazzi, M., *The Concept of International Obligations* Erga Omnes (1997, Oxford University Press)

Ressler, E., et al., *Unaccompanied Children: Care and Protection in Wars, Natural Disasters and Refugee Movements* (1988, Oxford University Press)

Robinson, N., *Convention relating to the Status of Refugees: Its History, Contents and Interpretation* (1953, Institute of Jewish Affairs)

Roth, A., *The Minimum Standard of International Law Applied to Aliens* (1949, A. W. Sijthoff)

Schachter, O., *International Law in Theory and Practice* (1991, Martinus Nijhoff)

Shaw, M., *International Law* (2003, Cambridge University Press)

Sieghart, P., *The International Law of Human Rights* (1983, Clarendon Press)
  The Lawful Rights of Mankind (1985, Oxford University Press)

Sinclair, I., *The Vienna Convention and the Law of Treaties* (1984, Manchester University Press)

Sohn, L., and T. Buergenthal, *International Protection of Human Rights* (1973, Bobbs-Merrill)
  The Movement of Persons Across Borders (1992, American Society of International Law)

Steiner, H., and P. Alston, *International Human Rights in Context* (2000, Oxford University Press)

Stenberg, G., *Non-Expulsion and Non-Refoulement* (1989, Iustus Fölag)

Takkenberg, A., and C. Tahbaz eds., *The Collected Travaux Préparatoires of the 1951 Geneva Convention relating to the Status of Refugees* (1989, Dutch Refugee Council)

Tiberghien, F., *La protection des réfugiés en France* (1999, Economica, Presses Universitaires d'Aix-Marseille)

UNHCR, *Handbook on Procedures and Criteria for Determining Refugee Status* (1979, reedited 1992, UNHCR)

Vierdag, E., *The Concept of Discrimination in International Law, with a Special Reference to Human Rights* (1973, Martinus Nijhoff)

Weis, P., *The Refugee Convention, 1951: The Travaux Préparatoires Analysed with a Commentary by Dr. Paul Weis* (posthumously pub'd., 1995, Cambridge University Press)

Zetterqvist, J., *Refugees in Botswana in the Light of International Law* (1990, Scandinavian Institute of African Studies)

Zieck, M., *UNHCR and Voluntary Repatriation of Refugees: A Legal Analysis* (1997, Martinus Nijhoff)

Articles and chapters

Acer, E., "Living up to America's Values: Reforming the US Detention System for Asylum Seekers," (2002) 20(3) *Refuge* 44

Alfredsson, G., "Article 17," in A. Eide et al. eds., *The Universal Declaration of Human Rights: A Commentary* 255 (1992)

Alston, P., "International Law and the Human Right to Food," in P. Alston and K. Tomasevski eds., *International Law and the Human Right to Food* 10 (1984)

Anderfuhren-Wayne, C., "Family Unity in Immigration and Refugee Matters: United States and European Approaches," (1996) 8(3) *International Journal of Refugee Law* 347

Arajäravi, P., "Article 26," in A. Eide et al. eds., *The Universal Declaration of Human Rights: A Commentary* 405 (1992)

Barutciski, M., "A Critical View on UNHCR's Mandate Dilemmas," (2002) 14(2/3) *International Journal of Refugee Law* 365

"Involuntary Repatriation when Refugee Protection is no Longer Necessary: Moving Forward after the 48th Session of the Executive Committee," (1998) 10(1/2) *International Journal of Refugee Law* 236

Barutciski, M., and A. Suhrke, "Lessons from the Kosovo Refugee Crisis: Innovations in Protection and Burden-Sharing," (2001) 14(2) *Journal of Refugee Studies* 95

Blay, S., and M. Tsamenyi, "Reservations and Declarations under the 1951 Convention and the 1967 Protocol relating to the Status of Refugees," (1990) 2(4) *International Journal of Refugee Law* 527

Bos, M., "Theory and Practice of Treaty Interpretation," (1980) 27 *Netherlands International Law Review* 135

Camus-Jacques, G., "Refugee Women: The Forgotten Majority," in G. Loescher and L. Monahan eds., *Refugees and International Relations* 148 (1990)

Castillo, M., and J. Hathaway, "Temporary Protection," in J. Hathaway ed., *Reconceiving International Refugee Law* 1 (1997)

Clapham, A., "UN Human Rights Reporting Procedures: An NGO Perspective," in P. Alston and J. Crawford eds., *The Future of UN Human Rights Treaty Monitoring* 175 (2000)

Clark, T., and J. Niessen, "Equality Rights and Non-Citizens in Europe and America: The Promise, the Practice, and Some Remaining Issues," (1996) 14(3) *Netherlands Quarterly of Human Rights* 245

Coles, G., "Approaching the Refugee Problem Today," in G. Loescher and L. Monahan eds., *Refugees and International Relations* 373 (1990)

Corliss, S., "Asylum State Responsibility for the Hostile Acts of Foreign Exiles," (1990) 2(2) *International Journal of Refugee Law* 181

Crawford, J., "The UN Human Rights Treaty System: A System in Crisis?," in P. Alston and J. Crawford eds., *The Future of UN Human Rights Treaty Monitoring* 1 (2000)

Crépeau, F., and M. Barutciski, "The Legal Condition of Refugees in Canada," (1994) 7(2/3) *Journal of Refugee Studies* 239

Dankwa, E., "Working Paper on Article 2(3) of the International Covenant on Economic, Social and Cultural Rights," (1987) 9 *Human Rights Quarterly* 230

Domb, F., "Jus Cogens and Human Rights," (1976) 6 *Israeli Yearbook of Human Rights* 104

Drzewicki, K., "The Right to Work and Rights in Work," in A. Eide et al. eds., *Economic, Social and Cultural Rights: A Textbook* 169 (1995)

Eide, A., "Article 25," in A. Eide et al. eds., *The Universal Declaration of Human Rights: A Commentary* 385 (1992)

"The Right to an Adequate Standard of Living, Including the Right to Food," in A. Eide et al. eds., *Economic, Social and Cultural Rights: A Textbook* 89 (1995)

Elles, D., "Aliens and Activities of the United Nations in the Field of Human Rights," (1974) 7 *Human Rights Journal* 291

Feller, E., "Carrier Sanctions and International Law," (1989) 1(1) *International Journal of Refugee Law* 48

Fitzmaurice, M., "The Law and Procedure of the International Court of Justice 1951–4: Treaty Interpretation and Other Treaty Points," (1957) 33 *British Yearbook of International Law* 203

Fonteyne, J.-P., "Illegal Refugees or Illegal Policy?," in Australian National University Department of International Relations ed., *Refugees and the Myth of the Borderless World* 16 (2002)

Fredriksson, J., "Reinvigorating Resettlement: Changing Realities Demand Changed Approach," (2002) 13 *Forced Migration Review* 28

Frelick, B., "Secure and Durable Asylum: Article 34 of the Refugee Convention," in US Committee for Refugees, *World Refugee Survey 2001* 42 (2001)

Fullerton, M.-E., "Hungary, Refugees, and the Law of Return," (1996) 8(4) *International Journal of Refugee Law* 499

Gandhi, P., "The Universal Declaration of Human Rights at Fifty Years: Its Origins, Significance and Impact," (1998) 41 *German Yearbook of International Law* 206

Gibney, M., "Kosovo and Beyond: Popular and Unpopular Refugees," (1999) 5 *Forced Migration Review* 28

Goldsmith, J., and E. Posner, "Understanding the Resemblance Between Modern and Traditional Customary International Law," (2000) 40(2) *Virginia Journal of International Law* 639

Goodwin-Gill, G., "Article 31 of the 1951 Convention relating to the Status of Refugees: Non-Penalization, Detention, and Protection," in E. Feller et al. eds., *Refugee Protection in International Law* 185 (2003)

"The Individual Refugee, the 1951 Convention and the Treaty of Amsterdam," in E. Guild and C. Harlow eds., *Implementing Amsterdam: Immigration and Asylum Rights in EC Law* 141 (2001)

"International Law and the Detention of Refugees," (1986) 20(2) *International Migration Review* 193

"*Nonrefoulement* and the New Asylum Seekers," in D. Martin ed., *The New Asylum Seekers: Refugee Law in the 1980s* 103 (1986)

"Refugee Identity and Protection's Fading Prospects," in F. Nicholson and P. Twomey eds., *Refugee Rights and Realities: Evolving International Concepts and Regimes* 220 (1999)

Grahl-Madsen, A., "Political Rights and Freedoms of Refugees," in G. Melander and P. Nobel eds., *African Refugees and the Law* 47 (1978)

Hailbronner, K., "*Nonrefoulement* and 'Humanitarian' Refugees: Customary International Law or Wishful Legal Thinking?," in D. Martin ed., *The New Asylum Seekers: Refugee Law in the 1980s* 123 (1986)

Hathaway, J., "The Emerging Politics of *Non-Entrée*," (1992) 91 *Refugees* 40; also published as "L'émergence d'une politique de non-entrée," in F. Julien-Laferrière ed., *Frontières du droit, Frontières des droits* 65 (1993)

"The Evolution of Refugee Status in International Law: 1920–1950," (1984) 33 *International and Comparative Law Quarterly* 348

"Harmonizing for Whom? The Devaluation of Refugee Protection in the Era of European Economic Integration," (1993) 26(3) *Cornell International Law Journal* 719

"The Meaning of Repatriation," (1997) 9(4) *International Journal of Refugee Law* 551; also published in European University Institute ed., *Legal and Policy Issues Concerning Refugees from the Former Yugoslavia* 4 (1997)

"A Reconsideration of the Underlying Premise of Refugee Law," (1990) 31(1) *Harvard International Law Journal* 129

"Review Essay: N. Nathwani, Rethinking Refugee Law," (2004) 98(3) *American Journal of International Law* 616

"What's in a Label?," (2003) 5 *European Journal of Migration and Law* 1

Hathaway, J., and A. Cusick, "Refugee Rights Are Not Negotiable," (2000) 14(2) *Georgetown Immigration Law Journal* 481

Hathaway, J., and C. Harvey, "Framing Refugee Protection in the New World Disorder," (2001) 34(2) *Cornell International Law Journal* 257

Hathaway, J., and A. Neve, "Fundamental Justice and the Deflection of Refugees from Canada," (1997) 34(2) *Osgoode Hall Law Journal* 213

"Making International Refugee Law Relevant Again: A Proposal for Collectivized and Solution-Oriented Protection," (1997) 10 *Harvard Human Rights Journal* 115

Helton, A., "Asylum and Refugee Protection in Thailand," (1989) 1(1) *International Journal of Refugee Law* 20

"Reforming Alien Detention Policy in the United States," in M. Crock ed., *Protection or Punishment: The Detention of Asylum Seekers in Australia* 103 (1993)

Humphrey, J., "Political and Related Rights," in T. Meron ed., *Human Rights in International Law: Legal and Policy Issues* 171 (1984)

Jacobsen, K., "Factors Influencing the Policy Responses of Host Governments to Mass Refugee Influxes," (1996) 30 *International Migration Review* 655

Kälin, W., "Supervising the 1951 Convention relating to the Status of Refugees: Article 35 and Beyond," in E. Feller et al. eds., *Refugee Protection in International Law* 613 (2003)

"Temporary Protection in the EC: Refugee Law, Human Rights, and the Temptations of Pragmatism," (2001) 44 *German Yearbook of International Law* 221

"Troubled Communication: Cross-Cultural Misunderstandings in the Asylum Hearing," (1986) 20 *International Migration Review* 230

Källström, K., "Article 23," in A. Eide et al. eds., *The Universal Declaration of Human Rights: A Commentary* 373 (1992)

Kiapi, A., "The Legal Status of Refugees in Uganda: A Critical Study of Legislative Instruments" (1993)

Kingsbury, B., "Legal Positivism as Normative Politics: International Society, Balance of Power and Lassa Oppenheim's Positive International Law," (2002) 13(2) *European Journal of International Law* 401

Koskenniemi, M., "'The Lady Doth Protest Too Much': Kosovo, and the Turn to Ethics in International Law," (2002) 65(2) *Modern Law Review* 159

Krause, C., "The Right to Property," in A. Eide et al. eds., *Economic, Social and Cultural Rights: A Textbook* 143 (1995)

Lauterpacht, E., and D. Bethlehem, "The Scope and Content of the Principle of Non-Refoulement," in E. Feller et al. eds., *Refugee Protection in International Law* 87 (2003)

Lawyers' Committee for Human Rights, "Review of States' Procedures and Practices relating to Detention of Asylum Seekers" (Sept. 2002)

Leckie, S., "The Inter-State Complaint Procedure in International Human Rights Law: Hopeful Prospects or Wishful Thinking?," (1988) 10 *Human Rights Quarterly* 249

McCrudden, C., "Equality and Discrimination," in D. Feldman ed., *English Public Law* (vol. XI, 2004)

"Institutional Discrimination," (1982) 2(3) *Oxford Journal of Legal Studies* 303

McGinley, G., "Practice as a Guide to Treaty Interpretation," [Winter 1985] *Fletcher Forum* 211

Maluwa, T., "The Concept of Asylum and the Protection of Refugees in Botswana: Some Legal and Political Aspects," (1990) 2(4) *International Journal of Refugee Law* 587

Mathew, P., "Australian Refugee Protection in the Wake of the *Tampa*," (2002) 96(3) *American Journal of International Law* 661

Melander, G., "Article 24," in A. Eide et al. eds., *The Universal Declaration of Human Rights: A Commentary* 379 (1992)

Meron, T., "Extraterritoriality of Human Rights Treaties," (1995) 89(1) *American Journal of International Law* 78

Motta, F., "Between a Rock and a Hard Place: Australia's Mandatory Detention of Asylum Seekers," (2002) 20(3) *Refuge* 12

Mtango, E., "Military and Armed Attacks on Refugee Camps," in G. Loescher and L. Monahan eds., *Refugees and International Relations* 92 (1990)

Noll, G., "Visions of the Exceptional: Legal and Theoretical Issues Raised by Transit Processing Centers and Protection Zones," (2003) 5(3) *European Journal of Migration Law* 303

North, A., and N. Bhuta, "The Future of Protection – The Role of the Judge," (2001) 15(3) *Georgetown Immigration Law Journal* 479

O'Connell, M.-E., "Re-Leashing the Dogs of War," (2003) 97(2) *American Journal of International Law* 446

Ohaegbulom, F., "Human Rights and the Refugee Situation in Africa," in G. Shepherd and V. Nanda eds., *Human Rights and Third World Development* 197 (1985)

Oppenheim, L., "The Science of International Law: Its Task and Method," (1908) 2 *American Journal of International Law* 313

Partsch, K., "Freedom of Conscience and Expression, and Political Freedoms," in L. Henkin ed., *The International Bill of Rights* 208 (1981)

Rao, T., "International Custom," (1979) 19 *Indian Journal of International Law* 515

Rehof, L., "Article 3," in A. Eide et al. eds., *The Universal Declaration of Human Rights: A Commentary* 73 (1992)

"Article 12," in A. Eide et al. eds., *The Universal Declaration of Human Rights: A Commentary* 187 (1992)

Ris, M., "Treaty Interpretation and ICJ Recourse to *Travaux Préparatoires*: Towards a Proposed Amendment of Articles 31 and 32 of the Vienna Convention on the Law of Treaties," (1991) 14(1) *Boston College International and Comparative Law Review* 111

Roberts, A., "Traditional and Modern Approaches to Customary International Law: A Reconciliation," (2001) 95(4) *American Journal of International Law* 757

Scheinin, M., "The Right to Social Security," in A. Eide et al. eds., *Economic, Social and Cultural Rights: A Textbook* 159 (1995)

Schmidt, M., "Servicing and Financing Human Rights Supervisory Bodies," in P. Alston and J. Crawford eds., *The Future of UN Human Rights Treaty Monitoring* 481 (2000)

Schwebel, S., "May Preparatory Work be Used to Correct, Rather than Confirm, the 'Clear' Meaning of a Treaty Provision?," in L. Makasczyk ed., *Theory of International Law at the Threshold of the 21st Century: Essays in Honour of Krzysztof Skubiszewski* 541 (1996)

Shacknove, A., "From Asylum to Containment," (1993) 5(4) *International Journal of Refugee Law* 516

Simma, B., "How Distinctive Are Treaties Representing Collective Interest? The Case of Human Rights Treaties," in V. Gowlland-Debbas ed., *Multilateral Treaty Making – The Current Status of and Reforms Needed in the International Legislative Process* 83 (2000)

Simma, B., and P. Alston, "The Sources of Human Rights Law: Custom, *Jus Cogens*, and General Principles," (1988–1989) 12 *Australian Year Book of International Law* 82

Skordas, A., "The Regularization of Illegal Immigrants in Greece," in P. deBruycker ed., *Regularization of Illegal Immigrants in the European Union* 343 (2000)

Slaughter, A.-M., "A Typology of Transjudicial Communication," (1994) 29 *University of Richmond Law Review* 99

Sohn, L., "The Human Rights Law of the Charter," (1977) 12 *Texas International Law Journal* 129

"Human Rights: Their Implementation and Supervision by the United Nations," in T. Meron ed., *Human Rights in International Law: Legal and Policy Issues* 369 (1984)

Sopf, D., "Temporary Protection in Europe After 1990: The 'Right to Remain' of Genuine Convention Refugees," (2001) 6 *Washington University Journal of Law and Policy* 109

Storey, H., "The Right to Family Life and Immigration Case Law at Strasbourg," (1990) 39 *International and Comparative Law Quarterly* 328

Tomasevski, K., "Health Rights," in A. Eide et al. eds., *Economic, Social and Cultural Rights: A Textbook* 125 (1995)

Trubek, D., "Economic, Social, and Cultural Rights in the Third World," in T. Meron ed., *Human Rights in International Law: Legal and Policy Issues* 205 (1984)

Verdirame, G., "Human Rights and Refugees: The Case of Kenya," (1999) 12(1) *Journal of Refugee Studies* 54

Verdross, A., "*Jus Dispositivum* and *Jus Cogens* in International Law," (1966) 60(1) *American Journal of International Law* 55

Walker, H., "Modern Treaties of Friendship, Commerce and Navigation," (1958) 42 *Minnesota Law Review* 805

Weis, P., "The 1967 Protocol relating to the Status of Refugees and Some Questions relating to the Law of Treaties," (1967) 42 *British Yearbook of International Law* 39

"The Concept of the Refugee in International Law," (1960) 87 *Journal du droit international* 928

Reports for the International Academy of Comparative Law

Addo, M., *International Academy of Comparative Law National Report for the United Kingdom* (1994)

Ahmad, N., *International Academy of Comparative Law National Report for Pakistan* (1994)

Allars, M., *International Academy of Comparative Law National Report for Australia* (1994)

Buttigieg, C., *International Academy of Comparative Law National Report for Malta* (1994)

Chimni, B. S., *International Academy of Comparative Law National Report for India* (1994)

Crépeau, F., *International Academy of Comparative Law National Report for Canada* (1994)

D'Orazio, G., *International Academy of Comparative Law National Report for Italy* (1994)

Einarsen, T., *International Academy of Comparative Law National Report for Norway* (1994)

Eriksson, M., *International Academy of Comparative Law National Report for Sweden* (1994)

Essuman-Johnson, A., *International Academy of Comparative Law National Report for Ghana* (1994)

Fraidenraij, S., *International Academy of Comparative Law National Report for Argentina* (1994)

Gionea, V., *International Academy of Comparative Law National Report for Romania* (1994)

Guimezanes, N., *International Academy of Comparative Law National Report for France* (1994)

Haines, R., *International Academy of Comparative Law National Report for New Zealand* (1994)

Hofmann, R., *International Academy of Comparative Law National Report for Germany* (1994)

Holterman, T., *International Academy of Comparative Law National Report for the Netherlands* (1994)

Kälin, W., *International Academy of Comparative Law National Report for Switzerland* (1994)

Khiddu-Makubuya, E., *International Academy of Comparative Law National Report for Uganda* (1994)

Kuosma, T., *International Academy of Comparative Law National Report for Finland* (1994)

Leus, K., and G. Vermeylen, *International Academy of Comparative Law National Report for Belgium* (1994)

Nkiwane, S., *International Academy of Comparative Law National Report for Zimbabwe* (1994)

Oikawa, S., *International Academy of Comparative Law National Report for Japan* (1994)

Papassiopi-Passia, Z., *International Academy of Comparative Law National Report for Greece* (1994)

Siwakoti, G., *International Academy of Comparative Law National Report for Nepal* (1994)

Thanh Trai Le, T., *International Academy of Comparative Law National Report for the United States* (1994)

Tharcisse, N., *International Academy of Comparative Law National Report for Burundi* (1994)

Vedsted-Hansen, J., *International Academy of Comparative Law National Report for Denmark* (1994)

Wiederin, E., *International Academy of Comparative Law National Report for Austria* (1994)

UNHCR documents

"Asylum Processes," UN Doc. EC/GC/01/12, May 31, 2001

"Declaration of States Parties to the 1951 Convention and/or its 1967 Protocol relating to the Status of Refugees," UN Doc. HCR/MMSP/2001/09, Dec. 13, 2001, incorporated in Executive Committee of the High Commissioner's Program, "Agenda for Protection," UN Doc. EC/52/SC/CRP.9/Rev.1, June 26, 2002

Detention of Asylum Seekers in Europe (1995)

"Families in Exile: Reflections from the Experience of UNHCR" (1995)

"Guidelines on International Protection No. 3: Cessation of Refugee Status under Articles 1(C)(5) and (6) of the 1951 Convention relating to the Status of Refugees (the 'Ceased Circumstances Clauses')," UN Doc. HCR/GIP/03/03, Feb. 10, 2003

Handbook on Procedures and Criteria for Determining Refugee Status (1979, reedited 1992)

"Handbook: Voluntary Repatriation: International Protection" (1996)

"Identity Documents for Refugees," UN Doc. EC/SCP/33, July 20, 1984

"Information Note on Implementation of the 1951 Convention and the 1967 Protocol relating to the Status of Refugees," UN Doc. EC/SCP/66, July 22, 1991

"Interception of Asylum-Seekers and Refugees: The International Framework and Recommendations for a Comprehensive Approach," UN Doc. EC/50/SC/CRP.17, June 9, 2000

"Local Integration," UN Doc. EC/GC/02/6, Apr. 25, 2002

"Note on Accession to International Instruments and the Detention of Refugees and Asylum Seekers," UN Doc. EC/SCP/44, Aug. 19, 1986

"Note on the Cessation Clauses," UN Doc. EC/47/SC/CRP.30 (1997)

"Note on Follow-up to the Earlier Conclusion of the Executive Committee on Travel Documents for Refugees," UN Doc. EC/SCP/48, July 3, 1987

"Note on Refugee Women and International Protection," UN Doc. EC/SCP/59, Aug. 28, 1990

"Note on Travel Documents for Refugees," UN Doc. EC/SCP/10, Aug. 30, 1978

"Protection of Refugees in Mass Influx Situations: Overall Protection Framework," UN Doc. EC/GC/01/4, Feb. 19, 2001

"Reception of Asylum-Seekers, Including Standards of Treatment, in the Context of Individual Asylum Systems," UN Doc. EC/GC/01/17, Sept. 4, 2001

"Refugee Children: Guidelines on Protection and Care" (1994)

"Refugee Resettlement: An International Handbook to Guide Reception and Integration" (2002)

"Revised Guidelines on Applicable Criteria and Standards Relating to the Detention of Asylum Seekers," Feb. 1999

INDEX

For references to treaties and other international instruments by article, reference should be made to the Table of Treaties and Other International Instruments. For jurisprudence by case, reference should be made to the Table of Cases.

absolute rights: *see* standard of treatment of aliens, evolution of regime, bilateral/FCN treaty regime; standard of treatment of refugees (CRSR Art. 7(1)), absolute rights

access to courts: *see* courts, access to (CRSR Art. 16); courts, access to (equality before) (ICCPR Art. 14(1))

acquired rights (CRSR Art. 7(3)), reciprocity, exemption (Art. 7(2)) 203

acquired rights dependent on personal status (CRSR Art. 12(2))
  as absolute right 237
  compliance with formalities required by the law 227–228
    1933 and 1938 Conventions and 227–228
  drafting history 221–228
  married women 221–222
  matrimonial status 221–222
  physical presence, relevance 163–164
  potential abuse of provision 222–223
  public policy and 225–227
  separation of refugee from law of country of nationality as objective 227
  succession and inheritance 223–225

acquired rights in first country of arrival, loss 331–332

adequate standard of living: *see* necessities of life, right to

administrative assistance (CRSR Art. 25): *see also* consular protection; protection of refugees (UNHCR Statute Art. 8)
  as absolute right 237
  affirmative action, need for 635–636
  consular role of high commissioners for refugees as predecessor 94
  documents or certifications: *see also* documentation (identity papers) (CRSR Art. 27); documentation (travel documents) (CRSR Art. 28); personal status (applicable law) (CRSR Art. 12(1))
    "credence in absence of proof to contrary" (Art. 25(3)) 643–644
    "documents" 642–643
    drafting history/rationale 639–644

1073

---

[1] Elsewhere in the Index normally referred to as *Handbook*